MATERNAL, NEONATAL, AND WOMEN'S HEALTH NURSING

MATERNAL, NEONATAL, AND WOMEN'S HEALTH NURSING

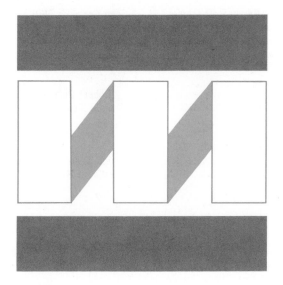

Susan M. Cohen, RN, DSN
Associate Professor
School of Nursing
The University of Texas
Health Science Center at Houston

Carole Ann Kenner, RN,C, DNS
Assistant Professor
College of Nursing and Health
University of Cincinnati

Andrea O. Hollingsworth, RN, PhD
Assistant Professor
School of Nursing, University of Pennsylvania
Philadelphia

SPRINGHOUSE CORPORATION
Springhouse, Pennsylvania

STAFF

Executive Director, Editorial
Stanley Loeb

Director of Trade and Textbooks
Minnie B. Rose, RN, BSN, MEd

Art Director
John Hubbard

Clinicial Consultant
Helene K. Nawrocki, RN, MSN

Editors
Kathy E. Goldberg, Catherine E. Harold, Nancy Priff (senior editors); Kathleen Cassidy, Tony DeCrosta, Keith de Pinho, Rafaela Ellis, Barbara Glasser, Jeffrey E. Heller, Dianne Herrin, Judd Howard, Kevin J. Law, Judith P. Lee, Deborah J. Lyons, Allison Walker

Acquisitions Editors
Margaret Belcher, RN, BSN, Betsy Steinmetz (associate)

Clinical Editors
Marlene Ciranowicz, RN, MSN; Lynne Hutnik Conrad, RN,C, MSN; Patricia Dillon, RN, MSN; Lauren A. Giannakopoulos, RN, BSN; Bernadette Handler, RN, CCRN; Sandi Nettina, RN,C, MSN, CRNP; Beverly Ann Tscheschlog, RN

Copy Editor
Elizabeth Kiselev

Designers
Stephanie Peters (associate art director), Lynn Foulk (book designer), Julie Carleton Barlow, Anita Curry, Elaine Ezrow, Donna Giannola, Lesley Weissman-Cook

Illustrators
John Carlance, Will Davidson, Jean Gardner, Frank Grobelny, Neal Hughes, Bob Jackson, Christine Jones, Debra Koenig, John Murphy, Bob Neumann, Judy Newhouse, Gary Phillips, George Retsick, Pierre Schnog, Wiley Searles

Art Production
Robert Perry (manager), Anna Brindisi, Nancy Frazier, Donald Knauss, Anet Oakes, Ann Raphun, Thomas Robbins, Robert Wieder

Typographers
David Kosten (manager), Diane Paluba (assistant manager), Elizabeth Bergman, Joy Rossi Biletz, Phyllis Marron, Robin Rantz, Valerie L. Rosenberger

Manufacturing
Deborah Meiris (manager), T. A. Landis, Jennifer Suter

Production Coordinators
Aline Miller, Maura Murphy

Photograph Credits
Lennart Nilsson, from *A Child Is Born,* for fetal development; Harriette Hartigan, Artemis, for birth sequence; Erica Freudenstein for unit opening pages.

Library of Congress Cataloging-in-Publication Data
Cohen, Susan M.
    Maternal, neonatal, and women's health nursing.
    Includes bibliographical references and index.
    1. Obstetrical nursing.   2. Pediatric nursing.   3. Family nursing.
I. Kenner, Carole.   II. Hollingsworth, Andrea O.   III. Title.
[DNLM: 1. Family—nurses' instruction.   2. Gynecology—nurses' instruction.
3. Nursing Process.   4. Obstetrical Nursing.   5. Pediatric Nursing.
WY 157 C678m]
RG951.C64   1991
610.73'678
ISBN 0-87434-258-9   90-10448

CONTENTS IN BRIEF

CONTENTS IN DETAIL

UNIT ONE ◆ Nursing the Childbearing Family: History, Concepts, and Practice

CHAPTER 1 ◆ Family Nursing Care: History and Trends   4

Sylvia A. McSkimming, RN, PhD; Carole Ann Kenner, RN,C, DNS

CHAPTER 2 ◆ Family Structure and Function   25

Christine A. Grant, RN, PhD; Gale Robinson Smith, RN, PhD, CS

CHAPTER 3 ♦ Nursing Process and the Childbearing Family

Gale Robinson Smith, RN, PhD, CS; Cynthia L. Armstrong, RN,C, MSN

CHAPTER 4 ♦ Nurse-Client Interaction

Florencetta Gibson, RN, MSN, MEd

Sarah D. Cohn, CNM, MSN, JD

UNIT TWO ◆ **Women's Health Care**

Constance A. Bobik, RN, MSN

Linda Wheeler, CNM, MN, EdD

Catherine Ingram Fogel, RN,C, PhD; Barbara C. Rynerson, RN,C, MS

Janet K. Williams, RN, PhD, CPNP

Bonnie Mauger Graff, RN, MSN, CRNP

CHAPTER 13 ◆ **Gynecologic Disorders** 282

Rosemary Theroux, RN,C, MS; Peggy Sherblom Matteson, RN,C, MS

CHAPTER 14 ◆ **Violence Against Women** 320

Rosemary J. McKeighen, RN, PhD, CMFT, FAAN

CHAPTER 15 ♦ **Women's Health-Compromising Behaviors**   **338**

Anne Myers Gudmundsen, RN, PhD

UNIT THREE ♦ **The Antepartal Period**

CHAPTER 16 ♦ **Conception and Fetal Development**   **364**

Leonard V. Crowley, MD; Susan M. Cohen, RN, DSN

CHAPTER 17 ✦ Physiologic Changes during Normal Pregnancy   391

Bernadine Adams, RN, BSN, MN

CHAPTER 18 ✦ Psychosocial Changes during Normal Pregnancy   406

Constance Sinclair, RN, MSN, CNM

CHAPTER 19 ✦ Care during the Normal Antepartal Period

Christabel A. Kaitell, RN, BN, MPH, SCM

CHAPTER 20 ✦ Nutrition and Diet Counseling

Ann Brodsky, MS, RD

CHAPTER 21 ◆ Family Preparation for Childbirth and Parenting

Joan Engebretson, RN, MS; Harriett Linenberger, RN,C, MSN, ACCE-R

480

Patricia Anne Mynaugh, RN, PhD

Catherine Dearman, RN, PhD

UNIT FOUR ◆ The Intrapartal Period

CHAPTER 24 ◆ Physiology of Labor and Childbirth   583

Lynne Hutnik Conrad, RN,C, MSN

CHAPTER 25 ◆ **Fetal Assessment**

Connie Marshall, RN, MSN

CHAPTER 29 ◆ **The Third and Fourth Stages of Labor**   **705**

Jan Weingrad Smith, CNM, MS, MPH

CHAPTER 30 ◆ **Family Support during the Intrapartal Period**   **727**

Virginia H. Kemp, RN, PhD; Tommie P. Nelms, RN, PhD

CHAPTER 31 ◆ **High-Risk Intrapartal Clients** 737

Aileen MacLaren, CNM, MSN; JoNell Efantis, RN, ARNP, MSN

CHAPTER 32 ◆ **Special Obstetric Procedures** 767

Peggy J. Drapo, RN, PhD; Charlotte R. Patrick, RN, MS, MEd

CHAPTER 33 ◆ Intrapartal Complications

788

Andrea O. Hollingsworth, RN, PhD

CHAPTER 36 ◆ **Care of the Normal Neonate**   871

Carole Ann Kenner, RN,C, DNS

Gail Blair Storr, RN, MN, MEd

Laurie Porter Gunderson, RN, PhD; Darlene Nebel Cantu, RN,C, MSN; Laura Rodriguez Vaello, RN,C, MSN, NNP

CHAPTER 39 ♦ **Care of the Families of High-Risk Neonates**   985

Ann E. Brueggemeyer, RN, MBA, MSN

CHAPTER 40 ◆ **Discharge Planning and Neonatal Care at Home** 1007

Brook Gumm, RN, MSN; Mary E. Lynch, RN, MS

CHAPTER 43 ◆ **Psychosocial Adaptation of the Postpartal Family** 1074

Sarah Elizabeth Whitaker, RN,C, MSN

CHAPTER 44 ◆ **Postpartal Complications**   **1095**

Paula Maisano Herndon, RN, MS

Annette Gupton, RN, MN

APPENDICES

MASTER GLOSSARY

INDEX

ADVISORY BOARD

CONSULTANTS

Senior Consultants

Leonard V. Crowley, MD
Codirector, Department of Pathology, Riverside Medical
Center; Visiting Professor, College of St. Catherine,
St. Mary's Campus; Clinical Assistant Professor of
Laboratory Medicine and Pathology, University of Minnesota
Medical School, Minneapolis

Aileen MacLaren, CNM, MSN
Clinical Assistant Professor, Nurse-Midwifery,
University of Miami

Bernadine Adams, RN, BSN, MN, Assistant Professor,
Northeast Louisiana University, Monroe

Marguerite C. Barbiere, RN, EdD, Assistant Professor/
Assistant Dean Undergraduate Program, Widener
University School of Nursing, Chester, Pa.

Cynthia Barnes-Boyd, RN, BSN, MSN, CCRN, Assistant Director
of Nursing, Parent-Child Health; Assistant Professor of
Nursing, Maternal-Child Health, College of Nursing,
University of Illinois Hospital, Chicago

Claudia Anderson Beckman, RN, PhD, Associate Professor,
University of Tennessee, Memphis

Linda A. Bernhard, RN, PhD, Assistant Professor, College of
Nursing, The Ohio State University, Columbus

Julie Boozer, RN, PhD, ACCE, Chairman, Division of Nursing,
Wesley College, Dover, Del.

Ann L. Boutcher, RN,C, MSN, Genetic Counselor, Genetics
Associates of North Carolina, Chapel Hill

Ina J. Bramadat, RN, MSN, Doctoral Candidate, Associate
Director, Undergraduate Programs, School of Nursing,
University of Manitoba (Canada), Winnipeg

Linda P. Brown, RN, PhD, Assistant Professor, School of
Nursing, University of Pennsylvania, Philadelphia

Felissa L. Cohen, RN, PhD, FAAN, FABMG, Professor, Medical-
Surgical Nursing; Acting Head, Department of Medical-
Surgical Nursing; Director, Center for Narcolepsy,
College of Nursing, University of Illinois at Chicago

Susan M. Cohen, RN, DSN, Associate Professor, The
University of Texas, Health Science Center at Houston

Judith B. Collins, RN,C, MS, OGNP, FAAN, Associate Professor,
Schools of Nursing and Medicine; Director, Health
Policy Office—Office of the Vice President for Medical
Services, Medical College of Virginia, Virginia
Commonwealth University (MCV/VCU), Richmond

Chandice Covington, RN, PhD, Assistant Professor, Wayne
State College of Nursing, Detroit

Leonard V. Crowley, MD, Codirector, Department of
Pathology, Riverside Medical Center; Visiting Professor,
College of St. Catherine, St. Mary's Campus; Clinical
Assistant Professor of Laboratory Medicine and
Pathology, University of Minnesota Medical School,
Minneapolis

Barbara Derwinski-Robinson, RN,C, MSN, Associate
Professor, Montana State University, Billings

Janet L. Engstrom, RN, CNM, PhD, Nurse Coordinator, Center
for Assisted Reproductive Technology, Michael Reese
Hospital, Chicago

Elaine Erhard, RN,C, MSN, Nursing Instructor, School of
Nursing, Good Samaritan Hospital, Cincinnati

Sandra A. Faux, RN, PhD, Assistant Professor; Coordinator,
Graduate Program, University of Western Ontario
(Canada), Faculty of Nursing, London

M. Josephine Flaherty, RN, PhD, Principal Nursing Officer,
National Health and Welfare, Ottawa, Ontario, Canada

Catherine Ingram Fogel, RN,C, PhD, Associate Professor,
University of North Carolina, Chapel Hill

Julie C. Fortier, RN, PhD, Assistant Professor, School of
Nursing, University of Maryland, Baltimore County
Campus

Sarah B. Freeman, RN,C, MS, Assistant Professor; Director
GONP Program, Emory University, Atlanta

Marilyn M. Friedman, RN, PhD, Professor, Department of
Nursing, California State University, Los Angeles

Sue Ellen Gaffney, RN,C, MSN, Perinatal Clinical Nurse
Specialist, University of Connecticut Health Center;
Assistant Clinical Professor, School of Nursing,
University of Connecticut, Farmington

Linda M. Gigliotti, MS, RD, Dietitian, Integrated Medical
Specialties, Phoenix, Ariz.

Barbara K. Hahnemann, RN, PhD, Director of Nursing,
Presentation College, Aberdeen, S.D.

Bridget A. Haupt, PharmD, Assistant Director of Pharmacy,
Department of Pharmacy, Thomas Jefferson University
Hospital, Philadelphia

CONTRIBUTORS

Bernadine Adams, RN, BSN, MN, Assistant Professor, School of Nursing, Northeast Louisiana University, Monroe

Cynthia L. Armstrong, RN,C, MSN, Perinatal Clinical Nurse Specialist, School of Nursing, University of Pennsylvania, Philadelphia

Constance A. Bobik, RN, MSN, Assistant Professor, Brevard Community College, Cocoa, Fla.

Ann Brodsky, MS, RD, Nutritionist, Women's Health Practice, Champaign, Ill.

Ann E. Brueggemeyer, RN, MBA, MSN, Instructor, School of Nursing, Good Samaritan Hospital, Cincinnati

Darlene Nebel Cantu, RN,C, MSN, Nurse Educator, School of Professional Nursing, Baptist Memorial Hospital System, San Antonio, Tex.

Susan M. Cohen, RN, DSN, Associate Professor, School of Nursing, The University of Texas, Health Science Center at Houston

Sarah D. Cohn, CNM, MSN, JD, Associate Counsel, Medicolegal Affairs, Yale New Haven Hospital, Yale School of Medicine, New Haven, Conn.

Lynne Hutnik Conrad, RN,C, MSN, Clinical Nurse Specialist, Maternal-Child Health, Rolling Hill Hospital, Elkins Park, Pa.

Leonard V. Crowley, MD, Codirector, Department of Pathology, Riverside Medical Center; Visiting Professor, College of St. Catherine, St. Mary's Campus; Clinical Assistant Professor of Laboratory Medicine and Pathology, University of Minnesota Medical School, Minneapolis

Debra C. Davis, RN, DSN, Associate Professor, Troy State University, Montgomery, Ala.

Deborah S. Davison, MSN, CRNP, Assistant Professor, La Roche College, Pittsburgh

Catherine Dearman, RN, PhD, Associate Professor, School of Nursing, Troy State University, Montgomery, Ala.

Peggy J. Drapo, RN, PhD, Professor, College of Nursing, Texas Woman's University, Denton

JoNell Efantis, RN, ARNP, MSN, Adjunct Instructor, School of Medicine, University of Miami

Joan Engebretson, RN, MS, Assistant Professor, The University of Texas, Health Science Center at Houston

Harriett W. Ferguson, RN,C, EdD, Associate Professor and Assistant Chairperson, Department of Nursing, Temple University, Philadelphia

Catherine Ingram Fogel, RN,C, PhD, Associate Professor, University of North Carolina–Chapel Hill

Florencetta Gibson, RN, MSN, MEd, Psychiatric Clinical Specialist, Assistant Professor, School of Nursing, Northeast Louisiana University, Monroe

Bonnie Mauger Graff, RN, MSN, CRNP, Clinical Faculty–Clinical Research, School of Nursing, University of Pennsylvania, Philadelphia

Christine A. Grant, RN, PhD, Clinical Coordinator, Mental Health Clinical Research Center, Department of Psychiatry, University of Pennsylvania, Philadelphia

Anne Myers Gudmundsen, RN, PhD, Director of Craniofacial Research and Publications, Humana Hospital–Medical City, Dallas

Brook Gumm, RN, MSN, Clinical Nurse Specialist, Discharge Planning and Apnea Team, Children's Hospital Medical Center, Cincinnati

Laurie Porter Gunderson, RN, PhD, Faculty, College of Nursing and Health, University of Cincinnati

Annette Gupton, RN, MN, Associate Professor, School of Nursing, University of Manitoba (Canada), Winnepeg

Kathleen Convery Hanold, RN, MS, Director, Women and Infant Services, Barnes Hospital, Washington University Medical Center, St. Louis

Paula Maisano Herndon, RN, MS, Education Specialist, Saint Francis Hospital, Tulsa, Okla.

Andrea O. Hollingsworth, RN, PhD, Assistant Professor, School of Nursing, University of Pennsylvania, Philadelphia

Christabel A. Kaitell, RN, BN, MPH, SCM, Assistant Professor, School of Nursing, Faculty of Health Sciences, University of Ottawa, Ontario, Canada

Virginia H. Kemp, RN, PhD, Associate Professor and Director, Center for Nursing Research, School of Nursing, Medical College of Georgia, Augusta

Carole Ann Kenner, RN,C, DNS, Assistant Professor, Parent Child Nursing, College of Nursing and Health, University of Cincinnati

Harriett Linenberger, RN,C, ACCE-R, MSN, Clinical Instructor, School of Nursing, The University of Texas, Health Science Center at Houston

Judy Wright Lott, ARNP, MSN, Assistant Professor, College of Nursing, University of Florida, Gainesville

Mary E. Lynch, RN, MS, Assistant Clinical Professor, Department of Family Health Care Nursing, University of California, San Francisco

Aileen MacLaren, CNM, MSN, Clinical Assistant Professor, Nurse-Midwifery, University of Miami

Connie Marshall, RN, MSN, Perinatal Clinical Specialist, Vice President, Conmar Publishing, Inc., Citrus Heights, Calif.

Peggy Sherblom Matteson, RN,C, MS, Doctoral Candidate, Boston College, Chestnut Hill, Mass.

Rosemary J. McKeighen, RN, PhD, CMFT, FAAN, Professor, College of Nursing, University of Iowa, Iowa City

Sylvia A. McSkimming, RN, PhD, Associate Director of Nursing, Research and Education, St. Vincent Hospital and Medical Center, Portland, Ore.

Patricia Anne Mynaugh, RN, PhD, Assistant Professor, College of Nursing, Villanova University, Philadelphia

Tommie P. Nelms, RN, PhD, Assistant Professor, School of Nursing, Georgia State University, Atlanta

Charlotte R. Patrick, RN, MS, MEd, Lecturer, College of Nursing, Texas Woman's University, Denton

Barbara C. Rynerson, RN,C, MS, Associate Professor, School of Nursing, University of North Carolina, Chapel Hill

Constance Sinclair, RN, MSN, CNM, Staff Nurse, Graduate Hospital, Philadelphia

Gale Robinson Smith, RN, PhD, CS, Assistant Professor, College of Nursing, Rutgers–The State University of New Jersey, Newark

Jan Weingrad Smith, CNM, MS, MPH, Clinical Nurse Specialist, Maternal–Child Health, Lawrence Hospital, Bronxville, N.Y.

Gail Blair Storr, RN, MN, MEd, Assistant Professor, Faculty of Nursing, University of New Brunswick (Canada), Fredericton

Rosemary Theroux, RN,C, MS, Coordinator, Women's Health Network, Leonard Morse Hospital, Natwick, Mass.

Laura Rodriguez Vaello, RN,C, MSN, NNP, Neonatal Nurse Practitioner–Clinical Nurse Specialist, Baptist Medical Center, San Antonio, Tex.

Donna J. van Lier, CNM, PhD, Nurse-Midwife, Private Practice, Atlanta OB/GYN Associates

Linda Wheeler, CNM, MN, EdD, Associate Professor, School of Nursing, Oregon Health Sciences University, Portland

Sarah Elizabeth Whitaker, RN,C, MSN, Instructor, College of Nursing and Applied Health, University of Texas at El Paso

Janet K. Williams, RN, PhD, CPNP, Lecturer, College of Nursing, University of Iowa, Iowa City

Nancy Fugate Woods, RN, PhD, FAAN, Professor, Parent and Child Nursing, University of Washington, Seattle

FOREWORD

Over the past decade, nursing's role in the health care of women and neonates has changed dramatically. Because of socioeconomic changes, women may bear their first child in their teens or mid-forties, requiring very different types of nursing care. As a result of consumer education, many women and their partners are concerned about the effects of preconception health on maternal and neonatal outcomes, increasing the demand for preconception nursing care. With scientific and technological advances, health care has become more complex, requiring expert nursing skills to monitor maternal, fetal, and neonatal health or help diagnose and treat problems. Also, early discharge from health care facilities has placed even greater value on the nurse's ability to teach a client to care for herself, her neonate, and her family.

To provide expert care to women and their families, the nurse needs current, accessible information on the following topics, among others:
- fetal monitoring
- genetic complications
- delivery options
- parental adjustment to an imperfect neonate
- family planning
- emergency interventions during labor
- neonatal assessment
- coping with the high-risk neonate
- parental and family teaching
- discharge planning.

Maternal, Neonatal, and Women's Health Nursing offers that—and more. It orients the nurse to mastering procedures, anticipating problems, identifying complications, responding to emergencies, and reviewing laboratory studies—as well as applying the nursing process to the client and her family.

The text is divided into six units. Unit One, Nursing the Childbearing Family: History, Concepts, and Practice, sets the stage for a holistic, family-centered approach to care. It surveys the changes that have affected the delivery of health care throughout history, explores the role of the nurse in a changing society, and predicts the changes that may be needed to improve family care. It presents a framework for analyzing family structure and function, and it guides the nurse through the delicate legal and ethical issues linked to rapid technological advances, the proliferation of malpractice lawsuits against physicians and nurses, and recent legal decisions affecting a woman's right in the outcome of pregnancy.

Unit Two, Women's Health Care, explores the basic health concerns that bring women into contact with health care professionals—sexuality; health promotion; reproduction and family planning; genetic, infectious, and gynecologic disorders; violence; and health-compromising behaviors. The unit emphasizes the multifaceted, unifying role of the nurse in promoting women's health within a health care system—and a society—undergoing continual and dramatic change. To provide the knowledge base essential to a thorough understanding of women's health issues, the unit surveys reproductive anatomy and physiology and provides basic information on integrating assessment findings and documenting nursing care.

Unit Three, The Antepartal Period, investigates the prenatal factors that enhance maternal health, promote a healthy intrauterine environment, and increase the odds for a healthy neonate. The nurse caring for the pregnant client must teach and counsel prospective parents about such factors as genetic disorders and maternal physical and psychological status—as well as provide specific care measures that promote maternal and fetal health.

This unit helps the nurse fulfill these roles by examining the events of pregnancy—from the moment of conception to the onset of labor—and by delineating the prenatal care required by the pregnant client and her family. It discusses fetal growth and development; surveys all facets of normal pregnancy, including the physiologic and psychosocial changes that it causes; outlines family preparation for childbirth and parenting; discusses the effect of nutrition on fetal outcome; and details the nurse's role in maintaining high-quality antepartal care. To ensure effective nursing care in high-risk as well as low-risk situations, this unit also discusses pregnancy-related medical problems.

Unit Four, The Intrapartal Period, prepares the nurse to anticipate the needs of the childbearing family, promotes holistic care by emphasizing childbirth as a family-centered event, and examines the personal and cultural factors that may affect the way the client and her family experience and perceive the intrapartal experience. Stressing health promotion as a nursing goal, the unit discusses various independent nursing roles, such as teaching, counseling, supporting, and advocating. It covers high-risk as well as low-risk labor and delivery situations.

Unit Five, The Neonate, prepares the nurse to care for normal and high-risk neonates and their families, presenting neonatal nursing from a family-centered perspective. The unit emphasizes adapting effective nursing strategies for individual neonates and their families. In addition to describing how the nurse functions as a member of an interdependent health care team, the unit discusses neonatal care within the home, where the nurse can gain valuable insight into the functioning, interrelationships, and resources of the family. The unit also identifies trends in neonatal health care and delineates the problems that pose an increasing threat to future generations—for instance, the growing number of children born with acquired immunodeficiency syndrome (AIDS) or suffering the effects of maternal substance abuse.

Unit Six, The Postpartal Period, explains how the nurse meets the physiologic, psychosocial, and teaching needs of the postpartal family by providing specific nursing measures, knowledge, counseling, and support. It describes the anatomic and physiologic changes that restore the body to a nonpregnant state, and it discusses nursing care to promote full postpartal recovery. Taking a family-centered approach, it explains how the nurse helps individual family members adjust to changes in their roles, tasks, and responsibilities and to the new family structure after childbirth. The unit also covers such trends as home nursing care for the postpartal client.

Useful appendices cover standards of nursing care required by NAACOG, the organization for obstetric, gynecologic, and neonatal nurses; the taxonomy of the North American Nursing Diagnosis Association; a conversion table for neonatal weights; temperature conversions; 1990 nutritional guidelines and weight table; selected resources for the disabled pregnant client; support resources for families with special-needs neonates; and guidelines for the prevention of HIV transmission. A master glossary of over 750 terms concludes the text. A thorough index allows easy access to all information.

Many features of this text make it an excellent resource. Its unit organization reflects its major concepts; it addresses issues, concerns, and trends for the student or nurse embracing maternal, neonatal, and family care; it relies on the nursing process to foster understanding of the dynamic connection between nurse and client; it applies nursing research to practice; and its chapter bibliographies group references by content concerns. These features produce a resource that encourages critical thinking and furthers professional and attentive care. Written for students and nurses by nurses with outstanding credentials and experience, *Maternal, Neonatal, and Women's Health Nursing* is practical, forward looking, and rich in details and appeal. In short, it sets high standards for the field.

Nancy Fugate Woods, RN, PhD, FAAN
Professor, Parent and Child Nursing
Director, Center for Women's Health
Research, University of Washington,
Seattle

PREFACE

The nurse who provides holistic maternal-neonatal care reaches beyond childbearing or reproductive concerns to comprehensive health care throughout the client's life. Such care is best administered within the context of the family because a client's health can affect—or be affected by—her family. To be appropriate and effective, the nurse's care must encompass the three universal standards of nursing specified by NAACOG, the organization for obstetric, gynecologic, and neonatal nurses: care that focuses on achieving optimum health potential within the framework of the nursing process; health education that encourages participation in and shared responsibility for health promotion, maintenance, and restoration; and policies, procedures, and protocols that clarify the scope of nursing practice and delineate the qualifications of those who administer care.

Maternal, Neonatal, and Women's Health Nursing helps today's nurses meet the challenges of these standards. Written for the undergraduate nursing student, this textbook is intended for use in nursing courses that cover physiology, clinical obstetrics, family-centered care, and neonatal care. It provides a balance of these content elements and also includes a women's health care component—a mix that is necessary to meet the growing demand for more comprehensive instruction in nursing care of women. It also accurately reflects the nursing model of care, highlighting its holistic nature and focus on health promotion.

This comprehensive textbook is practical, up-to-date, and easy to use. With its in-depth coverage of maternity and neonatal subjects and its inclusion of women's health outside the childbearing family, *Maternal, Neonatal, and Women's Health Nursing* is fully in step with today's nursing curricula and especially useful to those who must keep pace with rapidly evolving nursing skills, practice, and research. Because it presents basic and advanced nursing subjects, this text enriches students at every skill level.

The text consistently uses the nursing process as a format for each nursing care chapter. This presentation helps the student learn how to apply the nursing process to clinical practice. Each nursing care chapter begins with a discussion of pertinent physiologic principles, which is followed by assessment, nursing diagnosis, planning and implementation, and evaluation of care for the client and family. It concludes with documentation of the nursing process, reinforcing the need to assess and intervene accurately and thoughtfully.

Emphasizing its nursing process focus, the text distinguishes itself by integrating nursing diagnoses throughout. Each nursing care chapter contains an alphabetized list of representative diagnoses (including problem and etiology statements) appropriate for the types of clients the chapter addresses. In each of these chapters, nursing diagnoses also appear in emphatic dark type in the "Planning and implementation" section, explicitly linking nursing diagnoses and

appropriate interventions. The Appendix includes the complete list of nursing diagnostic categories by functional pattern, as approved by the North American Nursing Diagnosis Association (NANDA).

Maternal, Neonatal, and Women's Health Nursing is shaped by several key themes, including:
• Family-centered care. In addition to chapters devoted to the history, trends, and theories of family care, many other chapters highlight family considerations when caring for a client or her neonate.
• Health promotion. Addressed in every unit, often in the form of nursing care for the healthy client, client teaching handouts, and client self-care guidelines, health promotion reaffirms the nursing precept that all passages in a woman's life—from menarche to menopause—are essentially natural and normal.
• Care through advanced technology. Electronic fetal monitoring, laser surgery, in vitro fertilization, fetal extracorporeal membrane oxygenation, and other advanced technologies familiarize the student with these increasingly used options.
• Nursing's expanding role in maternal, neonatal, and women's health. Early chapters identify careers and advanced practice roles for nurses in these specialty areas. Later chapters highlight the contributions of nurse researchers, dramatizing the link between research and practice. All chapters recognize the nurse's key roles in health promotion, teaching, and family-centered nursing care.

As recommended by the Maternal-Infant Core Competency Project Regional Conferences, the text provides information in the three domains of learning—cognitive, psychomotor, and affective. It presents cognitive information clearly and logically with an emphasis on critical thinking. To address the psychomotor domain, it provides step-by-step instructions and illustrations for many clinical skills. For the affective domain, it includes a balanced presentation of various sensitive issues, such as abortion, in vitro fertilization, and antepartal diagnostic testing.

Maternal, Neonatal, and Women's Health Nursing is organized in six units—Nursing the Childbearing Family: History, Concepts, and Practice; Women's Health Care; The Antepartal Period; The Intrapartal Period; The Neonate; and The Postpartal Period. This organization encourages study of comprehensive and closely focused information, which also can be reviewed later with ease.

The first unit develops the relationship between the nurse and the childbearing family, highlighting family-centered care, use of the nursing process, and related ethical and legal issues. All subsequent units begin with chapters that present basic information about anatomy, physiology, and, when appropriate, psychosocial concerns. This sets the stage for the remainder of the chapters in the unit, and it helps the student differentiate clearly between normal and abnormal findings. The postpartal and neonatal units end with chapters on nursing care at home, a topic of increasing importance to nurses.

Useful pedagogical devices assist the reader throughout. Every chapter begins with learning objectives that focus the reader and with a glossary of important terms that acts as a ready reference. Each chapter's text emphasizes critical thinking in its systematic presentation and in the follow-up study questions. A summary restates and reinforces key information. Each chapter concludes with an up-to-date bibliography that is organized by the chapter's principal topics for the reader who wishes to explore a particular subject.

Throughout the text, charts and graphic materials hold the reader's attention, promote deeper understanding, and summarize data for easy recall. Vital nursing procedures and descriptions of anatomy and physiology are vividly illustrated. Bulleted lists and tables provide rapid review, and charts efficiently organize larger units of information.

Photographs illustrate noteworthy aspects of childbearing. These include award-winning photographs of fetal development by Lennart Nilsson and of a dramatic birthing sequence by Harriette Hartigan, a nurse-midwife. Unit-opening photographs capture major events in a woman's life with her child and family.

To highlight important themes and types of information and to promote access to and use of the information, many recurring features are included.

• *Psychomotor skills* presents illustrated, step-by-step instructions for detailed nursing assessment techniques, treatments, or other procedures.

• *Emergency alert* helps the nurse rapidly identify serious maternal or fetal problems, assess their severity, and intervene appropriately.

• *Family considerations* suggests appropriate nursing interventions for the client's family and demonstrates holistic, family-centered care.

• *Fetal status* and *Maternal status* assist the nurse in providing care for two clients at once through assessment reminders, special considerations, and nursing interventions.

• *Cultural considerations* provides a short list of assessment tips and special considerations or interventions for a nurse who is caring for a client—and family—from a culture other than the nurse's own.

• *Nursing research applied* summarizes a recent nursing research article and describes its application to nursing practice.

• *Client teaching* speaks directly to the client and provides useful instructions for self-care. After using this information to teach the client, the nurse can photocopy it for the client to take home.

• *Nursing diagnoses* presents an alphabetized list of appropriate nursing diagnoses based on the chapter's content and the NANDA taxonomy.

• *Applying the nursing process* describes how to perform nursing process steps for a client with a condition drawn from that chapter's content. A rationale for each nursing intervention assists student understanding.

Supplementary materials support teaching and learning with this text. For each text chapter, the *Instructor's Manual* includes a chapter overview, suggested lecture topics, suggested critical thinking activities, answers to study questions that appear in the text, and a test bank with answers and rationales. It also provides separate pages of test questions suitable for photocopying and overhead transparency masters on anatomy, physiology, assessment techniques, and clinical procedures. The *Student's Activities Book* presents various self-test materials, such as matching terminology and definitions, fill-in-the-blank questions, anatomic diagrams to label, values clarification exercises, and clinical simulations with questions.

The text and its supplements reflect years of nursing expertise through its contributors and consultants from the United States and Canada. All contributors are at least master's degree-prepared practicing clinicians, academicians, or researchers. Furthermore, a panel of experts in maternal, neonatal, and women's health has reviewed each chapter, and a distinguished advisory board has overseen the total effect of the book. The contributions of all these experts give the student a comprehensive view of this nursing specialty—and a well-illustrated, clinically applicable, and up-to-date text that its readers can continue to use through their years of clinical practice.

Nursing the Childbearing Family: History, Concepts, and Practice

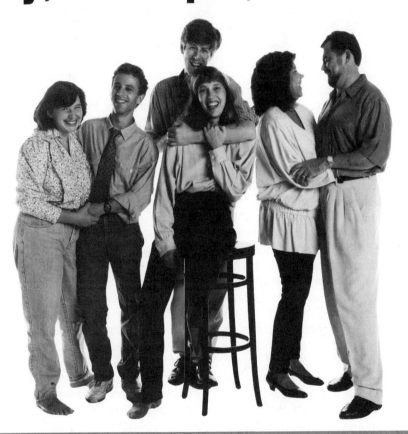

A s the twenty-first century approaches, the role of the nurse caring for the childbearing family becomes increasingly complex. Significant changes in both the health care system and family structure have dramatically altered the needs of childbearing families. To meet the challenge of caring for these families, nursing also must evolve.

This unit investigates important concepts in the nursing care of childbearing families, setting the stage for a holistic, family-centered approach to care. It surveys the changes that have affected the delivery of health care throughout history, explores the role of the nurse in a changing society, and predicts the changes that may be needed to improve family care. The unit presents a framework for analyzing family structure and function and shows how the nursing process can be applied to the family. It also guides the nurse through the delicate legal and ethical issues that have arisen in response to rapid technological advances, the proliferation of malpractice lawsuits against physicians and nurses, and recent legal decisions affecting a woman's right in the outcome of pregnancy.

Chapter 1
Family Nursing Care: History and Trends

Chapter 1 lays the foundation for family nursing care, placing it within the context of the changing social, economic, and political influences on the family throughout history. After tracing the evolution of the family from the traditional nuclear unit to the variations seen today, it discusses the family's basic functions. The chapter explores the history of family nursing care from ancient times to the early twentieth century. Then it identifies recent trends that have influenced families and their nursing care, such as reduced family size, increased numbers of working women, and two-career families. The chapter shows how women's changing roles and the consumer movement have enhanced client participation in health care, and touches on the ethical and legal concerns raised by expanded freedom of consumer choice. It describes the economic pressures that have turned health care facilities into competitive businesses and explores the ramifications of increased competition. It addresses the growing problem of increased health care costs and discusses the effects of cost-containment measures on the health care industry.

The chapter also explores the changing role of the nurse in providing family care. It describes the factors that have triggered a trend toward generalist maternity nursing but specialist neonatal nursing. It discusses the various roles and functions of the modern nurse in providing family care, with special focus on the growing importance of the nurse-researcher in providing a scientific basis for nursing care. The chapter describes career alternatives in family nursing, detailing the experience, education, and credentials required for specific nursing positions. It forecasts trends that will affect family nursing care, such as an increased emphasis on critical thinking and technical competency that will demand faster assimilation and application of new information by the nurse. It also discusses the importance of primary nursing to allow for greater individualization of nursing care, and predicts such trends as the continuation of early discharge for technology-dependent neonates and recommendations for the perinatal partnership model for regionalization. The chapter concludes with a discussion of current nursing research trends and predictions for research.

Chapter 2
Family Structure and Function

Chapter 2 defines and describes classic theories used to study and understand family structure and function, systems theory, structural-functional theory, developmental theory, interactional theory, and social exchange theory. The chapter explains how the nurse can apply each theory to a specific family to gain a broader perspective on the family's structure and function. Then it describes the various types of families found in Western society, from the traditional nuclear family to less conventional family types. The chapter elaborates on the functions of the family, from ensuring physical safety and providing sustenance to family members to helping members grow and develop psychologically and socially.

Next, the chapter explores family roles—the behavior patterns by which family members carry out their functions. After describing how family roles are assigned, it examines types of roles, both formal and informal, within a family. To help the nurse better understand family structure and function, the chapter investigates the four major family patterns—autocratic, patriarchal, matriarchal, and democratic.

Finally, Chapter 2 explores families in crisis. After identifying the various coping mechanisms a family may use in a crisis, the chapter examines family responses to crisis, detailing some factors that influence these responses.

Chapter 3
Nursing Process and the Childbearing Family

Chapter 3 presents a detailed examination of the nursing process, showing how the nurse applies the nursing process when caring for the childbearing family. It begins by discussing assessment, the first step in the nursing process, during which the nurse collects subjective and objective data. The chapter explains how to elicit information related to childbearing during the health history interview. To help ensure a holistic assessment, it highlights methods the nurse can use to assess a client's cultural, ethnic, religious, socioeconomic, and psychological background. Then the chapter briefly describes the components of physical assessment.

The chapter also explains how the nurse analyzes assessment data to formulate nursing diagnoses, the second step in the nursing process. It identifies nursing diagnosis categories established by the North American Nursing Diagnosis Association (NANDA) based on nine human response patterns, and it shows how the nurse assigns nursing diagnoses through a three-step process. This chapter includes a list of selected NANDA-approved diagnostic labels organized by human response pattern.

The chapter then addresses planning and intervention, the next step in the nursing process. It details the three phases of planning—setting and prioritizing goals, formulating nursing interventions, and developing a care plan. It presents examples of complete goal statements, details the categories of information that must be included in every nursing care plan, and provides a sample of a complete nursing care plan for a childbearing couple.

Chapter 3 then focuses on implementation, the next step in the nursing process, during which the nurse strives to accomplish the interventions specified in the care plan. The chapter identifies the four types of skills needed to implement nursing interventions effectively and offers guidelines for teaching adult clients—guidelines the nurse can use when implementing interventions that involve client teaching.

The chapter then addresses evaluation, the final step in the nursing process, explaining how the nurse uses assessment data to determine if goals have been met. It emphasizes the ongoing nature of evaluation and shows how evaluation is linked to and based on the goals developed for each nursing diagnosis. It also explains what to do if a goal remains unmet. Finally, the chapter discusses documentation, pointing out how documentation of nursing care promotes communication among members of the health care team and serves as a discharge planning tool and a legal record of care provided.

Chapter 4
Nurse-Client Interaction

Chapter 4 begins by describing the five interrelated phases of nurse-client interaction—preparation, initiation, consolidation and growth, development, and termination. It explores the roles of both nurse and client during each phase and explains how an emergency affects the duration and tasks of each phase.

The chapter then discusses the three skills most essential to nurse-client interaction. First it focuses on communicating, the skill through which the nurse determines the client's concerns and assesses her needs. The chapter elaborates on the steps that make the exchange of information between nurse and client easier and more effective, and details the special rights of the pregnant client.

Next, the chapter discusses teaching, the second skill essential to interaction. It examines how client age and readiness to learn affect teaching, explores outside influences that may pose obstacles to learning, and explains how the nurse can adapt teaching methods to the client's learning style. The chapter describes how the nurse can create an individualized teaching program and identifies the benefits and drawbacks of major teaching

strategies and tools. It also explains how the nurse evaluates the effectiveness of teaching.

Chapter 4 then discusses motivating, the third essential interactive skill. It illustrates how a caring attitude can help motivate a client to take charge of her own health care, and it examines various approaches to caring. The chapter concludes with a brief discussion of the benefits of self-care, in which the client actively and assertively participates in attaining her health care goals.

Chapter 5
Ethical and Legal Concerns in Family Care

Chapter 5 addresses the ethical and legal issues that the nurse may confront in caring for the family. It begins by defining ethics and identifying contrasting approaches to ethical decision making. It describes the principles that form the basis of ethical decisions, explains how financial and religious considerations may influence decisions, and presents a systematic decision-making model to help the nurse cope with ethical dilemmas.

The chapter shows how the nurse can use professional standards and guidelines to make ethical decisions with greater confidence and a decreased risk of liability, and it explains the importance of balancing these standards and guidelines against personal convictions, laws, and health care facility policies. It delineates the relationship between ethics and law and discusses the limitations of laws in defining personal ethical standards. Chapter 5 then addresses malpractice, detailing the four factors a plaintiff must prove to win a malpractice suit against a nurse or other health care provider and exploring recent trends in nurse malpractice cases. It identifies useful risk management strategies for maternal and neonatal nursing, including designation of a risk manager, use of incident reports and in-house attorneys, and accurate and thorough documentation of care.

The chapter then investigates specific ethical and legal issues in maternal and neonatal care. After discussing confidentiality and refusal of treatment, it presents a detailed exploration of the ethical issues particularly relevant to family nursing care—sterilization, infertility, surrogate motherhood, prenatal diagnosis, abortion, fetal research, fetal therapy, and fetal monitoring. The chapter concludes with a discussion of ethical issues surrounding the sick neonate, such as parental consent for potentially harmful procedures and withholding of treatment for the severely disabled neonate.

Family Nursing Care: History and Trends

Objectives

After reading and studying this chapter, the student should be able to:
1. Describe the functions of the family.
2. State key historic events that have affected nursing and women.
3. Trace the evolution of nurse-midwifery.
4. Describe recent social trends that have affected women and their families.
5. Define consumerism in health care.
6. Describe the relationship between women's changing roles and their active participation in health care.
7. List recent economic trends that have affected family health care in the United States and Canada.
8. Define current roles and careers in family nursing care.
9. State priorities for family nursing research.

Introduction

Family nursing care aims to deliver professional, quality health care to all family members based on their needs. To understand those needs, the nurse must apply various family theories and consider the family's culture and religion. (For more information, see Chapter 2, Family Structure and Function, and Chapter 3, Nursing Process and the Childbearing Family.)

When providing family nursing care to the client or her neonate, the nurse also cares for the client's family. For example, when providing postpartal home care, the nurse assesses how the client and her family function with the addition of a new member. Therefore, the nurse needs a working knowledge of family functions and dynamics.

A full understanding of family nursing care requires knowledge of the economic, social, and political influences on the family. To carry out nursing functions, the nurse must be responsive to societal needs, cultural values, financial constraints, and the political climate (American Nurses' Association [ANA], 1980). That means examining family nursing care in a social context to understand the family's nursing care needs for today and tomorrow.

To provide a foundation for care, Chapter 1 discusses the family and nursing care and presents the history of, recent trends in, and future projections for family nursing care in the United States and Canada.

The family

Until recently, the family was defined as a unit with a father, mother, dependent children, and possibly grandparents—known as the nuclear family. Today, however, that definition does not describe increasing numbers of family units. For example, today's family might be a couple with children, a single parent with children born before a divorce, a couple with children from previous marriages, a single parent (never married) with a child from a former or present partner, a single mother (never married) who was artificially inseminated, a married or unmarried couple with an adopted child, a married or unmarried couple with children, and so on. In short, many different combinations of people who live together may be a family. (For more information, see Chapter 2, Family Structure and Function.)

GLOSSARY

Diagnosis-related group (DRG): one of 470 groups of related diagnoses, each of which has an estimated length of hospital stay and cost. In the prospective payment system, DRGs are the basis for reimbursement by many private insurance companies and federal insurance programs.

Health care facility: service organization that provides health care services based on societal and client demands.

Health maintenance organization (HMO): group practice that charges a flat fee for each insured client, regardless of the extent or type of services the group provides. It emphasizes provision of government-mandated services that help maintain health and reduce inpatient hospital stays.

Preferred provider organization (PPO): group practice similar to an HMO, except that the insured client has the option of receiving care from a provider outside of the group for a somewhat higher fee. PPO services are not government-mandated.

Professional standards review organization (PSRO): organization that reviews the quality, usage, and type of services offered by a health care facility.

Prospective payment system (PPS): reimbursement system for health care services that allows a specific amount of money for a specific diagnosis, no matter how many days the client is hospitalized.

Regionalization of care: regional system that avoids costly duplication of services and ensures availability of essential services. Hospitals and special facilities, such as neonatal intensive care units and trauma units, are classified as primary, secondary, and tertiary health centers, depending on the facilities and personnel available, the population served, the number of beds in the facility, and other criteria.

Regardless of the family's composition, it performs most or all of the following functions.

• Affective. The family provides affection and understanding, which meets family members' psychosocial needs.

• Socialization and social placement. The family serves as the primary orientation for children to society. It also confers status on members based on their family roles.

• Reproductive. By conceiving and raising children, the family ensures its continuity and that of the species.

• Economic. The family provides financial resources and allocations to its members.

• Health. The family provides physical necessities, such as food, shelter, and health care (Friedman, 1986).

Nursing care

Families always have needed nursing care to fulfill their health care functions. Historically, female family members have provided this care; today, they continue this role, adding to it the role of health care broker (selecting the health care professional and facility for the family).

Because of today's family variations, family nursing care must address multiple needs and be open and nonjudgmental. Also, the nurse must be aware of family functions and help the client who provides and seeks health care for the family.

History of family nursing care

Throughout history, socioeconomic factors and technological advances have influenced the family and the development of nursing.

Early history

From the beginning of civilization to the fall of the Roman Empire around 500 A.D., women generally performed nursing tasks for family members or friends (Doheny, Cook, and Stopper, 1987). During this time, most people believed disease was the work of spirits.

The ancient Greek Hippocrates (c. 460 to c. 377 B.C.) began to move science and medicine from the supernatural realm to a more objective sphere by teaching that disease diagnosis was based on patient behaviors (Mitchell, 1968). For example, if the patient coughed up sputum, Hippocrates would diagnose the cause as a lung disease. He and his contemporaries recognized the need for trained nurses to care for the sick properly (Bullough and Bullough, 1978).

Around 300 B.C., the Romans initiated military nursing and built hospitals to treat the wounded. They also developed specialized attendants for civilian patients. Women known as midwives regularly attended births. (For more information, see *Developments in nurse-midwifery history.*)

From about 500 to 1500 A.D., a nurse was "any woman responsible for another's health" (Nightingale, 1859), and she could receive training from religious or military orders. As Christianity spread, the Roman Catholic church's influence on nursing began to grow. In the Mediterranean, convents and monasteries were used as treatment centers, and several orders of nuns started providing simple nursing care to meet patients' physical needs. During the Crusades, governments called on nurses to care for sick and wounded soldiers.

Society was primarily agricultural, and the family lived and worked together. Because families produced their own foods and goods and cared for their own sick, they were self-sufficient. Family members had the necessary skills because families had to maintain themselves or perish. Each member's activities contributed to the family's overall success.

As an outgrowth of these values, humanism began. This philosophy emphasized the individual's dignity and worth and capacity for self-realization. It continued to grow during the Renaissance.

Sixteenth to early nineteenth century

From about 1500 to the mid-1800s, Christianity was widespread, but internal struggles within the Catholic church caused deterioration of church-affiliated nursing care. Because of these struggles and because many Europeans still believed in supernatural powers, the church persecuted and burned as witches many nurses who practiced midwifery and healing. As nursing lost status and the church's support, only women of poor social standing continued to nurse (Palmer, 1977).

As late as the early 1800s, women were not allowed higher education. Most were prepared only for the socially acceptable roles of wife and mother. However, Florence Nightingale (1820 to 1910) pursued nursing, even though society viewed it with disdain. (Many people thought all nurses were like Sairey Gamp, the alcoholic, sadistic nurse in Dickens's 1844 novel, *Martin Chuzzlewit.*) The only nursing education available to Nightingale was on-the-job training in hospitals, which were little more than places where people died. This training was necessary, however, to prepare nurses to care for wounded soldiers. In the United States, wars aided the development of nursing for similar reasons—care for wounded soldiers (Bullough and Bullough, 1978). Even so, nursing did not make significant progress until after 1850.

Late nineteenth century

From the mid-1800s to the turn of the century, society changed rapidly in response to the Industrial Revolution (widespread change in the manufacture of goods through the use of power-driven machinery) and its major economic changes. The religious orders again established hospitals and called on women to become nurses. Because of the church's power and standing, this move made education acceptable for women and upgraded hospital facilities.

The Industrial Revolution affected family structure and roles. Many people left farming to work in factories where goods were mass-produced for resale rather than individually produced for family needs. However, family members who worked in factories earned meager salaries, worked long hours, and no longer could help the family produce all the goods its members needed. Those members who stayed at home could not meet the entire family's needs.

Two major classes developed in cities: the working class that performed the labor and the new middle class that enjoyed economic benefits from the new system. Poverty among workers was commonplace. Initially, most working class women remained at home to tend to family matters, while the rest of the family worked in factories. Even children were employed for 12 to 18 hours a day.

Gradually, however, women moved from work in the home to work in factories, hospitals, and schools. Jobs in hospitals and schools were considered particularly appropriate for women because they involved teaching children and caring for the sick—both related to the responsibilities of motherhood (Muff, 1988).

Women rarely had opportunities for advanced education, and the jobs open to them typically had lower status and earning potential than jobs that were open to men. Usually, jobs available to women were supervised by men and offered little opportunity for advancement. Nurses, in particular, found themselves in a male-dominated hierarchy in hospitals.

In Europe, Nightingale wrote her first book, *Cassandra* (1852, rev. ed., Stark, 1979), to speak against women's powerlessness. During the Crimean War in 1854, she established herself as an international figure. Nightingale studied the patient in the context of the environment. She observed that lack of light, warmth, cleanliness, ventilation, and proper nutrition were more responsible for war fatalities than were the combat wounds. She documented a decreased mortality rate after she and assisting nuns began caring for the injured; the mortality rate dropped from 42.7% to 2.2% in one year (Shealy, 1985). These dramatic results convinced skeptical physicians and the world of the advantages of

Developments in nurse-midwifery history

Throughout recorded history, midwives have provided competent maternal and neonatal care. However, their popularity has waxed and waned under the influence of socioeconomic factors, as described below.

Ancient times through 500 A.D.
Women known as midwives routinely attend births.

500 to 1500
British, French, German, and Greek records commonly refer to midwives at childbirth (Towler and Bramall, 1986).

1500 to 1700
Midwives typically are the only attendants at births in England, Germany, Italy, and Austria (Ehrenreich and English, 1973; Litoff, 1986).

1700 to 1800
Midwives attend births in the United States as immigrants adhere to the customs of their homeland. They continue to be valued and revered until the late eighteenth century.

Early 1800s
Physicians begin to manage childbirth in the United States and Britain. The medical profession emphasizes science, specialization, and formal standards for education and practice, which diminishes the role of nondegreed attendants at childbirth. Yet midwives continue to attend most births in Europe and about 50% of births in the United States (Litoff, 1986).

1800s to 1920
No formal education or practice standards exist for midwives. Instead, most learn their skills during informal apprenticeships. In England and the United States, male physicians usually care for upper class women; midwives usually care for poor and working class women.

Early 1900s
Scientific maternity care in the hospital is more common in the United States than in other countries, yet maternal and infant mortality rates are among the highest in the world (Litoff, 1986).
  Federal Children's Bureau established with assistance of Lillian Wald, who implemented the services to provide maternal-infant care by nurses and midwives.
  Shepherd Towner Act provided money for maternal-infant care, which was given by public health nurses and nurse-midwives.

1925-1932
Mary Breckinridge establishes the Frontier Nursing Service in Kentucky with British-trained nurse-midwives and American public health nurses. Her service boasts a maternal mortality rate of 0.68% when the national rate is 7% (Dye, 1983).
  The New York Maternity Center Association establishes a midwife school and clinic. Midwives trained here have a 0.1% maternal mortality rate when the average rate is 10.4% in New York City.

1940
Tuskegee Nurse-Midwifery School for black nurses opens in Alabama at a time when the maternal mortality rate is 8.5 per 1,000 live births and the fetal death rate in Macon County is 45.9 per 1,000 live births. Two years later, the county's maternal mortality rate is 0 and the fetal death rate drops to 14 per 1,000 live births for women under nurse-midwife care (Carnegie, 1986).

1945-1955
Catholic University of America and the Catholic Maternity Institute of New Mexico establishes the first university-affiliated master's degree nurse-midwife program.
  State University of New York and the Downstate Medical Center move the midwife school under the medical college.
  American College of Nurse-Midwives is established.

1970-1980s
Consumer movement causes an increase in the number of midwife-attended births, which leads to an increase in the number of midwife programs and positions.
  ACOG, NAACOG, and the ACNM develop a collaborative statement that formally recognizes nurse-midwives as members of the obstetric team.

Early 1990s
Nurse-midwives work in local health care facilities, health maintenance organizations, federal agencies, tertiary centers, birthing centers, home care agencies, as well as many in private practice.

expert nursing care. Nightingale's efforts promoted nursing and aided society's acceptance of it as a vocation.

After the war, Nightingale wrote *Notes on nursing: What it is and what it is not* (1859). In this book, she stated that nursing assisted nature, but that only nature could cure. Her ideas formed the foundation of modern nursing and its major concepts: nurse, patient, environment, and health. They also served as the basis of the nursing process used today.

In 1860, Nightingale set up the Nightingale School for Nurses at St. Thomas Hospital in London (Stark, 1979). This school marked the beginning of formal nursing education.

In the United States, Dr. Elizabeth Blackwell, the first woman to graduate from a U.S. medical school, attempted to train nurses using the Nightingale model (Bullough and Bullough, 1984). The Civil War (1861 to 1865) increased the demand for large numbers of nurses. Dorothea Lynde Dix, superintendent of the Female Nurses of the Union Army, directed nurse training. Clara Barton and Mother Bickerdyke also helped with the training, using many of Nightingale's concepts.

Sojourner Truth, a freed black slave, was a nurse during the Civil War. After the war, she nursed at Freeman's Hospital in Washington, met with President Lincoln, and lobbied Congress for funds to train nurses and physicians (Carnegie, 1986).

After the Civil War, the Nightingale model of training gained still wider acceptance in the United States. In 1872, the New England Hospital for Women and Children in Boston established the first training school in the United States. (In 1878, this hospital graduated Mary Eliza Mahoney, the first trained black nurse in the United States.) Implementation of the complete Nightingale model, including the issuance of diplomas, occurred in 1873 at the Bellevue Training School in New York, the New Haven Training School in Connecticut, and the Boston Training School in Massachusetts (Doheny, Cook, and Stopper, 1987).

Almost at once, the need arose for training in specialized skills. As a result, apprenticeships flourished in industry and health care. Historians say that hospitals of this period "owned" nurses because they trained women for work in their institutions, teaching them skills that were not easily transferable in a time of nonstandardized care. Most hospitals exploited nurses as cheap labor during their training.

The Industrial Revolution also brought a new set of health problems. As industry grew, cities expanded rapidly and factory wastes contaminated water supplies.

Combined with a lack of sanitation, these factors led to the spread of cholera, yellow fever, malaria, and typhoid fever (ANA, 1976). As a result, health care focused on sickness and disease rather than on natural occurrences, such as childbirth.

With the scientific advances that were made during this period, medicine and nursing grew, along with an increased knowledge of bacteria, microbes, species-specific diseases, and the development of X-rays. These advances helped reduce deaths from cholera and other communicable diseases. Public health nursing, which became popular in the 1880s, also helped reduce the death rate. Public health nurses typically provided home nursing care, which was vital to families who no longer felt able to meet health care needs by themselves.

To combat the spread of communicable diseases, such interventions as aseptic techniques and isolation wards became popular. Health care began to focus on expert skills, and hospitals became institutions of specialized health care delivery, replacing the home as a care setting.

With these technological changes, families felt even less able to provide care. Indeed, they looked to hospitals and health care experts if they could afford the services. As health care was increasingly institutionalized in hospitals, it became a commodity for purchase. Working class families had to depend on the wages they earned to purchase needed health care.

Early twentieth century

As health care became a commodity for purchase, the public began to demand the establishment of standards. In response, North Carolina passed a law in 1900 to create registration for nurses (Nahm, 1981), which helped improve the status of nursing. Over the next two decades, all states passed comparable laws. Nursing also responded to public concern over the infant mortality rate in the 1900s. For example, the Boston Lying-In Hospital began a home delivery program where a nurse visited a pregnant woman at home every 10 days before delivery (Arnold, Brecht, Hockett, Amspacher, and Grad, 1989). The program provided good prenatal care and decreased infant mortality.

From 1908 to 1917, the federal and state governments enacted laws to protect employees from harsh industrial working conditions. The status of women—and nurses—began to change also, primarily because more women joined the work force. As women contributed more to the family's resources from outside earnings, they developed a stronger power base in the family and in society.

This movement accelerated during World War I. To support the war effort, many women began working in factories and hospitals. After the war, many of these jobs were taken over by men, but the trend was already under way.

In 1923, the Goldmark Report increased the status of nursing. It called for revision of nurse training and an emphasis on education. By 1933, nursing had earned its place in higher education. The Association of Collegiate Schools of Nursing was formed and became a member of the American Council on Education (Dolan, Fitzpatrick, and Herrmann, 1983).

The Great Depression slowed the progress of nurses and other professional women during the 1930s. Because families had little money to spend on health care, nursing services were not in demand.

World War II re-energized the workplace. As the need for nurses grew, nursing training accelerated. In 1941 and 1942, the Bolton Bill provided federal assistance for nursing education. In 1942, the government founded the National Nursing Council for War Service, which enlisted the help of Dr. Esther Brown to study nursing education. Her report called for university schools of nursing and encouraged men to join the profession (Dolan, Fitzpatrick, and Herrmann, 1983).

As the civilian labor pool of men decreased during World War II, women entered higher paying fields, such as banking and manufacturing. At the end of the war, men reclaimed many of these jobs, but 15% to 20% of working women were in jobs and labor unions with higher pay. Labor unions dropped restrictions against women members and instituted an equal pay for equal work policy, increasing women's earning power.

Recent trends

In the late twentieth century, social, economic, and family nursing trends greatly affected families and their nursing care.

Social trends

Key social trends include decreased family size, an increased number of women in the work force and two-career families, and more active participation in health care.

Family size

Recent technological and economic changes have greatly affected family size, roles, and living environments. In 1970, the average U.S. family size was 5.79; in 1980, 2.75 (Santi, 1987). Although birth rates rose during the Baby Boom in the 1950s, the size of the U.S. household fell steadily through the 1970s because of high divorce rates, increased age at first marriage, changed household composition (such as an increased number of female-headed households), and an increased number of people of childbearing age who lived alone. In the early 1980s, the household size declined slowly (Santi, 1987).

Today's family has no need for members to produce its goods; rather, its first concern is with finances. In contrast to earlier times, a family is so expensive that in many cases both parents must work, making them unavailable to help socialize and care for children. When adult relatives are not available, parents may need to purchase child care services outside the family.

Women in the work force

Today, nearly two-thirds of all women in the United States work outside the home. Although their career options have expanded, most women work in only 20 occupations, including clerical and sales jobs. The average salary for women is 64% of the average salary for men. Men working in professions with the highest salaries earn about $100 more per week than women employed in their highest-paying professions (Sidel, 1987). Thus, in spite of fair labor practice laws, women commonly earn significantly less than men. The situation is similar in Canada, where men typically earn two-fifths more money than women for comparable jobs (Landsberg, 1986).

Because women generally earn less money than men for the same or equivalent work, they cannot contribute as much as men to a family's income and are more likely to have a lower standard of living if they head the household. These women also are less likely to have health insurance. More than 9 million childbearing women had no health insurance in 1984, and 5 million women with insurance had no maternity benefits (National Perinatal Association, 1989).

Along with lower income and inadequate health insurance, the high number of adolescent pregnancies has contributed significantly to infant mortality. In 1985, the birthrate was 52.5 per 1,000 women ages 10 to 19 (U.S Bureau of the Census, 1987). Moore (1989) reports that 115 adolescents become pregnant every hour in the United States. Many of these pregnancies result in premature births and subsequent neonatal complications. Currently, the United States ranks nineteenth among all industrialized countries in infant mortality (Arnold, Brecht, Hockett, Amspacher, and Grad, 1989).

Many women in the work force are mothers. For these women, key concerns include maternity leave, child care, stress, and the effects of their careers on their children.

Maternity leave. Although parents are increasingly seeking maternity or paternity leave after the birth or adoption of an infant, corporations contend that such leaves are too costly (Wisensale and Allison, 1989). Society, however, is demanding legislative changes to mandate such leaves to promote positive parent-infant interaction and role transition.

In 1987, 28 states and the federal government introduced maternity and paternity leave bills. However, only four states passed the legislation, and the laws differ greatly (Wisensale and Allison, 1989).

Child care. According to Shreve (1988), half of all women with children under age 3 are working outside the home. These women need affordable child care. Yet in the 1980s, cuts in funds for child care programs decreased the standards and the staff for many of these programs.

In response to these cuts and in recognition of the demands of child care and work, some corporations have started child care programs. Corporate child care programs reflect concern over the loss of productive hours when women must take work time to make child care arrangements.

Private child care services also are available. However, the cost of most private services exceeds the amount that most working women can afford, creating an economic barrier to employment for many mothers.

Affordable child care programs can help reduce stress for women who must balance their role in the work force and their role as a mother. Ross and Mirowsky (1988) found that women had high depression levels if child care was difficult to obtain and if their partner did not share in child care responsibilities. They had low depression levels if they encountered no difficulties with child care and their partner shared responsibility.

Stress. Working mothers typically report role stress, overload, and conflict that result from a full-time career and trying to meet the role demands of mother, homemaker, and partner. As a result of stress, women's health has declined. Smoking has increased among women, and more men than women have quit smoking since 1965 (Fiore, et al., 1989). As stress increases, so does risk-taking behavior, such as alcohol use (Bradstock, et al.,

1988). Sometimes this stress results from a perceived lack of control over job responsibilities. LaRosa (1988) found that women who perceive role stress or little control over the job are at significantly greater risk for illness, such as coronary heart disease.

Some women try to compensate by controlling an aspect of their lives, which can lead to an eating disorder, such as anorexia nervosa (characterized by prolonged refusal to eat) or bulimia (characterized by binge eating followed by purging). These problems are compounded by the perceived need to be thin at any cost (Akridge, 1989). (For more information about eating disorders, see Chapter 15, Women's Health-Compromising Behaviors.)

Perceived control over their lives can decrease women's stress. Perceived control over health outcomes can affect women's use of health promotion techniques, such as breast self-examination (BSE). In a recent study, Redeker (1989) found that women were more likely to perform BSE when they understood their susceptibility to breast cancer, learned about the benefits of screening techniques, and acquired this knowledge through self-paced learning.

Effects on children. Mothers in the work force also express concern about the impact of a career on their children. However, this concern is largely unsubstantiated. Research indicates some behavioral differences between children of working mothers and those of mothers who stay at home. Daughters of mothers who work outside the home exhibit more independence and autonomy than those of mothers who stay at home. They also have higher self-esteem and career goals (Shreve, 1988).

The differences between sons of working mothers and sons of mothers who stay at home is not as clear, perhaps because daughters see their mothers as role models and mirror the role they observe, whereas sons see their fathers as role models.

Two-career families

Many women in the work force are partners in two-career families. Stressors on the two-career family may be significant, especially if the family members' expectations about roles and family support are unmet. When each partner has minimum requirements to support the other in his or her career, then each has greater freedom to fulfill individual career or other goals. However, when one partner must repress goal achievements to support the other's goals, career stress is likely. Also, when the family must relocate to support one partner's career development, the other partner's career opportunities may be affected.

All two-career families with children share one

stressor in common: the need to balance parenting roles with career and partner roles. Stress is reduced in two-career families where income is sufficient to help balance these demands by allowing the partners to purchase child care and home care services. Stress may be greatly increased in two-career families where income is still insufficient.

Children of two-career families with adequate income do not seem to suffer from this arrangment. They do not report feeling cheated of time or attention. Rather, they report satisfaction with the family life-style, noting its positive aspects of financial security, self-sufficiency, and positive parental role models as benefits (Shreve, 1988).

The two-career life-style may delay childbearing. Many women want to establish a career before raising a family. This delay may put the woman's neonate at greater risk for a genetic defect, such as trisomy 21, or Down's syndrome (Creasy and Resnik, 1989). It also may increase the risk of workplace exposure to environmental substances, such as asbestos, radiation, pesticides, anesthetic gases, chemotherapeutic agents, organic solvents, and acids that may cause infertility or lead to health problems for a woman or fetus (Murphy, 1986). (For more information, see Chapter 11, Genetics and Genetic Disorders.)

Active health care participation

Two key factors account for more active participation by women in their health care: women's changing roles and the rise of consumerism. Although these factors have increased women's health care options, their effects also have posed concerns for the health care industry.

Women's changing roles. Throughout this century, women's roles have evolved greatly. This is evident in their perception and management of pregnancy and childbirth.

Traditional health care was paternalistic (Ashley, 1976). The physician told the woman what she needed and how she would receive health care. Today, except in emergencies, the pregnant woman generally has the economic power and personal freedom to choose among her health care options. She selects her health care facility and chooses her physician or nurse-midwife. She even may determine such things as delivery method, type of anesthesia to be used, and whether the neonate is located in the nursery or in her room. (For more information, see *Trends in childbirth care.*)

Consumerism. By the 1970s, women made up one-third of the work force. Greatly increased purchasing power gave them economic clout and greatly influenced how

Trends in childbirth care

Throughout most of the twentieth century, childbirth was viewed as a physician-dependent process and treated as an illness. During this time, women were heavily sedated to avoid labor pain.

Developments in the 1960s

In the 1960s, however, a more natural approach to childbirth came into vogue. Women began to take a stand on how and where childbirth should take place, and health care facilities responded by focusing on wellness rather than illness. Grantly Dick-Read (1959) wrote *Childbirth Without Fear,* and the Lamaze birthing method later became popular. Childbirth education classes offered prospective parents detailed instruction in childbirth preparation and delivery. Dr. Robert Bradley further aided the movement with his support of the partner's role in coaching during labor and delivery.

Developments in the 1970s

By 1978, however, an emphasis on convenience had been added to the prevailing model of care. Fetal monitoring, induced labor, and relatively safe cesarean delivery allowed labor and delivery to be planned (McBride, 1982), based on the family's, physician's, or health care facility's schedule. As a result, the cesarean birth rate nearly doubled between 1971 and 1978 (McBride, 1982).

After 1978, the trend again reversed. Reports of fetal damage or death related to maternal analgesia or anesthesia made women aware of and concerned about the fetal risks of modern medicine.

Today, natural childbirth is again an important approach to childbirth, with the revived popularity of midwives and homelike birthing rooms. This can be attributed to two key trends: women's changing roles and consumerism. These trends have given the pregnant client the power to choose her health care options.

they sought health care and how health care was provided.

Today, the pregnant woman has the right to assess the quality of service she receives and select future health care providers based on that assessment. During the antepartal, intrapartal, and postpartal periods, she and her partner have the right to be apprised of all information required to make a decision, have total control in making that decision, and challenge the authority of a health care professional or facility that puts them in a dependent position (Darling, 1988).

The pregnant woman can assess a health care provider before she receives care. She is no longer a patient but a client. Because of women's social and economic independence, health care professionals are paying more attention to women's desires. Consumerism is rising in the health care field.

A health care facility no longer can function as an authoritarian institution, but must operate as a business. To survive, it must create the right perception among consumers by creating an image and selling it to prospective clients (Peters and Austin, 1985).

Similarly, a health care professional no longer can take an authoritarian stance. To succeed, the professional must be a businessperson, market available services to prospective clients, and be responsive to their needs. Also, once the client selects a health care professional, that service must satisfy the client.

The woman's choice. The health care business has become a buyer's market; health care facilities have made great efforts to attract the business of pregnant clients. Instead of limiting birthing options to the hospital delivery room, they now may offer alternatives, such as delivery in a hospital, home, single-room maternity suite, labor-delivery-recovery-postpartal (LDRP) unit, or independent birth center.

Nurse-midwives are providing an option to pregnant clients who desire natural childbirth. They encourage the client to choose the position she wishes to be in during delivery. Besides the lithotomy position, she can squat, sit, or stand during delivery.

Many facilities also market their services to the pregnant client's family by providing family-oriented childbirth education classes. These classes may begin during the antepartal period and continue through the intrapartal and postpartal periods.

In response to demands for women's health care that does not focus solely on reproduction, women's health care collectives now offer another health care option: holistic care from a feminist perspective provided by nurse practitioners and nurse-midwives (Thomas, 1986). Most collectives offer routine Papanicolaou smears, breast examinations, stress management, counseling, and teaching. However, services vary from state to state, depending on the state's nurse practice act.

Today's pregnant client can select the health care facility, the professional who will assist her, and the health care itself. She can refuse drugs or medical procedures. She can opt to undergo genetic and other diagnostic tests on herself and her fetus. She can elect to terminate her pregnancy or prevent conception altogether.

Current concerns. The pregnant client's new freedom to choose has prompted concerns. Some physicians and facilities worry that this freedom will increase the number of malpractice cases if a client refuses technological interventions or opts for a nurse-managed, rather than a physician-managed, delivery. Some health care experts express concern about the client's right to make decisions that must weigh her best interests against those of the fetus, especially because the availability and legal ramifications of advanced technology can make such decisions extremely complex. For example, they wonder if the client should have the right to make a decision about the childbirth method and the use of electronic fetal monitoring (Afriat, 1987).

Because of these concerns and because the pregnant client can influence the childbearing process significantly, the client she must be armed with facts, know her options, and be an active participant in her health care decisions. She must possess sufficient data to make an informed decision for herself and her fetus. To assist the client, the nurse must provide information, be the client's advocate, and help her carry out her decision.

Economic demands

Health care has undergone dramatic changes in the past few years, primarily in response to economic demands. Not surprisingly, these changes have affected the nurse's role.

Hasenfeld (1983) describes the health care facility as a human service organization that must respond to social trends and client demands. Today's health care facility—once a traditional institution—has turned into a competitive business.

In local media, many health care facilities advertise free heart disease or cancer screenings or family health fairs. Some promote physician referral services or use physician testimonials to sell services. In all facets of medicine, including childbirth, advertising and promotional activities are becoming more common. They are signs of the growing competition among health care facilities in the United States.

Two key factors explain this growing competition: consumers and third-party payers. Increasingly sophisticated health care consumers are exercising options when they select services, which means that they may select one health care facility over another. Moreover, economic factors are changing the rules of the health care game. For example, all facilities compete for government funds, and those funds are not increasing as in earlier decades. Indeed, government and private insurance payers are trying to control reimbursements, even though costs are increasing. This makes operating a health care facility a greater financial challenge than previously.

In the past, only physicians could admit clients to a health care facility. This gave them economic power because they could take clients elsewhere if they were dissatisfied with the facility. Today, consumers choose their health care facility, health care professional, and method of health care delivery. For this reason, health care facilities market to clients as well as to physicians. They also may market to nurses and nurse-midwives who have admitting privileges.

Although partly spurred by increased consumerism in health care, the growing competition among health care facilities has been hastened by the increasing cost of health care. In 1903, consumers spent $29 million on hospital costs, which represented .08% of the U.S. gross national product (GNP). By 1983, this amount had risen to $3.7 billion, or 10.8% of the GNP (MacPherson, 1989). It has continued to rise. (For a comparison with the Canadian system, see *Economic factors in Canadian health care.*)

In response to these economic factors, the health care industry has embraced several cost-containment concepts, including prospective payment, alternative delivery systems, home health care, direct reimbursement, public health care, regionalization of care, and methods for reducing malpractice suits. These concepts have significantly changed client reimbursement, health care delivery, and facility operations.

Prospective payment

For many years, private insurance companies and the federal Medicare and Medicaid programs provided reimbursement based on the fees charged by physicians and health care facilities. They examined a client's health care costs after they had been charged and then used a complicated, nationwide averaging system to determine the reimbursable amount. This type of reimbursement was part of a retrospective payment system (reimbursement system based on services received and billed after the client received them).

The retrospective payment system changed with the Economic Stabilization Program of 1981 to 1984 (Hill, 1982). Over 3 years, this program attempted to bring rising health care costs under control by gradually moving to a prospective payment system (reimbursement system based on estimated costs for health care services before the client receives them).

To do this, policymakers organized disorders into 470 diagnosis-related groups (DRGs). Then they studied clients' diagnoses and average lengths of hospital stays. Based on this information, they determined the average number of hospital days and the average cost of care for clients with each of the 470 disorders. They began reimbursing most facilities at these levels in 1982.

Economic factors in Canadian health care

Canada's infant mortality rate of 0.8% is one-fifth lower than the U.S. rate of 1% (Brecht, 1989). Yet in 1983, Canadians spent only about 8.6% of their gross national product (GNP) on health care compared with U.S. expenditures of 10.8% of the GNP (Paxton, 1988). The chief reason for the success of Canada's health care is its government-mandated National Health Program, which provides free health care to every Canadian citizen.

National health program
Canada's National Health Program began in 1957 with passage of the Hospital Insurance and Diagnostic Services Act. Because of this act, 99% of all Canadians receive health insurance.

The program is governed by national standards of care but is administered by individual provinces. If the provinces meet the national standards of care, they receive federal funds to cover about 50% of their health care expenditures. These funds are provided under the Federal-Provincial Fiscal Arrangement and Federal Post-Secondary Education and Health Contributions Act (Paxton, 1988). The provinces provide the remaining funds from tax revenues.

Effects on health care
By assuming responsibility for providing health insurance for its citizens, the Canadian government guarantees universal access to care. This has affected Canada's infant mortality rate, making it one of the lowest among industrialized nations.

Canadian health care facilities experience as much pressure for early discharge as do facilities in the United States, primarily because hospital care is expensive. Alternative care settings are receiving more attention, as in the United States.

The Canadian system differs from that in the United States in two major ways: long waits for clients who want elective surgery or treatments, and limited expensive technologies, because a province may rule against duplicating costly machinery within certain geographical boundaries.

Under the DRG system, the health care facility must absorb the extra cost if a client's stay is longer than this average. If the stay is shorter, the facility may keep the difference.

Along with cost containment, DRGs have had two main effects on health care facilities. They prompted the formation of professional standards review organizations (groups within each facility that review the quality, usage, and type of services offered), and they encouraged facilities to discharge clients as early as possible. The latter effect has meant that some clients leave the facility less recovered than previously and require care at home.

Alternative delivery systems
Public demand, competitive pressures, and rising health

care costs have created a need for alternatives to the structured system of health care delivery. Two of the most common alternatives are health maintenance organizations (HMOs) and preferred provider organizations (PPOs).

HMOs. An HMO offers various health care services from one source for one price. Under this system, the client agrees to pay a regular fee to the HMO and to receive all health care services from HMO providers. In return, these providers agree to provide all necessary services to the client for a flat fee. HMO services are government mandated.

HMOs can reduce health care costs by placing physicians on a salary rather than by paying them on a fee-for-service basis. This payment system eliminates the incentive to increase the time and services used to provide care (Lancaster, 1982). HMOs also reduce costs by emphasizing services to prevent disease, which cost less than services to treat disease.

PPOs. A PPO offers a contracted, fixed-fee agreement between an individual and a group of health care providers and facilities for health care delivery. Like an HMO client, the PPO client pays a flat fee for health care and receives that care from a chosen group of providers. Unlike the HMO client, however, the PPO client can choose to receive care from a provider outside the group for a somewhat higher fee. Although PPO services are not government mandated, PPOs help control health care costs just as HMOs do.

Home health care

Private companies and public agencies may provide home health care services, which are important to postpartal clients and to other clients after discharge from a health care facility. Nursing care of postpartal clients and neonates at home has advantages and disadvantages.

Advantages. Follow-up home care for the postpartal client and her neonate is adequate and cost-effective for the client and insurer. In one study, neonates were randomly assigned to two groups. One group was discharged according to normal protocol at an average weight of 2,200 g (77.6 oz); the other was discharged about 11 days earlier at approximately 2,000 g (70.5 oz). The latter group received follow-up home care by a clinical nurse specialist, which cost an average of $576 per neonate—$18,560 less than the average cost per neonate in the first group. The researchers found no differences in the neonate's physical problems after discharge between the two groups (Brooten, et al., 1986).

Home care offers this cost advantage not only to healthy clients and neonates, but also to other clients. It also may be cost-effective for postpartal diabetic clients (York and Brown, 1989), clients who undergo unscheduled cesarean birth (Roncoli, 1989), and those who undergo hysterectomy (Cohen, Hollingsworth, and Rubin, 1989).

In these studies, clients were discharged 1 to 2 days earlier than usual and received follow-up care at home and by telephone for up to 8 weeks after discharge. The studies found that clients received more support and education under this system than was the norm for hospitalized clients. They also indicated that follow-up home care was satisfactory to clients because it allowed for individualized attention.

When follow-up home care is properly provided, it offers psychosocial support and increases client control over health care, which can benefit the client. One study found that parents who received follow-up home care during the first and fourth weeks after discharge benefited because they were able to ask the nurse questions on a one-on-one basis. It also indicated that low-income clients and neonates benefited when home care followed early discharge because the home visits eased the clients' concerns and used health care resources effectively (Norr, Nacion, and Abramson, 1989).

In fact, the trend toward early postpartal discharge and home care is consonant with the consumer's increasingly active participation in health care. After discharge, the client has more control over her health care. She can select her provider and obtain the information she desires.

Disadvantages. Several disadvantages of home care are related to early discharge. The client may be sent home too sick to receive sufficient self-care information and may suffer from this lack.

Another disadvantage is increased client responsibility with a neonate's early discharge and the anxiety that it may cause. Kenner (1988) found that parents were concerned about their ability to provide care for their neonate who had been discharged early from the neonatal intensive care unit (NICU). These clients admitted that they did not listen to or understand the discharge teaching because they believed that their neonate would not live to be discharged.

Kenner also found that these clients were afraid to leave their neonate with other caregivers; they felt they needed to provide care themselves. These anxieties can lead to social isolation, lack of social support, and increased stress for the client (Robinson, 1988). The nurse should discuss with antepartal and postpartal clients the need for and availability of social support.

Follow-up home care should ensure physical—and

psychological—well-being. Unfortunately, psychosocial support may be overlooked. For a client with little social support, the major disadvantage of home care is the burden of the care itself. Support from a partner, family, or friends should be available to prevent undue stress on the postpartal client (Kenner, 1988). According to McBride (1982), the nurse should meet with the client who lacks sufficient support and determine her concerns and needs.

Direct reimbursement

In health care facilities and home health care, direct reimbursement of nurses by third-party payers and some public health care programs can help contain costs. This is especially important because it separates nursing care costs from room and board charges or operating expenses in health care facilities. This allows hospital administrators to estimate nursing time required and money spent per client (MacPherson, 1989). It also demonstrates the cost-effectiveness of nursing care.

In providing home health nursing care, many nurses and midwives contract to accept a set fee. This allows reimbursement by third-party payers, promotes recognition of the nurse's contribution to health care, and helps contain costs by limiting the health care expenditure.

Public health care

The emphasis in public health care has shifted from illness treatment to health promotion through home teaching (Salmon and Peoples-Sheps, 1989). The economically disadvantaged consumer typically receives public health care at home or in a public health facility. Because the public health client lacks purchasing power, however, the availability of home health care depends greatly on the availability of public health nurses with appropriate education and experience.

Public health nurses have improved access to care for poor clients, performing home therapy for such conditions as hyperbilirubinemia and neonatal apnea, providing home antepartal care, and monitoring clients to control preterm labor (Harmon and Barry, 1989). (For more information, see Chapter 40, Neonatal Care at Home.)

Public health programs that provide home care for pregnant and postpartal clients are effective—and cost-effective. Economically disadvantaged clients who do not receive health care typically have a high risk of delivering premature and very-low-birth-weight neonates. Those who receive health care have much healthier outcomes. One study of antepartal testing and home monitoring of 156 public health clients showed that about 90% of the clients delivered after 35 weeks' gestation (Harmon and Barry, 1989). These results indicate that home care can delay delivery, which improves the neonate's chances for survival.

Moreover, this type of care saves money. Harmon and Barry found that home monitoring costs about $90 to $180 per week compared to hospital care, which costs $250 to $300 per day, making home care 36% to 60% less expensive.

Public health care is especially valuable for those poor clients at risk for premature delivery and delivery of low-birth-weight neonates. Public health nurses are becoming involved in case management of such clients (Salmon and Peoples-Sheps, 1989). They provide nursing care in the home, using established protocols of care.

Nurses also are beginning to administer public health programs designed to foster greater access to care and improve maternal and neonatal health (Salmon and Peoples-Sheps, 1989). This change is necessary because of the nation's relatively high infant mortality rate of about 10 per 1,000 live births, or 1% (Brecht, 1989).

Regionalization of care

New technology is helping premature neonates survive. For example, 240,000 to 350,000 premature neonates are born annually in the United States. Of those born at 28 weeks' gestation, technology is helping 90% of them survive; at 24 weeks, 10% (Otten, 1989). Yet the cost of specialized care for these neonates is millions of dollars annually. Many of them will have major disabilities that require costly, lifelong health care (Otten, 1989).

Such specialized care requires expensive equipment and highly skilled health care professionals, which make it costly. Because specialized care is expensive, not all health care facilities can afford to provide it. In 1976, the Committee on Perinatal Health published a report that defined levels of care that allowed facilities to focus on their areas of expertise while permitting access to all types of technology and care. This system, called regionalization, split the United States into regions, each having facilities that could provide a certain level of care. A Level I facility could provide care for mothers and neonates without illness or complications. A Level II or intermediate facility could offer care for neonates with short-term problems and for mothers with some complex obstetric problems. A Level III facility could provide care for high-risk clients. A client could be moved to a higher or lower level facility to provide appropriate care without duplication of costly services. (For more information on regionalization of care, see Chapter 38, High-Risk Neonates.) Regionalization helped facilities control costs by reducing their need to purchase expensive equipment. Yet it improved the quality of and access to care (Burkett, 1989).

Here is an example of how regionalization works. Extracorporeal membrane oxygenation (ECMO) is a highly effective, but extremely expensive, advancement in neonatal care. ECMO artificially oxygenates a neonate's blood by transporting blood out of the body via the right carotid artery, filtering it through a semipermeable membrane where gas exchange takes place, and returning the oxygenated blood to the body. Candidates for this treatment include near-term neonates with persistent pulmonary hypertension or diaphragmatic hernias. Before ECMO was available, these neonates had an 80% mortality rate. Now they have a 30% mortality rate in some centers (Kilbride, 1989).

Through regionalization of care, the neonate in need of ECMO would be transported from a community hospital to a tertiary care center for specialized care. As an alternative, a perinatal specialist could transport the mother to a high-risk perinatal center before delivery if a problem is suspected (Troiano, 1989). In either case, regionalization helps contain costs and promote better use of services.

Malpractice suits

Another economic trend in U.S. health care is the dramatic increase in malpractice suits involving childbirth. Between 1976 and 1986, the number of suits rose nearly 10%, and the average award increased from $17,600 to $70,000 (Cohn, 1987).

Social, technological, and economic factors have increased client expectations of health care and have created an environment that is conducive to malpractice suits. For example, today's consumers demand more participation in their care and continue to expect the best health care possible (Nosek, 1987). Technology has become so sophisticated that many families cannot believe that something could go wrong during childbirth. So when a problem occurs, the families are devastated. Also, maternal and neonatal clients are being discharged more quickly from hospitals, so they may be at risk.

Expensive malpractice suits have increased liability insurance rates. In some cases, rates are so prohibitive that many nurse-midwives, nurse practitioners, and obstetricians have left the field (Brecht, 1989).

In 1989, an Illinois state law began to protect health care professionals from unnecessary malpractice suits and bring the rising cost of malpractice insurance into check. The first Medical Malpractice Reform Act, enacted in Illinois, orders the attorney filing a malpractice suit to retain an impartial health care professional to review the medical records. Only if this health care professional finds evidence of malpractice and signs an affidavit to this effect can a jury trial take place (Nosek, 1987). This act also puts a ceiling on the award that the jury can make to the plaintiff. (For more information, see Chapter 5, Ethical and Legal Concerns in Family Care.)

Changes in family nursing care

Nursing is involved in many of the concerns the family seeks care for today, such as birth options, contraception, maternity care, neonatal care, women's health care, and infertility studies.

For the childbearing family, nursing care and health care delivery have changed in the past few decades. Before obstetric nursing was a specialty, nurses who worked in obstetrics usually took care of mothers during delivery as labor room nurses or after delivery as postpartal nurses. They were supported by nurses who took care of neonates in the nursery. Each of these nurses took care of their part of the process.

Rubin (1961) was the first to separate maternity and obstetric nursing. She saw the obstetric nurse's role as limited to assisting the obstetrician in the delivery of neonates. The maternity nurse's role, on the other hand, was to help the client fulfill the maternal role. As more parents wanted to take part in deliveries and have their neonate remain with the mother, nursing had to change to provide the care the consumer wanted.

Today's maternity nurse is more of a generalist, taking care of the pregnant client from labor to delivery and then caring for the client and neonate until discharge. Because many facilities have replaced the labor and delivery units and nurses with LDRP units and maternity nurses, the maternity nurse typically works in an LDRP unit. This nurse plays an independent and interdependent generalist role (Gay, Templeton, Edgil, and Douglas, 1988).

On the other hand, the nursery nurse has become more of a specialist. The new technologies have required the development of NICUs and nurses skilled in neonatal critical care. Although the healthy neonate usually receives care from the maternity nurse, the sick neonate needs care from a neonatal nurse specialist.

Nursing roles

Today's nurse may assume many roles in family care: direct caregiver, role model, client advocate, change agent, consultant, educator, manager, researcher, liaison, and innovator (Hamric and Spross, 1989; Ryan-Merritt, Mitchell, and Pagel, 1988). For example, if a client wants to keep good luck charms with her when giving birth, the nurse can be an advocate by getting other members of the health care team to accept the client's wishes. When a college sophomore asks about contraceptive choices, the nurse can act as an educator. As a change agent, the nurse might work on a quality assurance board or protocol committee to make changes that promote safe, satisfying childbirth. Many current childbirth practices have not yet undergone rigorous scientific analysis—an opportunity for the nurse-researcher. (For more information, see *Nurse-researchers*, pages 18 and 19.)

Growing numbers of studies are focusing on qualitative aspects of nursing care as nurse-researchers recognize that successful nursing care and client outcomes may involve more than quantifiable results. By studying women's experiences and perceptions of experiences within their environments, the nurse-researcher can help substantiate women's concerns (McBride and McBride, 1981). By providing a scientific knowledge base for maternity nursing care, research can help the nurse and the profession bring about necessary changes in nursing care.

Current topics in family nursing research typically focus on holistic care. They include public health issues, such as hospice care for neonates infected with acquired immunodeficiency syndrome (AIDS) and demographic studies to determine which factors affect maternal and neonatal health. They also include nursing care of clients at high risk for childbirth complications. (For an example, see *Nursing research applied: Certified nurse-midwife care and reduction in low-birth-weight neonates*, page 20.) Nurse-researchers also are studying the relationship between advanced technology and ethical questions for the nurse and family that can affect client care.

Family nursing careers

The nurse may decide to perform the following roles as a generalist or specialist in one of many family nursing careers. These career alternatives require different experience, education, and credentials.

Maternity staff nurse. A nurse with an RN license and appropriate work experience may work in a maternity unit. Duties may include labor and delivery care and care of the mother after delivery or of the mother and neonate, depending on the facility. The maternity staff nurse who desires additional preparation and professional recognition may take an examination to obtain certification as an inpatient obstetric nurse from the Nurses Association of the American College of Obstetricians and Gynecologists (NAACOG), the organization for obstetric, gynecologic, and neonatal nurses.

Perinatal staff nurse. A nurse with an RN license and appropriate work experience may work in a neonatal nursery. Typical duties depend on whether the nurse cares for healthy neonates in the well-baby nursery or for critically ill neonates in the NICU. For additional preparation and recognition, the perinatal staff nurse may obtain ANA certification in perinatal nursing by fulfilling requirements for clinical experience and education in the specialty. Alternatively, the nurse may obtain NAACOG certification by examination as a low-risk neonatal nurse.

Obstetric-gynecologic nurse practitioner. This career requires a master's degree in nursing. It focuses on primary care for healthy pregnant and nonpregnant women and emphasizes health promotion and maintenance. The nurse practitioner collaborates with a physician colleague and may diagnose and treat common problems, such as vaginitis, under standing protocols. In this career, the nurse may opt to receive NAACOG certification as an obstetric-gynecologic nurse practitioner.

Women's health nurse practitioner. With a master's degree in nursing, the women's health nurse practitioner can perform holistic assessment for women of all ages through health history, physical assessment, and diagnostic tests. Such a nurse commonly provides client education on women's health topics and can perform routine gynecologic examinations, provide family planning counseling, and insert and remove intrauterine devices.

Family nurse practitioner. This career requires a master's degree in nursing and allows the nurse to perform all the functions of the previous two nurse practitioners as well as other functions. Duties may include caring for neonates, children, adolescents, adult women, and possibly men. The family nurse practitioner focuses on continuing family assessment as its members adjust to new and different stressors.

Maternity clinical nurse specialist. With a master's degree in nursing and advanced clinical expertise, the maternity clinical nurse specialist can act as a consultant to other nurses, perform clinical research, and provide advanced care to the client. Frequently, the specialist educates the staff nurse formally and informally. The specialist also may provide primary care to members of the child-bearing family in any specialized clinical setting, such as a hospital, clinic, or independent birth center.

Neonatal clinical nurse specialist. This career requires a master's degree in nursing. It lets the nurse perform the

Nurse-researchers

Nurse-researchers have had an impact on nursing practice and family health care. For example, many have investigated ways in which nursing interventions can provide better, more cost-effective health care. The chart below lists only some of the many current nurse-researchers in maternal, neonatal, and women's health care and the topics of some of their research.

NURSE-RESEARCHER	RESEARCH TOPICS
Dyanne Alfonso, RN, PhD	Maternal role perception
Kathyrn Barnard, RN, PhD	Nursing assessment of infants, children, and parents
Susan Blackburn, RN, PhD	Perinatal environment, neonatal intensive care unit (NICU) environment
Dorothy Brooten, RN, PhD, FAAN	Postpartal care, early discharge, home care
Linda P. Brown, RN, PhD, FAAN	Home follow-up of very-low-birth-weight neonates, breast-feeding concerns
Marie Annette Brown, RN, PhD	Women's health
Anne Brueggemeyer, RN, MSN	Breast-feeding concerns of NICU mothers
Pricilla Butts, RN, MSN	Home follow-up of very-low-birth-weight neonates
Victoria Champion, RN, DNS	Health beliefs model and breast self-examination
Susan M. Cohen, RN, DSN	Premenstrual syndrome, women's health, early discharge after hysterectomy
Carol Ann Consolvo, RN, MS	Parental anxiety when neonate receives NICU care
Linda R. Cronenwett, RN, PhD	Prenatal care
Donna Dean, RN, MSN	Neonatal nursing, urine specific gravity in neonates
Mary Duffy, RN, PhD	Midlife women
Janet Engstrom, RN, PhD	Bottle-feeding and breast-feeding of preterm neonates
Linda Franck, RN, MSN	Neonatal pain
Jacqueline Fawcett, RN, PhD, FAAN	Self-image during pregnancy, cesarean birth
Susan Gennaro, RN, DSN	Very-low-birth-weight neonates and parental visits during hospitalization
Debbie Koniak-Griffin, RN, PhD	Maternal-fetal attachment in pregnant adolescents
Laurie Porter Gunderson, RN, PhD	Neonatal endotracheal suctioning
Andrea Hollingsworth, RN, PhD	Breast-feeding concerns, early discharge
L. Colette Jones, RN, PhD	Father-infant interaction
Carole Kenner, RN,C, DNS	NICU parent concerns, women's health
Gretchen Lawhon, RN, MSN	Infant development
Regina Lederman, RN, PhD	Maternal role attachment
Judy Wright Lott, RN, MSN, ARNP	Cerebral blood flow in the preterm neonate
Susan Luddington Hoe, RN, CNM, PhD	Kangaroo (skin-to-skin contact) care, underwater laboring

Nurse-researchers continued

NURSE-RESEARCHER	RESEARCH TOPICS
Kathyrn A. May, RN, PhD	Maternal-paternal attachment
Kathleen I. MacPherson, RN, PhD	Menopause
Paula Meier, RN, DNSc	Feeding of premature neonates
Ramona Mercer, RN, PhD	Maternal role attainment
Angela Barron McBride, RN, PhD, FAAN	Women's mental health
Helen Palisin, RN, PhD	Neonatal perception inventory
Nancy Reame, RN, PhD	Premenstrual syndrome
Paula Reams, RN, MSN	Neonatal nursing, urine specific gravity of neonates
Margaret Sandelowski, RN, PhD	Infertility
Joanne Stevenson, RN, PhD	Women's health
Sue Ann Thomas, RN, PhD	Father-infant interaction
Jacqueline N. Ventura, RN, PhD	Parental coping
Lorraine O. Walker, RN, EdD, FAAN	Maternal role attainment
Nancy Fugate Woods, RN, PhD	Women's health, human sexuality
Rosanne Perez Woods, RN, EdD	Perinatal and neonatal nurse specialist certification
Ruth York, RN, PhD	Very-low-birth-weight neonates, premenstrual syndrome, postpartal depression

same roles as the maternity clinical specialist, but emphasizes care of the high-risk neonate.

Neonatal nurse practitioner. With advanced preparation through a certificate program or a master's degree in nursing with a neonatal focus, this practitioner provides technical stabilization and care skills as well as comprehensive case management for the neonate and family.

Perinatal clinical nurse specialist. This master's-prepared nurse performs the same tasks as maternity and neonatal clinical specialists, but emphasizes care of the childbearing family at risk for maternal, fetal, or neonatal morbidity. Because of the trend to early discharge of mothers and neonates, this clinical specialist is finding new challenges as care shifts from the health care facility to the home.

Certified nurse-midwife. This career requires advanced preparation through either a certification or master's degree program in nurse-midwifery. The practice entails independent management of essentially healthy clients during antepartal, intrapartal, and postpartal periods as well as gynecologic health care. These practitioners work within a system with physician collaboration, consultation, and referral.

The future

In the future, families will continue to experience changes caused by socioeconomic and technological trends. As before, the nurse will need to adapt to care for the family. Key future trends for family nursing care are likely to be social, health care, and nursing research.

Social trends

In the book *Megatrends*, Naisbitt (1984) identifies social trends that influence American culture and health care today and are likely to influence it in the future. In the book *Megatrends 2000*, Naisbitt and Aburdene (1990) reconfirm the earlier observations and make additional predictions of the near future.

Informational society

The United States has changed from an industrial society to an informational society. The information pool has grown dramatically and become more available, especially via electronic information-retrieval devices, such as facsimile (FAX) and modulator-demodulator (MODEM) devices. In minutes, medical and scientific advances can be communicated throughout the world. In response to the availability and speed of global information, knowledge has increased rapidly.

In the informational society, the nurse will need to think critically and be technically competent to assimilate new information rapidly and apply it appropriately.

Because of rapid informational changes, the generalist in any profession may be much more useful to society than the specialist with a limited knowledge base who cannot adapt to change. This trend is supported by the medical profession's movement back to family medicine and general practice. However, the need for some specialists, such as in NICUs, will remain to meet the critical needs of vulnerable client populations.

High-tech, high-touch society

A second U.S. trend is the transition to a highly technical society that also requires high touch (personal caring and concerned behaviors). This trend is increasing the demands on nursing. For example, technological advances are prolonging the life of increasingly smaller premature neonates, sometimes through heroic measures. Yet the technology cannot offer the warmth, caring, and encouragement of a nurse. In addition, it can raise ethical dilemmas about the quality of life (Naisbitt, 1984).

In response to consumer demands for high-touch, individualized care, nursing has developed primary nursing, where the nurse consistently cares for certain clients and families. The primary nurse can individualize care based on in-depth knowledge of the clients' and families' needs.

Other high-touch options have resulted from increased use of technology in hospitals: alternative birthing methods, home health care, and decreased use of hospitals for natural occurrences, such as nonemergency birth and death. The movement toward a homelike hospital atmosphere is another answer to the need for high

---

NURSING RESEARCH APPLIED

Certified nurse-midwife care and reduction in low-birth-weight neonates

Studies from the past three decades have shown that neonates born to adolescent mothers have higher morbidity and mortality rates and more psychological and developmental problems. Low birth weight commonly is associated with poverty, limited access to or use of prenatal care, and poor nutrition, which may account for the poor neonatal outcomes.

A controlled study matched two groups of adolescents by age, race, socioeconomic status, and perinatal risk. The study group received care from nurse-midwives who saw the clients at every visit and coordinated additional care from a multidisciplinary team, as needed. This team consisted of nurses, social workers, nutritionists, obstetricians, and a psychiatrist. The control group received care at state-run maternity and child care clinics.

The researchers found that the nurse-midwives related to the clients in a nonauthoritative and nonthreatening manner. This increased client satisfaction with care as well as client compliance as evidenced by kept prenatal appointments and returns for postpartal follow-up care. This group of clients had lower rates of anemia, pregnancy-induced hypertension, low-birth-weight neonates, and perinatal mortality than predicted in numerous studies of this population. The control group had a higher incidence of low-birth-weight neonates.

Application to practice

The findings of this study support the nurse-midwife case management of this population, which the health care system frequently neglects. The nurse-midwife and nurses who taught the health education classes helped improve the outcome for these clients. This study clearly shows that nurses can make a difference. To improve their effectiveness, nurses who care for this population should add nonjudgmental teaching of prenatal nutrition, danger signs of pregnancy, childbirth preparation, infant nutrition, neonatal care, sexually transmitted diseases, and family planning into their care.

Piechnik, S., and Corbett, M. (1985). Reducing low birth weight among socioeconomically high-risk adolescent pregnancies: Successful intervention with certified nurse-midwife-managed care and a multidisciplinary team. *Journal of Nurse-Midwifery*, 30(5), 88-98.

---

touch as is the use of independent birth centers (Naisbitt, 1984).

Other social trends

Other trends include the movement from institutional care to self-care and from the either/or society to a society of multiple options (Naisbitt, 1984).

The trend toward self-care will continue the use of self-help groups, such as parent support groups, Alcoholics Anonymous, rape hotlines, and support groups for survivors of violence.

The move toward a multiple-option society will give

consumers more than one choice of life-style, career, and health care setting. Families will continue to take many forms, including those with single heads of households, two careers, and female breadwinners. Women will be free to postpone childbearing and enter the work force; men, to stay home with the children. Temporary employment services will grow, especially in such white-collar jobs as nursing. Families will want more control and active involvement in their health care.

More recently identified trends include the provision of day care and elder care as routine employee benefits, which can relieve stress for women working outside the home, and the rise of increasing numbers of women in leadership positions, which may bring about policy decisions in health care facilities, corporations, and government agencies (Naisbitt and Aburdene, 1990).

Health care trends

The economic and political pressures that have changed hospitals are likely to continue. More neonates who need ventilators or special feeding techniques or care will be discharged to home. For these technology-dependent neonates, the nurse must be prepared to provide care outside the hospital and accept the additional responsibility of high-technology home care.

Within the hospital, nursing responsibilities will change as legislation begins to regulate care for retarded or deformed neonates and the extension of life for increasingly smaller neonates. These clients will require highly skilled nursing care.

The health care delivery system also may change. According to the National Perinatal Information Center (NPIC, 1989), the regionalization of care needs to be revamped for several reasons. Perinatal regionalization has deteriorated over the past 5 years, competition has replaced cooperation among many participating health care facilities, differences in levels of care are blurring, and many facilities are upgrading their neonatal programs regardless of the number of high-risk neonates served.

For the future, the NPIC recommends a more competitive model for organizing services that:
• is client-centered, rather than facility-centered
• offers a flexible menu of hospital service options
• encourages coequal provider relationships as an alternative to centralized perinatal systems
• attempts to assure quality of care and systemwide efficiencies through establishment of minimal standards for patient volume and outcomes of care.

This model, known as the perinatal partnership, will need to be researched before it is implemented. When implemented, it should provide cooperative systems of care that keep the best aspects of centralized, regional care while addressing facility competition and the complexities of the modern health care environment.

Nursing research trends

Nurse-researchers will continue to investigate public health issues and conduct demographic studies to find the best ways to ensure maternal and neonatal health. They also will focus on nursing care for clients at high risk for childbirth complications to determine optimum care and the education necessary for healthy family outcomes. Brubaker, Teplick, and McAndrew (1988) predict that maternal-fetal intensive care units soon will be the best way to provide the care to the mother and fetus at risk.

With technological advances, nurses will raise questions about client outcomes and the effectiveness of new procedures. They will be concerned with ethical dilemmas that result from technology. For example, they may study pain suffered by NICU neonates from advanced technological procedures. With new technology available for fetal surgery, they may study ways to balance fetal needs against maternal outcomes. These issues and many others will need to be balanced with economic realities and will not be resolved easily.

Other research topics will include the effect of legislation on women's health, women's satisfaction with their decision to stay home with their children and not work outside the home, and the connections between women's health and job-related stress.

Chapter summary

Chapter 1 provided an overview of families and nursing care in the past and present and looked briefly to the future. Here are the chapter highlights.
• The traditional family (a nuclear unit of parents, children, and grandparents) has many variations today.
• The family performs affective, socialization and social placement, reproductive, economic, and health functions for its members.
• Throughout history, many social, economic, and technological factors have influenced the family, such as changes in resource production and use. These factors in turn have influenced the development of nursing.
• Recent social trends that have affected the family include decreased family size and increased numbers of women working outside the home. Working mothers commonly are concerned about maternity leave, child care,

stress, and the effect of their careers on their children.
• Other recent social trends include the increase of two-career families and the move toward active participation in health care.
• The following economic trends have influenced family health care: prospective payment, alternative delivery systems, home health care, direct reimbursement, public health care, regionalization, and malpractice suits.
• Current careers in family nursing include maternity staff nurse, perinatal staff nurse, obstetric-gynecologic nurse practitioner, women's health practitioner, family nurse practitioner, maternity clinical nurse specialist, neonatal clinical nurse specialist, neonatal nurse practitioner, perinatal clinical nurse specialist, and certified nurse-midwife. Each career has distinct requirements for education, experience, and certification.
• Future trends will involve social changes (such as the shift from an industrial to an informational society), new or modified forms of health care (such as the perinatal partnership), and new areas for nursing research.

Study questions

1. Which historic events were most influential in changing the status of women and nursing?

2. How have consumerism and women's changing roles affected maternity care in the United States?

3. Which techniques have helped reduce health care costs in the past 30 years?

4. What is the current scope of maternity nursing?

5. What are the future priorities for nursing research in maternity nursing?

Bibliography

American Nurses' Association. (1980). *Nursing: A social policy statement.* Kansas City, MO: Author.
Anderson, E., and McFarlane, J. (1988). *Community as client: Application of the nursing process.* Philadelphia: Lippincott.
Friedman, M. (1986). *Family nursing: Theory and assessment.* East Norwalk, CT: Appleton-Century-Crofts.
Hasenfeld, Y. (1983). *Human service organizations.* Englewood Cliffs, NJ. Prentice-Hall.
Lancaster, W. (1982). Health and health care delivery systems. In J. Lancaster and W. Lancaster (Eds.), *Concepts for advanced nursing practice: The nurse as a change agent* (pp.175-199). St. Louis: Mosby.
Paxton, J. (Ed.). (1988). *The statesman's year-book. World gazetteer* (3rd ed.). New York: St. Martin's Press.
U.S. Bureau of the Census. (1987). *Statistical abstract of the United States: 1988* (108th ed.). Washington, DC: U.S. Government Printing Office.

History
American Nurses' Association. (1976). *One strong voice.* Kansas City, MO: Author.
Bullough, V., and Bullough, B. (1978). *The care of the sick: The emergence of modern nursing.* Canton, MA: Watson Pub. Intl.
Bullough, V., and Bullough, B. (1984). *History, trends, and politics of nursing.* East Norwalk, CT: Appleton & Lange.
Carnegie, M. (1986). *The path we tread.* Philadelphia: Lippincott.
Committee for the Study of Nursing and Nursing Education. (1923). The Goldmark Report. New York: Macmillan.
Doheny, M., Cook, C., and Stopper, M. (1987). *The discipline of nursing: An introduction* (2nd ed.). East Norwalk, CT: Appleton & Lange.
Dolan, J., Fitzpatrick, M., and Herrmann, E. (1983). *Nursing in society: A historical perspective* (15th ed.). Philadelphia: Saunders.
Dye, N. (1983). Mary Breckinridge: The Frontier Nursing Service and the introduction of nurse-midwifery in the United States. *Bulletin of the History of Medicine,* 57 (4), 485-507.
Ehrenreich, B., and English, D. (1973). *Witches, midwives, and nurses: A history of women healers.* New York: Feminist Press.
Litoff, J. (1978). *American Midwives: 1860 to the present.* Westport, CT: Greenwood Press.
Litoff, J. (1986). *The American midwife debate.* Westport, CT: Greenwood Press.
Mitchell, O. (1968). *A concise history of western civilization.* New York: Van Nostrand Reinhold.
Nahm, H. (1981). History of nursing: A century of change. In J. McCloskey and H. Grace (Eds.), *Current issues in nursing* (pp. 14-25). Boston: Blackwell Scientific Publications.
Nightingale, F. (1859/1969). *Notes on nursing: What it is and what it is not.* New York: Dover Publications.
Palmer, I. (1977). Florence Nightingale: Reformer, reactionary, researcher. *Nursing Research,* 26(2), 84-89.
Shealy, M. (1985). Florence Nightingale 1820-1910: An evolutionary mind in the context of holism. *Journal of Holistic Nursing,* 3(1), 4-6.
Stark, M. (1979). *Florence Nightingale's Cassandra.* New York: Feminist Press.
Towler, J., and Bramall, J. (1986). *Midwives in history and society.* London: Croom Helm.

Recent trends
Afriat, C. (1987). Historical perspective on electronic fetal heart rate monitoring: A decade of growth, a decade of conflict. *Journal of Perinatal Neonatal Nursing,* 1(1), 1-4.
Akridge, K. (1989). Anorexia nervosa. *JOGNN,* 18(1), 25-30.
American Public Health Association. (1982). *Health of minorities and women chartbook.* Washington DC: Author.
Arnold, L., Brecht, M., Hockett, A., Amspacher, K., and Grad, R. (1989). Lessons from the past. *MCN,* 14(2), 75-82.

Ashley, J. (1976). *Hospitals, paternalism, and the role of the nurse.* New York: Teachers College Press.

Bradstock, K., Forman, M., Binkin, N., Gentry, E., Hagelin, G., Williamson, D., and Trowbridge, F. (1988). Alcohol use and health behavior life-styles among U.S. women: The behavioral risk factor surveys. *Addictive Behaviors,* 13(1), 61-71.

Brecht, M. (1989). The tragedy of infant mortality. *Nursing Outlook,* 37(1), 18-22.

Burkett, M. (1989). The tertiary center and health departments in cooperation: The Duke University experience. *Journal of Perinatal Neonatal Nursing,* 2(3), 11-19.

Centers for Disease Control. (1988). Progress toward achieving the 1990 objectives for pregnancy and infant health. *MMWR,* 37(26), 405-413.

Cohn, S. (1987). Trends in perinatal nursing professional liability. *Journal of Perinatal Neonatal Nursing,* 1(2), 19-27.

Committee on Perinatal Health. (1976). *Toward improving the outcome of pregnancy: A national report.* White Plains, NY: March of Dimes.

Creasy, R., and Resnik, R. (1989). *Maternal-fetal medicine: Principles and practice* (2nd ed.). Philadelphia: Saunders.

Darling, R. (1988). Parental entrepreneurship: A consumerist response to professional dominance. *Journal of Social Issues,* 44(1), 141-158.

Dick-Read, G. (1959). *Childbirth without fear: The principles and practice of natural childbirth.* New York: Harper & Row.

Flanagan, J., (1986). Childbirth in the eighties: What next? When alternatives become mainstream. *Journal of Nurse-Midwifery,* 31(4), 194-199.

Fiore, M., Novotny, T., Pierce, J., Hatziandreu, E., Patel, K., and Davis, R. (1989). Trends in cigarette smoking in the United States. *JAMA,* 261(1), 49-55.

Gay, J., Templeton, J., Edgil, A., and Douglas, A. (1988). Reva Rubin revisited. *JOGNN,* 17(6), 394-399.

Hamric, A., and Spross, J. (1989). *The clinical nurse specialist in theory and practice* (2nd ed.). Philadelphia: Saunders.

Harmon, J., and Barry, M. (1989). Antenatal testing, mobile outpatient monitoring service. *JOGNN,* 18(1), 21-24.

Hill, D. (1982). Economic constraints in the health care delivery system. In J. Lancaster and W. Lancaster (Eds.), *Concepts for advanced nursing practice: The nurse as a change agent* (pp. 200-215). St. Louis: Mosby.

Kilbride, J. (1989). ECMO basics: Questions and answers. *Perinatal Section News,* 14(1), 9.

Kopala, B. (1989). Mothers with impaired mobility speak out. *MCN,* 14(2), 115-119.

Landsberg, M. (1986). *Women and children first.* Markham, Ontario: Penguin Books.

LaRosa, J. (1988). Women, work, and health: Employment as a risk factor for coronary heart disease. *American Journal of Obstetrics and Gynecology,* 158(6), 1597-1602.

MacPherson, K. (1989). A new perspective on nursing and caring in a corporate context. *Advances in Nursing Science,* 11(4), 32-39.

McBride, A., and McBride, W. (1981). Theoretical underpinnings for women's health. *Women and Health,* 6(1-2), 37-55.

McBride, A. (1982). The American way of birth. In M. Kay (Ed.), *An anthropology of human birth* (pp. 413-429). Philadelphia: F.A. Davis.

Moore, M. (1989). Recurrent teen pregnancy: Making it less desirable. *MCN,* 14(2), 104-108.

Morris, B. (1989). *Legislative network for nurses.* Silver Springs, MD: Business Publishers, Inc.

Muff, J. (1988). *Socialization, sexism, and stereotyping: Women's issues in nursing.* Prospect Heights, IL: Wareland Press.

Murphy, D. (1986). Occupational health hazards. In J. Griffith-Kenney (Ed.), *Contemporary women's health: A nursing advocacy approach* (pp. 418-431). Menlo Park, CA: Addison-Wesley.

National Perinatal Association. (1989). *NPA Bulletin,* 4(1), Alexandria, VA: Author.

Norr, K., Nacion, K., and Abramson, R. (1989). Early discharge with home follow-up: Impacts on low-income mothers and infants. *JOGNN,* 18(2), 133-141.

Nosek, J. (1987). Expanded role liability in perinatal nursing. *Journal of Perinatal Neonatal Nursing,* 1(2), 39-48.

Otten, A. (1989, June 28). Technological advances in the science of birth alter the setting of high court's abortion rule. *The Wall Street Journal,* pp. 16-18.

Robinson, K. (1988). A social skills training program for adult caregivers. *Advances In Nursing Science,* 10(2), 59-72.

Roncoli, M. (1989). *Early hospital discharge and transitional care of women having unplanned cesarean births.* Paper presented at Seventh National Meeting of NAACOG, St. Louis.

Ross, C., and Mirowsky, J. (1988). Child care and emotional adjustment to wives' employment. *Journal of Health and Social Behavior,* 29(2), 127-138.

Rubin, R. (1961). Basic maternal behaviors. *Nursing Outlook,* 9(11), 683-686.

Ryan-Merritt, M., Mitchell, C., and Pagel, I. (1988). Clinical nurse specialist role definition and operationalization. *Clinical Nurse Specialist,* 2(3), 132-137.

Salmon, M., and Peoples-Sheps, M. (1989). Infant mortality and public health nursing: A history of accomplishments, a future of challenges. *Nursing Outlook,* 37(1), 6-7, 51.

Santi, L. (1987). Change in the structure and size of American households: 1970-1985. *Journal of Marriage and the Family,* 49(4), 833-937.

Shreve, A. (1988). *Remaking motherhood: How working mothers are shaping our children's future.* New York: Fawcett.

Sidel, R. (1987). *Women and children last: The plight of poor women in affluent America.* New York: Fawcett.

Thomas, D. (1986). The current health status of women. In J. Griffith-Kenney (Ed.), *Contemporary women's health: A nursing advocacy approach* (pp.48-72). Menlo Park, CA: Addison-Wesley.

Troiano, N. (1989). Applying principles to practice in maternal-fetal transport. *Journal of Perinatal Neonatal Nursing,* 2(3), 20-30.

Varney, H. (1987). *Nurse-midwifery* (2nd ed.). Boston: Blackwell Scientific Publications.

Wattenberg, M. (1989). *Birth dearth.* New York: Pharos Books.

Wisensale, S., and Allison, M. (1989). Family leave legislation: State and federal initiatives. *Family Relations,* 38(2), 182-189.

Yeaworth, R. (1976). Women and nurses: Evolving roles. *Occupational Health Nursing,* 24(8), 7-9.

York, R., and Brown, L. (1989). *Early hospital discharge and transitional care of childbearing diabetic women.* Paper presented at Seventh National Meeting of NAACOG, St. Louis.

Future trends

Brubaker, J., Teplick, F., and McAndrew, L. (1988). Developing a maternal-fetal intensive care unit. *JOGNN,* 17(5), 321-326.

Naisbitt, J. (1984). *Megatrends.* New York: Warner Books.

Naisbitt, J., and Aburdene, P. (1990). *Megatrends 2000: Ten new directions for the 1990's.* New York: William Morrow.

National Perinatal Information Center. (1989). *The perinatal partnership: An approach to organizing care in the 1990s.* Providence, RI: Author.

Peters, T., and Austin, N. (1985). *A passion for excellence: The leadership difference.* New York: Warner Books.

Rothman, B. (1989). *Recreating motherhood.* New York: Norton.

Nursing research

Brooten, D., Kumar, S., Brown, L., Butts, P., Finkler, S., Bakewell-Sachs, S., Gibbons, A., and Delivoria-Papadopoulos, M. (1986). A randomized clinical trial of early hospital discharge and home follow-up of very-low-birth-weight infants. *New England Journal of Medicine,* 315(15), 934-939.

Cohen, S., Hollingsworth, A., and Rubin, M. (1989). *Early hospital discharge and transitional care of women having hysterectomies.* Paper presented at Seventh National Meeting of NAACOG, St. Louis.

Kenner, C. (1988). *Parent transition from the newborn intensive care unit (NICU) to home.* Unpublished doctoral dissertation. Indiana University, Indianapolis.

Mercer, R., and Ferketich, S. (1988). Stress and social support as predictors of anxiety and depression during pregnancy. *Advances in Nursing Science,* 10(2), 26-39.

Piechnik, S., and Corbett, M. (1985). Reducing low birth weight among socioeconomically high-risk adolescent pregnancies: Successful intervention with certified nurse-midwife-managed care and a multidisciplinary team. *Journal of Nurse-midwifery,* 30(2), 88-98.

Redeker, N. (1989). Health beliefs, health locus of control, and the frequency of practice of breast self-examination in women. *JOGNN,* 18(1), 45-51.

Family Structure and Function

Objectives

After reading and studying this chapter, the student should be able to:

1. Explain the main aspects of each of these family theories: systems, structural-functional, developmental, interactional, and social exchange.
2. List and explain Duvall's eight stages of family development.
3. Describe various family types.
4. List functions fulfilled by the family.
5. Describe roles typically adopted by family members.
6. Explain the differences among autocratic, patriarchal, matriarchal, and democratic families.
7. Explain how coping mechanisms can help maintain family function and thwart crisis.

Introduction

The family is a basic unit of society. It is composed of two or more people who share emotional involvement and live in close geographical proximity (Friedman, 1986).

In the United States, the nuclear family—composed of married parents and their biologic children—has represented the traditional family structure. Its assignments of responsibilities has been linked to traditional sex-based roles. This family type, however, no longer adequately describes the American family. Contemporary families are changing dramatically in structure and function, adopting various arrangements that defy simple categorizing.

American families are not homogenous but regionally, ethnically, and organizationally diverse (White House Conference on Families, 1980). In "Households, Families, Marital Status, and Living Arrangements," The U.S. Bureau of the Census (1989) reported that women head one in six U.S. households. Other family types are becoming more common as well, including blended families, homosexual families, and cohabitation familes. Many members of such families have rejected traditional roles.

Because a family of any type involves close relationships, alterations in the health of one member commonly affects other members. Typically, the family plays a critical role in maintaining and promoting the health of its members, and one family member controls the interactions with health care professionals. The nurse, therefore, should take a family-centered approach, drawing on the resources of family members while caring for one of them. This approach can lead to holistic health care.

This chapter will help the nurse understand family structure and function along with some of the changes that have occurred in families recently. The chapter begins by describing some classic theories used by researchers and clinicians to study and describe the family. After describing the various types of families that the nurse is likely to encounter, it discusses the basic functions of all families, then looks within the family to examine typical roles of its members and relationships among them. Finally, the chapter briefly discusses family response to crises and the coping mechanisms used.

Glossary

Crisis: period of instability or disorganization that follows failure of normal coping skills; risk is highest when a stressful event coincides with a crucial stage in family development.

Empty nest syndrome: pattern of emotions that characterizes a family whose children have recently left home.

Family functions: purposes for which the family exists and tasks necessary to accomplish those purposes; includes physical survival, sustenance, personal nurturing, education, and the passing on of values and beliefs.

Family pattern: overall organization of family relationships regardless of roles adopted by each member.

Family theory: set of assumptions and hypotheses that provides a reference point for studying and understanding the family.

Maturational crisis: crisis linked to the developmental level of an individual or family.

Nuclear family: traditional family structure that includes father, mother, and their biologic children.

Role: set of repetitive behaviors adopted consciously or unconsciously that provides consistency in family relationships and accomplishment of tasks.

Self-differentiation: personal growth characterized by identification of one's abilities, actions, and relationships with others.

Situational crisis: crisis linked to a traumatic event.

Family theories

Many theories have been developed to describe family structure and function. These provide reference points from which to study and understand the family. Typically, sociologists view the family as an open social system in relation to other social systems, such as the church and school. Psychologists examine family interactions and relationships between selected individuals and as a whole. Anthropologists study the family in relation to its environment. Researchers from each of these disciplines use theories to consider the essential elements that define a family and provide a framework for organizing data on the family. The most important family theories include systems, structural-functional, developmental, interactional, and social exchange.

Systems theory

According to biologist Ludwig von Bertalanffy (1969), people are more than the sum of their parts and different from that sum also. Systems theory is the study of systems (individuals and families) as entities rather than as parts of a whole. Von Bertalanffy discovered several abstract laws that guide the behavior of all systems, including families. They encompass the following.

• Systems are organized complexities that reflect the influence of variables. Family behaviors are determined not by structural conditions but by relationships among the members.

• Systems interactions are dynamic and unique. Specific interactions have never occurred before and will never occur again.

• Changes that occur within persons, families, and environments proceed from the simple to the complex.

• Regular changes occur in the evolution of all systems in predictable—but not static—patterns of growth and development.

• People are living, open systems, and families are always evolving.

Numerous other family systems researchers and clinicians have added to von Bertalanffy's work. In the late 1960s and throughout the 1970s, the family movement came into its own and established major theories and treatments. Ackerman (1972) proposed that family problems begin with interpersonal conflict and that treatment should bring underlying conflicts to the surface to develop new family life patterns and encourage growth. Minuchin (1974) focused on family context and problems, emphasizing behavioral change through restructuring family boundaries and encouraging the family to observe and change unrewarding interaction.

Concepts integral to family systems theory include boundaries, structure, and functions. Boundaries are physical, emotional, or interpersonal spaces that separate family members. Every living system has boundaries; they maintain individual identity, regulate emotional intimacy, and define rules for relating, which provide the system's structure. Each family member must be allowed to function within personal boundaries but at the same time remain related to one another. Family boundaries must be clear and flexible. Within the family structure, members carry out role-related functions. Boundaries allow these functions to succeed.

Systems theory

An illustration of several key concepts of systems theory will help clarify the interactions involved. The diagram shows the elements of systems theory: input, throughput, output, and feedback. Input, the activator and operating material of the system, consists of energy, raw materials, or information; it may come from inside or outside the system. Throughput is the process by which the system converts input to make it usable. Output, in the form of energy, processed material, or information, results from the system's processes. A process that allows the system to monitor and evaluate itself, feedback is the return of output into the system, where it is throughput to produce new results.

In an example using a family as the system, input might be a 20-year-old daughter's sudden announcement that she is leaving home to live with her boyfriend. The throughput for each family member differs: the younger brother is pleased because he likes the boyfriend and hopes to move into his sister's room; the mother is resigned because she sees her daughter as an adult; and the father is angry with his daughter and her boyfriend because he disapproves of their living together. As the various members' feelings and thoughts are processed (throughput), the family eventually comes to a response (output). In this case, the family accepts the daughter as an adult who will act as she sees fit; however, the family is not proud of the manner in which she has broken from the primary unit. Over the next several months, feedback to the family shows that the daughter and boyfriend have established themselves as a stable couple and are considering marriage. This information increases the family's acceptance of the situation.

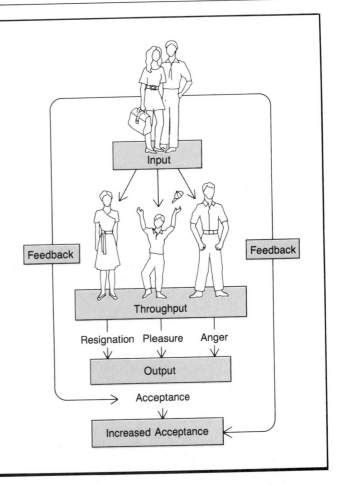

The concept of self-differentiation complements systems theory (Bowen, 1978). Self-differentiation involves the interaction between an individual's emotional system and cognitive system. The more one uses a cognitive system—which allows calm, logical decision making—the higher the level of self-differentiation. In times of crisis or stress, a person's capacity to reason or reflect may be compromised by emotions. Developmental, life-cycle, chronic, and situational stressors all can impinge upon normal functioning of individual, marital, and family systems.

Systems theory provides a holistic approach to individuals and families by viewing them in relation to the environment and accounting for change. Nurses with a holistic approach to patient care typically assess patients in the context of systems theory because it allows for intervention at many levels. (For more information, see *Systems theory.*)

Structural-functional theory

Originating in the nineteenth century, this theory focuses on social order and how it persists in society. The theory includes three basic premises.

• Society is a system made up of many subsystems (such as the family) that are typically called institutions.
• Each part of society affects every other part; therefore, a change in one part may affect another.
• Because society exists in a dynamic equilibrium, the system can function through most types of changes (Schulz, 1982).

The structural-functional theory assumes that the family, religion, and education are all part of the same social system, known as society. An equal exchange of resources and services exists between the family and society, which establishes equilibrium (Brown, 1931; Parsons and Bales, 1955; Malinowski, 1960; Winch, 1971). Society persists through marriage, integration of new members, and the actions of members to preserve or alter the established system. The family protects group survival (Brown, 1931) and meets the basic needs of individuals (Malinowski, 1960). Most children are reared to accept their society's values and goals and to pass these to their children.

Duvall's developmental stages

The following developmental stages reflect typical alterations in responsibilities that occur at certain times in life and correspond to physical maturation and altered cultural pressures and privileges (Duvall, 1984).

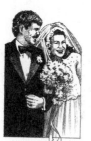

Stage 1: Beginning families
Marriage is associated with personal change and conflict as the partners move from independence to interdependence. Such factors as maturity, each partner's commitment to the other, and personal goals help determine success and satisfaction. Tasks at this stage include:
• clarification of marital roles and expectations
• decisions about parenthood.

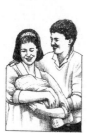

Stage 2: Families with infants
Integrating the first child into the family unit is the most significant developmental change in a marriage. Tasks at this stage focus on parental adaptation to the infant, including:
• provision of a safe, nurturing home environment
• adaptation of marital and other relationships to new roles and responsibilities.

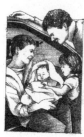

Stage 3: Families with preschool children
During preschool years, the child slowly shifts from dependence to self-reliance. At the same time, parents must begin teaching the child their and society's rules and demands. Tasks include:
• adjustment to new boundaries between the child and parents
• parental reinforcement of proper social behavior in the child.

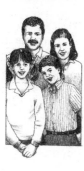

Stage 4: Families with school-age children
The child learns from people outside the family and develops a sense of self-identity. Peers become a major influence for a time; friendships become intimate and highly important. Tasks at this stage include:
• development of peer relations by the child
• parental adjustment to peer influences on the child.

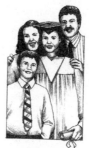

Stage 5: Families with adolescent children
Adolescence is characterized by rapid physical and emotional growth coupled with increased independence. Parents are faced with their child's growing need for autonomy; at this stage, the family no longer is primarily child-focused. Tasks include:
• parental accommodation to the child's increasing independence
• parents' revival of personal interests and issues.

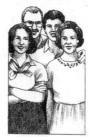

Stage 6: Families with young adult children
This stage begins when the first child prepares to leave home and ends after the last child has left. Parents establish new ties as each child departs. Tasks include:
• parental adjustment to each child's life-style choices
• parents' renegotiation of their marital relationship.

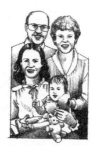

Stage 7: Families with adult children
This "empty-nest" period extends from the last child's departure to a spouse's retirement or death. This stage can be difficult for both partners, who may be unhappy with careers or home life and anxious about aging and death. Tasks include:
• re-establishment of the couple's bond
• acceptance of aging and eventual death.

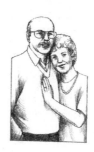

Stage 8: Aging families
Old age is a period of uncertainty and change. Activities alter, health and energy may decline, and family configurations change because of illness and death. Alternative living arrangements may be needed. Tasks during this stage include:
• redefinition of life-style to reflect financial and health status
• coping with altered self-esteem, status, and prestige.

In this theory, discrete family subunits function to perpetuate society. Families seek to maintain a stable societal structure by organizing around traditional, sex-based role relationships and by adopting largely conservative beliefs.

Developmental theory

This theory defines the family as beginning with marriage, increasing when children are born, diminishing when children leave home, and ceasing when the married couple dies. Throughout the family life-cycle, each member performs various roles and functions. Duvall (1984) categorized the family life-cycle and its associated tasks into eight stages that reflect major developmental steps in a family's life. (For more information, see *Duvall's developmental stages.*) Duvall's stages correlate with Erikson's (1950) eight-stage model of growth and development and Caplan's (1964) crisis theory. Rodgers (1962) expands Duvall's stages to include the individual developmental problems of each child.

Duvall defines developmental stages based on four considerations: (1) patterns of interaction that change with the size of the family, (2) the age of the oldest child, (3) the school placement of the oldest child, and (4) the function and status of the family before and after the parents bear children.

The developmental theory has benefits and drawbacks. Its major benefit is that it allows health care providers to assess the family's developmental level with some predictability. Its major drawback is that it addresses only the traditional, middle-class, nuclear family. As family types become more diversified, this theory will become less applicable.

Interactional theory

This theory views the family as an internal network of relationships (Friedman, 1986). Individual family roles develop from interaction between family members over specific situations. Those roles persist as long as family expectations remain constant in similar situations.

In this theory, families are primary social constructions (Schulz, 1982). Although members are expected to live up to certain social expectations, they may define and redefine their own roles. Roles are not static but change to some degree as family members interact. A married couple's relationship influences each individual in the family. This interaction, in turn, influences the marital relationship. Change in one partner affects the other, as does change in interactions with the rest of the family.

This theory emphasizes the extent to which people create their social realities through interaction. Mead (1967) suggested that the "I" is all but eliminated because individuals are determined more by their social situations than by themselves. The potential for personal development depends on interactions with others. No natural unfolding of potential occurs without the participation and involvement of others.

The major benefit of this theory is that, by emphasizing relationships, it facilitates identification of potential problems between family members. The major drawback is that, by failing to account for a family's interaction with its environment, the theory is self-limiting.

Social exchange theory

Although this theory encompasses a collection of explanations, propositions, hypotheses, and assumptions about social behavior, its central tenet is the reciprocal relationship between partners and the interplay of individual motives, perceptions, and behaviors.

Assumptions central to the social exchange theory include the following.
• A reciprocal, mutually dependent relationship can exist in which something of value is given by both partners.
• Rewarding certain behavior will encourage repetition of that behavior.
• Profit (the reward of a relationship minus its cost) is influential in maintaining a relationship.
• Exchange of rewards and costs may accommodate and maintain the relationship (Hollander, 1978).

In social exchange theory, the individual weighs the outcome of an interaction, considers the consequences, and chooses a behavior that will minimize costs and maximize rewards. This approach, although helpful in viewing relationships and behaviors, is limited. Like interactional theory, social exchange theory tends to emphasize the individual at the expense of the family and environment.

Putting theories into practice

Theories provide a basis for understanding the family; no one theory is completely right or wrong. Considering each theory gives the nurse various perspectives when assessing a family. For example, consider how these theories may be applied in the case of a young couple just after the birth of their first child.

A systems theory approach would define the birth of the child as a creation of a new subsystem, which changes the original system. Open family boundaries facilitate adjustment and adaptation to new roles.

When using a structural-functional approach, the nurse would identify the family as nuclear and would assess the couple's role relationships. New roles may be needed to fulfill additional family functions. The functions that need to be assessed include:
• provision of a safe environment for the child
• provision of sustenance and any needed economic adjustments
• socialization of the child, including the couple's preparation for child rearing
• affective needs of family members.

Using the developmental theory, the nurse would identify the family's developmental level and establish tasks to be completed. This family is in the second stage (families with infants). Assessment should focus on the family's developmental changes and should address:
• adjustment of the new family unit
• fulfillment of parental roles
• identification and ability to meet the child's needs
• adjustment to extended family relationships and role changes.

Using interactional theory, the nurse would explore the couple's perception of the child and the birth experience. The nurse also should establish how the couple expect family roles to change.

The social exchange theory also requires the nurse to examine interactions between family members but should include an investigation of perceived outcomes as well. The nurse should ask family members to consider the rewards, costs, and other effects of changes in their family structure and relationship.

Family types

Various family types, ranging from the traditional nuclear and extended families to single parent and alternative life-style families, have evolved in recent decades. The most common family types are described below.

Nuclear

The most readily recognized family type, the traditional nuclear family consists of a married couple and their biologic children. The classic nuclear family lives in a relatively independent household removed from grandparents and other relatives. The male partner functions primarily as provider and the female functions primarily as caretaker.

According to Friedman (1986), specific variations on the nuclear family include:
• nuclear dyad—a married couple with no children or whose children live elsewhere
• middle-aged or elderly couple—a married couple whose adult children have left home
• kin-network—a nuclear family who lives near other family members and engages in reciprocal physical and psychological support
• second-career family—a nuclear family in which the woman enters or returns to the work force.

The nuclear family has grown less common as economic and life-style trends have encouraged the development of alternative family types.

Extended

This family type includes the nuclear family and some or all of the members' relatives. Commonly included in the extended family are grandparents, siblings of the male or female partner, and children of those siblings. The extended family shares household responsibilities and provides an overall support system for family members. Extended families living with intact nuclear families are not as common in the United States as they once were.

Communal

This family type consists of cooperating groups of people committed to a larger community. Members of a communal family may be related by blood or marriage, or they may be unrelated. The family may include two or more monogomous couples and their children, for example, or several adults in a group marriage with their offspring. Typically, family members share resources and child rearing responsibilities. In most communes, members teach the next generation to maintain the commune's goals.

Single parent

Increasingly common in the United States, the single parent family typically originates from divorce, death, adoption, unwed motherhood, or a personal choice to forego marriage.

Over 90% of the children in single parent families live with the mother, while the remaining 10% live with the father, the grandparents, or other relatives (U.S. Bureau of the Census, 1989). A new twist to the single parent family is the number of children living with their grandparents. The Census Bureau predicts that more than 9.5 million children will be living apart from their parents in 1990. Most of these children will live with one or more of their grandparents. Several trends, such as the increasing divorce rate and decreasing numbers of grandchildren, portend that many grandparents will continue to take primary responsibility for their grandchildren (Cherlin and Furstenberg, 1986). For these families, the traditional grandparent role will change and tasks that these people faced in young adulthood will return to them. The assumption is that the single adult must perform the functions typically shared by two, including economic provision and emotional and psychological support for the children. Concurrently, the single parent receives reduced affection, communication, emotional support, and assistance. Stresses experienced by these parents include too many responsibilities, tasks, and emotional demands (Weiss, 1981).

Most women who head single parent homes live below the federal government's poverty line (Guttentag, Salasin, and Belle, 1980). These families may require financial assistance (Goodrich, Rampage, and Ellman, 1989).

Blended

Also known as a reconstituted family, the blended family arises when one or both partners lives with children from a previous partner. Thus, one or both partners becomes a stepparent.

Establishing roles and raising children in a blended family may be difficult. The stepparent may meet resistance from the spouse's biologic children. Resentments can appear quickly when members struggle to defend their biologic relatives or refuse to accept the changing family structure. Competition, rivalry, and everyday frictions may require constant attention, open communication, and honest expression of feelings. Typically, this family begins to function as an integrated unit only after spending much time and effort to establish acceptable roles.

Blended family relationships may become complicated through sheer numbers. Remarriage may add children, grandparents, siblings, and parents. Kinship lines may become confused, particularly in large families, creating conflict and anxiety among members of merging families. Continuity is best preserved when children in blended families can maintain the family relationships that existed before the blended family began.

Cohabiting

Also called a social contract family, a cohabiting family involves an unmarried couple living together in the same household (Cherlin, 1981). The typical cohabiting couple desire long-term intimacy without legal involvement. Sometimes called the "unmarried married," these cou-ples are increasingly common in the United States. They may encounter disapproval or ostracism from those who regard cohabitation as immoral.

People cohabit for many reasons, ranging from convictions to convenience. Some believe that intimate relationships are individual concerns and need not involve the state. Some cohabit to avoid future divorce or to test the relationship before marriage. Some oppose marriage in principle, believing that it demeans women. Some prefer to avoid the sentimentality, symbols, celebrations, and public nature of traditional marriages. By being more covert and private, cohabitation may allow the couple to remain more independent from society and from each other (Henslin, 1985). Also, many elderly couples cohabit for company and affection after the death of spouses. Some tax laws make marriage too expensive for them.

In a study of 23-year-olds, Thorton (1988) reported that half the women and two-thirds of the men cohabited before marriage or in lieu of marriage. Although living together may be an important transitional stage for many young people, most Americans eventually marry.

Homosexual

Gay and lesbian families resemble other types in that the partners make an emotional and economic commitment to each other. Although the homosexual family has no legal status in most states, some clergy will perform homosexual marriages. Some couples opt to perform their own marriagelike ceremonies.

Some homosexual couples choose to raise children as part of their families. Although research on the children in these families is limited, early findings suggest that measures of sexual identity for children raised by transsexual or homosexual parents do not differ appreciably from those of children raised by heterosexual parents (Green, 1978).

In recent years, the concept of homosexual parenting has become more accepted. However, homosexual parents still may experience sharp disapproval. According to Bozett (1988), this disapproval may envelop the family and friends of the homosexual couple as well as the couple themselves.

Family functions

Nathan Ackerman (1972), well known for his family theory, believes that the family has two basic functions: to assure the physical survival of the young, which requires providing food, clothing, and shelter; and to help family members grow and develop psychologically and socially. The basic functions—including physical safety, sustenance, personal nurturing, education, and socialization—apply to families everywhere and are essential for maintaining societies (Friedman, 1986).

Physical safety

Young children are helpless and vulnerable; they depend on adult family members to manage and maintain a safe environment. In some cultures, assuring physical safety may require weapons and physical barriers to protect family members from hostile forces. Although modern families do not face these overt threats, they may face the more subtle but no less hostile threats of drug abuse, interpersonal violence, and such health problems as contagious diseases.

Sustenance

The family provides sustenance to its members in the form of food, water, and shelter. Generations ago, most families provided that sustenance directly; they grew their own food, located and maintained their own water supplies, and built their own homes. With industrialization, however, many families shifted from an agrarian to an urban life-style and became consumers rather than producers. Currently, most families provide sustenance for members by purchasing goods and services. In fact, economic prosperity has become the focal point from which to define part of a family's success.

Personal nurturing

The family is responsible for providing affection, acceptance, and companionship to its members (Friedman, 1986); it is the primary source for personal acceptance, companionship, expression, self-esteem, and the fulfillment of individual goals. The need for love and belonging in a changing world is the foundation from which this family function emerges. Although the mother has traditionally assumed the primary role in providing attention and emotional support for the children, fathers increasingly are involved in this role. Family members demonstrate caring for one another by meeting individual needs for growth and personal fulfillment. The family also provides its members with psychological support, teaches younger members necessary social skills, and develops coping skills that benefit family functioning (Parsons and Bales, 1955; Hill, 1965).

Education

The family's educational function is multifaceted, incorporating classroom education, psychomotor skills, social functioning, and emotional and perceptual health. Although parents are not personally responsible for educating a child, they are responsible for ensuring that the child receives a formal education. In addition to formal education, families must prepare children to function in personal relationships and in society. This preparation involves teaching moral values, instilling a sense of purpose, and providing the direction and motivation needed to attain personal potential. The family's responsiveness to achievements is critical for a child and for building each member's desire to pursue new experiences throughout life.

Socialization

Families assume primary responsibility for teaching children how to be productive members of society. Schools, churches, and other institutions may assume some of this responsibility as well. Children receive their first and most intense socialization within the family, where they learn about values, culture, roles, and beliefs. This function perpetuates the family and prepares for the replacement of society's members. Participation in traditions and ceremonies helps families maintain their place in society and relationships within the family structure (Kertzer, 1989). Rituals may be linked to the family's changing developmental stage—such as graduations, marriage ceremonies, and funerals—and may serve to reinforce such family relationships as holiday celebrations. They may help maintain an ethnic consciousness, such as Bar Mitzvahs. Certain meetings and activities, such as the Girl Scouts, may help family members develop self-concept and personal identification.

Family roles

Family members typically carry out their family functions by adopting recurrent patterns of behavior, called roles. These maintain family stability by providing predictability in family functioning. Adoption of roles may be conscious or subconscious; at times, roles may overlap among family members, or they may be unique.

A family's culture, religion, socioeconomic status, and developmental stage influence how roles are assigned and how members function in their roles. According to Beavers (1982), families that function well—mature families—tend to balance roles and functions, communicate openly, respect each member's individuality, and use coping mechanisms that encourage constructive adaptation to everyday problems and periodic crises. (See *Family maturity* for more information.)

A successful family constantly monitors and responds to variables that affect its roles. The family assesses individual and group needs and acts to satisfy those needs through cooperation and healthy functional patterns. Members endeavor to fulfill role responsibilities, give and receive feedback, solve conflicts, and adjust roles as needed to allow each member to grow and develop in a safe, encouraging environment.

Assigning roles

Typically, roles correspond to a family's developmental stage, evolving as the family passes from one stage to the next. (For more information on developmental theory, see the "Family theories" section at the beginning of this chapter.) In the beginning family stage, for example, spouses typically collaborate on all roles. Working together, they provide all the family's needs, sometimes assigning primary responsibility for certain functions to one spouse. When children are born, the mother may assume most of the household and nurturing roles, and the father may control family finances. When children enter school, the mother may resume her career and the father may assume more household duties. As the children age, they typically take on roles that include increasing responsibility.

Family roles commonly reflect those the partners experienced in their families. For example, a man will tend to take control of family finances if his father had this responsibility. Role expectations for children also are guided, at least in part, by practices in the parents' families.

Differing role models and expectations in the parents' families may lead to conflict over acceptable roles for them and their children. Conflict between parents and children commonly arises as children begin to mature and assert opinions about their roles and functions within the family. Resolving role conflicts requires that family members sort out and identify problems, share possible solutions, and reach a workable compromise though negotiation. This can occur most successfully when family members communicate openly and honestly. (For more information, see *Family patterns,* page 34.)

Roles are most likely to succeed when they follow three steps: clarification, task allotment, and evaluation.

Family maturity

The way family members carry out their roles and relationships indicates the family's level of maturity. Members of mature families:
• view individuality as an asset, a trait to be encouraged
• express their thoughts and feelings openly and take responsibility for the actions that stem from these thoughts and feelings
• consider the opinions of other family members, respecting each person's perceptions.
Members of immature families:
• are intolerant of divergent ideas
• tend to communicate in a rigid, automatic manner both verbally and nonverbally.
Family maturity tends to develop over successive generations; however, no family reaches complete maturity, and specific circumstances may affect maturity in successive generations. For example, a family member who suffered serious, chronic illness as a child may as an adult expect an inordinate amount of attention and aid from other family members.

Role clarification involves detailing the tasks and expectations that accompany each role. The process should include dialogue, questioning, and negotiation among family members. Typically, roles and the tasks they include are established according to the family's priorities and work toward the family's goals.

After clarifying roles and tasks, the family must decide who will perform each task—that is, task allotment. Tasks for each member should be clearly defined, completely understood, and compatible with the individual's age, sex, and abilities (Beavers, 1982).

By evaluating role performance, family members can detect and discuss difficulties encountered in completing the tasks involved in each role. Inability or unwillingness to meet role expectations may create internal stress or conflict with other family members. Some types of role conflict include:
• interrole conflict—a family member assumes too many roles and, as a result, cannot fulfill the expectations of each one
• intersender conflict—role expectations differ among family members
• person-role conflict—a family member's internal values differ from those required to fulfill role responsibilities and expectations (Friedman, 1986).

Role transition may occur when the family experiences a life-cycle event, such as childbirth, illness, divorce, or death (Friedman, 1986). For example, a divorced mother may retain her responsibility for household maintenance and child rearing and also become responsible for family finances and record keeping. In another example, if a child becomes seriously ill, the mother may

Family patterns

Most families incorporate several roles into a family pattern. Family pattern refers to the overall way in which members relate, regardless of the roles they adopt. Examples of these patterns include the autocratic family, the patriarchal family, the matriarchal family, and the democratic family.

Autocratic family

In this pattern, relationships are rigid, one-sided, and tend to be defensive. Parents strive to control their children and direct their personal growth and development. The autocratic family adheres to rules and expectations; unmet expectations prompt fear and anxiety. Rarely is this family open to outside influences. Parents tend to emphasize the importance of the parental role, minimizing the potentially valuable contribution of children to the family.

The typical autocratic family has difficulty coping with change and loss, seeking instead to reinstate the past and preserve previous methods of relating. The leader may manipulate members to maintain that person's views. Individuals rarely become independent and rarely reach a high level of self-differentiation. The autocratic leader scrutinizes the outside environment to prevent children from being influenced by its thoughts and actions. Values in this family emphasize conformity and continuity rather than individuality and growth.

Patriarchal family

In this pattern, the male spouse assumes a dominant, rigid, sexually stereotypical role. Typically, the patriarch is financially successful, aggressive, work-oriented, and satisfied with his life. To the family, he provides material but not emotional support, assuming primary authority and making a majority of the family decisions. He retains financial control. Although his spouse may work, the man's career takes precedence.

Matriarchal family

In this pattern, the female spouse assumes primary authority; her male partner typically participates little in the family, abdicating his parental role. The matriarch displays intense involvement in the lives of her children, exhibiting a need to control and possess them. She makes all decisions pertaining to child rearing, imposing her values, morals, and beliefs on her children. In some matriarchal families, the male partner assumes the role of another child, submitting to punitive, patronizing behavior from his spouse.

Democratic family

In this pattern, adult partners function as equals and the children are respected individuals within the family. Adults strive to solve difficulties jointly with the children, placing emphasis on maintaining relationships. The democratic family is flexible and willing to change in an attempt to accommodate differing perceptions and needs. Partners solicit reactions and feelings from one another.

The democractic family recognizes the need for individual fulfillment, and each member is willing to give in exchange for receiving. This family has the ability to resolve conflicts and facilitate individual growth. Its members work together to negotiate compromises and identify expectations. Children raised in a democratic family are taught that communication is crucial and that equitable solutions usually can be reached.

Conflict may occur in the democratic family as frequently as it occurs in other families, but its members work through the conflict rather than avoid it. This family pattern requires individual strength and the willingness to work together.

---

spend more time caring for the child and the father may assume some of her usual roles as homemaker.

In a single parent family, the parent must assume all of the roles. If the parent cannot cope with the increased responsibility of these roles, parent-child relationships may suffer. In other cases, the parent compensates for lost spousal support by depending on the children for support, in effect transferring roles from the absent partner to the children. This can enhance the parent-child relationship by encouraging the parent to become more honest and direct with the children and involving them in family decisions at an early age.

Types of roles

Roles may be classified as formal or informal. Formal roles usually are associated with position, such as marital or parental roles. Informal roles may correspond to the family's emotional needs or help to maintain family stability, such as a family scapegoat role.

Although some roles may change and adapt throughout the life of any family, others usually remain consistent, such as that of provider, nurturer, decision maker, problem solver, tradition setter, value setter, and health supervisor (Friedman, 1986).

Provider

This person must ensure that the family has food, clothing, shelter, and money. Commonly in today's society, adult partners split this role.

Nurturer

This person has an affective role, offering love, support, care, reassurance, and comfort to each family member. The nurturer maintains or increases the other members' personal development. Although other family members may have nurturing qualities that overlap with this role, one person assumes the role of nurturer in the typical family.

Decision maker

This person assumes responsibility for family members' accountability. The person in this role may use an autocratic or democratic style to assign family tasks, delegate responsibilities, obtain information necessary to complete assignments, and follow through on outcomes of decisions. The decision maker reinforces joint family decisions and strives to make goals and dreams a reality.

Problem solver

This person assumes the job of family maintenance by setting standards of behavior. When standards are not met, family members approach the problem solver to assist in modifying behavior. Specific tasks include disciplinary actions, labeling of behavior as acceptable or unacceptable, identifying deviations in behavior, and monitoring daily interactions among family members.

Tradition setter

This person monitors and responds to anniversaries, birthdays, holidays, and family customs. Typical tasks include maintaining a family genealogy, taking photos at family gatherings, urging that children be named after old relatives, or seeking out birth certificates, gravestones, and family homesteads. The tradition setter strives to enhance the family's understanding of its place in history and society. By investigating the extended family, the tradition setter may create ways to bridge the past with the present and beyond. Most tradition setters care deeply about family origins and encourage other family members to participate.

Value setter

This person continually explores and clarifies the family's belief system and may try to control behavior based on a personal view of what family members should believe. Tasks include establishing standards and the latitude they allow and enforcing acceptable behavior. Depending on the value setter's personal beliefs, standards of acceptable behavior may range from strict to lenient. In many cases, behavior is judged on the specific circumstances involved, with judgments changing as the value setter's personal beliefs evolve. This role includes a significant management function in the typical family; maintenance of the family may fall largely to this person.

Health supervisor

This person examines the personal well-being of other family members. Tasks include suggesting or dictating standards for bathing, eating, dressing, and exercise; establishing responses to illness and health—for example, illness may be punished as weakness or cherished as a sign of need. Family health standards may be meticulous or lax, depending on the disposition of this person. Typically, the health supervisor controls the family's interaction with health care professionals.

Families in crisis

The typical family faces many potential crises during its life cycle. By learning healthy coping mechanisms, individuals and families can minimize or thwart most of these threats. When crisis does strike, families and health care professionals can help manage it with various intervention techniques.

Coping mechanisms

Individuals and families employ various skills and strategies to adapt to change and cope with stressors, which may range from minor variations in daily routines to major traumatic events. Children learn coping skills by watching other family members act and react and by sharing in their thoughts and feelings. Positive coping mechanisms include open, honest communication and reliance on an emotionally supportive network of family and friends.

Healthy families seek support in times of need from inside and outside sources. This support may provide buffering effects for the family (Nuckolls, Cassel, and Kaplan, 1972). It may reduce complications, as during pregnancy, labor, and childbirth. After childbirth, for example, spouses may want to participate in a support group or parent education class to build a sense of social support and help build parenting skills.

Schaefer, Coyne, and Lazarus (1981) describe three types of social support. Emotional support includes receiving reassurance, feeling emotional attachment, and being able to depend on another person. Tangible support involves direct help, such as lending money, doing chores, or caring for a sick family member. Informational support includes providing facts or advice and giving feedback. Nurses engage in all three types of support based on each client's needs.

Internally, coping involves concurrent noncognitive and cognitive processes classified as emotion-focused and problem-focused (Lazarus and Folkman, 1984). Emotion-focused coping involves subjective and emotional responses to a problem. Examples of emotion-focused coping include denying the problem or minimizing its importance, comparing the problem to that of someone else, or searching for a positive side to the situation. Problem-focused coping involves objective and rational responses to a problem. Typically, it includes identifying the problem, searching for possible solutions, determining the best solution, and then acting on it. The best solution depends on circumstances specific to the problem, the values and attitudes of family members involved, and the solution's feasibility.

Both aspects of coping affect how greatly a crisis upsets normal family functioning. To handle a crisis successfully, the family should follow a two-step process of identifying the problem and searching for acceptable solutions.

To identify the problem, family members should carefully and honestly appraise the situation and its potential for harm or loss. Some problems already will have caused harm or loss, such as delivery of a stillborn neonate. Other problems will threaten future harm, possibly prompting feelings of fear and anxiety along with the desire to solve the problem or handle the situation. For example, if amniocentesis reveals that a fetus has Down's syndrome (trisomy 21), the pregnant client and her partner may feel fear and anxiety about their ability to care for the child, while they simultaneously may share strong convictions that the child must have the best care.

Coping mechanisms that distort reality, interfere with personal relationships, or adversely affect work performance impair healthy family functioning. The nurse may be able to help families develop healthier coping mechanisms. For example, if the client's partner blames her for an unwanted pregnancy, the nurse can help guide the couple past blame and accusations and focus them on problem solving.

Crisis response

Most families experience crises from time to time. Typically, a family crisis occurs when a significant event coincides with a crucial stage of family development and threatens the family's stability. Crises are most likely when several stressful events occur simultaneously or in rapid succession, such as pregnancy, moving to a new home, and the death of a parent. Compounded stress generated by events of this significance can cause a crisis even in families with the best coping skills.

Typically, three conditions determine if a family responds well to a crisis: perception of the event, ability to use coping mechanisms, and participation in a social support system. Perception of a stressful event hinges on the client's opinion about its potential harm and the availability of solutions (Lazarus and Folkman, 1984). What one person considers a crisis another may not, based on such factors as age, emotional state, and life experience.

Most crises can be labeled as maturational, which are linked to the family's developmental level, or situational, which arise from traumatic events. Marriage, childbirth, and children leaving home may cause maturational crises. Dysfunction may occur if family members fail to adapt to these changes or misunderstand their implications (Carter and McGoldrick, 1988).

The sudden death of a family member, a violent crime, and financial failure are examples of situational crises, which may threaten the self-concept of the people involved. Typical reactions include shock, anger, hopelessness, and depression. Family health may be jeopardized if the crisis severely disrupts the individual's family role.

Crisis intervention strives in two ways to help clients regain normal function. The first involves assessment of factors that affect crisis development; the second, teaching the family to use internal capabilities and external aids.

Chapter summary

Chapter 2 presented the various aspects of family structure and function. Here are the chapter's key concepts.
• Modern families are diverse; no longer can the traditional nuclear family be considered the only norm.
• Family theories allow researchers and clinicians to understand the family by focusing on selected aspects, such as individual relationships and interaction with the environment.
• Duvall's eight-stage theory, perhaps the best known of the family theories, relates family development to life-cycle stages.
• The increase in single parent families represents a significant alteration in the Western family.
• The family's basic functions are to provide its members with physical safety, sustenance, personal nurturing, education, and socialization.
• Family members typically adopt certain roles—recurrent patterns of behavior—to allow families to function with some degree of continuity.
• Roles adopted by one or more family members include provider, nurturer, decision maker, problem solver, tradition setter, value setter, and health supervisor.
• Family pattern refers to overall family relationships and dominance; the democratic family displays the most healthy pattern.

• Healthy coping mechanisms can help families minimize or thwart crises.

• Family crisis is most likely to occur when several stressful events occur simultaneously or in rapid succession.

• Maturational crises are linked to the family's developmental level, whereas situational crises are caused by traumatic events.

• Although its structure is changing and diversifying, the family remains a vital social institution and a major stabilizing force for society.

Study questions

1. The Saru family consists of Mrs. Mary Saru, age 38, and her four children: Michael, age 17; Sandy, age 15; and the twins, Jerry and Jenny, age 4. Mrs. Saru has come to the family practice clinic because she has been eating and sleeping poorly and feels unable to make decisions. She also is worried about the children's reaction to their father's death.

How might the nurse use an understanding of coping mechanisms and crisis response to help the Saru family?

2. What changes in family patterns and roles might the nurse expect to see in the Saru family?

3. What input, throughput, and output might the nurse identify after considering the Saru family as a system? How could this information be used to help the family cope?

Bibliography

Ackerman, N. (1972). *Psychodynamics of family life: Diagnosis and treatment of family relationships.* New York: Basic Books.

Baltes, P.B., Reese, H.W., and Lipsitt, L.P. (1980). Life-span developmental psychology. *Annual Review of Psychology,* 31, 65-110.

Beavers, W.R. (1982). Healthy, midrange, and severely dysfunctional families. In F. Walsh (Ed.), *Normal family processes* (pp. 45-66). New York: Guilford Press.

Bowen, M. (1978). *Family therapy in clinical practice.* Northvale, NJ: Aronson.

Broderick, C.B. (1982). Adult sexual development. In B.B. Wolman and G. Stricker (Eds.), *Handbook of developmental psychology.* Englewood Cliffs, NJ: Prentice-Hall.

Caplan, G. (1964). *Principles of preventive psychiatry.* New York: Basic Books.

Doherty, W.J., and Jacobsen, N.S. (1982). Marriage and the family. In B.B. Wolman and G. Stricker (Eds.), *Handbook of developmental psychology.* Englewood Cliffs, NJ: Prentice-Hall.

Douglas, J.P. (1980). *Introduction to the sociologies of everyday life.* Boston: Allyn and Bacon.

Erikson, E. (1950). *Childhood and society,* New York: Norton.

Fowles, D.G. (1985). *A profile of older Americans: 1985.* Washington, DC: American Association of Retired Persons.

Friedman, M.M. (1986). *Family nursing, theory and assessment.* New York: Appleton & Lange.

Hayghe, H. (1986). Rise in mothers' labor force activity includes those with infants. *Monthly Labor Review,* 109, 43-45.

Hollander, E. (1978). *Leadership Dynamics.* New York: Free Press.

Kamerman, S.B. (1986). *Infant care usage in the United States.* Report presented to National Academy of Sciences Ad Hoc Committee on Policy Issues in Child Care for Infants and Toddlers, pp. 12-36. Washington, DC: National Academy Press.

Kamerman, S.B., and Hayes, C.D. (1982). The dimensions of change: Trends and issues. In S.B. Kamerman and C.D. Hayes (Eds.), *Families that work: Children in a changing world.* Washington, DC: National Academy Press.

Kerr, M., and Bowen, M. (1988). *Family evaluation: An approach based on Bowen theory.* New York: Norton.

Kertzer, D.I. (1989). Lasting rites. *Networker,* July, August, 21-29.

Logan, B., and Dawkins, C. (1986). *Family centered nursing in the community.* Menlo Park, CA: Addison-Wesley.

Malinowski, B. (1960). *A scientific theory of culture.* New York: Oxford University Press.

Maurin, J.T., Russell, L., and Memmott, R.J. (1989). An exploration of gender differences among the homeless. *Research in Nursing and Health,* 12(5), 315-321.

Mead, G.H. (1967). *Mind, self and society: From the standpoint of a social behaviorist.* Chicago: University of Chicago Press.

Minuchin, S. (1974). *Families and family therapy.* Cambridge, MA: Harvard University Press.

Murdock, G. (1949). *Social structure.* New York: Macmillan.

Murdock, G. (1965). *Social structure.* New York: Free Press.

Parsons, R., and Bales, R.F. (1955). *Family, socialization and interaction process.* New York: Free Press.

Rakel, R.E. (1977). *Principles of family medicine.* Philadelphia: Saunders.

Richards, E. (1989). Self-reports of differentiation of self and marital compatability as related to family functioning in the third and fourth stages of the family life cycle. *Scholarly Inquiry for Nursing Practice: An International Journal,* 3(3), 163-175.

Rodgers, R. (1973). *Family interaction and transaction: The development approach.* Englewood Cliffs, NJ: Prentice-Hall.

Rodgers, R. (1962). *Improvements in the construction and analysis of family life cycle categories.* Kalamazoo, MI: Western Michigan University Press.

Scanzoni, J. (1983). *Shaping tomorrow's family: Theory and policy for the twenty-first century.* Beverly Hills, CA: Sage.

Schaefer, C., Coyne, J. and Lazarus, R. (1981). The health-related functions of social support. *Journal of Behavioral Medicine,* 4(4), 381-406.

Schulz, D. (1969). *Coming up black: Patterns of ghetto socialization.* Englewood Cliffs, NJ: Prentice-Hall.

Sheehy, G. (1977). *Passages: Predictable crisis of adult life.* New York:

Bantam.

Spiro, M.E. (1954). Is the family universal? *American Anthropologist*, 56, 879-86.

U.S. Bureau of the Census. (1985). *Statistical abstract of the United States: 1984*. Washington, DC: U.S. Government Printing Office.

U.S. Bureau of the Census. (1989). *Households, families, marital status and living arrangements*. Washington, DC: U.S. Government Printing Office.

Whall, A.L. (1986). *Family therapy theory for nursing: Four approaches*. East Norwalk, CT: Appleton & Lange.

Wismont, J.M., and Reame, N.E. (1989). The lesbian childbearing experience: Assessing developmental tasks. *Image: Journal of Nursing Scholarship*, 21(3), 137-141.

White House Conference on Families. (1980). *Listening to America's families: Action for the 80s*. Washington, DC: U.S. Government Printing Office.

Zablocki, B. (1980). *The joyful community*. Chicago: University of Chicago Press.

Family theories

Carter, E., and McGoldrick, M. (1988). The family life cycle and family therapy: An overview. In E. Carter and M. McGoldrick (Eds.), *The family life cycle: A framework for family therapy* (2nd ed.; pp. 3-20). New York: Gardner Press.

Chadwick-Jones, J.K. (1976). *Social exchange theory: Its structure and influence in social psychology*. New York: Academic Press.

Duvall, E. (1984). *Marriage and family development* (6th ed.). New York: Harper & Row.

Horton, T.E. (1984). Conceptual basis for nursing intervention with human systems: Families. In J.E. Hall and B.R. Weaver (Eds.), *Distributive nursing practice: A systems approach to community health* (2nd ed.). Philadelphia: Lippincott.

Lidz, T. (1983). *The person: His and her development throughout the life cycle*. New York: Basic Books.

Rankin, S.H., and Weekes, D.P. (1989). Life-span development: A review of theory and practice for families with chronically ill members. *Scholarly Inquiry for Nursing Practice: An International Journal*, 3(1), 3-22.

Von Bertalanffy, L. (1969). *General systems theory*. New York: George Braziller.

Family types

Bassuk, E.L., Rubin, L., and Lauriat, A.S. (1986). Characteristics of sheltered homeless families. *American Journal of Public Health*, 76(9), 1097-1101.

Bozett, F.W. (1988). Social control of identity by children of gay fathers. *Western Journal of Nursing Research*, 10(5), 550-565.

Cherlin, A. (1981). *Marriage, divorce, remarriage*. Cambridge, MA: Harvard University Press.

Cherlin, A., and Furstenberg, F.F. (1986). *The new American grandparents: A place in the family, a life apart*. New York: Basic Books.

Goodrich, T.J., Rampage, C., and Ellman, B. (1989). Single parenthood. *Networker*. September-October, 52-56.

Green, R. (1978). Sexual identity of 37 children raised by homosexual or transsexual parents. *American Journal of Psychiatry*, 135(6), 692-697.

Grief, G.L. (in press). *Fathering alone: A guide for custodial dads*. Lexington, MA: Lexington Books.

Henslin, J.M. (1985). Cohabitation: Its context and meaning. In J.M. Henslin (Ed.), *Marriage and family in a changing society* (2nd ed.). New York: Free Press.

Hochschild, A., and Machung, A. (1989). *Second shift: Inside the two-job marriage*. New York: Viking Press.

Pitzer, M.S., and Hock, E. (1989). Employed mothers' concerns about separation from the first-and second-born child. *Research in Nursing and Health*, 12(2), 123-128.

Schulz, D. (1982). *The changing family: Its function and future* (3rd ed.). Englewood Cliffs, NJ: Prentice-Hall.

Thorton, A. (1988). Cohabitation and marriage in the 1980s. *Demography*, 25, 497.

Toman, W. (1976). *Family Constellation* (3rd ed.). New York: Springer.

Weiss, R.S. (1976). The emotional impact of marital separation. *Journal of Social Issues*, 32(1), 135-145.

Weiss, R.S. (1981). *Going it alone: The family life and social situation of the single parent*. New York: Basic Books.

Winch, R.F. (1971). *The modern family*. New York: Holt, Rinehart & Winston.

Families in crisis

Aquilera, D., and Messick, J. (1982). *Crisis intervention: Theory and methodology* (4th ed.). St. Louis: Mosby.

Glazer, G. (1989). Anxiety and stressors of expectant fathers. *Western Journal of Nursing Research*, 11(1), 47-59.

Guttentag, M., Salasin, S., and Belle, D. (1980). *The mental health of women*. New York: Academic Press.

Harkins, E.B. (1978). Effects of empty nest transition on self-report of psychological and physical well-being. *Journal of Marriage and Family*, 40(3), 549-556.

Hill, R. (1965). Generic features of families under stress. In H. Pared (Ed.), *Crisis intervention: Selected readings* (pp. 32-52). New York: Family Service Association of America.

Lazarus, R., and Folkman, S. (1984). *Stress, appraisal, and coping*. New York: Springer.

Nuckolls, K., Cassel, J., and Kaplan, B. (1972). Psychosocial assets, life crisis and the prognosis of pregnancy. *American Journal of Epidemiology*, 95(5), 431-441.

Cultural references

Brown, R. (1931). The organization of Australian tribes. *Journal of Oceania*.

Spiro, M.E., and Spiro, A.G. (1975). *Children of the kibbutz*. Cambridge, MA: Harvard University Press.

Nursing Process and the Childbearing Family

Objectives

After reading and studying this chapter, the student should be able to:

1. List the steps of the nursing process and discuss the purpose of each.
2. Describe important assessment areas for the childbearing family.
3. Explain the potential impact of cultural, socioeconomic, and psychological influences on the childbearing family.
4. List examples of nursing diagnoses commonly used for the childbearing family.
5. State the steps involved in developing a care plan.
5. Discuss approaches to evaluating nursing care.
6. Describe information necessary for adequate documentation.

Introduction

During the past 50 years, changes have radically altered family structure and function. Some of these changes, such as a significant increase in single-parent families, have had far-reaching consequences for social and health services. Nurses who care for childbearing families must fulfill numerous roles in today's health care settings.

The nurse's caring relationship with the client can be mapped out by using a simple, highly versatile tool: the nursing process. This process—a system for making nursing decisions that includes assessment, nursing diagnosis, planning, implementation, and evaluation—guides the nurse in providing quality care to the childbearing family in any setting. By following this process and backing it with thorough documentation,

the nurse can develop effective strategies to respond to current and potential needs and problems while promoting family health.

Family health—a family's ability to function constructively—depends on various factors. Cultural patterns, religious influences, socioeconomic status, and stage of family development shape each member's roles and functions within the family and also influence how the family perceives and copes with everyday problems and crisis situations.

The nurse promotes the health of the childbearing family by providing family-centered nursing care. This approach includes assessing each family member's health needs, identifying health deficiencies and strengths, and intervening with education and counseling to improve family health. The nurse also involves the client and her partner in health care decision making during pregnancy and after childbirth, such as where the delivery will take place—at home, in a hospital, or in a birth center—and how to participate in the delivery.

This chapter discusses each step of the nursing process, plus documentation of care, as it should be used by the nurse caring for the childbearing family.

Assessment

The first step in the nursing process, assessment involves the orderly collection and careful interpretation of information about a client's health status. Information that

GLOSSARY

Antepartal period: period during pregnancy and before labor and delivery. See *intrapartal period* and *postpartal period*.

Anthropometry: science that deals with measurement of the size, weight, and proportions of the human body.

Assessment: systematic collecting of subjective and objective data about a client's health status. See *nursing process*.

Clustering: process of grouping related assessment data to identify broad client needs; the nurse may then consult the NANDA taxonomy to choose an appropriate diagnostic category.

Coping: ways in which a person deals with stress and makes decisions.

Culture: integrated system of learned (not biologically inherited) beliefs, values, and behaviors characteristic of a society's members.

Ethnicity: affiliation with a group of people classified according to a common racial, national, linguistic, or cultural origin or background.

Ethnocentrism: belief that one's own cultural standards are superior.

Etiology: causal or contributing factor or factors.

Evaluation: determination of how successfully care plan goals have been met. See *nursing process*.

Goal: desired outcome of nursing care that guides formation and implementation of nursing interventions.

Implementation: nursing actions that carry out interventions described in the nursing care plan to achieve established goals. See *nursing process*.

Intervention: action performed by the nurse to implement the nursing care plan.

Intrapartal period: period during labor and delivery. See *antepartal period* and *postpartal period*.

Nursing care plan: written guide to a client's care encompassing the assessments, nursing diagnoses, planning, goals, and interventions throughout the course of care; the plan is revised and updated periodically.

Nursing diagnosis: descriptive statement identifying actual or potential client health problems that can be resolved or diminished by nursing care. See *nursing process*.

Nursing process: systematic problem-solving method that forms the framework for nursing practice; consists of five steps: assessment, nursing diagnosis, planning, implementation, and evaluation.

Objective data: information about a client's health status obtained through physical assessment and diagnostic study results.

Planning: involves setting and prioritizing goals for each nursing diagnosis, formulating interventions to help the client achieve these goals, and developing the nursing care plan. See *nursing process*.

Postpartal period: period after delivery. See *antepartal period* and *intrapartal period*.

Standardized nursing care plan: care plan developed for a group of clients with similar physical, emotional, or learning needs that reflects common standards of care.

Subjective data: assessment information obtained from the client and others with intimate knowledge of the client, typically through interviews.

comes from interviews with the client or family members is classified as *subjective* data. Information that comes from physical examination, medical records, diagnostic test results, and other medical or nursing sources is classified as *objective* data. Together, subjective and objective data give the nurse information essential for developing an effective care plan.

Assessment begins during the first meeting with a client and family and continues throughout the nurse-client relationship. Any change in the family—for example, in composition, socioeconomic status, health status, or relationships among members—requires reassessment and possible alteration in the nursing care plan. For a childbearing client, the nurse will find frequent reassessment necessary to identify the client's and family's changing needs during pregnancy, child-

birth, and the postpartal period. (For details, see *Assessing the pregnant client: An overview.*)

Assessment consists of two parts: health history (the major subjective data source) and physical assessment (the objective portion of the complete health assessment).

Health history

Giving insights into actual or potential problems, the health history provides the nurse with pertinent physiologic, psychological, cultural, and socioeconomic information in light of such factors as family life-style and relationships. The health history interview enables the nurse to determine client and family concerns, misconceptions, and other details related to bearing children.

Throughout the interview, the nurse must remain aware of verbal and nonverbal cues communicated by the client and family members. To interpret these cues accurately, the nurse must consider them in the context

Assessing the pregnant client: An overview

Providing effective nursing care for the pregnant client requires assessment by the nurse throughout the antepartal, intrapartal, and postpartal periods. Each period presents its own nursing challenges and focus.

Antepartal period

Quality nursing care during pregnancy goes far in assuring a positive outcome for client and neonate. Thorough, accurate assessment, an essential aspect of this care, begins with baseline data that will help guide subsequent assessment throughout pregnancy, labor, delivery, and the postpartal period.

Antepartal (prenatal) assessment focuses on physiologic, emotional, and socioeconomic considerations. Areas of particular importance include:
• nutrient intake, including unusual cravings
• extent of maternal discomfort and morning sickness
• learning needs related to preparation for labor and delivery
• fetal activity and uterine contractions.

The health history interview should explore the client's and family's attitudes toward the pregnancy and consider the physical, cultural, socioeconomic, genetic, and emotional factors affecting the client and family. If possible, antepartal interviews should include the client's partner, whose attitudes and adaptability may directly affect the client's attitudes toward her pregnancy, delivery, and childrearing.

Physical assessment centers on normal physiologic changes that occur during the stages of pregnancy as well as common indicators of problems that can occur at these stages.

Intrapartal period

Assessment during labor and delivery focuses on:
• the client's and family's psychological response to labor
• the client's and fetus's physiologic adaptation to labor
• any abnormal or unexpected findings during labor.

Relevant health history data include the client's preparation for and knowledge of labor and delivery, onset of labor (including rupture of membranes, bloody show, and other indicators), and frequency and duration of uterine contractions.

Physical assessment typically includes examining the cervix for effacement and dilation and assessing fetal heart rate and other fetal and maternal physiologic data.

Postpartal period

Assessment after delivery focuses on the client's and neonate's physiologic status and the family's adaptation to a new member. Important factors in postpartal assessment include:
• maternal bleeding and uterine involution
• the neonate's transition to extrauterine life (including skin color, respiratory effort, cardiac function, and other physiologic parameters)
• feeding and elimination patterns
• parent-neonate interaction.

---

of psychosocial, ethnic, and cultural influences on the client's life. These influences may affect the way a client or family responds to pregnancy, labor and delivery, neonatal care, and other aspects of childbearing.

Interviewing the client and family

During the health history interview, begin to establish a relationship with the client and family members based on trust and mutual respect. Convey a caring, nonjudgmental attitude, and question family members in a sensitive, respectful manner. Assure them that information they provide is confidential, noting who will have access to the client's record and how it may be used. (See *Family health assessment*, page 42, for more information.)

The following techniques help to ensure a successful interview:
• Provide privacy and minimize interruptions.
• Begin by making introductions and briefly explaining the purpose of the interview. Assure the client and family that notes taken during the interview will help in planning their care; emphasize that their answers will not be judged as right or wrong.
• Practice active listening. (For more information on active listening, see Chapter 4, Nurse-Client Interaction.)
• Ask open-ended questions that allow the client and family to express feelings and concerns. For a pregnant client, such questions might include, "Many women experience discomfort early in pregnancy. What kind of discomfort have you noticed?" For family members, such questions might include, "How do you feel about the pregnancy?"
• Use body language to convey interest and encourage the client and family to talk. Effective body language includes leaning forward, nodding periodically, and maintaining eye contact whenever possible. Inappropriate body language may include sitting with arms folded, glancing at the clock, and failing to make eye contact. This may inhibit a client from expressing true feelings or providing complete information.
• Note comments, facial expressions, and body language that may indicate areas requiring further exploration. For instance, if a client or family member physically tenses, avoids eye contact, or is reluctant to answer certain types of questions, change the topic and address these questions again later in the interview, after the client or family member seems more trusting and relaxed.

Throughout the interview, the nurse uses self-exploration to assess personal reactions to the client's and family's problems and perceptions, and refrains from making judgments about the client or family members based on personal values.

Family health assessment

The following format organizes the nurse's approach to assessment and ensures that all necessary information for planning and implementing care is included.

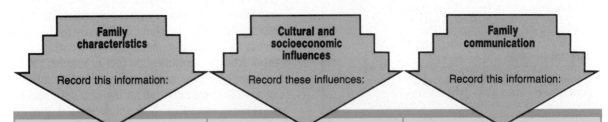

Family characteristics	Cultural and socioeconomic influences	Family communication
Record this information:	Record these influences:	Record this information:
• Family members (including parents, children, and grandparents), their ages, and how they are related. • Where each person lives. • How often family members contact each other and how contact is maintained (telephone, visits, letters, audio or video tapes). • Major life events (for example, miscarriage, death, genetic disease, divorce or separation, serious illness, employment change). • Closest and most distant family relationships. • Emotional barriers, if any, between family members (for example, a lack of communication about a past stressful event). • The family's developmental stage. • Issues that provoke intense emotional responses from family members (for example, alcohol abuse, money, sex, religion, death).	• The family's ethnic or racial background. • Level of education completed by each family member. • Each parent's occupation. • Which family members will care for the neonate. • The family's weekly, monthly, or annual income and income sources. • Anticipated change in expenses after the neonate's birth. • Family affiliation with a religious or spiritual organization, including denomination. • The family's social network (friends, neighbors, community activities, clubs) and its extent. • Family dietary habits and whether they meet the nutritional needs of individual family members.	• The attitudes of each family member about the impending birth and the extent of family discussions about these attitudes. • The family's level of knowledge and attitudes about health care and pregnancy care. • How the decision was made to have a child. • Which fantasies the parents have about their infant. • How the family has handled past major life changes and how the family copes with stress. • A subjective appraisal of how the birth will be managed by the family.

Influences on the family

In addition to information specific to the client's childbearing concerns, the health history interview should supply the nurse with information about cultural, ethnic, religious, socioeconomic, and psychological influences on the client and family as well as information about the family's coping patterns.

Cultural and ethnic background. A family's background may dictate appropriate behavior in many areas, including verbal and nonverbal language, religion and spirituality, family and societal roles and functions, coping methods, dress, and diet. Cultural and ethnic influences may have a great impact on how a client handles pregnancy and other aspects of family health. Keep in mind that *culture* refers to an integrated system of learned (not biologically inherited) behavior patterns characteristic of a society's members. *Ethnicity* refers to an affiliation with a group of people classified according to a common racial, national, linguistic, or cultural origin or background.

In North America, major ethnic groups include Asians, Blacks, Caucasians, Hispanics, and Native Americans. Among these groups, several cultural distinctions may exist. However, the nurse should avoid stereotyping or making assumptions about a client based on cultural or ethnic background. Each client is an individual and deserves a complete, open-minded assessment.

A common problem in providing care is a tendency to be ethnocentric—that is, to believe that one's cultural standards or beliefs are the best or most appropriate. For many nurses, beliefs regarding health and illness are influenced by the biomedical model, which emphasizes technology as a primary instrument for eradication of disease (Engel, 1977). Ignoring the effects of custom and culture on family behavior and perceptions can cause the nurse to overlook vital information. Moreover, the nurse must understand and value cultural data as a key adjunct in achieving the family's health care goals (Leininger, 1970).

To investigate these influences, begin by asking the client to describe her cultural and ethnic heritage. Her birthplace and living locations (countries or cities) may have influenced her beliefs. Assess the degree to which the client and family members embrace habits, values, beliefs, and behaviors that can be traced to their ethnic and cultural background. Identify barriers to communication (a modest knowledge of English, for example).

Question the client about any culturally imposed restrictions or expectations related to health care. Inquire about cultural healing practices and how they explain illness; ask whether the client consults healers. Investigate the client's food preferences and restrictions and the implications these have for teaching about nutrition.

Religious affiliation. In most cultures, religious beliefs play an important role in such significant life events as marriage, childbirth, and death. In fact, these beliefs may become so thoroughly ingrained in the culture that religion and culture become synonymous.

In many families, religious beliefs exert a major influence on the timing and circumstances of a woman's pregnancy. Most religions hold firm positions on such issues as contraception, abortion, and fertility services. Religions that forbid these family planning techniques typically assert that they tamper with God's natural order for conception and birth. During the health history interview, the nurse should attempt to determine the influence of a client's or family's religious beliefs on her pregnancy, labor and delivery, and postpartal care.

Socioeconomic status. Based on income, education, and occupation, a family's socioeconomic status affects many aspects of family life. Income influences the family's ability to provide basic needs, such as housing, food, clothing, health care, and education. A family with little income has limited options for meeting even basic needs. Health care may be sought only for emergencies.

Most low-income families lack private health insurance and must rely on public assistance. However, many are not eligible for assistance because their income, although low, exceeds the limit for eligibility. In the United States, recent federal budget cuts have eliminated public assistance programs for many families (Huey, 1988). Although various national health insurance programs continue to be proposed, an effective program has yet to be implemented (Harrington, 1988).

Socioeconomic status has special implications for a childbearing family, commonly influencing how the family uses health care services to maintain wellness and encourage a complication-free pregnancy and delivery.

NURSING RESEARCH APPLIED

Early discharge and home care of very-low-birth-weight infants

A study of 79 very-low-birth-weight infants was carried out to examine the safety, efficacy, and cost savings of early hospital discharge. Infants were randomly assigned to one of two groups: a control group discharged according to normal hospital routine and an experimental group discharged earlier but provided with instruction, counseling, home visits, and daily on-call availability of a hospital-based nurse specialist for 18 months after discharge.

The study revealed that the infants in the early discharge group (discharged an average of 11 days earlier) weighed 200 grams less and were 2 weeks younger at discharge than the control-group infants. Hospital expenses for the experimental group averaged 27 percent less than those for the control group. (The savings per infant was $18,560.) The two groups did not differ in the numbers of rehospitalizations, acute care visits, and physical or mental growth.

The study concluded that early discharge of very-low-birth-weight infants with follow-up care in the home by a nurse specialist is safe and cost-effective.

Application to practice
This study demonstrates that using the nursing process can improve the outcome for high-risk populations discharged early after hospitalization. The nurse specialist in this study began assessing the family and infant at delivery and began formulating goals, nursing diagnoses, and intervention strategies throughout the infant's hospitalization and for 18 months thereafter. The nurse was able to intervene appropriately and sometimes proactively to prevent serious problems. The nurse who begins working with the family at delivery and continues through discharge planning and beyond is the ideal health care provider for this population.

Brooten, D., Kumar, S., Brown, L., Butts, P., Finkler, S., Bakewell-Sachs, S., Gibbons, A., and Delivoria-Papadopoulos, M. (1986). A randomized clinical trial of early hospital discharge and home followup of very-low-birth-weight infants. *New England Journal of Medicine*, 315, 934-939.

One of the reasons low-income families may forgo prenatal care is lack of accessible, affordable services. A woman who receives no prenatal care is three times more likely to deliver a low-birth-weight infant than one who receives prenatal care. Partly because of deficient prenatal care, U.S. infant mortality has increased since 1982 in low-income sections of 20 states (Mundinger, 1986). (For related information on subsequent care of these high-risk infants, see *Nursing research applied: Early discharge and home care of very-low-birth-weight infants.*)

Low income also can affect a pregnant woman's nutritional status. Many low-income families cannot afford the varied diet needed by the mother to allow normal fetal growth and development. Maternal malnutrition and fetal abnormalities may result.

By remaining aware of and sensitive to these special problems, the nurse can be a positive influence for a family of low socioeconomic status. The nurse should care for and treat the family in a respectful manner.

During the health history interview, determine the family's principal wage-earner and the family's annual income. Assess the education levels of all family members to determine an appropriate vocabulary and level of teaching. Question the client about her network of social support and whether these individuals influence her health care practices. Ascertain how the family will be involved in the client's pregnancy and health care and whether community organizations will play any role in the client's health care.

Psychological influences. Assess the client's self-concept and perception of health care. Be alert for evidence that the client perceives discrimination in the health care system; this perception may increase client anxiety, prompt noncompliance with treatment, and cause future avoidance of the health care system. Attempt to determine how the pregnant client's cultural patterns affect her body image, coping ability, and self-esteem.

Coping. Assess the types of coping mechanisms used by the family, and, if necessary, help family members develop more positive coping strategies.

Coping refers to cognitive and behavioral efforts to manage problems and crises. The process has two components: noncognitive and cognitive. The noncognitive component comprises a person's emotional response to a problem. Trying to avoid thinking about a problem, blaming someone else for the problem, or reinterpreting the problem are examples of noncognitive responses. This type of coping typically occurs when a problem or threat cannot be resolved easily or immediately.

The cognitive component focuses on solving the problem through thinking, learning, and using decision-making skills (Lazarus and Folkman, 1984). Analyzing the problem, thinking about possible solutions, learning new skills, altering aspirations, and seeking professional help are examples of cognitive responses. This type of coping occurs when a solution seems feasible. (For more information on coping, see Chapter 2, Family Structure and Function.)

Poor coping skills may lead to abuse in some families. Note any signs of abuse to the pregnant client or to her children. (For a description, see *Family care: Child abuse assessment.*) In affected families, abuse typically increases during pregnancy with increased stress on the client, her partner, and other family members, who may feel neglected as they struggle with the demands of pregnancy.

FAMILY CARE

Child abuse assessment

Abuse in any form—physical, psychological, sexual—threatens the welfare of family members and the function of the family as a whole. When assessing family health, the nurse should be aware of abuse risk factors and the sometimes subtle signs and symptoms of abuse.

Family risk factors

- Minimal or nonexistent family social support
- Occurrence of multiple stress-producing life events
- History of poor parenting
- Parent who was sexually abused as a child
- Failure of parents to prepare for their infant by the last trimester
- Lack of eye contact with their infant

Signs and symptoms of abuse in younger children

- Nightmares
- Bed-wetting
- Excessive masturbation
- Regressive behavior
- Knowledge of explicit sexual language
- Withdrawal
- Frequent genital infections
- Irritability
- Loss of appetite

Signs and symptoms of abuse in older children

- Depression
- Poor self-image
- Withdrawal
- Substance abuse
- Staying away or running away from home
- Frequent complaints of infection, abdominal pain, dizziness, headache
- Self-mutilating behavior, such as burning or tattooing
- Attempted suicide
- Eating disorders, such as bulimia or anorexia nervosa
- Seductive or promiscuous behavior
- Attention-seeking or delinquent behavior

If an abused woman chooses to remain with her partner, her infant has a 30% chance of being abused as well (Kaufman and Zigler, 1987). If the woman chooses to leave her partner, she may have a different type of emotional hardship and may require financial help from social service agencies. (For more information on abuse, see Chapter 14, Violence Against Women.)

Physical assessment

After gathering the appropriate subjective information and establishing a rapport with the client during the health history, the nurse performs a physical assessment to collect objective data, which may substantiate or refute the nurse's or client's health concerns.

A physical assessment has three major components:
• general survey, including initial observations of the client's appearance and behavior
• vital signs, including temperature, blood pressure, pulse, and respirations; and anthropometric measurements, including height and weight
• physical examination, including assessment of body systems, organs, and structures. (For more information on physical examination, see Chapter 7, Women's Health Promotion, and Chapter 19, Care during the Normal Antepartal Period.)

Although the extent of physical assessment varies depending on the client's individual needs, the health care setting, the nurse's level of training, and other factors, the nurse must examine every client to obtain basic physiologic data. During any physical assessment, the nurse should pay particular attention to areas associated with current physical complaints and past problems that the client may have identified during the health history interview. Complete physical assessment involves evaluating all physiologic systems in an organized manner, typically from head to toe or from least invasive (general observation) to most invasive (such as pelvic examination) procedures. For many clients, diagnostic studies provide additional important assessment information.

Nursing diagnosis

After completing the assessment step, the nurse analyzes the subjective and objective data obtained. Such analysis allows the nurse to formulate nursing diagnoses, the next step in the nursing process.

A nursing diagnosis is a statement of an actual or potential health problem that nurses are capable of treating and licensed to treat (Gordon, 1987). Of course, appropriate treatments may involve collaboration with other health care professionals. Determining one or more applicable nursing diagnoses for a client provides the basis for formulating an individualized, effective nursing care plan. Each diagnosis must be supported by clinical information obtained during assessment.

Nursing diagnoses provide a common language to convey the nursing management necessary for each client among the many nurses involved in that client's care. To help ensure standardized nursing diagnosis terminology and usage, the North American Nursing Diagnosis Association (NANDA) has formulated and classified a series of nursing diagnosis categories based on nine human response patterns (NANDA, 1990). These patterns include:
• Exchanging (mutual giving and receiving)
• Communicating (sending messages)
• Relating (establishing bonds)
• Valuing (assigning worth)
• Choosing (selection of alterations)
• Moving (activity)
• Perceiving (reception of information)
• Knowing (meaning associated with information)
• Feeling (subjective awareness of information).

Within each pattern are NANDA-approved nursing diagnosis categories specific to that topic. For example, the human response pattern devoted to *relating* includes such diagnostic categories as "sexual dysfunction" and "parental role conflict." The complete list of NANDA diagnostic categories, arranged by human response pattern, is called the nursing diagnosis taxonomy. (For the complete list, see Appendix 2: NANDA Taxonomy of Nursing Diagnoses.)

Examples of the many nursing diagnosis categories that may apply to the childbearing family include:
• *knowledge deficit*, for a client who lacks adequate knowledge about self-care, physiologic changes that occur during pregnancy and labor, neonatal care, or various other areas
• *ineffective thermoregulation*, for a neonate who cannot adequately maintain body temperature after birth
• *ineffective breast-feeding*, for the client who has difficulty initiating or maintaining breast-feeding. (See *Nursing diagnoses: Family assessment*, page 48, and *Selected nursing diagnoses for the childbearing family*, pages 46 and 47, for additional nursing diagnoses. In addition, see appropriate chapters throughout the text for nursing diagnoses applicable to specific childbearing problems.)

Assigning specific nursing diagnoses involves several steps, including clustering assessment data, choosing the appropriate category, and adding specific client information.

Clustering assessment data. Designed to identify broad areas of client need, clustering begins with the nurse's review of assessment data for completeness and accuracy. Whenever possible, the nurse collects assessment data from all involved family members before making a

(Text continues on page 48.)

Selected nursing diagnoses for the childbearing family

Listed below under broad topics are examples of nursing diagnoses adapted to clients in maternal, neonatal, and women's health settings. These and other diagnoses appear together with related interventions in the "Planning and implementation" section of selected chapters throughout this text. For ease of recognition, nursing diagnoses appear in boldface italic type in individual chapters.

Sexuality concerns

Altered role performance related to fear of pregnancy

Altered sexuality patterns related to pregnancy

Anxiety related to sexual intercourse during pregnancy

Anxiety related to sexual misinformation

Body image disturbance related to mastectomy

Body image disturbance related to pregnancy

Knowledge deficit related to sexuality

Pain related to sexual position, secondary to pregnancy

Sexual dysfunction related to excessive alcohol ingestion

Sexual dysfunction related to inhibited female orgasm

Preconception planning

Altered family processes related to decision to conceive

Altered nutrition: less than body requirements, related to impending pregnancy

Altered role performance related to impending pregnancy

Anxiety related to the decision to conceive

Body image disturbance related to impending pregnancy

Health-seeking behaviors related to contraception

Knowledge deficit related to contraception and conception

Knowledge deficit related to self-care activities before conception

Personal identity disturbance related to the decision to conceive

Infertility

Altered family processes related to the stress of infertility

Anticipatory grieving related to infertility

Anxiety related to infertility tests

Body image disturbance related to infertility

Impaired adjustment related to childlessness

Ineffective family coping: compromised, related to infertility

Knowledge deficit related to factors that promote fertility

Pain related to endometrial biopsy

Powerlessness related to inability to control fertility

Social isolation related to lack of children

Genetic disorders

Altered parenting related to having a child with a genetic defect

Anxiety related to unknown future health of offspring

Health-seeking behaviors related to genetic testing

Ineffective family coping: compromised, related to fear of abnormality in offspring

Self-esteem disturbance related to awareness of having produced a child with a genetic defect

Social isolation related to perceived lack of support during decisions regarding pregnancy termination

Spiritual distress related to possibility of altering reproductive outcome

Violence against women

Altered sexuality patterns related to rape

Fear related to continuation of abuse

Impaired social interaction related to rape

Ineffective individual coping related to abuse

Post-trauma response related to abuse

Post-trauma response related to rape

Powerlessness related to abuse

Rape-trauma syndrome related to aftermath of rape

Self-esteem disturbance related to history of abuse

Spiritual distress related to rape

Women's health-compromising behaviors

Altered family processes related to drug abuse

Anxiety related to possible weight gain

Health-seeking behavior related to smoking cessation

Hopelessness related to morbid obesity

Ineffective family coping: compromised, related to alcoholism

Potential altered parenting related to alcohol's influence

Powerlessness related to binge-purge behavior

Powerlessness related to inability to control desire for drug

Social isolation related to decreased physical attractiveness

Social isolation related to longevity beyond that of friends and family

First stage of labor

Altered tissue perfusion: decreased placental, related to maternal position

Impaired gas exchange related to hyperventilation with increasing contractions

Impaired physical mobility related to electronic fetal monitoring equipment

Ineffective individual coping related to lack of family support

Knowledge deficit related to the labor process

Self-care deficit related to limited mobility during labor

Normal neonate

Altered parenting related to the addition of a new family member

Altered patterns of urinary elimination related to renal immaturity

Hypothermia related to cold stress

Ineffective breathing pattern related to transition to the extrauterine environment

Potential fluid volume deficit related to insensible fluid losses

Potential for infection related to umbilical cord healing

Potential for injury related to inability to process vitamin K

Infant nutrition

Altered family processes related to infant feeding

Altered sexuality patterns related to requirements of the breast-feeding infant

Anxiety related to the ability to properly feed the infant

Body image disturbance related to physiologic changes secondary to breast-feeding

Ineffective breast-feeding related to improper positioning at the breast

Potential for injury related to improper nipple care

Sleep pattern disturbance related to the infant's nutritional needs

Comfort promotion

Anxiety related to labor pain

Decreased cardiac output related to epidural anesthesia

Ineffective airway clearance related to general anesthesia

Knowledge deficit related to analgesia and anesthesia options

Pain related to frequency and intensity of uterine contractions

Self-esteem disturbance related to inability to cope with labor pain or negative perception of behavior

Urinary retention related to spinal anesthesia

diagnosis. Next, the nurse analyzes assessment data from different perspectives using standards of care, established physiologic norms, and information from other disciplines (psychology or social work to assess family relationships, for example, and sociology to assess cultural influences). Finally, the nurse determines how various data groups relate to one another, clustering them in appropriate groups. This step requires broad-based health care knowledge; the nurse should consult current literature or other health care professionals for help with unfamiliar subject areas.

Choosing nursing diagnosis categories. Using clustered assessment data to identify broad areas of client needs, the nurse chooses one or more appropriate nursing diagnosis categories from the NANDA taxonomy. Each category may address an actual or potential client problem.

Assigning specific nursing diagnoses. After choosing a nursing diagnosis category, the nurse appends specific client information to individualize the diagnosis. A complete nursing diagnosis has three segments: a problem, an etiology, and signs and symptoms (Gordon, 1987). The first segment is the nursing diagnosis category; for example, "ineffective breast-feeding." The second segment states the problem's etiology (causal or contributing factor or factors), introduced by the phrase "related

to" or "secondary to." A diagnosis of ineffective breast-feeding could be related to insufficient milk production, for example. The third segment identifies any signs or symptoms that help clarify and individualize the nursing diagnosis. Thus, "ineffective breast-feeding related to insufficient milk production secondary to intermittent bottle feedings" is an example of a complete nursing diagnosis.

In some cases, the nurse may need to formulate nursing diagnoses not yet included in the NANDA taxonomy. If this occurs, the nurse should attempt to maintain the three-part nursing diagnosis format.

Planning

After completing client assessment and formulating appropriate nursing diagnoses, the nurse develops a care plan appropriate for the client and family. Effective planning focuses on the client's specific needs, considers her strengths and weaknesses, incorporates her participation, sets achievable goals, includes feasible interventions, and is within the scope of the nursing practice setting.

Planning involves three basic steps: setting and prioritizing goals, formulating nursing interventions, and developing a care plan.

Setting and prioritizing goals

After establishing nursing diagnoses, the nurse sets one or more goals for each applicable diagnosis. A goal—the desired client outcome after nursing care—states what the nurse and client expect to achieve to minimize or eliminate a problem. Appropriate goals help guide the selection of nursing interventions and also serve as criteria for evaluating the effectiveness of the interventions. Goals should relate directly to the nursing diagnoses and reflect the desires of the client, family, and nurse, who work together to formulate them. Setting goals with the client helps ensure appropriate and realistic care planning, encourages her involvement, gives her a sense of control, and may improve compliance with the care plan.

An effective goal statement, or outcome criterion, is measurable, realistic, and stated so that the client and family understand it completely. It should include the desired client behavior and predicted outcome, measurement criteria, a specified time for attainment or reevaluation, and other conditions, if any, under which

---

NURSING DIAGNOSES

Family assessment

For family care planning, the nurse may find these nursing diagnosis categories helpful.

- Altered family processes
- Altered health maintenance
- Altered parenting
- Altered role performance
- Anticipatory grieving
- Anxiety
- Dysfunctional grieving
- Family coping: potential for growth
- Fear
- Hopelessness
- Impaired home maintenance management
- Impaired social interaction
- Ineffective family coping: compromised
- Ineffective family coping: disabling
- Ineffective individual coping
- Potential altered parenting
- Sexual dysfunction
- Spiritual distress

the behavior will occur. Examples of complete goal statements include: "The mother will demonstrate proper umbilical cord care by the first day after delivery," and "The father will demonstrate proper diaper changes before the neonate is discharged."

As appropriate, the nurse emphasizes that many health problems are interrelated and can be approached simultaneously; one problem need not be resolved before another is addressed. For example, a client may require meticulous perineal care to encourage healing of her episiotomy and, at the same time, require special assistance in learning to breast-feed her infant.

After goals are formulated, they must be prioritized. As in goal setting, the nurse should establish priorities together with the client and family. This involves ranking the nursing diagnoses and goals in order of importance, based on an accepted order, such as psychologist Abraham Maslow's hierarchy of human needs (the most frequently used order). Briefly, Maslow (1970) states that survival needs, such as food and water, must be met before less-life-threatening considerations, such as the need to be loved and the desire for self-actualization.

Goals may be short term or long term. Short-term goals may take priority over long-term ones. When prioritizing goals, the nurse and client should account for possible effects of the client's ethnic and cultural background, socioeconomic status, and other factors that can influence goal achievement.

Formulating interventions

After selecting and prioritizing goals, the nurse begins the next planning stage: formulating interventions to facilitate achievement of short- and long-term goals. Nursing interventions consist of strategies, actions, or activities intended to help the client reach established goals by diminishing or resolving problems identified in the nursing diagnoses.

The nurse and client should work together to formulate interventions, analyzing possible strategies and choosing those that seem most likely to achieve goals based on the client's particular circumstances. Interventions may be interdisciplinary, possibly including nursing and medical care, physical therapy, nutritional counseling, social services, and others.

Effective nursing interventions must be based on sound nursing practice, which stems from sound research. Such a knowledge base provides the proper rationales for nursing interventions. The body of knowledge addressing nursing interventions and their effectiveness is increasing; important nursing research studies and other current information can be found in nursing journals, textbooks, and other publications. If possible, the nurse also may consult maternal and neonatal health experts to obtain the latest information on aspects of practice.

Developing a nursing care plan

The nurse develops a nursing care plan by integrating each step of the nursing process: collecting and analyzing health history and physical assessment data, selecting nursing diagnoses, setting and prioritizing goals, formulating interventions, and evaluating outcomes. The care plan, which can be revised and updated as needed, acts as a written guide for and documentation of a client's care. Also, it helps ensure continuity of care when the client interacts with many nurses, and it facilitates collaboration by all involved health care providers.

The format of nursing care plans varies among health care facilities and sometimes among units in the same facility. All care plans, however, include written nursing diagnoses, goals, interventions, and evaluation criteria. Standardized care plans recently have evolved as a time-saving and efficient method of ensuring documentation of the nursing process approach to care. A standardized care plan incorporates the major aspects of nursing care required by clients with a similar problem, while allowing alterations to reflect individual differences. Such a care plan may be particularly valuable for a client undergoing a short hospitalization with only minor deviations from previous health status, such as a client who experienced uncomplicated labor and delivery. (For an example of a complete nursing care plan, see *Applying the nursing process: Client and partner knowledge deficit related to infant care,* pages 50 and 51. In addition, see nursing care chapters throughout the text for other examples of nursing care plans related to pregnancy and childbearing.)

Implementation

The next step in the nursing process, implementation involves working with the client and family to accomplish the designated interventions and move toward the desired outcomes. Effective implementation requires a sound understanding of the care plan and collaboration among the client, family, and other members of the health care team, as needed. The implementation phase begins as soon as the care plan is completed and ends when

Client and partner knowledge deficit related to infant care

After the birth of an infant, the nurse uses the nursing process to organize and guide discharge teaching. The table below shows how the nurse might use the nursing process when caring for the client described in the case history at right. The first column presents history and physical assessment data followed by a paragraph of mental notes. These notes help the nurse make important mental connections among assess-ment findings, aiding in development of the nursing diagnosis and planning.

The second column lists an appropriate nursing diagnosis; information in the remaining columns is based on this diagno-sis. Although not part of the nursing process, a rationale ap-pears for each intervention in the fourth column to explain how it contributes to the care plan.

ASSESSMENT	NURSING DIAGNOSIS	PLANNING
Subjective (history) data • Client and partner state that they need infant care instruction. • Client and partner state that they have special requests for ac-tivities surrounding circumcision. • Client and partner report that they are motivated to learn the specifics of infant care. **Objective (physical) data** • Client and partner maintain eye contact and speak softly and frequently to infant. • Client and partner ask many questions and express concerns regarding infant care. • Infant is to be circumcised the next day. • Client and partner use caution when lifting infant and hands shake slightly when caring for him. **Mental notes** *Client and partner express concerns about infant care at home. They would like to be present during circumcision. They are ea-ger to learn and "want to do what's best" for the infant. Both sets of grandparents live nearby and are available for assis-tance.*	Knowledge deficit related to infant care	**Goals** • The client and her part-ner will: • state the rationale be-hind infant care tech-niques by discharge • state they are comfort-able providing infant care before discharge • participate in their son's circumcision.

the established goals are achieved. Before and during implementation of any interventions, the nurse reas-sesses the client as needed to ensure that planned in-terventions continue to be appropriate. Periodic reassessment helps ensure a flexible, individualized, and effective care plan.

To implement nursing interventions effectively, the nurse needs four types of skills:
• cognitive skills, based on knowledge of current clinical practice and basic sciences
• affective skills, including verbal and nonverbal com-munication and empathy
• psychomotor skills, involving both mental and physical activity and encompassing traditional nursing actions

(for example, taking vital signs and administering med-ications) and more complex procedures (for example, fetal monitoring)
• organizational skills, such as counseling, managing, and delegating.

For interventions that involve client teaching, the nurse should use the methods by which most adults prefer to learn. The following principles offer guidelines for teaching adult clients:
• Many adults prefer certain learning formats over oth-ers; whenever possible, allow a client to choose from such varied formats as audiovisual presentations, small group discussions, and private sessions with the nurse.

CASE STUDY

Susan Schwartz, age 30, has delivered a healthy male. She and her partner, both from a Jewish background, have had no experience with infants and are eager to learn how to care for their son.

IMPLEMENTATION		EVALUATION
Intervention Demonstrate and provide such resources as written material, videotapes, and parental classes on infant bathing, circumcision, cord care, diapering, and feeding.	**Rationale** A demonstration allows for visual as well as verbal instruction. This provides an opportunity for the client and partner to obtain answers to their questions. Visual aids—such as videotapes—or parenting classes accommodate different learning styles and also allow interaction with other new parents.	Upon evaluation, the client and her partner: • demonstrated infant care with increased confidence and ease • provided loving and attentive infant care • expressed feeling more relaxed and confident when handling infant • attended the circumcision and kept the infant in client's room with proper instructions. Both expressed appreciation for the accommodation.
Request return demonstrations on consecutive days.	Return demonstrations allow for the client and partner to show mastery of new information and provide an opportunity to ask questions.	
Demonstrate and review importance of nurturing techniques and bonding.	This will promote normal parental interaction with infant and reduce anxiety. Effective bonding is directly related to infant development.	
Provide encouragement and positive reinforcement to client and partner. Involve grandparents or other family members at couple's request.	Positive feedback will promote relaxation and confidence in caring for infant. Involving grandparents or other family members may provide emotional support. Infant may benefit from a more relaxed environment.	
Explore requests for parents to be present at circumcision and to keep child in client's room immediately after procedure. (Compliance may be determined by health care facility policy.)	This experience supports the couple's cultural beliefs.	

• Participating in small group discussions allows adults to share their learning experiences.
• When motivated, adults usually will adopt the nurse's planned learning outcomes as their own.
• Adults want practical answers to their problems and typically enjoy practical problem solving.
• Adult learning is enhanced by opportunities to practice new skills and concepts, and by receiving performance feedback.
• Adults learn best and feel most free to express themselves in an atmosphere of trust and respect.

When the nurse uses these principles of adult learning, clients will perceive the educational value of the instruction and its application to their personal situations.

Evaluation

Through evaluation, the nurse obtains additional subjective and objective assessment data that relate to the goals identified in the nursing diagnoses. The nurse then uses these data to determine whether goals have been met, partially met, or unmet. Although evaluation comprises the final step in the nursing process, it actually occurs throughout, particularly during implementation, where the nurse continually reassesses the effect of interventions. Evaluation is directly linked to and must be based on the goals developed for each nursing diagnosis.

When all goals for a particular nursing diagnosis have been met, the nurse and client may decide that the diagnosis is no longer valid. The nurse then documents which goals were met and how and may delete the diagnosis from the nursing care plan. Alternatively, the nurse and client may judge a goal met but still feel that the nursing diagnosis is valid and decide to retain it in the care plan.

If goals have been unmet or only partially met by the target date for goal achievement, the nurse must reevaluate the care plan. Reevaluation involves deciding whether the initial plan was appropriate, whether the time assigned to the plan was realistic, whether the initial goals were realistic and measurable, and whether other factors interfered. Based on this information, the nurse can clarify or amend the assessment data base, reexamine and correct the nursing diagnoses as necessary, establish new goals reflecting the revised diagnoses, and devise new interventions for achieving these goals. The nurse then adds the revised care plan to the original document and records the rationale for these revisions in the nursing notes.

Documentation

Although not usually identified as a nursing process step, documentation of nursing care nevertheless is essential to effective care. Documentation serves several functions: It provides communication among members of the health care team, it functions as a discharge planning and quality assurance tool, and it establishes a legal record of care provided.

The nurse may document various care measures—including verbal communication, care plans, team meetings, and staff reports—in the client record. Commonly the primary data source for institutional quality assurance reviews, the client record also may be useful to nursing researchers investigating such issues as the effectiveness of certain interventions. Discharge planning relies on complete and accurate documentation to provide direction for follow-up home care. Third-party payers may examine the patient record to decide whether services provided were warranted and require reimbursement.

The client record also serves as legal documentation of the care provided by the health care team. The nurse is bound by law to document accurately and completely all nursing care provided as well as the client's response to that care. Patient records commonly are reviewed in litigation regarding alleged malpractice; in the eyes of the court, if a care measure is not documented on the patient record, it was not provided. (For more information, see Chapter 5, Ethical and Legal Concerns in Family Care.)

Documentation requirements vary among institutions; however, regardless of the format used, data must be documented according to these guidelines:
• Use the appropriate form and write only in ink.
• Write the client's name and identification number on each page.
• Record the date and time of each entry.
• Use only standard accepted abbreviations.
• Document symptoms in the client's own words.
• Be specific; avoid generalizations and vague expressions.
• Write on every line; leave no blank spaces.
• If a certain space does not apply to the client, write NA (not applicable) in the space.
• Do not backdate or squeeze new writing into a previously documented entry.
• Never document another nurse's work.
• Do not record value judgments and opinions.
• Sign every entry with the initial of your first name, last name, and title.

The complete client record must be readily accessible to all health care team members at all times. Each institution also must develop mechanisms for ensuring confidentiality of records (American Nurses' Association, 1976).

Regulations regarding the minimal frequency of documentation relative to client status may differ among states and institutions. In all cases, the nurse must use sound professional judgment and document all care provided to help ensure appropriate communication of information and provision of quality care.

Summary

Chapter 3 described the nursing process as it relates to the childbearing family. Here are the key concepts.
• The nursing process includes five steps: assessment, nursing diagnosis, planning, intervention, and evaluation. Documentation, although not technically a step, is

a crucial element. The nursing process is dynamic and ongoing, with steps typically occurring simultaneously.
• The first step, assessment, is the foundation for the other four steps. It involves collecting subjective and objective data about a client's health status.
• When assessing the health of a childbearing family, the nurse looks for cultural, religious, and socioeconomic factors that influence the client's perception of health and health care, life-style, and childbearing practices.
• The nurse organizes and analyzes assessment data to formulate nursing diagnoses—statements of actual or potential client health problems. Nursing diagnoses form the framework for the nursing care plan, which directs client care.
• Once nursing diagnoses have been developed, the nurse and family plan goals and interventions to achieve the desired outcomes.
• Planning and implementing interventions require the cooperation of the client, family, nurse, and other health care team members.
• The nurse teaches members of the childbearing family about family growth, development, and positive adaptations.
• Although evaluation is commonly viewed as the final step in the nursing process, it continues throughout client care. Evaluation reviews the client's status in relation to the established goals.
• Documentation of the nursing process must be accurate, thorough, concise, current, and in keeping with institutional policy.

Study questions

1. Explain the steps of the nursing process. How are they interrelated?

2. What are the two primary methods of data collection in nursing practice?

3. What are the implications of such influences as cultural, ethnic, and religious background; socioeconomic status; and psychological factors on the childbearing family?

4. Nursing diagnoses should include which three elements?

Bibliography

American Nurses' Association. (1976). *Code for nurses with interpretive statements.* Kansas City, MO: American Nurses' Association.

American Nurses' Association. (1980). *Nursing: A social policy statement.* Kansas City, MO: American Nurses' Association.

Doenges, M., Kenty, J., and Moorhouse, M. (1988). *Maternal/newborn care plans: Guidelines for client care.* Philadelphia: F.A. Davis.

Engel, G. (1977). The need for a new medical model: A challenge for biomedicine. *Science,* 196(4286), 129-136.

Gelles, R., and Straus, M. (1988). *Intimate violence.* New York: Simon & Shuster.

Harrington, C. (1988). A national health care program: Has its time come? *Nursing Outlook,* 36(5), 214-216.

Harris, L. (1989). Examine these myths of the '80s. *The New York Times,* May 19, 1989, p.35.

Huey, F. (1988). How nurses would change U.S. health care. *AJN,* 88(11), 1482-1493.

Kerr, M., and Bowen, M. (1988). *Family evaluation: An approach based on Bowen theory.* New York: Norton.

Leininger, M. (1970). *Nursing and anthropology: Two worlds to blend.* Ann Arbor, MI: Books On Demand, UMI.

Maslow, A. (1970). *Motivation and personality* (2nd ed.). New York: Harper & Row.

Mundinger, M. (1986). Health service funding cuts and the declining health of the poor. *New England Journal of Medicine,* 313(1), 44-47.

North American Nursing Diagnosis Association. (1990). *Taxonomy I—Revised, with official diagnostic categories.* St. Louis: NANDA.

U.S. Bureau of the Census. (1988). *Statistical abstract of the United States: 1989* (109th ed.). Washington, DC: U.S. Government Printing Office.

Nursing process

Alfaro, R. (1990). *Applying nursing diagnosis and nursing process: A step-by-step guide* (2nd ed.). Philadelphia: Lippincott.

Blair, C.L., Meyers, R., and Salerno, E. (1984). *Nursing assessment: Interview principles, procedures and tools.* New York: March of Dimes Birth Defects Foundation.

Carpenito, L. (1989). *Nursing diagnosis: Application to clinical practice* (3rd ed.). Philadelphia: Lippincott.

Gordon, M. (1987). *Nursing diagnosis: Process and application* (2nd ed.). New York: McGraw-Hill.

Morton, P. (1989). *Health assessment in nursing.* Springhouse, PA: Springhouse Corporation.

Popkess-Vawter, S., and Pinnell, N. (1987). Should we diagnose strengths? Yes—Accentuate the positive. *AJN,* 87(9), 1211-1216.

Stevens, K. (1988). Nursing diagnosis in wellness childbearing settings. *JOGNN,* 17(5), 329-335.

Stolte, K.M. (1986). Nursing diagnosis and the childbearing woman. *MCN,* 11(1), 13-15.

Family care

Lazarus, R., and Folkman, S. (1984). *Stress, appraisal, and coping.* New York: Springer.

Friedman M. (1986). *Family nursing: Theory and assessment.* New York: Appleton-Century-Crofts.

Hoff, L. (1989). *People in crisis: Understanding and helping* (3rd ed.). Redwood City, CA: Addison-Wesley.

Kaufman, J., and Zigler, E. (1987). Do abused children become abusive parents? *American Journal of Orthopsychiatry,* 57(2), 186-192.

Moleti, C. (1988). Caring for socially high-risk pregnant women. *MCN,* 13(1), 24-27.

Sarason I., Johnson, J., and Siegel, J. (1978). Assessing the impact of life changes: Development of the life experiences survey. *Journal of Consulting and Clinical Psychology,* 46(5), 932-946.

Telleen S., Herzog, A., and Kilbane, T. (1989). Impact of a family support program on a mother's social support and parenting stress. *American Journal of Orthopsychiatry,* 59(3), 410-419.

Nursing research

Brooten, D., Kumar, S. Brown, L., Butts, P., Finkler, S., Bakewell-Sachs, S., Gibbons, A., and Delivoria-Papadopoulos, M. (1986). A randomized clinical trial of early hospital discharge and home followup of very-low-birth-weight infants. *New England Journal of Medicine,* 315, 934-939.

Glazer, H., Francis, S., and Smith, C. (1987). Families' knowledge acquisition and written health materials. *Child Health Care,* 15(3), 152-155.

McLane, A. (1987). Measurement and validation of diagnostic concepts: A decade of progress...review of nursing diagnosis research, *Heart & Lung,* 16(6), 616-624.

Mercer, R., Ferketich, S., and DeJoseph, J. (1989). Effects of stress on family functioning during pregnancy. *Nursing Research,* 37(5), 268-275.

Shearer, E., Shiono, P., and Rhoads, G. (1988). Recent trends in family-centered maternity care for cesarean birth families. *Birth,* 15(1), 3-7.

Uphold, C., and Strickland, O. (1989). Issues related to the unit of analysis in family nursing. *Western Journal of Nursing Research,* 11(4), 405-417.

Nurse-Client Interaction

Objectives

After reading and studying this chapter, the student should be able to:

1. Describe five characteristic phases of nurse-client interaction.

2. Discuss significant methods to facilitate nurse-client communication.

3. Delineate teaching strategies that the nurse can use to meet each client's learning needs.

4. Describe differences between adolescent and adult learning patterns.

5. Define therapeutic empathy and self-care.

6. Describe the types of caring that can help motivate the client.

Introduction

When caring for a pregnant client, the nurse must provide various kinds of support and health care depending on the client's stated needs, her physical health, her view of pregnancy, and the amount of time available for interaction. Each client has special health care needs and desires. The ideal time for assessing those needs and desires, determining specific goals, and providing the care required is during the interaction between the nurse and the client.

Initiated and directed by the nurse, nurse-client interaction has five characteristic phases and requires active participation by both nurse and client. Typically, the relationship exists for a time agreed upon by both members at the outset. For a pregnant client, for example, nurse-client interaction might end with the client's discharge after a successful delivery. Within the various

phases of nurse-client interaction, the nurse may use as many skills and techniques as necessary to meet goals established with the client.

This chapter begins by describing the five phases of nurse-client interaction. It then examines important skills needed for successful interaction, including communicating, teaching, and motivating.

Phases of nurse-client interaction

For success, nurse-client interaction requires mutual participation and commitment. Although the length and content of each interaction varies with individual circumstances, all nurse-client interactions are based on specific goals; when goals are met, the interaction is complete.

When time and circumstances permit, nurse-client interaction typically includes five interrelated phases: preparation, initiation, consolidation and growth, development (working), and termination (Sundeen, Stuart, Rankin, and Cohen, 1989). The nurse and client perform certain roles during each phase, as described below.

Preparation

Ideally, the nurse begins the interaction in advance of the client's arrival by performing some or all of the following:

GLOSSARY

Accommodator: person who learns best from personal experience and hands-on demonstration.

Active listening: close evaluation of body language and voice inflection to supplement verbal communication.

Assimilator: person who learns best by assembling small bits of information gathered from various sources.

Body language: nonverbal signals, such as facial expression, gestures, and body position.

Contract learning: process in which the nurse and client agree on goals and anticipated outcomes before teaching begins.

Converger: person who learns best from applying abstract concepts to life experience.

Diverger: person who learns best by creating new ideas after sharing experiences with others.

Facilitator: person whose skill, aptitude, or experience eases the performance of a task.

Learning style: mode of learning preferred by the client; for example, memorization, observation, interaction, and experimentation.

Motivation: incentive or reason to act.

Noncompliance: failure to act in accordance with wishes, requests, demands, or requirements.

Operant conditioning: repeated rewards that encourage specific behaviors.

Programmed learning: teaching strategy where the nurse asks nonthreatening follow-up questions after each teaching session; may include computer-aided learning.

Self-care: active and assertive participation in attaining one's health care goals.

Therapeutic communication: interaction that focuses on attaining client goals rather than on the mutual pleasure received from social communication.

Therapeutic empathy: ability to view experiences, emotions, and thoughts from a client's perspective and to use that knowledge to build the client's awareness and help set goals.

• Evaluating the completeness of the client's record, including history and diagnostic information

• Identifying any previous, current, or potential problems, especially health and nursing issues

• Taking note of the client's cultural background and communication skills

• Preparing the environment for the meeting.

Insufficient or incomplete information in the client's record requires the nurse to collect additional data during or after the first meeting. These data should have a direct bearing on the client's current or anticipated needs. Collection of extraneous information could unduly increase the time needed to develop the nurse-client relationship (Sundeen, Stuart, Rankin, and Cohen, 1989), deprive the nurse of time needed for other tasks, and delay formation and completion of the client's goals.

The preparation phase is an especially important time for the nurse to consider if the client may encounter difficulties or complications. For example, the client's record may contain amniocentesis results that indicate Down's syndrome in the fetus. The nurse will need extra time to prepare special counseling to help this client accept the diagnosis and formulate goals for her pregnancy.

While evaluating the client's record, the nurse must keep an open mind and avoid making value judgments or reaching conclusions before meeting the client (Arnold and Boggs, 1989). Because personal impressions gained from reading a record may not represent the client accurately, collecting additional data at or after the first meeting may help to highlight her individuality and prevent the nurse from succumbing to stereotypes (Sundeen, Stuart, Rankin, and Cohen, 1989).

If circumstances permit, the nurse should attempt to locate a private, comfortable setting for the first meeting. It should contain adequate seating for the nurse, the client, and any family members who accompany the client. (For more on how environment may affect learning, refer to the "Teaching" section later in this chapter.)

Initiation

Nurse-client interaction can be affected greatly by first impressions. This is why the initiation phase—the first meeting between nurse and client—plays a key role in the success and outcome of the overall relationship. During the initiation phase, the nurse should orient the client, assess her needs, establish goals with her, and agree on a mutual commitment to the relationship.

After making introductions and assuring the client's comfort, the nurse begins with orientation. This includes explaining the phases of nurse-client interaction in lay terms, telling the client what will be expected of her while it exists, outlining the nurse's role, and introducing the client to any unfamiliar procedures and surroundings.

The nurse then should attempt to assess the client's needs based on her reasons for seeking nursing care, information contained in her record, and additional data, as necessary. If the preparation phase revealed gaps in the client's record, this may provide a convenient topic on which to start. Alternatively, the nurse may ask if the client has questions or concerns related to her need for health care. (For more on assessment, see Chapter 3, Nursing Process and the Childbearing Family.)

Assessing the client's needs allows the nurse to begin formulating goals. For example, the nurse may discover during this meeting that a pregnant client enjoys her job and fears losing it if she requests an extended maternity leave. This client's goals should include an investigation of her child-care options. As another example, the nurse may discover that a sexually active adolescent client displays confusion over contraceptive methods. Education is an initial goal for this client, either arranged for or provided by the nurse.

Most clients require multiple goals. For example, a pregnant client may have all of the following goals and more:
• Care for children at home while attending prenatal classes
• Transportation to prenatal classes
• Nutritional counseling
• Participation in a smoking cessation program
• Education in contraceptive methods available for use after delivery. (For a list of goals common to pregnant clients, see *Goals for the pregnant client.*)

The object of goal-setting is to help the client and nurse focus on meeting the needs that stem from the reason for seeking health care. Some goals may be more important than others. Some may require more time to complete than others. For a pregnant client, goals typically should include providing sufficient information, promoting wellness, working toward a successful pregnancy outcome, and cultivating the physiologic and psychological health of the client, neonate, and family for some period after delivery. (For more on setting and prioritizing goals, see Chapter 3, Nursing Process and the Childbearing Family.)

After making an initial assessment of the client's needs and working with her to establish goals, the nurse should schedule a time and place for subsequent meetings. Ideally, the meeting time and place should be convenient for the client. Typically, convenience adds significantly to a client's commitment and compliance (Sundeen, Stuart, Rankin, and Cohen, 1989). Some clients may be more committed to the relationship when they sign a written contract pledging participation. (For more on contracts, refer to the "Teaching" section later in this chapter.)

Goals for the pregnant client

According to Duvall (1984), the typical pregnant client requires goals that address the following issues.
• Acquiring knowledge about and planning for pregnancy, childbirth, and parenthood
• Adapting sexual patterns to pregnancy
• Adapting community activities to pregnancy
• Developing new patterns for earning and spending money
• Evaluating family roles, responsibilities, and authority
• Reorienting relationships with relatives, friends, and associates
• Expanding communication systems for present and anticipated emotional needs
• Arranging for physical care of the neonate
• Maintaining morale and an acceptable life-style during pregnancy and as a parent.

Consolidation and growth

In this phase, the nurse and client begin to implement the goals set in the initiation phase to map out a plan for the remaining goals, to initiate teaching sessions by the nurse or other health care provider, and to identify any additional goals that may be necessary. As a result, the nurse and client also clarify the intent and direction of interaction.

When a client reaches a stated goal, the nurse should offer strong support and encouragement. When a client has difficulty reaching a goal, the nurse should attempt to isolate obstacles to progress and help the client overcome them. If necessary, the nurse and client should revise unmet goals to provide the client with a greater sense of accomplishment and encouragement.

Development

During this phase, the nurse should evaluate the client's progress and help determine how well goals are being met. The nurse may accomplish this objectively by reviewing measurable data (weight loss, for example) and subjectively by soliciting verbal reports from the client. Reassessment of the client's needs and refinement of goals may be necessary.

Another goal of this phase is to strengthen the bond of trust between the nurse and client. In part, this trust is a natural outgrowth of the mutual effort to meet the client's goals successfully. The nurse should avoid reassuring the client falsely about unmet goals; this will only discourage her continued efforts and may make her doubt the nurse's sincerity—both stumbling blocks to continued development.

How an emergency changes nurse-client interaction

Because of today's rapid client movement and discharge, typical nurse-client interaction must be compressed and sometimes carried out without the client's active participation, such as during an emergency. However, despite these changes, nurse-client interaction still exists and should contain all the usual phases, even if in abbreviated form. For example, if a pregnant diabetic client arrives unconscious via rescue squad, nurse-client interaction might include the following steps, all of which are performed without the client's participation.

PREPARATION

May consist of a brief review of the client's record or a conversation with emergency personnel.

The nurse speaks to the ambulance crew and checks the client's record for pertinent information.

INITIATION

May include setting goals to manage life-threatening problems.

Goals for the unconscious client include I.V. blood glucose monitoring and insulin administration.

CONSOLIDATION AND GROWTH

May not evolve because of time constraints caused by an emergency. Nurse-client interaction may consolidate quickly; for example, the client must trust the nurse to help her breathe.

After initiation of insulin administration, the nurse should assess for additional goals, such as care for any injuries if the client fell.

DEVELOPMENT

May require evaluation of more objective signs than verbal reports from the client.

The nurse must gather data to determine the client's response to insulin administration.

TERMINATION

May create fewer feelings of abandonment and grief, especially if the client could not interact personally with the nurse.

The client may leave the emergency department before awakening, ending a nurse-client interaction that involved only nursing actions.

Termination

In this phase, nurse-client interaction ends. Depending on the client's initial reason for seeking nursing care and on the length and intensity of the relationship, separation may be emotionally distressing for both participants. To help ease the potential stress of this phase, the nurse should prepare the client during initiation and remind her periodically that termination is a planned phase.

As termination nears, the client may express feelings of abandonment and grief, and the nurse also may feel distressed. These feelings are normal and can be discussed, if the participants wish. (For a description of how circumstances may alter interaction, see *How an emergency changes nurse-client interaction.*)

Skills needed for nurse-client interaction

Although the phases of nurse-client interaction and the tasks included in each phase can be readily understood, the nurse may need some time to develop the skills necessary for success. The three most important skill areas are communicating, teaching, and motivating.

Communicating

The nurse must learn to discern the client's concerns and assess her needs. Many methods exist to make this exchange of information easier and more effective, including the following.

Establish a trusting relationship. Strive to make the client feel respected and accepted at her present level. This feeling helps to dispel her fears and free her to talk openly about her concerns (Arnold and Boggs, 1989).

Minimize distractions. Attempt to set a consistent time and place for each meeting, either verbally or in a written agreement. Eliminate distracting noise and exclude everyone but the client and chosen family members. Regulate the room temperature if possible, and arrange the seats in a manner conducive to communication.

Respect the client's rights. This includes both personal and legal rights applicable to each situation. All clients have the rights listed in the American Hospital Association's *Patient's Bill of Rights.* In addition, pregnant clients have the rights set forth in the International Childbirth Education Association's *Pregnant Patient's Bill of Rights* (Haire, 1975). These additional rights, which ensure the pregnant client's participation in decision making, include:
• the client's right to be informed in advance of any potential hazards to or direct or indirect effects on her or her child that may result from a drug or procedure prescribed or administered during pregnancy, labor, birth, or breast-feeding
• the client's right to be informed early in pregnancy of the potential benefits, risks, and hazards of the proposed therapy and of alternative therapy that can reduce or eliminate the need for drugs and obstetric intervention
• the client's right to be informed before the administration of any drug of its generic and brand names so she can advise health care professionals of any previous adverse reactions to it
• the client's right to decide without pressure from health care professionals whether to accept the risks inherent in the proposed therapy or to refuse a drug or procedure
• the client's right to know the name and qualifications of the individual administering a drug or procedure during labor or birth
• the client's right to be informed in advance whether a proposed therapy will directly benefit her and her child (medically indicated) or is an elective procedure performed for convenience, client choice, teaching, or research.
• the client's right to be accompanied throughout labor and birth by a person to whom she looks for emotional comfort and encouragement
• the client's right to choose, after medical consultation, a position for labor and birth that is least stressful to her and her child
• the client's right to have her child cared for at bedside (if the child is stable and without problems) and to feed her child according to the child's needs rather than hospital regulations
• the client's right to be informed in writing of the name and professional qualifications of the person who delivered the child (also should appear on birth certificate)
• the client's right to have her and her child's hospital medical records (including nurses' notes) complete, accurate, and legible and to have their records retained by the hospital until the child reaches at least the age of majority or to have the records offered to her before they are destroyed

• the client's right to have access during and after her hospital stay to her complete medical records and to receive a copy upon payment of a reasonable fee and without retaining an attorney.

These rights help prevent trauma or injury to the client and her child and help protect the health care professional and the hospital against litigation.

Look professional. Although appearance is not the most important element in the nurse's ability to interact, it does affect the client's perceptions. Appropriate clothing reduces distractions and may increase honest sharing. Depending on the environment, facility guidelines, the goals of the meeting, and personal choice, choose a uniform or appropriate street clothing.

Use appropriate terminology. The nurse should use vocabulary that the client can understand, which requires knowledge of her cultural and educational background. When introducing an unfamiliar term, define it clearly in lay terms but avoid using slang unless other words cannot communicate.

Recognize bias. If personal bias exists between the nurse and client, the relationship can never be trusting and open. In this case, do everything possible to resolve the problem. If resolution proves impossible, consider asking another nurse to care for the client.

Listen actively. By observing body language, listening for voice inflections, and attending to what a client has left unsaid, the nurse acts as a "detective," discerning the implications of a client's communication as well as its literal meaning. This close scrutiny demands the nurse's undivided attention and may be physically and mentally demanding.

Avoid "why" questions. To answer "why" may require a deep understanding and analysis of a problem. The client may not possess the knowledge or insight needed to answer such questions—especially in the early stages of the relationship—and may become frustrated (Arnold and Boggs, 1989).

Respect personal space. Every person requires a certain amount of space around the body into which only those who are known intimately may go. Typically, this space extends outward from the skin to about 18". The nurse who transgresses this space before the client is ready may produce intense discomfort and adversely affect nurse-client interaction. Because personal space requirements vary among individuals, the nurse should try to determine how close to sit to each client, how each client responds to touch, and how comfortable each client is with eye contact. Signs of discomfort may indicate a need for a wider personal space.

Consider cultural factors. The client's view of family, ethnic heritage, and religious beliefs may influence nurse-client interaction. In some cultures, extended families live in the same home and may participate in a client's health care, particularly when it concerns pregnancy (Whitman, Graham, Gleit, and Boyd, 1986). Explore tactfully the client's desire for family inclusion in nurse-client interaction.

Speak the client's language. If a language barrier makes communication difficult, refer the client to a colleague fluent in the client's language. A deaf client may require a nurse fluent in sign language.

Use therapeutic communication. Each conversation with the client should center on achievement of her goals. Strive to communicate in a way that is suitable and understandable to the client, focusing only on her needs. Sharing in the nurse's personal experience during therapeutic communication may facilitate the client's growth; however, the nurse should share personal information only when necessary to help the client achieve specific goals.

Use touch, as appropriate. Selective use of the touch of a hand or the squeeze of a shoulder may comfort the client, express compassion, and encourage the client's trust. Applied at the proper time and in the appropriate manner, touch may say more than words. Just as important as the client's perception of touch is the nurse's perception of it; both should be comfortable with this aspect of the interaction.

Teaching

Client teaching should take place as needed throughout nurse-client interaction and particularly during the consolidation and growth and development phases. To teach effectively, the nurse first should determine what the client already knows, her readiness to learn, the effect of her age on learning, obstacles to learning, and her preferred learning style. Then the nurse should create a teaching program that will help her attain the goals. Throughout, the nurse should adhere to important teaching principles and evaluate the effectiveness of the teaching program. (For tips on teaching, see *Principles of client teaching*.)

Principles of client teaching

While teaching, the nurse should adhere to important principles. These include:

Know the subject matter
The nurse must understand concepts before attempting to teach them. This principle helps reduce anxiety that the nurse may feel about teaching, and it helps the nurse provide the client with accurate information.

Be flexible in the relationship
The nurse should adopt the type of relationship that most helps the client. Some learners view the teacher as an authority; others view the teacher as an equal (Redman, 1984). Viewing the nurse as an authority may increase the client's motivation and desire to gain the nurse's approval.

Encourage mutual respect
Most clients will respect the nurse's knowledge; they also want the nurse's respect for their own knowledge or experience.

Use varied presentations
To help the client retain information, the nurse should present facts in logical blocks and also convey ideas that engage the client's imagination. Additionally, the nurse should use varied media in response to the client's stated learning style and preference. These differing approaches will accommodate different learning styles.

Allow bonding
When both nurse and client commit to a set of learning objectives, a bond forms between them that grows stronger with each successful teaching occasion (Redman, 1984).

Include others, as appropriate
The nurse should consider the needs of the client's partner and family members, as appropriate, in addition to the client's needs.

Readiness to learn

Before learning can occur, the client must have the desire and the ability to learn. Desire to learn may be heightened by awareness of a need, a social and cultural setting that encourages learning, a stress level that is neither too high nor too low, and ready access to a teacher or other information source.

As nurse-client interaction continues, the nurse will gain insight into the client's desire and ability to learn. In some cases, the nurse may benefit from giving the client a self-assessment questionnaire to clarify thought patterns and areas of uncertainty. The nurse also may benefit from assessing the client's feelings of control over life events. A client with an external locus of control believes that life is directed primarily by such external influences as luck, fate, and a diety. A client with an internal locus of control believes that life is directed primarily by the individual. The latter may have a stronger desire to learn than the former.

The effect of age

Another important consideration in creating a teaching program is the client's age. Knowles (1980) reports that adolescent learners are influenced by their developmental level and their need to use the information being taught. Many adolescents:
• take what is taught at face value (literally) and attempt to use it specifically in the manner it was taught
• retain knowledge best when given slow, organized, repetitive presentations
• require reteaching and reinforcement of information already learned. (For more on this topic, see *Teaching adolescent and adult learners.*)

Mature learners, on the other hand, typically:
• prefer lecture or group discussions over one-to-one sessions
• are self-directed, opting to set their own goals and direct their own learning based on personal insight and experience. When the nurse discourages self-direction, the client may become angry and withdrawn.
• are problem-oriented, experiencing optimal learning when they have identified a problem and must resolve it before going on to other goals
• equate learning with improved performance
• have other social priorities that demand their time and attention. A pregnant mother of two may not be able to spend each afternoon studying fetal growth and development. For this reason, teaching should be brief, clear, and to the point.

Obstacles to learning

The nurse also should consider the following outside influences that may impede learning.

Socioeconomic status. Low-income families may be preoccupied with the daily necessities and thus unable to devote themselves fully to learning. High-income families may be better educated and more motivated to learn.

Emotional problems. These may limit the client's ability to listen, concentrate, and learn. For such a client, offer brief, repetitive sessions with reinforcement and rewards.

Stress. Clients learn best when they are relaxed. Attempt to teach when the client's stress level is low.

Learning ability. Some clients naturally learn more slowly than others, a fact that may have no relation to intel-

---

Teaching adolescent and adult learners

To teach effectively, the nurse should consider characteristics common to adolescents and adults before adopting a specific teaching strategy.

CHARACTERISTICS	TEACHING CONSIDERATIONS DURING PREGNANCY
Adolescent	
• Learning affected by developmental stage • Information often not used until need becomes critical • Reteaching and reinforcement needed • Life experiences and knowledge limited	• Teaching should address effect of growing fetus on client and normal fetal development. • Client may wait until problem arises (such as bleeding or lack of weight gain) rather than seeking preventive health care. • Client may rely on nurse to monitor progress and reward appropriate behavior. • Lack of contraceptive education may have contributed to pregnancy, which is typically accompanied by insecurity and fear.
Adult	
• Learning driven by need and crises • Information may be used immediately or may be modified to suit needs • Little assistance or reinforcement required • Positive and negative experience used as guide for future actions	• Client is motivated to learn by physical, emotional, and relational changes. • Client will use learning to try to prevent health problems, such as edema and morning sickness. • Client is likely to attend prenatal classes and may need clarification of complex information from nurse. • Thorough history may reveal reason for client's moods and reactions.

---

ligence. Be alert for signs of learning disabilities and educational deficits, and be prepared to alter a teaching program in response to dyslexia, illiteracy, or other learning problems.

Learning style

Some people prefer to memorize information, others prefer to observe, and still others prefer trial and error. People tend to choose the learning style that has been successful for them in the past.

Kolb's research, described in Whitman, Graham, Gleit, and Boyd (1986), identifies four types of learners.
• The converger, who learns best when presented with abstract concepts and active experimentation, is the easiest client to teach. After hearing an abstract explanation

Learning styles and their applications

Many clients can be described by one of the following types. The nurse should follow the appropriate method after determining which learning style the client prefers.

CLIENT	LEARNING STYLE	TEACHING METHOD
Converger	Applies abstract concepts to life	Allow time for discussion after teaching sessions to help client formulate personal concepts from abstract ideas taught. Provide time for follow-up discussion of applications.
Diverger	Shares with other people and learns from their experiences	Arrange for client to attend interactive group sessions on pertinent topics.
Assimilator	Assembles abstract concepts and various information pieces into cohesive ideas	Incorporate various formats into teaching sessions, such as lecture, question and answer, audiotapes, slides, books, and group discussions.
Accommodator	Prefers personal experience and problem solving	If possible, allow the client to attend an appropriate laboratory session or workshop to test new ideas and skills.

of good nutrition, for example, the client will adjust her eating habits.

• The diverger, who creates ideas and learns best when sharing and learning from the experiences of others, understands abstract concepts but can apply them only with constant stimulation. This client typically learns best in group discussions.

• The assimilator, who prefers abstract ideas and assembling bits and pieces of information into one idea, may require supplemental information to drive the message home even when understanding what the nurse is teaching. Because this client may doubt the credibility of a single information source, combined media (books, audiotapes, and lectures, for example) may offer the most profitable learning experience.

• The accommodator, who learns best from personal experiences and solving problems through trial and error, is the most difficult to teach, because only personal experience offers adequate proof of validity. This client

typically learns best through hands-on demonstrations. (For a summary, see *Learning styles and their applications.*)

Teaching strategies
Throughout nurse-client interaction, the nurse may use any of several different teaching strategies. At times, the client may prefer to merge two or more strategies to achieve the desired outcome.

Individual teaching. Teaching clients one-to-one allows the nurse to provide long- or short-term teaching and continually assess progress. It also allows the nurse to address individual needs. This teaching strategy promotes a personal relationship that helps the client trust and confide in the nurse, further enhancing the teaching-learning process.

The major disadvantage of individual teaching is that the client cannot exchange ideas with anyone but the nurse, forfeiting the opportunity to share experiences with others in similar situations. (This strategy demands more of the nurse's time as a teacher because clients cannot be taught in groups. It also increases institutional expense.)

Group teaching. To maximize learning, members of a group should be similar in maturity, intelligence, and learning needs. Although many adults prefer small groups, most can learn in groups of almost any size. Adolescents typically require small groups because of their shorter attention span and tendency to become distracted. Groups also should be restricted in size when the teaching topic requires hands-on participation or when personal sharing will enhance learning.

Group teaching may reduce client expense and improve convenience (if classes are offered more frequently). Also, this method maximizes the nurse's time by providing services to multiple clients simultaneously.

Team teaching. By interacting with several health care providers, the client receives a range of viewpoints, expertise, and teaching styles. This versatility may prevent boredom and enhance learning. This approach may be appropriate for groups or individuals. Team members may have similar qualifications and professions, or they may represent various disciplines. (For further information, see *Team-teaching guidelines.*)

Contract learning. In this teaching strategy, the nurse and client agree on and pledge to work toward their goals before teaching begins. Some clients may benefit from a written contract that specifies goals. As appropriate, the contract may include a reward if the nurse believes it will enhance the client's compliance.

The contract should describe the roles of nurse and client, list the dates and times of future meetings, outline anticipated topics of discussion, encourage the client to take responsibility for herself (and her fetus, if she is pregnant), list goals as appropriate, and provide space for the signatures of both nurse and client. Both should receive copies.

When successful, the written contract has several advantages. It helps focus nurse-client interaction, specifies mutual goals and objectives, increases the client's motivation and commitment to strive for goals, and helps assure the client of the nurse's commitment to her and her care. Not all clients respond well to a written contract, however; the nurse should use judgment and sensitivity when considering this option to avoid raising the client's defenses.

Behavior modification. Based on the classic psychological principle of operant conditioning, the nurse may use rewards to reinforce and encourage desired behavior. As desired behavior becomes more frequent, rewards gradually become less frequent. When this technique succeeds, the desired behavior continues even though the rewards have diminished.

Although it may take several tries, behavior modification has worked for such varied goals as weight reduction, toilet training, and social behaviors. It is most effective when the client genuinely desires a behavior change. Three principles are central to the success of this technique:
- The reward must be granted immediately.
- The reward must be highly desirable to the client.
- The client must understand that the reward is given for specific behavior or performance of a specific task.
For example, a mother toilet-training her child will indicate the excreta and immediately praise (reward) the child for using the toilet properly. The child, enjoying the attention and praise, will tend to continue using the toilet correctly to keep receiving the reward.

Informal teaching. Occurring throughout nurse-client interaction and typically augmenting planned teaching strategies, informal teaching takes advantage of an optimal moment to convey an idea or concept. Such a moment may occur when a client or family member asks a direct question or makes an erroneous observation. One way to stimulate informal teaching opportunities is to hold discussions or question-and-answer sessions.

Audiovisual aids. Audiotapes, videotapes, and selected objects can improve a client's learning ability because they stimulate sight and touch as well as hearing. Helpful audiovisual aids include:
- charts and tables, which provide a concrete view of an abstract idea or depict relationships that may be unclear to the client
- physical objects, such as the equipment necessary for preparing infant formula
- pictures, which can help explain changes and define characteristics
- audiotapes and videotapes, which may help retain the client's interest.

Programmed learning. If a client shows inadequate learning or reports that she cannot understand the information presented, the nurse may opt for programmed learning, where each teaching session is followed by nonthreatening questions. The client answers the questions and provides rationales for her answers. For example, after teaching about nutrition, the nurse may ask the client to list meals that she consumed that day and identify which ones incorporated proper foods and which ones did not.

The nurse may allow the client to pace this program or may present the information at a predetermined rate. The instruction may be verbal or may include written material for the client to study at home.

Alternatively, the nurse may employ computer simulations and computer-assisted programmed learning. These programs interact with the client, presenting questions and indicating whether the client's responses are correct or incorrect and providing appropriate rationales. The nurse can use these programs, if facility policy allows, to teach such topics as infant feeding, postpartal care, and general infant care. Many computer-assisted programs for the childbearing family exist, allowing the nurse to choose one that is appropriate in topic and depth for each client.

Evaluating effectiveness

Throughout teaching sessions and especially at their conclusion, the nurse and client should evaluate each session's effectiveness (Whitman, Graham, Gleit, and Boyd, 1986). The nurse may wish to record teaching goals and then note which goals were met and which were not. This procedure helps reveal strengths and weaknesses in the teaching and the learning.

The most important measure of teaching effectiveness is how much the client has learned. However, the nurse also may learn by including self-evaluation of such teaching factors as clarity of presentation, diction, enthusiasm, and preparation. In evaluating client learning, the nurse should consider the client's educational level, emotional problems, cultural practices, personal values, and stress level. Although the nurse cannot control these factors, they may aid in developing future teaching strategies.

Motivating

In addition to developing skills in communicating and teaching, the nurse also must develop skills in motivating the client to assimilate and act on new information, thus taking charge of her own health care. Motivation is integral to each phase of nurse-client interaction. It requires a caring attitude and a commitment to encourage the client's responsibility and autonomy.

Caring for clients

A client who believes that the nurse cares for her will be more motivated to learn. Caring is a response in which the nurse acknowledges the emotional needs of the client or the client and her family. It enables the nurse to show concern, to feel a connection with the client, to isolate client problems, and to help the client find ways to solve them (Bonner, 1988). Through caring, the nurse can help meet the physiologic, psychological, and social needs of the client and her family.

In theory, caring for clients is simple. Clinically, however, genuine caring requires deliberate and constant consideration. To care effectively for—and thus motivate—a client, the nurse must be able to recognize needs not obvious to the client, help her recognize those needs, and then help fulfill them in an encouraging, uplifting manner. These achievements require the use of therapeutic empathy and various techniques designed to put caring into practice.

Therapeutic empathy allows the nurse to care for and motivate the client by recognizing and viewing experiences from the client's perspective in a sensitive yet professional manner. This ability encompasses more than simply the desire to help. (The desire to help may create feelings of sorrow or sympathy for the client—feelings that may eliminate objectivity and render the nurse ineffective.) Therapeutic empathy allows the nurse to draw upon personal experiences and feelings when attempting to understand the client's descriptions of health and learning concerns. Further, it helps the nurse recognize needs in light of the client's culture, social behavior, and attitude toward health care.

After recognizing a client's needs, the nurse uses one or more of the following approaches to caring:

• participative caring, in which the nurse encourages the client to take an active role in her own health, thus fostering a sense of control and confidence while also meeting health care needs

• problem-solving caring, in which the nurse detects client-specific problems and suggests solutions

• transformation caring, in which the nurse uncovers problems underlying the client's current needs and helps her find ways to change unhealthy behaviors

• advocacy caring, in which the nurse acts on the client's behalf by coordinating information, services, and referrals for the client's benefit

• healing caring, in which the nurse communicates caring through such physical demonstrations as massage and therapeutic touch

• reintegration caring, which may take such forms as encouragement, coaching, reprimands, or offering a shoulder to cry on; this type of caring often is effective for withdrawn or mildly depressed clients.

Interventions undertaken by the nurse also may communicate caring. Expressive interventions include those that build trust, sensitivity, acceptance of feelings, empathy, and nurturing. Instrumental interventions involve physical actions, fulfillment of the client's human needs, administering drugs and procedures, alleviating stress, and maintaining the physical environment.

Ideally, when the nurse successfully communicates a caring attitude, the client will gain confidence and control, thus becoming motivated to participate in her care.

Self-care

Active and assertive participation in attaining one's health care goals is the essence of self-care. By determining what the client needs to know to care for herself (and her fetus, if she is pregnant), the nurse can motivate the client by urging her to take charge of meeting those needs.

Poor self-care habits may raise risks for childbearing families. Studies have linked inadequate prenatal care in adolescent mothers with an increased incidence of such maternal and infant risks as toxemia, prolonged labor, infection, anemia, and prematurity (Herron, 1988;

Korenbrot, 1989; Mansfield, 1987; Mercer and Ferlstich, 1988; Mundiger, 1986; Reed and Leonard, 1989). Poor nutrition increases maternal mortality and morbidity. In contrast, clients who receive education in self-care and who are motivated show reduced obstetric risks.

Chapter summary

Chapter 4 outlined and explained the phases of nurse-client interaction and detailed three crucial skill areas. Important concepts include the following.
• Nurse-client interaction is initiated and directed by the nurse. It encompasses five phases: preparation, initiation, consolidation and growth, development, and termination.
• Although the structure of nurse-client interaction can be easily understood, the skills required for the nurse to make it successful may take years to develop. Important skills include communicating, teaching, and motivating.
• Communicating effectively with clients begins with specific efforts to encourage relaxation and trust; it includes such techniques as active listening and therapeutic communication.
• Teaching effectively depends on accurate assessment of the client's readiness to learn, developmental stage, obstacles to learning, and preferred learning style.
• The nurse should choose a teaching strategy that corresponds with the client's preferred learning style.
• Clients tend to be more motivated when they feel that the nurse genuinely cares for them and when they become actively involved in their health care.

Study questions

1. What are the five characteristic phases of nurse-client interaction and how do they interrelate?

2. Which methods can facilitate nurse-client communication?

3. Before teaching a client, which variables should the nurse assess?

4. Discuss individual client-teaching strategies appropriate for use with the childbearing family.

5. Connie and Nan-Sung, her husband, have come to the clinic for help because Connie has had two spontaneous abortions. They reside in a Chinese neighborhood in a large city. Which variables should the nurse consider when formulating teaching strategies for this couple?

6. Which two nursing traits are most helpful in motivating clients?

Bibliography

American Hospital Association. (1975). A patient's bill of rights (pamphlet). Chicago, IL: Author.

Arnold, E., and Boggs, K. (1989). *Interpersonal relationships: Professional communication skills for nurses*. Philadelphia: Saunders.

Beck, M., and Weathers, D. (1985, January 14). America's abortion dilemma. *Newsweek*, pp. 20-25.

Bonner, P., and Wruben, J. (1988). Caring is the candle that lights the dark, that permits us to find answers where others see none. *AJN*, 88(8), 1073-1075.

Bonner, P. (1984). *From novice to expert: Excellence and power in clinical nursing practice*. Menlo Park, CA: Addison-Wesley.

Bradshaw, M.J. (1988). *Nursing of the family in health and illness: A developmental approach*. East Norwalk, CT: Appleton & Lange.

Brophy, B. (1986, March 10). Expectant moms, office dilemma. *U.S. News and World Report*, pp. 52-53.

Bruess, C.E., and Poehler, D.L. (1987). What we need and don't need in health education. *Health Education*, 17(6), 32-36.

Davis, A.R. (1988). Developing teaching strategies based on new knowledge. *Journal of Nursing Education*, 27(4), 156-160.

Davis, J.H., Eyer, J., and Drott, P.M. (1987). Helping students assess parenting education needs. *Public Health Nursing*, 4(3), 141-145.

Duvall, E.M. (1984). *Marriage and family development* (6th ed.). New York: Harper & Row.

Fibich, S., and Yulsman, T. (1987, September). Modern midwifery: New childbirth options. *McCalls*. Vol.CXIV, No.12, pp. 92-93.

Gains, J. (1985). Health education content assessment. *Health Education*, 15(7), 6-8.

Grissum, M., and Spengler, C. (1976). *Woman power and health care*. Boston: Little, Brown.

Haire, H. (1975). The pregnant patient's bill of rights (pamphlet). Rochester, NY: International Childbirth Education Association, Inc.

Hembree, D. (1986, March). Reproductive risks. *Ms*, pp. 79-80.

Herron, M.A. (1988). One approach to preventing preterm birth. *Journal of Perinatal and Neonatal Nursing*, 2(1), 33-41.

Knowles, M.S. (1980). *The modern practice of adult education*. New York: Cambridge Book Co.

Korenbrot, C. (1989). Birthweight outcomes in a teenage pregnancy: A case management project. *Journal of Adolescent Health Care*, 10(2), 97-104.

Leino-Kilpi, H. (1989). Learning to care: A qualitative perspective of student evaluation. *Journal of Nursing Education*, 28(2), 61-66.

Mansfield, P.K. (1987). Teenage and midlife childbearing update: Implications for health educators. *Health Education*, 18(4), 18-23.

Mercer, R.T., and Ferlstich, S.L. (1988). Stress and social support as predictions of anxiety and depression during pregnancy. *Advances in Nursing Science*, 10(2), 26-39.

Moloney, M.M. (1986). *Professionalization of nursing.* Philadelphia: Lippincott.

Mundiger, M.O., (1986). Health service fundings cuts and the declining health of the poor. *New England Journal of Medicine*, 313(1), 44-47.

Office of Technology Assessment. (1986). Nurse practitioners, physician assistants and certified nurse-midwives: A policy analysis. Document No. 87-12139. Washington, DC: U.S. Government Printing Office.

Paskert, C.J., and Madara, E.J. (1985). Introducing and tapping self help mutual aid resources. *Health Education*, 16(4), 25-28.

Petosa, R. (1985). Promoting student learning of behavioral strategies. *Health Education*, 15(7), 39-45.

Rankin, S., and Duffy, K. (1983). *Patient education: Issues, principles, and guidelines.* Philadelphia: Lippincott.

Redman, B. (1984). *The process of patient education.* St.Louis: Mosby.

Reed, P.G., and Leonard, V.E. (1989). An analysis of the concept of self-neglect. *Advances in Nursing Science*, 12(1), 39-53.

Reverby, S. (1987). A caring dilemma: Womanhood and nursing in historical perspective. *Nursing Research*, 39(1), 5-11.

Riverby, S. (1987). *Ordered to care.* Cambridge, MA: Cambridge University Press.

Riehl-Sisca, J. (1989). *Conceptual models for nursing practice* (3rd ed.). East Norwalk, CT: Appleton & Lange.

Sundeen, S.J., Stuart, G., Rankin, E., and Cohen, S. (1989). *Nurse-client interaction: Implementing the nursing process* (4th ed.). St. Louis: Mosby.

Sutherland, M., and Fasko, D. (1987). Competencies of health education. *Health Education*, 18(5), 10-13.

Walker, R.A., and Bibeau, D. (1986). Health education as freeing (Pt. II). *Health Education*, 16(6), 4-8.

Weiss, E.H., and Kessel, G. (1987). Practical skills for health educators on using mass media. *Health Education*, 18(3), 39-41.

Whitman, N., Graham, B., Gleit, C., and Boyd, M. (1986). *Teaching in nursing practice: A professional model.* East Norwalk, CT: Appleton & Lange.

Wiist, W.H. (1988). Update on computer-assisted video instruction in health sciences. *Health Education*, 18(6), 8-12.

Young, W.B. (1987). *Introduction to nursing concepts.* East Norwalk, CT: Appleton & Lange.

Nursing research

Becker, H., and Sands, D. (1988). The relationship of empathy to clinical experience among male and female nursing students. *Journal of Nursing Education*, 27(5), 198-203.

Ethical and Legal Concerns in Family Care

Objectives

After reading and studying this chapter, the student should be able to:

1. Discuss the three principles on which a nurse should base ethical decisions.

2. Outline steps the nurse may take to help arrive at ethical decisions.

3. Name organizations that have issued ethics codes to guide nursing practice in maternal and child health care.

4. Describe the four elements that must be proven before a plaintiff may win a lawsuit.

5. Discuss the elements of informed consent.

6. List the three goals of risk management.

7. Explain why documentation of care is one of the nurse's most important risk management tools.

8. Describe the standard of care for intrapartal fetal monitoring.

9. Describe situations in which legal and ethical conflict may arise between the rights of a pregnant client and the rights of her fetus.

Introduction

As part of daily clinical practice, the nurse assesses clients and their situations, makes decisions based on acquired knowledge and experience, and takes appropriate action. Whether acting independently or interacting with families, physicians, other nurses, or health care agencies, the nurse always should take ethical and legal concerns into account.

Because ethical problems may occur more frequently in specialty practice, such as maternal and neonatal nursing, the nurse needs a sound knowledge of ethical principles and must know how they relate to laws. Such knowledge will facilitate ethical decision making and protect the nurse from unnecessary risk of liability.

This chapter presents guidelines for making ethical decisions, outlines the relationship between ethics and laws, provides methods to minimize legal risks, and offers some examples of the legal and ethical issues that attend maternal, neonatal, and women's health practice.

Making an ethical decision

Ethics is a discipline in which one attempts to identify, organize, analyze, and justify human acts by applying certain principles to determine the right action for a given situation. However, isolating principles on which to base an ethical decision can be difficult. Some people believe that ethical principles should be based on professional duty (the deontological approach). Others believe that they should be based on possible outcomes of the actions taken (the teleological approach). In either case, an ethical decision typically requires balancing conflicts between personal rights (Curtin and Flaherty, 1982).

Although the nurse's personal feelings play a part, they cannot compose the sole basis for ethical decisions. The nurse must learn how to reason morally, to identify the ethical dimensions of nursing practice, and to relate

GLOSSARY

Civil action: lawsuit addressing the rights and duties of private persons. Typically one person sues another for monetary damages.

Consent: voluntary act in which one person agrees to an action by another person. Not all consent given is informed consent.

Defendant: person against whom a lawsuit is brought.

Ethics: discipline that attempts to identify, organize, analyze, and justify human acts by applying certain principles to determine an appropriate response in a given situation.

Informed consent: legal rule in which a client is entitled to receive certain information about a proposed course of treatment or surgery. Usual required information includes risks, benefits, and alternatives.

Liability: obligation to pay monetary damages in a civil action.

Malpractice: form of negligence action brought against such professionals as nurses, physicians, lawyers, and accountants that alleges failure to meet applicable standards, thus causing harm.

Negligence: failure to act as a reasonable person would given similar training, experience, and circumstances.

Plaintiff: person who initiates a lawsuit.

Respondeat superior: legal rule under which an employer is held legally responsible for negligence or malpractice committed by an employee functioning within the scope of employment.

Risk management: steps taken to minimize either the chance of injury or the harm that occurs.

Standard of care: acts that a reasonable person would have performed or omitted under the circumstances; conduct against which the defendant's conduct is measured in a malpractice case.

ethical decisions to clinical practice (Thompson and Thompson, 1989).

The three ethical principles that can help the nurse meet these goals include:

• respect for the individual. The nurse must consider and support a client's rights to self-determination and autonomy, privacy, treatment refusal, truthfulness, and confidentiality. The client's ethical decisions take precedence over the nurse's convictions, even if the nurse finds the client's reasoning flawed. This is one of the more difficult aspects of ethics and nursing.

• beneficence. The nurse must avoid harming anyone and must try to prevent or remove harm and promote or do good.

• justice. The nurse must be fair and equitable in allocating services and resources to a client.

Ideally, these three principles provide the basis of ethical decisions. In some cases, however, other issues impinge. Financial, religious, medical, or legal issues may exert a significant influence. Consider the case of a pregnant client who develops vaginal bleeding. Her physician may confine her to bed for purely medical reasons. However, the client may find this judgment unsatisfactory because of the lack of care for her children, her financial situation, or her emotional capacity.

For the nurse, different kinds of ethical problems may arise. The nurse may confront a choice between equally desirable or undesirable conditions. The nurse's beliefs may conflict with the law, a professional code, or a health care facility policy. To address such problems, the nurse must identify the conflict, determine the underlying facts, consider possible options and their consequences (for the nurse, the other health care providers, the health care facility, and the client), and then use the ethical principles mentioned above in a thoughtful, step-by-step manner to decide on a course of action. (For specific guidelines, see *Model for ethical decisions.*)

Ethical conflicts between staff, clients, and within one's self are stressful both personally and professionally. If such conflicts become frequent or remain unresolved, the nurse may need to choose another nursing specialty or may choose to seek help from colleagues or a counselor.

Professional standards and guidelines

By knowing legal mandates, the nurse can make ethical decisions more confidently and minimize the risk of liability. A primary legal resource is the applicable nurse practice act, under which all nurses in a state function. (A few types of advanced practice—nurse-midwifery, for example—may function under a different statute in some states.) Each nurse practice act defines nursing in general terms, sets qualifications for licensure and grounds for discipline, and defines the powers of the board of nursing.

Rarely does a nurse practice act explicitly endorse or prohibit a specific nursing function, especially in a specialty practice area, such as maternal, neonatal, and women's health nursing. In many cases, professional standards offer more practical and ethical help than do laws, especially regarding practice standards.

Both the American Nurses' Association (ANA) and the International Council of Nursing (ICN) have published professional codes of ethics. (For ANA guidelines, see The *Code for Nurses,* page 70.) The ANA and ICN codes supplement ordinary professional standards by providing more specific actions that the nurse should embrace. For example, the ANA has defined maternal and child health nursing as a "specialized area of nursing focused on (1) health needs of women, their partners, and their families throughout their reproductive and childbearing years and (2) children through adolescence" (ANA, 1980). The ANA statement sets standards of practice and defines essential knowledge and skills required to practice. It also identifies two categories of maternal and child health nurses: the nurse generalist and the maternal and child health nurse specialist.

Other groups have published information that also could be helpful in determining practice standards. For example, NAACOG, the organization for obstetric, gynecologic, and neonatal nurses, has published standards for obstetric, gynecologic, and neonatal nursing and more specific "practice competencies and educational guidelines" for nurse providers of intrapartal care.

In situations that involve an ethical problem, the nurse must attempt to balance these various codes and statements with personal convictions, legal mandate, professional literature, and health care facility policies to arrive at an acceptable solution.

Ethics and the law

To help integrate ethical principles and decision making into practice, the nurse should understand the relationship between ethics and laws.

An ethical standard is an interpretation of right and wrong actions in a specific situation made by an individual or by designated persons or groups within a community or society and based on established traditions or widely held beliefs. Such an ethical standard is useful in guiding actions. Breach of an ethical standard may have professional or social penalties or consequences, but they are rarely as rigorous as legal penalties because ethical issues tend to be less clear-cut than legal issues.

Model for ethical decisions

Bunting and Webb (1988) proposed a model for decision making that relies on a systematic approach to ethical problems. When faced with an ethical dilemma, the nurse should consider the following questions before making a decision.

Which health issues are involved?

Which ethical issues are involved?

What further information is necessary concerning either of the above before a judgment can be made?

Who will be affected by this decision? (Include the decision maker and other caregivers if they will be affected emotionally or professionally.)

What are the values and opinions of the people involved?

What conflicts exist between the values and ethical standards of the people involved?

Must a decision be made and, if so, who should make it?

What alternatives are available?

For each alternative, what are the ethical justifications?

For each alternative, what are the possible outcomes?

Adapted from Bunting, S., and Webb, A. (1988). An ethical model for decision-making. *Nurse Practitioner,* 13(12), p. 32. Used with permission.

The *Code for Nurses*

The American Nurses' Association *Code for Nurses* provides ethical standards of conduct and guidelines for all aspects of nursing practice.

1 The nurse provides services with respect for human dignity and the uniqueness of the client, unrestricted by considerations of social or economic status, personal attributes, or the nature of health problems.

2 The nurse safeguards the client's right to privacy by judiciously protecting information of a confidential nature.

3 The nurse acts to safeguard the client and the public when health care and safety are affected by the incompetent, unethical, or illegal practice of any person.

4 The nurse assumes responsibility and accountability for individual nursing judgments and actions.

5 The nurse maintains competence in nursing.

6 The nurse exercises informed judgment and uses individual competence and qualifications as criteria in seeking consultation, accepting responsibilities, and delegating nursing activities to others.

7 The nurse participates in activities that contribute to the ongoing development of the profession's body of knowledge.

8 The nurse participates in the profession's efforts to implement and improve standards of nursing.

9 The nurse participates in the profession's efforts to establish and maintain conditions of employment conducive to high quality nursing care.

10 The nurse participates in the profession's effort to protect the public from misinformation and misrepresentation and to maintain the integrity of nursing.

11 The nurse collaborates with members of the health professions and other citizens in promoting community and national efforts to meet the health needs of the public.

Reprinted with permission of the American Nurses' Association, Kansas City, MO.

Laws, which are imposed on individuals by legislative and judicial bodies, tend to be specific, inflexible rules that stem from a historical interpretation of right and wrong; they typically change slowly. Laws impose specific penalties if breached and rarely are modified by an offender's personal convictions. An individual may not ignore a law with impunity, even if the individual believes the law is wrong.

A legal action (court case) may comprise a disagreement over the intent of a specific law. Usually, one party believes that another has failed to meet a law's requirements. The U.S. legal system minimizes the chance of one person (including a judge) imposing arbitrary standards on another by requiring, where possible, that legal arguments and decisions be supported by precedent (prior court decisions on similar disputes).

Ideally, a society's collective ethical standards relate closely to its laws. In fact, laws should directly reflect the personal, social, and professional ethics of the majority of the population at the time. Legislatures may enact laws to counter abuse of a particular ethical standard. In many cases, laws are enacted to protect personal rights.

Even though many laws are based on ethical principles, the nurse usually cannot depend on laws to define personal ethical standards. Not all ethical questions are addressed by laws. Furthermore, new laws typically lag behind the development of new technology. Additionally, although laws may represent a society's collective opinion, they cannot represent the individual beliefs of all of a society's members. So even if laws address a particular ethical point, the nurse still must arrive at a personal decision. The nurse also should allow each client to make personal ethical decisions.

Difficult questions arise when personal ethical standards differ from established laws or when laws have not yet addressed certain ethical issues. When such questions arise, the nurse should be prepared to make ethical decisions based on sound principles and established codes of ethics.

When laws are breached

The best defense against legal action is delivery of high-quality nursing care. However, even when practicing well within the state's nurse practice act, the nurse may incur a charge of malpractice, which is a form of negligence (a civil action). The principles of malpractice or professional liability are the same for nurses as for physicians and other health care providers. In order to win a lawsuit, the plaintiff (who is suing) must prove four elements.

First, the plaintiff must prove that a nurse-client relationship existed between the defendant and the plaintiff. This is rarely disputed because a nurse establishes such a relationship even when caring for a client outside the daily assignment.

Second, the plaintiff must prove that the nurse violated the applicable standard of care either by omission (failing to act) or by commission (acting inappropriately). The standard of care—the one in effect at the time of the incident, not when the case is filed or taken to trial—requires that the nurse do what a reasonable nurse with similar training and experience would have done under the same circumstances. Student nurses under the supervision of nurse-instructors are required to meet the same standard of care as graduate nurses. Expert nursing testimony verifies the standard of care and should be based on a review of medical records, professional standards, relevant health care facility policies, professional literature, and professional experience.

Third, the plaintiff must prove that acts committed or omitted by the nurse were causally related to the outcome.

Fourth, the plaintiff must prove damages. Although exceptions exist, the plaintiff typically must suffer physical injury before claiming monetary compensation for pain and suffering. Liability in a malpractice case requires that the defendant pay monetary damages. Malpractice is not a criminal offense; therefore, a defendant found guilty of malpractice will not be jailed.

Although the nurse who makes an error is personally and professionally liable, a principle of law called respondeat superior also holds the employer legally responsible for nursing negligence. Under this theory, many cases involving a nurse's care do not name the nurse as a defendant. Instead, the employing health care facility defends the action of an accused nurse. Even when the nurse is a named defendant, the employer's professional liability insurance company customarily defends the claim.

The nurse as defendant

A recent trend in some specialities, however, is for individual nurses to be named as defendants. This may result in increasing malpractice insurance premiums for nurses. Each nurse should stay informed of malpractice trends and monitor the amount of malpractice coverage recommended for individuals who are not insured through an employer or have inadequate coverage.

Some cases, such as medication errors and retained foreign bodies during surgery, offer clear examples of liability (although not necessarily by the nurse alone). Other cases may not incur liability even with a poor outcome; a principle of law asserts that a poor client outcome does not necessarily indicate negligent care. Even a mistaken professional judgment is not negligent if it was a reasonable decision under the circumstances.

Nelson v. Trinity Medical Center (1988), a recent malpractice case, demonstrates some of the liability problems in maternal and neonatal nursing. In this case, the client reported a sharp increase in contractions and abdominal pain just before being admitted in labor. Although the attending physicians had left standing orders for all clients to be placed on electronic fetal monitors, the nurse in charge believed incorrectly that all monitors were in use. Five hours later, when a monitor became available, it revealed fetal distress. The child was delivered by cesarean and suffered extensive brain damage.

When this case went to court, the jury found the health care facility (as employer of the nurse) liable and awarded more than $7 million in damages. The state supreme court later ruled the physicians (who had settled their part of the case out of court) not liable for the nurse's actions.

This case confirms that the nurse legally is required to use professional judgment in client care and also is required to follow reasonable physician orders. If the nurse cannot follow the orders, either because necessary equipment is unavailable or because the nurse believes the orders to be wrong or unsafe, the nurse must notify both a nursing supervisor and the responsible physician. Care provided and contacts with the physician must be documented; this documentation is the most important element in proving compliance with the legal standard of care.

Risk management

Risk management techniques have been particularly important in maternal and neonatal nursing. From a liability standpoint, obstetrics is a high-risk practice because it may involve both the client's health and the life-long health of her child. Legal action is relatively common with a poor birth outcome, and jury verdicts can specify substantial recompense.

Risk management has been developed to accomplish three main goals:
- Reduce the number and severity of client, visitor, and employee injuries.
- Ensure that client care is sufficiently documented so that any malpractice claim can be defended adequately.

• Protect the health care provider and health care facility against financial loss by ensuring adequate professional and general liability insurance.

Many states and organizations that accredit private health care facilities require them to designate a risk manager to work closely with quality assurance personnel. In some states, incidents resulting in client harm must be reported to state health authorities. Even without a state requirement, health care facilities require staff members to report client falls, medication errors, and unanticipated outcomes. Risk managers collect this information by reviewing discharge charts, incident reports (written or oral), or both.

Incident reports—a cornerstone of risk management—help health care facilities track patterns of errors and injuries. They aid nurses by providing an immediate opportunity to record an incident before memory fades. These reports should be written clearly and concisely and should contain no extraneous information. Incident reports do not substitute for medical record documentation about the incident; instead, they provide recorded facts along with extra information, such as the names of persons who witness a fall. When considering a malpractice action, the court may allow inclusion of an incident report in the case.

Some health care facilities have in-house attorneys to whom information about potential litigation can be directed. An individual's communications with the facility or personal attorney are privileged, and the contents of those communications need not be disclosed in any later legal action.

The other cornerstone of risk management is accurate and complete documentation of care. Besides offering excellent defense against malpractice, careful documentation encourages continuity of care among health care providers. Each health care facility maintains specific documentation requirements that correspond with its own forms and checklists. For maternal and neonatal health care, documentation always includes such characteristics as fetal heart rate, contraction patterns, and maternal vital signs. Documentation of other signs, such as the appearance of the fetus's head during the second stage of labor, may not be required unless an abnormality arises.

All documentation should be factual and written legibly. The nurse should never erase an error, but should draw a single line through it and initial the change. An entry inadvertently omitted should be added later in the record rather than squeezing it in where space is inadequate. A written explanation can justify why the entry appears out of sequence.

Ethical and legal issues

Various ethical and legal issues may arise for the nurse providing maternal and neonatal care. The following examples present representative issues.

Confidentiality

All clients, even those declared incompetent by a judge, have rights within the health care system. The scope of those rights depends upon the situation. Both ethics and law assure the confidentiality of medical information, and clients may take legal action if this confidentiality is breached. Nurses should know, however, that in some circumstances ethics or law may require the disclosure of what could be considered confidential information. For example, some argue that a client who tests positive for human immunodeficiency virus (HIV) should disclose this fact so that a sexual partner can take precautions to prevent transmission. By refusing to make this disclosure, the client forces the nurse or physician to decide whether to inform the sexual partner. As the law in many states stands currently, such disclosure could incur justified legal action; in other states, failure to disclose carries a greater legal risk.

Refusing treatment

With few exceptions (such as the court-ordered cesarean delivery discussed under "Concerns in later pregnancy" later in this chapter), competent clients may accept or refuse recommended treatment. To make this decision, every client is entitled to an explanation of the risks, benefits, and alternatives to the recommended treatment.

When a client refuses treatment, the nurse should notify the responsible physician and document the circumstances of the refusal. Forcing a client to undergo surgery or other refused treatment without court authorization opens the nurse and physician to a lawsuit.

Sterilization

In 1984, more than a million sterilization procedures were performed in the United States, 730,000 of them on women (Shapiro, 1988). Fewer than half the states have laws regulating sterilization; those that do require competent adult consent. States that allow sterilization of a minor require parental consent.

Many states have laws protecting mentally disabled clients who may not understand what they agree to in giving consent. These laws have developed in response to so-called eugenic sterilization laws passed before 1930. Eugenic sterilization laws permitted the sterilization of those judged insane, idiotic, moronic, or imbecilic (Gould, 1987), and thousands of people were involuntarily sterilized. Subsequently, many of these laws have been repealed.

Two types of protection have evolved for mentally disabled individuals: (1) some states prohibit sterilization of these clients; (2) other states require that the person requesting a client's sterilization obtain court permission.

Consent for sterilization should be in writing and signed by the client. Before giving consent, the client should receive a description of the procedure and be informed of alternatives, risks of the procedure, failure rates, and the probable permanency of the sterilization.

The physician who performs the sterilization is responsible for obtaining written informed consent. As with any client consent, the nursing staff has no independent legal obligation to verify the adequacy of the consent (by asking questions about what the client understands); but if the client indicates confusion or incomplete understanding, the nurse should call the physician, who should then review the procedure with the client.

Many lawsuits have resulted from sterilization procedures, a number of which involve some allegation of faulty consent. Some have alleged physician negligence in performing the procedure—a difficult allegation to prove—whereas others have claimed that the client was not told that the procedure could fail. This emphasizes the importance of documenting the discussion that preceeds procurement of the client's signature on the informed consent form.

Infertility

Defined as the inability to conceive after 12 months of unprotected and reasonably frequent intercourse, infertility affects an estimated 2.4 million couples and an unknown number of unmarried women who might wish to conceive (U.S. Congress, Office of Technology Assessment [OTA]—Infertility, 1988). This issue raises numerous legal and ethical questions, in part because many public and private insurance carriers refuse to pay for infertility services, claiming that infertility is not a disease. Instead, they classify infertility services as elective, thus unreimbursable. This distinction raises an ethical dilemma because it makes infertility services available only to clients who can afford expensive medical procedures. (See *Ethical issues in infertility treatment* for more information.)

Ethical issues in infertility treatment

According to Jansen (1987), infertility treatments raise ethical issues that commonly spark heated debate.

Cost of treatment
In the United States, some forms of health care depend on the client's ability to pay. Individuals from lower socioeconomic groups and those without health insurance typically cannot afford basic infertility treatment. Those who can afford it may feel compelled to try every available treatment until they conceive.

Every year, millions of dollars are spent on infertility research and technology that benefit only a small segment of the population. Some people argue that this money should be spent on more catastrophic health care concerns, such as acquired immunodeficiency syndrome (AIDS) or cancer research. Yet they disagree on who should determine the nation's health care priorities: the federal government, medical community, researchers, or other groups.

Procedures
Some procedures, such as in vitro fertilization (IVF), separate procreation from sexual intercourse and love. These procedures seem unnatural to some people. They believe, for example, that humans will be tempted to play God, implanting only embryos of a desired sex or genetic composition; or that people will try to use these procedures to their own advantage—such as having a child on their own schedule.

Embryo ownership and treatment
The fate of untransferred human embryos is complex. If parents die or separate, embryo ownership becomes a controversial issue.

Effects on children
Some people think that a child conceived through IVF or a donor's sperm or oocytes may develop adjustment or identity problems. They also worry that the parents will have reservations about sperm or oocyte donation.

Success rates
Some infertility centers report success rates based on signs of pregnancy, such as elevated levels of human chorionic gonadotropin, ultrasound detection of a yolk sac, and fetal cardiac activity. However, the actual birth rate may be much lower. Some individuals find this method of reporting success rates misleading because it may raise false hopes.

Rapid developments in infertility technology raise legal and ethical questions as well. Because technology has developed faster than statutory or case law, few precedents exist for evaluating specific situations concerning infertility. These situations typically involve artificial insemination, in vitro fertilization and embryo transfer, and surrogate motherhood.

Artificial insemination

In this process, fertilization of an ovum takes place not as a result of sexual intercourse but of deliberate placement of sperm in the vagina or uterus by another method (Ashley and O'Rourke, 1986). The oldest infertility technique, human artificial insemination using the partner's semen (homologous insemination or AIH) was first recorded in 1799; donor insemination (heterogenous insemination or AID) was first reported in the United States in 1909.

During a 12-month period in 1986-87, at least 65,000 births occurred from artificial insemination: 35,000 from AIH and the rest from AID. By comparison, 100 children were conceived via surrogate motherhood techniques and 600 by in vitro fertilization. Nearly 11,000 physicians in the United States use artificial insemination at least occasionally to treat infertile clients (U.S. Congress, OTA—Artificial insemination, 1988).

More than half the states have laws concerning some aspect of AID because this technique raises more legal questions than does AIH. These laws vary considerably. As of 1989, only three states addressed donor screening, although the medical literature confirms that infectious and genetic diseases can be transmitted via donor insemination. Many state laws require the written consent of the client and her partner before the insemination.

In vitro fertilization and embryo transfer

In this technique, a surgeon removes one or more ova from the client's ovary and combines each ovum with sperm in a sterile container. After a few days, the physician transfers one or more embryos from the container to the client's uterus. This technique can raise many of the same ethical and legal questions that AID raises. In most cases, the law has yet to answer them. For example, what should happen to a frozen embryo if the genetic parents divorce or die?

Embryo transfer raises even more complex questions because the procedure may involve an embryo genetically unrelated either to the woman who gestates it or to the man who will act as its father after birth. Further, donated gametes (reproductive cells) raise questions about the donor's legal liability if the child has a genetically transmitted disease.

Considering these possible combinations of circumstances, all participants in infertility programs should be screened in accordance with developing professional standards, and all gametes and embryos should be handled carefully. When a procedure involves gametes and conception, the consent form should state that the client has no guarantee of pregnancy or, if pregnancy occurs, that the child will be normal at birth.

Although in vitro fertilization takes place at many facilities in the United States, only a few states have laws that mention the technique. Of those, not all attempt to influence professional practice. Because few or no legal guidelines exist, health care providers who offer these services should take added precautions to inform prospective clients and to obtain written consent forms from clients and their partners. Both the discussion and the written consent form should describe the potential benefits and known risks of each procedure.

Surrogate motherhood

Several well-publicized legal cases have concerned children born under surrogate motherhood arrangements. In most of these cases, the surrogate was artificially inseminated by the partner of an infertile woman. The semen donor paid the surrogate mother's medical expenses and, upon release of the child, paid her an additional sum of money. This additional payment creates an ethical and legal dilemma. Many commentators claim that receiving payment for bearing a child qualifies as baby selling, which is ethically questionable and also illegal (Holder, 1988). Alternatively, they say that surrogacy arrangements involving no payment may be legally and ethically acceptable; a few courts have upheld this belief.

Laws concerning surrogacy arrangements remain uncertain. Despite considerable legislative activity, only a few states have passed laws governing surrogate motherhood contracts, and these vary considerably (Charo, 1988). The Baby M decision from the New Jersey Supreme Court is the only state high court case on the validity of a surrogacy contract, and the court invalidated the contract (In the Matter of Baby M, 1988).

When nurses and physicians who participate in surrogacy cases provide only prenatal and delivery services, liability is no different than in any other obstetric case. However, when they help to locate or match the prospective surrogate and semen donor, potential liability increases. In such a case, the nurse and physician assume obligations beyond those in the traditional provider-client relationship.

Concerns of early pregnancy

Two issues that arise early in pregnancy—prenatal diagnostic testing and abortion—may have far-reaching ethical and legal implications.

Prenatal diagnosis

In the early 1960s, researchers began aspirating desquamated fetal cells from amniotic fluid and analyzing them for fetal defects (amniocentesis). The American College of Obstetricians and Gynecologists (ACOG) now recommends that pregnant women age 35 or older —and younger women with a family history of neural tube defects—be offered amniocentesis services.

Because amniocentesis usually is performed after the sixteenth week of pregnancy, and because it raises the risk of miscarriage or fetal injury, researchers have worked to develop alternate techniques. Chorionic villus sampling (CVS), in use since 1980, is effective from the ninth to the twelfth week of pregnancy. Many conditions diagnosed with amniocentesis can be diagnosed with CVS providing an adequate tissue sample can be obtained. When percutaneous fetal umbilical blood sampling (PUBS) is necessary for fetal diagnosis (as in certain blood and metabolic diseases), it is done by amniocentesis. Although PUBS may be considered experimental in some facilities, neither amniocentesis nor CVS is considered experimental. Nevertheless, they are invasive and carry risk of injury to the mother and fetus.

The physician should obtain written informed consent for these procedures from the client. Before giving consent, the client should be informed of the risks, benefits, limitations, and alternatives (along with the risks associated with those alternatives) to the proposed diagnostic studies. A client may elect to refuse amniocentesis and other recommended testing. If she refuses, the nurse or physician must document the refusal along with statements made to the client regarding possible consequences of the refusal.

Now that ACOG and other professional groups recommend prenatal diagnostic testing for some clients, the courts have ruled that a nurse or physician must offer the testing even if the health care provider opposes the techniques on ethical grounds.

The nurse who chooses to participate in prenatal diagnostic testing should be sure to label specimens properly—so that each client receives proper results—and keep a log book to help assure timely results. The family may need referral to a genetics center for counseling and follow-up.

Abortion

Most laws applicable to health care originate at the state level. Regarding abortion, however, the law stems from federal constitutional principles as defined and refined by the U.S. Supreme Court. In 1973, the Court issued its opinion in *Roe v. Wade*, relying on the Fourteenth Amendment to the Constitution to protect privacy and, thus, procreative choice. States may regulate abortion availability and practice only as permitted by the U.S. Constitution.

Although abortion is legal in the United States, no law requires health care providers or facilities to provide the service. Nurses or other providers who are ethically or morally opposed to abortion cannot be forced to participate in the procedure.

Abortion may not be performed without the client's consent. Even when a state or health care facility does not require written consent, the physician responsible for the procedure may require it. The U.S. Supreme Court has held that spousal consent may not be required before a married woman aborts a pregnancy (*Planned Parenthood v. Danforth,* 1976). However, at least one state has introduced legislation that would require spousal notification.

Courts have held that neither a pregnant woman's parents nor the father of the child may compel the woman to undergo an abortion even if she is a minor. The law concerning abortion consent by minors is complex, but in the absence of any state law, a minor may consent to the procedure as long as she is considered capable of understanding the risks and benefits (Benshoof and Philpel, 1986).

In 1989, the U.S. Supreme Court upheld a Missouri law that prohibited the use of public facilities and personnel for abortion services and denied the use of public funds to pay for abortions (*Webster v. Reproductive Health Services*). The majority of the court chose not to overrule *Roe v. Wade,* but to abandon its trimester system. As a result of the 1989 Missouri opinion, state legislatures are now freer to regulate abortions, at least during certain stages of pregnancy.

The Canadian court decriminalized abortion in January 1988 (*Morgentaler, Smolin, and Scott v. The Queen*). Since then, Canada has been without an abortion law and provincial courts have responded in conflicting ways to a series of abortion cases. New national legislation is anticipated.

For the nurse, abortion presents a multidimensional issue. As client advocate, the nurse must encourage the client's autonomy and freedom of self-determination. As caregiver, the nurse must foster the client's physical and emotional well-being, providing the best care possible. (See Chapter 9, Family Planning, for more information.)

Concerns in later pregnancy

Although competent adults are legally permitted to refuse treatment and bear the consequences of their decision, precedent exists to force a woman to undergo a procedure for the benefit of her fetus.

One study revealed that court orders for cesarean deliveries have been sought in 11 states (Kolder, Gallagher, and Parsons, 1987). Only one such case, *Jefferson v. Griffin Spalding County Hospital Authority* (1981), has reached a state supreme court. A woman, who had been diagnosed with a complete placenta previa (the placenta covered the cervix), refused cesarean delivery before labor began. After a court hearing, the fetus was found to be neglected and was placed in the temporary custody of the Georgia Department of Human Resources. That agency was empowered to order the cesarean if necessary to save the life of the fetus. Some commentators view the use of child abuse and neglect laws to protect a fetus as a way to "correct" a woman's behavior during pregnancy. Others believe that these laws can be applied judiciously, maintaining respect for the woman's rights.

ACOG recommends that obstetricians refrain from performing procedures unwanted by a pregnant client. Nurses and physicians must make every effort to prevent situations in which the client and health care provider cannot maintain an acceptable relationship.

Fetal research

Embryonic and fetal research also presents ethical and legal dilemmas. Many states have laws addressing research on a live fetus: some prohibit it; others allow it if it poses no harm to the fetus or could preserve the fetus's life. Other state laws do not address research directly, but require maternal consent. Some of these laws impose severe criminal penalties for violation (Holder, 1985). Research on a dead fetus is addressed by state laws governing anatomic gifts.

Fetal therapy

Some conditions are potentially treatable in utero if no other potentially life-threatening congenital problem exists. These include erythroblastosis fetalis (a type of anemia), obstruction of the urinary tract, and diaphragmatic hernias. Although intrauterine transfusion to treat erythroblastosis fetalis has been used since 1963, many of the newer fetal therapies are considered experimental.

Some experts fear that therapies delivered to the fetus in utero will raise ethical and legal questions about a pregnant client's obligation to provide these treatments even if she opposes them. In 1987, a study reported that court orders for three intrauterine transfusions had been sought; courts granted the orders in two cases and refused in the third (Kolder, Gallagher, and Parsons, 1987). Once a therapy becomes a standard of care rather than an experimental treatment, the right to refuse therapy becomes an issue. As in the placenta previa case discussed above, the question of the mother's rights versus the fetus's rights arises.

Even when procedures are not considered experimental, the pregnant client must be thoroughly informed of the risks, limitations, benefits, and alternatives (including the effect of no treatment and of waiting until delivery for treatment) on her and on the fetus. The physician always should obtain written consent before the procedure. If a pregnant client refuses recommended in utero fetal therapy and the health care team decides to accept her refusal, nurses and physicians should document their discussions with the client, indicating what the client was told about the potential consequences of her refusal.

Fetal monitoring

A recent survey conducted by ACOG reported that nearly half of the obstetric claims against ACOG members involved fetal monitoring (ACOG, 1988). Data from NAACOG are similar (Brescia, 1985). Claims typically involve allegations of failure to monitor the fetus, failure to respond properly to monitor-generated data, and premature termination of fetal monitoring. Recently published professional standards state that the "method and intensity of fetal heart rate monitoring used during labor should be based on risk factors and delineated by department policy." Auscultation at 15-minute intervals during the first stage of labor adequately approximates continuous electronic fetal monitoring (ACOG and American Academy of Pediatrics, 1988; NAACOG, 1988).

Court cases clarify the standard for fetal evaluation during labor. In *Williams v. Lallie Kemp Charity Hospital* (1983), the fetus presented in a breech position. A medical student auscultated the fetal heart rate only twice before delivery. X-ray pelvimetry was improperly interpreted. The physician performed a complete breech extraction and had difficulty clearing the after-coming head from the birth canal. Asphyxiated at birth, the child was deaf, blind, and a spastic quadriplegic at the time of the trial. The jury awarded the child a total of $500,000 (the statutory maximum). An appeals court also found the health care facility at fault for its failure "to adequately monitor this child, either manually or mechanically, in accordance with clearly recognized standards of care."

Professional standards—such as the NAACOG statement about intrapartal fetal monitoring (NAACOG, 1988)—and court cases make clear that when an electronic fetal monitor is used, nurses (and physicians) must be competent to interpret the tracing. Nurses should record their interpretations of the tracing on the labor record and use the proper descriptive terms for patterns. When disagreement exists or could arise over the pattern interpretation (usually when the patterns are subtle), the record should describe the declines or should characterize the pattern seen.

Although fetal monitor strips may not be stored with the client's medical record (because they are bulky unless microfilmed), the staff should ensure that strips are properly labeled with the client's name and date and safely filed. The strips can be used for staff education sessions, but the staff must remember to return the strips to the proper file.

A threatening decline in fetal heart rate requires the nurse to take appropriate action (such as turning the client or administering oxygen) and to notify the responsible physician promptly. The medical record should reflect nursing interventions, physician notification, and the physician's response. If the physician does not respond to a serious problem, the nurse is legally obligated to notify a supervisor, who must then arrange appropriate emergency care for the client. In cases where the nurse considers a physician's management of a client unsafe, the nurse is obligated to try to convince the physician to change the orders. The nursing staff also is obligated to follow health care facility policy and summon another designated physician to review the case.

Concerns for the sick neonate

Congenital defects and diseases can range from minor to multiple and potentially fatal. Specific parental consent is not required for every procedure performed on a neonate. However, surgery and invasive radiology—either of which could harm the neonate—warrant written consent from a parent or legal guardian.

In most cases, parents may not decline standard medical care potentially helpful to their child. For example, if a child is born with a single, surgically correctable problem, a court most likely would order the procedure despite parental objection. However, before the state may override parental authority, it must show that the parents do not represent the child's best interest and that the child probably will suffer harm as a result.

If the child has multiple defects, the situation may differ somewhat. At the federal level, considerable controvery exists over treatment of severely disabled neonates. States must adhere to "Baby Doe" regulations if they expect federal funding under the Child Abuse Protection and Treatment Act. Only Pennsylvania and Indiana have refused funding, thus avoiding the federal regulations. These regulations typically require treatment for neonates with life-threatening conditions except when the neonate is chronically and irreversibly comatose or when treatment would be ineffective or merely prolong dying (Department of Health and Human Services, 1985).

A recent study of the usefulness of the federal regulations has revealed that many neonatologists believe the regulations interfere with parents' rights to determine the best interests of their child. The physicians also claim that the regulations pay too little heed to neonatal suffering (Kopelman, Irons, and Kopelman, 1988).

In addition to the federal regulations, professional organizations have developed statements intended to guide physicians and nurses in making decisions about disabled neonates. One of the most influential has been "Principles of Treatment of Disabled Infants," which was developed by several groups, including the American Academy of Pediatrics, the Association for Retarded Citizens, and the Spina Bifida Association of America. The statement opposes treatment decisions influenced by considerations of limited present or future resources or of limited individual potential. Further, the statement asserts that an infant's disability must not form the basis of a decision to withhold treatment (American Academy of Pediatrics, 1984).

Ethical discussion continues in the literature about whether and how to treat the multiply disabled neonate. Euthanasia is not now considered legally acceptable, but some commentators argue that it should be (Fletcher, 1987-88).

Chapter summary

Chapter 5 presented some of the ethical and legal concerns that attend maternal, neonatal, and women's health care. Here are the chapter highlights.

• Ethics attempts to identify, organize, analyze, and justify human acts by applying certain principles to determine what is right in a certain situation. Whether these principles are based on professional duty (deontological) or the possible outcomes of the actions taken (teleological), an ethical decision typically requires balancing conflicts between personal rights.

• Laws, which are imposed by legislative and judicial bodies, typically stem from historical interpretations of right and wrong. Ideally, laws reflect a society's collective ethical standards; however, not all ethical questions are addressed by laws, particularly questions related to new technology. Furthermore, laws cannot represent the individual beliefs of all of a society's members. Therefore, even when laws address an ethical point, the nurse still must make a personal decision.

• The nurse should base ethical decisions on three principles: respect for the individual (support of the client's right to decide ethical questions for herself), beneficence (avoiding harming anyone and actively promoting or doing good), and justice (fair and equitable allocation of services and resources).

• Because states' nurse practice acts rarely endorse or prohibit specific nursing functions, the nurse should look to professional standards for practical and ethical help. The American Nurses' Association and the International Council of Nursing have published professional codes of ethics that provide more specific actions for the nurse. Also, other groups have published information helpful in determining practice standards, such as the NAACOG (the organization for obstetric, gynecologic, and neonatal nurses) guidelines for nurse providers of intrapartal care.

• From a liability standpoint, obstetrics is a high-risk practice because it may involve both the client's health and the life-long health of her child. Legal actions against nurses are common, and the trend is for the individual nurse to be named as the defendant. Risk management has been developed to accomplish three main goals: to reduce the number and severity of client, visitor, and employee injuries; to ensure that client care is sufficiently documented so that any malpractice claim easily can be defended; and to protect the health care provider and health care facility against financial loss by ensuring adequate professional and general liability insurance. However, the best defense against legal action is delivery of high-quality nursing care.

• The nurse providing maternal and neonatal care may deal with various ethical and legal issues, such as confidentiality, treatment refusal, sterilization, and infertility and the related subjects of in vitro fertilization and embryo transfer and surrogate motherhood. Other ethical issues include those of early pregnancy, such as prenatal diagnostic testing and abortion, and of later pregnancy, such as client refusal of cesarian delivery, fetal research, and fetal therapy.

• Ethical issues may arise in the case of a sick neonate. Several professional groups have developed statements to guide physicians and nurses in the treatment of disabled neonates; one of the most influential, "Principles of Treatment of Disabled Infants," discourages basing treatment decisions on considerations of limited resources or individual potential and asserts that a disability should not form the basis of a decision to withhold treatment.

Study questions

1. To which three ethical principles should a nurse always attempt to adhere?

2. Which influencing factors should the nurse consider when making an ethical decision?

3. How do state nurse practice acts differ from codes or professional standards?

4. Which goals can risk management techniques help the nurse achieve?

5. Which risk management actions are necessary when the nurse cannot follow or refuses to follow physician orders?

6. Why are ethical issues involved in procedures currently used to counteract infertility?

7. Which risk management steps must the nurse take when engaged in fetal monitoring during labor?

Bibliography

American Fertility Society. (1988). Revised new guidelines for the use of semen-donor insemination. *Fertility and Sterility*, 49, 211.

American Nurses' Association. (1985). *Code for Nurses*. Kansas City, MO: Author.

American Nurses' Association. (1980). *A statement on the scope of maternal and child health nursing practice*. Washington, DC: Author.

Benshoof, J., and Philpel, H. (1986). Minor's rights to confidential abortions: The evolving legal scene. In J.D. Butler and D.F. Walbert (Eds.), *Abortion, medicine and the law* (3rd ed.; pp. 137-160). New York: Facts on File Publications.

Charo, R.A. (1988). Legislative approach to surrogate motherhood. *Law, Medicine & Health Care*, 16(1-2), 96-112.

Department of Health and Human Services. (1985). Child abuse and neglect prevention and treatment program. *Federal Register*, 50, 14878-14901.

Gould, S.J. (1987). *The flamingo's smile—Reflections in natural history*. New York: Norton.

Holder, A. (1988). Surrogate motherhood and the best interests of children. *Law, Medicine & Health Care*, 16(1-2), 51-56.

International Council of Nurses. (1973). *Code for Nurses. Ethical Concepts Applied to Nursing*. Geneva, Switzerland: Author.

Kolder, V., Gallagher, J., and Parsons, M. (1987). Court-ordered obstetrical interventions. *New England Journal of Medicine,* 316(19), 1192-1196.

Kopelman, L.M., Irons, T.G., and Kopelman, A.E. (1988). Neonatologists judge the "Baby Doe" regulations. *New England Journal of Medicine,* 318(11), 677-683.

Shapiro, H.I. (1988). *The new birth control book.* New York: Prentice-Hall.

Strong, C., and Schinfeld, J.S. (1984). The single woman and artificial insemination by donor. *Journal of Reproductive Medicine,* 29(5), 293-299.

Weaver, D. (1988). A survey of prenatally diagnosed disorders. *Clinical Obstetrics and Gynecology,* 31(2), 253-269.

Ethics

American College of Obstetricians and Gynecologists: Committee on Ethics. (1987) *Patient Choice: Maternal and fetal conflict.* Washington, DC: Author.

Applegate, M.L., and Entrekin, N.M. (1984). *Teaching ethics in nursing.* New York: National League for Nursing.

Ashley, B.M., and O'Rourke, K.D. (1986). *Ethics of health care.* St. Louis: Catholic Health Association.

Beauchamp, T. (1982). *Philosophical ethics. An introduction to moral philosophy.* New York: McGraw-Hill.

Bunting, S., and Webb, A. (1988). An ethical model for decision-making. *Nurse Practitioner,* 13(12), 30-34.

Closen, M.L., and Isaacman, S.H. (1988). The duty to notify private third parties of the risks of HIV infection. *Journal of Health and Hospital Law,* 21, 295-303.

Curtin, L., and Flaherty, J.M. (1982). *Nursing ethics, theories and pragmatics.* Bowie, MD: Brady Publications.

Jansen, R. (1987). Ethics in infertility treatment. In R. Pepperell, B. Hudson, and C. Wood (Eds.), *The infertile couple* (2nd ed.; pp. 346-387). Edinburgh: Churchill Livingstone.

Macklin, R. (1988). Is there anything wrong with surrogate motherhood? An ethical analysis. *Law, Medicine & Health Care,* 16(1-2), 57-64.

Thompson, J.B., and Thompson, H.O. (1981). *Ethics in nursing.* New York: Macmillan.

U.S. Congress, Office of Technology Assessment. (1988). *Artificial insemination.* Washington, DC: U.S. Government Printing Office.

U.S. Congress, Office of Technology Assessment. (1988). *Infertility: Medical and Social Choices.* Washington, DC: U.S. Government Printing Office.

Law

American College of Obstetricians and Gynecologists. (1988). *Professional liability and its effects: Report of a 1987 survey of ACOG's membership.* Washington, DC: Author.

Belitsky, R., and Solomon, R. (1987). Doctors and patients: Responsibilities in a confidential relationship. In H. Dalton and S. Buriss (Eds.), *AIDS and the law: A guide for the public* (pp. 201-209). New Haven, CT: Yale University Press.

Brescia, R. (1985). Statement of Nurses' Association of the American College of Obstetricians and Gynecologists. In *A forum on malpractice issues of childbirth proceedings.* Minneapolis: International Childbirth Education.

Creighton, H. (1986). *Law every nurse should know* (5th ed.). Philadelphia: Saunders.

Fletcher, J. (1987-88). The courts and euthanasia. *Law, Medicine & Health Care,* 15(4), 223-230.

Holder, A. (1985). *Legal issues in pediatrics and adolescent medicine* (2nd ed.). New Haven, CT: Yale University Press

In the Matter of Baby M., 525 A. 2d 1128, 217 N.J. Super. 313 (Superior Ct. Chancery Div. 1987), reversed on appeal 109 N.J. 396, 537 A. 2d 1227 (1988).

Jefferson v. Griffin Spaulding County Hospital Authority, 274 S.E. 2d 457 (Ga. 1981).

Morgentaler, Smoling, and Scott v. The Queen, 44 D.L.R. 4th (Canada, 1988).

Nelson v. Trinity Medical Center, 419 N.W. 2d 886 (n.D. 1988).

Planned Parenthood of Central Missouri v. Danforth, 428 U.S. 52 (1976)

Roe v. Wade, 410 U.S. 113 (1973).

Webster v. Reproductive Health Services. 109 S. Ct. 3040 (1989).

Williams v. Lallie Kemp Charity Hospital, 428 S. 2d 1000 (La. App. 1 Cir. 1983).

Standards

American Academy of Pediatrics, Joint Policy Statement. Principles of treatment of disabled infants. (1984). *Pediatrics,* 73, 559.

American College of Obstetricians and Gynecologists and American Academy of Pediatrics. (1988). *Guidelines for perinatal care* (2nd ed.).

NAACOG. (1986). Electronic fetal monitoring: Nursing practice competencies and educational guidelines. Washington, DC: Author.

NAACOG. (1988). Nursing responsibilities in implementing intrapartum fetal heart rate monitoring. Washington, DC: Author.

Nursing research

Anema, M.G. (1989). Ethical considerations in conducting nursing research. *Dimensions in Critical Care Nursing,* 8(5), 288-296.

Omery, A., and Caswell, D. (1989). Ethical perspectives. *Critical Care Clinics of North America,* 1(1), 165-173.

Price, B. (1989). The theory path of nursing research...ethical dilemmas. *Nursing Times,* 85(23), 62-63.

Renfrew, M. (1989). Ethics and morality in midwifery research. *Midwives Chronicles,* 102(1217), 198-202.

Women's Health Care

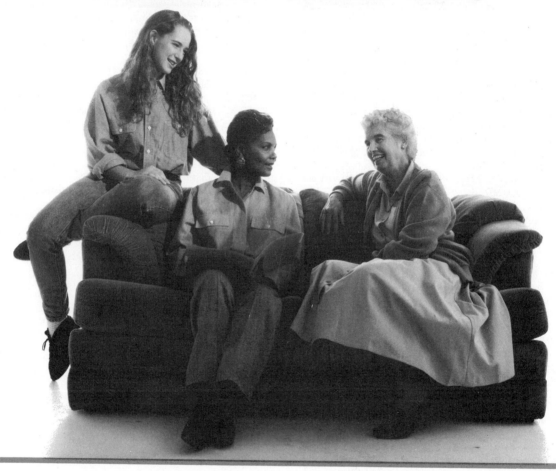

This unit explores the basic health concerns that bring women into contact with health care professionals—sexuality; health promotion; reproduction and family planning; genetic, infectious, and gynecologic disorders; violence; and health-compromising behaviors. One or a combination of these topics can affect a client's health and health needs.

To provide the knowledge base essential to a thorough understanding of the health issues discussed in this unit, the first chapter surveys reproductive anatomy and physiology. The remaining chapters provide basic information about a specific aspect of women's health, presenting this information in a nursing process framework. To demonstrate how to integrate assessment findings and document nursing care, these remaining chapters include charts that apply the nursing process to case studies.

Chapter 6
Reproductive Anatomy and Physiology

Chapter 6 reviews the anatomy and physiology of the female and male reproductive systems. It begins with the female, describing and illustrating the structure and function of the external and internal genitalia, bony pelvis, pelvic floor, and related pelvic structures. It then discusses breast development, innervation, and blood supply and traces the female reproductive cycle from menarche through menopause, describes the phases of the ovarian and endometrial cycles, and examines hormonal regulation of the reproductive cycle.

Chapter 6 then describes and illustrates the external and internal male genital structures and reviews sexual development, spermatogenesis, and hormonal regulation.

Chapter 7
Women's Health Promotion

Chapter 7 reviews the circumstances and attitudes influencing a client's contact with the health care system and investigates gynecologic needs across the life span, highlighting problems faced by the adolescent client approaching menarche and the adult client approaching menopause.

Next, the chapter presents a thorough discussion of assessment, posing health history questions that investigate health promotion and protection behaviors. It explains how to conduct the physical examination; notes the developmental variations to consider during assessment; and describes the educational pelvic examination (for the client who wants to learn about her reproductive anatomy). It includes illustrated procedures for examining the breasts and genitals and for bimanual palpation of the internal genitalia. The chapter reviews the diagnostic tests used to evaluate gynecologic status, including culture studies, mammography, transillumination, and colposcopy.

Chapter 8
Sexuality Concerns

Chapter 8 begins with the four-phase sexual response cycle described by Masters and Johnson and the response cycle described by the American Psychiatric Association. It then explores sexuality and its wide-ranging variations across the life span, highlighting sexual response and sexual activity during pregnancy and the postpartal period.

Next, Chapter 8 presents guidelines for reducing uneasiness during the health history interview; then it provides instructions for obtaining the sexual health history and exploring possible sexual dysfunction in a sensitive manner. It summarizes the physical and psychogenic causes of dysfunction, including sexual desire disorders, sexual arousal disorders, orgasmic disorders, and sexual pain disorders. After presenting relevant nursing diagnoses, the chapter provides appropriate planning and implementation information.

Chapter 9
Family Planning

Chapter 9 focuses on the role of the nurse in helping clients explore family planning goals and make decisions. The chapter explains how to keep personal beliefs from influencing nursing care for the client seeking family planning assistance, and it elaborates on the various roles of the nurse who assists with family planning—teacher, counselor, advocate, and researcher. The chapter features a comprehensive review of contraceptive methods and detailed client teaching information for many of these methods.

The chapter then addresses nursing care for the client requesting pregnancy interruption, describing abortion methods and pertinent preoperative and postoperative care. Finally, it discusses sterilization techniques and presents nursing care for female and male clients requesting sterilization.

Chapter 10
Fertility and Infertility

Chapter 10 prepares the nurse to assist clients with preconception planning and to care for clients who need help in conceiving a child or in coping with infertility. It begins by surveying the physiology of male and female fertility and exploring cultural myths and beliefs about fertility. Then, the chapter presents nursing interventions for the client who decides to conceive, including teaching about self-care, nutrition, and discontinuation of contraception.

Chapter 10 then addresses care for the infertile couple, highlighting diagnostic studies that determine the cause of infertility, describing infertility treatments for female and male clients, discussing artificial insemination, and outlining interventions for the couple for whom such treatments fail.

Chapter 11
Genetics and Genetic Disorders

Chapter 11 explains genetic factors that cause risk for the fetus, informs about the tests that identify some disorders, and helps the nurse improve parental understanding of the neonate with a genetic disorder. It focuses first on gametogenesis, the process through which genetic information is inherited, and then explains the Mendelian laws of inheritance. It highlights major characteristics of autosomal dominant, autosomal recessive, and X-linked recessive disorders. It presents a sample pedigree showing the occurrence of one or more genetic traits in different family members, illustrates the mechanisms of chromosomal abnormalities, and discusses the role of multifactorial inheritance in some congenital malformations. It also discusses genetic counseling, describing the roles of the nurse and specialists.

Chapter 12
Infectious Disorders

Chapter 12 prepares the nurse to help clients prevent or deal with an infectious disorder. It begins by describing the incidence of and transmission routes and risk factors for sexually transmitted diseases (STDs), gynecologic infections, and other genitourinary infections. It includes charts that compare clinical findings and treatments for various infections.

Chapter 12 shows the nurse how to integrate knowledge of infectious disorders into the nursing process. It offers a detailed discussion of areas to explore during the health history, such as sexuality and social support patterns. It discusses relevant diagnostic tests, including tests for the virus that causes acquired immunodeficiency syndrome. Turning to planning and implementation for the client with an infectious disorder, the chapter describes relevant teaching topics and strategies, and it provides information on other nursing interventions, such as infection control measures, referrals, emotional support, and family care. The chapter presents information on universal infection control precautions, provides charts on drugs used to treat STDs, and offers pertinent client-teaching aids.

Chapter 13
Gynecologic Disorders

Chapter 13 surveys common gynecologic disorders—those that represent normal variations as well as those arising secondary to infection, aging, or serious disease. First, it focuses on breast disorders, describing fibrocystic breast changes and other benign disorders. Then it discusses breast cancer, identifying its etiology and touching on associated clinical findings and treatments. It includes illustrations of breast surgery techniques and a chart of the stages of breast cancer.

Next, Chapter 13 discusses menstrual disorders, defining each disorder and showing how to apply the nursing process when caring for the client with such a disorder. It includes a chart comparing the etiology, clinical findings, and treatments for common menstrual disorders and provides teaching aids to help the client manage premenstrual syndrome. After reviewing and illustrating pelvic support disorders, Chapter 13 describes gynecologic cancer, elaborates on its treatments, and explains appropriate nursing care.

Chapter 14
Violence Against Women

Chapter 14 investigates nursing care for female survivors of abuse and rape, emphasizing ways the nurse can promote a healthier self-concept among such survivors. After defining and comparing abuse and rape and presenting related legal issues, it reviews myths about rape, explains the cycle of violence theory, and discusses rape-trauma syndrome.

Next, the chapter explains how to use self-assessment to screen for feelings that could prevent a therapeutic relationship with such a client. Then it shows how to tailor the assessment to the client's physical and emotional status, presenting a detailed description of physical examination of the rape survivor and emphasizing how to collect evidence in accordance with legal requirements.

Chapter 14 then discusses planning and implementation of care. For the survivor of abuse, it points out the need to involve the client in setting goals and to offer emotional support, then instructs the nurse in making referrals to appropriate sources of help and in providing care for the client's family. For the rape survivor, the chapter describes appropriate client teaching about pregnancy and STD prevention, and it explains how to provide rape counseling and family care.

Chapter 15
Women's Health-Compromising Behaviors

Chapter 15 investigates behaviors that threaten a woman's health, showing how the nurse can guide clients to promote their own health. It begins by exploring nutrition-related health issues, including inadequate diet, obesity, and eating disorders. Then it focuses on substance abuse, detailing the behaviors and defense mechanisms typical of substance-dependent clients and describing the properties of various addictive substances. The chapter presents charts clarifying the effects of smoking and comparing clinical features and treatment for each type of abused substance. Next, the chapter discusses the stressors that typically affect women and describes coping mechanisms for stress.

Chapter 15 then presents assessment questions that yield information about the client's nutritional concerns, substance abuse, or stress level. It offers guidelines for helping the client develop a self-care approach that increases her self-esteem. It explains how to teach the client about nutrition, exercise, smoking cessation, and stress management, and it offers guidelines for making appropriate referrals and caring for the client's family. It includes client-teaching aids on food, exercise, and tension relief.

Reproductive Anatomy and Physiology

Objectives

After reading and studying this chapter, the student should be able to:

1. Describe the structures and functions of the external and internal female genitalia.

2. Discuss hormonal regulation of the female reproductive cycle.

3. List the functions of estrogen and progesterone.

4. Describe the menstrual cycle.

5. Describe the structures and functions of the external and internal male genitalia.

6. Discuss hormonal regulation of the male reproductive system.

7. Describe spermatogenesis.

Introduction

Whatever the practice setting, every nurse will encounter clients concerned about reproduction and sexuality issues, such as family planning, contraception, fertility and infertility, premenstrual syndrome, sexually transmitted diseases, and sexual violence. The nurse will need in-depth knowledge of reproductive system anatomy and physiology to provide effective nursing care for such clients. This chapter reviews the structure, function, and hormonal control of the female and male reproductive systems and provides a nursing framework for assessing a client's reproductive and sexual health, identifying related problems, and developing an appropriate plan of care.

Female reproductive system

The female reproductive system includes the external and internal genitalia and the accessory organs, the breasts. (For illustrations of external and internal genitalia, see *Female genitalia,* pages 86 and 87.) The genitalia and their related structures respond to sexual stimulation, facilitate reproduction, and produce several hormones that regulate the development of female secondary sex characteristics, the reproductive cycle, and the physiologic changes associated with pregnancy and childbirth.

External genitalia

The *vulva* consists of the female external genitalia that are visible on inspection: the mons pubis, labia majora, labia minora, clitoris, ducts from Skene's (paraurethral) glands and Bartholin's (vulvovaginal) glands, vaginal orifice, hymen, fossa navicularis, and fourchette.

Mons pubis

Sometimes called the mons veneris, the mons pubis is a rounded cushion of adipose and loose connective tissue that covers the symphysis pubis (the anterior articulation of the four pelvic bones). Coarse hair begins to grow on the mons pubis at age 11 or 12, or approximately 2 years before menarche. The pattern of pubic hair growth (escutcheon) usually is triangular but may be diamond-

GLOSSARY

Androgens: class of hormone that stimulates the development of male secondary sex characteristics, such as facial hair and increased musculature.

Anovulatory: failure of the ovary to produce, mature, or release an ovum.

Climacteric: period of physiologic and psychological changes that occur toward the end of the female reproductive stage; may occur in males as sexual activity decreases with age.

Ejaculation: forceful expulsion of semen through the penile urethra.

Graafian follicle: mature ovarian vesicle located near the ovarian surface that contains an ovum. In response to hormonal stimulation during the menstrual cycle, the ovum matures and the vesicle ruptures.

Hymen: fold of membranous tissue that occludes or partially blocks the vaginal orifice.

Hysterectomy: surgical removal of the uterus.

Menarche: first menstruation; commencement of menstrual function.

Menopause: last menstruation; cessation of menstrual function.

Menstruation: cyclic discharge of blood and mucosal tissue from the uterus between menarche and menopause, except during pregnancy or lactation.

Ovaries: female gonads; glands located on each side of the pelvis that contain ova and secrete the hormones estrogen and progesterone.

Ovulation: maturation and discharge of an ovum from the ovary in response to hormonal stimulation during the menstrual cycle.

Papanicolaou smear: cytologic study of stained exfoliated cells to detect and diagnose certain conditions in the female reproductive tract, particularly premalignant and malignant conditions, such as cancer of the vagina, cervix, and endometrium.

Parity: obstetric classification of a woman by the number of births and stillbirths occurring after 28 weeks of gestation.

Puberty: developmental stage early in adolescence when reproductive ability begins and secondary sex characteristics develop.

Semen: white, viscous secretion of male reproductive organs consisting of spermatozoa and nutrient fluids that is ejaculated through the penile urethra.

Spermatogenesis: formation and maturation of spermatozoa.

Testes: male gonads; reproductive glands contained in the scrotum that produce sperm and the androgenic hormone testosterone.

shaped as growth extends to the umbilicus along the linea alba (the tendinous median line on the anterior abdominal wall). During the climacteric, the mons pubis becomes less pronounced with the loss of adipose tissue and thinning of pubic hair.

Labia majora

These two raised folds of adipose and connective tissue covered by skin taper down and back from the mons pubis to the perineum (muscle, fascia, and ligaments between the anus and vulva). After menarche, pubic hair covers the outer surface. The inner surface is pink and moist and resembles a mucous membrane. The labia majora of a neonate may appear engorged from maternal estrogen influence in utero. In a child and a nulliparous woman, the labia majora usually lie close together, completely covering underlying structures. However, the labia majora of a multiparous woman may lose tone and separate after childbirth. During the climacteric, the labia atrophy and become less prominent.

Because the labia majora are highly vascular, varicosities and hematomas commonly develop during pregnancy and childbirth as well as after obstetric or sexual trauma. The labia majora also contain many nerve endings, which make them sensitive to pain, pressure, touch,

temperature extremes, and sexual stimulation. Innervation originates in the S3 and L1 vertebral areas.

Labia minora

These two thin, pink, moist cutaneous tissue folds are situated between the labia majora. Each has an upper and lower section. Each upper section divides into an upper and lower *lamella*. The two upper lamellae join to form the *prepuce*, the hoodlike covering over the clitoris. The two lower lamellae form the *frenulum*, the posterior portion of the clitoris. The lower labial sections taper down and back from the clitoris to the perineum, where they meet to form the *fourchette*, a thin transverse tissue fold along the anterior edge of the perineum. Devoid of pubic hair, the labia minora contain sebaceous glands that secrete a lubricant that also acts as a bacteriocide.

The labia minora contain a rich vascular supply and many nerve endings, making them highly responsive to irritation and stimulation. In response to sexual stimulation, they swell and become more sensitive. This response stimulates other physiologic changes that prepare the genitalia for coitus.

In preterm neonates, the labia minora typically are larger than and protrude between the labia majora. In term neonates, children, and adults, the labia minora usually lie beneath the labia majora or protrude slightly. During the climacteric, they atrophy and become less pronounced.

Clitoris

The most sexually sensitive female genital structure, the clitoris is composed of highly vascular and innervated erectile tissue. It has two parts: the *glans*, highly innervated tissue at the tip of the clitoris, and the *corpus*, the body of the clitoris. Innervation for the clitoris stems from the pudendal nerve terminal branch next to the dorsal artery. Nerve branches terminate in the glans and prepuce. The glans is covered by stratified epithelium and contains a dense configuration of nerve endings, making it far more sensitive to stimulation than the corpus.

In its unstimulated state, the clitoris is almost totally covered by the prepuce. Sebaceous glands under the prepuce secrete smegma, a cheeselike, odorous substance.

When stimulated, the clitoris becomes engorged with blood and protrudes beyond the prepuce. In the neonate, the clitoris sometimes appears engorged—a normal consequence of maternal estrogen influence in utero.

Vestibule

This ovoid area of the external genitalia, bounded anteriorly by the clitoris, laterally by the labia minora, and posteriorly by the fourchette, is visible when the labia majora are separated. The thin vestibular floor is susceptible to irritation from chemicals, heat, discharges, or friction. Several internal structures open into the vestibule, including the urethra, the vagina, and ducts from Skene's and Bartholin's glands.

The *urethral meatus* is the opening through which urine leaves the body. This slitlike opening below the clitoris typically appears pink, puckered, and slightly elevated. Innervation stems from the sacral plexus along the perineal nerve.

Ducts from *Skene's glands*, located in spongy tissue on either side of the urethral meatus, open into the posterior wall of the urethra. Secretions from these glands help lubricate the vestibule during sexual stimulation.

Ducts from *Bartholin's glands*, the two small vulvovaginal glands located deep in the perineal structures, open into the lateral margins of the vaginal orifice. The alkaline mucus secreted by these glands lubricates the orifice and vaginal mucosa and provides a medium that promotes spermatozoa viability and motility during coitus.

The *vaginal orifice* lies in the center of the vestibule, between the urethral meatus and the fossa navicularis. A membranous fold, the *hymen* partially covers or occludes the vaginal orifice. Age, coitus, and parity affect its size and thickness. For example, the hymen of a neonate is vascular and projects beyond immediate structures, while the hymen of a virgin adult is avascular, has few nerve fibers, and is typically a circular or crescent-shaped partial covering of the vaginal orifice.

Although hymen rupture may occur during first coitus, many other factors can cause rupture, such as strenuous exercise or activity, tampon insertion, masturbation, or assault or injury. In rare instances, the hymen cannot be penetrated by the penis and must be broken by hymenotomy (surgical rupture of the hymen). After rupturing, the hymen forms irregular edges around the vaginal orifice known as hymenal tags (carunculae myrtiformes).

The *fossa navicularis* forms a slight depression or pitted area between the vaginal orifice and the fourchette.

Perineum

This complex structure of muscles, fascia, blood vessels, nerves, and lymphatics lies between the lower vagina and the anal canal. The base of the perineum rests between the fourchette and anus. During childbirth, the perineum may be stretched severely and may tear.

Internal genitalia

The female internal genitalia are highly specialized organs with one primary function: reproduction. They include the vagina, uterus, fallopian tubes, ovaries, and related structures. Hormones, especially estrogen and progesterone, regulate their development and function. Their blood supply passes through a network of arteries and veins, and innervation is provided through the autonomic nervous system. (For an illustration and details, see *Blood supply and innervation to the female pelvis*, page 89.)

Vagina

This highly elastic muscular tube extending up and back from the vaginal orifice to the uterus is situated between the bladder and rectum along the midline of the body. The vagina has several functions. During coitus, it accommodates the penis. During menstruation, blood and decidua discharged from the uterus pass through the vagina. During childbirth, it is the birth canal. Hormonal stimulation regulates most aspects of vaginal development and function.

(Text continues on page 88.)

Female genitalia

These illustrations show the external and internal genitalia of the mature female.

External genitalia

The vulva contains the external genitalia visible on inspection. The mons pubis is a cushion of adipose and connective tissue covered by skin and coarse hair. The labia majora border the vulva laterally from the mons pubis to the perineum. Two moist mucosal folds—the labia minora—lie within and alongside the labia majora and appear darker pink to red.

The introitus (vaginal orifice) and urethral meatus become visible when the labia are spread. Less easily visible are Skene's gland orifices. Bartholin's glands are located laterally and posteriorly on either side of the inner vaginal orifice. The hymen may partially or completely cover the vaginal opening.

Internal genitalia

The vagina, an elastic muscular tube, lies between the urethra and the rectum. The uterus lies between the bladder and the rectum. The uterine corpus is composed of three tissue layers. The *perimetrium*, part of the peritoneum, is the outermost layer.

The middle layer, the *myometrium*, contains three types of muscle tissue. First are longitudinal fibers that contract to help expel the fetus. Second are fibers that wrap around larger blood vessels and ligate them during placental separation. Third are fibers that encircle the fallopian tube exits and the internal cervical os to prevent regurgitation of menstrual flow.

The inner layer of the uterine corpus, the *endometrium*, contains columnar epithelial glands and stromal cells. The endometrium responds to hormonal stimulation and, from menarche to menopause, undergoes monthly degeneration and renewal except during pregnancy.

Two fallopian tubes attach to the uterus at the upper angle of the fundus. Usually nonpalpable, these slender tubes have distal fingerlike projections, called fimbriae, that partially surround the ovaries. Fertilization of the ovum usually occurs in the outer third of the fallopian tube.

Palpable, almond-shaped organs, the ovaries usually lie near the lateral pelvic walls, a little below the anterosuperior iliac spine.

EXTERNAL GENITALIA

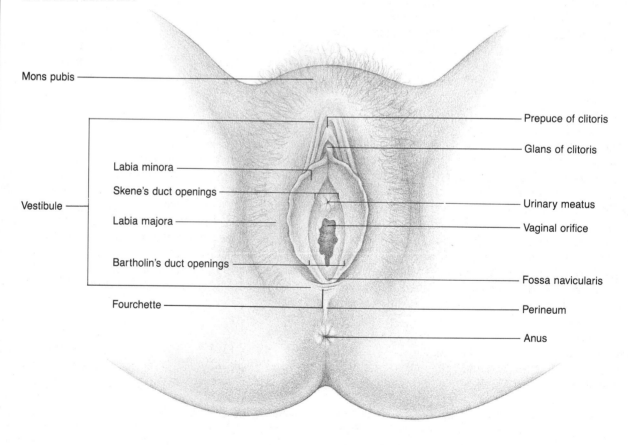

Mons pubis

Vestibule

Labia minora

Skene's duct openings

Labia majora

Bartholin's duct openings

Fourchette

Prepuce of clitoris

Glans of clitoris

Urinary meatus

Vaginal orifice

Fossa navicularis

Perineum

Anus

INTERNAL GENITALIA—LATERAL VIEW

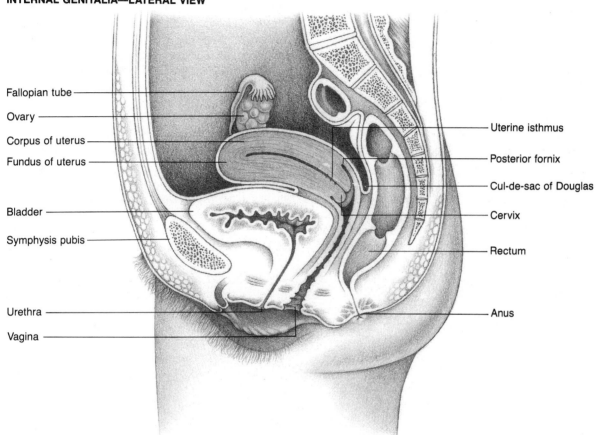

Fallopian tube

Ovary

Corpus of uterus

Fundus of uterus

Bladder

Symphysis pubis

Urethra

Vagina

Uterine isthmus

Posterior fornix

Cul-de-sac of Douglas

Cervix

Rectum

Anus

INTERNAL GENITALIA—ANTERIOR CROSS-SECTIONAL VIEW

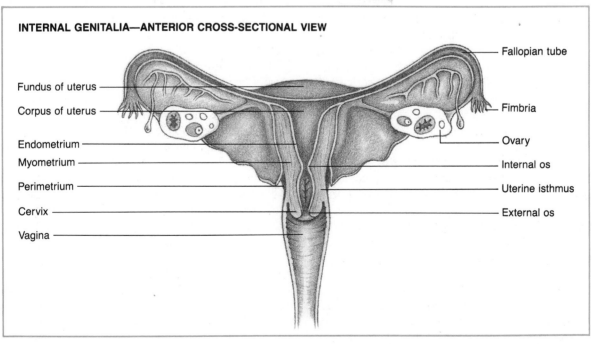

Fundus of uterus

Corpus of uterus

Endometrium

Myometrium

Perimetrium

Cervix

Vagina

Fallopian tube

Fimbria

Ovary

Internal os

Uterine isthmus

External os

Structure and function. The uterine cervix connects the uterus to the vaginal vault. Surrounding the cervix are four *fornices* or recesses in the vaginal wall: one anterior, two lateral, and one posterior. Thin connective tissue separates the fornices from surrounding organs. The deep posterior fornix aids impregnation by holding a reservoir of ejaculated semen close to the cervix.

The vaginal wall has three tissue layers: epithelial tissue, loose connective tissue, and muscle tissue. The epithelial layer is nonstratified squamous epithelium. Along the anterior and posterior vaginal walls, this layer contains rugae (transverse ridges), which allow the vagina to distend and stretch during coitus and childbirth.

Beneath the epithelium lies a thin layer of highly vascular connective tissue. The blood supply in this layer nourishes the underlying musculofascial layer and provides nutrients to the epithelial cells.

Two layers of smooth muscle, continuations of uterine superficial muscle fibers, form the inner musculofascial layer of the vaginal wall. The outer layer contains longitudinal muscle fibers; the inner layer, circular muscle fibers. The musculofascial layer firmly attaches the vaginal vault to the cervix.

Vaginal secretions should be slightly acidic. Acidity and alkalinity are measured on a pH scale of 0 to 14, with pH 7 as neutral. Values below 7 indicate increasing acidity; those above 7, increasing alkalinity. For example, pH 6.5 is slightly acidic, and pH 7.5 is slightly alkaline. The acidity of vaginal secretions is important because the incidence of pathogenic bacterial infections increases when the pH rises above 5.

Vaginal acidity is regulated by an interaction of lactobacillus and glycogen in the vagina. Secretions in the vagina begin neutral or slightly alkaline. When stimulated by hormones, glycogen is derived from the epithelial cells; it reacts with the lactobacillus to create lactic acid.

Age, menstrual cycle phase, and sexual activity affect vaginal acidity. Before menarche, normal vaginal pH ranges between 6.8 to 7.2. After menarche, vaginal pH ranges from 4 to 5 (Cunningham, MacDonald, and Gant, 1989). During the menstrual cycle, vaginal acidity is lowest at midcycle and highest just before menstruation. During sexual arousal, Bartholin's glands secrete an alkaline mucus which helps lubricate the vagina. During pregnancy, vaginal secretions increase and vaginal pH ranges between 3.5 and 6, significantly reducing the risk of infection. In a postmenopausal or elderly woman, vaginal pH is typically neutral or alkaline.

Support. The vagina is separated from adjacent structures by connective tissue. The *vesicovaginal septum* separates it from the bladder and urethra, and the *rectovaginal septum* separates it from the lower rectum.

Above the rectovaginal septum, a thin muscular wall separates the vagina from the cul-de-sac of Douglas, a pouch in the peritoneum between the rectum and vagina.

Ligaments and muscles attached to the vaginal wall by pelvic fascia support each section of the vagina. The levator ani muscle provides primary support and controls the vaginal orifice. The upper vagina receives added support from the transverse cervical, pubocervical, and sacrocervical ligaments. The middle vagina is supported by the urogenital diaphragm; the lower vagina, by the perineum.

Innervation and blood supply. Vaginal innervation is primarily autonomic. The vagina has relatively few specialized nerve endings. Sensory nerves begin in the vagina and terminate at the S2 through S4 level. The pudendal nerve provides minimal innervation to the lower vagina.

The upper, middle, and lower vaginal sections have separate vascularization. Blood flows to the upper vagina through branches of the uterine arteries; to the middle vagina through the inferior vesical arteries; and to the lower vagina through the hemorrhoidal and internal pudendal arteries. Venous blood returns through a vast venous plexus to the hemorrhoidal, pudendal, and uterine veins and then to the hypogastric veins. This plexus merges with the vertebral venous plexus.

Lymph drainage is similarly segregated. The upper vagina drains into the iliac lymph nodes; the middle, into the hypogastric lymph nodes; and the lower, into the inguinal lymph nodes. Separate drainage pathways for each section of the vagina influence how infections and cancerous cells spread to other areas.

Uterus

This hollow, pear-shaped organ with thick, muscular walls typically is situated along the midline of the body behind the symphysis pubis and bladder, above the vagina at the level of the pelvic brim, and in front of the rectum. During the reproductive cycle, hormones stimulate changes in the uterine lining that prepare it to receive a fertilized ovum. If ovum implantation occurs, the uterus maintains an environment conducive to fetal development. If implantation does not occur, the uterine lining is shed during menses. During childbirth, the uterine musculature provides the contractions that propel the fetus downward through the birth canal.

Structure and function. The uterus has three sections: the *corpus* or upper section; the *cervix*, the lower, constricted section that protrudes into the vagina; and the *isthmus*, a narrow segment connecting the corpus and cervix. The *fundus* is the rounded dome of the corpus that extends above the juncture with the fallopian tubes.

Blood supply and innervation to the female pelvis

Blood flows to and from the female pelvis via the ovarian artery and vein, uterine artery and vein, vaginal artery, inferior vesical artery and vein, and the hypogastric artery and vein. Innervation to the pelvis is provided through the autonomic nervous system. Sensory nerves begin in the vagina and terminate at the S2 to S4 level. The pudendal nerve provides minimal innervation to the lower vagina. Uterine innervation occurs through sympathetic nerve fibers that enter the pelvis through the hypogastric plexus and enter the uterus at the base of the uterosacral ligaments.

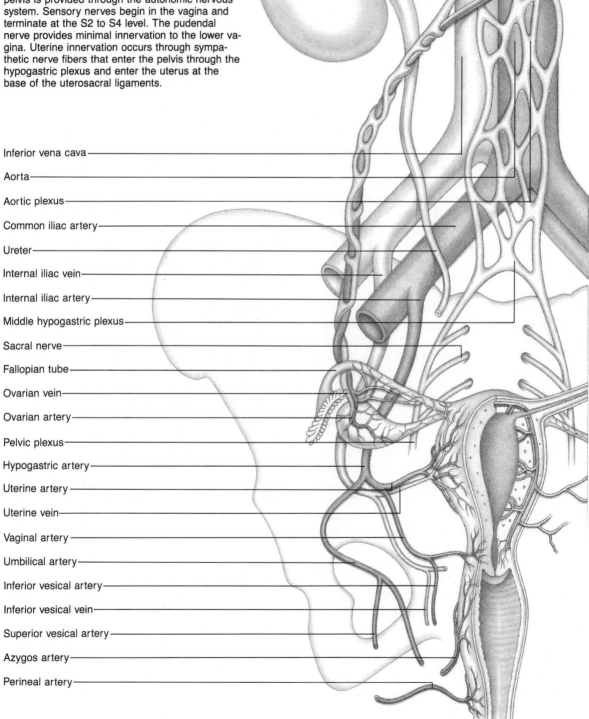

Inferior vena cava

Aorta

Aortic plexus

Common iliac artery

Ureter

Internal iliac vein

Internal iliac artery

Middle hypogastric plexus

Sacral nerve

Fallopian tube

Ovarian vein

Ovarian artery

Pelvic plexus

Hypogastric artery

Uterine artery

Uterine vein

Vaginal artery

Umbilical artery

Inferior vesical artery

Inferior vesical vein

Superior vesical artery

Azygos artery

Perineal artery

The corpus has three tissue layers: perimetrium, the outer, serosal layer; myometrium, the middle, muscular layer; and endometrium, the inner, mucosal layer. Each layer has a specific function.

The cervix, the part of the uterus that connects the uterine corpus and the vaginal canal, is composed of connective tissue, muscle cells, and elastic tissue. The fibrous and collagenous content of the supportive tissues and many rugae in the cervical canal lining make the cervix highly elastic, permitting the stretching necessary for fetal passage during labor.

The cervix projects into the upper portion of the vagina. The lower cervical opening is the *external os;* the upper one, the *internal os.* The channel between them is the cervical canal.

After menarche, the vaginal cervix is covered by stratified squamous epithelium, which is continuous with the vaginal lining. Tall, columnar cells that contain mucus-secreting glands line the supravaginal cervix. The squamous and columnar epithelium meet at a point known as the *squamocolumnar junction,* usually located at the external os or extending into the cervical area of the vagina, also known as the *transition zone.* Because the squamocolumnar junction is the site where cervical cancer usually begins, an examiner collects cells for the Papanicolaou (Pap) smear there.

Age and parity affect many uterine characteristics, including size, shape, weight, firmness, and the relative size of the corpus and cervix. The uterus of a neonate is 2.5 to 3.5 cm long. In a nulliparous woman, it is 5.5 to 8 cm long, 3.5 to 4 cm in diameter, and weighs between 50 and 70 g. In a multiparous woman, it is 9 to 10 cm long, 5.5 to 6 cm in diameter, and weighs 80 g or more (Cunningham, MacDonald, and Gant, 1989). After menopause, the entire uterus atrophies and shrinks.

In a child, the corpus makes up about one-third of the uterus; the cervix, two-thirds. In an adolescent, the corpus and cervix are of approximately equal size. In a multiparous adult, the corpus makes up two-thirds of the uterus; the cervix, one-third. (For more information and illustrations, see *Developmental changes in the uterus and cervix.*)

In an adult, the uterus normally is smooth, nontender, and firm to palpation. However, firmness varies with hormonal activity. For example, the uterus softens during the secretory phase of the menstrual cycle and during pregnancy, but becomes firmer during menopause.

The cervix is permanently altered by childbirth. In a nulliparous woman, the external os is a round opening about 3 mm in diameter; after the first childbirth, it becomes a small transverse slit with irregular edges.

Support. Although the cervix is anchored to the vagina, the corpus and fundus can move in the anteroposterior plane as well as laterally. The uterus is normally situated with the cervix pointing down and the isthmus bending forward and up 90 degrees so that the corpus lies at a right angle to the cervix. However, posture, parity, and bladder or rectal fullness influence its position. For example, the angle between the corpus and cervix decreases as the bladder fills, elevating the corpus and displacing the cervix.

The uterus is supported by ligaments, muscles of the pelvic floor, and the perineum. (See *Uterine ligaments,* page 92, for an explanation and illustration of these ligaments.)

Innervation. The autonomic nervous system provides uterine innervation. Sympathetic nerve fibers enter the pelvis through the hypogastric plexus and enter the uterus in ganglia near the base of the uterosacral ligaments. Sympathetic nerve fibers are joined at this juncture by the pelvic nerve, which is formed by parasympathetic nerve fibers from the second, third, and fourth sacral nerves. Parasympathetic nerves inhibit muscular contraction. Sympathetic nerves stimulate vasoconstriction and muscular contraction. Although innervation is important, the uterus exhibits adequate contractility for delivery even in the absence of innervation; for example, a paraplegic woman typically will have adequate uterine contractility for safe vaginal childbirth.

Most uterine nerve fibers control motor response; however, some sensory fibers also are present. Uterine stretching, ischemia, and chemical irritation can cause pain. Pain originating in the cervix and upper vagina is transmitted to the pelvic nerves. Uterine pain also is transmitted through the eleventh and twelfth thoracic nerve roots to the central nervous system.

Spinal or caudal anesthesia during labor is safe and effective because it affects sensory nerves only, not motor nerves. Many types of chronic pelvic pain can be relieved permanently by surgically severing the hypogastric plexus.

Blood supply and lymph drainage. The lower uterus receives blood through the uterine artery, which branches from the hypogastric artery, enters the base of the broad ligament, crosses the ureter, and divides into two arteries. The smaller branch supplies part of the cervix and upper vagina. The larger branch extends upward along the uterus, supplying the upper cervix before branching into many smaller arteries that penetrate the corpus.

Developmental changes in the uterus and cervix

Over a woman's lifetime, changes occur in the size of the uterus, the relative size of the corpus and cervix, and the shape of the external os. The illustration below shows the uterus in developmental stages from neonate to postmenopausal adult. For example, in a premenarchal woman, one-third of the uterus may be corpus and two-thirds may be cervix. In an adult multiparous woman, two-thirds of the uterus may be corpus and one-third may be cervix. The central opening of the cervix (the external os) is round and closed in a nulliparous woman. In a parous woman, the opening is an irregularly shaped slit.

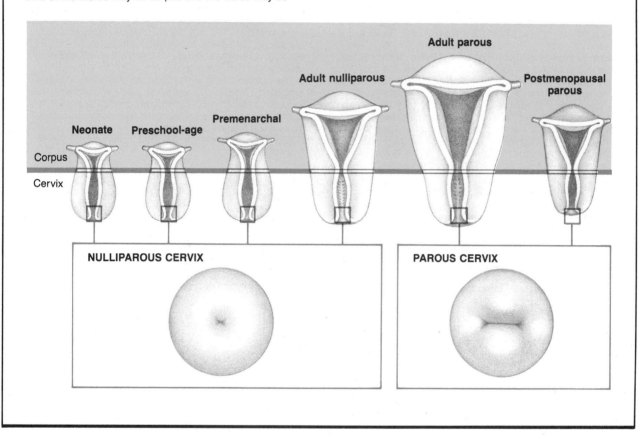

The upper uterus receives blood through the ovarian artery, which branches from the aorta, crosses the broad ligament, and merges with the ovarian branch of the uterine artery at the uterus.

The uterine vein carries venous return to the hypogastric vein, which in turn empties into the iliac vein. The ovarian veins carry venous return from the upper portion of the broad ligament and the ovaries. The right ovarian vein empties into the vena cava; the left ovarian vein, into the left renal vein.

Uterine lymphatic drainage is collected by three networks of lymphatic vessels: one located at the base of the endometrium, another within the myometrium, and one just below the perimetrium. Most lymphatic vessels that drain these networks follow the uterine and ovarian blood vessels. Uterine lymph drainage joins drainage from ovarian and tubule lymphatics near the uterine fundus and then empties into nodes near the aorta. This extensive drainage system has one flaw: it facilitates seeding into other areas if cancerous cells are present in the drainage.

Fallopian tubes

This pair of long, narrow tubes connects the ovaries and the uterus. Their functions include transporting ova, nourishing ova during the 2- to 3-day journey through the tubes, and providing a site for fertilization.

Structure and function. The fallopian tubes extend from the upper sides of the uterine corpus along the superior border of the broad ligament toward the pelvic wall. Before reaching the wall, each tube bends posteriorly and medially toward the ovaries. The tubes are flexible and approximately 8 to 13.5 cm long. (For an illustration, see *Fallopian tube and ovary,* page 93.)

Uterine ligaments

The uterus is a partially mobile organ supported by 10 ligaments. The broad ligament, cardinal ligaments, round ligaments, and uterosacral ligaments provide primary support while permitting limited movement; two ovarian ligaments and the infundibulopelvic ligaments provide ancillary support.

The broad ligament is a winglike fold of peritoneum that envelopes the uterus, extends to the pelvic walls, and divides the pelvic cavity laterally. It supports the uterus and keeps it positioned in the center of the pelvic cavity. The upper section of the broad ligament is loose connective tissue that encloses the fallopian tubes, ovaries, and the round and ovarian ligaments. The thick base of the broad ligament is continuous with pelvic floor connective tissue.

The cardinal ligaments (transverse ligaments also known as Mackenrodt's ligaments) are segments of dense connective tissue along the lower border of the broad ligament. These ligaments provide primary support for the uterus and attach it to the vagina. The posterior ligament extends from the uterus to the rectum and supports the supravaginal cer-

vix. Traction provided by this ligament also holds the uterus in its normal position.

Consisting of smooth muscle and connective tissue continuous with muscles of the uterine wall, the round ligaments extend from the uterus, below the fallopian tubes, and through the inguinal canal to merge with connective tissue in the labia majora. These ligaments help the broad ligaments hold the uterus in position, and they serve a special function during childbirth. As the uterus enlarges during pregnancy, the ligaments stretch and hypertrophy. When labor begins, they pull the uterus forward and downward, guiding the fetus into the cervix.

The uterosacral ligaments, strands of connective tissue and muscle covered by peritoneum, extend from the cervix, around the rectum, and into the fascia at S2 and S3. These ligaments help secure the uterus in its normal position by maintaining traction on the cervix.

The illustration below shows the location of the uterine ligaments.

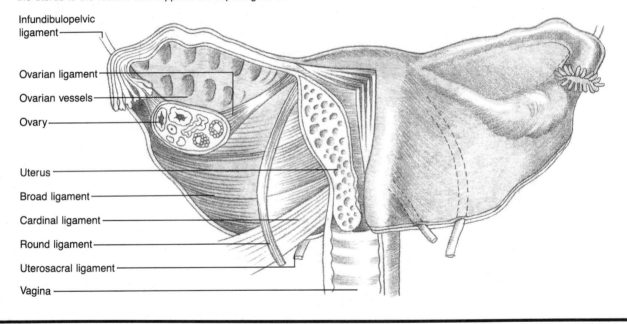

Infundibulopelvic ligament

Ovarian ligament

Ovarian vessels

Ovary

Uterus

Broad ligament

Cardinal ligament

Round ligament

Uterosacral ligament

Vagina

Each tube is composed of an *interstitial section, isthmus, ampulla,* and *infundibulum.* The short interstitial section has a diameter of 1 mm and is located within the uterine wall. The isthmus is a short, narrow (2 to 3 mm) section outside the uterine wall. Beyond the isthmus, the fallopian tube widens into the curved ampulla that makes up two-thirds of its length. The muscular walls of the ampulla are thin and elastic. Fertilization occurs here. The ampulla ends in the funnel-shaped infundibulum. Fimbriae (finger-like projections) within the infundibulum move in waves that sweep the mature ovum from the ovary into the fallopian tube.

Four separate tissue layers make up the fallopian tube wall. Peritoneal tissue, part of the broad ligament peritoneum that is continuous with the uterine and vaginal mucosa, forms the outer layer. Below the peritoneum, a subserous layer contains blood vessels and nerve fibers. Below this is a layer of longitudinal muscle tissue and circular, smooth involuntary muscle tissue, which generates the peristaltic motion that propels the ovum along the tube toward the uterus. The inner layer is mucosal tissue composed of ciliated and nonciliated columnar epithelium. Nonciliated cells secrete a protein-rich fluid that nourishes the ovum as it passes through the tube. Ciliated cells create currents in the fluid that augment the peristaltic action of the muscle layer.

Fallopian tube and ovary

The fallopian tube links the ovary and uterus. Each month, a mature ovum is pulled into the fallopian tube by fimbria in the ampulla. Peristaltic muscle action and wave motion of ciliated cells in the fallopian tube move the ovum toward the uterus. Nonciliated epithelial cells lining the fallopian tube secrete nourishment for the ovum during its 2- to 3-day journey. The illustration below shows major fallopian tube structures as well as surrounding structures.

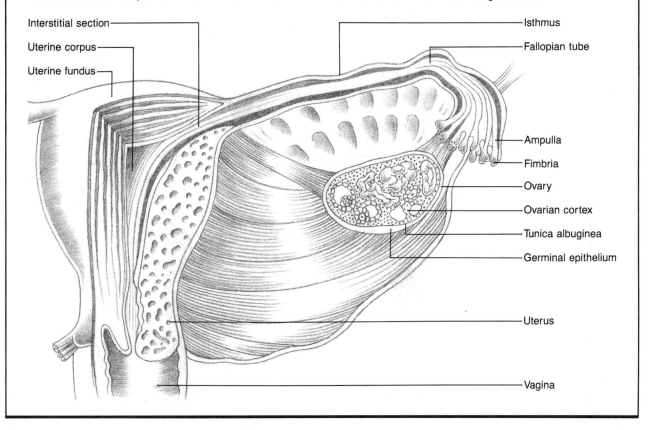

Interstitial section
Uterine corpus
Uterine fundus

Isthmus
Fallopian tube
Ampulla
Fimbria
Ovary
Ovarian cortex
Tunica albuginea
Germinal epithelium
Uterus
Vagina

Innervation and blood supply. Parasympathetic and sympathetic motor and sensory nerves from the pelvic and ovarian plexuses provide fallopian tube innervation. Pain originating in the fallopian tubes usually is referred to the area of the iliac fossa. The uterine and ovarian arteries supply the fallopian tubes with blood. Branches of the ovarian artery supply the ampulla; those of the uterine artery supply the isthmus. Venous blood returns through the uterine and ovarian veins. Vessels near the ureter carry lymphatic drainage to the lumbar nodes near the aorta.

Ovaries

These two almond-shaped organs are located on either side of the uterus. Their size, shape, and position vary with age. In a female fetus, the ovaries descend into the pelvis. At birth, they are small, round, smooth, and pink, and situated in the false pelvis. Between infancy and puberty, they grow larger, flatten, turn grayish, and descend into the true pelvis. During the childbearing years, they develop their almond shape and a rough, pitted surface. During pregnancy, they are displaced from the pelvis by the enlarging uterus. After childbirth, they return to their normal position. After menopause, they undergo rapid involution, shrinking to a diameter of 0.5 cm, wrinkling, and changing color from gray to white.

Structure and function. The ovaries are anchored close to the pelvic wall by three ligaments. The mesovarium ligament attaches the ovary to the back of the broad ligament, the ovarian ligament attaches it to the uterus, and the suspensory ligament attaches it to the lateral pelvic wall.

The ovaries have several structural layers but, unlike other structures of the internal genitalia, they have no peritoneal covering. Instead, they are covered by *germinal epithelium*, a single layer of epithelial cells that overlies the *tunica albuginea*—a protective layer of con-

The female bony pelvis

The bony pelvis is formed by the right and left innominate bones, the sacrum, and the coccyx. The innominate bones form the anterior and lateral portion of the pelvis. Each innominate bone consists of three bones: the ilium, ischium, and pubis, which fuse during puberty.

The pelvic brim (linea terminalis) divides the pelvis into two parts: the false pelvis and the true pelvis. The false pelvis, the broad upper portion of the basin above the pelvic brim, is bounded posteriorly by the lumbar vertebrae, laterally by the ilium, and anteriorly by the lower abdominal wall. The true pelvis, below the pelvic brim, is bounded by the sacrum and coccyx and the lower portion of the innominate bones. The true pelvis forms the bony limit of the birth canal.

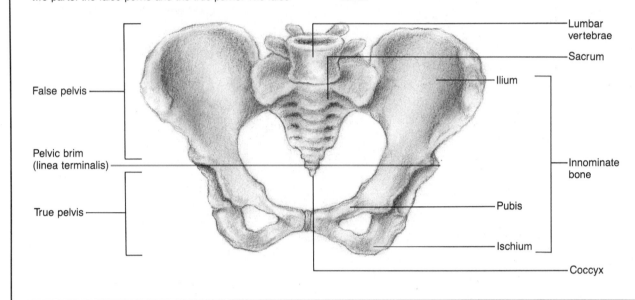

False pelvis

Pelvic brim (linea terminalis)

True pelvis

Lumbar vertebrae

Sacrum

Ilium

Innominate bone

Pubis

Ischium

Coccyx

nective tissue fibers. Under it lies the *ovarian cortex,* the primary functional layer, which contains graafian follicles containing the ova. The medulla, the central ovary layer, contains ovarian nerves, blood vessels, and lymphatics.

The primary function of the ovaries is the production of mature ova. At birth, each ovary contains approximately 500,000 *graafian follicles;* no additional follicles are produced later. During the childbearing years, one graafian follicle produces a mature ovum during the first half of each menstrual cycle. As the ovum matures, the follicle ruptures and the ovum is swept into the fallopian tube. The ovaries also produce estrogen and progesterone (hormones that regulate sexual development and the menstrual cycle) as well as a small amount of androgens.

Innervation and blood supply. Sympathetic and parasympathetic motor and sensory innervation originates in vertebral segments T10 to L1. The nerves serving the ovaries follow the ovarian arteries across the infundibulopelvic ligament to the ovary. However, the ovaries are relatively insensitive, unless they are distended. Mittelschmerz (mid-cycle pain) can result from irritation of the abdominal peritoneum by the blood or fluid escaping

with the ovum during ovulation. Blood is supplied through the ovarian arteries and returns through the ovarian veins. The left ovarian vein empties into the left renal vein; the right ovarian vein, into the inferior vena cava. Lymphatic drainage flows through the ovarian vessels into the iliac and periaortic nodes.

Bony pelvis

The female bony pelvis, which resembles a basin, supports the upper torso, protects pelvic structures, and forms the fixed axis of the birth canal. Age, sex, race, and heredity affect pelvic size and shape. The most significant differences between the female and male pelvis are the contours and thickness of the bones. The female pelvic bones are lighter and thinner, and the female pelvis is wider, shallower, and less ovoid.

Structure and function
The bony pelvis is formed by a right and left innominate bone (os coxae), the sacrum, and the coccyx. (See *The female bony pelvis* for an illustration.) Each innominate

bone is made up of three bones—ilium, ischium, and pubis—that fuse during puberty in a cup-shaped socket of the hip joint called the acetabulum. The ilium, the broad upper portion of the innominate bone, has an anterior prominence—the anterior iliac spine—and a convex portion—the iliac crest. The ischium, the strongest innominate bone, lies inferior to the ilium and below the acetabulum. The posterior end of this bone, the ischial tuberosity, is a marked protuberance that carries the body's weight in the sitting position. Two ischial spines project from the posterior border of the ischium into the pelvic cavity. The pubis extends from the acetabulum to the midpoint of the bony pelvis, forming the symphysis pubis.

The symphysis pubis is composed of fibrocartilage and the arcuate pubic ligament. The mobility of this ligament and the sacroiliac joint increases during pregnancy, allowing the pelvic outlet in the dorsal lithotomy position to increase by 1.5 to 2 cm. Beneath the symphysis pubis is a triangular space called the pubic arch. During delivery, the fetus's head passes under this arch.

The sacrum and coccyx form the back of the pelvis. The sacrum is a wedge-shaped bone formed by five fused vertebrae. The sacral promontory, located on the upper anterior portion of the first sacral vertebra, projects into the pelvic cavity. This projection, which can be palpated, is an obstetric landmark for pelvic measurements.

The coccyx, a small triangular bone formed by fused vertebrae, lies below and slightly forward of the lower border of the sacrum. The sacrum and coccyx meet at the sacrococcygeal joint. An intervertebral disc at this joint allows the coccyx to move backward during labor and provide additional space for the descending fetus.

The pelvic brim (linea terminalis) divides the pelvis into two parts: the false, or major, pelvis and the true, or minor, pelvis. The false pelvis has no specific obstetric significance. The true pelvis, below the pelvic brim, forms the bony limit of the birth canal. The diameter of the true pelvis is approximately 5 cm at the symphysis pubis and about 10 cm along its posterior wall.

Four basic pelvic types exist: gynecoid, android, anthropoid, and platypelloid. Pure pelvic types are unusual; most women have a combination of two basic types, with the features of one type predominating. (See *Pelvic types* for illustrations.)

Planes and diameters

The complex shape of the pelvis complicates determining and describing the exact location of the fetus during pregnancy, labor, and delivery. To facilitate assessment, obstetric specialists have designated specific pelvic planes (two-dimensional cross sections) to describe pel-

Pelvic types

Four pure pelvic types exist: gynecoid (the most advantageous for giving birth), android, anthropoid, and platypelloid. Variations in these basic pelvic types are described by the relationship between the anterior and posterior segments of the pelvic inlet. An imaginary line through the greatest transverse diameter of the inlet divides the pelvis into anterior and posterior segments. The posterior segment determines the pelvic type; the anterior segment defines the variation.

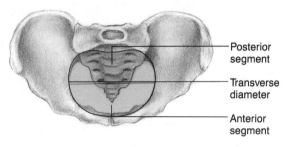

Posterior segment

Transverse diameter

Anterior segment

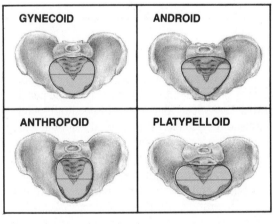

GYNECOID   ANDROID

ANTHROPOID   PLATYPELLOID

vic locations and openings. (For more information and illustrations, see Chapter 24, Physiology of Labor and Childbirth.)

During labor, the fetus descends into the birth canal. In most instances, the head presents first at a right angle to the plane of the inlet. The fetus descends slightly backward to the ischial spines in the midplane. At the ischial spines, the birth canal makes a near right-angle anterior bend. The descending fetus must rotate to pass between the spines and then contacts the musculature of the pelvic floor, which guides it into the vagina at the pelvic outlet.

Pelvic floor musculature

Muscles of the pelvic floor combine with the bony pelvis to provide support during pregnancy. These muscles stretch during delivery to allow passage of the fetus, then constrict afterward.

LITHOTOMY VIEW

Adductor muscle

Ischiocavernous muscle

Pubovaginal muscle

Urogenital diaphragm

Puborectal muscle

Pubococcygeal muscle

Iliococcygeal muscle

Coccyx

Femur

Vagina

Pudendal vessels

Transverse perineal muscle

Anus

Gluteus maximus muscle

Pelvic floor

Muscle pairs and deep fascia in the pelvic floor are accessory structures to the bony pelvis. The pelvic floor contains the upper and lower (urogenital) pelvic diaphragms and muscles of the external genitalia and anus. Pelvic diaphragm ligaments, fascia, and muscles are anchored to the perineal body. Perineal muscles protect pelvic viscera; perform the sphincter action of the urethra, vagina, and rectum; and contract during orgasm. (For an illustration, see *Pelvic floor musculature.*)

The upper pelvic diaphragm is bounded by the ischial spines, coccyx, and sacrum. This diaphragm contains deep fascia and the levator ani muscle, which is composed of four separate muscles (the iliococcygeal, pubococcygeal, puborectal, and pubovaginal) and supports abdominal and pelvic organs. During labor, these muscles help control relaxation periods and expel the fetus. The intricate weave of these muscles provides the elasticity that allows the vagina and surrounding structures to stretch during delivery and constrict afterward.

The lower pelvic diaphragm is located in the pelvic arch. Transverse perineal muscles originating at the ischial tuberosities enter the perineum to form the urethral and vaginal sphincters. These muscles work with the bulbocavernous muscle and the external anal sphincter to support the perineal floor and accommodate stretching during labor and childbirth.

Related pelvic structures

The pelvis contains urinary and intestinal structures as well as reproductive structures. These structures can be affected by changes in the reproductive tract.

Urinary structures

Urinary structures include the ureters, bladder, urethra, and urethral meatus. Two thin tubes, the ureters, originate at the kidney pelves, extend down along the posterior abdominal wall, pass over the pelvic brim beneath the uterine vessels, and enter the bladder at the level of the cervix. Pressure on the ureters from the enlarging uterus during pregnancy can cause urinary stasis, which may predispose to urinary tract infections. The bladder, a muscular sac that serves as a reservoir for urine, lies between the symphysis pubis and the uterus. When empty, it is situated entirely in the pelvis. When fully distended, it projects into the abdomen. The urethra carries urine from the bladder to the urethral meatus, the opening located in the vestibule between the clitoris and the vaginal orifice.

Intestinal structures

The pelvis contains four intestinal segments: the rectum, colon, cecum, and ileum. The highly vascular rectum lies behind the vagina and uterus. During pregnancy, the enlarging uterus presses against the rectum, causing veins in the lower rectum to engorge and possibly result in hemorrhoids. During labor and delivery, lacerations from the birth canal may extend to the rectum and anus.

The female breast

The illustrations below show the structure and lymph drainage of the mature female breast.

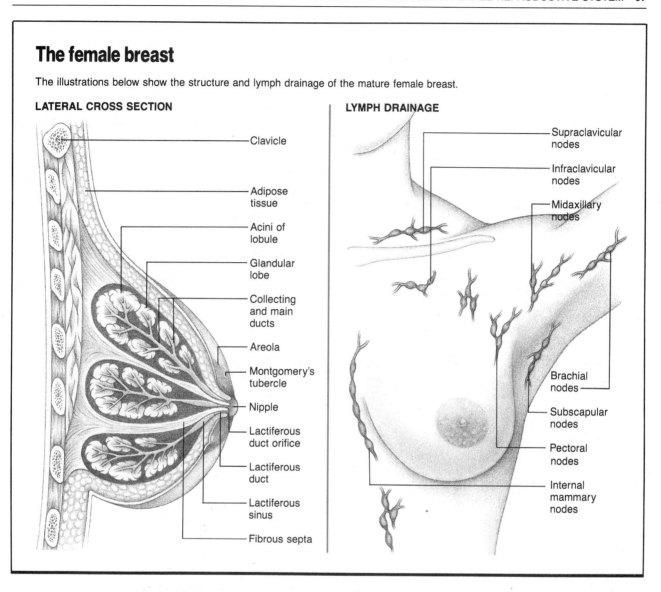

LATERAL CROSS SECTION

- Clavicle
- Adipose tissue
- Acini of lobule
- Glandular lobe
- Collecting and main ducts
- Areola
- Montgomery's tubercle
- Nipple
- Lactiferous duct orifice
- Lactiferous duct
- Lactiferous sinus
- Fibrous septa

LYMPH DRAINAGE

- Supraclavicular nodes
- Infraclavicular nodes
- Midaxillary nodes
- Brachial nodes
- Subscapular nodes
- Pectoral nodes
- Internal mammary nodes

The anus, the external opening of the rectum located behind the vaginal orifice and perineum, is surrounded by internal and external sphincter muscles, which anchor it to the coccyx and the perineum. Muscle contraction and relaxation controls the retention and expulsion of rectal contents.

Breasts

Highly specialized cutaneous, cone-shaped glands, the breasts are situated on either side of the anterior chest wall over the greater pectoral and the anterior serratus muscles. Vertically, they lie between the third and seventh ribs; horizontally, between the sternal border and the midaxillary line. A nipple is centrally located on each breast. A triangular-shaped portion of breast tissue known as the tail of Spence, or axillary tail, extends into the axilla. (See *The female breast* for illustrations of breast structure and lymph drainage.)

Structure and function

Each breast is composed of glandular (parenchymal), fibrous, and adipose tissue. Breast size and shape vary considerably among women, affected by such factors as heredity, nutrition, and parity.

Glandular tissue in each breast contains 15 to 20 lobes composed of clustered *acini*—tiny, saclike duct terminals that secrete milk. The breasts are supported by fibrous Cooper's ligaments and separated from each other by adipose tissue. The ducts draining the lobules converge to form *lactiferous ducts* and *sinuses* (ampullae), which store milk during lactation. These ducts drain onto the nipple surface through 15 to 20 openings.

Female breast development

This chart shows the sexual maturity stages of female breast development.

Stage 1
Preadolescent
Nipple elevation begins.

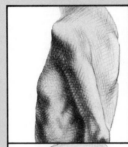

Stage 2
Breast budding
Breast and nipple form a small mound with areolar enlargement as elevation continues.

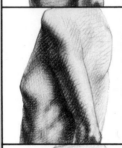

Stage 3
Continued enlargement
Breast enlargement continues with no distinct delineation of the areola.

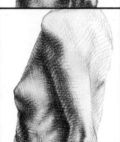

Stage 4
Secondary mound
A secondary mound forms beyond the original breast mound as the areola and nipple project.

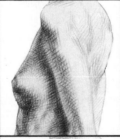

Stage 5
Breast maturity
The nipple projects from the areola, becoming part of the breast contour.

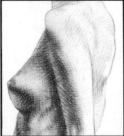

Adapted with permission of the publisher from Tanner, J.M. (1962). *Growth at adolescence* (2nd ed.). Oxford: Blackwell Scientific Publications, Ltd.

Centrally located on each breast, the nipple is composed of pigmented erectile tissue that responds to cold, friction, and sexual stimulation. In an adult, nipple diameter typically ranges between 0.5 and 1.3 cm. Surrounding the nipple is the areola, a more lightly pigmented circular area typically 2.5 to 10 cm in diameter. Sebaceous glands known as Montgomery's tubercles dot the areolar surface as small, round papules.

Development

The hormones estrogen and progesterone influence breast development and function throughout life. The breasts of a neonate may secrete a small amount of fluid for a few days after birth due to maternal estrogen stimulation in utero. During adolescence, estrogen production causes the breasts and nipples to enlarge and change contour. (See *Female breast development* for more information.) When ovulation occurs, progesterone production increases, stimulating development of the secretory cells in the breast.

Innervation and blood supply

Innervation of the upper breast stems from the third and fourth branches of the cervical plexus. Innervation of the lower breast arises in the thoracic intercostal nerve.

The breasts have an extensive vascular system. As the breasts enlarge during pregnancy, the superficial vascular pattern may be visible through the skin. Arterial, venous, and lymphatic vessels merge with internal mammary and axillary vessels. Lymphatics deep in the breast drain toward the axilla; other lymphatics drain into the jugular and subclavian veins. In breast cancer, this extensive lymphatic system facilitates metastasis of cancerous cells into the general circulation.

Female reproductive cycle

The female reproductive cycle, or menstrual cycle, actually involves two simultaneous cycles: the ovarian cycle and the endometrial cycle. (See *Female reproductive cycle* for more information.) A recurring menstrual cycle begins at menarche, continues throughout a woman's reproductive life, and ceases at menopause.

Menarche—onset of menses—typically occurs between ages 11 and 16 and marks the onset of reproductive function. After menarche, the breasts and other secondary sex characteristics become more pronounced. The ovarian hormones *estrogen* and *progesterone* stimulate and regulate most of these physiologic changes. Before menarche, the body inhibits estrogen production. At menarche, this inhibition ceases and estrogen levels in the bloodstream increase.

Female reproductive cycle

The female reproductive cycle, or menstrual cycle, typically lasts 28 days, although cycles from 22 to 34 days are normal. During the cycle, hormones influence the release of a mature ovum from a graafian follicle in the ovary. Hormones also stimulate changes in the endometrial layer of the uterus that prepare the uterus for ovum implantation. The hormones involved in this cycle are estrogen, progesterone, follicle-stimulating hormone (FSH), and luteinizing hormone (LH). The diagrams below illustrate all aspects of the cycle.

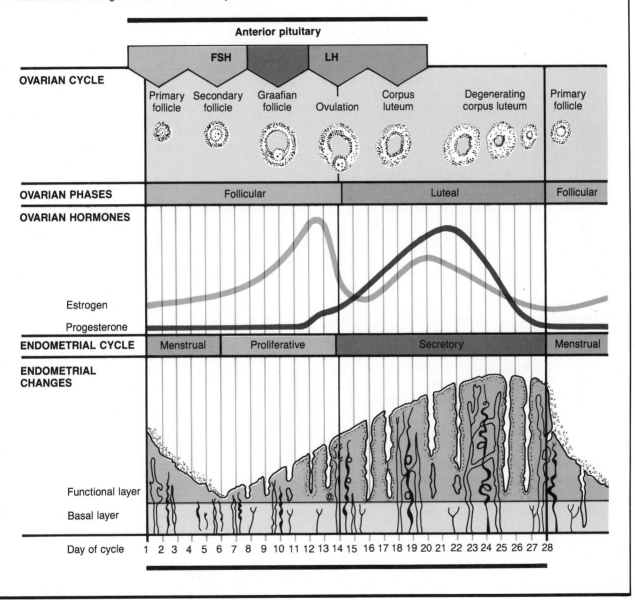

Menstrual flow may be irregular for up to 2 years after menarche because of anovulatory cycles associated with fluctuating estrogen levels and irregular shedding. When normal cyclic estrogen-progesterone interplay is established and consistent midcycle ovulation occurs, regular menstrual cycles are established.

Between ages 45 and 50, a woman typically begins the *climacteric* phase. Hormone production decreases, ovarian function declines, and menstruation becomes irregular. Declining estrogen production also may cause such symptoms as vasomotor instability (which causes hot flashes); atrophy of the skin, mucous membranes, and subcutaneous tissues; osteoporosis; and vaginal dryness. The climacteric ends at *menopause*—typically between ages 45 and 60—when reproductive ability ceases.

Ovarian cycle

This cycle begins as the corpus luteum of the previous phase degenerates and hypothalamic stimulation occurs. There are two phases in this cycle. The *follicular phase*, during which a graafian follicle develops and ruptures, begins on the first day of menstruation and usually lasts 14 days, culminating in ovulation. The *luteal phase* begins on day 15 and lasts through the end of the cycle. During the first 24 to 48 hours of this phase, the ovum is susceptible to fertilization. Variations in the length of the follicular phase account for variations in menstrual cycle length.

Follicular phase. On the first day of menses, primary follicles in the ovary begin to mature under the influence of pituitary gland hormones. Between days 5 and 7, a single follicle (graafian follicle) dominates and continues to mature while other follicles undergo involution. On day 12 or 13, hormonal influence triggers swelling of the graafian follicle. Around day 14, it ruptures and ovulation occurs, as the mature ovum emerges and enters the fimbriated (fringed) end of the fallopian tube.

Ovulation can produce several clinical signs. *Mittelschmerz*, abdominal pain in the ovarian region, signals ovulation in many women. Body temperature changes—typically a drop of 0.3° to 0.6° C (0.5° to 1.1° F) and then an increase above basal temperature—may signal ovulation. Evaluation of *spinnbarkheit*, the elasticity of cervical mucus discharge, can help pinpoint ovulation in many women. This involves aspirating a cervical mucus sample, placing it on a glass slide, pulling upward on the mucus with a forceps, and measuring the length of the resulting mucus threads. Before and after ovulation, cervical mucus threads usually are 1 to 2 cm long. On the day of ovulation, estrogen stimulation causes these threads to lengthen to 12 to 24 cm.

Luteal phase. After ovulation, the ruptured graafian follicle becomes a compact mass of tissue known as the *corpus luteum*. The corpus luteum produces small amounts of estrogen and progesterone, which stimulate changes in the uterine endometrium that prepare it to receive a fertilized ovum. The corpus luteum continues to secrete hormones for about 8 days. However, if the ovum is not fertilized, the output of estrogen and progesterone decreases as the corpus luteum degenerates. The decreased hormone levels cannot support the endometrium; menstruation then occurs in about 6 days, initiating the next cycle. If fertilization occurs, the gonadotropins produced by the trophoblast (outside layer of the embryonic cell) prevent the decline of the corpus luteum, stimulating it to produce large amounts of estrogen and progesterone.

Endometrial cycle

During this cycle, changes occur in the uterine endometrium that prepare it for implantation of a fertilized ovum. The endometrial cycle has three phases: *menstrual*, *proliferative*, and *secretory*.

Menstrual phase. During this phase, which begins on the first day of menses and lasts approximately 5 days, the compact, spongy layers of the endometrium that developed during the previous cycle are sloughed off and expelled. Menstrual flow is typically dark red from the daily loss of 50 to 60 ml of blood. Approximately 0.5 mg of iron is lost with each ml of blood. While endometrial tissue, cells, and mucus are being discharged, the endometrial basal layer regenerates.

Proliferative phase. This phase begins on day 5 and lasts until ovulation, typically on day 14 (9 days after cessation of menses). Early in this phase, the endometrium is 1 to 2 mm thick and undergoes few changes; cervical mucus is sparse and viscous. As estrogen secretion increases, the endometrium proliferates and the thickness of the uterine lining increases eight to ten times before ovulation.

Secretory phase. After ovulation, progesterone released by the corpus luteum increases endometrial vascularity and stimulates elongation of the glycogen-producing endometrial glands. The secretory phase lasts from day 14 to day 25. At the end of this phase, the endometrium is soft, velvety, edematous, and about 4 to 6 mm thick. Rich with blood and glycogen, it is ready to nourish an implanted fertilized ovum. When fertilization and implantation do not occur, endometrial circulation decreases as blood vessels constrict and then relax and bleed. Tissue necrosis follows ischemia. The subsequent sloughing of the compact and spongy endometrial layers marks the beginning of the next menstrual phase.

Hormonal regulation

Three endocrine structures—the hypothalamus, the pituitary gland, and the ovaries—produce the hormones that regulate the female reproductive cycle. These structures comprise a regulatory loop known as the *hypothalamic-pituitary-gonadal axis*, which generates physiologic changes through positive and negative feedback mechanisms. Prostaglandins, fatty acid derivatives present in many tissues, also affect the reproductive cycle.

Hypothalamus. The nervous system provides the hypothalamus with sensory data. The hypothalamus then stimulates the pituitary gland to release or suppress appropriate gonadotropic hormones (hormones that regulate gonadal function). Stimulation takes one of two forms. The hypothalamus stimulates or suppresses the release of follicle-stimulating hormone (FSH) or luteinizing hormone (LH) from the anterior pituitary by releasing gonadotropin-releasing hormone (GnRH) or gonadotropin-inhibiting hormone (GnIH). Nerve impulses from the hypothalamus stimulate the release of oxytocin by the posterior pituitary.

Pituitary gland. The anterior pituitary gland (adenohypophysis) produces the gonadotropic hormones FSH, LH, and prolactin. FSH and LH regulate ovarian hormone secretion, and prolactin stimulates milk secretion. The posterior pituitary gland (neurohypophysis) stores oxytocin, a hormone that regulates uterine muscle contractility and the release of milk into the mammary glands during lactation. The anterior pituitary does not produce gonadotropic hormones during early childhood; consequently, the ovaries receive no stimulation. Secretion of these hormones begins at approximately age 8 and eventually stimulates the onset of menses.

Ovaries. The ovaries produce estrogen, progesterone, and a small amount of testosterone. Estrogen and progesterone help regulate the reproductive cycle, testosterone increases the sex drive, and estrogen stimulates pubic and axillary hair growth and sebaceous gland secretion during puberty.

Prostaglandins. All cells in the body produce prostaglandins, but they are especially plentiful in the endometrium of females and the prostate gland of males. In females, prostaglandins affect ovulation, fertility, and uterine motility and contractility. During ovulation, prostaglandins and LH stimulate ovum release and corpus luteum regression. During labor and delivery, they help stimulate uterine motility and cervical dilation.

Hypothalamic-pituitary-gonadal axis function. On the first day of the reproductive cycle, low levels of estrogen and progesterone in the bloodstream stimulate the release of GnRH by the hypothalamus. GnRH stimulates the release of FSH and LH by the pituitary gland. During the first 5 or 6 days of the reproductive cycle, these hormones stimulate follicle development in the ovaries. The maturing graafian follicle releases a potent form of estrogen into the bloodstream, which stimulates the proliferation of uterine endometrium.

As the cycle approaches ovulation on day 14, the level of estrogen in the blood is maintained in a pulsatile manner, and the hypothalamus signals the pituitary to slow FSH secretion and increase LH secretion. A day or so before ovulation, LH production peaks and the follicle reduces estrogen secretion and begins secreting progesterone. LH and progesterone cause follicle swelling and then rupture during ovulation.

After ovulation, LH and prostaglandins stimulate corpus luteum regression. However, the corpus luteum continues to produce progesterone for several days. The high level of progesterone in the blood signals the hypothalamus to stimulate a reduction in FSH and LH secretion by the pituitary gland. Progesterone also stimulates secretory changes in the uterine endometrium that reduce contractility and prepare the uterus for ovum implantation, stimulates changes that prepare the fallopian tube mucosal lining to nourish the ovum, and stimulates lobule and acini development in the breasts and initiates their secretory phase.

The corpus luteum degenerates 8 to 12 days after ovulation, reducing the amount of progesterone in the blood. Unless fertilization occurs, the progesterone level quickly drops below that needed to sustain a fully developed uterine endometrium, and menstruation occurs.

Menstrual cycle variations

Although the normal menstrual cycle occurs roughly monthly, several variations can occur. Amenorrhea—absence of menses—is classified as primary (when cyclical menses is not established by age 18) or secondary (when menses cease for more than 3 months). Secondary amenorrhea can be caused by poor nutrition, strenuous athletic activity, and certain drugs, such as some types of tranquilizers.

Other menstrual cycle variations include:
• anovulation—failure of ovulation to occur
• hypomenorrhea—abnormally short menstrual cycle
• hypermenorrhea—abnormally long menstrual cycle
• menorrhagia—excessive menstrual flow
• metrorrhagia—uterine bleeding other than that caused by menstruation
• oligomenorrhea—abnormally light or infrequent menstrual flow
• polymenorrhea—abnormally frequent menstruation.
(For more information, see Chapter 13, Gynecologic Disorders.)

Male reproductive system

The male reproductive system is composed of external and internal genitalia. These organs and their related structures facilitate spermatogenesis, introduce mature spermatozoa into the female reproductive tract, and produce the hormones that regulate male sexual response, development of male secondary sex characteristics, and spermatogenesis. (For information about male sexuality, see Chapter 8, Sexuality Concerns.)

External genitalia

The male external genitalia include the *penis* and the *scrotum*. Sexual stimulation causes the normally flaccid penis to become erect, enabling it to penetrate the vagina and ejaculate semen during coitus. The scrotum contains and protects the testes, the male gonads. (For illustrations of these structures, see *Male reproductive system*.)

Penis
The penis, a pendulous, tubular structure, is attached to the front and sides of the pubic arch and is supported by the suspensory ligament that extends from the symphysis pubis to the deep fascia of the penis.

The penile shaft contains three layers of erectile tissue—two *corpora cavernosa* and the *corpus spongiosum*—and the urethra and is covered by fascia and a thin layer of skin. The glans, located at the end of the penis, is continuous with the mucous membranes of the urethra. Extending over the glans is a skinfold known as the prepuce, or foreskin.

During sexual arousal, sinuses in the corpora cavernosa fill with blood and cause penile erection. Parasympathetic nerve stimulation contracts the ischiocavernous muscles, preventing blood return and sustaining erection.

The urethra extends from the bladder through the prostate gland, urogenital diaphragm, and corpus spongiosum to the urinary meatus, a slitlike orifice in the glans penis. Mucus produced by Littre's glands along the urethra and the bulbourethral (Cowper's) glands at the base of the urethra moisten the urethral lining.

Sympathetic innervation of the penis originates in the hypogastric pelvic plexus. Parasympathetic innervation stems from the third and fourth sacral nerves. Blood flows to the penis through the internal pudendal artery and into the corpora cavernosa through the penile artery. Venous blood returns through the internal iliac vein to the vena cava.

Scrotum
This pouchlike structure, suspended from the perineal area below the penis, covers and protects the testes and spermatic cords and maintains the testes at a temperature conducive to spermatozoa production. The scrotum is composed of *dartos fascia*—connective tissue and smooth muscle fibers—and covered by a thin layer of deeply pigmented, wrinkled skin that is sparsely covered with sebaceous glands and pubic hair.

The dartos fascia gives the scrotal skin its wrinkled appearance. Wrinkling becomes less pronounced with age or in warm temperatures. Cold accentuates the wrinkled appearance by causing dartos contraction and cremasteric muscle shortening. This contraction helps maintain the temperature of the testes in cold temperatures by drawing them closer to the body.

Internally, the dartos fascia extends into a medial septum that separates the two testes and their related structures. A ridge (raphe) is visible on the surface of the scrotum where the two compartments meet.

Scrotum innervation stems from the genitofemoral, pudendal, posterior femoral cutaneous, and ilioinguinal nerves and the hypogastric plexus. (See *Blood supply and innervation to the male pelvis*, page 104, for more information.)

Internal genitalia

The male internal genitalia and related structures include the *testes;* a *duct system* composed of seminiferous tubules, epididymis, vas deferens, ejaculatory duct, and urethra; and *accessory structures*, including seminal vesicles, the prostate gland, bulbourethral glands, and urethral glands.

Testes
The testes—the male gonads—are two ovoid, glandular organs approximately 5 cm long and weighing 10 to 15 g located in the scrotum. They produce hormones (primarily testosterone) and mature spermatozoa.

Early in fetal development, the testes are situated in the abdomen. Testosterone stimulation during the first 7 months of development in utero causes them to descend into the inguinal canal. Complete descent of the testes into the scrotum usually occurs by birth. Complete descent is essential for spermatogenesis.

Male reproductive system

As shown in these illustrations, the male reproductive system consists of the penis, scrotum and its contents, the prostate gland, and the inguinal structures.

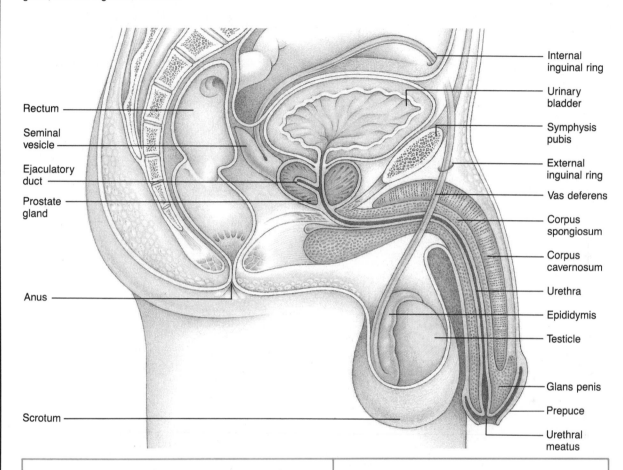

Rectum

Seminal vesicle

Ejaculatory duct

Prostate gland

Anus

Scrotum

Internal inguinal ring

Urinary bladder

Symphysis pubis

External inguinal ring

Vas deferens

Corpus spongiosum

Corpus cavernosum

Urethra

Epididymis

Testicle

Glans penis

Prepuce

Urethral meatus

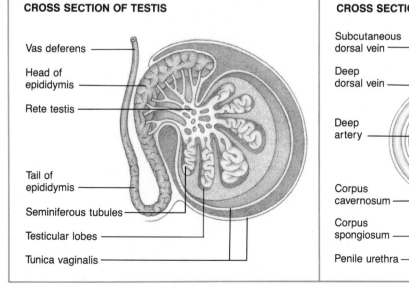

CROSS SECTION OF TESTIS

Vas deferens

Head of epididymis

Rete testis

Tail of epididymis

Seminiferous tubules

Testicular lobes

Tunica vaginalis

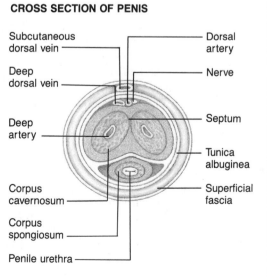

CROSS SECTION OF PENIS

Subcutaneous dorsal vein

Deep dorsal vein

Deep artery

Corpus cavernosum

Corpus spongiosum

Penile urethra

Dorsal artery

Nerve

Septum

Tunica albuginea

Superficial fascia

Blood supply and innervation to the male pelvis

The male pelvis is supplied by the internal iliac artery, which transports blood to the internal pudendal artery. This artery in turn supplies the external genitalia, including the corpora cavernosa, via the penile artery, enabling penile erection. Venous blood returns through the internal iliac vein to the vena cava.

The hypogastric plexus provides sympathetic innervation of the penis and scrotum. The testes receive parasympathetic innervation from the vagus nerve (cranial nerve X) and sympathetic innervation from the thoracic nerves.

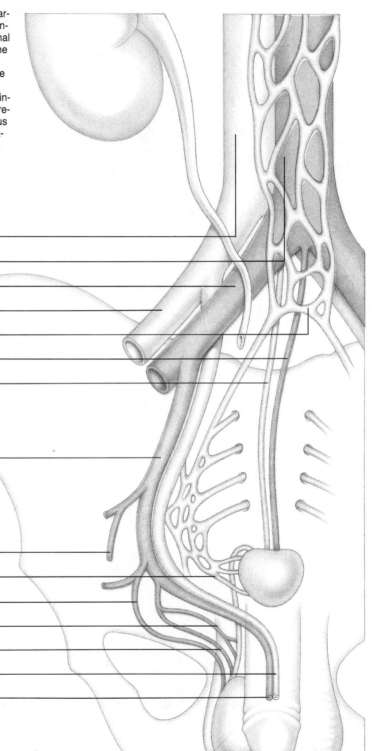

Inferior vena cava

Aorta

Right common iliac artery

Right common iliac vein

Hypogastric plexus

Sacral artery

Sacral vein

Internal pudendal artery

Right superior vesical artery

Lateral prostatic and vesical plexus

Perineal artery

Right vas deferens artery

Internal spermatic artery

Deep dorsal vein of penis

Dorsal artery of penis

The testes are covered partially by a serous membrane, the tunica vaginalis. Beneath this membrane lies the tunica albuginea, a tough, white, fibrous covering. Projections from the tunica albuginea extend into the testes and divide them into lobes, which are subdivided into lobules. Each testis has roughly 200 to 300 lobules, which contain coiled, convoluted seminiferous tubules surrounded by loose connective tissue. The connective tissue contains blood and lymph vessels and Leydig's cells—interstitial cells that produce testosterone. Leydig's cells typically are present only after puberty.

The testes receive parasympathetic innervation from the vagus nerve (cranial nerve X) and sympathetic innervation from the thoracic cord. Also, they contain extensive vascular and lymphatic systems.

Duct system

An extensive duct system composed of the seminiferous tubules, epididymis, vas deferens, ejaculatory duct, and urethra transports spermatozoa and other semen constituents through the male reproductive tract. Fertility problems can arise if injury or surgical intervention interrupts or blocks any part of this system.

Composed of spermatozoa and secretions from the seminal vesicles, vas deferens, prostate gland, and bulbourethral and urethral glands, semen is the transporting medium for spermatozoa during ejaculation. It also facilitates spermatozoa motility in the female reproductive tract.

Ejaculation forcefully expels approximately 3 to 5 ml of semen and millions of spermatozoa through the urethral meatus. Semen coagulates immediately after ejaculation and then liquifies under the influence of profibrinolysin (a clot-dissolving enzyme secreted by the prostate). Spermatozoa become highly motile as the coagulate dissolves. After entering the female reproductive tract, spermatozoa have a life span of 24 to 72 hours.

The most influential factor affecting male fertility is the number of spermatozoa released during ejaculation. If the spermatozoa count falls below 20 million/ml of semen, the male is classified as infertile. Other factors that affect fertility are spermatozoa size, shape, and motility and the composition of accessory gland secretions. (For more information, see Chapter 10, Fertility and Infertility.)

Seminiferous tubules. Seminiferous tubules within each testis lobule merge in a plexus called the rete testis. Along the upper border of the mediastinum of the testis are 10 to 15 efferent ducts that perforate the tunica albuginea and drain the rete testis into the epididymis.

Epididymis. The head of the epididymis, which stores immature spermatozoa until they mature, is located atop the testis. The tightly coiled body extends down the side of the testis, and the tail is continuous with the vas deferens. The entire structure is about 3.75 cm long.

Vas deferens. The vas deferens, or ductus deferens, extends through the scrotum and inguinal canal over the bladder to the prostate gland. Near the prostate, it enlarges into the ampulla. Peristaltic action propels spermatozoa and secretions through the vas deferens to the ampulla, where they are stored. There, sperm can survive for months. The vas deferens joins the seminal vesicle duct (a saclike gland lying against the posterior wall of the bladder) to form the ejaculatory duct, which empties into the prostatic urethra.

Innervation and blood supply. Duct system innervation stems from the hypogastric plexus of the autonomic nervous system. The portion of the vas deferens that lies within the scrotum contains pain receptors. The spermatic cord contains the nerve fibers and blood and lymphatic vessels that serve the duct system. The spermatic cord passes from the abdominal cavity through the inguinal canal to the scrotum.

Accessory structures

Male reproductive system accessory structures generate the medium that facilitates spermatozoa transport and survival after ejaculation.

Seminal vesicles. These lobular glands, located on either side of the prostate gland between the bladder and the rectum, merge with the vas deferens ampulla in the prostate to form the ejaculatory duct. During ejaculation, spermatozoa from the vas deferens and nutritive fluid from the seminal vesicles combine in the ejaculatory duct.

Columnar epithelium lining the seminal vesicles secretes a thick, alkaline fluid that is rich in prostaglandins, fibrinogen, proteins, fructose, and other nutrients. This fluid provides the nutrients essential for spermatozoa metabolism and motility in the female reproductive tract. Prostaglandins make the cervical mucus more receptive to the spermatozoa and encourage the uterine and fallopian tube peristaltic motion that moves the spermatozoa toward the ovaries.

Prostate gland. The urethra passes through the prostate gland, which is located below the bladder and the internal urethral orifice. Normally about 4 cm in diameter and weighing about 20 g, the prostate contains mucosal, submucosal, and external tubular glands. The 30 to 60 tubular glands secrete a thin, milky, alkaline fluid that contains high levels of zinc, calcium, citric acid, acid phosphate, and the clotting enzyme profibrinolysin. The alkalinity of this fluid offsets seminal fluid acidity, increasing semen pH to 6 to 6.5, the range necessary for spermatozoa motility.

Ducts from these glands open into the ejaculatory duct.

Bulbourethral (Cowper's) glands. The two pea-sized bulbourethral glands are located on either side of the urethra. When the male is sexually aroused, these glands secrete a clear, alkaline fluid that lubricates the penile urethra and neutralizes acidity there as well as in the vagina during coitus.

Urethral (Littre's) glands. Located along the membranous lining of the penile urethra, these tiny glands secrete lubricating mucus.

Male reproductive development and regulation

Hormones produced by the hypothalamus, pituitary, and testes control male sexual development and regulate spermatogenesis. The hypothalamic-pituitary-gonadal axis responds to positive and negative feedback to maintain hormonal balance.

Sexual development

The male hormone *testosterone* stimulates sexual development and regulates most aspects of reproductive ability. In the fetus, the Y chromosome stimulates testosterone secretion from the genital ridges, and the placenta secretes human chorionic gonadotropin, which stimulates testosterone secretion from Leydig's cells in the fetus's testes. Testosterone stimulates development of the penis, scrotum, seminal vesicles, prostate gland, genital ductal system, and descent of the testes through the inguinal canal. Shortly after the neonate's birth, testosterone production decreases.

Testosterone production remains low during childhood and increases during puberty, typically between ages 11 and 13. Influenced by testosterone, the penis, scrotum, and testes enlarge, and secondary sex characteristics —including hair growth on the genitalia, face, and chest and voice deepening—develop. Also, testosterone increases sebaceous gland secretion, which influences anabolism (cell-building) and results in increased male musculature, skeletal growth, and metabolism. In the adult male, testosterone affects sexuality and regulates the reproductive function. Interference with testosterone production will impair male libido and physiologic response to sexual stimulus.

Testosterone production continues throughout life, but decreases with age. Because of this decrease as a male ages, his sexual ability declines, muscle mass and hair growth decrease, skin loses elasticity, body fat distribution changes, and bones lose calcium.

Spermatogenesis

The process of spermatozoa formation, spermatogenesis occurs in the lobules of the testes and seminiferous tubules. (See *Spermatogenesis* for more information.) Hormones produced in the hypothalamic-pituitary-gonadal axis initiate spermatogenesis during puberty and regulate it thereafter.

Sertoli's cells in the lining of the seminiferous tubules provide nutrients for the spermatozoa for approximately 74 days. Immature spermatozoa enter the epididymis through the efferent ducts. At this point, spermatozoa lack motility and the ability to fertilize an ovum. They mature during the 2 to 10 days that they stay in the epididymis. During this time, the epididymal epithelium secretes fluid that nourishes the maturing spermatozoa. Most mature spermatozoa pass through the vas deferens and are stored in the ampulla; however, some are stored in the tail of the epididymis.

Hormonal regulation

Sexual development and spermatogenesis are initiated and regulated by the hypothalamic-pituitary-gonadal axis. Early in life, hormone production is inhibited. During puberty, inhibition ceases and the hypothalamus secretes GnRH, which stimulates the anterior pituitary to release LH and FSH. FSH stimulates the production of primary spermatocytes by germinal epithelial cells in the seminiferous tubules and influence the transformation of primary spermatocytes to secondary spermatocytes. At the same time, LH stimulates testosterone production by Leydig's cells in the testes. Testosterone stimulates the maturation of secondary spermatocytes and regulates the development of male secondary sex characteristics. (For additional information, see Chapter 16, Conception and Fetal Development.)

Spermatogenesis continues throughout life. The hypothalamus regulates testosterone production by monitoring blood testosterone levels. When levels fall, the hypothalamus signals the pituitary to increase LH production, which stimulates increased testosterone production in the testes. When levels rise too high, regulatory feedback mechanisms suppress further gonadotropin secretion, causing decreased testosterone production by the testes.

Spermatogenesis

Spermatogenesis, the formation of mature spermatozoa within the seminiferous tubules, occurs in four stages:
• Spermatogonia (primary germinal epithelial cells) grow and develop into primary spermatocytes. Both spermatogonia and primary spermatocytes contain 46 chromosomes, consisting of 44 autosomes and the two sex chromosomes X and Y.
• Primary spermatocytes divide to form secondary spermatocytes. No new chromosomes are formed at this stage; existing pairs divide. Each secondary spermatocyte contains half the number of autosomes (22). One secondary spermatocyte contains an X chromosome; the other, a Y chromosome.
• Secondary spermatocytes divide to form spermatids.
• Spermatids undergo several structural changes to become mature spermatozoa or sperm. Each spermatozoan is composed of a head, neck, body, and tail. The head contains the nucleus; the tail, a large amount of adenosine triphosphate, which provides energy for spermatozoa motility.

Spermatogonia (44 autosomes plus X and Y)

Primary spermatocytes (44 autosomes plus X and Y)

Secondary spermatocytes (22 autosomes plus X or Y)

Spermatids (22 autosomes plus X or Y)

Spermatozoa (22 autosomes plus X or Y)

Chapter summary

Chapter 6 described the structures and functions of the female and male reproductive systems. Key concepts are as follows.
• The organs and structures of female and male reproductive systems facilitate reproduction and provide sexual gratification. They also produce hormones that regulate the development of secondary sex characteristics and sexual response. In females, hormones also regulate the reproductive cycle; in males, spermatogenesis.
• External female reproductive structures include the mons pubis, labia majora, labia minora, clitoris, vaginal orifice, and the perineum. Internal structures include the vagina, uterus (corpus and cervix), fallopian tubes, and ovaries.
• External male reproductive structures include the penis (shaft and glans) and the scrotum. Internal structures include the testes, seminiferous tubules, epididymis, vas deferens, prostate gland, urethra, seminal vesicles, bulbourethral glands, and urethral glands.
• Hormonal stimulation in the hypothalamic-pituitary-gonadal axis initiates and regulates development of the reproductive system and secondary sex characteristics in both sexes.
• Menarche, the onset of cyclical menstrual periods, typically begins between ages 11 and 16. Menopause, the period when female hormone production and menstruation cease, typically occurs between ages 45 and 60. During the climacteric, the period preceding menopause, hormonal stimulation decreases and menses become irregular.
• The ovarian hormones estrogen and progesterone are the primary female hormones that regulate physiologic changes in the ovaries, uterus, and vagina during the female reproductive cycle.
• Specific diameters within the bony structure of the female pelvis determine whether normal vaginal delivery is feasible.
• The male hormone testosterone, produced in the testes, stimulates spermatogenesis and the development of male secondary sex characteristics.
• Spermatogenesis, the formation and maturation of spermatozoa, occurs in the lobules and seminiferous tubules of the testes. Spermatogenesis begins during puberty and continues throughout life.

Study questions

1. Discuss how pregnancy, labor, and delivery are aided by the structure and function of the vagina and uterus.

2. Jim and Ellie, a couple in their twenties, have tried to conceive for several months. Ellie does not understand why she cannot get pregnant. The health history interview reveals that her menses are irregular (ranging from every 34 to 45 days) and that she believes ovulation occurs 14 days after the start of her menstrual period. What would you teach her regarding ovulation during the female reproductive cycle? Include a discussion of how she might be able to detect when she is ovulating.

3. Explain the development and maturation of spermatozoa and the conditions that influence spermatozoa motility and male fertility.

4. Discuss the hormonal, anatomic, and physiologic changes that typically occur during the female climacteric and menopause.

5. Discuss the five stages of female breast development.

Bibliography

Ames, S., and Kneisl, C. (1988). *Essentials of adult health nursing*. Menlo Park, CA: Addison-Wesley.

Auvenshine, M., and Enriquez, M. (1985). *Maternity nursing: Dimensions of change*. Monterey, CA: Wadsworth.

Cohen, F., and Durham, J. (1986). *Nursing clinics of North America: Men's health*. Philadelphia: Saunders.

Cunningham, F., MacDonald, P., and Gant, N. (1989). *Williams obstetrics* (18th ed.). Norwalk, CT: Appleton & Lange.

Fogel, C. I., and Woods, N. F. (1981). *Health care of women: A nursing perspective*. St. Louis: Mosby.

Guyton, A. (1986). *Textbook of medical physiology* (7th ed.). Philadelphia: Saunders.

Morton, P.G. (1989). *Health assessment in nursing*. Springhouse, PA: Springhouse Corporation.

Sloane, E. (1985). *Biology of women* (2nd ed.). New York: John Wiley.

Spence, A., and Mason, E. (1987). *Human anatomy and physiology* (3rd ed.). Menlo Park, CA: Benjamin/Cummings.

Speroff, L., and Glass, R. (1988). *Clinical gynecology, endocrinology and infertility*. Baltimore: Williams & Wilkins.

Webster, D., and Huges, T. (Eds.). (1986). *Nursing clinics of North America: Women's health*. Philadelphia: Saunders.

Women's Health Promotion

Objectives

After reading and studying this chapter, the student should be able to:

1. Identify factors that may limit a woman's access to health care.
2. Compare health care needs for women of different ages.
3. Obtain appropriate health history information during a gynecologic assessment.
4. Describe gynecologic physical assessment techniques.
5. Discuss the benefits of an educational pelvic examination.
6. Describe common laboratory tests and other diagnostic studies used in health promotion for women.
7. Teach the client how to perform breast self-examination (BSE).
8. Identify women's health promotion topics.
9. Apply the nursing process to help a client understand health promotion activities.

Introduction

Health promotion is a key factor in women's health. Although women's health care focuses primarily on gynecologic care (care of the female reproductive system and related structures), it also addresses such factors as personal health habits and psychosocial concerns that can affect—or be affected by—a client's gynecologic health.

Because of this, the nurse must promote health and provide holistic care for the client by:
• interpreting health history, physical assessment, and diagnostic study data and evaluating their implications for the client's health
• assessing the client's risk for developing a health problem
• promoting the client's comfort and providing support during the gynecologic assessment
• addressing the client's psychosocial and cultural needs
• teaching the importance of regular gynecologic care and BSE
• advocating comprehensive health care for women of all socioeconomic groups
• modifying care, as needed, for clients of different ages
• screening for other health problems, such as substance abuse and smoking.

Chapter 7 describes how to meet these nursing responsibilities. It discusses the woman as a health care consumer and presents the factors that may influence her contact with the health care system. Then it explores the gynecologic assessment, including breast and pelvic examinations, noting variations for pediatric, adolescent, and adult clients. After exploring the gynecologic assessment, the chapter provides examples of nursing diagnoses and describes how to plan, implement, and evaluate client care.

GLOSSARY

Amenorrhea: absence of menses.

Anteflexed uterus: normal position in which the uterine corpus flexes forward at an acute angle.

Anteverted uterus: normal position in which the uterine corpus flexes forward at a less acute angle than an anteflexed uterus.

Atrophic vaginitis: inflammation in a short, dry, somewhat inelastic vagina, as may occur in a postmenopausal woman.

Bicornate uterus: Y-shaped or heart-shaped uterus.

Breast self-examination (BSE): procedure by which a woman assesses her breasts and accessory structures for signs of abnormality.

Climacteric stage: period from onset to end of hormonal and related changes that cease reproductive function. This developmental stage includes a premenopausal, menopausal, and postmenopausal phase and may last up to 20 years.

Colposcopy: examination of cervical and vaginal tissue using a colposcope for magnification.

Condyloma: wartlike growth on the external genitalia, vagina, cervix, or anus. It is caused by the human papilloma virus and may become an invasive cervical lesion; also known as a venereal wart.

Dimpling: breast skin puckering or depression, possibly caused by an underlying growth; also called retraction.

Dysmenorrhea: painful menstruation.

Dyspareunia: painful or difficult intercourse. May result from vaginal dryness associated with menopause.

Dysuria: painful or difficult urination.

Ectocervix: outer portion of the cervix lined with squamous epithelium.

Educational pelvic examination: assessment technique that allows the client to view her genitals and cervix through a hand mirror as they are identified by the examiner.

Endocervix: inner portion of the cervix.

Fibroids: benign, slow-growing uterine tumors.

Female circumcision: religious or cultural procedure that removes a portion of the clitoris and labia.

Hormone replacement therapy (HRT): use of estrogen by itself or with progestin to relieve menopausal symptoms.

Hot flash: transient sensation of warmth over the upper chest, face, and extremities caused by vasomotor disturbances associated with menopause.

Incontinence: inability to control urination or defecation. In a postmenopausal client, urinary incontinence may result from pelvic relaxation.

Mammogram: X-ray used to diagnose and evaluate breast lesions.

Menarche: onset of menses, usually occurring between ages 12 and 13.

Menopause: cessation of menses with the decline of cyclic hormonal production and function, usually between ages 40 and 60. Menopause may begin at an earlier age—for example, after surgical removal of the uterus, ovaries, or both.

Menorrhagia: increased menstrual bleeding.

Menstruation: cyclic discharge of blood and accumulated materials from the uterus.

Metrorrhagia: bleeding or spotting between menstrual periods.

Nipple inversion: inturning or depression of the nipple.

Osteoporosis: decreased bone mass, occurring most frequently in menopausal women.

Papanicolaou (Pap) test: cytologic study of a cervical tissue sample, performed most frequently to detect cervical cancer.

Peau d'orange: orange-peel-like appearance of breast skin, caused by edema.

Pelvic examination: assessment of the external and internal genitalia by inspection and palpation.

Perimenopausal: occurring during the climacteric stage.

Premenstrual syndrome (PMS): cyclic cluster of signs and symptoms, such as breast tenderness, fluid retention, and mood swings, that usually occurs after ovulation and before or during menses.

Puberty: developmental stage when secondary sex characteristics appear and reproductive ability begins.

Retroflexed uterus: normal position in which the uterine corpus flexes toward the rectum and the cervix lies in the normal position.

Retroverted uterus: normal position in which the uterine corpus flexes toward the rectum at a less acute angle than a retroflexed uterus.

Tail of Spence: extension of breast tissue, which projects from the upper outer quadrant of the breast toward the axilla; also called the axillary tail.

Toxic shock syndrome (TSS): severe illness caused by a bacterial infection. TSS has been associated with improper tampon use and typically causes sudden high fever, vomiting, diarrhea, myalgia, vaginal redness or discharge, skin rash, and sore throat.

Women and health care

Many factors can influence the client's perception of her health care needs. These include self-perception, body image, and developmental stage as well as cultural, religious, socioeconomic, and educational factors. Perceived societal norms also shape the attitudes of women and health care professionals about health care needs.

To provide holistic care for women, the nurse must understand the significance of these factors. For example, cultural and religious factors may influence a woman's choice of care and treatment. Her socioeconomic status may prohibit preventive care. Her educational level may cause a knowledge deficit about developmental changes such as menarche (onset of menses).

Because these factors can influence the client's health, the nurse must assess them and intervene appropriately—for example, by dispelling myths, advocating low-cost preventive care, and educating the client. To promote effective care, the nurse should be nonjudgmental and respectful of the client's values.

Women as health care consumers

Women are the primary consumers of health care. They visit physicians' offices more frequently and undergo more surgical procedures than men. These procedures, which include mastectomy (removal of one or both breasts) and hysterectomy (removal of the uterus), typically have long-term physical and emotional implications. In addition, more women than men live in nursing homes.

Several factors may account for women's higher health care consumption: society's historical association of reproductive function with illness and its view of menstruation and menopause as abnormal processes, increased health risks associated with pregnancy and contraception, increased life span, low status but high-stress employment, and stress caused by role conflict, single parenting, and careers.

Women also typically manage health care for their families. They establish family members' health care perceptions, identify their health care needs, and determine when members need professional health care (Griffith-Kenney, 1986). Factors that influence a woman's perception of her own health care needs probably will affect her perception of her family's needs. In fact, women's perceptions may be passed down through generations, making them an influential force in the health of our society.

Choice of primary care provider

A woman may obtain gynecologic care from a gynecologist, family physician, internist, or nurse practitioner. Ideally, she would choose a primary care provider based on the provider's philosophical approach to care. Influenced by the same variables that affect their perception of health care needs, women traditionally have chosen physicians, gynecologists, or internists as their primary care providers. Recently, however, more women have selected specially prepared nurse practitioners for primary care. Nurse practitioners who provide gynecologic care include nurse-midwives, women's health care nurse practitioners, family nurse practitioners, adult nurse practitioners, and geriatric nurse practitioners. They perform physical assessment, manage common health problems, and make referrals, as needed.

Factors influencing contact with the health care system

Access to health care and the attitudes of health care professionals can influence a client's contact with the health care system.

Access to care

Although access to health care facilities is essential to a woman's health, it may be limited by her socioeconomic status, cultural background, or sexual orientation.

Socioeconomic status. In the United States, access to health care is tied to ability to pay. Therefore, a woman in a lower socioeconomic group probably will have limited health care options. She may have to rely primarily on government-funded programs, such as Medicaid, to pay for health care. Yet many private practice physicians do not participate in Medicaid programs because of their relatively low payment levels and time-consuming payment procedures.

As an alternative, the woman may seek care at a public health clinic. However, many of these clinics maintain only daytime hours, with long waits, impersonal attention, and fragmented care. Also, they may offer only one type of service, such as well-child care, adult health, or prenatal care, forcing the client to visit several locations for complete services.

Yet health care is especially important to clients in lower socioeconomic groups, where survival rates for many diseases, such as breast and cervical cancer, are lower. Although Papanicolaou (Pap) tests and mammography can detect early signs of these cancers, some health insurers will not pay for these studies unless a problem or suspected disorder has been detected.

Even when screening programs are designed for high-risk, low-income individuals, women often do not take advantage of them (Funch, 1986), possibly because they lack knowledge about cancer and the value of prevention. More research is needed to identify features of prevention and early-detection programs that will attract and retain low-income women.

Cultural background. The client's cultural or ethnic background may limit her access to care, particularly if she speaks little English or is unaware of available health care services. When caring for a client from a different background, the nurse should provide culturally appropriate care. By talking to the client and to community leaders and traditional health care providers from the same cultural background, the nurse can gain an understanding of client behaviors and values that may affect gynecologic care. The nurse should try to obtain information about the following topics:
• Traditional sources of women's health care
• Cultural beliefs about the causes—and cures—of illness
• Major health problems in this group
• Importance of health care provider's sex
• Any charms or practices that are used to ensure good health and keep evil spirits away
• Issues that are considered inappropriate for discussion
• Behaviors of a health care professional that might go against traditional practices or customs
• View of time and importance of keeping appointments
• Role of women in this culture
• Decision-making processes
• Customs that mark major events, such as birth, menarche, menopause, and marriage
• Beliefs about contraception and sexuality
• Beliefs about preventive medicine, such as regular checkups, Pap tests, and BSEs.

Sexual orientation. Women who choose alternative sex roles may avoid traditional health care facilities for fear of discrimination. This may affect their care by limiting health care options. For example, lesbians report that, when their sexual preference becomes known to heterosexual health care professionals, responses include "ostracism, invasive personal questioning, shock, embarrassment, unfriendliness, pity, condescension, and fear" (Stevens and Hall, 1988).

Lesbians usually do not disclose sexual orientation unless they know that the health care professional is a lesbian. If the client fails to reveal her sexual preference, the health care professional may assess her improperly. If she reveals her sexual orientation, the health care professional may react with insensitive care or open hostility.

A lesbian adolescent is particularly vulnerable. She may suffer great personal conflict and emotional distress over sexual orientation, which may be compounded by lack of support from family, school, and community. A lesbian adolescent is likely to prefer a health care professional who is knowledgeable about the health care problems of lesbians. She also may appreciate a health care professional who does not assume that all adolescents are heterosexual and who can offer support about relating to family and peers (Paroski, 1987). She may benefit greatly from support groups and nonprejudiced health care (Gonsiorek, 1988).

Respecting individual differences and viewing people in the context of their environment can help the nurse provide appropriate care for a lesbian client. So can the following recommendations:
• Be aware of personal attitudes about homosexuality that could prejudice care.
• Develop interviewing techniques that acknowledge alternate life-styles.
• Seek information about lesbian culture and lesbian health concerns.
• Expand the definition of *family* to include the people who are most important to the client. (For more information, see Chapter 2, Family Structure and Function.)
• Recognize institutional policies that deny a lesbian's emotional needs. For example, some hospitals allow only parents, spouse, and adult children to visit a client in the critical care unit.
• Evaluate personal abilities to discuss lesbian health care sensitively.
• Avoid stereotyping.
• Recognize that confidentiality about sexual orientation may be critical to a lesbian (Johnson and Palermo, 1984).
• Request classes, workshops, or inservice programs about lesbians and their health care issues.
• Learn about community resources for lesbians.

Attitudes of health care professionals
A health care professional's attitude can influence the frequency and extent of a client's contact with the health care system. A supportive attitude can promote health care; a sexist or negative one may prevent it.

Supportive attitude. As a consumer, the client has the right to be informed and to participate actively in her health care decisions. As the client's advocate, the nurse must foster a supportive, nonjudgmental environment, provide the necessary information for the client's decisions, and respect the client's confidentiality and decisions. This promotes client participation and mutual cooperation in a therapeutic relationship, allowing the plan of care to be met more readily.

Sexist attitude. Because sexism is part of our culture, it also exists in the health care system. It may be reflected when health care professionals ignore some women's health complaints or write unnecessary prescriptions for women. Because sexist attitudes can negatively influence the client toward the health care system, the nurse must be alert for sexism and act as the client's advocate. Further, the nurse should take an objective, holistic approach when dealing with a client's health concerns.

Gynecologic needs across the life span

The client's gynecologic needs change across the life span, reflecting her physical and psychosocial development as well as her exposure to environmental influences.

Pediatric client (up to age 10)

The pediatric client's gynecologic needs usually stem from congenital anomalies, vaginal discharge, or trauma caused by sexual abuse or a foreign object in the vagina. Sexual abuse, including incest, affects 60,000 to 100,000 children annually in the United States (Lempert, 1986), with ten times more girls being affected than boys. It can cause physical effects, such as a sexually transmitted disease (STD), and long-term psychological effects, such as sexual dysfunction, depression, inadequate social skills, and difficulty with relationships.

Adolescent client (ages 11 to 19)

In addition to some continuing pediatric concerns, gynecologic needs for an adolescent client may include assistance with menarche (onset of menses), menstruation, contraception, STDs, and other problems.

Menarche. An adolescent needs preparation for the physical changes related to menarche and puberty. Menarche usually occurs between ages 12 and 13, but may occur as early as age 9 or as late as age 18. (For more information, see Chapter 6, Reproductive Anatomy and Physiology.)

An adolescent also may need psychological preparation for this developmental milestone. Some cultures celebrate menarche, giving the adolescent special attention. For example, an adolescent from southern India may receive a ritual milk bath while sitting on banana leaves and eating raw eggs in ginger. North Americans, however, tend to treat menarche as a biological event and either downplay its significance or send mixed messages about it (Weideger, 1976). To help the adolescent client adapt to menarche, the nurse should clearly explore its importance and meaning in her life.

Menstruation. After menarche, the adolescent may have many concerns about menstruation. She may worry about menstrual cycle irregularity—a common, normal variation that usually resolves 1 to 2 years after menarche. She also may be concerned about her rate of growth and development compared to that of her peers.

An adolescent client may need reassurance about the amount of menstrual blood loss, which is minimal and ranges from 30 to 100 ml. She also may appreciate learning that her cycle may take several months to stabilize.

The adolescent client may need information about the physiology of menstruation and external factors that may affect it, such as diet, exercise, sleep, climate changes, drug use, contraceptive use, stress, surgery, or illness. For example, a nutritional disorder, strenuous exercise, illness, or drug use may cause amenorrhea (absence of menses). Abnormal sleep patterns, stress, or climate changes may produce irregular menstrual cycles. The stress of surgery can make the menstrual period early or late. Oral contraceptives may cause metrorrhagia (bleeding or spotting between cycles); an intrauterine device (IUD), menorrhagia (increased menstrual bleeding). Such prescription drugs as anticoagulants and thiazides also may cause menorrhagia.

Because certain cultural myths and beliefs surround menstruation, the adolescent client may need accurate information to dispel them. (For more information, see *Cultural considerations: Menstruation*, page 114.)

Contraception. In one study, researchers found that about 19% of girls had had sexual intercourse by age 15; 50% by age 18; and 72% by age 19 (*Teenage Pregnancy in Industrialized Countries*, 1986). Many of these adolescents use contraceptive foams and condoms because they are easily available, cause few adverse effects, and prevent STDs. Many others choose an oral contraceptive, which requires medical supervision. The fewest number choose diaphragms and IUDs (Griffith-Kenney, 1986). (For more information, see Chapter 9, Family Planning.)

Sexual activity without contraception has far-reaching implications. The United States now has the highest

CULTURAL CONSIDERATIONS

Menstruation

When caring for a client from a different background, the nurse must keep the following representative cultural considerations in mind.

Menstruation as a negative force

Historically, people considered menstrual blood a volatile poison capable of wide-ranging destruction. For example, crops would not grow if a menstruating woman walked across a farmer's field, flowers would wilt if she passed by, and bread dough would not rise if she kneaded it.

Men believed that menstruating women were a threat to their potency. Because of this, they allowed no physical contact—especially sexual intercourse—during menses. Australian aborigines believed that if a man saw menstrual blood, his hair would turn gray and he would lose his vigor. To prevent this, they forbade menstruating women to touch anything that men used or to walk on paths that men traveled.

Some cultures housed women in separate quarters during menses where they were "cleansed" or "purified" before returning to their homes. Other cultures punished women for menstruating (Weideger, 1976).

In cultures where women were not segregated during menses, traditions arose for signalling or warning men. For example, in the lower Congo, if a menstruating woman was hailed by a man, she had to put her pipe in her mouth to signal she was "unclean." In other cultures, women were required to wear head bands during menstruation (Novak, 1921).

Menstruation as a positive force

Conversely, some cultures believed that menstrual blood had special powers. It has been used as a healant, an aphrodisiac, and as a method of securing fertility. The Wogeo men of New Guinea slit open the penis to allow blood to flow. They performed this "men's menstruation" because they thought of menstruation as a cleansing process (Bettelheim, 1962).

Menstruation as an energy drain

In the late nineteenth century, many physicians subscribed to the theory of bodily energy, which stated that the body functioned on a fixed amount of energy and that the woman's body had special energy needs related to menstruation and reproduction (Harlow, 1986). These special needs competed directly with those of other body systems for energy. Any physical or mental effort could cause several disorders. For these reasons, menstruating women were often excused from their responsibilities, and many people believed that physical and mental weakness were related to the normal functioning of the woman's reproductive organs.

Persistent myths about menstruation

Although few people still harbor myths about menstruation, some beliefs have persisted to the present day. Because of the bodily energy theory, some people believe that a woman is vulnerable to physiologic and psychological stress during menstruation. For example, they mistakenly believe that bathing, hair washing, and exposure to cold temperatures while menstruating can cause illness.

Because of the notion that menstrual blood is a source of contamination, many people still refrain from intercourse during menstruation. Even today, Orthodox Jewish women (a small percentage of the Jewish population) must take a ritual cleansing bath (mikvah) after menstruation.

As a result of long-standing beliefs about menstruation, many people still think it is personal and should be concealed from others. As a result, a woman may feel worry, anxiety, and fear about her ability to conceal her menstrual flow, to buy pads or tampons discretely, and to conceal them properly.

Nursing considerations

To help the client cope with detrimental myths and beliefs, the nurse should listen actively to the client's concerns, provide accurate information about menstruation, and discuss the positive aspects of this normal physiologic process.

For example, the nurse may point out that menstruation holds special meanings for most women. They may see it as a uniquely feminine experience, a reminder of their femaleness and reproductive potential. They may see regular menstrual cycles as a sign of health; disruptions, as a sign of illness (except during pregnancy). And although some women find menstruation bothersome, most view it as a normal part of life.

The nurse may tell the client that, although our society has become more open about discussing menstruation, research shows that some men feel excluded from this part of women's lives and frustrated with women's secretiveness about it. These men believe that sharing information about menstruation would help make them more understanding and supportive of women (Stern, 1986). Open discussion of menstruation and more research by nurses and others may promote a healthier view of menstruation and women.

---

adolescent pregnancy rate (1 million per year) in the industrialized world, with the highest rate among Black adolescents (Lempert, 1986). This creates health concerns for the adolescent and for society. An adolescent has a higher risk for pregnancy complications. Because adolescent pregnancy occurs most frequently in lower socioeconomic groups, it helps perpetuate poverty.

STDs. Increased sexual activity has increased the risk of STDs. Adolescents with multiple sexual partners and those who do not use barrier contraceptives, such as condoms, run the greatest risk.

In a study of 113 sexually active adolescents ages 13 to 19, 7.1% had gonorrhea and 27.4% had chlamydia. Few of them had sought health care because they suspected an STD; most had sought routine family planning and postpartal care (Smith, Phillips, Faro, McGill, and Wait, 1988). (For more information, see Chapter 12, Infectious Disorders.)

Other problems. The adolescent may face other problems, including:
• physical, emotional, or sexual abuse. Up to 35% of adolescent girls experience physical abuse while dating (NiCarthy, 1986).
• smoking. By the end of high school, 12.5% of students smoke at least half a pack of cigarettes a day (Johnston, O'Malley, and Bachman, 1988). Adolescent girls are the fastest growing group of smokers.
• alcohol use. Of 17,000 American high school seniors, 66% reported consuming alcohol sometime in the previous month and 5% reported drinking daily. Of the females, 28% consumed five or more alcoholic drinks in a row. Of all students, 37% said most or all of their friends get drunk at least once a week (Johnston, O'Malley, and Bachman, 1988).
• drug use. By the time they leave high school, 60% of all seniors have tried an illegal drug, probably marijuana, amphetamines, or cocaine. Almost 5% of all students reported daily marijuana use. About 20% reported that most or all of their friends smoke marijuana (Johnston, O'Malley, and Bachman, 1988).
• eating disorders. Anorexia nervosa (a disorder characterized by prolonged refusal to eat and abnormal fear of becoming obese) and bulimia (a disorder characterized by eating binges followed by self-induced vomiting or other purges) occur most frequently in middle-class adolescents, ages 13 to 20, and lead to death in 3% of all cases. The incidence of eating disorders in adolescents from lower socioeconomic groups is unknown.
• depression and self-destructive behavior. These are increasing problems in adolescents, as indicated by the U.S. adolescent suicide rate, which has tripled in the past 15 to 20 years. Depression and self-destructive behavior may be closely related to alcohol and drug use. (For more information about these problems, see Chapter 14, Violence Against Women, and Chapter 15, Women's Health-Compromising Behaviors.)

Adult client (childbearing years)

The adult client's gynecologic concerns may include contraception, infertility, stress-related disorders (such as amenorrhea or sexual dysfunction), and other concerns. (For information about a woman's needs during pregnancy, childbirth, and the postpartal period, see Units Three through Five.)

Contraception. The advent of contraception and recent changes in women's roles have affected traditional reproductive patterns—and women's gynecologic needs. Many women now plan their families. Some are deciding to postpone childbirth; others, to remain childless.

A client may select from various contraceptive methods. However, some contraceptive methods carry health risks. For example, long-term use of oral contraceptives may increase the risk of cardiovascular disease; use of an IUD increases the risk of pelvic inflammatory disease (PID), ectopic pregnancy, and other problems. (For more information, see Chapter 9, Family Planning.)

A client who postpones or prevents childbearing faces three other concerns: criticism for her decision, increased health risks (including breast cancer, some gynecologic disorders, and risks associated with pregnancy after age 30), and infertility.

Infertility. When a woman's life-style changes, she may change her mind about having children. If she has postponed childbearing until after age 30, infertility may occur, caused by physiologic decrease in fertility or a gynecologic disorder.

Infertility can be a crisis for any woman. Its assessment is time-consuming, treatment is costly, and the emotional impact can be devastating. However, it may place even greater stress on a woman who has postponed childbearing and has few remaining reproductive years. (For more information, see Chapter 10, Fertility and Infertility.)

Stress-related disorders. A woman may play many roles, ranging from home manager to child caregiver to employee. The demands of these roles can lead to stress and stress-related disorders. Yet the rewards of having multiple roles—increased family income, pension and health benefits, increased job-related skills, improved self-image, and stimulating social contact—may help improve a woman's health.

Other concerns. The increase in violent crimes against women is a major concern. Rape and other forms of abuse not only create immediate health care needs, but also can have long-term effects on a woman's health. (For more information, see Chapter 14, Violence Against Women.)

Such practices as smoking and drug or alcohol abuse can affect a client's health and are on the rise for women. (For more information, see Chapter 15, Women's Health-Compromising Behaviors.)

Adult client (perimenopausal years)

In this stage of life, the client's reasons for seeking gynecologic care may include menopausal signs and symptoms, sexual and cultural concerns, and post-menopausal disturbances.

Menopause, the cessation of menses, usually occurs between ages 40 and 60 (the climacteric). The climacteric is a developmental stage that includes a premenopausal, menopausal, and postmenopausal phase. During this normal physiologic event, reproductive function gradually diminishes and then ceases. (For more information, see Chapter 6, Reproductive Anatomy and Physiology.)

For many women, the postmenopausal years are joyful because they can have intercourse without contraceptives or fear of pregnancy, they do not have to carry menstrual hygiene products with them, and their children are old enough to care for themselves (McKeon, 1988).

For others, these years represent decline and debility. One reason for this negative perception may be that menopause traditionally has been viewed by predominantly male researchers as a time of estrogen withdrawal, characterized by such words as *failure, atrophy, decline,* and *breakdown* (Martin, 1987). Another reason may be that the experience of menopause is a relatively new phenomenon. Around 1900, the life expectancy for the average North American woman was just under 50 years. Now it is almost 80 years, meaning that a woman may live up to one-third of her life after menopause (National Institute on Aging, 1988).

Most of the research that characterizes menopause as a time of decline and debility is based on women who have sought medical or psychiatric help. Little research has been done on menopause in women who have had no significant complaints, so little is known about their perceptions of and feelings about menopause.

Menopausal signs and symptoms. The gynecologic needs of menopausal women typically result from menopause itself. Around age 40, most women experience physical and psychological symptoms of decreased estrogen and progesterone secretion, which last for 10 to 15 years. The onset and severity of these symptoms varies greatly with the individual.

Physical effects of menopause include irregular menses, hot flashes (transient sensations of warmth over the upper chest, face, and extremities), perspiration and chills, vaginal changes, and decreased bone mass. Combined physical effects of menopause and aging may include dysuria (painful urination), weight gain, decreased skin elasticity, atrophy of breast tissue and external

genitalia, and decreased levels of high-density lipoproteins (HDLs).

Irregular menses, which result from decreased estrogen levels, frequently signal the onset of menopause. The client typically notices a decrease in blood flow and frequency of periods until menstruation ceases.

Hot flashes result from autonomic vasomotor disturbances and vasodilation that accompany the neurohormonal changes of menopause. Usually followed by profuse perspiration and chills, hot flashes occur most frequently at night and last from several seconds to 5 minutes. (For more information, see *Nursing research: Hot flashes in menopause.*)

As estrogen levels decrease, vaginal changes may include atrophy, thinning of the mucosa, loss of rugae, decreased elasticity, and decreased secretions with increased alkalinity. These changes may produce vaginal dryness, burning, itching, and dyspareunia (painful or difficult intercourse). When low estrogen levels cause urethral atrophy, dysuria may result.

Loss of calcium can be caused by decreased estrogen levels, a sedentary life-style, and inadequate dietary calcium. It may lead to osteoporosis (demineralization of the bones and consequent decreased bone mass), which makes the bones more brittle, increases the risk of fractures, and may cause joint or bone pain.

Although decreased estrogen levels may affect fat distribution, weight gain usually results from poor diet and decreased exercise.

Decreased skin elasticity may result from reduced estrogen levels, aging, poor nutrition, smoking, sun exposure, or a combination of these factors. It may cause facial wrinkling accompanied by increased facial hair growth from the predominance of androgens.

A decrease in breast size and loss of elasticity may occur along with external genitalia atrophy. Pubic hair may thin and turn gray, particularly after menopause.

Decreased estrogen levels are associated with lower HDL levels, increasing the client's risk for cardiovascular disease.

Although researchers have not yet determined the extent to which psychological symptoms are caused by menopause or by sociocultural factors, these symptoms may include emotional lability, depression, irritability, decreased attention span, insomnia, headaches, and decreased energy. They may result, in part, from the effects of decreased estrogen on the central nervous system.

Sexual and cultural concerns. A client's sexual relationships may affect—or be affected by—the physiologic and psychological changes of menopause. Physiologic changes may be permanent (as with atrophic changes of the reproductive organs) or temporary (as with hot

NURSING RESEARCH APPLIED

Hot flashes in menopause

A study of 594 women between ages 35 and 60 investigated the prevalence of hot flashes and related variables, such as estrogen replacement therapy and age of menopause onset. For the purposes of this study, the researchers defined hot flashes as a vasomotor response to hormonal instability during menopause, characterized by a warm sensation and possibly by tingling, throbbing, a rush of blood, light-headedness, chills, and feelings of suffocation.

Using a structured questionnaire in telephone interviews, the researchers found that 88.4% of the women had experienced hot flashes. Most began after age 40 (89%), but one woman with a natural menopause (cessation of menses as a maturational process) reported her first hot flash at age 29. Frequency of hot flashes varied from too infrequent to count to 72 per day. The length of time women had experienced hot flashes ranged from 1 to 2 years in 35% of the subjects to more than 11 years in 10% of the subjects.

In this study, the hot flash prevalence rate (88%) exceeded that of comparable groups in previous studies (68%, 73%, and 75%). However, the number of women who reported one or more hot flashes per day (47%) was lower than the number reported in another study (70%). The discrepancy may be explained by the high percentage (42%) of women in the latest study who used estrogen. Of this group, 82% had surgically induced menopause, suggesting that this type of menopause produces more severe symptoms, which require estrogen use.

Application to practice
Results of this study support the prevalence of hot flashes in women during menopause. They also indicate that the frequency, duration, and severity of hot flashes can vary greatly among individuals and are affected by the cause of menopause and estrogen use.

Because the effects of menopause can vary so widely, the nurse must accurately assess the presence, frequency, and severity of hot flashes in each client. This assessment data can help the nurse individualize care to promote comfort, educate the client about the physiology of menopause, and facilitate her transition and adaptation to menopause and its physical effects.

For a client who chooses hormone replacement therapy, the nurse should explain its advantages, risks, and adverse effects to help the client make an informed decision about her health care.

Feldman, B., Voda, A., and Gronseth, E. (1985). The prevalence of hot flash and associated variables among perimenopausal women. *Research in Nursing and Health*, 8(3), 261-268.

flashes); psychological changes, such as emotional lability, are temporary. Nevertheless, they may affect a woman's self-image.

A woman's perception of menopause may affect her psychologically. For example, if she perceives menopause as a normal developmental stage, she is likely to experience it positively and view it as an opportunity for role redefinition and personal growth. If she believes reproduction is her main role, she may perceive menopause negatively and experience depression, guilt, frustration, or loss of purpose.

A woman's perception of menopause and associated changes can affect her sexual relationship, as can her partner's perceptions. Neither should think of menopause as the cessation of a woman's sexual drive or activity. In fact, drive and activity may increase with her freedom from contraception and fear of pregnancy.

Some changes, however, may adversely affect the sexual relationship. For example, vaginal changes may cause dyspareunia, which may reduce the frequency and enjoyment of intercourse. However, proper identification, treatment, and teaching should overcome most of these problems.

A culture's view of menopause may influence a woman's transition through this developmental stage. (For more information, see *Cultural considerations: Perceptions of menopause,* page 118.)

Postmenopausal disturbances. The major postmenopausal disturbances include atrophic vaginitis (inflammation in a short, dry, somewhat inelastic vagina), osteoporosis, and urinary incontinence. Several years after menopause, atrophic vaginitis may occur when the vaginal epithelium thins and vaginal secretions become scanty. It may cause dyspareunia and increase the risk of infection.

A major concern for postmenopausal women, osteoporosis may go undetected until a fracture occurs. In this debilitating, painful disease, the client experiences decreased bone mass that results in poor fracture healing, which may increase morbidity and mortality.

In postmenopausal women, osteoporosis may result from increased bone resorption at menopause, calcium store depletion that dates from pregnancy and lactation, a longer life span, less bone mass due to smaller body size, and insufficient calcium intake or absorption over a lifetime.

Although urinary incontinence does not result from menopause, it may occur in a postmenopausal woman with urethral structure atrophy and pelvic relaxation from menopause, multiple pregnancies, or obesity.

Elderly client
Older women have many health concerns, including such common age-related problems as loss of physical abilities, sensory and perceptual acuity, spouse, support systems, income, and home. These losses create additional health care needs, which may not receive treatment because a client's fixed income may restrict her access to health care.

Despite a growing elderly female population, health care professionals know little about their gynecologic needs, primarily because they typically are reluctant to seek gynecologic care. This is unfortunate because some gynecologic cancers occur between ages 60 and 70. Women over age 65 account for 25% of all cases of cervical cancer and 40% of deaths from invasive cervical cancer (Weintraub, 1989).

The elderly client also may need care for atrophic vaginitis, dyspareunia, osteoporosis, and especially incontinence.

Urinary incontinence may affect more than one-third of women over age 60, to the extent that one-third of these women must wear protective material (Diokno, Brock, Brown, and Herzog, 1986) and 10% are incontinent at least once a week. Yet only 20% of incontinent individuals seek medical help and two-thirds of these receive only symptomatic care rather than treatment of the underlying cause (Resnick, 1988).

This is unfortunate because incontinence is not a normal part of aging; it is a sign of an underlying abnormal condition. Moreover, several studies have found that, regardless of the cause, incontinence usually responds to treatment. It is curable in two-thirds of clients and manageable in most of the remainder (Resnick, 1988).

CULTURAL CONSIDERATIONS

Perceptions of menopause

When caring for a client from a different background, the nurse must keep the following representative cultural considerations in mind.

Not every culture perceives menopause in the same way. Typically, perception of menopause is related to perceptions of women's roles and aging. The Hispanic community, for example, has traditionally viewed a woman's primary role as childbearer and childrearer, even until late in the woman's childbearing years. Because her fertility is seen as a sign of her role fulfillment—and of her male partner's virility—she may suffer a loss of self-esteem during menopause (Orque, Bloch, and Monrroy, 1983).

For such a client, the nurse should anticipate coping problems and should talk to the client about her feelings. To build the client's self-esteem and help her cope, the nurse should help her take pride in the accomplishment of raising her children, should discuss other ways of perceiving this change, and should remind her that some childrearing may continue with her grandchildren.

On the other hand, many Asian cultures revere their elderly members, treating them with the deepest respect for their wisdom and experience. Because of these perceptions, an Asian woman is more likely to view menopause simply as a developmental phase—a normal part of life that brings new experiences—that requires no nursing interventions.

Women from a culture that glorifies youth and views menopause as a time of decline may benefit greatly from the nurse's help. The nurse should dispel or modify detrimental cultural myths and emphasize that menopause is a normal physiologic process. These actions may enable the woman to develop a greater sense of worth, redefine her roles, and secure her feminine identity.

Gynecologic care

Although many women seek gynecologic care as a routine part of health maintenance, others seek care for a specific health concern, such as premenstrual symptoms, menstrual discomfort, contraceptive information, pregnancy, an STD, infertility, sexual dysfunction, unexplained vaginal bleeding, menopausal symptoms, or urinary incontinence.

No matter what the client's reason for seeking care, the nurse should use the nursing process to provide appropriate gynecologic care, beginning with a comprehensive assessment. (For a case study that shows how to apply the nursing process when caring for a client seeking gynecologic care, see *Applying the nursing process: Client with knowledge deficit related to BSE and mammography*, pages 144 and 145.)

Assessment

The gynecologic assessment provides data about the client's health care needs, using a health history interview, physical assessment, and diagnostic studies. Because of its nature, the gynecologic assessment may cause embarrassment, discomfort, anxiety, fear, or stress in some clients. To minimize these problems, prepare the client properly, assess the least sensitive areas first, and develop a trusting relationship with the client.

Client preparation

To promote physical and psychological preparation and help establish a therapeutic relationship, provide instructions before the visit and information throughout the physical assessment. (For details, see the "Physical assessment section," pages 124 to 128.)

Preparation begins when the client schedules an appointment for gynecologic care. Ask a new client to review her and her family's health history and to bring copies of any medical records she may have. If the health care facility policy requires, send the client a health record and other forms to complete and bring to the visit. For any client, ask her to bring a menstrual record. (For an example, see *Client teaching: Menstrual and breast self-examination record*, page 120.)

Let the client know how long the visit will take. Advise her to avoid douching for 24 hours before the examination because douching may eliminate cells needed for diagnostic testing. Also tell the client to schedule her appointment for a time when she does not expect to be menstruating because blood can interfere with Pap test results. (If she has abnormal vaginal bleeding, however, reassure her that she can schedule an appointment anyway.) Finally, let the client know that she is welcome to bring a family member or friend to the visit and that she will have some private time with the health care professional whether or not she chooses to bring a companion.

Try to make the environment as pleasant and comfortable as possible. Avoid extremes in room temperature. Using a friendly tone, introduce yourself and assure the client that her privacy and confidentiality will be respected.

Health history

Conduct the initial health history interview in a private room with the client fully clothed, if possible. Ask one question at a time, using words that the client understands and giving her time to respond. If the client is elderly, ensure that she can hear you; speak respectfully and avoid familiarity and condescension.

Begin the interview with nonthreatening questions. Then, after establishing a rapport with the client, ask any difficult or potentially embarrassing questions. Because many questions may seem personal to the client, explain their importance to her care.

After introducing yourself and explaining your role, gather biographical data and assess the client's health status, health promotion and protection behaviors, and roles and relationships.

Biographical data. Obtain or confirm the client's name, address, and other biographical information required by the health care facility.

Particularly note the client's age, because it can affect her gynecologic needs. For example, an adolescent may need care for menstrual irregularities; an adult woman, for fertility counseling; an older woman, for management of menopausal symptoms. Knowledge of the client's age also provides a context for interpreting assessment data.

Health status. Next, evaluate the client's health, focusing on her current, past, and family health status.

Reason for seeking health care. Begin by asking the client, "Why are you here today?" Find out if she wants to ask any questions or needs any particular information.

The client's reason for seeking health care should guide the assessment. Asking if the client has any questions is helpful if the client is anxious or has questions she is afraid she will forget to ask. Identifying the client's information needs increases the likelihood that she will get that information.

Next, ask an open-ended question about the client's general health. This will ease her into the interview and give her a chance to bring up any problems.

Menstrual history. Ask questions about the client's menstrual history to investigate this important aspect of gynecologic health. For a menopausal or elderly client, ask only the questions that apply.

First, determine the client's age at menarche. Knowledge of menarche helps establish a menstrual pattern. Some clients have irregular menstrual periods up to 2 years after menarche.

Next, ask the client to specify the first day of bleeding of her last menstrual period (LMP). The client's answer indicates her current place in the menstrual cycle, which suggests appropriate care, such as examination with extra gentleness during the premenstrual phase. It also provides a context for evaluating physical findings. For example, breast tenderness may be normal in the premenstrual phase, but abnormal at other times of the cycle. An LMP longer than the client's normal cycle can suggest pregnancy or menopausal changes.

Continue by asking about the menstrual cycle length and the menstrual period duration. Normally, menstrual cycles vary in length by fewer than 7 days, and menstrual periods last 3 to 7 days. An irregular menstrual cycle or abnormally short or long menstrual period may indicate a gynecologic disorder. An abnormally long cycle in a client between ages 40 and 50 may indicate menopause, pregnancy, or a gynecologic disorder.

Then inquire about the blood flow during the menstrual period. If the client has difficulty describing her blood flow, ask such questions as, "How many tampons or pads do you use per day?" If she reports using six or more per day, find out to what extent they are saturated. A heavy blood flow may result from uterine fibroids and may cause anemia.

Ask about any menstrual or premenstrual symptoms. If the client suffers from dysmenorrhea (painful menstruation), determine its severity and document any treatments she uses to relieve it. If she reports premenstrual breast tenderness, bloating, headaches, nausea, vomiting, mood changes, anxiety, fatigue, restlessness, easy distractibility, irritability, or tension, document these symptoms and determine their effect on her. Such a client may have premenstrual syndrome (PMS), a cluster of physical and emotional symptoms that occur after ovulation and before or during menses. (For more information about assessment and treatment, see Chapter 13, Gynecologic Disorders.)

Identify the frequency and severity of any menopausal symptoms, such as menstrual irregularities and hot flashes, to aid in developing an effective plan for managing them.

Contraceptive history. For a client in her childbearing years, find out if she uses a contraceptive. If so, inquire about her satisfaction with the method, presence of adverse reactions, and any desire to change methods. If not, ask if she wants contraceptive information. Pregnancy may occur any time after menarche. A client who has problems with her present contraceptive or who does not use any may benefit from a discussion of contraceptive choices. Also, some contraceptive methods may alter menstrual patterns.

If the client has used contraception before, find out which method. Then determine how long she used it, if she had any problems, what she liked and disliked about it, and why she stopped using that method. The client's answers provide information that will aid in selecting an appropriate contraceptive method for her and may suggest areas for counseling. (For more information about assessment and care, see Chapter 9, Family Planning.)

Obstetric history. If the client is in her childbearing years, ask if she thinks she may be pregnant. Pregnancy is a possible cause of amenorrhea and may contraindicate mammography.

Then inquire about the client's previous pregnancies and their outcomes. Find out how many children the

---

CLIENT TEACHING

Menstrual and breast self-examination record

This chart offers an easy way to record the dates of your menstrual period and the amount of blood flow. It also serves as a reminder to examine your breasts every month. Fill in the dates of your menstrual period and your breast self-examination with these symbols: N (normal blood flow), L (light blood flow), H (heavy blood flow), and B (breast self-examination).

By reminding you to examine your breasts every month, this chart will help you develop a good health habit. By recording your menstrual periods, you will be able to give your doctor or nurse practitioner important information about your gynecologic health.

MONTH	DATE		
	1 2 3 4 5 6 7 8 9 10	11 12 13 14 15 16 17 18 19 20	21 22 23 24 25 26 27 28 29 30 31
January			
February			
March			
April			
May			
June			
July			
August			
September			
October			
November			
December			

client has and determine if she desires additional children.

This information will describe the client's family constellation and identify areas that need further exploration. A client who has had a miscarriage, stillborn infant, or some other perinatal loss may appreciate a chance to discuss it. So may a client who has had an elective abortion, especially if she underwent this procedure when it was illegal. In either case, determine the extent of loss and appropriateness of the client's grieving.

If a client has never been pregnant or has no living children, ask if children were or are desired. Some women have no children because they do not want them; others, because they are infertile. To differentiate, ask if she has been unable to become pregnant when she wanted to. An infertile client may experience severe emotional distress and need counseling. (For more information about assessment and care, see Chapter 10, Fertility and Infertility.)

If a client has relinquished a child for adoption, explore her feelings about it, possibly by asking, "Do you think about that child?" or "How do you feel about that?" Even when the birth mother feels the adoption was in the child's best interest, she may feel a great loss. Determine if she has completed her grieving and acknowledge her pain, if present.

Genitourinary problems. Ask if the client currently has any signs or symptoms of genitourinary infection, such as a fever or vaginal discharge or itching. These findings may warrant testing and treatment.

Inquire if the client has had a pelvic infection. Such an infection may leave scar tissue that causes ectopic pregnancy, pelvic pain, or infertility.

Also ask if the client has had an STD, such as syphilis, gonorrhea, herpes, chlamydia, or condyloma (anogenital warts). If so, document when it occurred and its treatment and follow-up. Also note the client's understanding of its consequences and transmission methods, and ask if her sexual partner received treatment and follow-up care. Because a client with a history of STDs runs a relatively high risk of reinfection, expect to obtain specimens for testing and provide information about protection against STDs.

If the client has had condyloma, ask if the warts were removed and if this treatment was effective. Because condyloma is associated with cervical cancer, the client should have a Pap test every year.

A client with a history of genital herpes may need counseling about the importance of annual Pap tests because herpes may increase the risk of cervical cancer and the risk of transmission to the neonate during delivery. The client whose lesions recur with stress, menstruation, or other activities may appreciate stress management and related information.

For a postmenopausal or older client, ask about any problems with urinary incontinence. In such a client, incontinence is a common but often-neglected problem that may respond to relatively simple interventions.

Additional medical history. Follow up by asking if the client has ever had seizures, migraine headaches, anemia, diabetes, urinary tract infections, cancer, hepatitis B, hypertension, a blood clot, a cerebrovascular accident (CVA or stroke), or a bleeding disorder. Also inquire about thyroid, heart, lung, gastrointestinal, or liver problems. This list of medical problems identifies areas that may disrupt the menstrual cycle, indicate a gynecologic disorder, influence the treatment plan, need attention during the current visit, or require a medical referral.

Ask if the client received any blood products between 1977 (when acquired immunodeficiency syndrome [AIDS] was first diagnosed in the United States) and March 1985 (when blood screening for the HIV antibody began). If so, she may have contracted a blood-borne disorder.

Surgical history. If the client has had surgery, determine the specific type. Reproductive tract surgery may alter normal functioning. For example, a hysterectomy or oophorectomy will halt menses and cause many menopausal signs and symptoms.

Allergies. Carefully document any allergies to drugs, foods, or environmental substances. If the client reports a drug allergy, ask her to describe it because she may be confusing side effects with an allergic reaction. Although undesirable, side effects do not necessarily contraindicate a drug's use. An allergic reaction, however, can be fatal and always contraindicates a drug's use. If the client reports a food allergy or an allergy to an environmental substance, inquire about its effects and usual method of treatment.

Family history. Ask the client if anyone in her family has or has had anemia, hypertension, cancer, diabetes, clotting problems, CVA, or a kidney, heart, or lung disease. Because these disorders are hereditary and may influence gynecologic health, a client with a positive family history may require special testing and health education.

Also determine if anyone in the client's family has had gynecologic or reproductive problems. Some gynecologic disorders, such as breast cancer and menstrual problems, have a familial tendency.

To identify other potential problems, ask if anyone in the client's family has any other illness that might influence her health or put her at special risk. If she is adopted, ask what she knows about her family medical history.

Health promotion and protection behaviors. To assess the client's health promotion and protective behaviors, pose questions about her personal habits (including use of drugs, alcohol, and tobacco); her sleep, rest, exercise, and nutrition patterns; stress; and health care activities.

Personal habits. Ask the client which prescription and non-prescription drugs she has used in the past year. Also find out why she took them and in what amounts. Prescription drug use may reflect treatment of a gynecologic or other problem or reveal inappropriate drug use. A client who takes mood elevators or tranquilizers, for example, may be under treatment for depression, or may be abusing these drugs. Use of some drugs, such as anticoagulants and phenothiazines, may cause menstrual irregularities or other gynecologic problems. (For more information, see Chapter 10, Fertility and Infertility.) Use of other drugs may influence the choice of treatment for gynecologic needs. A client taking medication for a cardiovascular disorder, for example, may not be able to use an oral contraceptive.

Follow up by asking which illicit drugs, such as cocaine or marijuana, the client has used in the past year. Such drug use may disrupt the client's menstrual cycle and endanger her health.

Inquire about the frequency and amount of alcohol use. Also determine if the client has ever had problems with or felt guilty about alcohol use. Her answers may indicate alcoholism, which can cause fetal alcohol syndrome, if she is pregnant.

If the client smokes, find out how many cigarettes per day. Strongly warn the client about health problems associated with oral contraceptive use. (For more information on assessment and treatment of substance abuse and smoking, see Chapter 15, Women's Health-Compromising Behaviors.)

Sleep and rest patterns. Ask how much the client sleeps at night and during naps. Lack of sleep can result from stress, depression, or an underlying disorder and may lead to irregular menstrual cycles and other gynecologic problems. In a menopausal client, sleep pattern disturbances may result from hot flashes, which typically occur at night.

Exercise. Have the client describe the amount and type of exercise she usually engages in. Although strenuous exercise may cause menstrual irregularities and other problems, regular moderate exercise can reduce menstrual cramping and can improve cardiovascular fitness, weight control, muscle strength, bone density, coordination, and mood (American College of Obstetricians and Gynecologists, 1985).

Nutrition. Using a 24-hour dietary recall, assess the nutritional value of the client's diet. Also determine if she takes any vitamins or minerals regularly. A poor diet may cause irregular menstrual cycles. A low-calcium diet may increase the client's risk for developing osteoporosis, especially after menopause; a high-cholesterol diet may increase her risk for developing cardiovascular disease. Also note any weight loss or dietary patterns that suggest an eating disorder, such as anorexia nervosa or bulimia, which can cause menstrual irregularities and other problems.

Stress. First, ask the client to estimate her current stress level and describe how she copes with it. This information may identify stress-related menstrual irregularities and be useful in planning appropriate support.

Next, find out if the client has experienced any major life changes in the past 3 years, such as the death of a loved one, a move, or a job change. A major loss, which is particularly common in older women, requires about a year of grieving to resolve.

Menstrual management. Find out if the client keeps a menstrual record. A client of childbearing age can use a menstrual record to predict the date of her next period and identify cycle length, intermenstrual bleeding, and amenorrhea. If she has brought the menstrual record with her, it can provide useful assessment data.

Ask if she has noticed any change in her menstrual cycle related to such factors as stress, drug use, diet, and climate changes. The cycle normally varies in response to these external factors.

Next, find out if she uses pads or tampons and determine her satisfaction with this method of menstrual flow control. Her comments may reveal a need for information about menstrual management. An adolescent client who has had little experience with menstruation is especially likely to have difficulty with its management.

Inquire whether the client uses a douche or vaginal spray. These products usually are not required for hygiene and may cause irritation or infection.

Investigate how the client feels about her menstrual periods. She may report feeling embarrassed, inferior, or unclean during menstruation, especially if she is an adolescent. Such a client may benefit from information about hygiene, pads, and tampons. She also may have fears or misconceptions that need to be addressed.

Health care activities. Ask the client for the date of—and reason for—her last physical examination. Determine if it included a pelvic examination and Pap test. This information helps evaluate the client's health status and gynecologic health practices. If the client has had an abnormal Pap test result, ask when it occurred and what kind of treatment and follow-up she received. An abnormal Pap test may be caused by many factors, including cervical cancer, an STD, or in utero diethylstilbestrol (DES) exposure.

Inquire how frequently the client performs BSE. Because BSE helps detect signs of breast cancer, all clients should perform it once a month. A client who forgets to practice BSE may find a combined menstrual and BSE record helpful.

Follow up by asking if the client has ever had a mammogram. If she has, find out when. A mammogram can detect breast cancer up to 5 years before it is detectable through BSE. To protect her health, the adult client should have a mammogram at regular intervals. (For more information, see *Client teaching: Health care activities.*)

Next, assess the client's understanding of the risk factors for AIDS: past or current I.V. drug use or blood transfusions, a past or current sexual partner who has used or is using I.V. drugs, a bisexual partner, a sexual partner who has had intercourse with prostitutes, a sexual partner with a history of blood transfusion, and being from or having intercourse with a person from an area where AIDS is endemic, such as Haiti or Central Africa. Knowledge of the risk factors can help the client avoid AIDS or identify the risk for AIDS and seek testing and treatment.

Ask the client about condom use to prevent STDs when she has intercourse with a new sexual partner or a partner who engages in unsafe sex. To reduce the risk of hepatitis B and AIDS transmission, the client should insist that any new sexual partner (or partner who engages in unsafe sex) wear a condom. The use of condoms coated with nonoxynol-9 affords the greatest protection.

Inquire whether the client thinks she should be tested for hepatitis B or AIDS. In an area with a high incidence of these diseases, the health care facility may offer routine testing. If not, refer the client to a facility that performs these tests.

Roles and relationships. Roles and relationships require careful assessment because health care needs may result from—or cause—role and relationship problems.

Cultural influences. Determine the client's cultural background and assess its effect on her beliefs about health, illness, menstruation, menopause, and related topics. A client's cultural background can affect her access to health care and her perceptions of menarche, menstruation, menopause, gynecologic health, and health promotion activities.

Sexuality patterns. First determine if the client is sexually active. A client who has never had sexual intercourse may require use of a smaller speculum and gentle reassurance during the pelvic examination.

If the client is sexually active, ask such questions as, "Do you have a regular sexual partner? Is this person your only sexual partner?" to avoid implying that she

---

CLIENT TEACHING

Health care activities

Certain tests and procedures can help you stay healthy. The following chart lists these activities and tells how often to have them done based on your age. However, if you are in a high-risk group, you may need to do these tests or procedures more frequently. Check with your doctor or nurse practitioner for more details.

TEST OR PROCEDURE	AGE TO START	FREQUENCY
Papanicolaou (Pap) test	18 (or after first sexual intercourse if under age 18)	Yearly
	After hysterectomy	Every 3 to 5 years
Breast self-examination	20	Monthly
Mammogram	35 to 39	Once
	40 to 49	Every other year
	50 and older	Yearly
Cholesterol screening	20	Every 5 years if less than 200 mg/dl
Fecal occult blood test	40	Yearly

Sources: American College of Obstetricians and Gynecologists (Pap test), American Cancer Society (breast self-examination and mammogram), Report of the Expert Panel on Detection, Evaluation, and Treatment of High Blood Cholesterol in Adults (cholesterol screening).

This teaching aid may be reproduced by office copier for distribution to clients. © 1991, Springhouse Corporation.

should be heterosexual or married. Her response not only will provide information about partners, but also will help determine which tests must be done and which counseling topics are most appropriate.

If the client has a regular partner, have her describe the relationship. If she responds with a single word, such as "Fine," investigate further by asking, "On a scale from 1 to 10, with 10 being terrific, how would you describe your relationship?" The client's answer should aid in understanding this relationship.

To complete this part of the health history, ask if the client has any questions or concerns about sex or sexuality. Follow up with a question such as, "What would you change about your sex life if you could?" The client's answer may lead to a discussion of sexual problems. For example, a postmenopausal or older client may report dyspareunia caused by atrophic vaginal changes. Many women have concerns that they hesitate to discuss, such as concerns about intercourse during menses. This question may identify specific information needs and anxieties that can be addressed in the nursing care plan.

Family. Begin by finding out how many people live with the client and their relationships with her. Then assess the nature of these relationships to determine the client's satisfaction with her living arrangements.

Find out if the client has been involved in arguments with her partner, children, or parents in the past month. If she has, inquire about their severity, including any instances of pushing or hitting. These questions may help identify an abusive relationship.

When the client reports physical, sexual, or emotional abuse, determine if she needs treatment or other care. If she is not currently in an abusive relationship, ask if she has been abused in the past. Any kind of abuse can have lasting effects. When a history of abuse is identified, she may need counseling. (For more information about assessment and treatment, see Chapter 14, Violence Against Women.)

For a client whose children live at home or one whose children have left home, ask her to describe her relationships with her children. This will help determine whether her family is a source of support or of problems.

Social support patterns. Inquire about the client's main sources of emotional support. Ask if she has a best friend or participates in church, club, recreational, or other social activities. Her answers will provide information about her social support systems.

Emotional health status. Ask the client about any recent emotional changes. Continue by asking if she has ever been depressed. A major health problem among women, depression may require referral to a mental health practitioner.

Then determine if the client has ever been in counseling or therapy. If so, find out when, why, and for how long. Knowledge of emotional problems will complete the client's clinical picture.

To conclude the health history, pose an open-ended question, such as, "Can you think of anything else I should know?" Such a question gives the client a chance to discuss any significant information not covered during the history.

Physical assessment

Before the physical assessment, gather the necessary equipment: blood pressure cuff, stethoscope, thermometer, scale, examination table with adjustable stirrups, a movable light, a vaginal speculum, material for collecting test specimens (spatula, cotton-tipped applicators, an endocervical brush, glass slides, cover slides, cytologic fixative, and culture bottles or plates), material to test stool for occult blood, hand mirror, water-soluble lubricant, and examination gloves.

This part of the gynecologic assessment includes measurement of vital signs, height, and weight; assessment of the breasts; and a thorough pelvic examination. It also may include thyroid gland or abdominal assessment if a thyroid or other disorder is suspected. When performing the physical assessment, take a systematic head-to-toe approach.

Vital signs, height, and weight. Begin the physical assessment by measuring the client's temperature, pulse, respirations, and blood pressure to obtain basic objective data. Particularly note hypertension, which may result from oral contraceptive use. Also watch for tachycardia (rapid pulse), which may indicate a need for cardiac and thyroid screening.

The client's height measurement will help evaluate the appropriateness of her weight. In an adolescent client, a height-weight chart can document growth and may provide reassurance about her growth pattern. In a menopausal client, it may uncover osteoporosis, which results in decreased height.

The client's weight reveals if she is underweight or overweight and offers an opportunity to discuss body image.

Breasts. Breast examination is an essential part of the annual gynecologic assessment. It helps identify these signs of cancer and other breast abnormalities: a lump or thickening in the breast or axillae, changes in breast size or shape, nipple discharge, and color or texture changes in the skin or areola (National Cancer Institute, 1988).

Breast examination includes inspection and palpation. (For an illustrated procedure, see *Psychomotor skills: Palpating the axillae and breasts,* pages 126 and 127.) While examining the breast, mentally divide it into four sections: the upper outer, upper inner, lower outer, and lower inner quadrants. (The upper outer quadrant includes the tail of Spence.) Then, picture the breast as a clock with the nipple as the center. Describe the location of any abnormality by its location on the clock and distance from the nipple in centimeters.

Inspection and palpation. Inspect the breasts with the client seated with arms at her sides, then with her hands on her hips, and finally with her arms overhead. If the client has large breasts, ask her to lean forward with her arms outstretched to free the breast tissue and allow more complete observation.

In each position, note the size, shape, and symmetry of the breasts. Normally, the breasts are conical and may vary slightly in size and shape. More extensive breast asymmetry, dimpling, or retraction (puckering or depression of localized breast tissue) may indicate a breast mass.

Observe the skin color and condition. Breast color should correspond with the rest of the client's pigmentation. Pronounced venous patterns that appear bilaterally in an obese, fair-skinned, or pregnant client may be normal. Pronounced unilateral venous patterns or pronounced bilateral patterns in a thin to normal-weight, dark-skinned, or nonpregnant client may be abnormal, possibly indicating breast cancer. The skin should look smooth. Peau d'orange (rough, orange-peel-like) breast tissue indicates edema and warrants further evaluation. Striae may be normal, especially in an obese client or a client with large breasts. Masses, skin lesions, or rashes warrant further evaluation.

Observe the size, shape, symmetry, and color of the nipples and areolae. Both normally appear round or oval and equal in size. The nipples should point symmetrically; asymmetric nipple direction may indicate a breast mass. Although darker than breast tissue, the nipples and areolae should correspond with the client's pigmentation. They normally darken during pregnancy.

Also note whether the nipples are inverted, everted, or flattened. These nipple shapes may be normal, but can indicate cancer if they occur suddenly or unilaterally. Document any rashes, fissures, ulcerations, or spontaneous discharge from the nipple—these may be signs of cancer.

Then inspect the axillae for rashes, masses, lesions, or discolored areas—these may indicate infection or cancer. Note axillary hair growth, which is normal after puberty.

Conclude the breast examination with palpation.

Pelvic structures. With special preparation, the nurse may perform the complete pelvic examination, which includes inspection and palpation of the external and internal genitalia as well as specimen collection.

Whether the nurse performs the pelvic examination or assists, two people besides the client should be present and one of them should be a woman. The second person offers the client emotional support, assists during the examination, and affords the examiner legal protection against accusations of sexual abuse.

Before the pelvic examination, ask the client about previous experiences with such examinations. Acknowledge any feelings of fear, dread, or embarrassment and plan to promote client comfort during the examination. If the client is undergoing this examination for the first time, explain what is going to happen, show how the speculum works, and describe the sounds and sensations that occur during the examination.

To prepare for the pelvic examination, adjust the height and distance of the stirrups from the examination table to match the client's height. If the client has not voided, ask her to do so. Then help her into the lithotomy position, make her as emotionally and physically comfortable as possible, and drape her so that her knees are covered and the examiner can see her face.

Remember to prepare the client properly for her age. An adolescent client may need extra guidance and support during the pelvic examination. An elderly client may need more time to respond to requests and may need help with undressing, moving to the examination table, and assuming the lithotomy position. All clients need to know what the examiner is doing at each step of the examination.

To perform the examination, put on gloves. Alert the client to the start of the examination by telling her to expect a touch on the back of the thigh. If the muscles around the vagina and rectum contract when the thigh is touched, proceed slowly and be especially gentle.

External genitalia assessment. Examine the external genitalia closely, particularly if the client reports vaginal itching or sores. To assess the external genitalia, use inspection and palpation.

Using words that the client understands, tell her that you will be touching and examining her external genitalia. Then observe the perineum and pubic hair. The perineum should be intact; the hair distribution should be consistent with the client's developmental age.

(Text continues on page 128.)

Palpating the axillae and breasts

Although the nurse can assess the axillae with the client sitting or lying down, the sitting position provides easier access for palpation. When the nurse palpates the breasts, the client should lie supine.

1 Begin with the client's right axilla. Ask the client to relax her right arm while you use your left hand to support her elbow or wrist. With your right middle three fingers cupped, reach high into the central axilla. Sweep the fingers downward and against the ribs and serratus anterior to try to feel the central nodes. Palpating one or two small, nontender, freely movable nodes is normal.

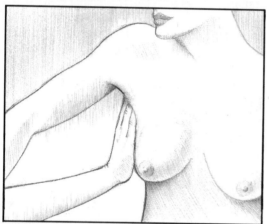

2 Assess the anterior nodes by palpating along the anterior axillary fold as shown. Next, assess the posterior nodes by palpating along the posterior axillary fold. Then palpate the lateral nodes by pressing your fingers along the upper inner arm, trying to compress these nodes against the humerus. Repeat the assessment on the client's left side.

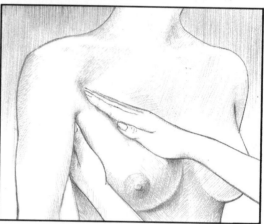

5 Choosing to palpate across or down the breast is satisfactory also, especially on a client with pendulous breasts. This is best done with the client seated.

While palpating, feel for masses or areas of induration (hardness). If a mass is suspected, move or compress the breast gently to look for dimpling. Also palpate for consistency and elasticity. The youthful breast is firmly elastic, with the glandular tissue feeling like small lobules. The mature breast may feel more granular or stringy. More nodularity and fullness may occur before

the menstrual period. The normal inframammary ridge at the lower edge of the breast is firm and may be mistaken for a tumor.

Also assess for tenderness, which can depend on the time in the menstrual cycle. The breasts may be tender the week before the menstrual period. Note where the client is in the menstrual cycle when breast assessment data are recorded and interpreted.

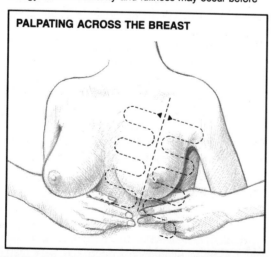

PALPATING ACROSS THE BREAST

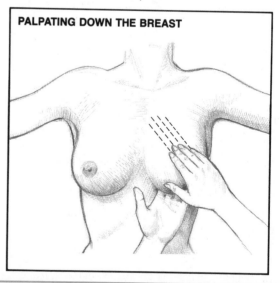

PALPATING DOWN THE BREAST

3 To palpate the breast, ask the client to lie supine with a small pad or pillow placed under her shoulder on the side being examined and with her arm on that same side placed above her head. This position allows the breast tissue to spread out evenly, facilitating the examination. Palpate large breasts with the client in the supine and seated positions.

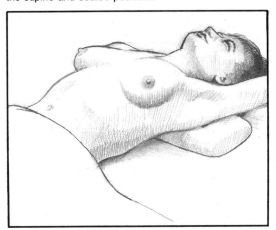

4 Using the middle three finger pads, palpate the breast in a systematic pattern, rotating the fingers gently against the chest wall. Palpate circularly from the center out or from the periphery in, being sure to palpate the tail of Spence. Repeat on the opposite breast.

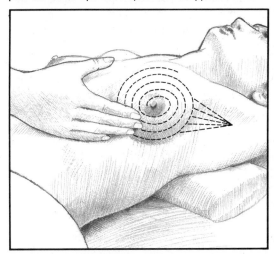

6 Palpate the areola and nipple. To palpate the nipple, gently compress it between the thumb and index finger. The nipple will become erect and the areola will pucker normally from the tactile stimulation. Repeat on the opposite breast.

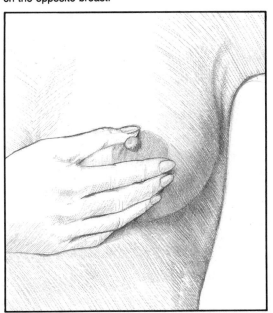

7 Gently milk the nipple for discharge by compressing it between the thumb and index finger. If discharge occurs, note the duct or ducts through which it appears. Repeat on the opposite breast.

8 Make a cytologic smear of any discharge not explained by pregnancy or lactation. Place a glass slide over the nipple, smear the discharge on it, and spray the slide with fixative immediately.

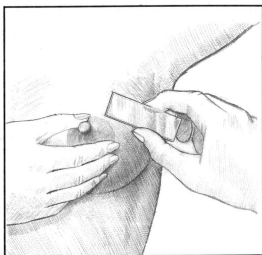

Abnormal distribution may suggest an endocrine disorder.

Next, inspect the labia and vaginal mucosa, separating the labia minora from the labia majora, as necessary, for close observation. The labia and vaginal mucosa should be pink and moist. Their size and shape, however, can vary greatly from client to client.

Note and characterize any vaginal discharge. A vaginal discharge may be normal or abnormal, depending on the client's age and timing in the menstrual cycle. A normal secretion is odorless and nonirritating. Before ovulation, it is clear and stretchy; after ovulation, white and not stretchy; during menstruation, bloody. Any other type of discharge is abnormal. If an abnormal discharge is present, obtain a specimen for culture.

While separating the labia, examine the vestibule, urethral orifice, vaginal orifice, and clitoris (if not hooded by tissue). Some countries practice female circumcision, including Sudan, Somalia, Ethiopia, Kenya, and Egypt (Cook, 1976). If the client grew up in one of these countries, carefully examine her genitals for keloid formation and the absence of the clitoris and labia minora.

Note any cystocele (bladder protrusion into the vagina), rectocele (rectum protrusion into the vagina), or scars, which may have been caused by vaginal childbirth. Also note any vulvar lesions (which may indicate cancer, herpes, or syphilis), growths (which may indicate cancer, condyloma, or cysts), or other abnormalities, such as signs of trauma or pediculosis.

After inspecting the external genitalia, palpate them. (For an illustrated procedure, see *Psychomotor skills: Assessing the female genitalia*, pages 129 to 131.)

Internal genitalia assessment. To assess the internal reproductive organs, begin with inspection via speculum. During this part of the assessment, collect specimens for the Pap test and tests for any abnormal cervical or vaginal discharge. (For specific guidelines, see *Obtaining specimens for culture*, page 132.)

Next, use bimanual palpation to assess the cervix, uterus, fallopian tubes, ovaries, and rectovaginal areas. (For an illustrated procedure, see *Psychomotor skills: Bimanual palpation*, pages 133 to 136.) Keep in mind that most women find the rectovaginal assessment uncomfortable and may feel like defecating or expelling flatus. To minimize discomfort, complete the procedure as quickly and gently as possible.

Educational pelvic examination. If the client wants to learn more about her reproductive anatomy, perform an educational pelvic examination, which allows the client to view her external genitalia and cervix through a hand mirror.

With the client in a Fowler's position, advise her to place the mirror between her legs so that she can see her external genitalia. While observing for abnormalities, point out major anatomic structures and features, such as the perineum, episiotomy scars (if present), labia majora and minora, vaginal opening, urethra, hymen, and clitoris. Mention the normal and usual asymmetry of the labia minora.

Use the technical terms for these structures and features only if the client understands them. Otherwise, use common terms such as outer lips (labia majora) and inner lips (labia minora). Keep in mind that common terms vary in different cultures and ethnic groups. If you are unfamiliar with these terms, teach the client a few simple medical terms or ask a member of the health care team who shares the client's background to supply terms that the client is likely to understand.

After pointing out the external genitalia, ask the client to relax with her hands on her abdomen. Insert the speculum. Then help the client hold the mirror so that it reflects the cervix through the speculum. If necessary, adjust the light and, if the cervix is in a posterior position, raise the speculum handle to make the cervix visible. After the client sees the cervix, ask her to relax again. Withdraw the speculum.

Developmental considerations

Normal assessment findings for the breasts and reproductive structures vary with the client's development. Understanding these developmental variations will help the nurse interpret physical findings.

Pediatric client. In an infant, assessment may reveal breast enlargement caused by maternal estrogen transfer at birth. This enlargement usually recedes within 2 weeks.

Examination of an infant or young child reveals softer and more resilient labia than in an adult. Labial agglutination (labia minora adhesions) may occur in an infant or toddler, causing urinary obstruction and requiring swift evaluation and treatment. Inflamed or edematous external genitalia in a child may indicate sexual abuse and require appropriate referrals.

Adolescent client. Between ages 8 and 13, the breasts begin to develop. (For more information, see *Female breast development* in Chapter 6, Reproductive Anatomy and Physiology.)

Pubic hair growth begins early in puberty. Initially, hair distribution is sparse, then increases and thickens as the adolescent reaches adulthood.

Assessing the female genitalia

A nurse practitioner or other nurse with special preparation may palpate the external genitalia and assess the internal genitalia using a vaginal speculum. To perform this part of the pelvic examination, first put on gloves. Do not palpate areas close to the anus until assessment completion, if at all. This will help prevent spreading fecal matter to the vagina and urethra. After touching the genitalia, ask an assistant to touch any equipment that will be handled by others: this examination requires medically aseptic technique. Then proceed as follows.

1 Explain each step of the procedure. To avoid startling the client, tell her that she will feel you touching her thigh and then she will feel you touching her external genitalia as you examine them. When examining the external genitalia, note any vulvar lesions, growths, discharge, edema, discoloration, varicosities, or trauma. Then gently spread the labia majora with the left hand, insert the right index finger into the vagina about 1½″ to 2″ (4 to 5 cm) and turn the finger pad upward.

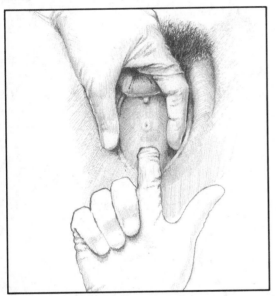

Milk the urethra and Skene's glands gently by exerting upward pressure on either side of the urethra and then directly over it. Culture any discharge.

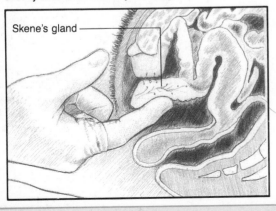

Skene's gland

2 Rotate the index finger downward and, using the thumb and index finger, palpate the areas of Bartholin's glands (at the 5 o'clock and 7 o'clock positions) in the vaginal walls at the introitus. The areas should feel smooth with no swelling, masses, or tenderness.

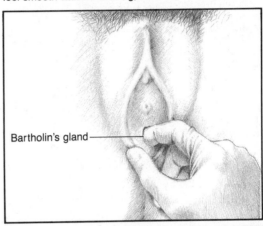

Bartholin's gland

3 Place the index and middle fingers on either side of the vaginal opening and spread the fingers to separate the opening. To check pelvic support, insert two fingers into the vagina and ask the client to bear down. Some slight muscle bulging is normal. Assess vaginal tone by having the client tighten her vaginal muscles around your two fingers. Tone should be greater in women who have not borne children vaginally. Then palpate the perineum between the index finger and thumb. The tissue should feel smooth and thick in a nulliparous client and thicker and rigid in a multiparous client who has had an episiotomy.

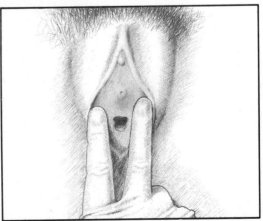

(continued)

Assessing the female genitalia continued

4 Select a speculum that has been warmed in a clean warming drawer, on a heating pad set on low, or under warm running water. (A cold speculum increases muscle tension.) Do not use any lubricant other than water on the speculum if a Papanicolaou (Pap) test will be obtained because lubricant can interfere with test results.

First, place the index and middle fingers of one hand inside the vaginal orifice to spread it apart about 1″ (2.5 cm). Exert downward pressure with the fingers. Simultaneously, use the opposite hand to introduce the closed speculum over the spread fingers. This maneuver bypasses the sensitive urethra adjacent to the anterior vaginal wall. Hold the blades closed with the index and middle fingers of the introducing hand. Make sure not to pinch or pull skin or hair.

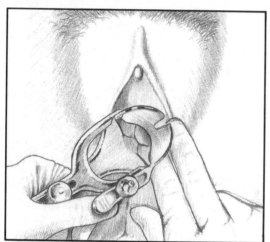

5 Once the blades have passed the introitus, remove the fingers, exerting downward pressure. Maintain downward and posterior pressure on the blades until the instrument is completely inserted.

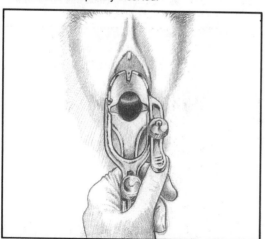

6 Open the speculum blades and look for the cervix. If you cannot see it, reposition the speculum more anteriorly, posteriorly, or laterally until the complete cervix appears. Occasionally, the speculum will need to be removed, the cervix located digitally, and the speculum reinserted. Tell the client when the speculum will be moved or reinserted.

To fix the blade of the metal speculum in the open position, tighten the thumbscrew. During speculum repositioning maneuvers, remind the client to relax. The cervix will be more posterior with the anteverted or anteflexed uterus and more anterior with the retroverted or retroflexed uterus.

The cervix should be shiny pink. However, it may be pale if the client is anemic or menopausal. Pregnancy gives it a bluish purple cast (Chadwick's sign). The cervix, with a diameter of about ¾″ to 1¼″ (2 to 3 cm) projects about ¼″ to 1¼″ (1 to 3 cm) into the vagina. The cervix position correlates with the position of the uterus; it should be midline.

Note the shape of the cervical os. An opening that looks like a horizontal slit usually means that the client has had a vaginal birth; a small, round opening usually means that she has not. Also assess for any abnormalities. Growths, lesions, mucopurulent discharge, or abnormal color require further evaluation.

VIEW THROUGH SPECULUM

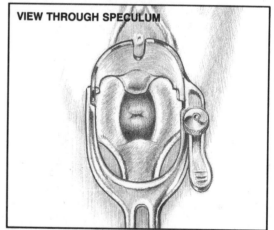

CROSS-SECTIONAL VIEW

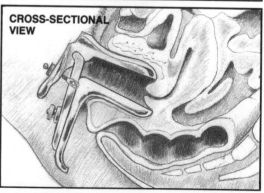

PSYCHOMOTOR SKILLS

Assessing the female genitalia continued

7 After inspecting the cervix, obtain an endocervical specimen for the Pap test by inserting a cotton-tipped applicator, an endocervical brush, or the longer serrated end of a spatula about ⅛" (0.5 cm) into the cervical os and rotating the instrument 360 degrees clockwise. Then smear the specimen onto a glass slide with a smooth, painting motion; too much pressure can destroy the cells. Spray the slide with cytologic fixative within 10 seconds of smearing it.

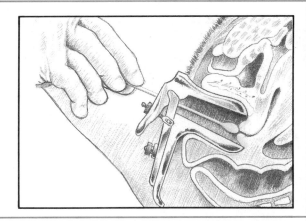

8 Retrieve a specimen from the ectocervix (the outer layer of the cervix) with the softly curved end of the spatula. Some health care facility protocols permit collecting both the ectocervical and endocervical smears simultaneously on the same slide (one on each end). Regardless, the procedure is the same: Place the curved end of the spatula in the os, apply pressure while turning it 360 degrees, transfer the scrapings to a slide, and spray the slide with fixative.

If the client has no cervix, as after a complete hysterectomy, scrape the vaginal cuff and obtain a vaginal pool specimen with a cotton-tipped applicator from the posterior vaginal area. If the client has dry mucosa, the applicator tip can be moistened with normal saline solution. Prepare the slide specimen as described previously; label the slide to indicate where the specimen came from.

A vaginal wall specimen may be needed to evaluate the maturation index (estrogen and progesterone influence on the cells). Take this specimen by scraping the blunt end of a spatula along the lateral middle third of the vaginal wall.

Transfer specimens from all cervical and vaginal areas to the slide and spray with cytologic fixative. (Note: If the specimen is too thick, it may be inappropriate for microscopic examination.)

When a client reports vaginal itching or a malodorous vaginal discharge, obtain a wet smear or wet prep. To do this, take a vaginal secretion specimen with a cotton-tipped applicator, place it on a glass slide, mix it with a drop or two of normal saline, and cover it with a cover slip.

9 After collecting all the specimens, unlock the speculum thumbscrew and begin to withdraw the speculum. Slowly rotating the blades 90 degrees in a moderately open fashion, inspect the anterior and posterior vaginal walls for abnormalities, such as lesions, discharge, swelling, abnormal color, and the presence or absence of rugae. (Speculum rotation is not necessary with a plastic speculum, because it allows observation through the clear plastic.) Women with adequate estro-

gen levels have pink, moist, rugose vaginal walls.

Finally close the speculum blades just before the distal ends reach the area adjacent to the urethral meatus and the introitus (to avoid trauma to the area), making sure that no mucosa, skin, or hair remains between the closed blades before withdrawing them. Place the speculum into a soaking solution or container or discard it if it is disposable.

Older client. On physical assessment, the menopausal or older client may exhibit fat redistribution, weight gain, increased facial hair growth, and such skin changes as dryness, loss of elasticity, and wrinkling.

Her breasts may atrophy and lose their elasticity. On palpation, they may feel more granular and less firm. Also, the inframammary ridge thickens and becomes easier to palpate, making it easier to mistake for a breast mass.

Assessment of the older client's external genitalia may reveal thinning and atrophy of the labia majora, reduction in size of the clitoris, and sparse, thin pubic hair that is brittle, gray, and straight. Examination of the internal structures may reveal a paler cervix, smaller uterus, and reduced vaginal secretions.

Diagnostic studies

Although some diagnostic studies are performed routinely on all clients, others may be prompted by the

Obtaining specimens for culture

This chart describes the equipment and techniques used to obtain specimens for culture studies that commonly are performed as part of the gynecologic assessment.

ORGANISM	SPECIMEN SITE	EQUIPMENT	PROCEDURE
Neisseria gonorrhoeae	Endocervix	• Cotton-tipped applicator • Thayer-Martin medium culture plate or bottle	• Insert a sterile cotton-tipped applicator ¼" (0.5 cm) into the cervical os, then rotate 360 degrees. Leave applicator in the os 10 to 30 seconds to absorb secretions. • Inoculate culture medium with specimen by simultaneously rotating the applicator and patterning a Z on the culture plate or in the bottle. • Place tightly capped bottle on its side or culture plate face up in a warm environment within 15 minutes of obtaining the specimen.
Chlamydia trachomatis	Endocervix	• Special swab (provided with test medium) • Special medium slide • Acetone	• Enzyme immunoassay: Collect specimen on a special swab, place in the medium provided, and send for analysis by spectrophotometer. • Monoclonal antibody test: Collect specimen with an endocervical brush (in a pregnant client, use a cotton-tipped applicator); apply specimen to a slide, allow to dry, and apply acetone.
Candida albicans, Trichomonas vaginalis, or organisms that cause bacterial vaginosis	Vaginal secretions from posterior vaginal pool	• Cotton-tipped applicator • Normal saline solution • Potassium hydroxide (KOH) solution • Glass slides and coverslips	• Dip the wooden end of a cotton-tipped applicator into the vaginal secretion pool without touching the mucosa, then into a drop of normal saline solution placed on a slide. If saline solution and KOH slides are needed, place the tip in the saline drop first, then in the KOH. • Apply glass coverslips and perform microscopic examination as soon as possible.
Treponema pallidum	Lesion on vagina, cervix, or external genitalia	• Cotton-tipped applicator • Glass slide and coverslip • Grease pencil • Normal saline solution • Gauze square	• Draw a dime- or nickel-size circle on a slide, using a grease pencil. • Place one drop of saline solution within the circle to keep the spirochete alive. • Wipe the lesion with a gauze square to remove mucus and crusts. • Squeeze the lesion to obtain serum. • Scrape the lesion with a cotton-tipped applicator. • Apply the specimen to saline on glass slide and cover with coverslip. • Send slide to the laboratory within 5 minutes. • As an alternate procedure for an external lesion, obtain a specimen by touching the dry slide to serum from the lesion and then add saline solution to the slide.

client's health history and physical assessment data. Studies may include laboratory tests, mammography, colposcopy, thermography, and transillumination.

Laboratory tests. The client may undergo various laboratory tests, including the Pap test, complete blood count (CBC), and many others. (For more information, see *Common laboratory studies,* page 137.) A client may need additional tests, such as thyroid function studies, to confirm a suspected endocrine disorder. Whenever a laboratory test is ordered, obtain the specimens or teach the client to collect the specimens, as needed. For example, teach the client to collect a midstream urine specimen for culture and sensitivity testing or a stool specimen for occult blood testing.

Mammography. Used to diagnose and evaluate breast lesions, this procedure usually requires two low-dose radiation X-ray exposures of each breast—anterior and oblique views.

If mammography is scheduled, prepare the client for it. Explain the procedure and tell the client that it can detect breast lumps as small as 1 mm, allowing earlier diagnosis than is possible with breast palpation, thereby increasing survival rates.

Advise the client that because mammography involves compressing the breast between two sheets of X-ray film, it may cause discomfort. To minimize discomfort, suggest that the client schedule mammography shortly after her menstrual period when the breasts are less tender. Also suggest that the client wear a two-piece outfit during the procedure, because she will need to undress to the waist.

Emphasize the value of mammography. According to one study of 62,000 women, early detection of breast cancer through mammography can decrease the mortality rate by at least 30% (Seidman, Gelb, Silverberg, LaVerda, and Lubera, 1987).

Remind the client that, even though mammography is valuable, it is not foolproof. Emphasize the importance of annual physical examinations and BSE in addition to mammography. (For more information, see Chapter 13, Gynecologic Disorders.)

Colposcopy. This procedure identifies epithelial abnormalities and areas for biopsy, using a binocular microscope with low magnification that allows detailed examination of the external genitalia, vagina, and cervix. It may be ordered to confirm intraepithelial or in-

(Text continues on page 137.)

PSYCHOMOTOR SKILLS

Bimanual palpation

A nurse practitioner or other nurse with special preparation may perform bimanual palpation after inspecting the cervix and obtaining a Papanicolaou smear and any other specimens. To perform this part of the pelvic examination, pal- pate the internal genitalia as follows. Use the dominant hand internally for the most comfortable approach, but try the other hand if this seems awkward.

1 Apply lubricant. Lubricant comes in a multi-use or single-use tube or a foil packet and may be squeezed onto a disposable gauze or paper square for easy use. Never touch a multi-use tube end with your gloved fingers; instead, allow the lubricant to drop freely onto the fingers. Discard a single-use tube or packet after one use.

After lubricating the index and middle fingers of the gloved hand, advise the client that you are going to place two fingers in her vagina to palpate her cervix, uterus, and ovaries. Then introduce the flexed fingers into the vagina using downward and posterior pressure. With the thumb abducted to avoid placing the thumb on the clitoris, palpate every aspect of the vaginal wall with the palmar surfaces of the fingers, rotating them as necessary. Rugae, a normal finding, feel like small ridges running concentrically around the vaginal wall. Note any nodules, tenderness, or other abnormalities. A client with a small vaginal opening may need to be examined with one finger.

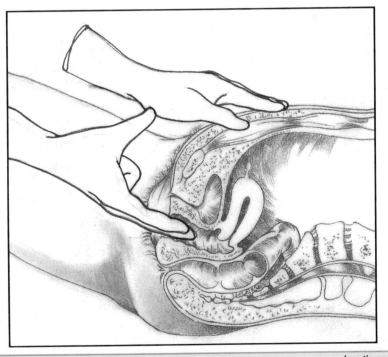

(continued)

Bimanual palpation continued

2 Insert your fingers deeper until the cervix is located with the palmar surface of the fingers. Feel its surface and run the fingers around its circumference. Gently move the cervix from side to side ½″ to ¾″ (1 to 2 cm; this should not hurt the client) and assess its shape, position, consistency, regularity of contour, and mobility. It should feel firm, smooth, mobile, and nontender when moved and touched. The cervix of an older woman is smaller and usually is recessed, as in a prepubertal girl; a pregnant woman's cervix typically is softened and enlarged by the third trimester.

The cervix, usually in the midline, points anteriorly, posteriorly, or midplane. Cervical position usually relates to uterine position. For example, a posterior cervix typically appears with an anteverted uterus; an anterior cervix, with a retroverted uterus. However, a cervix positioned to the right or left may indicate an abdominal mass shifting the uterus—and the cervix—to one side. Tenderness elicited by cervical movement may signal ectopic pregnancy or pelvic inflammatory disease.

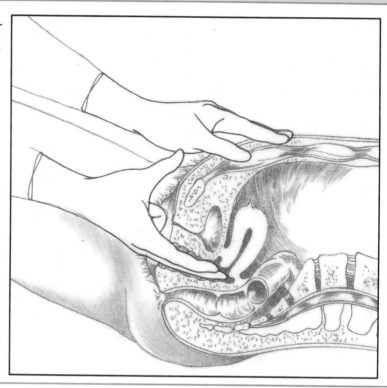

3 Position your hands for examination of the uterus. Place the external hand on the abdomen at a point midway between the symphysis pubis and the umbilicus. Leave the index and middle fingers of the examining hand in the vagina. Bring the external hand down toward the symphysis pubis and inward toward the internal hand to trap the uterus for examination.

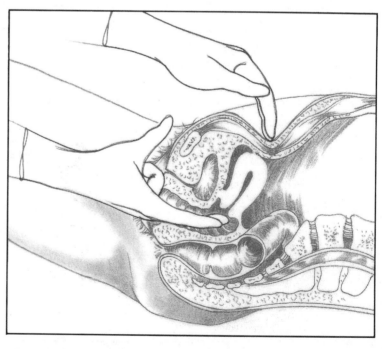

4 After trapping the uterus, examine it for position, size, shape, consistency, tenderness, mobility, and surface regularity. (Flexion indicates that the uterus is bent upon itself; version refers to a deflection of the long axis of the uterus from the long axis of the body, either anteriorly or posteriorly. Midplane position means the long axis of the uterus is parallel to the long axis of the body.) Also note whether the uterus lies midline or deviates to the left or right of the pelvis.

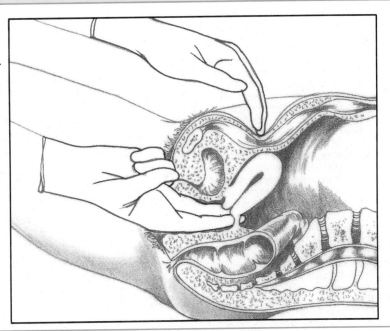

5 Determine whether the uterus is normal size or enlarged. The normal nonpregnant uterus is small and fits comfortably beneath the symphysis pubis in the pelvis; it is not palpable by abdominal examination. The postmenopausal uterus normally is smaller than before menopause. An enlarged uterus may result from pregnancy, fibroid tumors, or adenomyosis (uterine mucosal tissue growth into the uterine wall or oviducts). If the uterus is enlarged, estimate its size in weeks of gestation. For example, the size of a uterus enlarged by a tumor might be 12 weeks.

Unless an abnormality or pregnancy changes the shape of the uterus, it is pear-shaped and symmetrical. Note any deviations, such as a protruding mass on the fundal surface. A heart-shaped organ may indicate a bicornuate uterus, a congenital variant.

The muscular composition of the uterus typically makes it feel firm and smooth. A soft uterus suggests pregnancy; an irregular surface, fibroids. Severe tenderness may indicate infection or adenomyosis. The ligaments suspending the uterus in the pelvis allow it slight mobility. Limited mobility may indicate a pathologic condition, such as carcinoma, infection, or adhesions.

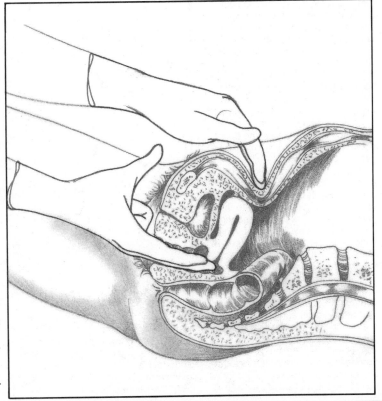

(continued)

Bimanual palpation   continued

6 Assess the right and left adnexal areas (ovaries and fallopian tubes). Place the internal fingers deeply into the cul-de-sac just under the external hand on the right lower abdominal quadrant. Then lift the internal fingers as the external fingers press down and inward toward the symphysis pubis. This maneuver allows the ovary and any masses to slip between the fingers. Repeat the maneuver on the left side.

   If palpable, the ovaries should be mobile, oval, somewhat flattened, firm, smooth organs shaped like 1¼″ x ¾″ x ¼″ (3 x 2 x 0.5 cm) almonds. They may be sensitive to palpation. The ovaries of a postmenopausal or prepubertal client should not be palpable. An ovary larger than 2″ (5 cm) is abnormal and requires further evaluation. Normal fallopian tubes usually are not palpable or sensitive.

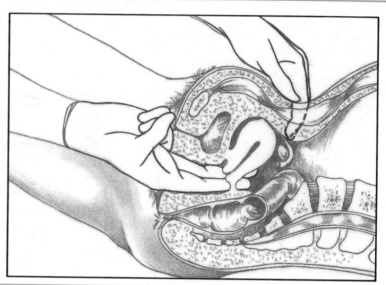

7 To prepare for rectovaginal examination, change the glove on the internal hand to prevent transfer of vaginal organisms into the rectum. The rectovaginal assessment is useful for examining a client with a small vaginal opening that permits only one finger to be introduced.

   Explain the procedure to the client, while lubricating the index and middle fingers of the gloved examining hand. To relax the client's anal sphincter and allow easier entry of the examining finger, ask her to bear down as if to have a bowel movement. (Assure her that she will not.) As she bears down, carefully insert the middle finger into the rectum.

   Inspect for hemorrhoids or other painful areas and avoid these lesions when inserting the finger. Next, as you insert the index finger into the vagina, tell the client to stop bearing down and to relax. Place the vaginal finger in under the cervix to keep it from being confused with a mass by the finger in the rectum.

   No masses or nodules should be felt by the rectal finger. A high percentage of rectal growths can be felt. The rectovaginal assessment provides a more complete evaluation of the posterior side of the uterus.

   After withdrawing the gloved finger from the rectum, check it for stool color and note any blood. Test for occult blood if the client is over age 40 or if you see tarry black stool (a possible sign of gastrointestinal bleeding) on the glove.

   When the examination is complete, clean the perineal area with tissue from front to back to remove excess lubricant. Give the client additional tissue for this purpose, if necesary. Help her to a sitting position. Wash your hands.

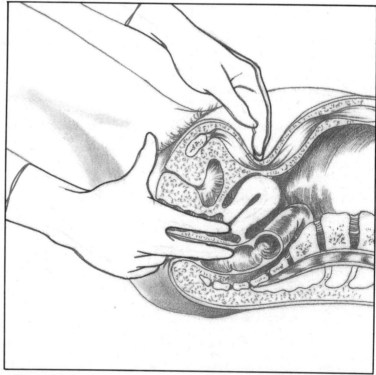

Common laboratory studies

Complete assessment data for a client include the results of various laboratory studies. The chart below lists commonly ordered studies and describes their significance.

BLOOD TESTS	URINE TESTS
Complete blood count (CBC) *Hemoglobin and hematocrit:* Screens for anemia, which may result from a menstrual disorder (such as menorrhagia) or a nutritional deficiency (such as anemia). *White blood cell (WBC) count with differential:* Identifies infection, which may be caused by a sexually transmitted disease (STD).	**Urinalysis** Evaluates the client's urine for glucose, protein, and infection.
	Urine culture and sensitivity Identifies the organism responsible for urinary tract infection and its susceptibility to antibiotics.
Rubella antibody test Determines if the client has antibodies to the disease, which is especially important because rubella infection in early pregnancy may cause fetal anomalies.	**OTHER TESTS**
	Papanicolaou (Pap) test Identifies preinvasive and invasive cervical cancer.
Total cholesterol Screens for hyperlipidemia, which commonly occurs after menopause, increasing the client's risk of cardiovascular problems. In a younger client, hyperlipidemia may influence her choice of contraceptive method.	**Wet smear** May detect infection with *Candida albicans, Trichomonas vaginalis,* or organisms that cause bacterial vaginosis.
VDRL test or rapid plasma reagin (RPR) test Screens for syphilis, which can cause congenital abnormalities if it is transmitted to a fetus.	**Cervical culture** May detect infection with *Neisseria gonorrhoeae* or *Chlamydia trachomatis.* Confirmation of either of these STDs requires treatment for the client and her partner.
HIV-III antibody test Detects antibodies to the AIDS virus. Many health care facilities offer this test for all high-risk clients.	**Fecal occult blood test (Hematest)** Detects minute quantities of blood in the feces, which can be caused by colorectal cancer.

vasive cervical cancer, evaluate a vaginal or cervical lesion, or assess a client whose mother received DES during pregnancy.

When colposcopy is needed, explain the procedure and its diagnostic value. Also, inform the client if biopsies will be obtained during the procedure.

Thermography. This procedure identifies heat patterns from inflammation or increased metabolism of malignant tumors. However, small or deep cancers may be missed, making thermography less comprehensive than mammography. Thermography is being replaced by ultrasonography and low-dose mammography. However, if thermography is scheduled, prepare the client by explaining the procedure and equipment. Its use should not preclude physical assessment and mammography.

Transillumination. Also known as diaphanography or light scanning, transillumination projects infrared light through breast tissue. A video camera photographs the light, which a computer transforms into images on a video screen. Lesions or areas of increased vascularity appear darker than surrounding tissue. Currently a pop-

ular supplement to mammography, this quick, safe, and painless procedure emits no radiation, making it useful for showing tumor changes without repeatedly exposing the client to radiation. When transillumination is scheduled, prepare the client by explaining the procedure and equipment.

Nursing diagnosis

After a review of assessment data from the health history, physical assessment, and diagnostic tests, formulate appropriate nursing diagnoses. (For a partial list of applicable nursing diagnoses, see *Nursing diagnoses: Women's health promotion,* page 139.)

Planning and implementation

Based on the client's health care needs, develop a plan that sets goals for the nurse and the client. Nursing goals may include:
• facilitating access to care
• establishing a therapeutic relationship

• minimizing anxiety about such concerns as developmental changes and gynecologic disorders
• enhancing the client's understanding of developmental changes and normal physiologic processes
• promoting successful completion of and adaptation to the developmental phase
• identifying health care needs and implementing treatment or making referrals
• establishing individualized teaching plans for health promotion and illness prevention
• encouraging the client to take personal responsibility for health care maintenance
• fostering a positive self-image in relation to menarche, menstruation, and menopause.

To implement this plan, intervene appropriately. Depending on the client's nursing diagnoses, listen actively, perform client teaching, provide information, and make necessary referrals.

Listen actively

Active listening is especially valuable for a client with *fear related to suspected gynecologic disorder, body image disturbance related to puberty,* or *anxiety related to menstruation.* In such a client, active listening can help identify misconceptions or knowledge deficits.

To listen actively, pay close attention to the client's words and assess the congruency between her words and her nonverbal messages. During the discussion, validate her correct assumptions, correct any misconceptions, give her time to formulate responses, express your concern, provide reassurance, and accept her values.

A client with a nursing diagnosis of *anxiety related to normal menopausal changes* or *body image disturbance related to menopausal changes* also may benefit from active listening. It may help her express fears and concerns and may enable her to identify needs more clearly. Keep in mind that the act of sharing feelings sometimes helps a client adapt to physiologic changes, such as menarche or menopause.

Teach about developmental changes

After identifying anxiety, a self-concept problem, or a knowledge deficit through assessment and active listening, provide the client with information about normal female anatomy and physiology and normal changes associated with menarche, adolescence, or menopause. This information should help minimize her anxiety, improve her self-concept, and correct any knowledge deficits or misconceptions.

Use diagrams, teaching models, or an educational pelvic examination to promote a better understanding of normal reproductive processes and changes. (For more information, see "Educational pelvic examination," page 128.)

Menarche. To help prepare the prepubertal client for menarche and to address a nursing diagnosis of *anxiety related to menarche,* take the following actions:
• Help the mother consider ways to prepare her daughter for menstruation. What attitudes does the mother want to communicate? What emphasis might convey a negative attitude? How can shame, embarrassment, or faulty communication be avoided? How can positive, open attitudes about menstruation be encouraged in all family members? Which cultural or family activities could celebrate menarche? Which books and other resources may be helpful?
• Discuss menstruation positively with the client, highlighting its importance in her life and its uniqueness to women.
• Discuss conditions that affect the menstrual cycle: weight, exercise, nutrition, stress, pregnancy, and disease.
• Emphasize that cycle length and frequency and amount of flow vary greatly from individual to individual.
• Be realistic in discussing the hygiene demands and possible discomfort of menstruation.
• Discuss menarche with the client as she experiences it.
• Discuss the menstrual cycle's role in reproduction, emphasizing the time when conception is most likely to occur.

Adolescence. An adolescent may have *anxiety related to menstruation.* To allay her anxiety, explain the physiology of menstruation. Tell her that her periods may be irregular, anovulatory, and painless at first. Explain that ovulation may not occur until 1 or 2 years after menarche, but that pregnancy is possible any time after menarche.

An adolescent also may have a nursing diagnosis of *anxiety related to normal growth patterns.* If so, explain that growth and development patterns normally vary from individual to individual. Reassure the client that her growth is normal for her and give her a height chart to record annual measurements.

Menopause. For a client with a nursing diagnosis of *anxiety related to normal menopausal changes* or *knowledge deficit related to the physiology of menopause,* provide information about the physiologic and psychological events of menopause and clarify any misconceptions.

NURSING DIAGNOSES

Women's health promotion

The following nursing diagnoses address problems and etiologies that a nurse may encounter when providing health care for a female client. Specific nursing interventions for many of these diagnoses are provided in the "Planning and implementation" section of this chapter.

- Altered health maintenance related to lack of exercise
- Altered health maintenance related to limited access to health care
- Altered health maintenance related to poor dietary habits
- Altered nutrition: less than body requirements, related to increased need for dietary calcium
- Altered nutrition: more than body requirements, related to decreased metabolic needs
- Altered nutrition: more than body requirements, related to decreased need for dietary cholesterol
- Altered role performance related to dysmenorrhea
- Altered sexuality patterns related to atrophic vaginal changes
- Anxiety related to diagnostic testing
- Anxiety related to menarche
- Anxiety related to menstruation
- Anxiety related to normal growth patterns
- Anxiety related to normal menopausal changes
- Anxiety related to role conflict
- Anxiety related to the gynecologic examination
- Body image disturbance related to menopausal changes
- Body image disturbance related to puberty
- Fear related to suspected gynecologic disorder
- Health-seeking behaviors related to preventive health care
- Impaired skin integrity related to aging
- Ineffective individual coping related to menopausal changes
- Ineffective individual coping related to menstruation
- Ineffective individual coping related to physiologic changes of puberty

- Ineffective thermoregulation related to hot flashes
- Knowledge deficit related to BSE
- Knowledge deficit related to factors that affect menstruation
- Knowledge deficit related to hormone replacement therapy
- Knowledge deficit related to management of menopausal changes
- Knowledge deficit related to menstrual self-care practices
- Knowledge deficit related to normal female physiology
- Knowledge deficit related to risk factors for gynecologic disorders
- Knowledge deficit related to the gynecologic examination
- Knowledge deficit related to the physiology of menopause
- Knowledge deficit related to women's health care activities
- Pain related to menstrual symptoms
- Pain related to premenstrual symptoms
- Potential for infection related to improper menstrual self-care practices
- Potential for infection related to unsafe sexual practices
- Potential for injury related to decreased bone mass
- Sexual dysfunction related to decreased vaginal secretions
- Sleep pattern disturbance related to hot flashes
- Social isolation related to recent divorce
- Stress incontinence related to pelvic relaxation

This should help develop the client's self-awareness, foster active participation in meeting her health care needs, and reduce anxiety, allowing her to deal effectively with these changes. If she is particularly concerned about the psychological changes of menopause, reassure her that they are normal, physiologic in origin, and temporary.

Teach health promotion activities

As needed, teach the client how to promote health through diet, exercise, health care activities, stress management, and risk factor identification.

Diet. If the client has a nursing diagnosis of *altered health maintenance related to poor dietary habits,* teach her

about a well-balanced diet. Provide information about the basic food groups and the number of servings required each day. Then ask her to keep a food diary to help reinforce positive nutritional habits and allow you to recommend diet changes at the follow-up visit. This is particularly important for a client with amenorrhea caused by weight loss or for one whose body image does not reflect her weight. (For more information, see Chapter 15, Women's Health-Compromising Behaviors.)

When a client has *pain related to premenstrual or menstrual symptoms,* diet changes may offer relief. A low-sodium diet may help reduce the bloating and weight gain associated with menstruation. Vitamin E, which is found in wheat germ, milk, eggs, meat, cereals, and leafy vegetables, may reduce cramping by inhibiting prostaglandins. Vitamin B_6 may lessen premenstrual moodiness and bloating by neutralizing the effects of increased estrogen. It is found in pork, egg yolks, and legumes. Calicum and magnesium also can help minimize menstrual symptoms. Dairy products contain high amounts of calcium; whole grain products and nuts provide magnesium.

For a postmenopausal client with *altered nutrition: less than body requirements, related to increased need for dietary calcium,* recommend a diet that provides 1 gram of calcium daily and 400 to 500 grams of vitamin D daily to promote bone mass.

For one with *altered nutrition: more than body requirements, related to decreased metabolic needs,* suggest regular exercise and a well-balanced diet with a daily caloric intake of about 14 calories per pound of body weight to prevent weight gain.

If the client has a nursing diagnosis of *sleep pattern disturbance related to hot flashes,* she may ask you about increasing her consumption of such things as B complex vitamins, vitamin E, and ginseng (an Oriental herb) tea or capsules, which consumer publications have reported to help control hot flashes. Advise her that she may try these methods, but that no studies support these anecdotal reports yet.

If she has *altered nutrition: more than body requirements, related to decreased need for dietary cholesterol,* teach her how to lower her cholesterol intake to minimize the risk of cardiovascular disease.

Exercise. When a client has a nursing diagnosis of *altered health maintenance related to lack of exercise,* teach her about the physical and psychological benefits of exercise and discuss an effective exercise program for her age and condition. A program that includes walking is appropriate for most clients as long as they have a safe neighborhood in which to walk. Regular walking can relieve tension and help protect against obesity and hypertension. For a client in good health, the program should include walking at a brisk but comfortable pace for 20 minutes at least four times each week.

For a client with a nursing diagnosis of *pain related to premenstrual or menstrual symptoms,* advise her that moderate exercise can improve the uterine blood supply, reducing cramping and discomfort. Remind her, however, that strenuous exercise over a long time can cause amenorrhea.

When a client's nursing diagnosis is *potential for injury related to decreased bone mass,* help her develop an exercise program that will meet her needs. Exercise not only improves overall health, but also may reduce the risk of osteoporosis. (For more information, see Chapter 15, Women's Health-Compromising Behaviors.)

Health care. A client with a *knowledge deficit related to BSE* may benefit greatly from instruction in BSE. (For more information, see *Client teaching: Breast self-examination,* pages 142 and 143.) BSE, which allows early detection of breast cancer, is especially important if the client cannot afford mammography or has limited access to health care.

After teaching BSE to the client, ask her to demonstrate it; then correct or reinforce her actions. Comment on the texture and consistency of the client's breasts to help her understand what is normal.

Many women who know how to perform BSE do not do it regularly. Of 230 undergraduate women in one study, less than 25% performed BSE monthly and about 30% rarely or never performed it (Hailey, 1987). Another study found that only 6% of high-risk women and 13% of low-risk women performed BSE monthly (Alagna, Morokoff, Bevelt, and Reddy, 1987).

A client who knows how to perform BSE may not do it regularly for several reasons: fear of finding an abnormality, lack of confidence in distinguishing between normal and abnormal findings, forgetfulness, fear of touching herself, embarrassment, or feeling it is not necessary. If a client does not practice BSE regularly, discuss her reasons. Then use this information to promote regular BSE. For example, if the client does not feel BSE is necessary, provide information about its benefits to help her accept it as a regular health care activity. If she has a partner and is fearful of touching herself, suggest that her partner learn and perform the procedure. If she is forgetful, show her how to use a menstrual and BSE record.

For a client with a *knowledge deficit related to women's health care activities* or *health-seeking behavior related to preventive health care,* tell her when gynecologic screening tests and procedures should be done and why they are important. Cite morbidity and mortality statistics, if necessary, to emphasize the importance of these tests and procedures. If she is at low risk and literate, provide standard written guidelines. If she is at high risk, give her an individualized schedule for screening tests and procedures and review it with her.

An older client may believe mistakenly that the need for gynecologic care ceases with menopause. To promote health care for this client, discuss the importance of having regular examinations and screening tests and procedures.

Stress management. For a client with a nursing diagnosis of *social isolation related to recent divorce* or *anxiety* *related to role conflict,* or with other stress-related problems, explain that stress can disrupt her menstrual cycle and increase her risk of illness. Then explore the cause of the client's stress and help her develop effective coping mechanisms. If she has used effective stress management techniques before, reinforce them. If she is unaware of the techniques, teach her about self-coaching, progressive relaxation, thought stopping, assertive behavior, and guided imagery. (For more information, see Chapter 15, Women's Health-Compromising Behaviors.) To develop the client's stress management skills further, suggest a stress management program or refer her for counseling.

Risk factor identification. For a client with a *knowledge deficit related to risk factors for gynecologic disorders,* alert her to them. Awareness of risk factors may motivate her to modify behaviors that put her at risk and to engage in behaviors—such as annual Pap tests and periodic physical examinations—that allow early detection of disorders.

Protection against STDs. If a client is not monogamous and has a nursing diagnosis of *potential for infection related to unsafe sexual practices,* advise her about practices that decrease the risk of STDs, such as using a condom, preferably coated with nonoxynol-9, each time she and her partner have intercourse.

Teach about tests

When assessment reveals abnormal findings and further testing is required, the client may develop a nursing diagnosis of *fear related to suspected gynecologic disorder* or *anxiety related to diagnostic testing.* To help her cope, explain the procedures, acknowledge her concerns, discuss complications that can occur, let her know when the test results can be expected, and establish a plan for follow-up. Encourage her to bring a relative or friend to the examination and discussion of findings.

Teach about menstrual management

For a client with *knowledge deficit related to menstrual self-care practices,* discuss preparation for menstruation, menstrual flow control, hygiene, sexual concerns, and comfort measures.

Preparation for menstruation. To prepare the client for menstruation, show her how to mark a calendar when her period begins and count forward to mark the expected date of her next period. Tell her to pay attention to signs of impending menstruation, such as minor facial blemishes, bloating, breast tenderness, weight gain, and food cravings. Also describe how external factors, such as diet, exercise, stress, and climate, can affect her menstrual cycle.

Menstrual flow control. Teach the client about products that are available to contain the menstrual flow. Discuss sanitary pads, which come in many sizes, absorbencies, shapes, styles, and types of packaging. Suggest that she try several to find the one most comfortable and best suited to her needs.

Also discuss tampons, which come in various absorbencies. Because improper tampon use has been associated with toxic shock syndrome (TSS, a severe illness caused by bacterial infection), teach the client how to use them properly. Advise the client to:
• Reduce her use of tampons.
• Change tampons at least every 4 hours.
• Alternate tampons with sanitary pads. At night, for example, she should use pads instead of tampons.
• Avoid using tampons when the menstrual flow is light. At this time, the vagina is relatively dry, making tampon insertion and removal more difficult.
• Never use more than one tampon at a time.
• Avoid using super-absorbent or deodorized tampons. Also avoid feminine deodorant sprays.
• Wash her hands and perineal area with soap and water before inserting a tampon. These actions help eliminate the bacteria that cause TSS.
• Stop using tampons and call her physician or nurse practitioner immediately if she develops fever, vomiting, diarrhea, muscle aches, vaginal redness or discharge, skin rash, or sore throat. These may be signs of TSS.

Hygiene. Teach the client that a douche or vaginal spray usually is not needed to maintain hygiene because natural secretions bathe the reproductive tract. In fact, excessive use of these products may wash away the normal protective vaginal secretions, increasing the risk of tissue trauma and infection.

Assure the client that daily bathing effectively promotes hygiene, especially during menstruation. Also discuss perineal hygiene. Suggest that she wear cotton underwear and avoid tight clothes to promote ventilation, and wipe from front to back after urination or defecation to prevent infection.

Sexual concerns. Advise the client that she may choose to have sexual intercourse during menses, based on her personal preference. Some women prefer to avoid or limit intercourse; others engage in it and report having their most erotic experiences.

Breast self-examination

Breast self-examination (BSE) is one of the most important health habits you can develop. By doing BSE once a month, you can detect breast problems quickly and get any necessary medical help to prevent more serious problems.

If you have not reached menopause yet, examine your breasts between the 4th and 7th day after menstrual bleeding begins. At this time, your hormones have the least effect on your breasts, making them easier to examine. If you have reached menopause, have had a hysterectomy, or are pregnant or breast-feeding and your periods have not returned yet, examine your breasts on the first day of every month or any other day that will help you remember this vital health habit.

When performing BSE, follow these steps.

1 Look at yourself in a mirror. With your arms at your sides, check for any obvious breast abnormalities. Look for dimpling, puckering, or breast flattening as you first raise your arms slowly, then press your hands against your hips, and finally, bend forward.

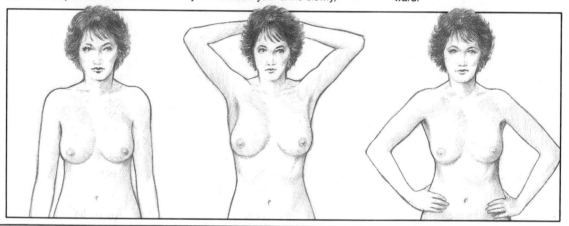

2 Stand with one hand behind your head. Using the pads of the middle three fingers on your opposite hand, examine each breast systematically by compressing it against your chest wall. Compress all parts of the breast in one of the three patterns shown: circular, vertical strip, or wedge. Repeat for your other breast. Examine your breasts when you are in the shower or standing before a mirror. Pay special attention to the upper outer areas of the breast.

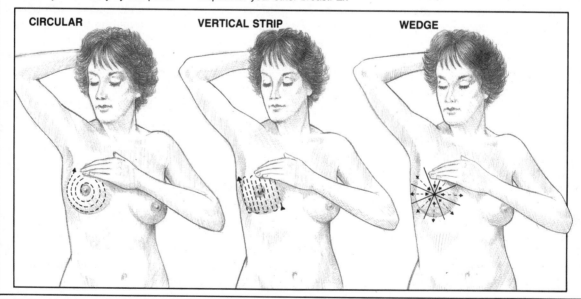

CIRCULAR   VERTICAL STRIP   WEDGE

Breast self-examination continued

3 Repeat the procedure lying down with a pillow or folded towel under your shoulder on the side you are examining. Repeat for your other breast.

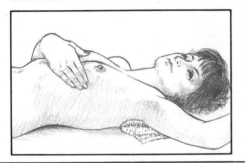

4 Next, squeeze the nipple gently between your thumb and index finger. Look for any drainage. Repeat for your other breast.

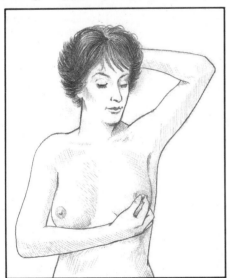

5 Report any of the following to your doctor or nurse practitioner:
- redness
- swelling
- lumps
- flattening
- puckering
- dimpling
- sunken areas
- nipples pointing in different directions
- drainage
- bleeding
- sores
- nipple rash

Comfort measures. If diet and exercise do not prevent or relieve premenstrual and menstrual discomfort, suggest over-the-counter analgesics, heat application or warm baths, and relaxation techniques. If these measures do not minimize the client's discomfort, refer her for further evaluation and treatment.

Teach about menopausal symptom management

Instruct a client with a nursing diagnosis of *ineffective thermoregulation related to hot flashes* to dress in layers. This will increase her comfort by allowing her to remove a layer or two of clothes when a hot flash occurs and to replace them when it passes. Reassure the client with a *sleep pattern disturbance related to hot flashes* that her discomfort may be unpreventable, but should be temporary. To prevent excessive fatigue, suggest frequent rest periods and the use of relaxation techniques. Also suggest appropriate diet changes, as discussed in the "Diet" section on pages 139 and 140.

A menopausal client with dyspareunia may have a nursing diagnosis of *altered sexuality patterns related to atrophic vaginal changes* or *sexual dysfunction related to decreased vaginal secretions.* If so, teach her to use a vaginal cream with estrogen, if prescribed, or advise her how to use a water-soluble lubricant, such as Lubrin, which is especially formulated for the menopausal woman. Also mention that increased sexual activity can improve vaginal lubrication and elasticity.

To manage menopausal symptoms, a client may need exogenous estrogen to compensate for decreased estrogen and progesterone production. From 1960 to 1975, physicians commonly wrote prescriptions for estrogen to relieve symptoms and prevent signs of aging. In 1975, the first studies documented the association between exogenous estrogen and endometrial cancer (Smith, Prentice, Thompson, and Herrmann, 1975; Ziel and Finkle, 1975). Since then, progestin (the synthetic equivalent of progesterone) with estrogen has been prescribed to treat menopausal symptoms. This combined hormone replacement therapy (HRT) greatly reduces the risk of endometrial cancer. However, more research is needed to document risks and benefits of estrogen and progestin HRT.

For menopausal symptoms, exogenous estrogen decreases hot flashes, restores vaginal moisture, and relieves dysuria, but does not relieve depression. It also prevents osteoporosis by blocking bone resorption, providing protection even when the woman begins estrogen therapy years after menopause—although protection is greatest when therapy starts soon after menopause and continues for 5 years.

If the physician prescribes HRT to control menopausal symptoms or prevent osteoporosis, the client will

APPLYING THE NURSING PROCESS

Client with knowledge deficit related to BSE and mammography

The table below shows how the nurse might use the nursing process to ensure high-quality care when caring for the client described in the case history at right. The first column presents history and physical assessment data followed by a paragraph of mental notes. These notes help the nurse make important mental connections among assessment findings, aiding in development of the nursing diagnosis and planning.

The second column lists an appropriate nursing diagnosis; information in the remaining columns is based on this diagnosis. Although not part of the nursing process, a rationale appears for each intervention in the fourth column to explain how it contributes to the care plan.

ASSESSMENT	NURSING DIAGNOSIS	PLANNING
Subjective (history) data • Client states, "I'm here for my yearly exam." • Client reports that she has never been taught breast self-examination (BSE), but would like to learn. • Client states she has never had a mammogram. • Client states her maternal grandmother died from breast cancer. • Client reports that her last menstrual period was 5 days ago and that her periods are regular, occurring every 28 days. • Client reports using oral contraceptives for the past 2 years. **Objective (physical) data** • Vital signs: temperature; 98.6° F; pulse, 80 beats/minute; respirations, 20; blood pressure, 120/80 mm Hg. • Breasts: symmetrical in size and shape, soft, and nontender with no dimpling, retractions, masses, or lesions. • Nipples: everted, pointing in same direction, nontender, and elastic with no retractions or discharge. • Axillae: no tenderness, masses, or lesions. • External genitalia: pink and moist with appropriate hair distribution, no lesions, inflammation, edema, or discharge. • Vagina: pink, without lesions or inflammation. • Cervix: parous, pink, firm, smooth, mobile, and nontender without lesions. Clear, odorless cervical discharge. • Uterus: midline, anteverted, firm, mobile, and nontender organ without masses. • Ovaries: oval-shaped organs, about 4 cm in size. Smooth, mobile, and slightly tender with no masses. • Rectum: No masses, nodules, or bleeding. • Stool specimen: negative for occult blood. • Pap test specimen: obtained and sent to laboratory. **Mental notes** *The physical examination reveals normal, healthy breast tissue, but the client has one risk factor for breast cancer: a maternal family history of breast cancer. To reduce her cancer risk, she will need reinforcement of BSE techniques and a system to remind herself to perform BSE. She also will need information about associated risk factors.*	Knowledge deficit related to BSE and mammography	**Goals** By the end of this visit, the client will: • describe the breast changes that normally occur during the menstrual cycle • demonstrate proper BSE technique • identify normal and abnormal breast changes on teaching model • explain how to use the menstrual and BSE record • consider scheduling an appointment for a baseline mammogram.

need extensive teaching, particularly if she has a *knowledge deficit related to hormone replacement therapy.* Tell such a client about common adverse effects, such as weight gain, breast and pelvic discomfort, headache, and vaginal discharge and bleeding. Advise her to report any of these effects immediately. She may need a dosage adjustment or assessment for cancer.

During menopause, a client may develop *potential for injury related to decreased bone mass.* If so, discuss calcium supplementation combined with low doses of estrogen, which can protect against bone loss (Ettinger, Genant, and Carr, 1987).

Other measures for preventing and treating osteoporosis may include weight-bearing exercise to strengthen the bones and smoking cessation to maxi-

CASE STUDY

Kathleen Kelly, age 37, is a married mother of three children and a part-time nursery school teacher. She has come to the health care clinic for her annual gynecologic examination.

IMPLEMENTATION		EVALUATION
Intervention Teach the client about normal breast anatomy and hormonal effects using illustrations or teaching models.	**Rationale** An understanding of normal breast anatomy and hormonal effects will help the client accurately evaluate her own breasts.	Upon evaluation, the client: • returned for scheduled mammogram • brought her menstrual and BSE record, which she used correctly • described the differences between normal and abnormal breast changes • reported performing BSE on the fifth day of her menstrual cycle • demonstrated correct BSE technique.
Describe and demonstrate BSE, differentiating between normal and abnormal breast changes.	This will enable the client to perform BSE and distinguish between normal and abnormal breast changes.	
Give the client a menstrual and BSE record and describe how to use it.	The menstrual and BSE record acts as a reminder to perform BSE and gives the client a place to document her efforts. It also documents the beginning of any menstrual problems.	
Provide written instructions on BSE.	Written instructions help reinforce learning and serve as a reference when the client performs BSE.	
Describe the purpose of mammography and advise the client about when it should occur.	Such information will emphasize the importance of a mammogram in early detection of breast cancer and other abnormalities.	
Instruct the client about risk factors related to breast cancer, such as family history of breast cancer.	Awareness of risk factors may prompt the client to make life-style changes that can reduce her risk of breast cancer.	

mize calcium retention. (For more information about the use of estrogen and calcium, see Chapter 15, Women's Health-Compromising Behaviors.)

A middle-aged or older client with a nursing diagnosis of *stress incontinence related to pelvic relaxation* may appreciate help in managing this troubling problem. Teach her to perform exercises that strengthen her pelvic muscles. (For more information, see *Client teaching: Kegel exercises*, page 146.)

Make referrals

If a client's needs exceed the health care team's ability to provide care, refer her to the appropriate community resources based on her nursing and medical diagnoses. For example, refer an adolescent with *ineffective individual coping related to physiologic changes of puberty* to a counselor. For other nursing diagnoses, consider referring her to a nutritionist, family therapist, or educator, as appropriate. Refer a client with *altered health*

Kegel exercises

You can help correct a problem with urine control by doing isometric exercises—called Kegel exercises—to strengthen your pelvic muscles. Here's how to do these exercises.

• Begin by sitting on the toilet with your legs spread. Then, without moving your legs, start and stop the flow of urine. The pubococcygeus (PC) muscle is the one that contracts to help control urine flow.
• Now that you've identified the PC muscle, you can exercise it. First, contract the PC muscle as you did to stop the urine flow. Count slowly to three, then relax the muscle.
• Next, contract and relax the PC muscle as quickly as possible, without using your stomach or buttock muscles.
• Finally, *slowly* contract the entire vaginal area. Then bear down, using your abdominal muscles as well as your PC muscle.

For the first week, repeat each exercise 10 times (1 set) for 5 sets daily. Then each week, add 5 repetitions to each exercise (15, 20, and so forth). Keep doing 5 sets daily. Keep in mind that Kegel exercises are like most isometric exercise. You can perform them almost anywhere—while sitting at your desk, lying in bed, standing in line, and especially while urinating.

After a week or two of practice, you should notice an improvement. To check your progress, insert one or two clean, well-lubricated fingers into your vagina so you can feel the PC muscle contract.

This teaching aid may be reproduced by office copier for distribution to clients. © 1991, Springhouse Corporation.

maintenance related to limited access to health care to a social worker who may be able to provide assistance. For a client with *ineffective individual coping related to menopausal changes* or *body image disturbance related to menopausal changes,* provide a referral to a mid-life support group or perimenopausal group. This type of self-help group usually consists of health care professionals and menopausal women and is designed to help the client adapt successfully to menopause.

Evaluation

To evaluate gynecologic care, determine if the goals were met and the care was effective. The following examples illustrate some typical evaluation statements:
• The client accurately described the physiologic changes of menarche.

• The client reported feeling confident about managing her menstrual flow and symptoms.
• The client openly discussed her anxieties about menstruation.
• The client demonstrated proper BSE techniques.
• The client scheduled an appointment for a mammogram.
• The client listed techniques she could use to decrease the effects of hot flashes.
• The client joined a mid-life support group.

In an ambulatory care setting where clients visit annually, evaluation of nursing care for every client may not be feasible. However, be sure to follow up with certain clients, such as those who require medication, have abnormal test results, will have or have had surgery, are starting or changing to a new contraceptive method, are in emotional turmoil, or have been referred. For such a client, telephone or write to determine (1) if the client took the recommended actions, (2) if procedures performed were effective, (3) if medications were purchased and taken as prescribed and if they relieved the symptoms, (4) if additional problems have developed, and (5) if any significant changes have occurred since the last visit.

If the care plan was not effective, reassess the client and determine why it did not achieve the desired goals. Then work closely with her to develop a more useful plan to meet her needs.

Documentation

Carefully record the assessment findings, the plan of care, and all other aspects of the nursing process. Keep in mind that this documentation will serve as the basis for evaluating the nursing care plan and will communicate your thoughts and activities to other members of the health care team.

Documentation of basic gynecologic care should include the client's:
• age
• reason for seeking care
• menstrual history
• contraceptive history
• obstetric history
• personal health history
• family history
• health habits
• sexual history
• psychosocial history

- vital signs, height, and weight
- other physical assessment findings, especially from the breast and pelvic examination
- test and procedure results
- response to teaching
- nursing care plan
- response to and understanding of the care plan.

Documentation also should include the nurse's plans for follow-up and evaluation of care.

Chapter summary

Chapter 7 described the health care needs of clients across the life span and discussed the components of gynecologic care, highlighting the nurse's role. Here are the key concepts.

- Gynecologic care focuses primarily on reproductive and related functions. It is a major portion of women's health care, which addresses all facets of a woman's life.
- As the largest group of health care consumers, women can influence the health care delivery system; they usually make health care choices for other family members.
- Two key factors influence a client's contact with the health care system: access to care, which may be influenced by the client's socioeconomic status, cultural background, or sexual orientation; and the attitudes of health care professionals.
- Two key events in a woman's life—menarche and menopause—are complex but normal biological, psychological, and social events.
- At different ages, women typically have different health concerns. For example, an adolescent client may be concerned with menstrual management and contraception; an older client, with atrophic vaginal changes and osteoporosis.
- The nurse must be sensitive to the client's developmental needs as well as her cultural background, sexual orientation, and socioeconomic status.
- To facilitate care, the nurse should prepare the client physically and psychologically before the gynecologic assessment.
- During the gynecologic assessment, the nurse should obtain information about the client's health status, in-

cluding her menstrual, contraceptive, obstetric, and family history as well as her history of genitourinary problems, other medical problems, surgery, and allergies.

- To assess the client's health promotion and protection behaviors, the nurse should ask about personal habits, sleep and rest, exercise, nutrition, stress, menstrual management, and regular health care activities, such as the Pap test and BSE. To assess the client's roles and relationships, the nurse should investigate her sexual, family, and other relationships and assess her emotional health status.
- During the physical assessment, the nurse measures the client's vital signs, height, and weight; inspects and palpates her breasts; and sometimes assesses her thyroid gland or abdomen. With special preparation, the nurse may examine the pelvic structures, inspecting and palpating external and internal genitalia and collecting laboratory specimens as needed.
- The nurse can incorporate an educational pelvic examination into the physical assessment to increase the client's understanding of her reproductive anatomy.
- Depending on the client's needs, diagnostic studies may include the Pap test, vaginal or cervical cultures, complete blood count, urinalysis, rubella titer, VDRL or RPR testing, HIV testing, mammography, and colposcopy.
- Active listening is an important part of nursing care, especially for a client distressed by a suspected gynecologic disorder or a normal physiologic change.
- A client who is entering menarche or menopause may benefit from teaching about normal female anatomy and physiology.
- Client teaching about health promotion activities is an important part of the nurse's plan of care. The nurse should teach all menstruating women to keep a menstrual record and all women over age 20 to perform BSE and keep a BSE record. The nurse also should provide information about screening tests and procedures, diet, exercise, stress management, risk factors for disease, and practices that protect against STDs.
- As needed, the nurse should provide information about protection against STDs.
- For a client in her childbearing years, the nurse may need to teach about menstrual management, including preparation, menstrual flow control, hygiene, sexual concerns, and comfort measures.
- For a menopausal client, the nurse may intervene by teaching her how to manage menopausal symptoms, including hormone replacement therapy, if prescribed.
- When the client's needs exceed the health care team's ability to provide care, the nurse should refer her to a

community resource, such as a therapist or support group.

• The nurse must evaluate and document all steps of the nursing process when providing care.

Study questions

1. How can the nurse increase access to health care for a lesbian? For a client from a different culture?

2. How are the health care concerns of an adolescent similar to and different from those of an older woman?

3. The nurse must orient Ms. Chris Beatty, the new receptionist at the Women's Health Center. What attitudes should the nurse help her develop? What information should the nurse tell Chris to give new clients when they make a gynecologic appointment? Why?

4. How should a nurse prepare Annie Gallagher, age 16, for her first pelvic examination?

5. Several screening tests and procedures are vital to a woman's health. What are these tests and procedures and how frequently should they be done?

6. What suggestions can the nurse offer to Mary Dwyer, age 55, to manage vaginal dryness related to menopause?

Bibliography

Cunningham, F., MacDonald, P., and Grant, N. (1989). *Williams obstetrics* (18th ed.). Norwalk, CT: Appleton & Lange.

Griffith-Kenney, J. (1986). *Contemporary women's health: A nursing advocacy approach.* Menlo Park, CA: Addison-Wesley.

Lewis, S., and Collier, S. (1987). *Medical-surgical nursing assessment and management of clinical problems* (2nd ed.). New York: McGraw-Hill.

Martin, E. (1989). *Woman in the body.* Boston: Beacon Press.

Morton, P. (1989). *Health assessment in nursing.* Springhouse, PA: Springhouse Corporation.

U.S. Congress, Office of Technology Assessment. (1986). *Nurse practitioners, physicians' assistants, and certified nurse-midwives: Policy analysis.* Washington, DC: U.S. Government Printing Office.

Adolescent care

Brooks-Gunn, J. (1988). Antecedents and consequences of variations in girls' maturational timing. *Journal of Adolescent Health Care, 9*(5), 365-373.

Coupey, S. (1984). The challenge of providing health care to adolescents. *Women and Health, 9*(2/3), 1-14.

Golden, N., Neuhoff, S., and Cohen, H. (1989). Pelvic inflammatory disease in adolescents. *Journal of Pediatrics, 114*(1), 138-143.

Gonsiorek, J. (1988). Mental health issues of gay and lesbian adolescents. *Journal of Adolescent Health Care, 9*(2), 114-122.

Irwin, C., and Vaughan, E. (1988). Psychosocial context of adolescent development: Study group report. *Journal of Adolescent Health Care, 9*(6S), 11S-19S.

Johnston, L., O'Malley, P., and Bachman, J. (1988). Psychotherapeutic, licit, and illicit use of drugs among adolescents. *Journal of Adolescent Health Care, 8*(1), 36-51.

NiCarthy, G. (1986). *Getting free* (2nd ed.). Seattle: Seal Press.

Paroski, P. (1987). Health care delivery and the concerns of gay and lesbian adolescents. *Journal of Adolescent Health Care, 8*(2), 188-192.

Stringham, P., and Weitzman, M. (1988). Violence counseling in the routine care of adolescents. *Journal of Adolescent Health Care, 9*(5), 389-393.

Tanner, J. (1987). Issues and advances in adolescent growth and development. *Journal of Adolescent Health Care, 8*(6), 470-478.

Teenage Pregnancy in Industrialized Countries: A Study Sponsored by the Alan Guttmacher Institute. (1986). New Haven: Yale University Press.

Adult care

Barrett-Connor, E. (1986). Postmenopausal estrogen, cancer, and other considerations. *Women and Health, 11*(3/4), 179-195.

Diokno, A., Brock, B., Brown, M., and Herzog, A. (1986). Prevalence of urinary incontinence and other urologic symptoms in the noninstitutionalized elderly. *Journal of Urology, 136*(5), 1022-1025.

Ettinger, B., Genant, H., and Carr, C. (1987). Postmenopausal bone loss is prevented by treatment with low-dosage estrogen with calcium. *Annals of Internal Medicine, 106*(1), 40-45.

McKeon, V. (1988). Dispelling menopause myths. *Journal of Gerontological Nursing, 14*(8), 26-29.

National Institute on Aging. (1988). *Health resources for older women.* Gaithersburg, MD: National Institute on Aging.

Older Women's League. (1989). The picture of health for midlife and older women in America. *Women and Health, 14*(3/4), 53-73.

Resnick, N. (1988). Urinary incontinence: A treatable disorder. In J. Rowe and R. Besdine (Eds.), *Geriatric medicine* (pp. 246-265). Boston: Little Brown.

Riis, B., Thomsen, K., and Christiansen, C. (1987). Does calcium supplementation prevent postmenopausal bone loss? *New England Journal of Medicine, 316*(4), 173-177.

Smith, D., Prentice, R., Thompson, D., and Herrmann, W. (1975). Association of exogenous estrogen and endometrial carcinoma. *New England Journal of Medicine, 293*(23), 1164-1167.

Voda, A., and Eliasson, M. (1983). Menopause: The closure of menstrual life. *Women and Health, 8*(2/3), 137-156.

Weintraub, N. (1989). Many elderly women not getting regular gyn exams. *OB/GYN News, 24*(4), 28.

Health concerns and promotion

Alagna, S., Morokoff, P., Bevett, J., and Reddy, D. (1987). Performance of breast self-examination by women at high-risk for breast cancer. *Women and Health, 12*(2), 29-46.

American Cancer Society (1988). *A personal plan of action for breast health.* Atlanta: American Cancer Society.

American College of Obstetricians and Gynecologists (1985). Women and exercise. *ACOG Technical Bulletin #87.* Washington, DC: American College of Obstetricians and Gynecologists.

Baker, L., Chin, T., and Wagner, K. (1985). Progress in screening for early breast cancer. *Journal of Surgical Oncology, 30*(2), 96-102.

Bassett, L., Bunnell, D., Cerny, J., and Gold, R. (1986). Screening mammography: Referral practices of Los Angeles physicians. *American Journal of Roentgenology, 147*(4), 689-692.

Fox, S., Klos, D., and Tsou, C. (1988). Underuse of screening mammography by family physicians. *Radiology, 166*(2), 431-433.

Frame, P. (1986). A critical review of adult health maintenance. Part 3: Prevention of cancer. *Journal of Family Practice, 22*(6), 511-520.

Freund, C. (1986). Nurse practitioners in primary care. In M. Mezey and D. McGivern (Eds.), *Nurses, nurse practitioners: The evolution of primary care.* Boston: Scott-Foresman.

Funch, D. (1986). Socioeconomic status and survival for breast and cervical cancer. *Women and Health, 11*(3/4), 37-54.

Gotto, A. (1988). Cholesterol: New approaches to screening and management. *Contemporary OB/GYN, 32*(1), 56.

Hendler, F. (1987). Southwestern internal medicine conference: Breast diseases and the internist. *American Journal of Medical Science, 293*(5), 332-347.

Landesman, S., Minkoff, H., Holman, S., McCalla, S., and Sijin, O. (1987). Serosurvey of human immunodeficiency virus infection in parturients. *JAMA, 258*(19), 2701-2703.

Mead, P., Cates, W., Jr., Minkoff, H., and Sever, J. (1988). AIDS: Looking ahead. *Contemporary OB/GYN, 32*(3), 76.

Johnson, S., and Palermo, J. (1984). Gynecologic care for the lesbian. *Clinical Obstetrics and Gynecology, 27*(3), 724-731.

Meisels, A., Morin, C., and Fortier, M. (1988). Rethinking common terminology for HPV. *Contemporary OB/GYN, 32*(2), 84.

Mullan, F. (1987). Rethinking public ambulatory care in America [sounding board]. *New England Journal of Medicine, 316*(9), 544-547.

National Cancer Institute. (1988). *What you need to know about breast cancer.* NIH Publication 88-1556. Washington, DC: U.S. Department of Health and Human Services.

Rimer, B. (1989). Single women found more likely to forgo mammography. *OB/GYN News, 24*(4), 13.

Schreiman, J. (1989). Early mammography in women with hereditary breast ca family. *OB/GYN News, 24*(4), 13.

Seidman, H., Gelb, S., Silverberg, E., LaVerda, N., and Lubera, J. (1987). Survival experience in the Breast Cancer Detection Demonstration Project. *CA—A Cancer Journal for Clinicians, 37*(5), 258-290.

Stevens, P., and Hall, J. (1988). Stigma, health beliefs, and experiences with health care in lesbian women. *Image: Journal of Nursing Scholarship, 20*(2), 69-73.

Cultural references

Bettelheim, B. (1962). *Symbolic wounds.* New York: Collier Books.

Harlow, S. (1986). Function and dysfunction: A historical critique of the literature on menstruation and work. In V. Oleson and N. Woods (Eds.). *Culture, society, and menstruation.* Washington, DC: Hemisphere Publishing Corp.

Novak, E. (1921). *Menstruation and its disorders.* New York: Appleton and Company.

Orque, S., Bloch, B., and Monrroy, L. (1983). *Ethnic nursing care: A multicultural approach.* St. Louis: C.V. Mosby.

Smith, P., Phillips, L., Faro, S., McGill, L., and Wait, R. (1988). Predominant sexually transmitted diseases among different age and ethnic groups of indigent sexually active adolescents attending a family planning clinic. *Journal of Adolescent Health Care, 9*(4), 291-295.

Stern, P. (1986). Women's social position as menstruating being. In V. Olsen and N. Woods (Eds.). *Culture, society, and menstruation.* Washington, DC: Hemisphere Publishing Corp.

Weideger, P. (1976). *Menstruation and menopause.* New York: Knopf.

Nursing research

Andrews, S. (1985). The experience of menarche: An exploratory study. *Journal of Nurse-Midwifery, 30*(1), 9-14.

Cook, R. (1976). *Damage to physical health from pharaonic circumcision (infibulation) of females: A review of the medical literature.* Alexandria, Egypt: World Health Organization, Regional Office for the Eastern Mediterranean.

Feldman, B., Voda, A., and Gronseth, E. (1985). The prevalence of hot flash and associated variables among perimenopausal women. *Research in Nursing and Health, 8*(3), 261-268.

Hailey, B. J. (1986). Breast self-examination among college females. *Women and Health, 11*(3/4), 55-65.

Lempert, L. (1986). Women's health from a woman's point of view: A review of the literature. *Health Care for Women International, 7*(3), 255-275.

Norbeck, J. (1984). Modification of life event questionnaires for use with female respondents. *Research in Nursing and Health, 7*(1), 61-71.

Pujanauski, A. (1989). *Homeless women and health care in an urban setting: Portland, Oregon.* Unpublished master's thesis, Oregon Health Sciences University School of Nursing, Portland, OR.

Redeker, N. (1989). Health beliefs, health locus of control, and the frequency of practice of breast self-examination in women. *JOGNN, (18)*1, 45-51.

Sexuality Concerns

Objectives

After reading and studying this chapter, the student should be able to:

1. Explain how feelings, beliefs, and attitudes about sexuality may affect the nurse's ability to provide related health care.

2. Summarize the physiology of sexual response for men and women.

3. Discuss the clinical significance of the human sexual response.

4. Characterize sexual concerns that occur during adolescence, adulthood, and older adulthood.

5. Explain the effects of the maternity cycle on sexual functioning.

6. Identify the components of a sexual health assessment.

7. Describe the major sexual dysfunctions.

8. Describe appropriate nursing interventions for sexual aspects of health care.

9. Apply the nursing process when caring for a client with sexuality concerns.

Introduction

Although experts do not agree on which sexual behaviors are normal or on a definition of sexual health, the definition developed by the World Health Organization (1975) serves as a guide:

Sexual health is the integration of physical, emotional, intellectual, and social aspects of sexual beings in ways that are positively enriching and that enhance personality, communication, and love. This

definition encompasses three essential elements: (1) capacity to enjoy and control sexual and reproductive behavior in accordance with a personal and social ethic; (2) freedom from shame, guilt, false beliefs, and other psychological factors that inhibit sexual response and impair sexual relationships; (3) freedom from organic disorders, diseases, and deficiencies that interfere with sexual and reproductive functions.

The topics of sex and sexuality almost always elicit strong personal reactions. Most individuals have deep convictions about sexuality and sexual practices that are based on moral and religious views, life experiences, and cultural influences. McCary and McCary (1984) note that our culture offers conflicting messages about sexuality, condemning many sexual relationships and practices while portraying sexuality as desirable and exciting.

Therefore, when the nurse addresses sexual aspects of health care with the client, both may feel uncomfortable. The nurse must ensure that personal attitudes do not interfere with objective interaction with the client and must create a caring and stress-free environment in which the client can talk honestly about sexuality. To create this environment, the nurse must be well informed about sexuality and sexual practices and must take care not to impose personal attitudes on the client.

To prepare the nurse to provide sensitive sexual health care, this chapter presents the physiology of sexual response, including the sexual response cycle and its clinical significance. It discusses the physical and

GLOSSARY

Androgyny: combination of male and female characteristics in the same individual.

Libido: psychic energy or instinctual drive associated with sexual desire, pleasure, or creativity.

Mid-life crisis: questions of self-esteem during middle adulthood related to the perceived loss of beauty, youth, and physical power.

Myotonia: increased muscular tension that causes voluntary and involuntary muscle contractions; a physiologic response to sexual stimulation.

Orgasmic platform: engorged lower third of the vagina during the sexual response cycle.

PLISSIT model: description of four levels of sexual counseling: permission, limited information, specific suggestions, and intensive therapy.

Refractory period: time after an orgasm when restimulation and orgasm are not possible for a man.

Sexuality: ongoing process of recognizing, accepting, and expressing oneself as a sexual being.

Spectatoring: phenomenon in which an individual imagines observing himself or herself during sexual activity.

Tumescence: swelling, as when the penis or breasts swell during sexual activity.

Vasocongestion: blood vessel engorgement and increased blood flow to tissues; a physiologic response to sexual stimulation.

---

psychosocial influences on human sexuality throughout life, exploring characteristics of healthy sexuality during each stage and highlighting the impact of the childbearing cycle on sexuality. Finally, the chapter shows how to use the nursing process to provide sexual health care.

Physiology of sexual response

The common phases of human sexual response were first identified in the early 1960s by Masters and Johnson. The most widely known approach for labeling and explaining physiologic response to sexual stimuli is the four-phase response cycle (Masters and Johnson, 1966). Another well-known approach is the response cycle described by the American Psychiatric Association (APA, 1987) in the *Diagnostic and Statistical Manual of Mental Disorders, DSM-III-R.*

Four-phase response cycle

The two principal physiologic responses to sexual stimulation are vasocongestion (blood vessel engorgement and increased blood flow to tissues) and myotonia (increased muscular tension that causes voluntary and in-

voluntary muscle contractions). Both responses build and resolve during the phases of the cycle.

In women, vasocongestion occurs primarily in the pelvic area and, to a lesser extent, in the breasts and other parts of the body. It produces vaginal lubrication, which prepares the vagina for penile penetration. In men, vasocongestion results in penile erection or tumescence (Kolodny, Masters, and Johnson, 1979).

In both sexes, myotonia is marked by such responses as the pelvic thrusts of orgasm, facial grimaces, and spasmodic contractions of hands and feet.

Masters and Johnson (1966) identified the following physiologic phases in the sexual response cycle.

• Excitement phase. Marked by vaginal lubrication in women and penile erection in men, excitement may develop from any bodily or psychic stimulus and increases in intensity in response to adequate stimulation. Distracting stimuli may interrupt, prolong, or end this phase.

• Plateau phase. In women, the vagina becomes engorged and the clitoris retracts under the clitoral hood. In men, the testes elevate until they are close to the body, and Cowper's glands release a few drops of mucoid substance. Distracting stimuli also may affect this phase.

• Orgasmic phase. Vasocongestion and myotonia peak in an involuntary climax that lasts only a few seconds and involves the entire body, although the focus is the pelvic area.

• Resolution phase. The body returns to its pre-excitement, or resting, state as vasocongestion resolves. When adequately stimulated, women may begin another sexual response cycle before sexual excitement has resolved completely. Men experience a refractory period (time after an orgasm when restimulation and orgasm are not

Physiologic changes in the four-phase response cycle

To provide appropriate care for a client with sexuality concerns, the nurse must understand the four-phase response cycle and its physiologic effects in women and men.

WOMEN	MEN
Excitement phase	
• Vaginal lubrication (in 10 to 30 seconds) • Thickening of vaginal walls and labia • Expansion of upper two-thirds of vagina and elevation of cervix and corpus • Clitoral tumescence • Nipple erection (in all women) • Sex flush (in about 25% of women), which appears over epigastric area and spreads over the breasts	• Penile erection (in 3 to 8 seconds) • Thickening, flattening, and elevation of scrotal sac • Partial testicular elevation and size increase • Nipple erection (in about 30% of men)
Plateau phase	
• Development of orgasmic platform (vasocongestion and engorgement of lower third of vagina) • Full vaginal expansion • Uterine and cervical elevation • Change of color of labia minora to purplish hue • Mucoid secretion, possibly from Bartholin's glands • Clitoral withdrawal • Sex flush (in 75% of women) • Carpopedal spasm • Generalized muscular tension • Hyperventilation • Tachycardia (100 to 160 beats/minute) • Increased blood pressure (20 to 60 mm Hg systolic; 10 to 20 mm Hg diastolic)	• Increase in penile coronal circumference • Testicular tumescence (50% to 100% enlarged) • Full testicular elevation and rotation (orgasm inevitable) • Purple hue to corona of penis (inconsistent) • Mucoid secretion from Cowper's gland • Sex flush (in 25% of men) • Carpopedal spasm • Generalized muscular tension • Hyperventilation • Tachycardia (100 to 160 beats/minute) • Increased blood pressure (20 to 80 mm Hg systolic; 10 to 40 mm Hg diastolic)
Orgasmic phase	
• Contraction of uterus from fundus toward lower uterine segment • Minimal relaxation of external cervical os • Contractions of orgasmic platform (0.8-second interval for 5 to 12 contractions) • External rectal sphincter contractions • External urethral sphincter contractions • Hyperventilation (up to 40 breaths/minute) • Tachycardia (up to 180 beats/minute) • Increased blood pressure (30 to 80 mm Hg systolic; 20 to 40 mm Hg diastolic)	• Ejaculation • Contractions of accessory reproductive organs (vas deferens, seminal vesicles, ejaculatory duct) • Relaxation of external bladder sphincter and contraction of internal bladder sphincter • Contractions of penile urethra (0.8-second interval for three to four contractions) • Anal sphincter contractions • Muscular contractions • Hyperventilation (up to 40 breaths/minute) • Tachycardia (up to 180 beats/minute) • Increased blood pressure (40 to 100 mm Hg systolic; 20 to 50 mm Hg diastolic)
Resolution phase	
• Ready return to orgasm with retarded loss of vasocongestion • Rapid loss of discoloration in labia minora and orgasmic platform • Slow disappearance of remainder of vasocongestion • Return of clitoris to normal size and position • Sweating reaction (30% to 40% of women) • Decreasing hyperventilation • Decreasing tachycardia	• Refractory period with rapid loss of vasocongestion • Loss of penile erection in a two-stage response: 50% rapid loss; 50% gradual loss • Sweating reaction (30% to 40% of men) • Decreasing hyperventilation • Decreasing tachycardia

Adapted from Fogel, C., and Lauver, D. (Eds.). (1990). *Sexual health promotion*. Philadelphia: W.B. Saunders (p. 49).

possible), the length of which varies with age and health. During this period, restimulation and further orgasm are not possible.

Individuals move progressively through the four-phase response cycle. Although no sharp divisions distinguish the phases, specific body changes will occur in sequence. (For more information, see *Physiologic changes in the four-phase response cycle*.)

DSM-III-R response cycle

The APA (1987) also has identified four phases of the sexual response cycle: appetitive, excitement, orgasm, and resolution. These phases incorporate biological and psychological components, making them useful in categorizing sexual disorders.

• Appetitive phase. This phase consists of sexual fantasies and desire for sexual activity. It recognizes a psychological dimension to sexual responsiveness and also identifies an area in which individuals may experience dysfunction.

• Excitement phase. In men, this phase is marked by penile erection and Cowper's gland secretion; in women, by pelvic vasocongestion with vaginal lubrication, external genitalia swelling, narrowing of the lower third of the vagina, lengthening of the upper two-thirds of the vagina, and breast tumescence. Men and women experience a sense of pleasure during this phase.

• Orgasm phase. In men, orgasm may be preceded by a sensation of ejaculatory inevitability. In women, the orgasm phase marks the peaking of sexual pleasure followed by a release of sexual tension and rhythmic contractions of the perineal muscles and reproductive organs. Women also may experience contractions of the lower third of the vagina.

• Resolution phase. In this phase, individuals experience general relaxation and a sense of well-being.

Clinical significance

In most cultures, myths and misconceptions surround sexuality and sexual function. In fact, many sexual problems can be traced to ignorance or misinformation about sexuality. The nurse who understands the sexual response cycle will be able to give the client more accurate information, thus dispelling myths and misconceptions.

The nurse may be asked about the differences between male and female sexual experiences, particularly the difference between the orgasmic patterns of men and women. Characteristic differences exist between men and women within the specific phases of the sexual response cycle, although the phases have a similar sequence.

Men experience a single sexual response cycle, characterized by a rapid excitement phase, a short plateau phase, an orgasm phase, and a resolution phase. The length of the refractory period varies with age, physical health, and emotional condition.

In nonpregnant women, the sexual response cycle may have three different patterns. In the first pattern, the woman has multiple orgasms with fairly rapid resolution. In the second pattern, the woman does not achieve orgasm, but experiences several peaks in the plateau phase and a longer resolution phase. In the third pattern, sexual excitement is interrupted more than once, followed by an intense orgasm and rapid resolution of sexual tension. The woman does not experience a refractory period; she may experience repeated orgasms before resolution.

Another difference between men and women is evident during the resolution phase. Men experience a refractory period, whereas women may experience repeated orgasms before resolution. Sherfey (1973) suggests that women have the capacity to experience orgasms until they are physically exhausted. The Hite (1987) data, in which several women reported experiencing multiple orgasms, support Sherfey's findings. Some women report their first experience of multiple orgasms during pregnancy, probably because of increased vasocongestion.

Many couples expect to achieve simultaneous orgasms and are concerned if they cannot. In fact, simultaneous orgasms are difficult to time. Men and women as a group progress through the sexual response cycle at differing rates, and individuals vary further in response. Many factors, including psychological state, illness, medication, sexual motivation, and environment, can influence an individual's sexual response.

Sexuality and the life cycle

Human sexuality is influenced by psychological, social, and cultural factors, and its nature changes throughout the life cycle.

Factors that influence sexuality

Attitudes about sexuality are influenced by moral, political, economic, cultural, and social values. Kinsey, Pomeroy, and Martin (1948, 1953) and Masters and Johnson (1966, 1970) are credited with helping society view sexuality scientifically by studying relationships among behavior, sexual repression, and childhood sexual expression. Many current experts recognize human individuality and the multiple purposes of sexual expression: procreation, pleasure, and expression of joy and love. They also recognize the importance of sexual liberation: the individual's need to express sexuality.

Pierson and D'Antonio (1974) report that two cultural norms are in transition. The first is a changing attitude toward masturbation, which is now acknowledged as a pleasurable sexual expression or a helpful technique for relieving sexual tension.

The second norm in transition is the attitude toward androgynous sexual behavior. (Androgyny refers to the combination of male and female characteristics in an individual.) Society is beginning to recognize that traits such as gentleness and aggressiveness are not unique to one sex and can be displayed by anyone, depending on the situation (Wallum, 1977; Bee, 1988).

Other cultures have different perspectives on sexuality, especially regarding behaviors that are considered masculine or feminine. Some cultures rigidly define sexual behaviors and roles; others accept a blend of traits in individuals. In many cultures and in some families in a particular culture, sex and sexuality are discussed openly; in others, these topics are discussed only privately. Therefore, the nurse's knowledge of the client's cultural beliefs, values, and practices is a prerequisite to carrying out the nursing process in relation to sexuality.

Myths about female sexuality prevail in the American culture, including the contradicting beliefs that women are less interested in and responsive to sex than men and, conversely, that women are sexually insatiable. Myths about male sexuality include the belief that men crave sex constantly.

When these myths conflict with a woman's personal experiences, she may feel alienated from her own experiences (Bernhard and Dan, 1986). Furthermore, the conflict between what a woman has been taught she should feel about her sexuality and what she actually feels can cause guilt and sexual anxiety and can lay the foundation for sexual dysfunction (Fogel and Woods, 1981; Bernhard and Dan, 1986).

When providing sexual health care to a female client, the nurse must pay attention to the client's sexual feelings and experiences. Such questions as, "What were you taught as a child about women and sex?" or "How do you think women should behave sexually?" will help clarify the client's attitudes toward sexuality.

Infancy and childhood

Constantine and Martinson (1981) indicate that several aspects of sexuality are established in early childhood and become fairly fixed: basic sexual identity, primary erotic orientation to the same or opposite sex, stimuli for sexual arousal, sense of security and comfort in being sexual, and sexual fears and preoccupations. Although most developmental theories presume the presence of two parents, child sexual development will progress normally in any family if adults communicate openly about sexuality.

Adolescence

In adolescence, rapid physical changes and psychosocial development affect sexuality. (For information about physical changes, see Chapter 6, Reproductive Anatomy and Physiology.)

A central issue for the adolescent is defining sexuality through such activities as dating. Dating prepares the adolescent for mate selection and adult competency in independent endeavors. It develops out of adolescent cliques of close friends to one-on-one same-sex friendships and then to formation of couple relationships (Chilman, 1983).

Dating allows the adolescent to select companions, test ideas about the self and others of the opposite sex, and ultimately experience sexual pleasure (Pierson and D'Antonio, 1974). However, sexual intimacy poses a central conflict for the adolescent because of the powerful emotions surrounding sexual intercourse. Attitudes about adolescent premarital intercourse vary. Some theorists believe that sexual experimentation is vital to adolescent development (Strean, 1983); others maintain that self-denial and anticipation, in themselves, are means of satisfaction and development (Pierson and D'Antonio, 1974).

The age for first intercourse declined during the 1970s from between ages 15 and 19 to between ages 13 and 15 (DeFries, Freedman, and Corn, 1985). Physical development and circulating levels of free testosterone prepare boys for sexual activity (Udry, Billy, and Morris, 1985). Social influences, especially the sexual behavior of close friends, are an important factor in a boy's sexual initiation. In girls, the presence of androgens and the behavior of friends are influential.

Risks associated with early sexual activity include acquired immunodeficiency syndrome (AIDS), other sexually transmitted diseases (STDs), and unplanned pregnancy. Because adolescents may engage in premarital sexual intercourse, health care professionals must educate them and their parents and teachers about these topics. According to a recent U.S. surgeon general, health care professionals should not instill fear about sex and AIDS, but should encourage adolescents to abstain from premarital sexual activity (Koop, 1987).

The delay between the onset of adolescent sexual activity and the first request for contraception information from a health care professional ranges from 9 to 12 months (Zabin and Clark, 1981). Furthermore, adolescents tend to use less effective contraceptive methods (Zelnik and Kantner, 1980). Younger adolescents are less apt to use contraception than are older ones. Of sexually active girls under age 15, 31% report using a contraceptive method; of those over age 15, more than 50% report using a contraceptive method (Zelnik and Kantner, 1980).

Adulthood

During early adulthood, developmental tasks include achieving maturity in sexual roles and in the relationship tasks begun in adolescence. For many, adulthood also is a time to marry and have a family.

For women, pregnancy and the postpartal period have physical and psychological influences on sexuality and sexual responsiveness. Proscriptions against sexual behavior during these times have existed for centuries, but some experts now encourage sexual activity for healthy couples who are comfortable with it (Mills, Harlap, and Harley, 1981; Flood and Naeye, 1984; Cunningham, MacDonald, and Gant, 1989). (For more information, see *Sexuality during pregnancy and the postpartal period,* page 156.)

Later in adulthood, physical and psychosocial changes occur in men and women as a result of the climacteric (menopause in women and reduction of sexual activity in men). Although individuals vary, men generally experience the climacteric during their fifties or sixties. It typically consists of emotional, physical, and sexual complaints, such as anxiety and depression, fatigue, poor appetite, and reduced libido (energy associated with sexual desire) or impotence (Weg, 1983). A gradual decline in androgen-dependent tissues results in decreased penile sensitivity and reduced testicular size and firmness. Women generally experience the climacteric between ages 40 and 60. It typically consists

of cessation of menses; body contour changes related to decreased muscle tone, skin elasticity, and fat accumulation; atrophic changes in genitourinary, muscular, and skeletal systems; and estrogen deficiency, which may account for affective and psychological changes. Although these physical changes alter sexual response capacity, the degree of alteration varies and depends in part on psychosocial factors. (For more information, see Chapter 7, Women's Health Promotion.)

According to Davis (1980), men and women may undergo a mid-life crisis (questions of self-esteem from a perceived loss of beauty, youth, and physical power). To make middle-age transitions less traumatic and relationships more satisfying, the individual must take respite as needed, examine facts, avoid blaming others, and accept needed help.

Older adulthood

Older adulthood refers to the period between the climacteric and death. The sexual response cycle changes during older adulthood. For men, the duration of each phase of the cycle increases. An erection takes longer to achieve and can be sustained longer before ejaculation, and ejaculate is expelled with less force. These factors may increase male sexual satisfaction in many cases (Woods, 1984; Weg, 1983). Many women, freed from the risk of conception, report heightened sexual satisfaction after menopause. However, thinner and dryer vaginal walls can cause discomfort, especially for women who do not engage in regular intercourse. For men and women, good physical health is a key to maintaining a positive sexual self-concept.

Weg (1983) summarizes that none of the physical changes that occur warrants the prevalent negative image of the sexless, loveless older adult. Sexual desire and activity can continue to be an integral part of life; in fact, older adults may be more responsible and considerate in interpersonal relationships than they were during earlier life stages.

Older adults may transcend gender-role stereotypes and engage in androgynous behaviors. After children leave home and the couple retires, the demands of nurturing and achieving decrease, allowing greater freedom and flexibility in sex-role development.

However, older adults remain vulnerable to the same stresses that affect relationships in middle age. In addition, the death of friends, spouses, or intimate partners during this period can affect sexuality. (For more information, see *Nursing research applied: Sexuality in older adults,* page 157.)

Sexuality during pregnancy and the postpartal period

Changes during pregnancy and the postpartal period can affect a woman's sexual response cycle and sexual activity.

PREGNANCY

Sexual response cycle

Masters and Johnson (1966) describe several changes in the sexual response cycle of pregnant women. During pregnancy, the progressive increase in pelvic vasocongestion may increase sexual desire. The excitement phase may be marked by pronounced breast tenderness, copious and rapid vaginal lubrication, engorgement of the labia majora, and a two- or three-fold increase in the size of the labia minora. During the plateau phase, localized vaginal engorgement occurs and the orgasmic platform develops more quickly.

During orgasm, the orgasmic platform contracts in the first two trimesters; contractions are minimized in the third trimester. Also during the third trimester, uterine spasms may last a half-hour (Engel-Sharts, 1990). The fetal heart rate may experience a transitory, nonproblematic slowing (Masters and Johnson, 1966). Although the resolution phase occurs, the pelvis is chronically vasocongested and orgasm does not clear the tissues. This may be experienced as heightened sexual tension.

Sexual activity

Some researchers report a gradual decrease in sexual interest and activity throughout the pregnancy (Ellis, 1980; Stegge and Jelovsek, 1982). Others report increased interest during the second trimester (Reamy, White, Daniell, and Levine, 1982) or no change in activity and desire (Masters and Johnson, 1966; Tolor and DiGrazia, 1976).

Several factors may contribute to increased sexual interest or activity during pregnancy: relief from pressure to conceive, elimination of the need to use contraception, loss of the fear of getting pregnant, increased awareness of the woman's body, celebration of their accomplishment, and increased desire and responsiveness because of the physiologic alterations of pregnancy (Engel-Sharts, 1990; Bing and Coleman, 1989).

Sexual activity may decrease during pregnancy because of the early symptoms of pregnancy, such as nausea and sleepiness or later discomforts, such as backache, fatigue, and increasing abdominal girth. Painful uterine cramping with orgasm, unsatisfactory resolution, discomfort or cervical bleeding associated with penetration, and vena cava compression in the supine position also may cause sexual activity to decrease.

Psychological factors, such as fear, cultural taboos, and negative self-image, also may contribute to decreased sexual activity during pregnancy. Some couples refrain from sexual activity because they fear it will harm the woman or the fetus.

The woman's image of her changing body also influences sexuality during pregnancy. She may feel that her increased breast size, altered pigmentation, and enlarged abdomen decrease—or increase—her attractiveness and heighten her sensuality. A woman also may view her weight gain positively or negatively.

POSTPARTAL PERIOD

Sexual response cycle

Masters and Johnson (1966) report a decrease in the speed and intensity of sexual responsiveness in the early postpartal period, although the subjective experience of sexual tension remains at prepregnancy levels. Physical reactions during sexual activity develop more slowly: vasocongestion with subsequent lubrication slows and decreases, as does vaginal distention. In the plateau phase, the orgasmic platform is less developed. Orgasmic contractions are shorter and less intense. By the end of the third postpartal month, the woman experiences a fairly complete return to prepregnancy patterns of sexual response.

Sexual activity

Most women report returning to prepregnancy levels of sexual activity in 2 to 12 months after delivery, with many resuming sexual activity 6 to 8 weeks after delivery (Masters and Johnson, 1966; Falicov, 1973; Fischman, Rankin, Soeken, and Lenz, 1986). Despite resuming sexual activity, however, some couples report declines in their desire for sexual activity when compared with prepregnancy desire.

Decreases in sexual activity and desire are related to physical and psychological factors. Physical factors may include vaginal or perineal pain, painful uterine contractions, lochia, weakness, fatigue, or breast engorgement. Episiotomy sites, postpartal hemorrhoids, or the effects of a complicated pregnancy, obstetric trauma, or cesarean delivery may affect a woman's sexuality. Some women also may fear injury or have concerns about the increased size of the vaginal introitus.

Psychological factors in decreased sexual activity may include dissatisfaction with one's appearance and fatigue from neonate care. Parents also may be preoccupied with incorporating new roles into their self-definitions, thus focusing all their attention on the neonate and neglecting their relationship with each other.

Another factor in delayed resumption of sexual activity may be traditional medical advice forbidding intercourse until the postpartal checkup (typically 6 weeks after delivery). Current recommendations, however, advise that the couple can resume intercourse after bleeding has stopped and the episiotomy has healed, usually 3 or 4 weeks after delivery. Some health care professionals suggest that sexual activity be resumed whenever the couple wishes as long as the woman experiences no discomfort (Cunningham, MacDonald, and Gant, 1989).

NURSING RESEARCH APPLIED

Sexuality in older adults

A 1988 study examined the behavior, knowledge, and attitudes of 28 volunteers, ages 60 and older, regarding sexuality and aging.

The subjects were divided into an experimental group and a control group. Both groups completed pretesting. The experimental group then participated in four educational sessions that included lectures and discussions about ageism, intimacy, physical changes of aging, diseases and physical problems in aging, nursing homes and privacy, and retirement marriages. The control group was given no such information. Subjects in both groups then participated in posttesting.

Results showed no significant pretest to posttest differences between the two groups in frequency of sexual activity or level of satisfaction. The experimental group showed a significant gain in knowledge of sexuality and aging from pretest to posttest and a slight increase in permissiveness. Conversely, the control group reflected a more conservative attitude.

Application to practice
These findings indicate the need for more education of older adults regarding various aspects of sexuality. The nurse must increase personal knowledge of, and be sensitive to, the attitudes and sexual experiences of older adults and the ways in which they express their sexuality. The nurse who understands and accepts older adult sexuality may help these clients achieve satisfaction within the scope of their beliefs and values.

Steinke, E. (1988). Older adults knowledge and attitudes about sexuality and aging. *Image*, 20(2), 93-95.

Nursing care for the female client with sexuality concerns

A client may express sexuality concerns and expect the nurse to provide sex education or counseling. The nursing process provides a systematic way of organizing sexual health care from assessment to evaluation.

Client assessment

To assess the client, the nurse gathers data through the health history, physical assessment, and laboratory tests.

Health history
The health history interview provides information about the client's basic and sexual health history. The primary source of this information is the client, although health records, family members, and friends also may supply data.

The client who senses that the nurse is uncomfortable discussing sexuality may become uneasy. The following guidelines will help the nurse approach the health history interview more comfortably.
• Choose a private location where the client will feel at ease sharing personal information.
• Arrange the seats comfortably apart.
• Observe carefully to determine if the client feels comfortable with direct eye contact. Listen closely and watch for nonverbal cues that indicate anxiety or discomfort.
• Note personal feelings. The nurse's embarrassment or negativity may prevent the client from being completely honest.
• Ask basic health history questions before obtaining a sexual health history, keeping in mind that various health concerns may affect sexuality and that sexuality may affect many aspects of life.
• Begin the interview with less sensitive questions, such as those related to menstrual history, and then proceed to more personal inquiries.
• Explain the reason for each question, and describe how the answer will help direct the client's care.
• Ask open-ended questions, such as, "Why are you here today?" to let the client tell her own story. Ask closed questions to collect a medical and menstrual history.
• Put the client at ease by demonstrating acceptance of various sexual behaviors and attitudes. Ask questions that demonstrate acceptance, such as, "Many women have erotic fantasies about someone other than their husbands. Has this happened to you?"
• Avoid using excessive medical terminology and euphemisms about sex. Clarify the meaning of slang expressions to ensure mutual understanding.
• Determine the client's sexual preference and sexual activities before suggesting interventions. Do not make assumptions about the client's sexual behavior; not all clients are sexually active or heterosexual.

Basic health history. After obtaining biographical data, determine the client's reason for seeking care. Gather information about her menstrual, contraceptive, gynecologic, obstetric, medical, and surgical history as well as her personal habits. (For detailed information, see Chapter 7, Women's Health Promotion.)

When gathering this information, note responses that could affect the client's sexuality or health care. Physical factors, such as bleeding between menstrual cycles in a client of childbearing age or menopausal changes in an older client, may affect sexuality patterns. The client's educational level, occupation, and religion may influence the choice of nursing interventions.

Sexual health history. When obtaining a sexual health history, begin by determining if the client is sexually active. If so, use a brief, screening history for sexuality concerns to determine if more extensive questioning is needed. Woods (1984) suggests asking these three questions as the screening history:
• Has anything, such as illness, pregnancy, or surgery, interfered with your being a sexual partner?
• Has anything, such as illness, medical treatment, surgery, or pregnancy, changed the way you feel about yourself?
• Has anything, such as surgery, medication, disease, or pregnancy, altered your ability to function sexually?

If the screening history indicates a sexuality concern, obtain a detailed sexual history to determine the client's level of sexual health and functioning.

Obtaining a sexual health history conveys the message that sexuality is a legitimate aspect of health. A sexual health history can have therapeutic as well as assessment value because it allows the nurse to provide information about sexuality and validate the client's concerns or sexual practices.

To begin the detailed history, ask the client to describe the frequency of her sexual activity. Inquire about her degree of satisfaction with her sexual activity, and determine if she has difficulty becoming aroused or having orgasms. Ask if she experiences vaginal lubrication during sexual intercourse or experiences pain. Her answers to these questions can provide information about her sexual satisfaction and can uncover problems that may need to be resolved.

Assess the client's sources of sex education and find out how old she was when she first learned about sexual intercourse. Ask how she reacted initially and if her values or beliefs have since changed. To gather specific information, ask such questions as, "What have you heard from family and friends about sex during and after pregnancy?" "How do you feel about sex during pregnancy?" and "How do you feel about masturbation and oral-genital sex?"

Evaluate the client's beliefs regarding appropriate sex role behaviors. Ask how she believes a woman should interact with men, and have her describe her dating patterns and the qualities she values in a partner. Keep in mind that religious, educational, social, and economic factors influence sex role orientation.

Continue by investigating the client's sexual desire and sexual interactions with her partner. Ask whether her sexual desire has increased, decreased, fluctuated, or otherwise changed over time. Investigate concerns about her sexual adequacy or body image, and assess the impact of these concerns on her desire for sexual activity.

Next, inquire about the client's sexual interactions with her partner. Determine the extent of communication between them and the characteristics of their sexual activity. Ask the client to describe their typical sexual behaviors, any behaviors that detract from the overall erotic encounters, and the sexual activities they employ other than intercourse. Ask her about the frequency and duration of any extramarital sexual experiences.

Ask the client to describe vaginal lubrication, including rapidity of lubrication, increased or decreased lubrication, and any vaginal pain during penile penetration. Also inquire about her orgasmic capacity: Does she achieve orgasm, and if so, how (by masturbation, penile penetration, or manual or oral stimulation by her partner)? How frequently does she achieve orgasm? Ask her to describe any situations that inhibit orgasm.

If the client states that her partner has a sexuality concern, explore the difficulty by asking her about his erectile functioning, including the quality of erections, situations that precipitate erectile failure, and satisfaction with penis size. Ask about his orgasmic experience, including frequency of ejaculation, how it is achieved (by vaginal penetration or manual or oral stimulation), any change in the quality of the orgasmic experience, and any concern over his partner and her orgasm. Also inquire about coital positions. If the client cannot answer these questions, suggest that her partner schedule an appointment for a detailed assessment.

Keep in mind that sexuality should be viewed on a continuum, ranging from adaptive to maladaptive, depending on its effect on the client, partner, and society. Because normality is difficult to define, consider these questions when evaluating a particular behavior:
• What does the behavior mean to the client?
• Does it enrich or impoverish the sex life of the client and her partner?
• Is it tolerable to society?
• Is it conducted between two consenting adults?
• Is it psychologically or physically harmful to the client or her partner?
• Does the behavior use coercion?

Sexual dysfunction. A client who describes a sexuality concern may have a sexual dysfunction. The nurse must be prepared to recognize disorders and refer the client to the appropriate health care professional.

Sexual dysfunctions may occur in one or more phases of the sexual response cycle, although they are less common in the resolution phase. Current research indicates that pathophysiologic causes are probably more common than psychogenic ones (Field, 1990). Although most sexual dysfunctions occur during sexual activity with a partner, they may occur during masturbation (Poorman, 1988). Sexual dysfunctions may be lifelong or may develop after a period of normal responsiveness. They may occur once or recur.

Sexual dysfunctions typically occur in clients in their late 20s and early 30s, a few years after establishing a sustained sexual relationship (APA, 1987). Sexual dysfunction may impair an individual's relationship with a partner, but it rarely interferes with occupational functioning (APA, 1987). (For more information, see *Summary of sexual dysfunctions*, page 160.)

Causes of sexual dysfunction. Sexual dysfunction can result from a physical cause, a psychological cause, or both.

Physical causes of sexual dysfunction vary. Fatigue, fever, and pain can limit sexual desire. Illness may cause fatigue, pain, or other systemic nonspecific effects and may interfere with neural, vascular, or hormonal components of sexual response. Generalized or localized infections and hepatic, pulmonary, and renal disease can decrease sexual desire and interfere with sexual performance (Livingston, McIntyre, and Fogel, 1984). Such medications as antihypertensive, antianxiety, and antidepressant agents also can cause sexual dysfunction.

Various diseases that affect the brain, spinal column, or peripheral nervous system also may affect sexual functioning. A history of mental disorders, chronic diseases, gynecologic infections, or STDs can cause sexual dysfunction. For example, as many as 60% of diabetic males experience erectile disorder (Manley, 1990). Vascular disorders that affect the genital blood supply also can impair erectile function, as can endocrine disorders, such as hypothyroidism. Endocrine disorders also may retard orgasmic responses in women (Manley, 1990). Certain types of prostatic or abdominal surgery may interfere with the autonomic and somatic innervation to the genital area, altering sexual performance.

Psychological causes of dysfunction include inadequate sexual knowledge, ignorance of sexual techniques, or misinformation. In a society that places strong prohibitions on sexual behavior, education, and discussion, partners may be ignorant of sexual anatomy or appropriate sexual techniques and may feel uncomfortable discussing their sexual desires.

Sexual problems may result from anxieties, including fear of sexual failure, fear of rejection by the partner, and fear of demand for sexual performance (Kaplan, 1974). Anticipatory anxiety can negatively affect sexual performance, as can spectatoring (phenomenon in which an individual imagines observing himself or herself during sexual activity). Furthermore, anxiety can produce a self-defeating cycle of fear and poor performance that confirms anxieties and fear of failure.

Another psychological cause of sexual dysfunction is an excessive need to please. Although the desire to give and share pleasure with a partner is important and healthy, a need to please the partner at all costs is not (Kaplan, 1974).

Poor communication between partners about sexual needs, feelings, and desires is another important factor in sexual dysfunction. Although poor communication may not cause dysfunction, it can further an unsatisfying sexual pattern or escalate sexual problems by limiting knowledge or restricting standards of acceptable sexual behavior.

Stress also may play a role in sexual dysfunction, resulting in anxiety that interferes with sexual responsiveness or fatigue that detracts from sexual interest. Anger, power struggles, and unresolved conflicts in the relationship also can contribute to sexual dysfunction.

Physical assessment and laboratory tests

Based on health history data, a physical assessment and laboratory tests may be performed. For example, if a client reports painful intercourse (dyspareunia) and heavy vaginal discharge, a pelvic examination and vaginal discharge evaluation should be conducted to check for vaginal infection. (For more information, see Chapter 7, Women's Health Promotion.)

Nursing diagnosis

After analyzing the assessment data, including the client's ideas about the problem, the nurse formulates appropriate nursing diagnoses. (For a partial list of possible nursing diagnoses, see *Nursing diagnoses: Sexuality concerns*, page 161.) Validate the diagnoses with the client before implementation to help ensure the effectiveness of the interventions.

Planning and implementation

After developing a plan of care for each diagnosis, the nurse establishes and clarifies the goals for intervention with the client. Based on the immediacy of the problem, establish priorities and list criteria by which to measure progress toward the goals. Then identify actions to help the client meet the goals. If possible, incorporate into the care plan any techniques that the client has used previously to cope successfully with similar problems.

The client with sexuality concerns may require various health services, ranging from education to intensive therapy with a specially trained health care professional. Expertise among nurses differs, and professional preparation will determine which nurse should intervene at each level of complexity.

Summary of sexual dysfunctions

Four categories of sexual dysfunctions exist: sexual desire disorders, sexual arousal disorders, orgasmic disorders, and sexual pain disorders. Each category includes several specific disorders, as described below. (Sexual desire refers to the frequency with which a person wishes to have sexual relations, whereas arousal is the subjective experience of sexual excitement as ascertained by the client's self-report [Poorman, 1988].)

Sexual desire disorders

Hypoactive sexual desire disorder
This disorder is characterized by a subjective lack of desire for sexual activity, a lack of sexual dreams or fantasies, and a lack of frustration if deprived of sexual activity. Sexual activity occurs infrequently or results only from reluctant compliance with a partner's desire for activity (Schover and LoPiccolo, 1982).

Sexual aversion disorder
This disorder is characterized by extreme repulsion by

and avoidance of almost all genital sexual contact with a partner (APA, 1987). Intense, irrational fear of sexual activity and a compelling desire to avoid sexual situations occur (Kaplan and Klein, 1987). The client attempts to avoid sexual encounters and, if pressured by a partner into having sex, experiences anxiety and escalating sexual fear. A mildly affected client may remain calm and enjoy a sexual experience, but this does not decrease phobic response in subsequent encounters.

Sexual arousal disorders

Female sexual arousal disorder
This disorder is characterized by partial or complete failure to attain or maintain vaginal lubrication and swelling or sexual excitement. A lack of a subjective sense of sexual excitement or pleasure is noticed during sexual activity (APA, 1987).

Male sexual arousal disorder
Previously known as impotence, male sexual arousal disorder is now called erectile disorder. It is

characterized by partial or complete failure to attain an erection or maintain one throughout sexual activity, accompanied by a lack of a subjective sense of sexual excitement or pleasure during sexual activity. Illness, extreme fatigue, alcohol consumption, medication, or anxiety may cause transient episodes of erectile failure. Occasional, transient episodes of erectile failure occur in approximately 50% of men and are not considered abnormal (Kaplan, 1974).

Orgasmic disorders

Inhibited female orgasm
The most common sexual problem among women, this disorder is characterized by a persistent or recurrent delay in or absence of orgasm despite a normal sexual excitement phase adequate in focus, intensity, and duration (Field, 1990). Subjects are otherwise sexually responsive, experiencing erotic feelings, genital swelling, and vaginal lubrication. Causes include a restrictive home environment, negative cultural conditioning, and unrealistic expectations about sexual performance. It is defined as a disorder only if the woman reports receiving sufficient stimulation.

Premature ejaculation
This disorder is characterized by ejaculation that

persistently or recurrently occurs with minimal stimulation or before, upon, or shortly after penetration and before the man desires to ejaculate. Age, the novelty of the sexual partner or situation, and frequency of sexual activity can affect the duration of the excitement phase and play a role in this disorder (APA, 1987).

Inhibited male orgasm
Characterized by a persistent or recurrent delay in or absence of orgasm after normal sexual excitement, this disorder commonly produces an inability to reach orgasm during vaginal intercourse (Poorman, 1988).

Sexual pain disorders

Dyspareunia
This refers to recurrent or persistent genital pain before, during, or after sexual intercourse. Physical causes include genitourinary tract infections, urethral or bladder diseases, diabetes, and anatomic defects. Emotional factors effecting this disorder can be divided into three categories: developmental factors, such as guilt, shame, fear, or religious taboos; traumatic factors, such as fear generated by previous painful coital experiences, such as rape; and relational factors, such as inadequate foreplay and distracting stimuli during early phases of the sexual response cycle (Poorman, 1988).

Vaginismus
Women with vaginismus experience involuntary spasms of the musculature of the lower third of the vagina, which interfere with intercourse (APA, 1987). Vaginismus can occur during any phase of the sexual response cycle when vaginal entry is attempted. Kaplan (1979) believes that the male analogue to vaginismus is psychogenic ejaculatory and post-ejaculatory pain.

A client with a complex sexual disorder may need intensive sex therapy. Most clients, however, will need only to express concerns and feelings, obtain information, and gain understanding and support. Basic nursing education allows intervention at this level, provided the nurse possesses accurate knowledge, is aware of personal values, has gained self-acceptance as a sexual being, and can communicate genuinely and therapeutically with the client.

The nurse performs many roles in providing sexual health care. As a sex educator, the nurse dispels myths, corrects misinformation, and provides accurate and appropriate information. The nurse also may help community groups develop sex education programs. As a sex counselor, the nurse attempts to help the client alter behavior to achieve goals and a more satisfactory level of sexual functioning. Although some nurses are sufficiently prepared to provide intensive therapy, most need to make referrals for this level of care.

Annon (1976) developed the PLISSIT model for intervening with clients experiencing sexual problems. This model describes four levels of sex counseling: permission, limited information, specific suggestions, and intensive therapy.

In this model, increasing knowledge and clinical skills are needed as interventions increase in complexity. The PLISSIT model is based on principles of learning theory and uses a behavioral approach to treat sexual problems.

Give permission

At the first level of the model, give the client professional permission to continue current sexual behaviors, and provide reassurance that such behaviors are normal. (Do not give permission for activities that are potentially harmful to the client or others.)

Giving permission allows the client to continue the behaviors and alleviates anxiety about normality. It also enables the client to incorporate sexual behaviors into a positive, accepting sexual self-concept.

Permission giving is particularly useful for the client with a nursing diagnosis of *anxiety related to sexual adequacy* or *sexual dysfunction related to guilt over enjoyment of sexual activities.* For example, a young woman may fear she is abnormal because she does not have orgasms during intercourse with her boyfriend, although she frequently has them during masturbation. Reassure her that young women do not have orgasms all the time, particularly during intercourse, and remind her that she is, indeed, capable of having orgasms. In other words, give her permission not to have orgasms all the time and reassure her that this is normal.

NURSING DIAGNOSES

Sexuality concerns

The following nursing diagnoses address representative problems and etiologies that the nurse may encounter when caring for a client with sexuality concerns. Specific nursing interventions for many of these diagnoses are provided in the "Planning and implementation" section of this chapter.

- Altered role performance related to fear of pregnancy
- Altered sexuality patterns related to inability to achieve orgasm
- Altered sexuality patterns related to perceived inadequate sexual performance
- Altered sexuality patterns related to pregnancy
- Anxiety related to sexual adequacy
- Anxiety related to sexual intercourse during pregnancy
- Anxiety related to sexual misinformation
- Body image disturbance related to mastectomy
- Body image disturbance related to pregnancy
- Knowledge deficit related to sexuality
- Pain related to sexual position, secondary to pregnancy
- Pain related to sexual position, secondary to recent mastectomy
- Sexual dysfunction related to excessive alcohol ingestion
- Sexual dysfunction related to guilt over enjoyment of sexual activities
- Sexual dysfunction related to inhibited female orgasm
- Sexual dysfunction related to psychogenic erectile dysfunction

---

Provide limited information

By providing limited information on facts directly related to the client's concerns, the nurse can help change potentially negative thoughts and attitudes about aspects of sexuality. Providing limited information is particularly helpful when the client has a nursing diagnosis of *knowledge deficit related to sexuality* or *anxiety related to sexual misinformation.*

Besides relieving concern and anxiety, information giving can help prevent temporary sexual behavior changes from becoming permanent ones. For example, a client who has recently undergone a stressful change in her life, such as moving or taking a new job, may complain that she and her partner are having sexual intercourse less frequently. If so, provide information about the effects of stress on sexual health and reassure the client that her response is fairly typical and probably temporary.

Client with altered sexuality patterns related to pregnancy

For a client with sexuality concerns, the nursing process helps ensure high-quality care. The table below shows how the nurse might use the nursing process when caring for the client described in the case history at right. The first column presents history and physical assessment data followed by a paragraph of mental notes. These notes help the nurse make important mental connections among assessment findings, aiding in development of the nursing diagnosis and planning.

The second column lists an appropriate nursing diagnosis; information in the remaining columns is based on this diagnosis. Although not part of the nursing process, a rationale appears for each intervention in the fourth column to explain how it contributes to the care plan.

ASSESSMENT	NURSING DIAGNOSIS	PLANNING
Subjective (history) data • Client says, "Sex feels different now that I'm pregnant." • Client says, "I don't see how Tom could want to make love with me. I'm so ugly now." • Client says, "I can't find a comfortable position for making love because I'm so big." • Client reports pain during intercourse and strong uterine contractions during orgasm. • Client asks, "Will my orgasms hurt the baby? He seems to move a lot after I have an orgasm. Could Tom's penis hit the baby's head? It really feels like the baby is right there." **Objective (physical) data** • Height: 5'1". • Weight: 128 lb (18-lb weight gain over her prepregnancy weight). • 32 weeks' gestation. • Pregnancy status within normal limits; no complications noted. **Mental notes** *Although Mary Sue is healthy and her pregnancy is progressing normally, she feels that the changes in her body have made her sexually unattractive. Body changes also have caused difficulty in finding a comfortable position for intercourse, and she fears that intercourse will jeopardize the safety of her fetus. For these reasons, Mary Sue may believe that she and Tom should stop having intercourse, although they had an active sex life before the pregnancy. Mary Sue may benefit from a discussion of sexual activity during pregnancy.*	Altered sexuality patterns related to pregnancy	**Goals** The client will: • decide what level of sexual activity she desires • learn alternative positions for sexual intercourse • use alternative modes of sexual expression. The couple will: • discuss their sex life and arrive at mutually satisfactory ways to express caring and intimacy.

Make specific suggestions

When the sexual problem is limited in scope and of sudden onset or brief duration, give the client specific behavioral suggestions that may relieve the problem. Reinforce existing positive behaviors and make simple suggestions for other positive behaviors. For example, for a client with a nursing diagnosis of *pain (sexual position) related to recent mastectomy* or *pain (sexual position) related to pregnancy*, suggest alternative positions, such as side-by-side or rear entry, so that she can continue sexual activity without discomfort.

Make referrals for intensive therapy

When the client's problems are not resolved by the first three levels of treatment and interfere with her sexual expression, make referrals for intensive therapy. Such a referral is necessary if the client has a nursing diagnosis of *sexual dysfunction related to inhibited female orgasm* or her partner has a diagnosis of *sexual dysfunction related to psychogenic erectile dysfunction*.

The most complex treatment level, intensive therapy is provided by a sex therapist with postgraduate education. At this level, sexual problem histories are used and interventions may include sex therapy, marital therapy, and psychotherapy.

CASE STUDY

During a routine prenatal visit, Mary Sue Grisholm, a primigravid client age 28, informs the nurse that she and her husband, Tom, do not have sexual intercourse as much as they did before her pregnancy, because sex seems different and she is uncomfortable during intercourse.

IMPLEMENTATION		EVALUATION
Intervention Discuss the client's feelings about sexual activity at this point in her pregnancy.	**Rationale** Open discussion helps the client clarify her feelings about sexual activity during pregnancy and decide which activities she wishes to experience.	Upon evaluation, the client: • reported satisfaction with her level of sexual activity • described increased comfort through the use of alternative positions for sexual intercourse • reported the use of other options for expressing caring and intimacy.
Facilitate communication between the client and her husband about their feelings and sexual desires.	Discussing issues with an impartial support person can enhance partner communication, relieve marital tension, and facilitate compromise.	
Reassure the client and her partner that the pregnancy and the desire to remain sexually active are normal.	*Giving permission* decreases anxiety and enhances the possibility of continuing mutually satisfying sexual behaviors.	
Provide accurate information and correct any misinformation about penile contact with the fetus.	*Providing limited information* corrects misinformation and decreases anxiety.	
Teach the couple alternative positions for sexual intercourse, such as the rear entry, side-by-side, or female-superior positions.	*Making specific suggestions* may relieve discomfort and increase the possibility that the couple will remain sexually active.	
Suggest other ways to express caring and intimacy, such as mutual masturbation, massage, or oral stimulation of the penis by the female (fellatio). However, advise the couple to avoid oral stimulation of the female by the male (cunnilingus) because of the rare possibility of an air embolus resulting from air blown into the vagina.	Additional specific suggestions make the couple aware of their options.	

Evaluation

During evaluation, the nurse assesses the client's response to interventions and progress toward, or achievement of, goals. Evaluation may identify the need to revise goals, obtain additional data, or modify nursing actions. The following examples illustrate appropriate evaluation statements:
• The client accurately described sexual functioning.
• The client communicated openly about sexual functioning.
• The client reported feeling reassured that her orgasmic pattern was normal.
• The client reported resumption of her usual sexual frequency.
• The client discussed alternative sexual positions with her partner.

Documentation

The nurse uses the nursing process to formulate nursing diagnoses based on all the assessment findings and then plans, implements, and evaluates the client's care. (For a case study that shows how to apply the nursing process when caring for a client with sexuality concerns, see *Applying the nursing process: Client with altered sexuality patterns related to pregnancy.*)

Document assessment findings and nursing activities thoroughly and objectively. Although each health care facility may require documentation of slightly different information, most require the nurse to record the following information about the client:
• history of a disorder that caused her to seek sexual health care
• history of a disorder or treatment that changed her feelings about herself
• history of surgery, pregnancy, or a disorder that altered her ability to function sexually
• contraceptive history
• STD history
• menstrual history
• sex education history
• sexual activity
• degree of satisfaction with sexual activities.

Chapter summary

Chapter 8 discussed sexuality concerns and sexual health care for clients and their partners. Here are the highlights of the chapter.
• Attitudes, beliefs, and values affect sexual health. To provide adequate sexual health care, the nurse must assess the client's values as well as his or her own.
• Cultural perspectives on sexuality vary. The nurse must understand the client's cultural background to provide appropriate sexual health care.
• The physiology of sexual response can be viewed through Masters and Johnson's four-phase response cycle or through the DSM-III-R response cycle.
• Physical, psychological, and social factors affect sexuality and sexual responsiveness. The nurse must assess the client's physical health, emotional state, and social background when providing sexual health care.
• The characteristics of healthy sexuality vary during each stage of life.
• Pregnancy, delivery, and the postpartal period affect the client's sexuality as well as that of her partner. The nurse can provide information and support to the childbearing couple.
• During client assessment, the nurse puts the client at ease by creating an open and caring environment for discussing sexuality concerns. Then the nurse obtains basic and sexual health history information and data from the physical assessment and laboratory tests.

• During the sexual health history, the nurse can uncover sexual dysfunctions, which may have physical or psychological causes or both.
• For a client with sexuality concerns, nursing interventions in the PLISSIT model include giving permission, providing limited information, making specific suggestions, and making referrals for intensive therapy.
• The nurse should evaluate all care to assess the client's response to interventions and progress toward goals. The nurse should document assessment findings and all nursing activities thoroughly and objectively.

Study questions

1. Why should the nurse clarify personal values about sexuality?

2. Mrs. Choi, a primigravid client age 35, is worried about her increased sexual desire. How might pregnancy alter a woman's sexual response? What should the nurse teach Mrs. Choi about her sexual response during pregnancy?

3. Which steps can the nurse take to make Mrs. Choi's sexual health assessment more comfortable for them both?

4. How do chronic disorders, such as diabetes or hypothyroidism, cause sexual dysfunction?

5. In the PLISSIT model, what is *permission giving?* How can it help the client with sexuality concerns?

Bibliography

American Psychiatric Association. (1987). *Diagnostic and statistical manual of mental disorders, DSM-III-R* (3rd rev. ed.). Washington, DC: American Psychiatric Press, Inc.

Andrist, L. (1988). Taking a sexual history and educating clients about safe sex. *Nursing Clinics of North America*, 23(4), 959-973.

Annon, J. (1976). The PLISSIT model: A proposed conceptual scheme for the behavioral treatment of sexual problems. *Journal of Sex Education and Therapy*, 2(1), 1-15.

Bee, H. (1988). *The developing child* (5th ed.). New York: Harper & Row.

Cunningham, F., MacDonald, P., and Gant, N. (1989). *Williams Obstetrics* (18th ed.). Norwalk, CT: Appleton & Lange.

Davis, A. (1980). Whoever said life begins at 40 was a fink or, those golden years—phooey. *International Journal of Women's Studies*, 3(6), 583-589.

Erikson, E. (1964). *Childhood and society*. New York: W.W. Norton.

Fogel, C., and Woods, N. (1981). *Health care of women: A nursing perspective*. St. Louis: Mosby.

Kolodny, R., Masters, W., and Johnson, V. (1979). *Textbook of sexual medicine*. Boston: Little, Brown.

Strean, H. (1983). *The sexual dimension: A guide for the mental health practitioner*. New York: Free Press.

Wallum, L. (1977). *The dynamics of sex and gender*. Skokie, IL: Rand McNally.

Sexuality

Bernhard, L., and Dan, A. (1986). Redefining sexuality from women's own experiences. *Nursing Clinics of North America*, 21(1), 125-136.

Constantine, L., and Martinson, F. (1981). *Children and sex: New findings, new perspectives*. Boston: Little, Brown.

Engel-Sharts, N. (1990). Sexuality during the reproductive years. In C. Fogel and D. Lauver (Eds.), *Sexual health promotion* (pp. 179-205). Philadelphia: Saunders.

Fogel, C., and Lauver, D. (Eds.) (1990). *Sexual health promotion*. Philadelphia: Saunders.

Hite, S. (1987). *The Hite report: A nationwide study of female sexuality*. New York: Dell Publishing.

Hogan, R. (1984). *Human sexuality: A nursing perspective* (2nd ed.). Norwalk, CT: Appleton & Lange.

Kilman, P. (1984). *Human sexuality in contemporary life*. New York: Newton, Allyn, and Bacon.

Kinsey, A., Pomeroy, W., and Martin, C. (1948). *Sexual behavior in the human male*. Philadelphia: Saunders.

Kinsey, A., Pomeroy, W., and Martin, C. (1953). *Sexual behavior in the human female*. Philadelphia: Saunders.

Masters, W., and Johnson, V. (1966). *The human sexual response*. Boston: Little, Brown.

Masters, W., and Johnson, V. (1970). *Human sexual inadequacy*. Boston: Little, Brown.

McCary, S., and McCary, J. (1984). *Human sexuality* (3rd brief ed.). Belmont, CA: Wadsworth Publishing.

Pierson, E., and D'Antonio, V. (1974). *Female and male: Dimensions of human sexuality*. Philadelphia: Lippincott.

Poorman, S. (1988). *Human sexuality and the nursing process*. Norwalk, CT: Appleton & Lange.

Sherfey, M. (1973). *The nature and evolution of female sexuality*. New York: Random House.

Weg, R. (1983). *Sexuality in the later years: Roles and behavior*. New York: Academic Press.

Woods, N. (1984). *Human sexuality in health and illness*. St. Louis: Mosby.

World Health Organization. (1975). Education and treatment in human sexuality: The training of health professionals. Report of a WHO Meeting, Technical Report Services. No. 572.

Adolescent sexuality

Burke, P. (1987). Adolescents' motivation for sexual activity and pregnancy prevention. *Issues in Comprehensive Pediatric Nursing*, 10(3), 161-171.

Chilman, C. (1983). *Adolescent sexuality in a changing American society* (2nd ed.). New York: Wiley.

Defries, Z., Freedman, R., and Corn, R. (1985). *Premarital pregnancy and childbirth in adolescents: A psychological overview in patterns of sexual activity*. Westport, CT: Greenwood Press.

Hayes, C. (1987). Adolescent pregnancy and childbearing. In S. Hoffeth and C. Hayes (Eds.), *Risking the future: Adolescent sexuality, pregnancy, and childbearing* (pp. 1-6). Washington, DC: National Academy Press.

Koop, C. (1987). Teaching children about AIDS. *Issues in Science and Technology*, 4(2), 67-70.

Udry, J., Billy, J., and Morris, N. (1985). Serum androgenic hormones motivate sexual behavior in adolescent boys. *Fertility and Sterility*, 43(1), 90-94.

Zabin, L., and Clark S. (1981). Why they delay: A study of teenage family planning clinic patients. *Family Planning Perspective*, 13(5), 205-17.

Zelnik, M., and Kantner, J. (1980). Sexual activity, contraceptive use, and pregnancy among metropolitan-area teenagers: 1971-1979. *Family Planning Perspectives*, 12(5), 230-237.

Sexuality during pregnancy and postpartal period

Bing, C., and Coleman, L. (1989). *Making love during pregnancy*. New York: Farrar, Straus, & Giroux.

Ellis, D. (1980). Sexual needs and concerns of expectant parents. *JOGNN*, 9(5), 306-308.

Falicov, C. (1973). Sexual adjustment during first pregnancy and postpartum. *American Journal of Obstetrics and Gynecology*, 117(7), 991-1000.

Flood, B., and Naeye, R. (1984). Factors that predispose to premature rupture of the membranes. *JOGNN*, 13(2), 119-122.

Mills, J., Harlap, S., and Harley, E. (1981). Should coitus late in pregnancy be discouraged? *Lancet*, 2(1), 136-138.

Reamy, K., White, S., Daniell, W., and Levine, E. (1982). Sexuality and pregnancy: A prospective study. *Journal of Reproductive Medicine*, 27(6), 321-327.

Stegge, J., and Jelovsek, F. (1982). Sexual behavior during pregnancy. *Obstetrics and Gynecology*, 60(2), 163-168.

Tolor, A., and DiGrazia P. (1976). Sexual attitudes and behavior patterns during and following pregnancy. *Archives of Sexual Behavior*, 5(6), 539-551.

Sexual dysfunction

Field, M. (1990). Psychosomatic sexual dysfunctions. In C. Fogel and D. Lauver (Eds.), *Sexual health promotion* (pp. 553-568). Philadelphia: Saunders.

Kaplan, H. (1974). The classification of the female sexual dysfunctions. *Journal of Sex and Marital Therapy*, 1(2), 124-138.

Kaplan, H. (1979). *Disorders of sexual desire and other new concepts and techniques in sex therapy*. New York: Brunner/Mazel.

Kaplan, H., and Klein, D. (1987). *Sexual aversion, sexual phobias, and panic disorder*. New York: Brunner/Mazel.

Livingston, C., McIntyre, and Fogel, C. (1984). Sexual dysfunction: Etiology and treatment. In N. Woods (Ed.), *Human sexuality in health and illness* (3rd ed., pp. 132-150). St. Louis: Mosby.

Manley, G. (1990). Endocrine disturbances and sexuality. In C. Fogel and D. Lauver (Eds.), *Sexual health promotion* (pp. 337-359). Philadelphia: Saunders.

Schover, L., and LoPiccolo, J. (1982). Treatment effectiveness for dysfunctions of sexual desire. *Journal of Sex and Marital Therapy*, 8(3), 179-197.

Nursing research

Fischman, S., Rankin, C., Soeken, K., and Lenz, E. (1986). Changes in sexual relationships in postpartum couples. *JOGNN*, 15(1), 58-63.

Guana-Trujillo, B., and Higgins, P. (1987). Sexual intercourse in pregnancy. *Health Care of Women International*, 8, 339-348.

Steinke, E. (1988). Older adults knowledge and attitudes about sexuality and aging. *Image*, 20(2), 93-95.

Family Planning

Objectives

After reading and studying this chapter, the student should be able to:

1. Identify the major goals and principles of family planning.
2. Describe the nurse's role in family planning.
3. Discuss the advantages, disadvantages, and special considerations of various contraceptive methods.
4. Identify cultural and physical factors that can affect a client's contraceptive choice.
5. Teach the client about specific contraceptive methods.
6. Understand the emotional and physical effects of pregnancy interruption and sterilization.
7. Apply the nursing process when caring for a client who seeks help with family planning, and document appropriately.

Introduction

Family planning allows control of reproduction for clients who plan to have children and for those who do not. In most cases, family planning decisions are made by both the female client and her male partner. However, because health care delivered by the nurse primarily affects the woman, this chapter will address only the female client unless otherwise noted. Family planning has two main goals:

1. To prevent or interrupt pregnancy. This goal allows the client to control her fertility and to reduce the fear of an unwanted or unplanned pregnancy.
2. To plan pregnancy. This goal can help a client maintain a certain interval between pregnancies, limit the total number of children in a family, regulate the timing

of births in relation to the parents' ages, and ensure the client's well-being and that of her child and family.

When helping a client reach either goal, the nurse should consider the following principles:

• Every client has the right to receive the necessary information to make an informed decision.
• The nurse should provide information in an open, nonjudgmental, respectful manner.
• The nurse should support the client's choice whether or not it is the choice the nurse would have made.
• The client's partner has the option to be involved in family planning.
• Family planning affects not only the client, but also the community and the world. Although population control is not the primary concern of family planning in this country, it can be a result.
• Family planning also should deal with identification and treatment of sexually transmitted diseases (Hatcher, 1988).

When assisting a client with family planning, the nurse functions as an important member of the health care team. Responsibilities vary, however, depending on the nurse's level of knowledge and comfort with the topic, specific job description and duties, and the work environment.

Before assuming any of these responsibilities, the nurse must carefully evaluate personal beliefs and attitudes about family planning, remembering that the ability to reproduce has many ethical, physical, emotional, religious, and legal implications. In all client contacts, the nurse must strive to avoid being influenced by personal beliefs. Family planning is a highly personal

GLOSSARY

Abortion: spontaneous or induced removal of the products of conception before the twenty-fourth week of gestation.

Basal body temperature (BBT) method: natural contraceptive method that predicts a client's fertile period by monitoring her daily BBT (the lowest body temperature of a healthy individual while awake).

Cervical cap: cup-shaped, flexible rubber device that fits over the cervix, is used with a spermicide, and acts as a barrier to sperm.

Cervical mucus method: natural contraceptive method that predicts a client's fertile period based on cervical mucus characteristics.

Chloasma: pigment changes that typically appear on cheeks, temples, and forehead during pregnancy. Also called melasma.

Coitus interruptus: natural contraceptive method in which the male withdraws his penis from the vagina immediately before ejaculation. Also called the withdrawal method.

Condom: sheath made of thin rubber, collagenous tissue, or animal tissue that is worn over the erect penis during intercourse to prevent sperm from entering the uterus.

Contraceptive sponge: doughnut-shaped device made of soft, synthetic material that contains spermicide.

Diaphragm: dome-shaped, flexible rubber device with a thick rim that contains a spring. It fits over the cervix, is used with a spermicide, and prevents pregnancy by blocking sperm passage into the uterus.

Dilatation and curettage (D & C): surgical method of pregnancy interruption that requires cervical dilatation and uterine scraping with a metal curette to remove the products of conception.

Dilatation and evacuation (D & E): surgical method of pregnancy interruption that requires extreme cervical dilatation and evacuation of uterine contents by large-bore suction equipment and crushing instruments.

Dysmenorrhea: painful menstruation; a possible contraindication to intrauterine device (IUD) use.

Endometriosis: ectopic growth and function of endometrial tissue; may be treated with an oral contraceptive.

Fertility awareness method: any of four natural contraceptive methods based on identification of fertile and infertile periods during the menstrual cycle and avoidance of intercourse during fertile periods.

Hysterectomy: surgical removal of the uterus. This procedure causes sterilization, but is not a preferred method because of its relatively high morbidity and mortality rate, high cost, and long recovery time.

Hysteroscopy: visual examination of the uterus through a hysteroscope (illuminated tube) that has been passed through the vagina. During this procedure, sterilization can be performed by passing silicone through the hysteroscope and using it to occlude the fallopian tubes.

Intrauterine device (IUD): plastic contraceptive device that contains copper or progesterone and is inserted in the uterine cavity. The IUD may prevent pregnancy by altering endometrial physiology and inhibiting implantation of the fertilized ovum.

Laminaria: Japanese seaweed used in some abortions to dilate the cervix.

Laparoscopy: visual examination of the internal abdomen through a laparoscope (illuminated tube) inserted in the abdomen via a 1″ (2.5-cm) subumbilical incision. During this procedure, female sterilization can be performed by ligating the fallopian tubes through the laparoscope.

Laparotomy: 4″ to 5″ (10- to 13-cm) abdominal incision below the umbilicus. During this procedure, female sterilization can be performed by crushing, ligating, banding, or electrocoagulating the fallopian tubes.

Menorrhagia: abnormally heavy or long menstrual periods; may be treated by an oral contraceptive.

Minilaparotomy: ¾″ to 1¼″ (2- to 3-cm) abdominal incision above the pubis. During this procedure, female sterilization can be performed by crushing, ligating, banding, or electrocoagulating the fallopian tubes.

Mittelschmerz: abdominal pain near the ovaries during ovulation; a symptom that may help predict fertile periods in the sympto-thermal contraceptive method.

Morning-after contraceptive: oral medication given 24 to 72 hours after sexual intercourse to prevent conception; typically used in emergencies, such as rape, condom breakage, or IUD expulsion.

Oral contraceptive: series of pills that contain estrogen, progestin, or both and inhibit ovulation.

Rhythm method: natural contraceptive method that predicts a fertile period by analyzing the length of eight previous menstrual cycles. Also called calendar method.

Spermicide: chemical substance that kills sperm. It is the active ingredient in contraceptive foams, creams, suppositories, and jellies.

Sterilization: process that terminates fertility, rendering a client unable to reproduce.

Sympto-thermal method: natural contraceptive method that predicts fertile periods based on BBT, cervical mucus changes, and such symptoms as mittelschmerz and changes in libido.

Vacuum curettage: surgical method of pregnancy interruption that requires cervical dilatation and suction equipment to evacuate the uterine contents.

Vasectomy: male sterilization procedure that requires cutting and tying or cauterizing of part of the vas deferens.

topic and must be handled professionally to ensure its success. A nurse who cannot offer nonjudgmental counseling about family planning must refer the client to another health care professional until the nurse can accept differing beliefs. If the client's choice is not medically supported, as when a client with hypertension wishes to use oral contraceptives, the nurse must make sure the client has all the information she needs to make her decision.

Whether working as a staff nurse in an inpatient setting or as a nurse practitioner in a private practice, the nurse who assists with family planning plays many roles: teacher, counselor, advocate, and researcher. The nurse acts as a teacher, for example, by educating the client about various contraceptive choices and, after helping her select the one most appropriate for her needs, by teaching her how to use it properly.

The nurse acts as a counselor by helping the client select the contraceptive method that best fits her lifestyle and needs. To do this, the nurse sensitively discusses such things as the importance of spontaneity in the couple's sexual expression and determines how comfortable the client is with touching her genitalia—factors that may make some methods more appropriate than others.

The nurse functions as an advocate by supporting the client's decision. This means abiding by the client's decision and defending her right to make that decision even if the nurse does not personally agree with it, such as the choice to have another child, interrupt a pregnancy, or undergo sterilization. For example, the nurse must ensure that the client—not the health care professional—has chosen the contraceptive method. If a health care professional pressures a client to use a particular method, the nurse must intervene on the client's behalf. The nurse also may become involved in advocacy at the governmental level, lobbying for universal access to family care (Kohnke, 1982).

In the field of family planning, the nurse's role as researcher is growing. The nurse can help expand the profession's knowledge by participating in research studies on such topics as factors that contribute to or detract from proper contraceptive use and cultural attitudes toward conception. In daily practice, the nurse also can identify additional research areas.

Although known attempts to control fertility date back about 5,000 years, conception was not understood until the mid-nineteenth century. Since then, scientists have searched for the perfect contraceptive method. Although they have not found it yet, they have produced many reliable methods.

Today, a client who wishes to control fertility faces many choices regarding contraception, pregnancy interruption (abortion), and sterilization. Each client or couple must evaluate the various options to decide which one best fits their physical, emotional, social, cultural, financial, and religious needs.

In many cases, this decision is based on the client's attitudes toward herself, her partner, intimacy, sexuality, and pregnancy. It also may be influenced by the client's developmental level and her social, cultural, and religious background.

Chapter 9 discusses the nurse's role in assisting the client with family planning decisions. It highlights client teaching about the wide range of contraceptive methods and demonstrates how to follow the nursing process steps—assessment, nursing diagnosis, planning, implementation, and evaluation—to individualize nursing care.

Assessing the female client

To obtain the information needed to plan client care, gather subjective data from the health history and objective data from the physical assessment and laboratory studies.

Health history

To help elicit adequate information, ask questions that investigate areas influential in contraceptive choices, such as the following:
• biographical data
• reason for seeking health care
• obstetric history
• menstrual history
• history of genitourinary disorders
• additional medical history
• surgical history
• family history
• previous contraceptive methods
• women's health care activities
• number of sexual partners
• frequency of intercourse
• involvement of partner
• culture and religion
• belief system.

During the interview, maintain a professional, self-confident, and nonjudgmental manner. Encourage the client's trust and responsiveness by posing open-ended questions in a comfortable, nonthreatening, and caring atmosphere.

Use the history interview to assess the client's knowledge of her anatomy and physiology and of contraception and conception, to evaluate her physical and emotional response to her menstrual cycle, to identify any mistaken ideas, and to assess her ability and motivation to use a particular contraceptive method.

Keep in mind that a client may need assistance even though she is already successfully using a particular contraceptive method. Her family planning needs may change as she ages or as she alters previous decisions about reproduction. Also, she may benefit from applicable research findings.

Health status

During this part of the health history, gather biographical data and information about the client's medical, menstrual, and obstetric history, and about her family's medical history.

Biographical data. Obtain the client's name, address, and other biographical information required by the health care facility.

Particularly note her age because it can influence contraceptive use. For example, a client over age 35 may prefer not to use an oral contraceptive because of the increased risk of cerebrovascular accident (CVA, or stroke). A client under age 15 may choose the same method her friends use without considering alternatives. (For more information, see *Nursing research applied: Influences on adolescent contraceptive use.*)

Reason for seeking health care. A simple question, such as, "Why are you here today?" can reveal the client's perceived need for contraception, pregnancy interruption, or sterilization, which will help direct the assessment's focus.

Obstetric history. Next, ask about previous pregnancies and their outcomes. Determine if and when the client has given birth or had an abortion. For a client wishing to use a diaphragm, the number of pregnancies and deliveries can provide a rough estimate of its size. If she has given birth recently, she will have to wait about 6 weeks to be fitted for a diaphragm to let her uterus and vagina return to normal. If she has had an abortion, she may have adhesions that would preclude use of an intrauterine device (IUD).

Menstrual history. First, determine the client's age at menarche (first menstruation). This helps establish a menstrual pattern. Some clients have irregular menstrual periods for the first several months to a year after menarche. Clients who take an oral contraceptive should have regular menstrual periods.

NURSING RESEARCH APPLIED

Influences on adolescent contraceptive use

A recent study of 76 adolescent women investigated how their parents, friends, and problem-solving abilities influenced the delay between beginning sexual intercourse and initiating oral contraceptive use. Based in an inner-city family planning clinic, the study used a structured questionnaire, semistructured interviews, and a problem-solving test to gather data from young women ages 13 to 19.

The study revealed that the adolescents were more likely to begin using contraceptives early if they lived with their mothers but not their fathers, had no older sisters, and thought their mothers approved of their having intercourse. The adolescents' contraceptive use did not seem to be influenced by their best friends' length of delay in seeking contraception or by their best friends' contraceptive use, except for Black adolescents. It also detected no relationship between problem-solving ability and length of delay. Most of the adolescents were good problem solvers who initiated contraceptive use after perceiving an internal cue, such as a late menstrual period, or an external cue, such as hearing about a classmate's unplanned pregnancy.

Application to practice

This exploratory study suggests that the nurse can easily cue an adolescent client's behavior by introducing—and nonjudgmentally discussing—sex and contraception. The nurse can help create an accepting environment where the staff is approachable and can help an adolescent substitute realistic thinking about sex and pregnancy for the "magical thinking" that makes her believe, "Pregnancy could never happen to me."

The study also suggests that the nurse can enhance the parents' role as their children's sex educators by working with the family to communicate openly and develop an accepting attitude. Further, the nurse can support and educate parents to help them feel secure about the knowledge they share with their children. Finally, the nurse may include knowledgeable peers in the counseling and teaching sessions, especially for Black adolescents.

White, J.E. (1987). Influence of parents, peers, and problem-solving on contraceptive use. *Pediatric Nursing*, 13(5), 317-60.

Next, ask about the length, regularity, and duration of her menstrual cycles. Irregular or long cycles may be associated with anovulation, suggesting an endocrine abnormality that could affect a physician's contraceptive prescription. Excessively long menstrual bleeding may be reduced with an oral contraceptive or increased with IUD use.

Finally, inquire about blood flow and the presence of blood clots or cramps during the client's menstrual period. Heavy blood flow in a client over age 30 may signify fibroids, which require further investigation. An oral contraceptive may help reduce heavy blood flow; an IUD could increase it and aggravate clotting or cramping.

History of genitourinary disorders. Ask the client if she has had pelvic inflammatory disease (PID). Such a client should not use an IUD because it increases the risk of reinfection.

Next, inquire about a history of toxic shock syndrome or recurrent urinary tract or vaginal infections. Because a diaphragm, cervical cap, or contraceptive sponge can increase the risk of toxic shock syndrome and urinary tract and vaginal infections, these contraceptive methods are contraindicated in a client with a history of any of these disorders. An oral contraceptive is contraindicated in a client with a history of vaginal, cervical, uterine, or breast cancer.

Also ask about previous sexually transmitted diseases (STDs). Condom use can dramatically decrease the risk of STD reinfection. If the client currently has an STD, it must be treated.

Additional medical history. Follow up by asking if the client has experienced migraine headaches, gallbladder disease, cardiac disease, liver disease, diabetes, clotting problems, or hypertension. A history of any of these disorders contraindicates oral contraceptive use, which increases their incidence.

Continue by finding out if she has a history of anemia, bleeding disorders, seizures, or depression. Common adverse effects of an IUD can increase a client's menstrual flow and spotting, which could complicate a bleeding disorder or anemia. An oral contraceptive may exacerbate seizures or depression, especially if it contains estrogen and progestin. Progestin-only pills are less likely to produce this effect.

Also ask about problems with the thyroid or adrenal glands. Endocrine problems can cause hormone imbalances that interfere with the action—and effectiveness—of oral contraceptives.

Surgical history. If the client has had reproductive tract surgery, determine the specific type. Some surgical procedures can alter the reproductive system, affecting the client's contraceptive choice. For example, a cervical biopsy may change the shape of the cervix, making a cervical cap difficult to fit.

Family history. Ask the client if anyone in her family has or has had a cardiac disease, hypertension, migraine headaches, a bleeding or clotting disorder, or a CVA. Oral contraceptives may exacerbate these disorders and should be used cautiously in a client with a family history of them.

Health promotion and protection behaviors

To evaluate the client's health promotion and protection behaviors, obtain information about previous contraceptive use and current health habits.

Previous contraceptive methods. If the client has used contraceptive methods, find out which ones. Then ask about their effectiveness and her satisfaction with them. The client's answers give clues to her previous experience and understanding of different contraceptive methods. They identify effective and ineffective methods and uncover problems, such as a client's inhibitions about touching her genitalia, that may interfere with proper use of other methods. They also help reveal misconceptions that may require correction.

Also ask how long the client used each contraceptive method. This allows further discussion of previous contraceptive methods and provides information about the client's long-term ability to use a particular method.

Finally, determine if the client had any problems with these methods, such as painful menstrual periods, trouble remembering to use a particular method, embarrassment, or reduced sexual enjoyment. A client who has had problems with a contraceptive method may not like it and may not use it effectively. If she has used several methods without satisfaction and is near the end of her childbearing years, she may want to discuss sterilization for herself or her partner as a permanent contraceptive method.

Health care activities. Ask the client for the date of her last routine checkup and her last gynecologic examination. This information indicates how highly the client values her health and how interested she might be in a method that requires several office visits, such as the cervical cap or IUD.

Also determine if the client knows how to examine her breasts. If so, inquire how frequently she does it. The client's answers provide information about her health habits and values. Monthly breast self-examination is particularly important if the client uses an oral contraceptive, which can cause breast changes.

Roles and relationships

To assess the client's roles and relationships, pose questions about her sexual habits and personal beliefs.

Number of sexual partners. Ask a question such as, "Do you have one or more than one sexual partner?" to obtain this information. A client with one sexual partner may want to involve him in the choice and use of a contraceptive method. A client with multiple sexual partners is at increased risk for STDs and cervical cancer and should take this into account when choosing a contraceptive method.

Frequency of intercourse. Ask the client if she has frequent sexual intercourse. Frequent intercourse could make some methods undesirable. For example, a client might not want to use a diaphragm if she has to add contraceptive jelly before each act of intercourse.

Involvement of partner. For a client interested in contraceptive methods, find out if she has discussed contraception with her partner to determine if it is a joint concern. Keep in mind that contraceptive effectiveness increases when the partner is supportive, when the relationship is long term, and when the partners share values.

For a client interested in pregnancy interruption or sterilization, ask if she has discussed it with her partner. If pregnancy interruption or sterilization is a joint decision, thoroughly explore each partner's concerns, motives, and desires, especially the desire to have children later.

Culture and religion. Ask the client to describe her culture and religion and discuss how they affect her view of birth, contraception, pregnancy interruption, and sterilization. A client's culture and religion may limit contraceptive use or forbid pregnancy interruption or sterilization. For example, a Catholic mother of seven may believe that contraception is forbidden by her religion, but her family may not be able to afford another child. In such a case, do not try to decide for the client or attempt to sway her. Instead, listen actively and let her work through the conflict between her beliefs and her finances. (For more information, see *Cultural considerations: Contraceptive choices*.)

Belief system. Assess for other beliefs that may influence the client's contraceptive choice by asking such questions as, "Does your family have beliefs or concerns about birth control (or abortion or sterilization) that are important to you?" These questions help identify factors that may facilitate or defeat successful use of a particular contraceptive method. They also can pinpoint areas of support or conflict for a client considering pregnancy interruption or sterilization.

Physical assessment

Perform a physical assessment and obtain additional data that will help the client make an appropriate contraceptive choice. Begin by measuring her height and weight and assessing her vital signs. Palpate her thyroid gland and auscultate her heart sounds. Then examine and palpate her breasts. The specially prepared nurse also will perform a gynecologic examination and obtain specimens for a Papanicolaou (Pap) test and cultures

---

CULTURAL CONSIDERATIONS

Contraceptive choices

A client's religious, ethnic, and cultural background may have a profound effect on her choice of contraception. When discussing contraceptive methods, the nurse should keep the following cultural considerations in mind.

• Some groups resist contraceptive use because they view it as an attempt by the majority to limit minority population growth. They may oppose pregnancy interruption and sterilization for similar reasons.

• Various religions, such as Roman Catholicism, teach that couples should engage in sex solely for procreation and that contraceptive use is against God's will. Members of these religions may, however, be free to use a natural contraceptive method that requires periodic abstinence. The Roman Catholic Church strictly prohibits abortions. It also prohibits sterilization unless sound medical indications exist. The Jewish faith permits therapeutic abortions if the mother's physical or psychological well-being is threatened.

• Some groups value the fertility that is demonstrated through childbirth. They show greatest respect for women and men who have had children and least respect for those who are childless. In a traditional Chinese family, for example, a woman's status improves after she bears a child, especially a male child. In Samoa, infertility is grounds for divorce. Members of these groups oppose any attempt to alter fertility.

• In some cultures, people believe that menstruation rids the woman of waste or unnecessary blood. Contraceptive methods that alter menstruation, such as oral contraceptives or IUDs, would be unacceptable because they interfere with this cleansing process. Other contraceptive methods, such as condoms or diaphragms, may be acceptable in these cultures.

---

for organisms that cause STDs. (For more information about gynecologic assessment procedures, see Chapter 7, Women's Health Promotion.)

Elevated blood pressure or body weight may contraindicate oral contraceptives. So may abnormal heart sounds, abnormal thyroid findings, or a breast mass or discharge, which would require further investigation.

The gynecologic examination may reveal an anatomic abnormality, such as a small cervix or short anterior vaginal wall, which would make diaphragm fitting and insertion difficult. It could also identify severe uterine retroflexion (tipping backward) or anteflexion (tipping forward), which would contraindicate IUD use.

Family planning

The following list of potential nursing diagnoses offers examples of the problems and etiologies that a nurse may encounter when caring for a client who needs help with family planning. Specific nursing interventions for many of these diagnoses are provided in the next four sections of this chapter.

- Altered sexuality patterns related to use of cervical cap
- Altered sexuality patterns related to use of diaphragm
- Altered sexuality patterns related to vasectomy
- Anticipatory grieving related to loss of fetus
- Anxiety related to discussing contraception with a stranger
- Anxiety related to effectiveness of current contraceptive method
- Anxiety related to pregnancy interruption
- Anxiety related to touching genitals to insert a barrier method of contraception
- Body image disturbance related to sterilization
- Decisional conflicts related to type of contraception
- Fear related to the sterilization procedure
- Health seeking behaviors related to contraception
- Ineffective family coping: compromised, related to desire to postpone childbearing
- Ineffective individual coping related to partner's use of condom
- Ineffective individual coping related to use of condom
- Ineffective individual coping related to vasectomy
- Knowledge deficit related to chosen contraceptive method
- Knowledge deficit related to contraceptive choices
- Knowledge deficit related to diaphragm insertion
- Knowledge deficit related to diaphragm use
- Knowledge deficit related to identification of fertile and infertile periods
- Knowledge deficit related to sterilization procedures
- Knowledge deficit related to use of vaginal sponge
- Pain related to sterilization procedure
- Pain related to use of an intrauterine device
- Potential for infection related to pregnancy interruption
- Self-esteem disturbance related to pregnancy interruption
- Sexual dysfunction related to difficulty in using current contraceptive method
- Spiritual distress related to conflict between religious beliefs and desire to use contraception
- Spiritual distress related to sterilization

Diagnostic studies

As the final assessment step, obtain information, as available, from the following baseline diagnostic studies: complete blood count (CBC), urinalysis, Pap test, Venereal Disease Research Laboratories (VDRL) test, endocervical culture for *Neisseria gonorrhoeae*, vaginal wet mount for *Trichomonas vaginalis* and *Candida albicans*, and cervical culture for *Chlamydia trachomatis*. If the client could be pregnant, also check the results of a pregnancy test, such as the serum or urine human chorionic gonadotropin test. (For more information about CBC and VDRL tests, see Chapter 19, Care during the Normal Antepartal Period. For information about pregnancy tests, see Chapter 17, Physiologic Changes during Normal Pregnancy. For information about the other tests, see Chapter 7, Women's Health Promotion.)

Using assessment data

After gathering the assessment data, review it carefully. Then identify pertinent nursing diagnoses for the client or couple. (For a partial list of applicable diagnoses, see *Nursing diagnoses: Family planning.*)

Based on the assessment findings and on nursing diagnoses that match the client's needs, develop and implement a care plan. For example, for a client with a nursing diagnosis of ***knowledge deficit related to diaphragm use***, plan what and how to teach her about this contraceptive method and then implement the plan. Depending on the client's abilities, include in the plan the use of pamphlets, diagrams, and models as well as a discussion of diaphragm care, spermicide use, and client demonstration of diaphragm insertion and removal.

Keep in mind that planning and implementation will vary greatly depending on whether the client requests assistance with contraception, pregnancy interruption, or sterilization.

The female client and contraception

When a client seeks help with contraception, first provide information about contraceptive methods. (For detailed information, see *Contraceptive methods.*) Then help the client decide which one is best for her and her partner,

(Text continues on page 179.)

Contraceptive methods

To help a client select the best contraceptive method, describe the methods available and discuss their advantages, disadvantages, and special considerations, including effectiveness. The following chart provides this information for the most common hormonal, mechanical barrier, chemical barrier, natural, and other methods of contraception. *Note:* The chart presents a range from use effectiveness (which reflects actual, sometimes inconsistent, use) to theoretical effectiveness (which reflects correct use of the method at all times.)

HORMONAL METHODS

Oral contraceptive

Description
This method may inhibit ovulation by blocking the action of the hypothalamus and anterior pituitary on the uterus. It consists of a series of pills that contain 50 mcg or less of estrogen and 1 mg or less of progestin; "minipills" contain progestin only.

Oral contraceptives are classified as monophasic, biphasic, or triphasic. Monophasic delivers a fixed amount of estrogen and progestin throughout the 21 days. Biphasic delivers a fixed amount of estrogen throughout the 21 days, but an increased amount of progestin on days 11 to 21. Triphasic delivers a progestin dose that changes every 7 days and an estrogen dose that remains fixed for 21 days or changes every 7 days, like the progestin dose.

Advantages
• Offers the lowest failure rate of nonsurgical contraceptive methods.
• Does not interfere with sexual spontaneity.
• Helps regulate menstrual cycle.
• May decrease the risk of endometrial and ovarian cancer, ovarian cysts, and noncancerous breast tumors.
• Decreases the incidence of anemia by decreasing menstrual blood flow.
• May decrease the risk of pelvic inflammatory disease (PID) and dysmenorrhea (painful menstruation).
• May decrease or eliminate premenstrual tension.
• May be used to treat menorrhagia (abnormally heavy or long menstrual periods) and endometriosis (ectopic growth and function of endometrial tissue).

Disadvantages
• May cause the following adverse effects: decreased libido (sexual desire), fluid retention, lethargy, depression, dizziness, nervousness, headache, increased appetite, nausea, vomiting, abdominal cramping, diarrhea or constipation, breast enlargement, breast tenderness, spotting or breakthrough bleeding, decreased or increased menstrual flow, vaginal yeast infection, photosensitization, and oily skin and scalp.
• Requires the client to remember to take the pill daily.
• Increases the risk of thromboembolic disorders, cerebrovascular accidents (strokes), and subarachnoid hemorrhage, especially if the client smokes or has hypertension.
• Increases the risk of myocardial infarction, especially in women over age 35 and in those with hypertension, diabetes, or obesity.
• May increase myopia and astigmatism, requiring contact lens refitting or new glasses.
• Increases risk of monilia vaginitis.
• Increases the risk of hepatic lesions, including hepatic adenomas.

Special considerations
• The effectiveness of oral contraception ranges from 98% to 99.5%.
• Oral contraception costs at least $5 per month.
• The benefits of oral contraception may outweigh the risks for healthy nonsmokers over age 40.
• Oral contraception is contraindicated in a client with a thromboembolic disorder, benign or malignant liver tumor, impaired liver function, known or suspected breast cancer or estrogen-dependent cancer, or coronary artery disease.
• Oral contraception must be used cautiously in a client with hypertension, epilepsy, asthma, diabetes, kidney disease, gallbladder disease, fibrocystic breast disease, systemic lupus erythematosus, a mental disorder, migraine headaches, or a family history of breast disease or genital carcinoma.
• Oral contraceptives may raise insulin requirements; enhance the metabolism of acetaminophen, lorazepam, and oxazepam; lower the efficacy of anticonvulsants, oral anticoagulants, antihypertensive agents, and hypo-glycemic agents; and impair the metabolism of caffeine, diazepam, chlordiazepoxide, metoprolol, propranolol, corticosteroids, imipramine, phenytoin, and phenylbutazone.
• The following drugs may lower the efficacy of oral contraceptives and increase the incidence of breakthrough bleeding: barbiturates, phenylbutazone, phenytoin, primidone, isoniazid, carbamazepine, neomycin, penicillin V, tetracycline, chloramphenicol, griseofulvin, sulfonamides, nitrofurantoin, ampicillin, antihistamines, antimigraine drugs, tranquilizers, and analgesics.
• To increase safety and decrease adverse effects, the physician may prescribe an oral contraceptive with 35 mcg or less of estrogen.
• To reduce the risk of blood clots, the client should discontinue her oral contraceptive 4 to 8 weeks before surgery or if an arm or leg needs a cast.
• A client who wants to become pregnant should discontinue her oral contraceptive, and use another contraceptive method, for 3 months before attempting to conceive, allowing hormone levels to return to normal.
• The client should avoid ultraviolet light and prolonged exposure to sunlight to reduce chloasma (pigment changes that may accompany pregnancy).
• The client should have a complete physical assessment, including a Pap test and breast examination, after the first three to six cycles of pills and every year thereafter.
• If a client who has taken all pills in the cycle misses a menstrual period, she should begin the next cycle on time. If a client misses a menstrual period and has not taken all the pills on time, or if she misses two consecutive menstrual periods in spite of taking all the pills, she should stop taking the pills and immediately have a pregnancy test. Estrogen and progestin use early in pregnancy has

(continued)

Contraceptive methods continued

Oral contraceptive continued

been associated with a higher risk of birth defects.
• Oral contraceptives should be kept in their original container and out of the reach of children.
• Many types and dosages of oral

contraceptives are available. A client who develops adverse reactions to one type may benefit from switching to another type.
• A client who cannot use estrogen can take the mini-pill, which works by

altering endometrial and cervical mucus and affecting sperm motility and survival. The pregnancy rate for mini-pill users is 2% to 3% compared to approximately 1% for users of pills containing estrogen and progestin.

Morning-after contraceptive

Description
This method prevents pregnancy after unprotected, mid-cycle intercourse. Medications include estrogen-progesterone combinations (Ovral) and diethylstilbestrol (DES). These medications work primarily by preventing implantation of the fertilized ovum.

Advantages
• Prevents pregnancy in unexpected occurrences, such as rape, condom breakage, diaphragm or sponge displacement, intrauterine device (IUD) expulsion, or loss or omission of oral contraceptive.

Disadvantages
• May cause mild nausea or vomiting for 1 to 2 days.

Special considerations
• The effectiveness of the morning-after contraceptive is 99%.
• Cost is at least $5 per course of therapy.
• The contraindications and cautions are the same as those for an oral contraceptive.
• Morning-after contraceptive use should begin within the first 3 days after intercourse, and preferably within the first 24 hours.
• Morning-after medication is intended only for emergencies, not for regular use.

• The usual DES dosage is 25 mg P.O. b.i.d. for 5 days, starting within 72 hours after intercourse. The usual Ovral or Lo/Ovral dosage is 2 tablets P.O. 24 to 72 hours after intercourse, and 2 more tablets 12 hours later; the usual d-norgestrel dosage, 0.6 mg P.O. up to 3 hours after intercourse; quingestanol acetate, 1.5 to 2 mg P.O. up to 24 hours after intercourse.
• Because a woman exposed to DES in utero has an increased risk of cervical and vaginal cancer, the client may be advised to terminate a pregnancy that DES has not prevented.

MECHANICAL BARRIER METHODS

Cervical cap

Description
A cup-shaped, flexible rubber device, the cervical cap fits snugly over the cervix and is used with a spermicide. Held in place by suction, the cap acts as a barrier to sperm. It is available in four diameters: 22, 25, 28, and 31 mm.

Advantages
• Does not alter hormones.
• Is more convenient than a diaphragm; can be inserted 8 hours before intercourse and requires no spermicide reapplication before repeated intercourse.

Disadvantages
• May cause toxic shock syndrome (severe *Staphylococcus aureus* infection).
• Increases risk of cervicitis and other cervical changes caused by prolonged exposure to spermicides, secretions, and bacteria in and around the cap.

• Requires client to touch her genitalia during insertion and removal.
• May be difficult to insert or remove.
• May produce an allergic reaction.
• May cause vaginal lacerations and abnormal thickening of the vaginal mucosa.
• May produce a strong odor if left in place for more than 36 hours.

Special considerations
• Effectiveness of the cervical cap ranges from 83% to 93%.
• The cervical cap costs at least $50, including visits for examination and fitting.
• The cap is not recommended for use by a client with a history of toxic shock syndrome, anatomic abnormalities of the cervix or vagina, acute cervicitis, or vaginal or pelvic infection or by a client who has undergone a cervical biopsy or cryosurgery. It also should not be used during menstruation and for at least 6 weeks postpartum.

• Because the cap is associated with cervical changes, the FDA recommends that it be used only by clients with normal Pap tests and that these clients have another Pap test after the first 3 months of use.
• Clients who are most likely to use the cervical cap include those who cannot be fitted for a diaphragm because of a severely retroverted uterus or decreased vaginal muscle tone, have previously used the diaphragm, or have developed frequent urinary tract infections when using the diaphragm. They also include clients who can no longer use oral contraceptives and those who are breast-feeding.
• The client must be rechecked for proper fit after a weight loss or gain of 15 pounds (6.75 kg) or more, recent pelvic surgery, recent pregnancy, or difficulty with the cap slipping out of place.

Contraceptive methods continued

Diaphragm

Description
The diaphragm is a dome-shaped, flexible rubber device with a thick rim that contains a spring. When placed over the cervix, it acts as a mechanical barrier to sperm. The diaphragm is used with spermicide to create a chemical barrier as well. It comes in different diameters (ranging from 50 mm to 105 mm with 75 to 85 mm most common) and types (coil spring, flat spring, arcing spring, and bow-bent spring).

Advantages
• Causes few adverse effects.
• Protects against sexually transmitted diseases (STDs) when used with a spermicide.
• Does not alter the body's metabolic or physiologic processes.
• Can be inserted up to 2 hours before sexual intercourse.
• Usually undetectable by either partner during intercourse, if properly fitted and inserted.

Disadvantages
• Requires insertion of additional spermicide in the vagina before each act of intercourse and if more than 2 hours have passed between diaphragm insertion and intercourse.
• Requires client to touch her genitalia during insertion and removal.
• Requires physical dexterity for insertion and removal.
• Increases the risk of toxic shock syndrome and urinary tract infections.
• May lead to vaginal ulceration, pelvic discomfort, cramping, or recurrent cystitis, if poorly fitted.
• May produce an allergic reaction, although this is rare.

Special considerations
• The effectiveness of the diaphragm ranges from 82% to 98%.
• The diaphragm costs at least $50, including the office visit, Pap test, fitting charge, and device.

• A diaphragm is contraindicated in a client with a history of toxic shock syndrome or recurrent urinary tract infections, an allergy to rubber or spermicides, or an anatomic abnormality, such as uterine prolapse, uterine retroversion, cystocele, or rectocele.
• It must be fitted by a health care professional because proper fit is essential for contraceptive effectiveness. A nurse practitioner or nurse-midwife can fit a diaphragm and provide the necessary client education.
• The client must be rechecked for proper fit after a weight loss or gain of 15 pounds (6.75 kg) or more, recent pelvic surgery, recent pregnancy, or difficulty with the diaphragm slipping out of place.
• The client should practice inserting and removing the diaphragm in the physician's office or clinic before its first use.

Condom

Description
The condom is a sheath made of thin rubber, processed collagenous tissue, or animal tissue that is worn over the erect penis during intercourse. It prevents sperm from being deposited in the vagina during intercourse.

Advantages
• Is available over the counter (OTC).
• Comes in an easy-to-carry packet.
• Is available in various textures, colors, and contours. A condom with a reservoir tip is recommended to hold the ejaculate.
• Ranges from 0.04 mm to 0.09 mm in thickness. A thicker condom is stronger; a thinner condom allows increased sensation.
• Helps prevent STD transmission, which can reduce infertility rates.

• May decrease the risk of cervical cancer.
• May help prevent premature ejaculation by decreasing glans sensitivity.
• Can help maintain an erection, especially in an older client, because the rim of the condom slightly constricts the penis.
• Can decrease vaginal friction and irritation, if a lubricated condom is used.

Disadvantages
• Decreases spontaneity during sexual activity.
• May produce an allergic reaction to rubber in either partner.
• May break during use, especially if it is used improperly or is of poor quality.

• May decrease sensation for the male client.
• Cannot be reused.

Special considerations
• The effectiveness of the condom ranges from 86% to 97%, but it can be increased to 98% by using it with a contraceptive foam, cream, or jelly.
• Although generally inexpensive, a condom may cost up to several dollars.
• Use of a condom actively involves the male client in contraception.
• A latex or other type of rubber condom prevents STDs— including acquired immunodeficiency syndrome (AIDS)—more effectively than a collagenous or animal tissue condom.
• A client allergic to rubber condoms may be able to use animal tissue condoms without problems.

CHEMICAL BARRIER METHODS

Vaginal spermicide

Description
This method may be a foam, cream, suppository, or jelly that contains a sperm-killing chemical.

Advantages
• Is easy to insert.
• Requires no prescription; is available OTC.
• Prevents STDs, such as gonorrhea,

trichomoniasis, herpes genitalis, and chlamydia infection.
• Decreases the risk of PID.

(continued)

Contraceptive methods continued

Vaginal spermicide continued

• May be used as a backup method during the first several months of oral contraceptive or IUD use.
• Can be used in an emergency, such as when a condom breaks.
• Enhances vaginal lubrication.

Disadvantages
• Can produce an allergic reaction in either partner.
• May leave an unpleasant taste for couples engaging in oral intercourse.

• Must be inserted before each act of intercourse.
• Requires the client to touch her genitalia for insertion.
• May leak from vagina.
• May be difficult for a physically or mentally disabled client to insert.
• May decrease either partner's sensations.

Special considerations
• The effectiveness of vaginal sper-

micide ranges from 80% to 98%—highest when spermicide is used with a diaphragm or cervical cap.
• Vaginal spermicide costs at least $2 per container.
• Vaginal spermicide is contraindicated in a client who is allergic to spermicides.
• The client should follow package directions for insertion time, which may vary from 15 minutes to 8 hours before intercourse.

Contraceptive sponge

Description
This method consists of a small, doughnut-shaped device made of a soft, synthetic material. It covers the cervix, creating a barrier to sperm, and contains a spermicide that inactivates them.

Advantages
• Does not require fitting by a health care professional; one size fits all female clients.
• Is available OTC.
• Is easy to remove by its attached loop.
• Maintains spermicidal effects for 24

hours, regardless of the frequency of intercourse.

Disadvantages
• Cannot be reused.
• May come apart during removal.
• Requires access to clean water because it must be inserted wet.
• Requires client to touch her genitalia during insertion and removal.
• May cause toxic shock syndrome, especially if left in place for more than 24 hours or during menstruation.
• May produce vaginal dryness by absorbing normal secretions.

• May produce an allergic reaction, although this is rare.

Special considerations
• The effectiveness of the contraceptive sponge ranges from 82% to 91%.
• A box of three contraceptive sponges costs at least $3.
• The sponge is contraindicated in a client who has had toxic shock syndrome.
• The client should not use the contraceptive sponge after an abortion or delivery until approved by her physician, nurse practitioner, or nurse-midwife.

Vaginal contraceptive film

Description
This barrier method consists of a small 2″ x 2″ semitransparent square of soluble contraceptive film that contains a spermicide.

Advantages
• Does not require fitting by a health care professional.
• Dissolves in normal vaginal fluids, forming a tenacious gel that renders sperm inactive.

• Washes away with natural body fluids.

Disadvantages
• Cannot be reused.
• Must be inserted 15 minutes to 1½ hours before intercourse.
• Must be inserted before each act of intercourse.
• Requires client to touch her genitalia for insertion.

Special considerations
• The effectiveness of the vaginal contraceptive film ranges from 80% to 90%.
• If vaginal irritation occurs, the client should stop using the contraceptive film for 48 hours. If irritation occurs with later use, she should consult her physician or nurse practitioner.

NATURAL METHODS

Rhythm (calendar) method

Description
This method predicts ovulation by mathematically analyzing the length of the client's eight previous menstrual cycles. By this formula, the fertile period extends from the eigthteenth day before the end of the shortest cycle through the eleventh day before the end of the longest cy-

cle. During the fertile period, the client should abstain from intercourse to prevent pregnancy.

Advantages
• Requires no drugs or devices.
• Is inexpensive.
• May be acceptable to members of

religious groups that oppose birth control.
• Encourages both partners to learn more about the functioning of the woman's body.
• Encourages communication between partners.
• Can be used to avoid or plan a pregnancy.

Contraceptive methods continued

Rhythm (calendar) method continued

Disadvantages
• Requires good record keeping before and during use of method.
• Restricts sexual spontaneity during the client's fertile period.
• Requires extended periods of abstinence from intercourse.

• It puts a client with irregular menstrual cycles at high risk for becoming pregnant.

Special considerations
• The effectiveness of the rhythm method ranges from 70% to 85%.

• The rhythm method costs little or nothing in dollars.
• This method may be unreliable if the client is affected by illness, infection, or other factors, such as stress.
• It requires a willingness and ability to monitor body changes.

Basal body temperature (BBT) method

Description
This method identifies ovulation by monitoring the client's daily basal temperature (the lowest body temperature of a healthy individual during waking hours). A client can determine the timing of ovulation after evaluating her BBT for 3 to 4 successive months. In many clients, the BBT drops slightly (0.2° F [0.1° C]) just before ovulation and rises noticeably (0.4 to 0.8° F [0.2 to 0.4° C]) 24 to 72 hours after ovulation. Because the temperature drop cannot be pre-

dicted, the client should avoid unprotected intercourse from the first day of her menses until the third day of temperature elevation.

Advantages
• Are the same as the advantages of the rhythm method.

Disadvantages
• Are the same as the disadvantages of the rhythm method.

Special considerations
• The effectiveness of the BBT method ranges from 70% to 75%.
• The BBT method costs few dollars, requiring only the purchase of a BBT thermometer, which is calibrated in tenths of a degree from 96° to 100° F (35.6° to 37.8° C).
• It may be unreliable if the client is affected by illness, infection, or other factors, such as stress.
• It requires a willingness and ability to monitor body changes.

Cervical mucus (ovulation or Billings) method

Description
With this method, the client can identify fertile and infertile days by her cervical mucus characteristics. During the preovulatory and postovulatory phases of the menstrual cycle, cervical mucus is normally yellow or white, sticky, and inelastic. During the ovulatory phase, the mucus becomes clear, thin, and elastic.

Advantages
• Are the same as the advantages of the rhythm method.

Disadvantages
• Are the same as the disadvantages of the rhythm method.

Special considerations
• The effectiveness of the cervical mucus method ranges from 70% to 75%.
• The cervical mucus method costs

little or nothing in dollars.
• It requires abstention from intercourse during the entire first cycle so the client can chart her mucus characteristics without confusion from semen or sexual lubrication.
• Mucus characteristics may be altered by semen, douches, lubricants, spermicides, or infections.
• The client should abstain from unprotected intercourse if she has any confusion about her mucus characteristics.

Sympto-thermal method

Description
This method combines several natural contraceptive methods to predict ovulation. The couple monitors BBT information and cervical mucus characteristics and watches for secondary signs of ovulation, such as mittelschmerz (ovarian pain during ovulation), increased libido, pelvic fullness, midcycle spotting, and vulvar swelling.

Advantages
• Are the same as the advantages of the rhythm method.

Disadvantages
• Are the same as the disadvantages of the rhythm method.

Special considerations
• The effectiveness of the sympto-thermal method ranges from 78% to 89%.
• The sympto-thermal method costs

few dollars, requiring only the purchase of a BBT thermometer.
• This method usually involves the client and her partner and emphasizes their dual responsibility for contraception or conception. For example, the client may identify the signs and symptoms; her partner may record them.
• Additional special considerations are the same as those of the BBT and cervical mucus methods.

(continued)

Contraceptive methods continued

Coitus interruptus (withdrawal) method

Description
One of the oldest contraceptive methods, coitus interruptus requires the male to withdraw his penis from the vagina immediately before ejaculation.

Advantages
• Requires no drugs or devices.

Disadvantages
• Has a high failure rate.

• Requires great control on the part of the male client.
• Can interfere with the sexual experience.

Special considerations
• Coitus interruptus is more effective than no contraception, but is not recommended because pre-ejaculatory fluid, which contains sperm, can be deposited in the vagina before ejaculation. When used with extreme care, this method may be up to 75% effective.
• This method costs nothing in dollars.
• After ejaculation, the man must urinate and wash the penis thoroughly before subsequent acts of intercourse.
• Only about 2% of all couples in the United States use this method; couples from other nations use it more frequently.

OTHER METHODS

Intrauterine device (IUD)

Description
An IUD, a plastic device that contains copper or medication (progesterone), can be inserted into the uterine cavity to prevent pregnancy. The exact mechanism of action of the unmedicated types is unknown, but they may work by creating a local, sterile, inflammatory reaction in the uterus. This reaction increases the number of uterine leukocytes, whose by-products are toxic to sperm and embryonic cells. Even if fertilization occurs, this reaction inhibits implantation.

Because many lawsuits are associated with IUD use, few IUDs are available in the United States. One brand, Progestasert, is a T-shaped device that contains 38 mg of progesterone released at a rate of 65 mcg/day, which acts locally on the endometrium to prevent conception. This device must be replaced annually. Another type is impregnated with copper, which is spermicidal.

Advantages
• Does not interfere with sexual spontaneity.
• Cannot be felt during intercourse.
• Produces no systemic metabolic effects.
• Does not require the client to touch her genitalia to use.

Disadvantages
• Must be inserted and removed by a physician or nurse practitioner.
• May cause dysmenorrhea and increased menstrual flow after insertion. These symptoms occasionally require IUD removal.
• Increases the risk of PID, especially if the client has frequent intercourse with multiple partners.
• May cause uterine cramping on insertion, especially in a nulliparous client.
• Is spontaneously expelled by about 5% to 20% of clients in the first year of use. These clients may benefit from insertion of another type of IUD.
• Increases the risk of ectopic pregnancy in a client who becomes pregnant with an IUD in place.
• Offers no protection against reproductive tract infections.
• Increases the risk of infertility.
• May cause uterine perforation, necessitating surgery, although this is rare.
• May result in sterility or death from septicemia, although this is rare.

Special considerations
• The effectiveness of an IUD ranges from 95% to 96%.
• An IUD costs at least $150, including the examination, insertion, and follow-up care.
• An IUD is contraindicated in a client with a history of ectopic pregnancy, bleeding disorders, anemia, severe dysmenorrhea, concern for future fertility, anatomic disorders that may interfere with proper insertion, abnormal Pap test results, abnormal uterine bleeding, and pelvic infection.
• An IUD usually is not recommended for a nulliparous client who wants to start a family later.
• An IUD should not be used after childbirth or an abortion until uterine involution is complete.
• Some authorities recommend that the client use an additional contraceptive method for the first 3 months after IUD insertion because of the risk of IUD expulsion.
• If the client becomes pregnant when using an IUD, the device should be removed by the seventh week of gestation to decrease the risk of spontaneous abortion, ectopic pregnancy, septic abortion, or premature labor.
• Infection may occur, especially in the first few weeks after insertion. It typically causes abdominal pain, vaginal discharge or bleeding, fever, and chills.
• The client should wait at least 3 months after IUD removal before trying to conceive to allow the uterine environment to return to normal.
• Researchers are studying the use of copper IUDs as "morning-after" contraceptives. They may prevent fertilized ovum implantation and would work most effectively if inserted 5 to 7 days after unprotected intercourse.

CLIENT TEACHING

Using an oral contraceptive

An oral contraceptive (birth control pills) contains two female hormones that prevent pregnancy by blocking release of an egg from the ovaries each month. Birth control pills are the most effective contraceptive method available and can almost completely prevent unplanned pregnancy, if taken correctly.

Birth control pill use
To take birth control pills properly, follow these directions:

- Swallow birth control pills whole.
- Take the pill at the same time each day—for example, with breakfast or at bedtime—to maintain constant hormone levels.
- Begin your first pill pack in one of three ways. Take the first pill on the first day of your period, or on the first Sunday after your period begins (to avoid having your menstrual period on the weekend), or on the fifth day of your period.
- Use another birth control method, such as a diaphragm, condom, or spermicidal foam, during the first cycle of pills.
- Take the pills as directed on the package insert. Your pills come in a pack that contains 21 or 28 pills. With the 21-pill pack, expect your period to begin a few days after you take the last pill in the pack. In the 28-pill pack, the last 7 pills are colored differently and are inactive. Expect your period to begin while taking these last 7 pills.
- If you forget to take a pill, take it as soon as you remember. If you don't remember until the next day, take both pills—the one you forgot and the one scheduled for that day.
- If you forget two pills in a row, take two pills for the next 2 days and use another birth control method for the rest of the cycle.
- If you miss three or more pills in a row, discard the rest of the pack and use another birth control method until your period begins. Then start a new pack of pills on your regular schedule.

Side effect prevention and identification
To prevent side effects and identify them properly, follow these directions:

- Have a gynecologic examination and Pap test every year (or every 6 months, if required by your doctor or nurse practitioner).
- Examine your breasts monthly for lumps, sores, discharge, and other abnormalities.
- If you smoke, try to stop. Smokers have a higher risk of blood clots and high blood pressure when they take birth control pills.
- Expect some spotting or bleeding during the first two cycles of birth control pills. However, if spotting or bleeding occurs after the second cycle, notify your doctor or nurse practitioner.
- Do not be alarmed if you gain a few pounds or develop skin blotches, nausea, or breast tenderness. These are common side effects.
- Notify your doctor or nurse practitioner immediately if you develop numbness, dizziness, severe headaches, vision changes, shortness of breath, severe depression, or pain in the chest, abdomen, arms, or legs.
- Notify your doctor or nurse practitioner if you miss a menstrual cycle or think you are pregnant.

This teaching aid may be reproduced by office copier for distribution to clients.
© 1991, Springhouse Corporation.

and teach her about the method she selects. If her partner wants to participate, include him in your discussions. Also make available appropriate client teaching aids. (See *Using an oral contraceptive,* above, *Using a cervical cap,* page 180, *Using a diaphragm,* pages 181 and 182, and *Using a condom,* page 183.)

Provide information
For a client with a nursing diagnosis of **knowledge deficit related to contraceptive choices,** begin by discussing the different classes of contraceptive methods and how they work. Explain that hormonal methods, such as an oral contraceptive, prevent pregnancy by using prescription drugs to alter the body's normal hormone balance. Provide an overview of mechanical barrier methods, which

use a cap or other device that physically blocks sperm passage through the cervix. Discuss chemical barrier methods, which halt sperm movement with a spermicide (sperm-killing chemical) that is inserted into the vagina. Also provide information about natural methods that use no drugs, devices, or chemicals, but require periodic abstinence from intercourse or penile withdrawal before ejaculation. Explain that other methods, such as an IUD, work in different ways.

Next, describe the specific contraceptive methods within each class, including their advantages, disadvantages, adverse effects, effectiveness, cost, contraindications, and other considerations (Zotti, 1987).

As new methods become available, provide information about them, too. Some researchers are working

(Text continues on page 183.)

Using a cervical cap

A cervical cap prevents pregnancy by covering your cervix (entrance to the womb), which stops sperm from entering the uterus (womb) and fertilizing the egg. To make sure that your cervical cap works effectively, you need to insert, remove, and care for it properly.

Insertion
To insert your cervical cap, follow these steps:

1 Fill the cap one-third full of spermicidal cream or jelly. Squat down or sit down and lean back. Spread your labia (outer lips of the vagina) with one hand.

2 Use the other hand to squeeze the sides of the cervical cap together between your thumb and forefinger. Insert the cervical cap into your vagina and push it up until it covers your cervix, as shown.

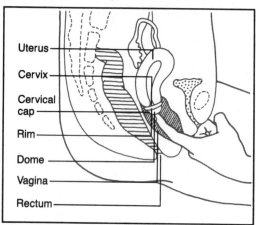

Uterus
Cervix
Cervical cap
Rim
Dome
Vagina
Rectum

3 Run your index finger around the rim, pressing it against the cervix to create a suction seal, as shown below. With your index finger, check the dome to make sure it covers the cervical opening. Behind the cap, the cervix will feel like the tip of your nose.

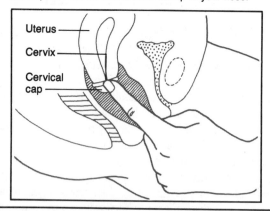

Uterus
Cervix
Cervical cap

Removal
The cervical cap must remain in place for at least 8 hours after intercourse but should be removed within 72 hours. When you are ready to remove the cervical cap, follow these steps:

1 Using your middle finger, lift the rim away from the back of the cervix, as shown below. Then pull the cervical cap out.

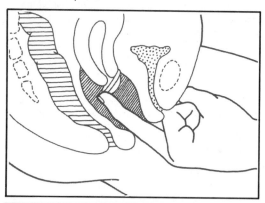

2 If you have difficulty reaching the back of the cervix, try squatting and pressing on your lower abdomen with your other hand. This action forces your cervix down so that you can reach and remove the cap.

Care
To care for your cervical cap, follow these directions:

• After you have removed the cervical cap, wash it with soap and water. Then rinse and dry it thoroughly.
• Store the cervical cap in its container away from heat.
• If the cervical cap develops an odor, soak it in isopropyl alcohol for 1 hour. Then rinse it in water and dry it thoroughly.
• Do not douche with a cervical cap in place.
• Use a different birth control method—instead of the cervical cap—during your period. Menstrual blood flow may interfere with the suction that keeps the cervical cap in place. Also, the cervical cap may interfere with your menstrual flow and cause an infection or more serious disorder.
• Have your cervical cap refitted after you lose or gain 15 pounds (6.75 kg) or more, or after childbirth, abortion, or cervical surgery.
• If you have difficulty inserting or removing your cervical cap or if it feels different than usual, ask your doctor or nurse practitioner to check it.

CLIENT TEACHING

Using a diaphragm

Your diaphragm prevents pregnancy by covering the cervix (entrance to the womb), which stops sperm from entering the uterus (womb) and fertilizing the egg. To make sure that your diaphragm works effectively, you need to insert, remove, and care for it properly.

Insertion by hand
To insert your diaphragm by hand, follow these steps:

1 Apply spermicidal cream or jelly to the rim of the diaphragm. Then place at least 1 tablespoonful of the cream or jelly inside the dome, and spread it all over the inner surface, as shown. If desired, spread some on the outside for added protection.

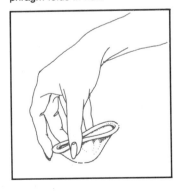

2 Get into a comfortable position for diaphragm insertion. You may squat, sit, lie down, or stand with one foot raised slightly and resting on a stool.

3 In your dominant hand, hold the diaphragm with the dome down. Squeeze the sides of the rim together so that the diaphragm folds in half.

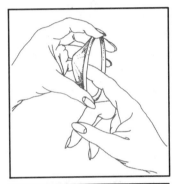

4 Spread your labia (outer lips of the vagina) with the other hand. Insert the diaphragm into your vagina as far as it will go. Be sure to tuck the front rim of the diaphragm behind your pubic bone, as shown.

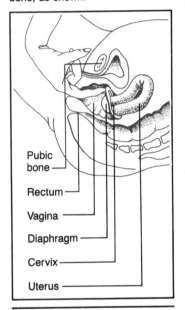

Pubic bone

Rectum

Vagina

Diaphragm

Cervix

Uterus

5 Check for proper placement by pressing the center of the diaphragm. Through the rubber, your cervix should feel like the tip of your nose.

6 Keep in mind that some experts say a diaphragm can be inserted up to 6 hours before intercourse. However, if more than 2 hours pass between diaphragm insertion and intercourse, insert more spermicidal cream or jelly into your vagina. Before each act of intercourse, insert additional cream or jelly, no matter how close together the acts occur.

Removal
The diaphragm must remain in place for at least 6 hours after intercourse to let the spermicidal cream or jelly work. When you are ready to remove your diaphragm, follow these steps:

1 Insert your index finger into the vagina and place it behind the front rim of the diaphragm. Then gently pull the diaphragm forward and out, as shown. Be careful not to tear the diaphragm, especially if you have long fingernails.

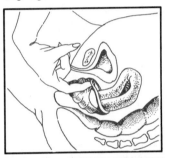

2 If the suction is too tight, try placing your index finger between your pubic bone and the diaphragm to break the suction. Then pull the diaphragm forward and out.

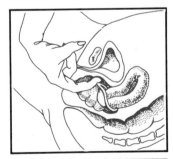

3 If you cannot reach the diaphragm, bear down as if you were having a bowel movement. This action forces the cervix down so that you can reach the diaphragm.

(continued)

Using a diaphragm continued

Insertion with introducer

If you prefer to insert your diaphragm with an introducer, follow these instructions.

1 Place 1 tablespoonful of spermicidal cream or jelly inside the diaphragm and spread it around. With the dome of the diaphragm against the palm of your hand, squeeze the sides of the rim together so that the diaphragm folds in half. Place one end of the rim over the grooved end of the introducer, as shown.

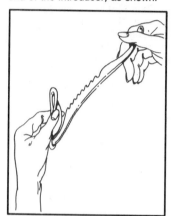

2 Fit the other end of the rim over the notch that it fits. Then place additional cream or jelly on the rim.

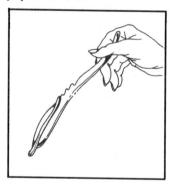

3 Get into a comfortable position for diaphragm insertion. Then spread your labia with one hand. Use the other hand to insert the introducer with the diaphragm as far back into the vagina as it will go, as shown.

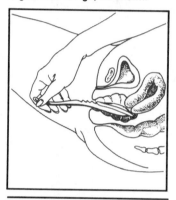

4 Gently twist the introducer to one side and remove it from your vagina. Wash it with soap and water. Then rinse and dry it thoroughly.

5 Check for proper diaphragm placement by using a finger to make sure its front rim is behind your pubic bone. Then press the center of the diaphragm. Through the rubber, your cervix should feel like the tip of your nose.

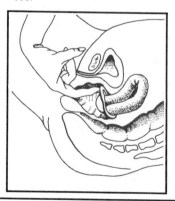

Care

To care for your diaphragm, follow these directions:

• Wash your diaphragm with soap and water after each use. Rinse and dry it thoroughly to keep the rubber in good condition.
• Store your diaphragm in its container in a cool, dry place.
• Before each use, hold the diaphragm up to a light and check for holes or tears. If you detect signs of wear or holes, make an appointment with your doctor or nurse practitioner to replace the diaphragm, and use another birth control method until you have a new diaphragm.
• Use a water-soluble jelly, such as K-Y jelly, or additional spermicidal cream or jelly, if you need vaginal lubrication. Do not use a petroleum jelly, such as Vaseline, because it can deteriorate your diaphragm.
• Have your diaphragm refitted after you lose or gain 15 pounds (6.75 kg) or more, or after childbirth, abortion, or pelvic surgery.
• If the diaphragm ever seems to fit differently, visit your doctor or nurse practitioner to check it.

on an oral contraceptive for men, called gossypol, originally developed in China. Derived from the cottonseed, this hormonal contraceptive inhibits spermatogenesis and is currently being evaluated in the United States for adverse effects, reversibility, and effectiveness. Other researchers are investigating antagonists to the gonadotropin-releasing hormone, androgen-progestin combinations that stop spermatogenesis, and inhibin—a drug to inhibit release of follicle-stimulating hormone.

Aid in decision making

During discussions, try to determine which factors are most likely to influence the client's proper use of—and satisfaction with—a contraceptive method. To do this, review her knowledge of human sexuality, commitment to pregnancy prevention, need for spontaneity in lovemaking, religious and cultural beliefs, life-style, finances, willingness to touch her genitalia, and pertinent contraindications.

If the client has a nursing diagnosis of **_anxiety related to discussing contraception with a stranger,_** she may be reluctant to speak frankly. If so, take special care to project a nonjudgmental, caring attitude. Reassure the client that the discussion is confidential and that she does not face a right or wrong contraceptive choice, just a personal preference.

Based on this discussion, guide the client to make sure she selects a method that is safe for her, suitable for her life-style, compatible with her religious and cultural beliefs and finances, and is one that she likes and

---

CLIENT TEACHING

Using a condom

A condom, or rubber, is a disposable birth control device that may be used for vaginal, oral, or anal sex. Designed for one-time use, a condom can protect against pregnancy, sexually transmitted diseases, and AIDS.

Many types of condoms are available, usually in drugstores. Most are inexpensive, and all are easy to use. They are generally reliable, as long as you do not store them for more than a year or keep them in your wallet or near heat. These actions can cause condoms to break or develop holes when you use them.

To use a condom effectively, follow these steps:

1 Put the condom over your erect penis before you enter your partner. To do this, hold the condom by the tip to squeeze out the air and make room for the semen when you ejaculate. Then place the unrolled condom on the end of your penis, as shown. (If you are uncircumcised, pull back your foreskin before putting on the condom.)

2 Hold the tip of the condom with one hand and unroll the condom onto your erect penis with the other hand, as shown. Be sure to unroll it until it touches your pubic hair. If you need extra lubrication, use a water-based lubricant, such as K-Y jelly, rather than a petroleum-based one, such as Vaseline.

3 After you ejaculate, firmly hold the edges of the condom as you withdraw from your partner. To reduce the risk of spilling any semen, withdraw while your penis is still erect.

4 Pinch the tip of the condom with one hand and unroll it off your penis with the other. Throw the condom away.

5 If the condom breaks or tears during vaginal intercourse, have your partner insert contraceptive foam, cream, or jelly into her vagina immediately.

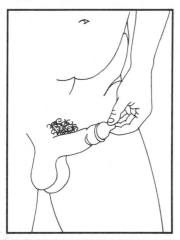

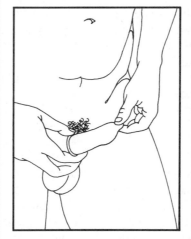

Using the rhythm method

The rhythm (or calendar) method requires you to count the days of your menstrual cycle and to avoid intercourse on certain days. This natural birth control method is based on the fact that ovulation (egg release) occurs roughly in the middle of your menstrual cycle and that your fertile period (the time when you are most likely to become pregnant) lasts from a few days before ovulation to a few days afterward. Although this birth control method is not precise, it can provide a rough estimate of your fertile and infertile days.

To use the rhythm method, follow these directions:

• Determine your fertile period by analyzing your menstrual cycles. To do this, list the length of each of the last eight cycles and identify the shortest and longest ones.
• Then subtract 18 from the shortest cycle and 11 from the longest cycle. For example, if your shortest cycle was 25 days, you would subtract 18 and get 7 days (25 − 18 = 7). If your longest cycle was 31 days, you would subtract 11 and get 20 days (31 − 11 = 20).
• Use these numbers as the days of your fertile period. In the example above, the fertile period would last from day 7 to day 20 of your cycle. (Remember to count day 1 as the first day of menstrual bleeding.)
• If you want to prevent pregnancy, avoid intercourse or use another birth control method during the fertile period. If you want to become pregnant, engage in intercourse during this period.

can learn to use properly. For example, if she is most concerned about preventing pregnancy, suggest methods with the highest effectiveness. Also remind her that no method but abstention is 100% effective and that maximum contraceptive effectiveness results from proper use. If the client is most influenced by religious beliefs that limit contraceptive choices, discuss natural methods in detail.

Teach about the method selected

Teaching is the most important intervention for a client who requests contraception, especially one with a nursing diagnosis of **knowledge deficit related to the chosen contraceptive method.** If a client does not use her contraceptive method properly, she could become pregnant.

Each method requires different information for client teaching. For a client who decides to use an oral contraceptive, for example, teaching focuses on when to take the pills and how to prevent and identify adverse effects.

(For detailed information, see *Client teaching: Using an oral contraceptive,* page 179.) If she needs a morning-after contraceptive, review the appropriate information with her.

If the client selects a mechanical barrier method of contraception, provide detailed instructions about its use and care. Also alert the client to any other important information. For example, if she wants to use a cervical cap, advise her to have another Pap test after the first 3 months of use to rule out cervical irritation or infection. Also teach her the signs and symptoms of toxic shock syndrome, such as sudden high fever, myalgia, rash, and peeling skin on hands and feet. Instruct her to stop using the cap and call the physician if these signs and symptoms occur.

If the client chooses a chemical barrier method of contraception, teach proper use and care of the vaginal spermicide or contraceptive sponge she has selected. For a vaginal spermicide, instruct her to read the package insert carefully, because some spermicides require insertion no longer than 15 minutes before intercourse, whereas others may be inserted up to 8 hours before intercourse. Tell her to insert the spermicide deep into her vagina and to remain supine after insertion. Advise her that she and her partner do not need to wait after spermicide insertion except when using a suppository or tablet, which takes 10 to 30 minutes to melt.

For a client who will be using a contraceptive sponge, instruct her to leave it in place for at least 6 hours after intercourse and not to douche between acts of intercourse or within 6 hours of the last act. Advise her that the sponge cannot be reused after removal.

When a client wants to use a natural contraceptive method, first explain the basic, common principles of the rhythm (calendar), basal body temperature (BBT), cervical mucus, and sympto-thermal methods. Each of these fertility awareness methods identifies fertile periods of the menstrual cycle so that the couple can avoid intercourse—and pregnancy—at that time. They calculate a client's fertile period based on these assumptions:
• Ovulation occurs around day 14, plus or minus several days depending of the length of the client's cycle.
• Sperm remain viable for 2 to 3 days.
• The ovum can survive for 24 hours (Britt, 1977).

Then teach the client how to use the specific method selected. (For detailed information, see *Client teaching: Using the rhythm method; Client teaching: Using the basal body temperature method;* and *Client teaching: Using the cervical mucus method,* page 186.) Keep in mind that the sympto-thermal method combines features of the BBT and cervical mucus methods.

If the client chooses to use an IUD, make an appointment for insertion. Then teach her related health promotion and protection behaviors. For example, advise

CLIENT TEACHING

Using the basal body temperature method

This natural birth control method requires you to take your temperature every day and avoid intercourse when your temperature reaches certain levels. It is based on the fact that ovulation (egg release) affects your temperature and allows you to predict your fertile period (the time when you are most likely to become pregnant). Although this method is not precise, it can roughly estimate your fertile and infertile days.

To use the basal body temperature method, follow these directions:

• Take your temperature at the same time every day as soon as you awaken and before you get out of bed. Ideally, you should take your temperature after 5 to 6 hours of sleep.
• Record your temperature for 3 or 4 months to establish your temperature pattern. Use another method of contraception during this time.
• After you establish a pattern, look for a recurring change in temperature. Every month, it should drop slightly (0.2° F) 24 to 36 hours before ovulation and rise (0.4° to 0.8° F) 24 to 72 hours after ovulation. Typically, the fertile period begins when your temperature starts to drop and ends after your temperature returns to normal after rising.
• Continue to record your temperature, and use it to guide your sexual activity. If you have a regular menstrual cycle and want to prevent pregnancy, avoid intercourse or use another birth control method during the fertile period. If you have an irregular menstrual cycle, avoid intercourse or use another birth control method from the first day of your menstrual period until after the third day of temperature elevation. If you want to become pregnant, engage in intercourse during this period.
• Remember that your temperature can be affected by illness, infection, fatigue, anxiety, sleeplessness, awakening later than usual, some medications, alcohol consumption before bed, use of an electric blanket, and sleeping in a heated water bed. If you are affected by any of these factors, note them on your records to help you interpret your temperature. If you cannot interpret your temperature readings or are worried about their accuracy, use another birth control method temporarily.

This teaching aid may be reproduced by office copier for distribution to clients. © 1991, Springhouse Corporation.

her to report the following signs and symptoms of infection to the physician immediately: abdominal pain, vaginal discharge or bleeding, fever, and chills. If the IUD is copper, instruct her to avoid abdominal X-rays and radiation or heat treatments to the abdomen or lower back because the copper may retain heat. Reassure her that she can safely use tampons with an IUD in place.

Also teach her to check for string placement at the end of each menstrual period, but never to attempt IUD removal herself.

The female client and pregnancy interruption

Interruption of pregnancy refers to the removal of the products of conception before the twenty-fourth week of gestation. A first-trimester interruption is performed within the first 13 weeks of gestation; a second-trimester interruption, between weeks 14 and 24.

A client may choose to interrupt her pregnancy for many reasons. These include preserving her own health or life, preventing the birth of an infant with a severe genetic or congenital disorder (such as Down's syndrome or Tay-Sachs disease), and terminating a pregnancy caused by rape or incest. She also may opt for pregnancy interruption for social or economic reasons.

The decision to interrupt a pregnancy has always been emotionally charged. Ethical debates about abortion were fueled by the legalization of abortion in 1973. Recent legal developments provide states with added power to impose restrictions. (For additional information, see Chapter 5, Ethical and Legal Concerns in Family Care.)

Requirements vary from state to state regarding parental notification for a minor who requests pregnancy termination. For these and many other reasons, the nurse should be familiar with applicable state laws.

When a client chooses to interrupt her pregnancy, provide information and preoperative and postoperative care. Nursing care should meet the client's physical—and emotional—needs before, during, and after the procedure. To help manage emotional needs, project a caring, nonjudgmental attitude and encourage the client to express her feelings.

Provide information

Be aware that an abortion can be performed by a surgical method (vacuum curettage, dilatation and curettage, or dilatation and evacuation) or by a medical method (prostaglandin injection or suppository, hypertonic saline injection, hypertonic urea injection, and other methods).

After the physician selects the appropriate method for the client's condition, explain the procedure and its potential complications. Then answer the client's questions and provide reassurance to help her cope with a nursing diagnosis of ***anxiety related to a pregnancy in-***

terruption procedure. Finally, ensure that informed consent is obtained. When answering her questions about a specific procedure, use the following information as a guide.

Vacuum curettage. This procedure, which requires a paracervical block, accounts for about 80% of all abortions. It should be performed 8 to 10 weeks after the last missed menstrual period.

For a vacuum curettage, the physician dilates the cervix by using metal dilators immediately before the procedure or by inserting laminaria (a hygroscopic Japanese seaweed) into the cervical canal beyond the internal os and keeping it in place with a tampon 6 to 24 hours before the procedure. When inserted into the cervix, laminaria gradually withdraws fluid from the cervical canal and expands, causing the cervix to expand gradually. Laminaria reduces the risk of cervical laceration and bleeding associated with metal dilators. However, it requires two visits to the physician: one for insertion and one for the procedure.

After the cervix is dilated, the physician inserts suction equipment into the uterus and evacuates its contents in 3 to 5 minutes. Then the physician scrapes the uterine wall with a uterine curette to remove any remaining tissue. The aspirated tissue requires careful evaluation to identify the placental villi, which validates pregnancy interruption.

The client may experience cramping during and after vacuum curettage. Complications may include uterine perforation, hemorrhage, cervical lacerations, and adverse reactions to the anesthetic agent.

Dilatation and curettage (D & C). This oldest surgical procedure for pregnancy interruption requires the physician to remove the products of conception by scraping the uterus with a metal curette. Because this procedure carries a relatively high risk of excessive blood loss, pain, cervical laceration, uterine perforation, and excessive cervical dilatation, it is used less frequently today than vacuum curettage.

Dilatation and evacuation (D & E). This procedure is most appropriate for use from the thirteenth to sixteenth week of gestation, although it may be used in the second trimester. Because of the increased size of the products of conception, the procedure may require greater cervical dilatation, large-bore suction equipment, and crushing instruments.

First, the physician uses laminaria to dilate the cervix. After removing the laminaria, the physician administers a paracervical block or general anesthetic, further dilates the cervix to about 2 cm, and removes

---

CLIENT TEACHING

Using the cervical mucus method

With this natural birth control method, you observe and chart the characteristics of your cervical mucus (the discharge that flows from the cervix down the vagina) and avoid intercourse on certain days based on these characteristics.

Cervical mucus changes during the menstrual cycle, especially during ovulation (egg release). By noting these changes, you can predict your fertile days (when you are most likely to become pregnant) and infertile days (when you are least likely to become pregnant). Although the cervical mucus method is not precise, it can provide a rough estimate of your fertile and infertile days.

To use the cervical mucus method, follow these directions:

- Every day, wipe yourself with bathroom tissue as you would after urinating. Then open the paper and observe the amount, color, thickness, stickiness, and stretchiness of the mucus that collects on it. Record your observations.
- Note the mucus changes during your cycle. For the first few days after your period, you should have little or no mucus. Intercourse should be safe on these infertile days.
- Over the next several days, the mucus should become thick, white or cloudy, and tacky. Abstain from intercourse on these potentially fertile days to avoid pregnancy.
- Over the next 4 to 6 days, the amount of mucus should increase so that you feel wet. The mucus should become thin, clear, and slippery. On the peak day, it should look and feel like egg white and be very stretchy. Ovulation occurs up to 24 hours later. During this entire fertile period and for 3 days after the peak day, avoid intercourse to prevent pregnancy.
- About 4 days after the peak day, the mucus should begin to thicken again and should continue to thicken until your period begins. During this infertile period, intercourse is less likely to result in pregnancy.
- Douches, semen, and contraceptive foams and jellies can change normal mucus. Avoid having them in your vagina for the first full menstrual cycle so that you can accurately characterize your cervical mucus. During later cycles, refer to your records to help predict the probable mucus characteristics, if these substances are in the vagina.
- Sexual arousal thins cervical mucus. Take this into consideration when you characterize the mucus. You may want to recheck it later in the day.
- A vaginal infection may change your normal mucus, making this birth control method unreliable. If you have an infection, you may want to use another method temporarily.

the uterine contents by vacuum curettage and other equipment. To prevent excessive blood loss, the physician may order I.V. oxytocin to cause vasoconstriction.

Prostaglandin suppository. A vaginal suppository of prostaglandin E_2 can be used to induce a second-trimester abortion or to complete an incomplete abortion. The 20-mg vaginal suppository takes 13 to 15 hours to work after the physician inserts it. Adverse effects of pregnancy interruption with prostaglandin E_2 may include nausea, vomiting, fever, and delivery of a live fetus.

Hypertonic sodium chloride injection. From the fourteenth to twenty-fourth week of gestation, an intra-amniotic injection of hypertonic sodium chloride can be used to interrupt pregnancy. In this procedure, the physician inserts an 18-gauge, 3″ (7.5-cm) needle into the amniotic sac, withdraws 150 to 250 ml of amniotic fluid, and injects an equal amount of hypertonic sodium chloride solution into the amniotic sac.

This procedure may work because sodium chloride releases the placental progesterone blockage, which normally prevents the onset of labor. Uterine contractions usually begin from 8 to 28 hours after sodium chloride injection, followed by fetal expulsion. If the contractions are weak and inconsistent or if other problems occur, the physician may repeat the procedure or augment the contractions with oxytocin. Complications of this procedure may include infection, disseminated intravascular coagulation, hypernatremia, increased blood volume, and—if infused directly into the circulation—cerebral edema and embolism.

Hypertonic urea injection. An intra-amniotic injection of hypertonic urea also may be used to interrupt a second-trimester pregnancy. This procedure resembles that of the hypertonic sodium chloride injection, except that the amniotic fluid is replaced with 80 g of urea in 200 ml of 5% dextrose in water. Although it may produce infection, this procedure causes fewer complications than the hypertonic sodium chloride procedure, costs less, and is feticidal. However, the hypertonic urea injection has a high failure rate when used alone. To overcome this disadvantage, it usually is combined with prostaglandin administration.

Other procedures. To ensure complete interruption of pregnancy, many health care professionals combine methods. They may use laminaria or prostaglandin suppositories to produce cervical dilatation, hypertonic sodium chloride or urea to achieve feticidal results, and prostaglandins or oxytocin to produce uterine contractions.

RU-486 (Mifepristone), a pill that induces abortion, has been used effectively in France and China. Not yet available in the United States, RU-486 works by blocking progesterone, a hormone vital for continuation of pregnancy. When followed by a prostaglandin injection to induce contractions, the drug allows a client who is less than 5 weeks pregnant to interrupt pregnancy without surgery. It decreases the risk of infection and uterine perforation but increases the risk of hemorrhage.

Provide preoperative care

Good preoperative care can help prevent complications after any type of abortion. To provide this care, remind the client that the pregnancy should be terminated as early as possible and that she should be in the best health possible. If she is Rh negative, administer $Rh_o(D)$ immune globulin (RhoGAM) to prevent an antibody response.

For a client with a nursing diagnosis of *anticipatory grieving related to loss of fetus, self-esteem disturbance related to pregnancy interruption,* or *anxiety related to pregnancy interruption,* provide preabortion counseling. Encourage the client to express her feelings and concerns. Facilitate the grieving process, if necessary, and work with the client to ensure that she is comfortable with her decision.

Provide postoperative care

Immediately after the procedure, the removed products of conception are inspected carefully to validate termination and rule out ectopic pregnancy (where the ovum implants outside the uterus, usually in a fallopian tube) or molar pregnancy (conversion of the ovum into a hydatid mole).

Tell a client who has undergone a first-trimester abortion that she is likely to experience mild cramping and slight bleeding. If her vital signs are stable, expect to discharge her a few hours after the procedure.

Advise a client who has had a second-trimester abortion via hypertonic sodium chloride injection or hypertonic urea injection that she will experience labor and delivery. For a client who has had a second-trimester abortion, monitor vital signs to detect hemorrhage or infection, monitor intake and output to assess hydration, and assist with perineal hygiene to check for excessive bleeding and to prevent infection. If the client remains stable, expect to discharge her 12 to 24 hours after the procedure.

Before the client is discharged, be supportive and employ therapeutic use of self to help her through this potentially troubling time. Adjust emotional support and care to the client's nursing diagnosis, which could be *self-esteem disturbance related to pregnancy interruption* or *spiritual distress related to pregnancy interruption.*

Usually, a client is discharged on the same day as the abortion unless a complication develops. Before she is discharged, be sure to teach her about the warning signs of complications. Instruct her to report bright red clots or bleeding that lasts longer than 7 days. Also advise her to report any signs of infection, such as a temperature above 100° F (37.8° C), foul-smelling vaginal discharge, severe uterine cramping, nausea, or vomiting. These interventions are particularly valuable for a client with a nursing diagnosis of *potential for infection related to pregnancy interruption.*

Teach the client with a nursing diagnosis of *knowledge deficit related to postoperative self-care* how to prevent complications. For example, instruct her not to use tampons or douches, and explain the importance of wiping her perineum from front to back. Advise her to avoid intercourse for 4 to 6 weeks. If she indicates that this is not possible, suggest that her partner use a condom.

Complete the postoperative care by informing the client that her menstrual period should return in 4 to 6 weeks, helping her select a contraceptive method if desired, and scheduling a follow-up appointment. Plan to reassess her health and emotional status at that time, being alert for a nursing diagnosis of *ineffective individual coping related to pregnancy interruption.* If necessary, refer her for counseling.

The female client and sterilization

For a client who wants to terminate fertility, provide information about sterilization procedures and provide preoperative and postoperative care.

Provide information
Before the client undergoes sterilization, explain the procedures and their effects in detail, especially for a client with a nursing diagnosis of *knowledge deficit related to sterilization procedures.* Inform the client that the most common female sterilization procedures require fallopian tube ligation or occlusion. These procedures, which may be performed via laparotomy, minilaparotomy, and laparoscopy, do not prevent ovulation or menstruation, but prevent ova from entering the fallopian tubes after ovulation. Additional procedures include hyster-

oscopy, which is currently under evaluation, and hysterectomy, which rarely is used today. After the physician and client select the most appropriate procedure, review it thoroughly with the client (Pool and Kohn, 1986). When describing the procedure, provide the following information (Pool and Kohn, 1986).

Laparotomy. During a laparotomy, the physician makes a 4″ to 5″ (10- to 13-cm) subumbilical incision with the client under general or local anesthesia. After the fallopian tubes are located, they are crushed, ligated, banded, or electrocoagulated. This procedure can be done during other abdominal surgery and easily is accomplished after a cesarean delivery.

Minilaparotomy. The basic procedure for a minilaparotomy is the same as that for a laparotomy. However, during a minilaparotomy, the physician makes a smaller (¾″ to 1¼″ [2- to 3-cm]) incision about 1¼″ (3 cm) above the symphysis pubis. Because the fallopian tubes and uterus lie just above the symphysis pubis after giving birth, sterilization via minilaparotomy easily is done within 72 hours after delivery. An obstetric client who has a minilaparotomy before hospital discharge can avoid a second hospital visit.

Laparoscopy. The most common surgical procedure for female sterilization, laparoscopy is performed with the client under general or local anesthesia. The physician makes a 1″ (2.5-cm) subumbilical incision and inserts a laparoscope (an illuminated tube that allows observation of the abdominal cavity and passage of coagulation and surgical equipment). Then the physician passes carbon dioxide or nitrous oxide through the laparoscope to displace the client's abdominal organs. With the organs out of the way, the physician ligates both fallopian tubes.

Hysteroscopy. For a hysteroscopy, the latest method used to perform a tubal occlusion, the client receives a local anesthetic. The physician passes a hysteroscope (an illuminated tube that allows observation of the uterine cavity and passage of instruments) through the vagina and uterus, into the fallopian tubes. Then the physician plugs the fallopian tubes with liquid silicone. Although the hysteroscopy may be reversed by removing the plugs, the success of reversal has not been documented.

Hysterectomy. This procedure requires surgical removal of the uterus through the abdominal wall or vagina. It is commonly performed to remove uterine fibroid tumors and to treat severe recurrent endometrial hyperplasia and uterine hemorrhage or cancer. Although the hysterectomy produces sterilization, it should not be used for this purpose alone because removal of the uterus is not necessary when a tubal ligation can provide the same results. Also, the morbidity and mortality rates, cost, and recovery time are greater for a hysterectomy than for a tubal ligation, and the irreversibility of a hysterectomy may have a greater psychological impact.

Provide preoperative care
A client who plans to undergo sterilization may have a nursing diagnosis of *anxiety related to the sterilization procedure, anticipatory grieving related to loss of fertility,* or *body image disturbance related to sterilization.* To help address these nursing diagnoses, provide sensitive preoperative care.

Because the decision to undergo sterilization is serious, allow the client time to consider it carefully without feeling rushed or forced. Thoroughly discuss the advantages and disadvantages of sterilization with her and her partner. Also explore the reasons for requesting permanent sterilization. Common reasons include dissatisfaction with reversible contraceptive methods, completion of the family, and numerous future years of pregnancy risk.

However, a client may request sterilization for other reasons, such as a troubled marriage or a desire to punish the partner, which may lead to additional difficulties. If she expresses a wish for sterilization for any of these reasons, encourage her to verbalize her anger or fears, arrange for her to speak with a nurse–family therapist, and advise the physician of her motives.

Make sure the client is comfortable with her decision and views the sterilization as final. Remind her that sterilization reversals are possible but not guaranteed. Also explore her feelings about the procedure and its effects, and encourage her to discuss her feelings openly. Discuss the possible consequences of a permanent change in fertility. The client's decision to undergo sterilization may violate a religious belief about procreation, or the loss of her ability to reproduce may trigger feelings of diminished self-worth and self-esteem.

Because of the permanence of sterilization procedures, give the client time to reflect and ask questions. Advise her that current federal and state regulations impose a waiting period of 30 to 60 days between the decision to be sterilized and performance of the procedure. Also note the federally mandated time limit that calls for expiration of the consent for sterilization after a certain time period.

When the client makes the final decision to undergo sterilization, advise her to stop taking her oral contraceptive 1 month before the procedure or to have her IUD removed. Tell her to use an alternate contraceptive method for that month.

Provide postoperative care
Instruct the client to expect abdominal tenderness for several days after a sterilization procedure. If she has had a laparoscopy, tell her to expect neck or shoulder soreness caused by nerve irritation from the injected gas. These interventions apply best to a client with *pain related to sterilization procedure.*

Although rare, complications from tubal ligations include infection, major vessel hemorrhage, and burns and bowel perforation from electrocautery equipment. Advise the client to watch for and report signs and symptoms of these complications, such as a temperature over 100° F (37.8° C), fainting, bleeding, or discomfort that increases or continues for more than 2 days.

Advise the client to avoid heavy lifting, strenuous exercise, and sexual intercourse for 7 days to promote healing of the surgical site.

For a client with a nursing diagnosis of *spiritual distress related to sterilization,* encourage her to express her feelings. If necessary, refer her to a member of the clergy or a local women's support group. Plan to reassess her emotional status during her follow-up visits.

The male client and sterilization

For a male client who wants to undergo sterilization, provide information about sterilization procedures and provide preoperative and postoperative care.

Provide information
For a client with a nursing diagnosis of *knowledge deficit related to sterilization procedures,* begin by explaining the vasectomy, a relatively simple procedure that interrupts the vas deferens, the pathway for sperm. Before the 30-minute procedure, which usually is done in the physician's office, the client receives a local anesthetic. Then the physician makes a small incision in both scrotal sacs and pulls the vas deferens through each incision. Next the physician occludes the vas deferens by cutting and tying it or coagulating it by cautery. Finally, the physician closes the incisions with absorbable sutures. The client usually can walk soon afterward.

A vasectomy commonly causes scrotal tenderness and swelling for a day or two but rarely produces severe adverse effects. Its effectiveness is high: less than 1% of all vasectomies fail to inhibit fertility. Although production continues after a vasectomy, sperm cannot travel

Client with spiritual distress related to conflict between religious beliefs and the desire to use contraception

During family planning sessions, the nurse can use the nursing process to help ensure high-quality care and appropriate decision making. The table below shows how the nurse might use the nursing process when caring for the client described in the case history at right. The first column presents history and physical assessment data followed by a paragraph of mental notes. These notes help the nurse make important connections among assessment findings, aiding in development of the nursing diagnosis and planning.

The second column lists an appropriate nursing diagnosis; information in the remaining columns is based on this diagnosis. Although not part of the nursing process, a rationale appears for each intervention in the fourth column to explain how it contributes to the care plan.

ASSESSMENT	NURSING DIAGNOSIS	PLANNING
Subjective (history) data • Client states, "I came here to find out about birth control methods, because I don't want to get pregnant. But I'm a strict Roman Catholic." **Objective (physical) data** • Vital signs: temperature 98° F, pulse 96/minute and regular, respirations 22/minute and regular, blood pressure 98/68 mm Hg. • Height: 5′2″, small frame. • Weight: 105 pounds. • Heart and breath sounds normal on auscultation. • Client behaves nervously and acts uncertain. She makes eye contact only briefly and quickly looks away. **Mental notes** *The client is restless and anxious. She seems distressed and may be torn between her need to prevent pregnancy and her religion, which forbids contraception. At this time, she will probably benefit most from help in dealing with her feelings and from factual information about contraception. She can return later—when she is calmer—for a complete assessment (including a pelvic and breast examination) and can obtain information about a contraceptive method, if she chooses.*	Spiritual distress related to conflict between religious beliefs and the desire to use contraception	**Goals** Before leaving the clinic today, the client will: • verbalize her concerns about using contraception • discuss her religious beliefs and their effect on her feelings • share what she feels are her contraceptive needs • learn about the various contraceptive methods available to her.

the normal pathway during ejaculation. Eventually, they are reabsorbed by the body.

As other male sterilization methods become available, describe them when providing client information. Chinese researchers are studying the use of a compound that can be injected into the vas deferens. This compound causes occlusion without scarring and can be removed, making the sterilization easy to reverse. Researchers also are investigating injection of a phenol mixture into the spermatic duct, which causes scar tissue that blocks the duct. Its reported effectiveness is 97%, and it causes fewer adverse effects than a vasectomy.

Provide preoperative care

To help a client with a nursing diagnosis of *fear related to the sterilization procedure,* encourage the client to ask questions and express his fears openly. Describe the advantages and disadvantages of a vasectomy to the couple, and reassure them that the procedure is simple, safe, and effective.

Explore the motives behind the desire for sterilization. Most clients choose sterilization as a permanent means of contraception. A client who seeks sterilization as a solution to a troubled marriage or a way to punish his partner may cause additional difficulties. If he chooses sterilization for such a reason, encourage him

CASE STUDY

Josephine Giovanni, a student age 18, visits the nurse practitioner at the college health clinic for family planning information. Ms. Giovanni is an Italian-American and was raised as a Roman Catholic.

IMPLEMENTATION		EVALUATION
Intervention Provide a private place to discuss the client's reasons for this visit. Assure the client that your discussion will be confidential.	**Rationale** A nervous, uncertain client will feel safer in a place that is private and has no distractions. Confidentiality should help the client feel safe about discussing her concerns.	Upon evaluation, the client: • discussed her conflicting feelings of loyalty to her family and religion and to her boyfriend • discussed her need to live her own life and make her own decisions • decided to read and think about the various contraceptive methods • scheduled a follow-up appointment for 1 week from today.
Allow time for the client to become comfortable enough to share her feelings, concerns, and fears.	Allowing adequate time prevents the client from feeling rushed and allows her to review her feelings and decide whether to share them.	
Project a nonjudgmental, caring attitude by listening actively.	A nonjudgmental attitude lets the client trust the nurse and share her confidence. The client may be used to being judged; perhaps she needs a chance to express her feelings without being judged.	
Explore the client's family and religious background and its effect on her contraceptive choices.	To be comfortable with her decision, the client needs to understand how it is affected by her family and religious background.	
Explain the various contraceptive methods to the client.	The client needs contraceptive information to make a choice that will be most suitable for her.	
Provide written information about contraceptive methods for the client to review.	The client can study printed information at home and keep it for reference.	
Allow time for the client to consider the various methods.	A follow-up visit will let the client know the nurse accepts her need for contraception and will give her the time to consider it fully.	

to verbalize his anger or fears, arrange for him to speak with a nurse–family therapist, and advise the physician of the client's motives.

Ensure that the client is comfortable with the decision for a vasectomy and views it as final. Advise him that a vasectomy may not be reversible. Although the vas deferens can be reconnected in 40% to 90% of attempts, fertility returns in only 18% to 60%. Factors that affect the success of a reversal attempt include the length of time between the vasectomy and reversal attempt, type of ligation material used, length of vas deferens removed, location of the original incision, and use of coagulation.

To help prevent a nursing diagnosis of *altered sexuality patterns related to vasectomy* or *ineffective individual coping related to vasectomy*, sensitively explore the client's feelings about the vasectomy. Help him evaluate the potential effects of a permanent change in fertility. Keep in mind that a vasectomy may violate his religious beliefs about procreation, diminish his sense of self-worth, and lower his self-esteem.

Provide postoperative care

To alleviate postoperative scrotal tenderness and swelling and help a client with a nursing diagnosis of *pain related to sterilization,* suggest that the client use a scrotal support, ice, and aspirin and get plenty of rest. For a client with a nursing diagnosis of *potential for infection related to sterilization procedure,* advise him to avoid intercourse and strenuous exercise for 7 days after the procedure.

Only a small percentage of clients who have had vasectomies develop such complications as hematomas, epididymitis (inflammation of the epididymis), or granulomas (granulation tissue masses) at the suture site. Nevertheless, teach the client to identify and report the signs of these complications, including scrotal swelling, lumps at the suture site, and fever.

Tell the client that sterilization does not occur immediately. It takes about 4 to 12 weeks or 6 to 36 ejaculations to clear the vas deferens of sperm. Advise the couple to use an alternate contraceptive method to avoid pregnancy, and tell the client to provide semen samples for a sperm count during this period. After sterilization has been achieved, advise the client to return for reevaluation after 6 months and again after 12 months to make sure the vas deferens remains occluded.

Evaluation

During this step of the nursing process, evaluate the effectiveness of the care plan. To do this, assess understanding of information and satisfaction with care by encouraging feedback from the client and her partner. When appropriate, ask the client to demonstrate a procedure, such as diaphragm insertion or care. Make arrangements for follow-up visits to obtain further evaluation data.

During the follow-up visits, determine if the client has reported danger signs promptly, is pregnant because of inconsistent contraceptive use, or is maintaining adequate records, such as a BBT chart. Avoid asking general questions, such as, "How are you doing with your diaphragm?" Instead, ask specific questions, such as, "What would you do if you forgot to take your pill tonight?" "How do you know when your diaphragm is in the proper place?" or "After intercourse, how long do you leave your diaphragm in place?" Such questions allow for indentification—and correction—of any erroneous information.

Be sure to state evaluation findings in terms of actions performed or outcomes achieved for each goal. The following examples illustrate appropriate evaluation statements:
• The client demonstrated proper use of the cervical cap.
• The client accurately recited the IUD's adverse effects that she must report to her health care professional.
• The client correctly listed the activities she should avoid for the first 7 days after her laparoscopy.
• The client and her partner expressed satisfaction with their contraceptive method.

Documentation

Be sure to document all steps of the nursing process as thoroughly and objectively as possible. Proper documentation allows evaluation of the effectiveness of the care plan; it also makes these data available to other members of the health care team, which helps ensure consistency of care. (For a case study that shows how to apply the nursing process to a client seeking help with family planning, see *Applying the nursing process: Client with spiritual distress related to conflict between religious beliefs and the desire to use contraception,* pages 190 and 191.)

When assisting a client with family planning, documentation should include:
• age and vital signs
• significant health history or physical assessment findings, such as a family history of genetic problems or a breast lump, that may affect contraceptive choices
• client's and partner's feelings and concerns about pregnancy and contraception
• client's menstrual history
• client's contraceptive history
• client's reproductive history
• client's sexual history
• partner's degree of involvement in family planning
• family planning information given to the client
• client teaching performed
• client's and partner's health habits that could affect a pregnancy or developing fetus.

Chapter summary

Chapter 9 described how to assist a client with family planning, which allows control of reproduction. Here are the chapter highlights.

• To be effective, family planning counseling requires the nurse to be nonjudgmental and to conduct discussions in a mature, professional manner.

• Family planning options include various contraceptive methods as well as procedures for pregnancy interruption (abortion) and termination of fertility (sterilization).

• For a client who desires contraception, the nurse assesses the client or couple to help identify the method that best fits their needs, beliefs, and life-styles. The nurse gives the client information about the advantages, disadvantages, effectiveness, cost, and other considerations related to the contraceptive method selected.

• For a client who requests pregnancy interruption, the nurse discusses surgical and medical procedures. The nurse also provides preoperative and postoperative care.

• For a female client who requests sterilization, the nurse describes possible procedures, such as a laparotomy, minilaparotomy, laparoscopy, and hysteroscopy. For a male client, the nurse discusses the vasectomy procedure. The nurse should emphasize that sterilization usually is a permanent contraceptive method, although a reversal may be possible. The nurse provides other related preoperative and postoperative care.

Study questions

1. What are the two major goals of family planning and their related principles?

2. What are the advantages, disadvantages, and effectiveness of the condom? IUD? Diaphragm?

3. Karen Berger, age 15, comes to the clinic for guidance in selecting a contraceptive method. She has irregular menstrual periods with heavy blood flow, a history of anemia, and a regular sexual partner. Which contraceptive methods might the nurse suggest? Why?

4. Ms. Grant, an attorney age 33, cannot decide between the cervical cap and an oral contraceptive. She asks the nurse to teach her about both to help her make a choice. What key factors should the nurse cover in a teaching plan for cervical cap use? Oral contraceptive use?

5. Which procedures may be used to interrupt a pregnancy or sterilize a client? What are their adverse effects?

Bibliography

Britt, S. (1977). Fertility awareness: Four methods of natural family planning. *JOGNN*, 6(2), 9-18.

Brokaw, A., Baker, N., and Haney, S. (1988). Fitting the cervical cap. *The Nurse Practitioner*, 13(7), 49-55.

Cervical cap enters North American market. (1988, September). *NAACOG Newsletter*, 15(9).

Donovan, P. (1987). AIDS and family planning clinics: Confronting the crisis. *Family Planning Perspectives*, 19(3), 111-114, 138.

Hatcher, R., Guest, F., Stewart, F., Stewart, G., Trussell, J., Cerel, S., and Cates, W. (1988). *Contraceptive technology 1988-1989* (14th rev. ed.). New York: Irvington Publishers.

Kohnke, M. (1982). *Advocacy, risk and reality*. St. Louis: Mosby.

Norris, A. (1988). Cognitive analysis of contraceptive behavior. *Image: The Journal of Nursing Scholarship*, 20(3), 135-140.

Orshan, S. (1988). The Pill, the patient, and you. *RN*, 51(7), 49-53.

Panzarine, S., and Gould, C. (1988). Knowledge about contraceptive use and conception among a group of urban, Black, adolescent mothers. *JOGNN*, 17(4), 279-282.

Pool, F., and Kohn, I. (1986). What to tell patients about sterilization. *RN*, 49(5), 55-61.

Youngkin, E., and Miller, L. (1987). The triphasics: Insights for effective clinical use. *Nurse Practitioner*, 12(2), 17-28.

Zotti, M. (1987). Nursing intervention to assist patients' decision making with respect to family planning. *Public Health Nurse*, 4(3), 146-150.

Nursing research

Forrest, J. (1988). U.S. women's contraceptive attitudes and practice: How have they changed in the 1980s? *Family Planning Perspectives*, 20(3), 112-118.

Hughes, C., and Torre, C. (1987). Health care issues: Predicting effective contraceptive behavior in college females. *Nurse Practitioner*, 12(9), 44-54.

Reis, J., and Herz, L. (1987). Young adolescents' contraceptive knowledge and attitudes: Implications for anticipatory guidance. *Journal of Pediatric Health Care*, 1(5), 247-254.

Strobino, B., Kline, J., and Warburton, D. (1988). Spermicide use and pregnancy outcome. *American Journal of Public Health*, 78(3), 260-263.

Swanson, J. (1988). The process of finding contraceptive options. *Western Journal of Nursing Research*, 10(4), 492-503.

White, J. E. (1987). Influence of parents, peers, and problem-solving on contraceptive use. *Pediatric Nursing*, 13(5), 317-321.

CHAPTER 10

Fertility and Infertility

Objectives

After reading and studying this chapter, the student should be able to:

1. Describe cultural myths and beliefs about fertility.
2. Identify risk factors detected during preconception assessment.
3. Describe nursing interventions that help promote preconception health.
4. Apply the nursing process in caring for a client who desires preconception planning.
5. Discuss female and male factors implicated in infertility.
6. Explain the emotional crisis of infertility.
7. Describe the nurse's role in caring for an infertile couple.
8. Describe infertility treatments.
9. Apply the nursing process in caring for an infertile client or couple.

Introduction

Most women assume that pregnancy and child rearing will be a natural part of their adult lives. As discussed in Chapter 9, Family Planning, many prefer to plan the number and timing of births in their family. When clients feel ready to have a child, they may seek help with preconception planning to pave the way for a normal pregnancy and a healthy child. Clients who discover that they cannot have a child may be devastated.

This chapter addresses the nurse's role in caring for clients who request help with preconception planning and for those who need help in conceiving or in dealing with their inability to conceive. It begins by describing the essential components of male and female fertility and the cultural myths and beliefs that surround it. Next, the chapter presents preconception planning for the fertile couple, highlighting nursing interventions that can promote preconception health and minimize risk factors during pregnancy. Then it explores factors that influence male and female infertility as well as diagnosis and treatment of this problem. Throughout, the chapter emphasizes nursing care for clients concerned about fertility and infertility.

Nursing responsibilities for such clients include:
• obtaining a thorough health history
• performing a detailed physical assessment
• obtaining appropriate diagnostic test data
• teaching about preconception health or infertility tests and treatments
• scheduling diagnostic tests at specific times for the infertile client
• performing certain diagnostic tests
• assisting with certain infertility treatments
• providing emotional support, when needed.

Essentials of fertility

Fertility results from complex interactions between the hypothalamus, central nervous system, gonads, and pituitary, thyroid, and adrenal glands. (For more information, see Chapter 6, Reproductive Anatomy and Physiology.)

For conception to occur, several events must take place in an environment conducive to ovum fertilization and embryo implantation and growth. The client's ovaries must produce an ovum, and her body must produce sufficient gonadotropic hormones to allow ovum matu-

GLOSSARY

Amenorrhea: absence of menses.

Anovulation: failure of the ovaries to produce, mature, or release ova.

Azoospermia: absence of sperm in semen.

Basal body temperature (BBT): lowest body temperature of a healthy individual while awake. Changes in BBT can be used to predict a woman's fertile period.

Biphasic pattern: sharp midcycle rise in BBT followed by a return to the baseline.

Cervical mucus test: examination of cervical mucus for color, consistency, stretchiness, and quantity—all of which normally change throughout the menstrual cycle in response to hormonal stimulation.

Cervical stenosis: narrowing of the canal between the cervical os and lower uterine corpus.

Corpus luteum: spherical yellowish tissue that grows within the ruptured ovarian follicle after ovulation and secretes progesterone.

Dysmenorrhea: painful menstruation.

Endometrial biopsy: test in which a sample of endometrial tissue is analyzed to determine the condition of the endometrium. This information helps identify the phase of the menstrual cycle.

Endometriosis: abnormal gynecologic condition in which endometrial tissue grows and functions outside the uterine cavity.

Follicle-stimulating hormone (FSH): anterior pituitary hormone. In women, FSH stimulates follicular growth; in men, it promotes spermatogenesis.

Gamete intrafallopian transfer (GIFT): procedure in which oocytes (incompletely developed ova) are taken from the ovary, mixed with sperm, and then instilled into the distal end of the fallopian tube. With GIFT, fertilization takes place in vivo (in the woman's own body).

Hirsutism: excessive body hair; in women, its distribution follows a masculine pattern.

Hysterosalpingography (HSG): X-ray film of the uterus and fallopian tubes to detect uterine abnormalities and assess tubal patency.

Infertility: inability to conceive after 1 year of regular intercourse without contraception or inability to carry a pregnancy to birth.

In vitro fertilization (IVF): procedure during which oocytes are taken from the ovary, mixed with sperm, and fertilized and incubated in a glass petri dish. Up to four viable embryos then are placed in the woman's uterus.

Laparoscopy: visual examination of the internal abdomen through a laparoscope (illuminated tube) inserted into the abdomen via a 1″ incision. During this procedure, a woman's reproductive organs can be assessed for causes of infertility.

Luteal phase: second half of the menstrual cycle from ovulation to menstruation.

Luteinizing hormone (LH): anterior pituitary hormone that stimulates ovulation and corpus luteum development.

Menarche: onset of menses.

Monophasic pattern: relatively flat BBT that does not vary more than .05° F each day.

Oligospermia: abnormally low number of sperm in semen.

Out-of-phase endometrium: discrepancy of 2 or more days between the ovulatory date, cycle date, and histologic date of the endometrium.

Ovulation: expulsion of an ovum from the ovary upon spontaneous rupture of a mature follicle.

Postcoital examination: assessment of sperm survival in cervical mucus after sexual intercourse.

Primary infertility: failure to conceive by a couple in which the woman has never been pregnant.

Secondary infertility: failure to conceive by a couple in which the woman has been pregnant before but now cannot conceive or carry a pregnancy to term.

Secretory phase: first half of the menstrual cycle from menstruation to ovulation.

Spinnbarkeit: stretchiness of cervical mucus at ovulation; caused by estrogen.

Ultrasonography: test with high-frequency sound waves to detect internal body structures.

---

ration and release. Her partner's testes must produce sufficient mature, motile spermatozoa (sperm), which must travel through his reproductive system and be ejaculated into her vagina. His reproductive system must produce secretions that permit sperm motility; her vaginal and cervical secretions must allow sperm survival. The ovum must enter a patent fallopian tube at the same time that sperm are present in the tube's distal end. The sperm must penetrate the ovum, and then the fertilized ovum must move through the fallopian tube to the uterus.

The client's endometrium must have had sufficient hormonal stimulation to allow implantation of the embryo. Her body must maintain appropriate hormone levels to create a uterine environment that allows the embryo to develop and the pregnancy to continue. If any of these events is interrupted or abnormal, fertilization will not occur or the pregnancy will not be sustained.

Cultural myths and beliefs

To respond properly to the couple's needs, the nurse needs an awareness of cultural beliefs about fertility. Throughout recorded history, people have been obsessed with fertility, perhaps because the species' survival has depended on the fertility of the people as well as the land. To explain aspects of fertility that they did not understand, people developed myths about natural phenomena and the meaning of life.

The ancient Greeks and Romans believed their gods had great potency and their goddesses had abundant fertility. Because of these beliefs, they built temples to these goddesses and called on them for help in matters of love and fertility (Bulfinch, 1987). They saw infertility as a punishment for a failing or wrongdoing.

The Bible has many references to fertility as well. For example, it states that God instructed Adam and Eve "to go forth and multiply." It also conveys the anguish of infertile women, such as Rachel and Elizabeth, and tells of their joy when they finally conceived and bore children after God heard their prayers. Even today, many people continue to view infertility as a punishment from God (Menning, 1988).

In different cultures, different symbols have represented fertility, and rituals have been conducted to encourage fertility. The ancient Chinese felt the sun and moon symbolized potency and fertility. In other cultures, fruits and vegetables have symbolized fertility: East Africans believed that bananas and figs were vessels for fertility spirits; West Africans gave coconuts to childless women to promote fertility. North Americans still throw rice at weddings, which is a vestige of an old ritual designed to ensure the couple's fertility (Binder, 1972).

Preconception care for the fertile couple

To help ensure a normal pregnancy and healthy fetus, the client should begin planning well before conception. Ideally, she should develop and maintain good health habits as soon as she decides to have a child. This is because the embryo's organs are especially sensitive during early development—when the client may not know she is pregnant. Also, pregnancy-related changes may distract the client from focusing on new health habits.

The nurse should pay close attention to the client's developmental status during the preconception stage for insights into the client's motivation and the likelihood of a successful pregnancy. An adolescent may want to become pregnant because she views pregnancy as a badge of adulthood. She may be influenced by her peers and their activities. Or she may seek pregnancy as an emotional response to situations at home.

A young adult's desire for a long-term relationship and parenthood may conflict with her desire for a career. Some young adults start families at this stage; others wait until later.

A more mature client may develop a now-or-never attitude toward pregnancy, especially if she knows that it will become more difficult to conceive and carry a child with age. This feeling may be complicated by ambivalence about having a child at all.

Whenever possible, the client's partner should be involved in decision making and in preconception planning. For any couple, the decision to become parents should be based on their desires and developmental status as well as their current demands and resources.

Assessment

To assess the couple's needs related to preconception planning, the nurse obtains a health history, performs a physical examination, and reviews the results of diagnostic studies.

Health history
A thorough health history of the client and her partner can provide data that will aid in planning a healthy pregnancy. It also can identify a client who is at high risk for maternal and fetal complications during pregnancy. Demographic data can help make this identification. For example, a client from a low socioeconomic group is more likely to have inadequate prenatal care, poor nutrition, and a poor overall health status. A neonate born to such a client is at high risk for low birth weight and prematurity. (For more information, see *Risk factor identification.*)

In the past, health care professionals focused only on the client's health history. Now, they also assess the partner because research suggests that the partner's health can affect a developing fetus. Also, his positive health habits can serve as a role model to the client and increase her motivation to maintain a healthful life-style before and during pregnancy.

When obtaining a health history from individuals who need help with preconception planning, ask questions about the following topics:
• biographical data
• gynecologic history
• obstetric history
• medical history
• health care activities
• nutrition habits
• personal habits
• exercise habits
• environmental health
• family roles and relationships.

Biographical data. Begin the history by obtaining biographical data from the client and her partner. Particularly note the client's age. A client over age 35 has an increased risk of giving birth to a child with a genetic defect. She and her partner may require genetic counseling. A client under age 16, who is still growing herself, may be ill-prepared physically and psychologically to handle a pregnancy.

Health status. To evaluate health status, assess the client's gynecologic and obstetric history and the couple's medical history.

Gynecologic history. Ask if the client has had pelvic inflammatory disease (PID) or if she or her partner has had a sexually transmitted disease (STD). PID or an STD may cause reproductive tract adhesions that interfere with fertility. For example, a recurrent STD may scar the fallopian tubes, blocking passage of the ovum.

Next, ask the couple which contraceptive method they currently use, how long they have used it, and what difficulties they may have had with it. A client should stop using oral contraceptives at least 3 months before conception to allow her hormone levels to return to normal. A client who has an intrauterine device (IUD) should have it removed at least 3 months before conception to let the endometrial lining of her uterus return to normal. During this 3-month period, the client should use another contraceptive method, such as a condom or diaphragm.

A client who has used an oral contraceptive for more than 3 years may take longer to become pregnant than one who has not used an oral contraceptive. A client who has had IUD problems, such as PID or heavy bleeding, may have developed uterine scar tissue that can inhibit implantation of a fertilized ovum. That also can cause difficulty in becoming pregnant.

Obstetric history. Determine if the client has had an abortion or miscarriage. A client with a history of spontaneous abortions may need a complete physical examination and extensive laboratory testing to identify and correct the cause. A client who has had an abortion may have adhesions that could cause problems during pregnancy.

Inquire if the client has given birth. If she has, have her describe it. Before conception, a client's obstetric history requires careful evaluation to identify and address any previous obstetric problems, such as premature delivery, perinatal death, or birth of a child with a congenital anomaly. A history of any of these problems increases their likelihood in subsequent births.

Risk factor identification

Certain demographic, obstetric, medical, nutritional, and other factors may place a client and fetus at risk for problems during pregnancy. When obtaining a client's preconception health history, the nurse should be especially alert for these factors to help prevent potential problems.

DEMOGRAPHY

- Age 15 or younger
- Age 35 or older
- Nonwhite
- Unmarried
- Low socioeconomic status
- Lack of transportation
- Location in rural or isolated area

OBSTETRIC HISTORY

- Previous spontaneous or elective abortion
- Previous premature neonate
- Previous perinatal death
- Previous neonate with a congenital anomaly
- Maternal anatomic difficulty, such as a severely retroflexed uterus or a pelvis too small for a normal delivery
- Previous pregnancy-induced hypertension
- Family genetic disorders

MEDICAL HISTORY

- Anemia
- Hypertension
- Cardiac, renal, thyroid, or psychological disorder
- Sexually transmitted disease or pelvic inflammatory disease
- Diabetes
- Epilepsy

NUTRITION

- 20% or more overweight
- 10% or more underweight

OTHER RISKS

- Cigarette smoking (one or more packs daily)
- Moderate to excessive alcohol consumption (from 2 ounces to more than 5 ounces daily)
- Drug use or abuse
- Exposure to teratogens at work or at home

If the client has been pregnant before, ask if she had an anatomic problem or pregnancy-induced hypertension (PIH). An anatomic problem, such as an extremely retroflexed uterus or small pelvis, could prolong labor or cause other delivery problems that would require cesarean birth. PIH may recur.

Follow up by asking if the client or any members of her family have given birth to a neonate with a genetic disorder. A family history of genetic disorders indicates the need for genetic counseling. (For more information, see Chapter 11, Genetics and Genetic Disorders.)

Medical history. To conclude this portion of the health history, ask if the client has been diagnosed with diabetes; anemia; hypertension; a heart, lung, thyroid, or kidney disorder; hepatitis; epilepsy; or psychological problems. Such conditions may worsen with the stress of pregnancy. To prevent exacerbation of an existing condition, the client will need to know or learn how to manage it. For example, a diabetic client will need to regulate her insulin levels carefully. Such a client also will need a complete physical examination to help determine if the disorder could interfere with her ability to conceive or carry the pregnancy to term.

Health promotion and protection behaviors. To assess the couple's health promotion and protection behaviors, ask questions about health care activities, nutrition habits, personal habits, exercise habits, and environmental and occupational health.

Health care activities. Ask the client for the date of her last routine checkup and her last gynecologic examination. Her answers will provide information about her level of self-care and will allow you to plan together for subsequent visits.

Inquire about the date of her last rubella (German measles) inoculation and tuberculosis (TB) test. Rubella and TB can cross the placenta, endangering the fetus. Even if she has had rubella or has been inoculated for it recently, she may be tested for immunity and receive a vaccination if she is not immune. A tuberculin test may be performed, if necessary.

Nutrition habits. Have the client perform a 24-hour dietary recall. Poor nutrition before pregnancy can jeopardize fetal well-being. For optimum health for the client and the fetus, the client's diet should include proper amounts of protein, vitamin C, vitamin B complex, folic acid, calcium, iron, and magnesium.

Personal habits. Ask the client how many ounces of alcohol she consumes daily or weekly. As her daily alcohol intake increases, so does the risk of giving birth to a neonate with congenital anomalies, such as intrauterine growth retardation, developmental delays, and craniofacial or limb defects (Rosen, 1983).

If the client or her partner smokes cigarettes, ask how many per day. A pregnant client who smokes one or more packs of cigarettes daily increases the risk of spontaneous abortion, intrauterine growth retardation,

premature birth, congenital abnormalities, and decreased neonatal length and head circumference. Secondhand smoke (smoke inhaled from those using cigarettes nearby) also may harm the developing fetus (Alexander, 1987).

Ask the client if she uses any prescription or over-the-counter (OTC) drugs. If she does, record which ones and how often she takes them. Prescription and OTC drugs may pass through her system to the fetus. Some are harmless, but others are dangerous and contraindicated during pregnancy. As part of preconception planning, the client needs to learn about drug use and its effect on a developing fetus. If she must take any drugs, advise her to ask her pharmacist, physician, or nurse about their safety during pregnancy.

Determine if the client uses illegal drugs, such as cocaine. These may be addictive to the fetus and cause additional stress to the fetus during labor and delivery. If these drugs are in the client's circulation during labor, the fetus may be at risk for toxic reactions if the client receives labor medication or anesthesia. Also, addicted neonates usually are ill at birth because they are experiencing drug withdrawal.

Cocaine may cause additional problems. During the first trimester, a cocaine user has an increased risk of spontaneous abortion; during the third trimester, of premature labor. A cocaine user's neonate is at a 15% greater risk for sudden infant death syndrome (SIDS). If the client uses cocaine shortly before giving birth, the fetus or neonate is at increased risk for perinatal cerebral infarction (Smith, 1988).

Exercise habits. Assess the client's exercise patterns. If she exercises regularly, find out what kind of exercise she does, how often, and for how long. Regular exercise before conception will help improve her circulation and muscle tone, preparing her body for a healthy pregnancy. Unless the client has an obstetric complication, such as placenta previa, she should continue moderate exercise throughout her pregnancy.

Environmental health. Have the client describe her job. Specifically inquire about occupational exposure to chemicals, toxic substances, or other environmental hazards. Substances in the workplace may be teratogens (substances that cause abnormal fetal development). Even past exposure to some substances can increase the risk of congenital birth defects in the child. If a client or her partner has been exposed to hazardous substances, she may need amniocentesis and other tests during the pregnancy to check for abnormalities.

Inquire about hobbies that may expose the client to hazardous substances, such as paint, furniture stripper, cleaning solvents, or glue. Also ask about exposure to other hazardous substances at home or in the community. Many common substances can act as teratogens and should be avoided during preconception and pregnancy. (For more information, see Chapter 11, Genetics and Genetic Disorders.)

Roles and relationships. Investigate roles and relationships to help assess the client's or couple's readiness for pregnancy and parenthood. Ask each partner a question such as, "What impact do you think a baby will have on your relationship with your partner?" Even a planned pregnancy can stress a relationship. To reduce this stress, the couple should communicate their feelings openly.

Conclude by asking the couple why they decided to have a child now. Certain motives, such as pressure to produce grandchildren, may place undue stress on the relationship. Through active listening, the nurse can help the couple explore their feelings and concerns and consider their own motives.

Physical assessment

Perform a physical assessment of the client to obtain baseline data, detect any problems, and provide information that can aid in preconception planning. Measure her height, weight, and vital signs. Palpate her thyroid, auscultate her heart and lungs, and examine her breasts. Finally, assist with a complete gynecologic examination. (For more information about gynecologic assessment procedures, see Chapter 7, Women's Health Promotion.)

For a client with a history of a particular disorder, assess additional areas. For example, palpate and percuss the liver of a client with porphyria (hereditary liver disease that affects porphyrin metabolism), which can worsen during pregnancy.

Diagnostic studies

During the gynecologic examination, obtain or assist with obtaining specimens for a Papanicolaou (Pap) test and STD cultures. Also obtain specimens for a complete blood count (CBC), urinalysis, and Venereal Disease Research Laboratory (VDRL) testing. (For information about the significance of these test results, see Chapter 7, Women's Health Promotion.)

If the client has a history of a particular disorder, expect to use additional screening tests. For example, plan to obtain blood for glucose testing if she has diabetes.

Nursing diagnosis

After performing a complete assessment, review the health history, physical assessment, and laboratory study findings. Then formulate appropriate nursing diagnoses based on these findings. (For a partial list of applicable diagnoses, see *Nursing diagnoses: Preconception planning.*)

NURSING DIAGNOSES

Preconception planning

The following nursing diagnoses address representative problems and etiologies that a nurse may encounter when caring for a client who is planning to conceive. Specific nursing interventions for many of these diagnoses are provided in the "Planning and implementation" section of this chapter.

- Altered family processes related to decision to conceive
- Altered nutrition: less than body requirements, related to impending pregnancy
- Altered role performance related to impending pregnancy
- Anxiety related to the decision to conceive
- Body image disturbance related to impending pregnancy
- Family coping: potential for growth, related to impending pregnancy
- Health-seeking behaviors related to contraception and conception
- Knowledge deficit related to contraception and conception
- Knowledge deficit related to self-care activities before conception
- Personal identity disturbance related to the decision to conceive

---

Planning and implementation

Based on assessment data and nursing diagnoses, plan care that meets the client's and her partner's needs. Nursing care consists primarily of preconception health promotion, which may require simple reinforcement of health habits or extensive education. It also includes care that helps family members cope with changing roles and relationships.

The prospect of pregnancy may strongly motivate a client to change poor health habits. However, remember to set realistic goals based on her abilities and motivation.

Preconception health

When the client decides to have a child, preconception health promotion is essential. She and her partner should maintain or enhance their health to help ensure the health of the fetus they hope to conceive. Assist them by teaching self-care activities, providing nutrition information, and discussing exercise, rest, and contraceptive discontinuation.

Teach self-care activities. For a client or couple with a nursing diagnosis of *knowledge deficit related to self-care activities before conception,* provide instruction and counseling on life-style changes that can improve their health and that of their fetus.

If the client smokes, explain the effects of smoking on the fetus. If her partner smokes, describe the dangers of secondhand smoke. Stress the importance of controlling the client's exposure to cigarette smoke, and suggest a smoking cessation program in the community.

Advise the client and her partner to limit their alcohol intake. Many authorities recommend consumption of no more than 1 ounce of alcohol a day; others advise consumption of no alcohol whatsoever. Explain that alcohol consumption can reduce male fertility and, if the client is pregnant, can cause fetal alcohol syndrome. For these reasons, alcohol bottles now display warning labels for pregnant women. If the client or her partner abuses alcohol and wants to stop, provide information about the local chapter of Alcoholics Anonymous or a similar program.

Instruct the client to avoid illegal drugs, such as cocaine, because they can harm the fetus. Tell her to check with her physician, nurse practitioner, or nurse-midwife before taking any prescription or OTC medications, because some of them may endanger the fetus.

If the health history revealed environmental hazards at work, at home, or in the community, help the couple plan ways to avoid them. For example, suggest consistent use of protective clothing and equipment in the workplace, substitution or discontinuation of dangerous substances at home, or relocation if the community has environmental hazards.

Provide nutrition information. For any client who wishes to conceive, explain the importance of nutrition to fetal health. Recommend a nutritionally sound diet that contains appropriate proteins, carbohydrates, fats, vitamins, and minerals.

When the nursing diagnosis is *altered nutrition: less than body requirements, related to impending pregnancy,* teach the client how to achieve a balanced diet. Instruct an adult client to include in her daily intake at least two servings from the milk group, two servings from the meat group, four servings from the fruit-vegetable group (including one good source of vitamin C and one of vitamin A), and four servings from the bread group. If the client is an adolescent, instruct her to follow the same daily diet except for the milk group, which should include at least four servings.

Before conception, the client's weight should be appropriate for her height. If her weight is too high, suggest a well-balanced reducing diet or membership in a weight-loss program. If her weight is too low, refer her to a dietitian for an appropriate diet.

Promote exercise and rest. Encourage the client to begin—or continue—an effective exercise program that will improve her overall fitness. This intervention is especially important for a client with a nursing diagnosis of *potential activity intolerance related to physiologic changes during pregnancy.* Help her select an enjoyable routine that meets her needs. Advise her to perform it at least three times a week for a minimum of 20 continuous minutes each session. For best results, teach her to maintain an exercise pulse rate of 70% to 85% of its maximum capability for her age.

Tell the client that rest and sleep patterns usually change during pregnancy, and encourage her to respond to her body's cues. If she feels tired, she should rest. If her nightly sleep is interrupted, she may benefit from an afternoon nap.

Discuss discontinuation of contraception. This intervention addresses a nursing diagnosis of *knowledge deficit related to contraception and conception.* Depending on the client's current contraceptive method, discuss how to discontinue it. If she uses an oral contraceptive, advise her to stop taking it 3 months before attempting to become pregnant. Tell her to rely on another contraceptive method during these months to prevent pregnancy while her body returns to its normal hormone levels.

If she has an IUD, urge her to schedule an appointment to have it removed 3 months before conception is desired. Instruct her to rely on a different contraceptive method during this time so that the endometrial lining of her uterus can return to normal before pregnancy.

Family care

When a client and her partner have a nursing diagnosis of *family coping: potential for growth, related to impending pregnancy* or *body image disturbance related to impending pregnancy,* plan to discuss the couple's concerns with them. During the discussion, listen actively and encourage open communication between the client and her partner.

Begin by sensitively exploring the couple's decision to conceive. Ask them how they have planned for this event. Candidly discuss potential changes in their life-style and relationship, helping them begin to see themselves as parents and understand the changes in their roles. Also allow them to express concerns about the body changes that will occur with pregnancy. If the client is worried about her body image, encourage her to talk openly with her partner about her fears. Remind her that many men find pregnant women attractive.

Evaluation

To complete the nursing process, evaluate the effectiveness of nursing care. Keep in mind that health promotion measures adopted before conception need continual evaluation before, during, and after pregnancy.

The following examples illustrate some appropriate evaluation statements:
• The client understood the importance of sound nutrition and has exhibited her ability to plan proper meals.
• The client described the importance of discontinuing her oral contraceptive and of using a different contraceptive method for 3 months before attempting to conceive.
• The client and her partner agreed to attend smoking cessation classes before conceiving.
• The client and her partner discussed their well-considered decision to have a child.

Documentation

Using the appropriate records, document all steps of the nursing process, including assessment data, nursing diagnoses, the plan of care, implementation activities, and evaluation findings. When caring for a couple who request client help with preconception planning, documentation should include:
• significant health history findings
• significant physical assessment findings
• results of diagnostic studies performed
• the couple's understanding of health habits that will prepare them for conception
• instructions given to the couple
• the couple's understanding of instructions
• the couple's emotional readiness for parenting.

Care for the infertile couple

The nurse preparing to provide appropriate care for an infertile couple must understand infertility, its factors, and its psychological effects.

Infertility

Infertility is the inability to conceive after 1 year of intercourse without contraception or the inability to carry a pregnancy to term (Speroff, 1987). Infertility may be primary or secondary. Those with primary infertility have never been pregnant; those with secondary infertility have been pregnant, but now cannot become pregnant or carry a pregnancy to term.

In the United States, infertility affects about one in every six couples. Its incidence appears to be increasing, possibly for the following reasons:
• More women are delaying intended pregnancies beyond age 30, when fertility decreases.
• STDs, which cause tubal scarring, are more common.
• Society now accepts the discussion of sexual problems, which allows more couples to discuss infertility openly and seek treatment (McCusker, 1982; Menning, 1988).

Twenty-five years ago, physicians could not diagnose the cause of infertility in 40% to 50% of people seeking treatment. Today, they can determine the cause in all but 5% to 10%. However, only about 50% of infertile couples can be treated successfully, leaving the others to deal with unfulfilled wishes for conceiving children (DeCherney, Polan, Lee, and Boyers, 1988; Siebel and Taymor, 1982). Those who do conceive may do so at high emotional cost caused by anxiety and frustration from the expense, time, and stress of infertility tests and treatments.

For most couples, infertility care requires extensive diagnostic studies and medical or surgical intervention to correct the problems. Advances in technology and research are improving the odds for conception; however, ethical dilemmas may intrude on who can conceive, how, and at what cost. (For more information, see Chapter 5, Ethical and Legal Concerns in Family Care.)

Infertility factors
The woman or man or both may be implicated in infertility. About 40% of infertility relates to the woman, 30% to the man, 20% to both, and 10% to unknown factors (Speroff, 1987).

Various factors may lead to female infertility. Structural abnormalities of the reproductive organs may block sperm from reaching the ovum or prevent the fertilized ovum from implanting in the uterus. Hormonal abnormalities may cause ovulatory disorders or create an environment hostile to pregnancy. Nonreproductive factors, such as occupational hazards and drug use, also may produce infertility.

Male fertility problems may affect spermatogenesis, relate to structural abnormalities, or disrupt sexual function. These factors may be congenital, genetic, or hormonal, or they may result from nonreproductive causes, such as occupational hazards or drug use.

Combined factors in both partners may influence infertility, such as male and female hormonal or structural factors, stress, or sexual misinformation. (For more information, see *Factors related to infertility.*)

Psychological effects

A reflection of the traditional nuclear family, most children begin playacting a parental role at an early age and grow up assuming they will have children of their own. Although some couples choose to remain childless, the decision for most is not *whether* to have children but *when.* The discovery that one is infertile and may never have children can evoke mild to profound psychological reactions (Menning, 1988).

Infertility is stressful for the couple who desire children. It can affect the infertile individual as well as the couple and their relationship (Menning, 1988). Infertility evaluation and treatment taxes the couple physically, emotionally, and financially because it can be uncomfortable, time-consuming, and costly.

Infertility evaluation and treatment focus on reproductive functioning, requiring the couple to share intimate information about sexual practices. Moreover, the timing of intercourse typically is determined by the treatment. Infertile individuals have reported feeling embarrassed because of having to share sexual information, anxious over the need to have intercourse on schedule, and frustrated because of the disruption in their lives (Menning, 1988).

Couples without adequate health care insurance or with policies that do not cover infertility treatments may not be able to afford therapy. However, an infertile couple may feel "driven" to continue treatment in spite of the inconvenience, cost, and discomfort (Olshansky, 1988).

Many complex feelings may accompany infertility. Initially, a man or woman may react with surprise or disbelief because the individual has assumed that he or she is fertile. Subsequently, the individual may experience all of the phases of grief (denial, anger, bargaining, depression, and acceptance) as well as other emotions, such as fear, anxiety, guilt, and disappointment. Before reaching acceptance or resolution of infertility, the individual may vacillate among all of these emotions (Menning, 1988).

For the infertile woman, emotions may fluctuate with the menstrual cycle. As ovulation approaches, she may feel hopeful and excited about the prospect of conception. After ovulation, she may feel anxiety as she awaits her next menstrual period. If menstruation occurs, she may feel disappointment, depression, and frustration (Davis, 1987).

The infertile man or woman may experience disturbances in self-concept and body image or a marked discrepancy between the present self and the ideal self (Platt, Fisher, and Silver, 1973). An infertile woman may feel empty, defective, incomplete, less desirable, and unworthy (Davis, 1984; Menning, 1988).

An infertile man may have similar feelings or may equate infertility with a defect in his masculinity. The discovery that he is infertile may even lead to impotence (Hirsch and Hirsch, 1989).

Infertility can cause discord (Hirsch and Hirsch, 1989) or can bring a couple closer together by giving them a common goal and a need to share their stresses and disappointments (Davis, 1984).

It can change the couple's relationship by making conception—rather than mutual affection or enjoyment—the goal of intercourse. After the discovery of infertility, a couple with previously normal sexual functioning may develop sexual problems, such as decreased frequency of intercourse, intercourse only during the woman's fertile period, orgasmic dysfunction, or decreased enjoyment. Ejaculatory failure frequently occurs in men who have to perform for postcoital examinations.

The woman's basal body temperature (BBT) chart, the basic monitoring tool in infertility treatment, serves as a record of menstrual cycle events. The couple may perceive this chart, which also has spaces for recording sexual intercourse, as a "report card" of their sexual behavior. Having to share the BBT chart and other sexual information with the health care professional can be stressful.

The infertile individual may feel powerless to control events. For the woman, her life may seem governed by her menstrual cycle. She may try to juggle social activities and work schedules to accommodate plans for conception. Feelings of powerlessness also may result from the realization that the individual cannot control fertility willfully and from the need to follow a rigid routine for infertility tests and treatments. (For more information, see *Nursing research applied: Responses to infertility treatments,* page 205.)

Infertility also may adversely affect the individual's or couple's relationships with family and friends. The couple without children may feel isolated or out of place at family functions. An infertile woman may feel depressed around pregnant family members or friends, especially when giving or attending a baby shower (Davis, 1984). Further, she may feel hurt by well-meaning family members or friends who give advice, such as, "Just quit trying so hard and you'll get pregnant."

Factors related to infertility

Female, male, or combined factors may be implicated in infertility. The following chart presents these factors by the structure or function that they may affect.

STRUCTURE OR FUNCTION AND EFFECTS	POSSIBLE CAUSES
Female factors	
Uterus • Structural changes	• Congenital abnormalities, such as an undersized or distorted uterus • Obstruction of the uterine cavity by a narrowed or divided endometrial surface, polyps, tumor, or Asherman's syndrome (scar tissue from vigorous curretage after abortion) • Infection that causes scarring, such as a sexually transmitted disease (STD), tuberculosis (TB), schistosomiasis, and infections associated with pelvic inflammatory disease (PID) or intrauterine device (IUD) use
Fallopian tubes • Partial or complete obstruction	• Congenital abnormalities that narrow or obstruct the tubes • Blockage of the tubes by tissue affected by endometriosis • Infection that causes scarring, such as acute salpingitis, which may result from such organisms as *Neisseria gonorrhoeae, Mycoplasma,* and *Chlamydia trachomatis*
Vagina and cervix • Alterations in vaginal or cervical secretions	• Infection that alters secretion pH or quantity, affecting sperm motility and viability • Use of spermicidal lubricants or douches • Poor cervical mucus from inadequate estrogen and progesterone production
• Alterations in vaginal or cervical structure	• Congenital structural abnormalities of the vagina, such as imperforate hymen • Congenital structural abnormalities of the cervical os, such as a stenosed (narrowed), malpositioned, or too-wide os
Hormones	
Ovulatory phase • Ovulatory dysfunction	• Use of oral contraceptives
• Anovulation from ovarian failure or faulty hormonal stimulation	• External factors, such as stress, exercise, and malnutrition • Adrenal or pituitary tumors • Adrenal hyperplasia (increased size of adrenal gland) • Hypothyroidism (insufficient thyroid output) or hyperthyroidism (excessive thyroid output) • Hyperprolactinemia (increased prolactin levels)
• Anovulation from ovarian abnormality	• Gonadal dysgenesis from a chromosomal disorder, such as Turner's syndrome, in which the individual has only one X chromosome instead of two • External factors, such as irradiation of the ovaries, cytotoxic drug use, or mumps oophoritis (inflammation of the ovaries) • Polycystic ovaries
Luteal phase • Progesterone level alterations	• Luteal phase deficiency (inadequate progesterone production by the corpus luteum, which leads to spontaneous first trimester abortion) • Progesterone receptor site abnormalities in the endometrium
Reproductive system • Altered physiology of ovaries and endometrium; adhesions that may obstruct reproductive tract	• Endometriosis (endometrial tissue that appears outside the uterus and responds to hormonal stimulation just as uterine tissue does)

(continued)

Factors related to infertility continued

STRUCTURE OR FUNCTION AND EFFECTS	POSSIBLE CAUSES
Male factors	
Spermatogenesis • Alteration in sperm production, maturation, mobility, or motility or interference with hormonal regulation of spermatogenesis	• Congenital abnormalities, such as Kleinfelter's syndrome (chromosome disorder that causes gonadal defects), testicular agenesis (congenital absence of testes) or dysgenesis (abnormal formation of testes), cryptorchidism (undescended testicle), or varicocele (abnormal veins in the scrotum) • Diseases, such as an acute or chronic illness, mumps during or after adolescence, orchitis (testicular infection), gonorrhea, TB, chronic nonspecific prostatitis or urethritis, diabetes, or endocrine, thyroid, or adrenal disease • Stress • Occupational hazards, such as heat exposure in a labor-intensive job or prolonged sitting as in truck driving • Increased intrascrotal temperature caused by such factors as obesity, tight underwear, and frequent use of hot tubs or saunas • Prescription drugs, such as chemotherapeutic agents, hormones, and specific drugs such as cimetidine, nitrofurantoin, and sulfasalazine (Corriere, 1986) • Nonprescription drugs or excessive caffeine, nicotine, or alcohol; illegal drugs, such as marijuana and narcotics (Behrman and Patton, 1988) • Nutritional problems, such as malnutrition • Polyspermia (abnormally high sperm count), which is associated with a high incidence of spontaneous abortion, although the exact cause is unknown • Hormonal disorders, such as hyperprolactinemia (abnormally high prolactin levels), which can lead to testicular atrophy • Autoimmunity (production of antibodies to sperm in the seminiferous tubules), which may occur after trauma or infection
Reproductive tract structures • Alteration of sperm flow	• Congenital abnormalities, such as hypospadias (location of urethra on underside of penis), urethral stricture, or anomalies of the epididymis or vas deferens • Infection that causes reproductive tract scarring and blockage, such as gonorrhea or prostatitis • Tumors • Surgery, such as a vasectomy
Sexual function • Alteration in ejaculation, preventing semen deposit deep in vagina at cervical os	• Surgery to widen the bladder neck, which can cause retrograde ejaculation • Such diseases as prostatitis, which can cause retrograde ejaculation, and diabetes or hypertension, which may cause ejaculatory problems • Drugs, such as antihypertensives, which may cause ejaculatory problems
• Alteration in erection	• Spinal cord lesions that cause sexual dysfunction
Combined factors	
Various structures and functions • Alteration in reproductive structures, hormones, or both	• Combined factors affect 20% of infertile couples. Alone, each factor may not affect fertility; together, they may produce infertility.
• Alteration in immune response	• Development of antibodies in female client to her partner's sperm, which would destroy them
• Anovulation or decreased spermatogenesis	• Stress
• Alteration in sexual function	• Misinformation about sexual practices, such as mistiming of intercourse or improper positioning • Physiologic problems, as described above, which may cause impotence, decreased libido, or ejaculatory disorders • Psychological problems, which may affect any aspect of sexual functioning • Illegal drug use, which may reduce libido

Assessment

In 85% to 90% of couples, pregnancy will occur within 1 year of regular (at least twice weekly) sexual intercourse without contraception (Speroff, 1987). Infertility investigation typically begins after the couple have been trying—unsuccessfully—to conceive for a year.

Determining the exact cause of the couple's infertility requires a thorough assessment. It must involve both partners because mutual cooperation and understanding are essential to successful treatment. It must evaluate the physical factors related to and the psychological effects of infertility. Assessment is time-consuming, expensive, and may take years to complete.

Health history

To assess infertility, the nurse must ask intimate questions. To make this easier, establish a rapport with the client. (Interview the female and male clients separately and then together.) Conduct the interview in a private area to maintain confidentiality. Begin the interview by introducing yourself, briefly describing the types of questions that you will ask, telling the client that the information is necessary for accurate diagnosis, and emphasizing that all information is confidential. Begin the interview by asking questions eliciting less intimate information before asking more personal questions, such as those concerning sexual practices.

For a comprehensive health history, be sure to obtain information about the following topics:
• biographical data
• menstrual history
• obstetric history
• fertility history
• environmental health
• contraceptive history
• infertility history
• medical history
• surgical history
• nutrition habits
• personal habits
• exercise habits
• sexual history
• cultural and religious background
• psychosocial status.

If the history reveals inadequate attempts to conceive, education and time may be indicated. If it reveals adequate exposure (intercourse at least twice weekly for 1 year without contraception) or if the couple report two or more pregnancy losses, then further investigation of both partners is warranted.

Female health history. When assessing the female client, obtain biographical data and evaluate her obstetric history as described in the section on "Preconception care for the fertile couple" earlier in this chapter. Also assess her menstrual history.

Biographical data. Particularly note the client's age because fertility decreases with age. For a woman over age 30, infertility investigation may begin after the couple have been trying to conceive for 6 months, instead of a year.

Menstrual history. Ask the client her age at menarche (onset of menses). Then focus on her current menstrual cycle, inquiring about its duration and regularity. Also ask her to describe the duration and amount of flow of her menstrual periods. Inquire if she experiences ovulatory pain or dysmenorrhea (painful menstruation). Menstrual irregularities may indicate hormonal problems that could affect ovulation and fertility. (For more information about the menstrual history, see Chapter 7, Women's Health Promotion.)

Obstetric history. The number of pregnancies, live births, and spontaneous and therapeutic abortions differentiates primary from secondary infertility. It also may indicate Asherman's syndrome (secondary sterility as a result of scarring caused by vigorous curettage during abortion).

Specifically ask the client about any births, pregnancies, or abortions in other relationships. Her answer may help rule out or identify female factors related to infertility. For example, if she has given birth before with a different partner, a male factor may be implicated in the couple's infertility. However, a female factor cannot be ruled out entirely because the client could have secondary infertility.

If the client has children, ask how long it took her to conceive, if she had any pregnancy complications, and how long she lactated. Difficulties with conception, pregnancy, or lactation may reflect hormonal problems.

Male health history. When interviewing the male client, explore his fertility history and environmental health patterns.

Fertility history. Ask about any pregnancies, births, and abortions in other relationships. A man who has impregnated a previous partner may be less likely as a cause of infertility.

Environmental health. Inquire about any occupational or other exposure to chemicals or excessive heat. Such exposure may affect spermatogenesis.

Combined health history. When assessing the couple, address the physical factors and psychological effects of infertility. Ask about their contraceptive, infertility, medical, surgical, and sexual histories; assess their nutritional, personal, and exercise habits; and evaluate their cultural and religious beliefs and psychosocial status.

Contraceptive history. Obtain contraceptive information as described in "Preconception care for the fertile couple" earlier in this chapter. Use of an oral contraceptive or an IUD can delay pregnancy by up to 3 months.

Infertility history. First, determine how long the couple have been trying to conceive. If they have had intercourse without contraception at least twice weekly for the past year, they may need to begin diagnostic and treatment procedures. If they have had less frequent intercourse, they may simply need instruction, encouragement, and more time.

Next, ask if they have received prior treatment for infertility. If so, have them describe the outcome. Knowledge of previous treatments may identify an existing infertility problem or rule out certain problems. It also may guide the choice of diagnostic tests and treatments.

Medical history. Obtain a complete history of illnesses and a family history of genetic and reproductive problems. Any of these factors may compromise fertility. For example, mumps, STDs, chronic disease, or recent febrile illness in the male client may affect spermatogenesis or sexual function, leading to infertility.

Surgical history. Investigate the couple's surgical history, particularly noting any abdominal, pelvic, or genitourinary surgery. Such surgical procedures may cause reproductive tract blockage and infertility.

Nutritional habits. As in the "Preconception care for the fertile couple" section, evaluate the female and male clients' diet. Malnutrition or vitamin deficiencies can cause anovulation or reduce spermatogenesis. Excessive intake of caffeine also can affect spermatogenesis.

Personal habits. As described in "Preconception care for the fertile couple," investigate the couple's use of alcohol and prescription, OTC, and illegal drugs. In the female client, drugs such as diethylstilbestrol (DES) can compromise fertility. In the male client, alcohol consumption and use of certain prescription, OTC, or illegal drugs may reduce spermatogenesis. Some prescription drugs, such as antihypertensives, may cause sexual dysfunction.

Exercise habits. As described in "Preconception care for the fertile couple," assess the couple's exercise habits. A female client who exercises excessively may develop anovulation. A male client who does not get regular exercise and has a sedentary job may develop reduced spermatogenesis.

Sexual history. Ask about the couple's libido (sexual desire), satisfaction with the sexual relationship, and frequency of orgasm. Reduced libido or satisfaction or lack of orgasms may lead to sexual dysfunction and infertility.

Also inquire about the frequency of intercourse and the positions used. Infrequent intercourse may decrease the chance of conception. So may too frequent (daily) intercourse or the use of certain positions, such as the female superior position. In couples who do not have regular intercourse or who are sexually inexperienced, subjecting them to a complete infertility investigation may be delayed for up to 2 years (Wheeler and Polan, 1988).

Have the couple describe their sexual practices. Find out if they use a lubricant during intercourse; that can have a spermicidal effect. Also determine if the female client gets up or douches immediately after intercourse, which can allow semen to flow out of the vagina. Any of these practices can reduce the chance of conception.

Ask them to describe their understanding of the most fertile period. Their answers may identify a knowledge deficit as a factor implicated in infertility.

Cultural and religious background. The couple's background can affect their view of infertility and degree of participation in diagnostic tests and treatments. (For more information, see *Cultural considerations: Infertility tests and treatments*.)

Psychosocial status. Thoroughly assess the couple's psychosocial status to evaluate stress related to infertility. If they seem to have problems communicating or sharing their frustrations for fear of disappointing or angering each other, plan to counsel them separately and then together.

During the psychosocial assessment, ask the couple why they want to have a child. This question may identify unrealistic expectations, such as a child rescuing a failing marriage, which would require further nursing action.

Then have the couple describe how they feel about their inability to have a child. An invitation to share feelings can help relieve some of the stress of infertility and can identify the need for stress management instruction.

Find out how infertility has affected the couple's relationship. If it has disrupted the relationship, they may need to explore ways to deal with the disruption.

Ask them to describe what they do to cope with infertility. If they are not coping well, they may need a referral to a support group for infertile couples or to another resource.

CULTURAL CONSIDERATIONS

Infertility tests and treatments

When caring for a client or couple from a different background, the nurse should keep the following cultural considerations in mind.

Because some cultures frown on masturbation, a male client may have difficulty providing a semen sample by masturbation. For such a client, the nurse can help by suggesting alternate ways to collect the sample, such as coitus interruptus or a special condom.

Some religions believe that interference with fertility is unnatural and wrong. They view artificial insemination by donor (AID), in vitro fertilization (IVF), and gamete intrafallopian transfer (GIFT) as particularly undesirable. When caring for clients who choose AID, IVF, or GIFT, the nurse must screen them carefully for emotional stability. The nurse also should help prepare them to withstand criticism from others and help them decide what to tell a child (if anything) about how he or she was conceived. Finally, the nurse should remind clients that a child conceived with donor oocytes or sperm legally is their child: A donor who signs appropriate legal documents should have no right or responsibility to the child.

Physical assessment

Perform a thorough physical assessment on each client, paying special attention to the reproductive and endocrine systems.

Female client. While performing the physical examination, be sure to note the development of the secondary sex characteristics. The breasts should be fully developed, and the distribution and amount of fat and pubic hair should be normal for the client's age. Abnormal growth in any of these areas may indicate a hormonal imbalance that could cause infertility.

Assess the client for hirsutism (excessive body hair in a masculine distribution), goiter (enlarged thyroid gland), or galactorrhea (lactation unrelated to childbirth or breast-feeding). These abnormalities also can indicate a hormonal dysfunction.

At the end of the complete physical assessment, perform a pelvic examination if you have had special training. (For information on pelvic assessment techniques and normal findings, see Chapter 7, Women's Health promotion.) Particularly note the size, shape, and position of the external genitalia. Abnormally large labia minora and clitoris suggest a hormonal imbalance.

When inspecting the vaginal introitus, evaluate the condition of the hymen. An intact hymen or a vaginal introitus that is too small could indicate a structural problem that might prevent full penile penetration and deposition of semen near the cervix.

Also check for signs of infection, such as thick, foul-smelling, or discolored vaginal or cervical secretions. A reproductive tract infection may alter the pH of the vagina and cervix, creating a spermicidal environment.

Using the speculum, inspect the cervix for size, shape, position, and the presence of tears or polyps. Cervical abnormalities can cause infertility. For example, the client may become pregnant but may not be able to carry the fetus to term because she has an incompetent cervix (mechanical defect that prevents the cervix from staying closed until the pregnancy reaches term).

During bimanual palpation of the uterus, determine its size, position, and mobility, documenting any structural abnormalities. (For an illustration, see *Uterine abnormalities.*) Note any lumps, which may be caused by tumors, or tenderness, which may suggest endometriosis. Also bimanually palpate the ovaries and adnexa. Lumpy, immobile structures may indicate adhesions.

Male client. Perform a complete physical assessment of the male client because any disorder that affects his overall health can affect spermatogenesis. During this assessment, pay close attention to the reproductive and endocrine systems, which are typically the source of an infertility problem.

To begin the physical assessment, observe the client's overall development and secondary sex characteristics. Small limbs and genitalia, sparse body hair, or gynecomastia (breast enlargement) may suggest an endocrine disorder and warrant evaluation for pituitary, thyroid, adrenal, or testicular problems.

While examining the penis, observe its shape and the placement of the urinary meatus. Abnormal penile curvature may be caused by Peyronie's disease (fibrous induration of the corpora cavernosa) or congenital chordee (downward curvature). A client with such a disorder may not be able to deposit semen near the cervix during intercourse, which can impede fertilization. Hypospadias (urinary meatus located on the ventral surface) or epispadias (urinary meatus located on the dorsal surface) may cause a similar problem.

Inspect and palpate the scrotum, noting the size, surface characteristics, and consistency of the testes, epididymis, and vas deferens. Abnormally large testes may result from varicocele (dilation of the pampiniform venous complex of the spermatic cord that causes swelling and pain), which may decrease sperm production by allowing blood to pool and increase the temperature of the scrotal area. Abnormally small testes suggest an endocrine problem. Irregularities or nodules may indicate tumors or adhesions.

To complete this part of the assessment, have the client stand. Then observe the veins at the junction of the scrotum and abdomen. Engorgement may indicate varicocele.

Diagnostic studies

Based on health history and physical assessment findings, diagnostic studies may be performed for the female client, male client, or both. Diagnostic evaluation is time-consuming, progressive, and may continue for years. Initial studies identify whether infertility is caused by factors in the female client, male client, or a combination; later studies rule out problems until the specific cause is identified.

Female client. Tests for infertility in the female client may include BBT recording, cervical mucus evaluation, blood and urine tests, other laboratory studies, sperm antibody agglutination studies, postcoital examination, endometrial biopsy, hysterosalpingography, pelvic ultrasonography, and laparoscopy.

BBT recording. The BBT is the lowest body temperature of a healthy individual while awake. In a woman, the BBT normally drops slightly (0.2° F [0.1° C]) 24 to 36 hours before ovulation and rises (0.4° to 0.8° F [0.2° to 0.4° C]) 24 to 72 hours after ovulation, when the corpus luteum of the ruptured ovary produces progesterone. Because of this, BBT recording usually is the first diagnostic study for the female client.

The biphasic pattern indicates normal ovulation and marks the most fertile period of the woman's cycle. It can be used to monitor infertility care, schedule further diagnostic tests, and plan intercourse during the most fertile period. (For a client who does not wish to become pregnant, it can be used as a natural birth control method.)

A monophasic pattern is abnormal and may reflect an ovulatory problem or luteal phase deficiency. A BBT that remains elevated may indicate pregnancy. (For samples, see *Basal body temperature patterns,* page 211.)

To measure the BBT, the client must take her temperature every morning before rising and record it on a special graph. She can use a BBT thermometer, which is calibrated in tenths of degrees, or a regular thermometer via the oral, rectal, or axillary route. On the graph, she also should record the date, menstrual period, sexual intercourse, cervical mucus characteristics, and any fac-

Uterine abnormalities

Bimanual palpation may detect a uterine abnormality. Unlike a normal uterus, the structurally abnormal uterus may interfere with the transport, implantation, or growth of an embryo. Structural abnormalities may include narrowed projections of the fundus (called horning) and septal deviations.

Normal uterus
Normally, the uterus is pear-shaped. The uterine neck (isthmus) joins the fundus to the cervix, the uterine part extending into the vagina. The fundus and the isthmus make up the corpus, the main uterine body.

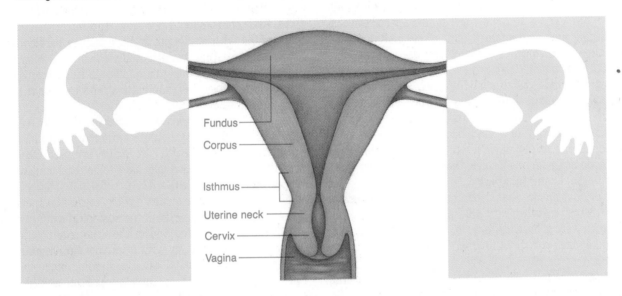

Fundus
Corpus
Isthmus
Uterine neck
Cervix
Vagina

Abnormalities

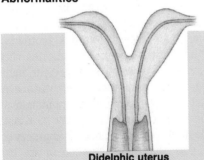

Didelphic uterus
Displays two cervixes
and vaginas

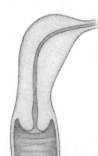

Unicornuate uterus
Displays single horn

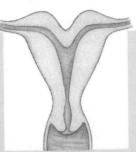

Partial bicornuate uterus
Displays partial horning

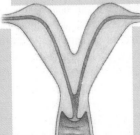

Complete bicornuate uterus
Displays horning all the
way down to the cervix

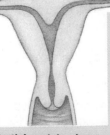

Partial septate uterus
Displays a small septum
(dividing wall) in the middle

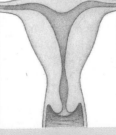

Arcuate uterus
Displays bow shape
at the top

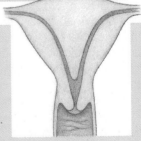

Complete septate uterus
Displays a large
septum in the middle

tors that may alter her BBT. (For more information about this method, see *Client teaching: Using the basal body temperature method of birth control* in Chapter 9, Family Planning.)

Cervical mucus evaluation. If estrogen and progesterone production is adequate, the quantity, color, thickness, stickiness, and stretchiness of cervical mucus normally change along with the BBT. Mucus normally is scant after menstruation. As ovulation approaches, it becomes more copious, has the consistency of raw egg white, and can be stretched 4 to 6 cm when pulled apart between the thumb and forefingers (spinnbarkeit). After ovulation, the mucus appears thick, cloudy, and pasty.

Cervical mucus that exhibits these characteristics indicates normal ovulation and can help guide an infertile couple's sexual intercourse. On the peak day, the mucus is stretchy and looks and feels like egg white. From the peak day to 3 days later (the fertile period), the couple should engage in intercourse every other day. If they do not wish to conceive, they should abstain from intercourse during this period.

Cervical mucus that does not change may indicate an ovulatory or other hormonal problem. (For more information, see *Client teaching: Using the cervical mucus method of birth control* in Chapter 9, Family Planning.)

Blood and urine tests. To assess hormone levels, several laboratory tests may be used, including blood tests for progesterone, estrogen, follicle-stimulating hormone (FSH), luteinizing hormone (LH), and thyroid hormones (protein-bound iodine, thyroxine, T_4, and T_3). Urine tests for hormone levels may include assays for 17-ketosteroids and 17-hydroxycorticosteroids. Abnormal levels in any of these tests suggest a hormonal problem.

Other blood and urine tests may include urinalysis, CBC, VDRL, Rh factor, and antibody titer tests. These tests screen for health problems that may affect fertility. For example, the urinalysis and CBC may detect an infection; the antibody titer test, a disorder such as mumps.

Special tests. A sex chromatin test may be done to screen for abnormalities in the number of sex chromosomes, which may indicate a genetic disorder that could cause infertility. Abnormal results indicate the need for a full chromosome analysis. (For more information, see Chapter 11, Genetics and Genetic Disorders.)

A client with amenorrhea may receive skull tomography to detect pituitary gland tumors that could interfere with hormone secretion.

Sperm antibody agglutination test. In this test, the client's serum is mixed with her partner's semen. The sample is tested periodically for sperm agglutination (clumping together), which normally does not occur. Agglutination indicates that the client has antibodies to her partner's sperm, which can cause infertility.

Postcoital examination. This test provides information about the interaction of sperm and cervical mucus. Timing of this examination is critical. It should occur just before ovulation and no more than 6 hours after intercourse. The BBT chart should not show the temperature rise associated with ovulation, and the client's cervical mucus should be thin, watery, and clear. Preparation also is important. The couple must abstain from intercourse for 3 days before the examination, and the client must not douche before being tested.

Scheduling the postcoital examination can be difficult. The client may ovulate earlier or later than expected or when the health care facility is closed. Because of this, the examination may have to be rescheduled and repeated several times.

If the health care facility's policy permits, a specially prepared nurse may perform the postcoital examination. With the client draped and in the lithotomy position, a plastic suction catheter with a narrow tip is gently inserted into her cervical canal and some mucus is aspirated. The mucus is then spread on a slide for microscopic evaluation.

Under high-power magnification, a normal postcoital specimen will reveal ferning (crystallization of cervical mucus into a fern-like pattern) and live, motile sperm. Thick mucus that shows no ferning indicates that the client was not ovulating or is estrogen deficient. Immobile or agglutinated sperm may result from various conditions, such as a cervical infection or an immune reaction. Absence of sperm in the specimen may be caused by azoospermia (lack of sperm in semen) or improper sexual technique, such as shallow ejaculation in the vaginal vault or rising or douching shortly after intercourse.

Endometrial biopsy. Performed by the physician, this outpatient procedure provides information about hormonal stimulation of the endometrium during the secretory (luteal) phase of the menstrual cycle. The luteal phase begins after ovulation (day 14 of a typical 28-day cycle) and continues until menstruation begins. Throughout the luteal phase, hormones stimulate the endometrial tissue, causing it to change slightly every day. Because of this, a biopsy of endometrial tissue is used to assess the menstrual date (the timing in the menstrual cycle determined by histologic evaluation of tissue development). The menstrual date is compared to the client's cycle date (timing in the menstrual cycle calculated from the be-

Basal body temperature patterns

The basic diagnostic tool in female infertility assessment, the basal body temperature (BBT) graph also may include a place to record cervical mucus characteristics and notes. When the client records her BBT on a standard graph, the resulting pattern can provide useful diagnostic information, as shown below.

Biphasic pattern

A BBT graph with a sharp midcycle rise (biphasic pattern), as shown in red below, indicates an ovulatory cycle. A chart with a sharp midcycle rise, prolonged temperature elevation, and absence of menses suggests pregnancy.

The lower portion of the graph may show cervical mucus characteristics and notes that help validate and interpret the BBT pattern.

Monophasic pattern

A BBT graph with a relatively flat (monophasic) pattern that does not vary more than .05° F each day, as shown in black below, suggests anovulation.

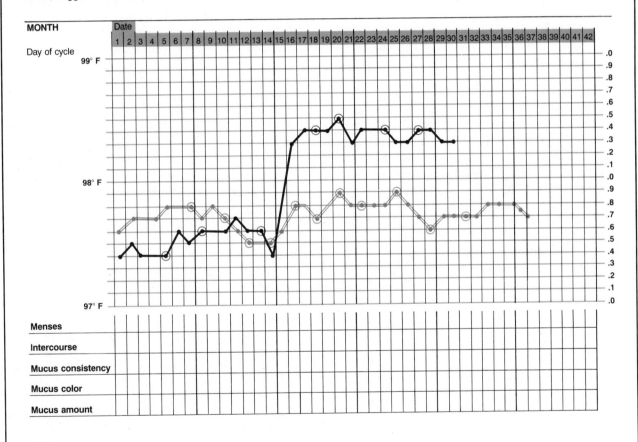

Notes

Key:

X	Menses	**W**	Wetness of external labia	**Y**	Yellow mucus	
•	Intercourse	**M**	Ordinary mucus consistency	**0**	No mucus	
P	Peak mucus symptom (last day of fertile-type mucus before it begins to dry up)	**T**	Tacky mucus	**+**	Slight amount of mucus	
		S	Smooth, slippery, stretchy mucus	**+ +**	Moderate amount of mucus	
		C	Clear mucus	**+ + +**	Large amount of mucus	
D	Dryness of external labia	**O**	Opaque mucus			

ginning of her last menses), which may or may not correspond. For example, the client's cycle date may be day 26, but her menstrual date may be day 21, indicating improper endometrial development and a possible hormonal imbalance.

Schedule the procedure 2 to 3 days before the expected onset of the client's next menstrual period. At this time, the endometrial tissue sample will have received the most hormonal stimulation. Help the client into the lithotomy position and drape her. Then explain each step of the procedure.

The physician exposes the cervix with a vaginal speculum and cleans it with povidone-iodine solution. Because the biopsy may cause cramping, the client may receive a paracervical block to relieve discomfort. After dilating the cervix, the physician passes a sounding instrument into the uterus to measure the depth of the uterine cavity. Then the physician inserts a cutting or aspirating instrument into the uterus and removes a small amount of endometrial tissue from the fundus.

In the laboratory, a pathologist evaluates the endometrial tissue histologically to assess the menstrual date. Then the histologic date is compared to the date of ovulation suggested by the BBT, cycle date, and subsequent onset of menses. Normally, the endometrium is in-phase: The histologic date of the endometrial tissue matches the cycle date within 2 days, indicating a normal luteal phase and hormonal balance.

The endometrium is out-of-phase if a discrepancy of 2 or more days exists between the ovulation date, cycle date, and histologic date. In other words, the endometrial tissue composition does not correspond to other indicators of the timing in the client's cycle. For example, the BBT chart may indicate that ovulation occurred 12 days ago, and the cycle date (based on last menses) is day 26. If the histologic date reveals an endometrium earlier than day 24 or later than day 28, the results are abnormal or out-of-phase.

An out-of-phase endometrium may result from inadequate progesterone, inadequate estrogen preparation and support, excess estrogen in relation to adequate progesterone, or endometrium nonresponse to hormonal stimulation.

Hysterosalpingography (HSG). A fluoroscopic X-ray of the uterus and fallopian tubes, HSG is used to detect structural abnormalities. It is done 2 to 6 days after menstruation to be relatively certain the client is not pregnant. To prepare for the procedure, the client is placed in the lithotomy position and draped, and a vaginal speculum is inserted. Because HSG can cause uterine cramps, a paracervical block may be given before the procedure. The physician inserts a cannula through the cervical os, instills dye into the uterus, and takes one or more X-rays.

The dye should fill a symmetrical uterine cavity, flow through normal-sized fallopian tubes, and spill freely into the peritoneal cavity. Abnormal findings may include a misshapen uterus or narrowed or occluded fallopian tubes. However, HSG sometimes clears the tubes of mucus, breaks up adhesions, and straightens kinked tubes.

Although uncommon, complications of HSG may include allergic reactions to the radiopaque dye, which may lead to embolization and death. Monitor the client for changes in level of consciousness or vital signs, and ask about any severe pain or dizziness. More commonly, the dye irritates the nerves, causing referred shoulder pain.

Pelvic ultrasonography. This diagnostic study can identify structural abnormalities in reproductive organs, ovarian cysts, uterine fibroids, masses, or foreign bodies. It also can be used to monitor follicular development and pregnancy.

The technician or a specially trained nurse may perform ultrasonography. Client preparation depends on the type of scanner used. If the client needs pelvic ultrasonography, she will need a full bladder to enhance visualization of the uterus and adnexa. Place the client on her back and drape her to expose only the lower abdomen. Because this noninvasive procedure is painless, anesthesia is not needed. (For more information about ultrasonography, see Chapter 22, High-Risk Antepartal Clients.)

Laparoscopy. Laparoscopy allows observation of pelvic organs and surgery for certain gynecologic disorders. In an infertile woman, common indications for laparoscopy include unexplained infertility, abnormal HSG results, signs of endometriosis, evaluation of ovarian dysfunction, tuboplasty (fallopian tube repair), and oocyte retrieval for artificial insemination (Siegler, 1988).

If the client needs laparoscopy, schedule it at the appropriate time, depending on its purpose. For example, schedule it to coincide with an endometrial biopsy if the client has unexplained infertility. If an oocyte must be retrieved for artificial insemination, schedule it when ultrasonography reveals a mature follicle. Also prepare the client for the procedure by teaching her about it and providing support. (For more information, see *Laparoscopy.*)

After laparoscopy, monitor the client by assessing vital signs and watching for excessive bleeding at the incision sites. Usually, recovery is uneventful and she

Laparoscopy

For an infertile client, laparoscopy may be used to examine the ovaries and fallopian tubes. It also may be used in diagnostic tests and treatments. For example, laparoscopy can be used to lyse adhesions, obtain biopsies, correct tubal occlusions, drain cysts, or obtain ova for gamete intrafallopian transfer (GIFT).

Before the procedure, the client is placed in the dorsal lithotomy position and her abdomen, perineum, and vagina are cleansed. If the client will receive general anesthesia, she is intubated for assisted ventilation.

During the procedure, the physician inserts the laparoscope (illuminated tube) into the abdomen via a 1″ (2.5-cm) subumbilical incision and instills carbon dioxide gas through the laparoscope to lift the abdominal wall away from the ab-

dominal organs. This creates a space for laparoscopic observation and exploration.

When laparoscopy is used to evaluate tubal patency, the physician injects methylene blue dye through a cannula into the vagina. As the dye passes through the uterus and fallopian tubes, the physician observes for blockage or other problems through the laparoscope, as shown. For more extensive observation, the physician may insert a manipulator into the uterus through the vagina or make a second puncture site above the symphysis pubis to insert forceps to manipulate the ovaries and fallopian tubes.

When laparoscopy is used to obtain ova in a treatment such as GIFT, the physician stabilizes the ovary with grasping forceps and penetrates the follicles with a needle to aspirate mature ova.

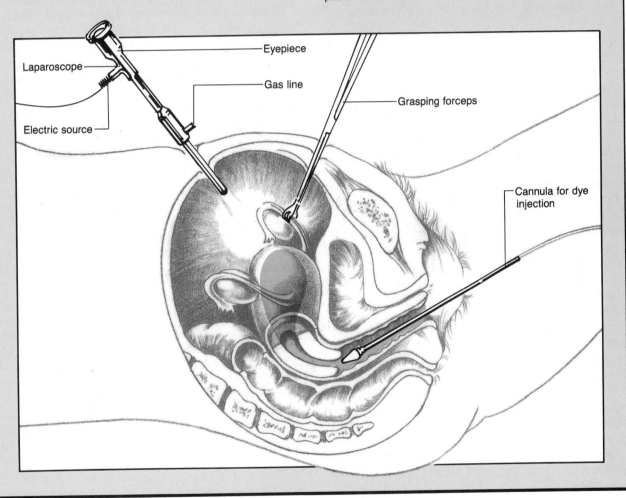

is discharged 4 to 6 hours later. Advise her to report signs of infection, such as fever, swelling, excessive abdominal pain, or discharge from the incision sites.

Male client. Physical assessment of the male client may require blood and urine tests, special tests, semen anal-

ysis, and the hamster zona-free ova test to assess for infertility.

Blood and urine tests. Blood tests may include assays of serum androgens (testosterone, androstenedione, and dehydroepiandrosterone [DHEA]), FSH, LH, T_3, T_4, and prolactin. Abnormal levels of any of these hormones may

Normal values for semen analysis

Commonly used to assess the male client for infertility, semen analysis evaluates several semen and sperm characteristics. Although the following values normally indicate fertility, a client with lower values may be able to father children.

CHARACTERISTIC	NORMAL RANGE
Semen liquefaction	Within 30 minutes
Semen volume	2 to 5 ml
Semen pH	7.2 to 7.8
Sperm morphology	More than 60% of the sperm are mature and normally formed
Sperm motility	More than 60% of the sperm are moving
Sperm count	More than 20 million/ml

indicate a problem in the hypothalamic-pituitary-testicular axis.

Other laboratory tests may be ordered, including urinalysis, CBC, and VDRL. Abnormal values may indicate an infection, which could cause scarring and structural blockage of the male reproductive system.

Special tests. As with the female client, a sex chromatin test and chromosome analysis may be ordered to identify a genetic disorder that can cause infertility, such as Kleinfelter's syndrome.

In a client with azoospermia, a testicular biopsy may be performed to determine if the problem is caused by nonproduction of sperm, blockage of the vas deferens or epididymis, or an endocrine disorder.

Other diagnostic studies may include venography (X-ray of veins after injection of a contrast medium), vasography (X-ray of blood vessels) to assess scrotal blood flow, and thermography (recording of infrared radiation) to assess the temperature in the scrotal area. These studies may detect a varicocele, which can interfere with ejaculation.

Semen analysis. Inexpensive and relatively simple, semen analysis usually is the first test performed on a male client to evaluate infertility. It evaluates semen liquefaction, volume, and pH as well as sperm morphology

(form and structure), motility (ability to move forward), and quantity. Because results can vary greatly, semen analysis should be repeated at least three times at 2- to 4-week intervals. (For details, see *Normal values for semen analysis.*)

When semen analysis is ordered, instruct the client to abstain from sex for 2 to 3 days before the test. Tell him to collect the specimen in a clean dry glass or plastic container, preferably through masturbation.

One alternative to masturbation is coitus interruptus (penile withdrawal from the vagina just before ejaculation). If the client uses coitus interruptus, advise him to place the ejaculate in a clean, dry container. For the semen analysis to be accurate, it must include the first portion of the ejaculate, which is the most concentrated.

Another alternative is a Silastic seminal fluid collecting device or a plastic condom. However, use of a plastic condom may affect sperm viability (Corriere, 1986). A regular condom cannot be used for specimen collection because it may contain a spermicide, powder, or other additive that can affect seminal fluid or damage sperm.

Ideally, the client provides a semen specimen while at the health care facility. As an alternative, he may collect it at home and bring it to the facility. However, such specimens frequently show decreased motility if the trip takes longer than 90 minutes or if the specimen is exposed to cold temperatures. To keep the specimen warm in cold weather, the client should hold the container next to his skin or in an inside pocket.

Upon analysis, the specimen should be within the normal ranges for semen liquefaction, volume, and pH and for sperm morphology, motility, and quantity.

Inadequate numbers of sperm, abnormal sperm morphology (such as double-headed sperm or sperm with abnormal heads or tails), inadequate sperm motility, or too much or too little seminal fluid points to the male client as the cause of infertility. For example, sperm with abnormal motility cannot travel through the uterus to the end of the fallopian tubes where fertilization occurs. A seminal volume below 2 ml may cause inadequate pooling of semen at the cervical os; a volume above 6 ml may dilute the concentration of sperm.

Hamster zona-free ova test. Even if the semen analysis is normal, the client may undergo the hamster zona-free ova test to assess sperm further. In this test, the client's sperm are mixed with hamster ova that have the zona pellucida (ova membrane) removed. Normally, the sperm easily penetrate the zona-free ova. Sperm that cannot penetrate may have an enzymatic defect, which would cause infertility.

Nursing diagnosis

After considering the assessment findings, formulate appropriate nursing diagnoses for each client. (For a partial list of applicable diagnoses, see *Nursing diagnoses: Infertile client.*)

Planning and implementation

The nurse plays an active role in the therapeutic management of infertility, especially in an infertility clinic. Here, the nurse answers questions, provides instructions, coordinates treatments, performs many diagnostic tests, and administers prescribed treatments. No matter what the setting, however, the nurse must be prepared to counsel the couple, making referrals as needed.

Based on assessment data and nursing diagnoses, develop an appropriate plan of care and establish goals to meet that plan. To achieve these goals, use such interventions as teaching about fertility and infertility, diagnostic studies, and treatments; coordinating care; counseling about sexual dysfunction; providing support; caring for the family; and making referrals.

Teach about fertility and infertility

To correct a **knowledge deficit related to factors that promote fertility,** candidly discuss fertility and all the factors that can promote it. (For more information, see *Client teaching: Actions that promote fertility,* page 216.) An understanding of these matters not only will promote health practices that favor fertility, but also may help minimize **anxiety related to infertility.**

Teach about diagnostic studies

The client or couple may have a nursing diagnosis of **anxiety related to infertility tests** or **knowledge deficit related to infertility tests.** If so, develop and conduct teaching sessions with the client or couple. (For details, see *Applying the nursing process: Clients with a knowledge deficit related to infertility tests,* pages 222 and 223.)

Teaching about tests can help the client or couple understand their role in the plan of care, promote self-care in infertility management, give them a sense of control over a situation that easily could make them feel powerless, and help ensure their active participation in the infertility tests.

Teach about treatments for the female client

For a female client with a nursing diagnosis of **anxiety related to infertility treatments** or **knowledge deficit related to infertility treatments,** plan one or more teaching sessions. Treatment depends on the structure affected and the underlying cause.

NURSING DIAGNOSES

Infertile client

The following nursing diagnoses address representative problems and etiologies that a nurse may encounter when caring for an infertile client or couple. Specific nursing interventions for many of these diagnoses are provided in the "Planning and implementation" section of this chapter.

- Altered family processes related to different goals concerning infertility
- Altered family processes related to the stress of infertility
- Anticipatory grieving related to infertility
- Anxiety related to infertility
- Anxiety related to infertility tests
- Anxiety related to infertility treatments
- Body image disturbance related to infertility
- Dysfunctional grieving related to infertility
- Impaired adjustment related to childlessness
- Impaired verbal communication related to relationship dysfunction
- Ineffective family coping: compromised, related to infertility
- Ineffective individual coping related to infertility
- Ineffective individual coping related to infertility treatments
- Knowledge deficit related to factors that promote fertility
- Knowledge deficit related to infertility
- Knowledge deficit related to infertility tests
- Knowledge deficit related to infertility treatments
- Knowledge deficit related to sexual practices that maximize the chance of conception
- Pain related to endometrial biopsy
- Powerlessness related to inability to control fertility
- Sexual dysfunction related to the need for sexual performance for diagnostic tests
- Sexual dysfunction related to the need for sexual performance on schedule
- Social isolation related to lack of children

Uterine treatments. About 25% of women with uterine anomalies have problems with fertility. Although these women usually can conceive, they may have difficulty carrying the pregnancy to term (Golan, Langer, Bukovsky, and Caspi, 1989). Surgical reconstruction of the uterus may restore fertility if the woman does not have ovarian agenesis (failure of ovaries to develop) or dysgenesis (abnormal ovary development). Uterine infections are treated with organism-specific antibiotics. However, if the infection is not treated early enough to prevent scarring, surgery also may be needed.

Tubal treatments. In the United States, about 1 million women are treated each year for acute salpingitis (fallopian tube infection). Of these, approximately 20% will

CLIENT TEACHING

Actions that promote fertility

To maximize the chance of conception, take these actions that promote fertility.

For the female client

- Always wipe from front to back after urinating or defecating. This keeps your perineal area clean and reduces the risk of vaginal and cervical infections that can cause infertility.
- Avoid using douches, irritating soaps, perfumed bubble baths, and feminine hygiene sprays to prevent genital irritation, which can lead to infection.
- Avoid tight clothing because it limits air circulation to the perineal area. These actions also prevent pH alteration that can compromise fertility.
- Be aware that your ability to become pregnant may be delayed for 2 to 3 months after you stop taking birth control pills or have an intrauterine device (IUD) removed.
- Remain supine with your hips elevated on a pillow and avoid urinating for 1 hour after intercourse to prevent sperm loss.

For the male client

- Avoid exposure to toxic substances and chemicals, which can alter your ability to make sperm.
- Avoid long, hot baths and tight underwear and pants, which can cause heat and decrease the sperm count over time. Instead, wear loose-fitting pants and underwear, such as boxer shorts.

This teaching aid may be reproduced by office copier for distribution to clients.
© 1991, Springhouse Corporation.

For the couple

- Eat a well-balanced diet that includes at least two servings from the milk group, two from the meat group, four from the fruit-vegetable group (including one good source of vitamin C and one of vitamin A), and four from the bread group.
- Exercise at least three times a week for a minimum of 20 continuous minutes each session. During your workout, maintain an exercise pulse rate of 70% to 85% of its maximum capability for your age.
- Limit your alcohol intake to no more than 1 ounce of alcohol a day. In men, alcohol can reduce fertility; in women, it can cause fetal abnormalities.
- Avoid using over-the-counter and illegal drugs, and discuss the use of prescription drugs with your doctor. Drugs may affect fertility.
- Avoid environmental hazards at work, at home, or in the community. To do this, use protective clothing and equipment, substitute less dangerous substances at home, or consider a job transfer, if necessary.
- Be alert for the most fertile period: the middle of the woman's menstrual cycle (day 14 of a 28-day cycle).
- Use the basal body temperature (BBT) recording and cervical mucus characteristics to help identify the fertile period.
- Have sexual intercourse every other day during the fertile period to increase the chance of conception.
- Do not use a lubricant during sexual intercourse because it could kill the sperm.
- Have sexual intercourse with the man on top to maximize penetration.

develop infertility from the infection. Treatment for tubal factors includes early diagnosis and antibiotic therapy to prevent tubal scarring and blockage. If blockage occurs, laparoscopic microsurgery may be used to divide and remove adhesions. If extensive repair is required, a laparotomy (4″ to 5″ abdominal incision below the umbilicus) may be performed.

In a client whose tubes cannot be repaired, in vitro fertilization (IVF) may offer hope. The first successful human IVF birth occurred in 1978 in England when Louise Brown was born. In IVF, the physician obtains oocytes from the client, mixes them with her partner's sperm, incubates them, and then returns the embryos to the uterus to grow and develop.

Although IVF success rates have increased, they are only 15% to 30% (National IVF-ET Registry, 1989; Testart, Belaisch-Allart, and Frydman, 1989). In addition, IVF requires time, money, and emotional commitment by the couple.

IVF initially was used for women with blocked fallopian tubes. Now it may be used for couples with infertility that does not respond to conventional treatments, men with oligospermia (inadequate number of sperm), women with endometriosis, and couples with abnormal results on postcoital examination.

Before IVF, the physician counsels and thoroughly examines the couple. Their diagnostic studies are checked to ensure a complete infertility evaluation was performed. In many IVF centers, a psychologist also interviews the couple to ensure they are psychologically stable and prepared for the procedure.

Then the client undergoes ovulation induction. (For a description of this procedure, see the discussion on the ovulatory phase under "Hormone treatments.") When the follicles are fully developed, she receives general anesthesia and the physician obtains mature oocytes using laparoscopic surgery or transvaginal retrieval with ultrasound guidance (Lopata and May, 1989). With transvaginal retrieval, the physician obtains occytes by going through the vagina, behind the uterus, and to the ovary. Then the physician aspirates each mature follicle, evaluates the oocytes microscopically, and assesses their maturity. About 8 hours later, the mature oocytes are mixed in a petri dish with the partner's prepared sperm. Then the mixture is incubated, and fertilization and division are assessed periodically.

Forty-eight hours after oocyte collection, the physician transfers up to four fertilized embryos to the uterine fundus using a special Teflon catheter inserted through the cervix. The client must remain supine for several hours after the embryo transfer. Untransferred embryos may be cryopreserved (stored under freezing temperatures) and transferred at a later date (Lopata and May, 1989).

For the next few weeks, serum levels of human chorionic gonadotropin (hCG) are closely monitored. A rise in hCG level indicates that pregnancy has occurred. The pregnancy is assessed at 6 to 8 weeks by ultrasound to document that the embryo is implanted in the uterus and to determine that fetal cardiac activity exists.

Vaginal and cervical treatments. The vaginal and cervical environments can be hostile to sperm. Vaginal fluid normally is acidic (pH < 5); cervical mucus, more alkaline (pH > 6). Because sperm fare better in an alkaline environment, those deposited near the cervical os have a better chance of surviving and ascending into the uterus and fallopian tubes. Because infections can alter this environment, they are treated with appropriate antibiotics. Cryosurgery (application of extreme cold to destroy damaged tissue) has been used to treat chronic cervical infections (Bayless and Boyers, 1988).

A stenosed (narrowed) cervical os can be widened by gentle dilation. A cervix that is too wide can be reduced by suturing or cryosurgery to prevent pregnancy loss. Cervical mucus that is not conducive to sperm transport and cannot be corrected may be bypassed with intrauterine artificial insemination.

Hormone treatments. Infertility caused by a hormonal factor may be treated with drugs or advanced technology. (For more information, see *Selected major drugs: Drugs used to treat infertility*, pages 218 and 219.)

Ovulatory phase. Ovulatory dysfunction, which accounts for 10% to 25% of female infertility (Boyers and Jones, 1988), usually can be treated successfully. When ovulatory dysfunction results from an oral contraceptive or IUD, the client must discontinue its use. When ovulatory dysfunction results from anovulation, treatment may include ovulation induction with various drugs.

With ovulation induction, treatment is progressive, usually beginning with clomiphene citrate (Clomid, Serophene). If the client does not ovulate, she receives a higher clomiphene dosage. Then if she fails to ovulate, she also receives an hCG injection at midcycle.

If the client still fails to ovulate, she may receive human menopausal gonadotropin (HMG, Pergonal) to stimulate follicular growth. Her HMG dosage depends on daily serum assays of estradiol, a hormone produced by maturing oocytes, and her follicular development is closely monitored by ultrasound. After HMG has successfully stimulated the follicles, she receives hCG to induce ovulation. The hCG mimics the LH surge in the body and causes ovulation within 36 hours. She should have intercourse 24 to 48 hours later. If estradiol levels exceed 2,000 pg/ml, hCG is withheld to prevent ovarian hyperstimulation syndrome. If more than four large follicles are present, hCG is withheld to prevent multiple gestation (Lightman, Jones, and Boyers, 1988).

A client who ovulates but does not become pregnant after ovulation induction may be a candidate for gamete intrafallopian transfer (GIFT). First described in 1984, this procedure transfers oocytes and sperm into the distal end of a fallopian tube. GIFT differs from IVF in that fertilization takes place in vivo (in the fallopian tube) rather than in vitro (in a petri dish). It is a major advance in infertility treatment related to endometriosis, unexplained infertility, sperm deficiencies, and cervical mucus hostility because its success rate (about 25%) is higher than that of IVF (National IVF-ET Registry, 1989).

Preparation for GIFT parallels that for IVF. It begins with an in-depth consultation with the physician about the procedure and its success rates. It continues with a thorough physical examination of both partners.

The GIFT procedure is similar to IVF. However, it takes only 40 to 60 minutes, and the client usually can be discharged the same day.

Some clinics use donor sperm and oocytes for GIFT. An English clinic reports a success rate of 35% with donor sperm and 40% with donor oocytes (Fincham, 1987). American clinics report about a 20% success rate with donor oocytes (National IVF-ET Registry, 1989).

Luteal phase. Luteal phase deficiency occurs in 3% to 5% of all infertile women and in up to 35% of women with recurrent first trimester abortions.

Treatments vary for luteal phase deficiency. Vaginal suppositories of hydroxyprogesterone may be prescribed.

(Text continues on page 220.)

SELECTED MAJOR DRUGS

Drugs used to treat infertility

Various drugs are available to treat female and male infertility. The chart below summarizes the major drugs currently in clinical use.

DRUGS	MAJOR INDICATIONS	USUAL ADULT DOSAGE	NURSING IMPLICATIONS
bromocriptine mesylate (Parlodel)	*Female:* Anovulation caused by hyperprolactinemia	2.5 mg P.O. b.i.d., increased every 3 to 7 days up to 15 mg daily until prolactin levels reach the normal range	• Advise the client to take the drug with meals to help prevent nausea and vomiting. • Instruct the client to record her basal body temperature (BBT) to determine when ovulation occurs. • Teach the client to report the following adverse reactions: nausea, vomiting, constipation or diarrhea, abdominal cramps, headache, fatigue, dizziness, light-headedness, or nasal congestion. • Advise the client that orthostatic hypotension may occur, especially at the beginning of the treatment. • Reassure the client that her period should return within 2 months. Advise her to use a barrier contraceptive method to prevent pregnancy until then because the risk of spontaneous abortion is increased during this period. • Discontinue the drug as soon as the client becomes pregnant.
	Male: Hypogonadotropic hypogonadism caused by hyperprolactinemia	2.5 mg P.O. b.i.d., increased every 3 to 7 days until prolactin is suppressed	• Advise the client to take the drug with meals to help prevent nausea and vomiting. • Teach the client to report the following adverse reactions: nausea, vomiting, constipation or diarrhea, abdominal cramps, headache, fatigue, dizziness, light-headedness, or nasal congestion. • Advise the client that orthostatic hypotension may occur, especially at the beginning of the treatment.
clomiphene citrate (Clomid, Serophene)	*Female:* Ovulation induction to stimulate follicle-stimulating hormone (FSH) production	50 to 200 mg P.O. daily on cycle days 3 to 7 or 5 to 9	• Teach the client when to take the drug. • Instruct the client to take and record her BBT daily to help determine if ovulation has occurred. • Advise the client that she may experience minor hot flushes, lower abdominal or pelvic pain, breast tenderness, visual disturbances, dizziness, or light-headedness. Tell her to report any severe pain or unusual symptoms. Severe abdominal pain may indicate ovarian cyst formation. • Caution against performing hazardous tasks requiring alertness or physical coordination. • Advise the client that the risk of multiple births—especially twins—is slightly higher than normal during clomiphene therapy.
	Male: Oligospermia caused by FSH deficiency	25 mg P.O. daily for 25 days, no medication for 5 days, then repeat	• Advise the client to take the drug at the same time every day to help him remember to do it.

SELECTED MAJOR DRUGS

Drugs used to treat infertility   continued

DRUGS	MAJOR INDICATIONS	USUAL ADULT DOSAGE	NURSING IMPLICATIONS
danazol (Danocrine)	*Female:* Endometriosis	200 to 400 mg P.O. b.i.d., beginning with menses and continuing for up to 6 months	• Teach the client how to take the drug, beginning with her next menses. • Advise the client that danazol may produce adverse reactions, such as weight gain, hot flushes, mood disturbances, skin eruptions, decreased breast size, and atrophic vaginitis. • Instruct the client to report any severe adverse reactions and to contact her physician if she cannot adjust to these reactions. • Advise the client not to take danazol during pregnancy.
dexamethasone (Decadron)	*Female:* Ovulatory disturbances caused by high levels of dehydroepiandrosterone	0.5 mg P.O. daily at bedtime	• Teach the client to take the drug nightly with clomiphene. • Advise the client to take the drug with food to avoid stomach upset.
gonadotropin-releasing hormone [GnRH] (Factrel)	*Female:* Ovulation induction in a client who has not ovulated in response to clomiphene citrate, HMG, or hCG therapy	20 to 40 mcg S.C. every 2 hours starting on cycle day 3	• Teach the client how to administer GnRH by infusion pump. • Use serum estradiol (E_2) levels and ultrasonography to monitor follicular growth beginning on cycle day 8. • Teach the client to report immediately any signs of ovarian hyperstimulation syndrome, such as abdominal pain or swelling.
human chorionic gonadotropin [hCG] (A.P.L., Pregnyl, Profasi)	*Female:* Ovulation induction to simulate the luteinizing hormone surge	10,000 IU I.M. given at midcycle	• Keep in mind that hCG may be administered with other drugs, such as clomiphene citrate and HMG, to induce ovulation. • Do not administer hCG if the client's E_2 levels exceed 2,000 pg/ml or if they fall between 1,500 and 2,000 pg/ml and rise more than 50% in 1 day. • Do not administer hCG if more than four fully developed follicles appear on ultrasonography. • Teach the client the signs of ovarian hyperstimulation syndrome and instruct her to report them immediately.
human menopausal gonadotropin [HMG] (Pergonal)	*Female:* Ovulation induction in hypogonadotropic amenorrhea, luteal phase deficiency that is unresponsive to other therapy, follicular stimulation for gamete intrafallopian transfer, or in vitro fertilization	150 IU I.M. on cycle days 3 to 7, followed by daily dosages based on E_2 levels and the number of maturing follicles detected by pelvic ultrasonography	• Teach the client how to administer the drug I.M. at home, if desired. • Inform the client that ovarian hyperstimulation syndrome can occur, causing ascites, pleural effusion, hypotension, dyspnea, electrolyte abnormalities, and possibly death. Instruct her to report abdominal pain or swelling immediately. • Advise the client that the chance of multiple births is increased with HMG therapy. • Teach the client about the treatment regimen and the importance of serial E_2 readings and pelvic ultrasonography.
	Male: Oligospermia caused by FSH deficiency	75 IU I.M. at least three times a week for 6 months; usually used with hCG 2,000 IU twice a week	• Teach the client to administer I.M. injections at home, if desired. • Advise the client that HMG may cause temporary gynecomastia (breast enlargement).

If necessary, clomiphene citrate may be used with hydroxyprogesterone to resolve the deficiency (Keenan, Hebert, Bush, and Wentz, 1989; Murray, Reich, and Adashi, 1989). When this combined drug therapy fails to produce normal endometrial development, hCG may be given alone or with HMG. These drugs facilitate ovulation and follicular stimulation, respectively. In clients with infertility caused solely by luteal phase deficiency, treatment produces pregnancy rates of up to 85% (Wentz, 1988). Those who do not respond to HMG therapy may undergo GIFT.

Endometriosis. The most effective drug for treating endometriosis is danazol (Danocrine), which creates pseudomenopause that aids in the regression of endometriosis by halting hormonal stimulation. Danazol therapy may precede or follow adhesion removal through surgery using laser vaporization, cauterization, or excision. Clients with mild endometriosis who undergo surgery and take danazol have the highest pregnancy rates. Unfortunately, danazol may produce adverse reactions, such as weight gain and mood swings, that the client may find unacceptable.

An experimental treatment for endometriosis is gonadotropin-releasing hormone agonist (GnRHa), which binds to the gonadotropin-releasing hormone receptor sites in the pituitary gland, interrupts the pituitary-ovarian feedback axis, and reduces estrogen production. When estrogen levels are reduced, endometriosis regresses. The client must take GnRHa intranasally by spray, 300 mcg t.i.d. for 6 months (Franssen, Kauer, Chadha, Zijlstra, and Rolland, 1989). For a client with normal fallopian tubes and mild endometriosis who does not conceive, GIFT may be used. (For more information see *Gamete intrafallopian transfer.*)

Teach about treatments for the male client

When a male client has a nursing diagnosis of *anxiety related to infertility treatments* or *knowledge deficit related to infertility treatments,* teach him about treatments for spermatogenesis, structural problems, or other treatments, as needed.

Spermatogenesis treatments. Treatment for idiopathic oligospermia (inadequate number of sperm in ejaculate from an unknown cause) is controversial and typically unsuccessful. However, oligospermia from environmental and toxic substance exposure usually corrects itself when exposure ends. Oligospermia caused by infection is treated with antibiotics.

Clomiphene citrate may correct spermatogenesis problems by stimulating FSH, which is necessary for spermatogenesis. Hormone therapy may be used for a client with an endocrine disorder. For example, a client with an FSH deficiency from hypothyroidism may receive thyroid replacement hormones and hCG or HMG. If the client has autoantibodies to sperm, he may receive prednisone (Behrman and Patton, 1988).

Structural treatments. When physical obstructions cause infertility, microsurgery usually is successful, especially for hypospadias and epididymal obstructions. Varicocelectomy (surgical removal of dilated veins in the spermatic cord) may raise sperm counts and improve motility.

Teach about treatments for combined problems

Treatment for combined problems with spermatogenesis, structure, and sexual function typically includes artificial insemination. Artificial insemination refers to instillation of the partner's sperm or a donor's sperm into the female client's vagina for conception. It may be conducted when the semen is abnormal.

Indications for artificial insemination with sperm from the partner (AIH, or homologous insemination) include impotence, retrograde ejaculation, and availability of cryopreserved sperm from a partner who later had a vasectomy. AIH also may be used if the female client has vaginismus, intense vaginal muscle contractions that tightly close the vaginal introitus (Lavy and Boyers, 1988). The success rate of AIH is low. However, couples who conceive with AIH usually do so in the first four cycles.

If the male client has a normal semen analysis with adequate sperm count and morphology, whole semen is used. If not, several split ejaculates can be combined to increase the sperm count. (A split ejaculate refers to the first portion of the ejaculate, which contains the largest concentration of sperm.)

Artificial insemination with donor sperm (AID, or heterologous insemination) is used when the client has azoospermia (lack of sperm in semen) or has oligospermia and has already tried AIH without success. Other indications for AID include abnormal sperm morphology; vasectomy with poor prognosis for reversal or with reversal failure and no cryopreserved sperm; a known genetic disorder; untreatable ejaculatory failure caused by trauma, drugs, surgery, neurologic disease, or spinal cord injury; or severe Rh-sensitization of the woman to her Rh-positive partner (Hummel and Talbert, 1989).

Donors are screened thoroughly for medical and genetic problems, and their semen is analyzed and tested for STDs. The American Fertility Society and the Centers for Disease Control recommend that the semen also be

Gamete intrafallopian transfer

Before the gamete intrafallopian transfer (GIFT) procedure begins, the female client receives drugs to stimulate follicle development. When daily serum estradiol (E₂) levels and ultrasonography indicate well-developed follicles, the client receives 10,000 IU of human chorionic gonadotropin (hCG) I.M. Because ovulation will occur within 36 hours, laparoscopic surgery for oocyte collection is scheduled within 30 hours after the client receives hCG. Just before surgery, ultrasonography is performed to ensure that the ovaries have not yet released the mature oocytes.

Under laparoscopic guidance, the physician collects the mature oocytes and sends them to the laboratory where they are mixed with the partner's prepared sperm. When the mixture is returned to the operating room, the physician loads a thin Teflon catheter with the mixture and places it inside a special cannula. Then the physician passes the filled cannula into the distal end of the fallopian tube and deposits the sperm and oocyte mixture ½″ to ¾″ (1.3 to 2 cm) inside the fallopian tube, as shown. This allows fertilization in vivo.

If the equipment cannot adequately enter the fallopian tube, the physician stops the GIFT procedure and returns the sperm and oocyte mixture to the laboratory for in vitro fertilization at a later date.

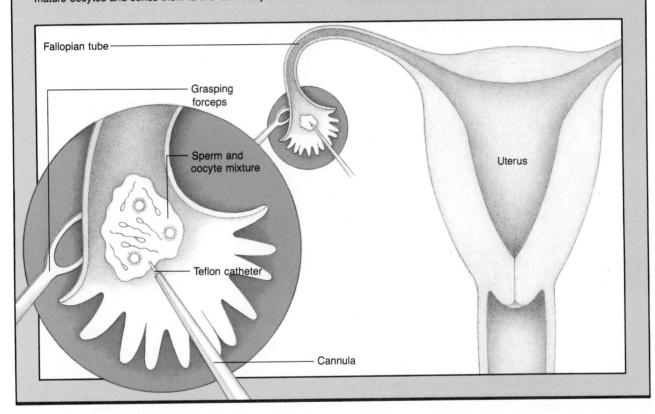

Fallopian tube

Grasping forceps

Sperm and oocyte mixture

Teflon catheter

Cannula

Uterus

tested for such diseases as hepatitis and cytomegalovirus or human immunodeficiency virus infection, frozen and quarantined for 6 months, and tested again before use. Freezing of semen has another advantage. Samples from the same donor can be stored and used when the couple desire a second child. Donors are matched to the client's race and physical characteristics (eye color, hair color, height, blood type, and Rh factor).

AIH or AID is scheduled to coincide with ovulation. The BBT should not have risen, the cervical os should be open with abundant clear mucus, and the LH levels should be increased. The female client is placed in the lithotomy position and draped. Then her cervix is exposed with a vaginal speculum. After drawing up the specimen into a long catheter attached to a syringe, the physician or specially trained nurse inseminates her by injecting the semen into the uterus or cervix or by dripping it across the cervical os and using a cervical cap to allow pooling. She remains in this position with her hips elevated for 20 to 30 minutes.

Dripping the specimen across the os simulates the natural depositing of semen during intercourse and is the preferred technique. Intracervical or intrauterine insemination may be used in a client with repeated abnormal postcoital examinations, scant cervical mucus, or cervical os stenosis. However, intrauterine insemi-

(Text continues on page 224.)

Clients with a knowledge deficit related to infertility tests

The table below shows how the nurse might use the nursing process to ensure high-quality care for the infertile couple described in the case history at right. The first column presents history and physical assessment data followed by a paragraph of mental notes. These notes help the nurse make important mental connections among assessment findings, aiding in development of the nursing diagnosis and planning.

The second column lists an appropriate nursing diagnosis; information in the remaining columns is based on this diagnosis. Although not part of the nursing process, a rationale appears for each intervention in the fourth column to explain how it contributes to the care plan.

ASSESSMENT	NURSING DIAGNOSIS	PLANNING
Subjective (history) data • Mrs. Iverson says that she has been trying to conceive for 1½ years. • Mrs. Iverson reports that she began menstruating at age 11. • Mrs. Iverson states that her menstrual periods occur every 29 days and last for 5 days with heavy flow on days 2 and 3, moderate-to-light flow on the other days, and occasional, mild cramps that are relieved with aspirin. • Mrs. Iverson states that her last menstrual period was 3 weeks ago. • Mr. Iverson states he was married to another woman at age 18 for 2 years and has one child from that union. • Mr. and Mrs. Iverson report understanding the menstrual cycle and the best time for conception to occur; they are not familiar with basal body temperature (BBT) or techniques that foster conception. **Objective (physical) data** *Mrs. Iverson* • 5'3", 132 lb. • Temperature 98.4° F, pulse 88 beats/minute, respirations 22/minute, blood pressure 120/84 mm Hg. • Well-developed female client with normal development of secondary sex characteristics and female hair distribution pattern. • Normal breast development for client's age and sex. Breast examination findings within normal limits. • Pelvic examination findings within normal limits. *Mr. Iverson* • 6'2", 198 lb. • Temperature 97.8°F, pulse 80 beats/minute, respirations 20/minute, blood pressure 128/86 mm Hg. • Well-developed male client with normal development of secondary sex characteristics and male hair distribution pattern. • Penis and scrotum assessment findings within normal limits. **Mental notes** *The physician has requested that Mrs. Iverson begin monitoring her BBT and cervical mucus and that Mr. Iverson provide a semen specimen for analysis. Because Mr. Iverson came with his wife today, now is the perfect time to obtain a fresh semen specimen. Like most infertile couples, Mr. and Mrs. Iverson seem anxious, but motivated, attentive, and ready to participate in the teaching process. To help them feel comfortable sharing concerns and telephoning with questions or problems, I will need to establish a therapeutic relationship with them.*	Knowledge deficit related to infertility tests	**Goals** By the end of this visit, the couple will be able to: • describe how to monitor BBT and cervical mucus • list techniques that promote conception • explain the steps in the diagnostic process.

CASE STUDY

Cindy Iverson, a secretary age 26, and her husband Tony, a real estate salesperson age 28, come to the clinic for diagnosis and treatment of infertility. They have been married for 5 years and have been trying unsuccessfully to conceive for 1½ years.

IMPLEMENTATION		EVALUATION
Intervention Explain the importance of monitoring BBT and cervical mucus.	**Rationale** An understanding of the importance of BBT and cervical mucus recordings may increase compliance with infertility treatments.	Upon evaluation, the couple: • described the importance of monitoring BBT and cervical mucus • demonstrated how to take the BBT and record it on the BBT graph • discussed techniques they could use to promote conception • described the next steps in the diagnostic process.
Teach Mrs. Iverson how to take her BBT and monitor cervical mucus.	Knowledge about these records can make the couple aware of the fertile period.	
Show her how to record the data on a BBT graph.	Accurate recording of data is necessary to schedule certain diagnostic tests and treatments.	
Describe to both clients those techniques that promote conception, including having intercourse every other day during the fertile period, ejaculating deep in the vagina, and elevating the hips on a pillow for 30 minutes after intercourse.	These techniques can increase the chance of conception.	
Discuss the steps in the diagnostic process.	An understanding of the diagnostic process may help relieve anxiety and give the couple a sense of control.	
Give the couple printed material about BBT recordings and other studies.	Printed materials can help reinforce the couple's learning.	

nation can stimulate prostaglandin release, causing painful cramping.

Artifical insemination, IVF, and GIFT offer new hope to many infertile men. Pregnancies have resulted with these procedures in couples with chronic infertility associated with the man.

When infertility results from combined hormonal or structural factors in both partners, each problem must be treated separately, as described earlier. When infertility is caused by other problems, the couple simply may need detailed instructions.

For example, if the female client has an immune response to her partner's sperm, teach her to avoid direct contact with his ejaculate by using a condom during intercourse. After 6 months, this practice should reduce the antibody level and allow conception to occur. If stress or lack of knowledge is causing infertility, teach the couple stress management techniques and provide information about fertility and sexuality. If sexual dysfunction is implicated, teach the couple to avoid drugs that can affect sexual functioning, provide counseling as discussed above, and make referrals, as needed.

Coordinate care

When caring for an infertile couple, expect to coordinate and manage their care. For example, maintain telephone contact with them between visits, help them interpret BBT recordings, and schedule tests according to the woman's cycle date.

When working on an IVF or GIFT team, act as the case manager. Coordinate tests and treatments and ensure that they occur at the appropriate time during the client's menstrual cycle. The timing of medications, monitoring procedures, and oocyte recovery is crucial to the procedure's success. Educate the couple about the procedure, listen to their frustrations, and provide encouragement.

Counsel about sexual dysfunction

A male client may develop *sexual dysfunction related to the need for sexual performance on schedule* or *sexual dysfunction related to the need for sexual performance for diagnostic tests.* Similarly, a female client may complain that sexual intercourse has become unsatisfying or that her libido has decreased. Impotence and other problems may result when the goal of intercourse becomes conception or specimen collection rather than affection or pleasure. To reduce anxiety and promote normal sexual functioning, counsel the female client to avoid informing her partner of her fertile period and then demanding intercourse. Encourage both partners to express feelings about sex on demand. Suggest that they explore ways to create a romantic atmosphere for sexual intercourse.

Provide support

If either client has a nursing diagnosis of *ineffective individual coping related to infertility treatments, ineffective family coping: compromised, related to infertility,* or *body image disturbance related to infertility,* provide emotional support. To help improve self-concept, listen actively to the couple's concerns and assure them that their frustrations are normal. To help establish effective coping mechanisms and facilitate adjustment, provide information and support to prepare them for each step of the evaluation and treatment process.

Keep in mind that infertility can become a crisis for the couple. Be alert for signs of a developing crisis, such as a marked change in behavior. Be prepared to use crisis intervention techniques and make referrals, as needed.

A client who perceives infertility as a loss may develop a nursing diagnosis of *anticipatory grieving related to infertility* or *dysfunctional grieving related to infertility.* If so, encourage the couple to express and deal with their feelings to help them cope with their grief. If they cannot cope, make a referral for individual or family therapy.

Stress may be the cause—or the result—of infertility. In either case, the couple may have a nursing diagnosis of *altered family processes related to the stress of infertility* or *impaired verbal communication related to relationship dysfunction.* To help them deal with stress, which can compromise treatment and perpetuate infertility, teach them to use stress management techniques and open communication. If necessary, refer them for additional help.

Care for the family

If infertility treatment is not successful, help the couple consider alternatives to conceiving their own child. This may allow them to review their options and adapt effectively to infertility. For example, the infertile couple may want to consider adoption. Those who decide to adopt typically believe that having a child is most important—not that a child be biologically theirs. However, a female client who adopts still may yearn for the pregnancy experience. If so, reassure her that these feelings are normal and common.

If the couple decide to adopt, prepare them for the process. Because healthy adoptable infants—especially Caucasian ones—are scarce, the decision to adopt requires a serious emotional commitment. The couple may have to deal with numerous adoption agencies and their requirements and cost. They may have to be investigated by an adoption agency and wait several years before they get a child. However, if they are willing to accept an older child or a disabled child, they may not have to wait as long.

Make referrals

When the couple's needs exceed the health care team's ability to provide care, refer them to the appropriate support group or other resource. Resources for an infertile couple may include Resolve (a national organization with support groups in 35 states), DES Action USA (an information and support organization for women exposed to DES), and the Endometriosis Association (an organization that offers support and education about endometriosis).

Evaluation

To evaluate nursing care, determine if the goals were achieved. Obviously, if the female client becomes pregnant and gives birth, the couple's most important goal has been met. However, because infertility treatment is not always successful, some couples will not be able to conceive their own child. For such a couple, evaluate their care in terms of how well they are coping with infertility. If they complete the grieving process and feel that life is meaningful and satisfying without the traditional family, then they have met their most important goal: carrying on with their lives.

Be sure to state evaluation findings in terms of action performed or outcomes achieved for each goal. The following examples illustrate some appropriate evaluation statements:
• The couple accurately described actions that promote fertility.
• The couple actively participated in infertility tests and treatments.
• The couple openly expressed feelings about infertility.
• The couple successfully coped with the stress of infertility tests and treatments.
• The couple reported resolution of grief related to infertility.
• The couple discussed alternatives to conceiving their own child.
• The couple reported little change in their relationship.

Documentation

Using the appropriate records, document all steps of the nursing process, including assessment data, nursing diagnoses, the plan of care, implementation activities, and evaluation findings. Also document other aspects of infertility care, such as diagnostic tests and treatments and the clients' response to them.

When caring for an infertile couple, documentation should include:
• significant health history findings
• significant physical assessment findings
• diagnostic studies performed and results
• the couple's understanding of fertility and related factors
• instructions given about infertility tests and treatments
• the couple's understanding of instructions
• the couple's emotional response to infertility and related tests and treatments
• referrals made.

Chapter summary

Chapter 10 described how to assist a client or couple with preconception planning or infertility. Here are the key concepts.
• Different cultures may have different myths and beliefs about fertility, but they all value it highly.
• Preconception planning can increase the chances of a successful pregnancy.
• During the preconception assessment, the nurse screens the client and her partner for factors that may place the client—or her fetus—at high risk for complications during pregnancy. The nurse also carefully evaluates the couple's current health habits, motives, and plans for having a child and the stability of their relationship.
• The nurse can promote preconception health by teaching self-care activities, providing nutrition information, promoting exercise and rest, and discussing discontinuation of contraception. The nurse also provides care for the family.
• Female or male problems or both can cause infertility.
• Female problems implicated in infertility can be structural or hormonal. Structural problems may affect the uterus, fallopian tubes, vagina, or cervix. Hormonal ab-

normalities may cause ovulatory or luteal phase problems or endometriosis.

• Male problems associated with infertility may affect spermatogenesis, reproductive tract structures, or sexual function.

• A couple's combined infertility problems may include immune response, stress, lack of knowledge, and sexual dysfunction.

• An emotional crisis for the couple who desire children, infertility can affect their relationship adversely.

• The nurse should obtain separate health histories from both partners. The female client's health history should cover biographical data and menstrual and obstetric history; the male client's health history should cover fertility history and environmental health. The combined health history should cover contraceptive, infertility, medical, surgical, and sexual history. It also should include evaluation of nutrition, personal, and exercise habits; cultural and religious background; and psychosocial status for both.

• During the physical assessment, the nurse should focus on evaluation of the reproductive and endocrine systems of each partner.

• Diagnostic studies for the female client may include BBT recording, cervical mucus evaluation, blood and urine tests, special tests, sperm antibody agglutination test, postcoital examination, endometrial biopsy, hysterosalpingography, pelvic ultrasonography, and laparoscopy. Studies for the male client may include blood and urine tests, special tests, semen analysis, and the hamster zona-free ova test.

• The nurse plays a crucial role in caring for the infertile couple. Key interventions include teaching about fertility and infertility, diagnostic studies, and treatments; managing care; counseling about sexual dysfunction; providing support; caring for the family; and making referrals.

• Infertility treatments can be costly, time-consuming, and sometimes ineffective. Treatments for male and female infertility include drugs to induce ovulation and spermatogenesis, and such procedures as AIH, AID, GIFT, and IVF.

Study questions

1. Ms. Berger, age 24, is a mother of two who occasionally uses cocaine. She smokes two packs of cigarettes daily and eats sporadically. Which health habits should the nurse evaluate before Ms. Berger conceives?

What difficulties may occur if this client fails to modify her health habits?

2. What is infertility and how may it affect a couple emotionally? How can the nurse help an infertile couple cope with their inability to have a child?

3. Which problems or dysfunctions may be implicated in infertility in a female client? A male client? Which diagnostic studies are likely to be used for each client?

4. What are the nurse's responsibilities in caring for an infertile couple?

5. How does IVF compare with GIFT? What is the nurse's role in these procedures?

Bibliography

Corriere, J. (1986). *Essentials of urology.* New York: Churchill Livingstone.

Cunningham, F., McDonald, P., and Gant, N. (1989). *Williams obstetrics* (18th ed.). East Norwalk, CT: Appleton & Lange.

Griffith-Kenney, J. (1986). *Contemporary women's health: A nursing advocacy approach.* Menlo Park, CA: Addison-Wesley.

Lewis, S., and Collier, I. (1987). *Medical surgical nursing assessment and management of clinical problems* (2nd ed.). New York: McGraw-Hill.

Speroff, L. (1987). The epidemiology of fertility and infertility. Presentation at the twentieth postgraduate course. Reno: American Fertility Society.

Yen, S., and Jaffe, R. (1986). *Reproductive endocrinology: Physiology, pathophysiology, and clinical management* (2nd ed.). Philadelphia: W.B. Saunders.

Preconception planning

Alexander, L. (1987). The pregnant smoker: Nursing implications. *JOGNN, 16*(3), 163-173.

Cranley, M. (1983). Perinatal risks. *JOGNN, 12*(6), 13s-18s.

Rayburn, W. (1984). OTC drugs and pregnancy. *Perinatology and Neonatology, 8*(5), 21-27.

Rosen, T.S. (1983). Infants of addicted mothers. In A. Fanaroff and R. Martin (Eds.). *Behrman's neonatal-perinatal medicine* (4th ed.; pp. 239-252). St. Louis: C.V. Mosby.

Smith, J. (1988). The dangers of prenatal cocaine use. *American Journal of Maternal Child Nursing, 13*(3), 174-179.

Infertility

Bayless, R., and Boyers, S. (1988). Cervicitis. In A. DeCherney, M. Polan, R. Lee, and S. Boyers (Eds). *Decision making in infertility* (pp. 54-55). St. Louis: C.V. Mosby.

Behrman, S., and Patton, G. (1988). Evaluation of infertility in the 1980s. In S. Behrman, R. Kistner, and G. Patton (Eds.). *Progress in infertility* (3rd ed.; pp. 1-22). Boston: Little, Brown.

Boyers, S., and Jones, E. (1988). Ovulatory function evaluation. In A. DeCherney, M. Polan, R. Lee, and S. Boyers (Eds). *Decision making in infertility* (pp. 10-11). St. Louis: C.V. Mosby.

Davis, D.C. (1987). A conceptual framework for infertility. *JOGNN*, 16(1), 30-35.

DeCherney, A., Polan, M., Lee, R., and Boyers, S. (1988). *Decision making in infertility*. St. Louis: C.V. Mosby.

Fincham, E. (1987). Gift of life. *Nursing Times*, 83(48), 51-53.

Franssen, A., Kauer, F., Chadha, D., Zijlstra, J., and Rolland, R. (1989). Endometriosis treatment with gonadotropin-releasing hormone agonist Buserelin. *Fertility and Sterility*, 51(3), 401-408.

Golan, A., Langer, R., Bukovsky, I., and Caspi, E. (1989). Congenital anomalies of the mullerian system. *Fertility and Sterility*, 51(5), 747-755.

Hummel, W., and Talbert, L. (1989). Current management of a donor insemination program. *Fertility and Sterility*, 51(6), 919-930.

In vitro fertilization/embryo transfer in the United States: 1987 results from the National IVF-ET Registry (1989). *Fertility and Sterility*, 51(1), 13-19.

Jansen, R. (1987). Ethics in infertility treatment. In R. Pepperell, B. Hudson, and C. Wood (Eds.). *The infertile couple* (2nd ed; pp. 346-387). Edinburgh: Churchill Livingstone.

Keenan, J., Herbert, C., Bush, J., and Wentz, A. (1989). Diagnosis and management of out-of-phase endometrial biopsies among patients receiving clomiphene citrate for ovulation induction. *Fertility and Sterility*, 51(6), 964-967.

Lavy, G., and Boyers, S. (1988). Artificial insemination: Husband. In A. DeCherney, M. Polan, R. Lee, and S. Boyers (Eds.). *Decision making in infertility* (pp. 148-149). St. Louis: C. V. Mosby.

Lightman, A., Jones, E., and Boyers, S. (1988). Ovulation induction: Human menopausal gonadotropins. In A. DeCherney, M. Polan, R. Lee, and S. Boyers (Eds.). *Decision making in infertility* (pp. 32-33). St. Louis: C.V. Mosby.

Lopata, A., and May, D. (1989). The surplus human embryo: Its potential for growth, blastulation, hatching, and human chorionic gonadotropin production in culture. *Fertility and Sterility*, 51(6), 984-991.

Menning, B. (1988). *Infertility: A guide for the childless couple* (2nd ed.). Englewood Cliffs, NJ: Prentice-Hall.

Murray, D., Reich, L., and Adashi, E. (1989). Oral clomiphene citrate and vaginal progesterone suppositories in the treatment of luteal phase dysfunction: A comparative study. *Fertility and Sterility*, 51(1), 35-41.

Platt, J., Fisher, I., and Silver, M. (1973). Infertile couples: Personality traits and self-ideal concept discrepancies. *Fertility and Sterility*, 24(12), 972-976.

Siegler, A. (1988). Endoscopy in infertility. In S. Behrman, R. Kistner, and G. Patton (Eds.). *Progress in infertility* (3rd ed; pp. 71-92). Boston: Little, Brown.

Testart, J., Belaisch-Allart, J., and Frydman, R. (1989). Relationships between embryo transfer results and ovarian response and in vitro fertilization rate: Analysis of 186 human pregnancies. *Fertility and Sterility*, 45(2), 237-243.

Wentz, A. (1988). Luteal phase inadequacy. In S. Behrman, R. Kistner, and G. Patton (Eds.). *Progress in infertility* (3rd ed; pp. 405-476). Boston: Little, Brown.

Wheeler, J., and Polan, M. (1988). Epidemiology of infertility. In A. DeCherney, M. Polan, R. Lee, and S. Boyers (Eds.). *Decision making in infertility* (pp. 2-3). St. Louis: C. V. Mosby.

Zion, A. (1988). Resources for infertile couples. *JOGNN*, 17(4), 255-258.

Cultural references

Binder, P. (1972). *Magic symbols of the world.* New York: Hamlyn Publishing.

Bulfinch, T. (1987). *The age of fable.* Philadelphia: Running Press.

Menning, B. (1988). *Infertility: A guide for the childless couple* (2nd ed.). Englewood Cliffs, NJ: Prentice-Hall.

Stern, P. (1986). Women's social position as menstruating beings. In V. Olesen and N. Woods (Eds.). *Culture, society, and menstruation* (pp. ix-x). New York: Hemisphere Publishing Corp.

Nursing research

Aaronson, L., and Macnee, C. (1989). Tobacco, alcohol, and caffeine use during pregnancy. *JOGNN*, 18(4), 279-287.

Davis, D.C. (1984). Actions and reactions of infertile women to infertility. *Dissertation Abstracts International*, 46(2B), 474. (University Microfilms No. DER85-07278.)

Frank, D., and Brackley, M. (1989). The health experience of single women who have children through artificial donor insemination. *Clinical Nurse Specialist*, 3(3), 156-160.

Hirsch, A., and Hirsch, S. (1989). The effect of infertility on marriage and self-concept. *JOGNN*, 18(1), 13-20.

McCusker, M. (1982). The subfertile couple. *JOGNN*, 11(3), 157-162.

Olshansky, E. (1987). Identity of self as infertile: An example of theory-generating research. *Advances in Nursing Science*, 9(2), 54-63.

Olshansky, E. (1988). Responses to high technology infertility treatment. *Image: Journal of Nursing Scholarship*, 20(3), 128-131.

Sarvatzky, M. (1981). Tasks of infertile couples. *JOGNN*, 10(2), 132-133.

Genetics and Genetic Disorders

Objectives

After reading and studying this chapter, the student should be able to:

1. Describe the basic principles of genetic inheritance, including the role of genes, deoxyribonucleic acid (DNA), and chromosomes.

2. Explain mitosis and meiosis.

3. Summarize the major causes of genetic disorders.

4. Describe autosomal dominant, autosomal recessive, X-linked dominant, and X-linked recessive inheritance patterns.

5. Give reasons why a dominant gene might not behave like a dominant gene.

6. Explain diagnostic tests used to identify risk factors or genetic disorders in a fetus, client, or other family member.

7. Apply the nursing process when caring for a client who has or is at risk for transmitting a genetic disorder.

Introduction

Successful transfer of genetic information from parents to offspring is a crucial step in normal human development. If a parent's genetic material contains an error or defect, or if an error arises during cell division, offspring may suffer profound deleterious effects. Because genetic factors are involved in many serious disorders, genetics is an important concern for the childbearing family.

Whether a client is considering pregnancy, is pregnant, or has delivered a neonate, the nurse can enhance health and well-being by assessing the risk of genetic disorders and providing information and services needed to address the client's problems and concerns. Primary

responsibilities include:

• assessing for genetic risk factors

• teaching prospective parents about genetic disorders before conception

• answering questions about genetic defects and disorders appropriately

• demonstrating sensitivity to ethical dilemmas faced by the couple at risk for having a child with a genetic disorder

• collaborating with other health care professionals when referring the family for evaluation and treatment of a genetic disorder.

• providing nursing care to the family whose neonate has a genetic disorder.

This chapter begins by introducing basic principles of genetic inheritance, including mitosis and meiosis. It then explains the major causes of genetic disorders, including monogenic factors, chromosomal abnormalities, and multifactorial influences. Finally, the chapter uses the nursing process to describe care appropriate for a client who has or is at risk for transmitting a genetic disorder.

Elements of genetic inheritance

Arranged in a linear fashion on double-stranded chains of DNA, genes are individual carriers of hereditary information. Each DNA chain is made up of a sugar (deox-

GLOSSARY

Alleles: a pair of genes that may be different from each other that occupy corresponding sites (loci) on homologous chromosomes.

Amniocentesis: prenatal needle aspiration procedure for obtaining amniotic fluid for analysis.

Autosome: general term for any chromosome except a sex chromosome.

Carrier: person who has one normal and one abnormal gene at corresponding loci, when the abnormal gene is not expressed phenotypically. Expression may occur in offspring if male and female carriers each transmit the abnormal gene.

Chorionic villus sampling (CVS): prenatal diagnostic procedure for obtaining fetal tissue from the villous area of the chorion.

Chromosome: microscopic, threadlike structure in the cell nucleus that contains genetic information arranged in a linear sequence.

Consanguinity: kinship; blood relationship.

Crossing-over: exchange of corresponding segments between homologous chromosomes while the chromosomes are paired during the first meiotic division.

DNA: deoxyribonucleic acid; the chemical that carries genetic information.

Diploid: having a full set of homologous chromosomes (46), as normally found in somatic cells.

Dominant: capable of expression when the gene is present on only one of a pair of homologous chromosomes.

Down's syndrome: disorder in which birth defects are caused by an extra number 21 chromosome; also called trisomy 21.

Expressivity: extent to which signs of a gene reveal themselves.

Gamete: male or female reproductive cell.

Gene: self-reproducing biological unit of heredity; located at a specific locus (site) on a particular chromosome.

Genotype: individual's genetic constitution; may refer to the total genetic constitution or to specific alleles present at a locus.

Haploid: having only one-half of a set of homologous chromosomes (23), as normally found in gametes.

Heterozygote: individual with two different alleles at a corresponding loci on homologous chromosomes.

Homozygote: individual with identical alleles (normal or abnormal) at corresponding loci on homologous chromosomes.

Homologous chromosomes: matching pair of chromosomes.

Index case: family member who brings a family under study; also known as proband or propositus.

Karyotype: chromosome complement arranged by relative size, centromere position, and staining pattern and depicted by photomicrograph.

Klinefelter's syndrome: disorder caused by an extra X chromosome in the male (XXY).

Linkage: association of genes located on the same chromosome, resulting in a tendency for some nonallelic genes to be associated in inheritance.

Locus: the specific site of a particular gene in a chromosome. Plural: loci.

Malformation: developmental defect.

Meiosis: specialized form of cell division that produces gametes.

Mitosis: cell division characteristic of all cell types except gametes.

Monosomy: absence of one chromosome of a homologous pair.

Mosaicism: two or more cell lines that differ genotypically but develop from a single zygote; an error that occurs during mitosis.

Mutation: any permanent inheritable change in DNA.

Nondisjunction: failure of homologous chromosomes or chromatids to separate during mitosis or meiosis, resulting in daughter cells that contain unequal numbers of chromosomes.

Pedigree: diagram of a family tree showing occurrence of one or more traits in the various family members.

Penetrance: frequency with which a gene manifests itself in phenotypes of individuals with that gene.

Phenotype: observable expression of a genetically determined trait.

Pleiotropy: multiple signs and symptoms caused by one or two genes.

Polar body: small, nonfunctional cell produced along with a functioning ovum during oogenesis.

Recessive: incapable of expression unless the responsible allele is carried on both members of a pair of homologous chromosomes.

Trisomy: presence of an extra chromosome in a diploid cell.

Zygote: diploid cell formed by the union of a haploid ovum and sperm; develops into an embryo.

---

yribose), an inorganic phosphate unit (phosphoric acid), and four types of nitrogen base (adenosine, thymine, cytosine, and guanine). Nitrogen bases are arranged randomly along the sugar-phosphate chains, each base bonding to a corresponding base on the adjacent chain. This arrangement forms the double helix structure char-

acteristic of DNA. (See *DNA structure*, page 230, for an illustration.) Varying combinations of nitrogen bases on each strand produce genetic differences among people.

Genes occur in pairs, one on each member (chromatid) of a paired set of homologous chromosomes. Genes at corresponding sites, or loci, on homologous chromo-

DNA structure

Depicted below is a schematic double helix structure of DNA. Nitrogen bases (adenine, guanine, thymine, and cytosine) bond in pairs between the two DNA strands. Adenine always bonds with thymine; guanine always bonds with cytosine. Variations in bonding order create genetic differences among people.

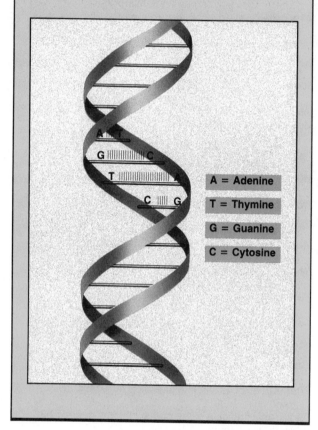

A = Adenine

T = Thymine

G = Guanine

C = Cytosine

somes are known as alleles. When alleles are identical at corresponding loci, the person is homozygous for the trait expressed. When alleles differ at corresponding loci, the person is heterozygous for the trait expressed.

All genes do not possess an equal probability of expression. In fact, when different genes occur at corresponding loci on homologous chromosomes, they must compete for expression. The gene expressed is *dominant.* The gene not expressed is *recessive.* Typically, when two recessive genes occur at corresponding loci, the trait for which they code will be expressed.

Precise replication and division of genetic information allow for normal cellular growth and function as well as accurate transmission to offspring. After replication and before cell division, DNA strands coil into short, thick strands known as chromosomes, which separate during cell division and produce two cells identical

to the original. In somatic cells, which make up most of the body, division takes place by mitosis. In reproductive cells, division takes place by meiosis.

Mitosis

Somatic cells contain 23 pairs of chromosomes and are known as diploid cells (because they contain a duplicate of each chromosome). When a somatic cell divides, the 23 pairs of chromosomes replicate and separate into two daughter cells identical to the parent cell. This complex event, known as mitosis, allows growth, development, and maintenance of an individual. It requires precise coordination and movement of cellular contents.

Mitosis typically is described in five phases: interphase, prophase, metaphase, anaphase, and telophase. (For illustrations and an explanation of these phases, see *Mitosis.*)

Meiosis

Also known as gametogenesis, meiosis produces gametes (germ cells) that contain half the chromosomes of somatic cells. They are known as haploid cells because they contain only one of each chromosome rather than a pair. Fertilization of two normal gametes, each with 23 chromosomes, restores the normal complement of 46 chromosomes in the zygote—a cell formed by the fusion of ovum and spermatozoon—and in its descendant cells. Mendelian laws of genetics govern the transmission of genetic information and the predictability of genetic traits inherited through generations.

Meiotic cell division occurs in two successive stages, with chromosome replication occurring at only one of those stages. Thus, four cells are produced with only twice the number of original chromosomes, meaning that each cell has half its original chromosome content. (For an illustration, see *Meiosis,* pages 232 and 233.)

Meiosis differs from mitosis in three major ways. In the first (which occurs during prophase I), chromosomes contributed by two different parents align so that matching genes are together. This is known as synapsis and occurs after chromosome replication. In this close alignment, genetic material "crosses over" between chromosomes, mixing the material provided by both parents.

The second event distinct to meiosis occurs when chromosomes move to opposite ends of the cell. Rather than separating at the centromeres as they do in mitosis, chromosomes remain attached at the centromeres and move as complete units to opposing poles. At the end of meiosis Stage I, each of two daughter cells contains

Mitosis

Through mitosis, the nuclear contents of a cell reproduce and divide. Mitosis occurs continuously in somatic cells for body growth and maintenance. The process is described in five phases: interphase, prophase, metaphase, anaphase, and telophase. The illustration below shows the various phases.

Interphase

Once thought to be a resting phase, interphase is a time of many normal cellular functions, including cellular respiration, protein synthesis, and chromosome DNA replication. Nuclear material is separated from the cytoplasm by a nuclear membrane during this phase. Chromosomes are long and thin and appear only as masses of granular chromatin. The nucleus of the cell is clearly visible. Centrioles (two small, cylindrical bodies) appear just outside the nucleus. Genetic material replicates in preparation for division.

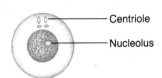

Centriole

Nucleolus

Prophase

Chromatin shortens and thickens into distinct chromosomes. Each chromosome consists of two strands, called chromatids. The chromatids are joined at a constricted area, the centromere. The centrioles separate and move to opposite poles of the nucleus, and protein microtubules coalesce to form a spindle structure. Microtubules attach to each centromere. The cell's nuclear membrane begins to break down.

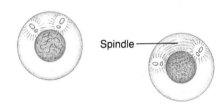

Spindle

Metaphase

The nuclear membrane completes its dissolution and the chromosomes, each attached to a microtubule, line up in the center of the cell in a flat plane.

Anaphase

Microtubules separate the sister chromatids (now referred to as daughter chromosomes) and draw them toward opposite poles of the cell.

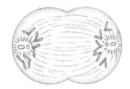

Telophase

When daughter chromosomes reach the poles, telophase begins. The chromosomes begin to uncoil, the spindle breaks down, a nuclear membrane forms around each group of chromosomes, and the nucleoli reform. The cytoplasmic portion of the cell divides, producing two daughter cells, each identical in chromosome and genetic composition. The daughter cells begin interphase, and mitosis begins again.

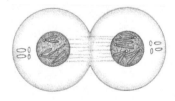

duplicate chromosomes attached by centromeres and composed of genetic material from both parents.

During meiosis Stage II, the third difference between mitosis and meiosis occurs: the two daughter cells divide into four without chromosome duplication. Centromeres separate as in normal mitosis and single chromosomes move to opposite poles in the cell. When the cell divides,

it contains a haploid number of chromosomes with genetic material from both parents.

Meiosis in the male (spermatogenesis) produces four viable spermatozoa. Meiosis in the female (oogenesis) produces one viable ovum and two nonviable polar bodies. Oocytes (developing ova) halt development after the

Meiosis

Meiosis, a two-phase reduction division, begins with a cell containing 46 chromosomes. During Stage I, two diploid cells, each containing 23 chromosomes, are formed. Stage II begins with these two diploid cells and ends with four haploid cells, each containing 23 chromosomes.

STAGE I

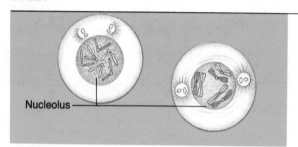

Nucleolus

Prophase I
Chromosomes condense and become visible. Although they have replicated during interphase, they may not appear as double strands early in prophase. The nuclear membrane breaks down and the spindle appears. Homologous chromosomes move together and intertwine (synapse) as they exchange genetic material. Double strands become visible. Late in prophase, paired chromosomes move as a unit to the center of the cell.

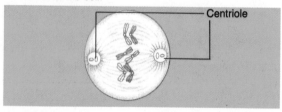

Centriole

Metaphase I
Spindle fibers become well established, with one microtubule attached to each chromosome pair; each chromosome consists of two joined chromatids that do not separate during the first meiotic division.

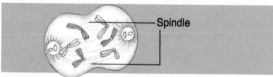

Spindle

Anaphase I
Chromatids do not separate. The homologous chromosomes of each pair, which have been altered by genetic material exchange at synapse, separate and move to opposite poles of the cell.

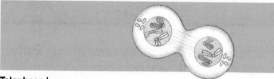

Telophase I
Two new daughter cells are formed. Each contains only one member of each homologous pair of chromosomes—half the total number in the parent cell.

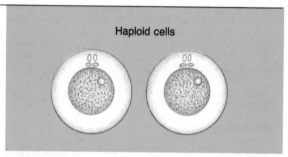

Haploid cells

Interkinesis
Each chromosome consists of two chromatids that do not replicate. The second meiotic division is like a mitotic division, but the cell entering the second division possesses only 23 chromosomes.

STAGE II

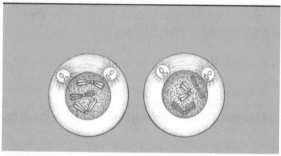

Prophase II
The double-stranded chromosomes appear as thin threads, the nuclear membrane disappears, and the spindle forms.

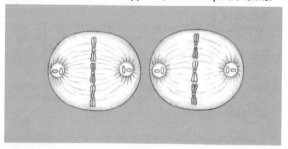

Metaphase II
During this phase, chromosomes line up in the center of the cell. Chromatids comprising each chromosome are still attached at the centromere; spindle fibers attach to the chromatids.

STAGE II (continued)

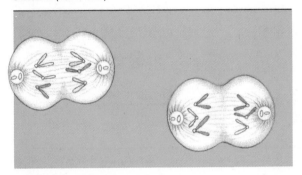

Anaphase II
Chromatids separate to form individual chromosomes and are pulled to opposite poles of the cell by the spindle fibers.

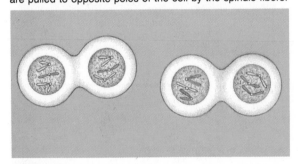

Telophase II
Cellular membranes begin to form around each group of chromosomes. The chromosomes uncurl, the spindle breaks down, and haploid cells result.

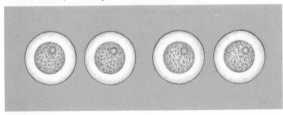

Haploid cells
Each daughter cell contains 23 chromosomes—one unduplicated member of each homologous chromosome.

first stage of meiosis and do not complete it until after fertilization. (For a diagram of how male and female meiosis differ, see *Gametogenesis*, page 234.)

Genetic disorders

When abnormalities arise in cell division and transmission of genetic information to offspring, genetic disorders may result. Ranging from benign alterations to fatal syndromes, genetic disorders number in the thousands and occur at a significant rate before and after birth. Approximately half of spontaneous abortions may be associated with chromosomal abnormalities. Many genetic disorders are apparent at or shortly after birth. Of all neonates, 2% to 3% have major congenital defects (caused by genetic factors, environmental factors, or a combination). By age 25, more than 5% of individuals develop a disease that has a genetic component (Baird, Anderson, Newcombe, and Lowry, 1988).

Genetic disorders may result from monogenic (single gene) factors, chromosomal abnormalities, or interactions between genetic alterations and the environment.

Monogenic disorders

Sometimes called Mendelian disorders, monogenic disorders follow specific inheritance patterns within families and typically occur in the fixed proportions described by Gregor Mendel, a pioneer in genetic research. About 1% of neonates display monogenic disorders, which may involve dominant or recessive genes on autosomes or sex chromosomes.

Specifically, monogenic disorders may be autosomal dominant, autosomal recessive, X-linked dominant, or X-linked recessive. Because autosomes outnumber sex chromosomes by 44 to 2, most monogenic disorders involve autosomes. One gene causes expression of a dominant disorder; two genes are needed for expression of a recessive disorder. Rarely, a monogenic disorder may arise as a new mutation. (For a summary, see *Inheritance patterns in monogenic disorders*, page 236.)

Autosomal dominant inheritance
Autosomal dominant disorders are expressed by one copy of an abnormal gene that appears on an autosome rather than on a sex chromosome. The affected individual is

Gametogenesis

In the male, meiotic division forms four spermatozoa. In the female, it forms one viable ovum and two nonviable polar bodies. All male and female reproductive cells (gametes) are haploid, containing 23 chromosomes—one member of each homologous pair. The letters shown (X or Y) indicate the sex chromosome within the cell.

	SPERMATOGENESIS	OOGENESIS
Meiosis Stage I	Primary spermatocyte *46 chromosomes (XY)*	Primary oocyte *46 chromosomes (XX)*
Meiosis Stage II	Secondary spermatocytes *23 chromosomes (X or Y)*	Secondary oocyte *23 chromosomes (X)* / First polar body
Cell differentiation	Spermatids *23 chromosomes (X or Y)*	Ootid *23 chromosomes (X)* / Second polar body
Reproductive cells	Spermatozoa *23 chromosomes (X or Y)*	Ovum *23 chromosomes (X)*

heterozygous—that is, has one normal and one abnormal gene at corresponding loci. The abnormal gene is dominant. Many autosomal dominant disorders are characterized by delayed manifestation of structural or physical malformations. Typically, an autosomal dominant disorder appears in a parent before it appears in a child, enabling health care professionals to predict the likelihood of transmittal to children.

Autosomal disorders may be difficult to trace when one of four factors comes into play, including penetrance, expressivity, pleiotropy, and mutation. Although these factors may occur in other modes of inheritance, they most often affect autosomal dominant disorders.

Penetrance. For an unknown reason, a dominant trait may not be expressed even though the gene is present. The extent to which a gene expresses a trait is known as its penetrance. For example, if expressed in all carriers, the gene has 100% penetrance. If expressed in 75% of carriers, the gene has 75% penetrance. Analysis of genetic risk factors can be difficult in cases of reduced penetrance because absence of a trait in parents does not necessarily mean absence of the trait in offspring.

Expressivity. Expression of a trait may vary among family members. For example, complications of Marfan's syndrome (which include abnormal length of extremities, subluxated optic lenses, and cardiovascular abnormalities) may vary in their presence and severity among family members.

Pleiotropy. In some cases, one or two genes may cause multiple clinical manifestations.

Mutation. Normally, genes line up in a specific order on specific chromosomes according to the trait they control. Variations in genes can cause permanent, inheritable changes in descendants. This is called mutation. The risk that parents will produce another child with a similar mutation is small. (For more information, see *Mechanisms and consequences of genetic mutation.*)

Autosomal recessive inheritance

Two expressed abnormal autosomal genes will cause an autosomal recessive disorder. The affected person inherits one copy of the altered gene from each parent, creating homozygosity for that trait. Typically, the parents are heterozygous for the disorder and may not know they are carriers until they bear an affected child. Heterozygosity in both parents may result from consanguinity.

For example, parents who have a child with cystic fibrosis typically have no signs of the disorder themselves. Other family members may show no signs as well, unless one or more siblings inherited two copies of the abnormal gene.

Many hundreds of disorders are attributed to autosomal recessive defects, which characteristically develop at an early age and may have similar clinical manifestations. Additionally, ethnic background may increase the risk for certain individuals to be carriers of autosomal recessive disorders.

X-linked disorders

Produced by an abnormal gene on the X chromosome, X-linked disorders always are expressed in males be-

---

Mechanisms and consequences of genetic mutation

A mutation is a permanent, inheritable change in gene sequence. Very rare, this type of change may occur in several ways and produce various consequences.

MECHANISMS

- Spontaneous change in nitrogen bases (substitution, addition, or deletion of one or more base pairs)
- Loss of a gene sequence during chromosome replication or as a result of chromosome breakage
- Addition of a gene sequence during chromosome replication or as a result of translocation
- Defective DNA-manufacturing enzymes
- Chemicals (mutagens) that modify or substitute for nitrogen bases
- Damage from radiation
- Elevated temperature

CONSEQUENCES

- Underproduction of a product
- Overproduction of a product
- No production of a product
- Production of an abnormal product

---

cause the male has only one X chromosome. Without the offsetting allele possessed by a female carrier, the defective X-linked gene behaves like a dominant gene when paired with a Y chromosome, leading to clinical manifestations. Because a male possesses only one X chromosome, he can be neither homozygous nor heterozygous for an X-linked trait; thus, the male is termed hemizygous.

Males with X-linked disorders will transmit the gene to all daughters. Transmission will not occur from father to son because the father transmits the unaffected Y chromosome to his sons.

Through a process known as X-inactivation, which occurs only in females, one X chromosome probably becomes inactivated early in embryonic life. If the chromosome carrying the abnormal gene becomes inactivated, the female carrier will show no clinical signs of the disorder. If the chromosome carrying the normal gene becomes inactivated, the female carrier may develop the disorder even though she has one normal gene. Although the latter situation is rare, it may occur in such disorders as hemophilia. (Although only one X chromosome in each somatic cell is assumed to be functional, two X chromosomes are needed during early female development. When an X chromosome is missing, altered development occurs.)

Inheritance patterns in monogenic disorders

Listed below are four groups of monogenic disorders and patterns for each group.

AUTOSOMAL DOMINANT

Disorders
• Achondroplasia—form of dwarfism characterized by short limbs and normal trunk
• Familial hypercholesterolemia—excess cholesterol in the blood
• Huntington's chorea—purposeless physical movements and progressive mental deterioration leading to dementia
• Marfan's syndrome—connective tissue disorder characterized by abnormally long extremities, subluxated optic lenses, and cardiac problems
• Myotonic dystrophy—sustained muscular contraction, muscular atrophy, cataracts, hypogonadism, balding, and cardiac anomalies
• Neurofibromatosis—developmental changes in the nervous system, muscles, bones, and skin, marked by multiple soft tumors known as neurofibromas

Patterns
• Male and female offspring are equally likely to be affected.
• One parent must transmit the abnormal gene for an individual to have signs of the disorder.
• With each pregnancy, the affected individual has a 50% chance of passing the gene to the offspring.
• Variable expression of signs may be apparent in affected individuals.
• Individuals in several generations may be affected.
• Pleiotropy produces multiple problems from the abnormal gene.
• Nonpenetrance occurs when an individual with an affected parent and an affected offspring appears to have no clinical signs of the disorder.

AUTOSOMAL RECESSIVE

Disorders
• Congenital adrenal hyperplasia—abnormal increase in number of adrenal cortical cells
• Cystic fibrosis—widespread dysfunction of exocrine glands in infants, children, and adolescents
• Alpha₁ antitrypsin deficiency—hereditary emphysema and other serious symptoms
• Phenylketonuria—phenylalanine accumulation resulting in mental retardation and neurologic anomalies.
• Tay-Sachs disease—inborn defect of lipid metabolism, more commonly affecting children of Jewish descent
• Sickle cell anemia—type of hemolytic anemia, more commonly affecting Blacks

Patterns
• Male and female offspring are equally likely to be affected.
• Each parent must transmit the abnormal gene for an individual to have clinical signs of the disorder.
• If both parents are carriers, an offspring has a 25% chance of receiving the abnormal gene from each parent and being affected with the disorder.
• Each offspring who receives an abnormal gene from

only one parent will be a carrier.
• Each offspring who receives a normal allele from each parent will be genetically normal.

X-LINKED DOMINANT

Disorders
• Hypophosphatemic rickets—abnormal bone ossification associated with low serum phosphorus
• Incontinentia pigmenti—abnormally pigmented lesions and abnormalities of the hair, eyes, skeleton, and central nervous system
• Ornithine transcarbamoylase deficiency—impaired urea formation and production of excess ammonia or its compounds in the blood

Patterns
• The abnormal gene exists on the X chromosome.
• One parent must transmit the abnormal gene for an individual to have signs of the disorder.
• Male and female offspring may show signs of the disorder, although female offspring may have milder manifestations because of the offsetting effect of the normal X chromosome.
• Some disorders caused by the abnormal gene may be lethal in the male fetus.
• A female carrier has a 50% chance of passing the abnormal gene to each offspring.
• A male will transmit the abnormal gene to each of his female offspring and none to his male offspring.

X-LINKED RECESSIVE

Disorders
• Color blindness—inability to distinguish certain colors
• Duchenne's muscular dystrophy—chronic, progressive weakness and pseudohypertrophy of muscles, followed by atrophy, lordosis, and peculiar swaying gait
• Glucose-6-phosphate dehydrogenase deficiency—metabolic error that produces severe hemolytic crises
• Hemophilia A and B—hemorrhagic disorders caused by deficiency of coagulation factors
• Testicular feminization—genotypic male appears female because of lack of receptors for testosterone and dihydrotestosterone

Patterns
• The abnormal gene exists on the X chromosome.
• One abnormal gene is not sufficient to cause a disorder in most females who carry it on one of two X chromosomes.
• One abnormal gene is sufficient to cause a disorder in males who have the abnormal gene on the X chromosome.
• A female carrier has a 50% chance to pass the abnormal gene to each offspring. A female offspring with the abnormal gene will be a carrier; a male offspring with it will be affected.
• No male-to-male transmission can occur because the abnormal gene is on the X chromosome and a male passes the Y chromosome to his male offspring.

X-linked dominant inheritance. In these rare disorders, one copy of a defective gene on an X chromosome produces clinical signs. Although both males and females can be affected, X-inactivation may produce milder clinical manifestations in females. Some X-linked dominant disorders are fatal in males.

X-linked recessive inheritance. Typically, X-linked disorders involve a recessive abnormal gene; this means that only males exhibit clinical signs of the disorder because they have no offsetting X allele. In rare cases, the disorder may appear in females through X-inactivation of the normal allele, as described above.

Chromosomal abnormalities

Genetic defects also can be caused by addition, loss, or rearrangement of part or all of an autosome or sex chromosome. Chromosomal abnormalities occur in about 0.6% of live births and in about 50% of early spontaneous abortions. Although no one knows the cause of chromosomal abnormalities, parental age seems to be significant.

Increased maternal age has been associated with a heightened risk for such fetal nondisjunction abnormalities as Down's syndrome and Klinefelter's syndrome. Because of this association, prenatal diagnosis is recommended for all women who will be age 35 or older when their neonates are born (Morgan and Elias, 1989).

Although no clear-cut correlation exists between paternal age and Down's syndrome, the incidence of autosomal dominant genetic defects increases with paternal age.

During normal cell division, chromosomes separate so that genetic information is split between resulting daughter cells. If chromosomes do not separate normally, daughter cells may receive too much or too little chromosomal material. Loss of an entire chromosome is known as monosomy; addition of an entire chromosome is known as trisomy. Both autosomes and sex chromosomes may be affected.

Several characteristics of chromosomal alterations have been isolated.
• When chromosomal alterations occur, they are present from conception.
• Individuals with alterations of a particular chromosome typically exhibit similar phenotypes (physical expression of genetic composition).
• Chromosomal rearrangements may manifest themselves sporadically or produce no clinical signs.

Although some patterns of chromosomal abnormalities are well recognized—for example, those in Down's syndrome—a karyotype usually must be performed to identify the specific alteration and to establish a diagnosis. (For a description of karyotype, see the "Prenatal detection" section later in this chapter.)

Chromosomal abnormalities may be numerical or structural, as described below.

Numerical changes

The normal cell contains 22 pairs of autosomes, numbered 1 through 22, and two sex chromosomes, making 23 chromosomal pairs. When paired chromosomes fail to separate, either in the first or second stage of meiosis, the resulting gamete has 24 chromosomes rather than the normal 23. This is known as nondisjunction. Conception then produces a fetus with one extra chromosome. The extra chromosome will match one of the chromosomal pairs and is called a trisomy, meaning three. The extra chromosome may be either an autosome or a sex chromosome. (For a diagram, see *Mechanism of nondisjunction*, page 238.)

Trisomy of large autosomes typically results in spontaneous abortion and has not been observed in live neonates. Trisomy of smaller autosomes—such as 13, 18, and 21—may allow delivery of a live neonate, but produces profound developmental disturbances in multiple organ systems. Trisomy of sex chromosomes allows embryonic development but produces developmental abnormalities.

When nondisjunction occurs during early embryogenesis, the daughter cell lacking a chromosome dies; the cell containing an extra chromosome proliferates, leading to a population of trisomic cells intermixed with populations of normal cells. This is known as mosaicism.

Autosomal abnormalities. Three examples of numerical autosomal abnormalities include Down's syndrome, Edwards' syndrome, and Patau's syndrome.

Down's syndrome (trisomy 21). The most common autosomal disorder, Down's syndrome results from an extra number 21 chromosome, typically produced through nondisjunction. Less commonly, translocation or chromosomal mosaic may produce an extra number 21 chromosome. Because Down's syndrome may result from one of several mechanisms, affected children should have a karyotype to identify the pertinent chromosomal alteration. Parents who bear a child with nondisjunction Down's syndrome have a 1% to 2% risk of the syndrome in any additional child (Morgan and Elias, 1989). Parents who bear a child with translocation Down's syndrome have a variable risk depending on the type of translocation involved.

Mechanism of nondisjunction

Nondisjunction in meiosis can lead to the formation of gametes with an extra or missing chromosome, as illustrated below. If a chromosomally abnormal gamete resulting from nondisjunction unites with a normal gamete during fertilization, the zygote will contain an abnormal amount of chromosome material that may lead to spontaneous abortion or a defective fetus.

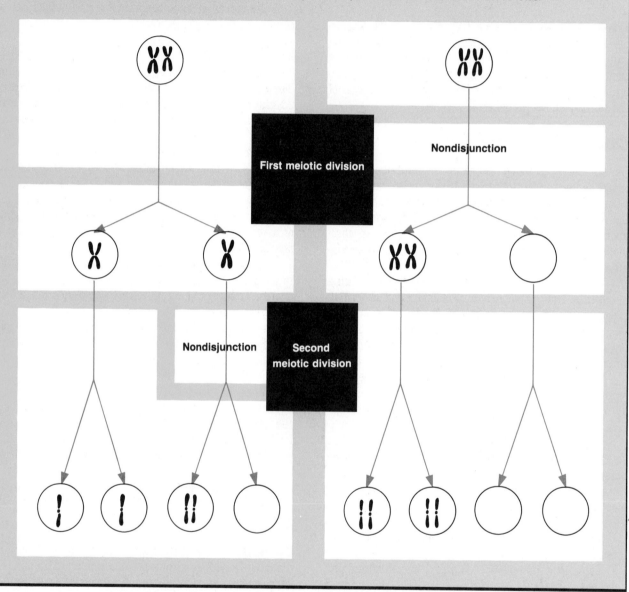

Clinical manifestations include mental retardation; a small head with flat profile; epicanthic eye folds; slanted, almond-shaped eyes; a perpetually open mouth with large, protruding tongue; low-set ears; and thick hands and feet, perhaps with webbing between the digits. Physiologic problems, which may be profound, typically include congenital heart defects and intestinal disorders. Increased susceptibility to various diseases shortens the life of some Down's syndrome individuals.

Edwards' syndrome (trisomy 18). Many fetuses with trisomy 18 are spontaneously aborted. Of delivered neonates, fewer than 10% live to age 1 (Thompson and Thompson, 1986). Heart and kidney defects are common, along with severe mental and developmental retardation. Clinical signs include small, defective eyes; a narrow, receding chin; rocker-bottom feet, and low-set, malformed ears. Muscle tone typically is exaggerated, leading to stiff joints and clenched fists with the index finger tightly folded across the third finger.

Patau's syndrome (trisomy 13). This syndrome is similar in many respects to Edwards' syndrome. Heart and kidney defects are common, along with severe mental and developmental retardation. Clinical signs may include cleft lip and palate, polydactyly, and deafness. Of those born alive, more than half die before age 1 month; fewer than 5% live to age 39 (Thompson and Thompson, 1986).

Sex chromosome abnormalities. Typically less severe than autosomal abnormalities, these account for about one-third of all chromosomal errors in neonates. Because sex chromosome alterations typically prevent puberty and cause infertility, many affected individuals are not diagnosed until they fail to undergo puberty.

Turner's syndrome. An X chromosome monosomy, Turner's syndrome produces a female phenotype. Only about 1 in 100 affected fetuses survive. Of those, about 60% lack an entire X chromosome; in mosaic Turner's syndrome, some cells could have 46 chromosomes and some could have 45 chromosomes. As with other chromosomal abnormalities, a karyotype documents the specific type of chromosomal abnormality present.

Some features of Turner's syndrome can be recognized in the neonatal period. These include a webbed neck and lymphedema of the hands and feet. Other abnormalities include coarctation of the aorta, renal anomalies, short stature, and learning disabilities involving deficits in visual and spatial skills. Usually, affected individuals have normal intelligence.

Because individuals with Turner's syndrome do not have normal ovarian tissue, they may not produce the hormones necessary to initiate puberty and will not produce ova. Exogenous hormone therapy at the time when puberty would ordinarily begin can produce development of secondary sex characteristics. However, it will not produce fertility.

Klinefelter's syndrome (XXY syndrome). The neonate with Klinefelter's syndrome typically looks like a normal male; diagnosis may not be made until the individual fails to undergo puberty. This individual tends to have increased height and an increased risk for learning disabilities involving expressive language skills. He has small testes and is almost always infertile. He may benefit from testosterone replacement therapy to promote normal pubertal development, although it will not make him fertile.

Other sex chromosome abnormalities. The *XXX syndrome* produces females who may have normal intelligence and fertility. The *XYY syndrome* produces males who typically are fertile and may be quite tall, prone to acne, and have reduced intelligence. The *fragile X syndrome,* in which an X chromosome breaks near the end of the long arm, produces males with mental retardation. Female carriers may have mild retardation.

Structural changes

Not all chromosomal alterations involve the whole chromosome. In some cases, part of a chromosome may be deleted, duplicated, or inverted. Such structural abnormalities can result from translocation, deletion, duplication, or inversion. Although chromosomal breakage and repair may occur without deleterious effects in an individual, they take on particular significance if they pass to the next generation in reproductive cells.

Translocation. By transferring a portion of one chromosome to another chromosome or to a different position on the same chromosome, translocation alters chromosomal material in the ovum or spermatozoon. In balanced translocation, genetic information is rearranged and maintains a normal amount of chromosomal material. Because of this rearrangement, however, gametes may receive too much or too little genetic information. In unbalanced translocation, a portion of a chromosome becomes attached to another chromosome, creating either partial trisomy or partial monosomy. Clinical manifestations depend on the size and location of chromosomal material added or lost and the chromosome affected.

Deletion. Loss of part of a chromosome may produce various clinical manifestations. For example, loss of part of the short arm of chromosome 5 produces a syndrome(known as cri du chat) marked by severe mental deficiency and a plaintive, catlike cry.

Duplication. A chromosomal segment may appear more than the normal number of times.

Inversion. A chromosomal segment may break off at either end, rotate 180 degrees, and rejoin the chromosome, causing the genes carried on one arm to be in a position and sequence different from those on the other arm. Inversion may contribute to infertility, increased spontaneous abortion, and genetic defects.

Multifactorial inheritance

Some congenital defects result from an interaction between multiple genes and environmental factors. For example, genetic information may predispose a developing fetus to cleft lip and palate, but the latent tendency may not develop unless adverse environmental factors prompt it.

Although multifactorial inheritance may be involved in many congenital malformations, other genetic factors may cause them as well. For example, cleft lip with or without cleft palate can be produced by monogenic, chromosomal, teratogenic, or multifactorial influences. Only after other causes have been ruled out can the defect be assumed to have a multifactorial inheritance pattern. However, if a client bears a child with a defect potentially linked to multifactorial inheritance, she should take pains to avoid potential environmental hazards in subsequent pregnancies—even if the first child's defect probably stemmed from a monogenic, chromosomal, or teratogenic cause.

Multifactorial disorders include neural tube defects (NTDs), urinary tract anomalies, congenital heart diseases, orthopedic anomalies, cleft lip and palate, abdominal wall defects, and pyloric stenosis. Prognosis depends on the severity and type of defect. Some defects are readily corrected; others cause neonatal death.

Errors in neural tube development, caused by failure of the neural tube to close before the twenty-eighth day of embryonic development, cause anencephaly (absence of skull and cerebral hemispheres), spina bifida (opening of lumbosacral vertebrae), or encephalocele. Severity can range from mild to extreme. Birth of one child with an NTD indicates increased risk of bearing subsequent children with the same disorder.

Urinary tract anomalies have high mortality rates and include renal agenesis (malformation or absence of kidneys) and urinary tract obstruction.

Congenital heart defects include patent ductus, coarctation of the aorta, septal defects, pulmonic stenosis, and tetralogy of Fallot.

Orthopedic anomalies include clubfoot and congenital hip dysplasia.

Abdominal wall defects include omphalocele and gastroschisis. Commonly associated with other congenital anomalies, these anomalies have a high mortality rate (Osband, 1989).

Assessment

Assessment for genetic birth defects can be performed at the preconception, prenatal, or postnatal stage. Ideally, genetic risk should be assessed before conception. Even if conception has occurred, however, nursing assessment should include a detailed health history, physical assessment, and review of diagnostic studies.

Health history

When screening for genetic defects, the nurse obtains an extensive health history from the client and her partner, emphasizing family history, exposure to teratogens, and cultural and ethnic background. Assessment questions also should address economic factors, such as the availability of funds to pay for genetic screening tests. Of even greater concern may be the cost of caring for a genetically impaired child. Assess the effect of these factors on family function and make referrals, as appropriate.

The family history can reveal the risk of genetic disorders and may aid in diagnosing genetic disorders. Risk factors include:
• previous birth of an affected child
• family history of genetic defects
• intrauterine exposure to known teratogens
• couples who belong to certain population groups at risk for known genetic disorders
• client over age 35
• client's partner over age 40
• history of three or more spontaneous abortions or stillbirths
• consanguinity
• single or multiple congenital abnormalities in a parent or previous offspring
• delayed or abnormal physical or psychological development in a parent or offspring
• mental retardation
• failure to thrive in infancy or childhood
• blindness
• deafness
• family history of neoplasms with known hereditary component, such as retinoblastoma

• infertility
• early onset of common diseases, such as coronary artery disease
• unexpected drug or anesthesia reaction.

To gather complete and accurate data, allow 30 to 45 minutes for the complete interview. Establish and maintain trust by being nonjudgmental about the family history data. Inform the client that all information will be included in the official health record, but none will be shared with others without the client's written permission.

After explaining the purpose of the family history, begin by constructing a three-generation pedigree—a diagram of relationships among family members that includes pertinent comments on each person's health status. (For further information, see *Constructing a three-generation pedigree*, page 242.)

During the health history, gather biographical data; medical, obstetric, and family history; health promotion and protection behaviors; drug use; health habits; environmental and occupational health; finances; ethnic background; and roles and relationships. These questions screen for any health or familial problems that may increase the risk of birth defects.

Biographical data
Record the client's age. The risk of autosomal chromosome anomalies increases with greater maternal age. Determine the ethnic backgrounds of the client and her partner. Some autosomal recessive disorders are more common in certain ethnic groups; individuals in these groups should be informed about their risks, appropriate screening, prenatal testing, and available counseling.

Medical history
The client's health status and that of her partner can help identify potential genetic disorders. Simple questions, such as, "Do you have any health problems?" or "Does your partner have any health problems?" may reveal important information.

Obstetric history
Ask the client how many times she has been pregnant and whether any pregnancies have ended in miscarriage, therapeutic abortion, stillbirth, or a child with birth defects. Ask the client to identify genetic variations in partners by whom she has become pregnant. Previous pregnancy loss may indicate increased risk for birth defects in offspring. Previous therapeutic abortion may have been related to genetic alterations discovered during prenatal diagnostic testing.

Certain infections contracted during pregnancy are known teratogens (such as rubella, toxoplasmosis, and herpes). Determine if the client has been exposed, infected, or vaccinated.

Family history
To begin drawing the pedigree, find out how many children the client has, the sex and age of each, and whether any have health problems. Asking about each child will elicit more complete health information.

Documentation of relatives in the client's generation and the client's parents constitutes minimal information for constructing a three-generation pedigree. Add more family members to the pedigree if they have pertinent health problems. Ask about the health of each of the client's siblings, nieces, nephews, and parents. Also ask if any family members are adopted, which could introduce genetic defects not otherwise present in family members.

Determine if any family members have had Down's syndrome, chromosomal disorders, NTDs, birth defects, hemophilia, cystic fibrosis, mental retardation, or other inherited disorders. Record each disease or disorder and the family member's relationship to the client.

Some information may be difficult to elicit because the client feels stigmatized by inherited disorders or family circumstances. Be alert for evidence of this discomfort when the family history includes such problems as mental retardation, mental illness, single parenthood, adoption, nonpaternity (when the man acting as a child's father is not the child's biological father), or elective abortion. Assurance of confidentiality also may help in obtaining a complete history.

Health promotion and protection behaviors
Assessment of these behaviors helps identify unhealthy practices or environmental factors that could increase the risk of multifactorial inheritance. This assessment also may reveal the family's economic constraints.

Drug use
Determine if the client takes any medications or illicit drugs. Some may influence multifactorial inheritance. Nonjudgmental attitudes are essential to obtain honest answers. Communicate that the client's honesty enhances the chances for a healthy infant.

Health habits
Because cigarettes are associated with intrauterine growth retardation, determine if the client smokes. Ask if she drinks because alcohol in sufficient quantity and

Constructing a three-generation pedigree

A pedigree can provide information useful for tracking and predicting the occurrence of genetic disorders. It should include at least three family generations and clearly indicate family members positive for the trait being monitored. For ease of communication with other health care professionals, the nurse must use consistent symbols, such as those shown below. Information displayed in the pedigree can be used for genetic counseling. This sample pedigree depicts a family in which the daughter and the father's relatives have a genetic disorder.

Male	☐	Index case (family member who initiates study)	☐
Female	○	Monozygous twins	
Sex undesignated	◇	Dizygous twins	
Married	☐—○	Individual with a genetic disorder	▨
Divorced	☐≠○	Carrier of a genetic disorder	⊙
Aborted		Age of individual	○₁₁ ☐₁₉
Pregnant		Number of individuals of the same sex	③ ③
Adopted	☐ ○	Consanguineous relationship	☐=○
Dead	⊘ ⊘	Unmarried	☐--○

SAMPLE PEDIGREE

at critical times is associated with birth defects. Start by asking about a specific amount consumed, such as one six-pack of beer a day, or a fifth of liquor a day. Suggesting an amount that seems high improves the chances of getting a more realistic estimate. This questioning should begin with nonthreatening topics; encourage and support the client to help her feel comfortable answering questions that could seem more threatening.

Environmental health

The unknown dangers of environmental agents make many pregnant clients fearful. A simple question such as, "Do you have any other concerns about things that might be harmful to your baby?" may reveal her feelings. Answer questions with factual information when specific risks are known and refer all other questions to specialists.

To find out more about the potential teratogenicity of an environmental agent, contact a genetic clinic or high-risk obstetric unit. Some have teratogen hotlines that can provide current information about many agents. Because such information changes rapidly, accurate and up-to-date facts are vital. Include several categories of teratogens in the risk assessment.

Occupational health

To identify occupational hazards or teratogens that could increase the risk of multifactorial inheritance or spontaneous genetic changes in genetic information, find out if the client works with dangerous substances and, if so, which ones. Determine if she has been exposed to toxic chemicals, radiation, or X-rays during pregnancy.

Finances

Economic considerations are an important part of the assessment. The cost of genetic testing and counseling may exceed the family's resources. When clients have a financial need, work with them to help find alternate resources, or refer them to a social service agency or genetic counseling unit to obtain needed services. This may be particularly important at the postnatal stage.

Roles and relationships

Assess the effect on the client of being a carrier or having a child with a genetic defect, and investigate the family's readiness and ability to care for a potentially disabled child.

Ask if the client and her partner are blood relatives. Consanguinity increases the chance that the couple will share abnormal genes.

Cultural values can influence decisions and attitudes toward genetic disorders and birth defects. Knowledge that one carries a genetic defect and may produce an abnormal child can threaten self-image. Individual reactions to and resolution of the internal conflict differ widely, even between partners.

After the health history interview, review the history data with the client and her partner, keeping in mind that most cannot answer all questions during the first interview. They may not know family details or may be reluctant to share sensitive information. However, this information is important and should be reviewed during later meetings.

Physical assessment

Genetic screening also includes a thorough physical assessment to determine if malformations (developmental defects) are present. The physical assessment also can help determine if a malformation is isolated or associated with other anomalies. If other anomalies are present, the pattern of abnormalities may have a common genetic cause.

Observations of physical appearance should be as accurate and objective as possible. Record measurements of any structures that appear abnormal (head circumference, for example). Take photographs whenever possible. Physical examination of family members may be necessary to determine if they have unusual features and if those features are associated with a genetic disorder.

Diagnostic studies

Various studies can be used during each stage of screening—preconception, prenatal, and postnatal—to help identify risks and differentiate among genetic disorders.

Screening tests are performed on healthy clients who show no signs of, but have increased risk for, a disorder. Teach the client about the purpose of selected tests and the meaning of results so that she understands what kind of information the testing will provide.

Screening tests must meet sensitivity and specificity criteria without undue false-negative or false-positive results. (False-negative results indicate absence of a particular disorder when the disorder exists. False-positive results indicate the presence of a particular disorder when the disorder does not exist.) Tests of appropriate sensitivity should be capable of identifying all clients with a specific genetic disorder or altered gene, thus minimizing false-negative results. Tests of appropriate specificity should be capable of isolating the factor in question, thus minimizing false-positive results. Because some screening tests overlap normal and abnormal ranges, the potential exists for both false-positive and false-negative results. Therefore, the client should be informed of the limitations of any specific test, and questionable results should be evaluated further.

Assure the client that test results will be kept confidential. Other persons or groups—such as relatives, employers, and insurance companies—should not have access to test results without her permission. Arrange genetic counseling after the screening, as appropriate.

Preconception detection

Screenings for Tay-Sachs disease and sickle cell disease have been available since the early 1970s. Individuals who wish to be screened receive a blood test and genetic counseling. A client who is a carrier will not necessarily develop the disease. However, if the client who carries the sickle cell gene or the Tay-Sachs gene marries a carrier, they will have a 25% (1:4) chance that each child will be affected by the disease. Be prepared to clarify these facts if the client has questions about them. Also, make sure that the client understands that heterozygote screening is voluntary.

Recent developments in DNA technology have made molecular detection of DNA alterations possible for a number of genetic disorders, and the list is enlarging. Two different types of DNA testing are performed. One is known as direct detection, because the test identifies the exact genetic alteration. Some cases of sickle cell disease and some of cystic fibrosis can be detected in this manner. Although DNA studies can be used for carrier detection or prenatal diagnosis, they are costly and not widely available.

Direct detection cannot identify most mutations that cause genetic disorders. Because markers in the DNA sequence sometimes are located near the altered gene, mutations can be detected indirectly by locating a marker that is linked to the abnormal gene and inherited with it.

Two key points limit the accuracy of indirect detection. First, the gene and marker may separate during meiotic recombination. When this happens, the marker is no longer an accurate indicator of the gene's presence. Therefore, test accuracy depends on the absence of recombination. Likelihood of recombination declines when the marker and gene are close together on the chromosome. Second, markers that seem to be linked to a gene may vary in different families. In most cases, a blood sample from the individual with the disorder and from several relatives is needed.

Prenatal detection

Many hundreds of disorders can be diagnosed prenatally. Examples include Down's syndrome, NTDs, and Tay-Sachs disease. Some prenatal tests are used for screening and others are diagnostic.

Maternal serum alpha fetoprotein (MSAFP) test. Designed to screen for fetal NTDs, this test measures alpha fetoprotein (AFP), a glycoprotein normally excreted by the fetus into the amniotic fluid. The protein crosses the placenta, enters the maternal bloodstream, and can be measured by blood test between weeks 15 and 20 of pregnancy. Although norms vary according to laboratory standards, values 2.5 times above the median indicate a need for further diagnostic evaluation (Myhre, Richards, and Johnson, 1989). Among fetuses with NTDs, this test correctly identifies approximately 85% of them.

Factors that could result in misleading MSAFP levels include:
• incorrect calculation of pregnancy onset (AFP levels vary with pregnancy stage)
• twin fetuses (both would excrete AFP, increasing the level)
• fetal death, including spontaneous abortion
• congenital disorders, such as abdominal wall defects, high-gastrointestinal obstructions, nephrosis, and polycystic kidneys
• other genetic disorders, such as Down's syndrome and trisomy 18
• hydatidiform mole
• choriocarcinoma.

An abnormal MSAFP level prompts a second diagnostic test, typically ultrasound, to document gestational age, assess fetal viability, and determine if more than one fetus is present. If the second test reveals no reason for elevated MSAFP, further testing typically includes high resolution ultrasound and amniocentesis.

Most pregnant clients with elevated MSAFP do not have neonates with birth defects. However, these pregnancies may have an increased risk of prematurity, low birth weight, spontaneous abortion, or stillbirth (Hamilton, Hossam, and Whitefield, 1985). MSAFP analysis should be part of a coordinated system of resources, including laboratory studies, counseling, and adequate follow-up.

Ultrasonography. Prenatal ultrasonography, which is fetal imaging with ultrasound waves, may be used to detect gross structural abnormalities. Ultrasonography also is used to guide certain prenatal diagnostic procedures, such as amniocentesis and chorionic villus sampling (CVS). In cases where ultrasonography is used to investigate unusual results of a previous diagnostic test, the ultrasonographer typically is skilled in detecting fetal abnormalities.

Amniocentesis. Usually performed between weeks 16 and 20 (occasionally as early as week 13) of pregnancy, amniocentesis provides a sample of amniotic fluid for chromosomal analysis, amniotic fluid AFP, and acetylcholinesterase levels (which may indicate NTD). The type of analysis performed on aspirated amniotic fluid varies with risk factors specific to the client. (For an illustration, see *Amniocentesis* in Chapter 22, High-Risk Antepartal Clients.)

One common reason for amniocentesis to detect chromosomal abnormalities in a fetus of a client age 35 or over. This requires a karyotype. Typically obtained from amniotic fluid (for a fetus) or a blood sample from a neonate, child, or adult, a karyotype depicts an individual's chromosomal structure in a photomicrograph. Because chromosomes appear only during active cell division, the process requires that white blood cells be placed in a culture medium and stimulated to undergo mitosis. When visible under a microscope, pairs of chromosomes can be matched using light and dark bands and structural differences as a guide. Then they can be counted, photographed, and arranged by size. (See *Normal karyotype* for an example.)

Because it may take several weeks before results are available (depending on the speed of culture growth) emotional support from the nurse is critical to minimize the client's anxiety. The relatively advanced gestational age at which amniocentesis is performed and the need to culture amniotic cells before testing are its two main disadvantages.

Normal karyotype

A karyotype like the one below can be performed during active cell division to allow analysis for certain chromosomal abnormalities. The examiner photographs the chromosomes and arranges them by number, looking for numerical and structural abnormalities. This configuration shows a normal chromosomal complement in a male: 22 pairs of autosomes and 2 sex chromosomes (one X and one Y).

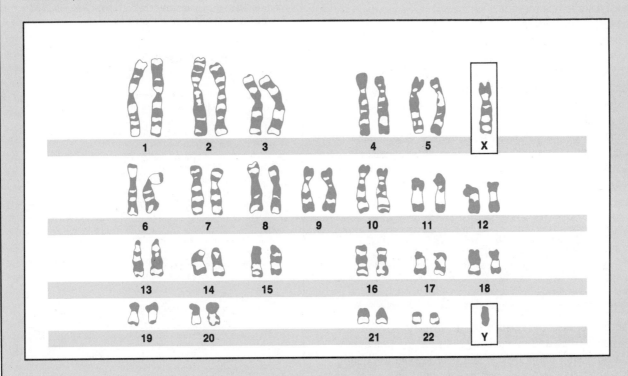

CVS. This test may be performed 9 to 12 weeks after the client's last menstrual period. (For an illustration, see *Chorionic villus sampling* in Chapter 22, High-Risk Antepartal Clients.) The main advantage of CVS over amniocetesis is that CVS allows testing earlier in fetal development. Excluding NTDs, disorders that can be identified by amniocentesis also can be identified by CVS. The procedure has two disadvantages compared to amniocentesis. First, pregnancy loss from CVS may exceed amniocentesis by approximately 0.8% (Rhoads, et al., 1989). Second, performing an amniotic fluid AFP test is impossible because CVS obtains no amniotic fluid.

Clients who have elected amniocentesis over CVS have done so to minimize fetal risk; those electing CVS preferred the test's earlier results (Lippman, Perry, Mandel, and Cartier, 1985).

Other procedures. *Fetoscopy* allows direct fetal visualization via a fiber-optic scope (fetoscope) inserted through the client's abdominal wall. This procedure may be required for obtaining fetal tissue samples, such as a skin biopsy. It can be used only during the second trimester. Risk of fetal loss, which ranges from 2% to 5%, exceeds that of amniocentesis or CVS.

Radiography allows visualization of fetal skeletal or limb malformations. However, because fetal exposure to ionizing radiation has been linked to abnormalities, radiography rarely is used.

Amniography allows X-ray visualization of the fetus after instillation of dye into the amniotic sac. Radiation dangers have limited use of this technique.

Magnetic resonance imaging eventually may provide detailed studies of fetal, uterine, and placental structures. Its safety in pregnancy currently is unknown.

In *cordocentesis,* which targets fetal circulation, the examiner inserts a needle through the client's abdomen using ultrasound as a guide, punctures the umbilical vein, and aspirates fetal blood. Fetal blood samples help in assessing fetal hemolytic disease. Risk of fetal death is unknown.

Postnatal detection

Testing programs now can screen for more than 10 genetic and metabolic disorders in neonates, some of which will lead to permanent disability or death if untreated. Postnatal identification of genetic disorders also allows for genetic counseling to the couple who are at an increased risk for conceiving other affected children. Although screening programs vary, each state must specify the following factors:
• disorders screened
• criteria for specimen collection
• criteria for laboratory analysis of specimens
• mandatory follow-up procedures after a positive result
• education required for health care professionals and the public.

Many states exempt neonates from screening that violates parents' religious beliefs. The nurse should know the procedures to follow for a family that does not want their neonate to have screening tests.

Nursing diagnosis

The nurse uses the client's health history, physical assessment data, and diagnostic studies to develop appropriate nursing diagnoses, which may involve the client, fetus, partner, and other family members. (For a partial list of possible nursing diagnoses, see *Nursing diagnoses: Genetic disorders.*)

Planning and implementation

The extent of the nurse's involvement in interventions for clients at risk for genetic abnormalities depends on acquisition of specialized training, charactertistics of the work setting (for example, in a clinic where the couple returns repeatedly, a specially prepared nurse may do much of the counseling), the type of genetic disorder involved, and individual needs of the parents and offspring. Specific genetic counseling may be carried out by the family's physician or a specially prepared practitioner. However, the nurse can and should provide interventions as part of the nursing care plan.

NURSING DIAGNOSES

Genetic disorders

The following are potential nursing diagnoses for problems and etiologies the nurse may encounter in clients concerned about genetic disorders. Specific nursing interventions for many of these diagnoses are provided in the "Planning and implementation" section of this chapter.

• Altered family processes related to a client's or partner's feelings about the presence of a genetic risk factor
• Altered family processes related to a physically or mentally disabled family member
• Altered family processes related to financial strains from genetic testing or treatment of a child with a genetic defect
• Altered parenting related to having a child with a genetic defect
• Altered sexuality patterns related to the risk of conceiving a child with a genetic disorder
• Anxiety related to the outcome of genetic evaluation
• Anxiety related to unknown health of offspring
• Grieving related to the anticipated or actual death of a child
• Ineffective family coping: compromised, related to fear of abnormality in offspring
• Ineffective individual coping related to fear of abnormality in offspring
• Knowledge deficit related to behaviors that can be harmful to the developing fetus
• Knowledge deficit related to genetic defects and their management
• Knowledge deficit related to genetic evaluation and counseling
• Knowledge deficit related to prenatal testing
• Knowledge deficit related to reproductive options
• Knowledge deficit related to the risk of having a child with a genetic defect
• Noncompliance related to ceasing personal behaviors that can harm a developing fetus
• Personal identity disturbance related to awareness of having produced a child with a genetic defect
• Social isolation related to a perceived lack of support during decisions about continuing a pregnancy
• Spiritual distress related to the possibility of terminating a pregnancy.

General interventions

Regardless of the nature of a specific genetic disorder, be prepared to address client concerns and problems with prompt management or referrals. To take an active role in managing these problems, implement a care plan focused on education, support, and counseling. Specific nursing goals typically include the following.

Provide information

The courts have established that health care professionals are legally responsible for informing clients of their risk of transmitting genetic disorders or birth defects based on family history, ethnicity, or teratogen exposure (Shaw, 1986). By extension, the nurse is bound to give clients complete and accurate information about diagnostic tests and their results.

Beginning before conception if possible, identify the client's risk of fetal genetic defects; provide appropriate information about genetic disorders, diagnostic tests, and reproductive alternatives; give emotional support to the client and involved family members; and—with special preparation—offer follow-up genetic counseling.

A client or partner may have a nursing diagnosis of *knowledge deficit related to the risk of having a child with a genetic defect.* Give each family member information about the risks of carrying the specific disorder, transmitting it to offspring, and the possible stigma associated with ethnically related disorders. Through actions and questions, reflect genuine concern for each family member's welfare.

In addition, the client or partner may have a nursing diagnosis of *knowledge deficit related to genetic evaluation and counseling* or *anxiety related to the outcome of genetic evaluation.* Communicate to each family member that screening is voluntary and that all results are confidential. A nurse-midwife, nurse practitioner, or physician will make appropriate referrals for screening tests for family members who wish to learn their specific risks of being carriers.

Inform any client nearing age 35 of the age-related risk for fetal chromosomal abnormality. Assure the client that this increased risk does not result from any deliberate action on her part. Explain the need for and function of appropriate prenatal diagnostic tests.

A client scheduled for prenatal testing, particularly with a nursing diagnosis of *knowledge deficit related to prenatal testing* or *anxiety related to outcome of genetic evaluation,* will need complete information about the procedure, its purpose, and the implications of its results. Be sure to explain that false-positive and false-negative results do occur and that possible follow-up testing presents little cause for alarm. Also explain that tests may miss a small percentage of abnormal fetuses. Emphasize that testing is voluntary. Provide emotional support to a client who receives abnormal results.

Aid decision making

After informing the couple about genetic risks for the client and her fetus, help them make decisions about pregnancy. If they fear bearing a genetically defective child, the couple may have a nursing diagnosis of *altered sexuality patterns related to the risk of conceiving a child with a genetic disorder.* If diagnostic tests reveal a genetically compromised fetus, the couple may have a nursing diagnosis of *spiritual distress related to the possibility of terminating the pregnancy.* To help the couple explore their feelings and concerns, be sensitive and open but avoid making judgmental observations.

The couple that understands the risks associated with transmission of a genetic disorder will be better equipped to make knowledgeable reproduction decisions. This understanding also may minimize their anxiety about genetic screening and the possibility of having a child with a genetic disorder. When caring for a family at risk for a genetic disorder, determine family members' understanding of the disorder and the risks of passing it to their children. For a family with a monogenic disorder, for example, nursing responsibilities include informing the couple that an autosomal dominant gene has a 50% chance of expression in offspring regardless of the child's sex and that the severity of autosomal disorders varies widely. Additionally, assess which risks may arise for the client during pregnancy. Some genetic disorders—such as Marfan's syndrome and cystic fibrosis—can increase the affected client's risk of health complications during pregnancy.

The client at increased risk for bearing a child with a genetic defect may need assistance in deciding on reproductive alternatives. Before becoming pregnant, she may need to choose among several options, including the following:
• accept the risk and attempt pregnancy
• avoid the risk and refrain from pregnancy
• minimize the risk by considering such alternatives as artificial insemination
• monitor the risk by undergoing prenatal diagnostic tests to identify an affected fetus.

Once pregnant, the client may need to choose among several other options, including the following:
• delivery of an affected fetus
• placement of an affected neonate with an adoptive family
• termination of the pregnancy.

Crisis intervention is useful in assisting families with their decisions (Kus, 1985). This approach includes helping the client identify the problem, generate and evaluate possible solutions, decide on a solution, and implement the decision. This approach is based on the nurse's ability to assist the client in making decisions.

For prospective parents, the decision to terminate the pregnancy when the fetus has genetic disorder will

Nursing goals for clients at risk for genetic disorders

The following nursing goals apply to any situation in which a risk of a genetic disorder arises. Specific clients may require more or fewer goals.

- Identify clients at risk for genetic disorders and make appropriate referrals.
- Provide support and counseling.
- Develop parents' understanding of inherited disorders, risk factors, and transmission modes.
- Develop parents' understanding of the genetic evaluation process.
- Minimize parents' anxiety about genetic testing and outcome.
- Provide an environment that allows parents to recognize and express their feelings.
- Facilitate grieving (anticipated or actual) related to genetic disorders or the death of a child from a genetic disorder or pregnancy termination.
- Provide assistance and information about alternatives to biological children when genetic disorders are present or probable.
- Minimize alterations in the client's life and relationships that may result from positive genetic testing or birth of a neonate with a genetic disorder.
- Provide resources or referrals to address the psychological or financial needs of a family with known carriers of a genetic disorder or an affected family member.
- Assist family members in developing effective coping mechanisms when a genetic disorder is identified in parents or offspring.
- Promote fetal health by helping the client eliminate environmental risks.

be difficult. An appropriate nursing diagnosis may be *grieving related to the anticipated or actual death of a child*. They will benefit from the nurse's sensitive support. When prospective parents learn that the outcome of prenatal testing has detected a genetic disorder, they have limited time in which to decide whether to continue or to terminate the pregnancy. Some will discuss the decision with family members, clergy, or others whose advice they value. Others make this decision alone. They may have a nursing diagnosis of *social isolation related to a perceived lack of support during decisions about continuing a pregnancy* or *spiritual distress related to the possibility of terminating a pregnancy*. The nurse who disagrees strongly with a client's decision about continuing a pregnancy should arrange for another nurse to assume client care responsibilities.

Few resources are available to the family deciding to terminate a pregnancy. The nurse's support and sensitivity are vital, especially in the unit where the termination occurs. For example, the client who has decided to terminate her pregnancy for genetic reasons may be upset about being in the same area with clients seeking termination for other reasons. Also, a client terminating her pregnancy for genetic reasons may experience a greater depression than one undergoing termination for another reason; follow-up counseling may be necessary.

Assist with pregnancy management

In certain cases, a fetal genetic disorder may require changes in pregnancy management. For example, galactosemia is an autosomal recessive disorder of galactose metabolism that leads to liver disease, cataracts, mental retardation and, in some cases, death. (See *Monogenic effects on mother, fetus, and neonate* for additional examples.) Prenatal diagnosis can determine if a fetus is affected. If so, the client's diet can be modified to restrict galactose intake, which may minimize harm to the fetus. An appropriate nursing diagnosis may be *knowledge deficit related to behaviors that can be harmful to the developing fetus*. A client who ignores interventions pertaining to pregnancy management may have a nursing diagnosis of *noncompliance related to ceasing personal behaviors that can harm a developing fetus*. (For a partial list of additional goals, see *Nursing goals for clients at risk for genetic disorders*.)

Genetic counseling

Genetic counseling provides testing, education specific to a particular disorder, presentation of alternatives specific to a particular disorder, and psychological support to help families adjust to genetic disorders. This process requires special educational preparation.

Clients who risk bearing children with genetic disorders or associated birth defects, or who have such disorders themselves, need counseling. This includes anyone with a history of birth defects, genetic disorders, alterations in growth, behavioral or learning disorders, alterations in sexual development, infertility, multiple spontaneous abortions, or stillbirths. Further, clients possibly exposed to teratogens (including alcohol) and clients age 35 or older should be informed about the availability of genetic counseling services.

Inform the client that genetic counseling is nondirective, meaning that she will not be told which decisions

Monogenic effects on mother, fetus, and neonate

A pregnant client who has a monogenic disorder may face increased health risks or may increase her fetus's or neonate's risk for complications. The chart below helps identify risk factors specific to these clients.

INHERITANCE PATTERN	DISORDER	MATERNAL COMPLICATIONS	FETAL OR NEONATAL COMPLICATIONS
Autosomal dominant	*Marfan's syndrome:* connective tissue disorder with tall stature, subluxated optic lenses, and dilation of the ascending aorta	With aortic dilation, increased risk of vascular rupture	Potential for premature birth
	Myotonic dystrophy: disorder of skeletal, cardiac, and smooth muscles characterized by sustained muscle contraction. Other characteristics include mental retardation, cataracts, and diabetes mellitus	Worsening of the disorder and increased risk of premature labor or spontaneous abortion	Increased risk of respiratory distress
	Achondroplasia: skeletal development disorder characterized by limbs with proximal shortening, large head, and prominent forehead	Symptoms of spinal compression may increase during pregnancy. Cesarean delivery is likely because of contracted pelvis.	Potential for respiratory arrest from narrow foramen magnum
Autosomal recessive	*Cystic fibrosis:* disorder involving exocrine secretions, including pancreatic and duodenal enzymes, sweat chlorides, and bronchial secretions	Increased risk of premature delivery and maternal mortality because of pulmonary infection	Potential for premature birth
	Phenylketonuria: impaired conversion of phenylalanine to tyrosine	Strict dietary modification required before conception to decrease risks of fetal damage	Risk of severe mental retardation, microcephaly, congenital heart disease, and low birth weight.
X-linked recessive	*Factor VIII deficiency (hemophilia A):* blood clotting disorder with prolonged bleeding following surgery, trauma, or dental work in some carriers	Increased risk of bleeding	Hemorrhagic symptoms during first week of affected male's extrauterine life, with implications for circumcision

to make or how to apply the information presented. Decisions about genetic testing, having children, or having prenatal diagnosis are personal. The genetic counseling team will help the family understand the information available and provide emotional support as family members consider their options.

Typically, genetic counseling services are provided by a team of specialists in medical genetics. This team may be located in a health care facility, at an outreach clinic, or in a health department program. Specialists include medical geneticists, specially prepared nurses, social workers, and counselors, as well as specialists in related diagnostic studies and treatments. These specialists are supported by all health care professionals who provide services to clients with genetic disorders—including nurses, physicians, and other health professionals who identify those at risk for genetic or birth defect disorders—educate them about risk factors, make referrals to genetic counseling units, and provide follow-up evaluation and support.

After such a support person recognizes a client's need for genetic counseling, the client and family are

Client with knowledge deficit related to genetic risk factors

The nursing process helps ensure high-quality care for the client who has genetic risk factors. The table below shows how the nurse might use the nursing process when caring for the client described in the case history at right. The first column presents history and physical assessment data followed by a paragraph of mental notes. These notes help the nurse make important connections among assessment findings, aiding in development of the nursing diagnosis and planning.

The second column lists an appropriate nursing diagnosis; information in the remaining columns is based on this diagnosis. Although not part of the nursing process, a rationale appears for each intervention in the fourth column to explain how it contributes to the care plan.

ASSESSMENT	NURSING DIAGNOSIS	PLANNING
Subjective (history) data • Client states that she is approximately 6 weeks pregnant. • Client says that she has just learned that her 35-year-old cousin gave birth to an infant with Down's syndrome. • Client expresses concern about her risk of having a child with Down's syndrome. • Client admits that she is afraid to talk to her cousin about her own fears. **Objective (physical) data** • Vital signs: pulse 96 beats/minute, respirations 32/minute, blood pressure 128/78 mm Hg • Well nourished, with no apparent abnormalities on head-to-toe physical examination. **Mental notes** *Client is afraid that she also will have a child with the same disorder. She may be afraid to ask her cousin for details because she does not want to give the impression that she does not love her cousin or does not accept the child. Client may want to know about prenatal diagnosis but having tests may or may not be consistent with values of her family and cousin.*	Knowledge deficit related to genetic risk factors	**Goals** The client will: • understand after this prenatal visit that two known risk factors related to having a child with Down's syndrome are chromosome type and maternal age • contact her cousin before genetic counseling evaluation to request specific information about the type of Down's syndrome present in her child • make arrangements for a genetic counseling evaluation as soon as possible and before her next prenatal visit.

referred to a genetic counseling unit. A team member meets with the family to obtain a family history, which will build on information already gathered by the nurse and others.

Before the first counseling visit, the nurse should urge family members to document health problems in their family, which may include birth or death cetificates, medical reports of health problems that relate to risk factors, and photographs of ancestors with genetic disorders or birth defects.

At the genetic counseling unit, the counseling team will review the family history, ask questions to clarify medical history, and examine family members who have genetic disorders or related birth defects. Diagnostic tests may be scheduled.

Next, the team will discuss their findings with family members, including the identity of any disorder and its causes, the likelihood that the disorder will occur in other or future family members, and the reproductive alternatives. This may require further genetic screening tests or prenatal diagnosis. In some situations, such as when both parents are carriers of an autosomal recessive disorder, artificial insemination may be discussed as a means to reduce the risk for future children.

According to the Ad hoc Committee on Genetic Counselling of the American Society of Human Genetics (1975), genetic counseling has the following goals:
• to understand the medical facts, including diagnosis, probable cause of the disorder, and management techniques available
• to understand how heredity contributes to the disorder and the risk of recurrence in specific relatives
• to understand the options for addressing the risk of recurrence

CASE STUDY

Annette Gray, a primigravid client age 35, has come alone to the obstetric clinic for her first prenatal interview.

IMPLEMENTATION		EVALUATION
Intervention Teach the client that Down's syndrome is associated with maternal age and a family history of chromosome translocation.	**Rationale** Specific information about genetic defects and their causes can decrease anxiety.	The client: • stated an understanding of the effect of maternal age and family history on her for having a child with Down's syndrome • demonstrated appropriate coping behaviors to address her fears about having a child with Down's syndrome • expressed willingness to ask her cousin about karyotype results before attending her first genetic counseling session • made and kept appointment at a genetic counseling unit before her next prenatal clinic appointment.
Encourage the client to express her fears and concerns about talking with her cousin and about her own risk of having a child with Down's syndrome.	Active listening communicates interest in the client's concerns and helps identify her fears.	
Facilitate referral to a genetic counseling unit.	Helping the client locate and obtain services can help relieve her sense of helplessness.	

• to choose appropriate action considering the risk involved and family goals, and to act in accordance with that decision
• to make the best adjustment possible to the disorder or to the risk of the disorder's recurrence.

Although genetic counseling requires special preparation, the nurse participates as a member of the clinical team. Besides reviewing family histories and providing information, support, and follow-up services, the nurse may coordinate counseling unit activities. (For a case study that shows how to apply the nursing process when caring for a client in need of genetic counseling, see *Applying the nursing process: Client with knowledge deficit related to genetic risk factors*.)

Genetic disorders or associated birth defects may place severe physical, psychological, and economic strains on the client and family. When a genetic or birth defect is identified, the nurse can assist the family in care management, referrals, and successful adjustment. The nurse's roles can include working with the client and family to:
• identify risk factors. The nurse may be the first person to whom the client voices a concern. Nursing responsibility includes understanding the significance of the client's information.
• identify physical or developmental abnormalities from physical assessment data.
• assess the need for referrals to specialty services for genetic evaluations, genetic counseling, or prenatal diagnostic studies.
• facilitate referrals for additional evaluations. The nurse who is acquainted with contact people in specialty clinics in the community is well equipped to assure that ap-

propriate services are obtained.
• demonstrate sensitivity to attitudes of the client with a genetic disorder, especially regarding reproduction.
• serve as the case manager, including helping family members find appropriate health services.
• prepare the family for the genetic counseling evaluation. The client's realization that something may be wrong can reduce self-esteem as well as create a fear that her children will not be normal.
• correct misconceptions about genetic counseling and its purposes. Some parents fear that they will be told to have no more children, will be blamed for genetic defects, or will be told to terminate a pregnancy.
• explain the typical outcomes from genetic counseling. Besides knowing what to expect, the family needs to understand that all information will be kept confidential. Tell them that they will receive a letter summarizing the conclusions of the genetic evaluation, and that this information can be sent to any other health care professionals they specify.

Documentation

Document all components of the nursing process. Information should include:
• risks for genetic disorders or associated birth defects identified through history, family pedigree, physical examination, and diagnostic tests
• results of diagnostic tests
• information provided to the client and her family regarding specific genetic disorders and their ramifications
• the client's response to information provided
• interventions applied and their outcomes
• decisions made by the client and her family, along with her stated reasons for those decisions
• referrals made for diagnostic tests or genetic counseling.

Evaluation

To complete the nursing process, the nurse evaluates the effectiveness of nursing care by reviewing the goals attained and the family's involvement and satisfaction with care received. Evaluate every step of the nursing process, including the care plan itself. As the client's situation changes, revise the care plan as necessary. The following examples reflect appropriate evaluation statements for a client and family at risk for genetic abnormality.
• The client and her family expressed understanding of the risk of transmitting a genetic disorder to their fetus.
• The client underwent prenatal diagnostic testing appropriate to her needs.
• Diagnostic testing revealed no genetic abnormality in the fetus.
• The client made an informed decision about continuing her pregnancy, based on probable neonatal outcomes specific to her situation.
• The client and her family attended genetic counseling sessions.

Chapter summary

Chapter 11 described the basic mechanisms of genetic inheritance, disorders related to genetic inheritance, and methods the nurse can use when caring for a client who has or who is at risk for transmitting a genetic disorder. Here are the key concepts.
• Somatic cells divide by mitosis and transmit identical genetic information to diploid daughter cells.
• Gametes divide by meiosis and transmit mixed genetic information to haploid daughter cells.
• Genetic disorders result from monogenic factors, chromosomal abnormalities, or multifactorial inheritance.
• Monogenic disorders may be inherited in one of four patterns: autosomal dominant, autosomal recessive, X-linked dominant, and X-linked recessive.
• A dominant gene may not behave like a dominant gene because of variations in its penetrance, expressivity, pleiotropy, or the occurrence of mutation.
• Chromosomal abnormalities may involve changes in chromosome number (as in trisomy or monosomy) or in structure (as in translocation, deletion, duplication, or inversion).

• Multifactorial inheritance occurs as a result of combined genetic and environmental factors.

• The health history of a client at risk for transmitting a genetic disorder should include biographical data, medical and obstetric history, family history, health promotion and protection behaviors, drug use, health habits, environmental and occupational factors, financial considerations, and roles and relationships.

• Various diagnostic studies can help detect and differentiate among genetic disorders, including the MSAFP test, ultrasonography, amniocentesis, and chorionic villus sampling.

• Nursing interventions typically required for a client at risk for transmitting a genetic disorder include providing information, helping with decision making, and assisting with pregnancy management.

• Typically, specific genetic counseling is undertaken by a team of specially prepared health care professionals.

Study questions

1. Which risk factors are associated with chromosomal abnormalities in children?

2. What may cause elevated results on an MSAFP test?

3. When taking a family history, the nurse learns that Mrs. Kern's father died of Marfan's syndrome. What information should the nurse elicit from the client?

4. When taking a family history, the nurse learns that the brother of Mrs. McPeak's husband has Factor VIII deficiency (hemophilia A). The client reports that her husband has tested negative for this disorder but asks if their children could inherit it. How should the nurse respond?

Bibliography

Ad hoc Committee on Genetic Counselling of the American Society of Human Genetics. (1975). Genetic counselling. *American Journal of Human Genetics*, 27, 240-241.

American Academy of Pediatrics, Committee on Genetics. (1989). Newborn screening fact sheets. *Pediatrics*, 83(3), 449-464.

Baird, P.A., Anderson, T.W., Newcombe, H.G., and Lowry, R.B. (1988). Genetic disorders in children and young adults: A population study. *American Journal of Human Genetics*, 42(5), 677-693.

Carpenito, L.J. (1987). *Nursing diagnosis: Application to clinical practice* (2nd ed.). Philadelphia: Lippincott.

Chervenak, F.A., Isaacson, G., and Mahoney, M.J. (1986). Advances in the diagnosis of fetal defects. *The New England Journal of Medicine*, 315(5), 305-307.

Clark, M.H., Frankel, M., and Trowbridge, D. (1989). A pedigree primer. *Journal of Pediatric Nursing*, 4(2), 112-118.

Hamilton, M., Hossam, I., and Whitefield, C. (1985). Significance of raised maternal serum-fetal protein in singleton pregnancies with normally formed fetuses. *Obstetrics and Gynecology*, 65(4), 465-470.

Harris, R. (1988). Genetic counseling and the new genetics. *Trends in Genetics*, 4(2), 52-56.

Helms, J. (1985). Active listening. In G. Bulecheck and J. McCloskey (Eds.), *Nursing interventions for nursing diagnoses* (pp. 328-337). Philadelphia: Saunders.

Hook, E., Cross, P., and Schreinemachers, D. (1983). Chromosome abnormality rate at amniocentesis and in live born infants. *JAMA*, 249(15), 2034-2038.

Jones, S. (1988). Decision making in clinical genetics: Ethical implications for perinatal nursing practice. *Journal of Perinatal and Neonatal Nursing*, 1(3), 11-23.

Kopala, B. (1989). Mothers with impaired mobility speak out. *MCN*, 14(2), 115-119.

Kus, R. (1985). Crisis intervention. In G. Bulecheck and J. McCloskey (Eds.), *Nursing interventions: Treatments for nursing diagnoses*. Philadelphia: Saunders.

Lippman, A., Perry, T., Mandel, S., and Cartier, L. (1985). Chorionic villi sampling: Women's attitudes. *American Journal of Medical Genetics*, 22(2), 395-401.

Mattison, D., and Angtuaco, T. (1988). Magnetic resonance imaging in prenatal diagnosis. *Clinical Obstetrics and Gynecology*, 31(20), 353-389.

Mor-yosef, S., Younis, J., Granat, M., Kedari, A,. Milgalter, A., and Schenker, J. (1988). Marfan's syndrome in pregnancy. *Obstetrical and Gynecological Survey*, 43(7), 382-385.

Morgan, C., and Elias, S. (1989). Prenatal diagnosis of genetic disorders. *Journal of Perinatal and Neonatal Nursing*, 2(4), 1-12.

Myhre, C., Richards, T., and Johnson, J. (1989). Maternal serum alpha-fetoprotein screening: An assessment of fetal well-being. *Journal of Perinatal and Neonatal Nursing*, 2(4), 13-20.

Osband, B. (1989). Multifactional inheritance: Implications for perinatal and neonatal nurses. *Journal of Perinatal and Neonatal Nursing*, 2(4), 43-52.

President's Commission for the Study of Ethical Problems in Medicine and Biomedical and Behavioral Research. (1983). Screening and counseling for genetic conditions: A report on the ethical, social, and legal implications of genetic screening, counseling and education programming. Washington, DC: U.S. Government Printing Office.

Rhoads, G., et al. (1989). The safety and efficacy of chorionic villus sampling for early prenatal diagnosis of cytogenetic abnormalities. *The New England Journal of Medicine*, 320(10), 609-617.

Schulman, J., and Simpson, J. (1981). *Genetic diseases in pregnancy: Maternal effects and fetal outcome.* New York: Academic Press.

Shaw, M. (1986). Editorial comment: Avoiding wrongful birth and wrongful life suits. *American Journal of Medical Genetics*, 25(1), 81-84.

Thompson, J., and Thompson, M. (1986). *Genetics in Medicine* (4th ed.). Philadelphia: Saunders.

Williamson, R., and Murray, J. (1988). Molecular analysis of genetic disorders. *Clinical Obstetrics and Gynecology*, 31(2), 270-284.

Cultural references

National Institutes of Health. (1987). Newborn screening for sickle cell disease and other hemoglobinopathies. *NIH consensus development conference statement*, April 6-8, 1987. Washington, DC: Author.

Wertz, D., and Fletcher, J. (1988). Attitudes of genetic counselors: A multinational survey. *American Journal of Human Genetics*, 42(4), 592-600.

Nursing research

Damarosch, S., and Perry, L. (1989). Self-reported adjustment, chronic sorrow, and coping of parents of children with Down syndrome. *Nursing Research*, 38(1), 25-30.

Heidrich, S., and Cranley, M. (1989). Effect of fetal movement, ultrasound scans and amniocentesis on maternal-fetal attachment. *Nursing Research*, 38(2), 81-84.

Strauss, S., and Munton, M. (1985). Common concerns of parents with disabled children. *Pediatric Nursing*, 11(5), 371-375.

Infectious Disorders

Objectives

After reading and studying this chapter, the student should be able to:

1. Describe selected sexually transmitted diseases (STDs) and their clinical findings and treatments.

2. Compare selected gynecologic infections, including their clinical findings and treatments.

3. Identify major urinary tract infections as well as their clinical findings and treatments.

4. Discuss TORCH (toxoplasmosis, others, rubella, cytomegalovirus, and herpes) infections and their importance in women of childbearing age.

5. Explain the clinical findings and treatments for human immunodeficiency virus (HIV) infection and acquired immunodeficiency syndrome (AIDS).

6. Identify factors that increase the risk of HIV infection.

7. Explain universal precautions for infection control.

8. Describe key areas to assess for a client with an infectious disorder.

9. Discuss common laboratory tests for a client with an infectious disorder.

10. List drugs commonly used to treat STDs along with their indications, major adverse effects, and nursing implications.

11. Summarize information the nurse can give a client to help prevent infection.

12. Apply the nursing process when caring for a client with an infectious disorder.

Introduction

Although hundreds of infectious disorders exist, this chapter focuses only on those that are likely to affect a woman's sexual health, genitourinary system, or ability to produce normal offspring. For discussion purposes, these disorders are divided into two groups: genitourinary infections (including STDs and gynecologic and urinary tract infections) and other infections (including TORCH and HIV infections).

STDs are relatively common in the United States. Of the reportable diseases, the number of cases of syphilis grew from 27,131 in 1983 to 40,117 in 1988; cases of gonorrhea decreased slightly from 780,905 in 1987 to 719,536 in 1988 (Centers for Disease Control [CDC], 1989b). For nonreportable diseases, official estimates for 1990 include 4 million cases of chlamydia, 1 million cases of condylomata acuminata, 3 million cases of trichomoniasis, and 200,000 to 500,000 cases of herpes genitalis (CDC, 1989b).

The incidence of HIV infection—and AIDS—is increasing rapidly. For example, 31,001 cases of AIDS were reported in 1988 (CDC, 1989c), but 10,563 cases were reported in the first 4 months of 1990 (CDC, 1990).

Many infectious disorders, especially STDs, can produce immediate physical problems as well as long-term effects, such as infertility. AIDS can lead to death. They also may cause emotional problems because they carry a social stigma and can affect intimate relationships. Therefore, in addition to providing physical care for the client, the nurse may need to offer emotional support to her, her sexual partner or partners, and family members.

This chapter describes some of the most common infectious disorders in women, highlighting their causes, clinical findings, and treatments. It also shows how to apply the nursing process when caring for a client with an infectious disorder.

GLOSSARY

Acquired immunodeficiency syndrome (AIDS): life-threatening disease that disables the immune system, rendering the body susceptible to opportunistic infection. AIDS is present when an individual with human immunodeficiency virus (HIV) infection develops Kaposi's sarcoma, extrapulmonary cryptococcosis, *Pneumocystis carinii* pneumonia, or other designated diseases.

Chlamydia: sexually transmitted disease (STD) caused by *Chlamydia trachomatis,* which is typically asymptomatic; the most common STD in the United States.

Condylomata acuminata: STD caused by human papillomavirus infection, which produces wartlike anogenital lesions.

Cryotherapy: therapeutic use of cold. It may be used to treat condylomata acuminata by freezing—and destroying—the lesions.

Cystitis: bladder inflammation, commonly caused by *Escherichia coli.* This lower urinary tract infection produces dysuria, urinary frequency and urgency, hematuria, and other urinary symptoms.

Dyspareunia: painful sexual intercourse.

Dysuria: difficult or painful urination.

Gonorrhea: STD caused by *Neisseria gonorrhoeae,* which may be asymptomatic or may produce vaginal discharge, urinary symptoms, dyspareunia, and menstrual irregularities.

Herpes genitalis: STD caused by herpes simplex virus, which is characterized by recurrent outbreaks of genital blisters that progress to shallow, painful ulcers.

Human immunodeficiency virus (HIV): retrovirus that can cause AIDS.

Pediculosis pubis: STD caused by *Phthirus pubis* (lice) infestation, which produces mild-to-severe pruritus in areas covered by pubic or other types of hair.

Pelvic inflammatory disease (PID): infection of the pelvic cavity; a common complication of an STD.

Pyelonephritis: acute inflammation of the ureters and kidneys, commonly caused by *E. coli.* It pro-

duces the effects of cystitis plus fever, chills, flank pain, and other signs and symptoms.

Scabies: STD caused by *Sarcoptes scabiei* (itch mite) infestation, which produces papular lesions and extreme pruritus along body creases in such areas as the axillae, breasts, and genitals.

Sexually transmitted disease (STD): disorder acquired through vaginal, anal, or oral intercourse.

Syphilis: STD caused by *Treponema pallidum,* which produces painless, papular lesions (chancres) and may progress through various stages to heart damage, seizures, and death.

T_4 lymphocyte: type of lymph cell that is vital to the body's immune response.

Tenesmus: persistent, ineffectual spasms of the rectum or bladder accompanied by the desire to empty the bowel or bladder.

TORCH infections: acronym for a group of infections that includes toxoplasmosis, other diseases (chlamydia, group B beta-hemolytic streptococcus, syphilis, and varicella zoster), rubella, cytomegalovirus, and herpesvirus. TORCH can harm an embryo or fetus.

Toxic shock syndrome (TSS): rare, potentially fatal, multisystem disorder caused by a toxin secreted by *Staphylococcus aureus.* TSS is associated with use of high-absorbency tampons.

Trichomoniasis: STD caused by *Trichomonas vaginalis,* which is characterized by vaginal discharge, urinary symptoms, and vulvar edema, pruritus, and tenderness.

Universal precautions: infection control measures that treat all blood and body fluids as potentially infectious.

Urethritis: urethral inflammation caused by a lower urinary tract infection, which produces the same effects as cystitis.

Vaginitis: vaginal inflammation, which may be caused by fungi, protozoa, or bacteria.

Vulvitis: vulvar inflammation, which may be caused by fungi, protozoa, bacteria, other organisms, chemical irritation, or allergic reaction.

Genitourinary infections

In women, common genitourinary infections include STDs, gynecologic infections, and urinary tract infections (UTIs).

Sexually transmitted diseases

Common STDs (infectious disorders acquired through vaginal, anal, or oral intercourse) include chlamydia, trichomoniasis, herpes genitalis, gonorrhea, syphilis, condylomata acuminata, pediculosis pubis, and scabies. Each STD varies in its cause, clinical findings, treatment, and implications during pregnancy. (For more information, see *Common sexually transmitted diseases,* pages 258 and 259. For information about their implications for pregnancy and fetal health, see Chapter 22, High-Risk Antepartal Clients.)

STDs pose a considerable threat to the health of women and their families. Since the 1960s, the overall incidence of STDs has increased. Many of the infecting organisms have developed resistance to antibiotics, making treatment more difficult. In addition, many STDs can leave lasting physical and emotional scars.

Chlamydia

Named after the infecting organism *Chlamydia trachomatis,* chlamydia is the most common STD in the United States (Bourcier and Siedler, 1987; CDC, 1989a; McElhose, 1988). It affects up to 4 million individuals annually (Swinker, 1986). However, about half of all infected women are asymptomatic and do not seek care; many develop pelvic inflammatory disease (PID).

The risk of contracting chlamydia is increased in women who are under age 30 (even higher in those under age 20), have multiple sexual partners, do not use a barrier method of contraception, and belong to a lower socioeconomic group (Loucks, 1987; Washington, Browner, and Korenbrot, 1987; Washington, Johnson, and Sanders, 1987; Marvin and Slevin, 1987; Corbett and Meyer, 1987). Chlamydia commonly coexists with gonorrhea, requiring dual treatment.

Transmission of *C. trachomatis* primarily follows mucosal contact with an infected person. Without treatment, the infection can ascend from the cervix to the fallopian tubes, causing scarring that can lead to infertility and ectopic pregnancy (Sanders, Harrison, and Washington, 1986).

Trichomoniasis

A common STD, trichomoniasis is caused by the flagellate, unicellular protozoon *Trichomonas vaginalis.* Annually, it affects about 180 million women worldwide and about 2.5 million women in the United States (Shesser, 1990). In women, many organisms must be present to produce symptoms (Benoit, 1988); otherwise, they may be asymptomatic. Trichomoniasis may be acute or chronic and may recur, especially if current sexual partners are not treated simultaneously.

Because *T. vaginalis* grows best when the vaginal mucosa is more alkaline than normal (a pH of about 5.5 to 5.8), factors that raise the vaginal pH may predispose a woman to trichomoniasis. These factors may include oral contraceptive use, pregnancy, bacterial overgrowth, exudative cervical or vaginal lesions, or frequent douching that disturbs normal vaginal lactobacilli that maintain acidity.

Trichomoniasis is transmitted primarily by sexual partners and secondarily by contaminated douche equipment or moist washcloths. Occasionally, an infected woman may pass *T. vaginalis* to her neonate during vaginal delivery.

Herpes genitalis

Herpes genitalis (genital herpes) is caused by the herpes simplex virus (HSV). HSV-1 is transmitted primarily through oral secretions, typically producing gingivostomatitis (gum and mouth inflammation) and oral labial ulcers (fever blisters). HSV-2 is transmitted chiefly through genital secretions and typically produces herpes genitalis. However, both HSVs commonly appear in genital infections. HSV transmission may result from sexual intercourse, oral-genital sexual activity, and such contact as kissing or hand-to-body contact. Also, a pregnant woman may transmit the infection to her neonate during vaginal delivery.

An acute, inflammatory disease of the genitalia, herpes genitalis is one of the most common recurring genitourinary infections. The initial or primary episode usually is self-limiting but may cause painful local or systemic disease. Recurrent episodes typically produce milder effects and may be triggered by stressors, such as fever, other infections, menstruation, emotions, and ultraviolet light exposure. Prognosis varies according to the client's age, immune defenses, and infection site.

Complications of chronic herpes genitalis include the spread of lesions to other sites, increased risk of cervical cancer, stiff neck, photophobia (light intolerance), and aseptic meningitis. Herpes genitalis also has been associated with an increased risk of HIV infection (Breslin, 1988; CDC, 1989a; McElhose, 1988).

Gonorrhea

Gonorrhea—an infection of the genitourinary tract (especially the urethra and cervix) and occasionally, the rectum, pharynx, and eyes—is caused by the gram-negative diplococcus bacteria, *Neisseria gonorrhoeae.* It affects 3% to 18% of sexually active women (Bell and Hein, 1984).

Transmission of *N. gonorrhoeae* typically results from sexual contact with an infected person. However, it also may be transmitted by direct contact with lesions or contaminated washcloths, towels, linens, and clothing. Also, neonates born of infected mothers can contract gonococcal ophthalmia neonatorum during passage through the birth canal. Children and adults with gonorrhea can contract gonococcal conjunctivitis by touching their eyes with contaminated hands.

Because gonorrhea produces symptoms in men more commonly than in women, men are more likely to seek treatment for it. About 50% of infected women are asymptomatic, so the nurse should urge all women to undergo routine screening.

(Text continues on page 260.)

Common sexually transmitted diseases

To understand various sexually transmitted diseases (STDs) in women, the nurse should be familiar with their clinical findings and treatments, as shown in the chart below. Unless otherwise stated, all treatments are recommended for the nonpregnant adult by the CDC.

DISEASE	CLINICAL FINDINGS	TREATMENT
Chlamydia	• Typically asymptomatic • Yellowish endocervical discharge • Dysuria (painful or difficult urination) • Spotting after intercourse or between menses • Pelvic inflammatory disease (PID), which produces pelvic pain and vaginal discharge and increases the risk of ectopic pregnancy and infertility (Bourcier and Seidler, 1987; McElhose, 1988; Whelan, 1988)	• Doxycycline hyclate (Vibramycin) or tetracycline (Achromycin, Tetracyn) for 7 days; alternatively, erythromycin base (E-Mycin, Robimycin) or erythromycin ethylsuccinate (E-Mycin E) for 7 days or sulfisoxazole for 10 days • Erythromycin base (E-Mycin, Robimycin), erythromycin ethylsuccinate (E-Mycin E), or amoxicillin trihydrate (Amoxil) for 7 days in a pregnant client • Concurrent treatment of all sexual partners, if possible
Trichomoniasis	• Thin, bubbly, yellow-green, malodorous vaginal discharge • Moderate to severe vulvar pruritus • Vaginal and cervical edema and tenderness • Dysuria and polyuria (excess urination) • Dyspareunia (painful intercourse) • Strawberry red vagina and cervix • Vaginal pH of 5.5 or higher	• Metronidazole (Flagyl, Protostat) P.O. in a single large dose or smaller doses for 7 days • Metronidazole P.O. in single dose during second and third trimesters (CDC, 1989a) • Concurrent treatment of all sexual partners, if possible
Herpes genitalis	*Primary outbreak* • Prodrome of influenza-like symptoms • Painful genital blisters that progress to macules, papules, vesicles, and then to pustules that develop into shallow, painful ulcers, which resolve in 2 to 6 weeks • Inguinal tenderness and lymphadenopathy (swollen glands) • Vaginal discharge, dyspareunia • Genital irritation, pruritus • Muscle pain, headache, fever, malaise, anorexia, dysuria *Recurrent episode* • Prodrome of pruritus, burning sensation in genitalia, tingling in legs, slight vaginal discharge • Fewer, less painful lesions that heal in 4 to 7 days (Breslin, 1988; McElhose, 1988)	• Acyclovir sodium (Zovirax) P.O. for 7 to 10 days during primary outbreak (contraindicated during pregnancy) • Symptomatic treatment, such as warm sitz baths • Adequate rest, balanced nutrition, and avoidance of stressors to help prevent recurrence • Infection control measures at home, such as conscientious hand-washing
Gonorrhea	• Typically asymptomatic • Yellow-green purulent discharge • Cervical tenderness • Dysuria, urinary frequency, or burning sensation on urination • Dyspareunia • Menstrual irregularities, spotting after intercourse • Swollen, painful labia; tender inguinal lymph nodes; PID • Profuse, purulent anal discharge, rectal pain, blood or mucus in stool, anal inflammation, pruritus, tenesmus (persistent spasms of the rectum or bladder), constipation • Sore throat and inflammation, if pharynx is affected • Arthritis, skin lesions, pericarditis, meningitis, septicemia (Fogel, 1988; McElhose, 1988)	• Ceftriaxone sodium (Rocephin) I.M. in one dose plus doxycycline for 7 days • Ceftriaxone in one dose plus erythromycin for 7 days during pregnancy • Concurrent treatment of all sexual partners, if possible • Report to public health authorities

Common sexually transmitted diseases continued

DISEASE	CLINICAL FINDINGS	TREATMENT
Syphilis	*Primary stage* • One or more painless chancres (papular lesions with a red base) on the genitalia, around the anus, or on the lips • Breakdown of chancres into indurated ulcers that develop a firm, elevated border and then disappear in about 3 weeks • Local lymphadenopathy that clears in 4 to 6 weeks *Secondary stage* • Nonspecific, symmetrical, nontender skin rash on trunk, extremities, or face that lasts 2 to 6 weeks • Condylomata lata (flat warts) on any moist skin surface *Latent stage* • Usually asymptomatic • Positive blood test, chancres *Tertiary stage* • Circulatory system effects, such as coronary artery disease, aneurysm, or heart damage that may lead to death • Central nervous system effects, causing convulsions and altered reflexes, sensorium, and speech • Bone weakness, skin rashes, and various other effects	• Penicillin G benzathine I.M. in one dose • Doxycycline or tetracycline P.O. for 2 weeks for the nonpregnant client who is allergic to penicillin (contraindicated during pregnancy) • Erythromycin for 2 weeks for the pregnant or nonpregnant client who is allergic to penicillin and tetracycline • Concurrent treatment of all sexual partners, if possible • Report to public health authorities
Condylomata acuminata	• Wartlike (painless, soft, fleshy) growths in the anogenital area • Chronic vaginal discharge • Pruritus • Dyspareunia	• No cure known • Topical application of podophyllum resin (Podoben) at weekly intervals (contraindicated during pregnancy) to remove warts • Topical application of trichloroacetic acid (80% to 90%) to remove warts • Topical application of fluorouracil (5-FU) for resistant condylomata • Cryotherapy (treatment using cold as a destructive medium) to remove warts • Electrodessication (form of electrosurgery that destroys tissue by burning it) to remove warts • Carbon dioxide laser therapy to destroy warts
Pediculosis pubis	• Tiny white specks (lice) close to base of hair shaft that resist removal • Lice in pubic hair, sometimes in hair of the axillae, on the trunk or legs, around the anus, or in the eyelashes • Mild to severe pruritus, skin irritation from scratching, small papules where lice nest and itching occurs	• Lindane (Kwell) shampoo (contraindicated during pregnancy) • Permethrin (1%) cream rinse • Pyrethrins and piperonyl butoxide • Crotamiton (Eurax) cream during pregnancy • Concurrent treatment of all sexual partners, if possible
Scabies	• Papular lesions at sites where mites burrow • Extreme pruritus (increasing at night) along body creases, such as the wrists, axillae, breasts, waistline, and genitalia	• Lindane shampoo or cream • Crotamiton cream during pregnancy • Second application if symptoms persist after 1 week • Concurrent treatment of all sexual partners, if possible

Untreated gonorrhea can spread through the blood to the joints, tendons, meninges, and endocardium and can lead to chronic PID and sterility. Most clients respond positively to adequate treatment, but reinfection is common.

Syphilis

A chronic, infectious STD, syphilis begins in the mucous membranes and, untreated, quickly becomes systemic, spreading to nearby lymph nodes and the bloodstream. The disease can progress through four stages: primary, secondary, latent, and tertiary. Primary syphilis appears approximately 21 to 90 days after the client is infected. Secondary syphilis appears weeks to months after the primary stage and lasts 2 to 6 weeks. The latent stage can last up to 30 years. Tertiary syphilis, the final stage, can last 1 to 40 years and can cause crippling or death. However, the client's prognosis is excellent if the disease is detected and treated in an earlier stage.

Syphilis is the third most prevalent reportable infectious disease. Incidence is highest among urban dwellers, especially between ages 15 and 39.

The spirochete *Treponema pallidum* causes syphilis after transmission primarily through sexual contact. Prenatal transmission from an infected mother to her fetus also is possible.

Condylomata acuminata

Infection with human papillomavirus (HPV) causes condylomata acuminata (venereal or genital warts). In the United States, its incidence has risen from 169,000 in 1966 to more than 2 million in 1987. This disorder rarely occurs before puberty or after menopause (CDC, 1989a).

The dry, wartlike growths of condylomata acuminata may appear on the vulva, vagina, cervix, or rectum. They may be large or small, multiple or single, and should be differentiated from condylomata lata (flat warts associated with second-stage syphilis) by a serology test.

Condylomata acuminata are highly contagious, and usually are transmitted through sexual contact. They grow rapidly in a warm, moist environment and their growth is increased by heavy perspiration, poor hygiene, or pregnancy. They may accompany other genital infections and predispose the client to cancer of the cervix, vagina, vulva, and anus (Bourcier and Seidler, 1987; Lucas, 1988; and McElhose, 1988).

Pediculosis pubis

Also called pubic lice, pediculosis pubis results from infestation by the parasite *Phthirus pubis*. Pubic lice use claws to cling to the hair shaft. They typically appear in pubic hair, but may spread to the hair of the axillae, trunk, anus, or legs as well as to the eyelashes.

Pediculosis pubis is transmitted through sexual intercourse or by contact with clothes, bed linens, or towels harboring lice. The lice feed on human blood and lay their eggs (nits) in body hairs or clothing fibers. The nits hatch in 7 to 9 days, and the young lice must feed within 24 hours or die. They mature in 2 to 3 weeks.

When a louse bites, it injects a toxin into the skin that produces mild irritation and a purpuric spot. Repeated bites cause sensitization to the toxin, leading to more serious inflammation. Treatment can eliminate lice effectively.

Scabies

Infestation with the parasite *Sarcoptes scabiei* (itch mite) causes scabies. Mites can live entire life cycles in the skin of humans, causing chronic infection. The female mite burrows into the skin to lay her eggs, from which larvae emerge to copulate and then reburrow, provoking a sensitivity reaction. The adult mite can survive without a human host for only 2 or 3 days.

Scabies transmission occurs through skin contact, sexual intercourse, or contact with infected bed linens or clothing.

Gynecologic infections

Women also commonly seek care for reproductive tract infections that are not STDs. These infections can cause troublesome symptoms and affect intimate relationships and long-term health. For example, a gynecologic infection can produce dyspareunia (painful intercourse), which may alter the client's sexual relationship. It also can ascend from a lower genital structure to the uterus, fallopian tubes, and peritoneal cavity, causing infertility, for example.

When the client develops symptoms of infection, she may develop feelings of anxiety, guilt, and fear. To understand the client's feelings and to differentiate normal and abnormal findings, the nurse must develop comprehensive knowledge about gynecologic infections, including vaginitis, vulvitis, PID, and toxic shock syndrome (TSS). (For more information, see *Common gynecologic infections*.)

Vaginitis

Vaginitis (inflammation of the vagina) can be caused by fungi or yeast (candidiasis), protozoa (trichomonas vaginitis), or bacteria (bacterial vaginosis). It typically results from overgrowth of normal vaginal organisms.

Common gynecologic infections

Because vaginal and other gynecologic infections can affect the client's long-term health, the nurse should be familiar with the clinical findings and treatment of these infections.

INFECTION	CLINICAL FINDINGS	TREATMENT
Vaginitis: candidiasis (moniliasis, a fungal or yeast infection)	• Thick, odorless, white or yellow vaginal discharge about the consistency of cottage cheese • Vaginal and vulvar pruritus • Vaginal and vulvar erythema, edema, and irritation • White or gray raised patches on vaginal mucosa • Dyspareunia • Dysuria	• Topical application of vaginal cream or suppositories of miconazole nitrate (Monistat), terconazole (Terazol-7), clotrimazole (Mycelex), butoconazole (Femstat), nystatin (Mycostatin), or tioconazole (Vagistat) • Oral antifungals and vaginal application of gentian violet (Genapax) for chronic, recurrent candidiasis
Vaginitis: bacterial (*Haemophilus*, *Gardnerella*, or nonspecific) vaginosis	• Thin, yellow-gray, scant vaginal discharge • Fishy vaginal odor, especially after intercourse • Vulvar irritation (rare) • Vaginal pH over 4.5 • Clue cells on microscopic examination of discharge	• Metronidazole (except during pregnancy) or clindamycin (Cleocin) P.O. for 7 days • Concurrent treatment of sexual partners, if possible (Shesser, 1990)
Vulvitis	• Vulvar pruritus and excoriation • Vulvar erythema and edema • Vulvar burning	• Treatment of any coexisting infection • Elimination of possible allergens
Pelvic inflammatory disease (PID)	• Bilateral, diffuse, lower abdominal pain that worsens with movement or intercourse • Fever and chills • Thick, yellow, purulent vaginal discharge • Irregular vaginal bleeding • Dysuria • Nausea, vomiting, and anorexia • Tenderness of the uterus and ovaries, especially with cervical movement • Infertility	Treatment regimens, consisting of broad-spectrum antibiotics, vary with the infecting organism. The following are examples only. • Cefoxitin or cefotetan I.V. plus doxycycline P.O. or I.V. for at least 48 hours after client improves; doxycycline P.O. for 10 to 14 days after discharge • Clindamycin I.V. plus gentamicin I.V. or I.M. for at least 48 hours after client improves; doxycycline or clindamycin P.O. for 10 to 14 days after discharge • If client is not hospitalized, cefoxitin I.M. and probenicid P.O. or ceftriaxone I.M. plus doxycycline or tetracycline P.O. for 10 to 14 days
Toxic shock syndrome (TSS)	• Sudden high fever and influenza-like symptoms (nausea, vomiting, diarrhea, sore throat, and headache) between days 2 to 4 of the menstrual period • Hypovolemia and hypotension within 48 hours • Erythematous macular rash on palms and soles that peels 1 to 2 weeks after onset • Myalgia (muscle pain), weakness • Marked hemoconcentration • Elevated blood urea nitrogen levels • Enzyme abnormalities (laboratory tests) • Disorientation and decreased level of consciousness followed by renal failure, disseminated intravascular coagulation, and circulatory collapse (Droegmueller, Herbst, Mishall, and Stencheur, 1987)	• Administration of I.V. beta-lactamase-resistant antibiotics, such as oxacillin, nafcillin, or methicillin, to treat the infection • Administration of vancomycin to treat the infection in a client with a penicillin allergy • Oxygen administration and mechanical ventilation to treat adult respiratory distress syndrome, if necessary • Administration of I.V. fluids, such as normal saline or lactated Ringer's solution; and colloids, such as plasmanate, blood, or blood products via large-bore needle, to correct circulatory collapse • Measurement of central venous pressure and pulmonary artery wedge pressure with a pulmonary artery catheter to monitor fluid volume • Use of antishock garments and vasopressors such as dopamine to maintain blood pressure, if necessary

The normal vaginal environment depends on a delicate balance of hormones and bacteria. Under the influence of estrogen, the vaginal epithelium is a thick, infection-free environment that promotes the growth of lactobacilli. By metabolizing glycogen, lactobacilli form lactic acid, which maintains an acidic environment (pH 4 to 5) that discourages bacterial growth.

Various factors can disrupt this normal balance, allowing overgrowth of normal flora and predisposing the client to infection: decreased lactobacilli (from use of antibiotics or douches), increased glycogen (from diabetes or excessive carbohydrate intake), increased estrogen (caused by pregnancy), and decreased resistance (caused by increased stress, poor nutrition, and use of feminine hygiene products, perfumed toilet paper, or tampons).

Vulvitis

Vulvitis (inflammation of the vulva) may coexist with vaginitis (vulvovaginitis) or occur alone. Because of the proximity of the vulva and vagina, inflammation of one easily precipitates inflammation of the other. Vulvitis, which may occur at any age and affects most women at some time, usually responds to treatment.

Vulvitis can result from the same organisms that cause vaginitis. It also may result from the organisms that cause gonorrhea, condylomata acuminata, herpes genitalis, pediculosis pubis, scabies, or molluscum contagiosum (skin and mucous membrane disease caused by a poxvirus); personal hygiene that allows contamination with urine or feces or vaginal secretions; and chemical irritations by—or allergic reactions to—feminine hygiene sprays, douches, soaps, vaginal spermicides, clothing, or toilet paper.

Pelvic inflammatory disease

A common complication of STDs, PID (infection of the pelvic cavity) can affect the uterus, fallopian tubes, ovaries, pelvic peritoneum, or the entire pelvis. This major gynecologic health problem affects about 1 million women each year in the United States. Its direct and indirect costs total about $3.5 billion annually (Droegemueller, Herbst, Mishall, and Stencheur, 1987).

PID typically results from sexually transmitted organisms, such as *N. gonorrhoeae, C. trachomatis, Mycoplasma,* and aerobic and anaerobic bacteria. However, it also can follow dilatation and curretage, hysterosalpingography, and intrauterine device (IUD) insertion. Other factors may contribute to PID, such as decreased resistance to infections and recurrent bacterial vaginosis.

Clients under age 30 and those who experience first intercourse at an early age or who have multiple sexual partners are at a higher risk of developing PID. Clients who are sexually inactive or are not menstruating rarely develop PID.

PID results from upward movement of organisms from the vagina and cervix to the uterus and fallopian tubes. Infection and inflammation spread through the open end of the tubes to the ovaries and peritoneal cavity.

In the fallopian tubes, the inflammation causes adhesions and scarring, which can decrease fertility. A single episode of PID increases the risk of ectopic (tubal) pregnancy about six times; tubal scarring causes infertility in approximately 60,000 women (Havens, Sullivan, and Tilton, 1986).

The client with PID may be acutely ill and later may experience chronic pelvic pain. The potential or actual loss of reproductive ability can damage the client's self-concept and generate considerable anxiety.

Careful follow-up is essential for the client with PID because she may develop complications, such as tubo-ovarian abscess or ectopic pregnancy, which may require surgery. Also, PID may recur, especially if the client's partners are untreated, if she becomes reinfected, or if her fallopian tubes sustain damage.

Toxic shock syndrome

TSS is a potentially fatal, multisystem disorder. It is caused by a toxin that is secreted by *Staphylococcus aureus* and enters the bloodstream. The toxin alters capillary permeability, causing intravascular fluid leakage and decreased circulating fluid volume, which may lead to hypotension and shock.

Relatively rare, TSS affected 390 women in 1988—far fewer than the 502 women affected in 1983 (CDC, 1989b). Since the early 1980s, the mortality rate associated with TSS has dropped from about 5% to less than 3% (Hoeprich and Jordan, 1989).

From 1% to 5% of women have TSS-producing strains of *S. aureus* in the vagina (Hoeprich and Jordan, 1989). Certain factors may increase the risk of TSS by giving the toxin a means of entry into the systemic circulation:
• use of high-absorbency tampons during menstruation
• use of a barrier method of contraception, such as a diaphragm, sponge, or cervical cap (rare)
• chronic vaginal infection, such as herpes genitalis
• postoperative or postpartal infection (Hoeprich and Jordan, 1989).

The greatest risk occurs in menstruating Caucasians around age 23 (Hoeprich and Jordan, 1989).

Although most women recover from TSS, some have mild recurrences with subsequent menstrual cycles, and a small percentage die from such complications as adult respiratory distress syndrome, intractable hypotension, and disseminated intravascular coagulation (Droegmueller, Herbst, Mishall, and Stencheur, 1987).

Urinary tract infections

UTIs include all bacterial infections of the lower urinary tract (urethra and bladder) and upper urinary tract (ureters and kidneys).

At least 10% of women will develop a UTI in their lifetime, making these infections the most common in women of all ages (Fogel and Woods, 1981). Women are at risk for infection because of the short length of the urethra, which is easily colonized by organisms, especially the normal rectal flora, *Escherichia coli*. These organisms progressively may colonize the perineum, urethral meatus, urethra, bladder, and possibly the kidneys.

In women between ages 18 to 24, sexual intercourse is a major cause of UTIs because it spreads organisms from the vagina, rectum, or perineum to the urethral meatus. In postmenopausal women, decreased estrogen levels make the urethra thinner and less resistant to bacterial invasion. Other factors that bring pathologic organisms into contact with the meatus are incomplete bladder emptying, use of a diaphragm or tampons, and urologic abnormalities.

The most common UTIs in women are cystitis, urethritis, and pyelonephritis.

Cystitis and urethritis

Cystitis (bladder inflammation) and urethritis (urethral inflammation) produce dysuria, burning on urination, urinary frequency and urgency, suprapubic pain, hematuria, low back discomfort, and bacteriuria. In a client with cystitis, bladder palpation and percussion produce pain.

Based on urine culture and sensitivity results, the nurse practitioner or physician selects appropriate antibiotics to treat the infection. If the client is not allergic to sulfa, she may receive co-trimoxazole (Bactrim, Septra) or sulfisoxasole (Gantrisin). Amoxicillin (Amoxil), tetracycline, norfloxacin (Noroxin), nitrofurantoin (Macrodantin), and cephalexin (Keflex) also may be used, depending on the infecting organism. A urinary analgesic such as phenazopyridine (Pyridium) may be prescribed to decrease dysuria.

Pyelonephritis

This acute inflammation of the ureters and kidneys is less common but more serious than cystitis, which may precede it. Pyelonephritis is more common in pregnant than nonpregnant clients because the ureters normally become dilated during pregnancy, which more readily admits ascending bacteria (Hoeprich and Jordan, 1989).

Pyelonephritis typically produces the signs and symptoms of cystitis plus general malaise, fever, shaking chills, costovertebral (flank) pain, lumbar pain, tenderness in the kidney and suprapubic areas, hematuria, nausea, vomiting, anorexia, and abdominal pain. Chronic pyelonephritis may develop from repeated infections and may produce kidney scarring and fibrosis.

Treatment calls for administration of antibiotics, such as a penicillin derivative or a cephalosporin, depending on the infecting organism. If the client develops a high fever and dehydration, hospitalization for intravenous antibiotics and fluids may be necessary. Other treatments include bed rest and increased fluid intake.

Other infections

Women also are at risk for other infections, including TORCH and HIV infections.

TORCH infections

The acronym TORCH includes toxoplasmosis, other diseases (chlamydia, group B beta-hemolytic streptococcus, syphilis, and varicella zoster), rubella, cytomegalovirus, and herpesvirus. These infections can harm an embryo or fetus. Because the client may be pregnant and not realize it, the nurse should pay close attention to these infectious disorders. (For more information about chlamydia, herpesvirus infection, and syphilis, see the "Sexually transmitted diseases" section of this chapter. For more information about the other infections in this group, see *TORCH infections*, page 264.)

HIV infection and AIDS

Infection with HIV can cause AIDS-related complex (ARC), a disease that produces fatigue, generalized lymphadenopathy, shortness of breath, weight loss, and rash. It also can cause AIDS, a disease that disables the immune system, rendering the body susceptible to life-threatening, opportunistic infections. Few disorders arouse more powerful emotions than AIDS. Those who contract AIDS suffer social stigma, chronic and debilitating illness, pain, and, typically, death. Because of

TORCH infections

The following chart compares the clinical findings and treatment for toxoplasmosis, group B beta-hemolytic streptococcus, varicella-zoster virus, rubella, and cytomegalovirus. (For findings and treatment of herpes genitalis, see *Common sexually transmitted diseases*.)

INFECTION	CLINICAL FINDINGS	TREATMENT
Toxoplasmosis	• Fever • Cervical lymphadenopathy • Myalgia • Malaise • Rash • Hepatosplenomegaly	• Sulfadiazine (Microsulfon) or pyrimethamine (Daraprim) with folic acid • Avoidance of eating raw meat and touching the litter or litter box of infected cats
Group B beta-hemolytic streptococcus	• Typically asymptomatic • Fever • Urinary urgency and frequency, dysuria • Fatal endocarditis (rare)	• Aqueous penicillin (Pfizerpen), ampicillin (Amcill, Polycillin), or gentamycin (Garamycin) with ampicillin
Varicella-zoster virus (herpes zoster, chickenpox)	• Painful lesions along the routes of cranial or spinal nerves in successive crops of macules, papules, vesicles with an erythematous base, and crusts • Gastrointestinal disturbances, malaise, fever, headache (early symptoms) • Pruritus • Varicella pneumonia with fever, cough, and chest pain (after the rash in an adult) • Encephalitis, hepatitis, nephritis, and myocarditis (rare complications)	• Bed rest and increased fluid intake • Acetaminophen (Tylenol) to relieve pain • Application of calamine lotion and bathing in colloidal oatmeal (Aveeno) in warm water to relieve pruritus • Prevention with varicella-zoster immune globulin (VZIG) for passive immunity or varicella-zoster vaccine (VZV, under clinical investigation in the United States)
Rubella (German measles)	• Diffuse, fine, red maculopapular rash • Fever • Malaise • Lymphadenopathy • Arthralgia • Sore throat • Cough	• Bed rest and increased fluid intake • Acetaminophen or aspirin to relieve discomfort • Prevention of disease by rubella vaccine
Cytomegalovirus	• Typically asymptomatic • Upper respiratory symptoms, such as cough, wheezing, and chest congestion • Extreme fatigue • Pneumonia with fever, chills, headache, productive cough, and chest pain • Retinitis (inflammation of retina)	• Bed rest and increased fluid intake • Acetaminophen or aspirin to relieve discomfort • Immunotherapy and administration of an antiviral agent to help control symptoms in an immunocompromised client; for example, ganciclovir (Cytovene) I.V. 5 to 7 days/week

this, the nurse must strive to provide sensitive, nonjudgmental care to the client with HIV infection, ARC, or AIDS.

Since the first case was reported in 1981, AIDS has spread rapidly, reaching epidemic proportions. From March 1987 to March 1988, approximately 23,000 people developed AIDS—58% more than the previous year. By the end of 1993, 390,000 to 480,000 people are expected to have AIDS in the United States (CDC, 1990).

Etiology

AIDS results from infection by the retrovirus HIV, which commonly infects T_4 lymphocytes (specific lymphocytes that are vital to the body's immune response). After infecting the T_4 lymphocyte host cells, HIV may become dormant or may replicate rapidly, disrupting T_4 lymphocyte functions and then destroying these cells.

When the number of T_4 lymphocytes decreases, the client becomes susceptible to opportunistic infections and malignancies, which the CDC uses as standards to confirm AIDS. These diseases include Kaposi's sarcoma, extrapulmonary cryptococcosis, *Pneumocystis carinii* pneumonia, herpes simplex, candidiasis, and toxoplasmosis of the brain (Gee and Moran, 1988; Grady, 1988; Rosenthal and Haneiwich, 1988).

Transmission

Although HIV has been isolated in amniotic fluid, blood, breast milk, cerebrospinal fluid, saliva, semen, vaginal secretions, tears, and urine, it is transmitted only through blood, semen, vaginal secretions, and possibly breast milk (CDC, 1987a; CDC, 1988a).

According to Lichtman and Papera (1990), HIV can be transmitted in several ways:
• sexual intercourse with an infected individual. Anal intercourse is particularly likely to cause transmission because penile penetration produces microhemorrhages in the thin anal mucosa (Peterman, Cates, and Curran, 1988).
• use of shared needles and syringes, as with illicit intravenous (I.V.) drug use
• transfusion of infected blood or blood products
• placental transmission from an infected client to her fetus
• transmission via breast milk from an infected client to her neonate (CDC, 1989a; Grady, 1988).
• artificial insemination by an infected donor
• needle sticks or exposure to infected body fluids.

Transmission does not occur through casual physical contact. The risk of transmission increases with the behaviors described above. However, the exact risk cannot be predicted. The following factors increase a woman's risk of contracting HIV infection and AIDS:
• having a bisexual male partner
• using illicit I.V. drugs or having a sexual partner who uses such drugs
• having numerous sexual partners
• having a sexual partner with an unknown drug or sexual history
• receiving, or having a sexual partner who received, blood or blood products (especially before HIV safeguards were established in April, 1985).

After a woman contracts HIV, she may pass it to a male partner, who may transmit it to a new partner, with or without knowing that the HIV infection is present. This chain of transmission can continue indefinitely. If the woman becomes pregnant, she may pass HIV to her fetus in utero or to her neonate in breast milk.

Clinical findings

Although other infections may affect the immune response, no other infection compromises the immune system as extensively as does HIV infection. After an incubation period of a few months to 10 years or more, HIV infection may produce various signs and symptoms. It may begin with weight loss, fever, night sweats, swollen glands, and diarrhea, and progress to symptoms of immunodeficiency. These mainly relate to specific opportunistic infections, such as Kaposi's sarcoma, pneumonia, or extrapulmonary cryptococcosis. For example, the client with *Pneumocystis carinii* pneumonia (PCP) also may display shortness of breath, tachypnea, and hypoxemia.

The signs and symptoms accelerate the longer a client has the HIV infection. A client with signs and symptoms of HIV has an increased chance of developing AIDS. However, the reason one HIV-infected person progresses to AIDS and another does not is unknown. The course of the HIV infection appears to be unaffected by pregnancy (Cates and Schulz, 1988; CDC, 1987a; CDC, 1989c; Peterman, Cates, and Curran, 1988).

The prognosis for the HIV-infected client is difficult to predict because the incubation period varies greatly. Typically, however, the prognosis worsens as the absolute T_4 count decreases (Cates and Schulz, 1988).

Treatment

Until researchers discover a cure for HIV infection, treatment is palliative and designed to combat opportunistic infections. Current treatment includes zidovudine (Retrovir), which also is known as azidothymidine (AZT). Prophylactic use of this drug decreases the mortality rate for the AIDS client by slowing virus replication. Zidovudine has been approved by the FDA for treating advanced ARC, AIDS, and asymptomatic clients with T_4 cell counts under 500/ml. Although research is being conducted on pregnant clients and neonates with HIV, prophylactic zidovudine is not approved for treating these groups. Other drugs may be prescribed in order to prevent opportunistic infections. Pentamidine isethionate for inhalation (NebuPent) is given prophylactically to the AIDS patient with a history of *P. carinii* pneumonia (PCP) or a peripheral T_4 cell count of less than 200/ml; pentamidine I.M. and I.V. is approved for the treatment of PCP. Researchers are attempting to develop more effective drugs and a vaccine for AIDS.

Additional treatment measures depend on the client's opportunistic infection and typically include fluid administration, parenteral nutrition, bed rest, and antibiotics.

Because no cure exists for HIV infection, prevention is key to stopping the spread of AIDS. A client can prevent HIV infection by avoiding high-risk activities and by abstaining from sexual intercourse, using condoms during intercourse, or having an exclusive sexual partner who has tested negative for HIV (CDC, 1989c).

Nursing care

A client with a genitourinary or other infection may feel anxious about its cause, treatment, and probable outcome. If the infection recurs, she may experience even more anxiety. Also, because some infections can affect her partner and alter sexuality patterns, the client may worry about her relationships.

In addition, the client with an STD, HIV infection, or AIDS may suffer from the social stigma and misinformation associated with the infection among the public. Because of this, the nurse's role as a nonjudgmental source of information is crucial. Factual information can make the difference between successful treatment or further transmission of infection.

When caring for a client with an infectious disorder, the nurse works to meet these general goals:
• Recognize the signs and symptoms of infection.
• Teach the client about the infection.
• Teach the client how to prevent infection.
• Teach the client about medications and other treatments.
• Stress the importance of compliance with the medication regimen and other treatments.
• Emphasize the importance of follow-up visits to ensure that the infection is controlled or eradicated.

To reach these goals, the nurse uses the nursing process for disease prevention, treatment, or symptom management in a client with an infectious disease. When providing care, the nurse can prevent self-infection or infection of other health care team members and clients by following infection control measures. (For more information, see *Universal precautions for infection control.*)

Assessment

During the assessment, gather subjective and objective data. Begin the assessment with a comprehensive health history and conclude with a thorough physical examination and a review of laboratory and other diagnostic tests.

Universal precautions for infection control

Using infection control measures only for clients with diagnosed infectious disorders can expose the nurse, other health care professionals, and clients to infection from those who are asymptomatic or undiagnosed. Because of this risk of exposure, the CDC recommends that *all* blood and other body fluids be treated as if they were infectious (CDC, 1987b; Peterman, Cates, and Curran, 1988; CDC, 1988b). To do this, the nurse should take the following universal precautions for infection control:

• Wear gloves during contact with any body fluid or in anticipation of such contact.
• Wear a disposable plastic apron or cover gown to prevent clothing from becoming soiled with blood or body fluids.
• Wear a mask and glasses or goggles to protect the eyes and oral and nasal mucous membranes from being splashed with body fluids.
• Immediately wash any exposed skin that accidentally has contact with body fluids.
• Wash hands immediately after removing gloves.
• Wash hands between clients.
• Discard used needles and other sharp instruments immediately in puncture-proof containers. Do not recap needles after use.
• Use resuscitation bags during resuscitation, whenever possible.
• Wear gloves to protect open hand lesions during direct client care or while handling instruments exposed to body fluids.
• Place linens in single, leak-proof (plastic or nylon) bags, and tie the bags securely.
• If a glove tears or a needle stick or other injury occurs during an invasive procedure, don new gloves as soon as client safety permits, and remove the needle or instrument from the sterile field.

Health history

Obtain a complete health history, gathering detailed information about the client's reason for seeking care and about related topics. Particularly note the client's menstrual and contraceptive history, history of genitourinary problems, and sexuality patterns because these may provide key information for a client with an infectious disorder. Also note factors that may alter immune response, such as age, nutritional status, environmental hazards, and life-style. (For more information about the complete health history, see Chapter 7, Women's Health Promotion.)

Conduct the interview in a nonjudgmental manner and reserve the most sensitive or personal questions for last when the client has developed a sense of trust and feels more relaxed.

Reason for seeking care. Determine which symptoms or concerns have made the client seek care. Her reasons can help guide the assessment and care plan. For example, if she reports a vaginal discharge or genital lesions or if her sexual partner recently developed an STD, assessment should include careful examination of her genitalia and the laboratory tests to help identify the infecting organism.

Menstrual history. Note any menstrual irregularities, which may be associated with an STD, such as gonorrhea, or other infectious disorder, such as PID. The menstrual history also can help rule out pregnancy, which is important because some drugs that are used to treat infectious disorders are contraindicated during pregnancy.

Also ask if the client uses tampons during her menstrual periods. Use of tampons, especially superabsorbent ones, increases the risk of TSS.

Contraceptive history. When obtaining the client's contraceptive history, keep in mind that some contraceptive methods can help protect the client from infection. For example, condoms can protect against HIV infection and some STDs. However, if the client is not comfortable with this method, she may not use it consistently, which would increase her risk of infection and pregnancy.

Other contraceptive methods may predispose a client to certain infections. For example, use of a diaphragm, contraceptive sponge, or cervical cap can increase the risk of TSS; IUDs may cause PID; and vaginal spermicides may produce vulvitis.

Genitourinary problems. Ask the client to describe her history of genitourinary problems, including STDs, vaginitis, and UTIs. These infectious disorders commonly recur. If the client has had any of these infections, inquire about precautions she has taken to prevent transmission or recurrence.

Additional medical history. Determine which childhood diseases the client had. This information will aid in understanding the client's immunity to certain diseases, such as rubella. Inquire about previous immunizations for the same reason.

For a client with AIDS, assess for effects in various body systems. For example, evaluate the respiratory system by inquiring about signs of *P. carinii* pneumonia, such as chronic dry cough and fever, which commonly is associated with AIDS. Assess the gastrointestinal system by asking about diarrhea, which may result from malabsorption, and constipation, which can be related to a Kaposi's sarcoma lesion or a malignant tumor. To assess for infection of the central nervous system, elicit a history of headaches, seizures, depression, or an unstable gait.

Surgical history. When obtaining a surgical history, particularly note gynecologic surgery, such as dilatation and curretage and hysterosalpingography, which may lead to PID.

Also ask if the client has received blood or blood product transfusions. The client who received transfusions before April 1985 may be at risk for HIV infection because blood was not screened for HIV before this date.

Allergies. Identify the client's allergies. Particularly note any sensitivity to antibiotics or other drugs that are likely to be prescribed for the client's complaint. Also assess for allergies to soaps or chemicals that may cause vulvitis or vaginitis.

Personal habits. Investigate the client's use of over-the-counter (OTC), prescription, and illegal drugs. Some OTC drugs, such as antacids, can interact with medications that may be prescribed to treat infection. Some prescription drugs, such as antibiotics, can alter the normal vaginal flora and predispose her to vaginitis. Use of illicit I.V. drugs increases the risk of HIV infection if the client shares needles with others.

Also inquire about the client's use of douches and feminine hygiene sprays. Use of these products can increase the risk of vaginitis and vulvitis.

Sleep and rest patterns. Evaluate the client's sleep and rest patterns, which may provide important information about the underlying disorder. For example, a client with scabies may not be able to sleep because of increased pruritus at night. The client with extreme fatigue may have HIV infection. She also may report chronic pain and malaise, which may lead to depression, fatigue, and altered sleep patterns (Gee and Moran, 1988; Grady, 1988; Rosenthal and Haneiwich, 1988).

Stress. Ask about the client's stress level and assess its effects on her life. Stress may trigger a recurrence of herpes genitalis or may predispose the client to vaginitis and other infections by suppressing her immune response.

Sexuality patterns. If the client is sexually active, ask her to state her age at first intercourse. Early sexual activity increases the client's risk of various STDs. Then determine the frequency of sexual intercourse and date of most recent sexual intercourse. If the client has an STD, she should notify her recent sexual partners. Also investigate types of sexual activity (vaginal, oral, or anal) and the number and regularity of partners. Anal intercourse increases the risk of HIV infection. A history of multiple sexual partners increases the risk of HIV infection as well as STDs.

Inquire about dyspareunia (painful intercourse), which could result from an undiagnosed STD or genitourinary infection, such as trichomoniasis or vaginitis.

Have the client describe high-risk factors in her partners, including a history of STDs, bisexuality, intercourse with multiple partners, and illicit I.V. drug use. These factors in a partner can increase the client's risk of contracting HIV infection or an STD.

Social support patterns. Find out who the client relies on for support. This information can be especially important for a client with AIDS who may grieve over her prognosis and feel socially isolated because of others' fear of the disease.

Physical assessment

After the health history, perform a complete physical assessment, beginning with recording the client's vital signs. Particularly note her temperature because fever is a common sign of many infections. A fever above 100° F (38° C) is especially likely in a client with PID, TSS, or pyelonephritis. Also be alert for decreased blood pressure, which is a characteristic sign of TSS.

Perform a head-to-toe assessment, paying particular attention to the skin and mucous membranes. Different types of skin lesions may suggest herpes zoster, toxoplasmosis, rubella, pediculosis pubis, scabies, TSS, and other infectious disorders.

Palpate the lymph nodes to detect lymphadenopathy, a common sign of many infections. Also palpate the abdomen and flank to identify tender areas, which may indicate PID or a UTI.

Finally, assist with a pelvic examination to assess the external and internal genitalia and to collect specimens for testing. (For more information and procedures, see Chapter 7, Women's Health Promotion.)

During the pelvic examination, paticularly note and characterize any lesions or discharge, which may aid in diagnosis of the problem. For example, soft, wartlike growths on the vulvar or vaginal mucosa may suggest condylomata acuminata. Detection of a yellowish endocervical discharge may indicate chlamydia or gonorrhea, which would require further investigation. (For more information, see *Nursing research applied: Routine chlamydia screening.*)

NURSING RESEARCH APPLIED

Routine chlamydia screening

To determine the incidence of chlamydia in female college students, researchers tested 419 family planning clients at a rural midwestern college clinic. To learn if clinical findings were reliable predictors of the need to test for *Chlamydia trachomatis*, they compared the students' history and physical assessment findings (such as mucopurulent cervical discharge or cervicitis) to their test results.

Nearly 13% of the students tested positive for chlamydia. Of these, 74% did not have signs or symptoms of the infection. Because the study found no significant relationship between the signs and symptoms and a positive test for chlamydia, it suggests that diagnosing chlamydia solely through signs and symptoms is inadequate.

Application to practice
This study indicates a high risk of chlamydia in asymptomatic female clients. Because chlamydia can cause permanent fallopian tube scarring and infertility, the need for routine screening becomes paramount. Because the number of people with asymptomatic chlamydia is unknown, the nurse should educate all clients about the importance of chlamydia testing and treatment.

Woolard, D., Larson, J., and Hudson, L. (1989). Screening for *Chlamydia trachomatis* at a university health service. *JOGNN*, 18(2), 145-149.

Also note any other abnormalities. Examination of pubic hair with an ultraviolet light may reveal pubic lice and confirm a diagnosis of pediculosis pubis (Benoit, 1988). Identification of itch mites with a magnifying glass should aid in diagnosis of scabies.

Diagnostic tests

Collect specimens for culture and other laboratory tests, as needed. (For details, see *Obtaining specimens for culture* in Chapter 7, Women's Health Promotion.) When the test results are available, review them and consider their implications. (For more information, see *Common laboratory studies* and Chapter 7, Women's Health Promotion.)

Keep in mind that the client will need counseling before, during, and after HIV testing (CDC, 1989a). Advise her before testing that a series of three tests must be performed to confirm HIV infection. First, an enzyme-linked immunosorbent assay (ELISA) is performed. If its results are positive, the ELISA is repeated. If the results of the second ELISA are positive, a western blot test is performed. If all three tests are positive, HIV infection is confirmed (Perdew, 1990).

During HIV testing, remind the client that a positive ELISA test does not necessarily indicate HIV infection but that it does suggest the need for further testing (Peterman, Cates, and Curran, 1988). In most cases, a

Common laboratory studies

The following laboratory studies may be performed to identify an infectious disorder. The nurse must consider the results of these studies along with other assessment data to provide appropriate care.

BLOOD TESTS

Complete blood count with differential
Evaluates hemoglobin, hematocrit, platelets, and red and white blood cells; lymphocyte count helps in evaluating T- and B-lymphocyte status.

Serum pregnancy
Rules out ectopic pregnancy when pelvic inflammatory disease (PID) is suspected.

Rubella antibody
Determines if the client has antibodies to the disease.

Cytomegalovirus (CMV)
Identifies infection by detecting CMV antibodies in serum.

Enzyme-linked immunosorbent assay (ELISA)
Screens for human immunodeficiency virus (HIV) by detecting antibodies against HIV.

Western blot
Confirms HIV infection in a client with a positive ELISA result.

Immunofluorescence assay
Confirms HIV infection in a client with a positive ELISA result.

VDRL test or rapid plasma reagin (RPR)
Screens for syphilis.

URINE TESTS

Urinalysis
Identifies the number of red and white blood cells in the urine to screen for urinary tract infections.

Urine culture and sensitivity
Identifies the specific organism causing urinary tract infection and its sensitivity to antibiotics.

CMV
Detects infection by isolating CMV in urine.

OTHER TESTS

Lesion culture
Identifies infecting organism.

Cervical culture
Identifies which organism is present in a client with PID symptoms.

Vaginal and cervical cultures for *Staphlococcus aureus*
Help identify toxic shock syndrome.

---

negative ELISA test indicates no infection. However, a negative test may occur in an infected client whose body has not yet developed HIV antibodies. This happens because the client can be infected for 6 to 12 weeks before her serum converts from HIV negative to HIV positive (Perdew, 1990). Advise the client who tests negative to avoid high-risk behaviors and to schedule a second test 3 months later. If that test is negative and if the client has not engaged in any high-risk behaviors, she is considered negative for HIV (CDC, 1988c).

If the client has positive results on all three tests for HIV infection, advise her that she is infectious and must take precautions to avoid HIV transmission to others. Reassure her, however, that the percentage of HIV-positive clients who develop AIDS is unknown and that these tests do not confirm AIDS or predict that the client will develop AIDS.

As needed, assist with or perform other diagnostic procedures. For example, assist with colposcopy for a client suspected of having condylomata acuminata because the growths may be so small that they can be identified only with a colposcope.

Nursing diagnosis

After obtaining the assessment data, review all health history, physical assessment, and diagnostic test findings. Based on these findings, formulate nursing diagnoses for the client. (For a list of possible nursing diagnoses, see *Nursing diagnoses: Infectious disorders*, page 270.)

Planning and implementation

For the client with an infectious disorder, plan interventions that address her specific disorder and meet her individual needs. The following nursing goals may be appropriate:
• The client will describe her infection, including its cause, transmission, treatment, and expected prognosis.
• The client will discuss the treatment plan and rationale with her sexual partner.
• The client will identify life-style factors that she can change to prevent further infection.
• The client will list signs and symptoms that indicate the need for further treatment.
• The client will comply with plans for follow-up care.
• The client will relate the importance of prompt treatment for future infections.
• The client will describe the sequelae of untreated infections.
• The client will describe proper tampon use. (For more information, see Chapter 7, Women's Health Promotion.)

NURSING DIAGNOSES

Infectious disorders

The following nursing diagnoses address representative problems and etiologies that a nurse may encounter when providing care for a client with an infectious disorder. Specific nursing interventions for many of these diagnoses are provided in the "Planning and implementation" section of this chapter.

SEXUALLY TRANSMITTED DISEASES

- Altered oral mucous membrane related to herpes lesion of lip
- Anxiety related to telling sexual partner about infection
- Fear related to pain
- Impaired tissue integrity related to podophyllum resin treatment
- Knowledge deficit related to preventive measures against STDs
- Knowledge deficit related to STDs
- Knowledge deficit related to STD treatment
- Noncompliance related to dislike of treatment regimen
- Pain related to herpes lesions
- Self-esteem disturbance related to STD reporting

GYNECOLOGIC INFECTIONS

- Altered patterns of urinary elimination related to dysuria
- Anxiety related to recurrent infection
- Body image disturbance related to infection
- Fear related to effects of recurrent pelvic infection on fertility
- Impaired tissue integrity related to vaginal pruritus and scratching
- Knowledge deficit related to infection
- Knowledge deficit related to infection prevention
- Pain related to infection
- Sexual dysfunction related to infection

URINARY TRACT INFECTIONS

- Altered patterns of urinary elimination related to bladder spasms
- Altered patterns of urinary elimination related to dysuria
- Knowledge deficit related to UTI prevention
- Pain related to kidney inflammation
- Urine retention related to dysuria

TORCH INFECTIONS

- Activity intolerance related to lethargy from cytomegalovirus infection
- Altered sexuality patterns related to painful herpetic lesions
- Fatigue related to cytomegalovirus infection
- Impaired tissue integrity related to syphilitic lesions
- Potential altered body temperature related to rubella

HIV INFECTION AND AIDS

- Altered nutrition: less than body requirements, related to nausea
- Altered oral mucous membrane related to Kaposi's sarcoma lesion on palate
- Altered parenting related to guilt feelings of transmitting HIV to neonate
- Altered role performance related to physical inability to care for the children's needs
- Altered thought processes related to AIDS drug therapy
- Anticipatory grieving related to partner's impending death
- Anxiety related to positive HIV test
- Anxiety related to stigma associated with AIDS
- Anxiety related to telling sexual partner about HIV infection
- Body image disturbance related to opportunistic infection
- Denial related to diagnosis of AIDS
- Diarrhea related to malabsorption caused by Kaposi's sarcoma
- Fatigue related to altered immune response
- Fear related to impending death
- Hopelessness related to lack of a cure for AIDS
- Impaired tissue integrity related to opportunistic infections
- Ineffective breathing pattern related to dyspnea and dry cough from pneumonia
- Ineffective family coping: compromised, related to inability of partner and children to provide emotional support
- Ineffective individual coping related to denial of AIDS
- Ineffective individual coping related to diagnosis of AIDS
- Knowledge deficit related to adverse effects of AZT
- Knowledge deficit related to AIDS
- Knowledge deficit related to HIV transmission
- Knowledge deficit related to support groups for HIV-infected people
- Noncompliance with infection prevention measures related to dislike of condoms
- Potential activity intolerance related to inadequate rest, malaise, and weakness
- Potential for infection related to AIDS
- Potential for injury related to unstable gait
- Powerlessness related to AIDS
- Self-esteem disturbance related to physical changes caused by AIDS
- Sexual dysfunction related to concerns about transmitting HIV infection to partner
- Social isolation related to socially unacceptable disorder

Make client participation a high priority when setting goals for the client with an STD or other infectious disorder. Because STDs can reduce a client's self-esteem and self-image, advocate self-care, which can help increase her self-esteem. Because these disorders can produce powerful psychological and emotional effects, involve family members and help them understand the illness.

Because AIDS involves a broad spectrum of potential diseases, plan specific, imaginative interventions for the client with AIDS. Keep in mind that each client's needs will differ, depending on the diseases that develop and her available support systems.

For a client with any infectious disorder, interventions commonly include teaching about infection, treatments, and prevention; taking infection control measures; providing support; making referrals; caring for the family; and promoting compliance.

Teach about infection

A client with an infectious disorder may have a nursing diagnosis of *knowledge deficit related to infection* or *anxiety related to telling sexual partner about infection*. To help the client, teach her about the cause of the infection and its transmission route, signs and symptoms, diagnosis, treatment, and prognosis.

Provide a confidential and private environment for the teaching session. During the session, offer clear, factual information to the client and, if possible, her partner. Encourage questions and participation by using a nonthreatening manner.

Provide written information about the infection for the client to review. This is particularly helpful for a client with a nursing diagnosis of *knowledge deficit related to AIDS* or *altered thought processes related to AIDS drug therapy* because she may have inaccurate information about the disorder or may have difficulty concentrating because of adverse drug effects. It also is valuable for any client who feels anxious during the teaching session.

Because the client may be at risk for other STDs, review the common signs and symptoms of STDs. Encourage her to seek health care immediately if any develop.

Teach about treatments

For a client with a *knowledge deficit related to STD treatment*, provide information about her prescribed therapy. (For more information, see *Selected major drugs: Drugs used to treat STDs*, pages 272 to 274.) For clients with other infectious disorders, teach about appropriate treatments. Also discuss any adverse effects. For example, advise the client with AIDS that zidovudine administration may cause anemia, cytopenia, headaches, myalgia, and nausea and requires close follow-up.

Stress the importance of completing the entire course of treatment as prescribed. Advise the client if a test-of-cure (follow-up test used to confirm that infection is no longer present) is required. For a client with syphilis or gonorrhea, for example, advise her that she must be reexamined 3 and 6 months after therapy to confirm cure (CDC, 1989c; McElhose, 1988; Whelan, 1988).

If the physician prescribes a therapeutic douche, teach the client how to use it properly. (For more information, see *Client teaching: How to douche,* page 275.)

Encourage the client to inform her sexual partners about the STD and to urge them to obtain testing and treatment. Inform a client with syphilis or gonorrhea that public health officials must be notified and that they will contact her sexual partners.

For specific disorders, provide information about self-care measures. For example, instruct a client with herpes genitalis to use the following techniques to manage symptoms and help prevent recurrence:

• Avoid stress, maintain balanced nutrition, and exercise regularly to promote overall health and minimize lesion outbreaks.
• Wash the genitals with mild soap and dry with a blow-dryer set on cool, except during pregnancy because this could cause an air embolus.
• Abstain from intercourse when lesions are active. Use a condom for the first year after the primary outbreak because viral shedding occurs then. (Some experts advise condom use indefinitely [CDC, 1989a; McElhose, 1988].)
• Apply hydrogen peroxide or another drying agent after vesicles rupture.
• Take aspirin to relieve pain during the primary episode.
• Use lidocaine or antiseptic spray if walking causes discomfort.
• Wear loose-fitting clothes without underpants to reduce discomfort.

Teach the client with condylomata acuminata to use the following self-care measures:
• Bathe in colloidal oatmeal solution (Aveeno).
• Dry the affected areas with a blow-dryer set on cool (contraindicated in pregnant clients).
• Wash off podophyllum resin as directed after application.

(Text continues on page 274.)

SELECTED MAJOR DRUGS

Drugs used to treat STDs

This chart supplies important information on the major drugs used to treat STDs and their effects on the client.

DRUG OR CLASS	INDICATIONS	USUAL ADULT DOSAGES	NURSING IMPLICATIONS
acyclovir (Zovirax)	Treatment of initial outbreaks of herpes genitalis Suppression of recurring herpes genitalis	200 mg P.O. every 4 hours while awake (5 doses daily) for 10 days 400 mg b.i.d. for up to 12 months	• Be aware that acyclovir is contraindicated in pregnant or breast-feeding clients. • Advise the client that common adverse reactions include nausea, vomiting, diarrhea, headache, dizziness, fatigue, and skin rash. • Advise the client to take the drug on an empty stomach 1 hour before or 2 hours after meals to prevent adverse gastrointestinal (GI) effects. • Stress the importance of avoiding sexual intercourse while active, visible lesions are present.
ceftriaxone (Rocephin)	Treatment of urinary tract and gynecologic infections caused by susceptible aerobic or anaerobic microorganisms, such as *Escherichia coli* Treatment of gonorrhea	1 to 2 g I.M. or I.V. once daily or in equally divided doses twice daily 250 mg I.M. in one dose	• Administer I.M. injections deep into large muscle mass. • Advise the client that common adverse reactions include hypersensitivity reactions, such as skin rash, pruritus, and fever; burning, redness, and pain at the injection site; and nausea, vomiting, and diarrhea. • Advise the client that her sexual partners should be treated simultaneously.
doxycycline hyclate (Doxychel, Vibramycin)	Treatment of chlamydia Treatment of primary or secondary syphilis in a client who is allergic to penicillin	100 mg P.O. b.i.d. for 7 days 100 mg P.O. b.i.d. for 14 days	• Administer cautiously to pregnant clients, neonates, children, and breast-feeding clients because of calcium-binding properties. • Advise the client that common adverse reactions include nausea, vomiting, diarrhea, photosensitivity, permanent discoloration and inadequate calcification of deciduous teeth, and nail discoloration. • Tell the client to take the drug on an empty stomach 1 hour before or 2 hours after meals. • Advise the client to avoid dairy products and antacids because they can decrease the drug's effectiveness. • Advise the client to avoid direct sunlight to prevent photosensitivity reactions.
erythromycin (E-mycin, Robimycin)	Treatment of chlamydia in a client who cannot take other antibiotics Treatment of acute pelvic inflammatory disease caused by *Neisseria gonorrhoeae*	500 mg P.O. q.i.d. for 15 days 400 mg P.O. every 6 hours for 7 days	• Tell the client to take the drug on an empty stomach. • This drug may be used in pregnant clients, neonates, and breast-feeding clients. • Advise the client that common adverse reactions include nausea, vomiting, diarrhea, abdominal cramping, heartburn, and skin irritation.
interferon alfa N3 (Alferon N)	Treatment of condylomata acuminata	0.05 ml per wart injected intralesionally twice weekly for 8 weeks; not to exceed 0.5 ml per session	• This drug is contraindicated in clients hypersensitive to interferon alfa and in those with a history of anaphylactic reactions to murine immunoglobulin, egg protein, or neomycin.

SELECTED MAJOR DRUGS

Drugs used to treat STDs continued

DRUG OR CLASS	INDICATIONS	USUAL ADULT DOSAGES	NURSING IMPLICATIONS
interfon alfa N3 (continued)			• Use drug cautiously in clients with debilitating illnesses (including unstable angina, coagulation disorders, or seizure disorders) because it may cause flulike syndrome. • Tell the client that signs and symptoms of hypersensitivity include hives, chest tightness, wheezing, and shortness of breath and to report such signs and symptoms immediately. • Explain that warts will continue to disappear after the 8-week treatment even without continued therapy.
lindane (Kwell)	Treatment of infestations of *Sarcoptes scabiei* Treatment of infestations of *Phthirius pubis*	Application of a thin layer of lotion or cream over entire skin surface of clean, dry body followed by washing off after 8 hours; second application in 1 week, if needed Application of a thin layer of lotion or cream over hair-covered areas of clean, dry body followed by washing off after 4 minutes; second application in 1 week, if needed.	• Instruct the client to scrub and then dry the entire body before application of lotion and then to apply to hair or affected areas; if shampooing, leave lather on for 4 minutes, and rinse thoroughly. • Advise the client that common adverse reactions include skin irritation, erythema, and signs of toxicity, such as dizziness and convulsions, if absorbed through skin or ingested. • Tell the client that all bed linens and clothes should be washed in hot water or dry-cleaned. • Inspect all family members and persons in close contact with the client for the parasites. • Tell the client to check herself for parasites. If she sees living parasites, advise her to repeat lindane application.
metronidazole (Flagyl, Protostat)	Treatment of trichomoniasis	2 g P.O. in a single dose or 500 mg P.O. b.i.d. for 7 days	• Advise the client that common adverse reactions include nausea, vomiting, anorexia, gastric distress, metallic taste, headache, vertigo, restlessness, rash, urticaria, pruritus, dyspareunia, and vaginal and vulvar dryness. • Tell the client to take the drug with meals, a snack, or milk to reduce GI distress. • Advise the client that sexual partners should receive treatment simultaneously. • Instruct the client to consume no alcohol during treatment because alcohol can produce antabuse-like reactions with severe nausea and vomiting. • Inform the client that the drug normally colors the urine dark or reddish brown.
penicillin	Treatment of syphilis and other infections caused by highly susceptible organisms	1 g probenecid; 30 minutes later, 4.8 million U penicillin I.M. in two divided doses in two injection sites	• If a solution, shake vial vigorously before administration. • Advise the client that common adverse reactions include hypersensitivity reactions, such as rash and pruritus; local pain, tenderness, and fever with I.M. injection; and nausea, vomiting, diarrhea, anorexia, and abdominal cramps, depending on drug form. • Monitor the client for signs of candidiasis, such as vaginal discharge and pruritus, because large doses of penicillin tend to increase yeast growth. • Clearly note any penicillin allergy on the client's chart.

(continued)

SELECTED MAJOR DRUGS

Drugs used to treat STDs continued

DRUG OR CLASS	INDICATIONS	USUAL ADULT DOSAGES	NURSING IMPLICATIONS
tetracycline (Tetracyn, Achromycin)	Treatment of chlamydia	500 mg P.O. q.i.d. for 7 days	• Administer cautiously to pregnant clients (only in last part of pregnancy), neonates, children under age 8, and breast-feeding clients because of the drug's calcium-binding properties.
	Treatment of gonorrhea in conjunction with ceftriaxone	500 mg P.O. q.i.d. for 7 days	• Advise the client that common adverse reactions include nausea, vomiting, anorexia, diarrhea, dizziness, photosensitivity, and permanent discoloration and inadequate calcification of deciduous teeth.
	Treatment of syphilis in a client who is allergic to penicillin	500 mg P.O. q.i.d. for 14 days	• Tell the client to take the drug on an empty stomach 1 hour before or 2 hours after meals.
			• Advise the client to avoid dairy products and antacids because they can decrease the drug's effectiveness.
			• Tell the client to avoid exposure to direct sunlight to prevent photosensitivity reactions.

• Urge sexual partners to be tested for HPV infection, even if they are asymptomatic.
• Use a condom during sexual intercourse until all warts are eradicated.

Teach the client with pediculosis pubis or scabies to wash all bed linens and clothing worn within 2 days of diagnosis in hot water and detergent or to have them dry-cleaned. Advise the client with scabies that pruritus may continue for several weeks after treatment.

Teach about infection prevention

For a client with a nursing diagnosis of *knowledge deficit related to infection prevention,* first teach general measures she can take to prevent infection or reinfection:
• Use conscientious hygiene, washing hands immediately after contact with infected areas.
• Wipe from front to back after urinating or defecating.
• Practice perineal hygiene, washing, rinsing, and drying the perineum regularly each day.
• Abstain from sexual intercourse or use a condom coated with a spermicide such as nonoxynol-9 during intercourse.
• Limit the number of sexual partners to reduce the risk of STDs.
• Avoid partners who have multiple sexual partners.
• Urge sexual partners to seek testing and treatment of infection.

After discussing general infection prevention measures, describe ones that are specific to the client's disorder. For a client with vulvitis or vaginitis, for example, advise her not to douche unless prescribed by the phy-

sician. Douching can reduce the normal vaginal flora and create an environment that makes the area susceptible to infection. Suggest that the client wear cotton underpants, which help keep the perineum dry, reducing the risk of infection. Advise her to avoid powders and perfumes because they can irritate the perineum.

Teach the client with a UTI measures for preventing recurrent infections. (For more information, see *Client teaching: Preventing urinary tract infections,* page 276.) This is particularly helpful for a client with a *knowledge deficit related to UTI prevention.* Remind the client that a follow-up urine culture should be performed after she completes her course of medication to ensure effective treatment of the UTI.

When the client has a *knowledge deficit related to HIV transmission,* explain the risk factors involved with HIV transmission. Counsel the client to modify behaviors that place her or her partners at risk. Also stress the importance of immediate and proper treatment.

Encourage the client to know her partner's sexual and drug history and HIV infection status before engaging in sexual intercourse. Advise her to use latex rather than animal membrane condoms during intercourse because some membrane condoms allow viruses to pass through them. Condoms coated with the spermicide may be effective against HIV transmission (American National Red Cross, 1989; Peterman, Cates, and Curran, 1988). Because HIV can be transmitted to the fetus, instruct the client to prevent pregnancy by using another contraceptive method along with the condom for extra protection.

How to douche

To treat your vaginal infection or irritation, your nurse practitioner or doctor has prescribed a douche. Read the instructions on the label carefully, and follow them. Use these guidelines to help you through the procedure.

Remember to douche only when prescribed by your doctor or nurse practitioner. Frequent douching can alter the normal vaginal pH, which can make you susceptible to vaginal infection. If you experience vaginal discharge, odor, or itching, contact your doctor or nurse practitioner.

1 Gather the equipment you will need: a douche bag, about 3 feet of tubing with a clamp and plastic nozzle, douche solution, and a water-soluble lubricant, such as K-Y Lubricating Jelly. To hang the bag, position a hook about 2 feet above your bathtub or use a straight-backed chair.

2 Urinate. Then wash your hands and prepare the solution according to the label instructions. After you have warmed the solution, sprinkle a few drops of it on the inside of your arm. If it feels warm enough, fill the douche bag with it.

Some douches come premixed in a container with a prelubricated nozzle. If the solution is cold, warm it by placing the container in a basin of warm water for about 20 minutes.

3 Because the solution will drain out of your vagina as you use it, position yourself comfortably reclining in a bathtub, sitting in a shower stall, or on the toilet.

If you're in a bathtub, recline with your feet toward the drain. Prop you back against the opposite end of the bathtub. Flex your knees and spread apart your legs, as shown.

If you sit in a shower stall, prop your back against the side at a 45-degree angle. Flex your knees and spread your legs.

If you prefer to douche while sitting on the toilet, seat yourself comfortably with your pelvis tilted and your knees flexed slightly.

4 Lubricate the nozzle with the water-soluble lubricant. Then use your fingertips to spread your vaginal folds (labia). With your other hand, unclamp the tubing and let a little solution run over your labia to reduce the risk of introducing bacteria into your vagina. Clamp the tubing.

5 While you spread your labia, gently insert the nozzle a short way. To do this, insert it upward at a 45-degree angle.

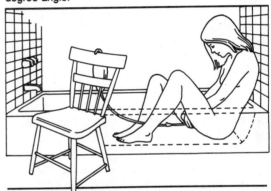

6 Open the clamp and allow gravity to draw the solution into your vagina. Slowly rotate the nozzle while advancing it 1 to 2 inches. Allow the solution to run out of your vagina freely. Continue until you have used all of the solution.

7 When the solution is gone, close the clamp and remove the nozzle.

8 Use a clean towel to pat yourself dry. Remember to dry yourself from front to back so you do not spread bacteria from your anus to your vagina.

Finally, wash the douche nozzle, tubing, and bag with soap and water. After rinsing and drying the equipment, store it in a clean, dry place.

Take infection control measures

In addition to universal precautions, take specific infection control measures, as needed. If a client with AIDS is hospitalized, she may need to be isolated to prevent an infection. Teach the client and her partner and family about isolation procedures.

Keep in mind that the client with AIDS probably will have a diagnosis of *potential for infection related to AIDS*. Also be aware that the risk of infection increases in a client with a nursing diagnosis of *fatigue related to altered immune response, anxiety related to stigma associated with AIDS, altered nutrition: less than body requirements, related to nausea,* or *impaired tissue integrity related to opportunistic infections.*

Because stress can reduce the body's immune response and fatigue, anxiety, and other factors can increase stress, teach the client how to reduce stress. Instruct her in deep-breathing and other relaxation techniques. Encourage her to engage in a hobby or activity that promotes a sense of well-being. Assess the client's nutritional status, and explain how her eating habits can promote health and reduce her susceptibility to infection.

Encourage cleanliness and thorough oral hygiene to prevent the breakdown of skin and mucous membranes. Advise the client to keep her fingernails short and avoid scratching herself. Teach the client how to monitor herself for infection and instruct her to avoid people with colds, influenza, or obvious signs of infection. Also, explain the importance of taking medications on time.

Provide support

Many emotions may surface in a client with an STD or AIDS because of the social stigma of these disorders. When a client learns of her diagnosis, she may express anger at her partner or health care provider. After the initial shock, she may experience such emotions as embarrassment, shame, guilt, or loneliness. She may have a nursing diagnosis of *fear related to pain, body image disturbance related to infection, self-esteem disturbance related to STD reporting,* or *social isolation related to socially unacceptable disorder.* If this occurs, provide emotional support and help her take steps toward accepting the disease.

The client with AIDS may be even more emotionally distressed. Because of the poor prognosis of AIDS, she may have a nursing diagnosis of *ineffective individual coping related to denial of AIDS, fear related to impending death, hopelessness related to lack of a cure for AIDS, powerlessness related to AIDS,* or *self-esteem disturbance related to physical changes caused by AIDS.*

To help such a client, encourage communication between her and her partner and between them and the health care team. Open communication provides opportunities for questions to be answered and permits clarification of concerns. Counsel the couple to help them deal with grief and ventilate their anger, fears, and feelings about themselves and each other.

Help the couple handle society's fear of disease transmission. Encourage them to obtain information about the disease and to adhere to all recommendations for disease prevention and transmission.

If the client is defensive, invite her to talk about her feelings in a nonthreatening environment. As she becomes better informed about her illness, she should feel less threatened. If she denies the illness, be supportive and allow her to work through this stage of grief. Never try to force the client to accept the reality of the disease if she is unprepared to do so.

Promote the client's self-esteem by allowing her to participate in and make decisions about her care. Help her plan short-term goals, such as accomplishing her

---

CLIENT TEACHING

Preventing urinary tract infections

To prevent recurring urinary tract infections, follow these guidelines:

- Drink at least ten 8-ounce glasses of fluid—especially water—daily. This helps flush bacteria from your urinary tract.
- Empty your bladder completely every 2 to 3 hours or as soon as you feel the urge to urinate.
- Wipe from front to back after urinating or defecating to prevent contamination with fecal material.
- Take showers instead of tub baths. If you must bathe, do not use bubble bath, salts, bath oil, or perfume because these can irritate you. Also avoid using feminine hygiene deodorants and douches, which can alter your normal vaginal environment.
- Avoid bladder irritants, such as alcohol, caffeine, tea, and carbonated beverages.
- Eat meats, eggs, cheese, nuts, prunes, plums, and whole grains, and drink cranberry juice daily. These foods acidify the urine, which helps decrease bacterial growth. Avoid foods that contain baking soda or baking powder, such as most baked goods.
- Clean the perineum before intercourse. Urinate before and after intercourse to wash away bacteria from the urethra.
- Allow time to become well-lubricated before intercourse. Apply a lubricant, if necessary.
- Urinate immediately before going to sleep and immediately upon arising, to decrease the time that urine remains in your bladder.
- Consider using a different birth control method if you use a diaphragm and have recurrent infections.
- Take all of the medication prescribed to treat your infection, even if your symptoms disappear.
- Return for a follow-up urine culture after you've taken all of your medication.
- Seek medical help for any unusual vaginal discharge, which suggests infection.

---

normal daily routine. Discuss the situation with the family, and enlist their emotional support for the client.

If the client is worried about who will care for her children if she dies of AIDS, help her consider her options and resolve this problem. If needed, refer her to a social service organization or support group that can help her make decisions about child care and draw up a will.

Individual and family counseling sessions should be instituted to help develop family unity. During these sessions, each family member's roles and responsibilities will be identified and modified, if needed.

Make referrals

Various referrals may be useful when a client's needs exceed the health care team's abilities to meet them. For example, the client who needs further counseling may benefit from referral to a nurse-counselor, psychologist, or social worker. A client with recurrent UTIs may need follow up with a urologist to investigate the cause. One who desires more information about HIV and AIDS prevention may appreciate referral to the National AIDS Information Line (1-800-342-AIDS in English or 1-800-344-SIDA in Spanish).

Care for the family

When a client develops HIV infection, her family and friends are likely to be concerned that they will become infected. Reassure them that, unless they engage in high-risk behaviors, their chance of contracting HIV is extremely low. Advise them that HIV cannot be transmitted by hugging, kissing, or shaking hands; making contact with utensils, clothes, telephones, or toilet seats used by the client; making contact with the client's saliva, sweat, tears, urine, or feces; swimming in a pool with the client; or eating food handled, prepared, or served by the client (Peterman, Cates, and Curran, 1988; CDC, 1988a).

Promote compliance

To promote compliance with the treatment regimen, schedule appointments at times that are convenient for the client and the health care team. Explain care recommendations in simple terms. Have the client identify reasons for adherence to the treatment regimen. This intervention is especially valuable when caring for a client with a nursing diagnosis of *noncompliance related to dislike of the treatment regimen*.

Evaluation

For many clients, evaluation may focus on cure of the infection and behavior changes. For a client with HIV infection or AIDS, however, evaluation cannot be based on disease resolution because a cure is not available. When evaluating such a client, focus on her understanding of the disease and its treatment, changes in sexual practices, and use of the health care system.

After implementing the nursing care plan, evaluate its effectiveness by comparing the actual outcomes with the goals. The following examples illustrate some appropriate evaluation statements:
• The client correctly described the characteristics and limitations of her illness.

• The client resolved negative feelings about her diagnosis.
• The client relied on her family for support.
• The client reported early signs of infection before complications occurred.
• The client reported recovery from the infection.
• The client described measures she has taken to prevent infection.
• The client returned for follow-up testing to assess treatment effectiveness.
• The client's partner scheduled an appointment to assess the need for treatment.
• The client followed the prescribed treatment plan.

Documentation

Based on the assessment findings, the nurse uses the nursing process to formulate nursing diagnoses and then plans, implements, and evaluates the client's care. (For a case study that shows how to apply the nursing process when caring for a client with an infectious disorder, see *Applying the nursing process: Client with knowledge deficit related to chlamydia treatment*, pages 278 and 279.)

Be sure to document assessment data and nursing activities as thoroughly and objectively as possible. Thorough documentation informs other health care team members about the client and her treatment and ensures that she receives comprehensive, accurate care. Keep in mind, however, that client care and documentation must remain absolutely confidential because many infectious disorders carry social stigma.

When caring for a client with an infectious disorder, documentation should include:
• health history findings, especially the reason for seeking care, menstrual and contraceptive history, history of genitourinary and other medical problems
• sexual history, including high-risk behaviors
• history of blood or blood product transfusion
• altered activities of daily living
• history of high-risk behavior, such as I.V. drug use
• support systems available
• physical assessment findings, especially those from a pelvic examination
• diagnostic tests performed and results
• diagnosis
• medications and other treatments prescribed
• client teaching performed
• client's understanding of instructions
• test-of-cure results, when applicable.

APPLYING THE NURSING PROCESS

Client with knowledge deficit related to chlamydia treatment

The nursing process helps ensure high-quality care for a client with an infectious disorder. The table below shows how the nurse might use the nursing process when caring for the client described in the case history at right. The first column presents history and physical assessment data followed by a paragraph of mental notes. These notes help the nurse make important connections among assessment findings, aiding in development of the nursing diagnosis and planning.

The second column lists an appropriate nursing diagnosis; information in the remaining columns is based on this diagnosis. Although not part of the nursing process, a rationale appears for each intervention in the fourth column to explain how it contributes to the care plan.

ASSESSMENT	NURSING DIAGNOSIS	PLANNING
Subjective (history) data • Client says that the abdominal pain began yesterday and has increased since. • Client reports no change in her menstrual periods; her last menstrual period started 1 week ago. • Client says that she takes an oral contraceptive daily. • Client states she has had only one partner for the past 9 months. To her knowledge, he does not have another partner or use illicit I.V. drugs. • Client reports, "I had a little discomfort the last few times we had sex." She and her partner engage in vaginal and oral intercourse. **Objective (physical) data** • Vital signs: temperature 100.8° F, pulse 82 beats/minute, respirations 24/minute, blood pressure 128/78 mm Hg. • Abdominal palpation: no adnexal masses. • Pelvic examination: friable, tender cervix; bilateral adnexal discomfort. **Mental notes** *Ectopic pregnancy can be ruled out as a cause of the client's pain because of her menstrual history, lack of adnexal masses, and correct oral contraceptive use. However, pelvic inflammatory disease related to chlamydia is a possible cause of her pain. The client will need to be tested for chlamydia and other STDs that can occur concurrently and should be given information about chlamydia treatment and prevention.*	Knowledge deficit related to chlamydia treatment	**Goals** Before leaving the clinic, the client will: • describe the proper administration of medication • describe behavior changes that are necessary during treatment • verbalize the understanding that her partner needs to be treated concurrently.

Chapter summary

Chapter 12 discussed various genitourinary infections, including STDs and gynecologic and urinary tract infections, as well as other infections, including TORCH and HIV infections. Here are the chapter highlights.
• STDs include chlamydia, trichomoniasis, herpes genitalis, gonorrhea, syphilis, condylomata acuminata, pediculosis pubis, and scabies. Many of these disorders produce such symptoms as vaginal discharge, lesions, and signs of inflammation, but many are asymptomatic.

• Gynecologic infections include vaginitis, vulvitis, PID, and TSS. Vaginitis and vulvitis commonly result from fungal, protozoal, or bacterial infection; PID, from untreated STDs; and TSS, from a toxin secreted by *Staphylococcus aureus.*
• UTIs include cystitis and urethritis (lower urinary tract infections) and pyelonephritis (upper urinary tract infections). UTIs commonly result from *Escherichia coli* infection and produce such effects as dysuria and urinary frequency and urgency.
• The acronym TORCH includes toxoplasmosis, other diseases (chlamydia, group B beta-hemolytic strepto-

CASE STUDY

Christine Binney, age 20, comes to the clinic for acute care because of bilateral lower abdominal pain. Ms. Binney has been using an oral contraceptive for 2 years.

IMPLEMENTATION		EVALUATION
Intervention Provide a confidential, private, unhurried environment for the teaching session.	**Rationale** The client will feel more at ease if the session is held in a private place without interruptions. An unrushed attitude communicates concern and decreases anxiety.	Upon evaluation, the client: • described proper administration of medication • discussed behavior changes necessary during treatment • verbalized the understanding that her partner must be treated concurrently.
Teach the client how to take the prescribed antibiotic and stress the importance of taking all of it.	Proper medication administration helps ensure successful treatment.	
Provide and review written information about the medication and its possible adverse effects.	The client can review written information at home and obtain answers to questions that may not have occurred to her during the session.	
Explain that the client's partner must be treated concurrently to prevent reinfection.	This explanation should increase compliance and comprehensive treatment.	
Encourage abstinence from intercourse or use of condoms until treatment is completed.	These measures can prevent reinfection of partners.	
Encourage questions.	Through answers to her questions, the client can understand the importance of chlamydia treatment and prevention.	

coccus, syphilis, varicella zoster), rubella, and cytomegalovirus and herpesvirus infections. These disorders can harm an embryo or fetus.

• Infection with HIV can progress to AIDS, a life-threatening immune system disorder. HIV invades and destroys T_4 lymphocytes, which are vital to the body's immune response. This compromises the immune system, making the body susceptible to opportunistic infections and malignancies. The HIV-infected client who develops one or more designated diseases has AIDS.

• When assessing the client with an infectious disorder, the nurse should obtain a complete health history, including the reason for seeking care, menstrual and contraceptive history, history of genitourinary and other medical problems, and sexuality patterns. The nurse also

should perform a physical assessment, paying close attention to the client's vital signs, skin and mucous membranes, lymph nodes, abdomen, and pelvic structures. Finally, the nurse should review the results of common laboratory tests and other diagnostic studies.

• When dealing with the client, the nurse must take universal precautions for infection control. These precautions require the nurse to treat all blood and body fluids as potentially infectious.

• To care for a client with an infectious disorder, the nurse may need to teach about the infection and its treatment and prevention, take infection control measures, provide support, make referrals, care for the family, and promote compliance.

Study questions

1. During a routine gynecologic visit, the nurse discovers a wartlike genital growth on Carrie Rundback, age 24. Which two STDs should the nurse suspect? How might the nurse differentiate between them?

2. Christine Pool, age 31, visits the clinic for treatment of intense perineal pruritus. Her health history reveals that her partner and children have pruritus in the same general area. What information should the nurse obtain to help differentiate pediculosis pubis from scabies?

3. At the college health clinic, Shirley Bond, age 19, reports itching, pain, and a burning sensation during urination. She has not had a Papanicoloau test in 2 years. Which health history questions and physical assessments are likely to provide the most information about Ms. Bond's condition?

4. Betty Webster, age 26, comes to the health clinic for treatment of chlamydia. She tells the nurse that the father of her two children was an I.V. drug user and that she has had another sexual partner for the past 3 years. Expressing concern for her children and herself, Betty asks if she could have AIDS. How should the nurse counsel Ms. Webster? What referrals would be most helpful?

5. Sarah Mitchell, age 26, has just tested positive for HIV infection. What information should the nurse provide for Ms. Mitchell?

Bibliography

Hacker, N., and Moore, J. (1986). *Essentials of obstetrics and gynecology.* Philadelphia: Saunders.

Hoeprich, P., and Jordan, M. (1989). *Infectious diseases* (4th ed.). Philadelphia: Lippincott.

Kee, J. (1987). *Laboratory and diagnostic tests with nursing implications* (2nd ed.). East Norwalk, CT: Appleton & Lange.

Kooker, B. (1987). 4 million female hospital workers face reproductive health hazards. *Occupational Health and Safety,* 56(4), 61-64.

Lichtman, R., and Papera, S. (1990). *Gynecology: Well-woman care.* East Norwalk, CT: Appleton & Lange.

Moses, M. (1987). Health workers and reproductive hazards. *Birth,* 14(3), 153-155.

Nurse's clinical library: Immune disorders. (1985). Springhouse, PA: Springhouse Corporation.

Thompson, J., McFarland, G., Hirsch, J., Tucker, S., and Bowers, A. (1989). *Mosby's manual of clinical nursing* (2nd ed.). St. Louis: Mosby.

Sexually transmitted diseases

Bell, T., and Hein, K. (1984). In K. Holmes (Ed.), *Adolescents and sexually transmitted diseases.* New York: McGraw-Hill.

Benoit, J. (1988). Sexually transmitted diseases in pregnancy. *Nursing Clinics of North America,* 23(4), 937-945.

Bourcier, K., and Seidler, A. (1987). Chlamydia and condylomata acuminata: An update for the nurse practitioner. *JOGNN,* 16(1), 17-22.

Breslin, E. (1988). Genital herpes simplex. *Nursing Clinics of North America,* 23(4), 907-915.

Centers for Disease Control. (1989a). 1989 Sexually transmitted diseases treatment guidelines. *MMWR,* 38(S-8), 1-43.

Centers for Disease Control. (1989b). Summary of notifiable diseases, United States 1988. *MMWR,* 37(54), 51-57.

Corbett, M., and Meyer, J. (1987). *The adolescent and pregnancy.* Boston: Blackwell Scientific Publications.

Enterline, J., and Leonardo, J. (1989). Condylomata acuminata (venereal warts). *Nurse Practitioner,* 14(4), 8-16.

Fogel, C. (1988). Gonorrhea: Not a new problem but a serious one. *Nursing Clinics of North America,* 23(4), 885-897.

Loucks, A. (1987). Chlamydia: An unheralded epidemic. *AJN,* 87(7), 920-922.

Lucas, V. (1988). Human papillomavirus infection: A potentially carcinogenic sexually transmitted disease (condylomata acuminata, genital warts). *Nursing Clinics of North America,* 23(4), 917-935.

Marvin, C., and Slevin, A. (1987). Chlamydia: Cause, prevention, and cure. *MCN,* 12(5), 318-321.

McElhose, P. (1988). The "other" STDs: As dangerous as ever. *RN,* 51(6), 52-59.

McQuiston, C. (1989). The relationship of risk factors for cervical cancer and HPV in college women. *Nurse Practitioner,* 14(4), 18-26.

Sanders, L., Harrison, H., and Washington, A. (1986). Treatment of sexually transmitted chlamydial infections. *JAMA,* 255(13), 1750-1756.

Staff. (1989). When is chlamydia screening necessary in family planning? *American Health Consultants' Contraceptive Technology Update,* 10(4), 45-49.

Swinker, M. (1986). Chlamydia trachomatis genital infections in college women. *Journal of American College Health,* 34(5), 207-209.

Washington, A., Browner, W., and Korenbrot, C. (1987). Cost-effectiveness of combined treatment for endocervical gonorrhea: Considering co-infection with *Chlamydia trachomatis. JAMA,* 257(15), 2056-2060.

Washington, M., Johnson, R., and Sanders, L. (1987). *Chlamydia trachomatis* infections in the United States. *JAMA,* 257(15), 2070.

Whelan, M. (1988). Nursing management of the patient with chlamydia trachomatis infection. *Nursing Clinics of North America,* 23(4), 877-883.

Gynecologic infections

Berkley, S. (1987). The relationship of tampon characteristics to menstrual toxic shock syndrome. *JAMA*, 258(7), 917-920.

Droegemueller, W., Herbst, A., Mishall, D., and Stencheur, M. (1989). *Comprehensive gynecology*. St. Louis: Mosby.

Havens, C., Sullivan, N., and Tilton, P. (Eds.). (1986). *Manual of outpatient gynecology*. Boston: Little, Brown.

King, J. (1984). Vaginitis. *JOGNN*, 13(2), 41s-48s.

Secor, R. (1988). Bacterial vaginosis: A comprehensive review. *Nursing Clinics of North America*, 23(4), 865-875.

Shesser, R. (1990). Common vaginal infections: A concise workup guide. *The Female Patient*, 15(2), 53-60.

Torrington, M. (1985). Pelvic inflammatory disease. *JOGNN*, 14(6), 21s-31s.

Wolf, P., Perlman, J., Fortney, J., Lezotte, D., Burkman, R., and Bernstein, G. (1987). Toxic shock syndrome. *JAMA*, 258(7), 908.

Urinary tract infections

Droegemueller, W., Herbst, A., Mishall, D., and Stencheur, M. (1989). *Comprehensive gynecology*. St. Louis: Mosby.

Fogel, C., and Woods, N. (1981). *Health care of women*. St. Louis: Mosby.

TORCH infections

Droegemueller, W., Herbst, A., Mishall, D., and Stencheur, M. (1989). *Comprehensive gynecology*. St. Louis: Mosby.

HIV infections and AIDS

American National Red Cross. (1989). HIV infection and AIDS (pamphlet).

Cates, W., and Schulz, S. (1988). Epidemiology of HIV in women. *Contemporary Ob/Gyn*, 32(3), 94-105.

Centers for Disease Control. (1989c). AIDS and human immuno-deficiency virus infection in the United States: 1988 update. *MMWR*, 38(S4), 1-38.

Centers for Disease Control. (1988a). How you won't get AIDS. (pamphlet).

Centers for Disease Control. (1988b). Acquired immunodeficiency syndrome and HIV infection among health care workers. Update. *MMWR*, 37, 229.

Centers for Disease Control. (1987a). Human immunodeficiency virus infection in the United States: A review of current knowledge. *MMWR*, 36(S-6), 1-20.

Centers for Disease Control. (1987b). Recommendations for prevention of HIV transmission in health care settings. *MMWR*, 36(2S), 3S-18S.

Centers for Disease Control. (1988c). What about AIDS testing? (pamphlet).

Centers for Disease Control. (1990). Division of STD, HIV prevention annual report. Washington, Author.

Gee, G., and Moran, T. (Eds.). (1988). *AIDS: Concepts in nursing practice*. Baltimore: Williams & Wilkins.

Grady, C. (1988). HIV: Epidemiology, immunopathogenesis, and clinical consequences. *Nursing Clinics of North America*, 23(4), 683-696.

Hendricksen, C. (1988). The AIDS clinical trials unit experience: Clinical research and antiviral treatment. *Nursing Clinics of North America*, 23(4), 697-706.

Perdew, S. (1990). *Facts about AIDS: A guide for health care providers*. Philadelphia: Lippincott.

Peterman, T., Cates, W., and Curran, J. (1988). The challenge of human immunodeficiency virus (HIV) and acquired immuno-deficiency syndrome (AIDS) in women and children. *Fertility and Sterility*, 49(4), 571-581.

Rosenthal, Y., and Haneiwich, S. (1988). Nursing management of adults in the hospital. *Nursing Clinics of North America*, 23(4), 707-718.

Nursing research

Woolard, D., Larson, J., and Hudson, L. (1989). Screening for *Chlamydia trachomatis* at a university health service. *JOGNN*, 18(2), 145-149.

Gynecologic Disorders

Objectives

After reading and studying this chapter, the student should be able to:

1. Discuss how a gynecologic disorder may alter a client's view of herself and her roles.
2. Compare the clinical findings and treatments for benign breast disorders with those of breast cancer.
3. Describe the etiology, clinical findings, and treatments of common menstrual disorders.
4. Discuss pelvic support disorders and their nursing implications.
5. Identify the clinical findings, diagnostic tests, and treatments associated with gynecologic cancer.
6. Describe appropriate support for the client with gynecologic cancer and for her family.
7. Apply the nursing process when caring for a client with a gynecologic disorder.

Introduction

A gynecologic disorder has physical, psychosocial, and sexual consequences that may affect a client's self-image and family interactions. Whether the disorder is a normal variation or is caused by aging, infection, or a serious disease, it can have a negative effect on the client's body image, sense of femininity, and role function.

The client's perception of a gynecologic disorder depends on her experiences, cultural beliefs, and role expectations. Conscious and subconscious factors influence her reaction and adaptation to a disorder and its effects on her work and recreation patterns, body function, appearance, and social and family roles.

Depending on the disorder, the client may worry about embarrassment, pain, surgery, disfigurement, changes in or loss of support, options for intimacy and reproduction, chronic disability, or death.

A client may seek care for a gynecologic disorder because she has noticed a change in her body, such as a breast lump or a change in her menstrual flow. Alternately, she may request care after a health care professional discovers unusual findings during a routine pelvic examination. These findings may indicate various causes. For example, abnormal Papanicolaou test results may be caused by inflammation (which can result from irritation or a sexually transmitted disease), herpes simplex, human papilloma virus infection, or cervical neoplasm. An ovarian mass may indicate a benign ovarian cyst, ectopic pregnancy, inflammatory lesion, functional (follicular) cyst, endometriosis, neoplasm, corpus luteum cyst (secreting progesterone), theca lutein cyst, serous cyst, mucinous neoplasms, endometrioid neoplasms, cystic teratoma, polycystic ovary disease (Stein-Leventhal syndrome), or parovarian neoplasm. Uterine masses may indicate myoma (fibromyoma, fibroid, or leiomyoma), adenomyosis, or endometrial polyps.

To provide appropriate care for a client with a gynecologic disorder, the nurse must possess knowledge, technical skills, and sensitivity to the client's emotional needs. Nursing care includes assessment and individualized support, intervention, and teaching to meet the needs of the client and her family.

To prepare the student for these functions, this chapter describes common gynecologic disorders, including breast disorders, menstrual disorders, pelvic support disorders, and gynecologic cancer. For each of these dis-

GLOSSARY

Adjuvant therapy: treatment in addition to the primary treatment.

Amenorrhea: absence of menses.

Anovulation: absence of ovulation.

Carcinoma: malignant epithelial neoplasm (cancer) that tends to invade surrounding tissue and metastasize to other body regions.

Carcinoma in situ: malignant neoplasm within surface epithelium that has not invaded deeper tissues.

Cervical conization: removal of a cone-shaped piece of cervical tissue for analysis or treatment; also called cone biopsy.

Cervical dysplasia: abnormal development of cervical tissue.

Chemotherapy: treatment with antineoplastic agents.

Colposcopy: examination of cervical and vaginal tissue using a colposcope for magnification.

Cryosurgery: treatment that destroys tissue by applying extreme cold.

Cystocele: herniation of the urinary bladder through a weakness in the vaginal wall.

Dyspareunia: painful or difficult intercourse.

Ectopic pregnancy: implantation of the fertilized ovum outside the uterine cavity.

Endometriosis: growth of endometrial tissue outside the uterine cavity.

Galactorrhea: flow of breast milk unrelated to breast-feeding.

Hysterectomy: surgical removal of the uterus through an abdominal or vaginal incision.

Laparotomy: incision through the abdominal wall.

Lumpectomy: breast cancer surgery that removes only the lump; usually followed by radiation therapy.

Lymphedema: excess fluid collected in tissues of the hand and arm when lymph nodes or vessels are removed or blocked.

Mammography: X-ray used to diagnose and evaluate breast lesions.

Mastectomy: surgical removal of a breast.

Menorrhagia: increased menstrual flow; also called hypermenorrhea.

Metastasis: transfer of disease from one part of the body to another, via the lymphatic system or bloodstream.

Metrorrhagia: uterine bleeding between menstrual periods.

Mittelschmerz: abdominal pain related to ovulation.

Neoplasm: benign or malignant growth with uncontrolled or progressive cell multiplication; also called tumor.

Omentectomy: removal of all or part of the fold of the omentum.

Oophorectomy: removal of one or both ovaries.

Pessary: device inserted into the vagina to support the pelvic structures; commonly used to treat cystocele.

Polycystic ovary disease: endocrine disturbance in which continued ovarian stimulation from luteinizing hormone causes anovulation and polycystic ovaries. Also called Stein-Leventhal syndrome.

Polymenorrhea: increased frequency of menstrual bleeding.

Premature ovarian failure: premature cessation of ovulation and menstruation.

Rectocele: herniation of the rectum into the vagina.

Salpingo-oophorectomy: surgical removal of the fallopian tubes and ovaries.

Staging: classification of neoplasms by their extent and spread from the original site to other body regions.

Uterine prolapse: downward displacement of the uterus from its normal position in the pelvis.

---

orders, it discusses how to assess the client, formulate appropriate nursing diagnoses, plan and implement effective nursing interventions, and evaluate and document client care.

Breast disorders

Wide variations exist in women's breasts, which may be large, small, saggy, firm, smooth, or lumpy; nipples may be large or small, prominent or inverted; left and right breasts may differ in size and shape. Throughout life, a woman's breasts undergo gradual changes from aging, menstruation, pregnancy, menopause, injury, and use of hormones as in oral contraceptives. During each menstrual cycle, most women also experience breast changes, including enlargement and tenderness 7 to 10 days before menses.

To become familiar with normal breast changes, every woman should perform a monthly breast self-examination (BSE). (For more information, see Chapter 7, Women's Health Promotion.) A woman who performs BSE may notice subtle, abnormal breast changes before they are obvious to a health care professional.

Most women discover early breast lumps through BSE. In fact, women discover 95% of all breast lumps themselves (Griffith-Kenney, 1986). Women familiar with their breasts have discovered lesions smaller than 1 cm, which are difficult or impossible for a health care professional to detect. Fortunately, only one of five early breast lumps is cancerous. When a lump is cancerous, early discovery and treatment greatly increase the chances for complete recovery.

Ignorance of individual differences and normal breast changes may cause a woman to assume that every change or pain is a sign of cancer, prompting needless anxiety. Even before a diagnosis is confirmed, the possibility of breast cancer threatens a woman's life-style, provoking fears about mutilating surgery, lost femininity, and relationship changes. A woman's responses to these fears determine when and if she will seek care and which treatment options she will choose.

Although nearly 75% of women seek medical care within a month after discovering a breast abnormality, about 20% delay seeking care for at least a year (Lierman, 1988). Factors that lead to delay are:
• denial of the abnormality
• lack of knowledge about breast disorders
• fear of breast surgery
• fear of altered body image and self-esteem
• fear of relationship changes
• reluctance to undergo invasive diagnostic tests and treatments (Griffith-Kenney, 1986).

Benign breast disorders

Several common breast disorders that are benign can provoke anxiety until cancer is ruled out. These conditions include fibrocystic breast changes, fibroadenoma, intraductal papilloma, and duct ectasia.

Fibrocystic breast changes

Also known as mammary dysplasia or chronic cystic mastitis, fibrocystic breast changes represent the most common benign breast condition. Previously, this hormonally induced, cyclic pain and lumpiness was called a disease. Today, however, many health care professionals feel this term is inaccurate because studies show that about 50% of all women have clinical signs—and nearly 90% have histologic signs—of fibrocystic changes, which suggests that fibrocystic breast changes are a normal variation. Therefore, many health care professionals call this condition fibrocystic breast changes or physiologic nodularity because the word disease causes needless anxiety (Love, Gelman, and Silen, 1982; Jones, Wentz, and Burnett, 1988).

This condition typically causes painful, multiple, bilateral breast masses (cysts) that change rapidly in size. The cysts are round, unfixed, and well-defined on palpation. Frequently, pain occurs or intensifies as the cysts enlarge during the premenstrual period. A large, fluid-filled cyst may cause localized pain as it distends; multiple small cysts may cause diffuse tenderness. The condition improves during pregnancy and lactation and resolves with menopause.

In many cases, an aspiration is performed to determine if a mass is a fluid-filled cyst or a solid neoplasm. The color of aspirated fluid indicates the age of the mass. Straw-colored fluid suggests a recently formed cyst; dark green fluid, an older cyst; dark red fluid, a recent trauma. If fluid cannot be aspirated or mammography indicates changes in the mass, surgical excision may be performed to rule out a neoplasm.

The most common treatments for fibrocystic changes are hormone administration and diet changes to exclude methylxanthines, particularly caffeine, and to include vitamins E, A, and B complex.

For some women, avoiding caffeine in coffee, tea, cola, chocolate, and related substances relieves symptoms caused by methylxanthines (Ellerhorst-Ryan, Turba, and Stahl, 1988; Russell, 1989). Some studies found that reducing caffeine provided greatest relief for women with constant, rather than cyclical, pain; others found no association between caffeine and fibrocystic breast changes. Still others have used megadoses of vitamins E, A, and B complex to control fibrocystic breasts with inconclusive results (Ellerhorst-Ryan, Turba, and Stahl, 1988).

Daily administration of a synthetic androgen, oral danazol (Danocrine), can significantly reduce or eliminate fibrocystic breast symptoms. However, the hormone can produce unpleasant adverse reactions, such as menstrual irregularities, weight gain, increased facial hair, and voice deepening. Also, its high price may make it prohibitive for many women; for this reason, most studies have provided the drug for only 6 months. In studies, women who stopped taking danazol noted a gradual increase in fibrocystic breast symptoms, but not to pretreatment levels.

Fibroadenoma

A common, painless, benign neoplasm, fibroadenoma occurs most frequently in women between ages 15 and 39. Multiple lumps in one or both breasts affect 10% to 15% of women (Griffith-Kenney, 1986).

The typical fibroadenoma ranges from 1 to 5 cm in diameter and is round, rubbery, firm, discrete, relatively mobile, and nontender. It is the most common benign breast neoplasm in women under age 25 (Griffith-Kenney, 1986). Because it is asymptomatic, a fibroadenoma typically is discovered during BSE, a routine checkup, or routine mammography.

In some cases, treatment is conservative; needle biopsy or surgical excision is performed only if the lump appears suspicious. The health care professional may choose to monitor the lump closely, postponing excision for as long as possible, especially if the client is young and excision could interfere with normal breast development. However, many health care professionals recommend needle biopsy or excision of all discrete lumps.

Intraductal papilloma

An intraductal papilloma—a neoplasm in the terminal portion of the duct system—may not be palpable. The most common early sign is unilateral, spontaneous serous or serosanguineous discharge from a single duct. Less common is a bloody discharge. Although an intraductal papilloma is benign, a papillary carcinoma (a malignant neoplasm) developing within the duct may produce similar symptoms.

Treatment for a benign papilloma is excision of the involved duct and mass (if present) with a wedge resection.

Duct ectasia

Sometimes called comedomastitis, duct ectasia refers to duct dilation or distention. Most common in women between ages 35 and 55 who have breast-fed infants, it causes a thick, sticky, nipple discharge accompanied by burning pain, pruritus, and inflammation. It also may produce a soft or firm, palpable, poorly delineated mass around the nipple.

Treatment typically is conservative and aimed at relieving symptoms. To minimize the risk of infection, the client should be instructed to keep her nipples clean and dry and take antibiotics, as prescribed.

Breast cancer

Breast cancer is the most common type of cancer and the second leading cause of death in women. Every year, about 130,000 women are diagnosed with breast cancer, and about 41,000 die from the disease (National Cancer Institute, 1988b; Droegenmueller, Herbst, Mishel, and Stencheur, 1987). (For information on classification of breast cancer, see *Breast cancer staging*.)

Etiology

Breast cancer affects women of all ages and also may affect men. Although its cause remains unknown, breast cancer has been linked to the following risk factors:
- age 50 or older
- family history of breast cancer
- cancer in one breast, an ovary, the uterus, or colon
- nulliparity
- pregnancy after age 30

Breast cancer staging

To understand the severity of the client's disorder and her probable treatment, the nurse should be aware of breast cancer staging. Through staging, the physician classifies a breast lump according to its size, nodal involvement, and metastatic progress, as described below.

CARCINOMA IN SITU

Very early breast cancer confined to mammary ducts or lobules and not extending into adjacent breast tissue.

STAGE I

The lump is less than 2 cm, and the cancer has not spread outside the breast.

STAGE II

The lump is less than 5 cm, or the cancer has spread as far as the axillary lymph nodes, or both.

STAGE III

The lump is greater than 5 cm, or the cancer has invaded the skin or become attached to the chest wall. The axillary nodes are affected primarily; the supraclavicular nodes also may be affected.

STAGE IV

The cancer has metastasized to other areas, which typically include the lungs, bones, liver, or brain (National Cancer Institute, 1988b).

- obesity
- diet high in animal fat
- exposure to high doses of X-rays before age 30.

The most important risk factor is a family history of breast cancer (Micozzi, Carter, Albanes, Taylor, and Licitra, 1989). A client's risk doubles if her mother, sister, or daughter has had breast cancer. Her risk also increases with a history of breast cancer in her father's family (Fitzsimmons, Conway, Madsen, Lappe, and Coody, 1989).

Clinical findings

In most cases, a client who seeks care for breast cancer has discovered a painless lump or thickened area in her breast. Less typically, she has observed a thickening or lump in the axilla, a change in breast size or shape, nipple discharge, or a color or texture change in the breast or areola. Palpation commonly reveals a nontender, firm or hard mass, 2 to 3 cm in diameter, with poorly delineated margins.

Treatment

The choice of breast cancer treatment depends on the cancer type, stage and location of the neoplasm, and the client's needs, age, menopausal status, general health, and body-image concerns. Depending on the extent of the disease, treatment may be curative or palliative.

Currently, four standard treatments exist for breast cancer: surgery, radiation therapy, adjuvant hormone therapy, and adjuvant chemotherapy. For breast cancer in Stage I or II, treatment usually is curative and calls for surgery with or without a systemic therapy (chemotherapy or hormone therapy). In most cases, Stage III breast cancer is treated with surgery, radiation therapy, or both, followed by at least one systemic therapy. When cancer reaches Stage IV, palliative treatment is used to control growth of the neoplasm and reduce pain and ulceration. It may include any or all of the four cancer treatments.

Surgery. The most common treatment for breast cancer, surgery may be a lumpectomy, partial mastectomy, subcutaneous mastectomy, simple mastectomy, modified radical mastectomy, or (less commonly) radical mastectomy. (For more information and illustrations, see *Breast surgery*, page 288.)

Cancer treatments commonly affect cancer cells as well as healthy cells, causing unpleasant adverse effects. Depending on the amount, type, and location of the removed tissue, surgery may cause numbness and tingling in the chest and axillae, skin tightness over the chest, stiff arm and shoulder muscles, weight imbalance, reduced strength, or limited movement. The lymph nodes are removed with most resections, including lumpectomy and partial mastectomy. Lymphedema (excess lymph fluid) may occur in the arm and hand, especially when radical mastectomy is performed. Lymphedema may be decreased if the client performs preventive exercises.

Radiation therapy. Also called radiotherapy, this treatment bombards malignant cells with ionizing radiation. It may be used to eradicate the cancer or to relieve its symptoms. It can be used preoperatively to shrink a large neoplasm or postoperatively to eliminate any malignant cells that remain after surgery. Each treatment causes cumulative damage to the cancer cells (Lewis and Levita, 1988).

The most common forms of radiation beams are X-rays, gamma rays, electrons, and neutrons. Radiation therapy usually consists of beaming radiation from an external source at the neoplasm several times.

Because radiation therapy damages normal as well as malignant cells, the treated breast may become firmer and change in size and shape, its skin pores may become enlarged, dermatitis may occur, and skin sensitivity may

increase or decrease (Rutherford, 1988). The client also may experience fatigue because of physiologic stress.

Hormone therapy. When breast cancer has spread to the lymph nodes or other parts of the body, the treatment plan should include systemic adjuvant therapy (treatment in addition to primary treatment) to destroy any undetected cancer cells remaining in the body. The choice of adjuvant hormone therapy over adjuvant chemotherapy depends on the client's menopausal status and whether the cancer is hormone-dependent—that is, has positive estrogen and progesterone receptors and therefore grows or shrinks in response to hormone stimulation.

Hormones influence the function and growth of normal—and cancerous—breast cells. About one-third of all breast cancers are hormone-dependent, and one-third of these respond to hormone therapy. Hormone therapy may be accomplished by administration of estrogens, antiestrogens, progestins, or androgens. The best results occur in hormone-dependent neoplasms.

Adjuvant hormone therapy can cause adverse reactions, including hot flashes, weight gain, nausea, vomiting, vaginal bleeding, edema, or a flare reaction (temporary worsening of the disease manifested by increased pain, swelling, erythema, and skin lesions; temporary increase in neoplasm size; increased skeletal pain; and mental confusion). Flare reaction occurs most commonly with estrogen and antiestrogen therapy.

Chemotherapy. Adjuvant chemotherapy combines oral or injectable cytotoxic drugs to eradicate micrometastasis after surgery. CMF (combination therapy with the alkylating agent cyclophosphamide [Cytoxan] and the antimetabolites methotrexate [Folex] and fluorouracil [Adrucil]) is used most frequently in premenopausal women with cancer that has spread to the lymph nodes, regardless of the degree of hormone-dependence of the neoplasm. Given every 28 days over 3 to 6 months, CMF significantly reduces mortality; 60% to 62% of the recipients have remained disease free for 4 years (Ludwig Breast Cancer Study Group, 1988).

The axillary lymph node status (determined through biopsy and examination of the axillary lumph nodes) and the results of the hormone receptor assay test determine the use of chemotherapy in postmenopausal women. Research shows that tamoxifen can reduce mortality by about 22% in postmenopausal women (Carbone, 1990).

No specific drug or drug regimen benefits all clients with breast cancer. Proponents of aggressive treatment believe that only systemic treatments, such as chemotherapy, are effective on a potentially systemic disease like breast cancer. Opponents agree that adjuvant chemotherapy benefits premenopausal women, but argue that few postmenopausal women receive equal benefit.

Furthermore, they note that drug toxicity and other adverse effects have not been duly considered (Doig, 1988).

Because chemotherapy damages all rapidly growing cells, it affects cancer cells as well as normal cells lining the gastrointestinal (GI) tract, hair cells, and blood-producing cells. Therefore, women who receive chemotherapy may suffer mouth sores, anorexia, nausea, vomiting, hair loss, fatigue, and lowered resistance to infection. Menstrual periods may become irregular or may cease, and infertility may develop. Although the incidence and severity of these effects vary with individual clients, more than 80% of women experience nausea, hair loss, and fatigue (Love, Leventhal, Easterling, and Nerenz, 1989).

Metastatic breast cancer

Metastatic disease occurs when cancer cells from the breast spread to other body areas. Metastatic neoplasm cells resemble those in the original cancer site and commonly spread to the lungs, bones, liver, or brain.

Confirmed metastasis places the breast cancer at Stage IV and shifts the goal of care from cure to relief from pain and maintenance mobility and functioning. To reach these goals, treatment typically is systemic and requires chemotherapy, hormone therapy, or both. Limited surgery or radiation therapy may control the breast neoplasm, relieve pain or obstruction, and treat the sites to which cancer has spread. The length of time a client with metastasis may live depends on which organs are involved and how her body responds to systemic therapy.

Symptoms of metastatic cancer vary depending on the organs affected. Bone metastasis increases the risk of fractures and causes extreme pain that is controllable only with constant serum levels of analgesia. Liver metastasis may cause ascites, requiring diuretic therapy and possibly paracentesis (surgical puncture of the abdominal cavity to aspirate peritoneal fluid). Lung metastasis results in pleural effusions and breathing difficulty. Brain metastasis causes memory loss, visual disturbances, headaches, seizures, and altered gait.

As the disease advances and the client loses the ability to function normally, palliative measures become less effective and increasingly complex management is required.

Nursing care

When a client seeks care because of a breast lump, the nurse uses the nursing process to provide individualized, holistic care. Using therapeutic communication, the nurse determines the significance of the client's breast condition to her self-esteem and evaluates her emotional status, coping mechanisms, and knowledge and beliefs about cancer. As the client expresses her anxieties, fears, and misconceptions, the nurse provides appropriate information and support.

The client whose breast lump is diagnosed as benign may wish to put the ordeal behind her. The nurse must encourage such a client to perform BSE monthly and to return for scheduled examinations.

Assessment

From the initial visit through the final evaluation of care, the nurse continually assesses the client to maintain a data base that provides insight into her physical, mental, emotional, and social status. By conducting holistic health assessments and maintaining an understanding, emotionally supportive atmosphere, the nurse can help decrease the client's apprehension and can provide emotional support.

Evaluation of a suspicious breast area includes a thorough health history, physical assessment, and review of diagnostic studies. (For more information and procedures, see Chapter 7, Women's Health Promotion.)

Health history. Determine the client's major reason for seeking health care. If she has noticed a breast lump or other changes, ask her to describe her finding. Have her pinpoint the onset, duration, and nature of the changes. Determine if they seem cyclic or constant, or if certain activities affect them. Also, ask the client to describe any previous breast changes or discomfort. This information can help differentiate between benign and cancerous breast changes.

Because breast cancer is linked to family history, obtain a complete family history of breast disorders. Specifically ask about breast cancer in both sides of the client's family.

During follow-up visits, determine whether the client knows and understands her diagnosis, proposed treatments, and their effects. If the client has cancer, ask her to describe her knowledge and beliefs about it. This discussion may reveal misconceptions that need to be corrected and may help in providing information she needs to cope with the disease and in preparing for informed consent.

Assess the client's daily activities and self-care level. Determine how her daily routine will be altered when she returns home after treatment. This information will help in planning ways to meet her needs.

Ask the client about her energy level and ability to relax and sleep. Have her describe situations or techniques that could help her feel more rested. This information will help in developing the client's care plan.

Assess the client's literacy level and ability to retain information. Ask how she learns best and how she prefers

Breast surgery

The client with breast cancer may need surgery, which can range from conservative to radical, as illustrated below. The choice of surgery depends on size and location of the neoplasm, cancer type, and the client's age and breast size.

Lumpectomy removes only the breast lump and a narrow margin of normal tissue surrounding it. It is suitable for lumps under 5 cm that have not spread to the axillary nodes and is followed by radiation therapy.

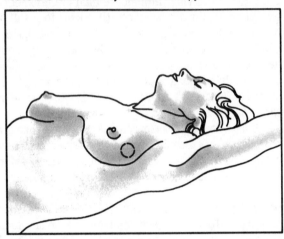

Partial (segmental) excision removes the lump, 2 to 3 cms of healthy tissue surrounding it, and the fascia over the chest muscles directly behind the lump. The axillary lymph nodes also may be removed. Some breast tissue remains. Radiation therapy may follow surgery.

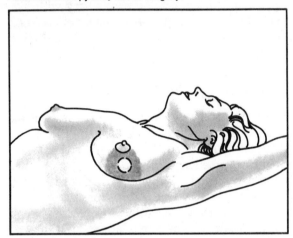

Total (simple) mastectomy removes the breast tissue and may remove the axillary lymph nodes closest to the breast. Radiation commonly follows.

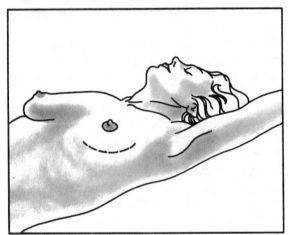

Modified radical mastectomy removes the breast, axillary lymph nodes, and chest muscle, but preserves the pectoralis major muscle. It is the most common surgery for breast cancer.

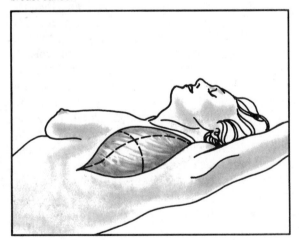

Subcutaneous mastectomy removes breast tissue while retaining breast skin. Tissue is examined histologically for invasive cancer. If cancer exists, more extensive surgery is scheduled. If staging was performed during an earlier biopsy, the subcutaneous mastectomy and breast implant insertion may take place during the same procedure.

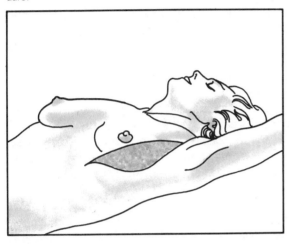

Radical mastectomy removes the breast, all of the axillary lymph nodes, chest muscles, and surrounding fat, tissue, and skin.

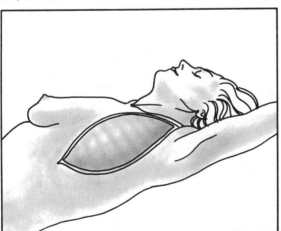

to have new information presented. Identify any difficulty she may have in communicating her thoughts and feelings. This information should help guide client teaching sessions.

Inquire about the client's perception of her identity, abilities, body image, and self-worth as well as the importance of her breasts to her self-image. Ask her to describe how she will look after treatment. Even a breast-saving procedure, such as a lumpectomy, can alter a client's self-concept and body image (Rutherford, 1988). Therefore, perform a psychosexual assessment of all clients who need breast surgery.

Ask the client to describe her condition and how it affects her daily activities. Ask if she experiences any constant or periodic pain. Determine her attitudes about the cause of her condition, the course she expects it to take, and possible treatments. Probe her perceptions of the effect of her condition and its treatment on her self-concept, sexuality, relationships, and sexual activity. This information reveals potential problems related to her body image and relationships.

Assess the client's roles and responsibilities in her family, work, and social environments. Discuss any relationship problems she anticipates because of illness or treatment. Assess family support, coping, and communication, and observe how family and friends interact with the client. This information will help in planning ways to meet the role change that may occur within her family and support system.

Determine the client's stressors and how she copes with them. Explore her internal and external resources for support. Breast cancer creates a crisis that may affect the client's coping and decision-making abilities. Plan to use information about her coping mechanisms and support systems to address her anxieties, fears, discomforts, and decision-making ability.

Ask the client about her religious and spiritual beliefs, values, and goals. Keep in mind that her beliefs may affect her care decisions.

Physical assessment. To obtain further information, perform a thorough physical assessment. Make special note of findings during breast inspection and palpation that may support a particular diagnosis. (For illustrated procedures, see Chapter 7, Women's Health Promotion.)

Diagnostic studies. When physical assessment reveals breast changes, the physician may order various diagnostic studies. For a client with fibrocystic breast changes, mammography may determine if other, non-palpable neoplasms are present. Other noninvasive imaging techniques may include ultrasonography, which can distinguish between a fluid-filled cyst and a solid mass; thermography, which discerns abnormal heat patterns on the breast surface, indicating possible cancer growth; and diaphanography, which uses a bright light to transilluminate the breasts, showing possible masses—but these techniques have been virtually replaced by mammography

Only microscopic examination of the neoplasm can identify cancer cells positively. Fine-needle aspiration removes cells for examination from a fluid-filled or solid lump; excisional biopsy, which removes the entire lump, permits comprehensive examination of a solid lump.

If the lump is benign, no further treatment is needed. If cancer is present, estrogen and progesterone receptor tests can determine if hormone treatment may be effective. Based on clinical findings and cellular analysis, the physician stages the cancer.

If the client has nipple discharge or bleeding, a cytologic examination of the discharge can identify malignant cells that indicate intraductal cancer. For this examination, a section of the lump is removed and examined to differentiate between benign papilloma and papillary carcinoma.

When assessment findings suggest metastatic disease, chest X-rays, liver function studies, complete blood count (CBC), and bone scans can help determine if and where metastasis has occurred.

Nursing diagnosis

Review health history, physical assessment, and diagnostic study data. Based on significant findings, formulate nursing diagnoses that address the client's needs as she moves from diagnosis through treatment. (For a partial list of possible nursing diagnoses, see *Nursing diagnoses: Gynecologic disorders.*)

Planning and implementation

By working with the client to set mutually agreeable goals, the nurse can develop a care plan that considers the client's individual strengths and weaknesses and addresses her concerns. The following examples illustrate appropriate goals.
• The client will express and cope with her anxieties, fears, and discomforts while a diagnosis is being determined.
• The client will prepare for therapy and move through the stages of grief if breast cancer is confirmed.
• The client will maintain optimal psychological and physical health before, during, and after surgery.
• The client will return to optimal functioning after treatment.
• The client will become comfortable with her altered body image.
• The client will continue to practice BSE.
• The client will function as well as possible if she develops advanced metastatis.

After goals have been established, the nurse can implement the care plan. Because individual client and family involvement in treatment will vary, the nurse should tailor interventions as needed. When caring for a client with a breast disorder, the nurse may provide support; teach about self-care, diagnostic tests, and surgery; assist with decision making; provide postoperative care; teach about reconstructive surgery and other therapies; administer care to the client with metastatic disease; and provide family care.

Provide support

Psychological support begins with the first nurse-client interaction. Any client seeking care for a breast disorder experiences distress. The nurse can reduce distress by helping the client clarify her values as she explores treatment options. After the client selects a care plan, the nurse functions as her advocate, supporting achievement of her goals.

Until a diagnosis is confirmed, the client may fear that she has cancer. She may have a nursing diagnosis of *anxiety related to discovery of a lump during BSE* or *fear related to the potential for breast surgery.* During this period, provide emotional support and reassure the client, if possible.

Discuss concerns with the client and her family, encouraging them to express feelings and providing time for the client and her partner to share their concerns privately. Provide support for the client facing surgery by showing concern for her feelings of loss, grief, and fear about her health status, change in body image, loss of a body part, and possible loss of sexual attractiveness. However, guard against offering false reassurances, which may give the client unrealistic expectations.

Emotional support helps prevent the client's new self-image and physical status from affecting her relationships negatively. When surgical dressings are removed and the client and her partner first observe the incision, provide special support. Allow them to grieve and encourage them to express feelings about the loss of a body part, disfigurement, and perceived loss of desirability. This is especially important for the client with a nursing diagnosis of *anticipatory grieving related to breast removal.*

Before the client views the incision, explain its expected appearance. When she sees the incision, make positive statements about her healing progress, such as "You seem to be healing well."

Teach the client to inspect the incision daily for signs of infection or drainage collection under the skin flap. Provide written instructions for incision care.

For a client with fibroadenoma, provide support by teaching her (and her mother, if the client is an adolescent) about the implications of diagnostic findings and

NURSING DIAGNOSES

Gynecologic disorders

The following nursing diagnoses address representative problems and etiologies that the nurse may encounter when caring for a client with a gynecologic disorder. Specific nursing interventions for many of these diagnoses are provided in the "Planning and implementation" section of this chapter.

BREAST DISORDERS

- Altered role performance related to breast cancer
- Altered sexuality patterns related to changes in breast tissue and sensations
- Anticipatory grieving related to breast removal
- Anxiety related to diagnostic tests
- Anxiety related to discovery of a lump during breast self-examination
- Body image disturbance related to alteration of tissue linked to sexual identity
- Decisional conflict related to breast cancer treatment
- Decisional conflict related to breast surgery
- Fear related to discovery of a breast lump
- Impaired physical mobility related to breast surgery
- Ineffective family coping: compromised, related to breast cancer
- Knowledge deficit related to breast cancer therapies
- Knowledge deficit related to breast care
- Knowledge deficit related to breast surgery
- Knowledge deficit related to diagnostic tests
- Knowledge deficit related to reconstructive surgery
- Pain related to breast cancer with metastasis
- Pain related to breast surgery
- Pain related to fibrocystic breast changes
- Potential for infection related to breast surgery

MENSTRUAL DISORDERS

- Anxiety related to abnormal menstrual pattern
- Anxiety related to management of premenstrual syndrome
- Body image disturbance related to androgenic effects of hormones
- Ineffective family coping: compromised, related to premenstrual anger and mood swings
- Ineffective individual coping related to abnormal menstrual patterns
- Ineffective individual coping related to invasive diagnostic procedures
- Ineffective individual coping related to mood swings

- Knowledge deficit related to normal menstrual cycle physiology
- Pain related to menstruation
- Sexual dysfunction related to dyspareunia

GYNECOLOGIC CANCER

- Altered nutrition: less than body requirements, related to nausea, vomiting, and anorexia caused by chemotherapy
- Altered role performance related to gynecologic cancer
- Altered sexuality patterns related to gynecologic surgery
- Altered urinary elimination patterns related to surgery
- Anxiety related to cancer treatment
- Anxiety related to cervical biopsy results
- Anxiety related to unmet informational needs about cancer and its treatment
- Body image disturbance related to loss of fertility
- Body image disturbance related to loss of organs associated with sexual identity
- Impaired tissue integrity related to vulvectomy
- Ineffective family coping: compromised, related to the client's gynecologic cancer
- Ineffective individual coping related to cancer
- Ineffective individual coping related to misconceptions about surgery
- Knowledge deficit related to cancer treatment
- Knowledge deficit related to gynecologic cancer
- Knowledge deficit related to treatment of abnormal Pap test results
- Noncompliance related to diagnostic tests
- Pain related to radiation therapy
- Potential for infection related to gynecologic surgery
- Self-esteem disturbance related to guilt about cancer
- Self-esteem disturbance related to radical gynecologic surgery
- Sexual dysfunction related to altered body structure
- Social isolation related to others' fear of cancer

the importance of returning for further observations as directed. When surgery is scheduled, address the client's questions and concerns about the effects of breast surgery.

When a client has intraductal papilloma, explain treatment procedures and provide concerned, listening support.

For a client with duct ectasia, provide information, emotional support, and reassurance that symptoms do not necessarily indicate cancer.

Teach self-care for benign breast disorders. The client with a benign breast disorder may have a nursing diagnosis of *knowledge deficit related to breast care* or *pain related to fibrocystic breast changes.* For such a client, suggest ways to increase her comfort, such as wearing a brassiere 24 hours a day, taking a mild diuretic premenstrually, applying ice packs to the breasts, restricting sodium intake, and taking salicylates or other anti-inflammatory drugs. Advise the client with fibrocystic breast changes that the moderate to severe pain may cease spontaneously within 1 year.

Teach other self-care activities, such as eliminating caffeine and adopting vitamin therapy. (For more information, see *Nursing research applied: Effects of caffeine restriction on breast pain*.)

While teaching self-care methods, encourage the client to perform BSE every month, schedule regular examinations with her health care professional, and return for care whenever she discovers breast changes. Remind the client with fibrocystic changes that her risk of breast cancer may be slightly increased (Love, Gelman, and Silen, 1982; Griffith-Kenney, 1986).

Teach about diagnostic tests. The client with a *knowledge deficit related to diagnostic tests* or *anxiety related to diagnostic tests* may benefit from explanations of diagnostic studies and their effects and significance. Be sure to explain that a biopsy for diagnosis and staging is performed separately from any necessary surgery.

Assist with decision making. A client who has difficulty in choosing a particular treatment plan may have a nursing diagnosis of *decisional conflict related to breast surgery* or *decisional conflict related to breast cancer treatment*.

As the client's advocate and educator, help her with decision making by providing emotional support as she clarifies her values and by offering information as she seeks knowledge and explores alternatives. Reassure her that you will support her decision, whatever it may be. Only the client can decide if the benefits of surgery outweigh its risks in her case.

Teach about surgery. The client may have a nursing diagnosis of *knowledge deficit related to breast surgery*. After the treatment plan has been agreed upon, support the client's decision and review her knowledge about the chosen surgery and possible future adjuvant therapies. Teach about pertinent routines and procedures and outline postoperative sensations and expectations. Carefully explain site preparation, NPO status, recovery room procedures, postoperative pain management, dressings, postsurgical ambulation, deep-breathing and coughing techniques, arm exercises, and diet.

Most clients will display high levels of hope, a preference for open communication, and a desire for information (Cassileth, Zupkis, Sutton-Smith, and March, 1980). Because high stress levels may interfere with the client's ability to absorb information, reiterate information, encourage questions, and provide time for expression of concerns.

Discuss recovery with the client, including her rehabilitation and gradual resumption of activities. If she desires, provide information on community resources and arrange a visit with a woman who has had a mastectomy.

NURSING RESEARCH APPLIED

Effects of caffeine restriction on breast pain

A recent study considered the effects of methylxanthines (caffeine, theophylline, and theobromine) on breast pain in women with fibrocystic breast changes. All 138 women in the sample experienced breast pain from fibrocystic breast changes, which were documented by mammography, physical examination, and a history of symptoms.

After reporting their caffeine consumption and degree of pain, the women were counseled about abstaining from or reducing caffeine consumption. They were provided with a list of common products that contain caffeine.

At the end of 1 year, 113 women (81.9%) had reduced their caffeine intake substantially. Of those, 69 (61%) reported a decrease in or cessation of breast pain.

Application to practice
This study suggests that women who limit caffeine consumption experience reduced pain associated with fibrocystic breast changes. Although not every woman in the study benefited from caffeine reduction, a statistically significant number reported lower pain levels. For a client with pain caused by fibrocystic breast changes, the nurse can suggest abstinence from caffeine as a conservative, yet possibly effective, treatment.

Russell, L. (1989). Caffeine restriction as initial treatment for breast pain. *Nurse Practitioner*, 14(2), 36-40.

Provide postoperative care. During the postoperative period, care goals include facilitating wound healing and minimizing lymphedema. To help achieve these goals, do not use the affected arm for blood pressure measurements, injections, I.V. therapy, or drawing blood.

After surgery, the client may have a nursing diagnosis of *potential for infection related to breast surgery*. Because of this, assess the client regularly for signs of hemorrhage, shock, and infection. Also check her vital signs, inspect the dressing, use sterile technique when changing dressings, and administer antibiotics, as prescribed. Monitor the drainage device and record output. Where applicable, assess other sites, such as the donor or graft site.

To decrease the risk of lymphedema, place the client in a semi-Fowler's position on her back or unaffected side. Position her arm with the wrist elevated above the elbow and the elbow above the shoulder. Monitor edema by measuring the circumference of the upper arm and forearm daily. Encourage the client to use her arm for simple tasks, such as eating, washing, and toothbrushing. Within 24 hours after surgery, initiate the prescribed forearm exercises. Help the client maintain full range of motion in the affected arm by teaching and encouraging progressively more difficult arm exercises.

This will help prevent a nursing diagnosis of *impaired physical mobility related to breast surgery.*

Every 2 hours, help the client change positions (between her back and unaffected side), cough while supporting her chest, and perform deep-breathing exercises, even though the pressure dressing may make deep breathing difficult.

For a client with a nursing diagnosis of *pain related to breast surgery,* minimize discomfort by positioning her arm to decrease muscle tension and preventing exposure to extreme heat or cold. Discuss phantom breast pain (pain that seems to emanate from the removed breast), reassuring the client that phantom pain is normal. To help relieve pain, provide backrubs and teach the client to perform imagery or progressive muscle relaxation. Encourage her to walk as soon as possible to improve ventilation and circulation and to maintain active range of motion in her legs.

Teach the client about infection risks to her affected arm caused by restricted circulation and lymph node removal. Explore methods that she may use to protect against infection. Encourage her to maintain good posture, holding her back straight, pulling her shoulders back, and letting her arms hang at her sides. Provide written instructions about long-term protection for the affected side. (For more information, see *Client teaching: Hand and arm care after a mastectomy.*)

Help the client resume her sexual expression. Recommend sexual positions that alleviate pressure on the chest wall or suggest the use of alternative sexual expressions until the site is no longer tender.

Discuss the client's gradual resumption of other normal activities, identifying her concerns about role fulfillment. Explore resources that might help meet her needs as she recovers. Help her select and adapt to a bra and prosthesis.

Before the client is discharged, discuss the disease, effects of surgery, and planned adjuvant therapy. Prepare her for continuing fatigue and encourage her to rest accordingly. Inform her of community exercise programs for women after mastectomies. Review and encourage regular monthly BSE of the remaining breast.

Teach about reconstructive surgery. The client who undergoes breast surgery may have a *knowledge deficit related to reconstructive surgery.* Before mastectomy, discuss the option of breast reconstruction, because it offers a focal point for psychological recovery. Most clients who undergo mastectomy are candidates for breast reconstruction, but many who are initially interested later change their mind.

Before surgery, assess the client's knowledge about breast reconstruction and determine her goals and priorities. Common reasons for electing reconstructive sur-

---

CLIENT TEACHING

Hand and arm care after a mastectomy

Lymph node removal during breast surgery increases the risk that your arm may swell or become infected. To decrease your risk of these problems, follow the suggestions below.

- Do not offer your affected arm for blood pressure measurements, injections, or intravenous treatments.
- Wear long sleeves and gloves if you garden.
- Use a thimble if you sew.
- Wear rubber gloves if you wash dishes or whenever your hands will be in water more than a minute or two
- Use pot holders to avoid burns if you handle hot pans.
- Avoid wearing a tight watch or bracelet or carrying a purse on your arm. These may impair circulation.
- Push back your cuticles rather than cutting them.
- Avoid lifting heavy objects with your affected arm.
- Avoid sunburn on your affected arm.
- Elevate your affected arm whenever you can.
- If you injure your hand or arm, wash the site with soap and water. Then apply an antiseptic cream and a bandage.
- Be alert for signs of infection, such as redness, heat, swelling, pain, drainage with pus, fever, or chills. If these signs occur, notify your doctor as soon as possible.

This teaching aid may be reproduced by office copier for distribution to clients. © 1991, Springhouse Corporation.

---

gery include restoring balance or self-esteem, feeling feminine or "whole," improving sexual relations, and becoming less preoccupied with one's physical state.

Offer realistic information about advantages and disadvantages of breast reconstruction. Advantages include a more balanced appearance that provides a psychological boost and improves body image and a natural breast shape without the limitations of a prosthesis. Disadvantages include the possible disparity in appearance between the reconstructed and the unaltered breast, the expense, and the risks of additional surgery, including the possibility of unsatisfactory results or surgical complications. Emphasize that reconstruction provides a substitute—not a replacement—for the removed breast.

Breast reconstruction involves one of two procedures. If sufficient skin and muscle tissue remain after cancer removal and radiation therapy, an implant made of silicone gel or inflated with normal saline may be inserted at the site. If the remaining skin and muscle tissue are insufficient, skin grafts may supply new tissue to hold the implants in place. Some reconstructive surgery also includes creating the appearance of a nipple by grafting a piece of tissue from the contralateral areola, upper medial thigh, ear lobe, toe pad, or skin flap onto the breast (d'Angelo and Gorrell, 1989).

Before surgery, instruct the client in postoperative coughing, deep-breathing techniques, and pain management strategies, such as proper positioning, massage, imagery, and use of medication. After surgery, maintain comfort and prevent complications. Assess skin tissue viability and observe for redness, swelling, drainage, odor, and tenderness. Also teach the client about the healing process and possible complications (d'Angelo and Gorrell, 1989).

Before discharge, instruct the client to wear a special brassiere 24 hours a day until healing is complete. This brassiere helps shape the reconstructed breast appropriately. Teach the client to limit activity on the affected side during recovery and to increase activity gradually. Stress the importance of complying with restrictions to achieve the best results with the fewest complications. If the client received an implant to be inflated with normal saline solution, review her schedule for return visits.

Teach about other therapies. If the client needs radiation therapy, hormone therapy, or chemotherapy, describe the typical adverse effects of these treatments and discuss comfort measures. This is particularly useful for a client with a nursing diagnosis of *knowledge deficit related to breast cancer therapies.*

Because the client is stressed and may not retain all the information presented, provide written materials for review and encourage a supportive family member to accompany her at teaching sessions. Review her therapy plan, addressing her questions and concerns. Prepare her to manage the adverse effects of treatment, keeping in mind that individuals differ greatly in their coping styles and responses to treatment (Hopkins, 1986).

Advise the client that radiation therapy may cause lethargy, fatigue, anorexia, nausea, and skin reactions, such as erythema followed by skin sloughing. Encourage her to counter these effects by resting, eating a balanced diet, and reporting nausea and skin reactions to her physician. Reassure her that the symptoms will subside gradually after treatment is completed.

For a client who will receive hormone therapy, discuss typical effects. Estrogens may cause fluid retention, breast tenderness, urinary incontinence (Griffith-Kenney, 1986), androgens, voice deepening, increased facial hair, clitoral hypertrophy, increased emotions, or libidinal changes (Dunne, 1988); and antiestrogens, nausea, vomiting, hot flashes, lightheadedness, headaches, vulvar itching, and vaginal bleeding. Because a client

who receives hormone therapy probably will take the medication at home, instruct her to report any reactions to her physician.

When a client is scheduled for chemotherapy, discuss its adverse effects, including alopecia (hair loss), GI disturbances, fluid retention, decreased appetite, and neuropathy resulting in decreased libido, impaired self-esteem, and negative body image. For such a client, reinforce the importance of balanced nutrition and encourage the family to assist her during chemotherapy by offering small, appetizing meals (Grindel, Cahill, and Walker, 1989).

Care for the client with metastatic disease. A client with metastatic disease experiences a gradual reduction in abilities. When caring for a client with a nursing diagnosis of *pain related to breast cancer with metastasis,* aim to maximize her remaining abilities while relieving pain and enhancing comfort. If the client has bone metastasis, teach proper body mechanics to reduce bone stress.

Provide emotional support to the client and her family as they grieve and face the inevitability of her death. When the client returns home, provide information on community resources, such as home health care and hospice services.

Provide family care. Breast cancer not only affects the client, but also her family and friends. As they face the prospect of altered plans, income loss, increased home management and medical expenses, and changes in sexual functioning and family roles, they may develop a nursing diagnosis of *ineffective family coping: compromised, related to breast cancer* or *altered role performance related to breast cancer.*

Partners of women with breast cancer report heightened anxiety, depression, and psychosomatic problems, such as headaches or anorexia. Although their mood changes and role problems typically resolve over time, their distress levels remain relatively constant for up to 18 months after the client's mastectomy. In one study, the partners' reported distress levels did not differ significantly from those of the clients (Northouse, 1989).

The client may fear a change in the way her family and friends feel about her. At the same time, family members and friends may avoid discussing the illness with the client for fear of upsetting her. To help all members adapt, encourage them to engage in an open dialogue about breast cancer and its treatments and physical effects.

Evaluation

The goals developed by the nurse and client serve as the basis for evaluation. By reviewing these goals, the nurse and client can evaluate which goals have been met and which have yet to be achieved. The following examples illustrate some appropriate evaluation statements.

• The client expressed an understanding of her surgery and asked appropriate questions about postoperative interventions and pain control.

• The client demonstrated growing acceptance of her new self-image by viewing the incision line.

• The client set realistic goals and actively participated in her chosen treatment plan.

• The client expressed reasons for keeping follow-up appointments.

A client achieves full recovery when she perceives her breast disorder as part of her history and resumes an activity level that matches her abilities and desires.

Documentation

Although each health care facility requires documentation of slightly different information, most expect the nurse to record the following:

• reason that the client seeks care

• history of the disorder, including changes in breast lump size, shape, or location

• related symptoms, including breast pain or heat

• results of breast inspection and palpation

• results of mammography

• client teaching performed by the nurse.

Menstrual disorders

The menstrual cycle results from a complex interplay between the endocrine and reproductive systems. The hypothalamus produces gonadotropin-releasing hormone (GnRH), which stimulates the pituitary gland to produce follicle-stimulating hormone (FSH) and luteinizing hormone (LH). FSH and LH, in turn, stimulate the ovaries to produce estrogen and progesterone. In response to these hormones, the uterus proliferates and then sheds its lining. (For more information, see Chapter 6, Reproductive Anatomy and Physiology).

Dysfunction may occur at any step in this process, making evaluation difficult. In addition, numerous factors—including hormonal imbalances, structural abnormalities, and life-style—can affect the menstrual cycle. To help a client with a menstrual disorder, the nurse must have a sound knowledge of normal menstrual variations, of treatment for menstrual disorders, and of life-style factors that affect the menstrual cycle.

The most common menstrual disorders include amenorrhea, dysmenorrhea, premenstrual syndrome (PMS), mittelschmerz, metrorrhagia, and endometriosis. (For a chart that summarizes etiology, clinical findings, and treatments, see *Common menstrual disorders*, pages 296 to 298.)

Amenorrhea

Amenorrhea (absence of menses) typically occurs during pregnancy, the postpartal period, lactation, and menopause, but it can occur at other times as well. The failure of menstruation to occur within 2 years of full secondary sexual development or by age 16 constitutes primary amenorrhea. A 6-month cessation of established menses represents secondary amenorrhea.

Although amenorrhea is not a disease, it can be a sign of one. Management of amenorrhea depends on its underlying cause and the client's desired outcome.

Dysmenorrhea

Like amenorrhea, dysmenorrhea (cramping pain before and during menstruation) may be primary or secondary. Primary dysmenorrhea consists of painful menstruation without evidence of an organic defect. It is most common in nulliparous and obese clients and frequently associated with prolonged menstrual flow. About 75% of women suffer from primary dysmenorrhea; 10% of these women experience severe symptoms for 1 to 3 days in each cycle (Droegenmueller, Herbst, Mishell, and Stencheur, 1987). Secondary dysmenorrhea is related to organic pelvic disease, such as pelvic inflamatory disease (PID), endometriosis, uterine fibroids, ovarian cysts, or pelvic masses.

Premenstrual syndrome

A relatively common problem, PMS is a physical and psychological disorder producing symptoms that recur during the luteal phase (days 14 to 28) of the menstrual cycle and resolve by day 3 of the menstrual phase. Possibly 95% of women experience PMS symptoms, and 5% to 10% of them experience severe symptoms (Severino and Moline, 1989). More than 150 physical and psychological symptoms have been associated with PMS, and these can vary by person and cycle. Most PMS sufferers seek treatment for mood swings that disrupt their personal and professional lives, causing despair and loss of self-esteem.

PMS tends to occur during periods of hormonal change: after giving birth, after a period of amenorrhea, when beginning or ceasing an oral contraceptive, at pu-

(Text continues on page 298.)

Common menstrual disorders

The following chart summarizes the etiology, clinical findings, and treatments for various common menstrual disorders.

Amenorrhea

Etiology
Primary amenorrhea
Chromosomal defects; lack of gonadal development; hormonal imbalances; systemic disease; congenital defects of the reproductive tract, such as imperforate hymen or absence of uterus; hypothalamic dysfunction; neoplasms of the pituitary or hypothalamus

Secondary amenorrhea
Medications, such as oral contraceptives and tranquilizers; systemic diseases, such as tuberculosis, hypothyroidism, and diabetes mellitus; ovarian cysts; uterine abnormalities; pituitary neoplasms; hypothalamic dysfunction caused by chronic stress or anxiety; nutritional factors causing decreased estrogen levels, such as anorexia nervosa or inadequate body fat; excessive exercise; polycystic ovary disease (Stein-Leventhal syndrome); premature ovarian failure (menopause before age 35); infection; anovulation (absence of ovulation)

Clinical findings
• Normal pelvic examination findings or ovarian cysts
• Lack of secondary sex characteristics
• Dark, coarse facial hair and obesity, indicating excessive androgen production
• Galactorrhea (milk flow unrelated to lactation), possibly indicating a pituitary tumor

Treatments
• Hormone replacement therapy if ovarian failure exists (For more information, see Chapter 7, Women's Health Promotion.)
• Administration of progesterone if a client does not menstruate during 6 months after discontinuing an oral contraceptive
• Administration of an ovulation-inducing medication (Clomid, Serophene) if pregnancy is desired
• Periodic administration of progesterone (three times per year) to induce bleeding and prevent endometrial hyperplasia in a client who does not menstruate monthly
• Use of an oral contraceptive to induce menses in a client who has a psychological need for menses, but does not desire pregnancy

Dysmenorrhea

Etiology
Primary dysmenorrhea
Excess release of prostaglandins during menstrual shedding of the decidua; increased smooth muscle contraction and vasospasm of uterine arterioles, leading to tissue ischemia and cramping pain

Secondary dysmenorrhea
Endometriosis; pelvic neoplasms; ovarian cysts; pelvic inflammatory disease; adenomyosis; uterine fibroids; cervical stenosis; cervical or endometrial polyps; uterine prolapse; endometrial carcinoma; use of an intrauterine device

Clinical findings
Primary
• Early adolescence, usually 1 to 2 years after menarche
• Mild cramps to severe, incapacitating pain
• Cramping several hours before menstrual flow begins
• Spasmodic cramping localized to the lower abdomen and radiating to the back and upper thighs
• Vomiting, diarrhea, headache, syncope, and leg pains
• Normal pelvic examination findings

Secondary
• Established pattern of relatively comfortable periods
• Pelvic congestion, masses, or inflammation from infections or adhesions
• Various pain locations
• Undiagnosed gynecologic disease

Treatments
• Administration of a nonsteroidal anti-inflammatory drug (NSAIDs), such as ibuprofin (Advil, Nuprin, Motrin, Rufen), naproxen (Naprosyn), mefenamic acid (Ponstel), naproxen sodium (Anaprox, Anaprox DS), or ketoprofen (Orudis)
• Use of oral contraceptives, except where contraindicated, in clients who obtain no relief from NSAIDs
• Balanced nutrition
• Administration of vitamin E (a mild prostaglandin inhibitor)
• Heat application
• Regular exercise
• Stress management
• Frequent rest
• Treatment of underlying disorder in client with secondary dysmenorrhea

Common menstrual disorders continued

Premenstrual syndrome (PMS)

Etiology
Exact cause unknown. Possible causes include a hormonal imbalance caused by estrogen excess or progesterone deficit; deficiency of the brain neurotransmitter serotonin; withdrawal from beta endorphins; prolactin or prostaglandin excess; a nutritional and vitamin B deficiency that lowers the threshold for stress.

Clinical findings
Luteal phase
- Aggression and anger
- Insomnia
- Anxiety, mood swings, depression, crying, panic attacks, poor concentration, decreased coping skills
- Fluid retention
- Migraine headaches
- Breast pain and tenderness
- Acne
- Food cravings and binges
- Rhinitis, asthma
- Backache, joint pain
- Alcoholic bouts
- Altered glucose tolerance
- Clumsiness
- Worsening of chronic medical problems
- Social withdrawal

Treatments
- Low sodium, high complex carbohydrate diet
- Other dietary changes
- Vitamin and mineral supplements
- Regular exercise
- Stress management techniques
- Medications, such as an oral contraceptive, diuretic, antidepressant, or natural progesterone, as prescribed

Mittelschmerz

Etiology
Increased follicular pressure before ovulation; leakage of small amounts of follicular fluid or blood into the peritoneal cavity, causing a mild peritoneal reaction

Clinical findings
- Moderate to severe midcycle lower abdominal pain
- Normal pelvic examination findings

Treatments
- Reassurance that mittelschmerz is a normal response to ovulation
- Administration of a mild analgesic or NSAID, such as ibuprofen, for pain

Metrorrhagia

Etiology
Anovulation or irregular ovulation; infection; breakthrough bleeding with an oral contraceptive; pregnancy disorders, such as ectopic pregnancy or threatened abortion; systemic diseases, such as hypothyroidism or blood dyscrasia; uterine fibroids; endometrial or cervical polyps; psychogenic (stress-related) disorders

Clinical findings
- Irregular bleeding or spotting between menstrual periods
- A gynecologic abnormality causing the intermittent bleeding, such as infection of the cervix or uterus, endocervical polyps, or uterine fibroids
- Normal physical and pelvic examinations

Treatments
- Change to another contraceptive method for metrorrhagia related to contraceptive use
- Antibiotic administration for metrorrhagia related to infection
- Surgery for metrorrhagia related to a uterine or adnexal mass
- Frequent observation and follow-up for dysfunctional uterine bleeding caused by anovulation
- Supplemental oral progesterone 10 days per month, beginning in the third week of the menstrual cycle, for chronic and heavy bleeding
- Use of an oral contraceptive to create a more regular menstrual flow, if pregnancy prevention is needed

Common menstrual disorders continued

Endometriosis

Etiology
Endometrial tissue in various locations in the pelvic cavity, including the ovaries, uterine ligaments, pelvic peritoneum, appendix, small intestine, and lymph nodes; movement of endometrial cells to other sites through vascular and lymphatic channels

Clinical findings
• Asymptomatic in about 30% of women (Garner and Webster, 1985)
• Secondary dysmenorrhea that worsens progressively and can be incapacitating
• Dyspareunia (painful intercourse)
• Infertility caused by pelvic adhesions that inhibit ovum transport through the fallopian tube
• Metrorrhagia
• Dull, cramping pain in the lower abdomen and back that may begin at ovulation and continue until menses
• Ovulatory pain
• Painful bowel movements

Treatments
• Administration of progesterone or a combination estrogen-progesterone oral contraceptive on a continuous schedule, causing amenorrhea and pseudopregnancy that shrink the ectopic endometrial tissue; high recurrence rate after therapy concludes
• Danazol (a synthetic androgen) therapy to decrease estrogen and progesterone secretion. Danazol (Danocrine) 400 mg given orally twice a day as continuous therapy for 6 months.
• Nasally administered, nafarelin acetate (Synarel), a gonadotropin-releasing hormone agonist, which suppresses the pituitary-ovarian axis, causes low levels of follicle-stimulating hormone and luteinizing hormone, and induces a menopausal state
• Laparoscopic surgery to lyse adhesions, remove small implants, and cauterize adhesion sites. Lasers recently have been combined with the laparoscope to vaporize endometrial implants.
• Hysterectomy for a client whose chronic severe pain does not respond to medical therapy and who has completed childbearing

berty when menses begins, before menopause as menses ends, and after tubal ligation. Although not hereditary, PMS is familial. Its symptoms can increase with each pregnancy and with age. PMS sufferers may have low tolerance for synthetic hormones (such as oral contraceptives) and may have higher rates of pregnancy-induced hypertension and postpartal depression (Dalton, 1984).

Mittelschmerz

Many women experience mittelschmerz (abdominal pain during ovulation) with each menstrual cycle. Lasting from a few hours to 2 days, mittelschmerz is marked by a sharp, localized pelvic pain (in a lower abdominal quadrant) that progresses to a dull ache. This discomfort is caused by peritoneal irritation, the result of blood escaping from the ovary at the site of the ruptured follicle. Pinkish vaginal spotting that resolves spontaneously may accompany the pain. In some cases, mittelschmerz may cause pain as severe as that of intense dysmenorrhea.

Metrorrhagia

Metrorrhagia (irregular bleeding or spotting between periods) is one of the most common reasons women seek health care. The volume with metrorrhagia varies from scant spotting to heavy bleeding. Although metrorrhagia

may suggest a benign disorder, such as anovulatory bleeding, it also may signal endometrial cancer or other serious disorders.

Abnormal uterine bleeding with no organic cause represents dysfunctional uterine bleeding (DUB), a form of metrorrhagia. Usually caused by anovulation or irregular ovulation, DUB is marked by scanty or profuse bleeding without accompanying pain. DUB is most common immediately after menarche or before menopause. In adolescents, irregular bleeding may be normal for up to 2 years after menarche.

Normally, estrogen and progesterone counterbalance each other. In DUB, estrogen causes the uterine lining to thicken as usual, but the lack of ovulation causes a progesterone deficiency. This "unopposed" estrogen results in irregular shedding of the endometrium, causing DUB.

Endometriosis

In endometriosis (growth of endometrial tissue outside the uterus), cyclic estrogen and progesterone fluctuations stimulate the ectopic endometrial tissue to grow, become secretory, and bleed, inflaming adjacent tissue and releasing prostaglandins. As a result, abdominal pain, adhesions, and fibrosis occur.

Endometriosis affects about 25% of all women and up to 40% of infertile women. It most often occurs in women ages 30 to 40 who have delayed childbearing (Garner and Webster, 1985). The disorder is familial.

Nursing care

The client with a menstrual disorder may be deeply concerned about the normalcy of her symptoms. The nurse can help such a client by using the nursing process to assess her symptoms; evaluate their impact on her job performance, sexuality, relationships, self-esteem, and other aspects of her life; and intervene appropriately.

Assessment

To obtain a complete picture of the client's health, perform a thorough health history and physical assessment and review the results of appropriate diagnostic studies.

Health history. Assess the client's reason for seeking care and her menstrual and sexual history. Also evaluate her support systems, responsibilities at home and on the job, current stressors, and usual nutrition and exercise patterns. (For more information, see Chapter 7, Women's Health Promotion.)

Obtain more detailed information, depending on the client's reason for seeking care. For a client with amenorrhea, for example, carefully evaluate her for use of medications, increased stress levels, recent weight loss or athletic training, or such signs of menopause as hot flashes. Also inquire about galactorrhea (flow of breast milk unrelated to lactation)—a sign of pituitary tumor, which could cause amenorrhea.

If the client reports dysmenorrhea, determine its onset, duration, and severity; its effect on her daily activities; the presence of other symptoms; and the type and effectiveness of her current pain management techniques. This information aids in diagnosis of the cause of dysmenorrhea and directs client teaching about medications.

Ask a client with PMS to describe her symptoms in detail, and determine their onset, duration, and severity. Inquire about the client's diet, stress level, sodium intake, use of medications and vitamins, and the effect of PMS on her activities and relationships. PMS has been linked to sodium and caffeine intake, high stress, and other life-style factors.

Because no tests can detect hormone alterations related to PMS, identification of this disorder relies on a menstrual record (Servino and Moline, 1989). Instruct the client to create a chart on which she records her symptoms in relation to her menstrual cycle each day for 2 or 3 cycles. The first day of the chart should correspond to the first day of her menstrual cycle. (For more information, see *Menstrual record for PMS*, page 300.)

During the follow-up visit, review the client's menstrual record. If symptoms occur in the luteal phase and resolve after menses begins, the client probably has PMS. If symptoms occur throughout the cycle, she may have another disorder. If she has a psychological problem, such as depression, refer her to a mental health professional for evaluation.

In a client with mittelschmerz, determine the amount of bleeding, if any, and the severity and timing of the pain in relation to her menstrual cycle. This information aids in diagnosis and directs client teaching. Pain that occurs in the middle of the client's menstrual cycle suggests a normal, physiologic cause.

If a client has metrorrhagia, evaluate the timing and amount of bleeding in relation to her usual cycle. Inquire about accompanying symptoms, such as cramping and vaginal discharge, use of medications, and presence of hot flashes. This information assists in making a definitive diagnosis.

When the client's symptoms suggest endometriosis, evaluate the onset and quality of pain, associated symptoms (such as pain during bowel movements or intercourse), and attempts to achieve pregnancy. Although increasingly intense pelvic pain suggests endometriosis, the symptom also may result from other gynecologic disorders, such as PID, ectopic pregnancy, ovarian cysts, or ovarian cancer.

Physical assessment. Perform a complete physical assessment, including breast inspection and palpation and assist with a pelvic examination. (For more information and procedures, see Chapter 7, Women's Health Promotion.) During the physical assessment, particularly note findings related to the client's reason for seeking care.

In a client with amenorrhea, the pelvic examination may reveal ovarian cysts. Observation may detect a lack of secondary sex characteristics—suggesting a hypothalamus or pituitary problem, chromosomal defects, lack of gonadal development, or congenital defects of the reproductive tract—or may reveal facial hair and obesity—indicating excessive androgen production. On breast palpation, galactorrhea may indicate a pituitary tumor.

In a client with primary dysmenorrhea, the pelvic examination commonly reveals no abnormalities. In a client with secondary dysmenorrhea, examination may reveal signs of ovarian cysts or endometriosis, such as tenderness when the sites are palpated.

In a client with PMS, a physical and pelvic examination may detect such gynecologic problems as ovarian cysts, which may cause symptoms of hormonal imbalances. However, the absence of abnormalities does not rule out PMS.

CLIENT TEACHING

Menstrual record for PMS

Premenstrual syndrome (PMS) causes many symptoms that resemble those of other disorders. To help your doctor or nurse practitioner make an accurate diagnosis and create an effective treatment plan, keep a record of your PMS symptoms. On the days your symptoms occur, fill in the boxes on the chart below, grading the severity of your symptoms and the amount of menstrual blood flow as shown. Day 1 of the cycle is the first day of your menstrual period.

DATE																												
DAY OF CYCLE	1	2	3	4	5	6	7	8	9	10	11	12	13	14	15	16	17	18	19	20	21	22	23	24	25	26	27	28

MENSTRUAL FLOW

BODY WEIGHT (LB)

WEIGHT GAIN OR LOSS

SYMPTOMS

- Nervous tension
- Mood swings
- Irritability, anger
- Anxiety
- Headache
- Increased appetite, food cravings

- Rapid heartbeat
- Fatigue, sluggishness
- Dizziness, faintness, or shakiness
- Depression, sadness
- Forgetfulness
- Crying spells

- Confusion
- Insomnia, sleep problems
- Arm or leg swelling
- Skin eruptions
- Breast tenderness or discomfort
- Abdominal bloating

- Lower abdominal cramps
- Backache
- General aches and pains
- Altered sex drive
- Clumsiness
- Desire to avoid people

Symptoms:

☐ none

◻ mild; symptoms exist but do not interfere with activities

◪ moderate; symptoms interfere with activities but are not disabling

◼ severe; symptoms are disabling

Menstrual blood flow:

◯ none

⦰ slight

◑ moderate

● heavy

◕ heavy with clots

This teaching aid may be reproduced by office copier for distribution to clients. © 1991, Springhouse Corporation.

In a client with mittelschmerz, a pelvic examination will reveal ovarian tenderness at midcycle but no abnormalities. In a client with metrorrhagia, examination may reveal signs of ovarian cysts, uterine fibroids, or other abnormalities (such as an enlarged uterus) when the sites are palpated.

During the pelvic examination, a client with endometriosis may display nodules on the uterosacral ligaments, ovarian enlargement and tenderness, and a fixed, retroverted uterus (because of adhesions from endometriosis) that can be palpated.

Diagnostic studies. For a client with amenorrhea, diagnostic tests should include a serum pregnancy test and an assay of thyroid-stimulating hormone (TSH) and prolactin levels. If premature ovarian failure is suspected, tests may be ordered to evaluate dehydroepiandrosterone (DHEA), testosterone, FSH, and LH levels.

If the prolactin and TSH levels are normal, a progesterone challenge test typically will be performed to determine the presence of sufficient estrogen to stimulate the endometrium. The physician may prescribe 100 to 200 mg of progesterone in oil intramuscularly or progesterone, 100 mg in the morning and 200 mg at bedtime for 10 days. If menstrual bleeding occurs within 2 weeks of progesterone therapy, the endometrium is functional and amenorrhea is caused by anovulation. If bleeding does not occur, the physician may prescribe oral estrogen (Premarin) and progesterone. Absence of menses after this second hormone administration indicates an endometrial problem; menses indicates a problem with the ovaries or hypothalamus. FSH and LH level testing can rule out ovarian failure.

If a client with dysmenorrhea displays abnormalities during the pelvic examination, further diagnostic studies (such as ultrasonography, gonorrhea and chlamydia cultures, or laparoscopy) may be ordered to determine the cause of the pain.

For a client with suspected PMS symptoms, laboratory studies, such as a CBC (to rule out anemia or infection), TSH and T_4-level tests (to rule out an underlying thyroid disorder), and a prolactin-level test (to rule out endocrine system abnormalities), will be performed.

If mittelschmerz persists, ultrasonography may be ordered to rule out an ovarian cyst.

The cause of metrorrhagia may be investigated more fully by a CBC, serum pregnancy test, ultrasonography, and chlamydia and gonorrhea cultures. Diagnostic dilatation and curettage or endometrial sampling also may be necessary. (For more information about dilatation and curettage, see Chapter 9, Family Planning.)

Although the client's history and physical assessment data may suggest endometriosis, only direct visualization of endometrial implants can confirm the diagnosis. Through a laparoscope, endometrial implants appear as brown or blue black nodules. Adhesions also may be seen. Biopsy samples commonly will be taken during laparoscopy.

Nursing diagnosis
After considering all assessment findings, formulate appropriate nursing diagnoses. (For a partial list of applicable diagnoses, see *Nursing diagnoses: Gynecologic disorders,* page 291.)

Planning and implementation
Based on the client's needs, develop appropriate goals for care, as in the following examples.
• The client will describe the normal menstrual cycle and explain how diet, stress, and exercise may affect it.
• The client will discuss the causes and treatments of dysmenorrhea.
• The client will identify life-style factors that she can modify to decrease her PMS symptoms.
• The client will describe mittelschmerz as a normal variation.
• The client will discuss the cause and treatment of metrorrhagia.
• The client will make an informed decision about treatments for her endometriosis.

To meet these goals, the nurse should provide support, teach about treatments, and provide family care.

Provide support. A client with a menstrual disorder may fear that she has a serious disease, such as cancer. She may have a nursing diagnosis of *anxiety related to abnormal menstrual pattern* or *ineffective individual coping related to abnormal menstrual pattern.* To help such a client, provide support. Reassure her that many so-called abnormalities are actually normal variations that life-style changes may help correct. Express confidence that testing will detect true abnormalities, which can be managed with appropriate treatment.

Offer information about normal menstrual cycle physiology and how various factors, such as diet and exercise, can affect it. Review her menstrual history to help her understand what is normal for her body. These actions may help reduce anxiety as well as address a nursing diagnosis of *knowledge deficit related to normal menstrual cycle physiology.*

Teach about treatments. Inform the client with irregular menstrual cycles to keep a menstrual chart, noting menses, spotting, and any symptoms of life-style decisions (such as excessive exercise, extreme weight loss, excessive stress, and unbalanced or insufficient nutrition) that may affect menstruation and cause amenorrhea.

The client with dysmenorrhea may have a nursing diagnosis of *pain related to menstruation,* which may be relieved through use of nonsteroidal anti-inflammatory drugs (NSAIDs). If so, advise her to take them, as prescribed, at the onset of cramping. These drugs may decrease menstrual flow and are contraindicated in clients with a history of ulcers, aspirin allergies, kidney or liver disease, or anemia. Teach the client about possible adverse reactions to NSAIDs, including GI irritation, dizziness, headache, nervousness, and fluid retention, and instruct her to report them to the physician, nurse practitioner, or nurse-midwife if they occur.

Teach about nonpharmacologic remedies for dysmenorrhea, including a well-balanced diet, heat application, regular exercise, stress management techniques, and frequent rest.

A client with PMS may have a nursing diagnosis of *ineffective individual coping related to mood swings* or *anxiety related to PMS management.* For this client, validate the legitimacy of PMS and involve her in planning treatment.

No single treatment relieves all PMS symptoms. Therefore, individualize treatment based on the client's personal situation and symptoms. Keye (1988) advocates a biopsychosocial (medical, psychological, and social support) approach. The most important components are client and family education, fear elimination, coping, life-style changes, and intervention with medication. As needed, teach the client about pharmacologic and nonpharmacologic treatments. (For more information, see *Client teaching: Managing PMS.*)

For the client with metrorrhagia, teach her to chart her periods, noting the amount of bleeding that occurs. If diagnostic tests are ordered, teach the client about them.

Reassure the client with mittelschmerz that her condition is a normal occurrence, not a disease.

Treatment for endometriosis depends on the client's age, desire for fertility, presence of adhesions, severity of symptoms, and interference with life-style. Teach her about the treatment that is appropriate for her. For example, if she will be treated with danazol, inform her about possible adverse reactions, including acne, weight gain, edema, hot flashes, spotting, and decreased breast size. Instruct her to contact her physician immediately if any of these reactions occur. Clients usually report fewer adverse reactions with GnRH agonist than danazol, making a nursing diagnosis of *body image disturbance related to androgenic effects of hormones* less likely.

CLIENT TEACHING

Managing PMS

By changing a few of your habits, you may reduce the severity and frequency of premenstrual syndrome (PMS) symptoms. Try the following changes. However, before taking vitamins, minerals, or other supplements, check with your doctor. Some doctors may advise that you take some or all of the vitamins, minerals, or other supplements listed below. No one can guarantee that these will help relieve the severity of PMS symptoms.

DIET

- Consume less refined sugar, red meat, alcohol, and caffeine.
- Eat more complex carbohydrates, such as legumes, whole grains, and cereals.
- For the 2 weeks before your menstrual period, eat small, frequent meals (five or six a day) to prevent low blood sugar.
- Limit your salt (sodium) intake for 2 weeks before your menstrual period.

VITAMIN, MINERAL, AND OTHER SUPPLEMENTS

- Take low doses of vitamin B_6, also called pyridoxine (up to 50 mg daily). High doses may be harmful.
- Limit vitamin E to 400 IU daily.
- Take magnesium supplements (up to 250 mg daily).
- Take the B vitamins together, as in a B-complex formula.

EXERCISE

- Do aerobic exercise (walk briskly, jog, bicycle, or swim) three times a week for at least 20 minutes.

STRESS MANAGEMENT

- Use relaxation techniques, such as progressive muscle relaxation and meditation, as needed.
- Limit your responsibilities for 2 weeks before your menstrual period, if possible.
- Rely on your family, friends, and others for support.
- Learn to delegate tasks and responsibilities.

OTHER

- Take medications as prescribed by your doctor.

Provide family care. Because a menstrual disorder can affect the client's body image, self-esteem, sexuality, and relationships, it can affect family members too. To address their needs, provide information about the disorder and its diagnosis, effects, and treatments. Assess family members' coping methods, reinforcing effective ones and

NURSING RESEARCH APPLIED

Coping responses of men whose partners have PMS

Although premenstrual syndrome (PMS) has been associated with divorce, child abuse, and alcoholism, little research has been done on the way PMS symptoms affect relationships and family functioning. A recent study interviewed 86 couples about the woman's PMS symptoms and her partner's coping strategies. Couples were divided into high- and low-symptom groups based on the intensity of the woman's symptoms. Both groups had similar demographics. However, couples in the low-symptom group had fewer children and were better educated.

Analysis revealed that partners used various coping responses. Men in the high-symptom group learned more about PMS and sought help with their partner more often than those in the low-symptom group. This led the researchers to conclude that men's coping responses were related to the severity of their partners' PMS symptoms. Some of the most common coping responses included, "I told myself that she can't help it, tried to learn more information about symptoms, went went with her to seek help, got angry at her, became afraid, and took on more household tasks."

Application to practice
The nurse must be aware that PMS symptoms clearly extend beyond the client, affecting family relationships. Nursing intervention must focus on the couple, providing men with information and counseling to help them develop positive coping strategies.

Cortese, J., and Brown, M. (1989). Coping responses of men whose partners experience premenstrual symptomatology. *JOGNN*, 18(5), 405-412.

suggesting additional ones. (For more information, see *Nursing research applied: Coping responses of men whose partners have PMS.*)

Evaluation
After implementing the plan of care, assess its effectiveness in reaching client goals. State evaluation findings in terms of actions performed or outcomes achieved for each goal. The following examples illustrate some appropriate evaluation statements.
• The client with amenorrhea reported decreased anxiety about her menstrual cycle changes related to lifestyle factors.
• The client with dysmenorrhea reported decreased school absences related to pain.
• The client with PMS reported increased self-esteem and decreased symptoms.
• The client with mittelschmerz recognized her problem as normal and relieved her pain with aspirin.

• The client with metrorrhagia correctly described her treatment plan and scheduled tests.
• The client with endometriosis reported decreased pain and minimal adverse reactions to the medication.

Documentation
Although each facility requires documentation of slightly different information, most require the nurse to record the following:
• reason that the client seeks care
• client's menstrual history
• results of diagnostic studies
• plan for follow-up care
• client teaching performed by the nurse.

Pelvic support disorders

Childbirth, pelvic trauma, stress, strain, and aging may weaken pelvic structures. This weakening may cause pelvic support disorders, including cystocele, rectocele, and uterine prolapse. (For information on clinical findings, treatments, and nursing considerations, see *Common pelvic support disorders,* page 304.)

Cystocele occurs when the posterior bladder wall prolapses (descends, protrudes, or projects) through a weakness in the upper anterior vaginal wall. It can range from small to large, producing minor symptoms or major discomfort. Cystocele may result from a congenital weakness or from laceration and excessive stretching of pelvic support tissue after prolonged labor or vaginal delivery of a large neonate. After menopause, atrophy of pelvic support tissue linked to decreased estrogen may produce this condition. Most parous women have a small, asymptomatic cystocele.

Rectocele, marked by a prominent bulging of the posterior vaginal wall, results from trauma to the fascia and levator ani muscles supporting part of the lower bowel—as when descent of the neonate's head during delivery weakens the rectovaginal septum. Heavy lifting, straining at stool, and pregnancy can aggravate this condition.

Most common in obese, multiparous, middle-aged women, uterine prolapse occurs when the uterus descends into the vagina. It may result from obstetric trauma to the pelvic ligaments, a postmenopausal weakening of the supporting pelvic muscles that is linked to decreased estrogen, or an abdominal mass or ascites that exerts pressure on the weakened muscles.

Common pelvic support disorders

Pelvic support disorders (cystocele, rectocele, and uterine prolapse) are relatively common in middle-aged and older clients and may coexist. To provide the best possible care, the nurse should be familiar with these disorders as well as their treatments and nursing considerations, as described below.

Cystocele

Description
Normally, pelvic muscles and connective tissue support the vagina, uterus, bladder, and rectum. In cystocele, however, the bladder protrudes through a weakness in the vaginal wall.

Clinical findings
The client with cystocele may complain of pelvic fullness, a bearing down sensation, backache, urinary frequency or urgency, incomplete bladder emptying, and urinary stress incontinence. Symptoms commonly worsen after prolonged standing.
The pelvic examination typically reveals a soft, bulging mass at the vaginal opening, which increases when the client bears down. A urine culture rules out infection.

Treatment
Treatment depends on the client's age, sexual activity, desire to bear children, and degree of prolapse.
For mild cystocele, Kegel exercises can increase pelvic muscle tone. In postmenopausal women, hormone replacement therapy (HRT) may decrease genitourinary atrophy and improve pelvic tone. (For more information, see Chapter 7, Women's Health Promotion.)
For an older client in whom surgery is contraindicated or for a client who is pregnant or has not completed childbearing, severe cystocele treatment may include inserting a pessary (device used to support pelvic structures) into the vagina. A pessary requires positioning the uterus and cervix in their usual locations in the pelvis; the perineum must be capable of holding the pessary in place. Pessaries are available in various sizes and shapes and should be fitted to the client.
Various surgical procedures can help a client who has completed childbearing and has significant pelvic relaxation. The most common is the anterior colporrhaphy (suturing of the pubocervical fascia to support the bladder and urethra). If a rectocele coexists, a posterior colporrhaphy (suturing of the fascia and perineal muscles in the midline to support the perineum and rectum) or anterior-posterior colporrhaphy is performed.

Nursing considerations
• Reassure the client that cystocele is a common, benign disorder.
• Teach the client Kegel exercises.
• Teach the client about HRT.
• Advise the client with a pessary that a nurse practitioner or physician must change it periodically and inspect the tissues for infection and ulceration.
• Teach about surgery, if indicated.

Rectocele

Description
In rectocele, the rectum protrudes into the vagina.

Clinical findings
The client may report fullness and pressure in the vagina, constipation, rectal fullness, and painful defecation. The pelvic examination reveals bulging of the posterior vaginal wall at the introitus.

Treatment
As with mild cystocele, Kegel exercises and HRT may increase pelvic tone and muscular support in a client with mild rectocele. A diet rich in fiber and fluids will help prevent constipation; stool softeners can prevent straining at defecation.

Nursing considerations
• Reassure the client that rectocele is a common, benign disorder.
• Teach the client Kegel exercises.
• Teach the client about HRT.
• Advise the client to increase her intake of high-fiber foods and water.
• Instruct the client to take stool softeners, as prescribed.
• Teach about surgery, if indicated.

Uterine prolapse

Description
In uterine prolapse, the uterus descends below its normal position in the pelvis. In first-degree prolapse, the uterus descends until the cervix appears at the vaginal opening; in second-degree prolapse, until the cervix protrudes through the vaginal opening; in third-degree prolapse (a rare condition), until the entire uterus is outside the vagina.

Clinical findings
The client may report feelings of heaviness, fullness, or "falling out" in the perineal area. She also may have a bearing-down sensation in the lower abdomen, dyspareunia (painful intercourse), urinary urgency and frequency, and low backache. The pelvic examination reveals that the uterus has descended into or outside the vagina.

Treatment
For first-degree prolapse, treatment is the same as that for cystocele and rectocele. For second- and third-degree prolapse, treatment may include anterior and posterior colporrhaphies and vaginal hysterectomy.
For older clients, surgery such as the Manchester-Forthgill operation (which combines an anterior and posterior colporrhaphy with cervical amputation and suturing of the cardinal ligaments) or Le Fort's operation (suturing the anterior and posterior vaginal walls to support the uterus) may be necessary.

Nursing considerations
• Same as for cystocele and rectocele.
• Teach about surgery, if indicated. Remember that certain procedures, such as Le Fort's partial colpocleisis, should be performed only on older clients with severe uterine prolapse.

Gynecologic cancer

Gynecologic cancer may affect the ovaries, fallopian tubes, endometrium, cervix, vagina, or vulva. Its chief warning signs are a change in bowel and bladder habits, unusual bleeding or discharge, and a thickening or lump. (For more information, see *Understanding gynecologic cancers*, pages 306 to 308.)

Ovarian cancer

This type of gynecologic cancer typically takes the form of epithelial, stromal, or germ cell carcinoma. Although its cause is unknown, risk factors for developing ovarian cancer have been identified. Factors that place a woman at high risk include nulliparity, a history of breast cancer, or exposure to high levels of environmental radiation or asbestos. Factors that place a woman at low risk include the use of an oral contraceptive (National Cancer Institute, 1987b; Pernoll and Benson, 1987).

Fallopian tube cancer

Adenocarcinoma represents the most common type of fallopian tube cancer. Nulliparous women are at highest risk for this disease (Pernoll and Benson, 1987).

Endometrial cancer

Almost all endometrial cancers are adenocarcinomas. Although the exact cause is unknown, unopposed estrogen stimulation of the endometrium, caused by postmenopausal estrogen therapy or other hormone treatments, is implicated.

The risk of endometrial cancer decreases with use of oral contraceptives that contain estrogen and progesterone. Risk increases with obesity, diabetes, infertility, and late menopause (National Cancer Institute, 1987a; Pernoll and Benson, 1987).

Cervical cancer

Most cervical cancers are squamous cell carcinomas. In many cases, they occur in women with a history of sexually transmitted diseases (STDs). They also commonly appear in those with the sexually transmitted human papilloma virus (HPV) infection, which produces cervical dysplasia (abnormal tissue development) that later may develop into cervical cancer (McQuiston, 1989).

Factors that increase the risk of developing cervical cancer include sexual intercourse before age 18, multiple sexual partners, a mother who took diethylstilbestrol (DES) while pregnant, smoking, and oral contraceptive use. Factors that decrease the risk include menopausal estrogen therapy, nulliparity, and use of a barrier method of contraception (Fullerton and Barger, 1989; Mandelblatt, 1989; McQuiston, 1989; National Cancer Institute, 1987a).

Vaginal cancer

Almost all vaginal cancers are epidermoid. The remainder are adenocarcinomas, sarcomas, or melanomas. Young women whose mothers took DES during pregnancy have an increased incidence of an unusual type of vaginal cancer called clear cell vaginal adenocarcinoma (Pernoll and Benson, 1987; Rubin, 1987).

Vulvar cancer

The most common vulvar cancer is squamous cell carcinoma, which arises from the epithelium of the vulvar mucosa. Less commonly, malignant tumors may arise from the urethral mucosa or glands associated with the vulva, such as the Skene's or Bartholin's gland.

Several disorders commonly accompany vulvar cancer, including obesity, hypertension, and chronic vulvar irritation secondary to diabetes mellitus, granuloma inguinale, or vulvar dystrophy. Also, herpes simplex virus or HPV infections correlate with an increased incidence of vulvar cancer in situ.

Vulvar cancer accounts for 3% to 5% of female genital carcinoma. The average age of affected women is 62. Risk factors are diabetic vulvitis and cervical cancer (Pernoll and Benson, 1987; Rubin, 1987).

Nursing care

The nurse who cares for a client with gynecologic cancer must consider the physical and psychological effects of the disorder as well as the effects of treatment, especially on the client's body image and sexuality.

A client's psychological response to gynecologic cancer depends on the functions she attributes to her reproductive organs and on her prognosis. The nurse must teach the client about her disease, treatment, and recovery process and must address her concerns about menstrual functioning, sexual and reproductive capacity, and physical condition, while supporting her as she grieves over her losses.

To provide the best care to a client with gynecologic cancer, the nurse should employ the nursing process.

(Text continues on page 308.)

Understanding gynecologic cancers

Gynecologic cancers include ovarian, fallopian tube, endometrial, cervical, vaginal, and vulvar. The nurse should be familiar with the clinical findings, diagnostic tests, staging, and treatments of these disorders, as described in the chart below.

Ovarian cancer

Clinical findings
• Usually asymptomatic
• Vague symptoms, such as intestinal upset or shoulder pain (referred pain)
• Abdominal swelling or bloating, lower abdominal discomfort, sensation of fullness, anorexia, urinary frequency, or constipation (as neoplasm increases in size)
• Flatulence, indigestion, nausea, and weight loss

Diagnostic tests
• Blood and urine tests, ultrasonography, X-rays including computed tomography (CT) scan, lymphangiography, intravenous pyelography (IVP), and barium enema (to check for metastasis)
• Laparoscopy or laparotomy to visualize the ovary and surrounding organs and tissues to confirm a diagnosis or obtain fluid and tissue samples by pelvic washing for analysis

Staging
• Stage I: cancer confined to the ovaries
• Stage II: cancer in one or both ovaries with extension to the uterus, fallopian tubes, or other pelvic tissues
• Stage III: cancer in one or both ovaries with extension to the abdominal lymph nodes or outer surface of other abdominal organs, such as the liver or intestines
• Stage IV: cancer in one or both ovaries with extension to the inside of the liver or other abdominal organs or to organs outside the abdomen (National Cancer Institute, 1989)

Treatments
• For Stage I, removal of only the affected ovary and fallopian tube if the client wishes to remain fertile and the cancer resides in an intact capsule and is limited to one ovary.

All other Stage I clients undergo total abdominal hysterectomy (removal of the uterus) and bilateral salpingo-oophorectomy (removal of the fallopian tubes and ovaries) with or without a partial omentectomy (removal of the peritoneum). If the capsule surrounding the cancer has ruptured, ascites is present, or pelvic washings find cancer cells, chemotherapy (usually cisplatin and cyclophosphamide) or intraperitoneal P32 radiation therapy follows surgery.
• For Stage II, total abdominal hysterectomy and bilateral salpingo-oophorectomy. Residual disease is treated with internal or external radiation therapy or combination chemotherapy with cisplatin as a base (National Cancer Institute, 1989).
• For Stages III and IV, abdominal hysterectomy and bilateral salpingo-oophorectomy followed by combination chemotherapy.
• Recurrent ovarian cancer may be treated with more surgery, new drugs, or new drug combinations as they are approved for use.
• "Second-look" laparotomy (including inspection of abdomen, pelvic and abdominal washings, and biopsies of abnormal areas) may follow chemotherapy to assess the degree of response. The laparotomy determines subsequent treatments and allows surgical removal of any remaining cancer. "Second-look" surgery after radiation therapy is not widely accepted because of possible surgical complications, such as tissue damage, in clients who have been treated with radiation.

Fallopian tube cancer

Clinical findings
• No specific classic signs or symptoms
• Postmenopausal bleeding
• Latzko's sign (intermittent serosanguineous discharge accompanied by colicky lower abdominal pain), suggesting occasional fallopian tube dilation and subsequent fluid discharge through the uterus
• Abdominal enlargement and intestinal obstruction (late manifestations)

Diagnostic tests
• Papanicolaou (Pap) test
• Ultrasonography to detect a semicystic mass in the adnexal region
• Preoperative chest X-ray and barium enema to check for metastases
• Exploratory surgery to confirm diagnosis

Staging
• Stage I: carcinoma confined to one or both fallopian tubes, with or without ascites
• Stage II cancer extension to the uterus, ovaries, or other intraperitoneal organs or tissues in the true pelvis
• Stage III: cancer extension to the uterus or ovaries and other intraperitoneal organs and tissues beyond the true pelvis
• Stage IV: metastasis to organs or tissues outside the peritoneal cavity (Jones, Wentz, and Burnett, 1988)

Treatments
• Total abdominal hysterectomy and bilateral salpingo-oophorectomy (primary treatment)
• Postoperative external or internal radiation therapy
• Intraperitoneal instillation of radioactive chromic phosphate (for early cases without microscopic residual neoplasms)

Understanding gynecologic cancers continued

Endometrial cancer

Clinical findings
• Abnormal vaginal bleeding after menopause (most common symptom)

Diagnostic tests
• Endometrial biopsy, dilatation and curettage (D&C), or both to diagnose cancer
• Blood tests, X-rays, endoscopy, CT scan, and ultrasonography to determine if cancer has metastasized

Staging
• Stage 0: carcinoma in situ (confined to surface epithelium)
• Stage I: cancer confined to uterine corpus
• Stage II: cancer of corpus and cervix, but no extension beyond uterus

• Stage III: cancer extension beyond the uterus, but not outside the pelvis
• Stage IV: cancer extension beyond the pelvis or within the bladder or rectum (National Cancer Institute, 1987a)

Treatments
• Abdominal hysterectomy with bilateral salpingo-oophorectomy
• External or internal radiation therapy as a primary or postoperative treatment
• Hormone therapy with synthetic progesterone, such as hydroxyprogesterone (Delalutin), medroxyprogesterone (Provera), and megestrol (Megace), for recurrent endometrial cancer not amenable to surgery or radiation therapy
• Chemotherapy (being tested)

Cervical cancer

Clinical findings
• Usually asymptomatic
• Abnormal vaginal bleeding and increased vaginal discharge

Diagnostic tests
• Inspection during pelvic examination to detect visible irregularities
• Pap test to detect irregular cellular structure
• Colposcopy, Schiller's test, cervical conization, or D&C to diagnose cancer
• IVP, complete blood count, barium enema, cystoscopy, lymphangiography, bone scan, or proctoscopy to determine the extent of cancer, if found

Staging
• Stage 0: carcinoma in situ
• Stage I: cancer confined to cervix
• Stage II: cancer extension beyond cervix, but not to pelvic wall
• Stage III: cancer extension to pelvic wall

• Stage IV: cancer extension beyond pelvis or within the bladder or rectum (National Cancer Institute, 1987a)

Treatments
• For Stage 0, cryosurgery, cauterization, or surgical conization for a client who wishes to remain fertile; hysterectomy for a client who does not wish to remain fertile
• For Stage I, radiation therapy or hysterectomy. A younger client may prefer surgery to save her ability to produce ovarian hormones. An older client may prefer a combination of internal and external radiation.
• For Stage II, radical hysterectomy or internal or external radiation therapy
• For Stage III, radiation therapy
• For Stage IV, various treatments, which may include pelvic exenteration (removal of all pelvic organs, lymph nodes, and peritoneum)
• Chemotherapy if cancer has spread extensively or reappears after initial treatment with surgery or radiation
• Chemotherapy as an adjuvant to radiation therapy for Stages III and IV (experimental)

Vaginal cancer

Clinical findings
• Usually asymptomatic
• Painless bleeding after sexual intercourse or vaginal examination
• Increased vaginal discharge and vulvar pruritus, dyspareunia
• Leg pain or edema, urinary frequency, or painful defecation (as disease develops)

Diagnostic tests
• Pap test to detect early signs of cancer
• Complete inspection of the vagina, with colposcopy, staining with Lugol's solution, Schiller's test, and biopsy

Staging
• Stage 0: cancer in situ
• Stage I: cancer confined to the vaginal wall

• Stage II: cancer extension to the subvaginal tissue, but not the pelvic wall
• Stage III: cancer extension to the pelvic wall
• Stage IV: cancer extension beyond the true pelvis to the mucosa of the bladder, rectum, or distant organs (Pernoll and Benson, 1987)

Treatments
• For Stage 0, laser surgery, radiation therapy, or intravaginal application of antineoplastic fluorouracil cream
• For Stages I or II, radical hysterectomy and removal of the upper vagina
• For Stage III, internal and external radiation therapy
• For Stage IV, pelvic exenteration

(continued)

Understanding gynecologic cancers continued

Vulvar cancer

Clinical findings
• Vulvar irritation with pruritus, localized discomfort, and possible discharge
• Early lesions similar to chronic vulvar dermatitis (most common sign)
• Late lesions that may appear as a lump in the labia, a large cauliflower-like growth, or a hard ulcerated area in the vulva
• Bloody discharge from lesion caused by necrosis, infection, and ulceration

Diagnostic tests
• Biopsy and histologic evaluation of lesions to differentiate between sexually transmitted diseases (syphilis, chancroid, or granuloma inguinale), basal cell carcinoma, squamous cell carcinoma in situ, and other conditions of the vulva
• Colposcopy and palpation of the primary lesion, urethra, vaginal mucosa, cervix, rectum, and inguinal lymph nodes to determine the extent of the lesion
• Chest X-ray, complete blood count, IVP, urinalysis, bone scan, or CT scan to detect metastatis

Staging
• Stage 0: cancer in situ, intraepithelial carcinoma
• Stage I: cancer (malignant neoplasm 2 cm or less in diameter) confined to the vulva with nodes that are not palpable or clinically suspicious of cancer
• Stage II: cancer (malignant neoplasm larger than 2 cm in diameter) confined to the vulva with nodes that are not palpable or clinically suspicious of cancer
• Stage III: cancer (malignant neoplasm of any size) with extension to the urethra, vagina, perineum, and anus, with nodes that are palpable and clinically suspicious in one or both inguinal areas
• Stage IV: cancer (malignant neoplasm of any size) with extension to the bladder mucosa, rectal mucosa, or both, with metastasis to the bone or to another distant point, and with fixed, ulcerated malignant neoplasms noted in one or both inguinal areas (Jones, Wentz, and Burnett, 1988).

Treatments
• For squamous cell carcinoma, wide excision of the neoplasm and removal of potential routes of metastasis. To reduce the incidence of infection, bowel cleansing with an antibiotic, especially if the perineal skin is ulcerated.
• For carcinoma in situ, removal of circumscribed lesions by wide local excisions. For multifocal and superficial lesions, vulvar skin removal and replacement by skin grafts. For extensive and diffuse hypertrophic disease, total vulvectomy.
• For extensive squamous cell carcinoma, radical vulvectomy and lymphadenectomy.
• For inoperable or locally recurrent lesions, internal radiation therapy.
• For small lesions of basal cell carcinoma, local excision. For more extensive lesions, deep and wide resection. Lymphadenectomy only if squamous cells are identified.

Assessment

Gather baseline data by obtaining a health history, performing a physical assessment, and reviewing the results of diagnostic studies. (For more information and procedures, see Chapter 7, Women's Health Promotion.)

Health history. Throughout the initial health history, note any risk factors for gynecologic cancer, including intercourse before age 18, multiple sexual partners, childbearing before age 16, STDs, and HPV infection (Fullerton and Barger, 1989; Mandelblatt, 1989; National Cancer Institute, 1987b).

Determine the client's reason for seeking health care and ask her to describe any changes in her vulva, vagina, or perineum. Have her describe any current or periodic pain. Assess her dietary habits and bowel and urinary patterns, noting any recent changes.

Assess her menstrual, contraceptive, and obstetric history. Also inquire about her sexuality patterns.

Evaluate the client's perception of her identity, abilities, body image, and self-worth. Her illness may affect her self-image.

Have the client describe her goals. Her philosophical, religious, and spiritual beliefs also may affect her care decisions.

Ask the client how she learns best (for example, whether she prefers to read or watch videos), and assess her for physical, psychosocial, cognitive, or developmental disabilities. Identify any difficulties she may have in communicating her thoughts and feelings. This information should help in planning effective client teaching sessions.

After a client receives a diagnosis of gynecologic cancer, assess her further. Ask if she understands her disease, the proposed treatment, and its probable effects. Review the information her physician has provided, and correct any misconceptions. Support the client with additional information she may need to cope.

Ask the client to describe the effect of her illness and treatment on her daily activities and on her ability to care for herself. If her daily activities have been altered, formulate strategies for meeting her needs when she returns home.

Investigate the client's perception of her energy levels and ability to relax and sleep. If she has difficulties in these areas, discuss ways to facilitate rest.

Determine her perception of her disease and any proposed treatments or surgery. Discuss her concerns about hospitalization and any anxiety about testing, surgery, and other treatments. Also assess for previous depression and investigate her perception of her stress level.

When a treatment is proposed, assess her understanding of it and its effects on her hormone status and sexuality. Discuss any fears she may have about losing attractiveness or femininity after surgery. Determine her level of satisfaction with her sexual partner if she has one, and discuss any sexual problems that her disease or treatment may cause.

Physical assessment. Perform a complete physical assessment, including assisting with a pelvic examination and bimanual palpation. (For procedures, see Chapter 7, Women's Health Promotion.)

Many physical assessment findings help confirm a diagnosis of gynecologic cancer. For example, visual inspection of the cervix through a speculum may reveal structural irregularities that suggest cervical cancer. Palpable fixed ovaries may signal ovarian cancer. Hard, ulcerated vulvar lesions may indicate vulvar cancer. On bimanual palpation, a slightly tender pelvic mass separate from the uterus and ovaries may indicate fallopian tube cancer, PID, or endometriosis.

Diagnostic studies. Review the results of laboratory tests and other diagnostic studies.

Papanicolaou (Pap) test. A common screening test for gynecologic cancer, the Pap test detects cervical cancer. Normal findings for the Pap test are Class I, indicating the absence of abnormal cells. Abnormal findings may be Class II (atypical, but nonmalignant cells present), Class III (dysplasia, a cell abnormality), Class IV (suggestive of, but inconclusive for, cancer), or Class V (conclusive for cancer).

However, this numerical grading system is gradually being superseded by one in which abnormal findings are described. An abnormal Pap test requires further testing. A colposcopy and biopsy must be performed before any definitive diagnosis or treatment plan can be formulated.

Although Pap tests are widely used, ineffective sampling techniques and difficulties in interpretation give Pap tests a false-negative rate of 10% to 20%.

Schiller's test. Although this test is not specific for any cancer, it can identify cervical lesions that need to be biopsied. During this test, the examiner applies an aqueous iodine solution to the cervix. The iodine stains the normal epithelium a deep brown, but does not stain abnormal epithelium.

Colposcopy. A diagnostic tool for comprehensive examination of the cervix and vagina, colposcopy is more accurate and more commonly used than Schiller's test. Performed in an outpatient setting by a physician or specially prepared nurse practitioner, colposcopy identifies atypical areas, which then can be biopsied.

A binocular microscope, the colposcope magnifies the cervix and its critical transformation zone in which metaplasia may have changed columnar epithelium to squamous epithelium. Most dysplasias and cancers originate in this area.

Through the colposcope, the examiner evaluates the cervix for surface pattern, clarity, demarcation, vascular pattern, color, tone, and opacity. If colposcopy reveals abnormal findings in the transformation zone, the examiner performs a punch biopsy and endocervical curettage (ECC) to obtain tissue samples for further testing.

Cervical conization. Also known as cone biopsy, cervical conization removes a cone-shaped portion of the cervix for diagnostic or therapeutic purposes. Although diagnostic cervical conization has been replaced by colposcopy in most cases, it may be used when colposcopy does not disclose the entire transformation zone, when the ECC is positive (indicating that dysplasia has extended upward), or when significant discrepancy exists between the Pap test and the biopsy. It also may be used to treat microinvasive squamous cell carcinoma.

Nursing diagnosis

Based on the assessment information, formulate appropriate nursing diagnoses. Each client will have individualized needs that may change throughout the treatment. (For a partial list of possible nursing diagnoses, see *Nursing diagnoses: Gynecologic disorders,* page 291.)

Planning and implementation

When developing a care plan, include the client and her family but keep in mind that the degree of client and family involvement may vary with different individuals and treatments. If possible, establish goals with the client. Appropriate goals may include:
• The client will cope effectively with her anxieties and discomforts during diagnostic studies.
• The client will describe the reasons for and expectations of diagnostic studies.
• The client will discuss diagnostic study results and treatment options.
• The client will begin to grieve after gynecologic cancer is confirmed.

• The client will describe proposed surgery and its expected effects on her hormone status and sexuality.
• The client will discuss common postoperative complications and methods to prevent them.
• The client will describe any special equipment she will use after surgery.
• The client will maintain optimal psychological and physical condition before, during, and after treatment.
• The client will return to optimal health after treatment.
• The client will describe her follow-up care schedule.
• The client will list symptoms of a problem or its recurrence and will discuss the importance of contacting her health care professional immediately.
• The client will describe temporary sexuality changes and will use alternative forms of sexual expression.

To help the client meet these goals, intervene by providing support and information about cancer, teaching about diagnostic tests and treatments, and providing family care.

Provide support. A diagnosis of cancer emotionally affects the client, her family, and her friends. The client may feel shame or guilt about developing the disease and putting her family through the turmoil and expense of treatment. This may cause her to feel angry, fearful, irritable, depressed, hopeless, or passive. At first, she may refuse to believe that this has happened to her; later, she may become irate, hostile, despairing, anxious, or withdrawn.

Such a client may develop a nursing diagnosis of *ineffective individual coping related to cancer.* To help her, explore her methods of coping with stress. Support existing coping skills and offer help if she cannot cope alone.

The client's family and friends also may experience trouble coping with cancer. Coworkers and friends may avoid the client out of an irrational fear of cancer, causing her to have a nursing diagnosis of *social isolation related to others' fear of cancer* or *self-esteem disturbance related to guilt about cancer.*

Isolation and guilt are especially likely to develop in a client who has heard that life-style factors can affect the risk of cancer. She may feel that she could have prevented cancer by living her life differently. Feeling guilty and isolated, she may keep her diagnosis a secret and withdraw from interactions with others. Encourage such a client to express her feelings openly, and refer her to a support group, if possible.

Provide information. As a consumer, the client has the right to seek information about her disease and participate in her health care decisions. Cancer clients who seek information about their disease gain a sense of control over it and feel better able to cope (Given and

Given, 1989). These findings underscore the importance of assessing the client's information needs and helping her establish priorities throughout her interactions within the health care system (Derdiarian, 1987).

Provide information about the client's disorder, diagnosis, tests, treatments, and prognosis. Explain diagnostic and therapeutic technical terms and jargon in words the client and her family can understand. Technical terms for equipment and procedures can produce anxiety and compromise cooperation and compliance unless the client understands what the equipment and procedures do and how they will be used. This is especially important for a client with a nursing diagnosis of *knowledge deficit related to gynecologic cancer, noncompliance related to diagnostic tests,* or *anxiety related to cancer treatments.*

Teach about diagnostic studies. Provide information about laboratory tests and other diagnostic studies, explaining the preparation, procedure, post-test care, and adverse effects that must be reported. Give the client time to ask questions, and if possible, provide written instructions for her to review at home. (For a sample, see *Client teaching: Colposcopy and biopsy.*)

Teach about treatments. To prevent a nursing diagnosis of *knowledge deficit related to cancer treatment* or *anxiety related to cancer treatment,* teach the client about proposed treatments.

Tell her that treatment depends on the stage (or extent) of the disease at diagnosis, the type of cancer cells, the rate of cancer growth, and her health and fertility concerns. Treatment for gynecologic cancer may include surgery, radiation therapy, chemotherapy, and hormone therapy.

Surgery. The primary treatment for gynecologic cancer is surgery. Because surgery causes anatomic and physiologic changes and because the client must adapt to these changes, surgery requires extensive nursing intervention. (For indications, procedures, and nursing considerations, see *Gynecologic surgery,* pages 312 and 313.)

If the biopsy reveals cervical intraepithelial neoplasia, treatments will be based on whether or not invasive cancer was found. Surgery aims to eradicate all abnormal cervical epithelium.

Conservative surgery may be used for a client who wishes to maintain her childbearing capacity. It may be cryosurgery, which destroys malignant tissue with extreme cold; cauterization, which destroys malignant tissue with extreme heat; or cervical conization. Less conservative procedures include hysterectomy (removal of the uterus), vulvectomy (removal of the vulva), radical vulvectomy (removal of the vulva, skin and fat of the

---

Colposcopy and biopsy

You have been scheduled for a colposcopy and biopsy. These tests are no more uncomfortable than a regular pelvic examination, and you should feel free to ask the doctor or nurse questions at any time. Here is some information that will help prepare you for these tests.

Colposcopy
Colposcopy is a way of viewing the cervix (the opening to the uterus) and vagina. Using a low-powered microscope called a colposcope, the doctor can examine magnified cells of the cervix and vagina and perform a biopsy (removal of a small tissue sample). A colposcopy and biopsy may be performed after an abnormal Pap test to differentiate precancerous from benign conditions, such as cervical warts.

Performed between menstrual periods, colposcopy and biopsy take about 20 minutes and are conducted in a doctor's office or clinic. During the tests, you will lie on an examination table just as you would for a pelvic examination. After inserting a speculum into your vagina, the doctor places the colposcope near the vaginal opening. Then the doctor or nurse washes your cervix with dilute acetic acid (vinegar) to make the cells easier to see.

Biopsy
After examining your cervix and vagina, the doctor performs a biopsy, taking a small amount of tissue from the cervix and endocervix (inside the cervical canal). The tissue is sent to a laboratory to determine if cell changes reflect a precancerous or benign condition. Based on the biopsy results, the doctor determines your treatment.

During a biopsy, no anesthesia is used because the cervix has few nerve endings that sense pain. You may feel some cramping and pinching, but the discomfort should end quickly. Afterwards, the doctor or nurse may apply a thick yellow medication to the biopsy areas to stop any bleeding. Then the doctor will insert a tampon into the vagina. You can remove it a few hours later. For a short time after the biopsy, you may wear a sanitary napkin to catch blood spotting.

To help the biopsy area heal, do not place anything into your vagina for 3 days. Do not have vaginal intercourse, douche, swim, or take tub baths. You may shower.

If you have unusual vaginal discharge, heavy bleeding, or pain, call your doctor immediately.

---

femoral triangle, and pelvic nodes) salpingo-oophorectomy (removal of the fallopian tubes and ovaries), omentectomy (removal of the omentum), and pelvic exenteration (removal of all pelvic organs, including the ovaries, fallopian tubes, uterus, cervix, vagina, pelvic lymph nodes, bladder, and rectum).

(For a case study that shows how to apply the nursing process when caring for a client with gynecologic cancer, see *Applying the nursing process: Client with impaired tissue integrity related to gynecologic surgery*, pages 314 and 315.)

Radiation therapy. Radiation therapy can be used preoperatively, intraoperatively, or postoperatively to treat gynecologic cancer. The type and stage of the disease, the proximity of vital organs to be protected, concomitant disease, the client's age, and the pelvic shape determine the use of this therapy. Radiation therapy may be external, provided by a beam of radiation from a machine located outside the body, or internal, provided by a temporary radioactive implant.

Adverse effects of radiation therapy include nausea, vomiting, diarrhea, fatigue, weakness, and alterations in CBC. Before treatment begins, make sure the client understands these effects, and address any fears she may have about burns, disfigurement, pain, sterility, or loss of sexual function. If necessary, help her arrange for financial assistance, transportation to treatments, and any support she may need at home.

For external radiation therapy (ERT), the most common radiation beams are X-rays, gamma rays, electrons, and neutrons. Treatment duration may vary from less than 1 minute to several minutes, depending on the amount of radiation to be delivered to the carcinoma (Lewis and Levita, 1988).

Typically provided on an outpatient basis, ERT typically is scheduled 5 days a week for several weeks. Before the first ERT treatment, the radiologist meets with the client to explain the procedure and, with indelible ink, marks the area to be treated. At this time, assess the client for gaps in information, and correct any misconceptions.

For the client who needs internal radiation therapy (IRT), describe all aspects of this treatment. IRT places radiation as close as possible to the malignant growth while sparing nearby healthy tissue. Because the client constitutes a radiation threat to others while the radiation implant is in place (48 to 72 hours), individuals near the client must take precautions.

IRT requires brief hospitalization and may be performed using one of two techniques. The health care professional may place the IRT source and its applicator in position simultaneously, or may insert the applicator first and later insert the radioactive source. Use of the applicator-first technique reduces staff exposure to radiation. With either technique, insertion takes place in the operating room with the client under a general anesthetic. Because of this, client preparation includes an enema to clear the GI tract, a douche to clear the vagina, a low-residue diet after enema administration, no food for 8 to 12 hours before the anesthetic, and an anesthesia work-up with on-call medications.

While the radium implant is in place, the client should restrict her movements to avoid dislodging it. Elevate the head of the bed to 35 degrees to help stabilize the client's position. Use an air mattress to prevent

Gynecologic surgery

The following chart describes the indications, procedures, and nursing considerations for the most common surgeries for a client with gynecologic cancer.

INDICATIONS	DESCRIPTION OF PROCEDURE	NURSING CONSIDERATIONS
Cryotherapy		
• Cervical intraepithelial neoplasia (CIN)—most common • Chronic cervicitis • Cervical erosion	The physician inserts a probe into the cervix and circulates carbon dioxide that freezes tissues, causing diseased tissue to become necrotic and slough off.	• Be aware that cryotherapy is relatively painless, causes few complications and minimal blood loss, and does not affect childbearing capacity. • Advise the client to expect a watery discharge for 2 to 3 weeks after the procedure. • Tell the client to place nothing in her vagina for 3 weeks after the procedure.
Cauterization		
• CIN (The physician might excise the lesion rather than cauterize it.)	A hot wire unit generates heat in the cervix, causing tissue to become necrotic and slough off.	• Be aware that the client will be anesthetized, which can pose risks and may cause cervical stenosis. • Advise the client to expect a vaginal discharge for 2 to 3 weeks after cauterization and not to place anything in her vagina during that period.
Laser therapy		
• CIN • Vaginal, vulvar, or cervical condylomata (warts)	A colposcope-directed laser beam is absorbed by the tissues, and vaporization destroys abnormal cells to various depths.	• Be aware that laser therapy can produce less cervical damage and scarring than traditional surgery. • Advise the client to expect a slight brown discharge for 1 week after laser therapy. • Tell the client to place nothing in her vagina for 2 weeks after laser therapy. • Remind the client that healing takes up to 3 months. She may need to limit sexual intercourse during that period.
Cervical conization (cone biopsy)		
• CIN detected by endocervical Curettage during colposcopy • To rule out invasive squamous cell carcinoma • Inability to visualize entire sguamo-columnar junction during colposcopy	The surgeon uses a cold scalpel (cold knife) or laser to cut a circular incision around the external os, removes a cone-shaped piece of tissue, takes biopsies at apex, sutures the cervix, and performs a D&C.	• Be aware that short-term complications may include heavy bleeding and infection. Long-term complications may include cervical stenosis, infertility, decreased cervical mucus, and premature labor in future pregnancies. • Advise the client that menstrual bleeding should be normal after conization, but may be heavier, with brownish premenstrual discharge.
Oophorectomy		
• Ovarian cancer • Severe pelvic inflammatory disease • Ectopic pregnancy • Ovarian cysts	The surgeon performs a laparotomy and removes one or both ovaries.	• Observe the hospitalized client for signs of hemorrhage, infection, atelectasis, and pulmonary embolism. • Monitor vital signs every 15 minutes during the first hour, then every 30 minutes thereafter. • Teach the client to turn, cough, and breathe deeply every 2 hours for 24 hours. • Administer I.V. fluids and medications as prescribed. • Advise the client that her hormone status will not change if one ovary is removed. If both are removed, the client will not secrete hormones and may need hormone replacement therapy.

Gynecologic surgery continued

INDICATIONS	DESCRIPTION OF PROCEDURE	NURSING CONSIDERATIONS
Radical hysterectomy		
• Cervical cancer in Stage I or II, to prevent spread to the lymphatic system	The surgeon removes the upper third of the vagina, uterus, pelvic lymph nodes, cardinal ligaments, and bladder pillars.	• Advise the client that the advantages of radical hysterectomy over lymphadenectomy with radiation therapy include prevention of recurrence, and avoidance of radiation exposure in normal tissue. Disadvantages include increased complications, shortening of the vagina, and urinary and vaginal fistulas (Fogel and Woods, 1981). • Tell the client that bladder dysfunction, the most common complication, may result from autonomic nervous system interruption. Although normal bladder function usually returns in 1 to 3 months, dysfunction can be prolonged and may be permanent. Deep venous thrombosis with pulmonary embolism is another, less common, complication. • Prepare the client preoperatively with bowel cleansing and administration of prophylactic antibiotics and heparin. • Prevent deep vein thrombosis with postoperative care, including early ambulation, low doses of subcutaneous heparin, and external pneumatic compression of the calf, as prescribed. Use a suprapubic catheter or retroperitoneal suction catheter to prevent infection and injury to the ureter, if prescribed. • Advise the client that hospitalization lasts from 1 to 2 weeks. • Caution the client that this surgery shortens the vagina, which may affect sexual intercourse.

pressure sores. Encourage active range of motion exercises for the arms and feet and deep breathing every 2 hours. Record vital signs every 4 hours, and assess the skin for rash or evidence of dehydration. Use an indwelling urinary catheter and fracture pan to meet the client's elimination needs while minimizing movement. Because radiation treatment causes rapid dehydration, encourage fluid intake. Administer pain medications, sedatives, and antiemetics as needed, and notify the physician immediately if vaginal or rectal bleeding or hematuria occurs.

Internal radiation therapy also may be used to control a pelvic malignancy. With this technique, transvaginal radium needles are implanted into the parametrium using a plastic template. Another technique, intraperitoneal radiation therapy, instills into the pelvic and abdominal cavities a liquid that contains radioactive phosphorus, 32P (known as P32). For both techniques, client care resembles that for IRT.

For health care professionals and visitors, radiation exposure can be controlled through distance, time, and the use of lead shields. During the procedure, health care professionals should work quickly and remain as far from the client as possible. Afterwards, those who come in contact with the client must wear protective garments. If no contact is permitted, her room must be prepared and fully stocked, and items must be placed within easy reach of the bed. The room also should be equipped with an intercom, telephone, radio, and television.

After the radium source is removed, give the client an enema or douche, if needed, and help her shower. Use special precautions when handling feces or urine; follow health care facility policy. Monitor bladder function and encourage fluid intake. Allow the client to be out of bed as desired, and provide a regular diet until she is discharged.

Before discharge, teach the client about maintaining nutrition and fluid intake, balancing rest and exercise, resuming sexual intercourse, keeping the vulva clean and dry while experiencing vaginal discharge, avoiding exposure to sunlight (which can cause skin damage), and obtaining treatment for pruritus.

Client with potential for impaired tissue integrity related to gynecologic surgery

The table below shows how the nurse might use the nursing process when caring for the client described in the case history at right. The first column presents history and physical assessment data followed by a paragraph of mental notes. These notes help the nurse make important mental connections among assessment findings, aiding in development of the nursing diagnosis and planning.

The second column lists an appropriate nursing diagnosis; information in the remaining columns is based on this diagnosis. Although not part of the nursing process, a rationale appears for each intervention in the fourth column to explain how it contributes to the care plan.

ASSESSMENT	NURSING DIAGNOSIS	PLANNING
Subjective (history) data • Client is 5 days postoperative. • Client reports decreased tenderness of incision. • Client states that she is not ready to look at the incision yet. • Client states that she feels depressed and worries whether her husband will still love her. • Client expresses anxiety about how the incision will look after it heals. **Objective (physical) data** • Temperature 98.4°F, pulse 88 beats/minute, respirations 34/minute, blood pressure 112/80 mm Hg. • Incision line clear and healing with no drainage, erythema, or edema. • Client appears depressed and anxious. • Client is verbalizing her fears. **Mental notes** *Although postoperative infection is the most common complication of this surgery, the client has not developed an infection and the wound appears to be healing well. Nevertheless, the incision site will need careful monitoring until discharge to ensure tissue integrity. Also will need to spend time with the client to encourage her to verbalize her feelings and to accept the incision.*	Potential for impaired tissue integrity related to gynecologic surgery	**Goals** By the time of discharge, the client will: • avoid postoperative infection of incision • assist with incision care • demonstrate home care of incision.

Instruct the client to report the following to her physician immediately: vaginal, rectal, or urinary tract bleeding; foul-smelling vaginal discharge; fever; abdominal distention or pain; or signs and symptoms of menopause, such as amenorrhea and hot flashes.

Because radiation therapy causes nutrient deficiencies, malnutrition can occur. Therefore, instruct the client to eat a well-balanced, high-protein diet complete with vitamins and minerals before therapy starts and to eat as much as possible during therapy. Because anorexia will increase as the day progresses, encourage her to eat at least one-third of the day's protein and calories at breakfast. Serve foods at room temperature; bland foods may offset therapy-induced taste alterations. If the client finds chewing difficult, chop or blend foods. If nausea interferes with nutritional intake, provide antiemetics, as prescribed. Maintain the client's fluid intake at 2,000 to 3,000 ml/day, unless contraindicated. Implement tube feedings only if all other interventions fail to provide adequate nutrition.

Chemotherapy. Combinations include two or more of the following: cisplatin (Platinol), cyclophosphamide (Cytoxan), doxorubicin (Adriamycin), and hexamethylmelamine (National Cancer Institute, 1989).

Before treatment begins, prepare the client for probable adverse reactions to chemotherapy, such as nausea, vomiting, alopecia (hair loss), weakness, and fatigue, discussing their meanings and management. Explore the emotional distress these reactions may cause (Love, Leventhal, Easterling, and Nerenz, 1989), and address irreversible ones, such as amenorrhea in younger women.

Nursing interventions for chemotherapy are similar to those for radiation, because physiologic responses are similar. However, chemical toxicity may cause pain during drug administration.

CASE STUDY

Jean Baxter, age 55, is married and has three children. Five days ago, she underwent a radical vulvectomy and lymphadenectomy for squamous cell cancer of the vulva.

IMPLEMENTATION		EVALUATION
Intervention Assess the incision site at each dressing change.	**Rationale** The most common complication of Mrs. Baxter's surgery is impaired wound healing due to infection.	Upon evaluation before discharge, the client: • had an incision site that was clear and free of infection • viewed the incision • demonstrated knowledge of appropriate wound care at home.
Follow aseptic technique when cleaning and irrigating the incision and changing dressings.	Frequent observation of the incision site is necessary to assess for signs of infection, such as erythema, tenderness, exudate, odor, and tension on suture lines. Cleansing, irrigation, and dressing changes remove exudate and facilitate healing.	
Encourage the client to view the incision. Encourage the client to become involved in her care when she feels ready to do so.	Viewing of the incision may help dispel misconceptions about the extent and the nature of surgery. It also helps the client accept the reality of the surgery.	
Monitor vital signs every 4 hours or as ordered by the physician.	Infection may elevate temperature, pulse, or both.	
Teach the client to inspect for signs of infection, and instruct her to contact her physician should infection occur.	Active participation in self-care may increase feelings of self-worth and help prepare the client for discharge.	

Nausea, vomiting, and altered taste may cause food aversions in a client receiving chemotherapy. At the first sign of nausea, provide antiemetics as prescribed. Keep in mind that cisplatin is a potent emetic and can cause severe nausea and vomiting. If anorexia develops, suggest small, frequent feedings. If diarrhea and GI disturbances occur, note the consistency, frequency, amount, and color of the stool. Provide or suggest a low-residue diet. Replace fluid and nutritional losses and administer camphorated opium tincture (Paregoric) or diphenoxylate with atropine sulfate (Lomotil), as prescribed.

Advise the client that chemotherapy may cause skin alterations. If she develops dermatitis, provide calamine lotion or diphenhydramine hydrochloride (Benadryl). If alopecia develops, suggest that she cover her head with a scarf or wig, and reassure her that hair usually grows back in 3 to 6 months.

Reduce stomatitis by suggesting that the client avoid irritating foods, such as citrus fruit and spicy foods. For mouth comfort, suggest that she use a soft toothbrush, avoid strong mouthwashes, and use peroxide or lidocaine (Xylocaine Viscous Solution) as a mouthwash before meals. If constipation occurs, advise her to increase her intake of fluids and fiber; provide cathartics and stool softeners, as prescribed.

Advise the client to look for signs of bone marrow depression, such as bleeding and infection. If bone marrow depression occurs, take precautions to protect her from injury.

Hormone therapy. Teach the client about hormone therapy and urge her to keep follow-up appointments. Hormone therapy may include synthetic progesterones, such as parenteral hydroxyprogesterone (Delalutin) and medroxyprogesterone (Provera) and oral megestrol (Megace). Response to this therapy depends on estrogen and progesterone receptor levels in the malignant tissue.

Provide family care. The client and her family may have a nursing diagnosis of *ineffective family coping: compromised, related to the client's gynecologic cancer* or *altered role performance related to gynecologic cancer.* If the diagnosis or treatment plan has affected the client's relationship with her partner, facilitate communication about grief, guilt, isolation, sexual dysfunction, dying, and death. Encourage family members to share their concerns, and refer them to a therapist or support group, if desired.

Evaluation

To evaluate nursing care, compare the outcomes of interventions with the goals established with the client. The following examples illustrate some appropriate evaluation statements.
• The client correctly described her disorder, the diagnostic tests, and the treatment plan.
• The client demonstrated self-esteem through self-care and expression of self-acceptance.
• The client discussed anatomic changes caused by her disorder.
• The client discussed alternative methods of sexual expression with her partner.
• The client listed ways to cope with the physical and emotional effects of her disease.
• The client discussed ways to protect herself from complications.
• The client expressed satisfaction with her physical and psychological comfort.
• The client identified ways to maintain her independence.
• The client adjusted her life-style to help cope with physical changes.
• The client maintained appropriate nutrition and hydration.
• The client kept all appointments.
• The client listed the signs and symptoms for which she should seek further care.
• The client maintained self-esteem during hospitalization and after discharge.
• The client expressed feelings of loss after the surgery.
• The client verbalized an understanding of sexuality changes caused by surgery.
• The client demonstrated acceptance of her new self-image by viewing her incision and participating in her care.

Documentation

Using the appropriate records, document all steps of the nursing process. Also document other aspects of care, such as diagnostic tests and treatments and the client's response to them.

Although each facility requires documentation of different information, most require the nurse to record the following:
• reason that the client seeks care
• results of diagnostic studies
• scheduled treatments
• follow-up care
• adverse effects of treatment, such as anorexia or skin discoloration
• client teaching performed.

Chapter summary

Chapter 13 described a broad range of gynecologic disorders, including breast, menstrual, and pelvic support disorders as well as gynecologic cancer. Here are the chapter highlights.
• Benign breast disorders include fibrocystic breast changes, fibroadenoma, intraductal papilloma, and duct ectasis. Before breast changes are diagnosed as benign, the nurse must provide information and support because many women assume that all breast changes signal cancer. After diagnosis, the nurse must provide information on treatment, self-care techniques, and life-style decisions affecting benign breast disorders.
• Breast cancer is the most common type of cancer in women and the second leading cause of their death. Treatments include surgery, radiation therapy, hormone therapy, and chemotherapy. When caring for a client with breast cancer, the nurse must teach about self-care, diagnostic tests, and treatments; assist with decision making; provide postoperative care; and provide information and support to the client and her family.
• Menstrual disorders include amenorrhea, dysmenorrhea, premenstrual syndrome, mittelschmerz, metrorrhagia, and endometriosis. They can affect the client physically and emotionally. The nurse can play a key role in supporting and educating the client about medications, treatments, and life-style factors—including stress, diet, and exercise—that can affect menstrual disorders.
• Pelvic support disorders include cystocele, rectocele, and uterine prolapse. The nurse who cares for a client

with these disorders must provide education and support to help the client understand the treatment options and make life-style decisions affecting her condition.

• Gynecologic cancers include ovarian, fallopian tube, endometrial, cervical, vaginal, and vulvar cancer. Treatments include surgery, radiation therapy, hormone therapy, and chemotherapy. When caring for a client with gynecologic cancer, the nurse must consider the physical and psychological effects of the disorder and the client's chosen treatment. The nurse must inform the client about self-care, and support the client and her family during decision making. For example, when the client faces surgery, the nurse must support her in her decision while respecting her right to choose her treatment and exercise control over her body.

• The nurse who cares for a dying client with metastatic cancer must provide information and support to the client and her family.

Study questions

1. Shelley Martinson, age 36, seeks care because she has noticed breast changes during BSE. What emotions are likely for her? How can the nurse help Ms. Martinson deal with these emotions?

2. Mary Gunther, age 42, is recovering from a modified mastectomy. Which key points should the nurse address when teaching Mrs. Gunther about her planned chemotherapy and radiation treatments?

3. What are the differences between primary and secondary amenorrhea? Primary and secondary dysmenorrhea?

4. Felicia Brownlee, age 22, tells the nurse she thinks she has premenstrual syndrome (PMS). What techniques should the nurse use to assess Ms. Brownlee? Which life-style changes might the nurse suggest for a client with PMS?

5. Margaret Smith, age 50, seeks care because she has discovered a lump in her left breast. What type of testing will the nurse prepare her for?

Bibliography

Droegemueller, W., Herbst, A., Mishell, D. and Stencheur, M. (1987). *Comprehensive gynecology*. St Louis: Mosby.

Dwyer, J. (1986). *Manual of gynecologic nursing*. Boston: Little, Brown.

Fogel, C., and Woods, N. (1981). *Health care of women: A nursing perspective*. St. Louis: Mosby.

Griffith-Kenney, J. (1986). *Contemporary women's health: A nursing advocacy*. Reading, MA: Addison-Wesley.

Havens, C., Sullivan, N., and Tilton, P. (Eds.). (1986). *Manual of outpatient gynecology*. Boston: Little, Brown.

Hawkins, J., and Higgins, L. (1982). *The health care of women: Gynecologic assessment*. Boston: Jones and Bartlett.

Hawkins, J., Roberto, D., and Stanley, J. (1987). *Protocols for nurse practitioners in gynecologic settings*. New York: Tiresias Press.

Jones, III, H., Wentz, A., and Burnett, L. (1988). *Novak's textbook on gynecology* (11th ed.). Baltimore: Williams & Wilkins.

National Cancer Institute. (1988a). *1987 Annual Cancer Statistics Review* (88-2789). Bethesda, MD: National Institutes of Health.

Neeson, J., and Stockdale, C. (1981). *The practitioner's handbook of ambulatory OB/GYN*. New York: John Wiley & Sons.

Speroff, L., Glass, R., and Kase, N. (1988). *Clinical gynecologic endocrinology and infertility* (4th ed.) Baltimore: Williams & Wilkins.

Breast disorders

Carbone, P. (1990). Adjuvant therapy of stage II breast cancer. *Cancer*, 65 (Suppl. 9), 2148-2154.

d'Angelo, T., and Gorrell, C. (1989). Breast reconstruction using tissue expanders. *Oncology Nursing Forum*, 16(1), 23-27.

Derdiarian, A. (1987). Informational needs of recently diagnosed cancer patients. *Cancer Nursing*, 10(2), 107-115.

Doig, B. (1988). Adjuvant chemotherapy in breast cancer. *Cancer Nursing*, 11(2), 91-98.

Dunne, C. (1988). Hormonal therapy for breast cancer. *Cancer Nursing*, 11(5), 288-294.

Ellerhorst-Ryan, J., Turba, E., and Stahl, D. (1988). Evaluating benign breast disease. *Nurse Practitioner*, 13(9), 13-28.

Fitzsimmons, M., Conway, T., Madsen, N., Lappe, J., and Coody, D. (1989). Hereditary cancer syndromes: Nursing's role in identification and education. *Oncology Nursing Forum*, 16(1), 87-94.

Love, S., Gelman, R., and Silen, W. (1982). Fibrocystic "disease" of the breast: A nondisease? *New England Journal of Medicine*, 307(16), 1010-1014.

National Cancer Institute. (1988b). *What you need to know about breast cancer* (88-1556). Bethesda, MD: National Institutes of Health.

Nettles-Carlson, B. (1989). Early detection of breast cancer. *JOGNN*, 18(5), 373-381.

Rice, M., and Szopa, T. (1988). Group intervention for reinforcing self-worth following mastectomy. *Oncology Nursing Forum*, 15(1), 33-37.

Rutherford, D. (1988). Assessing psychosexual needs of women experiencing lumpectomy. *Cancer Nursing,* 11(4), 244-249.

Schwartz-Appelbaum, J., Dedrick, J., Jusenius, K., and Kirchner, C. (1984). Nursing care plans: Sexuality and treatment of breast cancer. *Oncology Nursing Forum,* 11(6), 16-24.

Survival in early breast cancer. (1989). *Nurses' Drug Alert,* 8(3), 19.

Menstrual disorders

ACOG Committee. (1989). *Premenstrual syndrome: Opinion #66.* Chicago: American College of Obstetrics and Gynecology.

Connell, A. (1989). Abnormal uterine bleeding. *Nurse Practitioner,* 14(4), 40-56.

Chihal, H. (1989). *Premenstrual syndrome: A clinic manual* (2nd ed.). Amityville, NY: Essential Medical Information Systems, Inc.

Dalton, K. (1984). *Premenstrual syndrome and progesterone therapy* (2nd ed.). Chicago: Year Book Medical Publishers.

Frank, E.P. (1986). What are nurses doing to help PMS patients? *American Journal of Nursing,* 86(2), 136-140.

Garner, C., and Webster, B. (1985). Endometriosis. *JOGNN (suppl.),* 14(6), 10s-20s.

Keye, W. (1988). Premenstrual syndrome: Seven steps in management. *Postgraduate Medicine,* 83(3), 167-73.

Lauersen, N. (1985). Recognition and treatment of premenstrual syndrome. *Nurse Practitioner,* 10(3), 11-20.

Severino, S., and Moline, M. (1989). *Premenstrual syndrome: A clinician's guide.* New York: Guilford.

Treybig, M. (1989). Primary dysmenorrhea or endometriosis. *Nurse Practitioner,* 14(5), 8-18.

Wilhelm-Hass, E. (1984). Premenstrual syndrome: Its nature, evaluation and management. *JOGNN,* 13(4), 223-229.

Wilson, M. (1984). Menstrual disorders: Premenstrual syndrome, dysmenorrhea, amenorrhea. *JOGNN,* 13(2), 11s-19s.

Pelvic support disorders

Cashavelly, B. (1987). Cervical dysplasia: An overview of current concepts in epidemiology, diagnosis and treatments. *Cancer Nursing,* 10(4), 199-206.

Cohen, S. (1989). Another look at physiologic complications of hysterectomy. *Image—Journal of Nursing Scholarship,* 21(1), 51-53.

Hacker, N., and Moore, G. (1986). *Essentials of obstetrics and gynaecology.* Philadelphia: Saunders.

Pernoll, M., and Benson, R. (1987). *Current obstetric and gynecologic diagnosis and treatment* (7th ed.). East Norwalk, CT: Appleton & Lange.

Gynecologic cancer

Cohen, S., Hollingsworth, A., and Rubin, M. (1989). Another look at psychologic complications of hysterectomy. *Image: Journal of Nursing Scholarship,* 21(1), 51-3.

Finck, K. (1986). The potential health care crisis of hysterectomy. In D. Kjervik and I. Martinson (Eds.). *Women in health and illness* (pp. 200-217). Philadelphia: Saunders.

Fullerton, J., and Barger, M. (1989). Papanicolaou smear: An update on classification and management. *Journal of the American Academy of Nurse Practitioners,* 1(3), 84-90.

Given, B., and Given, C. (1989). Compliance among patients with cancer. *Oncology Nursing Forum,* 16(1), 97-103.

Lehr, P. (1989). Surgical lasers. *AORN,* 50(5), 972-977.

Lewis, F., and Levita, M. (1988). Understanding radiotherapy. *Cancer Nursing,* 11(3), 174-185.

Mandelblatt, J. (1989). Cervical cancer screening in primary care: Issues and recommendations. *Primary Care,* 16(1), 133-155.

National Cancer Institute. (1989). *Cancer of the ovary: Research report* (89-3014). Bethesda, MD: National Institutes of Health.

National Cancer Institute. (1988c). *What you need to know about cancer of the uterus* (88-1562). Bethesda, MD: National Institutes of Health.

National Cancer Institute. (1987a). *Cancer of the uterus: Research report* (87-171). Bethesda, MD: National Institutes of Health.

National Cancer Institute. (1987). *What you need to know about cancer of the ovary* (87-1561). Bethesda, MD: National Institutes of Health.

Rostad, M. (1988). The radical vulvectomy patient: Presenting complications. *DCCN,* 7(5), 289-294.

Rubin, D. (1987). Gynecologic cancer: Cervical, vulvar, and vaginal malignancies. *RN,* 50(5), 56-63.

Cultural references

Ludwick, R. (1988). Breast examination in the older adult. *Cancer Nursing,* 11(2), 99-102.

Skubi, D. (1988). PAP smear screening and cervical pathology in an American Indian population. *Journal of Nurse Midwifery,* 33(5), 203-207.

Willis, M., Davis, M., Cairns, N., and Janiszewski, R. (1989). Inter-agency collaboration: Teaching breast self-examination to Black women. *Oncology Nursing Forum,* 16(2), 171-177.

Nursing research

Cassileth, B., Zupkis, R., Sutton-Smith, K., and March, V. (1980). Information and participation preferences among cancer patients. *Annals of Internal Medicine,* 92(6), 832-836.

Champion, V. (1987). The relationship of breast self-examination to health belief model variables. *Research in Nursing and Health,* 10(6), 375-382.

Clarke, D. (1989). Factors involved in nurses' teaching breast self-examination. *Cancer Nursing,* 12(1), 41-46.

Cortese, J., and Brown, M. (1989). Coping responses of men whose partners experience premenstrual symptomology. *JOGNN,* 18(5), 405-412.

David, A., Roul, R., and Kuruvilla, J. (1988). Lessons of self-help for Indian women with breast cancer. *Cancer Nursing,* 11(5), 283-287.

Dodd, M. (1988). Patterns of self-care in patients with breast cancer. *Western Journal of Nursing Research,* 10(1), 7-24.

Doherty, M. (1989). The effect of circumvaginal muscle exercize. *Nursing Research,* 38(6), 331-335.

Grindel, C., Cahill, C., and Walker, M. (1989). Food intake of women with breast cancer during their first six months of chemotherapy. *Oncology Nursing Forum,* 16(3), 401-407.

Holmes, S. (1989). Use of a modified symptom distress scale in assessment of the cancer patient. *International Journal of Nursing Studies,* 26(1), 69-79.

Hopkins, M. (1986). Information-seeking and adaptational outcomes in women receiving chemotherapy for breast cancer. *Cancer Nursing,* 9(5), 256-262.

Jenkins, B. (1988). Patients' reports of sexual abuse after treatment for gynecological cancer. *Oncology Nursing Forum,* 15(3), 249-354.

Lauver, D. (1989). Instructional information and breast self-examination practice. *Research in Nursing and Health,* 12(1), 11-19.

Lierman, L. (1988). Discovery of breast changes: Women's experiences and nursing implications. *Cancer Nursing*, 11(6), 352-361.

Lilley, L. (1987). Human need fulfillment alteration in the client with uterine cancer: The registered nurse's perception versus the client's perception. *Cancer Nursing*, 10(6), 327-337.

Love, R., Leventhal, H., Easterling, D., and Nerenz, D. (1989). Side effects and emotional distress during cancer chemotherapy. *Cancer*, 63(3), 604-612.

Lovejoy, N., Jenkins, C., Wu, T., Shankland, S., and Wilson, C. (1989). Developing a breast cancer screening program for Chinese-American women. *Oncology Nursing Forum*, 16(2), 181-187.

Ludwig Breast Cancer Study Group. (1988). Combination adjuvant chemotherapy for node-positive breast cancer. *New England Journal of Medicine*, 319(11), 677-683.

McQuiston, C. (1989). The relationship of risk factors for cervical cancer and HPV in college women. *Nurse Practitioner*, 14(4), 18-26.

Micozzi, M., Carter, C., Albanes, D., Taylor, P., and Licitra, L. (1989). Bowel function and breast cancer in U.S. Women. *American Journal of Public Health*, 79(1), 73-75.

Northouse, L. (1989). A longitudinal study of the adjustment of patients and husbands to breast cancer. *Oncology Nursing Forum*, 16(4), 511-516.

Rudin, M., Martinson, I., and Gilliss, C. (1988). Measurement of psychosocial concerns of adolescents with cancer. *Cancer Nursing*, 11(3), 144-149.

Russell, L. (1989). Caffeine restriction as initial treatment for breast pain. *Nurse Practitioner*, 14(2), 36-40.

Violence Against Women

Objectives

After reading and studying this chapter, the student should be able to:
1. Describe the cycle of violence.
2. Identify indicators of abuse in the health history and physical assessment.
3. Describe common nursing interventions for an abused client.
4. Identify the phases of rape-trauma syndrome and its variations.
5. Describe how to assist during a rape examination and collect evidence from a client who has been raped.
6. Discuss nursing interventions for a client who has been raped.
7. Apply the nursing process when caring for a client who has been abused or raped.

Introduction

In the United States, violence against women is widespread and typically takes the form of repeated physical abuse, rape, and other forms of assault. The *Statistical Abstract of the United States: 1989* indicates that 2.1 million women in the United States are abused, raped, or murdered every year and that nearly one-third of them experience extreme violence more than once a year (U.S Bureau of the Census, 1988). Yet these incidence rates are conservative because social stigma, personal shame, and fear lead to underreporting of abuse and rape. Abuse

alone may affect about 4 million women (Centers for Disease Control [CDC], 1989a).

For the client who has been abused or raped, the nurse attempts to achieve these goals:
• Accurately assess the effects of the violence.
• Acknowledge the wide range of feelings that the client may express.
• Intervene appropriately for physical and psychological trauma.
• Protect the client from additional emotional trauma.
• Establish a trusting relationship to promote change in the family.
• Prevent violation of the client's rights.
• Provide a safe environment for the physical and psychological well-being of the client and her family.
• Discuss the client's options and strategies.
• Provide links to community resources.

The nurse must keep in mind that women who have been abused or raped have been viewed traditionally as victims by society—including the health care profession. Today, they are recognized as survivors rather than victims, to promote a healthier self-concept.

This chapter prepares the nurse to care for survivors of violence. It begins by comparing the types of violence against women. Then it explores nursing care for a client who has been abused or raped, highlighting use of the nursing process.

Abuse

Abuse refers to physical violence directed against one person by another who lives in the same household. Sometimes called domestic or family violence, it occurs between people who know each other intimately.

GLOSSARY

Abuse: physical violence directed against one person by another who lives in that household, typically resulting in serious physical and psychological damage to the woman. Also called battering or domestic or family violence.

Cycle of violence: common pattern of abuse. It has three phases (increasing tension, abusive episode, and kindness and contrition) and may vary in intensity and duration for each couple.

Learned helplessness: belief that one is powerless and unable to act independently.

Rape: sexual intercourse without consent, achieved through the use of threats, force, intimidation, or deception. It requires penile penetration of the vagina.

Rape examination kit: commercially prepared kit that includes everything needed for rape examination and evidence collection.

Rape-trauma syndrome: group of symptoms that results from rape and includes an acute phase, outward adjustment phase, and a reorganization phase. Also a nursing diagnosis approved by the North American Nursing Diagnosis Association.

Sexual assault: penetration of any orifice (other than the vagina) by the penis, other male appendage, or an object without consent, achieved through the use of threats, force, intimidation, or deception.

Spousal rape: sexual intercourse that results from threats, physical force, or intimidation by the woman's spouse or partner.

Somatic complaints: physical symptoms caused by psychological concerns.

Research suggests that wife abuse accounts for more injuries that require medical treatment than automobile accidents, rapes, and muggings combined (Stark and Flitcraft, 1987). Annually, more than 1 million women seek care for injuries caused by abuse (Stark and Flitcraft, 1982).

In many cases, homicide results from unchecked, long-standing violence, usually by a man against a woman. In 1986 and 1987, 37% of female homicide victims were killed by a spouse or partner (U.S. Department of Justice, 1987).

Factors that promote abuse include acceptance of violence in the culture, sexual inequality, exposure to violence as a child, use of alcohol or drugs, and poverty. For example, sex-role stereotypes and socialization patterns can produce learned helplessness (belief that one is powerless and unable to act independently) that furthers unequal relationship roles and fosters abuse. To reduce abuse, social scientists recommend elimination of (1) the idea of one sex as superior, (2) unequal pay for identical work, which can perpetuate financial dependence in a relationship, and (3) sex roles that assign child care to one parent.

Once abuse begins, it typically will continue and escalate. It may start with throwing things, pushing, grabbing, slapping, kicking, and biting. Then it may progress to beating with the fists and hitting with an object. It may escalate to threats with and eventual use of a knife or gun. Regardless of the level of abuse, however, it usually follows a cyclic pattern. (For more information, see *Cycle of violence,* page 322.)

Legal protection against abuse varies from state to state. Because of this, the nurse should be familiar with the laws that apply to the client. For example, in some states, a woman may obtain a civil injunction or restraining order to protect herself only after she files for divorce or leaves the abuser. In many states, domestic violence cases are handled by the family court, a judicial body that emphasizes reconciliation rather than deterrence of or punishment for abuse.

In every state, laws impose criminal penalties for assault, battery, rape, burglary, and kidnapping. Yet these laws may not be enforced if the suspect is a cohabitant and the damage inflicted is not severe. Therefore, the abused woman faces difficulties when she seeks redress through the legal system. With knowledge of the current laws, the nurse can provide general guidance and refer the client for legal assistance.

Rape

Legally, rape refers to sexual intercourse without consent, achieved through the use of threats, force, intimidation, or deception. Technically, rape requires penile penetration of the vagina. In contrast, sexual assault refers to penetration of any other orifice by the penis, other male appendage, or other object without consent, achieved through the use of threats, force, intimidation, or deception (Griffith-Kenney, 1986). Because legal definitions of rape vary from state to state, and because rape and sexual assault require similar clinical care, this chapter refers to any type of sexual attack as rape.

Cycle of violence

Walker's (1984) cycle of violence theory describes three separate phases of family violence, which can occur over several weeks or months and vary in intensity and duration for each couple. The cycle of violence shows that abuse is not constant or totally random and helps explain why a woman may not leave an abusive situation.

To provide sensitive care for an abused woman, the nurse should be familiar with the cycle of violence, as illustrated below.

**Phase I
Increasing tension**
In this phase, the man engages in minor abuse, such as dish throwing or grabbing the woman too tightly. In response, the woman typically acts compliant or passive and stays out of his way to pacify him and lessen her risk of injury. This phase may last for weeks or years.

**Phase II
Abusive episode**
This phase involves acute battering of the woman by the man in an explosion of violence. During this phase, which usually lasts 2 to 24 hours, the woman feels powerless and may try to protect herself or hide.

**Phase III
Kindness and contrition**
In this phase, the man promises to change, becomes kind and loving, and may ask for the woman's forgiveness. Because the woman wants to believe that he loves her and will not become violent again, she convinces herself that he will change. His loving behavior reinforces her beliefs, but the cycle usually repeats itself.

Rape is a violent criminal act. During a rape, the woman is overpowered and may fear injury or death. Afterwards, she may be physically, socially, and psychologically devastated. She may sustain short-term injuries from physical abuse and forceful intercourse, such as vaginal or rectal trauma. She also may develop short- and long-term emotional problems.

Rape generates extreme anxiety and stress for the woman, causing emotional and psychological reactions as well as somatic complaints (physical symptoms caused by psychological concerns) known as rape-trauma syn-drome. According to Burgess and Holmstrom (1979), this acute stress reaction usually has two phases: the acute (short-term) phase and the reorganization (long-term) phase. Some experts include an outward adjustment (intermediate) phase (Golan, 1978). (For more information, see *Rape-trauma syndrome.*)

Myths about rape profoundly affect the woman's view of herself as well as society's view of the rapist and the woman he attacks. One such myth is that rape occurs because a woman acts or dresses seductively, enticing the rapist and making him lose control. Other myths include the idea that women enjoy or secretly desire rape, that "nice girls" do not get raped, that rapes occur only in dark alleys, and that a woman cannot be raped unless she is willing.

The incidence of rape is high and increasing. Every year 1,000 out of every 100,000 women are raped in the United States (U.S. Department of Justice, 1987). Of these women, 1% to 15% need hospitalization, 3% to 4% need emergency department (ED) treatment, and 32% require some medical treatment for their injuries. The number of rape-related deaths is unknown because they typically are recorded as homicides. The risk of pregnancy from rape is low, about 1%; the risk of contracting a sexually transmitted disease (STD) is more than 4% and rising (U.S. Bureau of the Census, 1988).

Spousal rape also is increasing statistically. From 1970 to 1987, this form of rape increased from 18.7 to 37.4 per 100,000 women (U.S. Department of Justice, 1989). In 40 states, however, the laws provide no legal recourse for spousal rape because they assume that marriage gives permanent and irrevocable consent to all sexual approaches.

Even though rape is a crime with potentially devastating effects, it tends to be ignored as a public health problem. Health care professionals who are insensitive to a client's needs or who believe that she provoked her rape may treat her roughly, making the examination after the attack a "second rape." Also, they may allow her to leave the facility without providing information on STDs, pregnancy, or other physical or psychological effects of the rape. Because of this, the nurse must be aware of his or her feelings about rape and provide thorough, nonjudgmental care.

Nursing care

The nursing process provides a framework for all nursing care for a client who has been abused or raped. Typically, the nurse comes into contact with such a client in the ED. However, the nurse also may care for these clients in other health care settings. Depending on the setting and the client's needs and desires, the nurse may provide short-term or long-term care. For example, a client who seeks care in the ED for physical injuries needs immediate care, but may resist other offers of help. A client

Rape-trauma syndrome

A client who has been raped may develop rape-trauma syndrome. Although individuals show distinct variations in their response to rape, most pass through these three phases or their variations (Burgess and Holmstron, 1979).

Acute phase
In this phase, which occurs immediately after the rape and may last for several days to several weeks, the client may experience disorganization and a wide range of emotions, typically including shock and disbelief. Her emotional style may be *expressed,* in which she shows her fear, anger, and anxiety by crying, sobbing, smiling, or acting restless and tense, or it may be *controlled,* in which she hides her feelings and acts calm, composed, or subdued.

She may experience physical disturbances, such as vaginal pain or feelings of suffocation. She also may develop psychological effects, predominantly fear of physical injury, mutilation, death, or the rapist's return.

Outward adjustment phase
After the acute phase, the client may seem adjusted, returning to her usual roles. However, she is using denial and suppression to cope with the rape and regain control of her life.

During this phase, she may move, install new locks, get an unlisted telephone number, buy a weapon, or take a self-defense course. These actions force the rape trauma deeper into her subconscious.

Reorganization phase
When the denial and suppression of the outward adjustment phase no longer sustain the client, she enters the reorganization phase. During this phase, she may feel anxious and depressed and experience various difficulties. She may develop phobias, such as fear of being alone, fear of being with strangers or men, or fear related to some sensory input during the rape. For example, she may freeze with fear if she smells the cologne the rapist wore. These fears may prompt her to change her life-style.

During this phase, other problems may include menstrual or gynecologic disorders, sexual dysfunction, and sleep disorders, including violent nightmares in which she relives the rape or kills her attacker.

Variations
Rape-trauma syndrome has two major variations: the *compound* reaction and the *silent* reaction. In the compound reaction, a client with a history of physical, psychiatric, or social difficulties develops additional problems, which may include depression, psychotic behaviors (such as hallucination and regressive actions), or acting-out behaviors (such as cursing or throwing things). Or she may abuse alcohol or drugs or experience changes in sexual activity.

In the silent reaction, the client does not tell anyone about the rape or deal with her feelings about it. As a result, she develops a massive psychological burden. This reaction is particularly noteworthy because many women still do not report rape, especially spousal rape.

who obtains care from her physician or nurse practitioner for chronic sleep problems related to abuse or for emotional disturbances related to rape-trauma syndrome may need long-term care.

Assessment

The nurse varies the assessment depending on whether the client has been abused or raped.

Abuse

Before providing care, perform a self-assessment for feelings of inadequacy, horror, anger, or disgust; judgmental ideas about abuse; fear of violence; or an overwhelming desire to rescue the client. Such feelings can inhibit recognition of the client's feelings and thwart the development of a therapeutic relationship. If self-assessment reveals such feelings, ask another nurse to care for the client.

To assess a potentially abused client, modify the assessment based on her condition. For example, if she has been admitted to the ED with severe injuries, shorten the initial health history and focus the physical assessment on the injuries.

During the assessment, collect data systematically. Keep in mind that the client may be experiencing physical and emotional pain along with immobilizing fear. She may feel stigmatized and reluctant to share information unless she knows she is safe. To help the client relax, focus on her physical symptoms first. Next, try to discover if she has experienced physical abuse. Then, ascertain whether she views the abuse as a problem.

Obtain information from the health history, physical assessment, and diagnostic studies for later use in developing the plan of care.

Health history. To obtain useful information during the health history interview, maintain a professional, self-confident, and nonjudgmental manner. Ask general assessment questions, as described in Chapter 7, Women's Health Promotion, as well as some specific questions about abuse.

Reassure the client that her privacy will be respected and that confidentiality will be strictly enforced. This is important because she may be ashamed of the abuse, afraid of her partner, and fearful that he will be told. To help allay the client's feelings of aloneness, let her know that you are familiar with the problems of abuse.

Begin by obtaining general health history information, including the client's reason for seeking health care. Note any responses that suggest actual or potential abuse. (For more information, see *Health history indicators of abuse*.)

Then screen for abuse. Do this even with a client who has no overt injuries or signs of unhappiness in her relationship with her partner. To help identify a client who is abused, routinely ask such questions as, "How does your family deal with stress?" and "Have you ever been physically hurt by anyone?" when assessing a client's history of injuries.

Next, assess family dynamics to evaluate interpersonal relationships. For a client in an intimate relationship with a man, inquire about abuse. If a history of abuse exists, allow the client to talk about it without interrupting her. Also assess her dependence on her partner and note reports of psychological abuse and controlling behaviors, such as jealousy and enforced isolation.

To determine the potential danger to the client, assess the abuse pattern for a cyclic increase in severity. Using graph paper, mark the number and intensity of abusive episodes over time to document and help the client understand the pattern of abuse.

Evaluate the client's support systems. Also assess her perceptions of her children and the effects of abuse on them. Finally, explore the topic of sexual abuse. The client may reveal discomfort with the sexual relationship, which should be thoroughly assessed through further questioning. For example, she may not think of abuse as forced sexual intercourse or other undesired sexual activities.

Physical assessment. During the physical assessment, focus on areas or body systems that have sustained injury. For example, if the client has an injury in her lower leg, focus on the musculoskeletal system. If she reports sexual abuse, assist with a pelvic examination to evaluate for trauma. Carefully note and document all signs of injury, past and present. If the health care facility's policy allows, take photographs to help identify and document injuries.

Gently and carefully examine any other areas where the client reported sustaining abuse. During the examination, note the client's general appearance as well as her verbal and nonverbal behaviors, which can provide clues about how she deals with her feelings. For example, a client who displays a flat affect (no emotion in her facial expression) may be distancing herself from or denying her feelings.

Perform a complete mental status assessment, particularly noting low self-esteem, depression, and suicidal intent. A useful way to assess self-esteem is to have the client describe her strengths and weaknesses.

Health history indicators of abuse

During the health history, the nurse should be alert for responses that suggest actual or potential abuse. For each health history topic, the following chart lists findings that may indicate abuse.

Reason for seeking care
- Vague information about cause of injury or a delay in seeking treatment
- Inappropriate reaction by partner to client's injuries and emotional state
- Partner who provides all data and is reluctant to leave
- Request for emergency department treatment for vague stress-related symptoms, such as nausea, insomnia, headaches, and abdominal pain
- Intense fear, anxiety, or somatic complaints (physical symptoms caused by psychological concerns)
- Implausible explanation of trauma

Current health status
- Treatment for mental illness
- Frequent physical or somatic complaints, such as headaches or nausea

Health history
- Multiple fractures and other injuries
- Anxiety, substance abuse, or depression
- Injuries during pregnancy
- Spontaneous abortions
- Somatic complaints
- Frequent visits to physicians
- Suicide attempts or ideation
- Frequent hospitalizations, especially for physical injuries or depression
- Refusal to be hospitalized

Family health history
- Traditional values of male authority and dominance in family of origin
- Spousal abuse, child abuse, or both in family of origin

Review of physiologic systems
- Headaches
- Palpitations
- Gastrointestinal disturbances
- Inability to concentrate
- Aggressive sexual activity that causes pain and diminishes sexual desire
- Joint pain or other tender areas, especially in the extremities
- Chronic pain elsewhere

Sleep patterns
- Sleep disturbances
- Nightmares
- Insomnia

Nutrition
- Marked weight gain or loss
- Anorexia
- Marked increase in food intake

Socioeconomic status
- Membership in ethnic group that believes in male dominance

- Social isolation
- Control of finances by partner
- Conflict resolution through physical violence

Environmental health
- Guns in the home or otherwise readily available
- History of accidents in the home

Emotional health status
- Low self-esteem
- Feels trapped, helpless, or powerless
- Compliant or passive
- Chronic fatigue or low energy
- Strong commitment to marriage at all costs
- Zealous concern for children
- Major decisions made by partner
- Feels abuse is deserved and provoked

Social support
- Few friends and acquaintances
- Lack of external resources
- Minimal support system
- Unfamiliarity with social agencies

Partner characteristics
- Abusive courtship
- Alcohol or substance abuse
- Belief in male dominance
- Enjoyment of violent or aggressive recreational activities
- History of unsuccessful relationships
- Feels threatened by client's skills or abilities
- Possessiveness or jealousy
- Need for immediate gratification
- Low self-esteem
- Powerlessness in interpersonal situations
- Situational or developmental stressors, such as low income and need to provide for several children
- Hypervigilence about the client's activities
- Poor verbal skills
- Suppressed rage and anger, which may be expressed by quiet, tense behavior
- Poor impulse control, which may be expressed by easy loss of temper
- Demanding and physically forceful sexual behavior
- Unrealistic accusations of client's sexual infidelity

Parents' relationship with children
- Child abuse
- Use of corporal punishment
- Conflicts and disputes settled physically
- Lack of closeness
- Excessive television viewing
- Minimal interaction between father and children
- Unrealistic parental expectations

During the physical assessment, be alert for the following indicators of abuse.

• General appearance. Hyperresponsive behaviors, such as pulling away during the physical examination; extreme fatigue; poor grooming or inappropriate attire; hesitant or predominantly nonverbal communication; extremes of body weight; facial grimacing and slow or stiff movement, which may indicate pain.

• Vital signs. Hypertension or tachycardia.

• Skin. Tenderness, burns, bruises, edema, welts, or scars, especially on the face, breasts, abdomen, or genitalia.

• Head. Cuts, scars, or signs of subdural hematoma, such as reduced mentation over time and vital sign changes.

• Eyes. Periorbital swelling or discoloration, subconjunctival hemorrhage, tearing, or photosensitivity.

• Genitourinary system. Perineal edema, bruises, or tenderness; external bleeding; pain when pelvic area is touched.

• Rectum. Anal or rectal bruises, tenderness, bleeding, edema, or irritation.

• Musculoskeletal system. Signs of recent fractures (especially of facial bones, radius, ulna, or ribs), such as tenderness, edema, and limited range of motion; signs of old fractures, such as improper body alignment and reduced mobility; signs of pulling or twisting, such as spiral fractures of the radius or ulna or shoulder dislocation.

• Abdomen. Abdominal injuries, especially in a pregnant client, or signs of intra-abdominal injury, such as vomiting, abdominal tenderness, tympany, or rebound tenderness.

• Nervous system. Hyperactive reflex responses, areas of numbness from old injuries, inappropriate or flat affect, or selective recall.

Diagnostic studies. Obtain diagnostic studies, as ordered. Keep in mind that X-rays, ultrasound recordings, and other tests not only provide information about injuries but also may be needed as evidence.

Rape

Before performing the complete assessment, provide immediate care of injuries and prepare the client for examination and treatment. Then obtain a health history, perform or assist with a physical assessment that includes evidence collection, and obtain laboratory tests, as ordered. Be sure to follow health care facility protocol, document all findings, and handle all evidence carefully; these procedures may affect future legal proceedings.

Immediate care. Immediate medical care takes priority and usually begins in the ED. As needed, perform an emergency assessment and intervene appropriately. Help reduce the client's stress in the ED by giving her attentive care and providing support. Follow the health care facility's protocols and state regulations about reporting rape. When the client's physical stability is ensured, prepare her for a thorough assessment and rape examination.

Client preparation. Make the client feel as safe and comfortable as possible by moving her to a quiet, private room or area and assuring her that you or someone else (such as a community advocate or another nurse) will stay with her throughout the examination. Help her gain a sense of control by explaining each step of the examination and its importance. Ask her not to urinate, defecate, or drink until after specimens have been collected because these actions could remove evidence, such as semen or foreign materials. Inform her about the legal process, and explain that evidence must be collected in case she decides to bring charges against her attacker later.

Discuss treatments that may be ordered, and encourage her to ask questions about anything that she does not understand. The physician should obtain informed consent when necessary. If the client is a minor, consent may be obtained from her parent or guardian. Depending on health care facility policy, witness the signatures on the consent form.

Throughout the assessment, remember to act as the client's advocate. (For more information, see *Advocacy*.) If available, ask a volunteer advocate from a women's group or crisis center to assist by reviewing the client's rights; helping her notify family, friends, and authorities; and planning for the rape examination.

Health history. To help obtain all necessary information, establish a rapport with the client by explaining the reasons for the health history questions. Because the client's medical records may be subpoenaed, record all information objectively and, when possible, in the client's own words.

During the health history, show respect for the client's dignity and be alert for nonverbal clues to emotional distress or pain.

Description of the rape. Start by taking a history of the incident. The client may be embarrassed to state what happened or to have it written down. If so, ease her embarrassment by ensuring complete privacy during the health history and explaining that the information is vital to planning her care. Offer nonjudgmental emotional support during the history, and let her vent her feelings as she describes the incident.

The time and place of occurrence suggest the type of evidence to look for, such as fresh or dried semen, grass stains, or dirt. The use of a weapon during the attack could help explain the injuries, and more than one assailant could account for variations in evidence, such as several hair colors or blood types. The nature of the attack indicates where to obtain semen specimens and check for bruises and other signs of trauma. For example, if the rapist ejaculated in the client's face and hair, plan to obtain semen specimens from these areas rather than from the vagina.

If the client lost consciousness during the attack, determine the cause. Also note the client's use of drugs and alcohol and document it according to facility protocol.

Medical history. Obtain a brief medical history, noting any medications the client is taking and any drug allergies. If the client's treatment includes drugs, this information will help prevent drug interactions and adverse reactions.

Determine if the client had an STD at the time of the rape. Carefully record such information according to facility policy, because information unrelated to the rape could bias a jury if it is disclosed in the courtroom.

Gynecologic history. Inquire about the client's last menstrual period and, if she is sexually active, ask about her contraceptive use. Plan to discuss pregnancy prevention with a client who is in the fertile period of her menstrual cycle and does not use a continuous-acting contraceptive method, such as an oral contraceptive or an intrauterine device.

Also ask the client to specify the date and time of the last sexual intercourse before the rape. Motile sperm remain in the vagina for 6 to 12 hours; in the cervix, 3 days. So if the client had intercourse several days before the rape, expect to collect semen specimens from the vagina only—not the cervix—as evidence of rape.

Find out if the client was pregnant at the time of the rape. If so, she may need special medical care for herself and her fetus.

Physical assessment. A physician or nurse practitioner performs the rape examination, and the nurse assists. During this part of the assessment, preserve the client's dignity by having her meet the examiner while seated rather than in the lithotomy position.

Before the examination, obtain a sterile speculum and a rape examination kit. Although rape kits provided by health care facilities may differ, most facilities use

Advocacy

As the advocate for a client who has been raped, the nurse offers emotional support, provides information, and upholds the client's decisions. To do this, the nurse applies the following guidelines for general and legal advocacy.

GENERAL ADVOCACY GUIDELINES

- Emphasize the client's assets.
- Encourage the client to explore healthy aspects of herself.
- Emphasize the client's responsibility for her health.
- Help the client distance herself emotionally.
- Provide health information, such as prevention of pregnancy and sexually transmitted diseases.
- Support the client's decisions.

LEGAL ADVOCACY GUIDELINES

- Help the client notify the police.
- Ensure that the physician obtains informed consent. Witness the signatures on the consent form, according to health care facility policy.
- Remain with the client during interviews to provide support and ensure that legal, law enforcement, and other individuals treat the client properly.
- Act as an observer. Do not ask questions for the police officer or other interviewer.
- Ensure that no evidence is omitted.
- Document all information properly.
- Maintain the client's confidentiality. Do not discuss her case with unauthorized personnel.
- Provide general information about the legal process and refer the client for legal assistance.
- Arrange for a properly trained volunteer to accompany the client to all police interviews and legal proceedings.

commercially prepared kits that include everything required for examination and evidence collection. After the examination, mark unused rape kit items as such and return them with the evidence to the crime laboratory.

Put on rubber gloves to avoid contaminating the specimens to be collected. Help the client remove her clothes and save them to be analyzed for semen and blood stains. If her clothes are wet, allow them to dry. Circle any suspected blood or semen stains on the clothing with a laundry marker, and place each piece of clothing in a separate paper bag. (Do not use plastic bags: Airtight bags stimulate bacterial action that may alter the evidence.) As with all medical evidence, label these bags with the client's name, date, time of collection, health care facility name, and your name. Collect any debris from the client's body, label it in the same manner and note the body area from which it was obtained, and enclose it in separate paper envelopes.

General condition. Begin by assessing the client's general condition. Observe for bruises, punctures, lacerations, abrasions, redness, swelling, fractures, burns, and bleeding.

Examine the back and buttocks thoroughly, particularly if the client was forced to lie on the ground. Injuries and other signs of force refute the assailant's assertion that the sexual advance was invited. If indicated by facility protocol, take photographs of any visible injuries.

Skin, hair, and nails. In this part of the examination, collect fingernail clippings or scrapings, foreign or loose head hair and pubic hair, and samples of all dried semen from the skin for analysis by the crime laboratory.

Obtain fingernail clippings or scrapings because these may contain skin or blood specimens that will help identify the assailant. For each hand, collect the fingernail clippings or scrapings on a separate sheet of white paper. Then fold the papers and place them in separate, properly labeled envelopes.

To find hair that might belong to the assailant, collect all loose and foreign hair from the head and then from the pubic area. (Beginning with less private parts of the body helps make the client more comfortable.) Using the clean, unused comb from the rape kit, comb the hairs onto a clean sheet of paper. Then fold the paper and place it in a properly labeled envelope along with the comb. Be sure to place head hair and pubic hair in separate envelopes. Finally, pull out 15 to 20 hairs by the roots from different areas of the crown and perineum. The crime laboratory will analyze these hair strands for color and texture and compare them to the loose and foreign hairs and to those obtained from the assailant.

Using an ultraviolet light, check the client's skin for dried semen, which appears brittle, scaly, slightly yellow, and shiny. Remove the dried material by gently rubbing one or more saline-moistened cotton-tipped applicators over the area. Air dry the swabs before placing them into a properly labeled and sealed test tube. The crime laboratory uses these specimens to detect semen, acid phosphatase, and sperm.

Also under the ultraviolet light, check for fresh semen, which has a bluish white florescence. Examine the entire body for fresh semen, paying close attention to the thighs and perineum. If semen is matted in the client's hair, clip it, air dry it, and place it in a properly labeled envelope.

If blood or sputum is present on any parts of the body, use a cotton-tipped applicator to obtain specimens and make smears.

Head and neck. Carefully search for injuries to the head, neck, and throat. From 30% to 60% of rape clients are severely injured in these areas. When examining the client's mouth, note any loose or broken teeth, which may be evidence of use of force.

Obtain a saliva sample by having the client place saliva in the appropriate container. From the saliva specimen, the crime laboratory determines if the client secretes blood group (ABO) antigens. (Blood group antigens appear in saliva, blood, and semen.) Then the laboratory compares the client's saliva to that of the assailant. In a client who is a nonsecretor (has no specific blood group antigens in her saliva), the presence of antigens in her vagina or elsewhere suggest semen from the assailant.

Swab the client's oral cavity where the gums meet the teeth. Using separate swabs, make smears that will be tested for STDs and semen. Also inspect the oral cavity for signs of an existing STD, such as lesions.

Pelvic examination. The pelvic examination is performed to collect additional specimens and to assess the genitalia and rectal area for injuries. (For specific procedures, see Chapter 7, Women's Health Promotion.) Be sure to diagram and describe any genitourinary and rectal trauma carefully.

To assist the examiner who performs the pelvic examination, follow these guidelines. Before beginning, place the client in the lithotomy position. During the examination, maintain eye contact with the client, offer support, and explain each step. To minimize discomfort, especially for a client with inflamed genitals, lubricate the speculum with warm water. The examiner will not use a prepared lubricant, such as K-Y jelly, because it may alter test results. If muscle tension causes pain during the examination, note signs of pain on the medical record.

The examination includes assessment of the vulvar area, hymen, and vaginal walls for signs of injury. Bleeding or fresh blood clots suggest rupture of the hymen. Adult clients frequently sustain lacerations higher in the vagina; younger ones, closer to the introitus. Deep lacerations require surgical evaluation.

To obtain a vaginal specimen for semen testing, the examiner swabs in a circular motion over the entire vaginal area because ejaculatory emission is not uniform. (If the client had intercourse before the rape, only the lower portion of the vagina is swabbed.) Place air-dried swabs in a properly labeled test tube. In some states or counties, rape protocols require aspiration of vaginal contents for semen testing. If this is required, follow the health care facility's protocols.

Next, the examiner assesses the condition of the cervix, noting trauma, tears, bleeding, edema, abrasions, and tenderness. Swabbed cervix secretions provide a gonorrhea culture.

The examiner bimanually palpates the uterus, being alert for signs of pregnancy, tumors, masses, or tenderness. The examiner assesses the internal and external rectal areas, particularly noting any rectal masses or tenderness. Rectal abnormalities may indicate bleeding under the tissues due to trauma. A rectal specimen for semen testing is obtained by swabbing around the rectal orifice. Place the air-dried swabs in a properly labeled test tube. The rectal area also will be swabbed to obtain a specimen for a gonorrhea culture.

If required by health care facility protocol, a rectal wash follows the examination and specimen collection. Preserve the aspirated wash material in a sterile, properly labeled container for sperm analysis or acid phosphatase testing.

Laboratory tests. As prescribed, draw whole blood samples for blood typing, pregnancy testing, and screening for gonorrhea, syphilis, and *chlamydia*. The physician may request drug and alcohol tests, especially if the client appears to have been drugged before, during, or after the attack. Is so, obtain appropriate specimens. Also obtain a urine specimen for a pregnancy test to assess for pre-existing pregnancy. The test results will determine whether or not the client will be offered the morning-after pill, Ovral. (For information about these tests, see Chapter 7, Women's Health Promotion. For information about other tests, see *Common laboratory tests*.)

With special preparation, the nurse may examine the specimens for motile sperm. On a wet mount, sperm are present when a drop of a commercial stain turns light blue. Keep in mind that specimens must be examined immediately.

After examination of wet mounts for motile sperm, allow the client to shower. Give her fresh clothes if her family or friends have brought some to the health care facility, or offer her a gown. Give her time to rest or talk with her family or friends before beginning the next phase of her care.

Nursing diagnosis

Review all health history, physical assessment, and diagnostic findings. Based on significant findings, formulate nursing diagnoses. (For a partial list of applicable nursing diagnoses, see *Nursing diagnoses: Violence against women*, page 330.)

Common laboratory tests

In addition to analysis of evidence by the crime laboratory and tests for sexually transmitted diseases, several other tests may be performed for a client who has been raped. The nurse should be aware of the commonly ordered studies described in the chart below.

SEMEN TESTS AND SIGNIFICANCE

Acid phosphatase color test
Detects acid phosphatase, a group of phosphatase enzymes that appear primarily in semen. Acid phosphatase found in specimens taken from clothing or parts of the body confirms semen deposition.

Microscopic examination for sperm
Identifies whole spermatozoa or fragments, which helps confirm semen deposition. (A man who has had a vasectomy or who has azoospermia will have no sperm in his semen.)

Blood group substance test
Identifies A, B, and O substances in males who have the dominant secretor gene in a homozygous or heterozygous state. Thus, the male who has group A blood and is a secretor has soluble blood group A substance in his seminal fluid and group A substance on the surface of his red blood cells. The results of blood and enzyme groupings can demonstrate that a suspected rapist's semen is different from or consistent with semen found in or on the client's body.

SEMEN AND VAGINAL SECRETION TESTS AND SIGNIFICANCE

Phosphoglucomutase (PGM) test
Detects which one of the three possible patterns of PGM (an enzyme found in vaginal and seminal secretions) exists in the client and suspected rapist. If their patterns differ, identification of the rapist will be easier.

Planning and implementation

The nurse develops and implements a plan of care for the client who has been abused or raped.

Abuse

During the planning stage, work with the client to develop short-term and long-term goals, depending on the health care setting. For example, help the ED client formulate short-term goals and refer her to other health care professionals for long-term care. In other situations, help the client with both types of goals whenever possible.

Ensure that short-term goals are simple and concrete so that the client can solve some of her problems and feel encouraged to work on achieving long-term goals.

NURSING DIAGNOSES

Violence against women

The following nursing diagnoses address some of the problems and etiologies that a nurse may encounter when providing care for a client who has been abused or raped. Specific nursing interventions for many of these diagnoses are provided in the "Planning and implementation" section of this chapter.

ABUSE

- Anticipatory grieving related to separation from partner
- Anxiety related to life changes prompted by abuse
- Fear related to continuation of abuse
- Ineffective family coping: compromised, related to financial stress
- Ineffective individual coping related to abuse
- Post-trauma response related to abuse
- Potential for violence: directed at others, related to abuse
- Potential for violence: self-directed, related to abuse
- Powerlessness related to abuse
- Self-esteem disturbance related to history of abuse
- Sleep pattern disturbance related to fear of abuse
- Social isolation related to abuse

RAPE

- Altered family processes related to rape
- Altered sexuality patterns related to rape
- Anxiety related to rape
- Body image disturbance related to rape
- Decisional conflict related to discussing rape with the family
- Fear related to rape
- Impaired social interaction related to rape
- Ineffective family coping: compromised, related to rape
- Ineffective individual coping related to rape
- Knowledge deficit related to the risk of pregnancy from rape
- Knowledge deficit related to the risk of STDs from rape
- Post-trauma response related to rape
- Potential for infection related to rape
- Rape-trauma syndrome related to aftermath of rape
- Rape-trauma syndrome related to feelings of uncleanliness and humiliation
- Rape-trauma syndrome: silent reaction, related to inability to discuss rape
- Spiritual distress related to rape

Keep in mind that an abused client may have difficulty setting and achieving long-term goals. Because of her feelings of dependency, she may ask the nurse to plan goals for her. If the client is not ready to reflect on her future, temporarily delay discussion of long-term goals and encourage her to set simple, short-term goals, such as making a telephone call or discussing her problems with a family member.

Remember that this is the *client's* plan. Offer support and suggest alternatives, if needed, but do not impose goals on her; rather, encourage her to discover her own solutions. To enhance the client's self-esteem and confidence in her planning abilities, have her set goals and give her positive reinforcement when she achieves them. Identify and prioritize her health needs and work with her to develop a plan to meet them.

Depending on the health care setting, implement care by providing support, supplying information, assisting with grief, making referrals, and providing family care.

Before implementing any plans, however, discuss the client's strengths with her. For a client with a nursing diagnosis of *self-esteem disturbance related to history of abuse,* this discussion may begin to help improve her self-esteem, relieve her fear of being condemned for inciting the abuse or not ending the relationship, and enable her to take action.

Provide care and support. In addition to caring for the client's physical injuries, provide emotional support. Before an abused client can talk about her problems, she needs to feel safe physically and psychologically, especially if she has a nursing diagnosis of *fear related to continuation of abuse.* To help her feel safe, approach her in a concerned, nonjudgmental manner that promotes trust. Remember that an abused client may express repressed anger at health care professionals or the facility providing care.

The client with *self-esteem disturbance related to a history of abuse* may believe she deserves the beatings and assume that all men beat their partners. If so, help her examine her situation and explore the options. Support her attempts to make her own decisions, and avoid making them for her.

For a client with a nursing diagnosis of *post-trauma response related to abuse,* encourage her to discuss her feelings about the abuse. At first, she may not want to express repressed feelings because she may fear her potential for violence against her abuser if she vents her anger or rage. Gently remind her that abused women typically have a wide range of feelings, all of which are valid.

If the client is in a potentially fatal relationship, particularly if her abuser has a weapon or has threatened to kill her, urge her to take assertive action, such as contacting protective services, the police, or a shelter for abused women. If she cannot take action, contact community services for advice. Advise her to seek professional counseling to help her deal with the long-term effects of abuse.

For the abused pregnant client, provide specialized care. (For more information, see *Nursing research applied: Interventions for abused pregnant clients.*) Keep in mind that about one in every 50 pregnant women is beaten (U.S. Bureau of the Census, 1988). During pregnancy, she may be subjected to focused kicks and punches to her abdomen. Experts are not sure exactly how pregnancy engenders violence, but theorize that the pregnant woman may appear psychologically or sexually threatening to her partner or that her pregnancy may represent an additional financial burden that the family income cannot sustain.

Supply information. A client with a nursing diagnosis of *ineffective individual coping related to abuse* may need to feel some control over her environment. To help her gain a sense of control, inform her about the procedures that will be performed, the questions that will be asked, and the individual who will examine her. Also advise her that her record will be kept confidential.

Explain the cycle of violence and its effects on women and their children. This information may help the client understand the gravity of her situation and prompt her to take action.

Assist with grieving. An abused client may grieve over loss of the ideal relationship, of trust in her partner, of her body image, of self-esteem, of sense of safety, and of children—as well as physical losses. Her grieving may be complicated by a change in the abuser's behavior to being loving and contrite.

If the client has a nursing diagnosis of *anticipatory grieving related to separation from partner,* help her work through the stages of grief and remind her that grief is a healthy response to loss. Explain that grieving usually follows a pattern, but that its sequence, intensity, and duration may vary individually. Tell her that progress toward resolution is seldom direct and that many people vacillate between stages of grief. Throughout her grieving, provide support.

Make referrals. Many communities now are beginning to help women prevent abuse or deal with its effects. They

---

NURSING RESEARCH APPLIED

Interventions for abused pregnant clients

A major health problem, abuse during pregnancy not only affects the woman but also her fetus. Yet abuse commonly begins or escalates during pregnancy. To investigate this phenomenon, researchers interviewed 290 pregnant women. The sample included 43.1% Hispanic, 32.1% Caucasian, and 22.4% Black women whose average age was 25. Of the 23% who reported abuse before or during the pregnancy, 63.8% did not know of resources for abused women. The remainder cited the family as the primary resource, followed by shelters and police or legal assistance. Few identified health care professionals as a resource.

Application to practice
The nurse who gives perinatal care is in a particularly good position to detect indicators of potential abuse. To do this, the nurse should observe the couple for poor communication and lack of support in their interactions, particularly during childbirth education classes.

The nurse also should work to prevent violence at three levels. The first level, education, should include teaching about abuse in childbirth education and other classes, developing programs for families at risk for abuse, researching the problem, educating the community about it, and promoting legislative changes.

The second level, screening, should involve assessment of women for abuse, discussing abuse with men, detecting abuse, providing crisis intervention, referring abusers to therapists, and volunteering in abused women's shelters.

The third level, care, should include referring abused women to shelters; working with family members, lawyers, police, shelter personnel, and counselors; encouraging the media to dispel myths about abuse; providing follow-up care; and acting as an advocate for the abused woman in court.

Helton, A., and Snodgrass, F. (1987). Battering during pregnancy: Intervention strategies. *Birth,* 14(4), 142-147.

---

may do this through crisis centers, organizations against abuse, consciousness-raising groups, shelters, or self-defense groups. The judicial and health care systems also have taken steps that reflect society's movement toward prevention and treatment of violence. For example, they have set up educational programs to teach how to identify and treat abused women and have made connections with shelters and women's centers for hotline numbers and referrals.

Communities vary in their resources for abused women and how they provide aid. However, many have open shelters (protected environments available to any abused woman) and transition homes, where the woman can find safety for herself and her children and assistance in preparing to earn a living, if needed.

Although shelters differ, most provide individual and group counseling, assist in dealing with the police and legal and social services, offer child care, and provide help with future plans, such as employment counseling and coordination with housing authorities. Usually, they are run by combined professional and volunteer staffs. They may provide access to health care services in different ways. Many offer educational programs for students in the health care professions, which offer clinical experience and provide various services to abused women.

When an abused woman needs assistance from health care, law enforcement, and legal professionals, refer her to appropriate resources, such as peer support groups or professional counselors. This may be especially useful for a client with *anxiety related to life changes prompted by abuse.* To anticipate her future needs, give her telephone numbers for all community resources, such as abused women's shelters, legal aid societies, and social service agencies.

Provide family care. Because violence affects the abused, the abuser, and the rest of the family, assess and provide care for them, if possible. Keep in mind that abuse can stem from *ineffective family coping: compromised, related to financial stress* and other problems.

Try to evaluate the abuser's ability to handle stress. He probably will pose a continued threat to others until he receives help in understanding his behavior and how to change it. When talking with him or another family member, obtain answers to such questions as:
• Have you recently lost your job or other means of support?
• Do you have problems with alcohol or drugs?
• Is the woman pregnant with a child you do not want?

Suggest that the abuser seek regular support from a self-help group and call a telephone hot line in times of crisis. Commonly available through family service agencies and hospitals, these support systems can give him someone understanding to talk to and may help prevent further abuse.

Rape

Be alert to personal feelings when planning and implementing care for a client who has been raped. Keep in mind that the nurse's anxiety or anger at the client, rapist, or others can affect client care.

Develop goals with the client to maintain or restore her self-respect, dignity, integrity, and autonomy. Focus on goals that help her cope with the stress and life disruptions caused by the rape.

To provide care after a rape, teach about pregnancy and STD prevention and provide rape counseling and family care.

Teach about pregnancy prevention. A client who has been raped may have a *knowledge deficit related to the risk of pregnancy from rape.* If the client is in the most fertile period of her menstrual cycle and does not use a continuous form of contraception, advise her that pregnancy is possible. To prevent pregnancy in this case, she may receive two tablets of Ovral immediately and two tablets in 12 hours.

Advise the client to arrange for a pregnancy test several weeks after the rape if she suspects she is pregnant. Let her know that if she is pregnant, a health care professional will discuss options with her. (For more information, see Chapter 9, Family Planning.) Always provide written information because the client may be anxious and unable to remember all oral instructions.

Teach about STD prevention. The client is likely to have a nursing diagnosis of *potential for infection related to rape* or *knowledge deficit related to risk of STDs from rape.* Advise the client that she is at risk for contracting an STD if she sustained vaginal, oral, or anal penetration during the rape. Provide oral and written information about STDs and their treatment.

If the health care facility has a specific protocol for STD treatment and follow-up, describe it to the client so that she will know what to expect and will be more likely to follow the regimen. Typically, a client receives ceftriaxone, 250 mg I.M. followed by doxycycline 100 mg P.O. b.i.d. for 7 days or tetracycline hydrochloride 500 mg P.O. q.i.d. for 7 days (CDC, 1989b).

Because months may elapse between exposure to the human immunodeficiency virus (HIV) and seroconversion and because baseline testing at the time of exposure has little value, HIV testing usually is not done during the initial examination. However, the client should receive a topical (vaginal, oral, or rectal) preventive treatment with nonoxynol-9 or a 1:10 vinegar solution as soon as possible after the rape (Foster and Bartlett, 1989; Hicks, et al., 1985). Follow-up testing for HIV may be performed at a later date.

Provide rape counseling. When counseling the client, remember to avoid viewing her as a victim, because she may have difficulty abandoning the victim role and seeing herself as a capable, productive person. Initially, the client may have a nursing diagnosis of *ineffective individual coping related to rape* or *anxiety related to* *rape.* If so, she will need help addressing her crisis and the related fears, feelings, and issues. To help her, use crisis intervention techniques.

For example, encourage her to talk about the rape and express her feelings and fears in a nonjudgmental atmosphere where her privacy and confidentiality are assured. Listen actively and with concern. Monitor the actions of others who may be less sensitive to her psychological needs. Allow time for expression of feelings to help her regain a sense of control over the event and renew mastery over her life.

Keep in mind that a client who has been raped may develop a nursing diagnosis of *rape-trauma syndrome related to aftermath of rape.* To anticipate potential problems, advise the client that she will need time to confront the crisis and deal with her intense and varied feelings. Reassure her that resolution eventually will occur, especially if she takes one problem at a time. Also help her gain some understanding of the assault. If she questions her judgment before the attack, help her examine alternate behaviors that could be used in the future, and remind her that her behavior did not justify such violence.

When examining alternate actions for dealing with current problems, point out the need to use old and new sources of support. Remind the client that she may have delayed reactions to the rape, including phobias, nightmares, psychosexual distress, and increased motor activity. Explore different ways she might cope with her reactions, such as talking about her feelings with family and friends.

Refer the client for ongoing counseling to assess the appropriateness of her reactions and the nature and availability of her support systems. A client who needs help in eliciting the support of family and friends may have a nursing diagnosis of *decisional conflict related to discussing rape with family* or *rape-trauma syndrome: silent reaction, related to inability to discuss the rape.* Also give the client a list of rape resource telephone numbers and addresses.

Before discharging the client, ensure that she has a safe place to go and transportation to it. If she was raped at home, contact a rape crisis center or volunteer advocate to locate alternate housing and help with the transportation costs. If possible, have a family member, friend, or advocate meet her at the health care facility when she is discharged.

Provide family care. Every family responds differently to rape, but all are vulnerable to poor coping, inadequate resolution, and dysfunction, which can cause a nursing diagnosis of *ineffective family coping: compromised, related to rape.* If the client's family is present, provide care by assessing their reactions and setting goals that will promote their well-being and ability to cope. Keep in mind that, like the client, the family typically passes through the acute, outward readjustment, and reorganization phases in response to rape.

Evaluation

To complete the nursing process, evaluate the effectiveness of nursing care by reviewing the goals attained. (For a case study that shows how to apply the nursing process when caring for an abused client, see *Applying the nursing process: Client with potential for trauma related to increasing abuse,* pages 334 and 335.) State the evaluations in terms of actions performed or outcomes achieved for each goal. When caring for an abused client, evaluate her achievement of short-term and long-term goals. The following examples illustrate such evaluation statements:

• The client felt less fearful and verbalized her sense of loss.
• The client exhibited a feeling of control by asserting her willingness to contact a community resource.
• The client correctly stated the relationship of abuse and stress to somatic symptoms.
• The client understood the importance of maintaining her health by exercising regularly and eating a balanced diet.
• The client reported decreased tension and other symptoms after using stress management techniques.

When caring for a client who has been raped, also evaluate her progress. The following examples illustrate appropriate evaluation statements:

• The client disclosed the rape to her family.
• The client verbalized her feelings about the rape.
• The client called the local rape crisis center to join a support group.
• The client understood the importance of STD treatment and follow-up.
• The client agreed to visit her nurse practitioner for follow-up care in 2 weeks and 4 weeks.

Documentation

Thorough documentation of assessment findings and all nursing activities is critical for care of a client who has been abused or raped. It not only serves as a baseline for future care and evaluation, but also provides vital information to legal and social service professionals who may work with the client. Proper documentation also helps ensure consistency and completeness of care.

Each health care facility may require documentation of slightly different information. For an abused client, however, most require the nurse to record the following information:

APPLYING THE NURSING PROCESS

Client with potential for trauma related to increasing abuse

For an abused woman, the nursing process helps ensure high-quality care. The table below shows how the nurse might use the nursing process when caring for the client described in the case history at right. The first column presents history and physical assessment data followed by a paragraph of mental notes. These notes help the nurse make important mental connections among assessment findings, aiding in development of the nursing diagnosis and planning.

The second column lists an appropriate nursing diagnosis; information in the remaining columns is based on this diagnosis. Although not part of the nursing process, a rationale appears for each intervention in the fourth column to explain how it contributes to the care plan.

ASSESSMENT	NURSING DIAGNOSIS	PLANNING
Subjective (history) data • Client has been married for 3 years and had lived with her current partner for 3 years before that. • Client has three children, ages 4, 6, and 8. • Client has an eighth-grade education. • Client states abuse has occurred for the past 5 years. • Client states violence escalated from verbal to physical abuse, which now includes punching, kicking, pushing, and slapping. • Client expresses feelings of worthlessness and complains of headaches, soreness, insomnia, and anorexia. **Objective (physical) data** • Temperature 99° F, pulse 98, respirations 22, and blood pressure 116/88 mm Hg. • Height 5'10"; weight 120 lb. • Old and new bruises over back, chest, arms, and legs. • Sunken eyes surrounded by dark circles; does not maintain eye contact during conversation. **Mental notes** *Because the client has only an eighth-grade education and has never worked outside the home, she is deeply concerned about supporting her three children if she leaves or divorces her husband. She is obviously stressed by the abuse, as evidenced by insomnia and anorexia, which has caused her to be 10 pounds underweight. Escalation of abuse has reduced her self-esteem further and places her at risk for severe injury.*	Potential for trauma related to increasing abuse	**Short-term goals** The client will: • realistically assess the danger of her situation • identify her husband's behavior pattern. **Long-term goals** The client will: • identify the effects of violence on her children • identify the advantages and disadvantages of obtaining a divorce • use community resources, as needed.

• health history findings, including exact quotations of the client's description of the problem
• family history and other health history findings that suggest abuse
• physical assessment findings, including detailed descriptions and illustrations or photographs of the client's injuries
• diagnostic study findings
• legal issues explored with the client

• referrals to other health care professionals or agencies, such as a social worker or Child Protective Services
• instructions for follow-up care.

For a client who has been raped, most facilities require documentation of the following information:
• description of the rape
• pertinent medical and gynecologic history findings
• result of mental status examination

CASE STUDY

Susan Jacob, a married homemaker age 30, was admitted to the emergency department with vague, somatic complaints.

IMPLEMENTATION		EVALUATION
Short-term intervention Share facts about abuse with client.	**Rationale** Information about abuse gives the client a more comprehensive understanding of the behavior.	Upon short-term evaluation, the client: • stated the past abuse pattern and made projections for the future • listed five personal strengths • agreed to use a shelter or transitional home, as needed.
Discuss legal alternatives and the safety of shelters and transition homes.	Discussion of legal alternatives and shelters teaches the client that she can change her environment temporarily or permanently.	
Point out the client's strengths.	Identifying the client's strengths helps enhance her self-esteem and outlook.	Upon long-term evaluation, the client: • sought legal counsel • reported fewer headaches • reported less tension • stated that she sleeps 7 hours every night.
Provide appropriate resources and referrals.	Appropriate referrals and resources can help the client cope and make future plans.	
Provide positive reinforcement for problem-solving efforts.	Positive reinforcement enhances the client's outlook on herself and her future. Increased self-esteem will, in turn, make problem-solving more effective.	
Long-term intervention Discuss characteristics of abusive men and point out parallels to her husband's behavior.	**Rationale** Such a discussion may help the client understand factors that influence abuse and realize that other women may experience similar problems.	
Have client review her marriage and its effect on her and her children.	Through review, the client may gain insight into the home environment and its effects.	
Identify coping mechanisms and help the client learn to use them effectively.	Effective coping mechanisms will help decrease stress and promote a calmer family environment.	
Continue to explore her attitudes, feelings, and values.	Exploration allows the client to organize and understand her feelings and values, which will help her set priorities.	

• physical assessment findings
• evidence collected
• specimens taken and where they were sent
• plans for follow-up care
• names of others who questioned the client or were involved in her care.

Chapter summary

Chapter 14 discussed two major types of violence against women: abuse and rape. Here are the highlights of the chapter.

• In the United States, abuse and rape are underreported primarily because of social stigma, personal shame, and fear of reprisal.

• The cycle of violence has three phases: increasing tension, abusive episode, and kindness and contrition. Once abusive behavior begins, it typically continues and may escalate.

• The nurse may provide short-term or long-term care for an abused client.

• When assessing a client, the nurse should look for indicators of abuse during the health history, such as a history of somatic complaints and abuse in the family of origin. The nurse also should be alert for indicators of abuse during the physical assessment, such as signs of recent fractures and hyperactive reflex responses.

• For an abused client, the nurse can intervene by providing care and support, supplying information, assisting with grief, making referrals, and providing family care.

• Rape is a violent criminal act that can produce a range of physical and psychological effects.

• The rape-trauma syndrome has three phases: acute (short-term), outward adjustment (intermediate), and reorganization (long-term).

• To provide the best possible care for a client who has been raped, the nurse should act as her advocate and work closely with law enforcement and health care professionals on her behalf.

• Nursing care for the client who has been raped begins with immediate care for physical injuries followed by client preparation for the rape examination. While taking the history, the nurse obtains a description of the rape and a medical and gynecologic history. During the examination, the nurse performs or assists with physical assessment and specimen collection, obtaining evidence and documenting all findings.

• Laboratory tests for a client who has been raped include tests for saliva and blood, tests for semen, and smears for STDs. They also include evaluation of evidence by the crime laboratory.

• Nursing interventions for a client who has been raped include teaching about pregnancy and STD prevention and providing rape counseling and family care.

Study questions

1. What is the cycle of violence? How does it cause some women to stay in an abusive relationship?

2. Jenny Ostriker, age 25 and 4 months pregnant, was admitted to the emergency department with signs of trauma to the head and abdomen. Ms. Ostriker offers an implausible explanation for her injuries; she is anxious and hypervigilant. Which health history topics should the nurse use to investigate suspected abuse?

3. Which nursing interventions are likely to be most useful for Ms. Ostriker?

4. Anne Feldman, age 30, was raped 6 months ago. She tells her nurse practitioner that she thought she was "getting over the attack just fine," but now is beginning to feel anxious, depressed, and fearful of being alone. She also reports insomnia and nightmares. What phase of the rape-trauma syndrome is Ms. Feldman experiencing? How can the nurse help her?

5. Shelley MacIntyre, age 19, is brought to the emergency department after being raped on her way home from work. After making Ms. MacIntyre as comfortable as possible and obtaining history information, the nurse collects which evidence? How?

Bibliography

Centers for Disease Control. (1989a). Education about adult domestic violence in U.S. and Canadian medical schools 1987-88. *MMWR*, 38(2), 17-19.

Foege, W. (1986). Violence and public health. In *Surgeon General's workshop on violence and public health report* (DHHS Publication No. HRS-D-MC86-1). Washington, DC: U.S. Dept. of Health and Human Services.

Gellert, G., and Mascola, L. (1989). Rape and AIDS. *Pediatrics*, 83(4), 644-645.

Griffith-Kenney, J. (1986). *Contemporary women's health: A nursing advocacy approach*. Menlo Park, CA: Addison-Wesley Publishing.

Hurley, M. (Ed.). (1986). *Classification of nursing diagnoses: Proceedings of the sixth conference*. St. Louis: C.V. Mosby.

Klingebell, K. (1986). Interpersonal violence: A comprehensive model in a hospital setting—from policy to program. In *Surgeon General's workshop on violence and public health report* (DHHS Publication No. HRS-D-MC86-1). Washington, DC: U.S. Dept. of Health and Human Services.

Kohnke, M. (1982). *Advocacy: Risk and reality*. St. Louis: C.V. Mosby.

Rosenberg, M., and Mercy, J. (1985). Homicide and assaultive violence. In *Violence as a public health problem*. Atlanta: U.S. Public Health Service.

U.S. Bureau of the Census. (1988). *Statistical abstract of the United States: 1989* (109th ed). Washington, DC: U.S. Government Printing Office.

U.S. Department of Health and Human Services. (1985). *Health: United States.* (DHHS Publication No. PHS-86-1232). Hyattsville, MD: U.S. Public Health Service, National Center for Health Statistics.

U.S. Department of Health and Human Services. (1987). *Report of the Surgeon General's workshop on children with HIV infection and their families* (DHHS Publication No. HRS-D-MC, 87-1). Washington, DC: U.S. Government Printing Office.

U.S. Department of Justice. (1985). *Crime in the United States: Uniform crime reports, 1975, 77, 79, 81, 83, 85* (pp. 18-19). Washington, DC: U.S. Government Printing Office.

U.S. Department of Justice. (1987). *Uniform crime report for the United States.* Washington, DC: U.S. Government Printing Office.

U.S. Department of Justice. (1989). *FBI. Population at risk: Rates and selected crime indicators.* Washington, DC: U.S. Government Printing Office.

Abuse

Campbell, J. (1981). Misogyny and homicide of women. *Advances in Nursing Science,* 3(1), 67-85.

Campbell, J. (1984). Abuse of female partners. In J. Campbell and J. Humphreys (Eds.), *Nursing care of victims of family violence* (pp. 246-275). Norwalk, CT: Appleton & Lange.

Campbell, J. (1984). Nursing care of abused women. In J. Campbell and J. Humphreys (Eds.), *Nursing care of victims of family violence* (p. 102). Norwalk, CT: Appleton & Lange.

Campbell, J. (1986). Nursing assessment for risk of homicide with battered women. *Advances in Nursing Science,* 8(4), 36-51.

Centers for Disease Control. (1989a). Education about adult domestic violence in U.S. and Canadian medical schools 1987-88. *MMWR,* 38(2), 17-19.

Gelles, J., and Cornell, C. (1985). *Intimate violence in families.* Beverly Hills, CA: Sage Publications.

Gelles, R., and Straus, M. (1988). *Intimate violence: The definitive study of the causes and consequences of abuse in the American family.* New York: Simon & Schuster.

Goolkasian, G. (1986). *Confronting domestic violence: A guide for criminal justice agencies* (GDJ-28-23-V-81). Washington, DC: Office of Justice Programs, National Institute of Justice.

Gilbert, C. (1988). Sexual abuse and group therapy. *Journal of Psychosocial Nursing and Mental Health Services,* 26(5), 19-23.

King, M., and Ryan, J. (1989). Abused women: Dispelling myths and encouraging interventions. *Nurse Practitioner,* 14(5), 47-58.

McLeer, S., and Anwar, R. (1989). A study of battered women presenting in an emergency department. *American Journal of Public Health,* 79(1), 65-66.

Moehling, K. (1988). Battered women and abusive partners: Treatment issues and strategies. *Journal of Psychosocial Nursing and Mental Health Services,* 26(9), 8-11, 15-17, 39-40.

Stark, E. (April, 1981). Wife abuse in the medical setting: An introduction for health personnel. Monograph series #7. Washington, DC: National Clearinghouse on Domestic Violence, U.S. Government Printing Office.

Stark, E., and Flitcraft, A. (1982). Medical therapy as repression: The case of battered women. *Health and Medicine,* Summer-Fall, 29-32.

Stark, E., and Flitcraft, A. (1987). Violence among intimates: An epidemiological review. In J. van Haslett (Ed.), *Handbook of family violence,* (p.7). New York: Plenum Pub.

Walker, L. (1977). *The battered woman.* New York: Harper & Row.

Walker, L. (1984). *The battered woman syndrome.* New York: Springer.

Rape

Burgess, A., and Holmstrom, L. (1979). *Rape, crisis, and recovery.* Englewood Cliffs, NJ: Prentice-Hall.

Centers for Disease Control. (1989b). 1989 Sexually transmitted diseases treatment guidelines. *MMWR,* 38(S-8), 1-43.

Foster, I., and Bartlett, J. (1989). Anti-HIV substances for rape victims. *JAMA,* 261(23), 3407.

Gellert, G., and Mascola, L. (1989). Rape and AIDS. *Pediatrics,* 83 (4, Pt. 2), 644-645.

Golan, N. (1978). *Treatment in crisis situations.* New York: Free Press.

Hicks, D., Martin, L., Getchell, J., Heath, J., Francis, D., McDougal, J., Curran, J., and Voeller, B. (1985). Inactivation of HTLV-III/LAV-infected cultures of normal human lymphocytes by non-oxynol-9 in vitro. *Lancet,* 2(8469-70), 1422-1423.

Horos, C. (1985). *Rape.* New Canaan, CT: Tobey Publishing.

Keene-Payne, R. (1988). Serving as an expert witness in rape cases. *Nurse Practitioner,* 13(7), 59-62.

Koss, M., and Burkhart, B. (1989). A conceptual analysis of rape victimization. *Psychology of Women Quarterly,* 13(1), 27-40.

Osterholm, M., MacDonald, K., Danila, R., and Henry, K. (1987). Sexually transmitted diseases in victims of sexual assault. *New England Journal of Medicine,* 316(16), 1024.

Siegel, J., Sorensen, S., Golding, J., Burnam, M., and Stein, J. (1989). Resistance to sexual assault: Who resists and what happens? *American Journal of Public Health,* 79(1), 27-31.

Nursing research

Campbell, J. (1989). Women's responses to sexual abuse in intimate relationships. *Health Care for Women International,* 10(4), 335-346.

Cochrane, D. (1987). Emergency nurses' attitudes toward the rape victim. *AARN Newsletter,* 43(7), 14-18.

Damrosch, S., Gallo, B., Kulak, D., and Whitaker, C. (1987). Nurses' attributions about rape victims. *Research in Nursing and Health,* 10(4), 245-251.

Helton, A., McFarlane, J., and Anderson, E. (1987). Battered and pregnant: A prevalence study. *American Journal of Public Health,* 77(10), 1337-1339.

Helton, A., and Snodgrass, F. (1987). Battering during pregnancy: Intervention strategies. *Birth,* 14(3), 142-147.

McFarland, J. (1989). Battering during pregnancy: Tip of an iceberg revealed. *Women and Health,* 15(3), 69-84.

Newbern, V. (1989). Sexual victimization of child and adolescent patients. *Image,* 21(1), 10-13.

Tilden, V., and Shepherd, P. (1987). Increasing the rate of identification of battered women in an emergency department: Use of a nursing protocol. *Research in Nursing and Health,* 10(4), 209-215.

Ward, C. (1988). The attitudes toward rape victims scale: Construction, validation, and cross-cultural applicability. *Psychology of Women Quarterly,* 12(2), 127-146.

Women's Health-Compromising Behaviors

Objectives

After reading and studying this chapter, the student should be able to:

1. Discuss common nutritional concerns of women.

2. Explain the addictive properties and long-term effects of smoking.

3. Compare alcohol abuse with other forms of substance abuse.

4. List common causes and effects of stress in women.

5. Apply the nursing process when caring for a client with a health-compromising behavior.

6. Use appropriate nursing interventions for a client with a health-compromising behavior.

Introduction

During the past 30 years, dramatic changes have altered women's perceptions of their health needs and issues. Increases in the number of working women, working mothers, and single mothers have affected women's lifestyles and health behaviors and changed the demands they make on the health care system.

This chapter explores some of those concerns, including nutrition, substance abuse (nicotine, alcohol, and other drugs), and stress. Then it focuses on ways in which the nurse can help women adopt behaviors that prevent disease and promote health.

Nutritional concerns

Modern life creates nutrition-related health problems. Food manufacturing and packaging have decreased the vitamin and mineral content of the average diet and have added sugar, salt, fat, and artificial ingredients. Society's reliance on technology to perform physical labor has decreased physical activity and caloric expenditure among Americans, typically increasing obesity (body weight of 20% or more above the ideal).

Nutrition and disease

Despite increased knowledge about nutritional needs, many people do not eat a balanced diet. Rather, their food choices and eating patterns are influenced by socioeconomic and cultural factors, including:

• individual food preferences
• cultural preferences and traditions
• social associations (for example, large meals as social events)
• family demographics, including the age and number of family members
• product advertising and promotion
• established eating patterns
• allotted food preparation time
• number of meals eaten at home
• availability of prepared foods.

GLOSSARY

Alcoholism: pathologic pattern of alcohol use marked by cognitive, behavioral, and physiologic symptoms that indicate inability to reduce intake, continued use despite adverse consequences, tolerance, and withdrawal. Also called alcohol dependence.

Amphetamine: drug that stimulates the sympathetic nervous system.

Anorexia nervosa: eating disorder characterized by a morbid fear of weight gain and by self-starvation.

Barbiturate: nonnarcotic, sedative drug that can cause physical and psychological dependence.

Bulimia: eating disorder characterized by a binge-purge cycle, depression, and self-deprecation.

Cocaine: central nervous system stimulant derived from coca leaves that produces euphoria and anesthetizes nerve endings.

Delirium tremens (DTs): acute, sometimes fatal psychotic reaction to alcohol withdrawal that occurs in about 5% of withdrawing alcoholics and usually lasts 2 to 4 days; characterized by fever, tachycardia, hypertension or hypotension, vivid hallucinations, seizures, and combativeness.

Flashback phenomenon: auditory and visual hallucinations related to a previous frightening or pleasurable experience. May result from use of a psychoactive drug.

Hallucinogen: psychotomimetic drug that alters consciousness and causes hallucinations.

Hyperplastic obesity: obesity characterized by an increase in the number of fat cells.

Hypertrophic obesity: obesity characterized by an increase in the size of fat cells.

Marijuana: commonly abused drug obtained from the flowering tops, stems, and leaves of the hemp plant. Also called cannabis sativa, weed, grass, pot, or tea.

Methadone: synthetic narcotic used in detoxification programs to replace heroin.

Nicotine: addictive alkaloid found in tobacco.

Obesity: body weight of 20% or more above ideal weight.

Opiate: narcotic drug derived from opium (such as codeine, morphine, and heroin) that may relieve pain or induce sleep.

Polypharmacy: practice of taking different drugs simultaneously in varying dosages.

Scanning: technique for relieving stress by identifying and then relaxing tense muscles.

Substance abuse: maladaptive pattern of substance use marked by continued use despite knowledge of impaired social, occupational, psychological, or physical functioning caused or exacerbated by its use. Abused substances can include nicotine (in tobacco), alcohol, and legal and illegal drugs.

Substance dependence: cluster of cognitive, behavioral, and physiologic symptoms that indicate impaired control of substance use as evidenced by tolerance and withdrawal symptoms.

In response to recent reports from governmental and institutional boards about the effects of food on health, many Americans are trying to reduce their intake of fats, salt, and artificial additives while increasing their fiber intake. Unfortunately, these attempts can be made difficult for consumers of prepared foods. Many prepared foods, such as soups and high-fiber cereals, contain high levels of sodium, which can contribute to hypertension and cardiac disease, or sugar, which can affect body weight. Some women change their eating patterns to try to consume a more healthful diet; others may have altered eating patterns that have caused obesity or have resulted from an eating disorder, such as anorexia nervosa and bulimia. (For more information, see *Nutritional concerns*, page 340.)

Obesity

Current standards define obesity as a body weight that is 20% or more above the norm, or ideal. Based on insurance company actuarial tables, the norm is the range of weights (related to height and age) associated with the lowest mortality rate (Brownell and Foreyt, 1986).

Although morbidity and mortality statistics related to obesity are imprecise, many researchers believe that a weight of 20% to 30% above the norm increases an individual's risk for:

• cardiovascular disease, including congestive heart failure, hypertension, and thrombophlebitis
• gallbladder and biliary disease
• hyperlipidemia
• maturity-onset diabetes
• hernia
• arthritis
• pulmonary insufficiency
• pregnancy-induced hypertension.

As an individual's weight increases beyond 30% above the norm, so does the risk of developing these conditions.

Nutritional concerns

A common nutritional concern among women is obesity, but the eating disorders anorexia nervosa and bulimia are increasingly common problems. To provide appropriate care, the nurse should be familiar with the signs and symptoms, selected treatments, and prognosis for each of these concerns, as described in the following chart.

SIGNS AND SYMPTOMS	TREATMENTS	PROGNOSIS
Obesity		
• Significant long-term weight gain, skin thickening, pale striae, weakness, joint strain or pain • Pattern of overeating in relation to energy expenditure or history of endocrine abnormality (less common) • Weight-to-height ratio of more than 20% above normal • Triceps skinfold measurement indicating obesity	• A nutritionally balanced diet providing fewer calories than are expended daily (treatment of choice). May be particularly effective when the client learns to recognize environmental and psychological factors that prompt excessive eating (Long, 1989). • A medically supervised liquid diet containing protein, vitamins, and minerals, followed by establishment of a healthful diet and eating behaviors (for clients who are at least 40 pounds overweight). A liquid diet can provide rapid weight loss, averaging 40 pounds in 10 to 15 weeks. However, rapidly lost weight is three times as likely to be regained and may cause muscle loss (Gershoff, 1989). • Intestinal bypass. This last-resort measure for morbid obesity has a relatively high morbidity and mortality. The client eats less because overeating causes diarrhea, flatus, or abdominal distention (Gastric Restrictive Surgery, 1989).	The long-term (2 to 3 years) success rate for maintaining weight loss is only about 10% (only one in ten clients maintains weight loss) (Agras, 1989). The client who has been obese throughout childhood and adolescence may have fat cell hyperplasia, making significant weight loss difficult. Such a client must weigh the emotional stress of dieting against the likelihood of regaining lost weight. A client who is slightly (10 to 20 pounds) overweight and feels no stress related to weight may benefit more from accepting a decision not to diet than from searching for a weight-loss method. Nutritional counseling and a regular exercise program also may help.
Anorexia nervosa		
• Weight loss of more than 25% of body weight • Distorted body image, morbid fear of obesity, compulsion to be thin • Inadequate protein and caloric intake with avid exercising and refusal to eat • Abuse of laxatives or diuretics • Dental caries, amenorrhea, susceptibility to infection • Skeletal muscle atrophy, loss of fatty tissue, reduced bone density • Bradycardia, orthostatic hypotension • Blotchy skin, fine lanugo hair on arms and back, scalp hair dryness or loss • Repressed anger, poor self-concept	No single treatment approach has proved most effective. Treatments include: • total parenteral nutrition for an extremely malnourished client • psychiatric evaluation and therapy • behavior modification • isolation of the client from her family • modification of detrimental family dynamics • hospitalization • careful monitoring of body weight • photography before and after treatment • art therapy, which includes drawing oneself.	Prognoses vary. Some experts predict that many clients treated will increase their food intake substantially, others will increase food intake and then relapse, and some will continue to eat very little. Of the last group, a few will die. Other experts suggest that anorexia will continue because it allows her to control her family. A client who regains weight may resume menses and reverse the effects of malnutrition.
Bulimia		
• Weakness, flaccid paralysis, lethargy, convulsions from electrolyte imbalances • Uncontrollable binge eating followed by vomiting • Dieting, vomiting, or use of laxatives, enemas, and diuretics to lose weight • Exaggerated dread of weight gain • Muscle weakness • Dental staining and deterioration • Depression, self-deprecation • Irregular menses • Secretive behavior, such as hoarding food and laxatives and eating in private	Because bulimia has only recently been recognized as a disease, the most effective therapy is not yet known. Treatments include: • behavior modification • hospitalization if the client's physical or psychological condition continues to deteriorate • careful monitoring of body weight (Brownell and Foreyt, 1986) • psychiatric evaluation and therapy • art therapy • combined cognitive and behavioral therapies for 4 to 6 months.	Combined cognitive and behavioral therapies have had some success. In highly motivated bulimic clients, 60% have been able to stop binge eating (Agras, 1989). Continued bulimia may cause medical complications, such as gastric dilation, parotid swelling, esophagitis, pancreatitis, and dysrhythmias (Kirkley, 1986).

Obesity also may be related to social, emotional, and financial problems. Obese people may suffer discrimination, resulting in feelings of rejection, isolation, and loss of self-esteem (Burtis, Davis, and Martin, 1988).

According to actuarial tables, almost 50% of American men become overweight by mid-life, typically gaining most of this excess weight during their thirties. Up to 60% of women are overweight by mid-life, typically gaining weight during their forties and fifties. Between 2% and 15% of children and adolescents also are overweight (Burtis, Davis, and Martin, 1988).

Many people who try to lose weight become locked in a cycle of weight loss and weight gain. Women commonly try crash diets, which rob the body of nutrients. The body reacts to these diets as if it were undergoing starvation, slowing the basal metabolic rate by around 30%. This slowdown in caloric use continues after the dieter returns to normal eating, typically causing the dieter to regain any lost weight and possibly more.

Anorexia nervosa

Anorexia nervosa (an eating disorder characterized by preoccupation with food and an irrational fear of weight gain) affects adolescent girls and young women at least 10 times as often as young men. Societal pressure to be thin and cultural norms that equate slimness with beauty may play a part in anorexia nervosa.

This disorder leads to self-imposed dieting that continues in spite of weight loss, hunger, threats, and family members' pleas to eat. Although the exact cause is unknown, anorexia nervosa may stem from psychological problems related to identity and self-concept. Because the anorexic typically refuses to eat, this disorder can lead to severe weight loss, amenorrhea (absence of menstruation), and other problems. Family dynamics play an important role in treatment for this disorder.

Bulimia

With bulimia (an eating disorder characterized by insatiable food cravings that typically result in food binges followed by depression and self-deprecation), the client develops a binge-purge pattern, consuming large quantities of food and then purging the body by self-induced vomiting, laxatives, or other methods. Once thought to be a variant of anorexia nervosa, bulimia now is recognized as a distinct and much more common disorder.

The average bulimic client is a woman in her mid-twenties, although bulimia may begin at age 17 and extend beyond age 50. Between 10% and 25% of bulimic clients weigh below the norm; more than 50% weigh at least 10% over the norm. The precise cause of bulimia is unknown but may be similar to that of anorexia nervosa.

Experts have not yet identified all the disorder's ramifications and long-range effects. Because depression commonly accompanies changes in eating habits, health care professionals typically diagnose bulimia as a primary depressive disorder accompanied by dietary fluctuations.

Substance abuse

Substance abuse is a maladaptive pattern of substance use marked by continued use despite knowledge of impaired social, occupational, psychological, or physical functioning caused or exacerbated by substance use (American Psychiatric Association [APA], 1987). The abused substance may be nicotine, alcohol, or an over-the-counter, prescription, or illegal drug. According to the APA, any three or more of the following behaviors indicate abuse:
• ingesting the substance more frequently or in larger amounts than prescribed
• persistently desiring to quit or reduce use, or unsuccessfully attempting to quit or reduce use
• spending an inordinate amount of time seeking, taking, or recovering from the substance
• neglecting obligations because of intoxication or withdrawal symptoms
• reducing important occupational or social activities because of substance use
• continuing substance use despite knowledge of adverse effects
• developing a tolerance to the substance's effects
• manifesting characteristic withdrawal symptoms when not taking the substance
• taking the substance to relieve or prevent withdrawal symptoms.

When caring for a client, the nurse may uncover substance abuse or abuse-related conditions, such as trauma, malnutrition, sexually transmitted diseases, skin diseases, tuberculosis, or endocarditis. The nurse also may uncover use of more than one substance, such as alcohol and tranquilizers or polypharmacy (simultaneous use of several drugs). The nurse who cares for a substance abuser should keep the following points in mind.

• Addictive substances act on the brain, engaging brain circuits related to emotion, motivation, and behavior.
• Addictive behavior is motivated by the pleasure or reward the substance gives.
• Susceptibility to addictive drugs and the capacity to recover from addiction vary greatly among individuals.
• No single addictive personality exists, although personality traits may play a role in addiction (Cohen, 1988).

A substance abuser typically uses two key defense mechanisms: denial and isolation. When using denial, the abuser rejects the notion that the abused substance is causing a problem, thus impeding treatment and recovery. When using isolation, the abuser separates himself or herself from people, situations, information, or feelings that challenge the denial. Use of denial may prevent recovery or promote a relapse in a former substance abuser.

The denial-isolation pattern that enables the abuser to continue substance abuse also may induce guilt, shame, low self-esteem, and loneliness. The abuser may rationalize the dependence or project emotions onto others, resulting in dependence on others, lying about or making excuses for continued substance abuse, extreme withdrawal symptoms, social isolation, or loss of responsibility (Kozlowski, et al., 1989).

A substance abuse problem may be complicated by polypharmacy. Polypharmacy is a major cause of drug-related deaths.

After detoxification, former substance abusers may resume substance abuse in a search for the intense pleasure the substance brings or in response to extreme stress.

Inner city hospitals report soaring rates of neonates damaged by heroin, methadone, alcohol, and crack cocaine. Of 4,000 neonates studied, 10% to 17% were affected by their mother's substance abuse (Lewis, Bennett, and Schmeder, 1989).

The number of neonates born to crack-abusing women has increased 10% per year in the past 3 years (Lewis, Bennett, and Schmeder, 1989). One sign of crack or cocaine use is neonatal depression, in which the neonate does not look at the mother, does not respond to stimuli, and is poorly oriented. According to Lewis, Bennett, and Schmeder, crack- or cocaine-affected neonates also show subnormal stepping and walking reflexes on the Brazelton Neonatal Behavioral Assessment. (For information about substance abuse during the antepartal, intrapartal, and postpartal periods, see Chapter 22, High-Risk Antepartal Clients; Chapter 31, High-Risk Intrapartal Clients; and Chapter 38, High-Risk Neonates).

Smoking poses special risks for pregnant women. Nicotine causes vasoconstriction that can decrease the placental blood supply. This decreased blood supply in turn may decrease fetal growth and cause low birth weight. (For more information, see Chapter 16, Conception and Fetal Development.)

Properties of addictive substances

Cohen (1988) reports that addictive substances may share most or all of the same properties. They may:
• offer reward and reinforcement for use
• promote changes in brain function or mood that increase as drug amounts increase
• produce tolerance
• cause withdrawal symptoms when stopped.

Examples of addictive drugs include nicotine, alcohol, cocaine, cannabis sativa (marijuana), opiates, and such other drugs as barbiturates, amphetamines, hallucinogens, tranquilizers, and sedatives. (For more information about these drugs, see *Understanding substance abuse*.)

Nicotine

For many years, most people considered smoking tobacco a habit. Today, experts recognize that smoking is an addiction to nicotine, a clear to light-amber alkaloid found in tobacco and classified as a stimulant. When ingested, nicotine increases the heart rate and blood pressure.

Incidence

Although North American culture has begun to restrict smoking, up to 80% of Americans still are affected by it. About 50 million Americans smoke, and millions of others breathe second-hand smoke from others' cigarettes (Kozlowski, et al., 1989). The typical smoker begins with a few cigarettes a day in adolescence. One-third to two-thirds of adolescents who smoke two or more cigarettes daily eventually become habitual smokers of at least one pack per day.

Addictive properties

Milhorn (1989) noted that nicotine:
• causes addiction by altering brain chemistry and stimulating the brain to release dopamine, a chemical implicated in heroin, cocaine, and other addictions
• displays the common features of addictive substances, including escalating use and physical withdrawal symptoms with discontinuation of use
• is as addicting or more addicting than most other drugs.

Understanding substance abuse

The nurse who cares for a client who abuses alcohol or drugs needs to know the incidence, signs and symptoms, and treatments for each substance.

INCIDENCE AND SUBSTANCE	SIGNS AND SYMPTOMS	TREATMENT
Alcohol		
l0 million U.S. citizens are alcoholics (Hyman and Cassem, 1987)	• Depressed brain activity and respirations • Blood vessel dilation resulting in flushed skin, sweating, and clammy palms • Alcohol-related medical complications, such as cirrhosis, gastritis, pancreatitis, polyneuropathy, heart muscle disease, heart failure, and coronary artery disease • Alcoholic blackouts (amnesia of the time period when drinking) • Drinking bouts of 48 hours or more • Alcohol-related problems, such as arrests for drunken driving, work problems, drinking before breakfast, or controlling the alcohol craving by drinking mouthwash, antifreeze, or other forms of nonbeverage alcohol *Withdrawal symptoms* • Mild symptoms, including agitation, tremulousness, anorexia, disturbed sleep, and occasional hallucinations and seizures • Severe symptoms, including convulsions, hallucinations, and delirium tremens (acute psychotic reaction to alcohol withdrawal)	• Detoxification (process of freeing the client from alcohol dependency by lowering the blood alcohol level and controlling withdrawal symptoms) • Withdrawal over 3 or more days • Treatment of withdrawal symptoms with medications and support from a health care professional, friend, or family member • Total avoidance of alcohol and reliance on a supportive network after detoxification • Referral to an alcoholic rehabilitation program, such as Alcoholics Anonymous • Referral to a family support group
Cocaine		
More than 30 million U.S. citizens have tried cocaine, about 6 million use the drug several times a day, and half of those may be addicted (Rubenstein, 1989).	• Vasoconstriction, tachycardia, increased blood pressure • Euphoria, hallucinations, feelings of increased mental and physical prowess • Gaunt appearance • Maladaptive behavior, impaired judgment and social or occupational functioning • Postcocaine crash lasting several hours or days after drug binge (ingestion every 10 minutes), producing severe depression, anxiety, irritability and migrainelike headaches (Satel and Gawin, 1989) *Withdrawal symptoms* • Drug craving, irritability, shaking • Anorexia or hunger and nausea • Irregular sleep patterns • Lack of motivation, intense subjective feelings, depression, suicidal urges	• Detoxification • Withdrawal over 3 or more days • Treatment of withdrawal symptoms with medications and support from a health care professional, friend, or family member • Strict control over or total avoidance of cocaine use • Replacement of the cocaine addiction with activities that support positive human relationships and increase self-esteem (Hogan, 1990) • Referral to a drug rehabilitation program
Marijuana (cannabis sativa)		
Almost 60% of U.S. citizens have tried marijuana; about 20 million use it daily (Jenike, 1987).	• Dreamlike state, sense of contentment, improved social interaction, loss of inhibitions • Damage to nasal mucosa, alveolar cells, bronchioles, and airways *Acute panic reactions* • Flashback phenomenon, acute psychosis, paranoia • Abdominal discomfort, headache *Acute toxicity* • Impaired reflexes, short-term memory, and depth perception	• Treatment to improve disturbed interpersonal relationships (particularly helpful in adolescents, who may use marijuana to defy authority) • Time to outgrow the habit • Establishment of permanent relationships with nondrug users to help decrease drug use (Cohen, 1988) (continued)

Understanding substance abuse   continued

INCIDENCE AND SUBSTANCE	SIGNS AND SYMPTOMS	TREATMENT
Opiates		
More than 1.3 million U.S. citizens have used heroin; 500,000 to 750,000 persons currently use it (Ball, Corty, Bond, Myer, and Tommesello, 1988).	• Lethargy, nodding, warm, flushed skin • Lower abdominal sensation of intense pleasure • Sensation of pleasure lasting 2 or more hours *Withdrawal symptoms 8 to 12 hours after the last dose of heroin or morphine* • Dilated pupils, rhinorrhea, and lacrimation • Sweating, slight temperature elevation *Withdrawal symptoms 2 to 14 days after the last dose of heroin or morphine* • Insomnia • Nausea, vomiting, and diarrhea • Tachycardia and hypertension • Muscular weakness, twitches, joint pain, piloerection	• Correction of opiate overdose with naloxone or naltrexone • Detoxification with methadone • Referral to specific drug treatment center
Barbiturates		
Use is unknown because barbiturates are easily obtained by prescription.	• Slurred speech, unsteady gait • Vertical or horizontal nystagmus *Barbiturate overdose* • Respiratory depression, death *Withdrawal symptoms* • Seizures	• Detoxification with decreasing doses of pentobarbital until the drug is metabolized. This prevents seizures associated with rapid drop in blood levels of barbiturate.
Amphetamines		
Amphetamine use is estimated to be higher than opiate use in the United States.	• Rapid speech • Headache, anorexia or nausea • Elevated pulse and blood pressure • Fine tremors of the extremities • Dilated pupils with decreased light reactivity *Withdrawal symptoms* • Lethargy, severe depression	• Detoxification using benzodiazepine (Valium) to promote sedation and propranolol (Inderal) to counteract severe adrenergic hyperactivity • Hospitalization to control suicidal impulses, if post-amphetamine depression persists
Hallucinogens		
Use is probably high because hallucinogens are the easiest and least expensive to manufacture.	• Kaleidoscopic hallucinations • Tactile, visual, and auditory images • Strong feelings of introspection and disengagement • Feelings of superhuman powers • Extreme excitement, unpredictable destructive behavior, frightening hallucinations • Severe panic reaction or psychotic behavior with overdose (infrequent)	• Supportive management for undesirable adverse effects • Hospitalization for severe panic reactions or prolonged psychotic episodes
Tranquilizers and sedatives		
Use probably is very high because tranquilizers (especially diazepam [Valium] and sedatives are easily obtained by prescription.	• Drowsiness, fatigue, dizziness • Impaired motor coordination, reaction time, and cognitive reasoning • Dysarthria, slurred speech, tremors *Drug overdose* • Confusion, coma, diminished reflexes • Hypotension and depression *Withdrawal symptoms* • Hyperreflexia, seizures, hallucinations	• Gradual withdrawal under medical supervision • Rehabilitation to prevent recurrence of drug abuse

About 80% of those who stop smoking experience physical and psychological withdrawal symptoms, including tobacco craving, irritability, anxiety, poor concentration, restlessness, increased appetite, and decreased heart rate. These symptoms are most severe during the first 48 hours after smoking ceases. Although symptoms gradually subside after about 2 weeks, the desire to smoke may remain for years and peak during periods of high stress.

Like others who attempt to stop using addictive drugs, reformed smokers have a high relapse rate. More than 70% of those who stop smoking resume within 3 months, a relapse rate comparable to that for heroin and alcohol (Kozlowski, et al., 1989).

Nicotine use is associated with the use of other addictive drugs (Milhorn, 1989). Cross-addicted individuals state that nicotine cravings are as intense as those for other drugs.

Many smokers' nicotine addiction is linked with common daily behaviors, such as driving, watching television, and talking on the telephone. Also, smoking offers benefits that addicts find irresistible, including anxiety relief, appetite control, heightened alertness, and improved mental performance.

Long-term effects

Although nicotine causes addiction, more than 4,000 other substances in tobacco cause most of smoking's long-term effects (Surgeon General, 1988). (For more information, see *Effects of smoking*, page 346.) The most common long-term effects include:
• cancers of the lung, mouth, throat, pancreas, kidney, and bladder
• cardiovascular diseases, including cerebrovascular accident (CVA), myocardial infarction, and vascular disease
• respiratory diseases, including emphysema, bronchitis, asthma, and pulmonary infections.

According to the U.S. Surgeon General (1988), tobacco consumption is the major cause of lung cancer worldwide. Among American women, lung cancer is the third most common form of cancer, and its incidence continues to rise.

Smoking also contributes to cardiovascular disease, the principal killer of women over age 65. Of the 524,000 deaths from cardiovascular disease in 1986, 246,000 (47%) were women. Scientists once believed that estrogen protected women from cardiovascular disease, but a 1989 retrospective analysis of 12 studies found no conclusive evidence to support that belief. Further analysis has demonstrated that postmenopausal women with severe coronary artery disease who took estrogen lived longer than those who never took estrogen, but that estrogen had little effect on women with normal coronary arteries (Higgins, 1989).

Alcohol

A depressant or sedative drug, beverage alcohol (ethanol) depresses brain activity and dilates blood vessels. Although alcohol has been used widely since ancient times, modern society offers contradictions about its consumption. Alcoholic beverages are used during religious ceremonies, celebrations, cultural rites, and social events and are valued for their ability to relieve anxiety and induce relaxation. However, most societies value self-control in alcohol consumption. In fact, efforts to regulate alcohol use date from the Babylonian Code of Hammurabi, around 1700 B.C.

Although alcoholism is controllable, it is an incurable, chronic, and potentially fatal disease. Its medical complications include cirrhosis, neurologic disorders, cardiac disease, and coronary artery disease. An alcoholic's life expectancy is 10 to 12 years shorter than a nonalcoholic's. Alcohol consumption contributes to about 50% of fatal motor vehicle accidents, 33% of suicides, and 67% of homicides. Alcoholism and its effects cost U.S. society more than $60 billion annually (Hyman and Cassem, 1987).

Scientists have not yet identified the etiology of alcoholism, but they have uncovered its major risk factors: males with a family history of alcohol abuse. Men have a 3% to 5% chance of developing alcoholism; women, a 1% chance. Women with a family history of alcoholism, however, appear to be at greater risk for developing the disease. Although women typically begin drinking at a later age than men, they suffer the medical and psychosocial effects at the same age, suggesting that women need less alcohol to undergo its adverse effects (Hyman and Cassem, 1987).

Cocaine

A central nervous system stimulant found in coca leaves, cocaine produces effects similar to those of amphetamines. Although Peruvians have chewed coca leaves since 500 A.D., the active ingredient was not extracted from the leaf until 1855 and was not called cocaine until 1859. In the late nineteenth and early twentieth centuries, cocaine was widely used in beverages such as Coca-Cola and in medicines. Although cocaine is not a narcotic, the Harrison Narcotics Act of 1914 restricted its use in the United States.

Effects of smoking

The following chart illustrates the effects of smoking on active smokers (those who smoke) and passive smokers (those who breathe others' smoke) according to the Surgeon General (1988). By understanding the relationship between smoking and disease, the nurse can provide preventive care and recognize possible disease development.

EFFECTS	ACTIVE SMOKERS	PASSIVE SMOKERS
Cancerous	Oral cavity, pharynx, larynx, esophagus, lung, pancreas, kidney, bladder cancer	Lung cancer
Cardiovascular	Aggravation of exercise-induced angina, coronary artery disease, myocardial infarction, cardiac dysrhythmias, sudden cardiac death, cerebrovascular accident, aortic aneurysm, arteriosclerotic and peripheral vascular disease	Aggravation of exercise-induced angina, premature ventricular contractions
Respiratory	Impaired pulmonary function, emphysema, acute and chronic bronchitis, chronic cough, hoarseness caused by vocal cord irritation	Impaired pulmonary function in adults and children, asthma attacks, pulmonary infections, bronchiolitis, slowed lung growth
Perinatal	Increased risk of fetal mortality, low birth weight, spontaneous abortion, sudden infant death syndrome, congenital abnormalities, hyperactivity in childhood, cancer in later life	Low birth weight
Other	Peptic ulcer disease, erythrocytosis (red blood cell destruction), leukocytosis (white blood cell destruction), smoker's skin (pale, grayish cast caused by decreased blood flow to skin), decreased senses of taste and smell, abnormal sperm counts, chromosomal damage, decreased fertility, increased accident rate, altered drug metabolism, increased risk of cardiovascular disorders in women who take oral contraceptives	Increased hospital admissions of infants, middle ear infections and sinusitis in children, decreased growth rate

Cocaine's chief medical use today is as a local anesthetic for nose and throat surgery. It increases heart rate and blood pressure, constricts blood vessels, and stimulates mental awareness.

Once cocaine addiction develops, casual use becomes impossible. Some users become addicted and others die from cardiac effects on their first use. Most cocaine users snorted the powdered drug until 1986, when crack, a less expensive form of cocaine, became available. Produced by heating cocaine powder along with baking soda or another catalyst to produce a hard chunk of the drug, crack is smoked in glass water pipes or rolled in cigarettes and produces the immediate, intense euphoria associated with drugs abused through I.V. injections (Schnoll and Karan, 1989).

Because more women of childbearing age are using cocaine, the nurse must be alert to signs of its use, especially during pregnancy. Many women who use cocaine trade sex for the drug, increasing their risk of contracting a sexually transmitted disease. When used by pregnant women, cocaine causes abruptio placenta. Also, the vasoconstriction, tachycardia, and increased blood pressure caused by cocaine may harm the developing fetus. It can cause low birth weight, decreased neonatal interactive behaviors, congenital (especially urogenital) defects, and increased potential for sudden infant death and other apnea syndromes. When taken shortly before giving birth, cocaine may produce fetal CVA (Lewis, Bennett, and Schmeder, 1989).

Marijuana

A drug found in the flowering tops, stems, and leaves of the hemp plant, marijuana was first used as a drug in 2737 B.C., according to a Chinese medical text. Its use spread from China to India and North Africa, reaching Europe in 500 A.D. and the United States in the early twentieth century (Jenike, 1987).

In low doses, marijuana produces feelings of euphoria and well-being, relaxation, and altered perceptions. Short-term memory becomes impaired, and the user experiences difficulty performing complex motor tasks, such as driving. Balance, stability, information processing, and decision making also are impaired for 4 to 8 hours. Marijuana users report that the drug produces increased hunger, dry mouth and throat, altered sense of time, vivid visual imagery, and a keener sense of hearing. Increased heart rate and peripheral blood flow, reddening of the conjunctiva, and decreased intraocular pressure also occur. Higher doses of marijuana may produce paranoia, delusions, and psychosis. Performance of complex motor tasks is impaired, and reaction time is slowed (National Institute on Drug Abuse, 1981).

Chronic marijuana use may result in amotivational syndromes characterized by apathy, dullness, and impaired judgment, concentration, and memory. Severe abuse may result in loss of interest in personal appearance and the pursuit of personal goals. Other adverse effects may range from frequently occurring panic reactions to less frequently occurring episodes of toxic psychosis.

Physical dependence on marijuana does not develop in occasional users; the effect on long-term users is being studied, and genetic links are being explored. Abrupt discontinuation after long-term use produces withdrawal symptoms, which may include loss of sleep, irritability, restlessness, decreased appetite, weight loss, hyperactivity, and diaphoresis (National Institute on Drug Abuse, 1981).

Opiates

Opiates are narcotic drugs that contain or are derived from opium (found in Papaver somniferum, or poppy plants) or that produce opium's effects. They include morphine (the active ingredient in opium), heroin (a synthetic derivative of morphine and the most widely known opiate), codeine, meperidine (Demerol), methadone, hydromorphone (Dilaudid), and fentanyl (Sublimaze).

References to opium date from 4000 B.C., and the first descriptions of its effects were recorded around 300 B.C. Morphine was isolated from opium in 1805, and heroin was synthesized in 1875. Like cocaine, opiates were banned for nonmedical use in the United States by the Harrison Narcotics Act of 1914. Medical uses of opiates include pain relief, diarrhea and cough relief, and induction of drowsiness. An opiate overdose can cause asphyxiation and death.

Individuals who use opiates daily in regularly increasing doses can become addicted in fewer than 2 weeks. Contrary to popular belief, however, opiate dependence rarely develops from medical use (Chenitz, 1989).

Other drugs

Other types of abused drugs include barbiturates, amphetamines, hallucinogens, tranquilizers, and sedatives.

Barbiturates
Generally classed as sedative or hypnotic drugs, barbiturates can cause physical and psychological dependence. As tolerance for these drugs builds, increased dosages are needed to produce the desired effect. Rapid withdrawal from barbiturates can produce seizures; overdose can cause death.

Amphetamines
Commonly abused stimulants, amphetamines are considered sympathomimetic drugs because they stimulate the sympathetic nervous system. They produce feelings of euphoria and rebound depression.

Hallucinogens
These include lysergic acid diethylamide (LSD), mescaline, and phencyclidine (commonly called PCP or angel dust). Tolerance to hallucinogens builds but dissipates rapidly, and no evidence exists of withdrawal symptoms. However, these drugs can cause psychoses.

Tranquilizers and sedatives
Prescription tranquilizers and sedatives are easily obtained and abused. Women seek treatment for symptoms more frequently than men, and society sanctions relieving uncomfortable symptoms with medications. Together, these factors set the scene for abuse.

Stress

Stress is any emotional, physical, social, economic, or other positive or negative factor that demands a response or change. Men and women are exposed to different stresses and may react differently to them. To help women cope with stress, the nurse needs to recognize these differences. The nurse also must understand that each woman's reaction to stress depends on her experiences, socialization, and values.

Stressors

Stressors are biological, psychological, or social stimuli that strain a woman's resources. They can be specific threats to well-being, such as illness or physical abuse, or subtle demands, such as societal expectations that conflict with a woman's self-concept.

Some factors that particularly stress women include poverty, career and family demands, and aging.

Poverty

More than three-fourths of America's poor are women and children, and many of these women are single heads of households (Santi, 1987). (For additional information, see Chapter 1, Family Nursing Care: History and Trends.) Poverty may bring illness, reduced nutrition, inadequate housing, and limited access to health care, increasing women's stress.

Career and family demands

Women constitute 43% of the nation's labor force (Norris, 1986). The responsibilities of holding a job and managing a home and family may increase stress, causing emotional distress, ambivalence toward the maternal role, and physical ailments. On the other hand, some women may have improved self-esteem and physical health when balancing multiple roles.

Aging

American women live 7 to 8 years longer than American men. The longer a woman lives, the more likely she is to require long-term nursing care or chronic disease management. An older woman may face the stresses of caring for an ailing partner (Jacobs and McDermott, 1989), and she is more likely than a man to suffer the stresses of surviving a spouse, including loneliness and financial problems. An older woman also may experience the psychological stress of aging in a society that values youth.

Coping mechanisms

Every individual develops mechanisms for coping with stress, but some mechanisms are more successful than others. (For more information about coping, see Chapter 2, Family Structure and Function.)

A woman's responses to stress have been shaped since birth. If she felt valued and supported by her family, she probably has the resources to cope with change. If not, however, she may feel unable to handle stress. Ac-

cording to Griffith-Kenney (1986), the following factors can limit a woman's ability to manage stress.

• Powerlessness. Women traditionally have been socialized to be physically, emotionally, and economically powerless. This socialization conflicts with women's changing roles in society. For example, a woman who needs to support her family may be hampered by a belief that she is economically powerless and must rely on a man. Such a woman may respond by becoming depressed or feeling helpless. In turn, she may blame herself for these feelings, increasing her sense of powerlessness.

• Limited options. Women traditionally are taught to avoid confrontation, to seek the approval of others, and to respond to situations passively and submissively. If a woman has accepted this traditional role, she may feel incapable of accomplishing her goals. She may fear trying new coping methods and may deny herself permission to be assertive. She also may avoid making decisions for fear of upsetting others.

• Anger. Through socialization, women learn to be gentle, soft-spoken, and passive. They rarely learn skills for direct communication, negotiation, and confrontation. Society teaches that anger is an improper response for women. Women who express anger may be labeled as overemotional or hysterical, and their anger is trivialized or denied. As a result, women have found indirect outlets for their anger, expressing it through manipulation, depression, physical or sexual activity, and even household chores. Unresolved anger can lead to ineffective coping, including aggression against others and self-destructive acts, such as attempted suicide, substance abuse, alcoholism, or eating disorders.

• Failure to nurture oneself. Women are socialized to nurture and support others. Nurturing themselves and determining their own priorities proves difficult for many women. Typically, they cannot accept their own needs and feel guilty or selfish if they need time for themselves or desire support from others.

• Confusion of internal and external processes. Because women are socialized to respond to others' needs, they may have difficulty developing a clear self-concept. The absence of a clear self-concept produces confusion about the origin of problems, causing women to blame themselves for problems created by others or by the external world. Even some women who have been abused or raped blame themselves, adding self-oppression to the oppression imposed on them by others. Women who can distinguish between internal and external processes can eliminate this double oppression and assess their problems realistically.

Effects of stress

Stress may produce various effects, including:
- elevated blood pressure
- tension or migraine headaches
- sleep-onset insomnia or early morning awakening
- fatigue
- overeating or loss of appetite
- indigestion, nausea, or vomiting
- constipation or diarrhea
- neck, shoulder, or lower back pain
- hives
- increased drug and alcohol consumption
- hyperventilation
- irritability
- depression
- minor accidents
- cold hands or feet
- heart palpitations.

Nursing care

When a client seeks help with a health-compromising behavior, the nurse should use the nursing process to assess the client and intervene appropriately.

Assessment

Perform a thorough assessment, including a health history, physical assessment, and laboratory studies. (For more information and procedures, see Chapter 7, Women's Health Promotion.)

Health history

In addition to the basic history data described in Chapter 7, obtain detailed information about the client's reason for seeking care and related concerns. Also assess her perception of health. (For information about the effect of women's attitudes on their health, see *Nursing research applied: Women's views of health.*)

Nutritional concerns. If the client's basic history data suggest a nutritional concern, request her menstrual history and investigate her mental status. Record her highest and lowest weight during the past year and inquire about her satisfaction with her body weight. A client with a nutritional concern may not perceive her body weight accurately.

NURSING RESEARCH APPLIED

Women's views of health

In a recent study, researchers asked 528 Asian, Black, Caucasian, Hispanic, and Native American women, ages 18 to 45, the question, "What does health mean to you?" Although the women universally preferred exuberant well-being over the absence of disease or symptoms, their specific definitions of health varied greatly. Definitions included self-actualization, healthy life practices, positive self-concept, appropriate body image, social involvement, fitness, full cognitive function, positive mood, and harmony.

The women's answers appeared unrelated to age, education, income, ethnic background, or employment status. The variety of responses supports the assertion that health is a highly personal value that the individual defines.

Application to practice

As this study suggests, the nurse must view the client individually and not assume that demographic variables, such as age and race, define the client's concept of health. Instead, the nurse should assess the client's perception of health before suggesting interventions.

To help the client understand her attitudes toward health, the nurse should ask questions that relate to the client's well-being. Answers to such questions as, "What does health mean to you?" "How are you coping with stressful situations in your life?" and even, "How has your day been going?" will help the client explore her health image.

Woods, N., Laffrey, S., Duffy, M., Lentz, M., Mitchell, E., Taylor, D., and Cowan, K. (1988). Being healthy: Women's images. *Advances in Nursing Science,* 11(1), 36-46.

Using a 24-hour dietary recall or food diary, explore the client's nutritional patterns. Note her diet, eating habits, and use of vitamin and mineral supplements. Also assess her knowledge of nutrition by asking which items she eats from the four basic food groups and the size and number of servings.

Determine if the client has a disorder or cultural or religious beliefs that affect her diet. Note her food preferences and the significance of eating to family life. Also find out which family members buy the groceries and plan and cook meals.

Help the client gain insight into her eating patterns by asking the following questions: "Do you eat because you are hungry or because it is time to eat? Do food flavors influence your eating? Do you clean your plate regardless of whether your hunger is satisfied? What makes you stop eating?" Such questions may help the obese client become aware that she is using food as more than a source of sustenance.

Carefully assess socioeconomic data, including the primary source of income, the relationship of income to financial needs, other sources of assistance, and unmet needs because of financial constraints. A client from a lower socioeconomic group will have to plan carefully to provide a balanced diet on minimal funds.

Exercise and activity. Assess the client's exercise patterns. Exercise can help maintain ideal weight; improve musculoskeletal, cardiovascular, and respiratory fitness; and reduce stress, especially for a client with a sedentary, high-pressure job. Be sure to note any health risks related to exercise. A family history of coronary artery disease, hypertension, CVA, or sudden death suggests cardiovascular disease, which can put an exerciser at risk. A client who smokes or is obese, hypertensive, or sedentary also has increased exercise risks and may require further testing.

Determine the client's age and pregnancy status. An older client with limited joint movement may need an exercise program tailored to her range of motion. A pregnant client may need a modified exercise program.

Find out if the client has participated in an exercise program previously. If so, determine what she liked and disliked about it. Ask if she has a companion with whom exercising might be more motivating and enjoyable. Her answers can aid in creating a personalized exercise plan.

Assess the client's support systems. A client who enlists support from friends or family members is more likely to make permanent health habit changes.

Substance abuse. Assess the client for substance abuse at her annual gynecologic examination or initial prenatal visit. If she uses tobacco, determine the amount and duration of use. Also assess the influence of stress on her tobacco consumption. Identify her concerns about smoking and its effects, and determine if she previously has attempted to stop smoking.

If the client drinks alcohol, determine the amount and duration of use. Ask how her alcohol intake compares with that of others. Identify any relationship between stress and alcohol intake and note her concerns about drinking patterns. Determine how her drinking affects other aspects of her life.

If the client uses drugs, determine which over-the-counter, prescription, and illegal drugs she takes and why. Determine the amount, frequency, and duration of drug use, and inquire about polypharmacy.

Because the family plays such a vital role in substance abuse, assess the family's strengths. (For more information, see Chapter 3, Nursing Process and the Childbearing Family.) To provide individualized care to a substance abuser's family, the nurse must understand the family's dynamics. When assessing the family, identify the member who supports or makes excuses for the abuser most frequently. Determine which members try to help the abuser and which are affected by the abuse.

Assess how the family views the substance abuser: as a helpless victim or as a willful abuser. Evaluate the family's view of self-control and management of ambivalence and uncertainty. Identifying the family's coping mechanisms helps family members recognize their strengths and weaknesses.

If the client refuses to accept that she is a substance abuser, ask questions such as these to clarify the situation:
• "While under the substance's influence, does your behavior violate your normal rules of behavior?" Behavior changes are recognizable signs of a problem.
• "Do you break promises related to substance use?" Broken promises suggest dependence on a substance.
• "Does your version of your substance use differ from that of others?" Examining how her actions affect others helps the client assess behaviors realistically and recognize their causes.

Stress. If the client reports feeling stressed or complains of stress-related symptoms, identify her level of stress, coping mechanisms, and the effects of stress on her life.

First, ask how she knows when she is feeling stressed. Have her identify stressful situations and describe the stresses she has experienced during the past year.

To assess her coping mechanisms, evaluate how she deals with stressful situations, and determine whether her coping strategies are successful.

Ask about the client's physical response to stress. Find out if she perspires profusely, gets butterflies in her stomach, develops headaches, or becomes nauseated. Determine how stress or her response to it has affected her family or work. Ask if stress has significantly affected her life or health.

Physical assessment

Perform a physical assessment as described in Chapter 7, Women's Health Promotion, focusing on specific areas related to the client's life-style concerns.

For example, if the client seeks help with a nutritional concern, note her physical appearance and obtain her current weight, height, and other anthropometric data. Then determine the appropriateness of her body weight for her height, using standard weight tables. Also screen for risk factors, such as hypertension or other cardiovascular disease, that might affect an exercise program. Evidence of disease may require further testing.

Laboratory studies

Review any recent laboratory studies, such as a complete blood count and urinalysis, or other diagnostic tests to obtain baseline information. If risk factors are present, the client may undergo a urine drug screen, human immunodeficiency virus (HIV) test, blood glucose test, serum cholesterol assay, electrocardiography, stress test, and other age-appropriate tests. Test results provide further data for planning appropriate interventions.

Nursing diagnosis

After collecting and analyzing the assessment data, formulate appropriate nursing diagnoses for the client. (For a partial list of possible nursing diagnoses, see *Nursing diagnoses: Health-compromising behaviors*.)

Planning and implementation

After formulating the nursing diagnoses, help the client outline her goals and develop an individualized plan. Use appropriate nursing interventions to help her reach these goals.

NURSING DIAGNOSES

Health-compromising behaviors

The following nursing diagnoses address representative problems and etiologies that a nurse may encounter when helping a client with a health-compromising behavior. Specific nursing interventions for many of these diagnoses are provided in the "Planning and implementation" section of this chapter.

NUTRITIONAL CONCERNS

- Altered nutrition: less than body requirements, related to binge eating followed by purging
- Altered nutrition: less than body requirements, related to self-imposed fasting
- Altered nutrition: more than body requirements, related to binge eating followed by purging
- Altered nutrition: more than body requirements, related to caloric intake that exceeds caloric expenditure
- Altered nutrition: potential for more than body requirements, related to binge eating
- Altered sexuality patterns related to decreased libido
- Anxiety related to possible weight gain
- Anxiety related to refeeding program
- Body image disturbance related to weight gain
- Fear related to weight gain
- Hopelessness related to morbid obesity
- Ineffective family coping: compromised, related to need for control by specific family members
- Ineffective individual coping related to fear of failure
- Knowledge deficit related to nutrition
- Noncompliance related to instructions for increasing caloric intake
- Potential fluid volume deficit related to self-induced vomiting and use of laxatives
- Powerlessness related to binge-purge behavior
- Self-esteem disturbance related to self-perception as obese
- Sleep pattern disturbance related to depression
- Social isolation related to decreased physical attractiveness

SUBSTANCE ABUSE

- Altered family processes related to drug abuse
- Dysfunctional grieving related to loss of ideal family
- Health-seeking behaviors related to smoking cessation

- Hopelessness related to inability to stop alcoholic from drinking
- Ineffective airway clearance related to smoking
- Ineffective breathing pattern related to long-term effects of smoking
- Ineffective family coping: compromised, related to alcoholism
- Ineffective individual coping related to role changes caused by alcoholic family member
- Knowledge deficit related to inability to stop smoking
- Knowledge deficit related to nicotine gum use
- Knowledge deficit related to treatment for substance abuse
- Potential altered parenting related to alcohol's influence
- Potential for infection related to debilitated state of alcoholic
- Powerlessness related to inability to control desire for drug
- Self-esteem disturbance related to loss of control over drinking
- Sexual dysfunction related to consuming large amounts of beverage alcohol

STRESS

- Altered family processes related to changing family structure
- Anticipatory grieving related to aging and changing body image
- Anxiety related to changing role demands
- Knowledge deficit related to stress management
- Social isolation related to longevity beyond that of friends and family

When assisting a client with a health-compromising behavior, take a self-care approach. Self-care recognizes and emphasizes the individual's power over personal actions and encourages the client to act on her behalf to promote health and prevent, detect, and treat disease.

Develop an individualized diet program

For a client with a nursing diagnosis of *altered nutrition: less than body requirements, related to self-imposed fasting* or *altered nutrition: less than body requirements, related to binge eating followed by purging,* plan a refeeding program based on the client's caloric needs. Create a series of well-balanced menus that are acceptable to the client. Have her record her daily intake. To avoid encouraging binging or fasting, urge her to increase caloric intake gradually and to pay attention to any changes in eating patterns.

When a client has a nursing diagnosis of *altered nutrition: more than body requirements, related to caloric intake that exceeds caloric expenditure,* help her apply the following guidelines to develop a nutritious reducing diet.
• Avoid the empty calories found in many snack foods.
• Eat a balanced diet high in nutrients. (For more information, see Chapter 20, Nutrition and Diet Counseling.)
• Eat more calcium-rich foods, such as low-fat dairy products and dark-green vegetables.
• Reduce the amount of fat in the diet.
• Take small portions and chew slowly.
• Eat only when hungry.

Teach about nutrition

Have the client keep a food diary. (For a sample, see *Client teaching: Food and exercise chart.*) This record may serve as a form of behavior modification and a basis for client teaching about nutrition. This is particularly important for a client with a *knowledge deficit related to nutrition.* A diary provides a visual record of eating habits, helping the client decrease or improve food intake.

After the client has kept records for a week, review them together, pointing out healthful and unhealthful patterns and explaining appropriate food choices within the basic food groups. (For more information, see Chapter 20, Nutrition and Diet Counseling.)

Teach about exercise

For a client with a nursing diagnosis of *altered nutrition: more than body requirements, related to caloric intake that exceeds caloric expenditure* or *body image disturbance related to weight gain,* discuss the importance of exercise and a balanced reducing diet. Suggest that the client record exercise along with food intake.

To help motivate the client to exercise, explain its benefits. Aerobic exercise not only speeds weight loss, but also improves muscle tone, increases cardiovascular and respiratory stamina, inhibits bone loss, stimulates peristalsis and thereby reduces the need for laxatives, decreases stress, and enhances the general sense of well-being.

Explain that exercise can take many forms, from simple changes in one's routine, such as walking to work or using the stairs, to full-scale exercise programs. Regardless of the type of exercise chosen, teach the client to do it safely. (For details, see *Client teaching: Exercise safety,* page 354.)

Then explore any misinformation the client may have about exercise and correct it before planning an exercise program. (For more information, see *Exercise myths,* page 355.) Many clients hold mistaken beliefs about exercise, believing, for example, that it can replace a well-balanced diet.

Develop a personalized exercise plan

With the client's input, develop specific, realistic goals for exercise and weight loss. Consider the client's age, occupation, opportunities for exercise, and target weight when setting these goals.

Personalize the exercise plan by discussing the client's exercise preferences. The following questions can help determine her preferences for exercise type, frequency, and duration.
• "Do you prefer to exercise in the morning, afternoon, or evening?"
• "Do you plan to join an exercise class or to exercise on your own?"
• "Which physical activities do you enjoy?"
• "Do you have access to exercise equipment? If so, what kind?"
• "Would a weight-training program interest you?"

Develop a smoking-cessation plan

A client who smokes may have a nursing diagnosis of *health-seeking behaviors related to smoking cessation* or *knowledge deficit related to inability to stop smoking.* If so, help the client explore her smoking habits and develop a plan to stop.

A smoking-cessation plan should include:
• discussion of the client's smoking behavior
• assessment of her interest in smoking cessation

CLIENT TEACHING

Food and exercise chart

To help you and your health care professional understand your eating and exercise patterns, use this chart for 1 week. After eating or exercising, record information on the chart as shown in the sample below.

FOOD INTAKE CHART

	Sample
Time at start and end of eating	7:00 a.m. – 7:15 a.m.
Amount and types of food	4oz. orange juice, 8oz. black coffee
Location	bedroom
Mood	neutral
Body position	standing
Hunger at start Satiety (fullness) at end	none moderate

EXERCISE CHART

	Sample
Time at start and end of exercising	10:00 a.m. – 10:30 a.m.
Type of exercise	walking
Location	city street
Degree of fatigue at start and end	slight at start; none at end
Mood at start and end	neutral at start; happy at end

This teaching aid may be reproduced by office copier for distribution to clients. ©1991, Springhouse Corporation.

- a target date to quit smoking
- smoking-cessation strategies
- a follow-up plan (Milhorn, 1989).

For the client who wishes to stop smoking, follow these steps:
- Determine why the client wants to quit, encouraging her to express the reasons as clearly as possible. Ideally, the reasons should be the client's, not her family's or physician's.
- Help the client understand her habit by examining it thoroughly. Suggest that she keep a cigarette-by-cigarette record for 7 days, recording when, where, with whom, and during which activities she smokes. Have her note the events that immediately precede lighting a

CLIENT TEACHING

Exercise safety

If you walk or jog as part of your exercise plan, follow these tips to make your exercise as safe as possible.

• Have a physical examination (and a stress test, if needed) before beginning any exercise program.
• Wear comfortable, light-color, lightweight clothes in layers.
• Apply reflectors to the back, front, and sleeves of outer garments unless you always exercise during daylight.
• Purchase well-fitting shoes that cushion your feet.
• Select a comfortable surface on which to walk or jog. A school track is ideal.
• Carry water with you and drink 4 ounces every 15 minutes.
• If you must walk or jog along roads, avoid rush hour and stay as far to the side as you can.
• Familiarize yourself with the area in which you are walking or jogging.
• Know the location of telephones and police stations.
• Walk or jog with a friend or a group.
• Carry identification in several places. Sewing a pocket inside an inner garment creates a safe place for keys, money, and identification.
• Be alert at all times.
• Leave valuables at home.
• Tell someone where you are going and when you will return.
• Stop exercising when you tire or experience pain.
• Carry a stick to threaten unfriendly dogs.

This teaching aid may be reproduced by office copier for distribution to clients. © 1991, Springhouse Corporation.

cigarette and describe how she feels afterward. Record-keeping helps the client understand—and break—her smoking habit by identifying when and where she will be tempted to smoke. It also helps in planning specific strategies for handling temptations—for example, by changing routines or patterns associated with smoking.
• Have the client select a target date to quit smoking, based on personal circumstances. For example, if she smokes at work, she may quit on a Friday so that she can adjust to not smoking over the weekend. Planning to quit is more effective than quitting impulsively.
• Promote the client's determination to quit on the target date. Encourage her to remain vigilant, stressing that she should not become overconfident if she is successful initially.
• Have the client enlist help and cooperation from those around her. She needs people to support her decision to quit. Supporters can help by cooperating with the client's efforts to alter her routines.

• Remind the client that relapses are common and do not indicate an inability to quit. Continue to support her if she does suffer a relapse, assuring her that few ex-smokers have quit without a few relapses.

Develop a smoking prevention plan

To prevent smoking and potential nursing diagnoses of *ineffective airway clearance related to smoking* and *ineffective breathing patterns related to long-term effects of smoking,* develop a smoking prevention plan. Early intervention is especially important for adolescents, who are at high risk for smoking. The following strategies are useful:
• Provide information about the harmful effects of smoking. Emphasize effects that concern adolescents most, such as skin wrinkling, tooth and finger staining, and the unpleasant odor on hair and clothes.
• Discuss personal and social attitudes about smoking.
• Emphasize nicotine's addictive nature.
• Discuss the illusions presented in smoking advertisements.
• Hold discussions in a smoke-free environment.
• Involve teachers in the smoking prevention program, helping them understand and support its goals.

(For a case study that shows how to apply the nursing process when caring for a client with a health-compromising behavior, see *Applying the nursing process: Client with knowledge deficit related to inability to stop smoking,* pages 356 and 357.)

Teach about nicotine gum

For a client who wishes to stop smoking, the physician may prescribe nicotine gum, which substitutes for cigarettes much as methadone substitutes for heroin. A client who uses nicotine gum requires physician supervision and may have a nursing diagnosis of *knowledge deficit related to nicotine gum use.* To help such a client, explain the gum's uses and effects.

Nicotine gum may work best for those who smoke between 10 and 15 cigarettes per day. It contains 2 mg of nicotine per piece—not enough to satisfy heavy smokers, although they may find it helpful. The client should chew no more than 4 mg (2 pieces) of gum at a time. Chewing more can irritate the mucous membranes of the mouth and pharynx.

Because 10% of users become dependent on nicotine gum, the client should use it for no more than 3 months and should taper off its use over 3 to 4 weeks (Milhorn, 1989). Advise the client that, although nicotine gum provides some nicotine replacement, it may not be completely satisfying. The rapid nicotine blood levels obtained from smoking do not occur with gum chewing, and gum does not provide the relaxation or social interaction associated with smoking.

Teach about drug therapy

If the physician prescribes drugs to treat substance abuse, review their use and effects with the client. This is particularly important for a client with a nursing diagnosis of *knowledge deficit related to treatment for substance abuse.*

Teach stress-management skills

During the stress assessment in the health history, the client may have become aware of the stressors she faces and her means of coping with them. For a client with a nursing diagnosis of *knowledge deficit related to stress management,* the quest for self-awareness should continue. The nurse can facilitate self-awareness throughout these four phases:

• Initial appraisal. During this phase, help the client assess actual and potential stressors and discuss ways of reducing or reinterpreting them.

• Strategic thinking. Explore possible coping strategies with the client by improving problem-solving and decision-making skills, exploring alternatives, mobilizing other resources, and analyzing previous coping patterns.

• Implementation of coping efforts. Provide support and encouragement as the client adopts and experiments with coping strategies.

• Evaluation. Along with the client, evaluate the usefulness of these coping strategies, reinforcing successful ones, modifying or abandoning unsuccessful ones, and suggesting ways to deal with prolonged stress.

The client who needs help managing stress may benefit from assertiveness training, psychotherapy, individual or group support, exercise, and relaxation techniques, such as deep breathing. (For information about relaxation techniques, see Chapter 21, Family Preparation for Childbirth and Parenting.)

Make referrals

For a client with anorexia nervosa or bulimia, make referrals to other health care team members, such as a psychiatric clinical nurse specialist, psychiatrist, psychologist, social worker, or dietitian. A psychologist may explore the client's needs and family interaction patterns through individual counseling or group therapy. A dietitian may help the client establish and maintain a nutritious diet.

An obese client may benefit from referrals to a dietitian or a weight-loss support group, such as Weight Watchers. Although these groups may provide excellent support, their effectiveness depends on the individual's motivation and the group leader's skill (Brownell and Foreyt, 1986).

Smokers also may benefit from the support of a self-help group or from a referral to a psychologist or hypnotist.

Exercise myths

The nurse can help the client gain realistic expectations about exercise by dispelling common exercise myths with the facts below.

MYTH	FACT
The only reason to exercise is to burn calories.	Although exercise burns calories, it also benefits the entire body by increasing high-density-lipoprotein cholesterol and bone mass; relieving anxiety, stress, and constipation; enhancing cardiovascular fitness; and improving muscle strength, flexibility, and endurance.
No pain, no gain.	Excessive or improper exercise increases the chances of bone, joint, and muscle injury. Benefits are possible without pain.
Muscle will turn to fat if you stop exercising.	Unused muscle does not turn into fat. It breaks down and decreases in size.
Drinking liquids during exercise causes cramps.	Dehydration causes cramps. During exercise, cold drinks leave the stomach quickly and do not cause cramps.
If your body needs liquids while exercising, you'll feel thirsty.	Exercise blunts the body's thirst mechanism. Drinking 16 oz of liquid 15 minutes before exercising and 4 oz every 15 minutes during exercising will prevent dehydration.
Excess weight can be sweated off.	Weight loss immediately after exercise is actually fluid loss. Lost weight from fluids will be regained when they are replenished.
To build strong muscles, you need to eat extra protein.	Stressing the muscles through resistance exercises, such as weight lifting, builds them. No extra protein is required.
Extra vitamins and salt tablets are needed during vigorous exercise.	Extra vitamins provide no benefit and waste money. Because the body normally regulates its need for salt, salt tablets can cause dehydration by pulling water from body tissues. An adequate diet provides necessary salt.
In addition to diet and regular exercise, you need to use special products for cellulite.	Cellulite is an invented word that refers to fat deposits just under the skin. Regular exercise can help reduce some fat deposits, but others cannot be eliminated.
Spot reducing can cause fat loss in an isolated area.	Although exercise may tone a specific muscle group, it cannot remove fat from one spot only.

APPLYING THE NURSING PROCESS

Client with knowledge deficit related to inability to stop smoking

The nursing process can assist the client who needs help to stop smoking. The table below shows how the nurse might use the nursing process when caring for the client described in the case history at right. The first column presents history and physical assessment data followed by a paragraph of mental notes. These notes help the nurse make important mental connections among assessment findings and aid in development of the nursing diagnosis and planning.

The second column lists an appropriate nursing diagnosis; information in the remaining columns is based on this diagnosis. Although not part of the nursing process, a rationale appears for each intervention in the fourth column to explain how it contributes to the care plan.

ASSESSMENT	NURSING DIAGNOSIS	PLANNING
Subjective (history) data • Client states she has smoked since age 17. • Client says she smokes one pack (20 cigarettes) per day. • Client states she is concerned about her health. • Client states her father died from emphysema. • Client states she has bronchitis 3 to 4 times per year. • Client states she is developing an early-morning cough that does not clear until 2 hours after awakening. **Objective (physical) data** • Vital signs: temperature 98.2° F, pulse 72 beats/minute, respirations 16/minute, blood pressure 128/82 mm Hg. • Height 5' 4", weight 122 lb. • Lines around outer corners of eyes, cheeks, and upper lip. • Lungs clear. • Slight hoarseness. **Mental notes** *Client does not seem to be in physical distress, but seems to be serious about seeking help to stop smoking.*	Knowledge deficit related to inability to stop smoking	**Goals** By the next clinic visit, the client will: • explore her reasons for smoking • examine psychosocial reasons for smoking • plan a target date to quit smoking • seek a support group • be aware that relapses are common.

Alcoholism treatment is best handled by a specialized organization or institution. Alcoholics Anonymous, one of the best-known treatment programs, incorporates the following in its program:
• education about alcohol's effects
• use of a support network
• group forgiveness for relapse
• family involvement
• restoration of self-esteem
• promotion of a sense of belonging (feeling like one of a group, which establishes closeness)
• alleviation of loneliness or feelings of isolation
• atmosphere of free expression and catharsis
• sharing of experiences with others
• opportunities to help others.

Similar groups may be available for clients with other forms of substance abuse.

Care for the family
Family care, which may be necessary for nutritional concerns and other health-compromising behaviors, is perhaps most critical to the family of a substance abuser. Substance abuse by one family member involves all family members. Each family member becomes involved in complex interaction patterns that revolve around the abuser's behaviors, such as missing work, coming home late, and taking money to buy the substance. Treatment of a substance abuser's family calls for specialized skills and experience and usually requires a team effort.

For the family with a nursing diagnosis of *ineffective family coping: compromised, related to alcoholism* or *altered family processes related to drug abuse,* assess self-knowledge of these problems and consult with other health care team members, if necessary. Help the family members develop coping strategies and healthy responses to the disease of substance abuse. Promote self-discovery for the family members, helping them understand how they enable the substance abuser to maintain the addiction.

For the family of a substance abuser, the nurse may:
• help each family member detach emotionally from the abuser's behavior and carry on with life. A complex

CASE STUDY

Sarah Green, age 27, is concerned about her inability to stop smoking. She seeks counseling at the Women's Health Clinic.

IMPLEMENTATION		EVALUATION
Intervention Have the client keep a diary of her smoking pattern, recording the time and place of smoking.	**Rationale** Keeping a record may help the client recognize cues that trigger smoking behavior and may uncover a socially reinforced smoking pattern, such as smoking while socializing with friends.	At the next clinic visit, the client: • stated her reasons for smoking • planned a target date to quit smoking • selected a support person • expressed determination to stop smoking.
Help the client plan a target date to quit smoking.	A smoking-cessation plan that begins when the temptation to smoke is lowest can set a deadline and increase the chances of success.	
Encourage the client to seek help from friends who support her decision. Encourage her to continue with her plan.	Supporters can increase the client's resolve to quit and provide understanding and care when difficulties arise.	
Advise the client to telephone the Women's Health Clinic if she has difficulty quitting.	Even if a relapse occurs, encouragement reminds the client that quitting is possible. Clinic counselors can provide reassurance and reinforce the client's decision to quit smoking.	

process, emotional detachment requires a change in behavior toward the addicted family member (Gentry, 1987).

• help each family member develop coping strategies that allow a healthy response to the disease of substance abuse.

• help the family work through the seeming contradictions of recovery, such as harsh or uncaring treatment designed to aid in the abuser's recovery.

• help family members develop insight into their behaviors. For example, the nonaddicted partner may maintain the addiction by making excuses for the abuser, completing the abuser's tasks, or giving the abuser money. Other family members may perpetuate these behaviors as they assume responsibility for the abuser's or the abuser's partner's actions.

• provide information about resources available for treatment of the abuser and family members.

• help nonaddicted family members assume responsibility for themselves and for one another. This frees them from stereotyping as helpless victims or willing accomplices and allows the recovering abuser to resume previous roles gradually. As the abuser recovers, family members will need help acknowledging ambivalent feelings about changing family relationships.

Evaluation

After the plan is implemented, evaluate its effectiveness, comparing the client's behaviors to her goals. If the client has not complied with the plan, reanalyze the assessment data and confirm the nursing diagnosis with her. If necessary, modify the plan.

Increase the client's motivation to change her behaviors by asking for her assistance in the evaluation. For example, work together in reviewing her food diary and in planning weekly menus that include basic nutrients. Emphasize the importance of her weekly weight checks. To ensure correction of serious nutritional problems, work closely with the client and her dietitian.

Typical evaluation statements may include:

• The client kept food and exercise records for 2 weeks and brought them to her next clinic visit.

• The client helped plan an exercise program and followed it for 2 weeks.
• The client lost 4 pounds in 2 weeks.
• The client expressed an understanding of USRDA standards.
• The client expressed a feeling of self-worth and satisfaction with her exercise program.
• The client began a program of walking with a friend.
• The client set a target date to quit smoking.
• The client agreed to enter a rehabilitation program for cocaine users.
• Nonaddicted family members examined their past and present roles, identifying role changes.
• Nonaddicted family members acknowledged their ambivalence about change.
• Some family members expressed resentment toward agencies that treat alcoholics.
• The client identified stressful situations and her physical reactions to them.

Documentation

A client who seeks help for a health-compromising behavior probably will need follow-up care to help ensure long-term change. This requires regular use of the nursing process. Based on initial and follow-up assessment findings, use the nursing process to formulate nursing diagnoses and then plan, implement, and evaluate the client's care.

The client's health-compromising behavior will determine what specific information must be documented. However, typical documentation includes:
• client's vital signs
• client's height and weight
• nutritional status
• health history information pertinent to health-compromising behavior
• goals established with the client to address the specific behavior
• plan of care to address the specific behavior
• evaluation of the client's progress
• client's perception of progress.

Chapter summary

Chapter 15 described behaviors that may compromise a woman's health and explored the related nursing care. Here are the chapter highlights.
• Common nutritional concerns include obesity, anorexia nervosa, and bulimia. The nurse must consider the cultural and psychosocial meanings of food for a client with a nutritional concern.
• Smoking, an addictive habit, adversely affects the lungs, cardiovascular system, and fetal development. For this addiction, nursing interventions include developing smoking-cessation and prevention programs and teaching about nicotine gum.
• A client may abuse various substances, including alcohol, cocaine, marijuana, opiates, and nonnarcotic (nonopiate) drugs. For such a client, the nurse can intervene by teaching about drug therapy, making referrals for substance abuse programs, and helping the family members identify and cope with their feelings about the problem.
• Substance abuse by a pregnant client can adversely affect the fetus's health. The nurse must be alert to signs of substance abuse in a pregnant client.
• Exercise is an important intervention for obesity and stress. The nurse must individualize the client's exercise program to ensure safety and to meet the client's needs.
• Stress related to changing roles and responsibilities affects many women. The nurse can help a client cope with stress by suggesting stress-management skills, such as deep breathing and scanning for tension.
• For any health-compromising behavior, the nurse uses the nursing process to assess the client, formulate appropriate diagnoses, plan and implement interventions, and evaluate their effectiveness.

Study questions

1. Karen Murdoch, a 17-year-old senior in high school, has just received a diagnosis of anorexia nervosa. What is a possible cause of this eating disorder? What may be prescribed for Karen's treatment?

2. Sandy Hoffman, age 29, has gained 30 pounds (10 pounds after each of three pregnancies). She comes to the clinic for guidance on improving her eating habits and beginning an exercise program. How can the nurse help Ms. Hoffman?

3. Carol Freeman, age 42, has requested help in her attempt to stop smoking. She is newly divorced, has two teenage sons, and runs her own advertising agency. Which psychosocial aspects of smoking should the nurse consider when helping this client develop a smoking-cessation plan?

4. During her annual gynecologic examination, Anne Brownlee, age 22, says that she and her husband Jim are ready to start planning a family. Her history reveals that she uses cocaine "occasionally." What should the nurse tell Ms. Brownlee about cocaine's effects on her and the fetus she hopes to conceive?

5. Nora Sokolowski has returned to college at age 36. She feels stressed because she works full-time, is recently widowed, and wishes she had a child. Which nursing interventions may help this client cope better with her stress?

Bibliography

American Cancer Society. (1989). Cancer statistics 1989. *CA, A Cancer Journal for Clinicians*, 39(1), 3-20.

American Psychiatric Association. (1987). *Diagnostic and statistical manual of mental disorders, DSM-III-R* (3rd ed. rev.). Washington, DC: Author.

Gentry, J. (1987). Social factors affecting women's health. *Public Health Reports*, July-August (Suppl.), 8-9.

Hazzard, W. (1989). Why do women live longer than men? *Postgraduate Medicine*, 85(5), 271-283.

Higgins, L.C. (1989), Estrogen survival benefits split. *Medical World News*, page 56.

King, P. (1989). A woman of the land. *Image: Journal of Nursing Scholarship*, 21(1), 19-22.

Li, F. (1988). I. Cancer epidemiology and prevention, Oncology. *Scientific American*, Chapter 12, 1-8.

Pollner, F. (1989). Courting women. *Medical World News*, 30(8), 42-52.

Yankauer, A. (1989). Women's health: Special issue. *American Journal of Public Health*, 79(15).

Nutritional concerns

Agras, W. (1989). Obesity, bulimia nervosa, and anorexia nervosa. *Scientific American*, 4(9), 1-12.

Brownell, K., and Foreyt, J. (1986). *Handbook of eating disorders: Physiology, psychology and treatment*. New York: Basic Books.

Bruch, H. (1978). *The golden cage: The enigma of anorexia nervosa*. New York: Vintage Books.

Burtis, G., Davis, J., and Martin, S. (1988). *Applied nutrition and diet therapy*. Philadelphia: Saunders.

Gastric Restrictive Surgery. (1989). *JAMA*, 261(10), 1491-1494.

Gershoff, S. (Ed.). (1989). On Oprah and Optifast. *Tufts University Diet and Nutrition Letter*, 6(12), 1-2.

Herzog, D. (1982). Anorexia nervosa: A treatment challenge. *Drug Therapy (Hospital Edition)*, 7(3), 89-96.

Kirkley, B. (1986). Bulimia: Clinical characteristics, development, and etiology. *Journal of American Dietetic Association*, 86(4), 468-475.

Manson, J. (1990). A prospective study of obesity and risk of coronary heart disease in women. *New England Journal of Medicine*, 322(13), 882-890.

Mead, W. (1989). Is exercise tolerance testing indicated for diagnoses and/or screening in family practice? *The Journal of Family Practice*, 28(4), 473-476.

Simopoulos, A. (1989). Nutrition and fitness. *JAMA*, 261(19), 2862-2863.

Webster, J. (1989) Key to healthy aging: Exercise. *Journal of Gerontological Nursing*, 14(12), 8-15.

Substance abuse

Ball, J., Corty, E., Bond, H., Myer, S., and Tommesello, A. (1988). The reduction of intravenous heroin use and non-opiate abuse during methadone maintenance treatment: Further readings. *National Institute of Drug Monograph Service*, 81, 224-230.

Centers for Disease Control. (1987). *Smoking control among women: A Center for Disease Control community intervention handbook*. Atlanta: Author.

Chenitz, W. (1989). Managing vulnerability: Nursing treatment for heroin addicts. *Image: Journal of Nursing Scholarship*, 21(3), 210-214.

Cohen, S. (1988). *The chemical brain: The neurochemistry of addictive disorders*. Irving, CA: Care Institute.

Dixon, S. (1989). Effects of transplacental exposure to cocaine and methamphetamine on the neonate. *Western Journal of Medicine*, 150(4), 436-42.

Gritz, E., Marcus, A., Berman, B. Read, L., Kanim, L., and Reeder, S. (1988). Evaluation of a worksite self-help smoking cessation program for registered nurses. *American Journal of Health Promotion* 3(2), 26-35.

Hixson, J. (1989). Plague of drug-blighted newborns. *MedicaTribune*, April 13, p. 19.

Hogan, D. (1990). Cocaine intoxication. *Drug Therapy*, 20(2), 89-93.

Hyman, S., and Cassem, N. (1987). Alcoholism. In E. Rubenstein and D. Federman (Eds.), *Scientific American medicine* (pp. 1-12). New York: Scientific American.

Hynes, M. (1989). A school-based smoking prevention program for adolescent girls in New York City. *Public Health Reports*, 104(1), 83-87.

Jenike, M. (1987). Drug Abuse. In E. Rubenstein and D. Federman (Eds.), *Scientific American medicine* (pp. 1-8). New York: Scientific American.

Kozlowski, L., Jelinek, L., and Pope, M. (1986). Cigarette smoking among alcohol abusers: A continuing and neglected problem. *Canadian Journal of Public Health*, 77(3), 205-207.

Kozlowski, L., Wilkinson, A., Skinner, W., Kent, C., Franklin, T., and Pope M. (1989). Comparing tobacco cigarette dependence with other drug dependencies. *JAMA*, 261(6), 898-901.

Lewis, K., Bennett, B., and Schmeder, N. (1989). The care of infants menaced by cocaine abuse. *MCN*, 14(5), 324-329.

Milhorn, H. (1989). Nicotine dependence. *American Family Physician*, 39(3), 214-224.

National Institute on Drug Abuse. (1981). *Marijuana and Health: Report to the U.S. Congress from the Secretary of Health and Human Services*. Washington, DC: National Academy Press.

Overpeck, M., Moss, A., Hoffman, H., and Hendershot, G. (1989). A comparison of the childhood health status of normal birth weight and low birth weight infants. *Public Health Reports*, 104(1), 58-70.

Pike, R. (1989). Cocaine withdrawal: An effective three-drug regimen. *Postgraduate Medicine*, 85(4), 115-121.

Rubenstein, E. (1989). Intoxication by centrally acting agents. In E. Rubenstein and D. Federman (Eds.), *Scientific American medicine* (pp. 2-12). New York: Scientific American.

Satel, S., and Gawin, F. (1989). Migrainelike headache and cocaine use. *JAMA,* 261(20), 2995-2996.

Schnoll, S., and Karan, L. (1989). Substance abuse. *JAMA,* 261(19), 2890-2892.

Surgeon General. (1988). The health consequences of smoking: Nicotine addiction 1988. *The 1987 Report of the Surgeon General* (Publication CDC 88-88406). Washington, DC: U.S. Government Printing Office.

Stress

Barrett, N. (1979). Women in the job market: Occupations, earnings and career opportunities. In R. Smith (Ed.), *The subtle revolution: Women at work* . Washington, DC: Urban Institute.

Collier, H. (1982). *Counseling women.* New York: Free Press.

Griffith-Kenney (1986). *Nursing and women's health: A nursing advocacy approach.* Menlo Park, CA: Addison-Wesley.

Jacobs, P., and McDermott, S. (1989). Family caregiver costs of chronically ill and handicapped children: Method and literature revue. *Public Health Reports,* 104(2), 158-163.

Norris, J. (1986). Welcoming remarks: National Health Conference on Women's Health. *Journal of the U.S. Public Health Service,* Supplement to July-August issue, 4-6.

Rohrbaugh, J. (1979). *Women: Psychology's puzzle.* New York: Basic Books.

Santi, L. (1987). Change in the structure and size of American households. *Journal of Marriage and the Family*, 49(4), 833-937.

Nursing research

Duffy, M. (1988). Determinants of health promotion in midlife women. *Nursing Research,* 37(6), 358-362.

Woods, N., Laffrey, S., Duffy, M., Lentz, M., Mitchell, E., Taylor, D., and Cowan, K. (1988). Being healthy: Women's images. *Advances in Nursing Science,* 11(1), 36-46.

The Antepartal Period

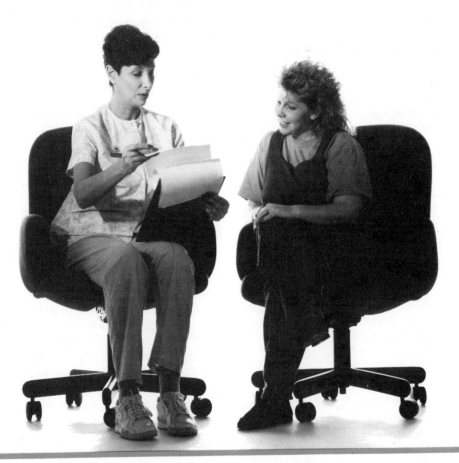

The quality of the environment in which a fetus grows affects childhood health significantly. Thus, the nurse who is familiar with the prenatal factors that enhance maternal health and promote a healthy intrauterine environment can increase the odds for a healthy childhood. The nurse caring for the pregnant client must teach and counsel prospective parents about such factors as genetic disorders and maternal physical and psychological status, as well as provide specific care measures that promote maternal and fetal health.

This unit helps the nurse fulfill these roles by examining the events of pregnancy—from the moment of conception to the onset of labor—and delineating the prenatal care required by the pregnant client and her family. It discusses fetal growth and development; surveys all facets of normal pregnancy, including the physiologic and psychosocial changes brought on by pregnancy; outlines family preparation for childbirth and parenting; discusses the effect of nutrition on fetal outcome; and details the nurse's role in maintaining high-quality antepartal care. To ensure effective nursing care for high-risk as well as low-risk situations, this unit also discusses pregnancy-related medical problems.

Four chapters in the unit provide the necessary theoretical framework for caring for the antepartal client. The remaining chapters follow a similar format, using the nursing process to guide antepartal nursing care. To demonstrate how to integrate assessment findings and document nursing care, these chapters include charts that apply the nursing process to case studies.

Chapter 16
Conception and Fetal Development

Chapter 16 explores development from fertilization of an ovum to the end of the fetal period. It discusses the preembryonic period (from fertilization through the subsequent 3 weeks), identifying the conditions necessary for fertilization. Then it elaborates on the second and third weeks of development, illustrating trophoblast differentiation, chorionic villi formation, and notochord development.

Next, Chapter 16 focuses on the embryonic period (weeks 4 to 8 of gestation). It describes germ layer development and the onset of cell differentiation and cell organization, and then it reviews development of the decidua and fetal membranes. After surveying the events of the fetal period (weeks 9 to 40 of gestation), the chapter elaborates on the placenta, detailing its circulation and endocrine functions and describing and illustrating the transfer of substances across the placenta. The chapter presents an essay of fetal development viewed through a camera's eye—remarkable and classic photographs of the early weeks of development.

Chapter 17
Physiologic Changes during Normal Pregnancy

Chapter 17 focuses on the dramatic physiologic changes, in each body system, that accompany normal pregnancy. It begins by explaining how pregnancy is diagnosed, offering a chart that compares presumptive, probable, and positive signs of pregnancy. Then it details pregnancy-related changes in the structure and function of each body system, with special focus on the reproductive and endocrine systems. It illustrates abdominal muscle migration and changes in fundal height and posture during pregnancy.

Chapter 18
Psychosocial Changes during Normal Pregnancy

Chapter 18 examines the psychosocial aspects of pregnancy and childbirth by discussing the challenges of the first trimester of pregnancy, exploring such topics as the client's ambivalence toward pregnancy and her partner's preparation for fatherhood. Then the chapter focuses on development of a mother image, a father image, and fetal bonding. It looks at psychosocial adaptation during the third trimester, describing the client's adaptation to activity changes and preparation for parenting and exploring the couple's ability to support one another. It specifies the coping mechanisms a pregnant client may use to deal with stress and explores preparing siblings and grandparents for the birth.

For each trimester, the chapter presents an examination of representative client feelings toward changes in her body image and sexuality and discusses typical dreams and fears experienced by women and men. It concludes by describing the psychosocial needs of special families dealing with pregnancy, including single-mother families, blended families, and lesbian families. The chapter includes a discussion of how cultural background affects psychosocial adaptation during pregnancy.

Chapter 19
Care during the Normal Antepartal Period

Chapter 19 surveys the nursing care essential to the health of the pregnant client and her fetus. First, it identifies the components of nursing assessment from the time pregnancy is suspected until delivery. It describes the health history information the nurse should gather, highlighting data about the current pregnancy and previous pregnancies. It explains how to elicit information about possible substance abuse that may pose a threat to the client or fetus. Then it presents how to conduct an appropriate physical examination, using a body systems approach to detect pregnancy-related physiologic changes. It features immunization guidelines for the pregnant client and charts the normal physiologic changes of pregnancy by trimester.

Chapter 19 then covers how to encourage family adaptation, minimize antepartal risks, aid client adaptation to pregnancy, and minimize client discomfort. It elaborates on client teaching during the antepartal period, covering such topics as rest, breast care, hygiene, childbirth exercises, sexual patterns, and preparation for childbirth.

Chapter 20
Nutrition and Diet Counseling

Chapter 20 describes the nutritional requirements of the pregnant client and identifies nutrition-related factors that may affect pregnancy outcome. First, it examines the effects of preconception body fat percentage, body weight, contraception, and alcohol use on the course and outcome of pregnancy. Then it looks at some antepartal nutritional concerns, including nutritional deprivation, nutritional supplementation, and weight gain. Next, it specifies nutritional needs during pregnancy, charting recommended dietary allowances and requirements for energy, water, vitamins, and minerals.

Chapter 20 then elaborates on factors that influence antepartal nutrition: maternal age, frequent pregnancies, socioeconomic status, unusual food patterns or diets, and other conditions that precede conception. It discusses nutrition-related effects of such antepartal risk factors as gestational diabetes, anemia, and multiple gestation. The chapter features client-teaching aids on increasing iron intake and absorption and modifying the diet to relieve constipation or reduce nausea or vomiting.

Chapter 21
Family Preparation for Childbirth and Parenting

Chapter 21 describes the goals and components of childbirth education and examines the nurse's role in preparing clients for childbirth and parenting. It begins with a historical perspective, describes current options in childbirth preparation, and charts the various nursing roles in childbirth education, specifying the education required and the organizations that certify nurses for each role. After reviewing the characteristics of adult learners, it describes how to assess an adult to determine learning ability and teaching needs and explains how to choose an appropriate teaching strategy and presentation method.

Next, Chapter 21 explores the common components of childbirth education classes. Focusing first on the physiologic aspects of pregnancy and childbirth, it surveys relaxation and breathing techniques, proper posture and body mechanics, and exercises to promote comfort during pregnancy and childbirth. It includes client-teaching aids on relaxation and massage during labor and delivery, and it features a chart comparing the components of childbirth education classes during the first, second, and third trimesters.

Then the chapter explains how to prepare a client for the transition to parenthood during the preconceptional, antepartal, and postpartal periods. It discusses preparing the client's partner for fatherhood and concludes by describing the philosophy and techniques of various childbirth methods and by elaborating on special childbirth preparation classes, including breast-feeding classes, expectant father classses, home birth classes, and adolescent- and single-parent classes.

Chapter 22
High-Risk Antepartal Clients

Chapter 22 prepares the nurse to provide optimal care for the high-risk antepartal client and her fetus. It explores the conditions that place the pregnant client at high risk—those that jeopardize maternal or fetal health or impede normal fetal development, childbirth, or the transition to parenthood. First, it focuses on the adolescent and mature client, elaborating on the physical and social risks these clients may face during pregnancy. Then it discusses the implications of cardiac disease, diabetes mellitus, anemia, infection, or substance abuse on pregnancy; it also explores the effects of pregnancy on these medical conditions. Next, Chapter 22 details the special management needs of the pregnant client who suffers trauma or requires surgery. It features charts showing how anemia, infection, and substance abuse affect the client, fetus, or neonate.

Chapter 22 then explores the components of a useful assessment data base and describes the invasive and noninvasive fetal tests that may be ordered for the high-risk client. It explains how to monitor the client's health status; teach her and her family about the high-risk condition and its management; promote rest, exercise, and adequate nutrition; prevent infection; provide support; monitor the fetus; and promote compliance.

Chapter 23
Antepartal Complications

Chapter 23 explains how to meet the physical and psychosocial needs of the client with an antepartal disorder or malfunction (one arising before the onset of term labor). The chapter describes the etiology and incidence of such problems as spontaneous abortion, ectopic pregnancy, gestational trophoblastic disease, incompetent cervix, premature rupture of the membranes, and preterm labor and delivery. Then it focuses on antepartal complications arising from multisystem disorders—hyperemesis gravidarum, hypertensive disorders, and Rh incompatibility.

Next, Chapter 23 illustrates techniques to diagnose ectopic pregnancy and pregnancy-induced hypertension (PIH) and offers nursing interventions to promote the client's well-being, prevent or control further complications or sequelae, and provide emotional support. Highlights include an illustration of cervical cerclage to treat incompetent cervix and charts detailing the mechanism of action, dosages, and nursing implications of drugs used to inhibit labor, treat hyperemesis gravidarum, and manage PIH.

Conception and Fetal Development

Objectives

After reading and studying this chapter, the student should be able to:

1. Describe fertilization.

2. Outline developmental events that occur between fertilization and implantation of an ovum.

3. List structures present in the pre-embryo 3 weeks after fertilization.

4. Describe the major developmental events of the embryonic period.

5. Describe the major developmental events of the fetal period.

6. Discuss the production and balance of amniotic fluid.

7. Explain placental function and hormone production.

8. Describe the special characteristics of fetal circulation.

Introduction

Development of a functioning human being from a fertilized ovum involves a complex process of cell division, differentiation, and organization. Development begins with the union of spermatozoon and ovum to form a composite cell containing chromosomes from both parents. This composite cell divides repeatedly; individual cells increase in size. Beginning approximately 4 weeks after fertilization, daughter cells differentiate—that is, develop specialized properties not possessed by the par-

ent cells, such as the ability to conduct nerve impulses or contract rhythmically. Finally, groups of differentiated cells organize into complex structures, such as the brain and spinal cord, liver, kidneys, and other organs that function as integrated units.

A precise timetable governs each developmental step concurrently with other related phases. During this time, the fetus and mother form a relationship via the placenta that provides an environment conducive to fetal growth and well-being.

The time from fertilization to birth is the period of gestation. Its length can be calculated by two methods. One method calculates from the last ovulation (called ovulation age): gestation length from last ovulation approximates 38 weeks. Because few clients know when ovulation occurs, however, the method using menstrual flow (called menstrual age) is used more commonly. In this method, gestation is calculated from the beginning of the last normal menstrual period: gestation length approximates 40 weeks.

This chapter begins at ovulation—when fertilization can occur—and describes fertilization and factors that can influence it. Three main periods of prenatal development are explained: pre-embryonic, embryonic, and fetal. Additionally, the chapter discusses the environment necessary for normal development throughout the three developmental periods. This discussion includes the decidua, fetal membranes, placenta, and fetal circulatory system.

GLOSSARY

Acrosome: membranelike covering on the head portion of a spermatozoon.

Allantois: diverticulum in the embryo's caudal end; allantoic blood vessels help form those of the umbilical cord.

Amniotic sac: membrane that surrounds the fetus, contains amniotic fluid, and eventually lines the chorion.

Blastocyst: embryo precursor just after the morula stage.

Blastomere: daughter cell formed by mitosis just after fertilization of an ovum.

Capacitation: process of spermatozoon activation that includes structural change in the acrosome.

Conception: act of becoming pregnant, starting with the fertilization of an ovum and ending with implantation of the ovum in the uterine wall.

Conceptus: products of conception, including fetal membranes, placenta, and pre-embryo, embryo, or fetus.

Corona radiata: layer of granulosa cells that adheres to the zona pellucida before fertilization of an ovum.

Ectoderm: outermost of the three primary germ cell layers of the embryo.

Embryo: developing organism after the pre-embryonic stage and before the fetal stage; most authorities consider it weeks 4 through 8.

Endoderm: innermost of the three primary germ cell layers of the embryo.

Fertilization: penetration of a female gamete by a male gamete.

Fetal-placental unit: umbilical cord, placental layers, and chorionic villus—through which placental transfer occurs.

Fetus: developing organism after the embryonic stage; most authorities consider it week 9 through delivery.

Gamete: male or female reproductive cell (spermatozoon or ovum).

Gametogenesis: developmental process by which spermatozoa and ova are formed.

Graafian follicle: mature ovarian vesicle located near the ovarian surface that contains an ovum.

Implantation: attachment of the blastocyst to the uterine wall; occurs 6 to 7 days after fertilization of the ovum.

Meiosis: specialized form of cell division that produces gametes.

Mesoderm: middle layer of the three primary germ cell layers of the embryo.

Mitosis: cell division characteristic of all cell types except gametes.

Morula: small mass of cells formed after a zygote undergoes several mitotic divisions.

Notochord: rod-shaped structure that defines the primitive axis of the body and forms the central developmental point of the axial skeleton.

Oogenesis: process by which ova develop.

Ovum: female gamete (plural ova).

Pre-embryo: developing organism from implantation through week 3, when—according to most authorities—the organism becomes an embryo.

Primitive streak: small aggregation of cells at the embryo's caudal end that offers early evidence of the embryonic axis.

Spermatozoon: male gamete (plural spermatozoa).

Spermatogenesis: process by which spermatozoa develop.

Trophoblast: layer of ectoderm on the outside of the blastocyst that implants the embryo in the uterine wall and forms the chorion, amnion, and chorionic villi.

Zona pellucida: noncellular layer covering the surface of a mature ovarian follicle.

Zygote: diploid cell formed by the union of a haploid ovum and spermatozoon; develops into an embryo.

Pre-embryonic period

Beginning with fertilization, the pre-embryonic period lasts for 3 weeks. During this crucial developmental stage, implantation occurs, cells divide rapidly and begin to differentiate, and the placenta and embryo begin to form.

Fertilization and implantation

Penetration of a female gamete (ovum) by a male gamete (spermatozoon) marks the beginning of conception. Called fertilization, this event requires coordination of a complex array of physical and chemical factors, some of which begin long before the spermatozoon and ovum join to form a zygote (the single cell resulting from the union of male and female gametes).

The first step needed for fertilization is gametogenesis, where gonadotropic hormones stimulate testicular and ovarian precursor cells to develop into mature gametes. (See Chapter 6, Reproductive Anatomy and Physiology, and Chapter 11, Genetics and Genetic Disorders, for additional discussion of gametogenesis.)

The second step necessary for fertilization is introduction of spermatozoa into the vagina, either through ejaculation or artificial means. In normal ejaculate, spermatozoa are suspended in seminal fluid, composed of viscous secretions from the seminal vesicles and from the prostate and bulbourethral (Cowper) glands. Ejaculate typically contains about 3 ml of seminal fluid and up to 100 million spermatozoa per ml. Many of the spermatozoa aggregate in the portion of fluid ejaculated first rather than in a uniform distribution throughout the fluid. Ejaculate volume may vary from less than 2 ml to more than 5 ml, depending primarily on the interval between ejaculations.

Only spermatozoa (not seminal fluid) migrate through the cervix and into the uterus. Passage through the cervix is accomplished primarily by active transport. The middle section of each spermatozoon's tail contains enzymes that catalyze energy needed for propulsion, resulting in a lashing motion that propels the spermatozoon forward. Rhythmic uterine contractions move spermatozoa passively through the uterus and toward the fallopian tubes. The spermatozoa spread diffusely over the endometrium and enter both fallopian tubes, where they retain their fertilizing capability for up to 48 hours after intercourse (Cunningham, MacDonald, and Gant, 1989).

Meanwhile, under the influence of follicle-stimulating hormone (FSH) and luteinizing hormone (LH), several ovarian follicles begin to mature during the female reproductive cycle. Granulosa cells surrounding the follicles proliferate, and a layer of acellular material called the zona pellucida forms on the surface of the developing follicle. Fluid accumulates within the layer of granulosa cells, eventually forming a central, fluid-filled cavity within the follicle known as a graafian follicle. At ovulation, the graafian follicle discharges its ovum, which is surrounded by the zona pellucida and several layers of adherent granulosa cells called the corona radiata. The ovum is swept into the adjacent fallopian tube by beating cilia that cover the tubal epithelium; peristaltic contractions of smooth muscles in the fallopian tube wall propel the ovum toward the uterus. (See Chapter 6, Reproductive Anatomy and Physiology, for additional information on the female reproductive cycle.)

Fertilization is possible only when a descending ovum meets an ascending spermatozoon that has spent several hours in the female reproductive tract.

Several conditions must be met before fertilization may occur, including the following.
• Seminal fluid, which is composed primarily of slightly alkaline secretions of the prostate and seminal vesicles, must protect spermatozoa from destructively acid vaginal secretions.
• Cervical mucus must be thin and conducive to spermatozoa passage. This occurs only during the midportion of the menstrual cycle. Later, cervical mucus thickens in response to progesterone stimulation.
• Spermatozoa count typically must exceed 20 million per ml of seminal fluid.
• Contact must occur between a spermatozoon and an ovum. Spermatozoa have no "guidance system" to direct them toward the ovum. Further, complex mucosal folds inside the fallopian tubes tend to impede and deflect spermatozoa.

When a spermatozoon penetrates an ovum, the spermatozoon's tail degenerates and the head enlarges and fuses with the nucleus of the ovum. This restores the cell's genetic component to 46 chromosomes—23 from the spermatozoon and 23 from the ovum. The fertilized ovum, known as a zygote at the one-cell stage, undergoes a series of mitotic divisions as it continues to travel down the fallopian tube toward the uterus. By the end of the first week after fertilization, the morula (small mass of cells) has begun to implant in the uterine wall. (See *Overview of conception* for a detailed description.)

Period of twos

During the second week of development, known as the period of twos, implantation progresses, the inner cell mass forms two germ layers, the blastocyst cavity develops into two cavities, and the trophoblast differentiates into two cell layers.

Period of threes

During the third week of development, known as the period of threes, the embryonic disk evolves into three layers, and three new structures are formed: the primitive streak, the notochord, and the allantois. The chorionic villi acquire central cores of mesoderm and now also consist of three layers. (See *Pre-embryonic development: Weeks 2 and 3*, pages 370 and 371 and *How germ layers develop*, page 372, for illustrations.)

(Text continues on page 372.)

Overview of conception

A complex process, conception requires the exact coordination of several steps, including gametogenesis, fertilization, and implantation.

Gametogenesis

The female gamete (ovum) is produced during the ovarian cycle. This cycle begins on the first day of menses, when primary follicles in the ovary start to mature. Soon a single follicle (graafian follicle) dominates and continues to mature while the other follicles undergo involution. Hormonal influences cause swelling of the graafian follicle, which eventually ruptures; the mature ovum emerges from the follicle and enters the fallopian tube, leaving behind the corpus hemorrhagicum.

After ovulation, the ruptured graafian follicle becomes a compact mass of tissue called the corpus luteum. It produces hormones that stimulate changes in the endometrium to allow implantation of a fertilized ovum. If the ovum is not fertilized, in about 8 days hormone production decreases and the corpus luteum degenerates into a fibrous mass known as the corpus albicans; the cycle then begins again in about 6 days. If fertilization occurs, hormone production continues until about the seventh week of pregnancy.

For a detailed description of male gamete production, see Chapter 6, Reproductive Anatomy and Physiology.

DEVELOPING OVUM

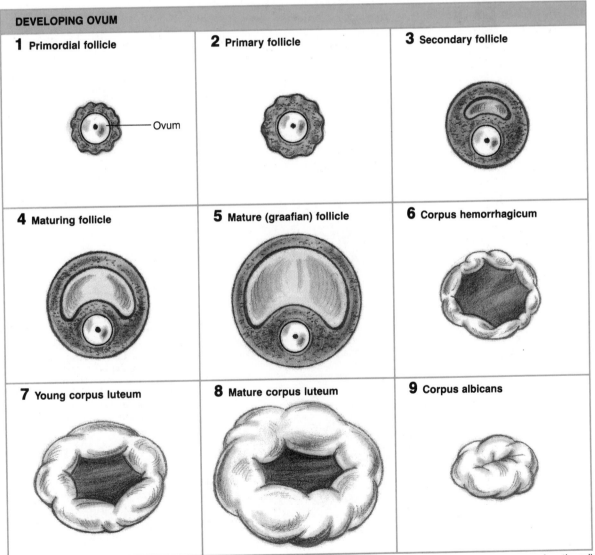

1 Primordial follicle — Ovum

2 Primary follicle

3 Secondary follicle

4 Maturing follicle

5 Mature (graafian) follicle

6 Corpus hemorrhagicum

7 Young corpus luteum

8 Mature corpus luteum

9 Corpus albicans

(continued)

Overview of conception continued

ANATOMY OF A SPERMATOZOON

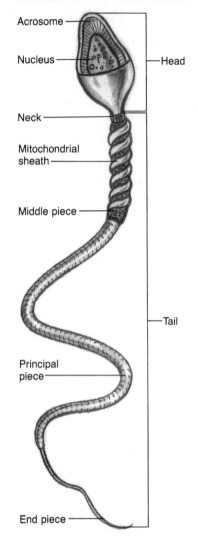

Acrosome

Nucleus

Head

Neck

Mitochondrial
sheath

Middle piece

Tail

Principal
piece

End piece

ANATOMY OF AN OVUM

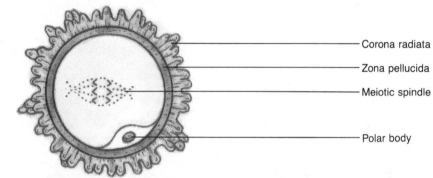

Corona radiata

Zona pellucida

Meiotic spindle

Polar body

FERTILIZATION

1 When a spermatozoon meets an ovum after several hours in the female reproductive tract, the spermatozoon undergoes activation (called capacitation).

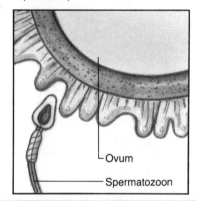

Ovum

Spermatozoon

2 The covering of its acrosome develops small perforations; enzymes released through these perforations disperse the ovum's granulosa cells (corona radiata).

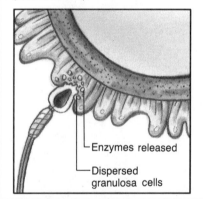

Enzymes released

Dispersed
granulosa cells

3 The spermatozoon then penetrates the zona pellucida. This triggers the ovum's second meiotic division, which makes the zona pellucida impenetrable to other spermatozoa.

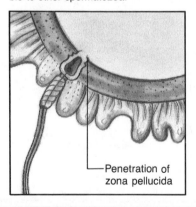

Penetration of
zona pellucida

4 After the spermatozoon penetrates the ovum, the nucleus is released into the ovum, the tail degenerates, and the head enlarges and fuses with the nucleus of the ovum. This fusion gives the fertilized ovum—called a zygote—a total of 46 chromosomes.

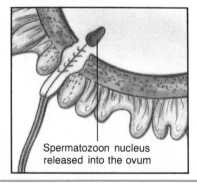

Spermatozoon nucleus
released into the ovum

Implantation

As the fertilized ovum travels through the fallopian tube toward the uterus, it undergoes mitotic divisions (called cleavage), forming daughter cells (initially called blastomeres). The first cell division is completed about 30 hours after fertilization, and subsequent divisions occur rapidly. The zygote develops into a small mass of cells called a morula, which reaches the uterus about the third day after fertilization. Fluid accumulates in the center of the morula, forming a central cavity. At this stage, the structure is called a blastocyst. Its cells differentiate into two groups:

• a peripheral rim of cells (the trophoblast) that will give rise to fetal membranes and contribute to placenta formation (early blastocyst)

• a discrete cluster of cells enclosed within the trophoblast, called the inner cell mass, that will form the embryo (late blastocyst).

For several days, the blastocyst remains within the zona pellucida and unattached to the uterus. Then the zona pellucida degenerates and, by the end of the first week after fertilization, the blastocyst attaches to the endometrium. The part of the blastocyst adjacent to the inner cell mass, called the embryonic pole of the blastocyst, is the first part to become attached. In contact with the endometrial lining, the trophoblast proliferates and invades the underlying endometrium by separating and dissolving endometrial cells.

During the following week, the invading blastocyst sinks below the surface of the endometrium and the site of penetration becomes sealed over, restoring the continuity of the endometrial surface.

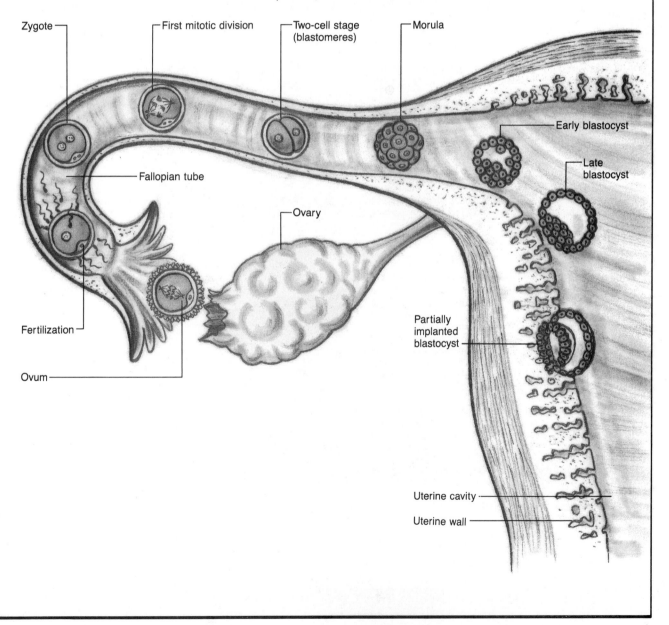

Zygote — First mitotic division — Two-cell stage (blastomeres) — Morula — Early blastocyst — Late blastocyst — Fallopian tube — Ovary — Partially implanted blastocyst — Fertilization — Ovum — Uterine cavity — Uterine wall

Pre-embryonic development: Weeks 2 and 3

8 days

Early in the second week after fertilization, a two-layered structure develops from the inner cell mass and separates slightly from the trophoblast, dividing the blastocyst cavity. Called the embryonic (or germ) disk, this structure forms the embryo. At this stage, it has two cell layers: columnar ectoderm facing the trophoblast and flat endoderm facing the blastocyst cavity.

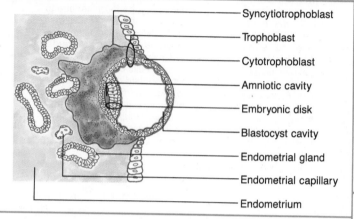

- Syncytiotrophoblast
- Trophoblast
- Cytotrophoblast
- Amniotic cavity
- Embryonic disk
- Blastocyst cavity
- Endometrial gland
- Endometrial capillary
- Endometrium

13 days

Clefts called the lacunar network form within this layer; blood from eroded endometrial vessels flows into the lacunar network.

The yolk sac lining separates and enlarges as the embryo develops, forming the extraembryonic coelom (or cavity). A layer of primitive connective tissue cells called extraembryonic mesoderm covers the interior of the enlarging coelom as well as the external surface of the amniotic and yolk sacs.

After the blastocyst cavity develops a mesodermal lining, it is known as the chorionic cavity; its wall is the chorion. The cavity with its enclosed amniotic sac, yolk sac, and embryonic disk is known as the chorionic vesicle.

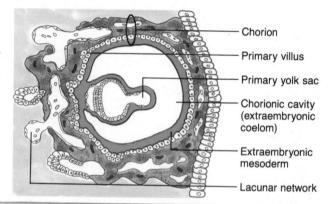

- Chorion
- Primary villus
- Primary yolk sac
- Chorionic cavity (extraembryonic coelom)
- Extraembryonic mesoderm
- Lacunar network

16 days

A thickened area called the primitive streak develops on the dorsal surface of the caudal half of the embryonic disk, giving rise to a layer of intraembryonic mesoderm. This layer spreads to the periphery of the disk and joins the extraembryonic mesoderm covering the amniotic and yolk sacs. It then differentiates and develops into a horseshoe-shaped channel (the intraembryonic coelom) that extends along the sides of the disk and curves across the midline of the cephalad (head end) to the prochordal plate. This channel is the forerunner of the pericardial, pleural, and peritoneal cavities.

Chorionic villi continue developing during the third week. At first, they become lined with mesoderm and are called secondary villi. Then their internal cells differentiate into connective tissue and blood vessels, at which point they are called tertiary villi. Newly formed blood vessels in the villi connect with those in the chorion and body stalk and, eventually, with the embryo's developing circulatory system. This establishes circulation between the embryo and placenta. Blood circulates through the villi when the embryo's heart starts to beat.

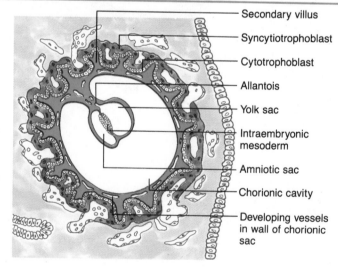

- Secondary villus
- Syncytiotrophoblast
- Cytotrophoblast
- Allantois
- Yolk sac
- Intraembryonic mesoderm
- Amniotic sac
- Chorionic cavity
- Developing vessels in wall of chorionic sac

12 days

As the embryonic disk separates from the trophoblast, the amniotic cavity forms between them. On the opposite side of the embryonic disk, a layer of cells derived from the trophoblast lines a larger cavity called the primary yolk sac. Its cells merge with the endoderm of the embryonic disk.

During the second week, the trophoblast differentiates into two layers: the cytotrophoblast and peripheral syncytiotrophoblast. The peripheral layer erodes the endometrium, facilitating implantation and initiating contact between the conceptus and uterine circulation.

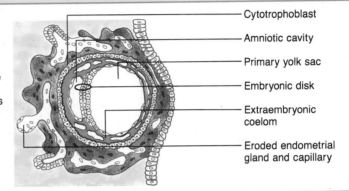

- Cytotrophoblast
- Amniotic cavity
- Primary yolk sac
- Embryonic disk
- Extraembryonic coelom
- Eroded endometrial gland and capillary

14 days

Late in the second week, part of the yolk sac pinches off, reducing its size and causing a corresponding increase in the size of the chorionic cavity. By the end of the second week, the embryonic disk and its surrounding amnion and yolk sac project into the chorionic cavity, suspended from the chorion by a mass of mesodermal tissue called the body stalk, which eventually develops into the umbilical cord.

Proliferating columns of cytotrophoblast extend into the syncytiotrophoblast layer, forming fingerlike extensions called primary chorionic villi. The blood-filled spaces between them—intervillous spaces—are derived from the trophoblast lacunae. Blood flow through these spaces near the end of the second week may cause some bleeding from the implantation site.

Ectodermal cells proliferate to form a mesodermal germ layer that separates the embryo's ectoderm and endoderm layers except in two small areas at the cephalic and caudal ends. The cephalic area of ectoderm-endoderm fusion, called the prochordal plate, eventually forms the oral cavity. The caudal area of fusion—the cloacal plate—eventually forms the urogenital and anorectal openings.

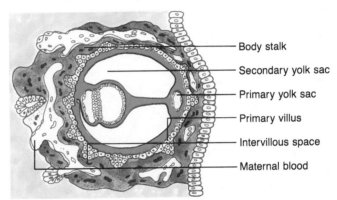

- Body stalk
- Secondary yolk sac
- Primary yolk sac
- Primary villus
- Intervillous space
- Maternal blood

21 days

A midline tubular column of cells extending from the cephalad along the primitive streak, the notochord is the structure around which the spinal column forms; it also induces nervous system formation from the embryonic disk's overlying ectoderm. The paraxial mesoderm beside the developing notochord thickens to form blocks of primitive connective tissue called somites, which look like bumps on the embryo's surface. Somite formation begins in the third week and extends into the fourth; the number of somites on an embryo is a relatively accurate indicator of age.

The allantois is a small diverticulum that projects from the caudal part of the yolk sac into the mesoderm of the body stalk. This structure plays a role in the development of the urinary system.

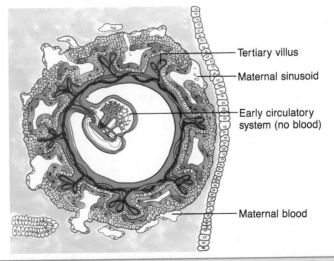

- Tertiary villus
- Maternal sinusoid
- Early circulatory system (no blood)
- Maternal blood

Embryonic period

Early in the fourth week, the flat, pre-embryonic structure becomes a cylindrical embryo that, over the following 4 weeks, nearly triples in size. Embryonic cells undergo complex differentiation and develop into primitive organ systems.

Two major events occur during this period.
- Cell differentiation begins.
- Cell organization begins.

Especially during this period, drugs ingested by the mother, some viral infections, radiation, and other environmental factors can seriously disturb embryonic development, possibly leading to congenital abnormalities. (See *System development: Weeks 2 to 8* and *Embryonic development: Weeks 4 to 8 (days 22 to 56)*, pages 374 and 375, for information about these developmental periods.) In addition, specialized structures that protect and nur-

How germ layers develop

Each of the three germ layers (ectoderm, mesoderm, and endoderm) will form specific tissues and organs in the developing embryo.

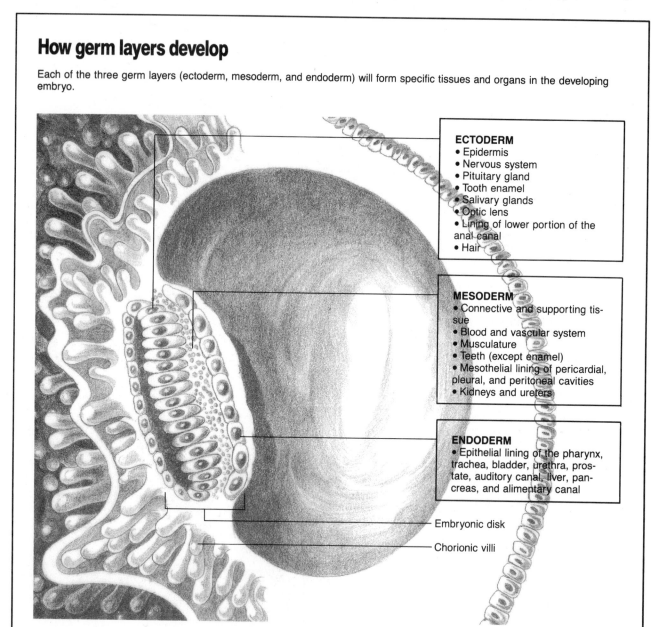

ECTODERM
- Epidermis
- Nervous system
- Pituitary gland
- Tooth enamel
- Salivary glands
- Optic lens
- Lining of lower portion of the anal canal
- Hair

MESODERM
- Connective and supporting tissue
- Blood and vascular system
- Musculature
- Teeth (except enamel)
- Mesothelial lining of pericardial, pleural, and peritoneal cavities
- Kidneys and ureters

ENDODERM
- Epithelial lining of the pharynx, trachea, bladder, urethra, prostate, auditory canal, liver, pancreas, and alimentary canal

Embryonic disk

Chorionic villi

System development: Weeks 2 to 8

The following chart highlights significant events during pre-embryonic and embryonic development and the times they occur.

CARDIOVASCULAR SYSTEM

2 to 4 weeks
- Heart begins to form
- Blood circulation begins
- Primitive red blood cells circulate
- Tubular heartbeat by 24 days

5 to 7 weeks
- Atrial division
- Heart chambers present
- Fetal heartbeat detectable
- Groups of blood cells identifiable

8 weeks
- Development of heart complete
- Fetal circulation follows two circuits: two intraembryonic and four extraembryonic

ENDOCRINE SYSTEM

4 weeks
- Thyroid can synthesize thyroxine

EXTERNAL APPEARANCE

4 weeks
- C-shaped body; pigment in eyes; auditory pit enclosed

8 weeks
- Flat nose, eyes far apart, digits well formed; recognizable eyes, ears, nose, and mouth

GASTROINTESTINAL SYSTEM

4 weeks
- Oral cavity and primitive jaw present
- Stomach, ducts of pancreas, and liver form

GENITOURINARY SYSTEM

4 to 7 weeks
- Rudimentary ureteral buds present

HEPATIC SYSTEM

4 weeks
- Liver function begins

6 weeks
- Hematopoiesis by liver begins

MUSCULOSKELETAL SYSTEM

4 weeks
- Limb buds appear

8 weeks
- First identification of ossification (mandible, humerus, occiput)

NERVOUS SYSTEM

4 weeks
- Well-marked midbrain flexure
- Neural groove closed
- Spinal cord extends the entire length of spine

8 weeks
- Differentiation of cerebral cortex, meninges, ventricular foramina, and cerebrospinal fluid circulation

REPRODUCTIVE SYSTEM

6 to 8 weeks
- Sex glands appear
- Differentiation of sex glands into ovaries or testes begins
- External genitalia appear similar

RESPIRATORY SYSTEM

4 to 7 weeks
- Primary lung, tracheal, and bronchial buds appear
- Nasal pits form
- Abdominal and thoracic cavities separated by the diaphragm

---

ture the embryo—including the maternal decidua and fetal membranes—become fully functional during this period. (See *Development of the decidua and fetal membranes,* pages 376 and 377, for a detailed discussion.)

Each of the germ layers derived from the inner cell mass will form specific tissues and organs within the embryo. In general, the ectoderm forms the embryo's external covering and the organs that come into contact with the environment. The endoderm forms the embryo's internal lining: the epithelium of the pharynx, the respiratory and gastrointestinal tracts, related organs, and parts of the urogenital tract.

The mesoderm, which is sandwiched between the other two cell layers, forms various supporting tissues, muscles, the circulatory system, and major portions of the urogenital system.

Cell differentiation in each germ layer depends more on location than on inherent characteristics. For example, ectoderm cells transplanted during early development into locations normally occupied by endoderm will differentiate as endoderm cells. The converse is true, too. These transplantations suggest that embryonic cells,

(Text continues on page 377.)

Embryonic development: Weeks 4 to 8 (days 22 to 56)

During this period, the embryo undergoes rapid growth and differentiation, as illustrated at right. The embryo develops organ systems, limbs, eyes, and ears; the amnion, yolk sac, and connecting stalk unite to form an umbilical cord with two arteries and one vein.

During the fourth week, the center of the embryonic disk grows more rapidly than the periphery as the nervous system begins to form. As a result, the embryonic disk flexes and bulges into the amniotic cavity. The amniotic sac, attached to the lateral margins of the embryonic disk, follows the changing contour of the embryo and bends around it. Part of the yolk sac also becomes enfolded within the embryo, and later will form the intestinal tract, among other important structures.

The lateral margins of the embryonic disk fuse in the midline to form the ventral (anterior) body wall. Fusion is incomplete in the middle of the body wall where the umbilical cord is attached. The portion of yolk sac not enfolded with the embryo protrudes, still connected to the embryo by a narrow duct. It persists for a time but eventually degenerates. The embryo begins to bend into a C-shape.

During the fifth week, the head and heart grow rapidly. The amnion, yolk sac, and connecting stalk unite to form the umbilical cord, containing two arteries and one vein. At this time, the embryo's four limb buds are most vulnerable to injury by teratogens (such as drugs or radiation).

During the sixth week, the head grows larger than the trunk and appears to be bent over the heart area. The eyes, nose, and mouth are more evident. The upper limbs have elbows and wrists. The hand plates develop ridges called finger rays.

During the seventh week, the head continues to enlarge and cerebral hemispheres appear. The face elongates, placing the eyes in a more frontal position. The areas over the heart and liver are prominent because these organs form earlier than others. Limbs continue to develop, especially the fingers.

During the eighth week, the head makes up half of the total embryonic mass. A face occupies its lower half. Eyelid folds have developed. The external ears look similar to their final shape. Arms, legs, fingers, and toes are distinct. Sexual differences may be observed. (For photographs of embryonic development, see pages 382 to 385.)

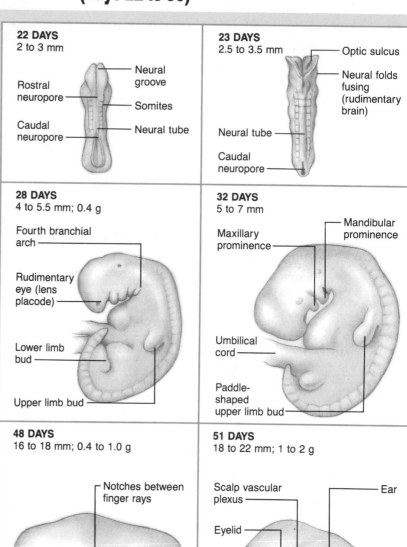

22 DAYS
2 to 3 mm

Rostral neuropore
Neural groove
Somites
Caudal neuropore
Neural tube

23 DAYS
2.5 to 3.5 mm

Optic sulcus
Neural folds fusing (rudimentary brain)
Neural tube
Caudal neuropore

28 DAYS
4 to 5.5 mm; 0.4 g

Fourth branchial arch
Rudimentary eye (lens placode)
Lower limb bud
Upper limb bud

32 DAYS
5 to 7 mm

Maxillary prominence
Mandibular prominence
Umbilical cord
Paddle-shaped upper limb bud

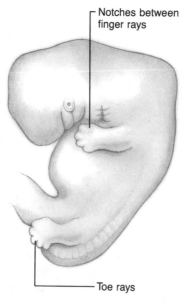

48 DAYS
16 to 18 mm; 0.4 to 1.0 g

Notches between finger rays
Toe rays

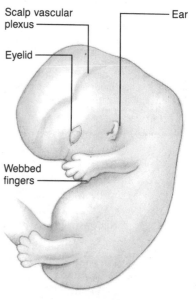

51 DAYS
18 to 22 mm; 1 to 2 g

Scalp vascular plexus
Ear
Eyelid
Webbed fingers

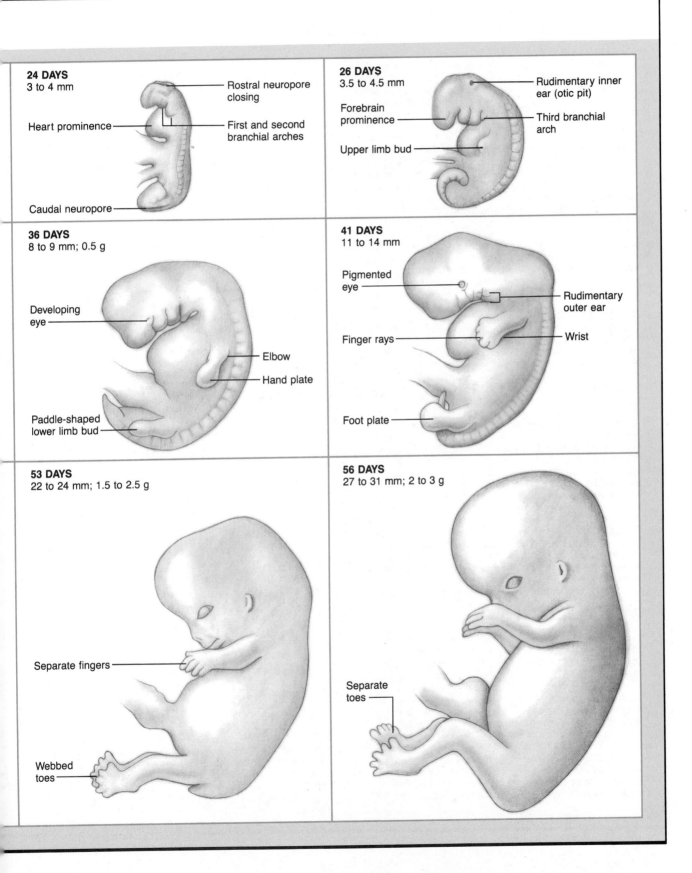

24 DAYS
3 to 4 mm

Rostral neuropore closing

Heart prominence

First and second branchial arches

Caudal neuropore

26 DAYS
3.5 to 4.5 mm

Rudimentary inner ear (otic pit)

Forebrain prominence

Third branchial arch

Upper limb bud

36 DAYS
8 to 9 mm; 0.5 g

Developing eye

Elbow

Hand plate

Paddle-shaped lower limb bud

41 DAYS
11 to 14 mm

Pigmented eye

Rudimentary outer ear

Finger rays

Wrist

Foot plate

53 DAYS
22 to 24 mm; 1.5 to 2.5 g

Separate fingers

Webbed toes

56 DAYS
27 to 31 mm; 2 to 3 g

Separate toes

Development of the decidua and fetal membranes

Specialized tissues support, protect, and nurture the embryo and fetus throughout its development. Among these, the decidua and fetal membranes begin to develop shortly after conception and contribute to a successful pregnancy. The illustrations highlight their development at approximately 4, 8, 16, and 32 weeks.

Decidua

During pregnancy, the endometrium is called the decidua. It provides a nesting place for the developing conceptus and has some endocrine functions. Decidual cells secrete prolactin (a hormone that promotes lactation) and relaxin (a hormone that inhibits uterine contractility). They also synthesize prostaglandin (a potent mediator of many physiologic functions).

Based primarily on its position relative to the embryo, the decidua may be known as:
• decidua basalis, which lies beneath the chorionic vesicle
• decidua capsularis, which stretches over the vesicle
• decidua parietalis, which lines the rest of the endometrial cavity.

Chorion and chorionic villi

The chorionic villi arise from the periphery of the chorion. However, as the chorionic vesicle enlarges, villi from the superficial part of the chorion (adjacent to the decidua capsularis) atrophy. This part of the chorion, which becomes smooth, is called the chorion laeve. In contrast, villi arising from the deeper portion of the chorion (adjacent to the decidua basalis) proliferate; this part of the chorion is called the chorion frondosum.

The villi of the chorion frondosum project into the large blood vessels within the decidua basalis through which the maternal blood flows. Blood vessels form within the villi as they grow, and become connected with blood vessels that form in the chorion, body stalk, and within the body of the embryo. Blood begins to flow through this developing network of vessels as soon as the embryo's heart begins to beat.

Amniotic sac

Enclosed within the chorion, the amniotic sac gradually increases in size and surrounds the developing embryo. As it enlarges, the amniotic sac expands into the chorionic cavity, eventually filling the cavity and fusing with the chorion. Additionally, the decidua capsularis stretches and thins, eventually fusing with the decidua parietalis on the opposite wall of the uterus.

Fluid in the amniotic sac provides a buoyant, temperature-controlled environment that protects the fetus during gestation. Amniotic fluid volume gradually increases from about 50 ml at 12 weeks to about 800 to 1,000 ml at term. Fluid is produced by filtration and by excretion. During the first part of pregnancy, amniotic fluid is derived chiefly by filtration from maternal blood. Some fluid is filtered from fetal blood passing through the placenta; some diffuses directly through the skin and respiratory tract of the fetus.

During the latter half of pregnancy, when the fetal kidneys begin to function, urine becomes a major source of amniotic fluid. Both filtration and excretion add to the fluid volume; these additions are counterbalanced by ingestion of amniotic fluid by the fetus. Normally, the fetus swallows up to several hundred milliliters of amniotic fluid daily. The fluid

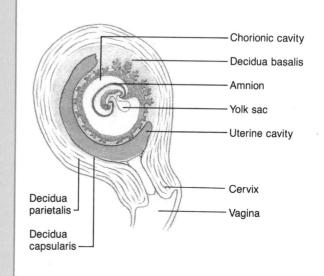

APPROXIMATELY 4 WEEKS

Chorionic cavity

Decidua basalis

Amnion

Yolk sac

Uterine cavity

Cervix

Vagina

Decidua parietalis

Decidua capsularis

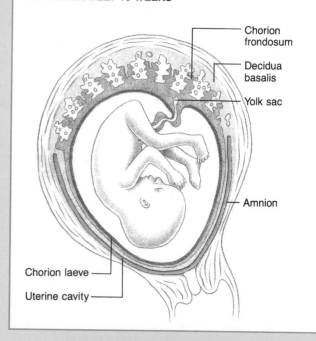

APPROXIMATELY 16 WEEKS

Chorion frondosum

Decidua basalis

Yolk sac

Amnion

Chorion laeve

Uterine cavity

is absorbed from the intestines into the circulatory system and transferred across the placenta to the mother's circulation. Eventually the mother excretes it in her urine.

Amniotic fluid volume adjusts to fluid produced by maternal and fetal sources and fluid lost through the fetal gastro-

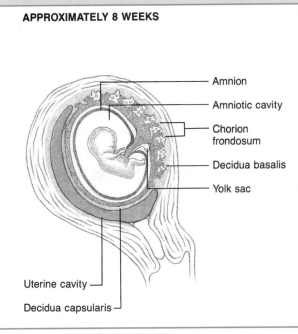

APPROXIMATELY 8 WEEKS

- Amnion
- Amniotic cavity
- Chorion frondosum
- Decidua basalis
- Yolk sac
- Uterine cavity
- Decidua capsularis

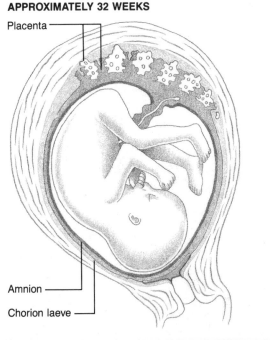

APPROXIMATELY 32 WEEKS

- Placenta
- Amnion
- Chorion laeve

intestinal tract. Although amniotic fluid quantity varies somewhat among women, extreme variations are abnormal and usually are associated with serious fetal abnormalities. The volume, source, and composition of amniotic fluid vary with the stage of gestation.

which may develop in various ways, are induced into specific development.

Induction apparently is accomplished by diffusion of a specific nucleoprotein (the inductor or organizer) from a group of cells to adjacent cells (the responding cells). The ability of cells to respond to inductive stimuli is called competence. Cells respond to inductors for a limited time during development; as they mature and differentiate, they lose competence. As cells differentiate, they become organized into complex systems that interact internally and with other body systems. For example, the notochord and adjacent mesoderm induce the overlying ectoderm to form the neural plate, which forms the nervous system. Formation of the allantois induces blood vessels to develop in the body stalk.

Many developmental processes result from a complex chain reaction. One tissue serves as a primary inductor, causing differentiation in adjacent tissues. In turn, these act as secondary inductors, directing differentiation in other groups of cells.

Many examples of chain reaction inductions have been described, the best known involving the neural tube and eye. The neural tube (precursor of the neural system) is induced initially by the notochord and adjacent mesoderm. Mesoderm surrounding the newly formed neural tube then causes outpocketings called optic vesicles (which eventually form the retina and optic nerve) to extend from the developing tube. Each vesicle differentiates and then induces lens formation from the adjacent ectoderm of the head. The lens induces the formation of the cornea, conjunctiva, and associated ocular structures from the surrounding mesoderm.

Fetal period

Lasting from weeks 8 to 40, the fetal period involves further growth and development of organ systems established in the embryonic period. When fully developed, fetal organs begin to function and supply part of the fetus's metabolic needs. (See *Fetal development: Weeks 9 to 40*, pages 378 and 379, and *System development: Weeks 8 to 40*, page 380, for illustrations and characteristics of this period.) In addition, the placenta continues to develop.

Fetal development: Weeks 9 to 40

In the ninth week, the eyelids fuse together, remaining so until the seventh month. The fetus's head remains disproportionately large. Limbs are disproportionately small at week 9, but by week 12 the arms have reached normal proportions. Legs and thighs remain small. The liver begins to produce red blood cells, a function taken over by the spleen at about 12 weeks. At 12 weeks, the placenta is complete and fetal circulation has developed.

By the end of week 16, the head makes up one-third of the total size of the fetus, and the brain is roughly delineated. The forehead is prominent, with lanugo (fine hair) growing on it. The chin is apparent, and the ears are placed higher on the head than previously. Fingernails begin to form. The kidneys function, secreting urine, and the fetus begins to swallow amniotic fluid. The lower limbs lengthen and the skeleton ossifies. The intestines withdraw from the umbilical cord to their normal position in the abdomen.

By week 17, the fetus's body is covered with lanugo, and sebaceous glands secrete sebum. This forms the vernix caseosa, a cheeselike material that covers the skin, protecting it from the drying action of the amniotic fluid. Many women feel movement, or quickening, between 16 and 20 weeks. Heart tones may be heard with a fetoscope placed over the symphysis pubis. By 20 weeks, the lower limbs are fully formed.

Although gaining weight steadily, the fetus between weeks 21 and 24 appears lean in comparison with a fetus at term. The wrinkled skin is covered with vernix caseosa. The lungs produce surfactant (a respiratory by-product); meconium (fetal excrement) is present in the rectum.

The face matures between 25 and 28 weeks; eyelashes and eyebrows form. Eyelids open and close. Skin is red. Most fetuses are considered viable by week 27 if given expert care.

Between 28 and 32 weeks, subcutaneous fat causes the fetus to grow more rounded. Vernix caseosa forms a thick coat on the skin. Cerebral fissures and convolutions appear. Born at the end of this period, the neonate has a good chance of survival if adequate care is provided.

Subcutaneous fat increases further during weeks 33 through 38. The fetus has hair and fully formed limbs with fingernails and toenails. Lanugo disappears from the face but remains on the head. Skin on the fetus's face and body becomes smooth. Amniotic fluid volume declines. The skull continues to be the largest body part. All organ systems are developed and can support extrauterine life. In males, the left testicle descends into the scrotum between 37 and 39 weeks. Both testicles are fully descended by 38 weeks.

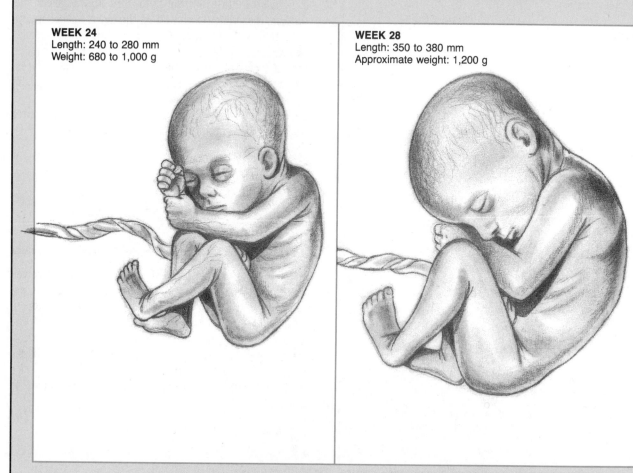

WEEK 24
Length: 240 to 280 mm
Weight: 680 to 1,000 g

WEEK 28
Length: 350 to 380 mm
Approximate weight: 1,200 g

WEEK 12
Approximate length: 70 mm
Approximate weight: 28 g

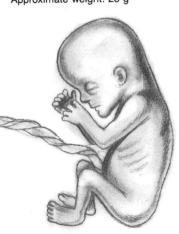

WEEK 16
Length: 100 to 170 mm
Weight: 55 to 120 g

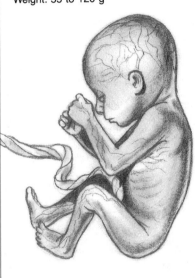

WEEK 20
Length: 160 to 250 mm
Weight: 223 to 310 g

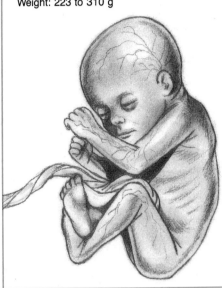

WEEK 32
Length: 380 to 430 mm
Weight: 1,700 to 2,400 g

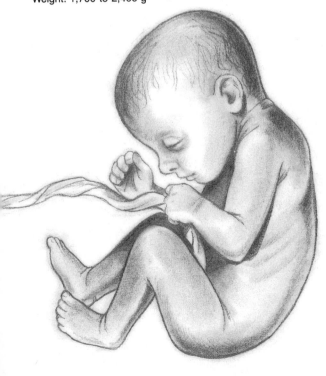

WEEK 38
Length: 480 to 520 mm
Weight: 2,800 to 3,200 g

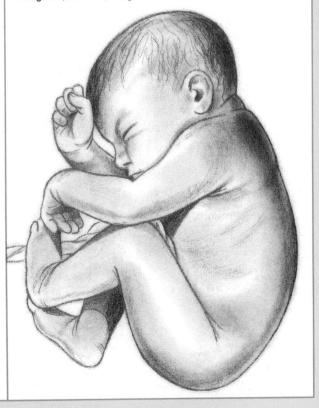

System development: Weeks 8 to 40

The following chart highlights significant events during fetal development and the times they occur.

CARDIOVASCULAR SYSTEM

16 to 20 weeks
- Fetal heart tone audible with fetoscope

ENDOCRINE SYSTEM

10 weeks
- Islets of Langerhans differentiated

12 weeks
- Thyroid secretes hormones
- Insulin present in pancreas

EXTERNAL APPEARANCE

12 weeks
- Nails appear
- Skin pink and delicate
- Lacrimal ducts developing

16 weeks
- Dominant head
- Scalp hair present
- Sweat glands developing

20 weeks
- Vernix, lanugo, and sebaceous glands appear
- Legs considerably lengthened

24 weeks
- Skin red and wrinkled
- Eyes structurally complete

28 weeks
- Eyelids open

32 weeks
- Increasing amount of of subcutaneous fat
- Pink, smooth skin

36 weeks
- Lanugo disappearing
- Soft earlobes with little cartilage

40 weeks
- Copious vernix
- Moderate to profuse hair
- Lanugo on shoulders and upper body
- Ear lobes stiffer with cartilage

GASTROINTESTINAL SYSTEM

8 to 11 weeks
- Intestinal villi form
- Small intestine coils in umbilical cord

12 to 16 weeks
- Bile is secreted
- Intestine withdraws from umbilical cord to normal position
- Meconium present in bowel
- Anus open

20 weeks
- Enamel and dentin are deposited
- Ascending colon appears
- Fetus can suck and swallow
- Peristaltic movements begin

GENITOURINARY SYSTEM

8 to 12 weeks
- Bladder and urethra separate from rectum; bladder expands as a sac
- Kidneys secrete urine

13 to 20 weeks
- Kidneys in proper position with definitive shape

36 weeks
- Formation of new nephrons ceases

MUSCULOSKELETAL SYSTEM

12 weeks
- Some bones well outlined
- Ossification continues

16 weeks
- Joint cavities present
- Muscular movements detectable

20 weeks
- Ossification of sternum
- Mother can detect fetal movements (quickening)

28 to 32 weeks
- Ossification continues
- Fetus can turn head to side

36 weeks
- Muscle tone developed; fetus can turn and elevate head

NERVOUS SYSTEM

12 to 16 weeks
- Structural configuration of brain roughly completed
- Cerebral lobes delineated
- Cerebellum assumes prominence

20 to 24 weeks
- Brain grossly formed
- Myelination of spinal cord begins
- Spinal cords ends at S-1

28 to 36 weeks
- Cerebral fissures appear
- Convolutions appear
- Spinal cord ends at L-3

40 weeks
- Myelination of brain begins

REPRODUCTIVE SYSTEM

12 to 24 weeks
- Testes descend into the inguinal canal
- External genitalia distinguishable

RESPIRATORY SYSTEM

8 to 12 weeks
- Bronchioles branch
- Pleural and pericardial cavities appear
- Lungs assume definitive shape

13 to 20 weeks
- Terminal and respiratory bronchioles appear

21 to 28 weeks
- Nostrils open
- Surfactant production begins
- Respiratory movements possible
- Alveolar ducts and sacs appear

38 to 40 weeks
- Pulmonary branching two-thirds complete
- Lecithin-sphingomyelin (L-S) ratio 2:1

Placenta

A flattened, disk-shaped structure that weighs about 500 g, the placenta is derived from the trophoblast and from maternal tissues. The chorion and the villi are formed from the trophoblast, and the decidua basalis, in which the villi are anchored, is derived from the endometrium. The fused amnion and chorion extend from the margins of the placenta to form the fluid-filled sac enclosing the fetus, which ruptures at birth. (See *Placental and membrane development in dizygotic and monozygotic twins*, page 387, for illustrations of how placental development may vary.)

Placental circulation

The placenta circulates blood between the mother and fetus so that oxygen and nutrients may be exchanged. This is accomplished through a specialized circulation system in which fetal and maternal blood do not mix.

The fetus is connected to the placenta by the umbilical cord, which contains two arteries and a single vein. The arteries follow a spiral course in the cord, divide on the surface of the placenta, and branch to the chorionic villi. Oxygenated arterial blood from the mother is delivered into large spaces between the villi (intervillous spaces) and delivered to the fetus through the single umbilical vein. Oxygen-depleted blood travels from the fetus to the chorionic villi through the two umbilical arteries. This blood leaves the intervillous spaces and flows back into the maternal circulation through veins in the basal part of the placenta.

Placental transfer

Substances are transferred across the placenta via four mechanisms: simple diffusion, facilitated diffusion, active transport, and pinocytosis. (See *Placental transfer*, page 386, for examples of these substances.) The fetal-placental unit (umbilical cord, placental layers, and chorionic villi) must have developed properly and be functioning for placental transfer to occur.

Requiring no energy, diffusion is a passive process that moves dissolved substances from an area of high concentration to one of lower concentration. Several factors influence its rate:
• Concentration gradient (the amount of difference in concentration of substances on either side of the placenta)
• Size of molecules (small molecules diffuse more rapidly than large ones)
• Solubility of molecules in the lipid layer of a cell membrane (more soluble molecules diffuse more rapidly).

Simple diffusion transfers oxygen, carbon dioxide, water, and most electrolytes across the placenta. Facilitated diffusion is similar to simple diffusion, but its rate of transfer is faster because carrier molecules transport substances without the use of energy. Glucose is transferred across the placenta in this way.

Requiring energy, active transport can move a substance from cells containing a lower concentration to ones containing a higher concentration by using carrier molecules that combine with the substance and carry it across the placenta. Amino acids, water soluble vitamins, and iron are transferred this way.

Pinocytosis is a mechanism through which placental membranes engulf intact droplets. Large molecules such as globulins and lipoproteins, which are too large to transport through diffusion or active transport, are transferred in this way. Gamma globulins are readily transported by pinocytosis.

Maternal protein hormones are not transferred through the placenta, with the exception of small amounts of thyroxin and triiodothyronine. Steroid hormones traverse the placenta freely. Viruses may cross the placenta and infect the fetus, as may some bacteria and protozoa.

Endocrine functions

In addition to providing the means by which the mother nourishes the developing fetus, the placenta also functions as an endocrine organ, producing various peptide, neuropeptide, and steroid hormones. The two major peptide hormones are human chorionic gonadotropin (hCG) and human placental lactogen (hPL). The neuropeptides include gonadotropin-releasing hormone (GnRH), thyrotropin-releasing factor (TRF), and adrenocorticotropic hormone (ACTH). Synthesized by the cytotrophoblast (outer layer of the trophoblast), they may regulate the synthesis and release of peptide hormones from the syncytial trophoblast. The two major steroid hormones are estrogen and progesterone.

Human chorionic gonadotropin

This hormone is a glycoprotein composed of two subunits designated alpha and beta. The alpha subunit also is present in three other glycoprotein hormones: FHS, LH, and thyroid-stimulating hormone. The beta subunit is unique to hCG. Produced by the syncytiotrophoblast (peripheral layer of the trophoblast), hCG can be detected in the mother's serum as early as 8 days after conception,

(Text continues on page 386.)

Photographic essay of embryonic and fetal development

Before the client knows for certain that she is pregnant, the embryo is growing rapidly in a cavity beneath the surface of the uterine wall. There, the embryo begins a development that the following classic photographs illuminate.

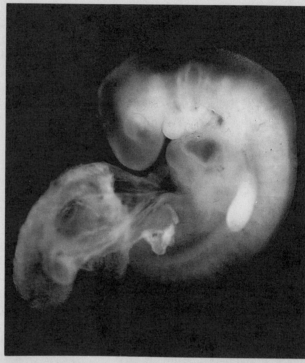

Week 4
Approximate length: 5 cm (0.2")
The embryo has no facial characteristics; the head and neck comprise half the body length.

Week 6
Approximate length: 1.5 cm (0.6")
The embryo floats freely in the fluid-filled amnion. The yolk sac and its stem are still attached but have ceased growing because the liver has begun producing blood cells.

Week 7
Approximate length: 2 cm (0.8")
The umbilical cord has formed, and the heart is beating.

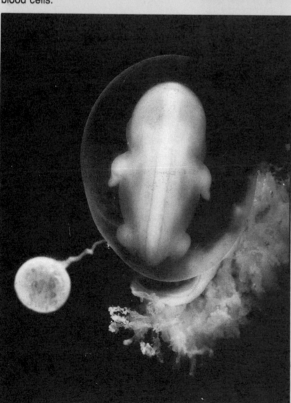

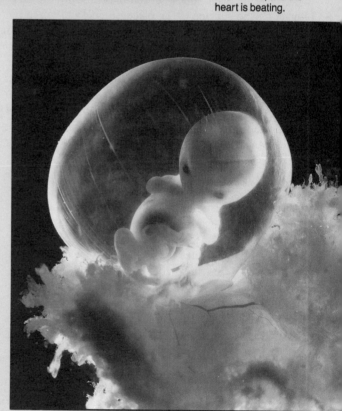

Photographs courtesy of Lennart Nilsson, from *A Child Is Born* (Revised Edition). New York: Dell Publishing, 1986.

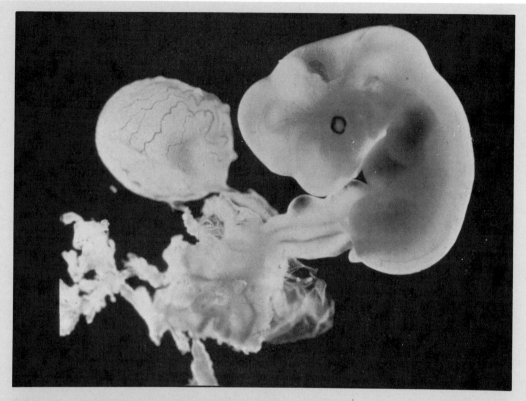

Week 5½
Approximate length: 1 cm (0.4")
Because no bone marrow exists at this stage, the yolk sac is the principal supplier of blood cells. Blood circulation is mostly outside the embryo.

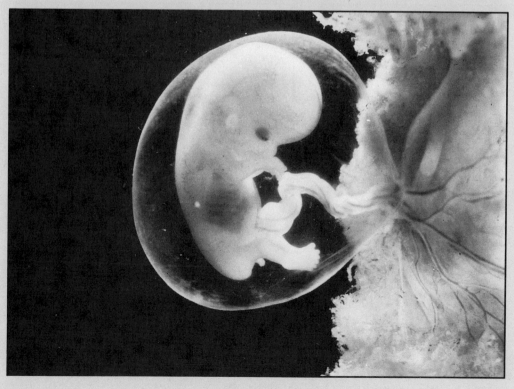

Week 9
Approximate length: 4.5 cm (2")
The placenta has grown where the blastocyst implanted itself in the uterine wall. The fetus receives nourishment through the umbilical cord.

(continued)

Photographic essay of embryonic and fetal development continued

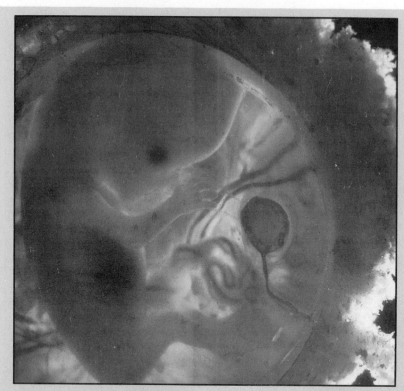

Week 11
Approximate length: 6 cm (2.4")
Blood cells are now produced in the liver and spleen, and the heart is functioning. The face has assumed a baby's profile, and the lips open and close. Although the mother cannot feel the weak legs and arms, they are in constant motion.

Week 18
Approximate length: 25 cm (10")
During constant movement, the fetus may pass a thumb across the mouth. The lips and tongue will respond with a suckling action.

Week 18
Approximate length: 25 cm (10")
Lanugo that follows the whorled skin pattern will be mostly shed before birth. The eyebrows are faintly apparent.

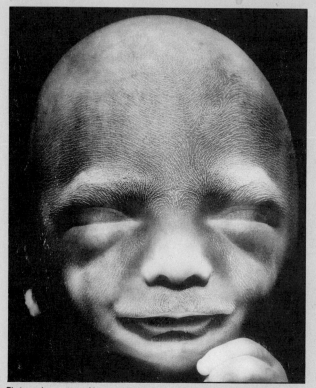

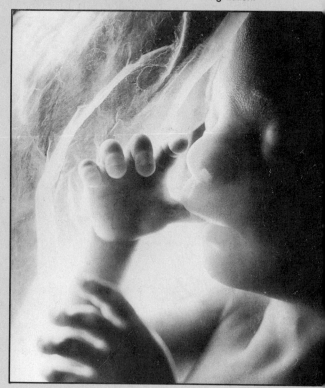

Photographs courtesy of Lennart Nilsson, from *A Child Is Born* (Revised Edition). New York: Dell Publishing, 1986.

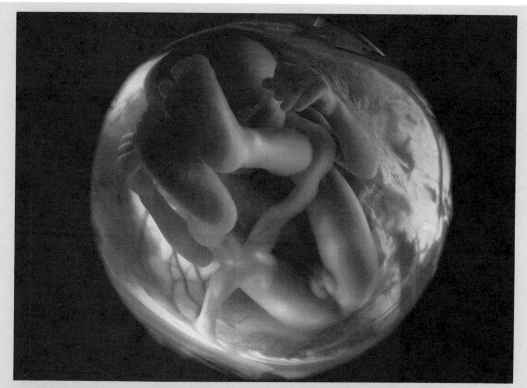

Week 16
Approximate length: 18 cm (7")
One half the length of a neonate, the fetus has ears that function. Although the eyes have grown shut, they will reopen later. The mother may now feel faint kicks as the fetus moves around.

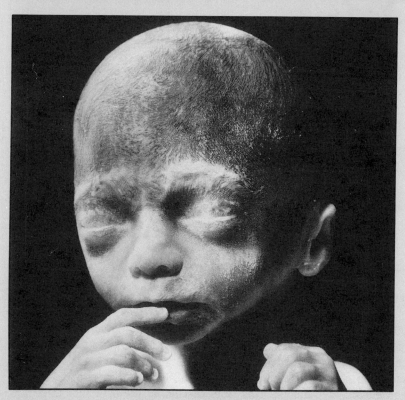

Week 20
Approximate length: 30 cm (12")
Vernix, a protective skin ointment that covers all body surfaces, is especially thick on the upper lip, eyebrows, and scalp.

Placental transfer

Many substances can be transported from mother to fetus and back through the placenta. The fetal-placental unit must have developed properly and be functioning for placental transfer to occur.

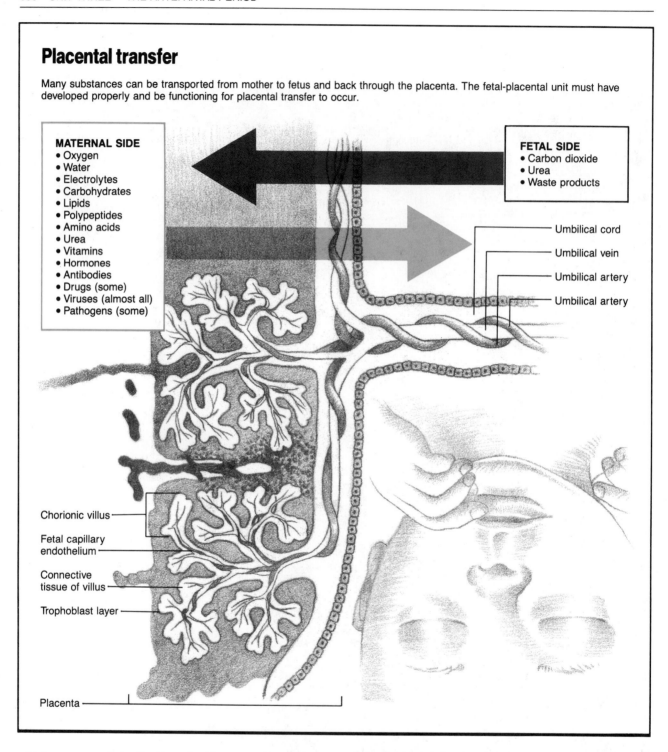

MATERNAL SIDE
- Oxygen
- Water
- Electrolytes
- Carbohydrates
- Lipids
- Polypeptides
- Amino acids
- Urea
- Vitamins
- Hormones
- Antibodies
- Drugs (some)
- Viruses (almost all)
- Pathogens (some)

FETAL SIDE
- Carbon dioxide
- Urea
- Waste products

Umbilical cord
Umbilical vein
Umbilical artery
Umbilical artery

Chorionic villus
Fetal capillary endothelium
Connective tissue of villus
Trophoblast layer
Placenta

which corresponds to the time the blastocyst is burrowing into the endometrium.

Levels of hCG rise rapidly to about 100 IU/ml at about the tenth week of gestation, and then gradually decline, reaching a low of about 10 IU/ml by the twentieth week and remaining at low levels for the remainder of gestation. For the first 8 weeks of pregnancy, hCG maintains the corpus luteum, which provides the progesterone essential to the pregnancy until the placenta takes over hormone production. This hormone also may regulate maternal and fetal synthesis of steroid hormones, and it stimulates testosterone production by the testes of a male fetus.

The detection of hCG in the blood and urine by immunologic tests specific for the beta subunit of hCG is the basis of widely used pregnancy tests. Highly sen-

Placental and membrane development in dizygotic and monozygotic twins

Born in about 1% of pregnancies, twins may be either dizygotic (fraternal) or monozygotic (identical). Seventy percent of twins are fraternal, resulting from two ova fertilized by two spermatozoa. Each zygote implants separately and forms its own placenta and fetal membranes. Although the placental margins may fuse together, each fetus remains enclosed within its own amnion and chorion. A fused placenta of this type is called a diamnionic dichorionic placenta. Genetically, the fetuses are no more alike than typical siblings.

Thirty percent of twins are identical—that is, they result from the division of a single fertilized ovum. Thus, the fetuses are genetically alike and must be of the same sex. In most identical twin pregnancies, the inner cell mass divides after the blastocyst has formed but before implantation occurs. Each half of the inner cell mass forms an embryo with its own amniotic sac, but both fetuses develop within the same chorionic cavity and share one placenta. This is known as a diamnionic monochorionic placenta. However, if the ovum splits before the inner cell mass forms, identical twins may have a diamnionic, dichorionic placenta.

Rarely, the inner cell mass divides after formation of the amniotic sac. Two embryos develop within a single amniotic sac, forming a monoamnionic monochorionic placenta. Incomplete division of the inner cell mass results in conjoined (Siamese) twins.

DIZYGOTIC TWINS

Two blastocysts implant separately and develop individual fetal membranes and two separate placentas.

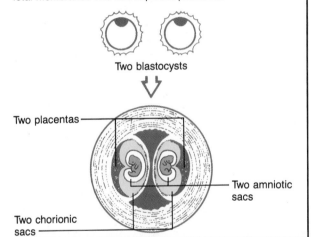

Two blastocysts implant close together and develop individual fetal membranes and two fused placentas.

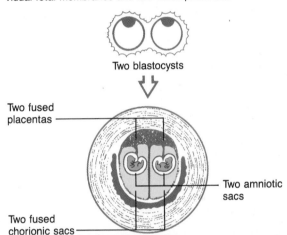

MONOZYGOTIC TWINS

One blastocyst implants with two inner cell masses, forming two amnions, one chorion, and one placenta.

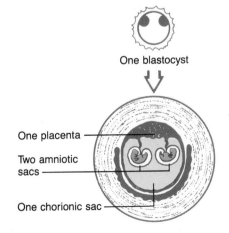

One blastocyst implants and the inner cell mass divides, forming one amnion, one chorion, and one placenta. Incomplete division results in conjoined twins.

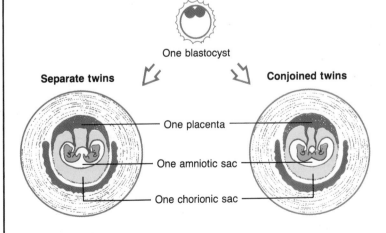

Fetal circulation

During development, three shunts operate to bypass the fetus's liver and lungs: the ductus venosus, foramen ovale, and ductus arteriosus.

Oxygenated blood returns from the placenta in the umbilical vein. Part of the blood passes through the sinusoids in the liver, but most is shunted into the inferior vena cava through the first bypass channel, the ductus venosus. Most of the blood flowing into the right atrium from the vena cava is directed into the left atrium through the second shunt, the foramen ovale, bypassing the lungs. Blood then flows from the left atrium to the left ventricle and is ejected into the aorta.

Some of the blood returning to the right atrium through the superior vena cava flows into the right ventricle and then is pumped into the pulmonary artery. Because the lungs are deflated, blood flowing into the pulmonary arteries encounters resistance. Consequently, most of the blood entering the main pulmonary artery bypasses the lungs and flows directly into the aorta through the ductus arteriosus.

The small amount of blood ejected from the right ventricle to the lungs returns to the left atrium through the pulmonary veins. This blood mixes with that passing from the right atrium to the left atrium through the foramen ovale, flows into the left ventricle, and is ejected into the aorta.

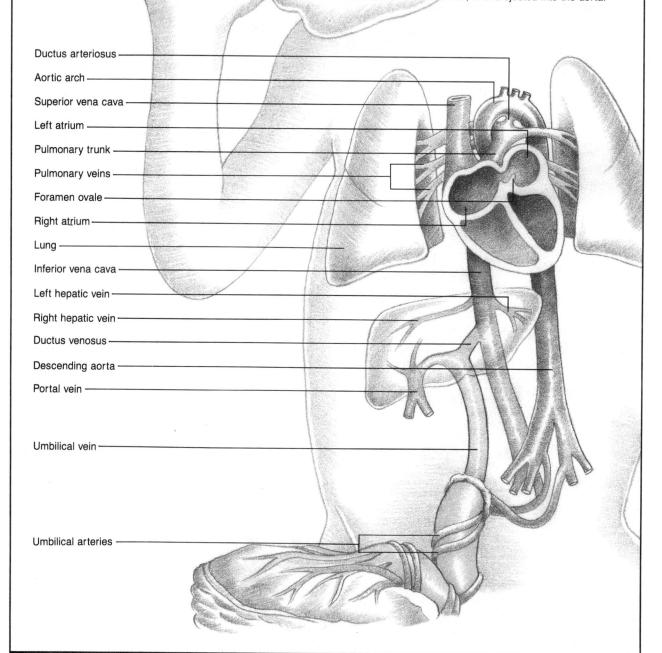

Ductus arteriosus

Aortic arch

Superior vena cava

Left atrium

Pulmonary trunk

Pulmonary veins

Foramen ovale

Right atrium

Lung

Inferior vena cava

Left hepatic vein

Right hepatic vein

Ductus venosus

Descending aorta

Portal vein

Umbilical vein

Umbilical arteries

sitive and specific pregnancy tests can detect hCG in blood and urine even before the first missed menstrual period, and sensitive tests almost invariably are positive if pregnancy causes a missed menstrual period.

Human placental lactogen

Also known as human chorionic somatomammotropin, hPL is a single-chain polypeptide hormone that is produced by the syncytiotrophoblast and has properties similar to pituitary growth hormone. HPL stimulates the maternal metabolism of protein and fat to ensure adequate amino and fatty acids for the mother and fetus. It may antagonize the action of insulin in the mother, decreasing maternal glucose use and making it available to the fetus. The hormone also stimulates the growth of the breasts in preparation for lactation. HPL levels rise progressively throughout pregnancy.

Other peptide hormones

The placenta also produces human chorionic thyrotropin, which has thyroid-stimulating properties, and human chorionic adrenocorticotropin, which has ACTH properties. The physiologic role of these placental hormones is not known. Another placental glycoprotein hormone called inhibin inhibits FSH secretion during pregnancy.

Estrogen

Three types of estrogen are produced by the placenta, differing chiefly in the number of hydroxyl groups attached to the steroid nucleus: estrone (E_1), estradiol (E_2), and estriol (E_3). Estrogen production (primarily estriol) and estrogen urinary output increase throughout pregnancy. Progesterone production also increases; progesterone is excreted in the urine as the metabolite pregnanediol.

In contrast to the ovary, which has all the enzyme systems needed for synthesis of both estrogen and progesterone from simple compounds, the placenta lacks important enzymes and is unable to synthesize these hormones completely. To synthesize estrogen, the placenta must be provided with compounds from the fetal and maternal adrenal glands. Most of the steroids produced by the placenta are secreted into the maternal blood.

Because estrogen production depends on an adequate supply of precursor steroids from the fetal adrenal gland, a reduced estrogen output in pregnancy can indicate insufficient fetal adrenal gland development. Anencephaly, a congenital abnormality in which the brain fails to develop, commonly is associated with failure of the adrenal glands to develop normally. In other instances, the fetal adrenal glands may undergo hyperplasia or excessive development. As would be expected, the estrogen output in the urine of a woman carrying an affected fetus is much increased because of the greater amount of precursor steroids provided to the placenta by the enlarged fetal adrenal glands.

Progesterone

Progesterone is synthesized by the placenta through hydroxylation of maternal cholesterol. Cholesterol is carried to the placenta in low-density lipoprotein particles that become attached to receptors on the surface of the trophoblasts and are carried into the cytoplasm of the cell where the lipoprotein is degraded. The cholesterol freed from the lipoprotein is converted first to pregnenolone and then to progesterone. Because the fetus plays no part in progesterone biosynthesis, progesterone levels are unaffected by fetal distress or fetal abnormalites.

Fetal circulation

Because lungs do not function in a fetus, blood is oxygenated by the placenta. Fetal circulation differs from neonatal circulation in that three shunts bypass the liver and lungs and separate the systemic and pulmonary circulations. Because of the shunts, the umbilical vein carries oxygenated blood and the umbilical arteries carry unoxygenated blood. The shunts are:
• the ductus venosus
• the foramen ovale
• the ductus arteriosus.
(See *Fetal circulation* for an illustration and description of this specialized system. For further discussion of fetal circulation, see Chapter 34, Neonatal Adaptation.)

Chapter summary

Chapter 16 described fetal development during normal gestation. Here are the chapter highlights.
• In vivo fertilization can take place only when a mature spermatozoon ascends through a fallopian tube, encounters a mature, descending ovum, and enters and fertilizes it.
• Implantation follows fertilization by about 1 week.
• Human development from fertilization to birth includes three distinct periods: pre-embryonic, embryonic, and fetal.
• All human organ systems are derived from three germ cell layers: ectoderm, endoderm, and mesoderm.
• All organ systems are formed by the eighth week of gestation.

• Specialized organs and tissues that develop shortly after conception support, protect, and nurture the fetus. These include the decidua, fetal membranes, amniotic fluid, and placenta.

• The placenta arises from the trophoblastic tissue layer and supports the fetus by providing the mechanisms for nutrition, respiration, and waste removal.

• Placental transfer of substances is accomplished by simple diffusion, facilitated diffusion, active transport, and pinocytosis.

• Fetal circulation includes three shunts that bypass the lungs and liver: the ductus venosus, foramen ovale, and ductus arteriosus.

Study questions

1. How is an in vivo ovum fertilized?

2. How and where is a fertilized ovum implanted?

3. Which major structures develop during the pre-embryonic period?

4. Which major developments occur during the embryonic period?

5. What are the three germ cell layers, and which organ systems arise from each layer?

6. By which mechanisms are substances transported across the placental barrier?

7. How does fetal circulation differ from neonatal circulation?

Bibliography

Battaglia, F., and Meschia, G. (1986). *An introduction to fetal physiology.* Orlando, FL: Academic Press.

Briggs, G.G., Freeman, R.K., and Yaffe, S.J. (1986). *Drugs in pregnancy and lactation* (2nd ed.). Baltimore: Williams & Wilkins.

Chapman, M.C., Chard, T., and Grudzinskas, G. (Eds.). (1989). *Implantation.* New York: Springer-Verlag.

Crowley, L.V. (1988). *Introduction to human disease* (2nd ed.). Boston: Jones and Bartlet.

Crowley, L.V. (1974). *An introduction to clinical embryology.* Chicago: Year Book Medical Publishers.

Cunningham, F.G., MacDonald, P.C., and Gant, N.F. (Eds.). (1989). *Williams obstetrics* (18th ed.). East Norwalk, CT: Appleton & Lange.

Danforth, D.N., and Scott, J.R. (Eds.). (1986). *Obstetrics and gynecology* (5th ed.). Philadelphia: Lippincott.

England, M. (1983). *A color atlas of life before birth: Normal fetal development.* Chicago: Year Book Medical Publishers.

Faber, J., and Thornburg, K. (1983). *Placental physiology: Structure and function of fetomaternal exchange.* New York: Raven Press.

Guyton, A. (1986). *Textbook of medical physiology* (7th ed.). Philadelphia: Saunders.

Hacker, N.F., and Moore, J.G. (Eds.). (1986). *Essentials of obstetrics and gynecology.* Philadelphia: Saunders.

Isaacson, G. (1986). *Atlas of fetal sectional physiology.* New York: Springer-Verlag.

Jones, C.T., and Nathanielsz, P.W. (1985). *The physiological development of the fetus and newborn.* Orlando, FL: Academic Press.

Moore, K.L. (1983). *Before we were born: Basic embryology and birth defects* (2nd ed.). Philadelphia: Saunders.

Moore, K.L. (1988). *The developing human: Clinically oriented embryology.* (4th ed.). Philadelphia: Saunders.

O'Rahilly, R., and Muller, F. (1987). Developmental stages in human embryos. Washington, DC: Carnegie Institute of Washington.

Page, E.W., Villett, C.A., and Villee, D.B. (1976). *Human reproduction* (text ed.). Philadelphia: Saunders.

Pansky, B. (1982). *Review of medical embryology.* New York: Macmillan.

Rana, M.W. (1984). *Key facts in embryology.* New York: Churchill Livingstone.

Roberts, D.F. (Ed.). (1976). *The biology of human fetal growth.* Symposia of the Society for the Study of Human Biology Series, vol. 15. New York: Taylor & Francis.

Rolfe, P. (Ed.). (1987). *Fetal physiological measurements.* Woburn, MA: Butterworth.

Sadler, T.W. (1985). *Langman's medical embryology* (5th ed.). Baltimore: Williams & Wilkins.

Speroff, L., Glass, R.H., and Kase, N.G. (1988). *Clinical gynecologic endocrinology and infertility* (4th ed.). Baltimore: Williams & Wilkins.

Physiologic Changes during Normal Pregnancy

Objectives

After reading and studying this chapter, the student should be able to:

1. Distinguish among presumptive, probable, and positive signs of pregnancy.

2. Describe the major signs and symptoms used to diagnose pregnancy.

3. Discuss physiologic changes that occur in the maternal reproductive, endocrine, respiratory, cardiovascular, urinary, gastrointestinal, musculoskeletal, integumentary, immune, and neurologic systems during pregnancy.

4. Relate the underlying causes for maternal physiologic changes.

Introduction

Physiologic changes that occur during pregnancy are among the most dramatic that the human body can undergo. They help the client adapt to pregnancy, maintain health throughout pregnancy, and prepare for childbirth. They also create a safe and nurturing environment for the fetus. Some begin even before the client becomes aware that she is pregnant.

Physiologic changes associated with pregnancy may range from subtle to overwhelming. Although these changes are normal and necessary, they may be uncomfortable and—especially for the primigravid client—even frightening. To care for pregnant clients properly, the nurse must understand the physiologic changes of normal pregnancy, when they occur, and how they are likely to affect the client. This chapter begins by outlining the presumptive, probable, and positive signs of pregnancy.

It then describes the physiologic changes that occur in each maternal body system, the role various hormones play in initiating and regulating body functions during pregnancy, and the signs and symptoms commonly caused by these changes. (For information on nursing care of the antepartal client, see Chapter 19, Care during the Normal Antepartal Period.)

Diagnosing pregnancy

Early pregnancy produces a constellation of physiologic changes (signs and symptoms) that the health care provider must evaluate as a group before reaching a tentative diagnosis of pregnancy. Some of these changes may be presumptive signs of pregnancy (those that allow an assumption of pregnancy until more concrete signs occur), such as amenorrhea; some may be probable signs of pregnancy, such as abdominal enlargement. Neither presumptive nor probable signs confirm pregnancy because both may be caused by medical conditions. They may suggest pregnancy, however, especially when several are present at once. Probable signs suggest pregnancy somewhat more strongly than presumptive signs. Positive signs, such as fetal heartbeat and palpable fetal movement, prove pregnancy because they cannot be caused by any condition. (For more details, see *Presumptive, probable, and positive signs of pregnancy*, pages 394 and 395.)

GLOSSARY

Amenorrhea: absence of menstruation.

Ballottment: passive movement of the fetus elicited during pelvic examination in the fourth and fifth months of pregnancy.

Basal metabolic rate: body's expenditure of energy, typically documented by measuring oxygen intake and use.

Braxton Hicks contractions: painless uterine contractions that occur at irregular intervals throughout pregnancy; do not cause cervical changes.

Chloasma: irregular, brownish blotches over the malar prominences (cheek bones) and forehead.

Colostrum: viscous, yellowish fluid expressed from the nipples during pregnancy, increasing as term approaches; high in protein, antibodies, and minerals but low in fat and sugar compared with mature human milk.

Decidua: name of the endometrium following implantation.

Fibrin: insoluble protein formed from fibrinogen and essential for blood clotting.

Fibrinogen: protein clotting factor in blood plasma that is converted to fibrin by the action of thrombin.

Funic souffle: blowing sound heard as fetal blood courses through the umbilical cord.

Hematocrit: volume percentage of red blood cells in whole blood.

Hemoglobin: protein in red blood cells that transports oxygen.

Hyperemia: increased amount of blood.

Hyperplasia: increase in cell number.

Hypertrophy: increase in cell size.

Linea nigra: dark line extending from the umbilicus or above to the mons pubis.

Meralgia paresthetica: tingling and numbness in the anterolateral portion of the thigh caused by entrapment of the lateral femoral cutaneous nerve in the area of the inguinal ligaments.

Mucus plug: protective mucus barrier that blocks the cervical canal during pregnancy; caused by estrogen stimulation.

Puerperium: 6-week period after childbirth.

Quickening: fluttering movements in the abdomen, typically felt after 16 to 20 weeks of pregnancy.

Striae gravidarum: pink streaks in the skin caused by separated connective tissue; typically appear on the breasts, abdomen, buttocks, or thighs and turn silvery after childbirth. Also called stretch marks.

Uterine souffle: blowing sound heard with a stethoscope as blood flows through the uterine arteries to the placenta.

Changes in body systems

Physiologic changes that help diagnose pregnancy make up only a small number of the changes that occur in a pregnant client. As the fetus grows and hormones shift, the client's body undergoes physiologic changes, primarily to adapt to the fetus and to prepare for childbirth. Physiologic adjustments occur in each body system.

Reproductive system

External reproductive structures affected by pregnancy include the labia majora, labia minora, clitoris, and vaginal introitus. These structures enlarge because of increased vascularity; the labia majora and labia minora also enlarge because of fat deposits. Although the structures reduce in size after childbirth, they may not return to their prepregnant state because of loss of muscle tone or perineal injury. For example, the labia majora remain separated and gape after childbirth. In addition, varices may be caused by pressure on vessels in the perineal and perianal areas.

Internal reproductive structures change dramatically to accommodate the developing fetus. Like their external counterparts, these internal structures may not regain their prepregnant states after childbirth.

Ovaries

Once fertilization occurs, ovarian follicles cease to mature and ovulation stops. The chorionic villi, which develop from the fertilized ovum, begin to produce human chorionic gonadotropin (hCG) to maintain the ovarian corpus luteum. The corpus luteum produces estrogen and progesterone until the placenta is formed and functioning. At 8 to 10 weeks of pregnancy, the placenta assumes production of these hormones and the corpus luteum—no longer needed—undergoes involution (reduction in organ size caused by a reduction in the size of its cells).

Uterus

The nonpregnant uterus is smaller than the size of a fist, measuring approximately 7.5 × 5 × 2.5 cm. It weighs approximately 60 to 70 g in the nulliparous client and 100 g in the parous client. In its nonpregnant state, the uterus can hold no more than 10 cc of fluid. Its walls are composed of several overlapping layers of muscle fibers that adapt to the developing fetus and aid in expulsion of the fetus and placenta during labor and childbirth. (For more information on uterine muscles, see Chapter 6, Reproductive Anatomy and Physiology.)

The uterus retains the developing fetus for approximately 280 days, or 9 calendar months, and undergoes progressive changes in size, shape, and position in the abdominal cavity.

Enlargement. In the first trimester, the pear-shaped uterus lengthens and enlarges in response to elevated levels of estrogen and progesterone. This hormonal stimulation primarily increases the size of myometrial cells (hypertrophy), although a small increase in cell number (hyperplasia) also occurs. These changes increase the amount of fibrous and elastic tissue to more than 20 times that of the nonpregnant uterus. Uterine walls become stronger and more elastic.

During the first few weeks of pregnancy, the uterine walls remain thick and the fundus rests low in the abdomen. The uterus cannot be palpated through the abdominal wall. After 12 to 16 weeks of pregnancy, however, the uterus typically reaches the level of the symphysis pubis and may be palpated through the abdominal wall.

In the second trimester, the corpus and fundus become globe-shaped, and as pregnancy progresses the uterus lengthens to become oval in shape. The uterine walls become thinner as the muscles stretch; the uterus rises out of the pelvis, shifts to the right, and rests against the anterior abdominal wall. At 20 to 22 weeks of pregnancy, the uterus may be palpated just below the umbilicus and reaches the umbilicus at 22 to 24 weeks. As uterine muscles stretch, Braxton Hicks contractions may occur, helping to move blood more quickly through the intervillous spaces of the placenta. (For more information on Braxton Hicks contractions, see Chapter 19, Care during the Normal Antepartal Period, and Chapter 27, The First Stage of Labor.)

In the third trimester, the fundus reaches nearly to the xiphoid process (also called the ensiform process). Between 38 and 40 weeks of pregnancy, the fetus begins to descend in the pelvis (lightening), which causes fundal height to drop gradually. (For an illustration, see *Changes in fundal height during pregnancy*.) The uterus remains

(Text continues on page 396.)

Changes in fundal height during pregnancy

During pregnancy, the fundus progresses from a position low in the abdomen, where it cannot be palpated through the abdominal wall, to one just under the xiphoid process. The illustrations below show how fundal height changes throughout pregnancy.

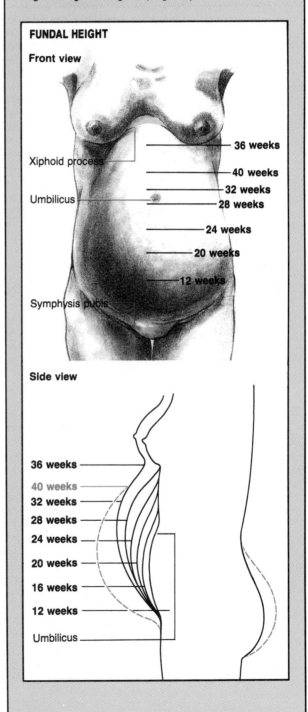

FUNDAL HEIGHT

Front view

Xiphoid process

Umbilicus

Symphysis pubis

- 36 weeks
- 40 weeks
- 32 weeks
- 28 weeks
- 24 weeks
- 20 weeks
- 12 weeks

Side view

- 36 weeks
- 40 weeks
- 32 weeks
- 28 weeks
- 24 weeks
- 20 weeks
- 16 weeks
- 12 weeks

Umbilicus

Presumptive, probable, and positive signs of pregnancy

The following chart lists and describes typical presumptive and probable signs of pregnancy and explains their pregnancy-related and possible other causes. The chart then describes positive signs of pregnancy.

SIGN	DESCRIPTION	PREGNANCY-RELATED CAUSES	POSSIBLE OTHER CAUSES
Presumptive			
Amenorrhea	Absence of menses. Usually the first indication of pregnancy in client with regular menstrual periods.	• Rising levels of human chorionic gonadotropin (hCG) hormone	• Anovulation, blocked endometrial cavity, endocrine changes (early menopause, lactation, glandular dysfunction), medications (phenothiazines), metabolic changes (anemia, malnutrition, long distance running), psychological disorder, systemic disease
Nausea and vomiting	Onset typically at 4 to 6 weeks, continuing through first trimester or occasionally longer.	• Rising levels of hCG • Emotional stress • Reduced gastric motility, reflux • Altered metabolism	• Gastric disorders, infections, psychological disorders (pseudocyesis, anorexia nervosa)
Urinary frequency	Begins during first trimester when enlarging uterus exerts pressure on urinary bladder; resolves during second trimester when uterus rises out of pelvis; resumes during third trimester when fetus descends into pelvis.	• Enlarging uterus exerts pressure on urinary bladder	• Emotional stress, pelvic tumor, renal disease, urinary tract infection
Breast changes	Enlargement begins early in first trimester. Breasts become tender and may tingle or throb. As pregnancy progresses, nipples enlarge, become more erectile, and may darken. The areolae widen. Veins become more visible beneath breast skin.	• Hormonal changes • Growth of secretory ductal system • Increase in glandular tissue	• Hyperprolactinemia induced by tranquilizers, infection, prolactin-secreting pituitary tumor, pseudocyesis, premenstrual syndrome
Fatigue	Malaise, general discomfort, lethargy with no apparent cause.	• Unexplained, although progesterone may play a role	• Anemia, chronic illness
Quickening	Client's first awareness of active movements of fetus, usually felt as fluttering movements in lower abdomen at 16 to 20 weeks.	• Movement of fetus	• Excessive flatus, increased peristalsis
Skin changes	May include linea nigra, chloasma, vascular markings, and striae. Because pigment changes may persist, they are not a reliable sign in multigravid clients.	• Increase in melanocyte-stimulating hormone • Increased estrogen • Stretching and atrophy of connective tissue	• Cardiopulmonary disorders, estrogen-progestin oral contraceptives, obesity, pelvic tumor
Probable			
Braun von Fernwald's sign (also called Piskacek's sign)	Fullness and irregular softness of fundus near area of implantation. Can be felt at 5 to 6 weeks of pregnancy.	• Local reaction to implantation; increased blood flow to pelvic organs	• Uterine tumor
Hegar's sign	Softening of uterine isthmus may be felt at 6 to 8 weeks via vaginal or rectovaginal examination.	• Increased blood flow to pelvic organs	• Excessively soft uterine walls

Presumptive, probable, and positive signs of pregnancy continued

SIGN	DESCRIPTION	PREGNANCY-RELATED CAUSES	POSSIBLE OTHER CAUSES
Goodell's sign	Softening of cervix at 6 to 8 weeks.	• Increased blood flow to pelvic organs	• Estrogen-progestin oral contraceptives
Chadwick's sign	Bluish coloration of mucous membranes of cervix, vagina, and vulva at 6 to 8 weeks.	• Engorgement caused by increased blood flow to pelvic organs	• Hyperemia of cervix, vagina, vulva
McDonald's sign	Easy flexion of fundus into cervix at 6 to 8 weeks.	• Increased blood flow to pelvic organs	• Oral contraceptives, uterine tumor
Ladin's sign	Soft, palpable area on anterior middle portion of uterus near junction of uterus and cervix.	• Increased blood flow to pelvic organs	• Oral contraceptives, uterine tumor
Abdominal enlargement	Softening of uterus and fetal growth cause uterus to enlarge and stretch abdominal wall.	• Enlarging uterus	• Ascites, obesity, uterine or pelvic tumor
Braxton Hicks contractions	Uterine contractions beginning early in pregnancy and becoming more frequent after 28 weeks.	• Possibly from enlargement of uterus to accommodate growing fetus	• Hematometra, uterine tumor
Ballottment	Passive movement of fetus felt during pelvic examination. Typically identified at weeks 16 to 18.	• Rebounding of fetus in response to pressure exerted on uterus	• Ascites, uterine tumor or polyps
Uterine souffle	Soft, blowing sound synchronous with maternal pulse as blood flows through uterine arteries.	• Increased vascularity as blood flows through placenta	• Large ovarian tumor, enlarging myoma
Funic souffle	Sharp, blowing sound synchronous with fetal pulse as blood flows through umbilical cord.	• Increased vascularity as blood flows through umbilical cord	• Aneurysm of abdominal aorta, iliac artery, or renal artery
Fetal outline	Fetus may be palpated through uterine wall after 24 weeks.	• Growing fetus	• Subserous uterine myoma
Positive pregnancy test	Based on detection of hCG secreted by chorionic villi. Levels of hCG begin to increase 6 to 8 days after conception, peak at 8 to 12 weeks, and gradually decline during second and third trimesters.	• Increased levels of hCG	• Luteinizing hormone is similar to hCG and may cross react in some pregnancy tests.
Positive			
Fetal heartbeat	May be detected as early as week 5 using ultrasound, week 10 using doppler ultrasound, week 12 using fetal electrocardiography, and week 16 using a standard fetoscope.	• Fetal cardiovascular development	• None
Fetal movement on palpation	May be felt as thump or flutter through abdomen after week 18; may be visible after week 20.	• Fetal growth	• None

oval in shape. Its muscular walls become progressively thinner as it enlarges, finally reaching a muscle wall thickness of 5 mm or less. At term (40 weeks), the uterus typically weighs approximately 1,100 g, holds 5 to 10 liters of fluid, and has stretched to approximately 28 × 24 × 21 cm.

Progressive abdominal enlargement (accompanied by amenorrhea) is the most observable sign of pregnancy, although posture and previous pregnancies will influence the type and amount of enlargement. Enlargement typically is more pronounced in the multigravid client because the uterus assumes a more forward position after previous pregnancies reduce abdominal muscle tone.

Endometrial development. During the menstrual cycle, progesterone stimulates increased thickening and vascularity of the endometrium, preparing the uterine lining for implantation and nourishment of a fertilized ovum. After implantation, menstruation ceases and the endometrium becomes the decidua, which is divided into three layers: decidua capsularis, decidua basalis, and decidua vera. The decidua capsularis covers the blastocyst (fertilized ovum). The decidua basalis lies directly under the blastocyst and forms part of the placenta. The decidua vera lines the remainder of the uterus. (To review the menstrual cycle, see Chapter 6, Reproductive Anatomy and Physiology.)

Vascular growth. As the fetus grows and the placenta develops, uterine blood vessels and lymphatics increase in number and size. Vessels must enlarge to accommodate the increased blood flow to the uterus and placenta. By the end of pregnancy, an average of 500 ml of blood may flow through the maternal side of the placenta each minute (Cunningham, MacDonald, and Gant, 1989). Maternal arterial pressure, uterine contractions, and maternal position affect uterine blood flow throughout pregnancy.

Elongation and softening of the isthmus. After 6 to 8 weeks of pregnancy, the isthmus softens and can be compressed during a vaginal or rectovaginal examination. This compression, known as Hegar's sign, offers one of the most important early signs of pregnancy. As pregnancy advances, the isthmus becomes part of the lower uterine segment. During labor, it expands further.

Cervical changes. In addition to softening, the cervix takes on a bluish color during the second month of pregnancy, becomes edematous, and may bleed easily upon examination or sexual activity.

Hormonal stimulation causes the glandular cervical tissue to increase in cell number and become more hyperactive, secreting a thick, tenacious mucus. This mucus thickens into a mucoid weblike structure, eventually forming a mucus plug that blocks the cervical canal and erects a protective barrier against bacteria and other substances that might enter the uterus.

Perhaps the outstanding characteristic of the cervix is its ability to stretch during childbirth, which is possible because of increased connective tissue, elastic fiber, and enfoldings in the endocervical lining.

Vagina

Estrogen stimulates vascularity, tissue growth, and hypertrophy in the vaginal epithelial tissue. Vaginal secretions—white, thick, odorless, and acidic—increase. The acidity of vaginal secretions helps prevent bacterial infections, but it fosters yeast infections, a common occurrence during pregnancy. This change in pH arises with increased production of lactic acid from glycogen in the vaginal epithelium; increased lactic acid results from the action of *Lactobacillus acidophilus*.

Other vaginal changes include:
• development of the same bluish color as the cervix and vulva due to increased vascularity
• hypertrophy of the smooth muscles and relaxation of connective tissues, which combine to allow the vagina to stretch during childbirth
• lengthening of the vaginal vault
• possible heightened sexual response.

Breasts

During the first trimester, increased levels of estrogen and progesterone enlarge the breasts and cause tenderness. They may tingle or throb. The nipples enlarge, become more erectile, and—along with the areolae—darken in color. Sebaceous glands in the areolae become hypertrophic, producing small elevations known as Montgomery's follicles. Areolae widen from a diameter of less than 3 cm (1½″) to 5 or 6 cm (2″ or 3″) in the primigravid client. Rarely, patches of brownish discoloration may appear on the skin adjacent to the areolae. These patches, known as secondary areolae, may be a sign of pregnancy if the client has never breast-fed an infant.

As blood vessels enlarge, veins beneath the skin of the breasts become more visible and may appear as intertwining patterns over the anterior chest wall. Breasts become fuller and heavier as lactation approaches. They may throb uncomfortably. Increasing hormones cause the secretion of a yellowish, viscous fluid from the nipples known as colostrum. High in protein, antibodies, and minerals but low in fat and sugar as compared with mature human milk, colostrum may be secreted as early as the first several months of pregnancy, but it is most common during the last trimester. It continues for 2 to 4 days after delivery and is followed by mature milk production.

Breast changes are more pronounced in the primigravid than in the multigravid client. In the latter, changes are even less significant if the client has breastfed an infant within the preceding year because her areola will still be dark and her breasts enlarged.

Endocrine system

Together with the nervous system, the endocrine system controls metabolic functions that promote maternal and fetal health throughout pregnancy. Estrogen stimulates and temporarily enlarges the pituitary, thyroid, and parathyroid glands. Other major endocrine changes occur as well.

Pituitary gland

Anterior pituitary hormones help to maintain the corpus luteum in early pregnancy. Two hormones secreted by the anterior pituitary—thyrotropin and adrenocorticotropic hormone (ACTH)—alter maternal metabolism so that pregnancy can progress. Prolactin, another anterior pituitary hormone, increases throughout pregnancy in preparation for lactation.

The posterior pituitary releases two hormones important in pregnancy. Vasopressin (antidiuretic hormone or ADH) helps regulate water balance through its antidiuretic action, and oxytocin stimulates labor and aids in lactation through its effect on breast tissue.

Thyroid gland

As early as the second month of pregnancy, thyroxine (T_4)-binding protein increases and total T_4 rises correspondingly. Because the amount of unbound T_4 does not increase, the client does not develop hyperthyroidism. However, thyroid changes do produce a slight increase in basal metabolic rate (BMR), cardiac output, pulse rate, vasodilation, and heat intolerance. The BMR increases about 15% during the second and third trimesters as the growing fetus places additional demands for energy on the client's system. By term, the client's BMR may have increased 25%. It returns to the prepregnant level within 1 week after childbirth.

In addition, estrogen increases circulating amounts of triiodothyronine (T_3). Because much of this hormone is bound to proteins and is thus nonfunctional (like T_4),

its elevation does not lead to a hyperthyroid condition during pregnancy.

Parathyroid gland

As pregnancy progresses, fetal demands for calcium and phosphorus increase. The parathyroid gland responds by increasing hormones during the third trimester to as much as twice the prepregnant level.

Adrenal gland

Increased estrogen raises the levels of cortisol and aldosterone. However, increased cortisol does not significantly increase the metabolism of carbohydrates, fats, and proteins (as it normally would) because much of the cortisol is bound by the cortisol-binding globulin transcortin. Elevated aldosterone minimizes the sodium-wasting effect of progesterone by promoting sodium resorption in the renal tubules.

Pancreas

Although the pancreas itself undergoes no changes during pregnancy, maternal insulin, glucose, and glucagon levels change. As pregnancy advances, fetal growth and development require increased glucose. For example, after ingesting oral glucose, the pregnant client has prolonged hyperglycemia, hyperinsulinism, and reduced glucagon levels. Although the reason for these level shifts is unknown, they probably provide a sustained supply of glucose to the fetus. The placenta secretes a hormone—human placental lactogen (hPL)—that promotes fat breakdown (lipolysis) and provides the client with an alternate source of energy.

However, hPL has a complicating effect. Along with estrogen, progesterone, and cortisol, hPL inhibits the action of insulin, which results in an increased need for insulin throughout pregnancy.

Respiratory system

Throughout pregnancy, biochemical and mechanical changes occur in the respiratory system in response to hormonal alterations. As pregnancy advances, these changes facilitate gas exchange, providing the client with increased oxygen.

Anatomic changes

The diaphragm rises by approximately 4 cm during pregnancy, which prevents the lungs from expanding as much as they normally do. The diaphragm compensates by increasing its excursion ability, and the rib cage compensates by flaring from approximately 68 degrees before pregnancy to about 103 degrees in the third trimester. In addition, the anteroposterior and transverse diameters of the rib cage increase by about 2 cm and the circumference increases by 5 to 7 cm. This expansion is possible because increased progesterone relaxes the ligaments that join the rib cage. As the uterus enlarges, thoracic breathing replaces abdominal breathing.

The upper respiratory tract vascularizes in response to increasing levels of estrogen. The client may develop respiratory congestion, voice changes, and epistaxis as capillaries become engorged in the nose, pharynx, larynx, trachea, bronchi, and vocal cords. Increased vascularization also may cause the eustachian tubes to swell, leading to such problems as impaired hearing, earaches, and a sense of fullness in the ears.

Functional changes

Changes in pulmonary function improve gas exchange in the alveoli and facilitate oxygenation of blood flowing through the lungs. The respiratory rate typically remains unaffected in early pregnancy. By the third trimester, however, increased progesterone may increase the rate by approximately two breaths/minute.

Tidal volume and minute volume. Tidal volume (the amount of air inhaled and exhaled) rises throughout pregnancy as a result of increased progesterone and increased diaphragmatic excursion. In fact, the pregnant client will breathe 30% to 40% more air than she does when not pregnant. Minute volume (the amount of air expired per minute) increases by approximately 50% by term. The difference between changes in tidal volume and minute volume creates a slight hyperventilation, which decreases carbon dioxide in alveoli. The resulting lower $PaCO_2$ in maternal blood leads to a greater partial pressure difference of carbon dioxide between fetal and maternal blood, which facilitates diffusion of carbon dioxide from the fetus.

Lung capacity. An elevated diaphragm decreases functional residual capacity (the volume of air remaining in the lungs after exhalation), and decreased functional residual capacity contributes to hyperventilation. Vital capacity (the largest volume of air that can be expelled voluntarily after maximum inspiration) increases slightly during pregnancy. These changes, along with increased cardiac output and blood volume, provide adequate blood flow to the placenta.

Acid-base balance. During the third month of pregnancy, increased progesterone sensitizes respiratory receptors and increases ventilation, leading to a drop in carbon dioxide levels. This increases pH, which might cause mild respiratory alkalosis, except that a decreased bicarbonate level partially or completely compensates for this tendency.

Cardiovascular system

Pregnancy alters the cardiovascular system so profoundly that, outside of pregnancy, the changes would be considered pathological and even life-threatening. During pregnancy, however, these changes are vital to a positive outcome.

Anatomic changes

The heart enlarges slightly during pregnancy, probably because of increased blood volume and cardiac output. This enlargement is not marked and reverses after childbirth.

As pregnancy advances, the uterus moves up and presses on the diaphragm, displacing the heart upward and rotating it on its long axis. The amount of displacement varies depending on the position and size of the uterus, the firmness of the abdominal muscles, the shape of the abdomen, and other factors.

Auscultatory changes

Changes in blood volume, cardiac output, and the size and position of the heart alter heart sounds during pregnancy. These changed heart sounds would be considered abnormal in a client who is not pregnant.

During pregnancy, S_1 tends to exhibit a pronounced splitting, and each component tends to be louder. An occasional S_3 sound may occur after 20 weeks of pregnancy. Definite changes tend not to occur in either the aortic or pulmonic components of S_2. Many pregnant clients exhibit a systolic ejection murmur over the pulmonic area.

Cardiac rhythm disturbances, such as sinus arrhythmia, premature atrial contractions, and premature ventricular systole, may occur. In the pregnant client with no underlying heart disease, these arrhythmias do not require therapy, nor do they indicate development of myocardial disease.

Hemodynamic changes

Pregnancy affects heart rate and cardiac output, venous and arterial blood pressure, circulation and coagulation, and blood volume.

Heart rate and cardiac output. During the second trimester, heart rate increases gradually until it may reach 10 to 15 beats/minute above the prepregnant rate. During the third trimester, heart rate may increase 15 to 20 beats/minute above the prepregnant rate. The client may feel palpitations occasionally throughout pregnancy. In the early months, they result from sympathetic nervous stimulation.

Increased tissue demand for oxygen and increased stroke volume raise cardiac output by up to 50% by the thirty-second week of pregnancy. The increase is highest at rest when the client is lying on her side and lowest when she is lying on her back. The side-lying position reduces pressure on the great vessels, which increases venous return to the heart. Cardiac output peaks during labor, when tissue demands are greatest.

Venous and arterial blood pressure. When the client lies on her back, femoral venous pressure increases threefold from early pregnancy to term. This occurs because the uterus exerts pressure on the inferior vena cava and pelvic veins, retarding venous return from the legs and feet. The client may feel lightheaded if she rises abruptly after lying on her back. Edema in the legs and varicosities in the legs, rectum, and vulva may occur.

Early in pregnancy, increased progesterone levels relax smooth muscles and dilate arterioles, resulting in vasodilation. Systolic and diastolic pressures may decrease 5 to 10 mm Hg. Blood pressure reaches its lowest during the second half of the second trimester and then gradually returns to first trimester levels during the third trimester. By term, arterial blood pressure approaches prepregnant levels.

Brachial artery pressure is highest when the client lies on her back, which causes the enlarged uterus to exert the greatest pressure on the vena cava, and lowest when she lies on her left side, which relieves uterine pressure on the vena cava.

Circulation and coagulation. Venous return decreases slightly during the eighth month of pregnancy and at term increases to normal levels. Blood clots more readily during pregnancy and the postpartal period because of an increase in clotting factors VII, IX, and X.

Blood volume. Total intravascular volume increases during pregnancy, beginning between the tenth and twelfth weeks and peaking at approximately a 40% increase between the thirty-second and thirty-fourth weeks. Volume decreases slightly in the fortieth week and returns to normal several weeks postpartum. The increase consists of two-thirds plasma and one-third red blood cells. The increased blood volume supplies the hypertrophied vascular system of the enlarging uterus, provides nutrition for fetal and maternal tissues, and serves as a reserve for blood loss during childbirth and puerperium.

Hematologic changes
Pregnancy affects red and white blood cells and fibrinogen levels.

Red blood cell mass. Bone marrow becomes more active during pregnancy, producing up to a 30% excess in red blood cells if sufficient iron is available. The client may require an iron supplement to increase hemoglobin synthesis.

The increase in plasma volume is disproportionately greater than the increase in erythrocytes, which lowers the client's hematocrit (the percentage of erythrocytes in whole blood) and causes physiologic anemia of pregnancy. The hemoglobin level also decreases. A hematocrit below 35% and a hemoglobin level below 11.5 g/dl indicate pregnancy-related anemia.

White blood cell count. Leukocytes increase for unknown reasons during pregnancy, and the white blood cell count rises, ranging from 10,000 to 12,000 mm³. The count may increase to 25,000 mm³ or more during labor, childbirth, and the early postpartal period.

Fibrinogen levels. Fibrinogen—a protein in blood plasma—is converted to fibrin by thrombin and is known as coagulation factor I. In the nonpregnant client, levels average 250 mg/dl. In the pregnant client, levels average 450 mg/dl, increasing as much as 50% by term. This increase plays an important role in preventing maternal hemorrhage during childbirth.

Urinary system

The kidneys, ureters, and bladder undergo profound changes in structure and function during pregnancy.

Anatomic changes
Significant dilation of the renal pelves, calyces, and ureters begins as early as the tenth week of pregnancy, probably caused by increased estrogen and progesterone. As pregnancy advances and the uterus becomes dextrorotated, the ureters and renal pelvis become more dilated above the pelvic brim, particularly on the right side. In addition, the smooth muscle of the ureters undergoes hypertrophy and hyperplasia; muscle tone decreases, primarily because of the muscle-relaxing effects of progesterone.

These changes retard the flow of urine through the ureters and result in hydronephrosis and hydroureter (distention of the renal pelvis and ureters with urine), predisposing the pregnant client to urinary tract infection. In addition, because of the delay between urine formation in the kidneys and its arrival in the bladder, inaccuracies may occur during clearance tests.

Hormonal changes cause the bladder to relax during pregnancy, permitting it to distend to hold approximately 1,500 ml of urine. However, hormonal changes and pressure from the growing uterus cause bladder irritation, manifested as urinary frequency and urgency, even if the bladder contains little urine. Bladder vascularity increases and the mucosa bleeds easily. In the second trimester, when the uterus rises out of the pelvis, urinary symptoms abate. As term approaches, however, the presenting part of the fetus engages in the pelvis—exerting pressure once again on the bladder—and symptoms return.

Functional changes
Pregnancy affects renal plasma flow, glomeruler filtration rate, renal tubular resorption, and nutrient and glucose excretion.

Renal plasma flow. Early in pregnancy, renal plasma flow (RPF) increases by an unknown mechanism, rising to 40% to 50% above the prepregnant level by the third trimester. RPF then declines slightly.

Glomerular filtration rate. By the beginning of the second trimester, glomerular filtration rate (GFR) increases as much as 50% by an unknown mechanism; it remains elevated to term. This increase in GFR produces a consequent decrease in some laboratory test values, including blood urea nitrogen and creatinine.

Renal tubular resorption. Acting to maintain sodium and fluid balance, renal tubular resorption increases as much as 50% during pregnancy. The sodium requirement increases because the client needs more intravascular and extracellular fluid. Total body water increases also, to a total of about 7 liters more than in the prepregnant state. The amniotic fluid and placenta account for about half of this amount; increased maternal blood volume and enlargement of the breasts and uterus account for the rest.

Late in pregnancy, changes in posture affect sodium and water excretion. The client will excrete less when lying on her back because the enlarged uterus compresses the vena cava and aorta, causing decreased cardiac output. This decreases renal blood flow, which in turn decreases kidney function. The client will excrete more when lying on her left side because, in this position, the uterus does not compress the great vessels. Thus, cardiac output and kidney function remain unchanged.

Nutrient and glucose excretion. The pregnant client loses increased amounts of some nutrients, such as amino acids, water-soluble vitamins, folic acid, and iodine. Glycosuria (glucose in the urine) may occur as GFR increases without a corresponding increase in tubular resorptive capacity. Proteinuria (protein in the urine) is considered abnormal in pregnancy. It may occur occasionally during and after difficult labors.

Gastrointestinal system

Changes during pregnancy affect anatomic elements in the gastrointestinal system and alter certain functions. These changes are associated with many of the most discussed discomforts of pregnancy.

Anatomic changes
The mouth and teeth, stomach and intestines, and gallbladder and liver are affected during pregnancy.

Mouth and teeth. The salivary glands become more active, especially in the latter half of pregnancy. The gums become edematous and bleed easily because of increased vascularity. The teeth are unaffected; they lose no minerals to the developing fetus.

Stomach and intestines. As progesterone increases during pregnancy, gastric tone and motility decrease, slowing the stomach's emptying time and possibly causing regurgitation and reflux of stomach contents. The client may complain of heartburn.

The enlarging uterus displaces the stomach upward. In late pregnancy, the uterus displaces the small intestine as well. Hormonal changes and mechanical pressure reduce motility in the small intestine. Reduced motility in the colon leads to greater water absorption, which may predispose the client to constipation. The enlarging uterus displaces the large intestine and puts increased pressure on veins below the uterus, which may predispose the client to hemorrhoids.

Gallbladder and liver. As smooth muscles relax, the gallbladder empties more sluggishly. This prolonged emptying time, along with increased excretion of cholesterol in the bile caused by increased hormone levels, may lead to bile that is supersaturated with cholesterol and predispose the client to cholesterol crystal formation and gallstone development.

The liver does not enlarge or undergo any major changes during pregnancy. However, hepatic blood flow may increase slightly, and the liver's work load increases as the basal metabolic rate increases. Factors within the liver and increased estrogen and progesterone decrease bile flow.

Some liver function studies show drastic changes, possibly caused in part by increased estrogen levels. These changes would suggest hepatic disease in a nonpregnant client.

• Alkaline phosphatase nearly doubles, caused in part by increased alkaline phosphatase isozymes from the placenta.

• Serum albumin levels decrease.

• Plasma globulin levels increase causing decreases in albumin globulin ratios.

• Plasma cholinesterase levels decrease.

Functional changes

Nausea and vomiting may affect appetite and food consumption, even while energy demand increases.

Appetite and food consumption. The client's appetite and food consumption fluctuate. Many women experience nausea and vomiting early in pregnancy. Nausea typically is more pronounced in the morning, beginning at 4 to 6 weeks and subsiding by the end of the first trimester. Some women experience this morning sickness at other hours and beyond the first trimester. Severity varies from a slight distaste for food to severe vomiting. Certain odors and the sight of food can trigger an occurrence. Peculiarities in taste and smell also may develop.

Although uncomfortable for the client, morning sickness has no deleterious effects on the fetus. In fact, research suggests that clients who vomit in early pregnancy have a decreased incidence of spontaneous abortion, stillbirth, and premature labor (Klebanoff, Koslowe, and Kaslow, 1985). Morning sickness should be considered abnormal if accompanied by fever, pain, or weight loss.

In addition to the appetite reduction caused by nausea and vomiting, the client's appetite may be reduced by increased hCG levels and changes in carbohydrate metabolism, which are suspected appetite suppressants. Once nausea and vomiting cease, the client's appetite increases along with increasing metabolic needs. However, the old adage of "eating for two" is erroneous. (See Chapter 20, Nutrition and Diet Counseling, for more information.)

Carbohydrate, lipid, and protein metabolism. The client's carbohydrate needs rise to meet increasing energy demands. The client needs more glucose, especially during the second half of pregnancy. Plasma lipid levels increase starting in the first trimester, rising at term to 40% to 50% above the prepregnant level. Cholesterol, triglyceride, and lipoprotein levels increase as well. The total concentration of serum proteins decreases, especially serum albumin and perhaps gamma globulin. The primary immunoglobulin transferred to the fetus—IgG—is lowered in the client's serum. (See Chapter 20, Nutrition and Diet Counseling, for a complete discussion of carbohydrate, lipid, and protein metabolism.)

Musculoskeletal system

The client's musculoskeletal system changes in response to hormones, weight gain, and the growing fetus. These changes may affect the client's gait, posture, and comfort.

Skeleton

The enlarging uterus tilts the pelvis forward, shifting the client's center of gravity. The lumbosacral curve increases, accompanied by a compensatory curvature in the cervicodorsal region. The lumbar and dorsal curves become even more pronounced as breasts enlarge and their weight pulls the shoulders forward, producing a stoop-shouldered stance. Increasing sex hormones (and possibly the hormone relaxin) relax the sacroiliac, sacrococcygeal, and pelvic joints. These changes cause marked alterations in posture and gait. Relaxation of the pelvic joints may cause the client's gait to change. Shoe and ring sizes tend to increase because of weight gain, hormonal changes, and dependent edema. Although these changes may persist after childbirth, they more nearly approach their prepregnant states.

Muscles

In the third trimester, the prominent rectus abdominis muscles separate, allowing the abdominal contents to protrude at the midline. The umbilicus may flatten or protrude. After childbirth, abdominal muscles regain tone but typically do not return to their prepregnant state.

Integumentary system

Skin changes vary greatly among pregnant clients. Of those who experience skin changes, Blacks and brunette Caucasians typically show more marked changes than blondes. Because some skin changes may remain after childbirth, they are not considered an important sign of pregnancy in the multigravid client. The client may need the nurse's help to integrate these skin changes into her self-concept. Skin changes associated with pregnancy include striae gravidarum, pigment changes, and vascular markings. (For illustrations of some of these changes, see *Common skin changes during pregnancy*, page 403.)

Striae gravidarum

The client's weight gain and enlarging uterus, combined with the action of adrenocorticosteroids, lead to stretching of the underlying connective tissue of the skin, creating striae gravidarum in the second and third trimesters. Better known as stretch marks, striae on light-skinned clients appear as pink or slightly reddish streaks with slight depressions; on dark-skinned clients, they appear lighter than the surrounding skin tone. They develop most often in skin covering the breasts, abdomen, buttocks, and thighs. After labor, they typically grow lighter until they appear silvery white on light-skinned clients and light brown on dark-skinned clients.

Pigment changes

Pigmentation begins to change at approximately the eighth week of pregnancy, partly from the melanocyte-stimulating hormone and ACTH and partly from estrogen and progesterone. These changes are more pronounced in such hyperpigmented areas as the face, breasts (especially nipples), axillae, abdomen, anal region, inner thighs, and vulva. Specific changes may include linea nigra and chloasma.

Linea nigra refers to a dark line that extends from the umbilicus or above to the mons pubis. In the primigravid client, this line develops at approximately the third month of pregnancy. In the multigravid client, linea nigra typically appears before the third month.

Called the mask of pregnancy, chloasma (or facial melasma) refers to irregular, brownish blotches that appear on the malar prominences (cheek bones) and forehead. Chloasma appears after the sixteenth week of pregnancy and gradually becomes more pronounced until childbirth. Then it typically fades.

Vascular markings

Tiny, bright-red angiomas may appear during pregnancy as a result of estrogen release, which increases subcutaneous blood flow. They are called vascular spiders because of the branching pattern that extends from each spot. Occurring mostly on the chest, neck, arms, face, and legs, they disappear after childbirth.

Palmar erythema, commonly seen along with vascular spiders, are well-delineated, pinkish areas over the palmar surface of the hands. Once pregnancy ends and estrogen levels decrease, these changes reverse.

Epulides, also known as gingival granuloma gravidarum, are raised, red, fleshy areas that appear on the gums as a result of increased estrogen. They may increase in size, cause severe pain, and bleed profusely. An epulis that grows rapidly may require excision.

Other integumentary changes

Nevi (circumscribed, benign proliferation of pigment-producing cells in the skin) may develop on the face, neck, upper chest, or arms during pregnancy. Oily skin and acne from increased estrogen may occur. Hirsutism (excessive hair growth) also may occur, but reverses when pregnancy ends. By the sixth week of pregnancy, fingernails may soften and break easily, a problem that may be exacerbated by nail polish removers.

Immune system

Ordinarily, a mature immune system rejects implanted tissue within 2 weeks. During pregnancy, however, the fetus and placenta are protected from the maternal immune system by a mechanism that is not fully understood. The cell layer covering the fetus and placenta may mask antigens, thus preventing detection by sensitized lymphocytes (Cunningham, MacDonald, and Gant, 1989). The placental hormones progesterone and hCG may suppress cellular immunity (Gusdon and Sain, 1981).

Neurologic system

Changes in the neurologic system are poorly defined and incompletely understood. For most clients, neurologic changes are temporary and cease once pregnancy is over. Functional disturbances called entrapment neuropathies occur in the peripheral nervous system from mechanical pressure.

• The client may experience meralgia paresthetica—tingling and numbness in the anterolateral portion of the thigh that is caused when the lateral femoral cutaneous nerve becomes entrapped in the area of the inguinal ligaments. This is more pronounced in late pregnancy, as the gravid uterus presses on these nerves and as vascular stasis occurs.

• In the third trimester, carpal tunnel syndrome may occur when the median nerve of the carpal tunnel of the wrist is compressed by edematous surrounding tissue. The client may notice tingling and burning in the dominant hand, possibly radiating to the elbow and upper arm. Numbness or tingling in the hands also may result from pregnancy-related postural changes, such as slumped shoulders that pull on the brachial plexus.

• Increased metabolism creates the need for greater calcium intake. If the client ingests insufficient calcium, hypocalcemia and muscle cramps may occur.

• Lightheadedness, faintness, and syncope may be caused by vasomotor changes, hypoglycemia, and postural hypotension.

Common skin changes during pregnancy

The illustrations below show striae gravidarum and linea nigra, the two most common skin changes in pregnant clients. Not all clients develop stria gravidarum; those who do show a varied pattern in the number, size, and distribution. Linea nigra may be prominent or only slightly darker than the surrounding skin.

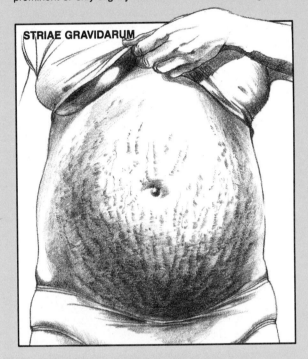

STRIAE GRAVIDARUM

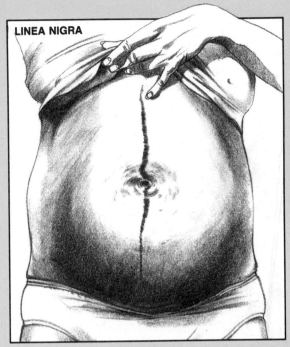

LINEA NIGRA

Chapter summary

Chapter 17 described the physiologic changes that take place during pregnancy and explained some of their reasons. The chapter includes the following key concepts.
• Some of the physiologic changes during pregnancy help in diagnosing it. Signs of pregnancy may be presumptive, probable, or positive. Presumptive and probable signs may be caused by conditions other than pregnancy; positive signs are caused only by pregnancy.
• Pregnancy alters every maternal body system, sometimes in ways that would be considered pathological in a nonpregnant client.
• Although normal, physiologic changes that occur during pregnancy may cause client discomfort and anxiety.
• Many pregnancy-induced physiologic changes stem from altered hormone levels, especially estrogen and progesterone.

• In the reproductive system, major physiologic changes include enlargement of external reproductive stuctures; cessation of ovulation and altered ovarian hormone production; uterine enlargement, vascularization, and migration; endometrial development; cervical softening and edema; development of a cervical mucus plug; vaginal vascularization, hypertrophy, and increased secretion; and breast enlargement and milk production.
• In the endocrine system, major physiologic changes include increased secretion of the pituitary hormones thyrotropin, ACTH, prolactin, vasopressin, and oxytocin; increased secretion of the thyroid hormones thyroxine and triiodothyronine; increased secretion of parathyroid hormones; increased secretion of the adrenal hormones cortisol and aldosterone; and increased secretion of insulin from the pancreas.
• In the respiratory system, major physiologic changes include flaring of the rib cage and a shift from abdominal breathing to thoracic breathing in response to the rising

diaphragm, vascularization of the upper respiratory tract, increased tidal volume and minute volume, decreased functional residual capacity, and development of mild respiratory alkalosis.

• In the cardiovascular system, major physiologic changes include enlargement and displacement of the heart; changes in heart sounds; increased heart rate and output, venous blood pressure, and blood volume; decreased arterial blood pressure and circulation; enhanced blood clotting; and increased levels of red blood cells, white blood cells, and fibrinogen.

• In the urinary system, major physiologic changes include dilation of the renal pelves, calyces, and ureters; elongation and relaxation of the ureters, which results in urinary stasis; relaxation of the bladder walls; bladder irritation, which results in urinary frequency and urgency; and increased renal plasma flow, glomerular filtration rate, and renal tubular resorption.

• In the gastrointestinal system, major physiologic changes include increased activity of the salivary glands; edema of the gums; decreased gastric tone and motility; displacement of the large and small intestines; increased gallbladder emptying time; liver function changes, including increased hepatic blood flow, decreased bile flow, and altered results of liver function studies; changes in appetite and food consumption; possible nausea and vomiting; and changes in carbohydrate, lipid, and protein metabolism.

• In the musculoskeletal system, major physiologic changes include a shift in the center of gravity, changes in posture and gait, and separation of the abdominal muscles.

• In the integumentary system, major physiologic changes include striae gravidarum, linea nigra, chloasma, vascular spiders, palmar erythema, epulides, oily skin, acne, hirsutism, and soft fingernails.

• In the immune system, physiologic changes prevent rejection of the fetus and placenta by a poorly understood mechanism.

• In the neurologic system, major physiologic changes include entrapment neuropathies; possible muscle cramping caused by insufficient calcium intake; and possible lightheadedness, faintness, and syncope.

Study questions

1. What are representative presumptive, probable, and positive signs of pregnancy? How do these three types of signs differ in their diagnostic value?

2. Which structural and functional changes take place in the respiratory system during pregnancy?

3. How do venous and arterial blood pressure change during pregnancy? Why?

4. Mrs. Mary Jones, age 26, is a primigravid client who is 28 weeks pregnant. She states that she perspires easily and feels hot off and on from doing minimal housework. Her temperature is 98.4° F; she shows no signs or symptoms of infection. What explanation might the nurse provide for Mrs. Jones?

5. Margaret Anderson, age 38, is a multiparous client whose hematocrit shows an appreciable drop at 24 weeks' gestation. What is the explanation for this decrease?

6. Miss Tanya Dover, age 15, is a primigravid client who complains of urinary frequency and burning. What physiologic changes in the urinary system during pregnancy can explain this complaint?

Bibliography

Beischer, N.A., and Mackay, E.V. (1986). *Obstetrics and the newborn: An illustrated textbook* (2nd ed.). Philadelphia: Saunders.

Bobak, I., Jensen, M., and Zalar, M. (1989). *Maternity and gynecologic care* (4th ed.). St. Louis: Mosby.

Brucker, M.C., and MacMullen, N.J. (1985). What's new in pregnancy tests? *JOGNN*, 14(3), 353-359.

Calvin, S., Jones, O.W., Knieriem, K., and Weinstein, L. (1988). Oxygen saturation in the supine hypotensive syndrome. *Obstetrics and Gynecology*, 71(6, Pt. 1), 872-877.

Clapp, J.F. (1985). Maternal heart rate in pregnancy. *American Journal of Obstetrics and Gynecology*, 152(6, Pt. 1), 659-660.

Cunningham, F., MacDonald, P., and Gant, N. (1989). *Williams obstetrics* (18th ed.). East Norwalk, CT: Appleton & Lange.

Danforth, D.N., and Scott, J.R. (Eds.). (1986). *Obstetrics and gynecology* (5th ed.). Philadelphia: Lippincott.

Engstrom, J.L. (1988). Measurement of fundal height. *JOGNN*, 17(3), 172-178.

Engstrom, J.L. (1985). Quickening and auscultation of fetal heart tones as estimators of the gestational interval: A review. *Journal of Nurse Midwifery*, 30(1), 25-32.

Gusdon, J.P., and Sain, L.E. (1981). Uterine and peripheral blood concentrations and human chorionic gonadotropin and human placental lactogen. *American Journal of Obstetrics and Gynecology*, 139(6), 705-707.

Guyton, A.C. (1986). *Textbook of medical physiology* (7th ed.). Philadelphia: Saunders.

Hart, M.V., Morton, M.J., Hosenpud, J.D., and Metcalfe, J. (1986). Aortic function during normal human pregnancy. *American Journal of Obstetrics and Gynecology*, 154(4), 887-891.

Hole, J.W., Jr. (1990). *Human anatomy and physiology* (5th ed.). Dubuque, IA: William C. Brown.

Klebanoff, M.A., Koslowe, P.A., and Kaslow, R. (1985). Epidemiology of vomiting in early pregnancy. *Obstetrics and Gynecology,* 66(5), 612.

Margulies, M., Voto, L., Fescina, R., Lastra, L., Lapidus, A., and Schwarcz, R. (1987). Arterial blood pressure standards during normal pregnancy and their relation with mother-fetus variables. *American Journal of Obstetrics and Gynecology,* 156(5), 1105-1109.

Munsick, R.A. (1985). Dickinson's sign: Focal uterine softening in early pregnancy and its correlation with placental site. *American Journal of Obstetrics and Gynecology,* 152(7, Pt. 1), 799-802.

Neeson, J.D. (1987). *Clinical manual of maternity nursing.* Philadelphia: Lippincott.

Niswander, K.R. (1987). Manual of obstetrics: Diagnosis and therapy (3rd ed.). Boston: Little, Brown.

Olds, S., London, M., and Ladewig, P. (1988). *Maternal newborn nursing* (3rd ed.). New York: Addison-Wesley.

Sztraky, K., and Roberts, G. (1986). A pharmacist's view of pregnancy testing. *Journal of Pharmacy Technology,* 2(May-June), 116-119.

Tierson, F.D., Olsen, C.L., and Hook, E.B. (1986). Nausea and vomiting of pregnancy and association with pregnancy outcome. *American Journal of Obstetrics and Gynecology,* 155(5), 1017-1022.

Willson, J.R., and Carrington, E.R. (1987). *Obstetrics and gynecology* (8th ed.). St. Louis: Mosby.

Psychosocial Changes during Normal Pregnancy

Objectives

After reading and studying this chapter, the student should be able to:

1. List principles that guide the nurse in promoting normal psychosocial adaptation to pregnancy.

2. Identify factors that affect the expectant parents' transition to parenthood.

3. Describe the expectant parents' psychosocial tasks, concerns, fears, dreams, and fantasies during each trimester of pregnancy.

4. Discuss the formation of a mother image and a father image during pregnancy.

5. Describe the development of prenatal bonding with the fetus.

6. Describe the effect of pregnancy on the couple's relationship.

7. Identify the primary characteristic of the parents' relationship that favors successful adaptation to pregnancy.

8. Describe the concerns and behaviors of siblings and methods that parents can use to prepare them for the new family member.

9. Describe the grandparents' role and involvement in pregnancy and childbirth.

10. Discuss the cultural and family variations that may affect the family's psychosocial experience of pregnancy.

Introduction

Pregnancy and childbirth are psychosocial events that deeply affect the lives of parents and families. Nothing defines the self-concept of most men and women more than the challenge of bearing and raising a child. Preg-nancy and childbirth change parents' lives irrevocably, presenting them with a long-term commitment that benefits from intellectual and emotional preparation.

The parents' response to pregnancy and childbirth is affected by psychological, social, economic, and cultural factors and by self-concept and attitudes toward sex-specific and family roles. All of these aspects of childbearing can affect their health and that of their children. Therefore, care of the expectant family presents the nurse with special responsibilities and challenges.

The nurse must promote the family's normal adaptation to and integration of the new family member. To achieve these goals, the nurse should perform these increasingly difficult functions as expertise allows.

• Promote each family member's self-esteem. Listen attentively, elicit questions and concerns, identify preferences and cultural influences, provide anticipatory guidance about emotional and psychological family changes, discuss as fully as needed each family member's necessary roles and tasks, affirm their efforts, inquire about and show concern for each family member's health care needs, and make referrals as needed.

• Involve all family members in prenatal visits, facilitate communication among family members, offer anticipatory guidance about family changes during pregnancy and the postpartal period, help mobilize the family's resources, offer sexual counseling, help the client maximize her family's positive contributions and minimize negative ones, praise the family's efforts, and offer books and other materials that address all family members.

• Promote the family's prenatal bonding (sometimes called attachment) with the fetus. During prenatal visits, share information about fetal development; help the fam-

GLOSSARY

Affirmation: technique used to reinforce a client's abilities, efforts, and self-esteem.

Ambivalence: conflicting feelings.

Body image: mental image of one's physical appearance, posture, gestures, personality, attitudes, and self-concept, and one's perception of others' reactions to that image.

Bonding: process through which an emotional attachment forms, which binds one person to another in enduring relationship, as between parents and infant. Sometimes called attachment.

Coping mechanism: conscious response to stress that allows an individual to confront a problem directly and solve it.

Couvade symptoms: pregnancy symptoms in an expectant father.

Defense mechanism: unconscious response to stress that distorts reality, allowing the individual to avoid, rather than directly cope with, an anxiety-producing situation.

Denial: defense mechanism that involves refusal to acknowledge thoughts, feelings, desires, impulses, or facts that are consciously intolerable.

Displacement: defense mechanism that transfers emotions from an anxiety-producing object to a less threatening object.

Father image: each man's concept of himself as a father, shaped from childhood memories of his own father, other role models, revision of his father image with other children, literature, and his imagination.

Fixation: defense mechanism that stops development at a particular stage because of inability to resolve an issue.

Mother image: each woman's concept of herself as a mother, shaped from childhood memories of her own mother, other role models, revision of her mother image with other children, literature, and her imagination.

Projection: defense mechanism that involves attributing to someone else traits that are unacceptable in oneself.

Rationalization: defense mechanism that involves creation of reasons to justify painful or unacceptable situations.

Reaction formation: defense mechanism that involves behaving in a way exactly opposite to an unconscious wish.

Regression: defense mechanism of retreat to an earlier developmental phase to reduce the demands of maturity.

Repression: defense mechanism of unconscious exclusion from the conscious mind of painful impulses, desires, or fears .

Self-esteem: degree to which one values oneself.

Sibling rivalry: competition between siblings for parental love and approval.

Womb name: nickname by which expectant parents refer to the fetus during pregnancy.

---

ily identify fetal heart tones, position, and movements; and reinforce bonding behaviors—such as patting the abdomen or talking to the fetus—by asking the client or her partner to note and report fetal movements.

• Facilitate resolution of conflicts related to pregnancy and childbirth. Help identify underlying conflicts through reflective communication, validation of feelings, and exploration of dreams and fantasies. Promote conflict resolution by teaching such techniques as personal affirmation and dream interpretation and by suggesting literature that helps identify and resolve conflicts. Refer for counseling any client who cannot resolve conflicts.

• Support adaptive coping patterns through realistic education of the family about pregnancy, childbirth, and the postpartal period. Discuss childbirth and human responses accurately and realistically. Frankly discuss the challenges of parenting. (For more information, see Chapter 21, Family Preparation for Childbirth and Parenting.)

• Deliver culturally sensitive nursing care. Gather information about the family's customs and beliefs to add to assessment data and to individualize care.

• Identify personal attitudes and feelings about childbearing. Avoid imposing personal values, feelings, and emotional reactions on others. Also, avoid making assumptions about the client and her preferences. Allow her to share her feelings freely.

• Act as an advocate for the expectant family in the health care facility, community, and society. In the facility, suggest more family-centered policies, such as sibling and grandparent visiting hours. In the community, expand childbirth options for expectant families by working to establish a birth center. At the national level, lobby for the health of poor mothers and neonates and for necessary changes in health care by writing to state representatives about laws that fund maternal-neonatal health care and other family services (Thompson, Oakley, Burke, Jay, and Conklin, 1989).

To prepare the nurse for these goals, this chapter discusses psychosocial adaptation in expectant parents. For each trimester of pregnancy, it defines the psychosocial tasks and concerns and explores variations that make each pregnancy unique. It explores grandparent and sibling roles and describes how parents can support them. The chapter also investigates cultural influences and family variations that can affect psychosocial adjustments.

Pregnancy: A time of transition

Three characteristics make childbearing a unique experience for the family: its sweeping changes, its unpredictable and uncontrollable nature, and its history as an ancient human experience, which is sometimes regarded as miraculous. Pregnancy is a time of profound psychological, social, and biological changes that affect the parents' responsibilities, freedoms, values, priorities, social status, relationships, and self-images. The events of the childbearing year (9 antepartal and 3 postpartal months) also may be unpredictable. Although expectant parents can control some events (for example, by obtaining early prenatal care) and can adopt positive attitudes, they cannot control all that happens during that year.

Some people regard pregnancy as a miracle and children as their parents' link to immortality. Repeating the ancient childbearing experience may cause parents to re-evaluate life's meaning, alter priorities, and consider their link with humanity—thus making pregnancy an exciting, yet unsettling, time of profound transition. Many factors can influence the smoothness of this transition:
• support from partner
• support from parents
• support from friends and others
• age
• planned or unplanned pregnancy
• socioeconomic status
• sexuality concerns
• previous childbirth experiences
• previous parenting experiences
• birth stories of family members and friends
• past experiences with health care facilities
• past experiences with health care professionals.

Stress and coping methods

The changes and challenges of pregnancy normally produce stress (psychological and physiologic tension that triggers an adaptive change). Ideally, the pregnant woman will cope realistically with the challenges and adapt to the changes, promoting her health. During pregnancy, stress may increase the incidence of neonatal complications by increasing sympathetic nervous system activity and catecholamine release, constricting uterine blood flow, and diminishing fetal oxygenation (Lederman, 1986; Mansfield and Cohn, 1986). During labor, maternal stress may decrease the neonate's Apgar score.

Overcrowding, geographic moves, disturbed personal relationships, concerns about the health of mother and neonate, and economic instability can increase stress during pregnancy, which has been associated with increased incidence of neonatal complications (Lederman, 1986). Expectant fathers commonly find the following concerns stressful: the neonate's health, normality, and condition at birth; the woman's pain during labor; and unexpected events during childbirth (Glazer, 1989).

Expectant mothers share these concerns and have others. In one study, Lederman (1984) found that all married primigravid women experienced some conflict about the role change to mother. (For more information, see *Nursing research applied: Causes and effects of anxiety.*) Lederman distinguished between adaptive and maladaptive anxiety. Adaptive anxiety promoted the woman's coping abilities because it increased her focus on the maternal role; maladaptive anxiety reflected ambivalence toward mothering and did not foster acceptance of the maternal role.

Reduced anxiety and better adaptation in early pregnancy relate to fewer and less severe pregnancy symptoms. They especially help reduce nausea, backache, dizziness, fatigue, and gastrointestinal distress (Grossman, et al., 1980).

When faced with a stressful situation, an individual may respond consciously, through coping mechanisms, or unconsciously, through defense mechanisms.

Coping mechanisms

An individual uses coping mechanisms to deal with problems by identifying strengths, mobilizing resources, and creating solutions. Coping mechanisms may include enlisting help from experts, family members, or friends; reading books or participating in classes or support groups, such as Alcoholics Anonymous; using spiritual resources, such as prayer or discussions with clergy members; exercising; keeping a journal; or meditating. The key to all these techniques is identifying and expressing feelings about the problem.

Defense mechanisms

These unconscious mechanisms distort reality, allowing an individual to avoid—rather than directly cope with—an anxiety-producing problem. Distorting reality and avoiding anxiety help maintain the individual's self-esteem and desired perception of reality. Defense mechanisms include denial (refusal to acknowledge thoughts, feelings, desires, impulses, or facts that are consciously intolerable), displacement (transfer of emotion from an anxiety-producing object to a less threatening object), fixation (becoming "stuck" at a lower level of maturity

NURSING RESEARCH APPLIED

Causes and effects of anxiety

In her classic research into the causes and effects of anxiety, Lederman (1984) studied 32 primigravid women with normal pregnancies. All were married and had attended childbirth classes. Predominantly middle class and college educated, 30 were Caucasian and 2 were Black. Each participated in prenatal interviews, completed a series of questionnaires, kept a dream record and diary, and was interviewed and physiologically evaluated during labor.

Lederman found that when these women reported feeling anxious, their serum epinephrine and cortisol levels were elevated. When the epinephrine level was elevated, the uterus was less active and fetal distress was more likely during labor. The elevated cortisol level also diminished uterine activity, although less dramatically than epinephrine. Women who were extremely anxious in early labor had longer second stages and were more likely to require forceps deliveries.

The study found a positive correlation between the following characteristics and anxiety and longer labor: difficulty accepting the pregnancy, difficulty identifying with the mother role, and fear of losing control.

Application to practice

Because anxiety and ambivalence can complicate labor and delivery, the nurse must observe the client during pregnancy, carefully noting her response to discomforts of pregnancy, reaction to fetal movement, attachment behaviors, and resolution of ambivalence about her pregnancy. The nurse should listen carefully to the client's comments about her closest relationships and the support she has received for the pregnancy and should observe the interactions of family members during prenatal visits.

If the client has difficulty resolving anxieties, the nurse should help her identify feelings, increase her self-awareness, and improve communication. Also, the nurse should support the client's role transition and the family's integrity as well as address the client's fear of losing control by discussing realistic expectations.

Lederman, R. (1984). *Psychosocial adaptation in pregnancy*. Englewood Cliffs, NJ: Prentice-Hall.

because of an inability to resolve an issue), projection (attribution to someone else of traits that are unacceptable to oneself), rationalization (creation of reasons to justify painful or unacceptable situations), reaction formation (behaving in a way that is exactly the opposite of an unconscious wish), regression (retreat to an earlier developmental phase to reduce the demands of maturity), and repression (unconscious exclusion of painful impulses, desires, or fears).

Everyone uses defense mechanisms to deal with stress. These mechanisms become harmful only if they are used to avoid responsibility in adult relationships. For example, a woman who denies her pregnancy will delay seeking health care and taking self-care measures.

A man who feels suffocated or overwhelmed by his pregnant partner's dependency may rationalize spending time away from her for seemingly important reasons, or he may regress, assuming fewer responsibilities than usual.

The individual whose coping mechanisms help solve problems and whose defense mechanisms do not prevent necessary psychological adjustments will adapt most easily and successfully to parenthood.

The first trimester

During the first trimester, the family's key psychosocial challenge is resolution of ambivalence. The mother copes with the common discomforts and changes of the first trimester; the father begins to accept the reality of the pregnancy. The couple may use dream examination to help deal with these psychosocial tasks.

Resolution of ambivalence

The first trimester is known as the trimester of ambivalence because parents experience mixed feelings.

Many women have unrealistic ideas about maternal instincts, expecting to feel only loving, happy thoughts about the fetus and motherhood. In fact, most women feel some ambivalence about pregnancy and motherhood. Pregnancy involves stressful changes that force a woman to think and behave differently than she has in the past (Kitzinger, 1984).

Ambivalence may reflect various fears: that the pregnant woman may not know how to act as a mother; that she cannot handle the added responsibility; or that the pregnancy may cause professional setbacks or financial concerns. She may dread miscarriage, especially if she has experienced one before, and labor and delivery, although they are months away. She may fear losing her individuality and becoming only a vessel or carrier for the fetus.

Also during the first trimester, a woman may grieve over abandoning old roles and dreams. She may regret giving up the spontaneity she enjoyed before her pregnancy. If she has other children, she may grieve over altering her relationship with them.

As the fetus grows, a woman may feel that she has lost control over her life. Her relationship with the father, which may not have seemed permanent before, now may seem like a lifelong bond. She may wonder how a baby will change that relationship further.

The pregnant woman's hormone levels and physical changes may cause emotional lability characterized by sensitivity, vulnerability, and heightened self-awareness. She may be more open about sharing dreams, fantasies, anxieties, and pleasures (Colman and Colman, 1977; Moore, 1978). A woman experiences this disequilibrium during each pregnancy (Stephens, 1985).

With each pregnancy, a woman explores a new aspect of the mother role and must reformulate her self-image as a pregnant woman and mother. Furthermore, each pregnancy has a unique meaning that is affected by its life context. For example, a baby may symbolically replace an important relative who recently died, or the parent may identify with a baby whose birth order is the same as his or hers (Colman and Colman, 1977).

Feelings of ambivalence are inevitable and normal, and partners who discuss them usually can resolve their grief and fears and enjoy the gratifications of expecting a child. When partners share feelings, they may find they are experiencing similar conflicts (Shapiro, 1987). Studies of married couples have shown that when the husband receives emotional support during pregnancy, his wife adjusts more easily and enjoys the pregnancy (Parke, 1981).

Coping with common discomforts and changes

In the early weeks of the first trimester, the woman watches for body changes that confirm her pregnancy. Her body image (her mental image of how her body looks, feels, and moves; of her posture, gestures, and physical abilities; and of others' impression of her physical appearance) changes as her breasts enlarge, her menses cease, and she experiences nausea, fatigue, waist thickening, and general weight gain. Depending on her acceptance of the pregnancy, the woman may enjoy or dread these changes.

In the first trimester, the woman typically perceives her ability to conceive as a positive reflection on her body image. However, some women may feel thwarted in their attempt to achieve the American ideal of thinness. Some complain of feeling fat and ugly; others enjoy their enlarging breasts (particularly in American society, which values large breasts). Although a woman may enjoy changes that bespeak her feminine reproductive role, she also may dread having a round pregnant shape, adding to her ambivalence.

Women's sexual responses during pregnancy vary widely. Some women are too uncomfortable during the first trimester to enjoy sexual intercourse; others, es-

pecially those who have had a spontaneous abortion, may fear fetal injury. Those who believe sex is for procreation only may feel guilty about sexual activity during pregnancy. Others may feel sexually stimulated by the freedom from contraception, the joy of conception, or the lack of pressure to avoid pregnancy or to have sex on schedule to achieve pregnancy. (For more information, see Chapter 8, Sexuality Concerns.)

A man's sexual response also may change during his partner's pregnancy. He typically will worry about how the pregnancy will change his relationship with his partner. He may feel personally rejected when his partner's fatigue, nausea, and other first trimester discomforts diminish her sexual interest. He may fear causing spontaneous abortion or fetal injury during intercourse.

Because of these fears and concerns, both partners may need extra affection during the first trimester. The nurse should encourage them to communicate and share their feelings and preferences about sexual activities.

Preparation for fatherhood

During the first trimester, the father typically finds the pregnancy unreal and intangible. The idea of the fetus may be abstract to him because he cannot observe physical changes in his partner. Accepting the reality of pregnancy is the father's main psychological task in the first trimester (Miller and Brooten, 1983).

In Western society, a man may suppress his feelings. His expected roles include supporting his partner, being in control, being strong, and not burdening his partner with his concerns. As a result, the father may suppress his concerns and may experience guilt if he has negative thoughts about the pregnancy. Also, he will notice that health care providers, family members, and friends rarely ask about his needs and concerns.

Nonetheless, pregnancy does have an emotional impact on the father, and the child will change his life dramatically. His attachment to the child can be as strong as the mother's, and he can be as competent as the mother in nurturing the child (Cronenwett and Kunst-Wilson, 1981).

A man's transition to fatherhood requires grieving for and abandoning old roles. His adjustment is affected by his readiness to end the childless period of the relationship, his desire to be a parent, his relationship with his father, his previous fathering experiences, and his comfort with his sexuality. It occurs more smoothly if the pregnancy was planned (Lemmer, 1987; May, 1987; Sherwen, 1987).

The expectant father typically feels nurturing toward his partner, particularly while the pregnancy remains a secret between them (Parke, 1981). He may enjoy her increased neediness and his new role as nurturer. Conversely, he may view his partner's emotionality as a sign of his inadequacy in meeting her needs. If the woman usually assumes a nurturing role, the man's adjustment may be especially difficult. Some men feel threatened because pregnancy brings permanence to the relationship.

The father may envy his partner's intimate link with the fetus, her position as the center of attention, or her ability to become pregnant. To express his own desire to create, he may undertake productive work projects or hobbies.

The father may believe pregnancy confirms his virility and masculinity or may irrationally fear that the fetus is not his (Shapiro, 1987; Colman and Colman, 1977). Because some men may view children as a kind of personal immortality, expectant fathers may ponder the meaning of life. Men in their thirties are especially prone to such ruminations.

Because he is not physically pregnant, the father can choose his degree and type of involvement in the pregnancy. May (1980) studied first-time expectant fathers and identified three fathering styles.

• Observer. The observer father thinks of himself as a bystander in the childbearing process.

• Expressive. The expressive father values mutuality in the relationship and feels like a full partner in the pregnancy. He experiences many emotions and may develop symptoms that mimic those of pregnancy.

• Instrumental. The instrumental father minimizes his emotions but manages the pregnancy, making appointments, asking questions during prenatal visits, watching his partner's diet, and playing a prominent role in labor and delivery.

None of these styles is more mature or competent than another. Although each father becomes more involved as the pregnancy advances, his fathering style usually remains consistent (May, 1980).

Regardless of fathering style, the man may experience two psychosocial phenomena during the pregnancy: obsession with his role as provider and couvade symptoms.

Provider role

Because society values a man's provider role, the expectant father usually ponders the increased financial responsibilities a child will bring. Financial concerns remain a major focus throughout pregnancy, and the man may exert tremendous effort to attain financial security. A disproportionate emphasis on finances may reflect deep doubts about his competence as a father. The more secure he feels about his family's economic status, the more open and nurturing he can be with his partner (Muenchow and Bloom-Feshbach, 1982).

Couvade symptoms

In the past in some cultures, an expectant father staged a loud demonstration of pain and anguish when his partner began labor (Meltzer, 1981). Its purpose was to distract demons from the mother and neonate and to establish the neonate's paternity (Bittman and Zalk, 1983).

A contemporary version of this phenomenon has become known as *couvade*, French for "to brood" or "to hatch." Today, couvade refers to the expectant father's experience of up to 39 symptoms of pregnancy, including nausea, weight gain, insomnia, restlessness, headaches, inability to concentrate, fatigue, and irritability (Clinton, 1987). Because these symptoms are not accepted by American society, which expects the father to be strong and supportive, American fathers rarely mention them. However, one study found that 70% of fathers reported one or more couvade symptoms (Strickland, 1987).

Couvade symptoms are not associated with the father's attachment to the fetus and are not limited to first-time fathers (Lemmer, 1987). However, they occur most frequently in fathers who are greatly involved in the pregnancy.

Dream examination

A dream is a symbolically coherent sequence of ideas, thoughts, emotions, or images that pass through the mind during rapid eye movement sleep. It differs from a daydream, or fantasy, in the amount of distracting sensory stimulation received from the outside world (Sherwen, 1987). During pregnancy, both partners may experience vivid dreams about the impending birth. The woman may recall her dreams with greater intensity because she typically is awakened more often at night by heartburn, fetal activity, or a need to urinate.

Dreams tend to follow a predictable pattern during pregnancy. By exploring them, expectant parents can better understand themselves and any subconscious conflicts they may have. (For more information, see *Dreams during pregnancy*, page 412.)

Dreams during pregnancy

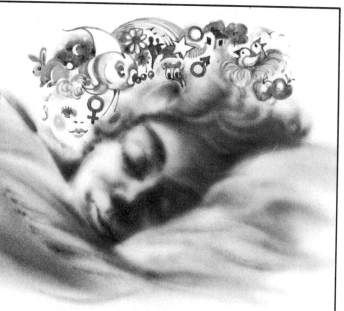

Many experts believe that dreams reflect an individual's suppressed conflicts, fears, and anxieties that are released into the subconscious during sleep. In *The Dream Worlds of Pregnancy*, Stukane (1985) suggested that dreams could enhance one's awareness of internal concerns and struggles and promote communication with a partner.

Stukane advised dreamers to record their dreams after awakening and to decipher each dream by having the partner ask the following questions.
• What do you think the dream is about?
• What is the dream's literal meaning?
• What is the dream's setting or mood?
• Describe each object in the dream, including details. What are the meanings of these objects for you?
• Describe the person in the dream. What is your relationship to him or her?
• What does the dream remind you of in waking life?

Dream themes vary with each trimester of pregnancy and depend on the dreamer's sex. The chart below illustrates common dream themes for women and men during each trimester of pregnancy.

TRIMESTER	WOMEN	MEN
First trimester	• Symbols that do not seem related to pregnancy • Fertility symbols, such as flowering plants, fruits, and vegetables • Cuddly small animals, such as birds or rabbits, which may represent the child-to-be • Fish, which may represent an embryo • Blood, which may symbolize fear of miscarriage	• Inner workings, such as plumbing and circuitry • Birds nesting or eggs hatching • Small animals (Sherwen, 1986) • Acts of sexual prowess or other comfortingly masculine behaviors that may compensate for nurturing, protective feelings for his partner (if the man perceives them as feminine and threatening)
Second trimester	• Beautiful babies who turn into monsters, reflecting worries about the baby's normalcy • Architectural symbols, such as houses with tunnels and secret passageways, which may represent the body housing the fetus • Misplacing the baby or missing or inadequate care equipment, which may reflect the woman's concern over her competence and ability as a parent • Toddlers, particularly if the woman perceives a baby as small and dependent in a threatening way • The baby's sex	• Intrusiveness of baby and aggression of father, possibly reflecting anxiety over the woman's seemingly divided loyalties (Sherwen, 1986)
Third trimester	• Giving birth alone • Giving birth and being the "star of the show" • Experiencing labor pain • Physical separation from the fetus • Labor and delivery • Shopping, which may reveal anticipation about the baby's sex • Malformed babies • Birth assistants • Being trapped in small places • Nightmares in which the partner rescues and protects the woman, representing labor and delivery fears	• Giving birth himself • Finding or being given a baby, often during elaborate initiation ceremonies (Stukane, 1985)

The second trimester

During the second trimester, psychosocial tasks include mother-image development, father-image development, coping with body image and sexuality changes, and development of prenatal attachment. To accomplish these tasks, the couple may examine their dreams and fears.

Mother-image development

As the second trimester begins, expectant parents have completed much of the first trimester's grieving. The woman has abandoned old roles and has begun to determine the sort of mother she wants to be (Varney, 1987). Her mother image is a composite of mothering characteristics she has gleaned from role models, readings, and her imagination.

As the woman becomes more dependent and yearns for warmth and security, she reviews the mothering she received as a child and her current relationship with her mother. She may contact her mother more frequently as she struggles to accept her pregnancy in relation to her mother.

The woman may experience guilt because her role as mother seems to compete with or usurp that of her own mother. As she recalls her childhood relationship with her mother, she may plan to adopt some of her mother's behaviors and avoid others. Making decisions that differ from her mother's may cause guilt, and she must differentiate between forming her own mother image and rejecting her mother.

Four aspects of the mother-daughter relationship will influence the woman's mother image:
• her mother's availability in the past and during the pregnancy
• her mother's reaction to the pregnancy, her acceptance of the grandchild, and her acknowledgment of her daughter as a mother
• her mother's respect for the daughter's autonomy and acceptance of her as a mature adult
• her mother's willingness to reminisce about her own childbearing and child-rearing experiences (Lederman, 1984).

Old conflicts in the mother-daughter relationship may resurface during pregnancy. The expectant woman may dwell on these conflicts, may feel unable to resolve old disappointments, and may carry a lack of trust into other relationships. Ideally, she will accept her mother's parenting and adjustment to the grandparent role.

When her mother is fully supportive, the expectant woman is more likely to welcome help without ambivalence and appreciate her teachings. When this occurs, both can tolerate each other's failings, and the woman may be able to approach childbirth and mothering with more self-confidence and less anxiety.

The mothering characteristics of sisters, friends, and other role models also help the woman form her mother image. If the woman has other children, she also may shape her mother image by reviewing her performance in mothering them and deciding how to alter it.

Her preoccupation with forming a mother image causes a period of introspection. As a result, she may show less affection, become more passive, or withdraw from her other children, who will react by becoming more demanding. Her partner also may feel neglected during this period.

Father-image development

While the woman develops her mother image, the man begins to form his father image based on his relationship with his father, previous fathering experiences, the fathering styles of friends and family members, and his partner's view of his role in the pregnancy.

As he starts to develop his father image, the man remembers his relationship with his father and sometimes increases contact with his parents. He may have difficulty viewing his father as a grandfather and coming to terms with his position as a father.

The man may have trouble envisioning himself as the father of a daughter because he has not experienced a father-daughter relationship. Conversely, he may hope to father a daughter to avoid reliving his relationship with his father (Colman and Colman, 1977).

If the man has other children, he may review the fathering he has done with them. He also may seek out the company of other men who are fathers, forming or revising his father image from a composite of their qualities.

Since the feminist movement of the 1970s, increasing numbers of men have participated in delivery and child care. However, most men were raised by fathers who experienced delivery from the waiting room and left child-rearing duties to their partners. Therefore, many have no role models for more involved fathering and must create a father image by piecing together ideas from friends, readings, classes, and especially from their partners.

Generally, the woman's expectations about her partner's involvement and the quality of their relationship predict the man's role in delivery and child rearing (Reiber, 1976). Some women desire privacy and modesty during childbirth and neither expect nor wish to involve their partners. Others expect their partner's full involvement in tracking fetal movements, attending prenatal visits, and acting as coach, advocate, and primary emotional support during labor.

Sociological factors also may affect the man's involvement in his partner's pregnancy and the development of his father image. In American society, for example, men are typically taught to be more rational than emotional and to act rather than to wait, even for a physiologic process to occur. Also, both sexes have conspired to portray birth as the ultimate female mystery. These cultural beliefs can influence a man's response to his partner's pregnancy.

Coping with body image and sexuality changes

The second trimester often is called a time of radiant health. Physical changes include a heightened sensuality with vasocongestion of the pelvis and increased vaginal lubrication, and 80% of women describe increased sexual gratification, even over prepregnant levels (Colman and Colman, 1977). However, studies show that women become increasingly dissatisfied with their body image as pregnancy progresses, feeling the most dissatisfied during the postpartal period (Strang and Sullivan, 1985).

One study showed that most men feel more positively about the physical changes of pregnancy than do their partners (Moore, 1978).

The way a woman and her partner view her body's changes will affect her sexual responsiveness and self-image. The woman who believes her changing body is achieving an important purpose may feel positive during pregnancy. However, American culture associates fatness with sloppiness, overindulgence, and an absence of self-control (Boston Women's Health Book Collective, 1985; Stern, 1987; Moore, 1978); therefore, some women may wear maternity clothes earlier than necessary to make clear that they are pregnant, not overweight.

The man may feel unnerved by his partner's now-unfamiliar body, intimidated by its workings, or uncomfortable having sexual intercourse with an unfamiliar element—the fetus—present. He also may perceive his partner as less sexually appealing or as a mother rather than a sexual being, thus losing sexual interest. He may perceive her sexual interest as demanding.

Development of prenatal bonding

A new phase begins at approximately 17 to 20 weeks, when the woman feels fetal movements for the first time. Because fetal movements are a sign of good health and may dispel the fear of spontaneous abortion, the woman almost always experiences the first flutter of movement positively, even when the pregnancy is unwanted. As a result, she becomes attentive to the type and timing of movements and to fetal responses to environmental factors, such as music, abdominal strokes, and meals.

After fetal movements begin, the woman and her partner may state a preference for the sex of the fetus. They may give the fetus a womb name (a nickname for the fetus during pregnancy). For example, they may call the fetus "Thumper" because of its kicking movements. Also, the woman may begin to imagine her child and fantasize about interacting with it. She may think about giving of herself to the child because giving is the essence of the maternal role (Lederman, 1984).

The woman may demonstrate bonding behaviors, such as stroking and patting her abdomen, talking to the fetus about eating while she eats, reprimanding the fetus for moving too much, engaging her partner in conversations with the fetus, eating a balanced diet, and engaging in other health promotion behaviors (Sherwen, 1987). Bonding is influenced by the woman's health, developmental stage, and culture, but not by obstetric complications, general anxiety, or demographic variables, such as socioeconomic level.

This prenatal bonding requires positive self-esteem, positive role models, and acceptance of the pregnancy. Social support improves this attachment (Cranley, 1981), which in turn increases the woman's feelings of maternal competence and effectiveness (Mercer, Ferketich, DeJoseph, May, and Sollid, 1988). One study demonstrated that women who displayed more bonding behaviors during pregnancy had more positive feelings about the neonate after delivery (Leifer, 1977).

Carter-Jessop (1981) designed a study in which pregnant women were instructed to palpate and identify the fetal position every day, to observe fetal reactions to the environment (such as being stroked), and to stroke, pat, and massage their abdomens briefly each day. They found that women who performed these actions demonstrated a more positive relationship with their neonates as measured by the amount of eye contact, smiling, talking, and touching.

Prenatal testing also may affect bonding. Many women undergo ultrasonography and keep the ultrasound recording as their fetus's first picture. Some researchers have found that ultrasonography increased the woman's bond with the fetus; others, that it increased the woman's health promotion behaviors, such as smoking cessation. However, others found no correlation between ultrasonography and maternal-neonatal bonding (Heidrich and Cranley, 1989).

Dream and fear examination

During the second trimester, the parents' dreams may reflect concerns about the normalcy of the fetus, parental abilities, divided loyalties, and related subjects. (For more information, see *Dreams during pregnancy*, page 412.)

Parents may experience various fears. Feeling dependent and vulnerable, the woman may fear for her partner's safety. In touch with mortality, the man may consider his death and how it would affect his family. He may recall risks he has taken, such as driving recklessly, and make a commitment to be more careful to avoid being taken from his partner and fetus.

The third trimester

As the third trimester begins, the woman feels a sense of accomplishment because her fetus has reached the age of viability. She may feel sentimental about the approaching end of her pregnancy, when the mother-child relationship will replace the mother-fetus relationship. At the same time, however, she may look forward to giving birth because the last months bring bulkiness, insomnia, childbirth anxieties, and concern about the neonate's normalcy.

During this trimester, psychosocial tasks include adaptation to activity changes, preparation for parenting, partner support and nurture, acceptance of body image and sexuality changes, preparation for labor, and development of birth plans. The technique of dream and fear examination may help the couple accomplish these tasks.

Adaptation to activity changes

The growing fetus makes daily activities more difficult for the woman and forces her to slow down. This change can affect her emotional state and her family relationships. For example, she may have to stop working outside the home, which can be painful if work is crucial to her identity and sense of self-worth, if she prides herself on controlling her life, or if finances are limited. Decreased social support for the woman on maternity leave can add to anxiety. Further, her increased dependence during pregnancy and decreased activities outside the home may change the family power structure.

Preparation for parenting

As the woman's body grows larger, the man typically catches up with his partner in anticipating and preparing for the neonate. To prepare for parenting, the couple now may focus on concrete tasks, such as preparing the nursery, making decisions about child care, and planning postpartal events.

The couple may discuss topics they never discussed before, such as religious upbringing, the degree to which the family should be child-centered, or financial obligations to the child (Shapiro, 1987). They also may decide how to divide the work of running a home with a child. These issues, which are vital to the parents' self-concept, require careful negotiations (Sherwen, 1987). If tasks are negotiated before delivery, postpartal adjustment will be easier.

Partner support and nurture

The couple's ability to support each other through the childbearing cycle is paramount. In a recent study, husbands and wives stated that 80% of their support during pregnancy came from their spouses (Brown, 1986). Other studies found that an egalitarian relationship (one not characterized by the dominance of either member) yields greater satisfaction, greater closeness during the pregnancy, and an easier transition to parenthood (Grossman, et al., 1980; Moore, 1983). Furthermore, relationships that allow flexibility, growth, and risk taking ease role transition.

Men and women express various needs and expectations during the last trimester. In one study, men expressed a need for more understanding and acceptance from their partners about their work schedules and changes in their sexual relationship; women wanted more help with infant preparations and more "thoughtful gestures" (Brown, 1986). Men and women wanted their partners to be more accepting of their need to "blow off steam." In another study, men attending Lamaze classes rated themselves very high on involvement in the pregnancy, but very low on talking to the partner's physician, spending extra time with the partner, doing extra housework, and reading about pregnancy and birth (Wapner, 1976).

In some cases, a spouse's attempt at support falls short of the partner's expectations or needs (Stichler, Bowden, and Reimer, 1979). For example, because the man takes longer to accept the fetus's reality, he may focus on protecting and nurturing his partner rather than the fetus. The woman may misinterpret this as failure to become attached to the fetus (Panuthos, 1984). Studies indicate, however, that men and women want to support their partners during the antepartal period and that communication is the key to doing so.

Highly satisfied couples discuss issues more often than do less satisfied couples. Expressing a positive regard for each other and a positive appraisal of the relationship creates an atmosphere in which the couple can share feelings, trust, and affection.

Acceptance of body image and sexuality changes

Some women are more comfortable with and confident in their bodies during pregnancy, feeling less concerned with each pound of weight gained. Others, however, feel sexually unattractive. They take up more space, are constantly aware of their large abdomen, feel awkward and fatigued, and suffer from backaches. Some women also feel their body is no longer their own. As the fetus begins to kick more vigorously, they may even fear for the safety of their internal organs.

The woman's body image and her partner's feelings affect her sexuality, sometimes diminishing her sexual interest. Some men also experience diminished sexual interest as pregnancy advances. Couples who desire sexual intimacy in the third trimester must be creative, using new positions and techniques. (For more information, see Chapter 8, Sexuality Concerns.) Whether or not the couple remains sexually active, the woman usually desires holding and reassurance.

Preparation for labor

Childbirth education classes can prepare the woman and her partner for labor and delivery. The partner's attendance at prenatal classes and participation in all aspects of pregnancy correlate with his degree of relationship satisfaction (Lederman, 1984). Women who feel supported by their partners during pregnancy and childbirth experience fewer complications and may make an easier postpartal adjustment (May, 1982).

Many men describe performance anxiety about labor and delivery. This anxiety is not unreasonable considering that the man is expected to support his partner physically and emotionally through a powerful, painful experience over which he has no control and about which he may have little understanding; to be an advocate for his partner in a sometimes intimidating medical world; and to witness birth without feeling queasy or faint or getting in the way (Panuthos, 1984; Clinton, 1985). By participating in prenatal visits and in the choice of health care professional, the man can reduce these anxieties.

Detecting labor is a major concern for most couples. Braxton-Hicks (false-labor) contractions may occur for several weeks before delivery, causing unnecessary loss of sleep. By making detailed practical arrangements in advance, the woman may ease concerns about identifying early labor.

Development of birth plans

A highly dependent woman may allow the health care team to make decisions about the birth plans, assuming that their decisions will be the wisest. A more independent woman may seek health care that is comfortable to her and that fits with her beliefs and knowledge, thus ensuring that her wishes will be honored during labor. A woman who shapes her childbirth experience and who develops realistic expectations of the event has dealt with her fears.

Jones (1987) stresses that the birth belongs to the parents, who have the right and responsibility to make decisions and who invite and pay for the services of birth assistants. He emphasizes that birth plans vary widely among individuals: one woman may insist on delivering in a facility with a neonatal intensive care unit; another may choose home delivery. Home birth statistics amassed by nurse-midwives attest to the safety of home births, giving women confidence in their choice of birth location.

Dream and fear examination

By revealing fears or hopes that parents may not acknowledge consciously, dreams can help defuse fears and prepare the parents more consciously for childbirth and parenting. (For more information, see *Dreams during pregnancy,* page 412.)

During the third trimester, a key psychosocial task is to overcome fears the woman may have about the unknown, labor pain, loss of self-esteem, loss of control, and death.

The unknown
Perhaps the most difficult aspect of pregnancy is awaiting labor. The primiparous woman wonders how contractions will feel; the multiparous woman, aware of the possibilities or recalling difficult moments from her last delivery, experiences anticipation also (Colman and Colman, 1977). All pregnant women become increasingly preoccupied with labor and delivery.

Labor pain
A woman who has prepared herself realistically will experience some anxiety about labor and delivery. Un-

fortunately, many women anticipate unbearable pain. The nurse can reassure each client that labor pain is intense but manageable. The gradually increasing discomfort reflects labor progress. The nurse also should review the risks and benefits of anesthesia and analgesia and should support the client's goals for pain management.

Loss of self-esteem

Many women value the childbirth experience, viewing it as joyous. For such a woman, self-esteem may be linked to her performance in labor and delivery. Her performance standards may be influenced by her partner, family members, friends, readings, films, childbirth educators, and the health care team. If a woman fails to meet the standards that she or others have set, she may lose self-esteem.

Loss of control

The intensity of labor may frighten women in a society that values control and rational thought and behavior (Lederman, 1984). If a woman's childbirth education class stresses rigid breathing patterns, reliance on a focal point, and quietness, she learns that control is paramount and that the mind must block physical sensations (Noble, 1983).

Such a woman may opt for the control of anesthesia, fearing that without it she will make noises during strong body sensations, act childishly, or lose control (Lederman, 1984). The nurse can help change the client's goal from rigidly defined "appropriate" behaviors, in which she tries to ignore her sensations, to less rigidly defined ones. To do this, the nurse should encourage the client to expect an intense experience in which she can perceive body sensations and participate in the birth process by working with her body, whether or not she makes noises, assumes unusual positions, or breathes differently than taught. The client also may benefit from information about childbirth techniques that place less emphasis on control. (For more information, see Chapter 21, Family Preparation for Childbirth and Parenting.)

Death

The American culture dismisses as irrational the fear of death during childbirth. However, many women fear death, and, rarely, some die from complications of childbirth. The woman's partner, the health care team, and others can help her cope with these fears by validating death as a real but remote possibility, exploring life-threatening circumstances, and discussing her wishes should she die during labor.

The father also may fear for the safety of his partner and child. He may be reluctant to share such fears with his partner, but sharing his feelings may help to defuse them.

Family considerations

Throughout the pregnancy, the expectant parents may need to prepare siblings for the new family member and involve the grandparents.

Sibling preparation

American parents typically assume that the neonate's birth will make siblings feel displaced and jealous. Siblings may sense this and act as they are expected to act. Rolfe (1985) suggests that parents share the news of an impending birth positively and deal with any feelings that arise. (For more information, see *Family care: Sibling preparation for a neonate,* page 418.)

Sibling attendance at the birth depends on the parents' values and beliefs and the health care facility's policies. Some parents may include siblings in the birth to eliminate feelings of exclusion and to avoid separating them from the mother. Their inclusion enhances their bonding with the neonate and may enhance their self-esteem. It also may help them accept childbirth and sexuality as normal aspects of life (DelGiudice, 1986).

Studies show that most siblings who attend a birth discuss it happily and positively, regarding it as a normal life event (DelGiudice, 1986). However, the sibling's preparation for the birth will determine the quality of the experience (Gomez, 1984).

During pregnancy, parents should involve siblings in decision making and should prepare them for the sights, sounds, colors, smells, sensations, and emotions of childbirth. During delivery, parents should provide a support person for each child, so that children can come and go as they please (Anderson and DelGiudice, 1985). Parents can help prepare siblings for the birth by using films, classes, home discussions, and audiovisual aids, such as a birthing doll (a doll containing a smaller doll that can be "delivered").

The family that excludes siblings from the birth can keep them involved by giving them a tour of the health care facility, explaining arrangements for their care during labor and delivery, and letting them visit the mother

Sibling preparation for a neonate

Awaiting the arrival of a new family member can be confusing or distressing for siblings. To help ease the transition for siblings and parents, the nurse can make the following suggestions to the parents.

• Express positive feelings through such statements as, "We love you so much we wanted another child."
• Deal with the siblings' expressed feelings, accepting these feelings without judgment and affirming the children's lovability.
• Avoid strong statements—positive or negative—about the new family member.
• Discuss which aspects of family life will be changed by the neonate and which will remain unchanged.
• Explain when the neonate is due by creating a calendar that shows the stages of fetal development during the seasons of the birth year. This will help siblings conceptualize the passage of time.
• Explain how the fetus was conceived and answer sex questions simply, truthfully, and individually. Ask for feedback and correct any misunderstandings siblings may have about conception.
• Devise household routines that involve both parents, so that the mother's absence during labor and delivery will not disrupt routines.
• Make bed and room changes early in pregnancy to prevent siblings from feeling displaced by the neonate.
• Involve siblings in preparations for the neonate, such as decorating the nursery or choosing a homecoming outfit.
• Involve siblings in health care. Encourage them to listen to fetal heart sounds, feel fetal movements, and attend childbirth education classes for siblings.
• Instill realistic expectations about the neonate's appearance, behavior, care, and feeding.
• Reminisce with siblings about their births and review baby photographs together.
• Include siblings in health care facility visits. Create a schedule for such visits that includes time for them to rest and be fed. Bring their pictures and toys to the health care facility. Spend time alone with them during visits.
• Plan the neonate's homecoming carefully to minimize sibling distress. Have the mother visit alone with siblings after arriving home, while the father holds the neonate.
• Reward mature behaviors and ignore immature ones.

and neonate after birth. Even when the child ignores the mother or cries at the end of a visit, such visits ease the separation for the child. A child's display of jealousy does not indicate the parents' failure; rather, it may indicate that the child feels well-loved and safe in expressing feelings.

Grandparent involvement

The grandparent-grandchild bond is second in importance only to the parent-child bond. Grandparents provide a sense of family continuity for their grandchildren, sharing family traditions and religious and moral values. They pass on the family history, provide older role models, and, ideally, affirm the vulnerable new parents' self-esteem.

Because the grandparent role is more flexible than the parent role, grandparents invest less ego in the relationship and can offer unconditional love. They may be able to discuss life issues more easily and may experience a new freedom to be themselves. Grandchildren may feel a similar freedom, accepting what grandparents offer without expectations.

Grandparents may view grandchildren as a self-extension into the future. They may reminisce about their own childhoods and parenthoods and attempt to remake their parental image or correct mistakes they made with their own children. They also may reexamine their values and religious heritage by sharing them with their grandchildren.

The grandchild's presence can help heal old rifts between grandparents or parents, or it can cause them to reenact old scenarios through criticism, competition, subtle undermining, or tests of loyalty. Some new parents may envy the amount of love and nurturing grandparents bestow on their grandchildren. Some grandparents may be ambivalent about their new role, feeling old or displaced from the parental role. Grandparents may be disappointed when their advice is ignored and may interpret their child's parenting style as criticism of their own.

Because the grandparent role is an imposed one, most grandparents have the right to decide what they will offer to grandchildren. Because the parents are in the central position, they must negotiate intergenerational relationships that are comfortable and satisfying for all three generations.

Special family needs

Families from different cultures, blended families, and those with single or lesbian parents may have special psychosocial tasks.

CULTURAL CONSIDERATIONS

Psychosocial aspects of pregnancy

Although each client has personal beliefs and values, her cultural background may influence her psychosocial adaptation during pregnancy as well as her self-care and health promotion measures, health-seeking behaviors, and interactions with health care professionals. When caring for a client from a different culture, the nurse should keep the following considerations in mind.

North American culture

Because the North American culture encompasses various ethnic and cultural backgrounds, no typical view of childbirth exists in America. However, widespread access to medical care and the movement toward family-centered childbirth permit a few generalizations about American attitudes toward pregnancy and childbirth.

In the United States, physicians typically manage a woman's pregnancy. Americans tend to rely heavily on medical intervention to ensure a healthy outcome for the mother and neonate. They usually emphasize technological intervention, including ultrasonography and other tests, to track fetal growth and health.

Americans consider health promotion activities an indication that the woman has accepted her pregnancy. They encourage the woman to get early prenatal care, to monitor her diet carefully, and to eliminate unhealthy practices, such as drinking alcohol and smoking. A pregnant woman who engages in unhealthy practices may meet with disapproval or disdain and may experience guilt and self-doubt.

American men participate in pregnancy and delivery to a greater extent than do men in many other cultures. A large percentage of American men attend childbirth education classes and are present during delivery. Many American men also are taking an increased role in infant care at home.

Asian culture

In the United States, Chinese, Japanese, and Korean clients may practice traditional beliefs or may adopt American customs and practices regarding childbirth.

The Chinese culture values maintaining a balance between the physical and spiritual aspects of life, especially during pregnancy. To help achieve this balance, a pregnant woman may avoid certain foods and drink herbal teas. After delivery, the woman may stay home and rest for 40 days, avoiding strenuous activity. She also may avoid contact with water for 40 days after delivery, believing that a postpartal chill can cause arthritis or body aches.

Japanese-Americans, who have the highest median income and educational level of any American minority group, tend to accept American practices. They view pregnancy as a normal state that requires few changes in the pregnant woman's daily routine. After delivery, the woman controls the neonate's care, although the extended family may participate.

Korean-American women believe that the pregnant woman or a family member experiences a *Tae Mong* (dream that predicts pregnancy). After she becomes pregnant, the Korean woman may read classical literature, view beautiful artworks, and adopt an optimistic and serene attitude to promote health and an easy delivery. Dietary restrictions include balancing hot and cold foods and restricting salty, spicy, or sour foods (Lee, 1989). Other restrictions include barring men and child-less women from the delivery area and keeping the neonate's father away from the mother and neonate for seven days after delivery.

The birth of a first child, especially a son, is an important event in a Korean family, integrating the mother into her partner's family and giving her status and economic security. In traditional Korean families, the mother-in-law is responsible for the pregnant woman's health and care. If she desires a grandson, the Korean mother-in-law will view care of her daughter-in-law as service to Samshin, the goddess of childbirth. Health care professionals should be aware that the Korean client may wish to involve her mother-in-law in decision-making discussions (Sich, 1988).

Southeast Asian culture

Southeast Asian (Vietnamese, Cambodian, and Laotian) women may hold what many Americans consider to be superstitious beliefs, such as the belief that sitting on a step in a doorframe can cause labor and delivery complications, or that a bath after sundown will result in an oversized neonate.

Some Southeast Asian women may see an herbalist or an acupuncturist before seeking Western health care and may refrain from expressing doubts about medications or procedures out of respect for authority. If the health care professional's advice conflicts with traditional beliefs, the Southeast Asian client may deal passively with this conflict, missing appointments or neglecting to fill prescriptions. The health care professional who is alert to such indirect messages can approach the client with an alternate plan (Lee, 1989).

Filipino culture

Filipino women share many traits with Southeast Asian women. They are taught to respect elders, defer to their partners, and avoid confrontation. The nurse who provides care to a Filipino client should be aware that she may wish to deal with issues indirectly and involve the family in health care planning (Stern, 1985).

Haitian culture

In Haiti, pregnancy is viewed as a matter-of-fact experience that does not need to be discussed. For this reason, Haitian women may not seek prenatal care (Harris, 1987).

Haitian women observe various practices after delivery. They may take a series of three herbal baths, conserve body heat, avoid white foods, and wear abdominal binders (Harris, 1987). The Haitian neonate's name may be chosen by a community leader or an older family member and may commemorate a family member who has died. The name of a deceased family member may signify that the dead person's unfinished business has been passed on to the neonate or that the neonate is expected to carry on a family business or profession (Meltzer, 1981).

Cultural considerations

Cultural beliefs about childbearing stabilize the emotional environment for both mother and neonate. Rites and rituals structure childbirth, supporting mother-infant bonding and integrating the mother and infant into the family and society (Sich, 1988). To maximize the family's resources and ability to enfold its new member, the nurse must note personal cultural biases and offer nonjudgmental support.

The cultural meanings of pregnancy and parenthood influence a woman's psychosocial experience of the childbearing year and her transition to parenthood. Respecting cultural traditions and beliefs maximizes the client's social support and personal integrity and the nurse's effectiveness. (For more information, see *Cultural considerations: Psychosocial aspects of pregnancy*, page 419.)

Blended families

A blended family (stepfamily) includes children from one or both parents' previous relationships. Stepparenting is more difficult than biological parenting for many reasons. Although most children feel emotional bonds that smooth over the deficiencies of biological parents, they may not feel close to stepparents and may judge them harshly. Also, blended families include a greater number of individuals with more complex relationships.

In a blended family, roles are nontraditional and ill-defined, which can engender ambivalence or competition between stepparents and stepchildren. Role uncertainty and feelings of insecurity add to the complexities of parenting.

When a neonate joins the blended family, family members must display tremendous sensitivity and commitment to pull the family together, integrate all members, and increase feelings of belonging in each child and each parent.

Single mothers

In 1984, 12 million children under age 18 lived in single-parent homes in the United States. About 90% of these homes were headed by women (Caplan and Caplan, 1984). A mother can be effective as a single parent and a mother's competence in child care is the most important influence on a child's growth and maturation. The father's absence from the family has not been proved to affect the child's psychosexual or intellectual development negatively (Friedman, 1981).

Single mothers experience special pressures, however. For a single adolescent mother, the psychological tasks of pregnancy and child care are compounded by the developmental aspects of adolescence. The mother may face stressful decisions, such as whether to keep or relinquish her neonate, and may suffer additional stress from minimal support systems, inadequate income, interrupted education, reduced vocational choices, and difficulty assuming the mother role. (For more information, see Chapter 22, High-Risk Antepartal Clients.)

An older women who decides to raise a child alone faces different psychosocial challenges. Although she typically plans carefully for child care and has greater financial resources and support systems than a single adolescent, she may experience role overload, role conflict, reduced flexibility, and reduced support in emergencies. She also may need to resolve the father's role in her life and the child's life.

Lesbian parents

Between 2% and 12% of American women are lesbians, and about one-third of them are mothers (Harvey, Carr, and Bernheine, 1989). Until recently, most of these women became mothers through heterosexual relationships, but today many lesbians are choosing to bear children through artificial insemination, adoption, or other means. Lesbians cite the same motivations for becoming parents as other parents do: love of children, desire to pass on their values, belief that they would be good parents, and desire to stabilize their lives (Olesker and Walsh, 1984).

A lesbian mother's status as a repressed minority member may complicate her psychosocial adaptation to pregnancy. She may have to negotiate the biological father's role, and she may have concerns about the legal status of her nontraditional family. Family members and others (including some health care professionals) may not be supportive and may be judgmental. Therefore, a lesbian may not be completely candid with the health care professional.

Chapter summary

Chapter 18 described psychosocial needs and tasks of expectant families. Here are the chapter highlights.
• Childbearing is vital to most individuals' self-concept and presents unique psychosocial tasks and challenges.
• The nurse who cares for the expectant family must promote normal adaptation and integration of the new member by promoting self-esteem, family integrity, pre-

natal bonding, conflict resolution, and adaptive coping.
• To provide appropriate care, the nurse must avoid imposing personal attitudes about childbearing on others.
• Various factors can affect an individual's transition to parenthood, such as socioeconomic status and support from the partner, parents, and friends.
• Stress and anxiety increase the discomforts of pregnancy and may complicate delivery. The nurse can help the client and her partner reduce stress by emphasizing coping mechanisms and facilitating open communication.
• In the first trimester of pregnancy, psychosocial tasks for expectant parents include resolving ambivalence; for the mother, coping with discomforts and changes; and for the father, beginning to accept the pregnancy and its implications for his provider role.
• In the second trimester, psychosocial tasks include developing a mother image and a father image, coping with changes in body image and sexuality, and developing prenatal bonding.
• In the third trimester, tasks include adapting to a slower pace, preparing for parenting, supporting and nurturing the partner, accepting body image and sexuality changes, preparing for labor, and developing birth plans.
• The expectant couple may use dream and fear examination to help accomplish psychosocial tasks.
• To prepare siblings to accept the neonate, the nurse can suggest ways for parents to involve them in the pregnancy and birth.
• Because parents are in the central position, they must negotiate intergenerational relationships that are acceptable to all three generations.
• Cultural views of pregnancy and childbirth vary. To provide culturally sensitive care, the nurse must understand the client's cultural background.
• Blended families and those with single or lesbian parents may have additional psychosocial concerns during pregnancy.

Study questions

1. Which factors affect a pregnant woman's transition to parenthood?

2. When does prenatal bonding begin? Which statements or behaviors indicate that a parent is forming this bond?

3. How does a woman form her mother image? How does this compare to the way a man forms his father image?

4. Which nursing interventions may help parents prepare siblings for a neonate?

5. John and Amy Hall, a married, two-career couple in their early thirties, are expecting their first child in 6 months. Which principles will help the nurse support them through the psychosocial changes during pregnancy?

Bibliography

Armstrong, P., and Feldman, S. (1990). *A wise birth.* New York: William Morrow.

Boston Women's Health Book Collective. (1985). *The new our bodies, ourselves.* New York: Simon & Schuster.

Friedman, M. (1981). *Family nursing: Theory and assessment* (2nd ed.). East Norwalk, CT: Appleton & Lange.

Grossman, F., Eichler, L., Winickoff, S., Anzalone, M., Gofseyeff, M., and Sargent, S. (1980). *Pregnancy, birth, and parenthood: Adaptations of mothers, fathers, and infants.* San Francisco: Jossey-Bass.

Jones, C. (1987). *Mind over labor.* New York: Viking Penguin.

Kitzinger, S. (1984). *The experience of childbirth* (5th ed.). New York: Penguin.

Miller, M., and Brooten, D. (1983). *The childbearing family: A nursing perspective.* Boston: Little, Brown.

Noble, E. (1983). *Childbirth with insight.* Boston: Houghton Mifflin.

Panuthos, C. (1984). *Transformation through birth: A woman's guide.* South Hadley, MA: Bergin & Garvey.

Sherwen, L. (1987). *Psychosocial dimensions of the pregnant family.* New York: Springer Publishing.

Stephens, C. (1985). Identifying social support components in prenatal populations: A multivariate analysis on alcohol consumption. *Health Care for Women International, 6*(5-6), 285-294.

Stichler, J., Bowden, M., and Reimer, E. (1979). Pregnancy: A shared emotional experience. In A. O'Connor (Ed.), *Nursing: The childbearing family.* New York: American Journal of Nursing Co.

Varney, H. (1987). *Nurse-Midwifery* (2nd ed.). Boston: Blackwell-Scientific Publications.

Parents

Baldwin, R., and Palmarini, T. (1986). *Pregnant feelings.* Berkeley, CA: Celestial Arts.

Bittman, S., and Zalk, S. (1983). *Expectant fathers.* New York: Ballantine Books.

Colman, A., and Colman, L. (1977). *Pregnancy: The psychological experience.* New York: Bantam.

Cranley, M. (1981). Roots of attachment: The relationship of parents with their unborn. *Birth Defects: Original Article Series, 17*(6), 59-83.

Leifer, M. (1977). Psychological changes accompanying pregnancy and motherhood. *Genetic and Psychological Monographs,* 95(1), 55-96.

Muenchow, S., and Bloom-Feshbach, J. (1982, February). The new fatherhood. *Parents,* pp. 64-69.

Parke, R. (1981). *Fathers.* Cambridge, MA: Harvard University Press.

Shapiro, J. (1987). *When men are pregnant: Needs and concerns of expectant fathers.* San Luis Obispo, CA: Impact Publishers.

Stern, E. (1987, January). "I'm Not Fat, I'm Pregnant." *American Baby,* pp. 63-68.

Stukane, E. (1985). *The dream worlds of pregnancy: A fascinating new area of dream research.* New York: William Morrow.

Wapner, J. (1976). The attitudes, feelings, and behaviors of expectant fathers attending Lamaze classes. *Birth and the Family Journal,* 3(1), 5-13.

Siblings

Anderson, S., and DelGiudice, G. (1985). *Siblings, birth, and the newborn.* Seattle, WA: Pennypress.

Caplan, T., and Caplan, F. (1984). *The early childhood years: The 2 to 6 year old.* New York: Bantam.

DelGiudice, G. (1986). The relationship between sibling jealousy and presence at a sibling's birth. *Birth,* 13(4), 250-254.

Gomez, D. (1984). Sibling preparation for childbirth. *Genesis* (Arlington), June/July: 16-17.

Rolfe, R. (1985). *You can postpone anything but love: Expanding our potential as parents.* Edgemont, PA: Ambassador Press.

Grandparents

Dodson, F. (1984). *How to grandparent.* New York: Harper & Row.

Kornhaber, A. (1987). *Between parents and grandparents.* New York: Berkley Books.

Cultural references

Choi, E. (1986). Unique aspects of Korean-American mothers. *JOGNN,* 15(15), 394-400.

Harris, K. (1987). Beliefs and practices Among Haitian American women in relation to childbearing. *Journal of Nurse-Midwifery,* 32(3), 149-155.

Lee, R. (1989). Understanding southeast Asian mothers-to-be. *Childbirth Educator,* Spring, 32-39.

Meltzer, D. (Ed.). (1981). *Birth: An anthology of ancient texts, songs, prayers, and stories.* San Francisco: North Point Press.

Sich, D. (1988). Childbearing in Korea. *Social Science Medicine,* 27(5), 497-504.

Stern, P. (1985). A comparison of culturally approved behaviors and beliefs between Pilipina immigrant women, U.S.-born dominant culture women, and western female nurses of the San Francisco Bay Area: Religiosity of health care. *Health Care for Women International,* 6(1-3), 123-133.

Nursing research

Carter-Jessop, L. (1981). Promoting maternal attachment through prenatal intervention. *MCN,* 6(2), 107-112.

Clinton, J. (1985). Couvade: Patterns, predictors, and nursing management: A research proposal submitted to the division of nursing. *Western Journal of Nursing Research,* 7(2), 221-243.

Clinton, J. (1987). Physical and emotional responses of expectant fathers throughout pregnancy and the early postpartum period. *International Journal of Nursing Studies,* 24(1), 59-68.

Cronenwett, L., and Kunst-Wilson, W. (1981). Stress, social support, and the transition to fatherhood. *Nursing Research,* 30(4), 196-201.

Glazer, G. (1989). Anxiety and stressors of expectant fathers. *Western Journal of Nursing Research,* 11(1), 47-59.

Harvey, S., Carr, C., and Bernheine, S. (1989). Lesbian mothers: Health care experiences. *Journal of Nurse-Midwifery,* 34(3), 115-119.

Heidrich, S., and Cranley, M. (1989). Effect of fetal movement, ultrasound scans, and amniocentesis on maternal-fetal attachment. *Nursing Research,* 38(2), 81-84.

Lederman, R. (1984). *Psychosocial adaptation in pregnancy: Assessment of 7 dimensions of maternal development.* East Norwalk, CT: Appleton & Lange.

Lederman, R. (1986). Maternal anxiety in pregnancy: Relationship to fetal and newborn health status. In H. Werley, J. Fitzpatrick, and R. Taunton (Eds.), *Annual Review of Nursing Research,* Volume 4 (pp. 3-19). New York: Springer Publishing.

Lemmer, C. (1987). Becoming a father: A review of nursing research on expectant fatherhood. *MCN,* 16(3), 261-275.

Mansfield, P., and Cohn, M. (1986). Stress and later life childbearing. *Maternal-Child Nursing Journal,* 15(3), 139-151.

May, K. (1980). A typology of detachment/involvement styles adopted during pregnancy by first-time expectant fathers. *Western Journal of Nursing Research,* 2(2), 445-453.

May, K. (1982). Three phases of father involvement in pregnancy. *Nursing Research,* 31(6), 337-324.

May, K. (1987). Men's sexuality during the childbearing year: Implications of recent research findings. *Holistic Nursing Practice,* 1(4), 60-66.

Mercer, R., Ferketich, S., DeJoseph, J., May, K., and Sollid, D. (1988). Effect of stress on family functioning during pregnancy. *Nursing Research,* 37(5), 268-275.

Moore, D. (1978). The body image in pregnancy. *Journal of Nurse-Midwifery,* 22(4), 17-27.

Moore, D. (1983). Prepared childbirth and marital satisfaction during the antepartum and postpartum periods. *Nursing Research,* 32(2), 73-79.

Olesker, E., and Walsh, L. (1984). Childbearing among lesbians: Are we meeting their needs? *Journal of Nurse-Midwifery,* 29(5), 322-329.

Reiber, V. (1976). Is the nurturing role natural to fathers? *MCN,* 1, 336-371.

Sherwen, L. (1986). Third trimester fantasies of first-time expectant fathers. *MCN,* 15(3), 153-170.

Strang, V., and Sullivan, P. (1985). Body image attitudes during pregnancy and the postpartum period. *JOGNN,* 14(4), 332-337.

Strickland, O. (1987). The occurrence of symptoms in expectant fathers: The couvade syndrome. *Nursing Research,* 36(3), 184-189.

Thompson, J., Oakley, D., Burke, M., Jay, S., and Conklin, M. (1989). Theory building in nurse-midwifery: The care process. *Journal of Nurse-Midwifery,* 34(3), 120-130.

Care during the Normal Antepartal Period

Objectives

After reading and studying this chapter, the student should be able to:
1. Summarize the major components of the antepartal health assessment.
2. Discuss antepartal risk factors that the nurse should assess.
3. Calculate or estimate the expected date of delivery.
4. Explain the importance of previous pregnancies and outcomes to the client's current pregnancy.
5. Describe interventions for common discomforts of pregnancy.
6. List danger signs of pregnancy.
7. Apply the nursing process when caring for a pregnant client and her family.

Introduction

During the antepartal period, members of the health care team strive to ensure the health of the client and her fetus. Nursing responsibilities typically include:
• Monitoring the pregnancy with other team members
• Gathering and interpreting health history data, physical assessment findings, and results of diagnostic studies
• Conducting regular prenatal assessments while encouraging the active participation of the client and her family in the pregnancy, labor, and birth
• Teaching the client about health risks and their prevention
• Teaching the client and family to recognize danger signals and seek care promptly
• Formulating goals for the prenatal period and intervening as necessary.

Of these responsibilities, the experienced, expert nurse or the advanced, prepared nurse practitioner, clinician, or nurse-midwife performs the full physical examination, interprets laboratory data, and takes pelvimetry measurements. The less experienced nurse may conduct the bedside history, take vital signs and weight, gather urine and blood samples, and teach the client and family members.

This chapter begins with client assessment, which is obtained through the health history and physical assessment. Both steps occur during the initial prenatal visit; selected aspects occur at scheduled follow-up visits. The assessment section includes instructions for determining the expected date of delivery (EDD). Client assessment is followed by nursing diagnoses applicable to many antepartal clients, followed by planning and implementing care for the healthy pregnant client. The chapter then presents interventions to help minimize client discomfort during pregnancy. Furthermore, it lists signs of impending danger to the client or fetus. Finally, the chapter discusses evaluation and documentation for the antepartal client.

Assessment

Ideally, antepartal assessment begins when a client seeks health care to confirm a suspected pregnancy and begin prenatal care. During the initial antepartal meet-

GLOSSARY

Breast shield: device worn late in pregnancy to draw out inverted nipples in preparation for breast-feeding.

Childbirth exercises: activities designed specifically to tone and strengthen muscles stressed during pregnancy, labor, and birth.

EDD: expected date of delivery.

Hoffman's exercises: areola-stretching technique designed to facilitate breast-feeding by breaking adhesions and allowing inverted nipples to become more protractile.

LMP: first day of the last menstrual period.

Lightening: subjective sensation the client may feel as the fetus descends into the pelvic inlet and changes the shape and position of the uterus near term.

Nagele's rule: method of calculating EDD using a client's LMP.

Pregnancy-induced hypertension: group of potentially life-threatening hypertensive disorders (also called toxemia of pregnancy) that usually develop late in the second trimester or in the third trimester; includes preeclampsia and eclampsia.

Preeclampsia: nonconvulsive form of pregnancy-induced hypertension characterized by the onset of acute hypertension, proteinuria, and edema after the twenty-fourth week of gestation. Called eclampsia when it includes seizures and coma.

Protractility: state of protrusion rather than inversion when referring to nipples.

Quickening: first awareness of fetal movement the client may have, typically at 16 to 20 weeks.

Varicosity: enlarged, tortuous area of a vessel; in pregnancy, typically venous varicosities of the legs, rectum, or vulva.

---

ing, the nurse gathers subjective and objective data pertinent to the client's pregnancy and general health. The initial antepartal meeting:

• provides background information and appropriate baseline data for care throughout pregnancy

• explores areas in which the client may face risks or require education

• begins the nurse-client interaction, out of which a trusting relationship may develop.

Assessment should continue regularly throughout the antepartal period. The client may schedule an examination every 4 weeks until the twenty-eighth week, every 2 weeks until the thirty-sixth week, and every week until delivery. However, the number of scheduled examinations depends on the client's overall condition.

Repeated contact between nurse and client enables the nurse to monitor the client's well-being, the fetus's development, and the onset of any problems. Also, it provides an opportunity for client teaching. If the client's partner or a family member attends these meetings, the nurse can provide supportive education to them, too.

Besides a health history and physical examination, antepartal assessment includes selected laboratory tests. Follow-up care focuses on maintaining the health and well-being of the client and fetus throughout pregnancy.

Health history

The health history interview should address all pertinent areas of the client's health—past, present, and potential. The nurse should consider the client's physical appearance and nonverbal communication as well as her verbal responses to questions.

Biographical data

Record the client's name, address, telephone number, birth date, and marital status. Ascertain her reason for requesting care, which may be suspected pregnancy. Pay special attention to her reason for her visit because she may reveal her feelings about a possible pregnancy.

The client's age will relate to possible risks she faces during pregnancy. Reproductive risks increase among clients under age 15 and over age 35. (For a discussion of these age-related risks, see Chapter 22, High-Risk Antepartal Clients.)

Investigating the client's marital status may give the nurse insight into family support systems, sexual practices, and possible stress factors.

Current pregnancy

After obtaining biographical data, focus on concerns directly related to the pregnancy. Record the client's reasons for believing herself pregnant, including the absence of one or more menstrual periods, nausea, vomiting, urinary frequency, breast tenderness, fatigue, or a positive result on a home pregnancy test. (For a complete description of possible, probable, and positive signs of pregnancy, see Chapter 17, Physiologic Changes during Normal Pregnancy.)

Ask if the client menstruates regularly, the typical length of her cycle, and the date of her last menstrual period (LMP). Knowing the LMP is useful in predicting gestational age and EDD.

EDD can be calculated using several methods, but Nagele's rule is used most commonly. By Nagele's rule, EDD equals the first day of the last normal menstrual period, minus 3 months, plus 7 days. For example, if the first day of the LMP was September 20, then the EDD will be June 27 of the following calendar year. Nagele's rule is based on a 28-day cycle and must be adjusted if the client has irregular, prolonged, or shortened menstrual cycles. An alternative method for determining the EDD uses an obstetric calculator wheel. However, these wheels vary from printing to printing, which may change the EDD by 2 or 3 days.

If the client cannot remember the date of her LMP, suggest special events or holidays as a way to reconstruct at least the month if not the date itself. If the client still cannot remember, record her LMP as questionable and rely on other methods—such as the date of quickening, uterine size and growth, and ultrasound—to help predict the EDD.

In addition to requesting the date of the client's LMP, ask her if her last menstrual period differed. Implantation of the fertilized ovum may produce a scant, bloody vaginal discharge at about the time of an expected menstrual period. If the client mistakes this discharge for her monthly flow, she will misinterpret her LMP. In addition, vaginal bleeding or spotting could indicate ectopic pregnancy or a problem with hormonal support of the endometrium. Cramping could indicate uterine fibroids or an intrauterine device (IUD).

Additional insight into the length of the pregnancy may be gained if the client has a good idea of when conception might have occurred, especially if she has regular menstrual cycles or was aware of the time of ovulation.

Ask if the couple planned the pregnancy. If so, they probably desire a child and have primarily positive thoughts about the pregnancy. If not, explore the client's and her partner's desire to maintain the pregnancy and explain options available to them. If the client had difficulty becoming pregnant, she may be apprehensive about her ability to maintain the pregnancy. If she had fertility therapy, she may worry about the possibility of multiple fetuses.

Begin assessing the client's educational needs (and her partner's needs, if possible) during the initial visit. Provide the couple with needed information or appropriate referrals. Education helps reduce fears associated with labor and delivery and with postpartal care of both client and neonate. Suggest childbirth education classes when appropriate. (See Chapter 21, Family Preparation for Childbirth and Parenting, for additional information.)

Documenting previous pregnancies

One method commonly used to document previous pregnancies is called the TPAL system. The first element, T, stands for the number of term neonates born (after 37 weeks' gestation). The second element, P, stands for the number of preterm neonates born (before 37 weeks' gestation). The third element, A, stands for the number of

T P A L

pregnancies ending in spontaneous or therapeutic abortion. The fourth element, L, stands for the number of children alive. Thus, a client with an obstetric history documented as gravida 4 para 1212 has been pregnant four times, delivered one neonate at term, two neonates prematurely, had one pregnancy end in abortion, and has two children alive.

Record the age, health status, and development of other children in the family. This information can suggest ways to help these children prepare for the neonate. Also, it may identify possible areas of family stress and dysfunctional coping behaviors.

After obtaining information on the current pregnancy, investigate possible pregnancy risk factors, which may stem from previous pregnancies and their outcomes, from the gynecologic history unrelated to previous pregnancies, from other aspects of the client's medical history, from family medical history, from a psychosocial problem, or from the client's education and occupation.

Previous pregnancies and outcomes

Discussion and documentation of the client's previous pregnancies may help the nurse, the client, and her family anticipate needs and expectations for the current pregnancy. (See *Documenting previous pregnancies,* and *Sample prenatal documentation form,* pages 426 and 427, for examples of documentation.)

Make note of birth weights, gestational ages, labor outcomes, and neonatal conditions for each of the client's other children, from the oldest to the youngest. Make special note of any problems or complications she encountered during each pregnancy, labor, and delivery. These may reveal increased risk for the current pregnancy. Such risk factors may warrant special education and guidance. Examples of risk factors include:
• possible cervical incompetence or adhesions resulting from previous abortion
• preterm or postterm labor in a previous pregnancy

(Text continues on page 428.)

Sample prenatal documentation form

The sample documentation form below illustrates the personal information, physical examination findings, and health history information that the nurse documents when assessing the pregnant client.

Prenatal Record

HOSPITAL:	
DOCTOR:	
CLIENT'S NAME:	
ADDRESS:	PHONE:
DATE OF BIRTH:	AGE:	MARITAL STATUS:
OCCUPATION:	PHONE:
FATHER'S NAME:	AGE:	OCCUPATION:
INSURANCE:	

PREGNANCY SUMMARY

MENSTRUAL HISTORY | CONTRACEPTION | FAMILY SITUATION | E.D.D. / REVISED E.D.D.

HISTORY OF PREGNANCY
- Bleeding
- Vomiting
- Pyrexia
- Smoking
- Alcohol
- Radiation

GRAVIDA	TERM	PREMATURE	ABNORMAL	LIVE	MULTIPLE PREGNANCY

OBSTETRIC HISTORY

NUMBER YEAR SEX GEST. AGE BIRTH WT. DUR. OF LABOR PLACE OF BIRTH TYPE OF DELIVERY COMMENTS

MEDICAL HISTORY

CLIENT HISTORY: Kidney Disease, Heart Disease, Hypertension, Diabetes, Infections, Thyroid Disease, Transfusions, Operations

FAMILY HISTORY: Hypertension, Diabetes, Heart Disease, Multiple Birth, Malformation, Genetic Disorder, Early Onset Deafness

PERSONAL INFORMATION

HEIGHT
PREPREGNANCY WT
PRESENT WT
BP

Head, neck, thyroid ☐ Abdomen ☐ Extremities ☐
EENT ☐ Vulva ☐ Varicosities ☐
Teeth Vagina ☐ Neurologic ☐
Chest Cervix ☐ Cytology ☐
Breasts ☐ Uterus ☐
Heart Vasc. Syst. ☐ Adnexa ☐

Prenatal Record

DOCTOR:	
CLIENT'S NAME:	
ADDRESS:	

RISK FACTORS IDENTIFIED IN INITIAL VISIT

LMP	E.D.D.	QUICKENING		PRE-PREG. WT.	BLOOD GROUP	RH FACTOR	RH ANTIBODIES	RUBELLA IMMUNE
VDRL	Hct	G	T	P	A	L		

SUBSEQUENT VISITS

Date	Wt	Cum. Wt. Gain	Gest. Age (wk)	SF Ht	Pres. Pos.	FHR	URINE			BP	TK GROUP	LAB
							PR	GL	AC			

COMMENTS

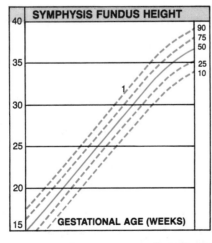

SYMPHYSIS FUNDUS HEIGHT

GESTATIONAL AGE (WEEKS)

REFERRED PAIN

Allergies	Medications

Discussion Topics

• inability to cope with labor pains
• adverse reactions to anesthetics and analgesics used during previous labor and delivery
• previous cesarean or forceps delivery.

The birth weights of the client's children and their modes of delivery provide information about maternal pelvic size. If any of the client's previous pregnancies ended with a stillbirth or with death during the neonatal period, carefully record factors contributing to the death.

Some risk factors may be linked to ethnic background. Examples include sickle cell disease among Blacks and Tay Sach's disease among Jews. Refer the couple for genetic counseling as needed. (For further discussion, see Chapter 11, Genetics and Genetic Disorders.)

Rh factor may raise the risk of complications for some clients. An Rh-negative client with an Rh-positive partner who previously delivered an Rh-positive neonate and did not receive RhoGAM is sensitized to the Rh factor and will need treatment to prevent complications in subsequent neonates.

Gynecologic history

The client's gynecologic history may include risk factors for the current pregnancy, independent of whether the client has ever been pregnant.

Ask if the client has had pain or discomfort during menstruation (dysmenorrhea). Primary dysmenorrhea, which usually involves spasmodic cramping in the lower abdomen, typically resolves after the first pregnancy. Secondary dysmenorrhea, which causes pain in various locations, may indicate such anatomic anomalies as cervical stenosis, which can complicate delivery.

Ask if the client has had a vaginal infection or a sexually transmitted disease, either of which could harm the fetus during development or delivery. For example:
• *Candida albicans* can cause thrush.
• Chlamydial infection can cause conjunctivitis and spontaneous abortion.
• Herpes genitalis can cause neonatal death.
• Gonorrhea can cause ophthalmia neonatorum.
• Syphilis and human immunodeficiency virus (HIV) can be transmitted to the fetus in utero. (See Chapter 12, Infectious Disorders, for more information on sexually transmitted diseases.)

Determine if the client used a contraceptive before becoming pregnant, and how long she used it. Pregnancy that results from contraceptive failure may raise special risks. For example, an oral contraceptive taken during the first trimester can be teratogenic. A failed IUD can cause spontaneous septic abortion and should be removed by the physician immediately after verification of pregnancy.

Medical history

Collect data about current and previous health factors that may be relevant to the current pregnancy.

Weight. An underweight or overweight client may reflect poor nutrition. An underweight client may deliver a low-birth-weight neonate; an overweight client may be at increased risk for gestational diabetes and pregnancy-induced hypertension (PIH). A client's dissatisfaction with her weight may influence her compliance with nutritional recommendations during pregnancy. (For more information on ideal wieght during pregnancy, see Chapter 20, Nutrition and Diet Counseling.)

Medications and allergies. Determine if the client has taken any prescription or over-the-counter drugs since becoming pregnant. Medications taken in the early weeks of pregnancy may adversely affect fetal development; for example, streptomycin can damage the eighth cranial nerve. Ask if the client has any medication allergies. A hypersensitivity reaction to a known allergen can precipitate anaphylaxsis, which could endanger both the client and her fetus.

Viral infections. Determine if the client has had any viral infections since becoming pregnant because they may have a teratogenic effect on the fetus.

Medical treatments or procedures. Inquire whether the client has had any dental treatments, surgery, or X-rays since her last menstrual period. If she had X-rays, was an abdominal shield used? X-rays may be harmful to the fetus, and noxious anesthetics may lead to abortion.

Substance abuse. Attempt to determine whether the client habitually uses substances known to cause or suspected of causing harm to the fetus or to herself.

If the client smokes, ask how many cigarettes per day. Women who smoke deliver, on average, smaller neonates than those who do not smoke. Further, intra-uterine growth retardation (IUGR) increases with the number of cigarettes smoked. IUGR was minimal or eliminated when smokers stopped smoking early in the pregnancy (Naeye, 1981). Smoking also may raise the incidence of preterm delivery (Shiono, Klebanoff, and Rhoads, 1986). If the client does not smoke, ask if she is exposed regularly to a smoke-filled environment, which also presents a risk.

If the client drinks alcohol, determine how much and how often. A safe level of alcohol intake during pregnancy has not been determined. However, excessive alcohol intake has serious harmful effects on the fetus, especially during the sixteenth to eighteenth week of pregnancy. Affected neonates demonstrate fetal alcohol syndrome, which includes microcephaly, growth retardation, short palpebral fissures, and maxillary hypoplasia. Alcohol intake may affect the client's nutrition and may predispose her to complications in early pregnancy, such as abortion. The combined effects of alcohol and cigarettes cause greater fetal anomalies than the sum of their individual effects (Brooten, et al., 1987).

Determine how many cups of caffeinated coffee, tea, and soda the client drinks daily. Although the effects of caffeine are not clearly understood in pregnancy, the client should exercise caution by limiting intake.

Determine if the client has used marijuana, cocaine, heroin, or other illicit drugs before and since becoming pregnant. These drugs pose serious threats to the health of both client and fetus. Marijuana use has been linked to short gestation and high incidence of precipitate labor; it may have effects similar to those of alcohol (Fried, Watkinson, and Willan, 1984). Cocaine use has been linked to increased spontaneous abortions, preterm labor, and abruptio placentae. Heroin and cocaine use create neonatal dependency and withdrawal trauma (Landry and Smith, 1987). Additionally, the HIV responsible for acquired immunodeficiency syndrome (AIDS) can be transmitted via shared needles used to inject drugs. The virus in a client can pass to the fetus.

Previous medical problems. Elicit information about the client's childhood disease profile, immunizations, past medical conditions and treatments, and surgical procedures.

Some diseases acquired in childhood may confer lifelong immunity. Of those that do not, some may endanger a fetus exposed at certain stages of development. Rubella, for example, may have teratogenic effects on the fetus if the client is exposed during the first trimester. Some immunizations may be recommended during pregnancy because of the client's increased susceptibility. (See *Immunization guidelines for pregnancy* for further information.) Other immunizations, such as rubella, are contraindicated during pregnancy because of the teratogenic effects of the attenuated live virus on the fetus.

Ask if the client has pets at home. Toxoplasmosis, contracted from organisms in cat feces, causes severe congenital anomalies in a fetus infected in the first trimester. Infections contracted from bird and dog parasites may put the client and fetus at risk as well.

Certain medical conditions could place a client at high risk or jeopardize the pregnancy. These include bleeding disorders, cancer, cardiac disease, diabetes, epilepsy, gallbladder disease, hepatitis, hypertension, phle-

Immunization guidelines during pregnancy

Some immunizations may be recommended during pregnancy because of the client's increased susceptibility. Others may be contraindicated because of their teratogenic effects. A list of recommendations follows.

IMMUNIZATION	RECOMMENDATION
Cholera	Killed bacterial vaccine given only to meet travel requirements
Diphtheria-tetanus	Toxoid given only after first trimester if no primary series or booster in 10 years
Hepatitis B	For postexposure prophylaxis, immune globulin given immediately and 1 month later
Influenza	Inactivated virus vaccines given only to pregnant clients with high-risk conditions (chronic cardiac disease, chronic asthma) after first trimester
Measles	Live attenuated virus vaccine contraindicated; pooled immune globulin given for postexposure prophylaxis
Mumps	Live attenuated virus vaccine contraindicated
Plague	Killed bacteria vaccine given selectively to exposed clients
Poliomyelitis	Live attenuated virus or inactivated virus vaccine given only during an epidemic or if the client will travel to endemic areas; oral form preferred
Rabies	Killed virus vaccine given with immune globulin for postexposure prophylaxis
Rubella	Live attenuated virus vaccine contraindicated
Typhoid	Killed bacterial vaccine given only if the client will travel to endemic areas
Varicella	Immune globulin not routinely indicated for healthy client exposed to varicella
Yellow fever	Live attenuated virus vaccine contraindicated unless exposure is unavoidable

Adapted from American College of Obstetricians and Gynecologists. (1982). Immunization during pregnancy. *ACOG Technical Bulletin*, No. 64. Washington, DC: Author.

bitis, psychiatric problems, renal disease, and urinary tract infection. (See Chapter 22, High-Risk Antepartal Clients, for more information.)

Symptoms not associated with possible or probable signs of pregnancy may signal disorders that could have an adverse effect on the pregnancy. Such symptoms warrant investigation.

Ask if the client ever had surgery and, if so, what surgery she had. Previous surgery on the uterus or vagina may have altered their structure, thus increasing the risk of adhesions, which can complicate delivery. Such clients may require a cesarean delivery.

Family health history

Because genetic anomalies and some medical and reproductive conditions are familial, gather family health data. Include the health history of the couple's grandparents, parents, and brothers and sisters.

Ask whether any member of the client's family or her partner's family has had any of the following:
• allergies
• bleeding disorders
• cesarean delivery
• children born with congenital diseases or deformities
• diabetes mellitus
• heart disease
• hypertension
• kidney problems
• multiple gestations (such as twins)
• PIH during a past pregnancy.

Psychosocial assessment

Important areas of psychosocial exploration include the client's attitude toward her pregnancy, her methods of coping with stress, and how cultural and religious beliefs may affect her pregnancy. (See Chapter 18, Psychosocial Changes during Normal Pregnancy, for further discussion.)

Pregnancy is physically and psychologically stressful. A client with problem-solving skills will be better equipped to cope with the changes brought on by pregnancy. If she planned for and desires her pregnancy, her adaptation will be less stressful. Also, emotional maturity and a high degree of self-esteem can ease the transition to motherhood. Conversely, pregnancy may unmask psychological problems, particularly in an adolescent client or one whose pregnancy is unplanned. For a client with a history of emotional or physical deprivation, pregnancy can be a time of crisis.

The client's partner may influence her attitude about pregnancy. If he has a negative attitude, she may experience additional stress that may adversely affect her health and, later, that of her neonate. Chemical or alcohol dependency in the client's partner may suggest under-lying psychological problems that could surface if pregnancy adds stress to the relationship.

Explore any concerns the client or her partner has about the pregnancy. Childbirth education classes may provide the couple with psychosocial support by giving them the opportunity to share concerns with other expectant couples.

Take note of the client's verbal and nonverbal communication patterns, which could reveal problems in adjusting to pregnancy or to impending parenthood. Watch for signs of increased anxiety, inappropriate responses or behavior patterns, difficulty managing stress, or refusal to accept the pregnancy. When necessary, refer the client for psychological assistance.

Assess the client's religious and cultural beliefs about pregnancy because they may affect her health practices during pregnancy and predispose her to complications. For example, an Amish woman may refuse recommended vaccinations.

Education and occupation

Educational level may influence the client's attitude toward pregnancy, the quality of her prenatal care and nutritional intake, her knowledge of neonatal care, and the psychosocial changes that accompany childbirth and parenting.

Identifying the client's occupation may help detect environmental hazards or exposure to teratogens, such as dry-cleaning fluids or X-rays. A client who must stand for long periods may develop backache during pregnancy. Her risk of falling increases during the second and third trimesters as her center of gravity changes. Lifting heavy objects may increase the risk of spontaneous abortion.

Ask if the client's employer provides maternity leave and, if so, its duration and financial coverage. Returning to work before postpartal physiologic and psychological adaptation occurs may adversely affect maternal health. Conversely, loss of income may pose a hardship for the client and may deny her services and supplies needed for her and her neonate's health. Also, lost income may increase stress and may affect the client's health.

Physical assessment

After collecting complete history data, the nurse assists with or continues the physical assessment. The initial examination provides baseline data against which subsequent changes can be evaluated. (See *Nurse's guide to pregnancy assessment* for a list of expected changes.) Follow-up client visits at regular intervals throughout pregnancy allow the nurse to monitor those changes and detect potential abnormalities. (See Chapter 17, Physiologic Changes during Normal Pregnancy, for more information.)

Nurse's guide to pregnancy assessment

This guide provides an overview of normal changes during pregnancy as seen from weeks 1 through 40.

FIRST TRIMESTER

Weeks 1 to 4

- Amenorrhea occurs.
- Breast changes begin.
- Immunologic pregnancy tests become positive; radio-immunoassay test is positive a few days after implantation of fertilized ovum; urine hCG test is positive a few days after occurrence of amenorrhea.
- Nausea and vomiting may begin between the fourth and sixth week.

Weeks 5 to 8

- Goodell's sign occurs (softening of cervix).
- Ladin's sign occurs (softening of uterine isthmus).
- Hegar's sign occurs (softening of lower uterine segment).
- Chadwick's sign appears (purple-blue vagina and cervix).
- McDonald's sign appears (easy flexion of the fundus over the cervix).
- Braun von Fernwald's sign (also called Piskacek's sign) occurs (irregular softening and enlargement of the uterine fundus at the site of implantation).
- Cervical mucus plug forms.
- Uterine shape changes from pear to globular.
- Urinary frequency and urgency occurs.

Weeks 9 to 12

- Fetal heartbeat may be detected using ultrasonic stethoscope.
- Nausea, vomiting, and urinary frequency and urgency lessen.
- Uterus becomes palpable just above symphysis pubis by 12 weeks.

SECOND TRIMESTER

Weeks 13 to 17

- Client gains approximately 10 to 12 lb (4.5 to 5.4 kg) during second trimester.
- Placental souffle heard on auscultation
- Client's heartbeat increases approximately 10 beats between 14 and 30 weeks' gestation. Rate is maintained until 40 weeks' gestation.
- By week 16, the client's thyroid gland enlarges by approximately 25%, and the uterine fundus is palpable halfway between the symphysis pubis and umbilicus.
- Client recognition of fetal movements, or quickening, occurs between 16 and 20 weeks' gestation depending on gravidity and obesity.

Weeks 18 to 22

- Uterine fundus is palpable just below the umbilicus at 18 weeks and is one fingerbreadth above by 22 weeks.
- Fetal heartbeats are heard with fetoscope at 20 weeks' gestation.
- Fetal rebound or ballottement is possible.

Weeks 23 to 27

- Umbilicus appears level with abdominal skin.
- Striae gravidarum usually become apparent.
- Uterine fundus shows evidence of increasing growth.
- Shape of uterus changes from globular to ovoid.
- Braxton Hicks contractions begin.

THIRD TRIMESTER

Weeks 28 to 31

- Client gains approximately 8 to 10 lb (3.6 to 4.5 kg) in third trimester.
- Uterine wall feels soft and yielding.
- Uterine fundus is halfway between the umbilicus and xiphoid process.
- Fetus's outline becomes palpable.
- Fetus is very mobile and may be found in any position.

Weeks 32 to 35

- Client may experience heartburn.
- Striae gravidarum become more evident.
- Fundal height measurement no longer is an accurate indication of gestational age.
- Uterine fundus is palpable just below the xiphoid process at term.
- Braxton Hicks contractions increase in frequency and intensity.
- Client may experience shortness of breath.

Weeks 36 to 40

- Umbilicus protrudes.
- Varicosities, if present, become pronounced.
- Ankle edema becomes evident.
- Urinary frequency recurs.
- Engagement (with or without lightening) occurs.
- Mucus plug is expelled.
- Cervical effacement and dilation begin.

Conduct all physical examinations in a private and comfortable room, and encourage the client to relax. Work efficiently but without rushing. Drape the client as appropriate to respect her modesty; remain alert for signs of discomfort. Explain pertinent examination steps as they occur.

Vital signs

Typically, the assessment begins with vital signs, followed by examination of the head, chest, abdomen, extremities, and pelvic area (when indicated). Alternatively, the examination may follow a body system progression.

At each return visit, ask the client to describe changes that have occurred since the previous visit. Compare these changes with those normally encountered by healthy, pregnant women. Question the client about any symptoms that seem abnormal, such as abdominal pain, vaginal bleeding, headache, or urinary tract pain.

Record the client's temperature, pulse, respirations, and blood pressure. Blood pressure normally remains within the client's prepregnant range. A rise of greater than 30 mm Hg in systolic pressure or 15 mm Hg in diastolic pressure may indicate PIH and should be investigated.

Record the client's height and weight, and compare them against norms for her age and activity level. Weight under 100 lb or over 200 lb may warrant investigation by the client's physician. Failure to gain weight during pregnancy suggests a serious abnormality. Excessive weight gain—more than 2 lb (0.9 kg) weekly—may result from excessive caloric intake, excessive sodium chloride intake, or PIH.

Body systems

When assessing the various body systems, keep the normal physiologic changes of pregnancy in mind.

Respiratory system. On the client's first visit, auscultate the anterior and posterior lung fields. A client in the third trimester may show increased respiratory effort during inspiration.

Musculoskeletal system. Observe the client's posture and gait. These will change later in pregnancy as her center of gravity shifts and hormones relax the pelvic structure.

Endocrine system. On the first visit, palpate the thyroid, which enlarges in about half of all pregnant women because of increased vascularity and hyperplasia.

Neurologic system. On the first visit, check the client's deep tendon reflexes for hyperreflexia, which is seen with PIH.

Cardiovascular system. Expect to hear accentuated heart sounds and, in about 9 out of 10 clients, systolic ejection murmur at 6 to 8 weeks' gestation. The point of maximum impulse may be displaced laterally as the heart moves in response to pressure exerted by the enlarged uterus.

Hematologic system. Observe the client's veins. Pelvic congestion predisposes her to venous varicosities in the legs, vulva, and rectum. Edema in the extremities, although common, may warn of PIH and deserves monitoring.

Gastrointestinal system. On the first visit, auscultate bowel sounds. Expect sounds to decrease during pregnancy as a result of reduced peristalsis.

Urinary system. On the first visit, palpate and percuss the bladder if uterus placement allows. Obtain a urine sample and test with a dipstick for glucose and protein.

Integumentary system. On the first visit, inspect the client's skin, particularly noting the appearance of pigment changes characteristic of pregnancy: chloasma, linea nigra, and hyperpigmentation of the areolae, nipples, and vulva. Inspect the client's abdomen, noting striae gravidarum as they appear. Progression of these changes should be documented during follow-up care.

Reproductive system. On the first visit, inspect and palpate the client's breasts, anticipating enlargement and increased nipple size and erectility by about the eighth week. Colostrum may be expressed as early as the twenty-fourth week. Striae on the breasts may become more visible as vascularity and venous engorgement increase throughout pregnancy.

During each visit, palpate the client's uterus for Braxton Hicks contractions, which occur more frequently, last longer, and are more intense later in pregnancy. During the second and third trimesters, palpation of the uterus through the abdominal wall may be affected by abdominal musculature, previous pregnancies, excess or inadequate amounts of amniotic fluid, and IUGR.

Monitor uterine growth to check the correlation between fetal growth and estimated gestational age. Fundal height is the characteristic used most commonly to monitor uterine growth. (See *Psychomotor skills: Measuring fundal height* for instructions.)

The nurse practitioner uses several measurements to help estimate the capacity of the client's pelvis. (For

Measuring fundal height

To monitor fetal growth between weeks 18 and 32, the nurse practitioner, nurse-midwife, or physician uses a flexible measuring tape to determine fundal height. The examiner places the client in a supine position and stands at her right side. With one hand, the examiner finds the point on the client's abdomen where soft tissue ends and the firm, round fundal edge begins and measures from that point to the notch at the inferior edge of the symphysis pubis. The length in centimeters equals approximate gestational age in weeks. For example, a fundal height of 20 cm corresponds with a gestational age of approximately 20 weeks, give or take 2 weeks. After week 32, fundal height measurement does not correlate as well with gestational age because of fetal weight variations.

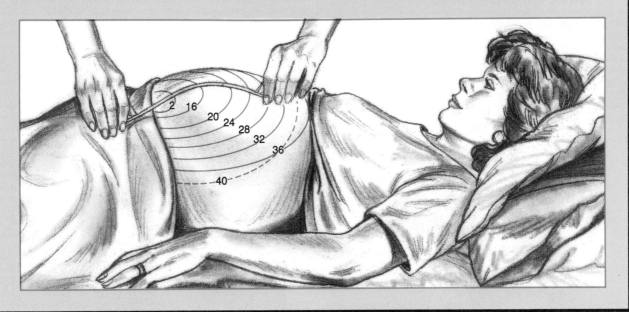

more information, see *Psychomotor skills: Taking pelvimetry measurements*, pages 434 and 435.) If possible, these measurements are taken during the first physical examination and again at 36 weeks' gestation; they indicate whether vaginal delivery will be possible.

Examine the client's breasts and internal pelvic organs only with special preparation and extreme caution, as described in Chapter 7, Women's Health Care. Because the pelvic examination is more tolerable with an empty bladder, ask the client to void before beginning the physical examination. Explain the proper technique for obtaining a clean-catch specimen, and test the client's urine to rule out glucose or protein.

Typically, a pregnant client undergoes a pelvic examination during the initial assessment and at least once during the final 4 weeks of pregnancy. Late in the pregnancy, the cervix will be soft and cervical dilation may have begun.

Fetal status

Document the client's first report of quickening (fetal movement), which usually occurs between weeks 16 and 20. At each subsequent visit, question the client about the fetus's activity level. If she reports that the fetus is less active, notify the physician immediately.

Assess fetal position using Leopold's maneuvers. (See Chapter 27, The First Stage of Labor, for instructions.) Fetal position may vary during pregnancy but, after week 36, it should remain unchanged until delivery.

Assess fetal heart tones, which can be heard with a Doppler device as early as week 10 and with an ordinary fetoscope as early as week 20. In the case of twins or an obese client, detection may be delayed. Early in the pregnancy, listen for fetal heart tones at the midline just above the client's symphysis pubis. Later in pregnancy, they can be heard most clearly through the fetus's back. (See Chapter 27 for a description of fetal heart auscultation.)

If suspected abnormalities arise, the nurse-midwife or physician may prescribe special tests to evaluate fetal

(Text continues on page 436.)

Taking pelvimetry measurements

Because of the advanced techniques required, pelvimetry measurements are performed by a nurse practitioner, nurse-midwife, or physician. The examiner asks the client to void before this procedure and explains that she may feel some discomfort. To determine pelvic capacity, the examiner estimates the subpubic arch, intertuberous diameter, interspinous diameter, and diagonal conjugate, as described below.

Pelvic outlet measurements

To palpate the subpubic arch—the inferior margin of the symphysis pubis—and to estimate its angle, the examiner turns both hands horizontally and places the thumbs in the arch, as shown on the left. Both thumbs should fit comfortably, forming an angle slightly more than 90 degrees. A narrower subpubic angle may cause dystocia.

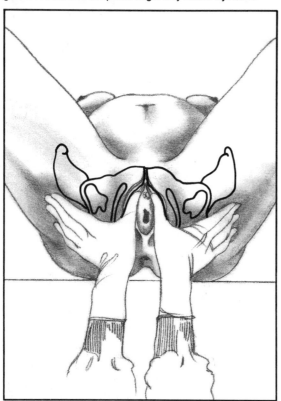

To estimate the intertuberous, or transverse, diameter, the examiner inserts a premeasured, clenched fist between the ischial tuberosities, as shown on the right. If the knuckles are a width of 8 cm or more and fit comfortably, the diameter is adequate. A Thom's pelvimeter can be used to take this measurement.

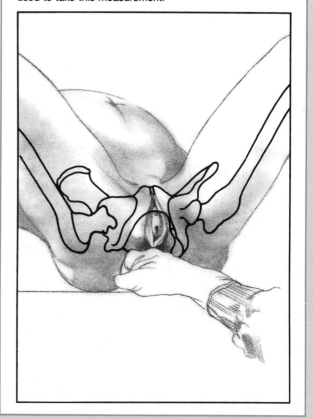

Midpelvis measurement

The interspinous diameter cannot be measured directly, but the examiner can estimate midpelvic capacity by inserting the examining finger or fingers into the vagina and palpating the ischial spines (which should be blunt), the side walls of the pelvis above and below the ischial spines (which should be straight and parallel), the sacrospinous ligament (which should be 2.5 to 3 fingerbreadths long), and the sacrum from below upward (which should be concave and hollow; only the last three sacral vertebrae can be felt without indenting the perineum). Finally, the examiner gently palpates the coccyx. It should move easily.

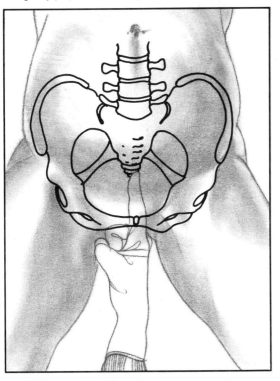

Pelvic inlet measurement

To estimate the diagonal conjugate, the examiner inserts two fingers into the client's vagina and attempts to reach the sacral promontory by indenting the perineum with the knuckles of the third and fourth fingers and then walking the fingers up the sacrum to the promontory. If successful, the examiner maintains contact with the promontory while raising the hand until it touches the lower margin of the symphysis pubis. With the other hand, the examiner marks this point as shown in the illustration. The examiner withdraws the hand from the vagina and measures the distance from the tip of the finger to the marked point. The measurement should be 11.5 cm or more. If the promontory is not reachable, the diameter is adequate. To obtain the obstetric conjugate, usually 10 cm, 1.5 cm is subtracted from the measurement of the diagonal conjugate.

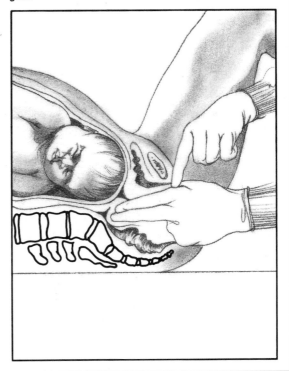

well-being. The Non-stress test and contraction stress test evaluate the oxygen transfer function of the placenta, predicting possible intrauterine asphyxia in high-risk pregnancies. Other tests of fetal well-being include amniocentesis, chorionic villus sampling, fetoscopy, fetal echocardiography and blood flow studies, percutaneous umbilical blood sampling, alpha-fetoprotein screening, computed tomographic scanning, and magnetic resonance imaging. (See Chapter 22, High-Risk Antepartal Clients, for more information.)

Diagnostic studies

Diagnostic tests that reflect the client's history and physical findings may include blood type and ABO group, complete blood count, rapid plasma reagent (RPR) test, sickle cell test, rubella test, urinalysis, cultures for sexually transmitted diseases, Papanicolaou (Pap) test, and others. (See Chapter 27, The First Stage of Labor, for a chart showing common laboratory studies.)

The nurse practitioner, nurse-midwife, or physician may decide the client will benefit from ultrasonography, which displays a two-dimensional echo image of the fetus and surrounding tissues. Ultrasound examination may be performed to:
• estimate delivery date
• evaluate fetal growth and condition
• investigate the possibility of ectopic pregnancy, hydatidiform mole, and other anomalies of pregnancy
• determine fetal presentation
• estimate fetal weight.

NURSING DIAGNOSES

Antepartal period

The following nursing diagnoses are examples of the problems and etiologies that the nurse may encounter when caring for a client in the antepartal period. Specific nursing interventions for many of these diagnoses are provided in the "Planning and implementation" section of this chapter.

• Altered family processes related to inclusion of an additional family member
• Altered fetal growth and development related to the effects of cigarette smoking
• Altered nutrition: less than body requirements, related to nausea and vomiting
• Altered patterns of urinary elimination related to compression of the urinary bladder
• Altered sexuality patterns related to fear of harming the fetus during intercourse
• Body image disturbance related to the discomforts of pregnancy
• Body image disturbance related to weight gain during pregnancy
• Constipation related to decreased peristalsis
• Impaired adjustment related to changes in body structure
• Knowledge deficit related to care measures required for optimal pregnancy outcome
• Potential for injury related to the effect of shifting center of gravity on exercise routine
• Sleep pattern disturbance related to increased fatigue

Nursing diagnosis

After completing the health history and physical assessment, the nurse analyzes the data and formulates appropriate nursing diagnoses. (For a partial list of nursing diagnoses applicable to healthy antepartal clients, see *Nursing diagnoses: Antepartal period.*) As much as possible, involve the client in determining appropriate diagnoses, which will increase their usefulness. Also, participation creates a sense of responsibility, retains the client's freedom of choice, and fosters her problem-solving ability.

Planning and implementation

The planning phase of the nursing process begins after nursing diagnoses are made. Together, the nurse, other members of the health care team, and the client set goals and work out ways to implement the plan of care to meet those goals. During the normal antepartal period, nursing goals typically include comfort promotion for the client, family adaptation to the addition of a new member, promoting maternal and fetal well-being, and relieving discomfort caused by the physiologic changes associated with pregnancy. (See *Applying the nursing process: Client with a knowledge deficit related to body changes typical of a first pregnancy*, pages 446 and 447, for a case study that shows how to apply the nursing process when caring for a pregnant client.)

Encourage family adaptation

Depending on experiences and coping abilities, family relationships may be strengthened or weakened by pregnancy, resulting in a nursing dagnosis of *altered family processes related to inclusion of an additional family member*. Family members may require confirmation that change is healthy or that interventions may be needed to maintain a sense of balance in the family. The nurse intervenes to help the family deal with the crises by being supportive and by providing necessary education for childbirth and parenting.

Partner

Ideally, the client's partner is her major source of support. Involve the partner in the plan of care, paying particular attention to his psychosocial adaptation to the pregnancy. Problems, if any, should be identified and discussed as they arise. The partner learns to adjust to the physical and psychological changes pregnancy imposes on the client as well as the impact these changes have on their daily interaction and sexual relationship.

Even if the client's partner welcomes the pregnancy, he may not wish to participate actively in labor and birth. This preference may stem from cultural traditions, personal feelings, or various other reasons. Respect the partner's wishes and help the client to accept them or to reach compromises.

Siblings

With the arrival of the neonate, each child's family position changes and new relationships develop. During the second trimester, when pregnancy becomes obvious, explore siblings' feelings about the forthcoming birth and encourage the couple to communicate openly with their children.

Sibling reactions vary, possibly including curiosity about babies and sex. This may provide a convenient opportunity for parents to discuss sexuality and reproduction with their children. Provide assistance and educational materials as appropriate. Siblings also may exhibit regressive behavior, acting out feelings of anger or frustration. Encourage parents to support and reassure children rather than punish them.

Some siblings may benefit from accompanying the client for antepartal visits, where they can listen to fetal heart tones and take part in activities that surround pregnancy. Some clients encourage their children to participate in labor and birth. If their inclusion is planned, arrange for them to attend prenatal classes designed specifically for children. Inform the couple that, even after attending preparatory classes, children may display unusual behaviors for a time after the birth of another child and require special understanding and attention from parents.

Grandparents

Although becoming grandparents typically produces positive feelings, it also may remind grandparents of their advancing age. Grandparents who adapt well to the pregnancy can be a source of emotional support for the couple and their children.

Minimize antepartal risks

The nurse has the opportunity and responsibility to teach the client and her family about potential risks during the antepartal period and care required to promote maternal and fetal well-being. In addition, without alarming the client, the nurse should urge her to report promptly any signs that could indicate danger to herself or the fetus. (See *Danger signs during pregnancy* for a list of such signs.)

Nutrition

Early in pregnancy, the client may have a nursing diagnosis of *altered nutrition: less than body requirements, related to nausea and vomiting.* Because pregnancy depletes nutrient stores, urge the client to maintain adequate intake of essential nutrients during pregnancy. Insufficient nutrition will not provide adequate nutrients to the fetus for growth and development, and may result in IUGR or other nutrition-related problems. (See Chapter 20, Nutrition and Diet Counseling, for in-depth discussion of this topic.)

Danger signs during pregnancy

The nurse should advise the pregnant client to report immediately any of the following signs and symptoms:
- Fever above 101° F (38.3° C)
- Severe headache
- Dizziness, blurred or double vision, spots before the eyes
- Abdominal pain or cramps
- Epigastric pain
- Repeated vomiting
- Absence of or marked decrease in fetal movement
- Vaginal spotting or bleeding (brown or red)
- Rush or constant leakage of fluid from the vagina
- Painful urination or decreased urine output
- Edema of the extremities and face
- Muscle cramps or convulsions

Exercise

A client should not start an exercise regimen during pregnancy. However, a client who exercises regularly may continue if she modifies her regimen to prevent a nursing diagnosis of *potential for injury related to the effect of shifting center of gravity on exercise routine.* Recommend the following guidelines:

• Warm up and stretch to help prepare the joints for activity.

• Exercise for shorter intervals. By exercising for 10 to 15 minutes, resting briefly, and then exercising for another 10 to 15 minutes, the client will decrease the risk of problems associated with shunting blood to the musculoskeletal system and away from the uterus and other vital organs.

• As pregnancy progresses, decrease the intensity of the exercise. This helps compensate for decreased cardiac reserve, increased respiratory effort, and increased weight during pregnancy.

• Avoid prolonged overheating. Strenuous exercise, especially in a humid environment, can raise the core body temperature. Especially in the first trimester, hyperthermia may increase the risk of teratogenesis. The client also should avoid hot tubs and saunas.

• Avoid high-risk activities that require balance and coordination, such as skydiving, mountain climbing, racquetball, and surfing. As pregnancy progresses, the client's changing center of gravity and softened joints may decrease balance and coordination.

• After exercise, cool down with a period of mild activity to help restore circulation and avoid pooling of blood.

• After cooling down, lie on the left side for 10 minutes to improve venous return from the extremities and promote placental perfusion.

• Wear appropriate sports shoes and a support bra.

• Stop exercising and contact the health care practitioner if any of the following occur: dizziness, shortness of breath, tingling, numbness, vaginal bleeding, or abdominal pain.

Substance abuse

Evidence continues to demonstrate that substance abuse represents great risk to the fetus, resulting in a nursing diagnosis of *altered growth and development related to the effects of cigarette smoking.* Encourage the client to stop smoking and avoid alcohol for the duration of pregnancy. Even a reduction in the number of cigarettes smoked daily may improve fetal condition (Naeye, 1981).

Caution the client against indiscriminate use of over-the-counter medications, especially during the first trimester. Inform her about the effect of illicit drugs on the developing fetus, and obtain professional counseling for an addicted client or habitual user.

Travel

Most pregnant clients can travel without undue risk to the fetus. However, the risk of accident increases with the amount of traveling. Recommend certain precautions:

• In moving vehicles, wear shoulder and lap belts to reduce injury in case of an accident.

• Do not remain seated for longer than 2 hours. Walk around for approximately 10 minutes to restore circulation.

• Airlines may require a note from a nurse-midwife or physician for customers in later stages of pregnancy. Also, carry a copy of recent medical records in case of emergency.

• As term approaches, determine the availability of medical care at the destination.

Occupation

The client may work throughout pregnancy, provided she faces no environmental hazards, has adequate rest periods, does not engage in hazardous physical activity (such as lifting heavy objects), and feels well.

During the last few weeks, she should avoid standing or sitting for long periods. Recommend that she elevate her legs whenever possible to relieve backache, improve venous return, and reduce edema in her legs. Suggest that she lie on her left side during work breaks, if possible, to enhance placental circulation.

Facilitate client adaptation

Especially during the second trimester when the fetus grows rapidly, the client may have difficulty adjusting to her changing body, resulting in nursing diagnoses of *impaired adjustment related to changes in body structure* or *body image disturbance related to weight gain during pregnancy.* Also, she may fear that her partner no longer finds her attractive.

Encourage the client to express her concerns and feelings about the fetus, changes in her body, and the pregnancy itself. Notice the tone and words the client uses to describe her body and the fetus. Determine how often the client interacts with the fetus; talking to the fetus, using a pet name, and similar behaviors indicate maternal-fetal bonding. (See *Nursing research applied: A comparison of maternal-fetal bonding in normal and high-risk pregnancies* for related information.) Take time to explore behaviors and feelings with the client and her partner. Find out if the client's partner relates to her differently than before, and encourage open communication between them to resolve the client's fears.

NURSING RESEARCH APPLIED

A comparison of maternal-fetal bonding in normal and high-risk pregnancies

This study sought to identify variables affecting maternal bonding in two types of pregnancy. The researchers defined maternal-fetal bonding as the extent to which the woman engaged in affiliation and interactive behaviors with the fetus, such as talking to the fetus, calling the fetus by a pet name, and maneuvering the fetus so that her partner could observe movement.

To investigate differences in bonding behavior, Kemp and Page (1987) conducted a study of 53 women with normal pregnancies and 32 women with high-risk pregnancies. The clients completed a prenatal bonding tool and a questionnaire that focused on the third trimester.

The researchers found no significant correlations in the scores of the normal and high-risk clients. Further, they found no significant correlations between bonding scores and education, age, race, unplanned pregnancy, whether the woman had a sonogram, or number of previous pregnancies.

Application to practice
The findings of this small study support the belief that maternal-fetal bonding occurs independent of risk level or demographic profile. Because it directly influences infant health and well-being, the nurse should assess all pregnant clients for development of bonding behaviors.

Some researchers have suggested that high-risk clients fear and resist bonding. This study disagreed with that hypothesis, possibly because high-risk clients who reached the third trimester may have become more hopeful of a positive outcome. A similar study should be carried out with clients in their first and second trimesters to address this issue.

Kemp, V.H., and Page, C.K. (1987). Maternal prenatal attachment in normal and high-risk pregnancies. *JOGNN,* 16(3), 179-183.

Minimize discomforts

Discomforts of pregnancy can cause varying amounts of distress for the client and her family, possibly resulting in a nursing diagnosis of *body image disturbance related to the discomforts of pregnancy.* These discomforts vary with the stage of pregnancy and the size of the uterus. How women respond to and feel about the changes and discomforts vary greatly. (See Chapter 17, Physiologic Changes during Normal Pregnancy, for a detailed discussion of these changes.)

Discuss the client's comfort level at each antepartal visit and recommend appropriate interventions if she reports problems. (See *Client teaching: Minimizing the discomforts of pregnancy,* pages 440 and 441, for specific interventions.)

Provide education

The nurse instructs the pregnant client on antepartal care measures in an effort to enhance client and fetal well-being. Although primigravid clients typically need more education, both primigravid and multigravid clients may have a nursing diagnosis of *knowledge deficit related to care measures required for optimal pregnancy outcome.* Education topics should include rest, breast care, clothing, personal hygiene, childbirth exercises, fetal activity monitoring, childbirth and parenting, and sexual activity.

Rest
Adequate rest during pregnancy is important for both physical and emotional health. Women need more sleep when pregnant, especially in the first and third trimesters when they may tire easily. Resilience and resistance to illness depend on adequate rest.

Sleeping becomes more difficult during the third trimester because of the enlarged abdomen, increased urinary frequency, and greater fetal activity. Finding a comfortable position becomes difficult. Encourage the client to try a left lateral position, which reduces uterine pressure on the other organs. Also, teach the client appropriate relaxation techniques to help prepare her for sleep. (See *Client teaching: Rest positions during pregnancy,* pages 442 and 443, for examples that encourage comfort.)

Breast care
Teach the importance of proper breast support to promote comfort, retain breast shape, and prevent back strain. This is especially important for the client with large breasts. Recommend that she wear a well-fitting support bra that has the following characteristics:
• wide straps that do not stretch (elastic straps lose their tautness quickly from the weight of the breasts and frequent washing).
• cups that hold all breast tissue comfortably.
• tucks or other devices that allow expansion, thus accommodating the enlarging chest circumference.
• a shape that holds the nipple line approximately midway between the elbow and shoulder. The back of the bra should not be pulled up by the weight of the breasts.

Emphasize the importance of cleanliness, especially as the client begins producing colostrum. Recommend that she use warm water to remove colostrum that crusts on the nipples. The client who plans to breast-feed should avoid using soap on her nipples because of its drying effect.

For the client who plans to breast-feed, teach nipple preparation techniques, which reduce soreness by distributing natural lubricants produced by Montgomery's

CLIENT TEACHING

Minimizing the discomforts of pregnancy

You may find that you suffer from different discomforts as your pregnancy progresses. The following list provides preventive measures that may help relieve these discomforts.

DISCOMFORT	POSSIBLE RELIEF
First trimester	
Nausea and vomiting	• Avoid smelling or eating foods that trigger nausea. • If early morning nausea occurs, eat plain crackers, dry toast, or other dry carbohydrates before getting out of bed. • Keep hard candy at the bedside. • Rise slowly from a lying or sitting position to avoid nausea. • Eat a small meal every 2 to 3 hours. • Avoid fatty or highly seasoned foods. • Eat a bedtime snack high in protein, such as cheese and crackers. • If you arise at night to urinate, drink 8 oz of a sweet beverage, such as apple juice. • Wait for 30 minutes after a meal to drink beverages. • Consult your doctor if vomiting occurs more than once daily or if it continues beyond the sixteenth week.
Urinary frequency and urgency	• Restrict fluids in the evening to reduce having to urinate during the night (daily intake should not go below eight 8-oz glasses). • Void every 2 to 3 hours during the day to reduce urgency and minimize the risk of urine staying in your bladder, which can lead to infection. • Consult your doctor if signs and symptoms of urinary tract infection arise, such as pain, burning, or blood in the urine. • Perform Kegel's exercises (tightening the muscles used to control urine flow) in sets of 10 several times a day to maintain perineal tone and control over urination.
Breast tenderness or tingling	• Wear a well-fitting support bra.
Fatigue	• Rest periodically during the day. • Allow more time for sleep at night.
Increased vaginal discharge	• Clean the perineum daily. • Wear cotton-crotch underwear, which allows air circulation. • Use talcum powder to help keep skin dry. Avoid douching, which can lead to infection.

DISCOMFORT	POSSIBLE RELIEF
Nasal stuffiness or bleeding	• Use a cool-air vaporizer, especially while sleeping.
Excessive saliva production	• Use an astringent mouthwash regularly.
Second and third trimesters	
Heartburn	• Eat smaller meals at shorter intervals. • Avoid fried or spicy foods. • Avoid lying down immediately after eating. • Maintain adequate fluid intake (six to eight 8-oz glasses daily, 30 minutes after meals). • Avoid citrus juices. • Avoid sodium bicarbonate (baking soda) because it disrupts the sodium-potassium balance. • Use an antacid as recommended by your nurse or doctor.
Ankle edema and varicose veins	• Avoid sitting or standing for long periods. • Avoid garters, knee-highs, or other restrictive bands around your legs. • Avoid crossing your legs. • Wear support or elastic stockings. • Exercise regularly to promote blood flow in your legs. • Elevate your feet and legs whenever possible; support your entire leg rather than simply propping up your feet. • Lie down with your feet elevated several times daily.
Enlarged veins in the groin	• Support your perineum with two sanitary pads worn inside your underpants. • When elevating your legs, elevate your pelvis as well to avoid pooling of blood in the pelvic area.
Hemorrhoids	• Avoid straining when having a bowel movement. • Use ice packs, warm soaks, and topical ointments and anesthetics. • Eat foods high in fiber to avoid constipation. • Maintain adequate fluid intake (six to eight 8-oz glasses daily, preferably water).

CLIENT TEACHING

Minimizing the discomforts of pregnancy continued

DISCOMFORT	POSSIBLE RELIEF	DISCOMFORT	POSSIBLE RELIEF
Hemorrhoids (continued)	• Insert hemorrhoids and lie on one side with your knees drawn up for several minutes. • Consult your doctor if hemorrhoids feel hard, are painful, or if rectal bleeding (more than few spots) develops.	Leg cramps (continued)	• Use a warm towel or leg massage to relieve discomfort. • Reduce milk intake as suggested by your doctor.
Constipation	• Increase fluid intake to more than eight 8-oz glasses daily, preferably water. • Increase dietary fiber by eating more fruits and vegetables. • Eat prunes, which are a natural laxative. • Exercise daily. • Take time for regular bowel movements. • Take laxatives only as prescribed by your doctor.	Faintness	• Avoid sudden changes in position (lying to sitting, for example). • Avoid standing for long periods. • Avoid crowds. • Lie on one side rather than on your back. • When feeling faint, sit down and place your head between your knees.
		Shortness of breath	• Use proper posture when standing. • Use pillows to support your back when sitting. • Stretch your abdomen by standing with your hands over your head and deep-breathing.
Backache	• Use proper body mechanics and good posture. • Perform exercises aimed at restoring body alignment. • Use leg muscles instead of back muscles when lifting objects. • Avoid lifting heavy objects. • Recline on a bed or lounge chair to rest back muscles.	Insomnia	• Lie on your left side with pillows supporting your back, under your abdomen, and between your legs. • Have a warm, caffeine-free drink or a backrub. • Perform relaxation techniques. • Attempt to alleviate distracting discomforts, such as lower back pain.
Leg cramps	• Stretch the calf muscle by standing up, pressing your foot firmly on the ground, and straightening your knee. • While lying face down, ask someone to press down on the back of your knee and flex your foot from the ankle toward your shin.	Abdominal discomfort, Braxton Hicks contractions	• Lightly massage the abdomen with a slow, circular motion. • Apply cream or lotion for dry skin. • Apply heat to the area.

This teaching aid may be reproduced by office copier for distrubution to clients. © 1991, Springhouse Corporation.

tubercles, stimulating blood flow to the breasts, and developing the protective layer of skin over the nipples. Begin teaching the client about nipple preparation in the third trimester. Tell her to avoid rubbing the nipples because this strips their protective lubricants. Instead, teach her to grasp the nipple between thumb and forefinger and gently roll and pull it. Oral stimulation of the nipple by the client's partner during sex play is also an excellent technique for toughening the nipple in preparation for breast-feeding. The couple who enjoys this stimulation should be encouraged to continue it throughout the pregnancy. (Because nipple stimulation triggers release of oxytocin, which can cause uterine contrac-

tions, do not recommend nipple preparation techniques for clients with a history of preterm labor.)

Nipple rolling is more difficult for women with flat or inverted nipples, but it still may be useful. With a truly inverted nipple, squeezing the areola between thumb and forefinger causes the nipple to retract. The normal or flat nipple protrudes. The client with inverted nipples can increase their protractility by performing Hoffman's exercises (Hoffman, 1953) or wearing special breast shields (such as Woolrich or Eschmann shields)

(Text continues on page 444.)

Rest positions during pregnancy

Finding a comfortable resting position during pregnancy can be difficult. Try the following suggestions.

Lying on your back

This position is most comfortable early in pregnancy, before the uterus grows large enough to place pressure on your internal organs. Avoid this position later in pregnancy.

Support your head with one or more pillows if you wish, especially if you experience shortness of breath, lower back pain, or rib pressure. Place the top pillow lengthwise to support your shoulders as well as your head. Place a pillow or folded blanket under your thighs to help relieve back pressure.

(Do not place it under your knees because it may impede circulation.) Relax your legs and feet so that they roll outward slightly. Rotating one leg so that the knee points outward may help relieve back pain. Rest your hands on your thighs or on the bed and bend your elbows slightly.

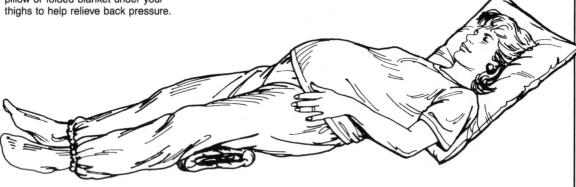

Lying on your side

The following steps describe lying on your left side, but you may lie on either side.

Support your head—but not your shoulders—with one or more pillows. (During the third trimester, place another pillow or a folded towel under your abdomen.) Rest your right arm on your hip. If your left arm becomes numb, place a rolled blanket or folded pillow lengthwise against your back and

lean gently against it, relieving some of the pressure on your arm. Flex your knees and keep them together. Place a pillow between your knees, if necessary, to help relieve back pain.

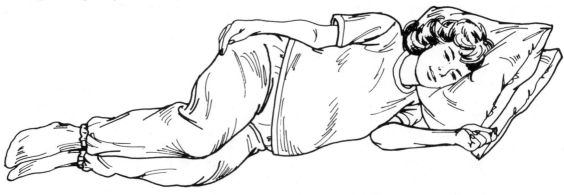

This teaching aid may be reproduced by office copier for distribution to clients. © 1991, Springhouse Corporation.

CLIENT TEACHING

Rest positions during pregnancy   continued

Lying in the supported front position

This position is similar to the side-lying position but may be more comfortable as pregnancy advances. You may lie on either side.

Place one or more pillows diagonally under your head, right breast, and right shoulder. Extend your left arm behind you and your right arm and leg in front, allowing your abdomen to be supported by the bed (place a small pillow or folded towel beneath it if necessary). If you have back or abdominal discomfort, try placing a pillow under your right leg.

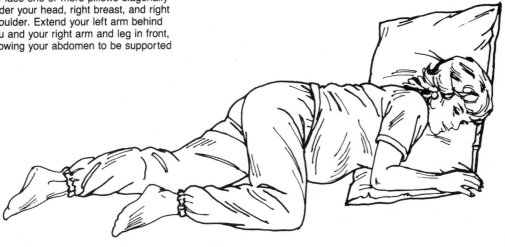

Sitting

When sitting, keep your back straight and use your leg muscles to lower yourself onto the seat. Slide back in the chair. Sit tall with your weight distributed evenly. Your back, buttocks, and shoulders should be supported by the back of the chair.

Place your feet flat on the floor or on a footstool. Let your legs relax and your knees separate naturally. Do not cross your legs, which can interfere with circulation. Let your arms rest on the chair arms or in your lap.

To rise, slide forward and lift yourself with your leg muscles, using your arms for support. Keep your back straight and avoid leaning forward.

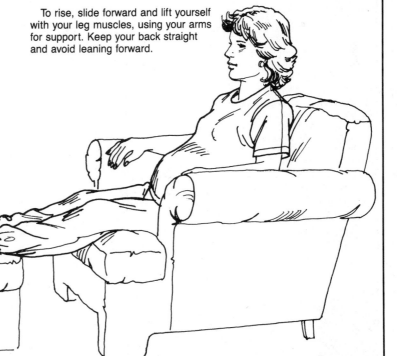

Increasing nipple protractility

A client who has inverted nipples can help them protrude by performing Hoffman's exercises or by wearing a special breast shield.

Hoffman's exercises

Teach the client to perform Hoffman's exercises by positioning her thumbs or index fingers on opposite sides of one areola, near the edge. She should then stretch the areola while pressing into the breast to help free any adhesions that could be causing the inversion. Instruct the client to repeat the exercise on the other breast.

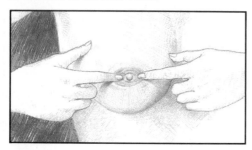

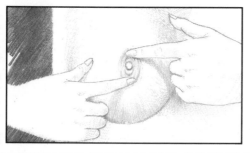

Breast shield

Breast shields, typically more successful than Hoffman's exercises, employ mild suction to draw the nipples out through a hole on the inside of each shield. Used during the third trimester and the postpartal period if necessary, breast shields should not be worn for more than a few hours at a time to minimize their drying effect.

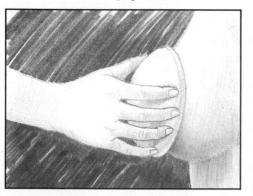

for the last 4 weeks of pregnancy. (See *Increasing nipple protractility* for an explanation of these two techniques.)

Clothing

Maternity clothes should be appealing to promote self-esteem and must be loose-fitting to allow for abdominal growth and client comfort. Instruct the client to avoid restrictive clothing, such as garters and tight waistbands, because they can impede venous circulation and encourage or aggravate varicose veins.

A maternity girdle may help a client who exercises during pregnancy or who has a pendulous abdomen that increases spinal curvature and causes backache. Advise against a girdle that has tight leg bands. Underwear should have a cotton lining to allow evaporation and absorption of increased secretions during pregnancy.

Shoes should fit properly, feel comfortable, and have a flat or low wedge heel. Instruct the client to avoid high-heeled shoes because they increase spinal curvature and aggravate backache.

Personal hygiene

The client should bathe daily to remove increased perspiration and vaginal discharge. The client with vaginal bleeding or ruptured membranes must avoid tub baths because of potential bacterial penetration. The client without such problems may shower or bathe, although she may need help getting in and out of the tub.

Remind the client that although her gums may be more tender and bleed during pregnancy, she must maintain good oral hygiene. She should have a dental examination early in pregnancy and any repairs should be done under local anesthesia only. X-rays and repairs that require systemic anesthesia should wait until after childbirth.

Childbirth exercises

Certain exercises help strengthen muscle tone in preparation for delivery and promote more rapid restoration of muscle tone after delivery. Additionally, some physical discomforts of pregnancy can be reduced considerably by faithful performance of body-conditioning exercises. (See Chapter 21, Family Preparation for Childbirth and Parenting, for more information on prenatal exercises.)

Fetal activity monitoring

Teach the client to assess her fetus's well-being by monitoring movement. Authorities differ on how many movements indicate health in the fetus. Freeman, et al. (1981) suggest that the client should notify her health care practitioner if she feels less than two movements per hour. Other suggestions include six or ten movements per hour; researchers currently are working to determine a reliable standard.

Some clinicians ask clients to use fetal movement records or a fetal activity diary. Keeping a written record of movements at particular times raises the client's awareness of her fetus's activity and her confidence that no problems exist. Further, a drop in fetal activity will be apparent immediately and signal the client to contact her health care practitioner.

Reassure the client that at times she will feel no movement. This may be because the fetus is asleep or because the client cannot feel the movements made. Ultrasound observations have revealed fetuses stretching, rolling, and moving limbs without detection by the mother. Factors that affect fetal activity include drugs, maternal hydration, cigarette smoking, glucose levels, and time of day.

Preparation for childbirth and parenting
Individual and group teaching allows couples to raise questions and seek clarification about any issue related to pregnancy, labor and delivery, the postpartal period, or parenting. Inform every couple of the nearest childbirth education classes. (See Chapter 21, Family Preparation for Childbirth and Parenting, for a detailed discussion.)

Sexual activity
The typical couple has many uncertainties about sexual intercourse during pregnancy. They may worry about harming the client or fetus or about starting labor before term. Additionally, the couple may worry about changes in their desire for each other. An applicable nursing diagnosis may be *altered sexuality patterns related to fear of harming the fetus during intercourse.*

Teach the client and her partner that during normal pregnancy they need not abstain from sexual activity (Reamy and White, 1985). If the client has vaginal bleeding, ruptured membranes, or other complications that could lead to preterm labor, the couple should consult their health care practitioner for advice.

Both partners may experience fluctuations in sexual desire. For the pregnant client, this typically stems from the normal discomforts of pregnancy. For example, nausea, fatigue, and breast tenderness may decrease desire in the first trimester. Resolution of many first trimester complaints may restore the client's interest in sex during the second trimester. In fact, increased pelvic vasocongestion may render intercourse more satisfying than before pregnancy.

Desire may decrease in the third trimester because of fatigue, dyspnea, urinary frequency, and general discomfort (Swanson, 1980). To minimize third trimester obstacles, suggest sexual positions that accommodate advanced pregnancy, such as side-by-side, female superior, or vaginal rear entry.

Tell the client that she need not worry about preterm labor being precipitated by intercourse as long as her pregnancy progresses normally (Klebanoff, Nugent, and Rhoads, 1984). During the third trimester, the client may experience longer contractions instead of the rhythmic contractions of orgasm, possibly accompanied by cramps and backache. Many women fear that these contractions could begin fetal descent.

The client's partner may experience changes in sexual desire as well, possibly related to concern over their changing relationship, his own feelings about the pregnancy, discomfort with his partner's changing body and family role, and concern about hurting the fetus. Some men have difficulty seeing their partner as both sexually attractive and a mother. Others find pregnancy arousing (Reamy and White, 1985). The nurse should help the couple communicate openly about these feelings.

Evaluation

In this step of the nursing process, the nurse evaluates whether nursing diagnoses have been resolved and goals met. Unmet goals may require modification.

Evaluation should take place at each antepartal visit. The nurse observes the client and questions her about problems identified previously. Evaluation statements should reflect actions performed or outcomes achieved for each goal. Examples of evaluation statements for the antepartal period include the following:
• Client accepts her changing body and has confidence in her partner's acceptance of it.
• Client has modified her strenuous exercise program to accommodate pregnancy.
• Client and her partner have enrolled in childbirth education classes.
• Client has joined a smoking cessation program.
• Client's weight gain and fundal height are consistent with the calculated EDD.
• Client understands which symptoms could indicate danger to her or her fetus.

Client with a knowledge deficit related to body changes typical of a first pregnancy

By using the nursing process, the nurse can help the primigravid client adjust to pregnancy with a minimum of stress. The table below shows how the nurse might use the nursing process when caring for the client described in the case history at right. The first column presents history and physical assessment data followed by a paragraph of mental notes. These notes help the nurse make important mental connections among assessment findings, aiding in development of the nursing diagnosis and planning.

The second column lists an appropriate nursing diagnosis; information in the remaining columns is based on this diagnosis. Although not part of the nursing process, a rationale appears for each intervention in the fourth column to explain how it contributes to the care plan.

ASSESSMENT	NURSING DIAGNOSIS	PLANNING
Subjective (history) data • Client reports that her last period was 3 months ago. • Client states that her breasts are sore and swollen and that she is gaining weight. • Client reports boyfriend does not want to have sex because she's getting fat. • Client admits to being fearful of the body changes that are occurring. **Objective (physical) data** • Vital signs: temperature 97.8° F, pulse 120, respirations 22, blood pressure 118/78 mm Hg. • Weight: 135 lb, up from 120 lb. • Age: 18. • Skin shows slight darkening of areolae and nipples. • Thyroid top normal size on palpation. • Fundal height just above symphysis pubis. • Pretibial edema +2 bilaterally. **Mental notes** *The client is young, frightened about body changes, has gained 15 lb, shows pretibial edema. Will need comprehensive information about pregnancy and fetal development. Also will need complete dietary assessment and follow-up. May be consuming primarily fatty, salty, fast foods typical of teenagers.*	Knowledge deficit related to body changes typical of a first pregnancy	**Goals** Before leaving the clinic, the client will: • discuss the physiologic changes that have occurred during the first trimester • explain changes expected during the second and third trimesters.

Documentation

The nurse documents all steps of the nursing process as thoroughly and objectively as possible. This allows more accurate evaluation and better communication between members of the health care team. The nurse must document the activities she performs. Therefore, documentation for the normal antepartal initial visit should include minimally:

• the client's vital signs, height, and weight
• age and occupation
• number of previous pregnancies
• danger signs encountered
• fetal activity
• relevant data about the client's other children
• allergies to medications
• psychological profile
• areas of concern
• client teaching accomplished
• date of next visit.

CASE STUDY

Sandy Tripper, age 18, is pregnant for the first time and comes to the clinic at 3 months' gestation for her first antepartal checkup. A girlfriend accompanies her.

IMPLEMENTATION		EVALUATION
Intervention Teach the client about physiologic changes that occur during the first trimester (such as breast changes, nausea and vomiting, and urinary frequency) using her experience as a model.	**Rationale** Using the client's experience will help her accept changes that have occurred as a normal part of pregnancy.	Upon evaluation, the client: • explained the changes that have occurred in her body and indicated that she felt comfortable with them • listed the changes she can expect during the second and third trimesters.
Teach the client about physiologic changes that occur during the second and third trimesters (such as weight gain, increased heart rate, shortness of breath, and Braxton Hicks contractions), using visual aids.	Helping her to anticipate impending changes may reduce her anxiety by reassuring her such changes are normal.	

The nurse-midwife or physician may perform and document EDD, LMP, and gestation in weeks; fundal height measurement; fetal heart rate (if gestation exceeds 12 weeks); date of quickening; and pelvic examination findings and collection of vaginal specimens for tests.

Some facilities have charts on which the client can document such data as weight changes, urine test results, and fetal activity during follow-up visits. The nurse should encourage client participation whenever possible.

Chapter summary

Chapter 19 outlined important aspects of nursing care during the antepartal period. Here are the chapter highlights.

• Assessment begins with the client's first antepartal visit and continues at regular intervals throughout pregnancy.

• The health history should include questions about the current pregnancy, past pregnancies, gynecologic history, medical history (including current symptoms), and family history.

• The initial physical assessment should include vital signs, weight, height, and a systematic, progressive assessment of the client's head and chest, abdomen, extremities, and pelvic area (as needed).

• Calculation of EDD is commonly performed using Nagele's rule or an obstetric calculator wheel.

• Laboratory tests performed routinely on pregnant clients include blood type and ABO group, complete blood count, Pap test, RPR test, sickle cell test, rubella test, urinalysis, and cultures for infectious diseases.

• Gestational age may be estimated between weeks 18 and 32 by measuring fundal height in centimeters or by using McDonald's rule. Either method should be augmented by the client's report of quickening and the nurse's auscultation of fetal heart tones.

• The nurse follows the nursing process to plan and implement antepartal care.

• Interventions typically focus on family preparation for a new family member, promotion of maternal and fetal well-being, and relief of common discomforts of pregnancy.

Study questions

1. What does "gravida 3 para 2012" reveal about the client to whom it applies?

2. How frequently should antepartal follow-up visits occur for the healthy client?

3. Mrs. Jones, a primigravid client age 21, reports that the first day of her last menstrual period occurred on March 18. What is her EDD?

4. When completing Mrs. Jone's antepartal history, what major components should be discussed?

5. Mrs. Jones's fundal height is 20 cm at the umbilicus. How many weeks pregnant is she?

6. Which interventions can help relieve the discomforts experienced by Mrs. Jones during the second trimester of pregnancy?

7. Which signs indicate imminent potential danger for Mrs. Jones and her fetus?

8. Devise a care plan for Mrs. Jones during her antepartal period.

Bibliography

Alexander, L.L. (1987). The pregnant smoker: Nursing implications. *JOGNN*, 16(3), 167-173.

American College of Obstetricians and Gynecologists. (1982). Immunization during pregnancy. *ACOG Technical Bulletin*, Number 64. Washington, DC: Author.

Andrews, S. (1988). Coping with the sexual health interview. *Journal of Nurse-Midwifery*, 33(6), 269-273.

Brown, M.A. (1987). How fathers and mothers perceive prenatal support. *MCN*, 12(6), 414-418.

Bush, J.J. (1986). Protocol for tuberculosis screening in pregnancy. *JOGNN*, 15(3), 225-230.

Cnattingius, S., Haglund, B., and Meirik, O. (1988). Cigarette smoking as risk factor for late fetal and early neonatal death. *British Medical Journal*, 297(6643), 258-261.

Cunningham, F., MacDonald, P., and Gant, N. (1989). *Williams obstetrics* (18th ed.). East Norwalk, CT: Appleton & Lange.

Durnin, J.V. (1987). Energy requirements of pregnancy. An integrated study in five countries: Background and methods. *Lancet* 2(8564), 895-896.

Freeman, R., Garite, R., Mondanlou, H., Dorchester, W., Rommal, C., and Devaney, M. (1981). Postdate pregnancy: Utilization of contraction stress testing for primary fetal surveillance. *American Journal of Obstetrics and Gynecology*, 140(2), 128-135.

Fried, P., Watkinson, B., and Willan, A. (1984). Marijuana use during pregnancy and decreased length of gestation. *American Journal of Obstetrics and Gynecology*, 150(1), 23-27.

Haddow, J.E. (1988). Second-trimester serum cotinine levels in nonsmokers in relation to birth weight. *American Journal of Obstetrics and Gynecology*, 159(2), 481-484.

Hellberg, D., Nilsson, S., Haley, N., Hoffman, D., and Wynder, E. (1988). Smoking and cervical intraepithelial neoplasia: Nicotine and cotinine in serum and cervical mucus in smokers and non smokers. *American Journal of Obstetrics and Gynecology*, 158(4), 910-913.

Kantrowitz, B. (1986, March 31) Changes in the workplace: Child care is now an item on the national agenda. *Newsweek*, page 57.

Kemp, V.H., and Page, C.K. (1987). Maternal prenatal attachment in normal and high-risk pregnancies. *JOGNN*, 16(3), 179-184.

Klebanoff, M., Nugent, R., and Rhoads, G. (1984). Coitus during pregnancy: Is it safe? *Lancet*, 2(8408), 914-917.

Kleinman, J.C., Pierre, M.B., Madans, J., Land, G.H., and Schramm, W.F. (1988). The effects of maternal smoking on fetal and infant mortality. *American Journal of Epidemiology*, 127(2), 274-282.

Kuhnert, B.R., Kuhnert, P.M., and Zarlingo, J.J. (1988). Associations between placental cadmium and zinc and age and parity in pregnant women who smoke. *Obstetrics and Gynecology*, 71(1), 67-70.

Kurth, A., and Hutchison, M. (1989). A context for HIV testing in pregnancy. *Journal of Nurse-Midwifery*, 34(5), 259-266.

Landry, M., and Smith, D.E. (1987). Crack: Anatomy of an addiction, Part 2. *California Nursing Review*, 9(3), 28.

Loveman, A., Colburn, V., and Dobin, A. (1986). AIDS in pregnancy. *JOGNN*, 15(2), 91-93.

Manning, F.A., Morrison, I., Lange, I.R., Harman, R., and Chamberlain, P.F. (1985). Fetal assessment based on fetal biophysical profile scoring: Experience in 12,620 referred high-risk pregnancies. *American Journal of Obstetrics and Gynecology*, 151(3), 343-350.

Merilo, K.F. (1988). Is it better the second time around? *MCN*, 13(3), 200-204.

Naeye, R. (1981). Influence of maternal cigarette smoking during pregnancy on fetal and childhood growth. *Obstetrics and Gynecology*, 57(1), 18-21.

Novak, S. (1988). In moments of crisis. *MCN*, 13(5), 349-351.

Preparation for Childbearing (4th ed.). (1972). New York: Maternity Centre Association.

Reamy, K., and White, S. (1985). Sexuality in pregnancy and the puerperium: A review. *Obstetrical and Gynecological Survey*, 40(1), 1-13.

Shepard, M.J., Hellenbrand, K.G., and Bracken, M.B. (1986). Proportional weight gain and complications of pregnancy, labor, and delivery in healthy women of normal prepregnant stature. *American Journal of Obstetrics and Gynecology*, 155(5), 947-54

Sherrod, R.A. (1988). Coping with infertility: A personal perspective turned professional. *MCN*, 13(3), 191-194.

Shiono, P., Klebanoff, M., and Rhoads, G., (1986). Smoking and drinking during pregnancy: Their effects on preterm birth. *JAMA*, 255(1), 82-84.

Smith, J. (1988). The dangers of prenatal cocaine use. *MCN*, 13(3), 174-179.

Swanson, J. (1980). The marital sexual relationship during pregnancy. *JOGNN*, 9(5), 267-270.

Wilson, D. (1988). An overview of sexually transmissable diseases in the perinatal period. *Journal of Nurse-Midwifery*, 33(3), 115-128.

Winslow, W. (1987). First pregnancy after 35: What is the experience? *MCN*, 12(2), 92-96.

Assessment

Clarke, E., Hatcher, J., McKeown-Eyssen, G.E., and Lickrish, G.M. (1985). Cervical dysplasia: Association with sexual behavior, smoking and oral contraceptive use? *American Journal of Obstetrics and Gynecology*, 151(5), 612-616.

Engstrom, J.L. (1988). Measurement of fundal height. *JOGNN*, 17(3), 172-178.

Friedrich, E.G. (1988). Current perspectives in candidal vulvovaginitis. *American Journal of Obstetrics and Gynecology*, 158(4), 985-986.

Gilson, G.J., O'Brien, M.E., Vera, R.W., Mays, M.E., Smith, D.R., and Ross, C.Y. (1988). Prolonged pregnancy and the biophysical profile. *Journal of Nurse-Midwifery*, 33(4), 171-177.

Kramer, M.S. (1987). Intrauterine growth and gestational duration determinants. *Pediatrics*, 80(4), 502-511.

Lewis, C., and Mocarski, V. (1987). Obstetric ultrasound: Application in a clinical setting. *JOGNN*, 16(1), 56-60.

Moore, L., Burns, A., Thomas, L., and Skaria, M. (1986). Self-assessment: A personalized approach to nursing during pregnancy. *JOGNN*, 15(4), 311-318.

Nichols, C. (1987). Dating pregnancy: Gathering and using a reliable data base. *Journal of Nurse-Midwifery*, 32(4), 195-204.

Wawrzyniak, M.N. (1986). The painless pelvic. *MCN*, 11(3), 178-179.

Willard, M.D., Heaberg, G.L., and Pack, J. (1986). The educational pelvic examination: Women's responses to a new approach. *JOGNN*, 15(2), 135-140.

Wilson, D. (1988). An overview of sexually transmissible diseases in the perinatal period. *Journal of Nurse-Midwifery*, 33(3), 115-128.

Wise, D., and Engstrom, J.L. (1985). The predictive validity of fundal height curves in the identification of small and large for gestational age infants. *JOGNN*, 14(2), 87-92.

Planning and implementation

Abrams, B.F., and Laros, R.K. (1986). Prepregnancy weight, weight gain and birth weight. *American Journal of Obstetrics and Gynecology*, 154(3), 503-509.

Brucker, M.C. (1988). Management of common minor discomforts in pregnancy. Part II: Managing minor pain in pregnancy. *Journal of Nurse-Midwifery*, 33(1), 25-30.

Brucker, M.C. (1988). Management of common minor discomforts in pregnancy. Part III: Managing gastrointestinal problems in pregnancy. *Journal of Nurse Midwifery*, 33(2), 67-73.

Chenger, P., and Kovacik, A. (1987). Dental hygiene during pregnancy: A review. *MCN*, 12(5), 344-343.

Davis, L. (1987). Daily fetal movement counting: A valuable assessment tool. *Journal of Nurse-Midwifery*, 32(1), 11-19.

De Grez, S.A. (1988). Bend and stretch. *MCN*, 13(5), 357-359.

Dohrmann, K.R., and Lederman, S.A. (1986). Weight gain in pregnancy. *JOGNN*, 15(6), 446-453.

Gantes, M., Schy, D.S., Bartasius, V.M., and Roberts, J. (1986). The use of daily fetal movement records in a clinical setting. *JOGNN*, 15(5), 390-393.

Hambridge, K., Krebs, N., Sibley, L., and English, J. (1987). Acute effects of iron therapy on zinc status during pregnancy. *Obstetrics and Gynecology*, 70(4), 593-596.

Honig, J.C. (1986). Preparing preschool-aged children to be siblings. *MCN*, 11(1), 37-43.

Humenick, S.S., and Bugen, L.A. (1987). Parenting roles: Expectation versus reality. *MCN*, 12(1), 36-39.

Johnson, P.A., and Gaines, S.K. (1988). Helping families to help themselves. *MCN*, 13(5), 336-339.

Maloney, R. (1985). Childbirth education classes: Expectant parents' expectations. *JOGNN*, 14(3), 245-248.

Maloni, J.A., McIndoe, J.E., and Rubenstein, G. (1987). Expectant grandparents' class. *JOGNN*, 16(1), 26-29.

Poole, C.J. (1986). Fatigue during the first trimester of pregnancy. *JOGNN*, 15(5), 375-379.

Slager-Earnest, S.E., Hoffman, S.J., and Beckmann, C.J. (1987). Effects of a specialized prenatal adolescent program on maternal and infant outcomes. *JOGNN*, 16(6), 422-429.

South-Paul, J., Rajagopal, K., and Tenholder, M. (1988). The effect of participation in a regular exercise program upon aerobic capacity during pregnancy. *Obstetrics and Gynecology,* 71(2), 175-179.

Taubenheim, A.M., and Silbernagel, T. (1988). Meeting the needs of expectant fathers. *MCN,* 13(2), 110-113.

Villar, J., Repke, J., Belizan, J., and Pareja, G. (1987). Calcium supplementation reduces blood pressure during pregnancy: Results of a randomized controlled clinical trial. *Obstetrics and Gynecology,* 70(3), 317-322.

Wallace, A.M., and Engstrom, J.L. (1987). The effects of aerobic exercise on the pregnant woman, fetus and pregnancy outcome. *Journal of Nurse-Midwifery,* 32(5), 277-290.

Nursing research

Aaronson, L.S., and MacNee, C.L. (1989). Tobacco, alcohol and caffeine use during pregnancy. *JOGNN,* 18(4), 279-87.

Brooten, D., Peters, M.A., Glatts, M., Gaffney, S.E., Knapp, M., Cohen, S., and Jordan, C. (1987). A survey of nutrition, caffeine, cigarette and alcohol intake in early pregnancy in an urban clinic population. *Journal of Nurse-Midwifery,* 32(2), 85-90.

Brown, J.E. (1988). Weight gain during pregnancy: What is optimal. *Clinical Nutrition,* 7, 181-90.

Gaffney, K.F. (1986). Maternal-fetal attachment in relation to self-concept and anxiety. *Maternal Child Nursing Journal,* 15(2), 91-101.

Gibby, N.W. (1988). Relationship between fetal movement charting and anxiety in low-risk pregnant women. *Journal of Nurse-Midwifery,* 33(4), 185-188.

Mercer, R.T., Ferketich, S.L., DeJoseph, J., May, K.A., and Sollid, D. (1988). Effect of stress on family functioning during pregnancy. *Nursing Research,* 37(5), 268-275.

Nutrition and Diet Counseling

Objectives

After reading and studying this chapter, the student should be able to:

1. Explain how physiologic changes during pregnancy affect nutritional needs.

2. Describe the effects of nutrient deficiencies or excesses on pregnancy outcome.

3. List nutritional risk factors affecting antepartal nutrition.

4. Assess nutritional status during pregnancy.

5. Set appropriate nutritional goals for the pregnant client.

6. Translate nutritional needs into food choices, taking the client's personal preferences and influences into account.

Introduction

The fetus, like every living organism, needs adequate nutrition to thrive. Encouraging the pregnant client to maintain proper nutrition during pregnancy helps ensure that the nutritional needs of the fetus are met.

Many factors influence the outcome of pregnancy, but few can be controlled as easily by the pregnant client as nutrition. Many pregnant clients want to know how to ensure the health of their fetus through proper nutrition. As a result, antepartal diet and nutrition information has increased dramatically during recent years, providing guidance for the pregnant client.

This chapter investigates how the physiologic changes of pregnancy affect the nutritional needs of the client and her fetus. It discusses the role of specific

nutrients in pregnancy as well as factors that may influence nutritional status. It then discusses how the nurse can recognize nutritional risk factors during pregnancy and provide appropriate nursing care. The chapter focuses on nutritional assessment (including history, physical assessment, and laboratory tests), goal-setting for the pregnant client, and interventions that help the client meet those goals through healthful food choices.

Nutrition and pregnancy

Nutrition before conception and during pregnancy is an important factor in the course and outcome of pregnancy.

Preconception nutrition

Such factors as degree of body fat, body weight, contraceptive method, and alcohol use can influence nutrition and pregnancy outcome.

Body fat

Fat normally contributes 26% to 28% to an adult woman's weight (Frisch, 1987). Low body-fat percentages—common in female athletes, chronic dieters, and women with anorexia nervosa—may interfere with regular menses and cause infertility. The body fat in a woman of average weight can provide approximately 144,000 calories, which can supply the additional energy

GLOSSARY

Amino acids: building blocks of protein; divided into 9 essential amino acids (those that the human body cannot make and must be provided in the diet) and 11 nonessential amino acids (those that the body can make from the essentials provided in the diet).

Anemia: blood disorder characterized by a change in red blood cells or decreased hemoglobin, which may be related to a deficiency of iron, vitamin B_{12}, or folic acid.

Calorie: measurement of heat (energy); also called kilocalorie or kcal.

Carbohydrate: energy source providing 4 calories/g; found in the diet in the form of starches, sugars, and fiber (which provides no calories).

Fat: energy source providing 9 calories/g; found in the diet in meat, dairy products, vegetable oils, and miscellaneous foods.

Gestational diabetes: type of diabetes first diagnosed during pregnancy, which may be asymptomatic except for impaired glucose tolerance test values. Also called gestational diabetes mellitus.

Lactose intolerance: condition in which an individual lacks sufficient lactase (the enzyme necessary to break down lactose, or milk sugar). Symptoms include diarrhea, abdominal cramps, and flatulence after ingesting milk or milk products.

Low birth weight: classification of neonates weighing less than 2,500 g at birth.

Megaloblastic anemia: blood condition in which immature blood cells become abnormally large, possibly because of nutrient deficiencies.

Minerals: nonorganic substances necessary for normal body functioning. Those needed in large amounts, such as calcium, phosphorus, sodium, and magnesium, are called macrominerals; those needed in small amounts, such as iron, iodine, zinc, and fluoride, are called microminerals, trace minerals, or trace elements.

Nutrient density: concentration of nutrients in relation to calories in a diet.

Pica: consumption of nonfood items.

Pregnancy-induced hypertension (PIH): group of potentially life-threatening hypertensive disorders that may develop in the second or third trimester; characterized by hypertension, extreme edema, and proteinuria; may lead to coma.

Protein: energy source, essential in various bodily functions, that provides 4 calories/g; can be complete (providing all 9 essential amino acids in the proportion needed for growth) or incomplete.

Recommended dietary allowances (RDAs): specific quantities of essential nutrients for different ages, sexes, and conditions judged adequate to maintain nutritional status of nearly all healthy people by the Food and Nutrition Board of the National Academy of Sciences.

Toxicity: quality or quantity of a substance that makes it poisonous.

Vegetarian: individual who avoids all animal products (vegan), all but eggs and milk (lacto-ovo vegetarian), all but poultry (pollo-vegetarian), or all but fish (pesco-vegetarian).

Vitamins: compounds needed in small amounts for normal body functioning. Vitamins may be fat-soluble (stored in fat) or water-soluble (incapable of being stored by the body).

---

the woman needs for pregnancy and 3 months of milk production even if she is unable to increase her nutrient intake.

Body weight

A woman should be within or near her ideal weight range before conception. (For more information on ideal weight range, see *Desirable weights for women*.) A woman weighing less than 85% of her ideal weight before pregnancy has a greatly increased risk of bearing a premature or low-birth-weight (less than 2,500 g) neonate (Van der Spuy, Steer, McCusker, Steele, and Jarvo, 1988). A woman weighing 35% above her ideal weight is at increased risk for gestational diabetes and pregnancy-induced hypertension (PIH)—conditions that can adversely affect pregnancy outcome (Frentzen, Dimperio, and Cruz, 1988).

Therefore, a woman planning a pregnancy should achieve her ideal body weight before conception. She should not attempt weight reduction during pregnancy because severely restricted food intake may cause maternal ketosis and adverse fetal effects.

Contraceptive method

Long term use of an oral contraceptive or intrauterine device (IUD) may alter a number of physiologic and metabolic processes. Oral contraceptives may interfere with the body's use of several vitamins, including riboflavin, pyridoxine, vitamin B_{12}, and folic acid. They also may decrease physiologic levels of zinc. However, most adult women maintain an adequate diet, and supplementation of these nutrients is not necessary (Tyler, 1984).

A woman using an IUD may experience increased blood loss during menstruation and therefore is more likely to develop iron-deficiency anemia (Borch-Johnsen, Meltzer, Stenberg, and Reinskov, 1990). Although iron intake can be increased through food choices, iron supplementation may be necessary.

Alcohol use

Habitual alcohol use typically leads to two nutritional problems: poor eating habits and interference with the body's use of nutrients. It also can have serious fetal consequences. Alcohol readily crosses the placenta, causing the greatest harm to the fetus during the first trimester when the major body systems are developing. Furthermore, a woman may not know that she is pregnant until several weeks after conception. Therefore, she should reduce her intake of alcohol or abstain if she is planning a pregnancy.

Habitual alcohol use during pregnancy may cause fetal alcohol syndrome, altered fetal growth that results in growth retardation, mental retardation, microcephaly, and other anomalies. (For more information on preconception considerations, see Chapter 10, Fertility and Infertility.)

Antepartal nutrition

Nutritional deprivation during pregnancy, which adversely affects pregnancy outcome and the fetus, can be avoided through nutritional supplementation. Inadequate weight gain, which frequently is used as a measure of nutrition during pregnancy, also may have adverse effects, although a recent study indicates that weight gain and nutritional adequacy are not as strongly related as previously believed (Aaronson and Macnee, 1989).

Nutritional deprivation

For obvious ethical reasons, researchers have limited to animal studies their investigations into nutritional deprivation during pregnancy. However, conclusions from animal studies must be applied with caution to human pregnancies. The human maternal-fetal relationship differs in many ways from the maternal-fetal relationship in other species. Most laboratory animals have more rapid growth and development than humans. They nourish more than one fetus, and the relative size of the fetuses may be much larger than those in human pregnancies. Also, the severe nutrient deficiencies examined in animal studies, such as a complete lack of a certain vitamin, rarely occur in human populations (Worthington-Roberts, Vermeersch, and Williams, 1989).

Data about the effects of food shortages provide some information on how nutritional deprivation affects human pregnancies. For example, World War II caused severe famines in several places, most notably in Leningrad for 6 months from 1941 to 1942. As a result, most live neonates weighed under 2,500 g (Stein, Susan, Saenger, and Marolla, 1975.) The birth rate also fell sharply, indicating decreased fertility and increased spontaneous abortions.

Desirable weights for women

The following chart shows the ideal range of body weight for women ages 25 to 59 based on height and weight. The chart assumes the client is wearing 1-inch heels and 3 pounds of indoor clothing.

HEIGHT		FRAME SIZE		
Feet	Inches	Small	Medium	Large
4	10	102-111	109-121	118-131
4	11	103-113	111-123	120-134
5	0	104-115	113-126	122-137
5	1	106-118	115-129	125-140
5	2	108-121	118-132	128-143
5	3	111-124	121-135	131-147
5	4	114-127	124-138	134-151
5	5	117-130	127-141	137-155
5	6	120-133	130-144	140-159
5	7	123-136	133-147	143-163
5	8	126-139	136-150	146-167
5	9	129-142	139-153	149-170
5	10	132-145	142-156	152-173
5	11	135-148	145-159	155-176
6	0	138-151	148-162	158-179

From 1944 to 1945, the Nazi embargo caused serious food shortages in Holland. Data from a landmark study of this period showed that neonates whose mothers had insufficient food intake during the second and third trimesters were significantly underweight at birth. Where intake was insufficient only during the first trimester, birth weight was normal (Stein, Susan, Saenger, and Marolla, 1975).

Low birth weight is undesirable because it commonly is linked to congenital defects or neonatal mortality. In fact, birth weight may indicate a neonate's overall condition. The lowest rate of neonatal mortality occurs for birth weights between 4,000 and 4,499 g; mortality rates rise for those born under 2,500 g (Brown, 1989).

Prenatal nutritional deprivation may have lasting effects, depending on the stage of development at which it occurs. If malnutrition occurs during the embryonic stage (2 to 8 weeks' gestation) when differentiation of major organs and tissues takes place, irreversible damage may occur. Because organ systems develop at different times during the embryonic stage, malnutrition may cause permanent damage in one organ and not another. If malnutrition occurs when cells primarily are increasing in size (after 8 weeks' gestation), the effects may be reversible (Worthington-Roberts, Vermeersch, and Williams, 1989).

Nutritional supplementation

Improving the pregnant woman's diet by increasing food intake or by adding missing nutritional elements can improve pregnancy outcome. The effects of supplementation depend on the severity of malnutrition. The more undernourished a woman, the greater benefit increased food or added elements will have on her pregnancy outcome.

In the United States, various food programs are available to low-income families who are at high risk for malnutrition. For example, the Special Supplemental Food Program for Women, Infants, and Children (WIC) provides nutrition education as well as coupons for purchasing highly nutritious foods (such as milk, cheese, eggs, iron-fortified cereals, and fruit juices). This national program provides assistance through pregnancy, lactation, and the first 5 years of childhood. Other food programs for eligible families include food stamps obtained from public assistance programs and local food banks when food needs are immediate.

Food supplementation between pregnancies also can be beneficial. One WIC study (Caan, Horgen, Margen, King, and Jewell, 1987) showed that neonates born to women receiving extra food for 5 to 7 months between pregnancies had higher birth weights (averaging 131 g more than neonates born to women not receiving extra food). Because 80% of perinatal deaths are associated with low birth weight (Wynn and Wynn, 1988), women at risk for inadequate nutrition should continue food supplementation programs as long as they are eligible.

Weight gain during pregnancy

Experts disagree on the amount of weight a woman should gain during pregnancy. However, general recommendations exist for the amount and pattern of weight gain.

Amount of weight gain. Recommendations for weight gain should take the woman's prepregnancy weight into consideration. For a woman entering pregnancy in her ideal weight range, a gain of 24 to 32 lb (11 to 15 kg) is adequate to meet the needs of the mother and fetus. The weight gain is caused by the weight of the fetus and placenta as well as increased adipose tissue, amniotic fluid, blood volume in the uterus, and fat and duct proliferation in the breasts.

Underweight women (less than 90% of ideal body weight) who gain the same amount of weight as ideal-weight women bear neonates at a younger gestational age and of lower birth weight and length. Ideally, an underweight woman should gain the recommended 24 to 32 lb plus the amount that she is underweight, or at least 15 kg (Seidman, Ever-Hadani, and Gale, 1989).

Controversy exists over the amount of gain appropriate for an overweight woman. Although weight gain exceeding the recommended amount is unlikely to harm the fetus, it does place more stress on the woman during delivery. Also, excessive gains may make the previously ideal-weight woman more prone to obesity after delivery. A recent study of body-weight changes between pregnancies found that 52% of those studied were significantly heavier in their second pregnancy than in the first, suggesting the need for exercise, attention to eating habits, and regular weight checks during the antepartal and postpartal periods (Samra, Tang, and Obhrai, 1988).

Recommendations for an overweight woman may range from no gain to a 30-lb gain. However, the most common recommendations for an overweight woman are 16 to 24 lb (7 to 11 kg). Neonatal birth weight increases with maternal weight gain even in overweight women, but the percentage of neonatal gain is not proportional (Seidman, Ever-Hadaini, and Gale, 1989).

Weight gains no greater than 16% to 25% of prepregnant weight are associated with fewer complications during pregnancy, labor, and delivery (Shephard, Hellenbrand, and Bracken, 1986). If weight gain is calculated as a percentage of prepregnancy weight, more individual recommendations can be made. For example, a 120-lb (55-kg) woman, at ideal weight for height, may be advised to gain 19 to 30 lb (9 to 14 kg), whereas a 140-lb (64-kg) woman, at ideal weight for height, would be advised to gain 22 to 35 lb (10 to 16 kg). The usual recommended gain is 20% of prepregnant weight.

An adolescent may need additional weight gain, depending on her stage of growth and development. During the first year after menarche, a nonpregnant adolescent normally gains approximately 8 lb (4 kg). This gain decreases each year; for example, 4 years after menarche, a weight gain of only 1½ lb (0.7 kg) is normal. These nonpregnant growth gains must be added to the expected weight gain of pregnancy. Adjustments also are necessary if an adolescent is underweight or obese (American Dietetic Association, 1989).

A woman carrying more than one fetus has higher nutrient needs and therefore should gain more weight. The optimal weight gain for a twin pregnancy is about 44 lb (20 kg) for a woman with an ideal prepregnant weight (Pederson, Worthington-Roberts, and Hickok, 1989).

Pattern of weight gain. During the first trimester of pregnancy, a woman normally should gain 3 to 5 lb (1 to 2 kg). Because of nausea and vomiting, however, she may gain no weight during this time. This does not harm the fetus; the weight gain during the first trimester goes largely to maternal changes, such as the growing uterus and breasts and increased blood volume.

During the second and third trimesters, weight gain is essentially linear, averaging 1 lb (0.5 kg) per week. For a woman with more than one fetus, the pattern of weight gain should parallel that for a single fetus until approximately 20 weeks. During the second half of the pregnancy, weight gain should average 1½ lb (0.7 kg) per week (Pederson, Worthington-Roberts, and Hickok, 1989).

Nutrient needs

During pregnancy, a woman's need for many nutrients increases the recommended dietary allowance (RDA)— the daily amount of a nutrient considered adequate for the needs of most healthy people, depending on sex, age, and reproductive status (for example, pregnant or lactating). These nutrients include carbohydrates, fats, and proteins (all energy sources) as well as water, vitamins, and minerals.

RDA standards

More than 50 nutrients are essential to human life. RDAs have been set by the Food and Nutrition Board of the National Academy of Sciences for 28 nutrients to inform the average, healthy person how much of each to consume daily. RDAs vary for different population groups and are revised periodically to reflect new nutritional knowledge. (For more information, see *RDAs for women of childbearing age*, page 456.)

Energy

Energy needs increase during pregnancy, and the caloric supply must increase to meet these needs while sparing protein for tissue building. (If calories from sources other than protein are insufficient, the body will burn proteins for energy.) A pregnant woman's energy needs increase 10% to 15%, or about 200 to 300 extra calories/day. (Additional calories may be needed for a woman who is underweight, large-framed, or unusually active). This number is derived by calculating the energy (number of calories) needed for the growth of the fetus and other tissues as well as the energy needed by the mother. The total additional energy needed during a 40-week pregnancy is 60,000 to 75,000 calories (Durnin, 1987).

Although the Food and Nutrition Board states an average increase of 300 calories/day is needed by a pregnant woman, caloric needs are not evenly distributed.

During the first trimester, a woman's needs are only slightly higher than for a nonpregnant adult woman. An increase of 150 calories/day for the first trimester and 350 calories/day for the remaining trimesters is recommended (National Research Council [NRC], 1989).

However, women may not need to follow these recommendations. A recent study of pregnant women from five countries showed that they did not increase their caloric intake significantly during pregnancy (Durnin, 1987). This study may indicate that the pregnant body uses energy more efficiently or that a pregnant woman reduces her activity level. Although more research in this area is necessary, health professionals should advise pregnant clients to eat a balanced diet according to appetite, making adjustments to promote proper weight gain.

Carbohydrates. The human body primarily uses blood glucose for fuel; because little transformation is required to turn carbohydrates into glucose, carbohydrates are the preferred energy source. Composed of carbon, hydrogen, and oxygen, carbohydrates are found in the diet as starches, sugars, and fiber. All carbohydrates, except fiber, provide 4 calories/g.

Despite the general public's impression that starches and sugars are fattening and unhealthy, both are necessary for a balanced diet. Nutrition experts recommend that 55% to 60% of dietary calories come from carbohydrates. This recommendation holds true during pregnancy.

Of the four food groups (milk, meat, grain, and fruits and vegetables), only the meat group is not a significant carbohydrate source. Carbohydrates in dairy products and fruits are mostly simple sugars in the form of lactose in milk and fructose in fruit. These simple carbohydrates are absorbed rapidly into the bloodstream because they require little or no breakdown. The grain group primarily supplies complex carbohydrates (starches). Made of several simple carbohydrates, complex carbohydrates are absorbed into the bloodstream over several hours, providing a steady source of energy. Vegetables contain simple and complex carbohydrates.

Grains, fruits, and vegetables are sources of fiber, the only carbohydrate that is not a calorie source. Recently, researchers have shown that fiber helps prevent colon cancer, control blood sugar levels, reduce blood cholesterol levels, and prevent constipation (Cooper, 1988).

Two types of fiber exist: soluble and insoluble. The soluble type, found in oats, beans, vegetables, and some fruits, is most effective at reducing cholesterol and controlling blood sugar levels. Insoluble fiber absorbs fluid as it passes through the intestine. Found in whole grain products, vegetables, and some fruits, it is noted more

RDAs for women of childbearing age

This table indicates the recommended dietary allowances of nutrients for healthy women in various U.S. age groups as well as for pregnant and lactating women. The amounts should represent average daily intake from a mixed diet.

NUTRIENT	AGE			PREGNANCY	LACTATING	
	15-18	19-24	25-50		1-6 MO.	7-12 MO.
Protein (g)	44	46	50	60	65	62
Vitamin A (mg)[1]	800	800	800	800	1,300	1,200
Vitamin D (mcg)[2]	10	10	5	10	10	10
Vitamin E (mcg α-TE)[3]	12	12	12	15	18	16
Vitamin K (mcg)	55	60	65	65	65	65
Cyanocobalamin (mcg)	2.0	2.0	2.0	2.2	2.6	2.6
Folic acid (mcg)	180	180	180	400	280	260
Niacin (mcg NE)[4]	15	15	15	17	20	20
Pyridoxine (mg)	1.5	1.6	1.6	2.2	2.1	2.1
Riboflavin (mg)	1.3	1.3	1.3	1.6	1.8	1.7
Thiamine (mg)	1.1	1.1	1.1	1.5	1.6	1.6
Vitamin C (mg)	60	60	60	70	95	90
Calcium (mg)	1,200	1,200	800	1,200	1,200	1,200
Phosphorus (mg)	1,200	1,200	800	1,200	1,200	1,200
Iodine (mcg)	150	150	150	175	200	200
Iron (mg)	15	15	15	30	15	15
Magnesium (mg)	300	280	280	320	355	340
Selenium (mcg)	50	55	55	65	75	75

[1]Retinol equivalents. 1 retinol equivalent = 1 mcg retinol or 6 mcg β-carotene.
[2]As cholecalciferol. 10 mcg cholecalciferol = 400 IU of vitamin D.
[3]α-Tocopherol equivalents. 1 mg d-α tocopherol = 1 α-TE.
[4]1 NE (niacin equivalent) is equal to 1 mg of niacin or 60 mg of dietary tryptophan.

Recommended Dietary Allowances, 10th ed., © 1989, by the National Academy of Sciences, National Academy Press, Washington, DC.

for its role in preventing colon cancer and reducing constipation by adding bulk to the stool, decreasing transit time.

Fats. Composed of carbon, hydrogen, and oxygen, fats are a more concentrated source of calories than carbohydrates, providing 9 calories/g. They are provided mostly through the meat and dairy food groups, although grain products also contain a small amount of fat. Fats often are found as a major ingredient in baked foods, such as cakes and cookies, and in candy. They also provide most of the calories in snack chips, salad dress-

ings, butter, margarine, and oils. Although a small amount of fat (providing 30% or less of total daily calories) is needed, this amount usually can be obtained in normal portions of meat, dairy, and grain products. Therefore, no extra fat is necessary during pregnancy.

Several types of fat exist. Saturated fats (primarily animal fat) raise blood cholesterol levels, which in turn contribute to heart disease. Saturated fat intake should be limited to no more than 10% of the total daily calories. Although such animal products as meats and dairy foods contribute the most saturated fat to a typical diet, some plant products, such as coconut and palm oils (so-called tropical oils), also are high in saturated fats.

Unsaturated fats (primarily plant sources of fat) include polyunsaturated and monounsaturated fats. Found in such foods as nuts and vegetable oils, polyunsaturated and monounsaturated fats can lower blood cholesterol. However, even these fats should be used in small amounts, providing no more than 20% of the total daily calories.

Although cholesterol is not a fat, it commonly is found in foods that are high in saturated fats—that is, in animal products. High-cholesterol foods include egg yolks and organ meats. Cholesterol levels rise during pregnancy, but researchers do not know whether this increase is caused by hormonal changes or dietary increases in saturated fat–containing products, such as milk and meats. Nutrition experts recommend a diet containing less than 300 mg of cholesterol daily for all people, including pregnant women.

Protein. This third source of energy supplies 4 calories/g. Protein is the only energy source for which an RDA exists. It is essential for tissue growth and maintenance, formation of essential body compounds (such as hormones and digestive enzymes), water balance regulation, nitrogen balance, antibody formation, and nutrient transport.

Proteins are complex molecules made of amino acids. Twenty amino acids exist, 9 of them essential (they cannot be synthesized by the human body and must come from an outside source) and 11 nonessential (they can be synthesized from essential amino acids by the body). All amino acids contain nitrogen, carbon, and hydrogen. They may contain other elements as well, but nitrogen distinguishes protein from fats and carbohydrates.

Depending on the combination of amino acids, a protein is complete or incomplete. A complete protein contains all 9 essential amino acids in the proportion needed for growth; an incomplete protein does not. With the exception of gelatin, all animal proteins (including milk, meat, fish, and poultry) are complete. Most plant proteins (such as grains, legumes, and some vegetables) lack one or more essential amino acids in the proportion needed for growth. An incomplete protein can be made into a complete protein by the body if it is eaten with a protein that contains the missing amino acids.

The RDA for protein increases from 50 g for a nonpregnant woman to 60 g for a pregnant woman. Although this increase is significant, the average American woman consumes more than 60 g of protein even when not pregnant. Therefore, many women will not need to increase protein intake further during pregnancy.

Because low-protein diets typically are low in total calories as well, the effects of protein deficiency are difficult to separate from those of caloric deficiency. Energy is the body's first priority. If energy needs are not met through carbohydrate and fat intake, the body will metabolize protein for energy, making it unavailable for other protein functions. Although estimates vary, a pregnant woman should consume 30 to 35 calories/kg of body weight (24 calories/kg if overweight) daily for optimal protein use.

Water

Another component essential for human life, water is an important part of the pregnant woman's diet. It is the major component of the fetus, placenta, breasts, and blood.

The human body typically contains 50% to 75% water. Water needs vary according to age, body weight, climate, and activity, but necessary intake is roughly 1 liter of water for each 1,000 calories consumed (NRC, 1989). Beverages provide about two-thirds of water intake; the remaining third comes from solid foods.

Vitamins and minerals

Vitamins are compounds that are needed in small amounts by the body for normal functioning; many serve as coenzymes in cellular reactions. They can be divided into two groups, fat-soluble and water-soluble. (For more information on the functions of vitamins and minerals and the effects of deficiencies or excesses, see *Vitamins and minerals,* pages 458 to 463.)

The fat-soluble vitamins—A, D, E, and K—are stored in body fat and usually are found in fat-containing products. However, water-soluble forms of these vitamins have been developed; therefore, they may be added to low-fat or nonfat foods, such as skim milk. Because fat-soluble vitamins can be stored in the body, toxicity is a greater risk with them than with water-soluble vitamins.

Water-soluble vitamins cannot be stored by the body and must be provided daily by the diet. They include the B vitamins and vitamin C. Folic acid (folacin) intake particularly is critical during pregnancy; the RDA for this B vitamin more than doubles, whereas the RDA for other B vitamins and vitamin C increases only slightly.

Minerals are nonorganic substances necessary for normal body functioning; they help maintain acid-base and water balance, act as catalysts in cellular reactions, transmit nerve impulses, and contribute to body structures. Minerals are divided into two categories: Those needed in high amounts (such as calcium, phosphorus, sodium, and magnesium) are called macrominerals; those needed in smaller amounts (such as iron, iodine,

(Text continues on page 464.)

Vitamins and minerals

Vitamins and minerals, which are essential for various body functions, can be found in various foods and in commercial preparations. The nurse should be familiar with the possible effects of deficiencies and excesses of each of these vitamins and minerals.

FUNCTION AND SOURCE	POSSIBLE EFFECTS	NURSING CONSIDERATIONS
Vitamin A		
Normal functions • Development of bones and teeth • Adequate night vision • Maintenance of healthy skin and membranes *Food sources* Liver, egg yolks, dairy products, fruits, and vegetables	*Deficiency* Prevention of conception; poor vision; eye defects in neonate (with severe deficiency) *Excess* Multiple birth defects from vitamin A toxicity caused by an intake greater than 25,000 IU/day during early pregnancy (American College of Obstetricians and Gynecologists, 1987)	• Advise the client that the recommended dietary allowance (RDA) for vitamin A does not increase during pregnancy. • Bright yellow and deep green foods typically have a higher vitamin A content than less richly colored foods. • Excessive vitamin A intake can be harmful. Prenatal vitamins should include no more than 8,000 IU of vitamin A. This amount of supplementation, plus the amount consumed with diet, is safe. • Caution a client of childbearing age to use a contraceptive method if she uses the anti-acne drug isotretinoin, a form of vitamin A, because of this drug's teratogenic potential.
Vitamin D		
Normal functions • Development of bones and teeth • Absorption and use of calcium *Food sources* Eggs, milk, butter, fish oils, and fortified foods, particularly milk	*Deficiency* Reduced availability of calcium for the client and fetus, which may affect fetal bone density and tooth enameling and lead to neonatal hypocalcemia *Excess* Hypercalcemia; hypercalciuria	• The RDA for vitamin D rises from 2.5 mcg/day to 10 mcg/day during pregnancy. • Results of a Finnish study, showing strong seasonal variation in vitamin D status, suggest that the pregnant client may need supplementation during the winter (Kuoppala, Tiumala, Parviainen, Koskinen, and Ala-Houhala, 1986). • Because of the possible effects of vitamin D excess, the client should avoid intakes of more than 25 mcg/day (1,000 IU) during pregnancy.
Vitamin E		
Normal functions • Poorly understood, but thought to act as an antioxidant in cell membranes, protecting them from destruction *Food sources* Vegetable oils, nuts, and seeds	*Deficiency* Sterility in males and decreased fertility in females (in animal studies). Although studies have shown that human reproduction is not affected by vitamin E deficiency, it is still thought of as the virility vitamin. *Excess* More research must be done before the consequences of deficiency or excess can be stated.	• The RDA for vitamin E during pregnancy is 10 IU/day, which can be obtained easily in a well-balanced diet.
Vitamin K		
Normal functions • Blood coagulation, protein biosynthesis *Food sources* Green, leafy vegetables (primary source), milk, meat, eggs, cereals, fruits, and vegetables	*Deficiency* Slower blood-clotting time *Excess* None observed	• The RDA for vitamin K during pregnancy is 65 mcg.

Vitamins and minerals continued

FUNCTION AND SOURCE	POSSIBLE EFFECTS	NURSING CONSIDERATIONS
Cyanocobalamin (Vitamin B$_{12}$)		
Normal functions • Formation of red blood cells (RBCs) • Maintenance of nerve and gastrointestinal tissue *Food sources* Animal products, especially meat and eggs	*Deficiency* Birth defects in animals; pernicious anemia *Excess* No problems from cobalamin excess reported in human pregnancies	• The RDA during pregnancy is 2.2 mcg, slightly higher than the 2 mcg recommended for nonpregnant needs. • A vegetarian who eats only fruits, vegetables, and grains may need B$_{12}$ supplementation.
Folic acid		
Normal functions • Synthesis of nucleic acid (essential for cell division) • Production of RBCs *Food sources* Wheat germ, organ meats, yeast, and mushrooms (richest sources); vegetables, especially such dark-green ones as broccoli and spinach; fruits, including oranges, bananas, berries, and melons	*Deficiency* Maternal megaloblastic anemia, in which megaloblasts (precursors to erythrocytes) develop into macrocytes (abnormally large erythrocytes) with a shorter life expectancy than normal erythrocytes. The fetal effects of folic acid deficiency are unclear; deficiency during early pregnancy may be associated with birth defects (Guthrie, 1988). *Excess* Unknown	• The RDA for folic acid during pregnancy is 400 mcg, compared with 180 mcg for nonpregnant needs. • Because folic acid deficiency during early pregnancy may be associated with birth defects, recommend a supplement containing 400 mcg of folic acid to the client attempting to conceive and advise her to continue this supplementation throughout her pregnancy (National Research Council [NRC], 1989).
Niacin		
Normal functions • Glycolysis, fatty acid metabolism, tissue respiration *Food sources* Meat, grain products	*Deficiency* Pellagra, characterized by dermatitis, diarrhea, and mucous membrane inflammation *Excess* Nicotinic acid ingestion (3 to 9 g) may cause flushing, increased use of muscle glycogen stores, decreased serum lipids, and decreased mobilization of fatty acids from adipose tissue during exercise	• Advise the client that the RDA increases from 15 mcg to 17 mcg during pregnancy.
Pyridoxine (Vitamin B$_6$)		
Normal functions • Production of RBCs and antibodies • Metabolism of protein *Food sources* Beef, ham, fish, egg yolks, spinach, bananas, and enriched cereals	*Deficiency* Convulsions, dermatitis, and anemia *Excess* Prolonged large doses can cause ataxia and sensory neuropathy (NRC, 1989)	• The current RDA during pregnancy (2.2 mg) is slightly higher than for nonpregnant needs (1.6 mg). • Pyridoxine intake often is supplemented, particularly in clients who formerly used oral contraceptives. Because oral contraceptives appear to alter pyridoxine metabolism, users may have had reduced levels at the onset of pregnancy (Bender, 1987). • Although some individuals report pyridoxine alleviates nausea during pregnancy, no proof exists of any relationship between nausea and pyridoxine intake. (continued)

Vitamins and minerals continued

FUNCTION AND SOURCE	POSSIBLE EFFECTS	NURSING CONSIDERATIONS
Riboflavin (Vitamin B$_2$)		
Normal functions • Synthesis of fatty acids and amino acids • Component of several enzymes necessary for growth *Food sources* Dairy products, liver, and meats	*Deficiency* Orobuccal cavity lesions, dermatitis, scrotal and vulvar skin changes, and anemia *Excess* No clear-cut consequences of riboflavin excess have been found.	• Riboflavin needs increase in proportion to carbohydrate intake. Therefore, the RDA for riboflavin during pregnancy increases from 1.3 mg to 1.6 mg.
Thiamine (Vitamin B$_1$)		
Normal functions • Metabolism of carbohydrates • Synthesis of acetylcholine • Normal growth and appetite *Food sources* Whole grain products or enriched grain products (primary sources), pork and organ meats, and legumes	*Deficiency* Congenital beriberi *Excess* None reported	• The need for thiamine is proportional to carbohydrate intake. Because of higher caloric needs, the pregnant client has a higher carbohydrate intake; therefore, the RDA for thiamine increases from 1.1 mg to 1.5 mg.
Vitamin C (Ascorbic acid)		
Normal functions • Formation and development of connective tissue and the vascular system • Formation of collagen (intercellular glue) • Aids in iron absorption *Food sources* Fruits and vegetables, especially citrus fruits and juices, tomatoes, peppers, potatoes, broccoli, strawberries, and melons	*Deficiency* Pregnancy-induced hypertension (PIH) and premature membrane rupture (with low dietary intake and low serum levels of vitamin C) *Excess* Rebound scurvy in neonates whose mothers' intake of vitamin C during pregnancy was excessive; the neonate continues to catabolize the vitamin at an excessive rate even after removal from the high levels of circulating vitamin C in the mother's body.	• The RDA for vitamin C during pregnancy is 70 mg/day, as opposed to 60 mg/day for nonpregnant needs.
Calcium		
Normal functions • Formation of bones and teeth • Mineralization of the fetal skeleton *Food sources* Milk, cheese, yogurt (primary sources), ice cream, ice milk, pudding, sardines (with bones), salmon (with bones), beans, oysters, shrimp, tofu, collards, bok choy, kale, mustard greens, turnip greens, and molasses	*Deficiency* Possibly related to PIH *Excess* Studies have shown no adverse effects in many healthy women consuming up to 2,500 mg/day of calcium; however, constipation and kidney stones may occur with doses above this level (NRC, 1989).	• Calcium needs increase greatly during pregnancy; mineralization of the fetal skeleton requires a large amount of calcium. Although the need for extra calcium is most acute during the last trimester (when the fetal skeleton calcifies), the RDA for calcium throughout pregnancy increases 50%, to a total of 1,200 mg/day, because calcium deposited in maternal bones early in pregnancy is transferred later to the fetus. • Calcium retention increases during pregnancy because increased estrogen production enhances calcium absorption from the intestines while decreasing urinary excretion of the mineral. • Clients who do not consume dairy products may need calcium supplements. However, encourage increased intake of calcium-rich foods, which provide other essential nutrients

Vitamins and minerals continued

FUNCTION AND SOURCE	POSSIBLE EFFECTS	NURSING CONSIDERATIONS
Calcium (continued)		that calcium supplements lack. The amount prescribed varies according to the client's dairy product intake. If the client consumes no dairy products, the usual recommendation is 1,200 mg. For each cup of milk, yogurt, or equivalent amount of other dairy products that she consumes, subtract 300 mg from the 1,200 mg total. • Absorption of calcium from supplements may be poor. Encourage the client to consume a dairy product when she takes a calcium supplement; the lactose, lactic acid, and vitamin D in dairy products enhances calcium absorption. (Some supplements contain vitamin D.) The supplement should be taken between meals to avoid interfering with calcium absorption.
Phosphorus		
Normal functions • Component in many vital substances, including the cell nucleus, cytoplasm, and the crystals of calcium phosphate responsible for rigidity and strength in bones and teeth *Food sources* Calcium-rich and protein-rich foods, such as milk, eggs, and meat	*Deficiency* Deficiency unlikely, but could cause leaching of calcium from mother's bones to form the fetal skeleton *Excess* Calcium-phosphorus imbalance; because phosphorus levels are inversely proportionate to calcium levels, excessive phosphorus intake decreases calcium absorption and increases calcium excretion, thereby creating an imbalance (Guthrie, 1988).	• The RDA for phosphorus increases from 800 to 1,200 mg/day during pregnancy • Because of the effects of excess phosphorus intake, discourage excessive consumption of meat during pregnancy.
Sodium		
Normal functions • Maintenance of extracellular fluid volume • Muscle contraction and neurotransmission • Amino acid uptake from the gastrointestinal tract *Food sources* Salt; found in varied amounts in most foods, especially processed foods	*Deficiency* Deficiency unlikely *Excess* Excessive sodium intake may not be harmful because the pregnant client's body is efficient at excreting sodium; however, a client who entered pregnancy with hypertension should follow sodium restrictions prescribed by her physician.	• Although sodium has no RDA, adequate intake during pregnancy has been set by the National Research Council at 3 mEq (69 mg) in addition to the normal dietary requirement of 2.4 g daily, an amount easily obtained in a well-balanced diet. Lactation increases sodium requirements by 6 mEq (135 mg) daily. • Although most dietary sodium is absorbed, the kidneys excrete excess sodium. In the past, sodium restriction was recommended during pregnancy in the mistaken belief that normal regulatory functions broke down and any sodium intake above minimum needs caused water retention and possibly hypertension. In fact, sodium requirements increase during pregnancy by 69 mg/day above non-pregnant levels (NRC, 1989).
Magnesium		
Normal functions • Formation and maintenance of teeth and bones • Catalyst in almost all reactions involving protein, carbohydrates, fats, and nucleic acids	*Deficiency* Possibly related to PIH, hypokalemia, and hypocalcemia (because magnesium affects potassium and calcium homeostasis)	• Because little is known about magnesium needs during pregnancy, the RDA is based on the amount of magnesium accumulated by the mother and fetus during pregnancy. A daily intake of 320 mg is recommended for pregnancy, as compared with 280 mg for non- (continued)

Vitamins and minerals continued

FUNCTION AND SOURCE	POSSIBLE EFFECTS	NURSING CONSIDERATIONS
Magnesium (continued) *Food sources* Vegetables, particularly the dark-green, leafy type (primary source), dairy products, legumes, meats, and grains	*Excess* Excess unlikely; effects on pregnancy are unknown	pregnant needs. • Data indicate that the magnesium intake of pregnant women in the United States is only 35% to 58% of the RDA (Perri and Franz, 1987).
Iron		
Normal functions • Essential component of hemoglobin, found in RBCs *Food sources* Liver, spinach, prunes, beef, pork, broccoli, legumes, whole wheat breads and cereals	*Deficiency* Iron-deficiency anemia *Excess* No reports of iron toxicity from food in healthy people without genetic defects, such as ideopathic hemochromatosis	• The RDA for iron during pregnancy is 30 mg/day, twice that for nonpregnant needs. This increase is caused by several factors. Blood volume increases about 50% during pregnancy, and iron is essential to RBCs. The placenta also stores a significant amount of iron. The fetus stores a 6-month supply of iron. Between 1,000 and 1,400 extra mg of iron are required over the course of pregnancy—60% going to the maternal plasma, 40% to the placenta and fetus (Winick, 1989). • The need for iron during pregnancy increases gradually; it is sharpest during the last trimester, when the fetus is storing iron. • The body typically absorbs only 5% to 10% of dietary iron. Although this absorption rate doubles during the last half of pregnancy (McGanity, 1987) through unknown mechanisms, dietary intake of iron commonly is insufficient, leading to iron deficiency. Because the fetus draws upon maternal iron reserves, the full-term neonate rarely is iron-deficient. • Because of the high dietary intake of iron needed to maintain iron stores during pregnancy (18 to 21 mg/day), and because most clients do not consume iron-rich foods regularly, the NRC (1989) recommends routine supplementation of iron. • Routine iron supplementation has several drawbacks. Iron causes nausea and constipation in one-fifth of women, which contributes to the noncompliance of about one-third of women. Also, iron can reduce the availability of zinc from the diet (Simmer, Iles, James, and Thompson, 1987). Despite these problems, iron-containing multivitamin supplements commonly are prescribed throughout pregnancy and 3 months postpartum.
Iodine		
Normal functions • Aids in thyroid gland function *Food sources* Iodized salt (primary source), salt-water seafood, animal and plant foods (depending on the iodine content of soil)	*Deficiency* • Cretinism (hypothyroid syndrome in which mental and physical development are arrested) with severe deficiency (rare since the introduction of iodized salt) • Restricted fetal development with mild to moderate iodine deficiency *Excess* None reported	• The RDA for iodine during pregnancy is set at 175 mcg/day, an increase of 25 mcg over nonpregnant needs. • In many highly developed countries, iodized salt is the only adequate source of iodine. Clients should not restrict salt intake during pregnancy without discussing it with their physician or nurse-midwife.

Vitamins and minerals continued

FUNCTION AND SOURCE	POSSIBLE EFFECTS	NURSING CONSIDERATIONS
Selenium		
Normal functions • Catalyzation of hydroperoxide breakdown *Food sources* Seafood, kidney, liver, meats, dairy products, fruits and vegetables (depending on selenium content of soil)	*Deficiency* Keshan disease *Excess* Doses of 27.3 g have caused selenium intoxication, characterized by nausea, abdominal pain, diarrhea, nail and hair changes, peripheral neuropathy, fatigue, and irritability	• The RDA for selenium rises to 65 mcg daily during pregnancy.
Zinc		
Normal functions • Nucleic acid synthesis, maintenance of tissue pH, and other functions *Food sources* Meat and seafood (primary sources), grains and legumes (from which less zinc is absorbed because of binding with other compounds)	*Deficiency* Zinc deficiency affects fetal growth. Severe zinc deficiency rarely is seen in humans; only neonates of women with acrodermatitis enteropathica, a zinc metabolism disorder, have shown high rates of mortality or severe malformation in live births (Worthington-Roberts, 1984). However, zinc metabolism also is altered by diabetes; data from diabetic pregnant women show a wide range of complications. *Excess* Stillbirth and premature birth from megadoses of zinc supplements	• The RDA for zinc is increased 3 mg over nonpregnant needs to 15 mg/day. Because this level of intake is difficult to reach without including animal proteins in the diet, vegetarians should be advised to take a zinc supplement. • Zinc intake may be supplemented by diabetic pregnant women (Hurley and Keen, 1988); however, megadoses should be avoided because of adverse fetal effects.
Fluoride		
Normal functions • Prevention of tooth decay *Food sources* Tea; various foods, depending on the fluoride content of the water supply where the food was grown and fluoride content of the water the food is cooked in	*Deficiency* None reported, but fluoride deficiency probably leads to caries-prone teeth *Excess* Mottling of the teeth, turning them brownish (Guthrie, 1988)	• Currently, an intake of 1.5 to 4 mg of fluoride/day is recognized as safe and adequate (NRC, 1989). No RDA has been set for pregnancy. Prenatal fluoride supplementation has a marked effect. In one study, women were given fluoridated water only or fluoridated water plus 1 mg of fluoride/day during pregnancy. When their children were examined (before age 10), only 3% of the group whose mothers received fluoride had caries, compared to 85% of the fluoridated-water-only group (Glenn, Glenn, and Duncan, 1982). • The physician may prescribe 2 mg of sodium fluoride/day for clients in areas without fluoridated water or with a family history of excess caries. • The levels of 1 ppm (part per million) at which water supplies are fluoridated, supplying the average adult with about 1.5 mg/day, will not lead to tooth mottling. However, some natural water supplies do have higher levels.

zinc, and fluoride) are called microminerals, trace minerals, or trace elements.

Increasing evidence suggests that multivitamin supplementation before and during the early weeks of pregnancy can reduce the risk of neural tube defect in neonates (Sheppard, et al., 1989). Women who have borne a neonate with neural tube defect should begin supplementation as prescribed by their physician before attempting to conceive again.

With the exception of iron and folic acid, a well-balanced diet, with foods from all four groups, needs no supplementation for a healthy pregnant woman; however, the woman may take vitamins and mineral supplements to ensure adequate intake. Whenever possible, nutrient deficiencies should be corrected by dietary changes. Health care professionals who routinely prescribe vitamin and mineral preparations should caution pregnant clients that the supplement is not a substitute for a balanced diet and that oversupplementation can cause problems. Such preparations contain only some of the approximately 50 recognized essential nutrients, and the nutrients in the supplement may not be well absorbed. Also, vitamin and mineral supplements do not contain the proteins, carbohydrates, fats, or water essential to life.

Factors influencing antepartal nutrition

A task force from the American College of Obstetricians and Gynecologists and the American Dietetic Association (1978) has identified factors that place a pregnant woman at risk for inadequate nutrition. Some precede conception; others come into play during pregnancy.

Risk factors before conception

These factors can place a woman at nutritional risk if she becomes pregnant: frequent pregnancies, abnormal reproductive history, socioeconomic factors, bizarre food patterns, substance addiction, chronic systemic disorders, prepregnant weight outside the ideal range, and age. Other risk factors identified since the task force include vegetarian diets and breast-feeding.

Frequent pregnancies
Pregnancy stresses a woman's body and commonly depletes stores of iron, folic acid, and vitamin B_6 until well after childbirth (Caan, Horgen, Margen, King, and Jew-

ell, 1987). When the interval between births is less than 1½ years, vitamin and mineral depletion is increased. The relationship of the interval between pregnancies and low birth weight illustrates the effects of frequent pregnancies. In 1987, 21% of neonates born within 1 year and 9% of those born within 1½ years of their mother's previous live birth were low birth weight, compared with 5% of those born 1½ to 5 years after their mother's previous live birth (National Center for Health Statistics, 1989).

Yet most research suggests that increased parity (number of pregnancies) is associated with *increased* birth weight (Caan, Horgen, Margen, King, and Jewell, 1987). These findings indicate that increased parity is not a risk factor when the interval between pregnancies is long enough to replenish nutrient stores (over 1½ years). However, health care professionals should emphasize the importance of a nutritious diet to a client expecting a child less than 1½ years after a previous birth.

Abnormal reproductive history
An abnormal reproductive history may include spontaneous abortion and stillbirth or bearing neonates of low birth weight or with birth defects. Although an abnormal reproductive history may not be explained by nutrition, a balanced diet typically improves the pregnancy outcome. If a client has borne a neonate with a neural tube defect, she may benefit from taking a multivitamin and mineral supplement. If she has borne a low-birth-weight neonate with no other identifiable cause, she should be counseled on caloric intake and acceptable weight gain during pregnancy, which appear to have the most effect on birth weight. A client who has had a spontaneous abortion or stillbirth in the last 1½ years also should take a multivitamin and mineral supplement and maintain a balanced diet because the previous pregnancy may have left her nutritionally depleted.

Socioeconomic factors
These factors include education, occupation, and income, each of which can have an impact on nutrition and pregnancy outcome. For example, a client with little education or whose English is not fluent may not understand traditional nutrition counseling. Also, if her occupation involves physical labor, her caloric expenditures will be higher, which complicates her dietary needs.

Low income is a significant risk factor because the client may be unable to purchase nutritious food in sufficient quantity. Nearly 1 million children are born each year in the United States to families whose incomes fall below the government's poverty line. Because socioeconomic class and birth weight are directly related, poverty must be considered a risk factor for pregnancy (Morrison, Najman, Williams, Keeprang, and Andersen, 1989).

To help minimize the effect of socioeconomic factors on pregnancy outcome, such programs as WIC provide nutrition education and food supplementation that increases protein, iron, calcium, vitamin C, and other nutrients (Rush, et al., 1988).

Bizarre food patterns

Food patterns leading to unbalanced food intake may be considered normal by a particular religion or culture. Besides being a source of nourishment, foods are associated with different emotional attributes, such as strength, beauty, and power. Eating patterns and food choices, therefore, vary widely among different cultures. Many myths about food and pregnancy are handed down from parent to child.

As long as the food intake is adequate, the individual's choices must be respected. Nutrient needs may be met working within the individual's beliefs. However, a client whose nutrient intake is inadequate must be educated about the risks of improper nutrition and encouraged to eat a balanced diet.

Substance addiction

Addiction to nicotine (in tobacco), alcohol, and other drugs can affect nutrition. For example, tobacco use reduces the oxygen-carrying capacity of the blood, which can lead to such problems as premature birth, stillbirth, and low birth weight. The pregnant client should be informed of these adverse effects and advised not to smoke during pregnancy (Federal-Provincial Subcommittee on Nutrition, 1987).

Several nutrients have been shown to be inefficiently used by smokers. These include vitamins A and C, folic acid, cobalamin, and calcium (Federal-Provincial Subcommittee on Nutrition, 1987). Nutrition counseling should emphasize intake of these nutrients.

Alcohol and drug abuse during pregnancy have well-documented adverse effects. The pregnant client should avoid using these substances, which can cause irreversible harm to the fetus. Drug and alcohol abusers typically suffer from poor nutrition. Although lack of attention to diet is one possible cause, the use of these substances may affect nutrient intake and the body's absorption and use of them, particularly B vitamins (Federal-Provincial Subcommittee on Nutrition, 1987).

Chronic systemic disorders

Such disorders as diabetes mellitus and various gastrointestinal, kidney, and cardiovascular diseases are treated with dietary modifications. With the stress of pregnancy, the client needs dietary management. For example, strict blood glucose control during early pregnancy may save a diabetic client from having a child with a birth defect. A diabetic client needs a strictly controlled meal plan as well as adjusted insulin and exercise routines. In some diseases where the diet is particularly limited (such as kidney disease, where protein, sodium, and potassium intake are reduced), nutrient supplementation may be required. The nurse should review possible drug-nutrient interactions if the client is taking medication for a disease.

Prepregnant weight outside the ideal range

A client under or over her ideal weight range is at risk during pregnancy. (For more information, see the section on body weight earlier in this chapter.)

Age

Pregnancy during adolescence poses several nutritional problems. If the adolescent is experiencing a rapid growth rate, her nutrient reserves already are being drawn upon. (Growth continues for about 4 years after menarche.) The adolescent's psychological state may make choosing nutritious foods difficult. Although she may say she is committed to having a healthy baby, she may not comply with nutritional advice. Many adolescents are so concerned with losing their figures that they intentionally limit weight gain by undereating or pursuing intensive physical activity, such as running daily. The extra stress that typically accompanies an adolescent's pregnancy may increase nausea, thus limiting food intake. Economics may come into play if her family situation is unstable; for example, an adolescent ostracized by her family because of the pregnancy may have no income. Finally, many adolescents rely on foods that are quick to prepare and eat, typically providing a limited range of nutrients.

Vegetarian diets

A true vegetarian (vegan) consumes no animal products whatsoever. The more common type of vegetarian, the lacto-ovo vegetarian, includes milk and eggs in the diet. Pollo-vegetarians allow poultry; pesco-vegetarians eat fish. Despite these restrictions on food intake, most vegetarians can meet their nutritional needs by taking extra steps to ensure adequate nutrients. For example, with proper combinations of proteins, the vegan can consume adequate complete proteins. However, health care professionals commonly encourage vegans to include milk and eggs in their diets during pregnancy to ensure sufficient complete protein consumption (Mutch, 1988).

Although protein intake is the greatest nutritional concern for vegetarians, low intakes of several other nutrients also are possible. Vegans may have diets deficient in calcium, riboflavin, and cobalamin. Although calcium is found in some green vegetables, such as collards and mustard greens, the availability of calcium is much lower in vegetables than in dairy products because of fiber and components that inhibit calcium absorption (Worthington-Roberts, 1984). Because meats are main contributors of iron and zinc and the only contributors of B_{12} to a non-vegetarian diet, intake of these nutrients may be insufficient as well.

Breast-feeding

A breast-feeding client who becomes pregnant typically is advised to wean her child, although she may choose to continue breast-feeding. Nutrient needs increase in a client who continues breast-feeding while pregnant. The extent of the increase varies according to the amount of milk that is being produced. Milk production may decrease and the taste of the milk may change because of pregnancy, possibly making the child receptive to weaning.

If the client plans to continue breast-feeding, she must eat a balanced diet with adequate calories, fluids, protein, vitamins, and minerals. A breast-feeding client theoretically needs an extra 500 calories/day; a pregnant client needs an extra 300 calories/day. A pregnant breast-feeding client therefore needs up to 800 calories/day over the typical requirement. Protein needs also increase greatly. A breast-feeding client needs an extra 15 to 20 g/day, whereas a pregnant client needs an extra 10 to 15 g/day. Totalling these brings the possible protein needs to an extra 25 to 40 g/day. Although these increases sound dramatic, protein and most caloric needs could be met by raising the recommended nonpregnant intake of 2 cups of low-fat milk/day to 4 to 6 cups/day in all (NRC, 1989).

Risk factors during pregnancy

Various factors can affect nutrition, including anemia, PIH, multiple gestation (more than one fetus), inadequate or excessive weight gain, pica, gestational diabetes, and lactose intolerance.

Anemia

Plasma volume typically increases 50% during pregnancy. This expansion begins early, peaks at the end of the second trimester, and remains at that level through the third trimester. The expansion lowers hemoglobin levels and hematocrit. This condition is called physiologic anemia, and normal laboratory values are adjusted during pregnancy to take it into account. However, nonphysiologic anemia also is common; it usually is caused by iron or folic acid deficiency.

About 95% of nonphysiologic anemia in pregnancy is caused by iron deficiency. Without adequate iron, hemoglobin levels cannot be maintained to transport adequate oxygen to fetal or maternal tissues. A hemoglobin level below 11 g/dl or a hematocrit less than 33% in-

dicates nonphysiologic anemia. Prevention of iron-deficiency anemia typically involves supplementation with 30 to 60 mg of elemental iron and emphasis on dietary sources of iron. If iron-deficiency anemia develops despite these measures, the physician may prescribe therapeutic levels of 180 mg elemental iron each day, commonly divided into three daily doses (McGanity, 1987).

In folic-acid-deficiency anemia, red blood cells become larger and are more immature than normal (megaloblastic). Folic acid deficiency is uncommon, but it may occur during pregnancy because of the increased requirements for folic acid. Prevention of folic acid deficiency involves emphasis on dietary sources or supplementation to provide at least 400 mcg of folic acid daily. Prenatal multivitamin and mineral formulations usually contain 1 mg, more than double the needed amount.

Pregnancy-induced hypertension

PIH characteristically occurs in the third trimester, near term. (For more information on PIH, see Chapter 23, Antepartal Complications.) Its cause has not been well-established, but it may be related to nutrition. Inadequate intake of calories, protein, sodium, and calcium all have been suggested as possible causes.

Past treatment of PIH has restricted sodium or caloric intake. However, restriction has not proved effective. Sodium restriction may worsen hypertension by stressing the body's mechanisms to conserve sodium. Caloric restriction is more likely to reduce birth weight than PIH.

Current treatment emphasizes optimal nutrition, particularly protein intake. Plasma protein deficiency from insufficient protein interferes with normal regulation of capillary fluid and circulating tissue fluid.

Some women enter pregnancy with hypertension. Sodium restriction may have been part of their treatment for prepregnancy hypertension. Continued sodium restriction may be appropriate in these cases, but sodium should not be severely restricted because of the delicate fluid and electrolyte balance required during pregnancy.

Multiple gestation

Twins occur in approximately 1 out of every 85 births. With the advent of fertility drugs, triplets, quadruplets, and higher multiple births have become more common. Many of the complications that accompany multiple births also are associated with nutritional factors. These complications include low birth weight, prematurity, anemia, and infections. Unfortunately, no guidelines exist for proper nutritional intake for a woman carrying more than one fetus. Specialists disagree how much calorie and protein needs are increased for a woman in her ideal weight range who is carrying twins; the most common recommendation is for a weight gain of 44 pounds (Pederson, Worthington-Roberts, and Hickok, 1989).

A common complaint from clients with two or more fetuses is fullness and heartburn after eating even small amounts. Therefore, they have difficulty consuming even the amounts recommended for a single fetus. Nutritional counseling should address this problem by suggesting smaller but more frequent meals each day. Low-bulk foods that are high in nutrients; for example, fruit juice is less bulky than a piece of fruit.

Inadequate or excessive weight gain

After the first trimester, if a client in her ideal weight range gains less than 2 pounds or more than 6 pounds in 1 month, dietary and medical evaluations should be performed. A client beginning the pregnancy underweight or overweight would be an exception to this rule. An underweight client may need to gain more than 6 pounds per month; an overweight client may have an adequate diet despite weight gains of less than 2 pounds per month.

Pica

The compulsive desire to eat nonfood items, pica typically includes clay, laundry starch, and freezer ice. Pica can influence the pregnant client's nutritional status in several ways. Because nonfood items replace nutritious foods, pica may decrease nutrient intake. Some substances, such as laundry starch, provide calories but few or no nutrients and may contribute to excessive weight gain. In addition, pica may contain toxins that could endanger the fetus. Lastly, some substances may interfere with nutrient absorption or adversely affect the gastrointestinal tract. For example, laundry starch or clay may interfere with iron absorption; large quantities of clay may cause fecal impaction.

Gestational diabetes

Gestational diabetes is associated with elevated blood glucose levels during pregnancy (late in the second trimester to delivery) and the return to normal glucose tolerance after delivery. Although estimates vary, gestational diabetes occurs in approximately 2% of all pregnancies, and some degree of glucose intolerance occurs in up to 15% of pregnancies (Gabe, 1986). (For more information on gestational diabetes, see Chapter 23, Antepartal Complications.)

Gestational diabetes is controlled by diet alone or by diet and insulin therapy. The nutrient and weight gain needs are the same for gestational diabetic women as for other women. However, the diabetic's diet differs in two major ways.

The first principle in this diet is the restriction of simple sugars. Sugar, whether white, brown, or pow-

dered, is the most common simple sugar; intake of foods containing sugar as a major ingredient, such as soft drinks, cakes, pies, and cookies, should be limited. Fruits are a source of the simple sugar fructose. In most cases, not enough fruit is eaten at one sitting to cause the glucose blood level to rise too high. However, fruit juices can be consumed in large enough quantities to warrant caution. Milk and yogurt contain the simple sugar lactose, but standard 1-cup portions do not dangerously elevate the blood glucose level. However, clients who typically consume 2 or more cups of milk or yogurt at one sitting should reduce these portions by half. Other simple sugars include glucose, honey, corn syrup, dextrose, and maltose. Gestational diabetic clients should read labels and use caution if these sugars are among the first three or four items in the list of ingredients, which may mean the product contains significant amounts of them.

The second principle of the gestational diabetic client's diet is to spread food intake evenly throughout the day. Even if meals exclude simple sugars, complex sugars (carbohydrates), fats, and proteins eventually are broken down by digestion into simple sugars. Carbohydrates in particular are broken down mainly into simple sugars. A large meal high in carbohydrates, such as spaghetti eaten with garlic bread, could cause the blood glucose level to rise significantly when the starches are broken down. Dividing food intake evenly into several meals and snacks helps maintain a steadier blood glucose level. Healthful snacks reduce hunger and the desire for high-sugar snacks. Small portions of some sweet foods may be allowed, depending on the severity of the condition and on the individual's willpower to stop with small portions (Franz, et al., 1987). A gestational diabetic client should be referred to a registered dietitian for an individualized meal plan and detailed instruction.

General guidelines for a diabetic diet include 55% to 60% of calories from carbohydrates, 30% or less from fat, and up to 20% from protein (Cooper, 1988).

Lactose intolerance

Milk and most milk products contain lactose, a natural sugar. The body uses the enzyme lactase to break down lactose for absorption. If the body lacks sufficient lactase to handle the lactose ingested, lactose intolerance results, with diarrhea, flatulence, cramping, and bloating. Lactose intolerance is fairly common in certain populations, with the greatest U.S. frequency among Blacks, Mexicans, and Asians.

Some individuals are lactose-intolerant from birth, particularly those born prematurely; however, most lactose intolerance develops later. Also, the degree of intolerance can vary so that some people can ingest small amounts of lactose without developing symptoms.

Although lactose intolerance does not affect the fetus directly, a pregnant client with lactose intolerance may have difficulty achieving calcium and vitamin D intake. Among the options available to the lactose-intolerant client are consuming dairy products that contain small amounts of lactose, such as cheese and cottage cheese; eating fermented dairy products, such as yogurt and buttermilk, where the lactose has been broken down by bacteria; drinking lactose-free milk; or using lactase replacement tablets or drops. The tablets are taken whenever milk or a milk product is consumed; the drops are added to a carton of milk 24 hours or more before it is consumed. Both break down the lactose as natural lactase would. Lactase replacement tablets and drops can be obtained without a prescription.

The client who chooses not to consume dairy products can take calcium supplements or drink calcium-fortified juices. However, this option does not provide the protein, vitamin D, riboflavin, and other nutrients that dairy products do. The lactose-intolerant client who does not consume dairy products should increase her daily servings from the meat group or drink soy milk to provide the necessary protein and other nutrients.

Nursing care

The nurse can identify a pregnant client's nutritional needs and help her meet them by using the nursing process. (For a case study that shows how to apply the nursing process when caring for a pregnant client, see *Applying the nursing process: Client with altered nutrition: less than body requirements, related to inadequate caloric intake,* pages 474 and 475.)

Assessment

Because nutrition is important throughout pregnancy, the nurse should assess it as early as possible—even before conception, if possible—and reevaluate it frequently. The initial assessment provides baseline information for the nursing care plan.

The initial and subsequent assessments include a health history, physical assessment, and review of laboratory tests.

Health history

To obtain information about nutritional status, gather health history data about the client's age, medical history, contraceptive history, obstetric history, personal habits, socioeconomic status, cultural and religious influences, and nutritional intake. (For more information, see Chapter 19, Care during the Normal Antepartal Period.)

Age. When collecting biographical data, note the client's age. An adolescent is more likely to be nutritionally at risk than an older client.

Medical history. Assess the client's history for chronic diseases (such as diabetes, cardiac disease, renal disease, and hypertension), and note their dietary implications. Also inquire about any other illnesses or conditions that may affect nutritional status by altering food intake or increasing nutritional needs, such as recent surgery that may increase the body's need for protein.

Ask the client if she has any food allergies or intolerances, such as lactose intolerance. These can affect her food choices and should be addressed during diet counseling.

Contraceptive history. Find out if the client was using contraception recently, and if so, determine which kind. An oral contraceptive or IUD can deplete the body's stores of several nutrients, including vitamin C and pyridoxine. If the client had been using contraception within 3 months of conception, her body may have insufficient stores of some nutrients.

Obstetric history. Record the number of children and their ages. Closely spaced pregnancies can deplete such nutrients as iron and folic acid. If this is the client's first pregnancy, she may require more detailed instructions on nutrition than a multigravid client.

Ask a multigravid client how close to the due dates her children were born and how much they weighed. A history of premature births or low-birth-weight neonates indicates the client may be at risk for poor nutrition; a history of neonates large for their arrival dates indicates she may be at risk for gestational diabetes.

Determine the client's weight gain during each previous pregnancy. Gains of less than 20 pounds or more than 35 pounds in a client in her ideal weight range suggest she needs encouragement to raise her nutrient intake or to control her caloric intake.

Ask the client if she had anemia, gestational diabetes, or other nutritional problems during previous pregnancies. Such problems are likely to recur in subsequent pregnancies. Stress the importance of iron-rich foods in preventing anemia during the current pregnancy.

Find out if the client breast-fed, and if so, her children's ages when she stopped. If she is still breast-feeding, emphasize the importance of increased caloric intake and adequate amounts of protein, calcium, and fluids.

Personal habits. Personal habits that could affect nutritional status include smoking, alcohol consumption, and over-the-counter, prescription, and illicit drug use. Ask about use of nonprescription vitamin and mineral supplements, which may be taken in excess of recommended doses.

Also assess the client's use of caffeine. Some evidence suggests that high caffeine intake is linked to low birth weight (Martin and Bracken, 1987).

Socioeconomic status. The client's occupation, income, educational level, and family may influence her exposure to educational materials, her awareness of community resources, or her knowledge of food and diets. Question the client about her intake of nutritious foods.

Cultural and religious influences. Find out if the client's culture or religion affects her through food restrictions, commonly chosen foods, and cooking methods. Cultural and religious factors may determine which foods the client is likely to include in her diet. Assess whether such factors interfere with proper nutrition.

Nutritional intake. To assess nutritional intake, obtain a diet history from the client using the dietary recall or dietary record methods. Both can be effective; therefore, use the method best suited to the situation and client. Perform a diet analysis after obtaining the information.

Dietary recall. With this method, tell the client to write down everything she ate and drank the previous day. Have her include portion sizes, preparation method (such as baking or frying), condiments (such as jelly or catsup), and where she ate (such as at home or in a restaurant).

The most common form of diet history, dietary recall has several advantages. It does not require previous instructions, making it appropriate for the client's first prenatal visit. It does not require her to bring anything with her or to expend any time outside the visit. Finally, it yields the foods she ate rather than ones she might choose if she knew her food choices would be examined.

The dietary recall typically covers the previous day's intake, which is as far back as most individuals can remember accurately. If the client is unsure about what she ate, having her think about her activities during that time may jog her memory. Ask about beverages and snacks, which commonly are omitted from the recall. Portion estimates are needed to judge nutrient adequacy, but most clients underestimate or overestimate portion sizes. Keep models of common servings available for comparison.

One major disadvantage of the dietary recall method is that the client's intake during the previous day may not reflect her typical eating habits. Therefore, when she has completed her list, use a food frequency checklist to determine how often she eats from each food group (daily, weekly, or rarely). Also ask if her diet differs on particular days, such as weekends or days off from work.

Dietary record. With this method, have the client document her food and drink intake for 1 or more days. In most cases, a 3-day record is sufficient to provide an accurate view of the client's eating habits. Advantages of the dietary record include accurate portion measurements and fewer forgotton items. However, the client may find diet records time-consuming or change her eating habits because she knows they are being examined.

Dietary records are most appropriate when a client has a particular nutritional problem, such as anemia, gestational diabetes, or excessive or inadequate weight gain. As with the dietary recall, ask the client if the recorded information is typical of her diet. If it is not, determine how her usual diet differs from the information she has recorded.

Diet analysis. After obtaining the diet history, analyze it for nutrient adequacy. Several analysis methods exist. The quickest method is to tally the servings from the four food groups in the diet because each contributes certain nutrients that are difficult to obtain from the other groups. If the diet contains four servings from the milk, grain, and fruit and vegetable groups and three servings from the meat group, it probably is adequate in most nutrients.

The computerized diet analysis method is gaining popularity. Specialized computer programs can determine the adequacy of many nutrients in 1 or more day's food intake. This method is precise and quick, although it may confuse the client who needs to improve her diet. For example, the printout may inform the client that her diet is low in thiamin, niacin, and riboflavin, which may be more confusing than stating that she should eat more grains. However, some computer programs include in the analysis lists of sources for particular nutrients in the analysis.

Another method, not commonly used because of time constraints, is nutrient calculation by hand. Nutrient values for specific foods can be found in books devoted to the subject, such as *Bowes and Church's Food Values of Portions Commonly Used* (Pennington and Church, 1989). Nutrient intakes can be compared to the RDAs during pregnancy. This method is useful when no computer analysis program is available and the client excludes one food group from her diet. For example, if the client were a vegan, calculating the protein, calcium, and iron content of her diet would be necessary before advising her how she can balance her intake.

Physical assessment

Besides measuring the client's vital signs, record her weight and height and determine the appropriateness of her weight for her height. Remember that height-weight tables apply to nonpregnant clients. However, they may be used as a baseline for evaluating the client's preconception weight and weight gain during pregnancy. If a client is obviously underweight or overweight, her eating patterns may not be optimal for health.

Although the condition of certain tissues, such as the eyes, skin, hair, and teeth, can give information on nutritional status, physical examination is of limited value. Changes in physical state typically do not occur until a particular deficiency is advanced. Dietary assessment and laboratory tests provide a more accurate view of nutritional status.

Laboratory tests

Blood tests exist for almost every nutrient, but the normal levels for many nutrients during pregnancy are unknown. A few nutritionally related blood tests typically are performed during pregnancy, including hemoglobin levels and hematocrit to identify anemia, mean corpuscular volume (MCV) and mean corpuscular hemoglobin concentration (MCHC) to differentiate folic acid and cobalamin (vitamin B_{12}) deficiencies from iron deficiency anemia, a fasting 1-hour glucose tolerance test (GTT) at 24 to 28 weeks' gestation to screen for gestational diabetes, a 3-hour GTT if the 1-hour GTT is elevated, and serum albumin level to detect possible protein deficiency or PIH (Winick, 1989).

Nursing diagnosis

After reviewing the client's health history data, diet analysis, physical assessment findings, and laboratory test results, the nurse formulates nursing diagnoses for the client. (For a partial list of applicable diagnoses, see *Nursing diagnoses: Nutrition and diet counseling*.)

Planning and implementation

Based on the client's assessment findings and nursing diagnoses, the nurse establishes goals and then plans and implements interventions to meet the client's needs.

Basic goals for nutrition throughout pregnancy include:
• Adjusting dietary intake to promote appropriate weight gain
• Increasing nutrient intake to meet the RDAs for pregnancy

NURSING DIAGNOSES

Nutrition and diet counseling

The following nursing diagnoses address representative problems and etiologies that a nurse may encounter when caring for a pregnant client. Specific nursing interventions for many of these diagnoses are provided in the "Planning and implementation" section of this chapter.

• Altered nutrition: more than body requirements, related to excessive caloric intake
• Altered nutrition: less than body requirements, related to food aversions
• Altered nutrition: less than body requirements, related to inadequate calcium intake
• Altered nutrition: less than body requirements, related to inadequate caloric intake
• Altered nutrition: less than body requirements, related to inadequate finances for food purchases
• Altered nutrition: less than body requirements, related to inadequate nutrient intake
• Altered nutrition: less than body requirements, related to nausea and vomiting
• Altered nutrition: less than body requirements, related to pica
• Altered nutrition: less than body requirements, related to strict vegetarianism
• Anxiety related to effects of food additives
• Anxiety related to weight gain
• Constipation related to insufficient fiber intake
• Knowledge deficit related to belief in food myths
• Knowledge deficit related to blood sugar control through food choices and distribution (for gestational diabetics)
• Knowledge deficit related to nutritional needs
• Knowledge deficit related to nutritional supplements
• Noncompliance with dietary intake recommendations related to desire to remain thin
• Pain related to heartburn and nausea

• Establishing appropriate food intake patterns for nutrition-related problems, such as anemia and nausea.

Monitor weight gain

Obtain the client's weight at every prenatal visit and compare it to her prepregnancy weight and her previous antepartal weight measurements. Variations from normal weight gain patterns may be associated with a nursing diagnosis of *knowledge deficit related to nutritional needs during pregnancy; altered nutrition: less than body requirements, related to increased nutritional needs during pregnancy;* or *noncompliance with food intake recommendations related to a desire to remain thin during pregnancy.*

If the client has inadequate weight gain and a nursing diagnosis of *altered nutrition: less than body requirements, related to nausea and vomiting,* suggest ways

CLIENT TEACHING

Altering diet to relieve nausea and vomiting

Two out of every three pregnant women experience some degree of nausea, yet relatively little is known about why nausea occurs or how to relieve it. Many researchers believe nausea is caused by rising estrogen levels early in pregnancy. Nausea typically resolves near the end of the first trimester and does not interfere with nutritional status.

However, excessive vomiting can be dangerous, especially if it continues past the first trimester. If excessive vomiting occurs, review your food and fluid intake to ensure adequate nutrition and prevent dehydration.

Although no solution works for everyone, the following recommendations may make you more comfortable.

• Keep crackers or dry toast near you at all times. Eat these when you feel nauseated.
• Eat several small meals instead of three large ones. An overly full or empty stomach may induce nausea.
• Have meals without a beverage. Save liquids for 30 to 60 minutes after the meal to keep your stomach from becoming too full.
• Limit high-fat foods, including oil, margarine, butter, whole-milk dairy products, fatty meats (such as bacon and sausage), salad dressings, and rich desserts. Fat causes higher production of stomach acid, which increases nausea risk.
• Limit spicy foods, particularly pepper-containing foods common in Oriental and Mexican dishes. Such foods also cause your stomach to produce more acid.
• Avoid alcohol, caffeine-containing beverages, and smoking, all of which increase nausea risk.
• Avoid any food that causes stomach discomfort. You may not be able to tolerate certain foods that others can.
• Take time to sit down for meals and chew food well. Eating on the run can lead to stress, which increases nausea risk; chewing your food well decreases the work your stomach must do.
• Look over this sample meal plan to see how these suggestions can be incorporated into your typical diet.

This teaching aid may be reproduced by office copier for distribution to clients.
© 1991, Springhouse Corporation.

MEAL OR SNACK	FOOD TO EAT
Upon awakening	2 crackers or ½ slice dry toast
Breakfast	1 egg 1 slice of toast with jelly ½ grapefruit
1 hour after breakfast	1 cup of low-fat milk
Mid-morning snack	6 crackers ½ cup of low-fat cottage cheese ½ cup of canned fruit
Lunch	1 bun 1 skinless chicken breast with lettuce, tomato, and mustard 1 cup of salad with 1 tbsp of dressing
1 hour after lunch	1 cup of milk
Mid-afternoon snack	½ bagel ¼ cup of tuna fish ½ cup of juice
Dinner	3 oz of roast beef ½ cup of green beans 1 baked potato 1 tbsp of sour cream 1 piece of angel food cake
1 hour after dinner	1 cup of milk
Evening snack	½ cup of pudding 1 banana

to reduce discomfort through food choices. (For more information, see *Client teaching: Altering diet to relieve nausea and vomiting.*)

If a client in her ideal weight range carrying one fetus gains less than 2 pounds per month, encourage her to increase her caloric intake. Conversely, if her gain is more than 6 pounds per month, evaluate her dietary intake to see if she is consuming excessive calories. Follow the same guidelines up to the twentieth week of gestation for a client with twins; after the twentieth week, evaluate her dietary intake if she gains more than 8 pounds per month.

However, verify certain variables recommending increased or decreased caloric intake. Appointments before or after meals may cause a weight difference of 3 to 4 pounds. Seasonal clothing changes also can vary scale weights by several pounds. Clients should schedule visits at approximately the same time of day and wear similar clothing to determine weight gain as accurately as possible.

A sudden large increase in weight after 20 weeks' gestation may be caused by excess fluid retention. Although some fluid retention is normal, it should occur gradually. A sudden shift in fluid balance can be a symptom of PIH, especially if blood pressure elevation and proteinuria are present.

Teach about nutrition

For a client with a nursing diagnosis of *knowledge deficit related to antepartal nutrition,* teach her about basic nutrients and the foods that contain them.

When developing a meal plan with the client, emphasize that the purpose of her diet is to promote fetal health, not to lose weight. Because the term *diet* may be associated with weight loss, use the term *meal plan* instead.

Explain which foods will help the client improve her nutrient intake. Based on the diet analysis, recommend specific foods and portion sizes. For example, instead of saying, "Your diet is low in calcium," explain that her diet is low in the milk group and give examples of foods she could consume, such as low-fat cottage cheese or milk.

When developing the client's meal plan, consider the forces that influence her food choices, including food allergies, food preferences, dietary restrictions related to disorders, and cultural, ethnic, and religious factors. Respect her preferences while helping her select appropriate foods to meet her nutritional needs.

Although foods can be chosen to meet nutritional needs for just about every culture or religion, specific nutrients or food groups still may need attention. Even within a given culture or religion, eating patterns vary greatly among individuals.

Discourage pica and encourage a balanced diet. Suggest foods that may offer similar textures or tastes as the nonfood items.

If the client is a vegan, use different food guides to develop the meal plan (Mutch, 1988). These guides may be particularly useful for a client with a nursing diagnosis of *altered nutrition: less than body requirements, related to alternative dietary patterns.* One food guide that meets all of the RDAs for most nutrients without including meat is one by the Seventh Day Adventists Dietetic Association (Heath, 1983). This guide calls for:
- four servings of soy milk or soy meat substitutes
- four servings of protein-rich legumes
- six servings of grains

CLIENT TEACHING

Selecting food to increase iron intake

Iron, an essential mineral, is needed in the blood to carry oxygen throughout the body. Without enough iron, you may look pale, feel tired, or easily become short of breath. However, you may have no obvious symptoms and will not know that you are anemic until after a blood test.

Only 5% to 10% of the iron in food is absorbed by the body. This rate increases to 10% to 20% when needs are high, such as during pregnancy. To cope with this problem, you must increase your intake of iron-rich foods and combine foods for maximum iron absorption.

Iron exists in food in two forms. Heme iron, which is absorbed most readily, is found in meat, fish, and poultry; non-heme iron is found in grains, dried fruits, and vegetables. The type of protein in meats can increase iron absorption from non-heme iron sources. Therefore, eating meat with spinach, an iron-rich vegetable, increases the amount of iron absorbed from the spinach.

Vitamin C has the same effect as meat: Having orange juice along with iron-fortified cereal increases the amount of iron you absorb from the cereal.

To get the maximum iron from your food, take the following steps:

- Eat poultry, fish, and meat often to provide easily absorbable iron and increase iron absorption from other foods.
- Have vitamin C–rich foods with meals. Good sources include oranges, grapefruits, tomatoes, peppers, broccoli, potatoes, watermelon, cantaloupe, and strawberries.
- Choose iron-fortified breads and cereals.
- Eat iron-rich vegetables, such as spinach, broccoli, asparagus, and other dark-green vegetables.
- Cook with iron pots and pans. Using iron cookware can dramatically increase the iron content of your meals. Acidic foods, such as tomato sauce, can leach valuable iron from iron cookware.
- Eat dried fruits or drink prune juice. Fruits usually do not contain iron, but they do pick up the mineral when dried on iron utensils.
- Avoid foods that decrease iron absorption, such as tea and coffee.
- If your doctor has prescribed an iron supplement, be sure to take it with meat or a source of vitamin C. Iron supplements can cause stomach discomfort. They also may darken your stools, which is not harmful. Taking your iron supplement with food should relieve some of the discomfort. Remember to take iron supplements regularly.
Note: Iron can be toxic if taken in large doses; remember to keep your iron supplements out of children's reach.

• eight servings of fruits and vegetables.

For an adolescent client, remember that various factors may place her at risk for inadequate nutrition. Whenever possible, include a member of the client's social support structure in the nutrition counseling to ensure outside reinforcement of good eating habits.

Prevent nutrition-related problems

If the client has a nursing diagnosis of **knowledge deficit related to methods of increasing iron intake and absorption during pregnancy,** teach her about iron-rich foods, foods that may increase or decrease iron absorption, cooking techniques to increase iron, and any prescribed iron supplements. Give her written instructions to follow at home. (For a sample, see *Client teaching: Selecting food to increase iron intake.*)

If the client has a nursing diagnosis of **constipation related to low-fiber intake,** encourage her to adjust her diet to help correct this problem. (For more information, see *Client teaching: Altering diet to relieve constipation.*)

Address nutrition-related concerns

If the client has a specific nutritional concern, use active listening to understand her concern fully. She may have a nursing diagnosis of **anxiety related to the effects of food additives on pregnancy.** If so, address her concerns. For example, teach her to read labels closely. Encourage her to consume organically grown fresh fruits and vegetables rather than processed foods. If organic produce is not available, encourage her to eat a wide variety of foods to limit the amount of chemicals from any one item.

If the client is concerned about caffeine intake, provide appropriate information. Some studies suggest that a high caffeine intake can cause a neonate to be smaller than average; however, an equal number of studies suggest that caffeine has no effect. To be safe, encourage her to limit caffeine intake to 200 mg/day and list the caffeine content of commonly consumed foods and beverages. For example, a 5-oz cup of automatic drip coffee has 137 mg caffeine, whereas a cola soft drink has 38 mg. If the client intends to breast-feed, recommend that she follow the same limit; caffeine readily crosses into breast milk and can keep her neonate awake.

Teach about weight control

For a client with excessive weight gain and a nursing diagnosis of **altered nutrition: more than body requirements, related to dietary intake that exceeds needs,** review her beliefs about antepartal nutrition. She may believe the myth that a pregnant woman must "eat for two." To dispel this myth, remind her that the second person for whom she is eating is very small and requires

---

---

only 150 extra calories a day during the first trimester and 350 during the second and third trimesters. If the client eats more than that, she may gain more than she needs for her pregnancy and have extra fat to lose after childbirth.

A small amount of food will supply 300 calories, such as two slices of bread with 1 tablespoon of peanut butter and 1 tablespoon of jelly or six crackers and 2 ounces of cheese. Although increases in food intake should be small to limit increases in calories, many of the client's nutrient needs increase substantially during pregnancy. Therefore, she must get the most nutrient value for the calories she consumes. A client who begins her pregnancy at ideal weight should gain between ½ and 1 pound each week. Overweight clients should gain slightly less, underweight clients slightly more.

(Text continues on page 476.)

APPLYING THE NURSING PROCESS

Client with altered nutrition: less than body requirements, related to inadequate caloric intake

The table below shows how the nurse might use the nursing process to ensure high-quality care for the pregnant client described in the case history at right. The first column presents history and physical assessment data followed by a paragraph of mental notes. These notes help the nurse make important connections among assessment findings, aiding in development of the nursing diagnosis and planning.

The second column lists an appropriate nursing diagnosis; information in the remaining columns is based on this diagnosis. Although not part of the nursing process, a rationale appears for each intervention in the fourth column to explain how it contributes to the care plan.

ASSESSMENT	NURSING DIAGNOSIS	PLANNING
Subjective (history) data • Client reports the following information in a 24-hour dietary recall: Breakfast—½ bagel, ½ grapefruit, 1 cup skim milk Lunch—2 cups lettuce salad, 2 tbsp reduced-calorie dressing, diet soft drink Dinner—2 ounces turkey meat, 1 plain baked potato, ½ cup green beans, 1 glass unsweetened iced tea. • Client states, "I can't believe that I've already gained 5 pounds!" • Education: college sophomore. • Marital status: single. • Client states, "I just take a vitamin every day so I don't have to worry about what I eat." **Objective (physical) data** • Height: 5'5". • Weight: 120 lb. • Frame: medium. • Age: 19. • 20 weeks into her first pregnancy. **Mental notes** *The nurse must remember that clients in this age group have acute awareness of body image. The nurse needs to explore with the client her feelings about weight gain and prevent attempts to diet during pregnancy.*	Altered nutrition: less than body requirements, related to inadequate caloric intake	**Goals** By the end of this visit, the client will: • verbalize her fears about gaining weight • describe how much weight gain is appropriate and the importance of adequate weight gain • understand that a vitamin supplement does not provide all needed nutrients and what a balanced prenatal diet is • develop a plan of changes she will make in her diet • list food assistance programs available to her.

CASE STUDY

Sally Klein, a college student age 19, arrives at the health center for a checkup. She is 5 months pregnant and is becoming increasingly concerned about her weight gain.

IMPLEMENTATION		EVALUATION
Intervention	**Rationale**	Upon evaluation, the client:
Establish rapport.	Establishing rapport is crucial in opening the client's mind to suggestions. A judgmental attitude may make the client shut out suggestions.	• verbalized her fears about gaining weight • explained how much weight gain is appropriate and the importance of adequate weight gain • discussed why a vitamin supplement does not provide all needed nutrients and why a balanced prenatal diet is important • developed a plan of changes to make in her eating habits • listed food assistance programs available to her.
Commend positive nutritional habits.	Almost any diet has something commendable about it. This client could be praised for her high intake of fruits and vegetables and abstention from alcohol and junk food. Commending good habits makes the client feel more positive about herself and more open to advice.	
Explore attitudes regarding weight.	The client needs to verbalize her concerns about her weight and how the pregnancy is affecting her life.	
Explain effects of diet on pregnancy, components of the recommended weight gain, components of a balanced prenatal diet, and limits of supplements.	The client needs information presented by a health professional. She may have heard it before from lay people, but she is more likely to take action after receiving advice from a professional.	
Explore financial situation.	Although the client's attitudes concerning weight seem to be the primary issue, her financial situation may compound the problem. She needs to verbalize her concerns about being unmarried and pregnant.	
Help client prioritize nutritional changes, individualized according to her preferences.	By prioritizing nutritional changes, the client is more likely to see the recommendations as possible. If she develops the timetable of changes herself, she is more likely to commit to making them. Working within the client's range of food preferences personalizes the food guide.	
Provide written information on topics discussed.	The client may be introduced to new information during the discussion. The nurse helps her by providing written information she can review later.	
Arrange for follow-up visit.	A follow-up visit is needed after the client begins implementing changes to evaluate her progress.	

Remind the client to eat at least four servings of milk, three of meat, four of fruits and vegetables, and four of grains each day. Check portion sizes to ensure she is not over- or underestimating serving sizes. If she gains weight too quickly, review her intake of miscellaneous foods. Foods high in sugar or fats, such as soft drinks, cookies, and snack chips, are considered miscellaneous foods; their intake should be reduced first. The client should limit servings from this group.

The client may limit weight gain by decreasing her use of certain miscellaneous foods in food preparation. For example, an average baked potato has about 150 calories, but 2 tablespoons of margarine raise the total calories to 350. Raw vegetable salads are virtually calorie-free, but salad dressing may contain 50 to 75 calories per tablespoon. Other miscellaneous foods that can drastically increase calories without adding many nutrients include oil, sour cream, cream cheese, mayonnaise, sauces, gravies, and sugar.

Besides eating less of these foods, the client can eat reduced-calorie versions of foods, such as light mayonnaise and diet margarine. Using these items can cut caloric intake from such foods by half.

The client also can check the fat content of required foods, such as dairy products and meat, and choose lower-calorie versions. For example, skim milk has about 7 grams less fat per cup than whole milk, which results in a difference of about 60 calories per cup. The client needs 4 cups of milk per day; therefore, she could decrease her caloric intake by 240 each day or 67,000 calories for the full pregnancy by drinking skim milk. Because approximately 3,500 calories will produce 1 pound of fat, this simple change theoretically could prevent 19 pounds of unnecessary weight gain during pregnancy.

If the client feels hungry after making these dietary changes, tell her to eat more fresh fruits, vegetables, and whole grain products. These high-fiber foods are filling without adding substantial calories.

Warn the client not to reduce her food intake below the minimum recommended number of servings from the four food groups. Maintaining a high-quality diet is important.

Make referrals

Some clients will need more in-depth nutrition education than a nurse can provide. In these cases, refer the client to a registered dietitian. Recognized as the nutrition experts in the health-care field, registered dietitians are found in private practices and hospital settings. Suggest that the client locate one by calling the American Dietetic Association.

If the client has a nursing diagnosis of *altered nutrition: less than body requirements, related to inadequate finances for food purchases,* refer her to appropriate social agencies or programs, such as WIC.

Evaluation

As with all nursing interventions, an evaluation is necessary to judge the effectiveness of nutritional guidance. State evaluation findings in terms of actions performed or outcomes achieved for each goal. The following examples illustrate some appropriate evaluation statements:
• The client accurately described her antepartal meal plan.
• The client agreed to seek financial assistance through WIC to obtain foods for a balanced diet.
• The client verbalized the basic principles of increasing iron intake and absorption to prevent iron-deficiency anemia.
• The client described ways in which she will decrease foods of low nutritional value to help prevent excessive weight gain.

Documentation

When assisting a pregnant client with nutrition and diet planning, documentation should include:
• age
• vital signs
• height, estimated prepregnancy weight, frame
• appropriateness of prepregnancy weight for height and frame
• current weight
• number of weeks pregnant
• appropriateness of weight gain for number of weeks pregnant
• significant attitudes concerning diet and weight
• significant health history findings
• dietary history
• adequacy of diet
• effects of attitudes on nutritional status
• significant physical assessment and laboratory test data
• client teaching performed
• nutrition information given to the client
• assessment of client's comprehension during teaching
• expectations of compliance
• plan for future visits.

Chapter summary

Chapter 20 described how to assist a client with nutrition and diet planning during pregnancy. Here are the chapter highlights.

• Nutrition education should begin before conception, if possible, or early in the pregnancy to ensure that the client understands the need for adequate nutrition.

• Various physiologic factors affect nutritional needs during pregnancy, including body fat and body weight.

• Specific nutrient deficiencies can adversely affect pregnancy outcome; however, nutritional supplements can improve nutritional status.

• Commonly used as an indication of nutritional status, optimal weight gain during pregnancy varies according to prepregnancy weight.

• To meet nutritional requirements, the client's diet should include adequate amounts of carbohydrates, fats, proteins, water, vitamins, and minerals.

• Many factors influence antepartal nutritional needs. Before conception, these factors include frequent pregnancies, abnormal reproductive history, socioeconomic status, bizarre food patterns, vegetarian diets, substance addiction, chronic systemic disorders, breast-feeding, prepregnant weight, and age. During pregnancy, risk factors include anemia, pregnancy-induced hypertension, more than one fetus, inadequate or excessive weight gain, pica, gestational diabetes, and lactose intolerance.

• A balanced antepartal diet consists of foods from the four food groups with calories adequate to promote desired weight gain. The client may need vitamin and mineral supplements to meet pregnancy needs in addition to a nutritionally sound diet.

• Nutritional assessment, which should be performed as early as possible, includes a health history (including a diet history), physical assessment, and review of laboratory tests.

• After establishing nutritional goals for the client, the nurse plans and implements appropriate interventions, which may include teaching about weight control and nutrition, developing a meal plan to prevent nutrition-related problems, discussing client concerns, and making any necessary referrals (such as to a food supplementation program or a dietitian).

Study questions

1. What is the appropriate weight gain for a pregnant client in her ideal weight range? An overweight client? An underweight client? A client expecting twins?

2. Which factors are most likely to affect antepartal nutrition?

3. Ms. Martinez, age 15, is 21 weeks pregnant. She has gained 20 pounds and reports that she often eats at fast-food restaurants and from vending machines. Which food choices should the nurse recommend to her and why?

4. Ms. Finney, age 26, is 32 weeks pregnant and is complaining of water retention and constipation. She states that she has eliminated all salty foods and table salt from her diet. What recommendations should the nurse make to her and why?

5. Which techniques are most helpful in assessing a pregnant client's nutritional status?

Bibliography

Bender, D. (1987). Estrogens and vitamin B_6: Actions and interactions. *World Review of Nutrition and Diet, 51,* 140-188.

Franz, M., Barr, P., Holler, H., Powers, M., Wheeler, M., and Wylie-Rosett, J. (1987). Exchange Lists: Revised 1986. *Journal of the American Dietetic Association, 87*(1), 28-34.

Frisch, R. (1987). Body fat, menarche, fitness, and fertility. *Human Reproduction, 2*(6), 521-533.

Guthrie, H. (1988). *Introductory nutrition* (7th ed.). St. Louis: Mosby.

Houts, S. (1988). Lactose intolerance. *Food Technology, 42*(3), 110.

Heath, P. (Ed.). (1983). *Diet manual including a vegetarian meal plan.* Loma Linda, CA: Seventh Day Adventist Dietetic Association.

Kaufman-Kurzrock, D. (1989). Cultural aspects of nutrition. *Topics in Clinical Nutrition, 4*(2), 1-6.

Mutch, P. (1988). Food guides for the vegetarian. *American Journal of Clinical Nutrition, 48*(Suppl. 3), 913-919.

National Center for Health Statistics. (1989). Advance report of final natality statistics, 1987. *Monthly Vital Statistics Report, 38*(3).

National Dairy Council. (1989). *Calcium: A summary of current research.* Rosemont, IL: Author.

National Research Council. (1989). *Recommended dietary allowances.* Food and Nutrition Board, Committee on Dietary Allowances. Washington, DC: National Academy Press.

Pennington, J., and Church, H. (1989). *Bowes and Church's food values of portions commonly used* (15th ed.). Philadelphia: Lippincott.

Perri, K., and Franz, K. (1987). Hypocalciuria in preeclampsia. *New England Journal of Medicine*, 317(14), 897-899.

Rush, D., Horvitz, D.G., Seaver, W.B., Leighton, J., Sloan, N.L., Johnson, S.S., Kulka, R.A., Devore, J.W., Holt, M., Lynch, J.T., Woodside, M., and Shanklin, D. (1988). The national WIC evaluation: Evaluation of the special supplemental food program for women, infants, and children. Study methodology and sample characteristics in the longitudinal study of pregnant women. *American Journal of Clinical Nutrition*, 48(Suppl. 2), 429-438.

Samra, J., Tang, L., and Obhrai, M. (1988). Changes in body weight between consecutive pregnancies. *Lancet*, 2(8625), 1420.

Shephard, M., Hellenbrand, K., and Bracken, M. (1986). Proportional weight gain and complications of pregnancy, labor, and delivery in healthy women of normal prepregnant stature. *American Journal of Obstetrics and Gynecology*, 155(5), 947-954.

Simmer, K., Iles, C., James, C., and Thompson, R. (1987). Are iron-folate supplements harmful? *American Journal of Clinical Nutrition*, 45(1), 122-125.

Smith, S., and Alford, B. (1988) Literate and semi-literate audiences: Tips for effective teaching. *Journal of Nutrition Education*, 20(6), 238B.

Stein, Z., Susan, M., Saenger, G., and Marolla, F. (1975). *Famine and human development: The Dutch hunger winter of 1944-45*. New York: Oxford University Press.

Winick, M. (1969). Malnutrition and brain development. *Journal of Pediatrics*, 74(5), 667-669.

Worthington-Roberts, B. (1984). Nutrition and maternal health. *Nutrition Today*, November/December, pp. 6-19.

Nutrition and pregnancy

American College of Obstetricians and Gynecologists. (1987). *Vitamin A supplementation during pregnancy*. American College of Obstetricians and Gynecologists Committee Opinion A, Number 52.

American Dietetic Association. (1989). Nutrition management of adolescent pregnancy: Technical support paper. *Journal of the American Dietetic Association*, 89(1), 105-109.

Borch-Johnsen, B., Meltzer, H.M., Stenberg, V., and Reinskov, T. (1990). Iron status in a group of Norwegian menstruating women. *European Journal of Clinical Nutrition*, 44(1), 23-28.

Brown, J. (1989). Improving pregnancy outcomes in the United States: The importance of preventive nutrition services. *Journal of the American Dietetic Association*, 89(5), 631-633.

Caan, B., Horgen, D., Margen, S., King, J., and Jewell, N. (1987). Benefits associated with WIC supplemental feeding during the interpregnancy interval. *American Journal of Clinical Nutrition*, 45(1), 29-41.

Dawson, E., and McGanity, W. (1987). Protection of maternal iron stores in pregnancy. *Journal of Reproductive Medicine*, 32(Suppl. 6), 478-487.

Durnin, J. (1987). Energy requirements of pregnancy: An integration of the longitudinal data from the five-country study. *Lancet*, 2(8568), 1131-1133.

Federal-Provincial Subcommittee on Nutrition. (1987). Nutrition in pregnancy: National guidelines. Montreal, Canada: Ministry of Supply and Services.

Franz, M. (1986). Is it safe to consume aspartame during pregnancy? A review. *Diabetes Educator*, 12(2), 145-147.

Glenn, F., Glenn, W., and Duncan, R. (1982). Fluoride tablet supplementation during pregnancy for caries immunity: A study of

the offspring produced. *American Journal of Obstetrics and Gynecology*, 143(5), 560-564.

Kuoppala, T., Tuimala, R., Parviainen, M., Koskinen, T., and Ala-Houhala, M. (1986). Serum levels of vitamin D metabolites, calcium, phosphorus, magnesium, and alkaline phosphatase in Finnish women throughout pregnancy and in cord serum at delivery. *Human Nutrition: Clinical Nutrition*, 40(4), 287-293.

Mardones-Santander, F., Rosso, P., Stekel, A., Ahumada, E., Llaguno, S., Pizarro, F., Salinas, J., Vial, I., and Walter, T. (1988). Effect of a milk-based food supplement on maternal nutritional status and fetal growth in underweight Chilean women. *American Journal of Clinical Nutrition*, 47(3), 413-419.

McGanity, W. (1987). Protection of maternal iron stores in pregnancy. *Journal of Reproductive Medicine*, 32(6 suppl.), 475-477.

Mitchell, M., and Lerner, E. (1987). Factors that influence the outcome of pregnancy in middle-class women. *Journal of the American Dietetic Association*, 87(6), 731-735.

Tyler, L.B. (1984). Nutrition and the pill. *Journal of Reproductive Medicine*, 29(7), 547-550.

Winick, M. (1989). *Nutrition in pregnancy*. Baltimore: Williams & Wilkins.

Worthington-Roberts, B., Vermeersch, J., and Williams, S. (1989). *Nutrition in pregnancy and lactation* (4th ed.). St. Louis, MO: Mosby.

Risk factors and antepartal nutrition

American College of Obstetricians and Gynecologists and American Dietetic Association (1978). *Assessment of maternal nutrition*. Washington, DC: Authors.

Cooper, N. (1988). Nutrition and diabetes: A review of current recommendations. *Diabetes Educator*, 14(5), 428-433.

Frentzen, B., Dimperio, D., and Cruz, A. (1988). *American Journal of Obstetrics and Gynecology*, 159(9) 1114-1117.

Gabe, S. (1986). Definition, detection, and management of gestational diabetes. *Obstetrics and Gynecology*, 67(1), 121-125.

Jovanovic, L. (1986). *A practical guide to the diagnosis and management of gestational diabetes*. Boerhinger Mannheim Corp. Indianapolis.

Lackey, C. (1982). Pica—Pregnancy's etiological mystery. In *Alternative dietary practices and nutritional abuses in pregnancy: Proceedings of a workshop* (pp. 84-96). Committee on Nutrition of the Mother and Preschool Child. National Research Council. Washington, DC: National Academy Press.

Leonard, T., Watson, R., and Mohs, M. (1987). The effects of caffeine on various body systems: A review. *Journal of the American Dietetic Association*, 87(8), 1048-1053.

Martin, T., and Bracken, M. (1987). The association between low birthweight and caffeine consumption during pregnancy. *American Journal of Epidemiology*, 126(5), 813-821.

Mills, J., and Graubard, B.I. (1987). Is moderate drinking during pregnancy associated with an increased risk for malformation? *Pediatrics*, 80(3), 309-314.

Morrison, J., Najman, J., Williams, G., Keeprang, J., and Andersen M. (1989). *British Journal of Obstetrics and Gynecology*, 96(3), 298-307.

Philpson, E., and Super, D. (1989). Gestational diabetes mellitus: Does it recur in subsequent pregnancy? *American Journal of Obstetrics and Gynecology*, 160(6), 1324-1329.

Raymond, C. (1987). Birth defects linked with specific level of maternal alcohol use, but abstinence still is the best policy. *JAMA*, 258(2), 177-178.

Tallarigo, L., Giampietro, O., Penno, G., Miccoli, R., Gregori, G., and Navalesi, R. (1986). Relation of glucose tolerance to complications of pregnancy in nondiabetic women. *New England Journal of Medicine,* 315(16), 989-992.

Van der Spuy, Z., Steer, P., McCusker, M., Steele, S., and Jarvo, H. (1988). Outcome of pregnancy in underweight women after spontaneous and induced ovulation. *British Medical Journal,* 296 (6627), 962-965.

Williams, E. (1986). Gestational diabetes mellites and diet control. *Diabetes Educator,* 12(1), 16-17.

Nutrition and fetal development

Harris, S. (1941) *Clinical pellagra.* St. Louis: Mosby.

Hurley, L., and Keen, C. (1988). Fetal and neonatal development in relation to maternal trace element nutrition: Manganese, zinc, and copper. In *Vitamin and Minerals in Pregnancy and Lactation.* Nestle Nutrition Workshop Series, Vol. 16. New York: Nevey/ Raven Press.

Overpeck, M., Moss, A., Hoffman, H., and Hendershot, G. (1989). A comparison of the childhood health status of normal birthweight and low birthweight infants. *Public Health Reports,* 104(1), 58-70.

Pederson, A., Worthington-Roberts, B., and Hickok, D. (1989). Weight gain patterns during twin gestation. *Journal of the American Dietetic Association,* 89(5), 642-646.

Rohr, F., Doherty, L., Waisbren, S., Bailey, I., Ampola, M., Benacerraf, B., and Levy, H. (1987). New England Maternal PKU Project: Prospective study of untreated and treated pregnancies and their outcomes. *Journal of Pediatrics,* 110(3), 391-398.

Seidman, D., Ever-Hadani, P., and Gale, R. (1989). The effect of maternal weight gain in pregnancy on birth weight. *Obstetrics and Gynecology,* 74(2), 240-246.

Sheppard, S., Nevin, N., Seller, M., Wild, J., Smithells, R., Read, A., Harris, R., Fielding, D., and Schorah, C. (1989). Neural tube defect recurrence after "partial" vitamin supplementation. *Journal of Medical Genetics,* 26(5), 326-329.

Wynn, M., and Wynn, A. (1988). Nutrition around conception and the prevention of low birth weight. *Nutrition and Health,* 6(1), 37-52.

Nursing research

Aaronson, L., and Macnee, C. (1989). The relationship between weight gain and nutrition in pregnancy. *Nursing Research,* 38(4), 223-227.

Brooten, D., Peters, M., Glahs, M., Gaffney, S., Cohen, S., and Jordan, C. (1987). A survey of nutrition, caffeine, cigarette and alcohol intake in early pregnancy in an urban clinic population. *Journal of Nurse Midwifery,* 32(2), 85-90.

Darby, W., McNutt, K., and Todhunter, E. (1975). Niacin. *Nutrition Review,* 33, 289-297.

Keshan Disease Research Group. (1979). Epidemiologic studies on the etiologic relationship of selenium and Keshan disease. Chinese Medical Journal, 92, 477-482.

Family Preparation for Childbirth and Parenting

Objectives

After reading and studying this chapter, the student should be able to:

1. Discuss the purpose of childbirth education.

2. Describe nursing roles in childbirth education.

3. Explain the learning principles that apply to childbirth and expectant parents' education.

4. Discuss common components of childbirth education.

5. Demonstrate breathing and relaxation techniques for the pregnant client and her partner.

6. Demonstrate exercises for correct posture and body mechanics for the pregnant client.

7. Describe the importance of role transition to parenthood.

8. Compare childbirth preparation methods.

Introduction

The purpose of childbirth education is to improve the health and well-being of the pregnant client, her fetus, and her family by providing information about conception, pregnancy, childbirth, and family life. Its overall goal is to enable the client or couple to:

• make informed choices about childbearing and child rearing based on accurate, scientific, and practical information

• follow an antepartal health regimen that includes appropriate nutrition, exercise, rest, health care, and psychological development

• cope effectively with pregnancy, labor, and childbirth

• deal positively with infant care and other demands of early parenthood.

NAACOG (1987), the organization for obstetric, gynecologic, and neonatal nurses, also notes that childbirth education helps couples make the transition from expectant parents to parents who are responsible for a neonate.

To achieve these goals, the client should receive childbirth education as soon after conception as possible (or even before conception for a client trying to become pregnant), continuing for about 3 months after delivery. The information provided should meet the needs of the entire childbearing family, which may include the partner, grandparents, siblings, and friends.

A client who begins childbirth education before pregnancy may wish information on decision making and such issues as combining a career with parenting or the effect of a new member on the family. In early pregnancy, education may focus on health habits and adaptation to pregnancy; in late pregnancy, on childbirth, neonatal care, and role transition.

In any setting, the nurse will find opportunities to teach the client and her family about childbirth and parenting. For example, the antepartal nurse can teach about discomforts of pregnancy, comfort measures, and hygiene while preparing the client for an examination. The postpartal nurse can teach the parents about neonatal behaviors while taking the neonate's vital signs. In addition, a nurse with advanced preparation may hold specialized childbirth education programs in a classroom setting.

GLOSSARY

Biofeedback: relaxation technique that uses electronic monitoring of the client's heart rate, temperature, and muscle contractions to teach her to gain control over involuntary physical responses to stress.

Cleansing breath: deep, relaxed breath before and after any patterned breathing during labor.

Conditioned response: reaction acquired through training and repetition, as employed in the psychoprophylactic method of childbirth education.

Doula: lay person who provides support during labor.

Effleurage: relaxation technique that uses light fingertip massage over the abdomen during labor.

Imagery: relaxation technique in which the client focuses on a mental representation of a real or imagined place. Also called visualization.

Kegel exercises: pelvic floor contractions taught antepartally to increase awareness of pelvic floor muscles and postpartally to restore function.

Meditation: relaxation technique that achieves an altered state of consciousness by slow deep-breathing and focusing on a single mental stimulus.

Montrice: trained professional support person during labor.

Music therapy: relaxation technique that uses musical sounds to alter physiologic responses to stress.

Neuromuscular dissociation: relaxation technique that uses tension and relaxation of specific muscle groups to develop awareness of muscle tension.

Paced breathing: learned breathing technique that aids relaxation and helps the client maintain control during labor contractions. May be slow, modified, or patterned.

Progressive muscle relaxation: systematic muscle contraction and relaxation to reduce tension.

Psychoprophylactic method (PPM): childbirth preparation technique developed by Ferdinand Lamaze that emphasizes concentration, relaxation, and education.

Touch therapy: relaxation technique that uses tactile stimulation to alter perceptions of discomfort during labor.

Historical perspective

For hundreds of years, childbirth took place in the home attended by family members and others who provided physical, psychological, and social support. Women prepared their daughters for the event and helped them make a smooth transition to the maternal role.

In the early twentieth century, physicians and hospitals increasingly assumed the duties of childbirth, thereby altering earlier traditions. They focused on the birth rather than on the transition to parenthood. Because hospitals dealt with birth as an isolated event, women recognized the need for formal and informal preparation for the entire birth experience.

Current options

Today, the nurse may be the pregnant client's primary source of education about childbirth and parenting. The nurse may provide educational services to individual clients or to groups of clients in classes. The client may obtain these services through health care facilities, national organizations, independent educators, or consumer-based community organizations.

Health care facilities. Hospitals and clinics may offer a range of classes. They also may provide information specific to the facility, including typical medical interventions and facility policies. Instructors may be nurses and members of national organizations.

National organizations. Such organizations as the American Society for Psychoprophylaxis in Obstetrics (ASPO) and the International Childbirth Education Association (ICEA) provide certification, conferences, information, and a network for childbirth educators. The client may contact the organization's national headquarters for referrals to local educators.

Independent educators. Many nurses and other independent health care professionals have private practices in childbirth education. They may emphasize individualized needs or special interests, such as home births or cesarean births. They may be associated with ASPO, ICEA, or the American Academy of Husband-Coached Childbirth (Bradley method) or may be independent.

Consumer-based community organizations. Many consumer-based groups encourage family-centered care, present nonmedical, alternative views of childbirth, and offer support groups, newsletters, and childbirth education classes as well as training for childbirth educators. Members may be affiliated with national groups, such as ASPO and ICEA. The organization establishes the criteria for instructors, class content, and format and monitors the quality and content of classes. (For more information, see *Nursing preparation for childbirth education*, page 482.)

Because childbirth options now are extensive, a match is particularly important between the family's

Nursing preparation for childbirth education

A registered nurse may teach a pregnant client about childbirth and parenting as part of her care. A registered nurse with additional education and certification can play various roles in preparation for childbirth and parenting, as described below. (In addition, a nurse practitioner, nurse-midwife, or clinical specialist may conduct special childbirth education classes. For more information, see Chapter 1, Family Nursing Care: History and Trends.)

Childbirth educator
The childbirth educator teaches preparation for childbirth and parenting. This position may require participation in continuing education programs and certification by an organization such as the International Childbirth Education Association (ICEA), American Society for Psychoprophylaxis in Obstetrics (ASPO), NAACOG (the organization for obstetric, gynecologic, and neonatal nurses), American Academy of Husband-Coached Childbirth (Bradley method), or a private organization.

Education coordinator
In this capacity, the nurse plans and implements educational programs, usually in a hospital. Programs may include early pregnancy information, classes for sibling or grandparent, and other topics in childbirth education. To prepare for this position, the nurse usually has completed continuing education programs or has a master's degree in nursing or a related field.

Lactation consultant
With continuing education credits and certification by the International Lactation Consultant Association, the lactation consultant provides information and support to pregnant and postpartal women who wish to breast-feed.

Montrice (trained professional support person for labor)
The montrice provides support to the client in labor. The position requires apprenticeship with a nurse or childbirth educator who is a montrice.

values, beliefs, preferences, and economic constraints and the childbirth preparation method, caregivers, and birth plan and location. To help the client select wisely, the nurse must assess his or her own values, beliefs, and feelings as well as those of the health care facility. Also, the nurse must be knowledgeable about childbirth techniques, preparation methods, and trends. Then the nurse will be prepared to help the client and her partner in their transition to parenthood.

To prepare the student for these vital nursing activities, Chapter 21 begins with an overview of learning principles. Then it discusses common components of

childbirth education, including preparation for the transition to parenthood. It concludes with a review of various childbirth preparation methods and classes for families with special needs.

Learning principles

Before attempting to teach, the nurse must be thoroughly familiar with the subject matter and learning principles and must have good communication skills. As a childbirth educator, the nurse must keep in mind that adults learn differently from children and that individual adults may learn in different ways. To be effective, the nurse must be familiar with general characteristics of adult learners as well as specific characteristics of the individual, such as low literacy, that may affect learning.

Knowles (1980) suggests five characteristics of adult learners. They:
• have a background of experiences that may facilitate learning
• have a self-directed learning style, as opposed to being dependent on the instructor for all information
• are interested in immediate application of knowledge
• value learning that facilitates mastery of current developmental tasks or is problem-focused and relevant to their situation
• value participation in learning.

For a client with poor communication skills or low literacy, Doak, Doak, and Root (1985) identify various characteristics that can affect learning. Such clients may:
• have a perspective that is limited to direct personal experiences
• perceive new information through its meaning to themselves only
• be unaware of the need to give information to health care professionals and may assume that others understand information the same way they do
• not think in terms of classifications or categories of information, but in specific and concrete terms
• give information in bits and pieces without identifiable patterns or logical connections.

To provide information that is appropriate for the family, the nurse first assesses each member's educational level, experience with childbirth education, perceived needs, and motivation to learn. This will provide data about the family's information needs and readiness for learning. The nurse also evaluates the family's cultural background and financial, social, developmental, and psychological status. (For more information, see *Cultural considerations: Birth beliefs.*) Much of this information can be obtained from the record of the couple's initial visit or from an interview with the client and her partner when they express interest in childbirth education.

To help tailor the teaching plan, the nurse also investigates the family's beliefs, values, and fears related to childbirth and parenting and assesses family dynamics and attitudes toward parenting.

Based on identified client needs, the nurse determines what should be taught and the most appropriate and efficient means of teaching it. After this decision, the nurse decides whether a large group, small group, or individualized approach is most appropriate. Then the nurse selects the appropriate presentation method, such as demonstration, discussion, or use of audiovisuals, based on such factors as the topic to be taught, the group's size, and the participants' educational background and previous childbirth education. Throughout the instruction, the nurse evaluates each participant's understanding and clarifies or corrects any misperceptions.

Common components of childbirth education

Whether childbirth education occurs in client-teaching sessions with individuals or in classrooms with groups of clients and their partners, it should include the following components:
• physiologic aspects of pregnancy and childbirth
• relaxation techniques
• breathing techniques
• posture and body mechanics
• exercise
• transition to parenthood.

The type of information varies with the trimester of pregnancy. (For more information, see *Childbirth education classes,* pages 484 and 485.)

Physiologic aspects of pregnancy and childbirth

To prepare the childbearing family for the physical changes of pregnancy, the nurse discusses early signs and symptoms and minor discomforts of pregnancy, stages of labor, and the physiology of lactation, depending

---

CULTURAL CONSIDERATIONS

Birth beliefs

In every culture, childbearing is surrounded by rituals, taboos, and prescribed behaviors. To provide culturally appropriate childbirth education, the nurse must learn about birth beliefs in different cultures and determine the degree to which the client and her family adhere to them. The following examples illustrate the importance of incorporating a cultural perspective into nursing care.

In the Mexican-American culture, the mother-daughter bond is typically extremely strong, particularly regarding such home-related activities as childbearing and child rearing (Griffith, 1982). Women care for family members who are ill or injured, and the women are modest about physical exposure. These factors can affect a Mexican-American woman's choice of a labor support partner and her family's preparation for childbirth.

For Orthodox Jews, family laws mandate physical separation of a husband and his wife during menstruation or any other nontraumatic uterine bleeding. Laws of modesty (Tznuit laws) prohibit a husband from observing his wife when she is immodestly exposed. Such cultural factors may limit an Orthodox Jewish husband's willingness or ability to provide his wife with verbal and psychological—rather than physical—support during labor (Lutwak, Ney, and White, 1988).

---

on the client's trimester of pregnancy. To provide appropriate information, the nurse assesses each individual or group for their knowledge of physiologic processes and tailors the presentation to their needs. (For detailed information, see Chapter 17, Physiologic Changes during Normal Pregnancy; Chapter 24, Physiology of Labor and Childbirth; and Chapter 41, Physiology of the Postpartal Period.)

Relaxation techniques

Childbirth education currently emphasizes relaxation and relaxation techniques. Various breathing techniques, exercises, and comfort measures during labor are used to promote relaxation. So is information about pregnancy, birth, and parenting, which promotes relaxation by reducing fear of the unknown. Relaxation during labor can help reduce tension, conserve energy, and increase the effectiveness of uterine contractions, resulting in more efficient labor.

During labor, a woman typically experiences fear of pain. This causes stress, which affects the sympathetic nervous system, resulting in a "fight or flight" response and elevated levels of epinephrine and norepinephrine.

(Text continues on page 486.)

Childbirth education classes

In a review of various studies, Lindeman (1988) found that childbirth education classes positively affected maternal and child health. The parents demonstrated positive attitudes toward labor and delivery. The client also required less medication in labor and delivery, decreased her alcohol and tobacco consumption, and continued breast-feeding for at least 6 weeks after birth. Lindeman also found that clients who participated in childbirth education classes knew more about labor and delivery than those who did not participate.

CLASS TYPE AND DESCRIPTION	PHYSIOLOGIC ASPECTS	RELAXATION
Early pregnancy (first trimester) classes These focus on physical and emotional changes, including nutrition, hygiene, management of discomfort, recognition of complications, sexuality, and family adaptation. They also address fetal development and teratogenic hazards and may teach relaxation techniques and body awareness through posture and body mechanics.	• Anatomy and physiology of pregnancy • Nutrition • Substance abuse and teratogens • Fetal development • Physical and emotional symptoms, such as fatigue, morning sickness, libido changes, urinary frequency, breast changes, and emotional lability • Diagnostic tests, such as chorionic villus sampling, alpha-fetoprotein screening, and amniocentesis • Sexuality • Importance and components of prenatal care • Warning signs of complications	• Introduction to relaxation techniques • Development of awareness of stress response
Mid-pregnancy (second trimester) classes These typically focus on self-care topics, including exercise, physiologic changes, comfort and hygiene measures, fetal development, infant-feeding decisions, and parenting.	• Fetal growth and development • Weight gain and nutrition • Minor discomforts • Quickening (first fetal movement felt) and fetal movements and positions • Neonate characteristics, such as reflexes, responsiveness, and sleeping and eating patterns	• Additional techniques, such as imagery, massage, and music. The parents are encouraged to begin working together to explore relaxation techniques that are most effective for them.
Late pregnancy (third trimester) classes These typically focus on the physiology of the third trimester, anatomy and physiology of labor, coping strategies for labor, medication, anesthesia, health care facility practices, the neonate's appearance and behaviors, early postpartal expectations, postpartal exercises, contraceptive options, and parenting. Ideally, third trimester classes build on earlier classes. In reality, many couples only take classes to prepare for labor and delivery, and these classes typically focus on techniques for coping with labor.	• Signs and symptoms of labor • Pelvic anatomy and the role of bony pelvis and pelvic floor muscles in labor and delivery • Fetal position and presentation • Differentiating between false labor and true labor • Physical symptoms at term, including dyspnea (shortness of breath), leg cramps, backache, urinary frequency, indigestion, and edema of the legs, hands, and feet • Warning signs of complications of late pregnancy • Progress of labor through all stages • Medical procedures during labor and delivery • Effects of medications and anesthetics • Nutrition, substance abuse, and teratogens • Postpartal self-care, breast care, and contraceptive methods	• Importance of relaxation • Relaxation techniques • Practice of relaxation

Other supporters claim these additional benefits from childbirth education classes: decreased duration of labor and delivery, increased maternal control of labor, faster recovery, fewer maternal and fetal complications, and increased maternal and paternal attachment to the neonate (Bennett, Hewson, Booker, and Holliday, 1985; Broome and Koehler, 1986).

Although the specific class content and order of presentation may vary, common components of all classes include physiologic aspects of pregnancy and childbirth, relaxation, breathing, exercise, and role transition.

BREATHING	EXERCISE	ROLE TRANSITION
• Awareness of normal breathing patterns • Awareness of situations that alter breathing patterns, such as anxiety or stress • Description of breathing patterns • Practice of slow paced breathing	• Posture • Body mechanics • Walking • Stretching • Kegel exercises • Pelvic tilt • Body toning	• Psychological responses to body changes • Consumer options about such things as health care providers and childbirth settings • Decision making about feeding method for neonate • Dealing with emotional lability • Exploring maternal and paternal roles • Communication skills to deal with expanding family
• Slow paced breathing to aid relaxation • Modified paced breathing • Patterned paced breathing	• Increasing repetitions of exercises • Modification of exercises because of physical changes, as needed	• Changes in body image • Identification of the fetus as separate from the mother • Prenatal attachment or bonding • Concerns of expectant fathers, such as role in labor and delivery, role as father and partner, financial concerns, and concerns for safety of client and neonate • Importance of support system • Sibling concerns • Neonatal care • Preparation of home and layette (clothing and equipment for neonate)
• Importance of breathing to promote relaxation • Slow paced breathing • Modified paced breathing • Patterned paced breathing • Expulsion breathing	• Posture • Body mechanics • Comfortable positions • Pelvic tilt • Kegel exercises • Tailor sitting (sitting on floor with legs crossed) • Body toning	• Emotional changes • Role of support person during labor • Importance of support systems, such as family members, friends, and even members of the childbirth education class • Normal characteristics of neonates • Effect of neonate on life-style • Infant safety measures, such as car seats • Sexuality • Siblings • Major life transition • Maternal role attainment • Paternal role attainment • Family planning

These catecholamines decrease the uterine blood supply, slowing labor and possibly causing fetal hypoxia.

Relaxation techniques attempt to reverse these effects by inducing muscle relaxation, lowering the heart rate and blood pressure, and increasing parasympathetic response. Techniques taught during childbirth education classes not only are effective during pregnancy and labor, but also during parenthood, especially when dealing with young children. In addition, they can help reduce anxiety, reduce symptoms of various health problems, and improve general well-being.

For the pregnant client and her partner, the nurse teaches such relaxation techniques as progressive muscle relaxation, neuromuscular dissociation, imagery, meditation, biofeedback, music therapy, and touch therapy. A combination of techniques usually is more effective than one method. (For information about relaxation techniques during childbirth, see Chapter 26, Comfort Promotion during Labor and Childbirth.)

Progressive muscle relaxation

This technique is based on the client's ability to receive internal feedback on muscle tension and relaxation. By learning to release muscle tension, the client increases oxygenation to her muscles (especially those in the uterus) and decreases her perception of pain.

To accomplish progressive muscle relaxation, the couple practices systematic contraction and relaxation of specific muscle groups. As the client works through each muscle group, her partner observes for tension and touches tense areas to help her achieve overall relaxation.

Neuromuscular dissociation

This technique teaches the couple to differentiate between tension and relaxation. It usually is taught after progressive muscle relaxation techniques in childbirth education classes. With this technique, the client tenses some muscles while simultaneously relaxing others. Her partner checks various muscle groups for tension or relaxation, gives her feedback, and helps her relax by using such phrases as, "Release your right arm."

Imagery

With this technique, the client focuses on a mental representation of a real or imagined place, using as many senses as possible. Imagery is a form of conscious daydreaming.

Applied consciously, imagery can relieve pain and anxiety. Some researchers have experimented creatively with imagery to see if it can benefit clients with such disorders as headaches, hypertension, and cancer (Simonton, 1982). However, the uses of imagery need further research.

In childbirth preparation, the client uses imagery primarily for relaxation. During labor, she may use it to imagine the cervix opening or the uterus contracting.

When teaching imagery to a client, advise her that each individual performs imagery differently and that no single correct way exists to do it. Some people form mental pictures; others feel or sense things. Gawain (1982) describes two basic types of imagery: active, programmed, or direct, in which the person pictures a specific situation; and passive, receptive, or permissive, in which the person allows the mind to wander and observes whatever appears. (For more information about progressive muscle relaxation, neuromuscular dissociation, and imagery, see *Client teaching: Relaxation techniques.*)

Meditation

With this technique, the client achieves an altered state of consciousness accompanied by physiologic responses associated with relaxation. To teach the basics of meditation, instruct the client to take slow, deep breaths and focus on a single mental stimulus, such as a flickering candle or the repetition of a single sound, word, or phrase.

Biofeedback

Traditionally, this relaxation technique has used electronic monitoring of the client's heart rate, temperature, muscle contractions, and other physical responses to give her feedback about her usually involuntary physical responses to stress and teach her to gain control over them.

In many cases, however, childbirth education classes teach biofeedback without machinery. In these classes, the client learns to become aware of her body responses, such as breathing and muscle tension, through external feedback (tactile or verbal) from her partner who regularly assesses her degree of relaxation. She also learns to identify internal feedback, such as changes in respirations and sensations of tension.

Internal feedback recognition can help the client have a sense of active control. Humenick (1981) proposed that a client who has participated actively in her child's birth may have increased control over her life and self-esteem, which can influence her approach to parenting.

Music therapy

Used for centuries as a therapeutic agent, music may be used during pregnancy to enhance relaxation and during childbirth to decrease tension and pain.

Suggest to the client how music can make her feel comfortable and relaxed. Music with a smooth flowing rhythm, low pitch, and low volume typically is most

CLIENT TEACHING

Relaxation techniques

During childbirth, relaxation techniques can help you reduce anxiety, tension, and discomfort. Throughout life, they can help anyone relax and cope better with stress. Many relaxation techniques exist. You can use one or more of them, as desired. Here are three of the most common ones that use the mind and body to achieve a comfortable state of relaxation.

Progressive muscle relaxation

This technique helps you identify various muscles and feel the difference between muscle tension and deep relaxation. It also reduces physical tension.

Perform the following tensing and relaxing exercises in a systematic pattern, such as starting with your feet and moving up to your head. Repeat each step at least once, tensing each muscle group for a few seconds.

1 Prepare your environment for relaxation by dimming the lights, adjusting the temperature to a comfortable level, and playing soothing music.

2 Sit comfortably or lie on your back or side. Use pillows to support your neck, knees, and lower back, if desired.

3 Concentrate on relaxing a specific muscle group. Start with your feet and work up to your calves, thighs, upper body, hands, arms, shoulders, neck, face, and head.

4 Tense and then relax a specific muscle group. Note the sensations of tension and relaxation in these muscles. Start with your feet and work up to your head as in Step 3.

Neuromuscular dissociation

After mastering progressive muscle relaxation, you may use this technique to further your awareness of relaxation in specific muscle groups. For each muscle group, concentrate on the difference in sensation between muscle tension and relaxation.

1 Tense your right leg by flexing your right foot toward your face. Hold for 3 to 7 seconds. Allow the rest of your body to remain relaxed. Have your partner check different body areas for relaxation. Release the tension in your right leg.

2 Tense your left leg by flexing your left foot toward your face. Hold for 3 to 7 seconds, and then release.

3 Repeat this process through each muscle group moving to the trunk, arms, neck, and face. In each group, tense your muscles, hold, and then release.

4 Now, tense your right arm and left leg, hold, and then release. Try tensing, holding, and then relaxing other combinations of muscle groups. Remember to keep the other muscle groups relaxed.

Imagery

You can use imagery by itself or with progressive muscle relaxation. With this technique, you imagine a special place where you feel deeply relaxed. Follow this procedure.

1 After loosening your clothing, lie down in a quiet place and close your eyes.

2 Relax your muscles as much as possible, moving systematically from toe to head. Think about each muscle as you will it to relax.

3 Form a mental image, using your sense of sight, hearing, smell, touch, and taste. For example, imagine the sights of a secluded stretch of beach with the clear water, white clouds, and pale gray sand. Then add sounds, such as rolling waves and seabirds calling. Feel the sand under your toes and the sun warming your skin, smell the suntan lotion, and taste the salt in the air.

4 Repeat short, positive statements that reinforce your relaxation, such as, "I am letting go of tension," "I am relaxing at will," and "I am in harmony with life."

5 If you like, write a description of your special place and tape-record it. Then play it back to help you concentrate on that place and relax.

6 During labor *only,* you may imagine your cervix opening and the baby moving down the birth canal.

This teaching aid may be reproduced by office copier for distribution to clients.
©1991, Springhouse Corporation.

relaxing. For this reason, classical or new age music may be more effective for relaxation than rock music. Keep in mind, however, that personal preference is important in selecting specific music tapes.

Touch therapy

As a relaxation technique, touch uses tactile stimulation to alter the client's perception of pain. During childbirth education, teach the client and her partner to use touch in various ways. For example, show them how to stroke muscle groups or use abdominal effleurage (light fingertip massage) for relaxation. (For more information, see *Client teaching: Effleurage.*)

Also suggest that they use massage of the back, neck, feet, and legs to reduce muscle tension during labor. If the client and her partner desire, teach them about acupressure (pressure point massage) to promote comfort and relaxation.

Keep in mind that touch can be soothing or upset-ting. Because of this and because individuals respond to touch differently, advise the client's partner to watch for feedback cues, such as facial grimacing or pulling away, and to modify the touch to meet the client's needs.

Breathing techniques

A single breathing technique that effectively relieves discomfort during labor does not exist. Each client needs to become familiar with various breathing techniques to discover those that prove most effective.

Each childbirth preparation method originally included its own breathing techniques and terminology. Eventually, differences in terminology caused confusion as families and instructors moved from one area to another, which indicated a need for universal terminology. In 1983, the ASPO redefined the breathing patterns to establish consistent terminology and adopted the term "paced breathing" (learned breathing techniques for use

---

CLIENT TEACHING

Effleurage

Effleurage is a massage technique that has helped many women relax during labor and reduce their discomfort. You can do this massage on yourself or ask your partner to do it. Although various effleurage patterns exist, use whichever pattern gives you the greatest comfort. Two common patterns are shown below.

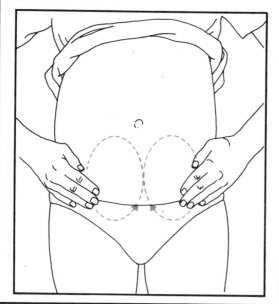

1 Using the fingertips of both hands, lightly stroke the abdomen in a slow, circular pattern, beginning at the navel, as shown.

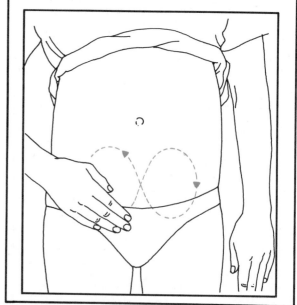

2 As an alternative method, use the fingertips of one hand and stroke lightly in a figure-eight pattern, as shown.

in response to labor contractions).

When teaching about breathing techniques, the nurse should encourage the client and her partner to use whichever tools will help them during labor while ensuring maternal and fetal safety. Because the exact terms and techniques may not be used by all childbirth educators or in all childbirth settings, the nurse should determine what the client and her partner already know and try to use or build on terms and techniques that are familiar to them. These techniques can be adapted for any childbirth setting because they are based on scientific principles and have been proven effective. Also, breathing techniques increasingly are viewed as relaxation techniques.

When preparing the client and her partner for labor, the nurse should encourage them to become familiar with normal breathing patterns at rest and under stress. This becomes the basis for breathing adaptation because the normal respiratory rate of 12 to 16 breaths/minute typically increases with stress and decreases with relaxation. This awareness of variations will enable the client to choose the breathing technique that will help her cope with the stress of labor.

Paced breathing

The current breathing patterns include slow paced breathing, modified paced breathing, and patterned paced breathing.

When teaching the client and her partner about paced breathing patterns, include these key points.
• Use paced breathing as a relaxation technique.
• Begin and end each breathing pattern with a deep cleansing breath.
• Use an external or internal focal point to help concentrate on breathing and relaxation.
• Use chest or abdominal muscles for breathing.
• Breath through the nose or mouth.

Cleansing breath. Described as a deep, relaxed breath, a cleansing breath should be used at the beginning and end of each labor contraction. It encourages relaxation and may improve oxygenation. When teaching this technique, advise the client to inhale and exhale slowly and deeply through the nose or mouth. Tell her to alter the depth and pacing of the cleansing breath, as needed, based on her comfort level.

Slow paced breathing. This type of breathing promotes—and results from—relaxation, making it a good tool to assess the client's effectiveness in coping with labor. Teach the client to breath comfortably at about half of her normal respiratory rate, or approximately six to nine breaths/minute. Reassure her that slow paced breathing provides adequate oxygenation for the fetus and encourage her to use this breathing pattern as needed throughout labor.

Formerly called slow chest breathing, this type of breathing no longer emphasizes chest breathing because it can cause tension in the neck, facial, and intercostal muscles.

Modified paced breathing. In reponse to mental or physical stress, the body normally increases the respiratory rate, pulse, and blood pressure. During the stress of labor, modified paced breathing (a modification of slow paced breathing) allows for this normal increase. Similar breathing patterns have been called rapid-shallow panting, accelerated-decelerated breathing, or hee-hee breathing.

Teach the client to use modified paced breathing as a relaxation technique when slow paced breathing no longer is effective. Because modified paced breathing is tiring, advise her to return to slow paced breathing as desired. Instruct her to increase her respiratory rate to no more than twice her normal rate because higher rates may interfere with maternal and fetal oxygenation and because hyperventilation or fatigue may occur if respirations are too rapid or deep. For greatest effect, tell her to increase her respiratory rate at the peak of the contraction and decrease it at the end.

Patterned paced breathing. Previously called rapid-shallow-blow, transition, hee-hoo, or pant-blow breathing, this technique uses a rhythmic breathing pattern that requires mental focus and practice. It enhances relaxation and helps the client cope with labor when other measures are no longer effective.

Teach the client to take a series of three to six modified paced breaths followed by a soft exhalation or blow to mark the end of the pattern. Encourage her to breathe in time to music or to vary the pattern as desired.

Advise the client to remain relaxed while breathing and to maintain a constant respiratory rate. Tell her not to force any particular sound when breathing. Although she should accentuate the exhalation every three to six breaths, her breathing pattern may be noticeable to her partner only.

Advise her not to exhale too forcefully or breathe too rapidly or she may hyperventilate. Ask her to report any symptoms of hyperventilation, such as dizziness and tingling in the hands, feet, or face. Should she hyperventilate, suggest that she can relieve her symptoms by breathing into cupped hands or a small bag.

Breathing techniques for pushing

Two types of breathing may be used for expulsion (pushing): traditional (closed glottis or breath-holding) and physiologic (open glottis or gentle breathing).

Traditional. Instruct the client to take two deep cleansing breaths when the contraction begins. Then advise her to inhale deeply, assume the pushing position, and bear down by tightening her abdominal muscles and relaxing her pelvic floor muscles. She should hold her breath for no more than 6 seconds as she pushes. Suggest that she take a short breath in the pushing position if needed. Tell her to take one or two deep cleansing breaths and relax as much as possible when the contraction ends.

Physiologic. Tell the client to take two deep cleansing breaths as the contraction begins. Instruct her to assume the pushing position with the third breath and to bear down while blowing out through pursed lips. Because this type of pushing emphasizes prolonged bearing down without breath-holding, advise her to take breaths as needed.

Proponents of physiologic breathing believe it is more effective than the traditional method because it allows the abdominal muscles to tighten and promotes pelvic floor relaxation naturally.

Posture and body mechanics

Good posture and body mechanics improve the client's comfort and safety, which are typically endangered by the extra weight and its distribution during pregnancy. Expect to teach these topics to clients in early pregnancy. (For details, see *Client teaching: Posture during pregnancy,* and *Client teaching: Body mechanics during pregnancy,* page 492.)

Exercise

Exercise helps minimize the discomforts of pregnancy and prepare the body for labor. In addition, women who exercise regularly during pregnancy report that they look and feel better (American College of Obstetricians and Gynecologists [ACOG], 1985). Although no conclusive evidence supports the idea that exercise can affect the length or quality of labor, experts agree that it helps maintain strength, build muscle tone, and protect the back—all of which are important during labor.

With the client, review the following recommendations about exercise during pregnancy (ACOG, 1985).
• Avoid exercise that increases the heart rate above 140 beats/minute because the cardiovascular system is already stressed by the increased blood volume during pregnancy.
• Avoid back-lying exercises after the fourth month of pregnancy because the enlarged uterus can reduce blood flow through the vena cava in this position.
• Avoid extreme joint flexion and jerky motions during exercise because hormonal changes of pregnancy can affect the connective tissue, making the joints less stable.
• Use the pelvic tilt exercise frequently to decrease lower back strain.
• Keep in mind that breathlessness is more common during pregnancy because the enlarging uterus presses up toward the diaphragm.
• Do not perform high-intensity aerobics or exercises that greatly increase oxygen consumption because pregnancy increases oxygen needs and decreases oxygen reserve.
• Limit vigorous exercise to 15 minutes and avoid exercising with a fever or in hot, humid weather. Such exercise raises the body temperature, which is transmitted to the fetus and may cause developmental abnormalities.
• Be aware that exercise may cause premature labor by stimulating production of hormones that increase uterine activity.
• Increase caloric intake to offset calories burned by exercise and to maintain normal blood glucose levels.
• Drink fluids before, during, and after exercise, as needed, to maintain adequate hydration.

One of the easiest ways to exercise during pregnancy is to take brisk walks. Walking can improve cardiovascular and respiratory functioning. If the client expresses an interest in walking, suggest that she wear loose-fitting clothes and comfortable shoes. Advise her to begin walking slowly for 10 to 15 minutes a day and to gradually increase the pace to a comfortable speed and a duration of 30 to 45 minutes a day. Teach her to squeeze her buttocks together while walking to help maintain an erect posture and support the lower back. If the weather does not permit outdoor activity, suggest that she walk in an indoor shopping mall.

CLIENT TEACHING

Posture during pregnancy

Posture is the position of the body, described by alignment of body parts to one another. Good posture is always important. During pregnancy, it's even more important because your extra weight and its distribution can make you feel off balance or uncomfortable. For your safety and comfort, begin using these techniques in the first trimester and continue them throughout your pregnancy.

Standing

To stand correctly, hold your head erect and tuck in your chin. Let your shoulders fall back gently and your arms hang relaxed at your sides. With your knees slightly bent, tuck in your buttocks and flatten your lower back.

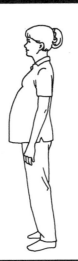

Lying on your back

Lie on your back with a pillow or rolled towel under your head for comfort. Use a pillow under your knees to elevate both legs and place a small pillow under the right side of your back. If you feel any back discomfort, use additional pillows or rolled towels under your head or legs.

   Caution: Do not lie flat on your back after the fourth month of pregnancy because the heavy uterus can compress certain veins, blocking blood flow to the fetus. After the fourth month, lie on your left side for uninterrupted blood flow. As an alternative, lie on your right side.

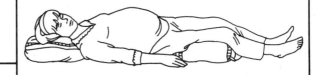

Sitting

Sit with your knees level with or higher than your hips. To achieve this posture, you may have to elevate your feet on a footstool or use a pillow under your upper legs. If needed, use a small cushion to support your lower back.

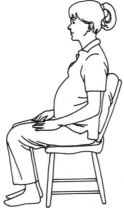

Lying on your side

Roll onto one side so that your abdomen is supported on a flat surface. Bend your uppermost leg forward and support it on a pillow. Keep your other leg straight or slightly flexed. This position may be most comfortable for sleep or relaxation.

   As your abdomen enlarges, place a small pillow under it for support. If desired, add another pillow under your uppermost leg for comfort.

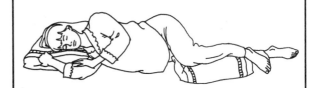

Lying on your side (alternative position)

Lie on one side with your head and upper arms supported on a pillow. Put pillows lengthwise between your slightly flexed legs for support. Also use pillows to support your feet.

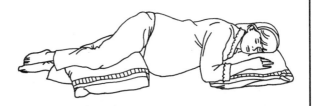

Body mechanics during pregnancy

Body mechanics describes the alignment of different parts of your body when you move. Like good posture, proper body mechanics is vital during pregnancy because your extra weight and its distribution can make you feel unbalanced, jeopardizing your safety. To modify your body mechanics during pregnancy, use the following techniques.

Lying down from a standing position
To lie down, first sit with your knees bent. Turn to one side. Using your arms to support your upper body, lower yourself until you are lying on one side.

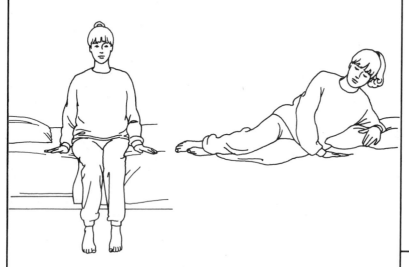

Rising from a lying position
To rise from a lying position, bend your knees and roll from your back to one side. Then use one or both arms to push yourself up.

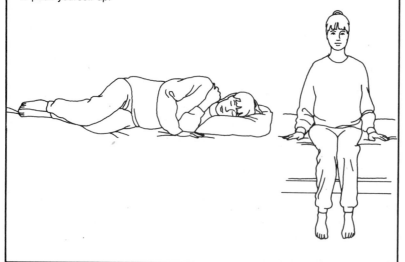

Lifting
To lift an object, stand with your feet 1½' to 2' apart; then bend both your knees until you squat, keeping your back straight. Use both hands to hold the object close to your body. Keeping your back straight, rise slowly by straightening your legs.

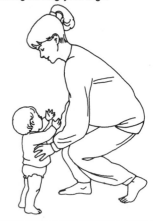

Lifting (alternative method)
First, kneel on one knee. Then bend your other leg as you keep that foot flat on the floor. Use both hands to hold the object close to your body. Keeping your back straight, rise slowly by straightening both legs.

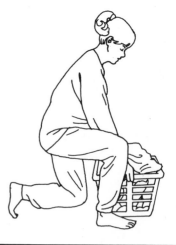

If the client expresses an interest in other forms of exercise, encourage her to try a program designed for pregnant women. (For an example, see *Client teaching: Prenatal exercises*, pages 494 to 497.) As an alternative, suggest a videotaped program of exercises for the childbearing woman. Before making any suggestions, however, screen the program carefully because ACOG recommendations for exercise change periodically as new information becomes available.

Before allowing a pregnant client to begin an exercise program, check her rectus muscles for diastasis (separation). To do this, have her lie on her back with her knees bent. Then ask her to raise her head and shoulders. This tightens the rectus muscles and allows measurement of the separation. If the muscles are separated more than 1″, she will need to support them during exercises by crossing her hands over her abdomen and pulling the muscles toward the midline.

Transition to parenthood

Discussion about the transition to parenthood can occur during the preconception, antepartal, and postpartal periods. It can help the client and her partner assess their support systems, mobilize support, identify ways to strengthen support, and anticipate the types of support they will need during the transition to parenthood.

Preconception period
Whenever possible, perform an in-depth assessment of the client's and partner's readiness for parenthood before conception. Then discuss life-style changes and assist the couple with decision making. (For more information, see Chapter 10, Fertility and Infertility.)

Antepartal period
During the antepartal period, work with the client to help her achieve a smooth transition to parenthood. Provide information and help her complete the tasks of pregnancy and resolve role development and role conflicts—activities that set the psychological stage for adaptation to her role as mother. Also prepare her for the postpartal period.

Completion of tasks of pregnancy. During each contact with the client, carefully note her ability to deal with prenatal tasks, such as accepting the pregnancy, seeking prenatal care, and preparing for the neonate. According to Rubin (1976), four specific tasks prepare the woman for the maternal role: seeking safe passage for herself and the child, ensuring the acceptance of the child by significant others, bonding with the unknown child, and learning to give of herself. Rubin states the successful accomplishment of these tasks during pregnancy leads to effective mothering after childbirth. (For more information, see Chapter 18, Psychosocial Changes during Normal Pregnancy.)

Also discuss the possibility of unexpected outcomes, such as preterm labor and delivery, cesarean delivery, and death of the fetus or neonate. Discussion should help the couple anticipate potential problems, options, and emotional responses, which may include anger, guilt, helplessness, and grief. If the client has a high-risk pregnancy, provide individual counseling or refer her and her partner to a support group.

Role development and role conflict resolution. To help the client make a successful transition to parenthood, promote appropriate role development and help her resolve any conflicts with the maternal role.

Conflicts can arise from her concept of a good mother, which commonly stems from her perceptions of her mother and her experience of being mothered. If the client perceives her mother unrealistically or idealistically, she may have difficulty imagining herself functioning as a good mother. Conversely, if she perceives her mother as a poor or inadequate model, she may have fears and anxieties about her own ability as a mother.

Role conflict also can result from inexperience. In our fast-paced, mobile society, the client may lack exposure to or knowledge about the maternal role. She may not find clear cultural guidelines or consistent role models for mothering. Help the client acquire child care skills and experience to promote a sense of competency and reduce this type of role conflict.

With more than 50% of women active in the work force, conflicts also can arise between pursuing a career and being a parent. If a client feels this type of role conflict, guide her in examining the meaning of her career and of her being a mother. Encourage her to assess the demands of each role and the resources she has to meet those demands.

Choice of infant feeding method is an important issue in the transition to parenthood and one that may cause conflict for the client. In a study of low-income Black mothers, Aberman and Kirchhoff (1985) discovered that over 50% had chosen a feeding method by the end of the first trimester; 82%, by the end of the second trimester. Therefore, plan to introduce the topic of infant feeding early in pregnancy, clearly discussing the advantages and disadvantages of breast- and formula-feeding. (For more information, see Chapter 37, Infant Nutrition.)

(Text continues on page 498.)

Prenatal exercises

During pregnancy, moderate exercise can increase your physical and mental well-being, minimize discomfort, and help prepare your body for labor without any risk to yourself or your baby. If you are in good health and your doctor, nurse-midwife, or nurse practitioner permits, use these exercises to tone the following muscle groups.

Neck, shoulder, and upper torso muscles
These exercises will help maintain good posture and relieve tension and rib cage pressure

Neck stretch
Turn your head from side to side, pausing as you look over each shoulder. Hold for a count of 5 in each direction. Then tilt your head from side to side, as if you were trying to touch your ear to your shoulder. Hold for a count of 5 in each direction. Do not extend your neck far enough to feel any strain. Repeat neck stretch movements 5 times at first. Build up to 10 repetitions.

Chin extension
Push your chin forward and hold for a count of 5. Then tuck your chin to your chest. Repeat the chin extension 5 times at first. Build up to 10 repetitions.

Shoulder roll
Roll your shoulders forward and up while you inhale slowly. Roll them back and down while you exhale slowly. Repeat the shoulder roll 5 times at first. Build up to 10 repetitions.

Elbow circles
While sitting in the tailor position (cross-legged on the floor), place your fingertips on your shoulders and make circles with your elbows. Do 5 elbow circles in each direction at first. Build up to 10 circles in each direction.

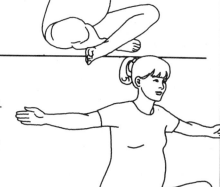

Flying exercise
While sitting in the tailor position, extend your arms straight to either side of your body at shoulder height. While keeping your arms straight, move them backward and forward. Repeat this exercise 5 times at first. Build up to 10 repetitions.

Pectoral stretch
Sit in the tailor position with your pelvis tilted forward slightly. Extend your arms straight before you and lift them to shoulder height. Then bend your elbows and pull your arms back as if you were trying to touch your elbows behind your back. Hold for a count of 5. Stretch your arms straight forward again. Repeat the pectoral stretch 5 times at first. Build up to 10 repetitions.

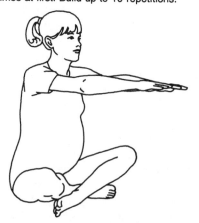

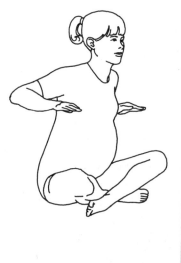

CLIENT TEACHING

Prenatal exercises continued

Pelvic muscles

Pelvic exercises can relieve lower back strain and promote good posture. They also will improve abdominal muscle tone, which helps support your growing uterus, deliver your baby, and protect your lower back during pregnancy and throughout life.

Pelvic floor muscles support your pelvic organs (the intestines, bladder, and uterus) and help control your urethra, vagina, and anus. During pregnancy, exercise of pelvic floor muscles can increase their strength, giving you greater control and ability to relax during delivery. They can improve healing, strength, and bladder control after childbirth.

Lying pelvic tilt

Lie on your back with your knees bent and both feet flat on the floor. Tighten your stomach muscles, pulling the front of your pelvis up toward your rib cage. Your buttocks should lift slightly off the floor. Hold for a slow count of 5, then release. Repeat this pelvic tilt 5 times at first. Build up to 10 repetitions.

Caution: Do not hold your breath during this exercise, and do not perform this exercise after the fourth month of pregnancy.

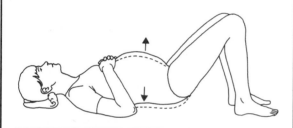

Pelvic tilt on all fours

Position yourself on your hands and knees with your head and back parallel to the floor. Tighten your stomach muscles and tuck your buttocks under to round the lower back. Hold for a slow count of 5, then release. Do not hold your breath. Repeat this pelvic tilt 5 times at first. Build up to 10 repetitions.

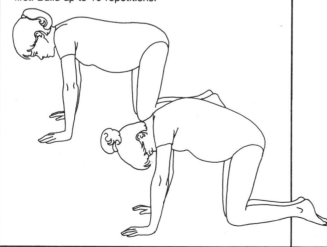

Pelvic floor or Kegel exercises

Tighten your pelvic floor muscles by squeezing the urethral and vaginal openings. (You can identify these muscles by trying to stop your urine flow.) You should feel the pelvic floor rise. Hold for a count of 5 and release. Repeat 5 times for a set, and perform a set 8 to 10 times each day.

Standing pelvic tilt

Stand with your back against a wall and your feet about 6″ away from the wall. Press your lower back against the wall by tightening your abdomen and tucking your buttocks down and in. Hold for a slow count of 5, then release. Repeat this pelvic tilt 5 times at first. Build up to 10 repetitions.

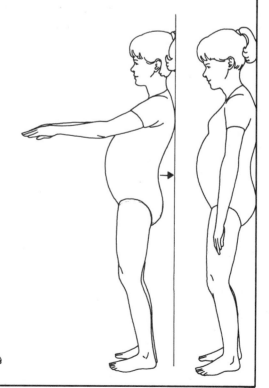

(continued)

Prenatal exercises continued

Abdominal muscles
These exercises will strengthen your abdominal muscles, which support your back, assist with your pushing during childbirth, and promote recovery after childbirth. Before doing any abdominal exercises, however, check with your doctor, nurse-midwife, or nurse practitioner.

Caution: After the fourth month of pregnancy, avoid doing exercises while lying flat on your back. Resume these exercises after your baby's birth.

Abdominal tightening while exhaling
Lie on your back or side with your knees bent. Take a deep breath through your nose and let your abdomen rise. Then forcefully blow out through your mouth while you tighten your abdominal muscles. Repeat this exercise 5 times at first. Build up to 10 repetitions.

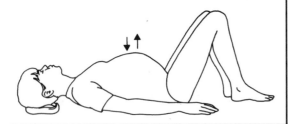

Resisted knee to chest
Lie flat on your back with your knees bent and your feet flat on the floor. Start with a pelvic tilt and then lift your head toward your chest as your raise one knee toward your abdomen. Grab your leg just below the knee using both hands. Using your leg muscles, try to push the knee toward your feet while your hands pull the knee toward your abdomen. Hold for a count of 5, then release. Repeat on the opposite knee. Do this exercise 5 times at first. Build up to 10 repetitions.

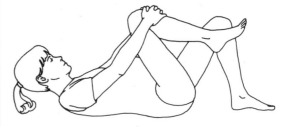

Head lift
Lie flat on your back with your knees bent and feet flat on the floor. Raise your head and look between your knees while you exhale forcefully through pursed lips. Tilt your pelvis slightly when exhaling. Hold for a count of 5, then release. Repeat the head lift 5 times at first. Build up to 10 repetitions.

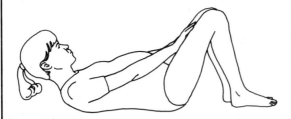

Straight curl up
Lie flat on your back with your knees bent and feet flat on the floor. Bring your chin to your chest as you exhale, continuing forward for about 8″. Be sure to curl your back without raising your waist. Then roll back down. Repeat this curl up 5 times at first. Build up to 10 repetitions.

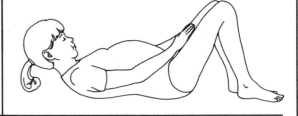

Diagonal curl up
Lie flat on your back with your knees bent and feet flat on the floor. While you exhale, reach both arms to the outside of your left knee and raise your upper body forward as you roll slightly toward your left. Then roll back down. Repeat on the right side. Do this curl up 5 times at first. Build up to 10 repetitions.

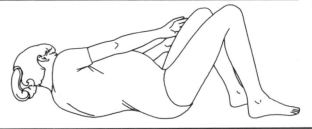

CLIENT TEACHING

Prenatal exercises   continued

Lower back and thigh muscles

Exercises for these muscles will help improve your posture and back stability and increase comfort during childbirth. During these exercises, be careful not to stretch too far because pain may result from separation of the pelvic joints. Because of this potential problem, the tailor stretch and extended leg stretch are optional.

Tailor (Indian style or cross-legged) sit and stretch

Sit on the floor with your knees out and ankles crossed. Hold your back erect to avoid slouching. While in this position, place your hands under your knees. Then press your knees toward the floor while resisting this movement with your hands. Hold for a count of 5, then release. Do this stretch 5 times at first. Build up to 10 repetitions.

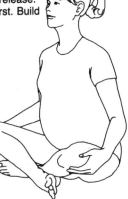

Extended leg stretch

Sit on the floor with your legs extended as far apart as comfortable. Gradually stretch your upper body forward without jerking or bouncing. Lead with both hands. Hold for a count of 5, then resume an upright position. Repeat this stretch 5 times at first. Build up to 10 repetitions.

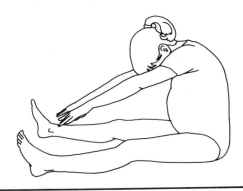

Lower leg muscles

Exercises for your lower leg muscles will promote good circulation, prevent swelling, and increase leg strength.

Calf stretch

Facing a wall, stand with one foot about 12″ in front of the other. Keep your farther leg straight and press your heel to the floor. Bend your nearer knee and lean forward to stretch the calf of your farther leg. Steady yourself with your hands (or arms) against the wall, if desired. Hold for a count of 5, then release. Switch legs and repeat. Do this stretch 5 times at first. Build up to 10 repetitions.

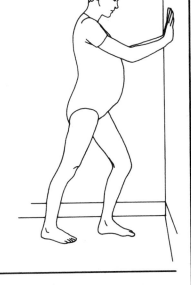

Ankle rotation

Sit on the floor with your legs straight out. Holding your legs still, make clockwise circles with your toes. Then make counterclockwise circles. Repeat the rotation 5 times in each direction at first. Build up to 10 repetitions in each direction.

Foot exercise

Sit or lie down. While holding your legs still, bend your ankles up and then down, pointing your toes. Repeat this exercise 5 times at first. Build up to 10 repetitions. If cramps result with downward extension, flex your foot upward and take a brief rest.

To help the client resolve role conflicts, use conflict resolution techniques. (For more information, see *Managing role conflict*.) Keep in mind that unresolved conflicts can interfere with labor and delivery. Tension and anxiety can inhibit relaxation, and communication problems can hamper the partner's ability to support the client in labor.

Preparation for the postpartal period. To help prepare the client for parenthood, provide information about possible postpartal physical and emotional changes, such as involution, fatigue, depression, and changes in libido. (For more information, see Chapter 41, Physiology of the Postpartal Period.) By learning about these normal changes, the client may be less anxious about them and may have more energy to devote to her role as a mother.

Prepare the client for the possibility that the neonate may have a different temperament or appearance or may be a different sex from the one she has anticipated. For most women, fantasies about the expected infant begin in early pregnancy as images of an older child and gradually progress to images of younger infants. At the time of birth, the fantasized infant usually is older than a neonate.

Also prepare the client to reconcile reality with expectations. The client may expect a perfect, beautiful neonate and expect herself to look radiant after childbirth. Let her know that real life may fall short of her ideal and that she occasionally may feel exhausted and frustrated or may feel like harming the neonate. To help her deal with the conflict between reality and expectations, provide anticipatory guidance, such as reminding her that even good parents occasionally have such feelings, but that they do not act on them. Also, tell her about coping strategies, such as removing herself from the situation, taking some quiet time, exercising, or enlisting help from a support person.

Help her plan ways to fit the neonate into the family structure and schedule. Remind her to include all family members in these plans because they, too, will need to make adjustments. To facilitate adjustment, suggest that the family assess tasks and reassign them differently. Encourage the family to explore the availability of support systems. Remind them that the goal of redefining the family is to incorporate the new member while meeting each individual's needs.

Postpartal period

If the client has not resolved role conflicts earlier, her postpartal adaptation will be more complicated. Besides role transition and adjustment to neonatal care, she also must restore herself physically and emotionally, reconcile reality with her expectations, and redefine family relationships. (For more information, see Chapter 43, Psychosocial Adaptation of the Postpartal Family.)

Fatherhood

Labor support and paternal role development can smooth the transition of the expectant father to parenthood.

Labor support. The expectant father commonly fills the role of labor support person, instructing, managing, and directing the client during labor. He also may play the role of client advocate while she is in labor—a dependent and vulnerable position. These roles require an understanding of the childbirth process and the client's individual needs. They demand psychomotor skills, such as assisting in comfort measures, relaxation techniques, and physical support. They also call for affective behaviors, such as encouragement, listening, reassurance, anticipatory guidance, clarification of feelings, and a supportive, caring attitude.

A labor support person offers many benefits to the woman in labor, such as increased overall satisfaction with the birth, greater self-esteem, and reduced feelings of helplessness; these in turn reduce pain and the need for anesthestics and analgesics. The father as the support person typically experiences increased satisfaction and self-esteem, assumes more caregiving activities with the neonate, and develops closer and more involved feelings for the neonate (Broome and Koehler, 1986).

In a study of fathers' participation in birth, May (1982) found that men with detached coping styles tended to assume the role of observer during labor. Because of this, allow the father a wide range of roles. Do not push him into active participation; if he is pushed beyond his competence or ability to function, he may suffer from guilt, feelings of inadequacy, and inhibited movement into the paternal role.

According to Nichols and Humenick (1988), fathers who are preparing to be labor support persons commonly fear not meeting the expectations of the birthing staff, being unable to protect the client from undesired intervention, doing something stupid or incorrect, and feeling timid, self-conscious, or inadequate.

Be sure to address the unique fears and needs of the father during childbirth education. To help prepare him, use role-playing, encourage him to practice relaxation techniques, share basic information about labor, and provide an orientation to the facility's labor and childbirth unit.

Managing role conflict

Certain behaviors usually accompany role conflict. As a childbirth educator, the nurse may be the first to become aware of them in a client.

Assessment
Sherwin (1987) suggests assessment for the following behaviors when working with a pregnant client.

• Lack of role models for motherhood. Assess the client's experience with maternal role models and isolation from other women during her pregnancy.
• Absence of or alienation from her mother or a mother figure. Past and present availability of the client's mother may indicate how easily she will move into the maternal role.
• Inability to fantasize about the neonate. Fantasy allows practice for the maternal role and assists in bonding with the neonate.
• Inability to resolve grief over loss of previous roles. A client who cannot accept life with a neonate as compensation for lost or greatly modified roles may experience role conflict.
• Inability to visualize life changes necessitated by the neonate's birth. A client who does not perceive the need to change her life-style after the birth may have difficulty with the maternal role.
• Inability to ensure a safe birth. A client with a high-risk pregnancy may feel guilty or feel that she may not be a good mother.
• Absence of support systems. If others do not accept the client's pregnancy, her future neonate, and her expected maternal role behaviors, the client may be insecure about her new role.
• Evidence of rejection of the fetus, such as lack of planning for the neonate. Because development of affectionate bonds parallels maternal role assumption, a client's rejection of the fetus can seriously jeopardize her maternal role attainment.
• Poor motivation for motherhood. If the pregnancy is unplanned and the client lacks motivation to be a mother, role conflict is likely.
• Lack of preparation for motherhood. If the client makes no preparation for the neonate or for childbirth, she may harbor some conflicts about taking on the role of mother.
• Inadequate conflict resolution. By the time of birth, if the client has not resolved her multiple role conflicts or has made no attempts at resolution, role crisis is possible.

Interventions
Use the following interventions to facilitate role conflict resolution (Sherwin, 1987).

• Encourage fantasy. Encourage the client to daydream or to remember and discuss her night dreams. Also, foster her imagination by discussing her plans for her neonate.
• Inform the client. Provide information directly to the client or suggest that she join a childbirth preparation class that will expose her to more information and to other women who may serve as role models.
• Encourage communication and support. The client can benefit from communication with and support from her family as well as support groups. Childbirth education classes may be a source of social support, especially if their format incorporates the sharing of feelings.
• Help the client clarify the problem. By helping the client discuss her problem or conflict, the nurse can help her resolve her difficulty and prepare for her maternal role.
• Support conflict resolution activities. For example, help the client list the positive and negative aspects of a career and motherhood to determine if one role is more important or if they are equally important. Then offer concrete suggestions about role modification, such as finding child care during working hours or modifying her job to accommodate both roles.
• Make referrals. If the client needs more intense or specialized help for a problem, such as a deep-seated ambivalence toward her mother, refer her to another member of the health care team, such as a psychologist.

Although the father is the most common labor support person in the United States, the montrice (a professional who provides labor support and is knowledgeable about prepared childbirth) is gaining in popularity. The montrice is usually a childbirth educator or a nurse who contracts with the family to support them through delivery. Sometimes a doula (lay person experienced in childbirth) acts as the support person for the couple during labor. If the couple choose to use another labor support person, involve the father in other aspects of childbirth, according to the couple's desires.

Role transition. Although the role of labor support person is an important one, do not encourage the father to focus solely on labor and delivery—a brief time in a lengthy process (May, 1988). Such a narrow focus would distract from other significant aspects of role transition. According to Sherwin (1987), the paternal role evolves through developmental and situational aspects, participation in the childbearing cycle, and father-neonate interactions.

Developmental and situational aspects. Developmentally, a man typically expects to become a father. Through the experience of being mothered, he is exposed to the maternal or nurturing aspects of parenthood. Through identification with his father, he has learned the paternal or provider-protector aspects. His relationship with his father may help in his transition to parenthood or complicate it in ways similar to the expectant mother's relationship with her mother. The expectant father may prejudge his paternal performance positively or negatively, depending on his view of his father.

Participation in the childbearing cycle. A father's active participation from preconception planning to labor and delivery promotes his adaptation to the paternal role and attachment to the neonate. Like the mother, the father may engage in fantasies and dreams about the neonate, aiding or complicating role transition.

Father-neonate interactions. Interactions with the neonate play a major part in the father-neonate relationship and the assumption of the paternal role. Paternal attachment is associated with caregiving, emotional investment, and stimulating play between the father and neonate.

Interventions to promote paternal role transition. To help the expectant father, prepare him for the feelings, conflicts, and fantasies he may have, for the changes in his pregnant partner, and for labor and delivery. (For more information, see Chapter 18, Psychosocial Changes during Normal Pregnancy.) Assess the father carefully to detect clues that may complicate the transition to parenthood, and intervene appropriately. For example, if assessment reveals financial concerns, suggest forms of financial assistance to promote assumption of the provider-protector role.

Allow the father to seek his own level of involvement in the birth of his child. Support both parents during the antepartal period, and include the father in all neonatal care teaching.

Special methods and classes

With special preparation, the nurse may teach specialized childbirth preparation methods and classes.

Childbirth preparation methods

Since the 1950s, various childbirth preparation methods have evolved, based on the work of different researchers. (For more information, see *Childbirth preparation methods*.)

Because these methods vary in their philosophies and techniques, the nurse should review the appropriate options with the client and her partner.

Special classes

At times, a client may have additional or different educational needs because of her knowledge level, physical health, or other factors. Also, her family may desire special education in preparation for the new family member. When this occurs, the client and her family may benefit from referral to one or more of the following classes.

• Breast-feeding classes. In the first trimester, an introductory class usually focuses on the importance of making a feeding decision and on the benefits of breast-feeding. Later in the pregnancy, classes highlight preparation for, mechanics of, and common problems during breast-feeding.

• Cesarean birth classes. These classes provide physical, mental, and emotional preparation for cesarean delivery, emphasizing the special procedures and risks and an orientation for the support person.

• Classes for hospitalized high-risk clients. Instruction may be highly individualized to meet the client's need for bed rest or deal with other restrictions. Education usually includes relaxation techniques that may be used during hospitalization and labor, basic reproductive anatomy and physiology, discussion of possible cesarean birth, and general parenting preparation information.

• Classes for parents with communication problems. For such parents, antepartal classes are taught in other languages or are geared for hearing- or vision-impaired clients.

Childbirth preparation methods

Various childbirth education methods emphasize different philosophies and techniques, as described below.

METHOD	PHILOSOPHY	TECHNIQUES
Dick-Read Childbirth without fear method (Dick-Read, 1933, 1987)	Knowledge about childbirth reduces fear, breaking the fear-tension-pain cycle and allowing a natural childbirth. Exercise and breathing promote relaxation during labor. "Unnatural aids," such as anesthetics and analgesics, should be avoided.	• Slow abdominal respirations followed by rapid-shallow chest breathing during contractions • Breath-holding for pushing
Lamaze Psychoprophylactic method (PPM) (Lamaze, 1987; Karmel, 1959; Chabon, 1966; Bing, 1982)	Psychoprophylaxis (psychophysical training technique used to reduce pain during normal childbirth) emphasizes active mental and physical conditioning and a controlled birth. Relaxation and breathing exercises promote mental control over pain. Through conditioned response techniques (response acquired through training and repetition), the client learns to respond to pain with breathing and relaxation.	• Slow chest breathing for early labor, rapid-shallow breathing for active labor, and rapid-shallow-blow breathing with breath-holding for pushing • Use of an external focal point to aid concentration, relaxation, and breathing
Bradley Husband-coached childbirth method (Bradley, 1981)	Birth is a natural occurrence, and the client's husband is the best person to support her during labor. He should be fully involved in childbearing from antepartal class attendance to active participation in the birth.	• Relaxation and slow deep-breathing similar to the Dick-Read method • Husband as coach • Use of a quiet environment for labor and delivery
Kitzinger Psychosexual method (Kitzinger, 1984)	The client focuses on internal sensory experiences so that she can respond to her body signals. Body awareness enhances the sensuality of childbirth, which is similar to orgasm.	• Relaxation based on imagery and an inward focus to promote comfort during labor • Breathing as a relaxed response to contractions • No predetermined breathing pattern • No forced pushing until the client feels the urge to push
LeBoyer Birth-without-violence method (LeBoyer, 1975)	The external environment surrounding the birth is important to neonatal adaptation.	• Use of soft lights, gentle music, and a warm, comforting environment to ease the neonate's transition to extrauterine life • Warm water bathing of the neonate by the father immediately after birth
Noble Gentle pushing method (Noble, 1982, 1983)	Labor is a normal physiologic process. The client should maintain awareness of body feelings and rely on her ability to cope with labor.	• Physical and self-awareness exercises • Spontaneous pushing during exhalation, typically with a grunt or groan and partial closure of the glottis • No forceful pushing or structured breathing
Odent Instinctive birth method (Odent, 1986)	Women can be self-reliant during childbirth because they have an instinct for and innate knowledge of the process. Childbirth is a sexual experience that should be experienced with spontaneity and freedom.	• Use of pools of warm water, music, and dim lights for relaxation • Use of any comfortable position during labor and birth • Immediate contact between mother, father, and neonate, possibly including a warm bath for the neonate

• Expectant father classes. Usually led by men, these classes help the father define his role in the changing family.

• Grandparent classes. Typically, these classes include changes in childbirth practices, changes in parenting practices, and helpful tips about grandparenting and supporting the client in labor.

• Home birth preparation. These classes prepare the client, her partner, and her family for home delivery.

• Infant cardiopulmonary resuscitation (CPR). Typically taught in health care facilities or community centers, these classes teach CPR techniques for infants. They are helpful for all parents of neonates and infants.

• Multipara classes. In these classes, the family learns how to cope with a new family member and make smooth role transitions. Topics may include infant care, mobilization of support at home, sibling rivalry, and the importance of adequate rest.

• Multiple birth preparation classes. Antepartal classes help prepare parents for multiple birth. Postpartal classes provide continuing support.

• Nutrition classes. These classes provide information about basic nutrition and special nutritional needs during pregnancy and breast-feeding. Infant feeding choices may be introduced.

• Parenting classes. These classes serve as a support group for new parents, focusing on child development and time-saving tips for integrating parenting and adult life-styles.

• Postpartal breast-feeding classes. These classes promote early breast-feeding to establish good feeding patterns. They highlight nutrition for the breast-feeding client, introduction of solid foods, and family nutrition. They also may address other topics, such as returning to work while continuing to breast-feed.

• Postpartal classes. Commonly held in the health care facility, these classes teach infant care skills, such as cord care, circumcision care, bathing, feeding, handling, dressing, and well-child care. They also teach maternal self-care, including hygiene, perineal care, breast care, and the need for comfort, rest, and exercise.

Some postpartal classes provide information about gynecologic follow-up and contraception. Others address parental role adaptation, infant growth and development, sexual readjustment, and the use of support systems.

• Refresher classes. For families who have participated in childbirth education classes before, refresher classes review prepared-childbirth techniques. They frequently include sibling adaptation.

• Sibling classes. These classes help prepare siblings for the mother's absence (during hospitalization) and the neonate's arrival. They attempt to reduce anxiety about the hospital and help siblings cope with separation from the mother. They expose the siblings to neonates and encourage them to play with dolls to prepare them for dealing with a neonate. Therapeutic play strategies help siblings recognize and express feelings. Also, parents are prepared to cope with sibling rivalry and an additional child.

• Single parent classes. These classes address the special issues of single parents and typically assist in forming a social support group.

• Specialized classes and support groups for clients with maternal, fetal, or neonatal risks. These classes offer group support for clients with specific problems, ranging from neonates with Down's syndrome, to premature neonates, to mothers with gestational diabetes.

• Teen pregnancy classes. These classes use group dynamics to relate to the adolescent's need for peer group support. They typically cover nutrition, feelings, preparation for childbirth, physical and psychological changes, and plans for infant care.

• Vaginal birth after cesarean (VBAC) classes. For the client who has had a cesarean delivery and wants to have a vaginal birth, VBAC classes provide special preparation.

Chapter summary

Chapter 21 provided an overview of common and special childbirth and parenting preparation methods and classes. Here are the chapter highlights.

• When preparing to teach about childbirth and parenting, the nurse takes into consideration the characteristics of adult learners, the effectiveness of various teaching methods, and the family's cultural background.

• Common components of childbirth education include the physiologic aspects of pregnancy and childbirth, relaxation techniques, breathing techniques, posture and body mechanics, exercise, and transition to parenthood. Specific information varies with the trimester of pregnancy.

• Commonly taught relaxation techniques include progressive muscle relaxation, neuromuscular dissociation,

imagery, meditation, biofeedback, music therapy, and various forms of touch.
• Commonly taught breathing techniques for labor include deep, cleansing breaths and slow paced, modified paced, and patterned paced breathing. Breathing techniques for pushing may be traditional or physiologic.
• Education about the transition to parenthood occurs from the preconception to postpartal periods.
• For the pregnant client, the transition to parenthood is eased by completion of tasks of pregnancy, resolution of role development and role conflicts, and preparation for the postpartal period.
• For the expectant father, the transition to parenthood is enhanced by labor support and other aspects of paternal role transition.
• Based on the work of different researchers, various childbirth preparation methods exist. They include the Dick-Read, Lamaze, Bradley, Kitzinger, LeBoyer, Noble, and Odent methods.
• For clients and families with special needs, the nurse may make referrals to special classes, such as sibling, grandparent, vaginal birth after cesarean, nutrition, and breast-feeding classes.

Study questions

1. Which learning principles should the nurse apply when teaching a couple about childbirth and parenting?

2. What are the common components of childbirth education and their significance?

3. Patty LeBram, age 25, has just been admitted to the labor and delivery area. She is in the first stage of labor and is accompanied by her husband, Pete. Which relaxation techniques may be helpful to Mrs. LeBram during labor?

4. The director of nursing has asked you to set up a preparation for parenting program. Which types of information would you include and why?

5. Marci Klein, age 22, complains of low back pain during her second trimester of pregnancy. Which exercises would you recommend to her?

Bibliography

American College of Obstetricians and Gynecologists. (1985). *Pregnancy exercise program.* Los Angeles: Feeling Fine Programs, Inc.

Austin, S. (1986). Childbirth classes for couples desiring VBAC...Vaginal birth after cesarean. *MCN,* 11(4), 250-255.

Avery, P., and Olson, I. (1987). Expanding the scope of childbirth education to meet the needs of hospitalized high-risk clients. *JOGNN,* 16(6), 418-421.

Biondillo, N., Gleeson, P., MacNeill, B., Norton, T., and Schick, P. (1988). *The H.O.P.E. handboook: A concise guide to pregnancy and birth* (3rd ed.). Garden City Park, NY: Avery Publishing Group.

Broome, M., and Koehler, C. (1986). Childbirth education: A review of effects on the woman and her family. *Family and Community Health,* 9(1), 33-44.

Brouse, A. (1988). Easing the transition to the maternal role. *Journal of Advanced Nursing,* 13(2), 167-172.

Bull, M., and Lawrence, D. (1985). Mothers' use of knowledge during the first postpartum weeks. *JOGNN,* 14(4), 315-320.

Doak, C., Doak, L., and Root, J. (1985). *Teaching patients with low literacy skills.* Philadelphia: Lippincott.

Gawain, S. (1982). *Creative visualization.* New York: Bantam.

Horn, M., and Manion, J. (1985). Creative grandparenting: Bonding the generations: Participation in the birth experience. *JOGNN,* 14(3), 233-236.

Humenick, S. (1981). Mastery: The key to childbirth satisfaction? A review. *Birth and the Family Journal,* 8(2), 79-83.

Humenick, S. (1981). Mastery: The key to childbirth satisfaction? A study. *Birth and the Family Journal,* 8(2), 84-90.

Johnsen, N., and Gaspard, M. (1985). Theoretical foundations of a prepared sibling class. *JOGNN,* 14(3), 237-242.

Knowles, M. (1980). *The modern practice of adult education: From pedagogy to andragogy.* New York: Cambridge Books.

Lindell, S. (1988). Education for childbirth: A time for change. *JOGNN,* 17(2), 108-112.

May, K. (1982). The father as observer. *MCN,* 7(5), 319-322.

May, K. (1988). Is it time to fire the coach? *Childbirth Educator,* 8(2), 30-35.

McKay, S., and Phillips, C. (1984). *Family centered maternity care: Implementation strategies.* Rockville, MD: Aspen Systems.

NAACOG. (1987). *Competencies and program guidelines for nurse providers of childbirth education.* Washington, DC: Author.

Nichols, F., and Humenick, S. (1988). *Childbirth education: Practice, research, and theory.* Philadelphia: Saunders.

Rubin, R. (1976). Maternal tasks in pregnancy. *Journal of Advanced Nursing,* 1(9), 367-376.

Sherwin, L. (1987). *Psychosocial dimensions of the pregnant family.* New York: Springer Publishing.

Simonton, P. (1982). Getting well again. New York: Bantam.

Sosa, R., Kennell, J., Klaus, M., Robertson, S., and Urrutia, J. (1980). The effect of a supportive companion on perinatal problems, length of labor, and mother-infant interaction. *New England Journal of Medicine,* 303(11), 597-600.

Vadurro, J., and Butts, P. (1982). Reducing the anxiety and pain of childbirth through hypnosis. *AJN,* 82(4), 620-623.

Childbirth education methods

Bing, E. (1982). *Six practical lessons for an easier childbirth.* New York: Bantam.

Bradley, R. (1981). *Husband-coached childbirth* (3rd ed.). New York: Harper & Row.

Chabon, I. (1966). *Awake and aware: Participating in childbirth through psychoprophylaxis.* New York: Delacorte Press.

Dick-Read, G. (1933). *Natural childbirth.* London: W. Heineman.

Dick-Read, G. (1987). *Childbirth without fear: The original approach to natural childbirth* (5th ed.). H. Wessel and H. Ellis (Eds.). New York: Harper & Row.

Karmel, M. (1959). *Thank you, Dr. Lamaze.* New York: Harper & Row.

Kitzinger, S. (1984). *The experience of childbirth* (5th ed.). New York: Penguin.

Lamaze, F. (1987). *Painless childbirth: The Lamaze method* (rev. ed.). Chicago: Contemporary Books.

LeBoyer, F. (1975). *Birth without violence.* New York: Alfred A. Knopf.

Noble, E. (1982). *Essential exercises for the childbearing year* (rev. ed.). Boston: Houghton Mifflin

Noble, E. (1983). *Childbirth with insight.* Boston: Houghton Mifflin Co.

Odent, M. (1986). *Birth reborn.* New York: Pantheon.

Wright, E. (1966). *The new childbirth.* New York: Pocket Books.

Cultural references

Griffith, S. (1982). Childbearing and the concept of culture. *JOGNN,* 11(3), 181-184.

Lutwak, R., Ney, A., and White, J. (1988). Maternity nursing and Jewish law. *MCN,* 13(1), 44-46.

Nursing research

Aberman, S., and Kirchhoff, K. (1985). Infant feeding practices: Mothers' decision making. *JOGNN,* 14(5), 394-398.

Bennett, A., Hewson, D., Booker, E., and Holliday, S. (1985). Antenatal preparation and labor support in relation to birth outcomes. *Birth,* 12(1), 9-16.

Brown, M., and Hurlock, J. (1985). Preparation of the breast for breastfeeding. *Nursing Research,* 34(2), 226-232.

Davis, J., Brucker, M., and MacMullen, N. (1988). A study of mothers' postpartum teaching priorities. *MCN,* 17(1), 41-50.

Giblin, P., Poland, M., and Sachs, B. (1986). Pregnant adolescents' health information needs. *Journal of Adolescent Health Care,* 7(3), 168-172.

Leff, E. (1988). Comparison of the effectiveness of videotape versus live group infant care classes. *JOGNN,* 17(5), 338-344.

Lindeman, C. (1988). Patient education. *Annual Review of Nursing Research,* 6, 29-60.

Hiser, P. (1987). Concerns of multiparas during the second postpartum week. *JOGNN,* 16(3), 195-203.

Maloney, R. (1985). Childbirth education classes: Expectant parents' expectations. *JOGNN,* 14(3), 245-248.

McKay, S., and Roberts, J. (1985). Second stage labor: What is normal? *JOGNN,* 14(2), 101-106.

Snyder, M. (1988). Relaxation. *Annual Review of Nursing Research,* 6, 111-128.

Tomlinson, P. (1987). Spousal differences in marital satisfaction during transition to parenthood. *Nursing Research,* 36(4), 239-243.

Weiss, S. (1988). Touch. *Annual Review of Nursing Research,* 6, 3-27.

High-Risk Antepartal Clients

Objectives

After reading and studying this chapter, the student should be able to:

1. Compare antepartal risks for adolescent and mature clients and describe appropriate interventions.
2. Discuss the effects of cardiac disease on a pregnant client and her fetus or neonate.
3. Describe the maternal, fetal, and neonatal effects of diabetes mellitus.
4. Compare the clinical findings for various anemias and their maternal, fetal, and neonatal risks.
5. Identify the maternal, fetal, and neonatal implications of various infections.
6. Describe the dangers of antepartal substance abuse to the client and her fetus.
7. Identify the risks of trauma and surgery for the client and her fetus.
8. Apply the nursing process when caring for a high-risk antepartal client.
9. Teach the antepartal client self-care measures that can reduce health risks for her and her fetus.

Introduction

Although pregnancy is a normal biologic event for most women, it represents a high-risk situation for those with conditions that threaten maternal or fetal health or interfere with normal fetal development, childbirth, or the transition to parenthood.

High-risk conditions include medical problems, such as diabetes and anemia; socioeconomic factors, such as poverty and substance abuse; and age-related concerns, such as childbearing during adolescence or maturity. They may exist before conception, as in cardiac disease or infection, or may occur suddenly during pregnancy, as in trauma or an acute condition—like appendicitis—that requires immediate surgery. Unlike complications of pregnancy, which also can place the mother and fetus at risk, high-risk conditions do not result from pregnancy. (For more information, see Chapter 23, Antepartal Complications.)

When caring for a pregnant client, the nurse's goal is to provide optimal prenatal care and promote the safe birth of a healthy neonate. To meet this goal for the high-risk antepartal client, the nurse must work closely with the rest of the health care team. Expert care can promote health for the client and her fetus and can decrease the risk of maternal, fetal, and neonatal morbidity and mortality.

This chapter investigates nursing care for the high-risk antepartal client. It begins by presenting background information about underlying conditions and their causes and treatments, highlighting their maternal, fetal, and neonatal effects. It describes how to assess existing or potential problems, formulate nursing diagnoses, plan and implement appropriate interventions, and evaluate nursing activities. It includes a discussion of nursing care and support for the client and her family.

GLOSSARY

Cephalopelvic disproportion: condition in which the size, shape, or position of the fetus's head prevents passage through the maternal pelvis.

Congenital anomaly: abnormality present at birth; particularly, a structural abnormality that may be genetically inherited or acquired during gestation.

Congenital heart defect: one of five common defects: atrial septal defect or ventricular septal defect, tetralogy of Fallot, patent ductus arteriosus, valvular abnormality, or coarctation of the aorta.

Diabetes mellitus: endocrine syndrome in which heterogenous chronic disorders are characterized by altered carbohydrate metabolism; caused by inadequate insulin secretion by the beta cells of the islets of Langerhans in the pancreas or by ineffective use of insulin at the cellular level.

Dystocia: difficult delivery caused by abnormalities in the fetus, client's pelvis, or uterine expulsive powers.

Folic acid deficiency anemia: blood disorder in which immature red blood cells (RBCs) fail to divide, become enlarged, and decrease in number.

Gestational diabetes: type of diabetes first diagnosed during pregnancy; may be asymptomatic except for impaired glucose tolerance test values. Also called gestational diabetes mellitus.

Human immunodeficiency virus (HIV) infection: condition that may lead to acquired immunodeficiency syndrome (AIDS), a life-threatening disease that affects the body's immune system, rendering it susceptible to opportunistic infections.

Hydramnios: excess amniotic fluid (usually over 1,500 ml) associated with congenital neonatal disorders and such maternal disorders as diabetes mellitus; also called polyhydramnios.

Hyperglycemia: abnormally high serum glucose level.

Hypoglycemia: abnormally low serum glucose level.

Iron deficiency anemia: blood disorder in which a lack of iron leads to production of smaller (microcytic) RBCs, reducing oxygen transport throughout the body.

Ketosis: condition characterized by an abnormally high concentration of ketone bodies in body tissues and fluids; also called ketoacidosis.

Macrosomia: excessively large fetus, typically weighing over 4,000 g.

Mitral valve prolapse: cardiac disease in which the mitral valve leaflets prolapse into the atrium during ventricular systole because of inadequate support from the chordae tendinae.

Peripartum cardiomyopathy: cardiac disease in which the left ventricle dilates and fails during the last month of pregnancy or first 6 postpartal months.

Polydipsia: excessive thirst; a characteristic symptom of diabetes mellitus.

Polyphagia: excessive hunger; a characteristic symptom of diabetes mellitus.

Polyuria: excessive urine excretion; a characteristic sign of diabetes mellitus.

Rheumatic heart disease: cardiac disease in which an untreated streptococcal infection leads to bacterial invasion and alteration of the mitral or tricuspid valve.

Sickle cell anemia: autosomal recessive blood disorder in which hemoglobin molecules become sickle- or crescent-shaped, which affects their oxygen-carrying capacity and causes vessel obstruction.

TORCH infections: acronym for a group of infections, including toxoplasmosis, other infections (chlamydia, group B beta hemolytic streptococcus, syphilis, and varicella zoster), rubella, cytomegalovirus, and herpesvirus type 2.

Age-related concerns

Most women give birth between ages 20 and 34. Various age-related factors can place an adolescent client (under age 19) or a mature client (over age 34) at risk during pregnancy. (For more information, see *Age-related risks during pregnancy.*)

Adolescent client

Adolescence, the period between puberty and adulthood, is characterized by physical, sexual, social, and psychological development and typically marks the initiation of sexual activity. Because many adolescents lack knowledge about contraception or simply feel that they will not become pregnant, their sexual activity may cause pregnancy. Although total births among adolescents have remained fairly stable, the rate for older adolescents has decreased and that for younger adolescents has increased. For example, the number of live births per thousand women increased between 1960 and 1985 from 0.8 to 1.3 in those ages 10 to 14. During the same period, the number decreased from 43.9 to 33.8 in those ages

Age-related risks during pregnancy

The following chart compares the physical and psychosocial risks of pregnancy and their nursing considerations for adolescent and mature clients.

PHYSICAL RISKS	PSYCHOSOCIAL RISKS	NURSING CONSIDERATIONS
Adolescent client		
• Inadequate intake of protein, calories, vitamins, and minerals (especially calcium and iron) for fetal development • Increased risk of maternal, fetal, and neonatal morbidity: pregnancy-induced hypertension (PIH), iron deficiency anemia, cephalopelvic disproportion, sexually transmitted diseases, premature birth, low-birth-weight neonate • Increased maternal, fetal, and neonatal mortality rate	• Arrested psychosocial development or identity confusion • Denial of pregnancy, leading to inability to cope • Avoidance of visits to health care professionals • Late or no prenatal care • Lack of adequate information about pregnancy • Increased desire to sever parent or family ties caused by mistaken beliefs about pregnancy; for example, that pregnancy will punish parents or worsen unstable family relationships or stressful living conditions • Difficulty assuming an adult identity • Failure to complete the tasks of adolescence, such as finishing school • Failure to establish a stable family • Failure to become self-supporting • Failure to bear a healthy neonate • Lack of social, physical, psychological, and financial assistance during and after pregnancy and birth • Lack of parental support • Usurpation of mother role by maternal grandmother, producing role confusion	• Provide prenatal education about pregnancy, fetal development, birth, and infant care, preferably in a setting that makes the client comfortable. (For example, some health centers schedule specific days for adolescent clients, which gives them the comfort of peer support.) • Emphasize the importance of early and continual prenatal care. • Discuss other options, such as adoption and abortion, as the client requests. • Encourage the client to continue formal schooling to help her mature and increase her career opportunities. • Help the client adjust to parenting through individual counseling sessions that identify and plan ways to meet her parenting needs. • Suggest that the client join in peer group discussions to seek help and suggestions from others in similar circumstances. • Help the client obtain financial aid from federal and state programs, such as the Special Supplemental Food Program for Women, Infants, and Children and Aid to Families with Dependent Children. • Promote the client's self-esteem and assist with decision making and problem solving. • Teach the client to recognize and report signs of pregnancy complications. • Teach about tests that should be performed during pregnancy. • Arrange for family counseling to discuss problems and maintain family unity.
Mature client		
• Increased risk of PIH • Increased risk of cesarean delivery • Increased risk of fetal and neonatal mortality • Increased risk of trisomies	• Increased stress level as the pregnancy advances • Difficulty adjusting to work restrictions for a career woman whose identity and self-worth are strongly tied to her work • Isolation from family, friends, and fellow professionals • Encountering ridicule, scorn, rejection, and sympathy instead of congratulations • Loss of support from peers, which may threaten self-esteem and satisfaction with personal and professional decisions	• Encourage the client to maintain her health before and during the pregnancy. • Inform the client and her partner about the availability, benefits, and risks of prenatal tests, such as amniocentesis, chorionic villus sampling, and alpha fetoprotein testing, and about genetic counseling. • Identify the client's concerns about the antepartal, intrapartal, postpartal, and parenting periods. Reduce her anxiety about these periods by teaching about expected changes. • Counsel the client during pregnancy and prepare her for labor, birth, and parenting. • Teach the client to recognize and report signs of pregnancy complications, such as PIH.

Chorionic villus sampling and amniocentesis

As a part of antepartal care, a mature client may elect to have various tests to detect genetic and other fetal abnormalities. Two commonly performed tests for such clients—chorionic villus sampling and amniocentesis—are illustrated here. Clients who are Rh-negative typically receive $Rh_o(D)$ immune globulin to prevent sensitization from either procedure.

Chorionic villus sampling

The procedure for transcervical aspiration of a chorionic villus sample is illustrated. Although this procedure may be performed transabdominally, this route is used rarely. With ultrasound as a guide, the examiner passes a plastic catheter through the cervical canal into the uterus. Tissue aspirated from the developing placenta may undergo chromosomal analysis, biochemical testing, or DNA studies.

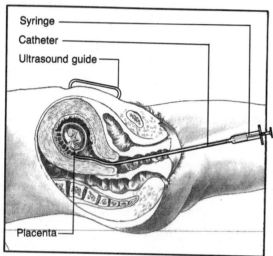

Amniocentesis

This diagram illustrates the procedure for aspirating a sample of amniotic fluid. Using ultrasound, the examiner passes a needle through the abdomen into the uterus and removes 25 to 35 ml of fluid. If fetal bleeding occurs, fetal blood cells may enter the maternal circulation, possibly causing Rh isoimmunization.

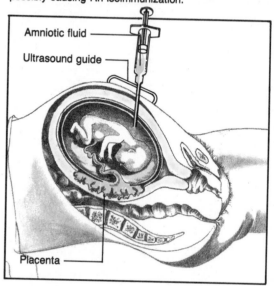

15 to 17 and from 166.7 to 81.7 in those ages 18 to 19 (U.S. Department of Health and Human Services, 1988).

Pregnancy poses risks to adolescents because of their physical and psychological immaturity, potential for pregnancy complications, lack of prenatal care, and lack of social and economic support systems. The pregnant adolescent may not finish school, which eventually can affect her quality of life, job opportunities and advancements, and economic stability.

Mature client

During the early 1980s, pregnancy and birth rates rose for women in their thirties, indicating that many women chose to postpone childbearing (Ventura, Taffel, and Mosher, 1988). The rates for women over age 34 also increased, possibly because of later marriages, relaxation of contraceptive measures, or desires to delay childbearing until after the establishment of a career. Mature women report emotional readiness for pregnancy, presence of a partner, and career and financial stability as reasons for a later pregnancy (Robinson, Garner, Gare, and Crawford, 1987).

An older woman who is healthy before pregnancy can reasonably expect a healthy pregnancy, as long as she receives appropriate antepartal care. She also may want genetic counseling and special antepartal testing for certain physiologic and psychosocial risks. (For illustrations of two of the most common antepartal tests in mature clients, see *Chorionic villus sampling and amniocentesis*. For details about their purpose, timing, and nursing considerations, see *Fetal testing for high-risk antepartal clients*, pages 528 to 531.)

Cardiac disease

Pre-existing cardiac disease places about 1% of pregnant women at risk (Gilstrap, 1989). A cardiologist may predict difficulties posed by cardiac conditions after evaluating the functional capacity of the client's heart. (For more information, see *Functional classifications for cardiac clients.*) Common cardiac diseases affecting pregnant clients include rheumatic heart disease, congenital heart defects, mitral valve prolapse, and peripartum cardiomyopathy. (For more information, see *Common cardiac diseases*, page 510.)

Rheumatic heart disease is the most common cardiac disorder among pregnant women (McAnulty, Metcalfe, and Ueland, 1988). Although the availability of penicillin and improvements in the standard of living have decreased the incidence of this disease, it nevertheless poses serious risks during pregnancy.

Congenital heart defects also pose risks during pregnancy. However, recently introduced techniques for early diagnosis and treatment have allowed women with congenital defects to lead normal, healthy reproductive lives.

Mitral valve prolapse is a common adult cardiac condition, occurring in 6% to 10% of women of childbearing age (Cruikshank, 1986d). Peripartum cardiomyopathy affects about 1 out of 1,300 to 4,000 pregnant women, posing the greatest risk for Black women, mature women, and those with multiple gestation (more than one fetus), pregnancy-induced hypertension (PIH), or postpartal hypertension (Homans, 1985).

With any cardiac disorder, cardiac decompensation may occur, challenging maternal and fetal health. Rarely, it may lead to maternal or fetal death. Careful medical, obstetric, and nursing care before and during pregnancy can minimize maternal and fetal risks.

Effects of pregnancy on cardiac disease

If the client's heart maintains adequate output through all the physiologic changes of pregnancy and through delivery, she should be free from cardiac complications. If she maintains her health and prevents complications, her functional classification should not change during pregnancy.

However, physiologic changes of pregnancy may cause cardiac stress, especially during the second trimester. These changes include increased plasma volume and expanded uterine vascular bed, which increase heart rate 10 to 15 beats per minute by the end of pregnancy and boost cardiac output by about 30% be-

Functional classifications for cardiac clients

This classification system from the New York Heart Association identifies the client's physical response to her cardiac disease. Before conception, the client's functional capacity should be assessed by a cardiologist to serve as a baseline. After conception, it should be reassessed and compared to the baseline to evaluate the effect of pregnancy on the client's heart.

CLASS	DESCRIPTION
Class I Uncompromised	No limitation of physical activity. A class-I client has no symptoms of cardiac insufficiency or anginal pain.
Class II Slightly compromised	Slight limitation of physical activity. A class-II client is comfortable at rest, but may experience excessive fatigue, palpitations, dyspnea, or anginal pain when engaging in ordinary physical activity.
Class III Markedly compromised	Marked limitation of physical activity. A class-III client is comfortable at rest, but experiences excessive fatigue, palpitations, dyspnea, or anginal pain with slight activity.
Class IV Severely compromised	Inability to perform any physical activity without discomfort. A class-IV client at rest may have symptoms of cardiac insufficiency or anginal syndrome, including choking, spasmodic pain, and shortness of breath. If she performs any physical activity, her discomfort increases.

tween 28 and 32 weeks' gestation. A client who experiences this cardiac stress needs weekly evaluation and may require bed rest, fluid restrictions, or such drugs as digitalis preparations, diuretics, antiarrhythmics, antibiotics, or anticoagulants (usually heparin).

Cardiac stress may intensify in the third trimester and may be severe enough to cause persistent pulmonary effects, such as crackles, tachycardia, tachypnea, dyspnea, or orthopnea. A client who experiences severe cardiac stress should adhere to prescribed treatments and should be monitored weekly for changes in pulmonary effects. To prevent complications, she may need to be placed on bed rest.

Common cardiac diseases

The chart below lists the clinical findings and treatments for common cardiac diseases that may affect a pregnant client.

DISEASE AND DESCRIPTION	CLINICAL FINDINGS	TREATMENT
Rheumatic heart disease		
Streptococcal infection leading to acute or chronic systemic rheumatic fever and, if untreated, to bacterial invasion of the mitral or tricuspid valve	• Inadequate cardiac functioning (classes I to IV) • Possible signs of right-sided heart failure, such as pitting dependent edema, weight gain, decreased urine output, and jugular vein distention • Possible signs of left-sided heart failure, such as crackles, dyspnea, coughing, tachycardia, tachypnea, and decreased urine output	• If damage is substantial, surgical correction before pregnancy through valvular repair or replacement (preferred) • After surgery, warfarin (Coumadin) or heparin (for the pregnant client) to prevent emboli at the valve prosthesis site • Close monitoring of the pregnant client if functional limitations remain after surgery because pregnancy will further strain her body • Daily supplementation with 300 mg of ferrous sulfate and 0.2 to 0.4 mg of folic acid to maintain hemoglobin levels at or above 12 g/100 ml during pregnancy (Brady and Duff, 1989) • Restriction of sodium intake to 2 g daily to prevent excess fluid retention • Depending on the client's functional classification, revision of her medical regimen, which includes digitalis preparations, diuretics, resting in semi-Fowler's position, and proper nutrition
Congenital heart defect		
One of five common defects: **1.** Atrial septal defect or ventricular septal defect (VSD). Abnormal opening between right and left atrium or right and left ventricle. **2.** Tetralogy of Fallot. Anomaly consisting of four defects, including pulmonic stenosis, VSD, malpositioning of the aorta so that it arises from the septal defect or the right ventricle, and right ventricular hypertrophy. **3.** Patent ductus arteriosus. Abnormal communication between the pulmonary artery and the aorta. **4.** Valvular abnormality. Abnormality of any heart valves, such as narrowing or widening. **5.** Coarctation of the aorta. Abnormal narrowing of the aorta, which causes increased aortic pressure and the need for increased ventricular pressure during systole.	• Minor functional limitations after mandatory surgical correction	• Surgical repairs early in life to improve cardiac functioning • If minor functional limitations remain after surgery, close monitoring of the client during pregnancy • Depending on the client's functional classification, revision of her medical regimen, which includes digitalis preparations, diuretics, resting in semi-Fowler's position, and proper nutrition
Mitral valve prolapse		
Lack of support from the chordae tendinae, causing mitral valve leaflets to prolapse into the atrium during ventricular systole	• Typically asymptomatic, but may cause arrhythmias, palpitations, lightheadedness, dizziness, and fatigue	• Life-style adjustments as necessary, such as paced activity and rest periods • Propranolol (Inderal) to treat associated tachyarrhythmias • Close monitoring for signs of complications
Peripartum cardiomyopathy		
Left ventricular dilation and congestive heart failure occurring in the last month of pregnancy or first 6 postpartal months	• Similar to congestive heart failure • Fatigue, weakness, dyspnea, orthopnea, angina, chest pain, palpitations, cough, hemoptysis, and abdominal pain	• Digitalis preparations, diuretics, anticoagulant (heparin), furosemide (Lasix), and bed rest

Effects of cardiac disease on pregnancy

Different cardiac conditions affect pregnancy differently. For rheumatic heart disease, maternal mortality increases with active heart disease at the time of pregnancy (Brady and Duff, 1989) and with functional classification. The mortality rate is higher for functional classes IV (6%) and III (5.5%) and decreases significantly with each class, dropping to 0.1% for class I.

Congenital heart defects should pose no problems by themselves during pregnancy. However, pulmonary hypertension associated with a defect, such as Eisenmenger's syndrome (ventricular septal defect with pulmonary hypertension), carries a 30% to 70% maternal mortality rate during pregnancy and the postpartal period. Therefore, the nurse must take steps to prevent circulatory overload (Ramin, Mayberry, and Gilstrap, 1989).

The client with mitral valve prolapse should not have difficulty continuing her pregnancy. However, her obstetrician should monitor her for complications and consult a cardiologist if symptoms worsen.

In the United States, peripartum cardiomyopathy leads to death in 25% to 50% of affected women (Homans, 1985). In others, it may resolve spontaneously, leaving no effects. A client with this disorder should consider future pregnancies carefully because relapses may occur.

Diabetes mellitus

The most common endocrine disorder in obstetrics, diabetes mellitus occurs in 1 out of approximately every 300 pregnancies (Hibbard, 1988). Although the introduction of insulin therapy for diabetes has reduced fetal mortality from 33% to less than 5% (Swislocki and Kraemer, 1989), the risk of congenital anomalies remains high in clients with insulin-dependent diabetes mellitus (IDDM). However, strict control of maternal serum glucose levels before conception and especially during the first trimester can help reduce this risk. Also, careful medical and nursing care can help the client manage her disorder successfully and deliver a normal, healthy neonate.

Pathophysiology

Diabetes mellitus results from inadequate insulin secretion by the beta cells of the islets of Langerhans in the pancreas or from ineffective use of insulin at the cellular level. Insulin regulates glucose and its transfer from the blood to body cells, all of which use glucose for energy. It also stimulates protein synthesis and free fatty acid storage in the fat deposits.

Insulin deficiency compromises access to essential nutrients for all body tissues. Without insulin, glucose circulates in the blood stream, unable to enter the cells. The energy-starved cells catabolize fats and proteins for energy, causing ketosis from fat wasting and negative nitrogen balance from protein breakdown and muscle tissue wasting.

The high level of circulating glucose leads to hyperglycemia, which exerts an osmotic force, pulling intracellular fluid into the blood and causing cellular dehydration. When the circulating glucose level exceeds the renal threshold, glucose spills into the urine, causing glycosuria. The urine's high osmotic level prevents reabsorption of water into the renal tubules, causing extracellular dehydration.

These changes produce the four classic signs and symptoms of diabetes:
• polyuria (frequent urination), which develops because the renal tubules do not reabsorb water
• polydipsia (excessive thirst), which is caused by the dehydration of polyuria
• polyphagia (excessive hunger), which results from tissue catabolism and inadequate cellular use of glucose
• weight loss, which occurs when the body burns fat and muscle tissues for energy.

Classifications

The National Diabetes Data Group (1979) classifies diabetes and other types of glucose intolerance as follows.
• Diabetes mellitus. This disorder may take three forms: type I, insulin-dependent diabetes mellitus (IDDM); type II, non-insulin-dependent diabetes mellitus; and secondary diabetes, or diabetes resulting from another condition, such as a pancreatic, hormonal, or insulin-receptor disorder.
• Impaired glucose tolerance (IGT). Formerly called latent or borderline diabetes, this asymptomatic disorder is characterized by normal or slightly elevated fasting levels of plasma glucose but abnormal glucose tolerance test values.
• Gestational diabetes mellitus (GDM). This disorder begins or is first diagnosed during pregnancy. A client with GDM may be asymptomatic except for impaired glucose tolerance. GDM has great implications for pregnancy because even mild diabetes increases the risk of fetal or neonatal morbidity and mortality. GDM may resolve after childbirth or may become IGT or type I or II diabetes mellitus.

Effects of pregnancy on diabetes

All pregnant women experience dramatic changes in carbohydrate, lipid, and protein metabolism. A pregnant diabetic woman is susceptible to hypoglycemia (abnormally low serum glucose level) and hyperglycemia (abnormally high serum glucose level). In some women, however, the growing fetus stresses maternal glucose production and use, disrupting normal carbohydrate metabolism and causing GDM. (For more information, see Chapter 17, Physiologic Changes during Normal Pregnancy.)

In a diabetic client, pregnancy can affect insulin needs. Early in pregnancy, estrogen and progesterone serum levels increase, causing hyperinsulinemia (increased maternal insulin secretion). At the same time, morning sickness may decrease food intake. These changes substantially decrease the need for insulin. Later in pregnancy, human placental lactogen (hPL) levels increase. This hormonal antagonist reduces insulin's effectiveness, stimulates lipolysis, and increases the circulation of free fatty acids. At the same time, the client's food intake usually improves, and maternal and fetal glycogen storage increases. Together, these changes increase the need for insulin (Mestman, 1985). By the third trimester, insulin requirements increase.

Pregnancy also can hasten vascular changes associated with diabetes. Because of this, the diabetic client must be evaluated for hypertension, nephropathy, and retinopathy throughout her pregnancy.

Effects of diabetes on pregnancy

If diabetes is not adequately managed before conception and during pregnancy, it increases fetal and neonatal risks. Preconception diabetic management maintains the client's health and prepares her for pregnancy, allowing fetal development to proceed normally. Blood glucose control throughout pregnancy reduces the risk of congenital anomalies and complications to the same level as that of the general population.

Maternal effects

The severity of the diabetes determines the degree of maternal effects. Uncontrolled diabetes or diabetes associated with vascular damage increases the risk of complications. However, comprehensive health care can control and lessen these risks.

Uncontrolled diabetes causes maternal hyperglycemia, increases the amount of circulating ketones from fatty acid metabolism, and results in ketosis. Decreased gastric motility (a normal change of pregnancy) and hPL's antagonistic effect on insulin further increase circulating glucose, predisposing the client to increased

ketosis. Without treatment, she may become comatose, and she or her fetus may die.

Hydramnios (excess amniotic fluid) occurs in about 10% of pregnant diabetic women. Amniotic fluid volume increases to more than 1,500 ml. Although the exact cause of hyramnios is unknown, it may result from increased maternal and fetal circulating blood sugar, which increases fetal urine in the amniotic fluid. The added fluid may increase maternal discomfort later in pregnancy. Also, it occasionally leads to premature rupture of the membranes and premature labor. Although amniocentesis may reduce fluid volume, it is not commonly used for this purpose because it increases the risk of infection, labor stimulation, and placental injury.

The vascular changes of diabetes produce PIH in 20% to 30% of pregnant diabetic clients. (For more information about PIH, see Chapter 23, Antepartal Complications.)

Glycosuria predisposes the pregnant diabetic client to infections, especially monilia vaginitis and urinary tract infections. These non-life-threatening infections usually can be controlled with perineal hygiene, increased fluid intake, and anti-infective agents.

Fetal and neonatal effects

Maternal diabetes may have many adverse effects on the fetus and neonate. It increases the incidence of fetal anomalies and neonatal morbidity and predisposes the neonate to diabetes. Without careful management, it increases the risk of fetal or neonatal death. Neonates born to women with advanced diabetes may display intrauterine growth retardation (IUGR).

Neonates born to mothers with poorly controlled diabetes usually have macrosomia (large body size and birth weight), causing cephalopelvic disproportion and uterine dystocia and requiring cesarean delivery. Macrosomia can affect all fetal organs except the brain. The degree of macrosomia appears to correlate with the degree of maternal hyperglycemia and lack of maternal vascular disease.

Maternal hypoglycemia also leads to life-threatening situations, including lack of fetal nutrition and possible hypotension leading to fetal distress if the mother loses consciousness.

Neonatal hyperbilirubinemia and hypoglycemia also are possible effects of maternal diabetes. Hyperbilirubinemia results when the neonate's immature liver does not metabolize bilirubin. Hypoglycemia may occur after the umbilical cord is severed at delivery because the neonate's pancreas may continue to secrete insulin for a brief time after the maternal glucose supply stops.

Treatment

Because selective screening may miss previously undiagnosed diabetes, all pregnant clients should be screened for glucose intolerance with a 1-hour (50-gram) diabetes screening test. If screening reveals glucose intolerance, treatment should begin.

For known diabetic clients, treatment may include diet changes, increased exercise, home glucose monitoring, and insulin administration before and during pregnancy to help ensure maternal and fetal health. During pregnancy, it also should include regular fetal evaluations.

Diet

A pregnant client with IDDM should ingest 35 calories/kg of her ideal body weight, or 2,200 to 2,400 calories daily; one with gestational diabetes should ingest 2,000 to 2,200 calories daily. Of these calories, 20% should be from proteins, 50% to 60% from complex carbohydrates, and 25% to 30% from fats (Samuels and Landon, 1986). The client should divide her daily intake into three meals and three snacks, with 25% of calories ingested at breakfast, 30% at lunch, 30% at dinner, and 15% in snacks, especially at bedtime to prevent hypoglycemia during sleep (Gabbe, 1985). The goal of this diet is to regulate blood glucose levels even though protein, carbohydrates, and fats are metabolized at different rates.

Exercise

A diabetic pregnant client should exercise because exercise helps reduce the need for insulin and helps regulate post-meal glucose levels (Schneider and Kitzmiller, 1989). If she exercised before pregnancy, she should continue her usual program. If she did not exercise before pregnancy, she should ease into nonstressful activities under her physician's guidance.

Because muscles use glucose for energy, exercise can decrease blood glucose levels. To correct any glucose deficiencies, the client must report pre- and post-exercise glucose levels to her physician, who can suggest compensatory dietary or insulin dosage changes.

Home glucose monitoring

Home glucose monitoring is an accurate, convenient way to determine the diabetic client's response to treatment. The nurse should provide the client with guidelines for acceptable blood glucose ranges and instruct her to report abnormal values to her physician.

An insulin-dependent diabetic client should monitor her glucose level four times a day, usually after fasting and meals. A client with any other type of diabetes should monitor her blood glucose as prescribed by her physician.

Insulin administration

The goal in diabetes treatment is to keep blood glucose levels within the normal range for pregnancy. If diet management cannot accomplish this goal, insulin therapy should be initiated (Gabbe, 1986). Results of home glucose monitoring enable the physician to prescribe insulin dosages that will meet the client's needs. Insulin therapy for the diabetic pregnant client uses highly purified animal or human insulin preparations, which are less allergenic than synthetic preparations and decrease the risk of maternal allergic reactions. Oral hypoglycemic agents cause prolonged hypoglycemia in the fetus if exposed near term and should not be used during pregnancy.

Insulin is administered subcutaneously. Typically, the client needs a mixture of intermediate-acting (NPH) and short-acting (regular) insulin in the morning and evening. Usually, two-thirds of the total insulin dosage is taken at breakfast, with the remaining third at dinner. Some physicians may prescribe continuous insulin therapy using an insulin pump and regular insulin to maintain blood glucose levels throughout pregnancy.

Fetal evaluation

For a diabetic client, regular fetal evaluations are particularly important. Tests for fetal well-being typically include ultrasonography, biophysical profile, fetal movement count, non-stress test, nipple stimulation contraction stress test, and oxytocin contraction test.

Anemia

Various anemias may predate the pregnancy or develop during it, including iron deficiency, folic acid deficiency, and sickle cell. They may affect the client and her fetus or neonate in different ways. (For more information, see *Maternal, fetal, and neonatal effects of anemias*, page 514.) However, an anemic client may complete an uneventful pregnancy if her condition is managed carefully with adequate nutrition and effective health care.

Iron deficiency anemia

This form of anemia results from an inadequate supply of iron for optimal formation of red blood cells (RBCs), producing smaller (microcytic) cells. Insufficient iron stores lead to a depleted RBC mass and, in turn, to a decreased concentration of hemoglobin, which normally transports oxygen throughout the body.

Maternal, fetal, and neonatal effects of anemias

Iron deficiency anemia, folic acid deficiency anemia, and sickle cell anemia can produce various maternal, fetal, and neonatal effects as described in the chart below.

ANEMIA	MATERNAL EFFECTS	FETAL AND NEONATAL EFFECTS
Iron deficiency anemia	• Poor tissue integrity • Tissue damage at birth • Antepartal or postpartal infection with impaired healing • Excessive bleeding after delivery	• Spontaneous abortion, stillbirth, or small-for-gestational-age (SGA) neonate • Intact fetal iron stores • Fetal distress from hypoxia during later pregnancy and labor, when hemoglobin fails to carry sufficient oxygen to the mother and fetus
Folic acid deficiency anemia	• Urinary tract and other infections • Bleeding complications during delivery • Pancytopenia (reduction of all cellular components of the blood) resulting from immature red blood cell production	• Spontaneous abortion and abruptio placentae complications
Sickle cell anemia	• Pregnancy-induced hypertension • Pulmonary emboli • Pneumonia • Urinary tract infection • Postpartal uterine infection	• Abruptio placentae complications • Intrauterine growth retardation • Prematurity • SGA neonate • Compromised fetal safety that can cause stillbirth and neonatal death when client's crises interfere with general vascular supply

Etiology

Pregnancy greatly increases the body's need for iron, and a client may not have adequate iron stores to meet the greater need. Without iron supplementation, the client may develop iron deficiency anemia.

Clinical findings

A client with iron deficiency anemia may tire easily and be susceptible to infection and postpartal bleeding. Even minimal blood loss during childbirth may cause an already anemic client to experience difficulty, including decreased blood pressure and dizziness. Other signs and symptoms may include weakness, headache, shortness of breath on exertion, anorexia, pica (craving to eat nonfood substances), irritability, and pallor.

Anemia is diagnosed by blood tests after a thorough health history and physical examination. When iron deficiency anemia is present, the hemoglobin level is below 11 g/liter, and the hematocrit drops below 32%.

Treatment

Supplemental iron should be administered to an anemic client before conception to maintain normal hemoglobin concentration. It should be continued during pregnancy. Daily oral doses of 200 mg of elemental iron, supplied in 1 g of ferrous sulfate or 2 g of ferrous gluconate,

provide the necessary requirements for a pregnant client with anemia. Divided doses help prevent or decrease adverse gastrointestinal (GI) effects, such as nausea and constipation.

An anemic client also should receive diet counseling. The nurse should teach her about iron-rich foods and encourage her to include them in her diet. (For more information, see Chapter 20, Nutrition and Diet Counseling.)

Folic acid deficiency anemia

Also known as megaloblastic anemia, pernicious anemia of pregnancy, or macrocytic anemia, folic acid deficiency anemia is rare in the United States (Cunningham, MacDonald, and Gant, 1989). Women with multiple gestation and those with hemoglobinopathies or other hemolytic disorders are especially susceptible to developing folic acid deficiency anemia (Cruikshank, 1986b).

Etiology

The body uses folic acid to break down and use proteins and to form nucleic acids and heme for hemoglobin. A deficiency may result from inadequate intake of animal protein and uncooked fresh vegetables, malabsorption, or a metabolic abnormality. When deficiency occurs, immature RBCs fail to divide and are released as enlarged cells (megaloblasts). Because they are fragile, many cells are destroyed before they are released into the bloodstream.

During pregnancy, the need for folic acid increases because of tremendous cell multiplication and accelerated erythropoiesis and deoxyribonucleic acid synthesis by the fetus and placenta (Cruikshank, 1986a). This places the pregnant client at risk for folic acid deficiency.

Clinical findings

Folic acid deficiency anemia gradually produces clinical findings, such as decreased hemoglobin levels despite sufficient iron intake, GI distress (including anorexia, nausea, and vomiting), fatigue, weakness, and pallor. In advanced stages, dyspnea and edema may appear.

Treatment

To prevent folic acid deficiency anemia, the client should take 400 mcg of folic acid daily during pregnancy. To treat anemia, she should receive 1 mg of folic acid three times daily. Because iron deficiency anemia almost always coexists with folic acid deficiency anemia, the client also should receive iron supplements.

The nurse should encourage the client to eat foods high in folic acid. (For more information, see Chapter 20, Nutrition and Diet Counseling.) The nurse also should teach the client to use little or no water in cooking because folic acid is a water-soluble vitamin that can be removed from foods as they cook.

Sickle cell anemia

Sickle cell anemia is characterized by recurring acute, painful, vaso-occlusive attacks known as crises. This disorder can cause organ damage and death. Some pregnant clients with sickle cell anemia can carry to term safely, if they receive careful management. However, nearly one-half the pregnancies of clients with sickle cell anemia end in abortion, stillbirth, or neonatal death. Yet maternal mortality from sickle cell anemia has decreased since 1972 from about 6% to about 1% (Cunningham, MacDonald, and Gant, 1989).

Etiology

This autosomal recessive disease (inherited from both parents) occurs almost exclusively among individuals of African or Mediterranean descent, especially Blacks. Between 6% and 13% of Black Americans carry the sickle cell trait (heterozygous state of the recessive disorder); 0.2% have sickle cell anemia (Kelton and Cruickshank, 1988).

Sickle cell anemia causes a structural abnormality in hemoglobin molecules (hemoglobin S), causing RBCs

to roughen and become sickle- or crescent-shaped. This shape affects the oxygen-carrying capacity and survival of the hemoglobin. It also causes RBC tangling that obstructs blood flow in small blood vessels and organs of high oxygen extraction, such as the spleen, bone marrow, and placenta.

Various factors may precipitate vessel obstruction and subsequent sickle cell crisis. These include infection, stress, dehydration, trauma, fever, fatigue, and strenuous activity. Crisis produces blood stasis, platelet aggregation, local hypoxia, edema, extreme pain, and tissue infarction.

Clinical findings

A pregnant client with sickle cell anemia is likely to experience crises during the second half of her pregnancy, although they may occur at any time. Sickle cell crises are characterized by acute, painful, recurring vaso-occlusive attacks that affect the extremities, abdomen, chest, and vertebrae. The client also may experience fever, dehydration, debilitation, hypertension, anemia, pulmonary problems, and osteomyelitis (bone infection).

Sickle cell anemia is diagnosed through laboratory testing with hemoglobin electrophoresis, which can distinguish between sickle cell anemia and sickle cell trait.

Treatment

The client can reduce the frequency of sickle cell crises by avoiding the precipitating factors. During a crisis, the client may need hydration, analgesics, and treatment of infection. Acetaminophen (Tylenol) relieves mild pain; meperidine (Demerol) with a sedative controls severe pain. She also may need a transfusion of RBCs.

During a sickle cell crisis, fetal status should be monitored. Unless the client is in labor or has an arterial oxygen level below 70 mm Hg, antepartal oxygen administration is not necessary.

Infection

Throughout pregnancy, the client should take measures to avoid infection. (For general information, see Chapter 12, Infectious Disorders. For antepartal information, see *Maternal, fetal, and neonatal effects of infections,* pages 516 to 520.) If infection occurs despite these measures, the client should be evaluated and treated promptly to prevent maternal and fetal complications. The most common

(Text continues on page 521.)

Maternal, fetal, and neonatal effects of infections

The following chart compares the maternal, fetal, and neonatal effects of TORCH, human immunodeficiency virus, and selected genitourinary infections as well as their nursing considerations.

MATERNAL EFFECTS	FETAL AND NEONATAL EFFECTS	NURSING CONSIDERATIONS
TORCH: Toxoplasmosis		
Spontaneous abortion (with widely disseminated infection in early pregnancy) and possibly fatal complications (in an immunosuppressed client)	Stillbirth, premature birth, microcephaly (abnormally small head), hydrocephaly (abnormally large head with accumulation of cerebrospinal fluid in the brain), hypotonia, seizures, coma, mental retardation, blindness, deafness, or chorioretinitis (choroid and retina inflammation)	• Evaluate each client at risk for the disease to ensure prompt identification. • Instruct the client to cook meat thoroughly to kill bacteria. • Teach the client to avoid contact with cat box filler, especially if the cats roam outside. Advise the client to wear gloves while gardening. Infected cat box filler or soil may come into contact with hand cuts or contaminate food during preparation.
TORCH: Other—chlamydia		
Pelvic inflammatory disease, dysuria, spontaneous abortion, placental inflammation, and postpartal endometritis 2 to 6 weeks after delivery	Stillbirth, premature birth, neonatal mortality; pneumonia, conjunctivitis (7 to 15 days after birth), or otitis media (Benoit, 1988; CDC, 1989; McElhose, 1988)	• Advise the infected client that her partner also must be examined and treated. • Teach the client that the risk of chlamydia increases with the number of sexual partners and decreases with the use of a barrier method of contraception.
TORCH: Other—group B beta hemolytic streptococcus infection		
Increased risk of septic abortion, chorioamnionitis, postpartal endometritis, arthritis, pyelonephritis, pneumonia, meningitis, and endocarditis	Stillbirth or fetal infection; neonatal infection from delivery (McCracken and Freij, 1987); neonatal susceptibility to pneumonia and septicemia; invasive disease within 7 days of birth, which can lead to death; meningitis within about 24 days, which can lead to death (Simpson, Gaziano, Lupo, and Peterson, 1988)	• Be aware that risk factors include premature labor, premature rupture of membranes, and a prolonged period between membrane rupture and labor. • Remind the client that failure to report signs and symptoms or to appear for prenatal follow-up visits increases the risk of undiagnosed infection. • Be aware that treatment before delivery significantly reduces maternal and neonatal infections (Merenstein, Todd, Brown, Yost, and Luzier, 1980). • Be alert for signs of neonatal infection. Be prepared to intervene by notifying the physician and preparing for blood transfusion and I.V. antibiotic administration.
TORCH: Other—syphilis		
Second trimester spontaneous abortion	Stillbirth, premature labor and birth, congenital infection, and anomalies (if mother is untreated)	• Tell the client that treatment for syphilis typically includes benzathine penicillin G (Bicillin). If she is allergic to penicillin, she may be referred for desensitization before treatment begins. • Be aware that erythromycin is not recommended because of a high failure rate in curing fetal infection. Tetracycline is contraindicated in pregnant clients because of adverse effects on fetal teeth and bones, increased incidence of fetal inguinal hernias, and increases in maternal liver toxicity (Sharp, 1986). • Advise the client to return every month to be checked for reinfection. To assess the client, expect to use quantitative non-treponemal serologic tests, such as Venereal Disease Research Laboratories and rapid plasma reagin tests. • Advise the client that if she receives adequate antibiotic treatment during pregnancy, the risk to her neonate is low. • Instruct the client to observe for signs and symptoms of premature labor.

Maternal, fetal, and neonatal effects of infections continued

MATERNAL EFFECTS	FETAL AND NEONATAL EFFECTS	NURSING CONSIDERATIONS
TORCH: Other—varicella-zoster (herpes zoster, chicken pox) infection		
Possible death from severe varicella pneumonia	Congenital abnormalities, including limb deformity, cortical atrophy, eye abnormalities, skin lesions, and pneumonia (when varicella occurs in the first trimester); neonatal varicella that may lead to pneumonia, encephalitis, and possibly neonatal death (South and Sever, 1986)	• Be aware that maternal infection in the last 4 days of pregnancy and within 48 hours after delivery can cause neonatal varicella. (During its incubation period, the infection is contagious.) • Be aware that vaccines usually are not given during pregnancy. However, varicella-zoster vaccine is under investigation for use in pregnant clients. • Be aware that the disease is uncommon in adult women because 95% of them are immune to varicella (South and Sever, 1986). • Be aware that varicella-zoster immune globulin (VZIG) may be given prophylactically to a pregnant client.
TORCH: Rubella—German measles		
Spontaneous abortion	Congenital anomalies, including cardiac defects (pulmonary artery stenosis and patent ductus arteriosus), intrauterine growth retardation (IUGR), deafness, cataracts, glaucoma, and mental retardation (Pritchard, MacDonald, and Gant, 1985); delayed effects (possibly for decades), such as insulin-dependent diabetes mellitus, sudden hearing loss, glaucoma, and encephalitis (South and Sever, 1986)	• Advise the pregnant client to prevent this disease by avoiding contact with anyone known to have rubella. • Be aware that a negative antibody titer indicates that the client is not immune to rubella. An antibody titer of 1:16 or greater indicates immunity; of less than 1:8, susceptibility to rubella infection; between 1:16 and 1:8, low resistance to infection. A nonpregnant client with low resistance should be vaccinated. • Advise the client to obtain rubella vaccination after she has delivered. Advise her not to become pregnant for at least 3 months after receiving the vaccine, which contains the live, attenuated virus.
TORCH: Cytomegalovirus infection		
Transplacental transmission of disease to the fetus or transmission to the neonate during vaginal delivery	Severe, permanent damage in about 10% of infected neonates (Cunningham, MacDonald, and Gant, 1989); neonatal hepatosplenomegaly, jaundice, thrombocytopenia, microcephaly, hearing loss, mental retardation, cerebral palsy, epilepsy, blindness, and possibly death	• Be aware that cytomegalovirus can be transmitted by any close contact, including kissing, breastfeeding, and sexual intercourse. • Advise the infected client that she should not breast-feed her neonate because the virus can be transmitted through breast milk. • Be aware that the disease may be fatal to a fetus, although it usually is innocuous in adults and children. • Be aware that accurate diagnosis in a pregnant client is made by detecting cytomegalovirus in the urine, noting a rise in IgM levels, and identifying cytomegalovirus antibodies in a serum IgM fraction. • Advise the client that although no treatment exists for cytomegalovirus infection, her physician may prescribe immunotherapy or an antiviral agent. • Expect to isolate the mother and neonate after birth.
TORCH: Herpesvirus type 2 infection		
Discomfort from lesions during the pregnancy, increased inci-	Spontaneous abortion or stillbirth if herpesvirus type 2 becomes	• Be aware that the safety of systemic acyclovir (Zovirax) in pregnant clients has not been established. (continued)

Maternal, fetal, and neonatal effects of infections continued

MATERNAL EFFECTS	FETAL AND NEONATAL EFFECTS	NURSING CONSIDERATIONS
Herpesvirus (continued) dence of secondary infection, and increased likelihood of cesarean delivery because the virus can be transmitted to the neonate during vaginal delivery	active before 20 weeks' gestation (Stagno and Whitley, 1985); premature labor if the virus becomes active later in pregnancy; local infection of the skin, eyes, or mucous membranes (Whitley, et al., 1988); symptoms that develop after birth, such as fever or hypothermia, poor feeding, seizures, and jaundice	Therefore, acyclovir should be used only in a pregnant client with a life-threatening, disseminated infection, such as encephalitis, pneumonitis, or hepatitis. • Expect a vaginal delivery for a client with genital herpes but no lesions. On the day of delivery, obtain a herpesvirus culture from the client and the neonate. • Expect a client with active genital lesions at the time of labor or membrane rupture to have a cesarean delivery to reduce the risk of virus transmission to the neonate. Although cesarean delivery should be performed within 6 hours of membrane rupture, it may prevent neonatal herpes regardless of the duration of membrane rupture. • For a client with genital lesions at or near term but before labor or membrane rupture, collect cultures every 3 to 5 days to monitor viral activity and assess appropriateness of vaginal delivery, as prescribed. • Be aware that the mother and neonate need not be isolated from each other, although intimacy carries a small risk (about 0.1%) of neonatal infection. • Allow the infected mother to care for her neonate as long as she washes her hands thoroughly before and after touching the neonate. • Reassure the client that she may safely breast-feed her neonate because herpesvirus type 2 is not present in breast milk. • Be aware that the incubation period is 2 to 12 days. A neonate who is symptom-free at birth may display symptoms later.
Human immunodeficiency virus (HIV) infection		
Transplacental transmission of HIV to the fetus or transmission to the neonate through breast-feeding	Possibility of abandonment by parents who leave the neonate in the health care facility permanently, death within a few years (Minkoff, 1988)	• Identify the client at risk for HIV infection and expect serum HIV studies. Risk factors include sexual intercourse with an HIV-positive individual or contact with the infected blood, blood products, body fluids, or used needles from an HIV-positive individual. • Counsel the client about disease transmission to her fetus and partner. • Educate the client and staff about disease transmission to reduce its spread. • Take precautionary measures to prevent contamination from infected body fluids and blood during testing and hospitalization. Alert caregivers to blood and body fluid precautions. • Be aware that diagnosis may be made during pregnancy. Provide support and referrals to counseling for the client faced with the devastating information that she has a terminal illness and her fetus has a 50% probability of contracting the disease transplacentally. • Expect cord blood tests for maternal HIV antibodies at delivery, which indicate maternal infection. Also expect the neonate's blood to be tested for HIV antibodies after delivery and regularly thereafter. If the neonatal titer decreases after delivery, the neonate has not been infected. If it increases, the neonate is infected.

Maternal, fetal, and neonatal effects of infections continued

MATERNAL EFFECTS	FETAL AND NEONATAL EFFECTS	NURSING CONSIDERATIONS
Genitourinary infection: Trichomoniasis		
Possible premature rupture of membranes, postpartal endometritis	Neonatal pneumonia	• Be aware that trichomoniasis has been identified in 10% to 25% of childbearing women. • Advise the client to avoid sexual intercourse or to use condoms. • Reevaluate the couple to assess treatment effectiveness. • Test for gonorrhea and chlamydia, as prescribed, which commonly accompany this infection. • Tell the client to practice thorough perineal hygiene. • Inform the client that unless her partner has been treated effectively, the infection may recur.
Genitourinary infection: Gonorrhea		
Dysuria, urinary frequency and urgency; premature rupture of membranes associated with peripartal fever and chorioamnionitis	IUGR; neonatal sepsis, meningitis, or arthritis; ophthalmia neonatorum (from vaginal delivery); anal, vaginal, and nasopharyngeal infection	• Expect to conduct laboratory tests to rule out other sexually transmitted diseases and to retest late in the third trimester. • Treat the client as prescribed, usually with ceftriaxone I.M., followed by erythromycin for 7 days. Also treat her partner, typically with ceftriaxone and doxycycline. Re-evaluate them to assess treatment effectiveness.
Genitourinary infection: Condylomata acuminata		
Increased reproduction of genital warts; possible obstruction of birth canal by warts	Epithelial tumors of mucous membranes on larynx, genital warts, and laryngeal papillomatosis (rare)	• Expect to prepare the client for cryosurgery or laser treatments to remove warts because topical podophyllum resin can be toxic to the fetus. • Expect vaginal delivery except in a client whose condyloma obstruct the birth canal. Because the route of transmission of the infection is unknown, routine cesarean delivery has no preventive value for a client with condylomata acuminata. • Instruct the client to report recurrence of warts after treatment.
Genitourinary infection: Pediculosis pubis		
Skin irritation	Neurotoxicity if maternal condition is treated with lindane (Kwell) during pregnancy or breast-feeding	• Expect to substitute crotamiton (Eurax) for lindane to treat pediculosis pubis in a pregnant or breast-feeding client.
Genitourinary infection: Vaginitis (candidiasis)		
Increased discomforts of pregnancy caused by vaginal itching and discharge	Thrush from delivery if vaginal organisms enter the neonate's mouth	• Be aware that candidiasis commonly occurs in pregnant clients with diabetes mellitus. • Teach the client about candidiasis and support her during occurrences. • Expect to provide local anticandidal preparations for the client and her partner if he has candidal balanitis. • Tell the client to practice thorough perineal hygiene. • Reevaluate the client and her partner to assess treatment effectiveness and to detect recurrence. • Assess the neonate after delivery for signs of thrush, such as creamy, white, slightly elevated plaque inside the mouth, primarily on inner cheeks and tongue.

(continued)

Maternal, fetal, and neonatal effects of infections continued

MATERNAL EFFECTS	FETAL AND NEONATAL EFFECTS	NURSING CONSIDERATIONS
Genitourinary infection: Vaginitis (bacterial vaginosis)		
Alteration in normal cervical-vaginal environment	Teratogenic effects if the mother is treated with metronidazole (Flagyl) during the first trimester	• Instruct the client to practice thorough perineal hygiene. • Reevaluate the client to assess treatment effectiveness and to detect recurrence. • Be aware that metronidazole should not be administered during the first trimester but may be used in the later trimesters. Evaluate the client for possibility of pregnancy before treatment begins. • Be aware that treatment of the client's partner is not necessary because no counterpart of bacterial vaginosis is recognized in men.
Genitourinary infection: Vulvitis		
No specific effects	No specific effects	• Support the client through the gynecologic examination and diagnostic studies. • Teach her how to use medications, including vaginal creams and oral medications. • Reevaluate the client to assess treatment effectiveness and to detect recurrence. • Provide additional nursing care depending on the infecting organism.
Genitourinary infection: Pelvic inflammatory disease (PID)		
Sterility from tubal infection and scarring; other effects, depending on the infecting organism	Various effects, depending on the infecting organism	• Be aware that PID is rare in pregnancy because the cervical mucus plug prevents infection from ascending into the uterus. However, it may occur in the first weeks of pregnancy. • Instruct the client to receive treatment and take precautions to prevent reinfection. • As prescribed, test the client for chlamydia and herpes, which commonly are associated with PID. • Provide additional nursing care, depending on the infecting organism.
Genitourinary infection: Pyelonephritis		
Increased genitourinary and abdominal discomfort, possibly premature labor	Possible teratogenic effect if the mother is treated with sulfonamides, but evidence is not conclusive; because sulfonamides can cause increased free bilirubin and kernictus if given to a neonate, do not administer them to a client near term.	• Be aware that the incidence of pyelonephritis increases because of the urinary stasis that occurs during pregnancy. Those at highest risk are primigravid clients, clients with difficult labors, diabetic clients, and clients with sickle cell anemia. • Do not administer sulfonamides to a pregnant client near term. • Encourage the client to maintain bed rest, drink plenty of fluids, and report worsening of symptoms. • Reevaluate the client to assess the effectiveness of treatment with antibiotics, fluids, and rest and to detect recurrence. • Recommend urologic consultation after delivery to assess for permanent genitourinary changes caused by the infection. • Evaluate for preterm labor and expect treatment with tocolytics, if necessary. • Assess the neonate for elevated bilirubin levels after birth.

or potentially harmful infections during pregnancy are TORCH, human immunodeficiency virus (HIV), and genitourinary infections.

TORCH infections

The acronym TORCH refers to toxoplasmosis, other infections (chlamydia, group B beta hemolytic streptococcus, syphilis, and varicella zoster), rubella, cytomegalovirus, and herpesvirus type 2 infections. These infections can cause major congenital anomalies or death of the embryo or fetus.

HIV infection

HIV infection can cause acquired immunodeficiency syndrome (AIDS), a life-threatening disease that affects the body's immune system, rendering it susceptible to opportunistic infections.

In the first 6 months of 1988, women accounted for more than 10% of reported HIV cases (Cates and Schulz, 1988). The percentage may be higher because many women who carry the virus are asymptomatic.

Genitourinary and other infections

Genitourinary infections include sexually transmitted diseases (STDs), gynecologic infections, and urinary tract infections. Some of these infections, such as gonorrhea and herpes, can be passed to the fetus as it traverses the birth canal.

Substance abuse

When a pregnant woman abuses a substance, it can affect her as well as her fetus and neonate. (For more information, see Chapter 15, Women's Health-Compromising Behaviors and *Maternal, fetal, and neonatal effects of substance abuse,* pages 522 and 523.)

Maternal risks

A pregnant client who abuses substances may suffer physical, psychological, social, and economic consequences. In addition, she may have a spontaneous abortion or premature delivery, or she may develop PIH, hemorrhage, or abruptio placentae.

A pregnant substance abuser is likely to neglect prenatal care because she fears admonishment from health care professionals, lacks the self-esteem to make personal health care a priority, or views prenatal care as unimportant and unnecessary. Yet such a client has a greater need for care because of possible exposure to HIV, STDs, hepatitis, malnutrition, and infection from injection sites—as well as risk of hypertension, antepartal bleeding, abruptio placentae, spontaneous abortion or stillbirth, and preterm labor (Finnegan and Wapner, 1987; Ronkins, Fitzsimmons, Wapner, and Finnegan, 1988). These factors and risks may arise from poor health, inadequate nutrition, infection, shared needles, multiple sex partners, and drug abuse and its effects.

Fetal and neonatal risks

First-trimester substance abuse has teratogenic effects on the fetus and increases the risk of spontaneous abortion. Use of cocaine may cause chromosomal abnormalities, leading to major genitourinary malformations (Chasnoff, Burns, and Burns, 1987; Chasnoff, Griffith, MacGregor, Dirkes, and Burns, 1989).

Maternal substance abuse may cause problems for the neonate as well, including IUGR, premature birth, and withdrawal symptoms. (For more information, see Chapter 38, High-Risk Neonates.)

Treatment

If a pregnant substance abuser seeks health care, the nurse should obtain baseline data and suggest ways to correct her health deficits. For example, the nurse may encourage her to join a drug rehabilitation program to control her substance abuse or may provide nutrition counseling and information about vitamin and iron supplements that may be prescribed. The nurse should encourage her to schedule appointments, as necessary, and inform her that she may have to provide a urine specimen for drug screening at each visit to identify the presence, type, and amount of drug abused.

For a client with an opiate or heroin addiction, a controlled substance withdrawal method with methadone administration may be recommended. "Cold turkey" withdrawal is not recommended during pregnancy because of the risk of fetal seizures, hypoxia, and death. A client receiving methadone also should participate in group counseling sessions. A multidisciplinary approach provides comprehensive physical, psychological, social, and economic care to the pregnant substance abuser.

Maternal, fetal, and neonatal effects of substance abuse

Many abused substances can affect the client and her fetus or neonate, as described in the chart below.

SUBSTANCE	MATERNAL EFFECTS	FETAL AND NEONATAL EFFECTS
Depressants		
Ethanol (alcohol)	Spontaneous abortion	Stillbirth, intrauterine growth retardation (IUGR), short palpebral fissures, microcephaly, mild to moderate mental retardation, irritability, poor coordination, fetal alcohol syndrome (Rodgers and Lee, 1988)
Narcotics heroin, methadone hydrochloride (Dolophine)	Spontaneous abortion, premature rupture of membranes, preterm labor, infections of the placenta, chorion, and amnion	Low birth weight, IUGR, withdrawal symptoms (vomiting, tremors, sneezing, increased muscle tone), seizures, respiratory distress, meconium aspiration with abrupt drug withdrawal, perinatal morbidity and mortality (Finnegan, 1986; Rodgers and Lee, 1988)
Barbiturates phenobarbital (Luminal)	Drowsiness, lethargy, and other reactions such as vertigo, headache, and CNS depression; benefits from use in pregnancy acceptable despite fetal risks if used for serious disorders, such as seizures	Central nervous system depression, seizures, withdrawal symptoms, hyperactivity, decreased sucking reflex, possible teratogenic effects, delayed lung maturity (Wapner and Finnegan, 1982)
Tranquilizers chlordiazepoxide (Librium), diazepam (Valium)	If client overdoses, prolonged hypoxia, malnutrition, poor weight gain, cross-dependence on alcohol and barbiturates	Same as for barbiturates, plus tremors, irritability, tachypnea, poor weight gain, sudden infant death syndrome (SIDS), decreased sucking reflex, hypotonia, hypothermia (Wapner and Finnegan, 1982)
Mixed narcotic agonist-antagonists pentazocine (Talwin)	Cellulitis, abscesses of arms resulting in infections	Low birth weight, IUGR, addiction (Wapner and Finnegan, 1982)
Stimulants		
Amphetamines amphetamine sulfate (Benzedrine)	Malnutrition, possible ventricular tachycardia and asytole during obstetric anesthesia	Congenital abnormalities, especially cardiac defects and oral clefts (Rodgers and Lee, 1988)
dextroamphetamine sulfate (Dexedrine)	Insufficient nutrition; serious cardiac arrhythmias, ventricular tachycardia, and withdrawal symptoms, including lethargy and profound depression	Withdrawal symptoms, low birth weight, IGUR from poor maternal nutrition, congenital heart defects (Rodgers and Lee, 1988)
Cocaine	Vasoconstriction leading to tachycardia, hypertension, dilated pupils and muscle twitching; myocardial infarction; cardiac and respiratory arrest; increased spontaneous abortion, abruptio placentae, preterm labor	Stillbirth; genitourinary problems, including prune-belly syndrome (congenital absence of abdominal musculature, causing distended, flabby abdomen that is creased like a prune) and hydronephrosis (Chasnoff, Griffith, MacGregor, Dirkes, and Burns, 1989); SIDS; depressed interactive behaviors (Rodgers and Lee, 1988)

Maternal, fetal, and neonatal effects of substance abuse continued

SUBSTANCE	MATERNAL EFFECTS	FETAL AND NEONATAL EFFECTS
Nicotine	Increased risk of neonatal mortality (20 or fewer cigarettes daily); decreased placental perfusion, abruptio placentae, placenta previa, functional anemia, premature rupture of membranes, preterm labor, spontaneous abortion (more than 20 cigarettes daily)	Reduced fetal breathing movements, small for gestational age, low birth weight, increased risk of SIDS, possible death (Rodgers and Lee, 1988)
Psychotropics		
Cannabis sativa (marijuana)	Cross-dependence on nicotine and alcohol	Possible teratogenic effects, prematurity, potential for meconium in amniotic fluid and for meconium aspiration (Wapner and Finnegan, 1982)
lysergic acid diethylamide (LSD)	Possible spontaneous abortion	Possible prematurity, chromosomal damage or anomalies (Rodgers and Lee, 1988)

Trauma or need for surgery

A pregnant client suffering from trauma or requiring surgery needs special management. The nurse must be aware of special considerations to provide appropriate care for such a client. (For more information, see *Effects of trauma on pregnancy*, page 524.)

Trauma

Trauma may result from accidental injury, physical abuse, or other factors. If the injury is major, it can endanger maternal and fetal health. Therefore, a pregnant client who suffers trauma needs immediate, expert health care.

Accidental injury is a major cause of trauma during pregnancy, occurring in 6% to 8% of all pregnancies (Neufeld, Moore, Marx, and Rosen, 1987). For a client who suffers accidental injury, the nurse should focus on maintaining the pregnancy and ensuring maternal and fetal health.

Physical abuse is another common cause of trauma during pregnancy. (For more information, see Chapter 14, Violence Against Women.) For an abused client, the nurse should focus on detecting any evidence of damage to the pregnancy, such as vaginal bleeding.

Surgery

Baden and Brodsky (1985) report that between 25,000 and 50,000 pregnant women undergo surgery each year in the United States for nonobstetric problems. (For more information, see *Nursing considerations for the pregnant client requiring surgery*, page 525.) Common surgeries during pregnancy include ovarian cyst removal, acute appendectomy, breast surgery, repairs of incompetent cervix, and surgery for cholecystitis (Rice and Pellegrini, 1985; Willson and Carrington, 1987).

Because of the risks, surgery should be postponed until after delivery, whenever possible, and nonsurgical interventions should be used. Such interventions may include rest, I.V. therapy, antibiotics, and gastric decompression via nasogastric tube. If these measures fail to control the client's condition, they may be used to provide relief until further evaluation is completed and surgery can be performed.

If surgery becomes necessary, the health care team should take a multidisciplinary approach to client preparation. Before surgery, consultants from anesthesiology, perinatology, cardiology, and internal medicine may evaluate maternal and fetal risks to reduce the probability of complications.

Then preoperative care may begin. Chest X-rays and electrocardiography (ECG) may be required if concerns exist about the client's cardiopulmonary status. During a chest X-ray, the client will wear a shield over her abdomen to protect the fetus from radiation.

Effects of trauma on pregnancy

Common causes of trauma during pregnancy include accidental injuries and physical abuse and its psychological stress. The chart below details typical injuries, their effects on pregnancy, and nursing considerations.

COMMON INJURIES	EFFECTS ON PREGNANCY	NURSING CONSIDERATIONS
Accidental injury		
• Falls resulting from too-flexible joints and a displaced center of gravity (Falls may cause fractures of the ankles, legs, or arms, but usually leave the fetus unharmed.) • Blunt abdominal trauma • Crushing injuries from vehicular accidents	• Depending on injury severity and gestational age, maternal and fetal death or fetal death from abruptio placentae • With blunt abdominal trauma during the third trimester, uterine and fetal injury • With fractured pelvis, abruptio placentae, ruptured bladder, retroperitoneal hemorrhage, and shock • With severe head trauma or internal injury hemorrhage, possible maternal death • With severe abdominal trauma sustained during a vehicular accident, uterine rupture and placental separation from the abdominal wall, spontaneous membrane rupture, premature labor, and severely jeopardized fetal health	• Be aware that any trauma may be fatal to the pregnant client and her fetus. Promptly assess and treat the injury as prescribed to decrease the maternal and fetal morbidity and mortality probability. • Ensure an adequate airway and provide oxygen as necessary. • Obtain an accurate clinical and obstetric history to evaluate maternal health. • Assist with a thorough physical assessment and review pertinent diagnostic studies to evaluate maternal health further. • Use electronic fetal monitoring to assess fetal status, as prescribed. • Assess the client's orientation, and inform her of treatment measures and plans for her care. • Position the client on her left side if possible, or insert a wedge under her right hip to decrease aortocaval pressure from the gravid uterus and to increase vascular volume. • Administer I.V. fluids and insert an indwelling urinary catheter, as prescribed. Follow other standard protocols of the health care facility. • Provide continual support throughout the initial period to calm an anxious client. • Perform comfort measures to decrease the amount of pain medication required. Consult with the obstetrician and surgeon about the best pain medications for the client.
Physical abuse		
• Burns • Lacerations • Contusions • Fractures • Head injuries • Dislocations • Penetrating injuries, such as stab or gunshot wounds • Stress-related disorders, such as headaches, insomnia, depression, and suicidal thoughts	• In early pregnancy, possibly no fetal harm because uterus is low in abdominal cavity and protected by amniotic fluid, organs, muscles, and bony pelvis • During late pregnancy, fetal harm because the uterus is protected less by the thinner abdominal wall (Amniotic fluid protects the fetus, unless substantial trauma occurs.) • Compromised fetal development if the client cannot eat or has multiple areas of bleeding • Spontaneous abortion from uterine rupture or placental separation	• Same as for accidental injury. • Remember that late in pregnancy, the gravid uterus is most likely to sustain injury from penetrating abdominal wounds (Slater and Aufses, 1985). • Advise the physically abused client that any physical or psychological abuse is abnormal and harmful to her mental and physical well-being.

Nursing considerations for the pregnant client requiring surgery

Certain physiologic changes of pregnancy may make surgery difficult. The chart below shows how the nurse can overcome these difficulties when caring for the pregnant client who requires surgery.

PHYSIOLOGIC CHANGE OF PREGNANCY	EFFECT ON THE CLIENT	NURSING CONSIDERATIONS
Decreased gastric motility	Increased risk of gastric regurgitation and chemical pneumonitis from pulmonary aspiration of acidic gastric contents	• Expect to administer an antacid to increase gastric pH and decrease the risk of chemical pneumonitis if the client vomits and aspirates during surgery. • Insert a nasogastric tube, as prescribed, for gastric decompression before and during surgery. • Assist with endotracheal intubation, rapid anesthesia induction, or use of regional anesthesia, as prescribed
Weight gain	Difficulty with endotracheal intubation	• Perform a presurgical examination to assist with pulmonary assessment.
Decreased functional pulmonary residual capacity, which can impair oxygenation	Further decrease in functional capacity with general anesthesia and remaining in the supine position	• Oxygenate the client, as prescribed, before anesthesia. • Expect to place a pillow under the client's right hip or tilt the operating room table to the left. • Expect the client to receive regional anesthesia, which reduces hyperventilation, improves maternal oxygenation, and benefits the fetus. This is preferred to general anesthesia in cases where increased cardiac work load is detrimental to the client.
Increased blood volume	Tolerance to blood loss during surgery	• Be aware that the pregnant client may not need blood transfusions as readily as the nonpregnant client.
Aortocaval compression by gravid uterus when the client lies supine	Impaired blood circulation and perfusion	• Expect to place a pillow under the client's right hip or tilt the operating room table to the left to displace the uterus, decreasing vessel compression and maintaining adequate perfusion to the heart, uterus, and placenta. • Use electronic fetal heart rate monitoring during and after surgery to evaluate for fetal distress, as prescribed.
Organ displacement	Difficulty in locating the appendix in a client with appendicitis	• Be aware that after the fifth month of pregnancy the appendix lies at the iliac crest level and continues to rise above it during the last trimester.

Laboratory tests can rule out some potential problems, such as anemia and infection, and provide preoperative baseline data.

When surgery is needed, the risk of maternal, fetal, and neonatal morbidity and mortality depends on the stage of the pregnancy and the surgical procedure. Because controversy exists over the fetal risks of various anesthetics in the first trimester, non-emergency surgery should be postponed until the second trimester, which also protects against spontaneous abortion and possible teratogenic effects from medications. Even for abdominal surgery, the second-trimester uterus should not be large enough to interfere with the operative site. Although surgery may induce premature labor, no evidence suggests that a higher incidence of fetal malformations is associated with anesthesia and surgery.

Nursing care

Ideally, all clients should be evaluated for disease and abnormalities before they conceive. Then, nursing care could strive to correct deficiencies and avoid complications. Sometimes, however, the client is first seen after she is pregnant and has a disease that complicates her pregnancy or endangers her fetus. Whether the nurse first sees the client before she is pregnant or during her pregnancy, the nurse can use the nursing process to deliver high-quality care.

Assessment

To build a useful, current assessment data base, obtain a detailed health history, perform a thorough physical examination, and review appropriate diagnostic studies. (For detailed information, see Chapter 19, Care during the Normal Antepartal Period.)

Health history

Begin by assessing the client's present health status and comparing it with her personal and family health history. This may uncover a previously undetected problem and suggest the need for specific tests. For example, the client with a history of recurring infections (mainly pneumonia and urinary tract infections), bleeding, increased fatigue, poor healing, and general poor health may have undiagnosed anemia. A primigravid client who reports the classic symptoms of diabetes (polyuria, polydipsia, polyphagia, and weight loss) and has a family history of diabetes should receive the 3-hour glucose tolerance test.

Next, ask the client to identify any problems for which she is receiving care, such as a cardiac disease or diabetes. Then investigate signs and symptoms caused by this problem. Note any change in the degree of signs and symptoms, such as increased fatigue, decreased activity tolerance, increased dependent edema, and increased shortness of breath, which may occur during the second and third trimester in a client with cardiac disease. Also, determine if these signs and symptoms resolve with rest. The stress of pregnancy can exacerbate the effects of some disorders, requiring treatment adjustments.

Evaluate the effectiveness of the client's current regimen in managing any previously diagnosed condition. For example, if the client has a congenital heart defect, determine if her treatment has corrected arrhythmias and signs of heart failure. This information may require treatment modifications.

Inquire into the client's past and present obstetric history. Particularly query any obstetric problems, such as spontaneous abortion or stillbirth, that may have been related to an undiagnosed or uncorrected condition. Obstetric problems may recur unless the client is properly tested and treated. For example, a client with a history of hydramnios, unexplained stillbirth, a large-for-gestational-age neonate, or a neonate born with congenital anomalies should receive the 3-hour glucose tolerance test and, if diabetes is confirmed, modify her diet and possibly receive insulin.

Because many infections recur, assess the client's history of infection. Inquire about past treatments and about her and her partner's overall health. Ask about contact with cats, which may expose her to toxoplasmosis. Inquire about childhood diseases and immunizations, which may now protect her from certain infections.

To identify the client's risk of contracting HIV infection and other diseases, question her about drug and substance use, sexual contacts, and blood or blood product transfusions.

If she uses drugs or abuses substances, obtain a complete drug history. If she hesitates to discuss details, assure her that her answers are confidential and are used only to help plan health care for her and her fetus. Combined with the obstetric history, the client's drug history helps determine which drugs the client has taken and if and how they have affected earlier pregnancies and may affect this one. Information about current drug use also guides the health care team toward a treatment plan.

Physical assessment

Obtain the client's vital signs and weight. Document these baseline data and compare them to preconception measurements to detect significant changes. Keep in mind that fever may be associated with anemia or TORCH, HIV, or genitourinary infections. Tachycardia also may be linked to anemia. Hypertension may be related to anemia or diabetes.

Then perform a head-to-toe physical assessment, including assisting with a pelvic examination. Note any abnormalities, which can provide clues to the client's underlying disorder or its progress. For example, pallor, thinness, and poor skin integrity suggest anemia. Renal complications, and other signs of vascular impairment signal advanced diabetes with vascular complications. Skin rash or lesions, enlarged glands or lymph nodes, muscle aches, and joint pain may be associated with a TORCH infection. Urinary frequency or urgency, nausea or vomiting, and vaginal discharge or itching suggest a genitourinary infection. Malaise, weight loss, diarrhea, lymphadenopathy, or evidence of Kaposi's sarcoma (purple or blue lesions) point to HIV infection. Skin abscesses and infections may indicate substance abuse.

Diagnostic studies

Obtain additional assessment data from routine prenatal laboratory tests, including complete blood count (CBC), coagulation studies, blood glucose levels, electrolyte and cardiac enzyme levels, and urinalysis. Because some infections are asymptomatic, check culture specimen results obtained during the pelvic examination.

Also expect to evaluate the fetus and check the results of any fetal diagnostic studies that were performed. (For more information, see *Fetal testing for high-risk antepartal clients,* pages 528 to 531.) If the fetus is monitored regularly, compare the results of each test to all others and to the baseline data to identify significant trends.

Perform or assist with other diagnostic studies, depending on the client's condition.

Tests for cardiac disease. For a client with cardiac disease, expect to monitor the results of the CBC, electrolyte levels, and if complications arise, cardiac enzyme levels.

Tests for diabetes. Expect to see the following diagnostic tests used to detect diabetes.

Urine glucose testing. Using a urine dipstick (Dextrostix), test the client's urine for glucose at each visit. This test should not be used to determine dietary management or insulin administration. Dextrostix detects glucose in the urine; Ketostix, ketones in the urine.

1-hour (50-gram) diabetes screening test. This oral glucose screening test is recommended for each pregnant client at 24 to 28 weeks' gestation. Advise the client that she does not need to fast before the test. Inform her that a blood sample for glucose testing will be drawn 1 hour after she ingests 50 grams of oral glucose solution. If her plasma glucose level is abnormally high, expect to prepare her for a 3-hour oral glucose tolerance test (Gabbe, 1986).

3-hour oral glucose tolerance test (OGTT). The OGTT may be used to diagnose gestational diabetes. Advise the client to eat a high-carbohydrate diet (more than 200 grams daily) for 2 days before this test. Also tell her to fast from midnight until the test time. When she arrives for her test, explain that a blood sample will be drawn to obtain a fasting plasma glucose level. Then after she ingests 100 grams of oral glucose solution, blood samples for plasma glucose levels will be drawn at 1, 2, and 3 hours. If two or more of the samples show abnormally high glucose levels, the client has gestational diabetes (Gabbe, 1986).

Glycosylated hemoglobin. Used to evaluate diabetic control, this test measures the percentage of glycohemoglobin (hemoglobin with a glucose molecule attached) in the blood, reflecting the blood glucose level during the previous 6 to 8 weeks. When performed monthly, it assists in diabetic management. Elevated glycohemoglobin levels indicate uncontrolled diabetes.

Blood glucose levels. In gestational and insulin-dependent diabetes, this test can be used to manage diabetes. It measures the blood glucose level, which is used to determine dietary changes and insulin dosage (Hollingsworth, 1988; Coustan and Felig, 1988).

Tests for anemia. For an anemic client, expect to monitor the results of hemoglobin electrophoresis, CBC, folic acid levels, and serum iron measurements.

Tests for infection. For a client with an infection, laboratory data reveal antibody titers and immune status. An abnormally high white blood cell count signals infection. Cultures taken from lesions or drainage samples can be used to identify a specific infecting organism.

Tests for substance abuse. Review the results of appropriate laboratory tests for the substance abuser. Urine drug testing provides information about substances abused. Biophysical profile testing assists with fetal health evaluation.

Nursing diagnosis

After considering all assessment findings, formulate appropriate nursing diagnoses for the client. (For more information, see *Nursing diagnoses: High-risk antepartal clients,* page 533.)

Planning and implementation

Nursing care of the high-risk antepartal client is holistic and encompasses the client, her fetus, and her family. The nurse monitors client health; teaches about the condition, its management, and effects; promotes adequate rest, exercise, and nutrition; prevents infection; provides support; promotes family well-being; monitors fetal health; and promotes compliance.

(Text continues on page 532.)

Fetal testing for high-risk antepartal clients

The high-risk client may benefit from antepartal testing, which may be noninvasive (occurring outside the body) or invasive (requiring entry into the body). The chart below describes various antepartal tests, including their purposes, timing, and nursing considerations.

NONINVASIVE TESTS

Ultrasonography

Description
The examiner applies conducting gel to the client's abdomen and moves a transducer across the area. The transducer transmits high-frequency sound waves to a screen, where they are displayed as images.

Purpose
• To determine position of the uterus and cervix, size and position of the developing fetus, area of placental formation, and cord insertion site
• To differentiate between a normal and abnormal fetus
• To determine number of fetuses, congenital abnormality, ectopic pregnancy, and amniotic fluid volume
• To diagnose fetal death through absence of fetal heart sounds and fetal movements or by identifying overlapping of fetal skull sutures
• To take fetal measurements (late in pregnancy), including the fetal skull biparietal diameters (BPD), femur length, and crown-rump length (CRL); to verify the presence of fetal organs; to verify cord insertion site and size of placenta; and to determine amniotic fluid volume, which identifies such abnormalities as intrauterine growth retardation and macrosomia
• To estimate gestational age by measuring CRL, BPD, and femur length, calculating the ratios between them, and comparing these measurements and ratios to those expected for various gestational ages
• To provide a baseline that allows meaningful interpretation of fetal growth during the pregnancy

Timing
As early as 5 weeks after the first day of the client's last menstrual period (LMP) to confirm pregnancy (Filly, 1988; Kurtz and Needleman, 1988); at 20 to 24 weeks' gestation (if client's first visit takes place at this time) to correlate the pregnancy dates with fetal gestational age and size

Nursing considerations
• Encourage the client to drink four to six glasses of fluid—but not to void before testing—to increase bladder fullness. Ultrasound waves will not traverse air; the fluid-filled bladder displaces the small bowel and provides a medium that sound waves readily penetrate.
• Be aware that from 24 weeks' gestation to term, estimates of gestational age based on ultrasonography may vary from the actual gestational age. At term, this variation may be 2 to 4 weeks (Kurtz and Needleman, 1988).

Fetal movement count

Description
The client identifies the presence and frequency of fetal movements. Normally, fetal movements average 200/day at 20 weeks' gestation, 575/day at 32 weeks' gestation, and 282/day at term (Sadovsky, 1985). Usually, normal fetal movement counts suggest a healthy fetus; decreased counts, possible fetal compromise.

Purpose
• To provide a rough index of fetal health

Timing
At 27 weeks' gestation and afterward

Nursing considerations
• Teach the client to record the number of fetal movements during 30 minutes, counted three times daily. Advise her to select times when she can relax and sit down to count these movements, and also when she knows the fetus is active. (Fetal movements normally decrease during fetal sleep periods, when maternal serum glucose levels are low, and during maternal use of tobacco or a central nervous system depressant.)
• Suggest that the client stimulate fetal movements by lying on her left side, eating a light snack, drinking orange juice, touching or moving her abdomen, or making a sudden noise, such as clapping her hands.
• Tell the client to stop counting if she notes five to six movements in each 30-minute period. Advise her to continue counting for an hour or more if she fails to note three movements in 30 minutes (Chez and Sadovsky, 1984).
• Advise the client to contact her health care provider if she notes fewer than 10 movements in two 1-hour periods spaced 12 hours apart, no movements in the morning, fewer than three movements in 8 hours, or if she becomes concerned for any reason. Changes in fetal activity patterns may require additional evaluation.
• Remind the client that wide variations in normal fetal movement exist in each woman and each pregnancy. However, the pattern of movement should not change greatly during her pregnancy.
• Tell the diabetic client to note fetal movements over 6 to 8 hours and emphasize the importance of becoming familiar with her fetus's activity pattern. Decreased movement occurs with decreased maternal serum glucose levels.

Fetal testing for high-risk antepartal clients continued

Biophysical profile (BPP)

Description
Through ultrasonography, the BPP evaluates fetal health by assessing five variables: fetal breathing movements (FBM), gross body movements (FM), fetal tone (FT), reactive fetal heart rate (non-stress test), and qualitative amniotic fluid volume (AFV) (Manning, Morrison, Lange, Harman, and Chamberlain, 1985). Each variable receives 2 points for a normal response; 0 points for an abnormal response. A fetus scoring 8 to 10 points is considered normal, with a low risk of oxygen deprivation. One scoring 6 or fewer points is at risk for asphyxia and premature birth.

Purpose
• To predict perinatal asphyxia
• To assess fetal risks
• To detect fetal anomalies

Timing
At 28 weeks' gestation or later

Nursing considerations
• Instruct the client undergoing BPP scoring about its purposes.
• Interpret BPP results for the client and reinforce instructions as the client's care alters.
• Provide psychological support, especially if testing will continue throughout the pregnancy.
• Advise the client that a low score, which may be evidence of fetal compromise, warrants detailed investigation.

Non-stress test (NST)

Description
The examiner places a tocodynamometer (TOCO) over the uterine fundus to record fetal movements while a Doppler ultrasound attachment, placed over the fetus's back, records the fetal heart rate (FHR). Both devices are secured to the client's abdomen and connected to an electronic fetal monitoring machine, which records a tracing of the FHR and fetal movement. The heart rate tracing is evaluated for accelerations (increases) during fetal movement. This test may be used immediately before, after, or independently of the BPP.

Purpose
• To assess fetal well-being

Timing
At 28 weeks' gestation or later. May be repeated weekly if results are normal and daily if they are abnormal or uninterpretable.

Nursing considerations
• Advise the client to eat a snack before the test to help ensure recordable fetal movements.
• Advise the client of the test results. Reactive (favorable) results show two to three FHR increases of 15 or more beats per minute (bpm), lasting for 15 or more seconds over 20 to 30 minutes. These increases occur with fetal movement. Nonreactive (unfavorable) results occur when the FHR response does not rise by 15 or more bpm over the specified time. A nonreactive NST may indicate fetal hypoxia. An uninterpretable NST may result from a poor tracing or insufficient fetal activity.
• Instruct the client to touch or rock her abdomen to move the fetus or to drink orange juice if minimal fetal movement occurs during the NST.
• Tell the client with persistent, uninterpretable test results that a nipple stimulation contraction stress test (NSCST) may be needed.

Nipple stimulation contraction stress test (NSCST)

Description
For the NSCST, the nurse places the TOCO and Doppler as described for the NST. Warm, moist towels may be applied to nipples for several minutes to increase suppleness and blood supply. Then the client brushes her palm across one nipple (through her clothes) until uterine contractions begin (up to 2 minutes). She stops this stimulation until the uterus relaxes, then repeats the stimulation for 2 minutes and rests for 5 minutes. She repeats this cycle for 40 minutes. If no contractions occur, she brushes both nipples. An electric breast pump may be used instead of nipple rolling for nipple stimulation. The FHR is monitored as for the NST because contractions may cause changes in the FHR.

Purpose
• To evaluate the FHR in response to uterine contractions

Timing
At 30 weeks' gestation or later, usually after an NST

Nursing considerations
• Be aware that the NSCST is not recommended for clients with a history of premature labor, premature rupture of membranes, abruptio placentae, placenta previa, cesarean delivery with a classical uterine incision, or with current multiple fetuses.
• Advise the client of test results. With negative (favorable) results, late FHR decelerations do not occur with contractions; with positive (unfavorable) results, they do.
• Be aware that the absence of late FHR decelerations indicates proper blood flow. Presence of late FHR decelerations demonstrates potential impairment in blood flow and possible fetal intolerance of labor. However, a client with a positive NSCST can deliver a healthy neonate.
• Be aware that positive results usually correlate with BPP results.

(continued)

Fetal testing for high-risk antepartal clients continued

Fetal acoustical stimulation (FAS)

Description
This antepartal test evaluates FHR acceleration during fetal movement. An acoustical stimulus is applied to the client's uterus several times to stimulate the fetus while the client undergoes an NST. The FHR is recorded on an electronic fetal monitor and evaluated for accelerations.

Purpose
• Same as NST

Timing
Same as NST

Nursing considerations
• Describe the test results, which are the same as for the NST.
• Advise the client that the test may be repeated within 24 hours or within a week if no FHR acceleration is detected.

INVASIVE TESTS

Chorionic villus sampling (CVS)

Description
For this early antepartal test, a sample of placental material is obtained and analyzed to detect fetal abnormalities.

Purpose
• To diagnose fetal karyotype, hemoglobinopathies, (sickle cell anemia, alpha and some beta thalassemias), alpha$_1$-antitrypsin deficiency, phenylketonuria, Down's syndrome, and Duchenne muscular dystrophy (Hogge, Hogge, and Golbus, 1986)

Timing
From 9 to 12 weeks' gestation

Nursing considerations
• Advise the client that complications of CVS include bleeding, spontaneous abortion, intrauterine infection, membrane rupture, and Rh isoimmunization (Elias, et al., 1985).

• Tell the client that other problems with CVS include inability to obtain a sample, sampling of maternal cells instead of fetal cells, and inaccurate prediction of fetal health.
• Assess the client after the procedure for complications and stabilization. An Rh-negative client should receive Rh$_0$(D) immune globulin to prevent sensitization from CVS.
• Remind the client to return for follow-up studies for continued evaluation of fetal well-being, such as ultrasonography, for laboratory tests for maternal infection, and for amniocentesis, as recommended.
• Assure the client that CVS does not cause neonatal malformations.

Alpha-fetoprotein (AFP) test

Description
A fetal serum protein, AFP may be tested in maternal serum (MSAFP) or in amniotic fluid (AFAFP). The examiner performs venipuncture each time a specimen is requested for MSAFP testing. An amniocentesis is required to determine AFAFP.

Purpose
• To predict open neural tube defects (NTD), such as spina bifida and anencephaly

Timing
Between 16 and 18 weeks after the LMP, when AFP levels are most stable (Schwager and Weiss, 1987). If AFP levels are elevated, another sample should be taken and tested.

Nursing considerations
• Be aware that clients at risk for fetal NTDs are those with a history of having a child with an NTD or with a strong family history of NTDs, those living where NTDs are prevalent (such as England, Ireland, and Wales), and those who are pregnant diabetics (Queenan, 1985; Lemize, 1989).
• Assess the client's understanding of testing procedures and the implications of test results.
• Discuss test results with the client. Elevated MSAFP and AFAFP levels are associated with NTDs; decreased levels, with trisomy 21 (Down's syndrome). However, Schwager and Weiss (1987) found that more than 40% of women studied had elevated AFP levels and delivered normal neonates.
• Provide psychological support throughout the pregnancy. If an abnormal neonate is born, recommend further client evaluation and counseling.

Amniocentesis

Description
This test evaluates a sample of amniotic fluid aspirated transabdominally from the amniotic sac.

Purpose
• To detect genetic disorders
• To diagnose various fetal defects, including chromosomal

anomalies, skeletal disorders, infections, central nervous system disorders, blood disorders, inborn errors of metabolism, miscellaneous metabolic disorders, and porphyrias
• To assess fetal lung maturity during the third trimester by evaluating the lecithin/sphingomyelin (L/S) ratio in the amniotic fluid

Fetal testing for high-risk antepartal clients continued

Amniocentesis (continued)

Timing
At 16 weeks' gestation to detect genetic disorder; at 30 weeks' gestation or later to assess L/S ratio

Nursing considerations
• Be aware that prime candidates for genetic screening by amniocentesis are clients over age 35 and those with a chromosomal or metabolic abnormality in an older child, chromosomal abnormalities in either parent, history of a sex-linked genetic disorder, or a family history of chromosomal or enzymatic abnormality or of NTDs (Willson and Carrington, 1987).
• Advise the client that test results take 2 to 4 weeks because of the complexity of fetal chromosomal diagnosis.

• Advise the client that complications related to amniocentesis include trauma to the client, fetus, umbilical cord, and placenta; premature labor or spontaneous abortion; infection; and maternal isoimmunization with hemolytic disease of the neonate.
• Monitor the client electronically for uterine irritability and alteration in FHR patterns for a few hours after the procedure. Vital signs should remain unchanged.
• Caution the client to observe for decreased fetal movement, persistent uterine contractions, or any abdominal discomfort after the procedure. If these occur, tell her to return immediately for evaluation.

Percutaneous umbilical blood sampling (PUBS)

Description
PUBS requires intrauterine aspiration of a fetal blood sample from the umbilical cord. It allows fetal transfusions in utero and access to fetal circulation for diagnostic tests and treatments.

Purpose
• To diagnose fetal blood disorders, such as coagulopathies, hemoglobinopathies, and hemophilias; congenital infections, such as rubella and toxoplasmosis; and chromosomal abnormalities (Ludomirski and Weiner, 1988)
• To treat Rh isoimmunization through blood transfusions (Dunn, Weiner, and Ludomirski, 1988)

Timing
After 16 weeks' gestation

Nursing considerations
• Before the procedure, prepare the client's abdomen by applying a povidone-iodine solution and sterile drapes.

• When assisting with the procedure, maintain sterile technique.
• Teach the client that PUBS can be used to assess, diagnose, and treat fetal anemia. Blood transfusions may be given through direct vascular access. Prompt treatment of the fetus in utero can maintain pregnancy, decreasing prematurity and the risk of death.
• Advise the client that complications of PUBS include chorioamnionitis, premature labor and rupture of amniotic membranes, abruptio placentae, bleeding, laceration or thrombus of an umbilical vessel, and transient fetal arrhythmias (Dunn, Weiner, and Ludomirski, 1988).
• Monitor the fetus with an NST after PUBS. Notify the physician if uterine contractions or FHR decelerations occur. An emergency delivery may be necessary if fetal distress continues.
• Perform a biweekly NST and BPP for fetal assessment until delivery. Inform the client of the importance of these follow-up studies.

Oxytocin contraction test (OCT)

Description
Oxytocin (Pitocin) is administered to stimulate uterine contractions to evaluate FHR. The nurse applies the TOCO and the Doppler as for the NST. As prescribed, the nurse performs an NST first and then begins an I.V. solution of 1,000 ml of dextrose 5% in water with 5 to 10 units of oxytocin (5 to 10 milliunits per 1 ml). An infusion pump regulates the solution, which is increased as prescribed, until three contractions occur in 10 minutes.

Purpose
• To evaluate the FHR in response to uterine contractions

Timing
Around 30 weeks' gestation

Nursing considerations
• Be aware that the physician gives standing orders for the nurse to intervene if fetal or maternal problems develop.

• Be aware that the contraindications for this test are the same as those for the NSCST. After three uterine contractions occur, the oxytocin is turned off and the main I.V. line is continued until FHR activity has been evaluated in relation to the contractions.
• Discontinue the infusion if no late FHR decelerations occur.
• If late FHR decelerations occur and do not return to baseline, notify the physician. Turn off the oxytocin, increase the main I.V. line rate, position the client on her left side (to move the gravid uterus away from her inferior vena cava), and administer oxygen. If this positioning does not return the FHR to normal, help the client onto her right side or place her on her hands and knees with her head and chest resting on the bed.
• Be aware that if client repositioning does not return the FHR to baseline, emergency cesarean delivery may be indicated, although this is rare.
• If late FHR decelerations do not occur, or if the decelerations return to baseline immediately after emergency treatment, evaluate fetal well-being further via electronic FHR monitoring for several hours.

Monitor health status

The high-risk antepartal client may have a nursing diagnosis of *decreased cardiac output related to valvular dysfunction, potential for infection related to metabolic and vascular abnormalities, potential for infection related to altered RBC structure and tissue perfusion,* or *impaired tissue integrity related to substance abuse and needle sharing.* To monitor her status, obtain her vital signs and weight at each prenatal visit. Obtain an ECG periodically, as prescribed. Monitor fluid intake and output. If a client develops pulmonary complications, be aware that a pulmonary artery catheter may be inserted to provide pulmonary pressure measurements.

Teach the client to monitor herself and report significant changes, especially signs and symptoms of potential complications. For example, teach the client with cardiac disease to note increased limitation of activity; presence of or increase in dyspnea, orthopnea, tachypnea, and edema; development of palpitations; significant increase or decrease in heart rate; and chest discomfort.

Inform the client of the need for regular examinations and tests. Advise her of all test results.

Teach about the condition, its management, and effects

Depending on the client's disorder or problem, provide information about its treatment and care and about the effects they should produce.

Cardiac disease. The client with cardiac disease may have a nursing diagnosis of *knowledge deficit related to cardiac disease management during pregnancy* or *impaired gas exchange related to decreased cardiac output.* If so, encourage her to assume a semi-Fowler's or a left side-lying position to promote fetal oxygenation by shifting the weight of the pregnant uterus off the major abdominal blood vessels. Suggest ways to arrange pillows for comfort so that her head, neck, and arms are supported in the semi-Fowler's position, and her back, uterus, and legs are supported in the left side-lying position. If the client is hospitalized, administer oxygen, as needed.

Diabetes. For a client with diabetes, nursing diagnoses may include *knowledge deficit related to the effects of diabetes on pregnancy* or *knowledge deficit related to diabetes management during pregnancy.* For such a client, provide information about diabetes, its effects on her and her fetus and neonate, and the treatment. Reassure her that careful managment during pregnancy can prevent fetal and neonatal problems. Also, advise her to avoid smoking because of its vasoconstrictive effects on the fetus and herself.

Instruct the client and her partner about diabetes mellitus, home glucose monitoring, and insulin, high-lighting the drug's purpose, types, dosage, and administration. Also review the signs and symptoms of hypoglycemia and hyperglycemia.

Reinforce the physician's recommendations for home glucose monitoring, insulin administration, and dietary management. Teach the client about acceptable glucose values, and encourage her to record these levels accurately along with the amount of insulin she self-administers.

If blood glucose cannot be regulated with intermittent insulin administration, a continuous infusion pump may be used or the client may be hospitalized during pregnancy for adjustment of insulin dosages.

Anemia. Teach the client about her disorder and its effects. This is particularly important for a client with a nursing diagnosis of *knowledge deficit related to the effects of anemia on pregnancy.* Inform her that she should report any evidence of bleeding, especially vaginal bleeding. Identify special needs for the anemic client during pregnancy, such as compliance with iron supplementation. Teach her that iron is absorbed best when taken with an acidic juice, such as orange juice, and absorbed poorly when taken with dairy products. Also inform the client that iron supplements may cause stool darkening and constipation. If constipation occurs, advise her to include more fluids, fruits, and fiber in her diet. If it persists, let her know that her physician can prescribe a stool softener.

Teach the client with sickle cell anemia about precipitating factors. Advise her to maintain proper nutrition and hydration. Also instruct her to avoid crowds and individuals with colds or infections to decrease the risk of infection. Stress the importance of noting and reporting signs and symptoms of impending infection to the physician.

Infection. The client with an infection may have a nursing diagnosis of *knowledge deficit related to disease transmission and prevention.* If so, teach her about the causes of infections, transmission routes, and prevention techniques. Describe the signs and symptoms of common infections, and help her identify predisposing factors. Encourage her to seek medical help if she suspects infection.

Care for the client with an infection involves all family or household members in controlling the infection, assuring satisfactory health for these individuals, and protecting the family caregivers. To accomplish these goals, educate the family about the infection, its risks, and preventive measures. These measures may include:
• sexual abstinence during the active phases of the disease

NURSING DIAGNOSES

High-risk antepartal clients

The following nursing diagnoses address representative problems and etiologies that a nurse may encounter when providing care for a high-risk antepartal client. Specific nursing interventions for many of these diagnoses are provided in the "Planning and implementation" section of this chapter.

CARDIAC DISEASE

- Activity intolerance related to altered cardiac function and decreased tissue oxygenation
- Altered family processes related to inability to maintain level of functioning within the family
- Altered tissue perfusion: cardiopulmonary, related to decreased cardiac output
- Decreased cardiac output related to valvular dysfunction
- Impaired gas exchange related to decreased cardiac output
- Ineffective breathing pattern related to decreased cardiac output
- Knowledge deficit related to cardiac disease management during pregnancy
- Potential for infection related to altered cardiac status
- Sleep pattern disturbance related to cardiac fatigue

DIABETES MELLITUS

- Activity intolerance related to rapid weight gain and fluid retention
- Altered nutrition: less than body requirements, related to altered carbohydrate metabolism
- Altered nutrition: less than body requirements, related to inadequate intake and excessive exercise
- Altered tissue perfusion: peripheral, related to vascular impairment
- Anxiety related to maternal, fetal, and neonatal effects of diabetes
- Knowledge deficit related to diabetes management during pregnancy
- Knowledge deficit related to the effects of diabetes on pregnancy
- Noncompliance related to specified diet, schedules for serum glucose testing, or insulin administration
- Potential for infection related to metabolic and vascular abnormalities

ANEMIA

- Altered nutrition: less than body requirements, related to increased need for iron-rich foods
- Altered tissue perfusion: peripheral, related to inadequate blood supply
- Anxiety related to maternal and fetal effects of anemia
- Fatigue related to decreased oxygen-carrying capacity of the blood
- Knowledge deficit related to prenatal care and anemia
- Knowledge deficit related to the effects of anemia on pregnancy
- Pain related to vascular occlusion of sickle cell anemia
- Potential for infection related to altered RBC structure and tissue perfusion
- Powerlessness related to frequency of sickle cell

INFECTION

- Altered family processes related to concern over adverse pregnancy outcomes
- Anticipatory grieving related to potential for congenital anomaly or death of fetus or neonate
- Ineffective individual coping related to possibility of delivering a neonate with a congenital anomaly or fatal infection
- Knowledge deficit related to disease transmission and prevention
- Knowledge deficit related to fetal and neonatal effects of maternal infection
- Noncompliance related to incomplete administration of prescribed medication
- Social isolation related to others' fear of disease transmission

SUBSTANCE ABUSE

- Altered nutrition: less than body requirements, related to limited food intake from continued substance abuse
- Altered parenting related to performance of neonatal care while under the influence of a substance
- Impaired tissue integrity related to substance abuse and needle sharing
- Knowledge deficit related to fetal effects of substance abuse
- Noncompliance with drug rehabilitation program related to continued substance abuse
- Potential for infection related to self-administered I.V. drugs
- Self-esteem disturbance related to dependence on a chemical substance

TRAUMA

- Altered family processes related to unexpected change in maternal health status
- Decreased cardiac output related to blood loss from trauma
- Fear related to the effects of trauma on the fetus
- Impaired gas exchange related to respiratory effects of chest trauma
- Pain related to traumatic injury

SURGERY

- Fear related to concerns that surgery may harm the fetus
- Impaired gas exchange related to surgery and preoperative and postoperative pain
- Knowledge deficit related to effects of surgery on the pregnancy
- Pain related to incision site
- Potential for infection related to complications of surgery

• use of a condom during sexual intercourse as recommended by health care professionals
• simultaneous treatment of the client and her partner
• evaluation for reinfection, as indicated by health care professionals
• careful adherence to perineal hygiene measures
• careful attention to proper disposal of body fluids and contaminated needles
• thorough hand-washing after contact with infected areas and before contact with the neonate and others.

Substance abuse. The pregnant substance abuser needs early prenatal care to decrease the risk of congenital anomalies in her neonate. During her early prenatal visits, help her control the type and amount of drugs that she takes. If she appears for care late in the pregnancy or misses appointments, continue to provide sensitive care at every opportunity during the antepartal, intrapartal, and postpartal periods.

The substance abuser may have a nursing diagnosis of **knowledge deficit related to fetal effects of substance abuse.** If so, teach her about the adverse effects of various substances on her and her fetus and neonate. Help her recognize that substances affect her fetus. Inform her that her neonate will have to undergo withdrawal and will be treated as an addict after birth.

After teaching about the fetal and maternal effects of substances, encourage her to seek treatment or to join a drug-counseling program.

Promote adequate rest and exercise

When the client has a nursing diagnosis of **activity intolerance related to altered cardiac function and decreased tissue oxygenation, fatigue related to decreased oxygen-carrying capacity of blood,** or **activity intolerance related to rapid weight gain and fluid retention,** stress the importance of obtaining adequate rest and limiting sodium and fluid intake.

For the client with cardiac disease, identify reasons for limiting activity and benefits of resting before or after activities. Help her find acceptable adjustments to professional and personal activities and to plan ways to modify her family's schedule to include rest periods. Also, encourage her to sleep at least 10 hours each night and to take morning and afternoon rests, particularly if she has a nursing diagnosis of **sleep pattern disturbance related to cardiac fatigue.**

Encourage the diabetic client to obtain adequate rest, including 8 to 10 hours of sleep each night and daily rest periods. Management of the client should include guidelines for effectively incorporating exercise into her daily regimen. The diabetic client may have a nursing diagnosis of **altered nutrition: less than body requirements, related to inadequate intake and exces-**

sive excercise. Suggest that she exercise about 1 hour after meals, when her blood glucose level is elevated, and inform her that she may need the added sugar in hard candy during exercise. Also advise her to monitor her glucose level before and after exercising.

For a client with sickle cell anemia, emphasize rest and pain-relief measures, such as hot showers or warm baths.

Promote adequate nutrition

The high-risk antepartal client may have a nursing diagnosis of **altered nutrition: less than body requirements, related to increased need for intake of iron-rich foods** or **altered nutrition: less than body requirements, related to altered carbohydrate metabolism.** To help such a client, evaluate her food preferences, needs, and restrictions, and estimate the nutritional value of the foods she eats. Incorporate these evaluations into a balanced diet that fulfills nutritional requirements, meets food preferences, and is economical. For any client, outline a pattern of ideal weight gain during pregnancy.

Depending on the client's underlying disorder, make specific dietary recommendations. To reduce fatigue for a client with a cardiac disease, suggest that she divide her daily intake into five or six meals throughout the day. To help control glucose levels for a diabetic client, advise her to divide her daily intake into three meals and three snacks. To prevent or correct iron deficiency or folic acid deficiency anemia, suggest foods that are rich in these nutrients.

A substance abuser may have a nursing diagnosis of **altered nutrition: less than body requirements, related to substance abuse.** When evaluating her dietary habits, also assess her financial status to determine if she has enough money to buy food. Such a client may spend more money on drugs than on basic needs. If necessary, consult a social worker who will determine the client's eligibility for food stamps and Women, Infants, and Children assistance. (For more information, see Chapter 20, Nutrition and Diet Counseling.)

Prevent infection

The high-risk antepartal client may be at increased risk for infection. For example, the client with a cardiac disease has an increased risk for upper respiratory tract infections, which can lead to subacute bacterial endocarditis. Her nursing diagnosis may be **potential for infection related to altered cardiac status.**

To help such a client, discuss the reasons for preventing infection. Encourage her to obtain sufficient rest and recommend that she avoid crowds, drafts, and people with viral infections. Stress the importance of healthful nutrition and adherence to prescribed vitamin and iron supplementation. Arrange for follow-up appointments at mutually agreeable times.

The diabetic client is likely to have a nursing diagnosis of *potential for infection related to metabolic and vascular abnormalities.* Teach such a client to watch for signs of infection, such as redness, warmth, swelling, and fever. Also instruct her to look for broken skin, bleeding, bruises, or slow healing and to report these findings to her physician. Advise her to trim her fingernails and toenails carefully to avoid accidental cuts. Teach her to maintain adequate peripheral circulation by avoiding constricting clothing on her legs. Adequate circulation, especially to the lower extremities, helps decrease the risk of ulceration and infection.

The client who abuses I.V. drugs risks infection from needles. She may have a nursing diagnosis of *potential for infection related to self-administered I.V. drugs.* Teach such a client the reasons, causes, signs, and symptoms of infections related to I.V. drug abuse. Explain how such infections can harm her and her fetus.

Good skin integrity decreases the chances of local and systemic infections. Depending on the route of drug administration, the client may have open areas or abscesses on her extremities. Help her maintain skin integrity by evaluating these sites and providing care to prevent systemic infection.

Provide support

The high-risk antepartal client may have a nursing diagnosis of *anxiety related to possible maternal, fetal, and neonatal effects of diabetes; anxiety related to maternal and fetal effects of anemia;* or *fear related to concerns that surgery may harm the fetus.* To help such a client, identify her concerns and expect an experienced nurse clinician to provide psychological support and counseling during and after the pregnancy.

Clearly inform the client of the risks for delivering a stillborn, abnormal, or infected neonate. Maintain honesty and confidentiality through pregnancy testing and discussion of results. Initiate counseling sessions to discuss the client's concerns and fears and provide guidance for future care. If necessary, refer her to a support group or mental health professional.

Promote family well-being

The high-risk antepartal client may have a nursing diagnosis of *altered family processes related to inability to maintain level of functioning within the family.* To help the client and her family cope, begin by teaching them about the physiologic changes of pregnancy and the effects of her condition on the pregnancy. Help them understand her needs so that they can provide support. Then evaluate the family's schedule and identify possible adjustments that incorporate family and client needs.

Suggest that the client consider ways to accomplish her tasks while resting.

As appropriate, foster communication between the client and her partner and between the family and health care team. Encourage family members to participate actively in family decision making. Provide opportunities for individual and group discussion and arrange for individual and family counseling sessions, if necessary.

Provide anticipatory guidance by preparing the client and her family for intrapartal, postpartal, and parenting responsibilities. Determine support needs after the discharge of the client and neonate.

Prepare the diabetic client and her partner for the possibility of cesarean delivery, which may be necessary if maternal and fetal complications develop.

For the client with an infection, help the couple identify the neonate's needs as a member of their family. Also, help them identify ways to handle society's fear of disease transmission. Encourage them to obtain information about the disease so that they can prevent transmission.

A client who abuses substances is especially likely to have a nursing diagnosis of *altered parenting related to performance of neonatal care while under the influence of a substance.* This client may benefit from neonatal care instruction during individual counseling sessions or peer group sessions. Coordinate care planning sessions for the client with the physician, nurse specialist, social worker, counselor, and nutritionist.

Monitor the fetus

During each prenatal visit, monitor fetal status by assessing fetal movement and fetal heart rate and by performing a non-stress test and nipple stimulation contraction stress test, if necessary.

In addition, inform the client and her partner about other diagnostic tests to determine fetal health, including ultrasonography, biophysical profile, oxytocin contraction test, and amniocentesis. Careful examination of the fetus assures the couple that optimum care is being provided and may relieve a client with a nursing diagnosis of *anxiety related to maternal, fetal, and neonatal effects of diabetes.* Allow time for questions and discussion of test results.

Promote compliance

To promote compliance with the medical regimen, invite the client to participate in her health care planning. Help her identify her needs throughout the pregnancy, and allow her to become a member of the health care team. Consider the client's educational level and daily schedule. Respect her judgments and incorporate her prescribed regimen into a workable daily plan.

Client with knowledge deficit related to diabetes control during pregnancy

For a high-risk antepartal client, the nursing process helps ensure high-quality care. The table below shows how the nurse might use the nursing process when caring for the client described in the case history at right. The first column presents history and physical assessment data followed by a paragraph of mental notes. These notes help the nurse make important connections among assessment findings, aiding in development of the nursing diagnosis and planning.

The second column lists an appropriate nursing diagnosis; information in the remaining columns is based on this diagnosis. Although not part of the nursing process, a rationale appears for each intervention in the fourth column to explain how it contributes to the care plan.

ASSESSMENT	NURSING DIAGNOSIS	PLANNING
Subjective (history) data • Client reports excessive hunger, increased urination especially at night, extreme thirst, and elevated blood glucose levels. • Client has a history of diabetes mellitus, which has been controlled. • Client's obstetric history includes one unexplained stillbirth at 36 weeks' gestation. **Objective (physical) data** • Temperature 98° F, pulse 100 beats/minute, respirations 24 breaths/minute, blood pressure 146/88. • Weight increase totals 6 pounds, beyond expectations for gestation. • Fundal height greater than expected for gestation. • Blood glucose level 150 mg/dl, urine sugar and acetone (S/A) +3/trace. **Mental notes** *The client's current signs and symptoms, history of diabetes, and laboratory test results indicate that her diabetes is not being controlled adequately. The client may not be aware of the effects of pregnancy on diabetes or of how to manage them.*	Knowledge deficit related to diabetes control during pregnancy	**Goals** By the end of this visit, the client will: • describe the importance of knowing the signs and symptoms of hypoglycemia and hyperglycemia • explain the importance, purpose, and effects of insulin on her fetus • demonstrate the proper method for home glucose monitoring • explain how to adjust her insulin regimen to correct changes in blood glucose levels.

Be sure to schedule appointments at times that are convenient for the client and health care team. Explain care recommendations in simple terms. Ask the couple to identify reasons for adhering to the medical regimen, and advise them that compliance with appointments promotes maternal and fetal health and alerts the physician to potential problems. This is particularly important for a client at risk for a nursing diagnosis of *noncompliance to a drug rehabilitation program related to continued substance abuse.*

Evaluation

Care of a high-risk antepartal client requires a multidisciplinary approach throughout the preconception, antepartal, intrapartal, and postpartal periods. The general goals are maintenance of client health and safe delivery of a healthy neonate.

To evaluate nursing care, determine if specific goals were achieved. State evaluation findings in terms of actions performed or outcomes achieved for each goal. The following examples illustrate some appropriate evaluation statements:
• The client accurately described her condition and its limitations on her health.
• The client correctly described the potential effects of her condition on herself and on her fetus and neonate.
• The client and her family actively participated in planning care and activities during and after the pregnancy.
• The client correctly listed the signs and symptoms of complications in her condition or pregnancy.
• The client endorsed a care regimen that affords her optimum health and functioning.
• The client planned for neonatal care.
• The client's family demonstrated support and concern.

CASE STUDY

Ellen Rawa, age 23, is G2 P0100 at 30 weeks' gestation. Although she is a diabetic, her glucose levels have been well controlled. At her regular prenatal visit, she complains of excessive hunger; increased urination, especially at night; and extreme thirst. She states her blood glucose levels over the past week have ranged from 120 mg/dl to 200 mg/dl.

IMPLEMENTATION		EVALUATION
Intervention Teach the client about the signs, symptoms, and interventions for hypoglycemia and hyperglycemia.	**Rationale** Information may decrease the client's fear and anxiety and help prevent severe hypoglycemia and hyperglycemia.	Upon evaluation, the client: • listed signs and symptoms of hypoglycemia and hyperglycemia • asked questions about her illness, its treatment, and its effects on her and her fetus • demonstrated proper technique for monitoring her blood glucose levels • stated how to adjust her insulin dosage regimen according to her blood glucose levels.
Teach the client about insulin and its purpose and effect on her and her fetus.	Increased knowledge will help make the client more cooperative and better able to manage her condition.	
Teach the client how to adjust her insulin regimen to compensate for changes in her blood glucose level.	Increased knowledge of changes in insulin requirements allows the client to achieve more certain control of her diabetes and better health for her and her fetus.	
Evaluate the client's accuracy in monitoring her glucose level at home.	Proper glucose monitoring, appropriate insulin dosage, and regular reporting to the health care team should ensure appropriate management.	

• The client identified changes in her pregnancy caused by the disease.
• The client planned nutritious meals.
• The client reported a change in her condition as soon as it occurred.
• The client made an appointment for counseling.
• The client and her family joined a support group.
• The client kept all appointments for prenatal care and laboratory tests.
• The client identified the changes in her body caused by her condition and her pregnancy.
• The client began a regular exercise program.
• The client and her partner attended individual and family counseling sessions.
• The client and her partner made an informed decision about fetal diagnostic testing.

Documentation

Using appropriate records, document all steps of the nursing process, including assessment data, nursing diagnoses, the plan of care, implementation activities, and evaluation findings. (For a case study that shows how to apply the nursing process when caring for a high-risk antepartal client, see *Applying the nursing process: Client with knowledge deficit related to diabetes control during pregnancy.*)

When caring for a high-risk antepartal client, documentation should include:
• baseline and current assessment data for the client
• baseline and current assessment data for the fetus
• the client's physical and psychological response to treatment

• the client's physical and psychological response to the limitations caused by her condition

• the family's response to and support of the client.

Chapter summary

Chapter 22 identified clients who are at risk during pregnancy. The goals for these clients are health maintenance throughout the pregnancy and safe delivery of a healthy neonate. Here are the chapter highlights.

• A pregnant adolescent is at risk physically and psychosocially because of immaturity, potential for pregnancy complications, lack of prenatal care, and lack of social and economic support systems. Prenatal care and counseling, support groups, and financial assistance can help assure a healthier start for the pregnant adolescent and her fetus.

• A mature client who gives birth after age 34 is likely to be prepared for her pregnancy physically, emotionally, and economically. Her needs include sensitive prenatal care and information about genetic testing. The nurse must counsel the mature client and her partner about the reasons for testing and support them after the results have been interpreted.

• A client with a cardiac disease, such as rheumatic heart disease, a congenital heart defect, mitral valve prolapse, or peripartum cardiomyopathy, can carry to term safely and give birth to a healthy neonate. She must be monitored regularly throughout her pregnancy and may benefit from such treatments as bed rest, fluid restrictions, proper nutrition, and administration of digitalis, diuretics, antiarrhythmics, antibiotics, and anticoagulants.

• Care for the client with diabetes mellitus should begin before conception to normalize serum glucose levels and replace oral hypoglycemic agents with insulin. Optimally, the client should achieve normal blood glucose levels before conception and maintain them throughout pregnancy. The nurse should promote diet regulation, insulin therapy, and careful glucose monitoring throughout pregnancy, as prescribed.

• Anemia may influence pregnancy and threaten the health of the client and her fetus. Iron deficiency anemia, folic acid deficiency anemia, and sickle cell anemia may worsen with pregnancy. Care for a client with iron or folic acid deficiency anemia includes diet counseling and nutritional supplements. Care for the client with sickle cell anemia includes counseling on crisis prevention,

treatment with hydration and analgesics, and infection care.

• TORCH infections include toxoplasmosis, other infections (chlamydia, group B beta hemolytic streptococcus, syphilis, and varicella-zoster), rubella, cytomegalovirus, and herpesvirus. They can be devastating to the fetus and neonate. Human immunodeficiency virus—and the risk of AIDS—can be transmitted from the mother to the fetus and neonate, even if the mother is asymptomatic. Genitourinary infections, such as trichomoniasis, gonorrhea, vaginitis, pelvic inflammatory disease, and pyelonephritis, also may influence fetal and neonatal health.

• Substance abuse harms the client and her fetus and neonate. It increases the client's risk of other diseases, such as hepatitis B and HIV infection, and commonly is associated with STDs. The nurse should counsel the client and provide information and referrals to educational programs to help her recover from substance abuse.

• The client may sustain trauma from accidental injuries or physical abuse during pregnancy. The type and timing of the injury influence pregnancy outcomes. Prompt assessment and treatment of injuries can improve maternal and fetal health. Abused clients need counseling to increase feelings of self-worth and provide support.

• Surgery should be avoided during pregnancy, if possible. If surgery cannot be postponed, intervention during the second trimester is preferred. Common surgical procedures performed during pregnancy include operations for ovarian cysts, appendicitis, breast tumors (lumps), incompetent cervix, and cholecystitis. A multidisciplinary approach reduces the risks for the client and her fetus.

• When caring for a high-risk antepartal client, the nurse should obtain a complete health history, perform a thorough physical assessment, and assist with and review diagnostic studies. Depending on the client's needs, the nurse monitors the client's health; teaches about the condition, its management, and effects; promotes adequate rest, exercise, and nutrition; prevents infection; provides support; promotes family well-being; monitors the fetus; and promotes compliance. Evaluation determines if the goals of maintaining client health and safely delivering a healthy neonate were achieved.

Study questions

1. When Judy Thompson, age 15, makes her first visit to the prenatal clinic, she is at 30 weeks' gestation with her first pregnancy. What guidelines will the nurse use in planning Judy's care?

2. Sandy Barrows, a primigravid client age 28, is 32 weeks pregnant. She has a history of rheumatic fever. What physiologic changes is she likely to experience at this time and why? What measures can the nurse use to provide her with the best care?

3. Edie Mason, age 24, has had insulin-dependent diabetes mellitus for 6 years. She is 20 weeks pregnant with her first child. What information must the nurse review with her about her glucose maintenance?

4. Arlette Jenkins, age 22, is 20 weeks pregnant. At her regular prenatal visit, she expresses concern about the effects of her sickle cell anemia on her fetus. What should the nurse tell her about these effects? What suggestions can the nurse make to help Ms. Jenkins avoid these effects?

5. Jessica Carter, age 18, is 24 weeks pregnant when she arrives for her first clinic appointment. She uses marijuana and cocaine and reports that a previous pregnancy ended in spontaneous abortion. Which questions should the nurse ask Jessica about her drug use? What teaching should the nurse undertake on this first visit?

Bibliography

Braunwald, E., Isselbacher, K., Petersdorf, R., Wilson, J., Martin, J., and Fauci, A. (Eds.). (1987). *Harrison's principles of internal medicine* (11th ed.). New York: McGraw-Hill.

Chez, R., and Sadovsky, E. (1984). Teaching patients how to record fetal movements. *Contemporary OB/GYN, 24*(4), 85-86.

Cruikshank, D. (1986a). Medical and surgical complications of pregnancy: Diseases of the alimentary tract. In D. Danforth and J. Scott (Eds.), *Obstetrics and gynecology* (5th ed.; pp. 523-527). Philadelphia: Lippincott.

Cruikshank, D. (1986b). Medical and surgical complications of pregnancy: Neurologic disease. In D. Danforth and J. Scott (Eds.), *Obstetrics and gynecology* (5th ed.; pp. 509-516). Philadelphia: Lippincott.

Cruikshank, D. (1986c). Medical and surgical complications of pregnancy: Urinary tract disease. In D. Danforth and J. Scott (Eds.), *Obstetrics and gynecology* (5th ed.; pp. 505-509). Philadelphia: Lippincott.

Cunningham, F., MacDonald, P., and Gant, N. (1989). *Williams obstetrics* (18th ed.). East Norwalk, CT: Appleton & Lange.

Dunn, P., Weiner, S., and Ludomirski, A. (1988). Percutaneous umbilical blood sampling. *JOGNN, 17*(5), 308-313.

Elias S., Simpson, J., Martin., A., Sabbagha, R., Gerbie, A., and Keith, L. (1985). Chorionic villus sampling for first-trimester prenatal diagnosis: Northwestern University Program. *American Journal of Obstetrics and Gynecology, 152*(2), 204-213.

Erikson, E. (1968). *Identity, youth, and crisis.* New York: Norton.

Filly, R. (1988). The first trimester. In P. Callen (Ed.), *Ultrasonography in obstetrics and gynecology* (2nd ed.; pp. 19-46). Philadelphia: Saunders.

Gabbe, S., Niebyl, J., and Simpson, J. (Eds.). (1986). *Obstetrics: Normal and problem pregnancies.* New York: Churchill Livingstone.

Hibbard, B. (1988). *Principles of obstetrics.* Stoneham, MA: Butterworth and Co.

Hogge, J., Hogge, W., and Golbus, M. (1986). Chorionic villus sampling. *JOGNN, 15*(1), 24-28.

Hollingsworth, D., and Resnik, R. (Eds.). (1988). *Medical counseling before pregnancy.* New York: Churchill Livingstone.

Jackson, L., and Wapner, R. (1984). Chorionic biopsy. *The New England Journal of Medicine, 311*(8), 539-540.

Kochenour, N. (1982). Estrogen assay during pregnancy. *Clinical Obstetrics and Gynecology, 25*(4), 659-672.

Kurtz, A., and Needleman, L. (1988). Ultrasound assessment of fetal age. In P. Callen (Ed.), *Ultrasonography in obstetrics and gynecology* (2nd ed.; pp. 47-64). Philadelphia: Saunders.

Ledbetter, D., Martin, A., Verlinsky, Y., Pergamant, E., Jackson, L., Yang-Feng, T., Schonberg, S., Gilbert, F., Zachary, J., Barr, M., Copeland, K., DiMaio, M., Fine, B., Rosinsky, B., Schuette, J., de la Cruz, F., Desnick, R., Elias, S., Golbus, M., Goldberg, J., Lubs, H., Mahoney, M., Rhoads, G., Simpson, J., and Schlesselman, S. (1990). Cytogenic results of chorionic villus sampling: High success rate and diagnostic accuracy in the United States collaborative study. *American Journal of Obstetrics and Gynecology, 162*(2), 495-501.

Lemize, R. (1989). Neural tube defects. *JAMA, 259*(4), 558-562.

Ludomirski, A., and Weiner, S. (1988). Percutaneous fetal umbilical blood sampling. *Clinical Obstetrics and Gynecology, 31*(1), 19-26.

Manning, F., Morrison, I., Lange, I., Harman, C., and Chamberlain, P. (1985). Fetal assessment based on fetal biophysical profile scoring: Experience in 12,620 referred high-risk pregnancies. *American Journal of Obstetrics and Gynecology, 151*(3), 343-350.

Marshall, C. (1986). The nipple stimulation contraction stress test. *JOGNN, 15*(6), 459-462.

Queenan, J. (Ed.). (1985). *Management of high-risk pregnancy* (2nd ed.). Oradell, NJ: Medical Economics Co.

Roberts, N., Dunn, L., Weiner, S., Godmilow, L., and Miller, R. (1983). Midtrimester amniocentesis: Indications, technique, risks and potential for prenatal diagnosis. *The Journal of Reproductive Medicine, 28*(3), 167-188.

Rodman, M., and Karch, A. (1989). *Pharmacology and drug therapy in nursing* (4th ed.). Philadelphia: Lippincott.

Sadovsky, E. (1985). Fetal movements. In J. Queenan (Ed.), *Management of high-risk pregnancy* (2nd ed.; pp. 183-193). Oradell, NJ: Medical Economics Co.

Schwager, E., and Weiss, B. (1987). Prenatal testing for maternal serum alpha-fetoprotein. *American Family Physician, 35*(4), 169-174.

Short, E. (1988). Genetic disorders. In G. Burrow and T. Ferris (Eds.), *Medical complications during pregnancy* (3rd ed.; pp. 136-179). Philadelphia: Saunders.

U.S. Department of Health and Human Services. (1988). *Health, United States, 1987,* Pub. No. (PHS 88-1232). Hyattsville, MD: National Center for Health Statistics.

Ventura, S., Taffel, S., and Mosher, W. (1988). Estimates of pregnancies and pregnancy rates for the United States, 1976-1985. *American Journal of Public Health, 78*(5), 506-511.

Willson, J., and Carrington, E. (1987). *Obstetrics and gynecology* (8th ed.). St. Louis: Mosby.

Zlatnik, F. (1987). Obesity in pregnancy. *Contemporary OB/GYN, 29*(1), 16-21.

Age-related concerns

Dryfoos, J. (1985). School-based health clinics: A new approach to preventing adolescent pregnancy? *Family Planning Perspectives*, 17(2), 70-75.

Friede, A., Baldwin, W., Rhodes, P., Buehler, J., and Strauss, L. (1988). Older maternal age and infant mortality in the United States. *Obstetrics and Gynecology*, 72(2), 152-157.

Heller, R. (1988). School-based clinics: Impact on teenage pregnancy prevention. *Pediatric Nursing*, 14(2), 103-106.

Hook, E., and Lindsjo, A. (1978). Down syndrome in live births by single year maternal age interval in a Swedish study: Comparison with results from a New York state study. *The American Journal of Human Genetics*, 30(1), 19-27.

Johnson, O. (1988). *The 1988 information please almanac* (41st ed.). Boston: Houghton Mifflin.

Kirz, D., Dorchester, W., and Freeman, R. (1985). Advanced maternal age: The mature gravida. *American Journal of Obstetrics and Gynecology*, 152(1), 7-12.

Kisker, E. (1984). The effectiveness of family planning clinics in serving adolescents. *Family Planning Perspectives*, 16(5), 212-218.

Makinson, C. (1985). The health consequences of teenage fertility. *Family Planning Perspectives*, 17(3), 132-139.

Mansfield, P., and Cohn, M. (1986). Stress and later-life childbearing: Important implications for nursing. *Maternal-Child Nursing Journal*, 15(3), 139-151.

Resnik, R. (1988). Pregnancy in women aged 35 years or older. In D. Hollingsworth and R. Resnik (Eds.), *Medical counseling before pregnancy* (pp. 14-18). New York: Churchill Livingstone.

Robinson, G., Garner, D., Gare, D., and Crawford, B. (1987). Psychological adaptation to pregnancy in childless women more than 35 years of age. *American Journal of Obstetrics and Gynecology*, 156(2), 328-333.

U.S. Department of Health and Human Services. (August 15, 1990). *Monthly Vital Statistics Report*, 39(4), Supplement.

Cardiac disease

Brady, K., and Duff, P. (1989). Rheumatic heart disease in pregnancy. *Clinical Obstetrics and Gynecology*, 32(1), 21-40.

Cruikshank, D. (1986d). Medical and surgical complications of pregnancy: Cardiovascular disease. In D. Danforth and J. Scott (Eds.), *Obstetrics and gynecology* (5th ed.; pp. 492-502). Philadelphia: Lippincott.

Gilstrap III, L. (1989). Heart disease during pregnancy. *Clinical Obstetrics and Gynecology*, 32(1), 1.

Homans, D. (1985). Peripartum cardiomyopathy. *New England Journal of Medicine*, 312(22), 1432-1437.

Lee, W., and Cotton, D. (1989). Peripartum cardiomyopathy: Current concepts and clinical management. *Clinical Obstetrics and Gynecology*, 32(1), 54-67.

McAnulty, J., Metcalfe, J., and Ueland, K. (1988). Cardiovascular disease. In G. Burrow and T. Ferris (Eds.), *Medical complications during pregnancy* (3rd ed.; pp. 180-203). Philadelphia: Saunders.

Nora, J., and Nora, A. (1987). Maternal transmission of congenital heart diseases: New recurrence risk figures and the questions of cytoplasmic inheritance and vulnerability to teratogens. *American Journal of Cardiology*, 59(5), 459-463.

Ramin, S., Mayberry, M., and Gilstrap, L. (1989). Congestive heart disease. *Clinical Obstetrics and Gynecology*, 32(1), 41-47.

Sachs, B., Brown, D., Driscoll, S., Schulman, E., Acker, D., Ransil, B., and Jewett, J. (1988). Hemorrhage, infection, toxemia, and cardiac disease, 1954-85: Causes for their declining role in maternal mortality. *American Journal of Public Health*, 78(6), 671-675.

Diabetes mellitus

Coustan, D., and Felig, P. (1988). Diabetes mellitus. In G. Burrow and T. Ferris (Eds.), *Medical complications during pregnancy* (3rd ed.; pp. 34-64). Philadelphia: Saunders

Cruikshank, D. (1986e). Medical and surgical complications of pregnancy: Endocrine and metabolic diseases. In D. Danforth and J. Scott (Eds.), *Obstetrics and gynecology* (5th ed.; pp. 516-523). Philadelphia: Lippincott.

Gabbe, S. (1985). Management of diabetes mellitus in pregnancy. *American Journal of Obstetrics and Gynecology*, 153(8), 824-828.

Gabbe, S. (1986). Definition, detection, and management of gestational diabetes. *Obstetrics and Gynecology*, 67(1), 121-125.

Granados, J. (1984). Recent developments in the outpatient management of insulin-dependent diabetes mellitus during pregnancy. *Obstetrics and Gynecology Annual*, 13, 83-98.

Hollingsworth, D. (1988). Diabetes. In D. Hollingsworth and R. Resnik (Eds.), *Medical counseling before pregnancy* (pp. 271-316). New York: Churchill Livingstone.

Mestman, J. (1985). Medical management of diabetes mellitus. In J. Queenan (Ed.), *Management of high-risk pregnancy* (2nd ed.; pp. 351-360). Oradell, NJ: Medical Economics Co.

National Diabetes Data Group. (1979). Classification and diagnosis of diabetes mellitus and other categories of glucose intolerance. *Diabetes*, 28(12), 1039-1057.

Ray, D., Yeast, J., and Freeman, R. (1986). The current role of daily serum estriol monitoring in the insulin-dependent pregnant diabetic woman. *American Journal of Obstetrics and Gynecology*, 154(6), 1257-1263.

Samuels, P., and Landon, M. (1986). Medical complications. In S. Gabbe, J. Niebyl, and J. Simpson (Eds.), *Obstetrics: Normal and problem pregnancies* (pp. 865-977). New York: Churchill Livingstone.

Schneider, J., and Kitzmiller, J. (1989). Medical management of diabetes mellitus during pregnancy. In S. Brody and K. Ueland (Eds.), *Endocrine disorders in pregnancy* (pp. 313-343). East Norwalk, CT: Appleton & Lange.

Spellacy, W. (1987). Diabetes mellitus. In J. Queenan and J. Hobbins (Eds.), *Protocols for high-risk pregnancies* (2nd ed.; pp. 140-143). Oradell, NJ: Medical Economics Co.

Swislocki, A., and Kraemer, F. (1989). Maternal metabolism in diabetes mellitus: Pathophysiology of diabetes in pregnancy. In S. Brody and K. Ueland (Eds.), *Endocrine disorders in pregnancy* (pp. 247-272). East Norwalk, CT: Appleton & Lange.

White, P. (1978). Classification of obstetric diabetes. *American Journal of Obstetrics and Gynecology*, 130(2), 228-230.

White, P. (1986). Classification of diabetes complicating pregnancy. The American College of Obstetricians and Gynecologists, *Technical Bulletin No. 92*, May 1986.

Anemia

Arthur, C., and Isbister, J.. (1987). Iron deficiency: Misunderstood, misdiagnosed, and mistreated. *Drugs*, 33(2), 171-182.

Cruikshank, D. (1986f). Don't overdo nutritional supplements during pregnancy. *Contemporary OB/GYN*, 27(2), 101-119.

Kelton, J., and Cruickshank, D. (1988). Hematologic disorders of pregnancy. In G. Burrow and T. Ferris (Eds.), *Medical complications during pregnancy* (pp. 65-94). Philadelphia: Saunders.

Martin, J., and Morrison, J. (1984). Managing the parturient with sickle cell crisis. *Clinical Obstetrics and Gynecology*, 27(1), 39-49.

Smithells, R., Seller, M., Harris, R., Fielding, D., Schorah, C., Nevin, N., Sheppard, S., Read, A., Walker, S., and Wild, J. (1983). Further experience of vitamin supplementation for prevention of neural tube defect recurrences. *The Lancet*, 1(8332), 1027-1031.

Solano, F., and Councell, R. (1986). Folate deficiency presenting as pancytopenia in pregnancy. *American Journal of Obstetrics and Gynecology*, 154(5), 1117-1118.

Winick, M. (1989). *Nutrition, pregnancy, and early infancy*. Baltimore: Williams & Wilkins.

Infection

Amstey, M. (1985). Herpes simplex. In J. Queenan (Ed.), *Management of high-risk pregnancy* (pp. 435-437). Oradell, NJ: Medical Economics Co.

Benoit, J. (1988). Sexually transmitted diseases in pregnancy. *Nursing Clinics of North America*, 23(4), 937-945.

Cates, W., and Schulz, S. (1988). Epidemiology of HIV in women. *Contemporary OB/GYN*, 32(3), 94-105.

Centers for Disease Control. (1989). 1989 Sexually transmitted diseases treatment guidelines. *MMWR*, 38(S-8), 1-43.

Centers for Disease Control. (1989). Update: Acquired immunodeficiency syndrome—United States, 1981-1988. *MMWR*, 38(14), 229-236.

Centers for Disease Control. (1985). 1985 STD treatment guidelines. *MMWR*, 34 (Suppl.), 75S-108S.

Cowan, M., Hellmann, D., Chudwin, D., Wara, D., Chang, R., and Ammann, A. (1984). Maternal transmission of acquired immune deficiency syndrome. *Pediatrics*, 73(3), 382-386.

Eschenbach, D. (1988). Infections and sexually transmitted diseases. In D. Hollingsworth and R. Resnik (Eds.), *Medical counseling before pregnancy* (pp. 249-269). New York: Churchill Livingstone.

Gibbs, R., Amstey, M., Sweet, R., Mead, P., and Sever, J. (1988). Management of genital herpes infection in pregnancy. *Obstetrics and Gynecology*, 71(5), 779-780.

Isada, N., and Grossman, J. (1986). Perinatal infections. In S. Gabbe, J. Niebyl, and J. Simpson (Eds.), *Obstetrics: Normal and problem pregnancies* (pp. 979-1048). New York: Churchill Livingstone.

Marion, R., Wiznia, A., Hutcheon, R., and Rubinstein, A. (1986). Human T-cell lymphotropic virus type III (HTLV-III) embryopathy. *American Journal of Diseases of Children*, 140(7), 638-640.

McCracken, Jr., G. and Freij, B. (1987). Bacterial and viral infections of the newborn. In G. Avery (Ed.), *Neonatology: Pathophysiology and management of the newborn* (3rd ed.; pp. 917-943). Philadelphia: Lippincott.

McElhose, P. (1988). The "other" STDs: As dangerous as ever. *RN*, 51(6), 52-59.

Merenstein, G., Todd, W., Brown, G., Yost, C., and Luzier, T. (1980). Group B Beta-hemolytic streptococcus: Randomized controlled treatment study at term. *Obstetrics and Gynecology*, 55(3), 315-318.

Minkoff, H. (1988). Managing AIDS in pregnant patients. *Contemporary OB/GYN*, 32(3), 106-114.

Murphy, P. (1989). Hepatitis B screening. *Journal of Nurse-Midwifery*, 34(1), 35.

Pritchard, J., MacDonald, P., and Gant, N. (1985). *Williams obstetrics* (17th ed.). East Norwalk, CT: Appleton & Lange.

Saltzman, R., and Jordan, M. (1988). Viral infections. In G. Burrow and T. Ferris (Eds.), *Medical complications during pregnancy* (3rd ed.; pp. 372-388). Philadelphia: Saunders.

Scott, J. (1986). Immunobiologic aspects of obstetrics and gynecology. In D. Danforth and J. Scott (Eds.), *Obstetrics and gynecology* (5th ed.; pp. 194-215). Philadelphia: Lippincott

Sharp, H. (1986). Reproductive tract disorders. In D. Danforth and J. Scott (Eds.), *Obstetrics and gynecology* (5th ed.; pp. 561-568). Philadelphia: Lippincott.

Simpson, M., Gaziano, E., Lupo, V., and Peterson, P. (1988). Bacterial infections during pregnancy. In G. Burrow and T. Ferris (Eds.), *Medical complications during pregnancy* (3rd ed.; pp. 345-371). Philadelphia: Saunders.

South, M., and Sever, J. (1986). Viral and protozoal diseases. In D. Danforth and J. Scott (Eds.), *Obstetrics and gynecology* (5th ed.; pp. 551-561). Philadelphia: Lippincott.

Stagno, S., and Whitley, R.J. (1985). Herpesvirus infections of pregnancy, Part II: Herpes simplex virus and varicella-zoster virus infections. *The New England Journal of Medicine*, 313(21), 1327-1330.

Whitley, R., Corey, L., Arvin, A., Lakeman, F., Sumaya, C., Wright, P., Dunkle L., Steele, R., Soong, S., Nahmias, A., Alford, C., Powell, D., Joaquin, V., and NIAID Collaborative Antiviral Study Group. (1988). Changing presentation of herpes simplex virus infection in neonates. *Journal of Infectious Diseases*, 158(1), 109-116.

Substance abuse

Chasnoff, I., Burns, K., and Burns, W. (1987). Cocaine use in pregnancy: Perinatal morbidity and mortality. *Neurotoxicology and Teratology*, 9(4), 291-293.

Chasnoff, I., Bussey, M., Savich, R., and Stack, C. (1986). Perinatal cerebral infarction and maternal cocaine use. *The Journal of Pediatrics*, 108(3), 456-459.

Chasnoff, I., Griffith, D., MacGregor, S., Dirkes, K., and Burns, K. (1989). Temporal patterns of cocaine use in pregnancy: Perinatal outcome. *JAMA*, 261(12), 1741-1744.

Finnegan, L. (1986). Neonatal abstinence syndrome: Assessment and pharmacotherapy. In F. Rubaltelli and B. Granati (Eds.), *Neonatal therapy: An update* (pp. 122-146). New York: Elsevier Science Pubs.

Finnegan, L., and Wapner, R. (1987). Narcotic addiction in pregnancy. In J. Neibyl (Ed.), *Drug use in pregnancy* (pp. 203-222). Philadelphia: Lea & Febiger.

Kallen, B., and Tandberg, A. (1983). Lithium and pregnancy: A cohort study on manic-depressive women. *Acta Psychiatrica Scandinavica*, 68(2), 134-139.

Kozel, N., and Adams, E. (1986). Epidemiology of drug abuse: An overview. *Science*, 234(4779), 970-974.

Loudon, J. (1987). Psychotropic drugs. *British Medical Journal*, 294(6565), 167-169.

Neerhof, M., MacGregor, S., Retzky, S., and Sullivan, T. (1989). Cocaine abuse during pregnancy: Peripartum prevalence and perinatal outcome. *American Journal of Obstetrics and Gynecology*, 161(3), 633-638.

O'Malley, P., Bachman, J., and Johnston, L. (1988). Period, age, and cohort effects on substance use among young Americans: A decade of change, 1976-1986. *American Journal of Public Health*, 78(10), 1315-1321.

Rodgers, B., and Lee, R. (1988). Drug abuse. In G. Burrow and T. Ferris (Eds.), *Medical complications during pregnancy* (3rd ed.; pp. 570-581). Philadelphia: Saunders.

Ronkin, S., Fitzsimmons, J., Wapner, R., and Finnegan, L. (1988). Protecting mother and fetus from narcotic abuse. *Contemporary OB/GYN*, 31(3), 178-187.

Wapner, R., and Finnegan, L. (1982). Perinatal aspects of psychotropic drug abuse. In R. Bolognese, R. Schwarz, and J. Schneider (Eds.), *Perinatal medicine: Management of the high-risk fetus and neonate* (2nd ed.; pp. 384-417). Baltimore: Williams & Wilkins.

Trauma and surgery

Baden, J., and Brodsky, J. (Eds.). (1985). *The pregnant surgical patient.* Mt. Kisco, NY: Futura Publishing.

Franger, A., Buchsbaum, H., and Peaceman, A. (1989). Abdominal gunshot wounds in pregnancy. *American Journal of Obstetrics and Gynecology,* 160(5, Part 1), 1124-1128.

Hammond, T., Mickens-Powers, B., Strickland, K., and Hankins, G. (1990). The use of automobile safety restraint systems during pregnancy. *JOGNN,* 19(4), 339-343.

Hillard, P. (1985). Physical abuse in pregnancy. *Obstetrics and Gynecology,* 66(2), 185-190.

Neufeld, J., Moore, E., Marx, J., and Rosen, P. (1987). Trauma in pregnancy. *Emergency Medicine Clinics of North America,* 5(3), 623-640.

Rice, S., and Pellegrini, M. (1985). Basic principles of teratology. In J. Baden and J. Brodsky (Eds.), *The pregnant surgical patient* (pp. 1-28). Mt. Kisco, NY: Futura Publishing.

Slater, G., and Aufses, A. (1985). Surgical aspects of pregnancy. In S. Cherry, R. Berkowitz, and N. Kase (Eds.), *Rovinsky and Guttmacher's medical, surgical, and gynecologic complications of pregnancy* (pp. 656-663). Baltimore: Williams & Wilkins.

Nursing research

Smith, J. (1988). The dangers of prenatal cocaine use. *MCN,* 13(3), 174-179.

Winslow, W. (1987). First pregnancy after 35: What is the experience? *MCN,* 12(2), 92-96.

Antepartal Complications

Objectives

After reading and studying this chapter, the student should be able to:

1. Recognize the signs and symptoms of antepartal complications.
2. Gather health history information for a client with antepartal complications.
3. Describe physical assessment techniques for a client with antepartal complications.
4. Interpret laboratory and diagnostic test data about the client with antepartal complications and her fetus.
5. Describe nursing care for a client with antepartal complications.
6. Discuss comfort and support measures for the client and her family.
7. Identify common needs of clients experiencing antepartal complications.
8. Understand the significance cultural background and family support may have on the childbearing process.
9. Apply the nursing process when caring for a client with antepartal complications and document that care.

Introduction

A normal pregnancy under ordinary circumstances is accompanied by multiple physiologic and psychological changes. If complications develop, however, the client can be negatively affected, as can the entire family. An antepartal complication is a disorder or malfunction that occurs before the onset of term labor (classified as 37 to 42 weeks' gestation). The discovery of such a complication can change a natural, joyful experience into a time of stress and anxiety. The client and her family may no longer look forward with unchecked enthusiasm to the birth of a child. Instead, fear may alter their expectations. In addition to worrying about the future, one or more family members—typically the client or her partner—may feel responsible for the problem.

Although normal, these reactions can lead to a breakdown in communication, worsening the situation. The nurse must assess the family accurately and offer information and support that will prevent or dispel feelings of guilt and blame.

Nursing care must meet physical, psychological, and sociocultural needs. During antepartal complications, the client and her family may need significant emotional support. The nurse's responsibilities include:
• interpreting health history, physical assessment, and laboratory and diagnostic test findings
• assessing the client's needs and adapting nursing care accordingly
• maintaining client safety and promoting client comfort
• recognizing changes in client health status and intervening as necessary
• teaching the client and her family about the antepartal complication she is experiencing, including discussing signs, symptoms, potential sequelae, and an overview of the treatments that may be required
• integrating the psychosocial and cultural needs of the client and her family and adapting antepartal care to include ethnic and cultural beliefs, whenever possible.

GLOSSARY

ABO incompatibility: condition in which the mother's blood type is O and the neonate's blood type is either A, B, or AB.

Abortion: termination of pregnancy at any time before the fetus reaches the age of viability.

Abruptio placentae: premature separation of part or all of the placenta from the uterine wall after the twentieth week of pregnancy and before delivery; hemorrhage and shock are common complications.

Antibody: protein produced in the body in response to a foreign substance (antigen) that reacts specifically with the antigen.

Antigen: foreign substance that stimulates the immune system to form antibodies to fight against it.

Chronic hypertension: hypertension that is present and observable before pregnancy, diagnosed by 20 weeks' gestation, or that extends past 42 days postpartum.

Chronic hypertension with superimposed preeclampsia: hypertension that is present and observable before pregnancy and is complicated by the hypertensive syndrome associated with preeclampsia.

Culdocentesis: needle puncture or incision to remove intraperitoneal fluid (blood, purulent drainage) by way of the vagina.

Dependent edema: edema in the lowest portion of the most dependent parts of the body.

Dilatation and curretage (D&C): surgical procedure that includes dilatation of the cervix and insertion of a curette to scrape the uterine walls and remove uterine contents. May be used as part of the treatment for endometriosis or as follow-up to an incomplete abortion.

Disseminated intravascular coagulation (DIC): abnormal clotting disorder characterized by hypoprothrombinemia, hypofibrinogenemia, and a subnormal platelet count. Caused by a major insult to the body, such as abruptio placentae.

Eclampsia: gravest, convulsive form of pregnancy-induced hypertension, affecting 1 of every 200 clients with preeclampsia, characterized by generalized tonic-clonic seizures, coma, hypertension, proteinuria, and edema; occurs between the twentieth week of pregnancy and the end of the first postpartal week.

Ectopic pregnancy: implantation of the fertilized ovum outside the uterine cavity.

Elective abortion: termination of pregnancy by choice before the age of viability.

Gestational edema: generalized interstitial accumulation of fluid (face, hands, sacrum, abdomen, ankles, tibia) after 12 hours of bed rest or a weight gain in excess of 2 kg (4 to 4½ lb) per week.

The presence of edema may be less significant than the weight gain.

Gestational hypertension: elevation of systolic and diastolic blood pressure equal to or exceeding 140/90 mm Hg; rise of 30 mm Hg systolic or 15 mm Hg diastolic above the client's baseline values. Elevated blood pressures must be present on two occasions at least 6 hours apart.

Gestational proteinuria: presence of protein in the urine during pregnancy. The urine specimen must be clean-catch or catheter-obtained. The protein must be 300 mg/liter or greater in a 24-hour specimen, or greater than 1 g/liter in a random daytime sample; it must be present on two or more occasions at least 6 hours apart.

Hyperemesis gravidarum: abnormal antepartal condition characterized by excessive nausea or vomiting leading to dehydration and starvation.

Incompetent cervix: condition in which the cervix will not maintain a pregnancy to term.

Isoimmunization: development of antibodies in response to isoantigens, which in this context are blood group antigens.

Laparotomy: incision through the abdominal wall.

Laparoscopy: insertion of an illuminated tube into the abdominal cavity to examine the contents.

Nonpitting edema: collection of fluid in the interstitial space of tissues.

Pitting edema: edema that when compressed leaves a small depression or pit.

Placenta previa: abnormally low implantation of the placenta so that it encroaches onto the internal cervical os.

Preeclampsia: nonconvulsive form of pregnancy-induced hypertension characterized by the onset of acute hypertension after the twenty-fourth week of gestation.

Pregnancy-induced hypertension (PIH): group of potentially life-threatening hypertensive disorders that may develop in the second or third trimester; includes preeclampsia and eclampsia.

Spontaneous abortion: abrupt termination of pregnancy from natural causes before the age of viability.

Therapeutic abortion: termination of a pregnancy for medical reasons (physiologic or psychological) before the age of viability.

Ultrasound: diagnostic device in which sound waves are projected through the body to obtain a scan of body parts and contents.

Viability: age and weight at which the fetus is capable of surviving outside the uterine environment (usually 24 weeks and over 500 g).

Bleeding disorders

Approximately 25% of all pregnant clients develop minimal vaginal bleeding, or spotting, during the first trimester. If the fetus is healthy, as determined by ultrasound, the client with first-trimester bleeding who complies with prescribed care will maintain the pregnancy in about 90% of all cases (Scott, 1986a).

The pregnant client with bleeding and pain is a diagnostic and management challenge because of the wide range of conditions associated with these symptoms, including normal pregnancy, spontaneous abortion, embryonic death, ectopic pregnancy, gestational trophoblastic disease, and many nonobstetric conditions (Deutchman, 1989).

Bleeding during pregnancy constitutes a medical emergency. It requires teamwork among health care professionals to minimize detrimental effects. The nurse must be aware that hemorrhage and shock could develop and be prepared to act immediately to combat those complications.

The most common causes of excessive bleeding during the antepartal period are spontaneous abortion and ectopic pregnancy. Near term, abruptio placentae (the premature separation of a normally implanted placenta) or placenta previa (abnormally low placement of the placenta) may cause hemorrhage or disseminated intravascular coagulation (DIC). For more information on abruptio placentae, placenta previa, and DIC, see Chapter 33, Intrapartal Complications.

Nursing care
The client and her family will need support during any emergency, but especially during a hemorrhagic episode. Even small amounts of visible blood can be frightening. Because it is associated with loss of life, severe bleeding causes fear and anxiety. Provide the client and her family with frequent, complete information on her care, its rationale, and her progress.

Nursing goals for the client with a bleeding problem are to:

- prevent or control severe hemorrhage
- sustain the pregnancy if reasonable or possible
- promote physical well-being of the client and her fetus
- provide emotional support for the client and her family
- prevent sequelae
- teach the client about self care
- assist in grieving for the loss of a fetus or the loss of the client's positive self-concept.

This chapter describes how the nurse should manage the care of a client with antepartal complications. These complications may be caused by reproductive system or multisystem disorders. For each disorder, it describes etiology, incidence, and nursing care. (For information on conditions associated with vaginal bleeding, see *Bleeding disorders*.)

Reproductive system disorders

Antepartal complications may be caused by such reproductive system disorders as spontaneous abortion, ectopic pregnancy, gestational trophoblastic disease, incompetent cervix, premature rupture of the membranes, and preterm labor and delivery.

Spontaneous abortion

Abortion is the termination of a pregnancy at any time before the age of viability. Viability is reached at about 20 to 24 weeks' gestation and a weight of over 500 grams, when the fetus is able to survive in an extrauterine environment (Beischer and MacKay, 1986). An abortion may be spontaneous, or the pregnancy may be terminated for medical or therapeutic reasons or for other elective reasons.

The nurse should keep in mind the negative connotations of "abortion" for many people. For this reason, people commonly refer to a spontaneous abortion as a "miscarriage."

An early spontaneous abortion is one that occurs before 12 weeks' gestation; a late abortion, between 12 and 20 weeks' gestation. Births after 20 weeks are considered preterm (Creasy, 1989). Almost 80% of all spontaneous abortions occur before 12 weeks' gestation; of those, the majority occur before 8 weeks (Scott, 1986b). Recurrent or habitual abortion is the loss of three of more pregnancies before the age of viability. Such repeated losses can be caused by genetic factors (chromosomal aberrations), anomalies of the reproductive tract (double uterus and its variants), an incompetent cervix, endocrine imbalances (such as hypothyroidism or diabetes mellitus), or systemic disorders (such as lupus erythematosus).

Etiology
Nearly 80% of spontaneously aborted fetuses display an abnormal genetic or chromosomal makeup that is not compatible with life; the remaining spontaneous abortions result from maternal causes (Beischer and MacKay, 1986). The latter may occur because of an acute infection, such as syphilis, pyelonephritis, or *chlamydia trachomatis* infection. Abnormalities of the reproductive system are common maternal causes of pregnancy loss during the second and third trimesters. A woman whose mother took diethylstilbestrol (DES) during pregnancy may have spontaneous abortions.

Anything that might interfere with normal ovum implantation and placental development may be related to spontaneous abortion. For example, implantation of the fertilized ovum and placental development can be inhibited by scar tissue on the endometrium, which could result from dilatation and curettage (D&C), previous childbirth, or severe infection. Alterations in hormones, such as progesterone, also may be related to pregnancy loss (Key, 1989).

The risk of early pregnancy loss is increased in women who have a history of first trimester pregnancy loss, uterine defects, chronic infections, or cigarette or alcohol abuse (Deutchman, 1989).

Little can be done to avoid genetic causes of spontaneous abortion. Certain other causes, however, can be prevented. Prepregnancy correction of maternal disorders, immunization against infectious diseases, proper early prenatal care, and prompt treatment of complications of pregnancy can prevent many spontaneous abortions.

Incidence

The exact incidence of spontaneous abortion is difficult to calculate because many early pregnancies are lost for unknown reasons before they are clinically evident. At least 15% of all pregnancies are known to end in spontaneous abortion. However, recent research into the first few days and weeks after conception indicates that the spontaneous abortion rate is far higher than 15%. Researchers postulate that if every woman were continually monitored, the rate might approach 50% (Key, 1989; Scott, 1986b).

Classification

According to Key (1989), abortions can be classified according to weight; that is, whether the fetus weighs 500 grams or less. (For a complete classification, see *Assessing different types of abortion*.)

Ectopic pregnancy

In ectopic pregnancy, the fertilized ovum is implanted in tissue other than the endometrium (lining of the uterus). More than 95% of ectopic pregnancies occur in the fallopian tubes, usually in the ampullary and isthmic segments. Less than 3% of all ectopic pregnancies are intra-abdominal, and less than 1% of these are implanted in cervical or ovarian tissues (Droegemueller, 1986).

Etiology

The majority of extrauterine pregnancies result from impeded progress of the fertilized ovum through the fallopian tube. The primary causes are tubal obstruction and delayed tubal transport (Osguthorpe and Keating, 1988).

A previous episode of pelvic inflammatory disease with accompanying salpingitis (inflammation of the fallopian tubes) commonly is implicated in cases of tubal obstruction. Salpingitis results in mucosal damage, tubal narrowing, diverticula (sacs or pouches in the tubal wall), and also may impair tubal motility (Osguthorpe and Keating, 1988).

Other conditions that predispose a woman to ectopic pregnancy include:
• previous therapeutic abortion or previous abdominal surgery (presence of scar tissue may affect tubal motility)
• use of an intrauterine device (IUD) for more than 2 years, which can cause a low-grade inflammatory response within the fallopian tubes
• in vivo exposure to DES, which can adversely affect tubal motility
• congenital anomalies that interfere with passage of the fertilized ovum or with implantation
• altered hormonal status that affects tubal motility.

Ectopic pregnancy results from fertilization of the ovum before it migrates to the fallopian tube. This delayed transport may leave the zygote in the fallopian tube at the time of implantation.

Incidence

Ectopic pregnancy is the leading cause of maternal death in the first trimester. In the United States, it occurs in 10.8 of every 1,000 pregnancies, and it accounts for 11% of all maternal deaths (CDC, 1990; Lawson, et al., 1988). The majority of ectopic pregnancies occur in women ages 25 to 34 (Loffer, 1986).

The incidence of ectopic pregnancy has increased fourfold over the past 21 years (CDC, 1990). The risk is 1.6 times greater for nonwhite women, and maternal mortality is 3.5 times higher for these women.

Common predisposing factors other than age include infertility and a previous ectopic pregnancy. A woman who has an ectopic pregnancy in one fallopian tube is at increased risk for developing an ectopic pregnancy in the opposite tube. Only 1 in 3 women who experience an ectopic pregnancy will give birth to a live neonate in a subsequent pregnancy (Osguthorpe and Keating, 1988).

Early diagnosis and management of an ectopic pregnancy helps reduce such potential complications as tubal rupture or hemorrhage, thereby improving the woman's chance for a successful subsequent pregnancy (Osguthorpe, 1987; Osguthorpe and Keating, 1988).

Assessing different types of abortion

The nurse must assess the different types of abortion accurately to provide adequate nursing care and emotional support.

TYPE AND DEFINITION	PHYSICAL FINDINGS	MANAGEMENT
Threatened		
Appearance of signs and symptoms of possible loss of embryo	*Bleeding:* slight *Cramping:* mild and intermittent *Expelled tissue:* none *Internal cervical os:* closed *Uterus size:* varies according to length of gestation	Bed rest; sedation; decreased stress; no sexual intercourse, douches, or cathartics. Further treatment depends on specific signs and symptoms. (Blood replacement therapy, I.V. therapy, and antibiotics may be indicated.)
Inevitable (Imminent)		
Signs and symptoms indicate certain loss of embryo	*Bleeding:* slight *Cramping:* mild and intermittent *Expelled tissues:* none *Internal cervical os:* open *Uterus size:* varies according to length of gestation	Prompt termination of pregnancy by dilatation and curettage (D&C)
Incomplete		
Part of the products of conception retained in the uterus	*Bleeding:* heavy *Cramping:* severe *Expelled tissues:* some *Internal cervical os:* open *Uterus size:* smaller than expected for length of gestation	Prompt termination of pregnancy by D&C or suction curettage
Complete		
All products of conception expelled from uterus	*Bleeding:* slight to moderate *Cramping:* mild to moderate *Expelled tissues:* all products of conception *Internal cervical os:* closed *Uterus size:* smaller than expected for length of gestation	No intervention needed unless hemorrhage or infection develops
Missed		
Nonviable fetus and other products of conception retained in uterus for 2 months or longer	*Bleeding:* slight *Cramping:* none *Expelled tissues:* none *Internal cervical os:* closed *Uterus size:* smaller than expected for length of gestation	If spontaneous evacuation of the uterus does not occur within 1 month, pregnancy will be terminated. Method of termination will depend on the length of gestation. Client must be monitored for signs of disseminated intravascular coagulation, which may develop if the products of conception remain in the uterus after 5 weeks.
Septic		
Infection of products of conception and endometrial lining of uterus, which may result from attempted interference early in pregnancy	*Bleeding:* varies; malodorous *Cramping:* varies *Expelled tissue:* varies, depending on whether tissue fragments remain *Internal cervical os:* usually open *Uterus size:* varies but will be tender *Other:* fever	Immediate termination of pregnancy by D&C; cervical cultures and sensitivities performed; broad spectrum antibiotic administered; temperature monitored

Classification

Ectopic pregnancies are classified by the site of implantation, such as tubal or ovarian, because the uterus is the only organ capable of maintaining a term pregnancy. Abdominal pregnancies occur once in approximately 15,000 live births; however, the delivery of a live, term neonate from an abdominal pregnancy occurs only once in approximately 250,000 live births. Intra-abdominal pregnancies also are associated with increased maternal mortality caused by uncontrolled hemorrhage and sepsis.

Gestational trophoblastic disease

Gestational trophoblastic disease (GTD) may be benign (hydatidiform mole) or malignant (choriocarcinoma). In GTD, trophoblastic cells covering the chorionic villi proliferate, and the villi undergo cystic changes.

In benign GTD, a neoplasm forms on the chorion (outer layer of the membrane containing amniotic fluid) when the chorionic villi degenerate and become transparent vesicles that hang in grapelike clusters (Hilgers and Lewis, 1986). These vesicles contain a clear fluid and may involve all or part of the decidual lining of the uterus. Usually no embryo is present because it has been absorbed.

In malignant GTD—a serious, rapidly developing, but rare carcinoma—neoplastic trophoblasts proliferate without cystic villi and may metastasize.

Etiology

The cause of GTD is unknown. (Several theories relate GTD to a nutritional deficit, specifically an insufficient intake of protein. These theories, however, have not been substantiated.) Because no specific etiology has been determined, prevention techniques are unknown.

Incidence

GTD is reported to occur in about 1 of every 2,000 pregnancies. Recent research indicates, however, that the incidence would be much higher if all cases of the disorder were identified. Some cases are not recognized because the pregnancy is aborted early and the products of conception are not available for analysis.

In most cases, GTD occurs in women who have had ovulation stimulation with clomiphene (Clomid), in women from lower socioeconomic groups, and in older women. The disorder is much more common in the Orient than in the West; for example, it occurs in appproximately 1 of every 200 pregnancies in the Philippines. The reason for the increased incidence among Oriental women is unknown, but nutrition may play a role (Berman and DiSaia, 1989).

Classification

The classification of GTD depends on whether it is localized or disseminated. A benign neoplasm is well localized in the uterus, whereas a malignant neoplasm may metastasize. The most common site of metastasis is the lungs. However, metastasis to the brain and liver may occur if the disease is allowed to progress (Berman and DiSaia, 1989).

A diagnosis of benign GTD does not denote a benign long-term prognosis, nor does a diagnosis of malignant GTD definitely indicate an unfavorable prognosis. For both diagnoses, close monitoring and thorough follow-up care is vital. (For more information, see the "Planning and implementation" section in this chapter.)

Incompetent cervix

Incompetent cervix (or premature dilation of the cervix) is characterized by painless dilation of the cervix without labor or uterine contraction. Depending on the length of gestation, spontaneous abortion or premature delivery may result.

Up to 40% of all perinatal deaths occur in association with pregnancies that terminate between 20 and 28 weeks' gestation. Cervical incompetence is a major contributor to those losses (Beischer and MacKay, 1986).

Etiology

Cervical incompetence may be caused by a previous traumatic delivery or a forceful D&C of the cervix (Scott, 1986b). Other etiologic factors may be congenital, such as a short cervix or an anomalous uterus (such as a double uterus or other altered shape).

Incidence

Incompetent cervix occurs in approximately 1 of every 1,000 deliveries, 1 of 100 abortions, and 1 of 5 habitual abortions, where the client has had three or more abortions (Beischer and MacKay, 1986).

Premature rupture of the membranes

Premature rupture of the membranes (PROM) is any rupture of the amniotic sac before onset of labor, independent of length of gestation. PROM presents a management challenge because of the divergent opinions surrounding its treatment. It is associated with maternal morbidity and mortality, primarily because of increased incidence of infection. Fetal and neonatal risks include sepsis, preterm delivery, anoxia, respiratory distress syndrome, cord prolapse, and traumatic delivery (Gibbs and Sweet, 1989).

Etiology

Although the etiology of PROM usually is unknown, many conditions predispose a woman to this disorder. Possible factors include incompetent cervix, amnionitis, placenta previa, fetal malpresentation, hydramnios, more than one fetus, and trauma (Gibbs and Sweet, 1989). Besides being a complication of PROM, infection also may be a cause. Some researchers have proposed a link among coitus, inflammation, and PROM. A woman with PROM before term is more likely to have microorganisms present on the cervix than one who does not have PROM (Gibbs and Sweet, 1989).

Incidence

Between 3% and 19% of all deliveries are preceded by PROM (Gibbs and Sweet, 1989). The percentage is significantly higher in preterm pregnancies.

Preterm labor and delivery

Defined as any delivery, regardless of the neonate's birth weight, that occurs between 20 and 37 weeks after the client's last menses. Preterm labor and delivery has been a significant cause of perinatal morbidity and mortality for many years (Creasy, 1989). Advances in technology have enhanced medical management of small neonates, but no significant decrease in low-birth-weight, preterm neonates has been documented (Creasy, 1989). The problem of preterm delivery is one of the most significant to be overcome in attempting to improve pregnancy outcome.

Etiology

Many factors can contribute to the onset of preterm labor and delivery, including pneumonia, appendicitis with sepsis, other acute infections, multiple gestation (more than one fetus), poverty, smoking, alcohol abuse, drug addiction, grand multiparity (five or more previous births), teenage pregnancy, and uterine anomalies. Psychological trauma also may be a contributing factor, as may significant adverse events or chronic stress during the second and third trimesters (Omer and Everly, 1988).

Incidence

Preterm labor and delivery accounts for 5% to 10% of all births in developed countries. Although the percentage is relatively small, this condition accounts for most neonatal deaths. The incidence almost doubles for Black clients (Creasy, 1989).

Maternal age under 19 or over 34 is a significant factor also. A previous preterm labor and delivery is associated with a risk of recurrence of 17% to 30%, with the incidence increasing significantly after two or more preterm labors and deliveries (Creasy, 1989).

Women in lower socioeconomic groups have an increased incidence of preterm labor and delivery. This may be related to nutritional status during pregnancy. A woman who weighs less than 50 kg (112 lb) at the start of her pregnancy is at a higher risk than one who weighs 57 kg (125 lb) or more.

Multisystem disorders

Antepartal complications may be caused by such multisystem disorders as hyperemesis gravidarum, hypertensive disorders, and Rh incompatibility.

Hyperemesis gravidarum

Sometimes called "pernicious vomiting," this complication of pregnancy involves dehydration and malnutrition. Because hyperemesis begins as simple nausea and vomiting, a definitive diagnosis can be difficult. The client's tolerance for nausea and vomiting, the degree of hydration, her electrolyte balance, and her level of disability all affect the diagnosis. The nurse should realize that every case of nausea and vomiting during pregnancy can be serious.

Mild nausea and vomiting, commonly called "morning sickness," occurs in approximately 50% of all pregnant women during the first trimester. Its physiologic basis is not completely understood. Theories link it to progesterone deficiency, hyperadrenalism, hyperthyroidism, or human chorionic gonadotropin (hCG) in the mother's blood (Key, 1989), but no one theory adequately explains the symptoms. "Morning sickness" is considered a minor, self-limiting nuisance that appears 4 to 6 weeks after a missed menses and disappears after about 14 to 16 weeks of gestation (Key, 1989). (For more information on mild nausea and vomiting during early pregnancy, see Chapter 18, Physiologic Changes during Normal Pregnancy.)

Etiology

The cause of hyperemesis gravidarum is not known. Etiologic theories embrace hormonal alterations, allergic conditions (possibly an autoimmune response to the pregnancy), or a psychosomatic condition (Key, 1989).

Hormonal alterations occur frequently in pregnancy. Progesterone produced by the placenta relaxes the smooth muscle of the uterus to help maintain pregnancy. Progesterone also slows gastric and intestinal motility, which may predispose pregnant clients to emesis. However, hyperemesis has not been directly related to progesterone activity.

Human chorionic gonadotropin levels also may affect emesis during pregnancy. Levels of hCG are elevated in clients with GTD and, according to Berkowitz and Goldstein (1984), many women with GTD develop hyperemesis. (For more information, see "Gestational trophoblastic disease" in the "Nursing care" section of this chapter.) Furthermore, hCG levels increase proportionately with placental size and the number of fetuses, and emesis is more probable in clients who are pregnant with more than one fetus. Despite these implied correlations, however, no clear relationship has been established between hCG levels and hyperemesis.

The autoimmune response (allergy) theory has been postulated because hyperemesis terminates with labor.

The psychosomatic theory is based on the fact that nausea unrelated to pregnancy can be psychological. An obnoxious odor, a repulsive sight, or even the recollection of such an odor or sight can cause nausea and vomiting. However, current research findings fall far short of demonstrating a psychosomatic cause of hyperemesis.

Other factors that could be related to hyperemesis are elevated thyroxine (T_4) levels and increased triiodothyronine (T_3) uptake. Another possible explanation is that some clients have a stress reaction pattern that involves gastrointestinal disturbances, such as nausea, vomiting, and diarrhea. Pregnancy could activate that stress pattern.

Incidence

Hyperemesis gravidarum occurs in 7 to 16 of every 1,000 pregnant women (Key, 1989). Its incidence appears to vary with life-style, race, amount of stress, number of gestations, marital status, and age; however, demographic factors are difficult to separate from cultural, sociologic, and environmental ones.

Hypertensive disorders

Hypertension is the third leading cause of maternal mortality in the United States, preceded only by hemorrhage and infection. About 7% of all pregnancies are affected by hypertension; 6% to 10% of perinatal deaths are associated with hypertensive episodes. According to Hacker and Moore (1986), the hypertensive episode may result directly from the pregnancy itself (pregnancy-induced hypertension), or it may predate the pregnancy and result from cardiovascular or renal disease. (For information on how PIH affects major body systems, see *Pathophysiology of pregnancy-induced hypertension*.)

The American College of Obstetricians and Gynecologists accepts the following terms in association with gestational hypertension: preeclampsia and eclampsia,

---

Pathophysiology of pregnancy-induced hypertension

Pregnancy-induced hypertension (PIH) affects major body systems, including the kidneys, lungs, liver, and uterus. Many of the PIH-induced changes in these systems—such as tissue ischemia and fibrinogen deposits in the vessel walls—can be identified only through postmortem studies.

Effects on kidneys
Low protein levels cause decreased plasma colloidal pressure and allow fluid to shift from intravascular to interstitial spaces, causing edema. Blood flow to the kidneys is decreased by the fluid shift. The decreased blood flow diminishes renal perfusion, which in turn triggers the release of renin that leads to the formation of the potent vasopressor angiotensin. These work to increase the blood pressure to offset the effects of diminished renal perfusion. Renal function becomes inefficient and the glomerular filtration rate decreases. Vascular spasms also decrease glomerular blood flow and constrict glomerular capillaries. Diminished renal function results in albuminuria and increased blood urea nitrogen.

Effects on liver
Vascular spasms result in vessel compression and, in some cases, extravasation (hemorrhage under the liver and in the intra-abdominal cavity). Fibrin clots also may form from elevated plasma fibrinogen levels in gestational hypertension (Ballageer, et al., 1989).

Effects on lungs
Pulmonary changes resulting from PIH include pulmonary edema and diffuse intrapulmonary bleeding, which could predispose the client to bronchopneumonia.

Effects on placenta
Placental changes from PIH affect the uteroplacental perfusion. These changes include premature aging, degeneration and calcification of tissues, congested intervillous spaces, and arteriolar thromboses. Shanklin and Sibai (1989) have identified extensive endothelial injury in placental biopsy samples of women with PIH. The integrity of uterine vessels and coagulation capabilities also were altered in those women. Rodgers, Taylor, and Roberts (1988) found that serum from preeclampsic women was toxic to endothelial cells maintained in vitro.

---

chronic hypertension, pregnancy-induced hypertension (PIH), chronic hypertension with superimposed preeclampsia, and transient hypertension (Gilbert and Harmon, 1986). PIH is characterized by hypertension, proteinuria, and edema. It has two basic forms: preeclampsia (a nonconvulsive form marked by the onset of acute hypertension after 24 weeks' gestation) and eclampsia (a convulsive form that occurs between 20 weeks' gestation and the end of the first postpartal week). This syndrome may develop at any point after 20 weeks' gestation or in the early postpartal period. (Hypertension before 20 weeks' gestation usually is associated with GTD.) Typically, the syndrome appears in the last trimester and disappears after 42 postpartal days. PIH may be difficult to distinguish from hypertensive states that predate the pregnancy. In addition, a definitive diagnosis of PIH may be impossible unless the client's blood pressure returns to baseline after pregnancy.

Chronic hypertension is present and observable before the pregnancy and is diagnosed by week 20 of gestation or extends 42 days after delivery. Chronic hypertensive disease may occur alone or with superimposed PIH.

Other terms that have been used or are used to define hypertension associated with pregnancy are toxemia, preeclampsia-eclampsia, and metabolic disease of late pregnancy.

Etiology

The exact cause of PIH is unknown; however, several theories explain aspects of the disorder. Geographic, ethnic, racial, nutritional, immunologic, and familial factors may play a role in its development, as they do in the development of hypertension in other periods of life.

PIH originally was thought to be caused by a circulating toxic substance. That theory, which is responsible for the term "toxemia of pregnancy," has not been proven; therefore, the term is factually incorrect even though it is frequently used (Cunningham, MacDonald, and Gant, 1989).

Incidence

The incidence of PIH ranges from 7% to 10% (Rodgers, Taylor, and Roberts, 1988). Factors that predispose a woman to PIH are:
• Primigravidity. Most women who develop PIH are pregnant for the first time. The incidence is especially high in those under age 17 or over age 35 (Gavette and Roberts, 1987).
• Multiple gestation. The incidence of PIH increases with the number of fetuses.
• Vascular disease. Especially associated with PIH are diabetes mellitus, hypertensive renal disease, or essential hypertension.
• GTD (hydatidiform mole). The hypertensive syndrome usually appears before 20 weeks' gestation if associated with GTD.
• Malnutrition or dietary deficiencies. Deficiencies in proteins and in water-soluble vitamins frequently are associated with the development of PIH (Belizian and Villar, 1980; Brewer, 1974; DeAlvarez, 1978).

As noted, PIH is one of the three major causes of maternal morbidity. Mortality figures in developing countries are 5% to 17% for the mother and 15% to 37% for the fetus. Mortality figures for developed countries are 0.5% to 1% for the mother and 8% to 10% for the fetus when eclampsia, a complication of PIH, occurs (Zuspan and Zuspan, 1986).

Rh incompatibility

Hemolytic disease of the newborn, also called erythroblastosis fetalis, is a progressive disorder of the fetal blood and blood-forming organs characterized by hemolytic anemia and hyperbilirubinemia. Erythroblastosis fetalis results from the transfer of red blood cell (RBC)-destroying antibodies from the mother to the fetus.

The more severe forms of isoimmune hemolytic disease are associated with $Rh_o(D)$ group incompatibility. (For more information, see *Rh factor*.) Before prophylactic $Rh_o(D)$ human immunoglobulin (RhIg) became available in 1968, this disease occurred in 0.5% to 1% of all term pregnancies in North America. Since immunization with RhIg began, however, the incidence of severe hemolytic disease of the newborn has been reduced drastically (Scott, 1986a).

Rh factor

During the 1940s, scientists discovered that when red blood cells (RBCs) from rhesus monkeys were injected into rabbits they produced an antiserum that, when injected back into the monkeys, caused agglutination (clumping) of some RBCs. The agglutinated RBCs contained the rhesus (Rh) antigen (the substance that stimulates production of antibodies) and were designated *Rh positive*. The RBCs that did not contain the antigen could not be agglutinated; these were designated *Rh negative*. Subsequent research revealed that the Rh factor is not a single antigen but a complex blood system with a number of variants.

The six common Rh antigens are identified as C, D, E, c, d, and e. Antibody formation results from the presence of one or more of these antigens. However, d is not a true antigen and does not induce antibody formation. Because 23 pairs of homologous chromosomes—one set from each parent—are present in each cell, an individual's genetic constitution in terms of these antigens might be, for example, DD, dd, or Dd. Different combinations allow eight Rh genotypes from a single Rh chromosome (CDe, cDe, and so forth).

The degree to which each antigen will induce antibody formation—known as *antigenicity potency*—varies (Scott, 1986a). No specific antiserum (serum that contains antibodies specific for the antigen) has been found for d; therefore, *d* is used to represent the absence of a discernable antibody (Lloyd, 1987).

In 1946, a "new" factor was isolated in a donor's blood and was labeled D^u. Researchers subsequently determined that a client who is genetically D^u positive does have a weak D antigen on the red blood cells and should be classified as Rh positive (Lloyd, 1987).

Etiology

Hemolytic diseases of the newborn, such as erythroblastosis fetalis, hydrops fetalis, and icterus gravis, were found to be linked to the Rh factor. These hemolytic disorders are caused by the hemolysis of fetal RBCs by maternal antibodies. Later research indicated that approximately 90% of clinical cases of hemolytic diseases in neonates followed maternal sensitization (isoimmunization) by Rh antigens (Scott, 1986a). The Rh-negative mother was sensitized by her fetus's Rh-positive RBCs, inherited from the Rh-positive father. (For more information on other hemolytic diseases, see *Other RBC antigen incompatibilities.*)

Theoretically, maternal isoimmunization also could be caused by a transfusion with Rh-positive or D^u-positive blood. This type of isoimmunization is rare, however, because typing and crossmatching are performed routinely before blood administration. A positive D^u factor would be identified at initial screening and that blood would be labeled as Rh positive (Lloyd, 1987).

Incidence

Almost 65% of the neonates of Rh-incompatible couples are Rh positive. Ten percent to 15% of Caucasian couples will be affected by Rh incompatibility. About 5% of Black couples will be Rh incompatible, and only rarely will an Oriental couple be affected (Scott, 1986a). This difference of incidence among races is related to the proportion of Rh positive and Rh-negative individuals in each group. For example, Caucasians have a higher proportion of Rh-negative individuals than do Blacks, so they have a greater chance of Rh incompatibility.

The risk of maternal sensitization is less than may be expected. The factors involved include the antigenicity of the antigen, the amount of antigen infused, and the mother's immunologic response to the antigen (Lloyd, 1987). Some clients have a greater antigenic response to the Rh factor. Only about 0.1% of mothers are sensitized during a first Rh-positive pregnancy. The risk of isoimmunization increases with the number of pregnancies if treatment with RhIg is not instituted. About 5% of Rh-incompatible pregnancies produce affected neonates (Scott, 1986). (For more information, see *Rh isoimmunization.*)

Maternal effects from Rh incompatibility have not been identified; however, severe Rh incompatibility results in erythroblastosis fetalis. When fetal blood reacts to the Rh-positive antibodies of the mother, fetal RBCs are destroyed (hemolysis) and fetal hemolytic anemia results. The released blood pigments, or bilirubin, are transported across the placenta, processed by the maternal liver, and excreted in the bile. When the amount of pigments is greater than the maternal liver can process, the neonate will be icteric (jaundiced) at birth.

Other RBC antigen incompatibilities

Fetal-maternal incompatibility of ABO groups also may cause hemolytic disease. The blood type of a person who has red blood cells (RBCs) with neither the A antigen nor the B antigen is designated as group O. Blood of individuals with group O contains anti-A and anti-B antibodies. Therefore, the group O mother who is pregnant with a fetus whose blood group is A, B, or AB has anti-A and anti-B antibodies that may be stimulated by the pregnancy and may be transferred across the placenta to her fetus. In ABO incompatibility, even the first child can be affected.

The largest percentage of neonates who are affected by ABO incompatibility has blood group A and mothers with blood group O. Black neonates are more likely to develop ABO incompatibility than Caucasian neonates (Cunningham, MacDonald, and Gant, 1989).

The clinical manifestations of fetal-maternal ABO incompatibility typically are mild and short-lasting. However, severe hemolysis with resultant hyperbilirubinemia and kernicterus is possible. No preventive agent is known for use in ABO incompatibility. Treatment of affected neonates is symptomatic, involving phototherapy and increased fluids. (For more information on phototherapy as a treatment for hyperbilirubinemia, see Chapter 38, High-Risk Neonates).

Other, less common RBC antigens also are capable of transplacental isoimmunization. Fortunately, isoimmunization related to these antigens is not common, and serious fetal injury from these factors is unlikely.

Hyperplasia of the bone marrow and extramedullary (spleen) hematopoiesis occur as fetal compensatory mechanisms to offset fetal anemia, which can lead to cardiac decompensation, cardiomegaly, hepatomegaly, and splenomegaly. A syndrome of generalized edema and ascites known as hydrops fetalis may result. At this point, the fetus will be at serious risk for intrauterine or early neonatal death.

The placenta of the seriously affected fetus is enlarged. The amniotic fluid may be stained a yellowish color from bile pigments. Following delivery, the erythroblastotic neonate becomes icteric because the neonate cannot excrete the bile pigments resulting from RBC hemolysis. Icterus neonatorum (jaundice in the neonate) can occur soon after birth in severe cases.

Generalized pigmentation of brain cells (kernicterus) commonly develops when the serum bilirubin rises to levels that are toxic to the neonate and can lead to death. Serious central nervous system abnormalities, such as choreoathetoid cerebral palsy, may develop and persist if the neonate survives.

Rh hemolytic disease of the neonate occurs once in approximately 150 to 200 full-term pregnancies in the United States (Scott, 1986a). At least 200,000 children are affected each year; 5,000 of these are stillborn. In cases of untreated severe hemolytic disease, about 10%

Rh isoimmunization

An Rh-negative woman will develop anti-Rh-positive antibodies when carrying an Rh-positive fetus. The progression of her sensitization is illustrated below.

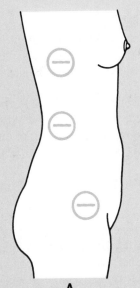

A
Rh-negative woman before pregnancy or other contact with positive antigen.

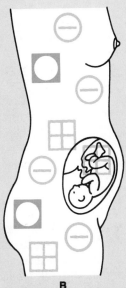

B
Rh-negative woman pregnant with Rh-positive fetus. Some Rh-positive blood passes into the maternal circulation during gestation.

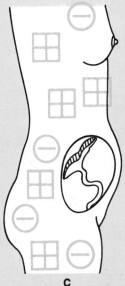

C
During placental separation, more fetal blood enters the maternal circulation.

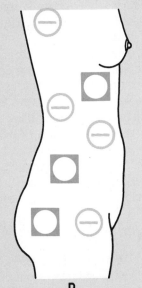

D
Maternal sensitization occurs after approximately 72 hours, and subsequent contact with Rh antigen induces formation of Rh antibodies (if RhIg has not been administered).

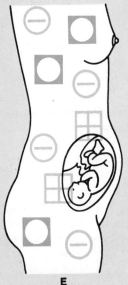

E
Subsequent pregnancies with Rh-positive fetuses are jeopardized because maternal anti-Rh-positive antibodies are formed, which cross the placenta and attack the RBCs of the fetus.

of affected neonates will develop kernicterus. With intrauterine (fetal) transfusions, however, that number can be reduced by about 40%. Amniocentesis studies, early delivery of affected fetuses, and exchange or replacement transfusions have decreased the mortality rate.

Complete recovery can be expected in neonates who do not develop kernicterus. If hyperbilirubinemia is treated promptly and effectively, most neonates recover without residual effects or sequelae. (For more information on neonatal hyperbilirubinemia, see Chapter 38, High-Risk Neonates.)

Assessment

The types of antepartal complications vary widely, as shown by the preceding discussions of their presentation and etiology. The nursing care of clients with antepartal complications therefore varies as well. Because the nursing process is a systematic method for providing flexible, varied care, it is used as a framework for providing nursing care to these clients.

The nurse begins with assessment, using data from the health history, physical assessment, and laboratory and diagnostic test results to make appropriate nursing diagnoses and provide holistic, humanistic care to the client.

Spontaneous abortion

Signs and symptoms of spontaneous abortion depend on the development of the implantation site, determined by the length of gestation. The three stages of development of the implantation site are:
• Early (or decidual). The fertilized ovum, surrounded by decidua, is poorly attached to the uterus. The early stage covers the first 6 weeks of gestation.
• Intermediate (or attachment). Chorionic villi in the basal plate of the decidua attach moderately well to the decidua basalis. The intermediate stage extends from 6 to 12 weeks of gestation.
• Late or (placental). After 12 weeks of gestation, the placenta is fully formed and firmly attached to the decidua basalis.

During the early stage of placental development, the symptoms of abortion are not severe; bleeding and cramping are minimal. During the intermediate stage, moderate cramping and blood loss are expected because the ovum and its surrounding tissues are larger and more firmly attached to the uterus. Severe pain is associated with a late abortion because the fetus must be expelled. Abdominal cramping, similar to labor, is usual. The amount of bleeding, however, is less than with an intermediate-stage abortion because the placenta remains attached until after the fetus has been delivered. Bleeding is more controlled because of strong uterine contractions.

A client who has a late-stage abortion may experience breast engorgement and lactation. Alterations in hormonal levels subsequent to pregnancy also may be responsible for a labile emotional state (Beischer and MacKay, 1986).

A pregnancy may have been terminated for several days before signs and symptoms become definite. For this reason, the exact date of termination can be difficult to determine. The following laboratory findings are characteristic of abortion.
• Urine. A negative or weakly positive urine pregnancy test.
• Blood. If blood loss is excessive or prolonged, anemia is probable (hemoglobin level below than 10.5 g/dl or hematocrit less than 32 g/dl). If sepsis occurs following a missed or incomplete abortion (in which portions of the products of conception remain in the uterus), the white blood cell (WBC) count will be greater than 12,000/mm^3. (The sedimentation rate will increase with abortion, anemia, or infection and therefore is not useful for diagnostic purposes.)
• Endocrine. hCG, estrogen, and progesterone titers can be minimal in abortions (Cunningham, MacDonald, and Gant, 1989).

A detailed, accurate history focusing on the client's recent health, menstrual, gynecologic, and obstetric history, contraceptive method used, and possible date of conception is necessary for a complete diagnostic evaluation. In addition to obtaining the health history, gather all pertinent information related to the client's physical state. Assess the amount and consistency of blood to determine whether any products of conception have been passed. To help refine the diagnosis, obtain complete pain information, including location, type, and duration.

Ectopic pregnancy

Gather and record such relevant history as occurrence of abdominal surgery, spontaneous or voluntary abortion, or ectopic pregnancy. Note religious preferences should baptism be requested or administration of blood or blood products be necessary.

Observe for abdominal pain, amenorrhea, and abnormal vaginal bleeding. Abdominal pain is the most consistent finding, occurring in over 90% of cases. The quality of pain varies markedly but usually is described as cramplike. Nausea and vomiting also may occur, along with urinary frequency. Signs of ruptured ectopic pregnancy may occur, including pallor, tachycardia, hypotension, and temperature elevation. Adnexal (lower right or left quadrant near ovary) tenderness occurs unilaterally in about 50% of clients. (For additional details, see *Unruptured and ruptured ectopic pregnancy: Comparing the signs and symptoms,* page 556.)

Complicating ectopic pregnancy diagnosis are the numerous disorders that share many, and possibly all, of the same signs and symptoms. These disorders include appendicitis, salpingitis, abortion, ovarian cysts, and urinary tract infections. Because definitive diagnosis is difficult, the condition may become an obstetric emergency if the ectopic pregnancy is unrecognized until the tube ruptures. Many emergency departments admit clients with a ruptured tubal pregnancy without previous signs or symptoms.

Recently developed tests, like the serum test for beta-subunit human chorionic gonadotropin (beta-hCG), have facilitated the diagnosis of ectopic pregnancy. Beta-hCG, a hormone produced by the trophoblastic cells of the developing placenta, can be detected in minute amounts by radioimmunoassay of the hormone in a blood sample 9 days after ovulation (Romero, 1986). It also can be detected quickly, accurately, and inexpensively by sensitive home urine tests for pregnancy.

Physical signs and laboratory tests other than those for beta-HCG have limited diagnostic value unless tubal rupture occurs. A missed period, adnexal tenderness, or a small adnexal mass, for example, may indicate ectopic pregnancy but also can indicate an ovarian or corpus luteum cyst (Osguthorpe and Keating, 1988).

Once a positive pregnancy test has been obtained, an ultrasound can be performed. If a gestational sac is not visible 5 to 6 weeks after the last menstrual period, an ectopic or abnormal intrauterine pregnancy can be suspected. Although ultrasound can be helpful, it is not a definitive diagnostic tool. First, a pseudogestational sac in the uterus occurs in 10% to 20% of clients with ectopic pregnancy. In addition, intrauterine and ectopic pregnancies can coexist (although rarely) so that the identification of one does not automatically rule out the other. Finally, because of their relatively small size, few ectopic pregnancies can be detected by ultrasound (Osguthorpe and Keating, 1988). Ultrasound has been more effective in ruling out an intrauterine pregnancy than in confirming an ectopic one.

A relatively new assessment development for ectopic pregnancy, endovaginal ultrasound may alter the typical approach (Jain, Hamper, and Sanders, 1988). It is performed by placing a transducer at the external opening of the vagina and directing sound waves into the pelvic cavity (For an illustration, see *Endovaginal ultrasonography,* page 557.) In comparison studies, endovaginal ultrasonography has been more sensitive than traditional transabdominal ultrasound in detecting ectopic pregnancies.

A laparoscopy can be performed to confirm a suspected ectopic pregnancy. Because blood is present in the abdominal cavity in about 65% of clients with unruptured ectopic pregnancies and other conditions not requiring laparotomy, laparoscopy is especially helpful in identifying the bleeding sites. (For more information on laparoscopy, see Chapter 10, Fertility and Infertility.)

The most effective diagnosis of an ectopic pregnancy combines these three diagnostic tools. Serum hCG levels in conjunction with ultrasonography and laparoscopy provide accurate information without using an invasive procedure.

Culdocentesis—aspiration or incision through the posterior vaginal fornix—also can be performed to detect intraperitoneal bleeding. (For an illustration, see *Culdocentesis,* page 558.) Retrieval of nonclotting blood is a positive indication of ectopic pregnancy or other peritoneal bleeding (Romero, 1986). Be aware, however, that a negative (clear fluid) or nondiagnostic (no fluid) result does not ensure the absence of an ectopic pregnancy.

A recent study of a single serum progesterone level as a diagnostic tool in ectopic pregnancy indicated a positive predictive index of about 90% (Buck, Joubert, and Norman, 1988). Certainly a single diagnostic test is preferable to numerous ones; however, further study is indicated before serum progesterone levels are used exclusively to diagnose ectopic pregnancy.

Gestational trophoblastic disease

Question the client about nausea, vomiting, and vaginal discharge (continuous or intermittent). Also ask her about the size of her abdomen. Because GTD typically is accompanied by rapid uterine growth, she may tell you, "I've gotten so big so quickly!"

Assess the client's vaginal discharge, which usually is brownish red. Send a specimen to the laboratory. Measure fundal height; usually the uterus is enlarged out of proportion to the weeks of gestation. A vaginal examination shows thinning and softness of the lower uterine segment. No fetal heart tones are heard nor can any fetal body parts be palpated. Laboratory studies show a reduced hemoglobin level, hematocrit, and RBC count and an increased WBC count and sedimentation rate. Human chorionic gonadotropin titers are extremely elevated. Urinalysis probably will show proteinuria. An ultrasound performed after the third month will show grapelike clusters rather than a fetus.

Unruptured and ruptured ectopic pregnancy: Comparing the signs and symptoms

To act decisively, the nurse must be able to distinguish between the signs and symptoms of unruptured and ruptured ectopic pregnancy.

Ovulation and implantation of intrauterine and ectopic gestations

Ovulation followed by fertilization of an ovum by a spermatazoon leads to pregnancy. In this illllustration, a fertilized ovum is implanted in the fallopian tube (ectopic); the other, in the uterine cavity indicates a normal implantation. Most ectopic pregnancies occur in the fallopian tubes.

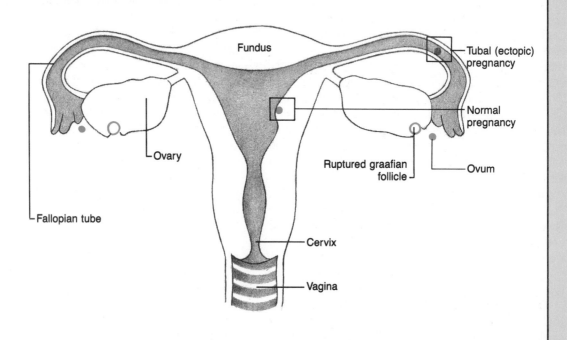

IF UNRUPTURED	Additional signs and symptoms IF RUPTURED
• Unilateral abdominal cramps and tenderness • Menstrual changes, such as spotting or a missed period • Low-grade fever (99° to 100° F [37.2° to 37.7° C]) • Normal pulse • Nausea and vomiting	• Abdominal discomfort from blood accumulation in the peritoneal cavity • Sudden onset of abdominal pain from blood accumulation in the peritoneal cavity or from tubal rupture • Shocklike state from ruptured tube or excess blood loss • Shoulder pain from irritation of the diaphragm from blood accumulation • Rapid, thready pulse from blood loss and hypovolemia • Cold extremities from excessive blood loss and decreased blood pressure

Endovaginal ultrasonography

The use of endovaginal ultrasonography may help identify an intrauterine pregnancy earlier in gestation than a traditional transabdominal ultrasonography can. In this illustration, *V* indicates the vertical distance assessed by ultrasound. *H* indicates the horizontal area assessed.

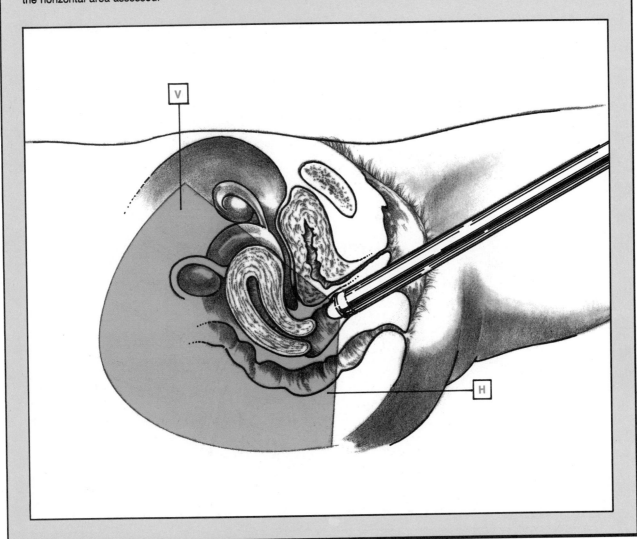

Incompetent cervix

The client with this condition does not have uterine contractions or other signs and symptoms of labor. A pelvic examination reveals other signs and symptoms of a dilated cervix possibly accompanied by a congenital problem, such as a short cervix, a double uterus, or a uterus with an altered shape. The client may report a previous traumatic delivery, incompetent cervix, or D&C.

Premature rupture of membranes

A pelvic examination discloses whether PROM has occurred. Using aseptic technique, a physician or specially prepared nurse uses a speculum to observe the cervix. Direct observation of amniotic fluid seeping from the cervical os confirms PROM. If this fluid is not visible, the practitioner may elect to test with nitrazine paper, which will indicate an alkaline substance by turning blue. (The vaginal area normally is acidic and amniotic fluid is alkaline.)

Nitrazine paper has about a 95% accuracy rate (Gibbs and Sweet, 1989). False-negative results may occur if

Culdocentesis

In culdocentesis, peritoneal fluid is aspirated through a puncture of the posterior vaginal fornix. As shown, the uterus is stabilized with a tenaculum during the procedure. A positive culdocentesis (aspiration of nonclotting blood) indicates ectopic pregnancy.

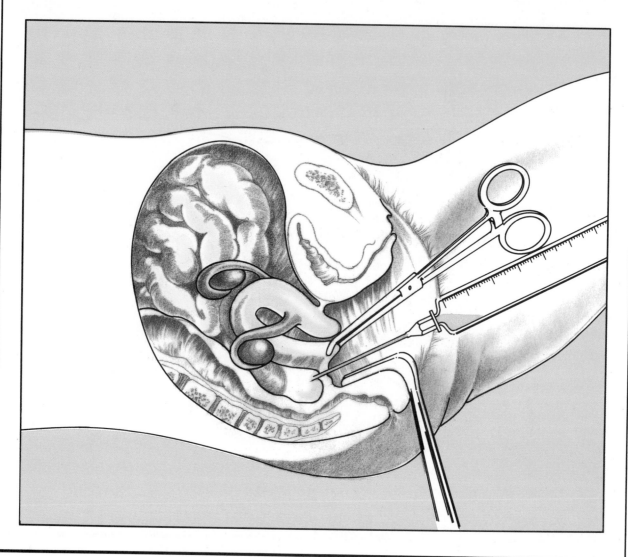

several hours have elapsed since rupture of the membranes or if the vaginal area has been contaminated with blood, urine, or antiseptic solutions.

Other tests to determine if fluid is amniotic include a smear on a clean slide (amniotic fluid makes a distinctive ferning pattern when it dries), a study of cell structure, and a staining technique to identify fetal fat cells. Because no laboratory or clinical test is foolproof, however, a combination of tests is necessary for an accurate diagnosis.

Ultrasound may be useful in identifying PROM if oligohydramnios (scant amount of amniotic fluid) can be identified on the scan. Once a diagnosis of PROM has been confirmed, the age of the fetus must be determined. If the client cannot remember the exact date of her last menstrual period, ultrasound can be useful in determining fetal age.

Preterm labor

The early symptoms of preterm labor are so subtle that they may be overlooked by the client and the medical and nursing staffs. Because of missed early symptoms, fewer than 25% of clients in preterm labor are candidates for long-term therapy to prevent preterm births (Creasy, 1989). Such therapy is contraindicated by PROM (30% to 40%), advanced cervical dilation (4 cm or more), maternal hemorrhage, and evidence of severe fetal compromise (decelerations in fetal heart rate).

Because the onset of preterm labor is insidious, a primary goal of obstetric care is to prevent it. Many of the factors contributing to preterm labor are reliable indicators and can be used to identify the client at risk. (For more information, see *Identifying the client at risk for preterm labor*.)

Regardless of the client's problem, assess the fundal height, weight, and vital signs and listen for the fetal heart rate. If the membranes are intact, the physician or nurse-midwife usually will perform a digital pelvic examination of the cervix. Progressive cervical changes may indicate that labor is proceeding; nevertheless, in some cases the physician or nurse-midwife may choose to wait for progressive cervical changes before beginning therapy (Creasy, 1989).

Because urinary tract infections commonly are associated with preterm labor, a urinalysis should be performed to determine whether bacteria are present.

Hyperemesis gravidarum

Unremitting nausea and vomiting that persist beyond the first trimester are characteristic of hyperemesis gravidarum. Vomitus ranges from undigested food, mucus, and bile early in the disorder to a "coffee-grounds" appearance in later stages.

Continued vomiting leads to dehydration, ultimately decreasing the circulating blood volume (hypovolemia). Laboratory studies may reveal hemoconcentration and, in severe cases, loss of hydrogen, sodium, potassium, and chloride. Signs of progressive dehydration and impending hypovolemia are weight loss, increased pulse rate, decreased blood pressure, changes in skin turgor, and dry mucous membranes. Dehydration also can lead to confusion and coma as well as to hepatic and renal failure.

The loss of gastric juices from vomiting can lead to metabolic alkalosis. Simultaneously, the client's altered nutritional state can cause metabolic acidosis. The acidosis may partially obscure the alkalosis and result in a mixed acid-base disorder.

Severe malnutrition also may cause hypoproteinemia and hypovitaminosis with resulting hypoprothrombinemia from severe malnutrition and possible hemorrhage.

In severe, long-term cases of hyperemesis gravidarum, the kidneys may cease concentrating urine effectively, causing increased serum levels of urea nitrogen and creatinine.

Identifying the client at risk for preterm labor

Several factors in the development of preterm labor are of reliable predictive value. Any factor from the high-risk category or any two from the low-risk category call for increased antepartal surveillance.

HIGH-RISK CATEGORY

History factors

- Cone biopsy
- Uterine anomaly
- At least one abortion during the second trimester
- DES exposure
- Preterm delivery
- Preterm labor

Factors in current pregnancy

- Placenta previa
- Hydramnios
- Abdominal surgery
- More than one fetus present
- Cervical dilation
- Effacement greater than 50%
- Uterine irritability

LOW-RISK CATEGORY

Socioeconomic factors

- Low socioeconomic status
- Age: less than age 19 or over age 34
- Single parent
- Work outside the home
- Height: less than 5' 3" (160 cm)
- Weight: less than 100 lb (45 kg)
- Cigarettes: more than 10/day

History factors

- Febrile illness
- Pyelonephritis
- First trimester abortion (fewer than 3)
- Less than 1 year since last delivery

Factors in current pregnancy

- Bleeding after 12 weeks' gestation
- Weight gain less than 7 lb (3.2 kg) by 22 weeks
- Albuminuria
- Hypertension
- Bacteriuria
- Weight loss of 5 lb (2.3 kg)
- Febrile illness
- Fetal head engaged at 32 weeks' gestation

Hypertensive disorders

Question the client with a hypertensive disorder about the length of her pregnancy because PIH typically occurs after 20 weeks' gestation. Also ascertain if in a previous pregnancy she had elevated blood pressure, proteinuria, or edema in her face, hands, feet, or legs. Ask her if she has vascular spasms, headaches, epigastric pain, visual disturbances, or irritability.

Physical examination will disclose the three classic signs of PIH: elevated blood pressure, proteinuria, and edema—especially of the face (evidenced by puffy eyes, coarse features, and a broad nose). When assessing a client with preeclampsia, weigh her daily, measure urine output every 8 to 12 hours (hourly if necessary), and assess for proteinuria using a reagent strip. Also assess for other indicators of PIH. (For a discussion of some of the factors, see *Nursing research applied: Factors associated with pregnancy-induced hypertension.*)

Evaluate the client for edema in her legs, hands, and face. To assess for edema, depress the client's skin over a bony prominence, such as the shin bone. In pitting edema, a depression remains in the skin and subcutaneous tissue after the pressure has been removed. The depth of the depression indicates the degree of pitting, which is classified as 1+, 2+, 3+, or 4+. A minor depression that disappears rather quickly indicates 1+ pitting; 4+ indicates a deep depression (approximately 2 cm) that remains for an extended period.

Assessment of deep tendon reflexes (DTRs) may indicate hypo- or hyperreflexia. Elicit the patellar (knee-jerk), biceps, and ankle reflexes. (For additional information on eliciting DTRs, see *Psychomotor skills: Deep tendon reflexes and ankle clonus.*) Reflexes should be checked every 4 to 8 hours, depending on the client's condition.

Rh incompatibility

Gather data focusing on previous pregnancies, especially those that ended in abortion. Note any blood replacement therapy the client has received previously.

The physical assessment may not be significant for a client with Rh incompatibility, but diagnostic studies are important. Blood type for ABO and Rh factor is established early in pregnancy to identify a client at risk for isoimmune hemolytic disease. Maternal isoimmunization is probable when antibody screening tests on maternal serum at around 20 weeks' gestation are positive. If the first test is negative, it should be repeated at 32 to 36 weeks. For the indirect Coombs' test, maternal blood serum is mixed with Rh-positive RBCs. In a positive test, the red cells become coated with Rh antibodies. The dilution of the blood at which this occurs determines

---

NURSING RESEARCH APPLIED

Factors associated with pregnancy-induced hypertension

A primary aim of optimal prenatal care is early detection of pregnancy-induced hypertension (PIH). A study was conducted to see if the development of PIH was significantly related to pregravid-to-ideal weight ratio, total weight gained during the first 2 trimesters of pregnancy, or maternal age. The antepartal records of 76 women were reviewed for age, weight before conception, weight and blood pressure readings at each visit, and demographic data. The pregravid-to-ideal weight ratio, mean arterial pressure (MAP), and weight gains at each visit then were calculated. The determination of PIH was based on subtracting the first calculated MAP from the highest recorded MAP. If the difference was 20 mm Hg or higher, PIH was considered to be present.

Low maternal age was the only factor significantly related to PIH. Pregravid weight and total prenatal weight gain were not found to be associated with PIH development in this study; however, because these are multifaceted variables, they cannot be discounted.

Application to practice

This study supports the previously demonstrated relationship between low maternal age and PIH development. It reinforces the need to educate young women about the complications of pregnancy. In addition, it underscores the importance of monitoring MAP changes throughout pregnancy. Analysis of MAP changes could prove to be an effective, low-cost, and low-risk predictive test for the development of PIH.

Remich, M.C., and Youngkin, E.Q. (1989). Factors associated with pregnancy-induced hypertension. *Nurse Practitioner*, 14(1), 20-24.

---

the titer or level of maternal antibodies, and the titer indicates the degree of maternal sensitization. If the titer reaches 1:16, an amniocentesis to measure the amount of bilirubin in the amniotic fluid is performed after 36 weeks' gestation.

Nursing diagnoses

After gathering assessment data, the nurse reviews it carefully to identify pertinent nursing diagnoses for the client with antepartal complications. (For a partial list of applicable diagnoses, see *Nursing diagnoses: Antepartal complications*, page 562.)

Deep tendon reflexes and ankle clonus

The deep tendon reflexes (DTRs) and ankle clonus provide an important physical sign for the client with pregnancy-induced hypertension. Abnormal DTRs and positive ankle clonus are precursors of seizures and must receive immediate intervention. If reflexes are 4 +, the client will need anticonvulsant therapy; notify the physician immediately. A 3 + reflex indicates that the client is responding to therapy; however, she still will need to be assessed every 4 hours. A 2 + response is normal, indicating that a therapeutic level of medication has been reached. A 1 + reflex should

prompt the nurse to notify the physician of medical treatment changes. Anticipate reduction of anticonvulsant therapy. An absent reflex (0) indicates that a toxic level of anticonvulsant (usually magnesium sulfate) has been reached. Stop the infusion, change the I.V. to "keep vein open" (I.V. rate to maintain patency of I.V. therapy with a solution, such as dextrose 5% in water), notify the physician immediately, and prepare an antidote (50 ml of 10% calcium gluconate) for injection.

To elicit the patellar reflex, have the client sit on the bed with one knee flexed and the lower leg dangling over the side. Tap the patellar tendon directly with a reflex hammer. A negative response may indicate depression of reflexes or that the client is not sufficiently relaxed. If she is unable to sit up, place an arm under her knees and raise. She must remain relaxed for an accurate tendon response.

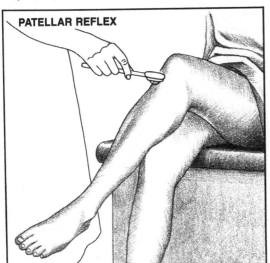

PATELLAR REFLEX

To elicit the biceps reflex, flex the client's elbow and place a thumb across the tendon in the antecubital space while supporting her arm with the fingers of the same hand. The reflex hammer will strike the nurse's thumb directly over the tendon. A positive reflex is a slight flexion of the elbow; the nurse will feel a contraction of the tendon under the thumb.

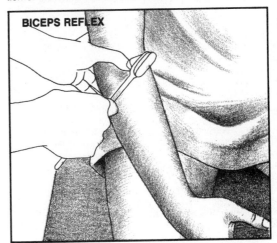

BICEPS REFLEX

To assess ankle clonus, use one hand to support the client's leg with the knee flexed. With the other hand, sharply dorsiflex the foot. Hold in position for a moment, then release. The normal (negative clonus) response is no rhythmic jerking of the foot while it is being dorsiflexed or after release. An abnormal (positive clonus) response is rhythmic jerking of the foot while dorsiflexed as well as when the foot returns to a plantar flexion upon release.

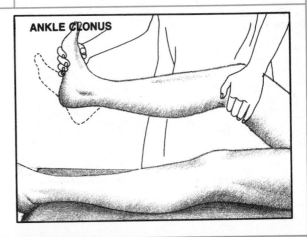

ANKLE CLONUS

NURSING DIAGNOSES

Antepartal complications

The following nursing diagnoses address problems and etiologies that the nurse may encounter when caring for a client with antepartal complications. Specific nursing interventions for many of these diagnoses are provided in the "Planning and implementation" section of this chapter.

- Altered health maintenance related to skipping medication doses
- Anticipatory grieving related to loss of pregnancy
- Anticipatory grieving related to potential loss of a fetus through abortion as manifested by expressions of anger
- Anticipatory grieving related to potential loss of a fetus through incompetent cervix
- Anxiety related to the unknown
- Constipation related to bed rest
- Decreased cardiac output related to bleeding at the site of ectopic pregnancy rupture
- Denial related to impending loss of pregnancy
- Denial related to tubal pregnancy as manifested by minimization of symptoms and use of home remedies to relieve symptoms
- Fear related to unknown effect of blood incompatability on the fetus
- Fluid volume deficit related to persistent vomiting
- Impaired physical mobility related to prescribed bed rest
- Ineffective family coping: compromised, related to inability to verbalize feelings
- Ineffective family coping: compromised, related to ineffective support as manifested in the partner's expressed frustration with the client
- Ineffective family coping: compromised, related to prolonged bed rest of the mother
- Knowledge deficit related to at-home uterine monitoring
- Knowledge deficit related to hypertensive condition
- Knowledge deficit related to necessary follow-up care
- Pain from abdominal cramping related to cerclage to repair an incompetent cervix
- Pain related to persistent vomiting
- Potential fluid volume deficit related to intra-abdominal hemorrhage upon rupture of tubal pregnancy
- Potential for infection related to I.V. therapy.
- Situational low self-esteem related to diagnosis of incompetent cervix
- Situational low self-esteem related to persistent vomiting
- Situational low self-esteem related to the inability to maintain pregnancy as manifested by crying and by verbalizing guilt

Planning and implementation

After assessing the client with antepartal complications and formulating nursing diagnoses, the nurse develops and implements a plan of care centering on the following common nursing goals:
- promoting the physical well-being of the client and her fetus
- preventing or controlling further complications
- preventing sequelae
- providing emotional support to the client and her family.

Spontaneous abortion

A client with suspected abortion should be referred to a physician immediately because emergency medical intervention may be needed to decrease complications. The client may have a nursing diagnosis of *denial related to impending loss of pregnancy.* To care for this client, save all expelled tissues and clots; maintain a calm, confident, and sympathetic manner; alert the physician to pertinent signs and history (for example, vital signs and amounts of bleeding); and encourage bed rest. Expect to administer sedatives and analgesics. Rest will decrease bleeding, and the medications will ease the client's anxiety. Try to stay with the client, and provide comfort measures usually associated with labor (such as a back rub and a cool cloth for her forehead). The client may be sensitive to any suggestion that she has somehow caused the abortion. The nurse will need to be sensitive to this feeling of vulnerability and be cautious when caring for the family to avoid increasing anxiety. Prepare the client physically and emotionally for D&C, if indicated.

After an abortion, the client may have a nursing diagnosis of *anticipatory grieving related to loss of pregnancy.* To care for this client, provide emotional support, and answer all questions or clarify any information for the client and her family. Question the client and family about family needs and coping mechanisms. Notify clergy to visit and baptize the products of conception, if the client wishes. Religious beliefs directly influence the client's and her family's expectations of care. Accommodating such needs within the facility's constraints enhances care.

Teach the client to wear a comfortable support bra to reduce discomfort from breast engorgement, which may produce anxiety and also will need appropriate intervention (dependent on the physician's orders and the client's preference.) Administer RhIg within 72 hours if the client is Rh negative and has not formed Rh antibodies from a previous Rh-positive pregnancy. This medication prevents the formation of maternal anti-Rh antibodies and thereby protects against sensitization from an Rh-positive fetus in future pregnancies. Monitor I.V. infusion and vital signs before, during, and after this procedure. Assess the hemodynamics of the client to maintain her optimal health.

Be aware that hormonal changes during pregnancy, combined with the circumstances of an abortion, may cause the client to exhibit symptoms of emotional strain. This can lead to a nursing diagnosis of *situational low self-esteem related to the inability to maintain pregnancy as manifested by crying and by verbalizing guilt.* Another appropriate nursing diagnosis may be *anticipatory grieving related to potential loss of a fetus through abortion as manifested by expressions of anger.*

Management of an abortion depends on its type and on the extent of the client's symptoms. An incomplete abortion may be followed by a D&C to remove the remaining tissues. The physician uses dilators to open the cervix and then performs suction curettage. Analgesics or general or local anesthetics may be used. Intravenous oxytocin, in a dextrose 5% in water intravenous solution, may be required to induce uterine contractions. Because retained placental fragments can cause the uterus to remain relaxed following the abortion, the uterine muscles may not constrict uterine vessels, causing hemorrhage during or after the procedure. Additional oxytocin infusion may be required to prevent hemorrhage.

Ergot products, such as methylergonovine, that cause uterine and cervical contractions are contraindicated until the uterus is empty. This reduces the chance of retaining placental fragments. After the procedure, however, the physician may order three or four doses of ergonovine, orally or intramuscularly, if the client's blood pressure is normal. Blood or antibiotics may be ordered in cases of extreme blood loss, anemia, or infection (Beischer and Mackay, 1986; Scott, 1986b).

If the cause of the abortion can be determined and eliminated, the chance for a future normal pregnancy is excellent. If no complications (such as infection or hemorrhage) occur, the abortion probably will have no detrimental physical effects on the client.

Ectopic pregnancy

A client who exhibits the signs and symptoms of ectopic pregnancy may have a nursing diagnosis of *denial related to tubal pregnancy as manifested by minimization of symptoms and use of home remedies to relieve symptoms.* This client also may have subsequent bleeding and

a nursing diagnosis of *decreased cardiac output related to bleeding at the site of ectopic pregnancy rupture.* Contact the physician immediately if signs and symptoms occur, and assess vital signs every 15 minutes or as prescribed. Appropriate laboratory data should be gathered, including blood type, CBC, Rh, crossmatch, and serum hCG. Take the following steps for emergency care:

• Prepare for I.V. fluids with port for medication and a large-bore needle to accommodate blood transfusions if needed.

• Have oxygen at hand to prevent hypoxia related to hypovolemia.

• Gather emergency medications and equipment in case of shock.

• Prepare the client for surgery by explaining the procedure, checking to see if her consent has been obtained, administering prescribed preoperative medication, and completing the surgical checklist.

• Keep the client and her family informed.

• Contact clergy to baptize the fetus if desired by the family, and document their wishes.

After surgery, the client may have a nursing diagnosis of *anticipatory grieving related to loss of pregnancy.* If the client is Rh negative, check to determine if antibodies are present in her blood, and prepare to administer RhIg if she has not formed Rh antibodies from an earlier pregnancy with an Rh-positive fetus. Administer fluids, medications, and treatments as prescribed and based on the client's preference and tolerance. Inform the client and her family if the fetus was baptized. Clarify, if necessary, the physician's explanation of cause, managment, and recovery, including chances for future pregnancies. For this situation, an appropriate nursing diagnosis may be *ineffective family coping, compromised: related to inability to verbalize feelings.* Encourage discussions of feelings by the client and her family to promote grieving. Encourage the client to return as indicated for follow-up care.

Effective management of ectopic pregnancy is complex. Hemorrhage is the major problem; bleeding must be controlled quickly and effectively. Because extreme blood loss can lead to shock, ensure that sufficient blood is available for transfusions.

Immediately after an ectopic pregnancy is diagnosed, a laparotomy can be performed to remove the products of conception, control blood loss by evacuating blood and clots, and cauterize bleeding vessels. However, according to Silva (1988), a laparoscopy is preferable to an incision because of lower cost and decreased morbidity.

New developments in laparoscopic surgery allow conservative approaches, including using lasers through the laparoscope to excise the affected area of the fallopian tube. Laser surgery decreases damage to the tube and provides a beneficial hemostatic effect (Huber, Hosmann, and Vytiska-Binstorfer, 1989; Modica and Timor-Tritsch, 1988). In many cases, the affected fallopian tube can be repaired and left in place. Salpingectomy, formerly the treatment of choice, now is reserved for cases in which the tube is significantly damaged or when the client does not wish to maintain fertility.

An interstitial ectopic pregnancy—a pregnancy occurring within a segment of the fallopian tube closest to the uterus—presents a diagnostic and management challenge. This rare form of ectopic pregnancy occurs in about 2.5% of all cases. Because of its location and lack of specific signs and symptoms, interstitial ectopic pregnancy typically is diagnosed through laparoscopy after tubal rupture and hemorrhage. With advances in ultrasonography, however, an eccentric location of the gestational sac can be identified (Weissman, Fishman, and Gal, 1989). Laparoscopic surgery to remove the products of conception can be successful if interstitial pregnancy is identified early, before rupture. If identification occurs concurrently with or after rupture, salpingectomy usually is required. Because the location is adjacent to the uterus, damage may result that will require removal of the uterus.

An ovarian pregnancy requires the removal of the affected ovary. An adherent fallopian tube also may require removal (Cunningham, MacDonald, and Gant, 1989).

An advanced ectopic pregnancy, which typically is abdominal, requires a laparotomy as soon as the client is stable and able to withstand surgery. If the placenta in an abdominal pregnancy is attached to a vital organ such as the liver, no attempt is made to separate or remove the placenta. The umbilical cord is cut flush with the placenta and the placenta is left in situ. Degeneration and absorption of the placenta usually occurs without complications. However, placental degeneration can lead to disseminated intravascular coagulation in some individuals.

Gestational trophoblastic disease

Monitor the client's vital signs, vaginal discharge, and urine for proteinuria. The client may have a nursing diagnosis of *anxiety related to the unknown,* in which she, and probably her partner, will require support when they are given the diagnosis and teaching in the necessary steps of management. If she has to wait for the uterine wall to become firmer before having a D&C, she will be going home knowing that she is not carrying a fetus. Give her time to work this through and verbalize her feelings. Be sensitive to her ability to cope, and assess her family support. After the D&C, routine postoperative care is necessary. The client may have a

nursing diagnosis of *knowledge deficit related to necessary follow-up care.* GTD can be malignant, making follow-up care extremely important.

Management of GTD involves evacuation of the uterine contents. An induced abortion may be followed by D&C; however, a D&C cannot be performed until the uterine wall becomes firmer and less friable (less easily torn or perforated). Tissue obtained from curettage must be examined by a pathologist for residual trophoblastic cells.

Vacuum suction also may be used to evacuate the uterus. As with a D&C, vacuum suction requires dilatation of the cervix. Whatever the treatment, blood replacement may accompany it (Hilgers and Lewis, 1986).

Because GTD can be malignant, follow-up care must continue for at least 1 year. Recommended care includes:
• hCG levels—once weekly until titers are negative for 3 consecutive weeks; then once monthly for 6 months; then every 2 months for 6 months.
• chest X-ray—once monthly until hCG titers are negative, then every 2 months for 1 year
• no pregnancy—for at least 1 year after all titers and X-rays are negative; an oral contraceptive is indicated to prevent pregnancy.

Continued high or rising hCG titers may indicate recurrent GTD. If the uterus is still intact, a secondary D&C can be performed to evacuate its contents (trophoblastic tissue, which produces the hCG). Curetted tissues are examined to identify signs of progression to choriocarcinoma, which requires a rigorous program of chemotherapy with methotrexate or dactinomycin. If chemotherapy is delayed, the choriocarcinoma has a tendency to rapid and widespread metastasis.

If hCG levels remain within normal limits for 1 year, the couple can anticipate a normal subsequent pregnancy. In this instance, probability of a recurrence of GTD is relatively low, especially if the client is age 40 or younger.

The nurse must be aware of the many options available for dealing with GTD in order to respond to the client's and family's questions about the procedures and probable outcomes.

Incompetent cervix

Provide basic preoperative and postoperative care for the client undergoing a cerclage of the cervix, paying special attention to vaginal bleeding. Frequently assess for the presence and quality of fetal heart tones. Cervical cerclage may lead to a nursing diagnosis of *pain from abdominal cramping related to cerclage to repair an incompetent cervix.* Decisions about the type of delivery the client will have usually depend on the position of the suture when she begins labor. Many physicians believe that if the suture is maintaining cervical closure, a cesarean delivery should be performed to preserve the suture, thereby maintaining cervical closure in future pregnancies. However, others believe that a cesarean delivery places the client unnecessarily at risk for maternal morbidity when the suture could easily be removed transvaginally (Parisi, 1989). Of course, a suture that has loosened or has become displaced will not maintain cervical closure in subsequent pregnancies. In that case, the suture is clipped and removed when labor begins and vaginal delivery may proceed (Beischer and MacKay, 1986).

Because incompetent cervix usually is not diagnosed until after one or more abortions, this probably is not the first time the client and her partner have had to face delivery complications or the loss of a fetus. Therefore, she and her family will need much support. Applicable nursing diagnoses in this situation include *anticipatory grieving related to potential loss of a fetus through incompetent cervix,* and *situational low self-esteem related to diagnosis of incompetent cervix.* Incompetent cervix can be corrected and the pregnancy maintained by wedge trachelorrhaphy (removal of a wedge from the anterior segment of the cervix with its closure) or by cervical cerclage. The procedure most frequently used is the transvaginal cervical cerclage (McDonald procedure), in which a band of nonabsorbable ribbon (Mersilene) is placed around the cervix beneath the mucosa to constrict the opening. The suture works much like the string on a drawstring bag. (For an illustration, see *Cervical cerclage.*) The key to the success for the procedure is placing the suture high enough on the cervix so that it will remain in place (Beischer and MacKay, 1986).

The physician typically will wait until 14 to 16 weeks' gestation, if possible, before performing the procedure to avoid having to remove the suture for a spontaneous first trimester abortion.

The pregnancy usually is maintained after cerclage, provided the membranes remain intact and the cervix was not more than 3 cm dilated or more than 50% effaced at the time of the correction. The procedure also may be performed transabdominally if necessary (Parisi, 1989).

Premature rupture of the membranes

An inaccurate diagnosis of PROM may lead to unnecessary induction of labor, cesarean delivery, or preterm delivery. Therefore, the physician must make every effort to make an accurate diagnosis of the disorder.

Management of PROM usually involves two distinctly different approaches based on the assessment of risks to both mother and fetus. In active management,

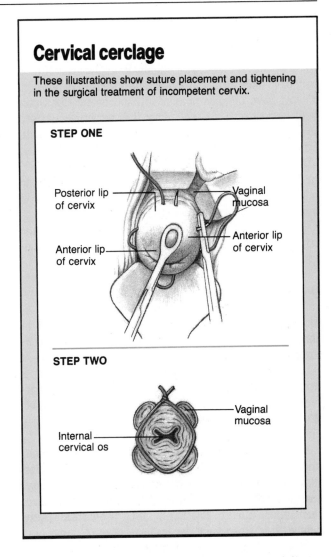

Cervical cerclage

These illustrations show suture placement and tightening in the surgical treatment of incompetent cervix.

STEP ONE

Posterior lip of cervix

Vaginal mucosa

Anterior lip of cervix

Anterior lip of cervix

STEP TWO

Vaginal mucosa

Internal cervical os

labor is induced and, if not effective, a cesarean delivery is performed. In expectant management, no action is taken to speed the onset of labor except in cases of amnionitis or fetal distress.

Because the client may have a nursing diagnosis of *potential for infection related to PROM,* prophylactic antibiotics also may be used. Little agreement exists, however, on their value if labor begins within 24 hours after PROM.

Respiratory distress syndrome (RDS) develops in 10% to 40% of neonates born to clients with PROM. Neonatal sepsis is identified in approximately 10% of neonates, and amnionitis occurs in 4% to 30% (Gibbs and Sweet, 1989). Other neonatal complications include asphyxia, malpresentation, and cord prolapse. Maternal complications include cesarean delivery and endometritis (inflammation of the uterus lining), occurring in 3% to 30% of clients with PROM.

Maternal mortality related to PROM is rare. Neonatal mortality is caused by RDS in 30% to 70% of cases. Anomalies account for 10% to 30% and infection for 3% to 20% (Gibbs and Sweet, 1989).

Infections following PROM are common and potentially severe. A client with oligohydramnios after PROM may have more clinically evident infections than one who did not have oligohydramnios. Amniocentesis for Gram stain and culture of the amniotic fluid sometimes is used to identify infection. Some problems are associated with this diagnostic tool, however. First, amniotic fluid is not always available for testing after PROM. Second, 20% to 30% of clients identified by amniocentesis as having infections do not have clinical signs or symptoms of infection (Gibbs and Sweet, 1989).

Other procedures to identify infection include maternal serum C-reactive protein and fetal movement studies.

Preterm labor and delivery

Management of preterm labor begins with bed rest in the lateral decubitus position and external uterine monitoring of fetal status.

Because the onset of preterm labor is insidious, a primary goal of obstetric care is to prevent its occurrence. Many of the factors contributing to preterm labor are reliable indicators and can be used to identify a client at risk.

Certain hormones—serum estradiol, progesterone, and prostaglandin or its metabolites—have been studied to determine their effect on preterm labor. Serial measurements of these hormones have provided data on their fluctuation, but no relationship has been consistently demonstrated between the levels of any of these hormones and the incidence of preterm labor.

Tocolysis (inhibition of uterine contractions) is a primary tool in caring for a client with preterm labor. Tocolytic drugs are 60% to 88% effective in stopping uterine contractions; however, many of the drugs have adverse effects on both the mother and the fetus. Furthermore, little is known about the cumulative effect of tocolytic drugs used in early gestations and continued over long periods (Givens, 1988). Absolute contraindications to tocolytic drugs include severe PIH, severe bleeding from any cause, chorioamnionitis, fetal death, a fetal anomaly that is incompatible with life, and severe fetal growth retardation. Relative contraindications include mild chronic hypertension, stable placenta previa, uncontrolled diabetes mellitus, fetal distress, and cervical dilation greater than 5 cm (Creasy, 1989).

Tocolytic drugs may be used with success to inhibit labor until term, interrupt labor long enough to transport the mother to a high-risk health care facility, or inhibit labor until prenatal steroids (to increase fetal lung ma-

turity) can become effective. (For an overview of tocolytic agents, see *Drugs used to inhibit labor*.)

Beta-adrenergic agents (isoxsuprine hydrochloride, ritodrine, and terbutaline sulfate) inhibit the contractility of the myometrium. A client taking one of these drugs may have a nursing diagnosis of *altered health maintenance related to skipping medication doses*. The client may believe that labor will stop without the drugs.

Magnesium sulfate, used for years to treat hypertensive episodes in pregnancy, is growing in popularity as a tocolytic agent. It has fewer adverse effects than beta-adrenergics and can be used in conjunction with beta-adrenergics or when they are contraindicated. Absolute contraindications to magnesium sulfate include myasthenia gravis, impaired renal function, and recent myocardial infarction.

Oral magnesium, such as magnesium sulfate, also may be used to provide safe, long-term tocolysis although the Food and Drug Administration has not approved it for this use.

Calcium antagonists, agents that regulate the flow of calcium within the cells of the myometrium, are under investigation for use as tocolytic agents. Because calcium is the key element in uterine contractility, calcium antagonists would seem to be the perfect tocolytic agent. However, their use in the inhibition of labor is experimental.

Prostaglandin synthetase inhibitors, such as salicylates, indomethacin, and naproxen, relax the gravid uterus and have been linked to the incidence of postmaturity (overly developed neonate). However, concern about bleeding, prolonged labor, and the potential fetal and neonatal effects has limited their use in preventing preterm labor.

The development in 1985 of a lightweight, highly sensitive tocodynamometer has allowed outpatient monitoring of uterine activity. This in-home monitoring capability is marketed with an intensive perinatal nursing service that incorporates 24-hour nurse availability, daily transmission of recorded uterine activity, weekly physician update, and ongoing client teaching and reinforcement of the treatment plan. An appropriate nursing diagnosis for an outpatient client is *knowledge deficit related to at-home uterine monitoring*. The cost of these programs varies, but many are covered under health insurance plans.

These services were designed exclusively for the high-risk preterm labor group. Monitoring usually is initiated at around 20 weeks' gestation and continues until 36 weeks' gestation. The client is taught to monitor herself for 1 hour each morning and each evening and to recognize early labor signs and symptoms.

Contact the client daily to assess compliance, teach her about preterm labor, and evaluate signs and symp-

Drugs used to inhibit labor

This chart summarizes the major tocolytic drugs in current clinical use.

DRUG AND MECHANISM OF ACTION	USUAL DOSAGE AND EFFICACY	NURSING IMPLICATIONS
magnesium sulfate		
Direct-acting calcium antagonist; affects uterine contractility by competing with calcium both inside and outside the cell.	I.V. bolus of 4 grams over 15 to 20 minutes plus 4 to 5 grams I.M. into each buttock, followed by a constant infusion of 2 grams/hour. Stable level is difficult to maintain because of rapid excretion through the kidneys. May work slower than beta-adrenergic agonists. Contractions may not stop immediately.	• Toxicity signaled by a respiratory rate below 15 breaths/minute, hyporeflexia, and urine output below 30 ml/hr. May cause neonatal lethargy, poor sucking reflex, and delayed motility of the gastrointestinal tract. • Monitor respiratory rate, deep tendon reflexes, and urine output every hour. Keep 10% calcium gluconate at bedside as antidote for overdose.
beta-adrenergic agonists (ritodrine and terbutaline sulfate)		
Stimulate beta-adrenergic receptors, which activate an enzyme (adenylate cyclase) that produces cyclic adenosine monophosphate (cAMP). cAMP inhibits the junction of myosin and actin (agents necessary for muscular contractility).	Initially, 50 to 100 mcg of ritodrine/minute by I.V. infusion, increasing by 50 mcg/minute every 10 minutes up to the minimum effective dose. Usual dose is 150 to 350 mcg/minute. Initially, 10 mcg of terbutaline sulfate/minute by I.V. infusion, increasing by 5 mcg/minute every 10 minutes up to 80 mcg/minute. After contractions cease, taper to the least effective dose by decreasing by 5 mcg/minute.	• May cause tachycardia, hypotension, bronchial dilation, increased plasma volume, increased cardiac output, arrhythmias, myocardial ischemia, reduced urine output, restlessness, headache, nausea, and vomiting. • Place the client in a left lateral position to minimize hypotension. • Monitor the maternal and fetal heart rates constantly. • Pulmonary edema is a serious but rare adverse reaction. Monitor weight daily to detect fluid overload.
calcium antagonists (nifedipine)		
Block the flow of calcium through calcium-specific channels in the myometrial cells. Nifedipine appears to target the uterus and has limited cardiac effects.	Initially, 10 mg orally t.i.d.; some patients may require up to 30 mg q.i.d. Maximum daily dosage is 180 mg. Onset of action is within 20 minutes. Use of these medications to inhibit labor remains experimental.	• May cause facial flushing, transiently elevated heart rate, palpitations, headache, dizziness, nausea, and hypotension.
prostaglandin synthetase inhibitors or nonsteroidal anti-inflammatory agents (indomethacin, salicylates, naproxen)		
Inhibit prostaglandin synthetase to decrease the amount of prostaglandins, which interfere with labor.	Dosage varies with drug used. May be used orally or rectally.	• *Fetal effects:* premature closure of ductus arteriosus. *Neonatal effects:* hyperbilirubinemia, altered platelet function, decreased urine output. *Maternal effects:* epigastric pain, rectal intolerance if suppositories are used, interference with platelet function, bleeding. • Monitor client with ruptured membranes carefully. These drugs can mask infection through antipyretic effect.

toms. The client transmits monitoring data by telephone to the nurse, who evaluates the number of contractions. If more than three contractions occur in 1 hour, instruct the client to force fluids immediately, empty her bladder, lie on her left side, and monitor her responses. If a second transmission of the same uterine activity follows, notify the physician or nurse-midwife (Givens, 1988).

Part of the trend to offer services outside the health care facility whenever possible, at-home uterine monitoring is more cost-effective and less complicated for the client than hospitalization. In addition, it allows the client to participate actively in her own health care. This trend also offers new opportunities for the nurse, whose role includes assessing client needs, planning interventions, and evaluating the effectiveness of those interventions. The nurse provides the educational and emotional support that are essential to this new prenatal care for high-risk clients.

Hyperemesis gravidarum

For the client with a nursing diagnosis of *fluid volume deficit related to persistent vomiting and decreased fluid intake,* expect to administer parenteral fluids, electrolytes, vitamins, and proteins as prescribed to counteract dehydration and loss of nutrients. Also be prepared to administer antiemetics as prescribed to decrease vomiting and promote rest. Expect oral intake to be restricted for the first 48 hours followed by cautious resumption of small, dry meals and then by clear liquids. This allows the gastrointestinal system to rest from overstimulation.

For a client with a nursing diagnosis of *pain related to persistent vomiting,* keep the room quiet, pleasant, and well-ventilated to promote rest and relaxation; maintain excellent daily hygiene, especially oral hygiene following vomiting episodes, to promote comfort; and limit visitors to promote client rest.

A client who appears clinically stable may be managed as an outpatient with close follow-up. Hydration with isotonic fluids is essential. In addition, teach the client how to assist with her own treatment—in nutrition, for example. Teach her that small, frequent meals that contain easily digested, high-carbohydrate foods will help to reestablish adequate vitamin and protein levels. Heartburn and reflux esophagitis are common and typically are treated symptomatically.

Antiemetics, a mainstay in treating hyperemesis, also have a mildly sedating effect. (For an overview of antiemetics, see *Drugs used to treat hyperemesis gravidarum.*)

Many clients report episodes of emesis in connection with a particularly stressful incident or aspect of their lives—a difficult relationship with a partner, for example. This could lead to a nursing diagnosis of *ineffective family coping: compromised, related to ineffective support as manifested in the partner's expressed frustration with the client.* If possible, a client with hyperemesis should try to avoid or resolve situations that aggravate the condition or increase stress.

An essential aspect of outpatient care is reassurance and support. A debilitated client who is worried about her pregnancy may experience a severe emotional crisis. Make a special effort to give the client emotional support.

For a hospitalized client with severe symptoms, treatment goals are to eliminate vomiting, restore hydration, reestablish electrolyte balance, and supplement vitamin intake. To achieve thses goals, restrict oral intake, expect to begin parenteral administration of fluids with electrolytes and supplementary vitamins and minerals, and administer antiemetics. This treatment plan allows rest for the overstimulated gastrointestinal tract while providing necessary nutrients to the body.

Persistent weight loss, acidosis, and malnutrition require total parenteral nutrition to provide adequate protein intake for mother and fetus.

Prolonged hospitalization can have a negative effect on the client's self-concept (Loos and Julius, 1989), resulting in a nursing diagnosis of *situational low self-esteem related to persistent vomiting.* Focus on positive behavior and provide distractions, which can provide psychological support to offset the client's negative feelings. The client who is receiving I.V. drugs may have a nursing diagnosis of *potential for infection related to I.V. therapy.* Change the I.V. site if infiltration occurs (or according to health care facility protocol) to decrease the chance of tissue damage and infection.

Before, during, and after hospitalization, the client needs a quiet, aesthetically pleasing environment. Maintain a calm, accepting attitude. A perceived lack of tolerance may indicate to the client that the nurse feels the disorder is psychosomatic and that the client does not need hospitalization.

Hypertensive disorders

Bed rest is prescribed for the client with a hypertensive disorder. Instruct the client to assume a left lateral position to increase renal and uterine perfusion. Increased renal perfusion facilitates diuresis. Other positions may compromise renal and uterine blood flow through compression of the vena cava and aorta. (For more information, see *Drugs used to treat pregnancy-induced hypertension,* page 570.)

Mild preeclampsia
Nursing care is aimed at improving or stabilizing the client. (See *Applying the nursing process: Pain related to*

Drugs used to treat hyperemesis gravidarum

This chart summarizes the major antiemetic agents in current clinical use to treat hyperemesis gravidarum.

DRUG AND MECHANISM OF ACTION	USUAL DOSAGE	NURSING IMPLICATIONS
promethazine (Phenergan)		
Depresses central nervous system and inhibits acetylcholine	I.M.:12.5 to 25 mg every 4 hours as needed. Also available in oral and rectal forms.	• May cause drowsiness and impair platelet aggregation; observe for bleeding in the fetus. • Safety during pregnancy has not been established.
prochlorperazine (Compazine)		
Blocks dopamine receptors in medullary chemoreceptor trigger zone	Oral: 5 to 10 mg t.i.d. I.M.: 5 to 10 mg every 3 to 4 hours	• May cause glycosuria, dry mouth, nasal congestion, restlessness, insomnia, anorexia, dizziness, postural hypotension, blurred vision. • Safety during pregnancy has not been established.
metoclopramide (Reglan)		
Blocks dopamine receptors in medullary chemoreceptor trigger zone	Oral: 10 mg q.i.d.	• May cause restlessness, anxiety, drowsiness, lassitude, extrapyramidal symptoms. • Safety and efficacy have not been established for therapy that continues longer than 12 weeks. • Safety during pregnancy has not been established.

effects of vasospasm and edema, pages 572 and 573.) The client may remain at home as long as edema and proteinuria do not increase. A physician, clinical specialist, or nurse practitioner must assess the client at least weekly to determine changes in her condition. As term approaches, data about fetal maturity and cervical status are required in case labor must be induced. For a nursing diagnosis of *knowledge deficit related to hypertensive condition,* teach the client to keep an accurate daily record of weight. She should report a weight gain of more than 1 lb/day. In addition, carefully explain to the client and her family the signs that indicate a deterioration in her condition, such as severe headache, rapid rise in blood pressure, epigastric pain, hyperreflexia (muscle twitching), edema, decreased urine output, or visual disturbances. Instruct her to report such signs to the physician immediately. The client may have a nursing diagnosis of *impaired physical mobility related to prescribed bed rest* or *constipation related to bed rest.* She must remain on bed rest and maintain a well-balanced, high-protein and high-fiber diet. Protein requirements are 70 to 80 g of protein/day (1 g/kg of body weight/day). The diet must contain adequate fiber and fluids because limited exercise can cause constipation.

The prescribed regimen may become boring and stressful for the client. Family members need to be involved because home management and child care must be assumed by someone else for the remainder of the pregnancy. Diversion is necessary for both the client and young children in the family. Preschoolers cannot understand why their mother stays in bed all day. Ensure that the client and her family understand all aspects of the regimen and why they are necessary. A nursing diagnosis of *ineffective family coping: compromised, related to prolonged bed rest of the mother* may be appropriate in this situation.

Severe preeclampsia

Treatment includes bed rest in a left lateral position. Keep the environment quiet, with minimal stimulation and dim lighting, and follow these procedures.
• Assess vital signs and deep tendon reflexes at least every 4 hours. Record weight daily; measure urine output every 1 to 4 hours according to the client's status. The client should maintain a high-carbohydrate, low-fat, 70- to 100-g protein diet with 2 g of sodium/day.
• Perform fundoscopic examinations daily to detect arteriolar spasms, edema, and hemorrhage. Administer

Drugs used to treat pregnancy-induced hypertension

This chart summarizes the major drugs in current clinical use to treat pregnancy-induced hypertension.

DRUG AND MECHANISM OF ACTION	USUAL DOSAGE	NURSING IMPLICATIONS
methyldopa (Aldomet)		
Stimulates central inhibitory alpha-adrenergic receptors; reduces plasma renin activity	Oral: 250 mg t.i.d.; may increase to 500 mg I.V.: initially, three 5 mg boluses 2 minutes apart	• May cause false-positive direct Coombs' test result, sodium retention, constipation, drowsiness
propranolol hydrochloride (Inderal)		
Nonselective beta-adrenergic blocking agent; principally affects myocardial (beta$_1$), bronchial, and vascular smooth muscle (beta$_2$) receptors; may block renin release	Initial I.V.: bolus 0.5 to 3 mg, slow push (do not exceed I mg/minute); may repeat initial dose after 2 minutes Maintenance I.V.: infuse at 2 to 3 mg/hr	• May cause bradycardia, hypotension, short-term memory loss, emotional lability, nausea, vomiting, dry mouth • May potentiate effects of insulin; effects potentiated by furosemide
magnesium sulfate		
Anticonvulsant; prevents and controls seizures in preeclampsia and eclampsia	I.M.: 4 to 5 grams of 50% solution in each buttock I.V.: 4 grams in 250 ml D$_5$W.	• May cause hypotension, drowsiness, sweating, absent or diminished reflexes, oliguria, respiratory paralysis • Observe deep tendon reflexes every 4 hours. If absent, discontinue medication and notify physician immediately.
labetolol (Trandate, Normodyne)		
Nonselective beta-adrenergic blocking agent	Initial I.V. or oral: 200 mg/day in 2 doses Maintenance: 400 to 800 mg/day in 2 doses	• May cause orthostatic hypotension and dizziness • Check hourly urine output. If below 30 ml/hour, notify physician.
atenolol (Tenormin)		
Selective inhibition of cardiac and lipolytic beta-adrenergic receptors	Oral: 50 mg/day; may increase to 100 mg/day	• May cause bradycardia, hypotension, congestive heart failure • Teach patient to take drug at regular time every day. Monitor blood pressure frequently.

sedatives as prescribed. Use a fetal and uterine contraction monitor for signs of labor and fetal well-being.
• If the client's condition improves within 3 to 5 days (for example, if urine output increases or weight decreases by 2 kg or more), further therapy will depend on the gestational age of the fetus. If the fetus is at 38 weeks' gestation or less, the client can be discharged to home care. Instruct her to record the frequency of fetal movement for 1-hour periods, 2 to 3 times daily.

If no improvement is noted, hyperreflexia occurs, the fetus is at 38 weeks' gestation or more, or the lecithin/sphingomyelin (L/S) ratio is appropriate, the physician may elect delivery. (For more information on L/S ratio and delivery procedures, see Chapter 33, Intrapartal Complications.)

Nursing care for the client with severe preeclampsia is aimed at:
• preventing eclampsia and seizures
• maternal survival with minimal morbidity
• birth of as mature a neonate as possible
• no significant postdelivery complications.

Continue to provide the same monitoring and care that the client received before she was hospitalized. In addition, prepare emergency equipment as soon as the client is admitted in case eclampsia occurs. Emergency equipment should include medications, suctioning apparatus, and in some cases, padded side rails on the client's bed.

Keep emergency anticonvulsant and antihypertensive medications available; these include magnesium sulfate, methyldopa, hydralazine, and propranolol hydrochloride. Be aware of the mechanism of action, usual dosage, and special considerations for each of these medications.

Eclampsia

Hyperreflexia is common just before seizures in the client with preeclampsia. Eclampsia is a complication of PIH. It is preceded by the signs of severe preeclampsia and one or both of the following:

• Tonic (normal tone of muscles) and clonic (alternating between involuntary muscle contraction and relaxation in rapid succession) seizures.

• Hypertensive crisis, in which blood pressure is elevated to such a degree that the client has an increased chance of developing a cerebrovascular accident or shock.

Tonic-clonic seizures are followed by hypotension and collapse and, in many cases, nystagmus, muscle twitching, and coma. Oliguria or anuria also may occur. Disorientation and amnesia delay immediate recovery.

The nurse's first priority during seizures is to ensure a patent airway, then to provide adequate oxygenation.

Rh incompatibility

Prophylaxis for Rh isoimmunization requires the use of RhIg. RhIg is not a treatment for isoimmunization because it has no effect against antibodies present in the maternal bloodstream. It provides passive immunity, which is transient and therefore will not affect a subsequent pregnancy. RhIg also prepares RBCs containing the Rh antigen for destruction by phagocytes before the client's immune system is activated to produce antibodies (active immunity). Antibodies formed by an active immune response remain within the individual's bloodstream, presumably for life. RhIg given to an Rh₀(D)-negative client who already is sensitized would accomplish nothing. Therefore, RhIg is recommended only for Rh-negative clients at risk for developing Rh isoimmunization. It should not be given to an Rh-positive client because the Rh antibodies could destroy her Rh-positive RBC. (For more information, see *Neonatal status: Monitoring when the client and neonate have an Rh incompatibility*.)

The American College of Obstetricians and Gynecologists (1986) recommendations for RhIg are as follows:

NEONATAL STATUS

Monitoring when the client and neonate have an Rh incompatibility

When a client has an Rh incompatibility, neonatal status must be monitored closely through neonatal blood studies and physical assessment, including assessment of the placenta.

NEONATAL CORD BLOOD STUDIES AT DELIVERY

• Blood type and Rh. These tests indicate the need, if any, for further assessment of maternal antibody formation.
• Direct Coombs' test on neonatal cord blood. This test determines the presence of maternal antibodies attached to the neonate's red blood cells (RBCs). A washed suspension of the neonate's RBCs obtained from the umbilical cord is mixed with Coombs' serum (serum containing antiglobulin). The test is positive—that is, maternal antibodies are present—if the neonate's RBCs agglutinate (clump).
• Hemoglobin level and hematocrit. Progressive hemolytic anemia reflects increased production of RBCs (erythropoiesis) as indicated by shifts in hemoglobin level and hematocrit as well as by an increased number of immature RBCs.
• Blood glucose level. Increased erythropoiesis increases blood glucose use. Hypoglycemia in the neonate must be recognized and treated early.
• Indirect or direct serum bilirubin level. Elevated levels of indirect bilirubin indicate hemolysis of RBCs, which frees bilirubin in the serum. (For more specific information on neonatal laboratory assessments, see Chapter 38, High-Risk Neonates.)

POSTDELIVERY ASSESSMENT

• Yellow-stained vernix (cheeselike covering on the neonate) or umbilical cord. Evidence of edema (hydrops fetalis), respiratory distress (nasal flaring, intercostal retractions), and alterations in heart rate (bradycardia, tachycardia) or rhythm (arrhythmias) may indicate pleural or pericardial effusions. Pleural or pericardial effusions and ascites indicate cardiac failure.
• Placental enlargement. The weight of the placenta is normally one-sixth that of the neonate. In hemolytic disease, the placenta may weigh as much as one-half to three-quarters that of the neonate.
• Hepatosplenomegaly. Liver and spleen enlargement indicates increased demands for disposal of bilirubin and increased erythropoiesis.
• Neonatal pallor with jaundice. Pallor is caused by RBC hemolysis; jaundice, by increased bilirubin levels. Jaundice typically appears within 24 to 36 hours of birth.
• Central nervous system manifestations of kernicterus. These include twitching, irritability, and high-pitched cry.

APPLYING THE NURSING PROCESS

Pain related to effects of vasospasm and edema

The nursing process helps ensure high-quality care for the preeclamptic client. The table below shows how the nurse might use the nursing process when caring for the client described in the case history at right. The first column presents history and physical assessment data followed by a paragraph of mental notes. These notes help the nurse make important connections among assessment findings, aiding in development of the nursing diagnosis and planning.

The second column lists an appropriate nursing diagnosis; the information in the remaining columns is based on this diagnosis. Although not part of the nursing process, a rationale for each intervention appears in the fourth column to explain how it contributes to the care plan.

ASSESSMENT	NURSING DIAGNOSIS	PLANNING
Subjective (history) data • Client states that this is her first pregnancy and that her husband has been very supportive. • Client says that she gets headaches; states, "My whole head hurts." • Client says she has dizzy spells. • Client reports that her legs ache. • Client states that her feet swell. Says they are sometimes "still swollen when I get up in the morning." **Objective (physical) data** • 32 weeks' gestation. • T 98.6° F, P 88, R 18, B/P 140/90. • 5-pound weight gain in 4 weeks. • No glucose in urine. • Trace protein in urine. • 2 + pitting edema in feet. **Mental Notes** *Generalized headaches and dizziness can indicate cerebral edema and vasospasm. Her husband is supportive and concerned about her headaches and will be helpful in providing comfort and support.*	Pain related to effects of vasospasm and edema	**Goals** The client will: • experience less pain within 24 hours • exhibit no pitting edema after 72 hours • walk about her room without headaches or dizziness after 72 hours.

• RhIg is given after delivery or abortion only to a client who is Rh negative and D^u negative, has not already developed isoimmunization, and whose fetus is $Rh_o(D)$ positive or D^u positive. (In a D^u-positive individual, RBCs display a weak positive reaction when tested with standard Rh-typing serums.) RhIg is *never* given to the neonate or the neonate's father.
• RhIg is not useful for a client who has Rh antibodies.
• RhIg should be administered intramuscularly, not subcutaneously or intravenously.

Assure the Rh-negative client with a nursing diagnosis of *fear related to unknown effect of blood incompatibility on the fetus* that in over 95% of cases, administering RhIg within 72 hours of evacuation of the uterus (by delivery or abortion) prevents isoimmunization to the Rh factor in her fetus.

Rh sensitization also is possible during pregnancy if the cellular layer separating the maternal and fetal

CASE STUDY

Marie Conner, a primagravid client age 27 at 32 weeks' gestation, comes to the medical clinic accompanied by her husband John. After a routine checkup, she is diagnosed as preeclamptic. Her vital signs are T 98.6° F, P 88, R 18, B/P 140/90. She has gained 5 pounds since her last visit 4 weeks ago. Her urine specimen is negative for glucose and contains a trace of protein. She has 2+ pitting edema of her feet.

IMPLEMENTATION

Intervention	Rationale
Provide comfort measures, such as a quiet environment, darkened room, and cool cloth to the head.	A dark, quiet environment will soothe the client.
Maintain client on bed rest in a left lateral recumbent (decubitus) position, but allow bathroom privileges.	Bed rest with bathroom privileges allows the client to rest while maintaining some self-care and facilitates kidney perfusion, thereby decreasing edema. Decreased movement also can ease headaches.
Administer analgesics as prescribed.	Analgesics can ease headaches and leg aches and will relax the client, allowing her to rest.
Clarify any misconceptions the client may have after discussing the disorder and its treatment with the physician. Answer all questions calmly and accurately, and provide emotional support.	Answering questions and clarifying misconceptions can put the client at ease, furthering rest and relaxation. Providing emotional support for the family assists in reducing anxiety and fear.
Encourage client compliance with the prescribed regimen.	Client compliance with the prescribed regimen can prevent any worsening of her condition and can facilitate recovery.
Assess vital signs (pulse, respiration, and blood pressure) every 4 hours unless otherwise ordered by the physician.	Serial measurements of vital signs will indicate the client's condition.
Check deep tendon reflexes (DTRs), especially hyperreflexia of the ankles, every 4 hours.	DTRs provide data on status of the central nervous system. Hyperreflexia precedes seizures. Absent reflexes may indicate magnesium sulfate toxicity.

EVALUATION

Upon evaluation:
• the client's blood pressure returned to baseline (130/80) within 12 hours; must continue to monitor closely to ascertain any changes in her condition
• no pitting edema noted; will continue to assess every 4 hours
• deep tendon reflexes 2+; will continue to assess every 4 hours
• negative clonus of ankle; will continue to assess every 4 hours
• the client had no complaints of headaches, leg aches, or dizziness.

circulations is disrupted and fetal blood enters the maternal bloodstream. The cellular layer may be disrupted during amniocentesis or by abruptio placentae.

For the client who is $Rh_o(D)$ negative and D^u negative and who has not already formed Rh antibodies, RhIg administered at about 28 weeks' gestation and again within 72 hours after delivery can help prevent Rh isoimmunization.

Evaluation

During this step of the nursing process, the nurse evaluates the effectiveness of the care plan against subjective and objective criteria. Evaluation findings should be stated in terms of actions performed or outcomes achieved for each goal. The following examples illustrate appropriate evaluation statements for clients with antepartal complications.

• The client has responded to small, frequent feedings by a reduced emesis.

• The client has verbalized understanding of the necessity for having a D&C after a spontaneous abortion.

• The client's ectopic pregnancy rupture site pain has been controlled with an analgesic agent.

• The client has listed the necessary follow-up for monitoring of GTD.

• The client's vital signs are stable after cervical cerclage.

• The client with mild preeclampsia shows a 2-pound weight gain, no proteinuria, and a diastolic blood pressure of 84 mm Hg this visit.

• The client has given a return demonstration of proper use of an at-home uterine monitor.

Documentation

All steps of the nursing process should be documentated as thoroughly and objectively as possible. Thorough documentation allows the nurse to evaluate the effectiveness of the care plan; it also makes this information available to other members of the health care team to ensure consistency of care.

Documentation for the client with antepartal complications should include:
• vital signs
• history and physical assessment findings of significance
• fetal heart rate
• laboratory and diagnostic test results
• client's and family's response to events
• medications given and their effectiveness
• Pre- and postprocedure care.

Chapter summary

Chapter 23 described antepartal complications and related nursing care for the affected client and her family. Here are the chapter highlights.

• Pregnancy, a significant life event that affects the client and her family physiologically and psychologically, can be accompanied by significant complications.

• Antepartal complications may result from reproductive system disorders, such as spontaneous abortion, ectopic pregnancy, GTD, incompetent cervix, PROM, and preterm labor and delivery. They also may be caused by multisystem disorders, such as hyperemesis gravidarum, hypertensive disorders, and Rh or ABO incompatibility.

• Spontaneous abortion, also called a miscarriage, can occur at any time before the age of fetal viability (20 to 24 weeks' gestation and a weight of over 500 grams). It typically causes bleeding and pain and is treated with rest, medications, emotional support, and other interventions, as needed.

• In ectopic pregnancy, the fertilized ovum is implanted in tissue other than the endometrium. This complication causes bleeding and abdominal pain. If rupture occurs, shock may ensue. The nurse must be prepared to control bleeding, administer transfusions, provide emotional support, and assist with removal of the products of conception.

• In GTD, trophoblastic cells covering the chorionic villi proliferate, and the villi undergo cystic changes. GTD may be benign, as in hydatidiform mole, or malignant, as in choriocarcinoma. It is characterized by rapid uterine growth, brownish red vaginal discharge, and a lack of fetal heart tones. Treatment calls for D&C or a similar procedure and at least 1 year of follow-up to detect signs of malignancy.

• Incompetent cervix refers to premature cervical dilation. This painless antepartal complication may lead to spontaneous abortion or premature delivery. When caring for a client with an incompetent cervix, the nurse should prepare her for cerclage, provide postoperative care, and offer emotional support.

• PROM, which occurs in 3% to 19% of all pregnancies, has an unknown etiology; however, several factors predispose a client to the condition. These factors include trauma, infection, hydramnios, and fetal malpresentation. Fetal morbidity and mortality rates are high following PROM, and RDS occurs in 30% to 70% of neonates. A key assessment finding includes amniotic fluid leakage. Depending on the risk to the mother and fetus, PROM may be treated with labor induction, cesarean delivery, or antibiotics.

• Preterm labor and delivery, which has been a significant cause of perinatal morbidity and mortality for many years, has responded to new technologies with increased survival rates and decreased complications.

• Hyperemesis gravidarum is a disorder of pregnancy in which excessive nausea and vomiting threaten the continuation of the pregnancy. Dehydration and electrolyte disturbances are common, and hospitalization may be necessary.

• PIH, a relatively common antepartal complication, causes increased blood pressure, edema, and proteinuria. Clients at risk include primigravid clients, elderly multigravid clients, teenagers, and those of low socioeconomic status. PIH is a major cause of maternal and fetal morbidity and mortality. Treatment includes bed rest and prevention of seizures.

• Hemolytic disease of the newborn can result from Rh incompatibility or ABO incompatibility. Rh incompatibility results when an Rh-negative client and an Rh-positive partner conceive a fetus with Rh-positive blood. Because of the potential for fetal and maternal blood mixing when the placenta separates after delivery, subsequent pregnancies are at risk for isoimmunization. In most cases, Rh isoimmunization can be prevented with RhIg. ABO incompatibility occurs when a client with blood group O becomes pregnant with a fetus with blood group A, B, or AB.

Study questions

1. Sandy Kravitz, a 23-year-old gravida 1 client, has been admitted to the hospital with hyperemesis gravidarum. Which actions can the nurse take to increase Ms. Kravitz's comfort level and promote rest?

2. Sharon Mason, a 26-year-old gravida 2, para 0, ab 2 client, is admitted to the unit with severe abdominal pain and bright red vaginal bleeding. After initial assessment, the nurse suspects spontaneous abortion (LMP was 8 weeks ago). Which nursing actions should the nurse initiate before calling the physician?

3. Mr. Evans brings his wife Sherry, age 21, to the emergency department because she has severe lower right quadrant pain. He thinks she has appendicitis. Assessment of her vital signs reveals a temperature of 99° F, a pulse rate of 92, respiration of 20, and blood pressure of 130/90. What other assessments are required before the nurse notifies the physician?

4. In the admission area of the labor and delivery unit, Susan Kelly, a 25-year-old primigravid client complains of generalized headache, dizziness, and swelling of her feet. What steps should the nurse take to assess Mrs. Kelly and her fetus?

5. Mrs. White, an Rh-negative 20-year-old primigravid client, has reached 28 weeks' gestation. Her partner is Rh positive. Her physician has told her she would receive RhIg at this prenatal visit. She tells the nurse she is afraid of needles and plans to refuse the medication. What are the nurse's responsibilities?

6. Cathy Pugh, a 23-year-old primigravid client at 28 weeks' gestation, is admitted to the labor and delivery unit in possible preterm labor. She suddenly complains of "feeling wet, like I just urinated." How can the nurse differentiate between rupture of the membranes and urine incontinency?

7. Sandy Allison, a 39-year-old multigravid client at 31 weeks' gestation, is admitted to the health care facility for preterm labor. Her physician orders an I.V. infusion of magnesium sulfate at 2 g/hour and an I.V. bolus of 6 g STAT. Several hours later, Sandy's deep tendon reflexes are 1+. What actions, if any, are appropriate before the nurse notifies the client's physician?

Bibliography

American College of Obstetricians and Gynecologists (1986). Management of isoimmunization in pregnancy. ACOG Technical Bulletin, No. 90.

Amon, E., Lewis, S.V., Sibai, B.M., Villar, M.A., and Arheart, K.L. (1988). Ampicillin prophylaxis in preterm premature rupture of the membranes: A prospective randomized study. *American Journal of Obstetrics and Gynecology*, 159(3), 539-543.

Beischer, N.A., and MacKay, E.V. (1986). *Obstetrics and the newborn* (2nd ed.). Philadelphia: Saunders.

Beth Israel Hospital Staff. (1982). *Obstetrical decision making*. St. Louis: Mosby.

Cunningham, F., MacDonald, P.C., and Gant, N. (1989). *Williams obstetrics* (18th ed.). East Norwalk, CT: Appleton & Lange.

Dahlberg, N.L.F. (1988). A perinatal center based antepartum home care program. *JOGNN*, 17(1), 30-34.

Delfs, E. (1957). Quantitative chorionic gonadotropin. *Obstetrics and Gynecology*, 9(1).

Deutchman, M. (1989). The problematic first-trimester pregnancy. *American Family Physician*, 39(1), 185-198.

Fossum, G.T., Davajan, V., and Kletzky, O.A. (1988). Early detection of pregnancy with transvaginal ultrasound. *Fertility and Sterility*, 49(5), 788-791.

Gibbs, R.S., and Sweet, R.L. (1989). Clinical disorders. In R.K. Creasy and R. Resnick (Eds.), *Maternal-fetal medicine: Principles and practice* (2nd ed.; pp. 656-662). Philadelphia: Saunders.

Gorrie, T.M. (1989). *A guide to the nursing of childbearing families.* Baltimore: Williams & Wilkins.

Hanson, F.W., Zorn, E.M., Tennant, F.R., Marianos, S. & Samuels, S. (1987). Amniocentesis before 15 weeks' gestation: Outcome, risks, and technical problems. *American Journal of Obstetrics and Gynecology,* 156(6), 1524-1531.

Henshaw, S.K., and Silverman, J. (1988). The characteristics and prior contraceptive use of United States abortion patients. *Family Planning Perspectives,* 20(4), 159-168.

Interim report of the Medical Research Council/Royal College of Obstetricians and Gynaecologists Multicentre Randomized Trial of Cervical Cerclage. (1988). *British Journal of Obstetrics and Gynecology,* 95(5), 437-445.

Jain, K.A., Hamper, U.M., and Sanders, R.C. (1988). Comparison of transvaginal and transabdominal sonography in the detection of early pregnancy and its complications. *American Journal of Roentgenology,* 151(6), 1139-1143.

Koonin, L., Atrash, H., Rochat, R., and Smith, J. (1988). Maternal mortality surveillance, United States, 1980-1985. *CDC Surveillance Summaries, MMWR,* 37(5), 19-29.

Lloyd, T. (1987). Rh-factor incompatibility, a primer for prevention. *Journal of Nurse-Midwifery,* 32(5), 297-307.

Modica, M.M., and Timor-Tritsch, I.E. (1988). Transvaginal sonography provides a sharper view into the pelvis. *JOGNN,* 17(2), 89-95.

Nyberg, D.A., Filly, R.A., Filho, D.L., Laring, F.C., and Mahoney, B.S. (1986). Abnormal pregnancy: Early diagnosis by US and serum chorionic gonodotropin levels. *Radiology,* 158(2), 393-396.

Nyberg, D.A., Mack, L.A., Laing, F.C., and Jeffrey, R.B. (1988). Early pregnancy complications: Endovaginal sonographic findings correlated with human chorionic gonadotropin levels. *Radiology,* 167(3), 619-622.

Parisi, V.M. (1989). Cervical incompetence. In R.K. Creasy and R. Resnick (Eds.), *Maternal-fetal medicine: Principles and practice* (2nd ed.; pp. 447-462). Philadelphia: Saunders.

Pussell, B.A., Peake, P.W., Brown, M.A., Charlesworth, G.A. (1985). Human fibronectin metabolism. *Journal of Clinical Investigation,* 76(1), 143-148.

Rayburn, W.F., and Schad, R.F. (1986). Antiemetics, iron preparations, vitamins and OTC drugs. In W.F. Rayburn and F.D. Zuspan (Eds.), *Drug therapy in obstetrics and gynecology* (2nd ed.; pp. 24-26). East Norwalk, CT: Appleton & Lange.

Sachs, B.P., Brown, D.A.J., Driscoll, S.G., Schulman, E., Acker, D., Ransil, B.J., and Jewett, J.F. (1988). Hemorrhage, infection, toxemia, and cardiac disease 1954-1985: Causes for their declining role in maternal mortality. *American Journal of Public Health,* 78(6), 671-675.

Scott, J.R., Branch, D.W., Kochenour, N.K., and Ward, K. (1988). Intravenous immunoglobulin treatment of pregnant patients with recurrent pregnancy loss caused by antiphospholipid antibodies and Rh immunization. *American Journal of Obstetrics and Gynecology,* 159(5), 1055-1056.

Scott, J.R. (1986a). Isoimmunization. In D.N. Danforth and J.R. Scott (Eds.), *Obstetrics and gynecology* (5th ed.). St. Louis: Mosby.

Ectopic pregnancy

Buck, R.H., Joubert, S.M., and Norman, P.J. (1988). Serum progesterone in the diagnosis of ectopic pregnancy: A valuable diagnostic test? *Fertility and Sterility,* 50(5), 752-755.

Centers for Disease Control. (June 22, 1990). Ectopic pregnancy—United States, 1987. *MMWR,* 39(24), 401-403.

Droegemueller, W. (1986). Ectopic pregnancy. In D.N. Danforth and J.R. Scott (Eds.), *Obstetrics and gynecology* (5th ed.). St. Louis: Mosby.

Fedele, L., Acaia, B., Parazzini, F., Ricciardiello, O., and Candiani, G.B. (1989). Ectopic pregnancy and recurrent spontaneous abortion: Two associated reproductive failures. *Obstetrics and Gynecology,* 73(2), 206-208.

Huber, J., Hosmann, J., and Vytiska-Binstorfer, E. (1989). Laparoscopic surgery for tubal pregnancy utilizing laser. *International Journal of Gynecology and Obstetrics,* 29(2), 153-157

Kadar, N., and Romero, R. (1988). Further observations on serial human chorionic gonadotropin patterns in ectopic pregnancies and spontaneous abortions. *Fertility and Sterility,* 50(2), 367-370.

Kuczynski, H.J. (1986). Support for the woman with an ectopic pregnancy. *JOGNN,* 15(4), 306-310.

Lawson, H., Atrash, H., Saftlas, A., Franks, A., Finch, E., and Hughes, J. (1988). Ectopic pregnancy surveillance, United States, 1970-1985. *MMWR,* 37 (SSS-5), 9-18.

Lindblom, B., Hahlin, M., and Sjoblom, P. (1989). Serial human chorionic gonadotropin determinations by fluoroimmunoassay for differentiation between intrauterine pregnancy and ectopic gestation. *American Journal of Obstetrics and Gynecology,* 161(2), 397-400.

Loffer, F.D. (1986). The increasing problem of ectopic pregnancies and its impact on patients and physicians. *The Journal of Reproductive Medicine,* 31(2), 74-77.

Makinen, J.I., Salmi, T.A., Nikkanen, V.P.J., and Juhani-Koskinen, E.Y. (1989). Encouraging rates of fertility after ectopic pregnancy. *International Journal of Fertility,* 34(1), 46-51.

Mecke, H., Semm, K., and Lehman-Willenbrock, E. (1989). Results of operative pelviscopy in 202 cases of ectopic pregnancy. *International Journal of Fertility,* 34(2), 93-100.

Osguthorpe, N.C. (1987). Ectopic pregnancy. *JOGNN,* 16(1), 36-41.

Osguthorpe, N.C., and Keating, K. (1988). Care of the client with ectopic pregnancy. *JOGNN,* 17(1), 32-38.

Pouley, J.L., Mahnes, H., Mage, G., Canis, M., and Bruhat, M.A. (1986). Conservative treatment of ectopic pregnancy. *Fertility and Sterility,* 46(7), 1093.

Romero, R. (1986). The diagnosis of ectopic pregnancy. In A.H. DeCherney (Ed.), *Ectopic pregnancy* (pp. 15-34). Rockville, MD: Aspen Publications.

Schenker, J.G., and Evron, S. (1983). New concepts in the surgical management of tubal pregnancy and the consequent postoperative results. *Fertility and Sterility,* 40(6), 709-723.

Silva, P.D. (1988). A laparoscopic approach can be applied to most cases of ectopic pregnancy. *Obstetrics and Gynecology,* 72(6), 944-947.

Stock, R.J. (1988). The changing spectrum of ectopic pregnancy. *Obstetrics and Gynecology,* 71(6), 885-888.

Timor-Tritsch, I.E., Yeh, M.N., Peisner, D.P., Blesser, K. and Slavik, T.A. (1989). The use of transvaginal ultrasonography in the diagnosis of ectopic pregnancy. *American Journal of Obstetrics and Gynecology,* 161(1), 157-161.

Vermesh, M., Silva, P.D., Sauer, M.V., Vargyas, J.M., and Lobo, R.A. (1988). Persistent tubal ectopic gestation: Patterns of circulating beta-human chorionic gonadotropin and progesterone, and management options. *Fertility and Sterility,* 50(4), 584-588.

Weissman, A., Fishman, A., and Gal, D. (1989). Interstitial pregnancy: A diagnostic challenge. *International Journal of Gynaecology and Obstetrics,* 29(4), 373-375.

Gestational trophoblastic disease

Berman, M.L., and DiSaia, P.J. (1989). Pelvic malignancies, gestational trophoblastic neoplasia, and nonpelvic malignancies. In R.K. Creasy and R. Resnick (Eds.), *Maternal-fetal medicine: Principles and practice* (2nd ed; pp. 1122-1149). Philadelphia: Saunders.

Fine, C., Bundy, A.L., Berkowitz, R.S., Boswell, S.B., Berezin, A.F., and Doubilet, P.M. (1989). Sonographic diagnosis of partial hydatidiform mole. *Obstetrics and Gynecology, 73*(3), 414-418.

Hilgers, R.D., and Lewis, J.L. (1986). Gestational trophoblastic disease. In D.N. Danforth and J.R. Scott (Eds.), *Obstetrics and gynecology* (5th ed.). St. Louis: Mosby.

Khazaeli, M.B., Buchina, E.S., Pattillo, R.A., Soong, S.J., and Hatch, K.D. (1989). Radioimmunoassay of free beta-subunit of human chorionic gonadotropin in diagnosis of high-risk and low-risk gestational trophoblastic disease. *American Journal of Obstetrics and Gynecology, 160*(2), 444-449.

Schlaerth, J.B., Morrow, C.P., Montz, F.J., and d'Ablaing, G. (1988). Initial management of hydatidiform mole. *American Journal of Obstetrics and Gynecology, 158*(6), 1299-1306.

Hypertensive disorders

Ballegeer, V., Spitz, B., Kieckens, L., Moreau, H., Van Assche, A.V., and Collen, D. (1989). Predictive value of increased plasma levels of fibronectin in gestational hypertension. *American Journal of Obstetrics and Gynecology, 161*(2), 432-436.

Belizian, J.M., and Villar, J. (1980). The relationship between calcium intake and edema, proteinuria and hypertension gestosis: A hypothesis. *American Journal of Clinical Nutrition, 33,* 2202.

Brewer, T. (1974). Metabolic toxemia of late pregnancy in a county prenatal nutrition education project. *Journal of Reproductive Medicine, 13*(5), 175.

Cotton, D.B., Longmire, S., Jones, N.M., Dorman, K.F., Tessem, J., and Joyce, T.H. (1986). Cardiovascular alterations in severe PIH: Effects of intravenous nitroglycerin coupled with blood volume expansion. *American Journal of Obstetrics and Gynecology, 154*(5), 1053-1059.

De Alvarez, R. (1978). Pre-eclampsia, eclampsia and renal disease in pregnancy. *Clinical Obstetrics and Gynecology, 21,* 881.

Gavette, L., and Roberts, J. (1987). Use of mean arterial pressure (MAP-2) to predict pregnancy-induced hypertension in adolescents. *Journal of Nurse Midwifery, 32*(6), 357-364.

Gilbert, E.S., and Harmon J.S. (1986). *High-risk pregnancy and delivery.* St. Louis: Mosby.

Gudson, J.P., Jr., Buckalew, V.M., Jr., and Hennessy, J.F. (1984). A digoxin-like immunoreactive substance in preeclampsia. *American Journal of Obstetrics and Gynecology, 150*(1), 83-85.

Hacker, N., and Moore, G. (9186). *Essentials of obstetrics and gynecology.* Philadelphia: Saunders.

Risch, H.A., Weiss, N.S., Clarke, and Roberts, J.M. (1989). Pregnancy-related hypertension. In R.K. Creasy and R. Resnick (Eds.), *Maternal-fetal medicine: Principles and practice* (2nd ed.; pp. 777-823). Philadelphia: Saunders.

Rodgers, G.M., Taylor, R.N., and Roberts, J.M. (1988). Preeclampsia is associated with a serum factor cytotoxic to human endothelial cells. *American Journal of Obstetrics and Gynecology, 159*(4), 908-914.

Shanklin, D.R., and Sibai, B.M. (1989). Ultrastructural aspects of preeclampsia: Placental bed and uterine boundary vessels. *American Journal of Obstetrics and Gynecology, 161*(3), 735-741.

Zuspan, F.P., and Zuspan, K.J. (1986). Acute and chronic hypertension during pregnancy. In W.F. Rayburn and F.P. Zuspan (Eds.), *Drug therapy in obstetrics and gynecology* (2nd ed.; pp. 73-92). East Norwalk, CT: Appleton & Lange.

Preterm labor

Brar, H.S., Medearis, A.L., DeVore, G.R., and Platt, L.D. (1988). Maternal and fetal blood flow velocity waveforms in patients with preterm labor: Effects of tocolytics. *American Journal of Obstetrics and Gynecology, 72*(2), 209-214.

Creasy, R.K. (1989). Preterm labor and delivery. In R.K. Creasy and R. Resnick (Eds.), *Maternal-fetal medicine: Principles and practice* (2nd ed.). Philadelphia: Saunders.

Givens, S.R. (1988). Update on tocolytic therapy in the management of preterm labor. *Journal of Perinatal Neonatal Nursing, 2*(1), 21-32.

Gupta, R.C., Foster, S., Romano, P.M., and Thomas, H.M. (1989). Acute pulmonary edema associated with the use of oral ritodrine for premature labor. *Chest, 95*(2), 479-481.

Iams, J.D., Johnson, F.F., and O'Shaughnessy, R.W. (1988). A prospective random trial of home uterine activity monitoring in pregnancies at increased risk of preterm labor, Part II. *American Journal of Obstetrics and Gynecology, 159*(3), 595-603.

Koehl, L., and Wheeler, D. (1989). Monitoring uterine activity at home. *AJN, 89*(2), 200-203.

McLendon, M.S. (1988). Home ambulatory uterine activity monitoring: A new tool in the management of women at risk for preterm birth. *Journal of Perinatal Neonatal Nursing, 2*(1), 1-9.

Milos, M., Aberle, D.R., Parkinson, B.T., Batra, P., and Brown, K. (1988). Maternal pulmonary edema complicating beta-adrenergic therapy of preterm labor. *American Journal of Roentgenology, 151*(5), 917-918.

Morales, W.J., Angel, J.C., O'Brien, W.F., Knuppel, R.A., and Finazzo, M. (1988). A randomized study of antibiotic therapy in idiopathic preterm labor. *Obstetrics and Gynecology, 72*(6), 829-833.

Moise, K.J., Huhta, J.C., Sharif, D.S., Ou, C.N., Kirshon, B., Wasserstrum, N., and Cano, L. (1988). Indomethacin in the treatment of premature labor: Effects on fetal ductus arteriosus. *New England Journal of Medicine, 319*(6), 327-331.

Omer, H., and Everly, G.S., Jr., (1988). Psychological factors in preterm labor: Critical review and theoretical synthesis. *American Journal of Psychiatry, 145*(12), 1507-1513.

Rayburn, W.F., DeDonato, D.M., and Rand, W.K. (1986). Drugs to inhibit premature labor. In W.F. Rayburn and F.P. Zuspan (Eds.), *Drug therapy in obstetrics and gynecology* (2nd ed.; pp. 172-183). East Norwalk, CT: Appleton & Lange.

Wilkins, I.A., Lynch, L., Mehalek, K.E., Berkowitz, G.S., and Berkowitz, R.L. (1988). Efficacy and side effects of magnesium sulfate and ritodrine as tocolytic agents. *American Journal of Obstetrics and Gynecology, 159*(3), 685-689.

Spontaneous abortion

Berkowitz, R.S., and Goldstein, D.P. (1984). Molar pregnancy: Etiology. In E.S. Hafez (Ed.), *Spontaneous abortion* (pp. 363-372). Hingham. MA: Kluwer Academic Publishers.

Glass, R.H., and Golbus, M.S. (1989). Habitual abortion. In R.K. Creasy and R. Resnick, R. (Eds.), *Maternal-fetal medicine: Principles and practice* (2nd ed.; pp. 437-446). Philadelphia: Saunders.

Hafez, E.S. (1984). Early embryonic loss: Physiology. In E.S. Hafez (Ed.), *Spontaneous abortion* (pp. 99-114). Hingham, MA: Kluwer Academic Publishers.

Key, T. (1989). Gastrointestinal disturbances. In R.K. Creasy and R. Resnick (Eds.), *Maternal-fetal medicine: Principles and practice* (2nd ed.). Philadelphia: Saunders.

McDonald, A.D., Armstrong, B., Cherry, N.M., Delorme, C., Diodati-Nolin, A., McDonald, J.C., and Robert, D. (1986). Spontaneous abortion and occupation. *Journal of Occupational Medicine*, 28(12), 1232-1238.

Michel, M., Underwood, J., Clark, D., Mowbray, J.F., and Beard, R.W. (1989). Histologic and immunologic study of uterine biopsy tissue in women with incipient abortions. *American Journal of Obstetrics and Gynecology*, 161(2), 409-414.

Neidhardt, A. (1986). Why me? Second trimester abortion. *AJN*, 86(10), 1133-1135.

Risch, H.A., Weiss, N.S., Clarke, E.A., and Miller, A.B. (1988). Risk factors for spontaneous abortion and its recurrence. *American Journal of Epidemiology*, 128 (2), 420-430.

Scott, J.R. (1986b). Spontaneous abortion. In D.N. Danforth and J.R. Scott (Eds.), *Obstetrics and gynecology* (5th ed.). St. Louis: Mosby.

Cultural references

Choi, E.C. (1986). Unique aspects of Korean-American mothers. *JOGNN*, 15(5), 394-400.

Lee, R.V. (1989). Understanding Southeast Asian mothers-to-be. *Childbirth Education*, 5(2), 32-34, 36, 39.

Roberson, M.H.B. (1987). Home remedies: A cultural study. *Home Healthcare Nurse*, 5(1), 35-40.

Nursing research

Loos, C., and Julius, L. (1989). The client's view of hospitalization during pregnancy. *JOGNN*, 18(1), 52-56.

Remich, M.C., and Youngkin, E.Q. (1989). Factors associated with pregnancy-induced hypertension. *Nurse Practitioner*, 14(1), 20-24.

Risch, H.A., Weiss, N.S., Clarke, E.A., and Miller, A.B. (1988). Risk factors for spontaneous abortion and its recurrence. *American Journal of Epidemiology*, 128(2), 420-430.

The Intrapartal Period

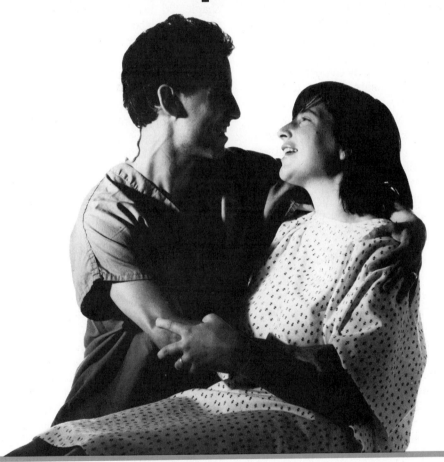

Childbirth is among the most exciting—yet stressful—events in the lives of the childbearing client and family. The nurse providing intrapartal care must have a thorough understanding of current theory and practices regarding labor and delivery to help the childbearing client and her fetus or neonate achieve optimal health. This unit provides the conceptual and clinical knowledge base to help the nurse attain such understanding. It prepares the nurse to anticipate the needs of the childbearing family, promotes holistic care by emphasizing childbirth as a family-centered event, and examines the personal and cultural factors that may affect the way the client and her family experience and perceive the intrapartal experience. Stressing health promotion as a nursing goal, this unit discusses various independent nursing roles, such as teaching, counseling, supporting, and advocacy. It covers high-risk as well as low-risk labor and delivery situations.

The first two chapters in the unit provide a theoretical framework, focusing on the physiology of labor and childbirth and fetal assessment during the intrapartal period. The remaining chapters follow a similar format, using the nursing process to guide nursing care. To demonstrate how to integrate assessment findings and document nursing care, these chapters include charts that apply the nursing process to case studies.

Chapter 24
Physiology of Labor and Childbirth

Chapter 24 addresses physiologic changes during the intrapartal period—from the onset of labor to immediately after delivery—to help the nurse anticipate and meet the needs of the intrapartal client. It reviews theories of labor onset, such as oxytocin stimulation and progesterone reduction, and describe its signs and symptoms, such as lightening and Braxton Hicks contractions. Next, the chapter elaborates on the mechanism of labor, illustrating the cardinal movements of labor from engagement through expulsion.

After specifying the physiologic changes during each stage of labor, the chapter examines the essential factors that affect labor—the fetus, the pelvis, uterine contractions and bearing-down efforts, placental position and function, and psychological response. It illustrates normal fetal skull characteristics and skull molding; fetal attitude, presentation, and position; and pelvic planes and diameters.

Chapter 25
Fetal Assessment

Chapter 25 specifies the concepts and methods used to evaluate fetal status during the intrapartal period. First, it describes the physiologic basis of fetal monitoring—uteroplacental-fetal circulation and fetal heart rate (FHR) regulation. Then it examines the monitoring techniques that help ensure prompt detection of problems. The chapter explores the use of the fetoscope and the ultrasound stethoscope. Then it discusses the use, benefits, and disadvantages of external and internal electronic fetal monitoring (EFM) and summarizes related controversies. It explains how to monitor uterine activity through manual palpation, an external tocodynamometer, an internal intrauterine pressure catheter, and telemetry. It also presents illustrated procedures showing how to apply external and internal electronic fetal monitors.

Next, Chapter 25 describes FHR patterns, providing the knowledge base necessary to recognize fetal distress patterns. It explains how to use the baseline FHR as a reference for subsequent FHR readings, describes how to identify baseline tachycardia and bradycardia, and discusses FHR variability and its components. Then it

elaborates on the periodic changes caused by uterine contractions and fetal movements, emphasizing early, late, variable, and prolonged decelerations. The chapter explains how to read a fetal monitor strip and features charts showing possible causes, clinical significance, and nursing interventions for FHR variations and common decelerations. After reviewing fetal scalp blood sampling and other fetal assessment techniques, the chapter outlines nursing responsibilities related to fetal assessment, including legal responsibilities, client teaching and support, and documentation of EFM.

Chapter 26
Comfort Promotion during Labor and Childbirth

Chapter 26 describes the characteristics and causes of pain during labor, and it prepares the nurse to promote physical and psychological comfort for the client experiencing labor pain. After describing the types of pain arising during the first, second, and third stages of labor, it explains how various physical and psychosocial factors affect pain perception and how the nurse determines a client's comfort promotion needs.

Next, Chapter 26 describes the essential components of assessment for a client experiencing labor pain—health history, physical assessment, and follow-up assessment to gauge the effectiveness and safety of comfort promotion measures. After presenting relevant nursing diagnoses, the chapter discusses comfort measures to reduce anxiety, promote hygiene, and aid relaxation. Then it explains how to care for the unprepared client by providing adequate information and initiating simple relaxation techniques early in labor. Next, the chapter examines the role of nonpharmacologic pain control measures, such as hypnosis and acupuncture and explores pharmacologic pain control through the use of analgesics, regional anesthetics, and general anesthetics. Charts delineate the indications and nursing considerations for analgesics, tranquilizers, and anesthetics during labor and the benefits and disadvantages of common administration routes for analgesic agents. It illustrates administration sites and methods used for regional anesthesia and describes how to identify and manage hypotensive crisis after spinal or epidural anesthesia.

Chapter 27
The First Stage of Labor

Chapter 27 describes nursing care that meets the physical, psychosocial, and cultural needs of the client during the first stage of labor—from onset of regular uterine contractions to complete cervical dilation. It explains how to conduct an initial assessment to determine if a client is in true labor or has a medical problem that could affect her or her fetus during labor and delivery. It illustrates auscultation of fetal heart tones, palpation of uterine contractions, and Leopold's maneuvers to determine fetal position. It explains how to assess and intervene for variations in the first stage of labor, how to distinguish true labor from false labor, and how to determine if the client should be admitted to the labor and delivery unit.

Chapter 27 then explains how to orient the client and her support person to the unit and tells how to conduct ongoing assessment to obtain data needed to formulate a care plan. It discusses assessment of the client's psychosocial status and admission tests and prenatal tests that may be ordered for the client in labor. The chapter provides nursing diagnoses for the client in the first stage of labor, then discusses initial planning and implementation of routine admission procedures, such as fluid infusion and skin preparation. Next, it presents ongoing planning and implementation, focusing on monitoring of vital signs, uterine contractions, fetal response to labor, labor progress, and urinary functions. It describes appropriate comfort and support measures, illustrates the steps of a vaginal examination, provides a client teaching aid showing alternate labor positions, and details nursing interventions that promote involvement of the client's family in her labor experience.

Chapter 28
The Second Stage of Labor

Chapter 28 explores the characteristics and progression of the second, or expulsive, stage of labor and outlines relevant nursing care. It begins by describing the signs that mark onset of the second stage, comparing and contrasting the two phases of this stage and discussing the diverse factors that affect its duration.

Next, Chapter 28 specifies the components of ongoing assessment during the second stage, explaining how to evaluate cervical dilation, contractions, bearing-down efforts, and factors related to fetal status. After providing nursing diagnoses, the chapter focuses on nursing interventions, such as providing emotional support, coordinating bearing-down efforts, assisting with hydration, and preparing for delivery. It discusses alternative ways of bearing down, compares the benefits and disadvantages of various labor positions, and offers step-by-step instructions on preparing the perineum for delivery. Then the chapter summarizes the essential steps of nursing care for the neonate immediately after delivery, including how to assign an Apgar score. The chapter includes a photographic essay on labor and delivery, beginning with crowning and concluding with the neonate and client sharing a moment of bonding.

Chapter 29
The Third and Fourth Stages of Labor

Chapter 29 prepares the nurse to care for a client and her neonate during the third and fourth stages of labor—a period extending from the neonate's delivery to approximately 1 hour after delivery of the placenta. It begins by discussing nursing care during the third stage. Describing assessment, it emphasizes the importance of evaluating maternal vital signs, the placenta, the perineum, and the fundus. After presenting nursing diagnoses for the third stage, the chapter focuses on nursing measures that promote hygiene, client repositioning, neonatal care, and parent-infant bonding. It discusses neonatal assessment, touches on relevant cultural considerations, illustrates placental and umbilical cord variations, and provides instructions on palpating and massaging the uterus after delivery. It concludes by presenting guidelines on evaluating and documenting care provided during the third stage.

Next, Chapter 29 describes nursing care during the fourth stage. It emphasizes the need for frequent, careful assessment; explains how to assess the client for discomfort and recovery from anesthesia and analgesia; and describes client evaluation for fatigue, hunger, thirst, and response to childbirth. The chapter provides appropriate nursing diagnoses, then it elaborates on such crucial interventions as maintaining maternal position, activity, hygiene, and comfort; preventing hemorrhage; ensuring proper fluid and nutritional status; and promoting parent-infant bonding.

Chapter 30
Family Support during the Intrapartal Period

Chapter 30 discusses the role of support for the intrapartal client in reducing emotional stress and physical discomfort during labor and delivery. First, it investigates the principles of support during labor and delivery, pinpointing the benefits of support from the client's family and friends. It examines the types of support a client may need, including perceived support, emotional support, and informational support. Next, it reviews the various sources of support that may be available to a client, examining the supportive roles of the client's partner, her or her partner's parents and children, and her family and friends.

Chapter 30 then discusses assessment, explaining how to identify the client's preferences regarding anesthesia, birth position, support person, and family involvement during labor and delivery. It describes how to assess the needs and concerns of the client's support person by evaluating this person's knowledge about childbirth, goals for and feelings about labor and delivery, and individual needs. The chapter emphasizes the special needs and expectations of the expectant father who serves as support person and reviews assessment of the client's cultural beliefs related to labor and delivery. After presenting relevant nursing diagnoses for the client's support person, Chapter 30 identifies nursing interventions to assist the client's family and support person and to balance the client's needs against theirs. It focuses on measures that help orient the support person to the labor and delivery unit, keep the support person informed of the client's progress, and provide sensitive care for the family.

Chapter 31
High-Risk Intrapartal Clients

Chapter 31 describes selected conditions that may jeopardize a client, fetus, or neonate during labor and delivery and explores the specialized nursing care these conditions necessitate. It examines the many stressors affecting the high-risk intrapartal client, such as fear of an uncertain pregnancy outcome, loss of confidence in her ability to give birth naturally, and anxiety about lack of control over labor and delivery; touches on the perinatal problems that may result from inadequate prenatal care; then outlines the general responsibilities of the nurse caring for the high-risk intrapartal client and her family.

Next, Chapter 31 identifies the maternal, fetal, and neonatal risk factors associated with selected conditions that may cause high-risk status—age-related concerns, cardiac disease, diabetes mellitus, infection, substance abuse, pregnancy-induced hypertension (PIH), and isoimmunization. Then it explains how to obtain a health history and conduct a physical assessment for the client with a high-risk condition and reviews the laboratory tests that help diagnose and monitor the client's status. After providing relevant nursing diagnoses, Chapter 31 explains how to tailor normal intrapartal care to meet the special needs of the high-risk client and discusses management of such intrapartal emergencies as diabetic ketoacidosis and PIH.

Chapter 32
Special Obstetric Procedures

Chapter 32 describes obstetric procedures and related nursing care for the client who requires special assistance to ensure normal delivery. First, it discusses the criteria, benefits, and disadvantages of nonsurgical obstetric procedures—version, labor induction, forceps delivery, vacuum extraction, and vaginal birth after cesarean delivery. Besides illustrating many of these procedures, the chapter reviews the use of prostaglandin (PGE$_2$) gel to induce labor. Then it investigates surgical obstetric procedures (episiotomy and cesarean delivery) and illustrates the various incisions used for cesarean delivery.

Next, the chapter presents nursing care for clients requiring special obstetric procedures. It explains the essentials of initial assessment, pointing out the importance of the psychosocial history to determine the client's and family's anxiety level and outlining the six crucial categories of baseline physical data to collect. Then it presents guidelines for ongoing assessment during and after labor, focusing on how to adapt the assessment to the specific procedure performed. After reviewing nursing diagnoses for the client, fetus, or selected family members, the chapter describes nursing measures that help maintain fluid balance, promote uterine contractions, prevent infection, prepare the client for cesarean delivery, and provide psychological support.

Chapter 33
Intrapartal Complications

Chapter 33 explores the complications that can arise during the intrapartal period and identifies the nurse's role in detecting and managing these problems. First, it describes the pathophysiology of complications arising from reproductive system disorders, specifying the various uterine, pelvic, placental, membrane and amniotic fluid, and umbilical cord factors that may be involved. It shows how to gauge progression of labor and provides a step-by-step procedure for emergency delivery. Next, the chapter reviews the systemic disorders (such as hemorrhage and shock) and fetal complications (such as malpresentation, malposition, and shoulder dystocia) that can cause intrapartal complications. Special features include discussions on assessment of and emergency nursing management for umbilical cord prolapse and fetal distress.

Chapter 33 then discusses nursing care for the client with an intrapartal complication. After explaining how to assess for each complication, it presents relevant nursing diagnoses. It discusses planning and implementation, then tells how to evaluate the client with an intrapartal complication and how to document nursing care.

Physiology of Labor and Childbirth

Objectives

After reading and studying this chapter, the student should be able to:

1. Describe maternal, fetal, and placental factors that may initiate labor.
2. Discuss the physiologic changes that commonly signal labor onset.
3. Explain the physiologic changes associated with uterine contractions and cervical effacement and dilation.
4. Explain the cardinal movements of labor.
5. Explain the four stages of labor, discussing what occurs in each stage.
6. Define the five essential factors of labor, and discuss how each affects the physiology of labor and childbirth.
7. Describe maternal physiologic and psychological changes associated with each stage of labor.
8. Explain fetal physiologic responses to labor.

Introduction

Impending labor and childbirth typically trigger both excitement and apprehension in a pregnant client. Whether about to give birth for the first time (a primiparous client) or experienced from previous childbirth (a multiparous client), she will have many physical and psychological needs. To meet these needs, the nurse must understand the labor process and how it affects the client and fetus.

This chapter begins with a discussion of the factors that may initiate labor, which still are poorly understood. It then describes physiologic changes that commonly signal labor onset, called premonitory signs and symp-

toms. Subsequent sections explain the mechanisms of labor, including cervical effacement and dilation and fetal cardinal movements; the four stages of labor; and factors affecting the labor process. The chapter concludes with discussions of physiologic changes that affect the client and the fetus during labor and childbirth.

Theories of labor onset

Although several theories of labor onset have been proposed, the exact mechanism has eluded researchers. Instead of a single initiating factor, several maternal, fetal, and placental factors probably interact to initiate labor. These include oxytocin stimulation, progesterone reduction, estrogen stimulation, fetal cortisol production, and the effects of fetal membrane phospholipids, arachidonic acid, and prostaglandins.

Oxytocin stimulation

Oxytocin, a hormone produced by the hypothalamus and stored in and released from the posterior pituitary gland, seems to play an important role in labor. As pregnancy progresses, the amount of maternal oxytocin increases, as do the number of oxytocin receptor sites within the uterine myometrium and decidua.

In the third trimester, the uterus becomes increasingly sensitive to the effect of oxytocin. At the time just

GLOSSARY

Asynclitism: state of lateral flexion of the head of the fetus toward either the symphysis pubis (anterior asynclitism) or sacrum (posterior asynclitism).

Attitude: relationship of the parts of the fetus to one another.

Biparietal diameter: greatest transverse distance between the two parietal bones.

Bloody show: blood-tinged vaginal discharge that occurs at the onset of labor when the cervical mucus plus is dislodged and small cervical capillaries break.

Braxton Hicks contractions: painless uterine contractions that occur at irregular intervals throughout pregnancy but become more noticeable as term approaches; major cause of false labor.

Breech presentation: fetal position in which the buttocks or feet present first.

Cardinal movements of labor: series of positional changes that occur as the fetus passes through the pelvis; progression includes descent, flexion, internal rotation, extension, external rotation (restitution and shoulder rotation), and expulsion.

Contraction: involuntary and intermittent tightening or shortening of uterine muscle fibers that leads to cervical dilation, effacement, and fetal descent.

Dilation: progressive widening of the external cervical os; also called dilatation.

Effacement: progressive thinning and shortening of the cervix during labor.

Engagement: state in which the widest diameter of the fetal presenting part reaches the level of the ischial spines.

Fetal lie: relationship of the long axis of the fetus to the long axis of the mother.

Fetal position: relationship of the landmark on the fetal presenting part to the front, back, and sides of the maternal pelvis.

Fontanel: nonossified area of connective tissue between the skull bones where the sutures intersect; allows molding of the skull for passage through the pelvis during delivery.

Labor: process that occurs from the onset of cervical effacement and dilation to delivery of the placenta.

Lightening: subjective sensations caused by descent of the fetus into the pelvis.

Oxytocin: hormone produced by the posterior pituitary gland that triggers uterine contractions.

Pelvis: bony structure made up of the sacrum, coccyx, and innominate bones; passageway through which the fetus travels during labor.

Presenting part: portion of the fetus that first enters the pelvic passageway.

Station: relationship of the presenting part to the ischial spines.

Synclitism: state in which the fetus's biparietal diameter is parallel to the plane of the mother's pelvic inlet.

---

before the onset of labor, the uterus becomes extremely sensitive to even small doses of oxytocin.

Whether oxytocin directly initiates labor remains unclear. At least indirectly, maternal oxytocin causes the release of bound calcium from the sarcoplasmic reticulum of the uterine myometruim, which in turn triggers uterine contractions. According to Cunningham, MacDonald, and Gant (1989), any role oxytocin may play is limited to the expulsive stage of labor and the postpartal period; at these periods, oxytocin enhances uterine contractions and prevents postpartal hemorrhage. Although researchers have concentrated their attention on maternal oxytocin, fetal oxytocin also may play a role in initiating labor.

Progesterone reduction

In animal studies, withdrawing progesterone has triggered labor and administering progesterone has delayed labor, prolonging gestation beyond normal periods. Controversy still exists, however, regarding the role of progesterone reduction in the pregnant woman. During pregnancy, progesterone blocks myometrial activity by helping to keep calcium bound and unavailable for muscle contraction. Tulchinsky and Giannopoulus (1983) reported decreased numbers of progesterone receptors in the myometria of pregnant women near the end of pregnancy as compared to nonpregnant women. Also, decreased progesterone levels have been found in women who experienced spontaneous abortion. Cunningham, MacDonald, and Gant (1989) reported that maternal progesterone blood levels do not decrease before labor begins.

Some researchers believe that progesterone produced by the fetal membranes decreases as term approaches. This decrease may be caused by a progesterone-binding protein in the amnion and the chorion. Decreased progesterone production may trigger the production of prostaglandins, which stimulate uterine contractions. Although disagreement exists on the role of progesterone, many researchers believe a shift in the estrogen-progesterone ratio plays a major role in increasing uterine contractility.

Estrogen stimulation

Maternal estrogen levels rise throughout pregnancy. Researchers believe estrogen may stimulate and affect labor in several ways. First, by sensitizing the uterine lining, estrogen increases the production of adenosine triphosphate and contractile proteins. Next, estrogen helps impulses pass among myometrial cells, causing the sensitized uterine muscle to contract.

Estrogen may stimulate prostaglandin production in the decidua and fetal membranes and may make the uterus more sensitive to oxytocin (Hariharan, Takahashi, and Burd, 1986).

Fetal cortisol production

In sheep, labor is associated with a sharp increase in cortisol production by the fetal adrenal gland. Cortisol causes the placenta to inhibit progesterone production and increase estrogen and prostaglandin production (Cunningham, MacDonald, and Gant, 1989). Clinical studies, however, have not yielded comparable results.

Researchers as far back as 1898 have recognized the association among fetal anencephaly (fetus that does not develop a brain), fetal adrenal hypoplasia (fetus that has small adrenal glands), and prolonged gestation. The adrenal glands in an anencephalic fetus typically weigh only 5% to 10% of the adrenal glands in a normal fetus (Cunningham, MacDonald, and Gant, 1989). At this time, however, the precise role the fetal adrenal glands play in labor onset is uncertain.

Fetal membrane phospholipids, arachidonic acid, and prostaglandins

Some researchers link labor onset to a complex interaction of maternal estrogen and progesterone and fetal membrane phospholipids, arachidonic acid, and prostaglandins. Estrogen acts on fetal membranes to increase their storage of arachidonic acid (compound made of an alcohol and an acid), a precursor in the biosynthesis of prostaglandins. Meanwhile, decreasing progesterone levels stimulate the production of phospholipase A_2, which in turn hydrolyzes (uses water to split a compound) phospholipids to convert the esterified arachidonic acid into a nonesterified form. Nonesterified arachidonic acid then undergoes biosynthesis to form prostaglandins, which stimulate uterine contractions (Hariharan, Takahashi, and Burd, 1986; Cunningham, MacDonald, and Gant, 1989).

Premonitory signs and symptoms of labor

Although the exact mechanism that triggers labor remains unclear, certain physiologic signs and symptoms (called premonitory) typically predict the onset of true labor. Some of these signs and symptoms may occur up to 3 weeks before labor onset; others coincide with the beginning of labor.

Lightening

Lightening, subjective sensations experienced by many clients late in pregnancy, occurs as the fetus settles lower in the pelvis, leaving more space in the upper abdomen. In primiparous clients, lightening normally occurs 2 to 3 weeks before labor begins; in multiparous clients, it may not occur until labor actually begins. This downward fetal movement decreases pressure on the diaphragm, easing respiratory effort and allowing the client to breathe more deeply. It also reduces compression of the stomach, allowing the client to eat more at each meal. Accompanying these sensations are a change in abdominal shape and a visible decrease in fundal height, at which time the fetus is commonly said to have "dropped." Lightening also has been associated with a reduction in amniotic fluid volume (Cunningham, MacDonald, and Gant, 1989).

Along with these beneficial effects, however, lightening also may cause discomfort. In some clients, the frequent urge to urinate experienced early in pregnancy returns because the uterus, lower in the pelvis after the fetus has dropped, pushes against the bladder. The client may feel fetal movements much lower in the abdomen, producing a sensation of pressure.

Also, downward pressure on deep leg veins from the enlarged uterus may cause pelvic pressure and edema of the legs. Increased pelvic pressure can lead to or aggravate hemorrhoids or varicose veins; this pressure may cause leg cramps or pain when it impinges on nerves.

Braxton Hicks contractions

Throughout pregnancy, the uterus undergoes a series of painless, irregular contractions known as Braxton Hicks contractions. These help prepare for labor by causing cervical changes late in pregnancy.

Braxton Hicks contractions have been described as pulling or tightening sensations focused primarily over the pubic bone. Although these contractions may occur every 5 to 20 minutes throughout pregnancy, they typically become most noticeable during the last 6 weeks of gestation in primiparous clients and the last 3 to 4 months in multiparous clients (Knuppel and Drukker, 1986). They are the primary cause of false alarms that bring pregnant clients to the hospital thinking that labor has begun. The nurse should assure the client that these contractions are normal, explain that they may become stronger during and following intercourse, and advise rest and relaxation techniques if they produce discomfort.

Cervical changes

Late in pregnancy, the cervix begins to change in preparation for dilation and onset of labor. Braxton Hicks contractions move the cervix upward as the lower uterine segment is formed. As a result, the fibrous connective tissue of the cervix loosens, causing the cervix to become softer, thinner, shorter, and more pliable—a process known as effacement. Prostaglandins also may contribute to cervical effacement.

As the cervix undergoes its prelabor changes, the mucus plug—which blocks the cervix throughout pregnancy—becomes dislodged. At the same time, some of the cervical capillaries rupture; blood mixes with the mucus, producing what is known as "bloody show." The client will detect a blood-tinged mucus discharge anytime from several days before labor to the onset of labor. Normally, only a few drops of blood mix with the mucus plug. The nurse should advise the client to notify the physician or nurse-midwife if she passes a larger amount of blood.

Rupture of membranes

Approximately 12% of all pregnant clients experience a spontaneous rupture of membranes (SROM) before labor begins. Within 24 hours, labor will spontaneously begin in about 80% of these clients. The time between SROM and labor initiation depends on the length of gestation. For example, a client at 33 weeks of gestation may not begin labor for several days after SROM, but one at term (at least 38 weeks of gestation) most likely will begin within 24 hours of SROM. A client who does not deliver within 24 hours after SROM is considered to have prolonged rupture of membranes, a condition that puts her and the fetus at increased risk for infection.

When the rupture occurs, the amniotic fluid may flow profusely or it may dribble. A client may confuse rupture of membranes with urinary incontinence caused by uterine pressure on the bladder. Testing of vaginal discharge with nitrazine paper allows the examiner to distinguish between the two conditions. Normal vaginal discharge and urine are both acidic, but amniotic fluid is alkaline (pH 7.2), which turns yellow nitrazine paper a deep blue upon contact.

Another simple test performs the same function. When allowed to dry on a microscopic slide, amniotic fluid assumes a characteristic fernlike pattern called ferning. Neither urine nor vaginal secretions assume this same pattern.

Another way to identify amniotic fluid is by directly observing pooled fluid within the vagina. The examiner inserts a sterile speculum and then asks the client to cough or bear down. If the membranes have ruptured, the examiner will observe fluid leaking into the vagina. (See Chapter 25, Fetal Assessment, for more details on assessing amniotic fluid.)

Other signs and symptoms

Clients have reported other signs and symptoms shortly before labor onset. A weight loss of 1 to 3 pounds, representing water loss, may result from changes in electrolyte concentrations of body fluids, which are linked to altered estrogen and progesterone levels. The effect of relaxin on pelvic joints may cause or increase sacroiliac discomfort. (Relaxin is a hormone secreted only during pregnancy that seems to soften the sacroiliac, sacrococcygeal, and pubic joints and increase their mobility.) Increased vaginal secretions, resulting from congestion of vaginal mucous membranes, also may occur.

In the last few days before labor onset, the client may experience a burst of energy known as the "nesting instinct." She may feel compelled to clean house and otherwise ensure that everything is ready for the neonate's arrival. The nurse should caution such a client against overexertion and encourage her to rest and build up energy reserves for labor and childbirth.

Mechanism of labor

For most clients, labor follows a consistent pattern. As uterine contractions intensify, the cervix effaces (thins and shortens) and dilates. Propelled by uterine contractions and the client's voluntary bearing-down efforts, the fetus descends through the birth canal via a series of passive movements known as cardinal movements.

Cervical effacement and dilation

Myometrial activity at the onset of labor leads to full cervical effacement and dilation. Effacement refers to a progressive shortening of the vaginal portion of the cervix and thinning of its walls as it is stretched by the fetus during labor. Effacement is described as a percentage, ranging from 0% (noneffaced and thick) to 100% (fully effaced and paper thin). With the cervix fully effaced, the constrictive uterine neck is obliterated, and the cervix becomes continuous with the lower uterine segment.

Cervical dilation refers to progressive enlargement of the cervical os from less than 1 cm to about 10 cm (full dilation) to allow passage of the fetus from the uterus into the vagina. Because uterine muscle fibers remain shortened even after a contraction ceases, the uterus elongates and the uterine cavity decreases in size. These actions force the fetus downward toward the cervix. Cervical dilation results from this pressure—referred to as fetal axis pressure—plus the upward pulling of longitudinal muscle fibers over the fetus. Typically, effacement and dilation occur more quickly in multiparous clients than in primiparous clients.

Cardinal movements

Cardinal movements refer to the typical sequence of positions assumed by the fetus during labor and childbirth. These positions are most commonly designated as descent, flexion, internal rotation, extension, external rotation (which includes restitution and shoulder rotation), and expulsion. (See *Cardinal movements of labor*, page 588, for illustrations of these positions.)

Descent

Descent refers to the downward movement of the fetus into the pelvic passageway. In a primiparous client, this process may begin several weeks before labor, but further descent usually does not occur until the second stage of labor.

In a multiparous client, descent usually begins with engagement. This downward motion results from one or more forces: contraction of the abdominal muscles, pressure from the amniotic fluid, direct fundal pressure upon the fetus (fetal axis pressure), and the extension and straightening of the fetus. The progression of this downward movement is described as follows:
• Floating. The presenting part (the portion of the fetus that enters the pelvic passageway first) moves freely above the pelvic inlet.
• Fixed. The presenting part has entered the pelvic inlet and no longer moves but is not yet engaged.

• Engaged. The widest part of the presenting part has reached the level of the ischial spines.
• Midpelvis. The presenting part has descended halfway to the pelvic floor.
• On the pelvic floor. The presenting part has descended to the perineum.

Two other considerations involved in fetal descent are synclitism and asynclitism. These are related to the diameter between the fetal parietal bones and the plane of the maternal pelvic inlet. The measurements and the position of the two can ease or disrupt labor. (For more information, see *Synclitism and asynclitism*, page 589.) Fetal descent can be enhanced by alternating changes from posterior to anterior asynclitism.

Flexion

Resistance from the cervix, pelvic walls, or pelvic floor can flex the head of the fetus. When the head flexes downward so that the chin rests against the chest, the smallest diameter of the head will approach the client's pelvis. In this position, the suboccipitobregmatic diameter (normally about 9.5 cm) will enter the birth canal. If neither flexion nor extension occurs, the occipitofrontal diameter (normally about 11.75 cm) will reach the pelvis first. (See "Factors affecting labor" later in this chapter for more on fetal head diameters.)

Internal rotation

In most cases, internal rotation occurs during the second stage of labor—sometimes during one contraction. During internal rotation, the anteroposterior diameter of the head comes in line with the anteroposterior diameter of the pelvic outlet. When the head meets resistance from the pelvic floor, it rotates approximately 45 degrees left of the midline of the anterior abdominal wall under the symphysis pubis. Internal rotation, caused by twisting of the neck, does not involve movement of the shoulders. The shoulders remain oblique (between a parallel and a perpendicular position).

Although most fetuses assume an occiput anterior position following internal rotation, some rotate instead to an occiput posterior or occiput transverse position. These positions occur primarily in clients with abnormal pelvic configurations, such as android or anthropoid pelvises. Approximately 70% of fetuses in either position rotate spontaneously to the anterior position (Danforth, 1982). However, failure of the fetus to assume an anterior position can lead to prolonged labor caused by the inability of the fetal occiput to fill the pelvic cavity adequately or to exert equal pressure around the cervical os. (See Chapter 33, Intrapartal Complications, for more information on prolonged labor.)

Cardinal movements of labor

For a fetus in the vertex (crown or top of head) presentation, labor follows a typical sequence. Inset boxes show a schematic of the relationship of the fetal skull to the maternal pelvis.

1 Engagement, descent, flexion. The widest diameter of the head passes the level of the pelvic inlet; as the fetus moves downward toward the ischial spines, the head flexes on the chest.

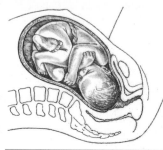

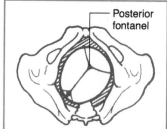

Posterior fontanel

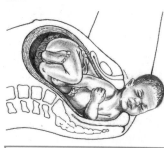

2 Internal rotation. The anteroposterior diameter of the head comes into line with the anteroposterior diameter of the pelvic outlet.

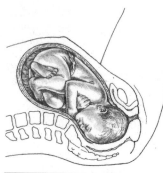

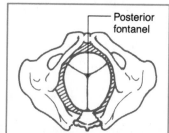

Posterior fontanel

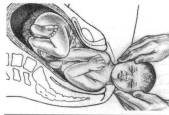

3 Extension. The head extends from the perineum after passing under the symphysis pubis.

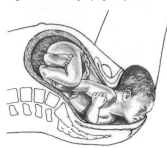

Anterior fontanel

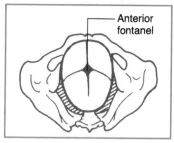

4 External rotation (restitution). The head rotates 45 degrees back to its original position.

Posterior fontanel

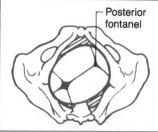

5 External rotation (shoulder rotation). The head rotates an additional 45 degrees to a transverse position; the anterior shoulder passes the perineum.

Posterior fontanel

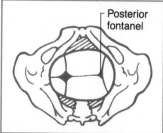

6 Expulsion. The rest of the body is easily delivered by lateral flexion.

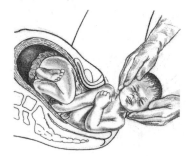

Extension

The head of the fetus remains in a flexed position until it passes under the symphysis pubis and reaches the perineum. The head then extends in response to pressure from uterine contractions, resistance from the pelvic floor, and intra-abdominal pressure from the client's bearing-down efforts.

Extension places the back of the fetus's neck in direct contact with the inferior margin of the symphysis pubis. As the head extends, it passes over the anterior margin of the perineum; then the head drops down, and the chin lies over the client's perineum.

External rotation

Once the head passes the perineum, it rotates 45 degrees, returning to the position it originally assumed during engagement. This is called restitution. Next, the fetus rotates an additional 45 degrees to assume a transverse position as the delivery proceeds. This movement positions the shoulders in line with the anteroposterior diameter of the client's pelvis. The anterior shoulder usually appears first, under the symphysis pubis; the posterior shoulder follows.

Expulsion

Once the shoulders pass the perineum, the remainder of the body is easily pulled upward and away from the perineum, following the natural curve of the pelvic passageway.

Stages of labor

Labor consists of four distinct stages. Understanding what occurs during each stage will help the nurse anticipate and meet the client's needs in labor. What follows is a brief discussion of each stage; for a more detailed description of each stage, see Chapter 27, The First Stage

Synclitism and asynclitism

Synclitism occurs in a normal labor when the biparietal diameter of the fetus becomes parallel to the plane of the pelvic inlet and the sagittal suture lies halfway between the symphysis pubis and the sacrum. Posterior asynclitism occurs when the head is flexed laterally toward the symphysis pubis; with this condition, the client's abdomen protrudes less than usual for her gestational period. Flexion toward the sacrum causes anterior asynclitism, in which the client's abdomen protrudes more than usual for her gestational period. Some degree of asynclitism is normal in labor. However, labor can be disrupted when asynclitism becomes fixed because of cephalopelvic disproportion.

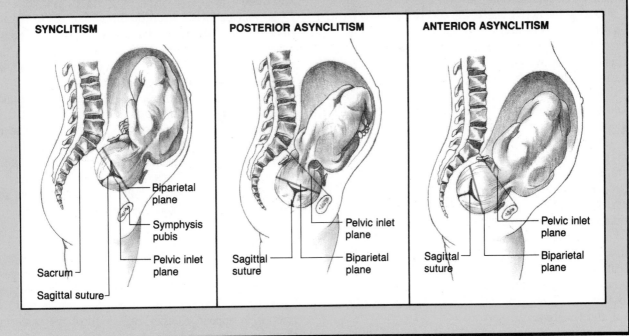

of Labor; Chapter 28, The Second Stage of Labor; and Chapter 29, The Third and Fourth Stages of Labor.

First stage of labor

The first stage is divided into latent, active, and transitional phases. Cervical dilation and fetal descent begin slowly during the latent phase, then accelerate during the active and transitional phases.

Latent phase

First described by Friedman (1954), the latent phase precedes active labor. In primiparous clients, this phase averages 8.6 hours; in multiparous clients, 5.3 hours. During this time, irregular, short, and mild contractions occur, and the cervix dilates to 3 or 4 cm.

The client may remain at home during the early part of the latent phase. When she enters the hospital, she may complain of abdominal cramping and lower back discomfort. Client behavior typically displays various degrees of excitement and apprehension. If she has not yet passed the mucus plug, she commonly will do so during the latent phase.

Active phase

Transition from the latent to the active phase occurs when the cervix dilates faster than 1.2 cm/hour in primiparous clients and 1.5 cm/hour in multiparous clients. In about 90% of clients, labor has progressed to the active phase by the time cervical dilation reaches 5 cm (Peisner and Rosen, 1986).

During the active phase, the cervix dilates to 7 cm. Contractions occur every 2 to 5 minutes, last 40 to 50 seconds, and are moderately intense. In primiparous clients, the active phase averages 5.8 hours; in multiparous clients, 2.5 hours.

Fetal descent continues throughout the active phase and into the transitional phase. The rate of descent is at least 1 cm/hour in primiparous clients and 2 cm/hour in multiparous clients.

Transitional phase

Occurring when the cervix is dilated between 8 and 10 cm, the transitional phase is the shortest, averaging less than 3 hours for primiparous clients and less than 1 hour for multiparous clients (Friedman, 1978). However, this phase is the most difficult for the client. Intense contractions lasting between 45 and 60 seconds occur every 1½ to 2 minutes. The client may thrash about, lose control of breathing techniques, and experience nausea and vomiting.

In total, the first stage of labor—including the latent, active, and transitional phases—lasts 3.3 to 19.7 hours for primiparous clients and 0.1 to 14.3 hours for multiparous clients. Using the Friedman graph, the nurse can follow the rate of cervical dilation and fetal descent. Then, by plotting dilation and station, the nurse can identify normal and abnormal labor patterns.

Second stage of labor

The second stage begins with complete cervical dilation and ends with birth. Intense contractions occur every 2 to 3 minutes and last 60 to 90 seconds. For primiparous clients, this stage averages 1 hour; for multiparous clients, 15 minutes. In either case, a second stage longer than 2 hours is considered abnormal.

The beginning of this stage is characterized by an increase in bloody show, rupture of membranes (if this has not already occurred), severe rectal pressure, and a reflex bearing-down with each contraction. As the fetus approaches the perineal floor, the perineum bulges and flattens. As the labia spread, the head appears at the vaginal opening. At this time, the client should assume an active role and push with each contraction. Roberts, Goldstein, Gruener, Maggio, and Mendez-Bauer (1987) report that labor progress and outcome can be enhanced if the nurse discourages the client from sustained breath-holding and encourages pushing, which reinforces the involuntary bearing-down reflex.

The head

To prevent maternal lacerations and damage to the fetus's intracranial area, the nurse or other birth attendant must control the speed at which the head passes the perineum. When necessary, applying pressure over the perineum can maintain flexion of the head.

Once the head emerges, the physician or nurse-midwife must check for the umbilical cord. If the cord is loose around the neck, it should be slipped over the head. If the cord is very tight, fetal hypoxia may occur; therefore, the attendant must clamp and cut the cord while it is still around the neck. The oral and nasal pharynx then are suctioned with a bulb syringe to remove secretions that may be blocking the airway.

The shoulders

Following external rotation of the head, the shoulders pass through the pelvic inlet. After the head emerges, the attendant applies slight downward traction to free the anterior shoulder. After it emerges, gentle upward traction is applied on the head to allow the posterior shoulder to emerge.

The body and extremities

Once the shoulders emerge, the rest of the body, which is narrower than the shoulders, slides out with little or no traction needed.

Third stage of labor

The third stage begins immediately after birth and ends with the separation and expulsion of the placenta. Strong but usually less painful contractions continue during this stage; their frequency may decrease to every 5 minutes. Normally, the placenta emerges about 5 minutes after the neonate's delivery.

Placental separation

Placental separation usually begins within minutes of birth. As labor nears completion and birth becomes imminent, the uterus begins to contract forcefully. By the time the neonate is delivered, the uterus consists of an almost solid mass of muscle with walls several centimeters thick above the lower segment. This mass differs greatly from the large cavity that previously housed the fetus. The fundal portion lies immediately below the umbilicus.

This decrease in uterine capacity causes the central portion of the placenta to pull away from the uterine wall. Bleeding from blood vessels in the area helps form a retroplacental hematoma. As this hematoma grows, the placenta further separates from the uterine wall. A placenta will not easily separate from a relaxed or boggy uterus because the decreased uterine muscles must first diminish the placental implantation site.

Signs indicating placental separation include lengthening of the umbilical cord, a sudden gush of dark blood from the vagina, and a change in uterine shape from disc-like to globular (which the nurse can palpate or see as a visible bulge above the symphysis). The client may have a sensation of vaginal fullness.

Placental delivery

The placenta is expelled through one of two mechanisms. In the Schultze mechanism, the central portion of the placenta separates from the uterine wall before the outside edges do. Then the central portion folds or buckles outward, away from the retroplacental hematoma. When the placenta is expelled, the shiny fetal side (commonly called "shiny Schultze") is visible.

In the Duncan mechanism, the placental edges separate first, followed by the central portion. Then the central portion rolls up and is expelled sideways, so that the rough-surfaced maternal side (commonly called "dirty Duncan") is visible. In the Duncan mechanism, separation may be incomplete, leaving placental fragments that may lead to infection or bleeding. Immediately after delivery, the placenta must be evaluated carefully for completeness, and the client must be assessed for excessive bleeding or a relaxed uterus.

Fourth stage of labor

Beginning with delivery of the placenta and extending through the first 4 hours after childbirth, the fourth stage allows the client's body to adjust to the postpartal stage. She should be assessed carefully for uterine atony, postpartal hemorrhage, and urine retention.

Ideally, the client and her partner should now hold and examine the infant and begin parent-infant bonding.

Factors affecting labor

Successful labor and childbirth requires coordination of five essential factors, sometimes termed the "five p's":
• passenger (the fetus)
• passageway (the pelvis)
• powers (uterine contractions and bearing-down efforts)
• placental position and function
• psychological response.
For the fetus to move successfully through the pelvis, the contractions and bearing-down efforts must be of adequate intensity and frequency, the placenta must be properly positioned and provide adequate oxygen to the fetus, and the client must be psychologically prepared. Problems involving any of these essential factors may jeopardize safe labor and childbirth and require medical or surgical intervention.

Fetus

Fetal factors affecting labor and childbirth include size and shape of the head, lie, attitude, presentation, position, and station. (See *The fetal skull and its adaptation to birth* on pages 592 and 593 for more information.)

Head

The skull is composed of several small, thin, incompletely developed bones, including two frontal bones, two parietal bones, two temporal bones, and one occipital bone

(Text continues on page 594.)

The fetal skull and its adaptation to birth

At term, the skull is composed of several thin, incompletely developed bones connected by membranous joints called sutures, which intersect at areas called fontanels. Responding to pressure exerted by the maternal pelvis and the birth canal during labor and delivery, sutures allow the cranial bones to shift, molding the head and easing the passage of the fetus. The type of molding that occurs is determined by fetal attitude—the overall degree of body flexion or extension.

Skull characteristics

In the normal fetus, the skull includes the landmarks and diameters (in color) shown in the illustrations below. The diameter measurements are averages for term neonates; individual measurements vary with fetal size, attitude, and presentation.

Biparietal diameter: measured between the parietal eminences; the widest transverse diameter of the head, 9.5 cm.
Bitemporal diameter: measured between the lateral sides of the temporal bones; the shortest transverse diameter of the head, 8 cm.
Occipitofrontal diameter: measured from the external occipital protuberance to the glabella; 11.5 cm.
Occipitomental diameter: measured from the external occipital protuberance to the chin; 12.5 cm.
Suboccipitobregmatic diameter: measured from the

underside of the occipital bone to the middle of the bregma; the anteroposterior diameter that presents when the head is well flexed, 9.5 cm.
Submentobregmatic diameter: measured from the junction of the neck and lower jaw to the middle of the bregma; the diameter that presents in face presentations when the head is fully extended, 9.5 cm.
Verticomental diameter: measured from the chin to the middle of the sagittal suture; seen in brow presentations, 13.5 cm. A normal-sized head cannot pass through a normal-sized pelvis in this position.

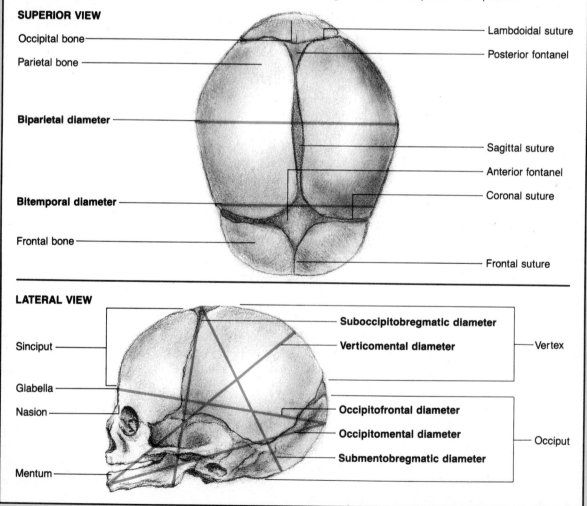

SUPERIOR VIEW

Occipital bone
Parietal bone
Biparietal diameter
Bitemporal diameter
Frontal bone

Lambdoidal suture
Posterior fontanel
Sagittal suture
Anterior fontanel
Coronal suture
Frontal suture

LATERAL VIEW

Sinciput
Glabella
Nasion
Mentum

Suboccipitobregmatic diameter
Verticomental diameter — Vertex
Occipitofrontal diameter
Occipitomental diameter
Submentobregmatic diameter — Occiput

Fetal attitude

Fetal attitude—the relationship of fetal body parts to one another—is important to successful labor and delivery. Classified according to the degree of overall body flexion or extension, fetal attitude ranges from full flexion to complete extension and determines the type of molding that occurs.

FLEXION

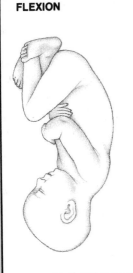

MILITARY ATTITUDE

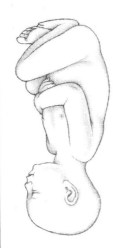

PARTIAL EXTENSION

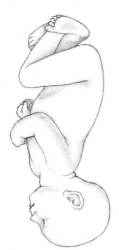

COMPLETE EXTENSION

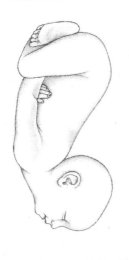

Molding

In a cephalic presentation, the skull molds to adapt to an unyielding maternal pelvis. The degree of flexion or extension of the head dictates which head diameter enters the pelvis first. The illustrations below depict some examples of molding based on various head positions.

OCCIPITAL ANTERIOR PRESENTATION

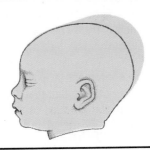

OCCIPITAL POSTERIOR PRESENTATION

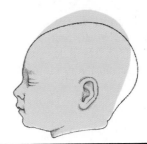

FACE PRESENTATION

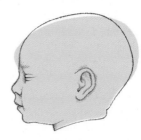

BROW PRESENTATION

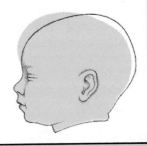

in the back, which eventually fuse to form the rigid cranial cavity characteristic of the adult. The largest part of the fetus, the skull also is the least compressible part. However, the skull bones are connected by flexible, membrane-occupied spaces called sutures, which allow alterations in skull shape (called molding). During labor, the skull bones are pressed together and may overlap, reducing the size of the head and facilitating passage through the unyielding pelvis.

Besides allowing for molding, the sutures separating these bones aid in identifying fetal position during labor. The sagittal suture, which runs in an anteroposterior direction, separates the two parietal bones. The frontal suture, an extension of the saggital suture, separates the two frontal bones. The coronal suture separates the parietal bones from the frontal bones. The lambdoidal suture separates the parietal bones from the occipital bone.

Sutures intersect at membranous spaces called fontanels. The anterior fontanel (also called the bregma) is located at the junction of the sagittal, coronal, and frontal sutures. Diamond-shaped, the anterior fontanel measures 3 to 4 cm long and 2 to 3 cm wide. By remaining open until the infant is about 18 months old, this fontanel gives the brain space to grow. The posterior fontanel is located at the junction of the sagittal and lambdoidal sutures. This triangular-shaped fontanel, approximately 2 cm wide, normally closes within 6 to 8 weeks after birth.

During labor, the head goes through movements designed to ensure that its smallest diameter enters the pelvis first. The head can flex or extend about 45 degrees and can rotate about 180 degrees. This ability to flex, extend, and rotate allows its smallest diameters to move down the birth canal and pass through the maternal bony pelvis.

Lie

Fetal lie refers to the position of the fetal spine in relation to the maternal spine . When the two spines are parallel, the fetus is in a longitudinal lie. When the spines are perpendicular, the fetus is in a transverse lie. When the fetal spine is at an angle between the parallel and perpendicular position, the fetus is in an oblique lie. Typically, a fetus in an oblique lie will convert either to a longitudinal or a transverse lie before birth.

Unless the fetus is positioned in a longitudinal lie, a vaginal birth is impossible, and surgical intervention becomes necessary.

Attitude

Fetal attitude refers to overall body flexion or extension, which determines the relationship of fetal parts to one another. The usual fetal attitude in the uterus is vertex,

with the head flexed so that the chin rests against the chest, the legs and arms folded in front of the body, and the back curved slightly forward.

The fetus normally exhibits varying degrees of flexion and extension throughout pregnancy, with no ill effects; however, fetal attitude becomes significant during labor and childbirth. With the fetus in a cephalic (head-first) presentation, a fully flexed attitude enables the smallest head diameter to enter the pelvis. As the degree of extension increases, the diameter of the head entering the pelvis also increases, making labor and chilbirth more difficult.

Position

Fetal position refers to the relationship of the presenting part to the front, back, or side of the maternal pelvis. The nurse establishes fetal position by determining three factors: a landmark on the fetal presenting part, whether this landmark faces the right or left side of the maternal pelvis, and whether the landmark faces the front, back, or side of the maternal pelvis. (See *Determining fetal position* for more information.)

Presentation

Fetal presentation refers to the manner in which the fetus enters the pelvic passageway. Presentation is classified according to the presenting part—the portion of the fetus that enters the pelvic passageway first—as:
• cephalic (head-first)
• breech (buttocks-first)
• shoulder
• compound.
(See *Classifying fetal presentation*, pages 596 and 597, for illustrations and descriptions of these presentations.)

Approximately 95% of all births occur with the fetus assuming a cephalic presentation. A shoulder presentation occurs when the fetal spine is perpendicular to the maternal spine. Unless the fetus in this presentation moves to a longitudinal lie, cesarean delivery is necessary. Predisposing factors in a shoulder presentation include placenta previa, neoplasms, fetal anomalies, hydramnios (excess of amniotic fluid), preterm labor, uterine atony, multiple gestation, and premature artificial rupture of membranes.

Before the twenty-eighth week of gestation, approximately 25% of fetuses are in a breech presentation. By the thirty-fourth week of gestation, however, most fetuses move to a cephalic presentation. Nevertheless, 3% to 4% of all term pregnancies involve breech presentation (Oxorn, 1986).

In most cases, the cause of breech presentation cannot be pinpointed; however, numerous maternal, placen-

Determining fetal position

Fetal position is determined by the relationship of a specific presenting part to the front, back, or side of the maternal pelvis. A notation system identifies three features: a landmark on the presenting part (O for occiput, M for mentum, S for sacrum, A for acromion process, and D for dorsal); whether this landmark faces the right (R) or left (L) side of the pelvis; and whether the landmark faces the front (A for anterior), the back (P for posterior), or a side (T for trans-

verse) of the pelvis. Thus, for a fetus with the occiput (O) as the presenting landmark, positioned facing the right side (R) and front (A) of the maternal pelvis, the nurse would identify the position as ROA.

In a vertex presentation (by far the most common), the fetus may assume one of the six positions illustrated below: LOP, LOT, LOA, ROP, ROT, or ROA.

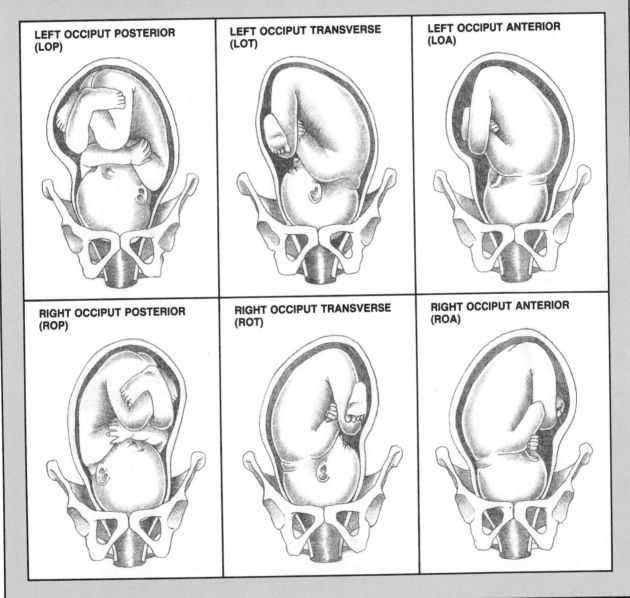

LEFT OCCIPUT POSTERIOR (LOP)

LEFT OCCIPUT TRANSVERSE (LOT)

LEFT OCCIPUT ANTERIOR (LOA)

RIGHT OCCIPUT POSTERIOR (ROP)

RIGHT OCCIPUT TRANSVERSE (ROT)

RIGHT OCCIPUT ANTERIOR (ROA)

tal, and fetal predisposing factors have been identified. Maternal factors associated with breech presentation include uterine anomalies, uterine relaxation resulting from previous childbirth, myometrial neoplasm, contracted pelvis, oligohydramnios (in which the fetus is restricted to the position it assumed during the second trimester), and hydramnios (in which the fetal position changes easily because of excessive amniotic fluid). Placental factors include the implantation of the placenta

Classifying fetal presentation

Fetal presentation may be broadly classified as breech, cephalic, shoulder, or compound. Cephalic presentations comprise almost all deliveries. Of the remaining three, breech deliveries are most common.

Breech

In the head-up presentation, the position of the fetus may be further classified as frank, where hips are flexed and knees remain straight; complete, where knees and hips are flexed; footling, where the knees and hips of one or both legs are extended; kneeling, where knees are flexed and hips remain extended; and incomplete, where one or both hips remain extended and one or both feet or knees lie below the breech.

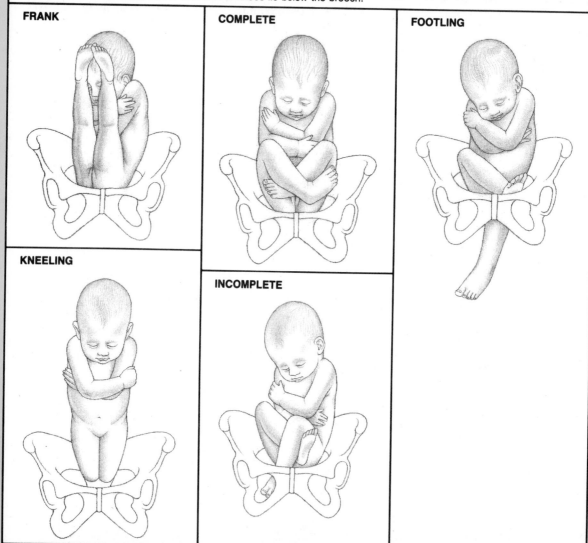

FRANK   COMPLETE   FOOTLING

KNEELING   INCOMPLETE

in either cornual-fundal region (the horns on either side of the fundus). Also reported to cause a higher incidence of breech presentations is placenta previa, a condition in which the placenta partially or totally covers the cervical os and blocks the fetus from leaving the uterus (Oxorn, 1986). Fetal factors include prematurity, multiple gestation, anencephaly, hydrocephaly (dilation of the cerebral ventricles after obstruction of the flow of cerebrospinal fluid), intrauterine fetal death, and other fetal anomalies.

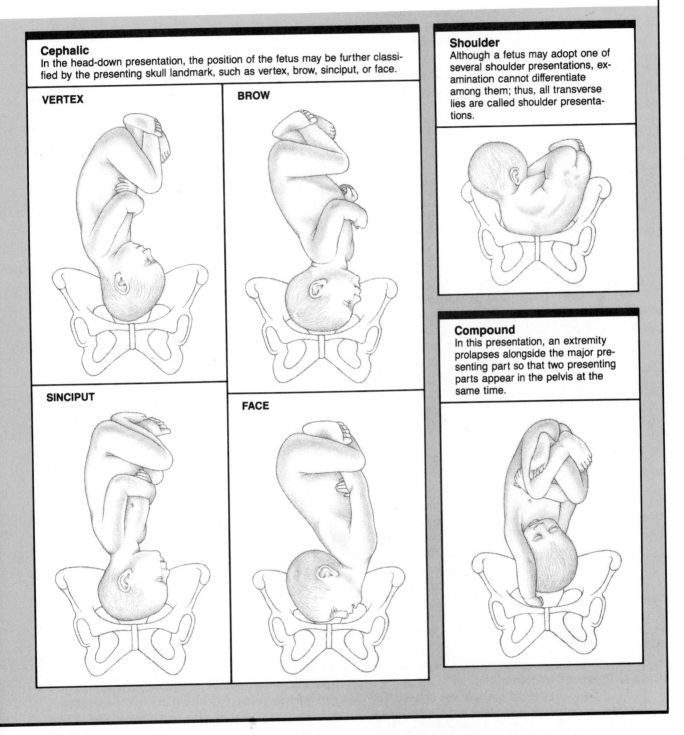

Cephalic
In the head-down presentation, the position of the fetus may be further classified by the presenting skull landmark, such as vertex, brow, sinciput, or face.

VERTEX

BROW

SINCIPUT

FACE

Shoulder
Although a fetus may adopt one of several shoulder presentations, examination cannot differentiate among them; thus, all transverse lies are called shoulder presentations.

Compound
In this presentation, an extremity prolapses alongside the major presenting part so that two presenting parts appear in the pelvis at the same time.

Station

Fetal station refers to the relationship of the presenting part to the maternal ischial spines. The ischial spines, located at midpelvis, form the narrowest portion of the pelvis through which the fetus must pass. When the largest diameter of the presenting part (usually the biparietal diameter of the head) is level with the ischial spines, the fetus is at station 0. Numbers from 1 to 3 indicate how many centimeters the presenting part is above or below the ischial spines. Thus, a presenting part above the ischial spines is designated as −1, −2, or −3; a presenting part below this point, +1, +2, or +3. When the presenting part is classified as being at greater than +3 station, it is at the pelvic outlet and visible on the perineum.

Successful vaginal birth requires progressive fetal descent from a minus station to 0 and then to a plus station during labor. Lack of this progressive descent with effective uterine contractions may indicate cephalopelvic disproportion or an inappropriately short or tangled umbilical cord. In such cases, cesarean delivery may be necessary.

Pelvis

The passageway through which the fetus must travel during labor consists of the pelvis and soft tissues. Pelvic types and diameters affect labor and childbirth.

The pelvis is partly ligamentous and partly bony. (See Chapter 6, Reproductive Anatomy and Physiology, for detailed information on pelvic anatomy.) Although Caldwell and Moloy (1933) first categorized four basic pelvic types—gynecoid, android, anthropoid, and platypelloid—a client usually has features of two or more types.

The true pelvis contains three levels, or planes: the pelvic inlet, the midpelvis, and the pelvic outlet. Diameters measured in these three planes indicate the amount of space available for the fetus during birth. (See *Pelvic planes and diameters*, pages 600 and 601, for more information and illustrations.)

The pelvic inlet has four diameters: the anteroposterior diameter, the bi-ischial (or transverse) diameter, and two oblique diameters. The pelvic inlet's anteroposterior diameter is further divided into the obstetric conjugate, the true conjugate, and the diagonal conjugate diameters. The diagonal conjugate can be measured during a pelvic examination; the other two diameters are estimated from this measurement.

The pelvic diameters can be affected by the client's position during labor, by relaxin (a hormone produced by the placenta) in the system, and by the amount of fat or soft tissue surrounding the pelvis. Assuming a squatting or lateral Sims' position may help increase the pelvic diameters. Relaxin helps to relax the pelvis and increase the pelvic diameters.

Pelvic tilt also may affect the progress of labor. The angle formed by the pelvic inlet plane and the horizontal plane is termed the pelvic plane inclination. When a client is standing, the angle between the inlet and horizontal planes is approximately 60 degrees. Decreasing the lumbar curve decreases this angle; increasing the lumbar curve increases the angle.

Contractions and bearing-down efforts

The third of the five essential factors in successful labor and childbirth, involuntary uterine contractions and voluntary bearing-down efforts must be adequate in intensity and frequency.

Uterine contractions

Rhythmic tightening of the upper uterine segment musculature, uterine contractions serve several purposes during labor and childbirth. Coordinated and effective uterine contractions promote fetal descent and rotation, cervical effacement and dilation, separation and expulsion of the placenta, and constriction of the uterine vasculature to prevent postpartal hemorrhage.

A uterine contraction begins in response to a change in electrical activity. This change, referred to as a wave of excitation, originates in pacemakers located near the uterotubal junctions. The downward movement of the electrical charge from the upper segment of the uterus to the cervix is known as fundal dominance. Contraction intensity and duration are both greater in the upper uterine segment than in the lower uterine segment.

These three characteristics—fundal dominance, intensity, and duration—help create a coordinated uterine contraction that produces maximum expulsive force. The muscular structure of the uterus (the myometrium) is unique because the fibers remain shortened even after the contraction is over instead of reverting to their precontraction size—that is, the fibers shorten progressively during labor. This is known as retraction or brachystasis. As labor continues, this progressive shortening of fibers results in a thickening of the upper uterine segment and a decrease in uterine size, which impels fetal descent.

For uterine contractions to propel the fetus through the birth canal effectively, several biochemical interactions must occur. First, adequate amounts of adenosine triphosphate and the contractile proteins actin and myosin must be present to provide energy. Second, proper levels of electrolytes—specifically calcium, sodium, and potassium—must be present for uterine muscles to contract. Third, proper amounts of oxytocin, prostaglandins, and acetylcholine must be present to ensure conduction of the uterine contraction wave as it moves downward from the fundus. Finally, the proper number and size of gap junctions (narrow channels in the intracellular spaces linking adjacent cells and transmitting electrical impulses) must be present in the myometrium to promote synchronous uterine smooth muscle contractions (Cunningham, MacDonald, and Gant, 1989).

Throughout pregnancy, the myometrium contains few or no gap junctions; they appear at the onset of labor,

Phases of a uterine contraction

As shown in the diagram below, a uterine contraction occurs in three phases: increment (building up), acme (peak), and decrement (letting down). Between contractions is a period of relaxation. The two most important features of

contractions are frequency and duration. Frequency refers to the elapsed time from the start of one contraction to the start of the next contraction. Duration is the elapsed time from the start to the end of one contraction.

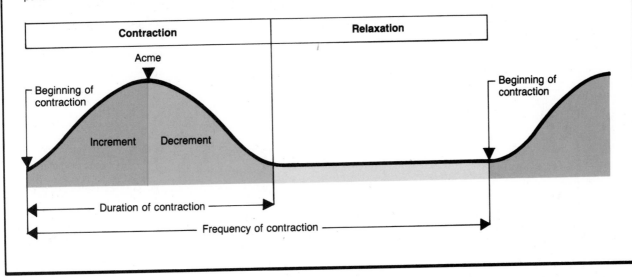

increase in number and size as labor progresses, and then begin to disappear within 24 hours after childbirth. Gap junction formation is promoted by estrogen, protein synthesis, and prostaglandins and is inhibited by progesterone. Because gap junctions are present in labor, whether spontaneous or induced, uterine contractions may not be reversible once they begin, even in premature labor.

A uterine contraction occurs in three phases: increment, acme, and decrement. (See *Phases of a uterine contraction*.) During the increment and acme phases, waves of excitation, initiated in the pacemakers, induce contractions. As the waves subside, contractions decrease in intensity and duration and conclude in the decrement phase.

During labor, the nurse evaluates the duration, frequency, and intensity of contractions. (See Chapter 27, The First Stage of Labor, for details on evaluating uterine contractions.) The duration of a contraction refers to the time between the beginning and end of the contraction. Duration usually ranges from 15 to 30 seconds in early labor to 45 to 90 seconds in later stages. The frequency of contractions is measured from the beginning of one contraction to the beginning of the next. In early labor, frequency ranges from 20 to 30 minutes; in the later stages, it ranges from 2 to 3 minutes.

The duration and frequency of contractions affect both the client and the fetus. Duration greater than 90

seconds and frequency less than 2 minutes increase the risk of uterine rupture and also put the fetus at high risk for hypoxia from uterine vasoconstriction. Excessively long and overly frequent contractions also sap the client's energy and strength during labor, hindering her voluntary bearing-down efforts.

The intensity of a contraction refers to its strength during the acme phase. Intensity can be measured directly with an intrauterine catheter and indirectly by palpation or external monitoring. The normal resting pressure of the uterus between contractions measured via intrauterine catheter is 10 mm Hg; this pressure can increase to 50 mm Hg during acme. When the pressure reaches 15 to 20 mm Hg, blood supply to the uterus and placenta is compromised, and the client begins to feel pain.

Bearing-down efforts

Once uterine contractions have fully effaced and dilated the cervix, the second stage of labor begins and the client's voluntary bearing-down efforts take over. In these efforts, she contracts the diaphragm and abdominal muscles to increase intra-abdominal pressure. This action, which applies pressure to the uterine walls, adds to the pressures from uterine contractions and aids fetal descent and expulsion. The client also experiences a great

(Text continues on page 602.)

Pelvic planes and diameters

During labor, the fetus descends into the birth canal through the complex bony structure of the pelvis. The true pelvis contains three planes: the plane of inlet, the mid-plane, and the plane of outlet. Fetal size and position in relation to several specific dimensions in these planes determines whether the fetus can pass safely through the birth canal. The illustrations below show the three pelvic planes and the important dimensions used to describe them; individual client measurements will vary. The inset illustrations show the level of each plane in the pelvis.

Plane of inlet

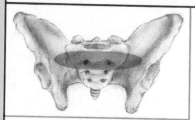

Important dimensions in the plane of inlet include:

Oblique: distance from the right or left sacroiliac joint to the opposing iliopectineal prominence, typically 12.8 cm or longer.

Transverse: greatest distance across the pelvic brim, forming at a right angle to the obstetric conjugate and typically measuring 13.5 cm or longer. This diameter alone does not accurately reflect the space available to the fetus; the presence of the colon in the left pelvis and the sacral promontory also must be considered.

Anteroposterior: distance from the symphysis pubis to the sacral promontory. This dimension may be measured as one of the following.

• True conjugate, from the upper limit of the symphysis to the sacral promontory. Typically 11 cm or longer, this dimension most often is determined by X-ray.

• Obstetric conjugate, from the posterior surface of the symphysis pubis to the sacral promontory. Typically 1.5 cm shorter than the diagonal conjugate, this dimension most often is determined by X-ray or ultrasonography.

• Diagonal conjugate, from the lower limit of the symphysis to the sacral promontory. Typically 12.5 to 13 cm, this dimension is the only superior strait measurement that can be obtained clinically.

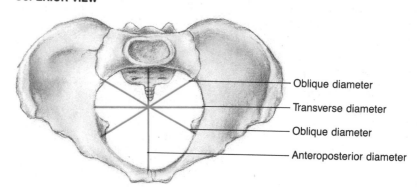

SUPERIOR VIEW

— Oblique diameter
— Transverse diameter
— Oblique diameter
— Anteroposterior diameter

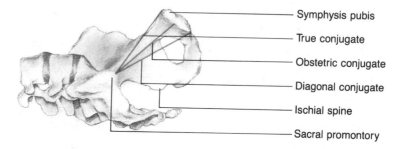

CUTAWAY LATERAL VIEW

— Symphysis pubis
— True conjugate
— Obstetric conjugate
— Diagonal conjugate
— Ischial spine
— Sacral promontory

Midplane

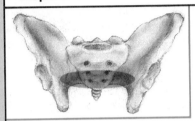

Important dimensions in the mid-plane include:

Anteroposterior: distance from mid-symphysis to the sacrum at the fused second and third vertebrae, typically 12.8 cm or more.
Posterior sagittal: segment of the anteroposterior diameter behind an imaginary line that extends between the ischial spines, typically 4.5 cm long.
Transverse: distance from the top of one acetabulum to the other, typically 12.5 cm or longer.
Ischial interspinous: distance between the ischial spines, typically 10.5 cm. This is the shortest diameter in the pelvis and an important obstetric measurement. The ischial spines can be palpated during vaginal examination to evaluate the descent of the fetus during labor.

CUTAWAY LATERAL VIEW

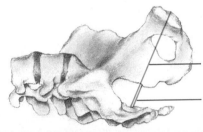

Anteroposterior diameter

Posterior sagittal diameter

ANTERIOR PELVIC TILT VIEW

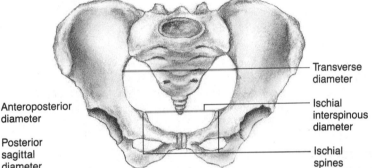

Transverse diameter

Ischial interspinous diameter

Ischial spines

Plane of outlet

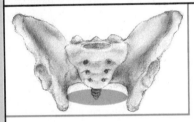

Important dimensions in the plane of outlet include:
Anteroposterior: distance from the lower border of the symphysis to the tip of the sacrum, typically 11.9 cm or longer. The coccyx can be displaced during labor and therefore is an unsuitable reference point.
Transverse: distance from the inner edge of one ischial tuberosity to the other, typically 11 cm or longer. Because this diameter becomes progressively smaller as the pubic arch narrows, it has great significance during labor. The fetus may not be able to pass beneath an arch that is too narrow.

Posterior sagittal: distance from the sacral tip to a line extending between the ischial tuberosities.
Subpubic angle: angle formed by the apex of the walls of the pubic arch that establishes the width of the passage beneath the pubic arch; a small angle results in a narrow passage, and a greater angle results in a wider passage. A narrow arch forces the head of the fetus backward toward the coccyx, making head extension difficult. This increases the risk of outlet dystocia (labor difficulty at the pelvic outlet), which may necessitate forceps delivery and increases the risk of injury to the client and fetus.

LITHOTOMY VIEW

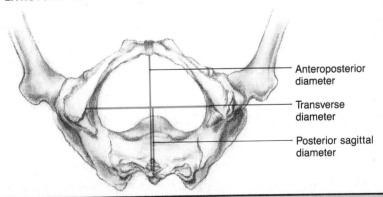

Anteroposterior diameter

Transverse diameter

Posterior sagittal diameter

involuntary urge to push as the head of the fetus descends and pushes against the sacral and obturator nerves. (See Chapter 28, The Second Stage of Labor, for details on pushing.)

Positions for labor

The optimal position for labor has been debated since the 1600s. Although Mauriceau (1637-1709) is credited with introducing the recumbent (lying-down) position for childbirth, he intended its use only to facilitate the use of forceps in delivery. In fact, Mauriceau's writings show that he encouraged pregnant women to walk about their chambers during labor so that pressure from the weight of the fetus would hasten cervical dilation and shorten labor.

Throughout most of the world today, labor and childbirth most often occur with the woman in an upright position. In contrast, the recumbent position remains a Western tradition (Rossi and Lindell, 1986).

The number and type of positions assumed independently by women during labor were studied by Carlson, et al. (1986). Suggesting their desire for change and mobility, the women in the study group assumed an average of 7.5 positions during labor. When allowed to change their position whenever they desired, they did so most frequently in the latent stage—an average of three times, with the left lateral position most commonly assumed. During the active stage, multiparous clients walked around in many instances.

Position during labor can affect the frequency and intensity of contractions. For a client in the supine position, contractions may be less intense but more frequent. For one in the lateral position, contractions tend to be more intense but less frequent.

Studies that evaluate the effect of an upright position and walking around during the first stage of labor have yielded inconclusive results (Rossi and Lindell, 1986). However, many women find walking during labor a positive experience. Lupe and Gross (1986) concluded that neither the assumption of various positions nor walking seems to harm the pregnant woman or the fetus or inhibit the progress of labor. Although not conclusive, data suggest that walking, standing, or sitting may shorten labor.

Placental position and function

Throughout pregnancy and during labor, the fetus depends on the placenta for oxygenated blood and nutrients. Placental malposition or malfunction can hinder labor and childbirth and may compromise the well-being of the fetus. In most cases, the placenta is attached to the upper uterine segment. However, 1 in every 200 to 300 pregnancies involves placenta previa—implantation of the placenta in the lower uterine segment, where it partially or totally covers the cervical os. Besides blocking the os, placenta previa causes the placenta to separate from the uterine wall partially or totally as the cervix dilates, typically causing hemorrhage.

Other conditions can cause placental malfunction. For example, in abruptio placentae, occurring in about 1 in 250 pregnancies, the placenta prematurely separates from the uterine wall. Another condition, uteroplacental insufficiency, impairs the ability of the fetus to withstand the rigors of labor. (For more information on placenta previa and abruptio placentae, see Chapter 33, Intrapartal Complications; for more information on uteroplacental insufficiency, see Chapter 31, High-Risk Intrapartal Clients.)

Psychological response

The role that a pregnant woman's mental and emotional state plays in labor and childbirth has received increasing attention over the last several decades. In 1961, Rosengren identified a relationship between a woman's perception of her health state during pregnancy and her behavior during labor. He found that those who adopted a "sick role" during pregnancy had a higher incidence of prolonged, difficult labor. More recent studies point to a relationship between anxiety and the length and difficulty of labor. In particular, researchers have found that high epinephrine levels triggered by maternal anxiety can lead to diminished uterine activity and longer labors (Lederman, 1977). Other researchers have found that women who experienced severe pain or distress-related thoughts may be more likely to experience an inefficient labor (Wuitchik, Bakal, and Lipshitz, 1989).

These and other studies indicate the importance of an appropriate psychological response to the physiologic and emotional demands of labor. Factors that may influence a client's psychological response include preparation for labor, support systems, and coping mechanisms.

Preparation for labor

Preparing for labor usually means seeking and absorbing information on childbirth. Many couples attend childbirth classes to learn about physiologic changes that occur during labor and delivery and techniques to help the client during this process. (See Chapter 21, Family Preparation for Childbirth and Parenting, for more information on childbirth education.)

Support systems

A client needs other individuals, such as her partner, to whom she can turn for emotional and physical support during labor and childbirth. Experts know that a client tends to be less fearful, more comfortable, and more likely to view her childbirth experience positively when a support person is present during labor (Cranley, Hedahl, and Pegg, 1983; Mercer, Hackley, and Bostrum, 1983). Clients whose partners coach them through labor and childbirth may report less pain, require less medication, and experience shorter labor than those whose partners are not present (Berry, 1988).

Coping mechanisms

The pregnant client brings to labor various coping mechanisms she has used previously. Examples include confrontation, control, avoidance, and optimism. The nurse must recognize these mechanisms and evaluate how they will help or hinder the client. Even when a client's coping skills differ dramatically from the nurse's, the nurse must not make judgments or attempt to alter the coping mechanisms as long as they are successful for the client and do not interfere with her safety or that of the fetus.

Maternal systemic response to labor

Labor produces significant changes in many body systems. Understanding these changes will help the nurse provide better care for the client during labor.

Cardiovascular system

In the first and second stages of labor, cardiovascular system changes primarily affect blood pressure. Cardiac output increases dramatically between contractions as labor progresses, rising 10% to 15% in the first stage of labor and 30% to 50% in the second stage. Contractions during the first stage of labor raise systolic blood pressure readings about 10 mm Hg and diastolic readings from 5 to 10 mm Hg. Because of this fluctuating increase, blood pressure readings between contractions will be the most reliable ones.

Contractions in the second stage raise systolic and diastolic readings an average of 30 mm Hg and 25 mm Hg, respectively. Between contractions, blood pressure may remain elevated by 10 mm Hg systolic and 5 to 10 mm Hg diastolic. This persistent elevation puts a client who already has hypertension at increased risk for complications, such as cerebral hemorrhage (Beischer and Mackay, 1986).

The client's position during labor also can affect blood pressure. The inferior vena cava of a supine client is less compressed as the fetus descends, whereas the aorta remains compressed until delivery, resulting in possible hypertension. (For an illustration, see Chapter 27, The First Stage of Labor.) Although approximately 90% of clients at term experience supine hypotensive syndrome, only 10% to 15% exhibit signs and symptoms, such as lightheadness (Albright, Joyce, and Stevenson, 1986). Factors that may increase a client's risk of supine hypotensive syndrome include dehydration, hypovolemia, obesity, multiple gestation, and hydramnios.

A strong contraction reduces blood flow through the uterine artery into the intervillous spaces. Consequently, blood flow is redirected into the peripheral circulation, leading to increased peripheral resistance. This in turn leads to increased blood pressure and decreased pulse rate.

The client's voluntary bearing-down efforts in the second stage of labor greatly alter intrathoracic pressure. As the client performs Valsalva's maneuver (holds her breath and tightens her abdominal muscles), intrathoracic pressure increases, venous return decreases, and venous pressure increases. As blood from the lungs is forced into the left atrium, cardiac output, blood pressure, and pulse pressure all increase, and bradycardia temporarily occurs. These processes reverse when Valsalva's maneuver ceases; however, the nurse must be aware of the long-term effect on the client with a history of cardiac disease. Also, the fetus may experience hypoxia during this time.

Other factors that may alter blood pressure during labor include anxiety, pain, and certain medications. For example, hypotension may result from administration of a narcotic, such as meperidine (Demerol), because of its vasodilating effects or from a regional anesthetic because of its sympathetic blocking effects.

A slow, progressive rise in pulse rate typically occurs during labor. Factors that may exacerbate this rise include pain, anxiety, hemorrhage, infection, certain medications (such as tocolytics), dehydration, increased cardiac output, and decreased plasma volume.

Gastrointestinal system

During labor, gastric motility and absorption decrease and gastric emptying time (the time required for the stomach to empty) increases. As a result, a client in labor may vomit food she consumed as long as 24 hours before labor began (Danforth, 1982). These normal physiologic responses are enhanced by narcotic administration, which also slows labor.

Solid foods usually are withheld during labor to prevent the risk of aspiration if an emergency arises and general anesthesia is needed. For similar reasons, some physicians advocate giving the client antacids to neutralize gastric acid either during labor or immediately before anesthetic administration. Because gastrointestinal absorption of fluids is not altered, sipping water or chewing ice chips is allowed during labor.

Respiratory system

Oxygen consumption increases dramatically during labor, from a normal rate of about 250 ml/minute up to approximately 750 ml/minute during contractions (Knuppel and Drukker, 1986). Both during and between contractions, oxygen consumption increases progressively throughout labor. By the second stage of labor, a client's oxygen consumption may be twice that before onset of labor. This dramatic increase is especially likely in an unmedicated client experiencing extreme anxiety. Resulting hyperventilation can lead to respiratory alkalosis, hypoxia, or hypocapnia. The nurse must monitor the client for signs of such problems and intervene promptly to avoid endangering the fetus.

Hematopoietic system

The normal leukocyte count of 5,000 to 11,000 mm³ may increase to about 25,000 mm³ during labor. This rise occurs particularly during prolonged labor, leading some researchers to link it with strenuous muscle activity or increased stress. Other significant hematologic changes include increased plasma fibrinogen levels and decreased plasma glucose levels and blood coagulation times.

Renal and urologic system

During labor, decreased sensory perceptions may impair the client's ability to feel bladder fullness and the urge to void. Also, compression of the ureters by the uterus may impede urine flow. Either of these factors can lead to urinary stasis and, if bladder fullness is profound, possibly impede fetal descent. For this reason, the nurse should encourage the client to empty her bladder every 2 hours during labor.

When engagement occurs and the presenting part of the fetus enters or passes the pelvic inlet, the base of the bladder is pushed upward and forward. Pressure from the presenting part may interfere with blood and lymph drainage from the base of the bladder, leading to tissue edema.

During labor, trace amounts of protein in urine commonly occur because of muscle breakdown. However, levels above trace amounts should alert the nurse to the possibility of pregnancy-induced hypertension. (See Chapter 31, High-Risk Intrapartal Clients, for more information on pregnancy-induced hypertension.)

Fluid and electrolyte balance

Labor can have several effects on the client's fluid and electrolyte balance. Increased muscular activity increases body temperature, which in turn causes fluid and electrolyte loss through diaphoresis. Increased respiratory rate and resultant hyperventilation increase fluid loss through evaporation. Vomiting, which may occur during the transitional phase of active labor, also can cause fluid and electrolyte loss. For these reasons, careful monitoring of fluid intake and output is essential during prolonged labor to prevent dehydration and related problems.

Fetal systemic response to labor

Understanding the normal fetal response to labor helps the nurse quickly identify variations from normal and intervene promptly to prevent further complications.

Cardiovascular system

The normal fetal heart rate ranges from 120 to 160 beats/minute. A rate greater than 160 beats/minute is considered tachycardia; a rate of 120 or less, bradycardia. According to Beischer and Mackay (1986), normal rhythm is fairly constant, with the baseline reflecting a fluctuation of ± 5 to 10 beats over a selected time interval. (See Chapter 25, Fetal Assessment, for a detailed description of these changes.)

Fetal blood pressure is one of several factors responsible for ensuring an adequate exchange of gases and nutrients to and from the fetal capillaries and the intervillous space. Adequate placental and fetal reserve ensures that the fetus can withstand the stresses of anoxia brought on by uterine contractions.

Respiratory system

The fetus's breathing activity decreases sharply during labor (Beishcher and Mackay, 1986). Through ultrasonography, an examiner can study these breathing movements and distinguish true preterm labor from false labor.

Acid-base status

During pregnancy, the fetus is at risk for both respiratory and metabolic acidosis. Because a major role of the placenta is to function as a fetal lung, any conditions interrupting normal blood flow to or from the placenta will increase fetal $PaCO_2$ and decrease fetal pH (Knuppel and Drukker, 1986).

Since the technique of monitoring fetal capillary blood pH was introduced in the early 1960s, it has gained widespread clinical acceptance because it indicates how adequately tissues are being supplied with oxygen. Measuring PaO_2 indicates the status of the fetus at the time of sampling; however, compared to the pH, PaO_2 may be difficult to measure correctly and may fluctuate rapidly. Because the blood pH is influenced by respiratory and metabolic factors, both rapid (respiratory) and prolonged (metabolic) changes can be detected (Knuppel and Drukker, 1986).

During the first stage of labor, the fetal scalp capillary blood pH is approximately 7.35; during the second stage, approximately 7.25 (Korones, 1986). Values below 7.2 indicate fetal distress. This decrease results from uterine contractions, which inhibit placental exchange, and from decreased maternal pH. Decreased values become more evident during the second stage of labor because the hypoxia associated with pushing leads to metabolic acidosis.

Fetal activity

The term fetus moves between 20 and 50 times per hour. These movements remain largely unchanged during labor until the membranes have ruptured; then the movements decrease (Beischer and Mackay, 1986).

Using ultrasound to study movement during labor, Griffin, Caron, and van Geijn (1985) found that fetal behavioral states present during pregnancy continue during labor. The fetus periodically changes from quiet to active sleep states, in spite of ruptured membranes and uterine contractions that progressively increase in frequency, duration, and intensity.

Vital signs

During the fetus's quiet sleep state, which normally lasts about 40 minutes, the heart rate variability may decrease. A decrease lasting more than 40 minutes, however, may indicate fetal hypoxia and requires further investigation. (For details, see Chapter 34, Neonatal Adaptation.)

A low maternal temperature has been shown to lead to fetal bradycardia; however, the fetal heart rate returns to normal as maternal temperature rises (Jadhon and Main, 1988). Researchers believe that the temperature of amniotic fluid and the fetus parallel the client's temperature. The fetus responds to lower temperatures with decreased metabolic requirements and a decreased pulse rate.

Chapter summary

Chapter 24 described the physiologic and psychological changes that trigger labor and occur during it. Here are the chapter highlights.

• Although researchers have not identified the exact mechanism that triggers labor, current theories include the effects of oxytocin stimulation, progesterone withdrawal, estrogen stimulation, the action of fetal cortisol, and the interaction of phospholipids, arachidonic acid, and prostaglandins.

• Premonitory signs and symptoms of labor include lightening, Braxton Hicks contractions, cervical changes, bloody show, rupture of membranes, and a burst of energy.

• In most clients, labor follows a consistent pattern. As uterine contractions intensify, the cervix undergoes effacement and dilation to allow passage of the fetus from the uterus into the vagina.

• Propelled by uterine contractions, the fetus maneuvers downward through the pelvis via a series of steps known as cardinal movements: descent, flexion, internal rotation, extension, external rotation (restitution and shoulder rotation), and expulsion.

• The first stage of labor—comprising latent, active, and transitional phases—extends from the beginning of true labor to complete cervical dilation.

• The second stage of labor starts with complete cervical dilation and ends with birth.

• The third stage of labor extends from birth to separation and expulsion of the placenta.

• The fourth stage of labor encompasses the first 4 hours after childbirth or until the client is stable.

• Successful labor and childbirth require coordination of five essential factors, commonly known as the "five p's": the passenger (fetus), passageway (pelvis), powers (uterine contactions and the client's bearing-down efforts), placental position and function, and the client's psychological response.

• In about 95% of clients, the fetus assumes the cephalic (head-first) position. Flexibility of the fetal skull bones allows the skull to adapt to the pelvic passageway, a process known as molding.

• The client's pelvic type and diameters influence the labor process.

• Uterine contractions are involuntary and involve intermittent tightening and relaxing of uterine muscle fibers in response to electrical activity. In the second stage of labor, the client's voluntary bearing-down efforts augment uterine contractions and aid fetal descent and expulsion.

• The placenta must be properly positioned to ensure successful childbirth and fetal well-being.

• The client's psychological response has a significant effect on labor and childbirth. Factors that may influence this response include preparation for labor, support systems, and coping mechanisms.

• Labor causes many physiologic changes in the client's body systems, especially the cardiovascular, gastrointestinal, respiratory, hematopoietic, and renal and urologic systems.

• During labor, the fetus experiences significant changes in cardiovascular and respiratory responses, acid-base status, physical activities, and vital signs.

Study questions

1. Describe the five essential factors of labor and explain how each affects labor.

2. Describe maternal physiologic responses to labor according to body system.

3. Describe the major fetal physiologic responses to labor.

4. Define the four stages of labor and describe physiologic and psychological changes that occur during each stage.

5. Discuss the notation used to identify three features that help determine fetal position.

Bibliography

Albright, G., Joyce, T., and Stevenson, D. (1986). *Anesthesia in obstetrics; Maternal, fetal, and neonatal aspects* (2nd ed.). Boston: Butterworth.

Berry, L. (1988). Realistic expectations of the labor coach. *JOGNN*, 17(5), 354-355.

Burroughs, A. (1986). *Bleier's maternity nursing* (5th ed.). Philadelphia: Saunders.

Conrad, L. (1988). *Maternal-newborn nursing.* Springhouse, PA: Springhouse Corporation.

Cunningham, F.G., MacDonald, P.C., and Gant, N.F. (1989). *Williams obstetrics* (18th ed.). East Norwalk, CT: Appleton & Lange.

Danforth, D. (Ed.). (1982). *Obstetrics and gynecology* (5th ed.). Philadelphia: Lippincott.

Korones, S. (1986). *High-risk newborn infants: The basis for intensive nursing care* (4th ed.). St. Louis: Mosby.

Knuppel, R., and Drukker, J. (1986). *High-risk pregnancy.* Philadelphia: Saunders.

Malinowski, J., Pedigo, C., and Phillips, C. (1989). *Nursing care during the labor process* (3rd ed.). Philadelphia: F. A. Davis.

Mercer, R., Hackley, K., and Bostrum, A. (1983). Relationship of psychosocial and perinatal variables to perceptions of childbirth. *Nursing Research*, 32(4), 202-207.

Morishima, H., Pedersen, H., and Finster, M. (1978). The influence of maternal psychological stress on the fetus. *American Journal of Obstetrics and Gynecology*, 131(3), 286-290.

Peisner, D., and Rosen, M. (1986). Transition from latent to active labor. *Obstetrics and Gynecology*, 68(4), 448-451.

Roberts, J. (1979). Maternal positions for childbirth. *JOGNN*, 18(1), 24-32.

Rosengren, W. (1961). Some social psychological aspects of delivery room difficulties. *Journal of Nervous Mental Disorders*, 132, 515.

Schuster, C., and Ashburn, S. (1986). *The process of human development: A holistic life-span approach* (2nd ed.). Boston: Little, Brown.

Maternal response

Bassell, G., Humayun, S., and Marx, G. (1980). Maternal bearing-down efforts—Another fetal risk? *Obstetrics and Gynecology*, 56(1), 39-41.

Caldwell, W., and Moloy, H. (1933). Anatomical variations in the female pelvis and their effect on labor with a suggested classification. *American Journal of Obstetrics and Gynecology*, 26, 479.

Carlson, J., Diehl, J., Sachtleben-Murray, M., McRae, M., Fenwick, L., and Friedman, E. (1986). Maternal position during parturition in normal labor. *Obstetrics and Gynecology*, 68(4), 443-447.

Cranley, M., Hedahl, K., and Pegg, S. (1983). Women's perceptions of vaginal and cesarean deliveries. *Nursing Research*, 32(1), 10-15.

Lederman, R., McCann, D., and Work, B. (1977). Endogenous plasma epinephrine and norepinephrine in last trimester pregnancy and labor. *American Journal of Obstetrics and Gynecology*, 129(1), 5-8.

Lowe, N. (1987). Parity and pain during parturition. *JOGNN*, 16(5), 340-346.

Lupe, P., and Gross, T. (1986). Maternal upright posture and mobility in labor—A review. *Obstetrics and Gynecology*, 67(5), 727-734.

Roberts, J., Goldstein, S., Gruener, J., Maggio, M., and Mendez-Bauer, C. (1987). A descriptive analysis of involuntary bearing-down efforts during the expulsive phase of labor. *JOGNN*, 16(1), 48-55.

Rossi, M., and Lindell, S. (1986). Maternal positions and pushing techniques in a nonprescriptive environment. *JOGNN*, 15(3), 203-208.

Fetal response

Beischer, N., and Mackay, E. (1986). *Obstetrics and the newborn* (2nd ed.). Philadelphia: Saunders.

Boylan, P., and Lewis, P. (1980). Fetal breathing in labor. *Obstetrics and Gynecology*, 56(1), 35-38.

Griffin, R., Caron, F., and van Geijn, H. (1985). Behavioral states in the human fetus during labor. *American Journal of Obstetrics and Gynecology*, 152(7, Pt. 1), 828-833.

Hughey, M. (1985). Fetal position during pregnancy. *American Journal of Obstetrics and Gynecology*, 153(8), 885-886.

Jadhon, M., and Main, E. (1988). Fetal bradycardia associated with maternal hypothermia: 2. *Obstetrics and Gynecology*, 72(3, Pt. 2), 496-497.

Labor: Stages and mechanisms

Friedman, E. (1954). The graphic analysis of labor. *American Journal of Obstetrics and Gynecology*, 68, 1568-1575.

Friedman, E. (1978). *Labor: Clinical evaluation and management* (2nd ed.). East Norwalk, CT: Appleton-Century-Crofts.

Oxorn, H. (1986). *Oxorn-Foote human labor and birth* (5th ed.). East Norwalk, CT: Appleton & Lange.

Tulchinsky, D., and Giannopoulus, G. (1983). Estrogen/progesterone eceptors and parturition. In P. MacDonald and J. Porter (Eds.), *Initiation of parturition: Prevention of prematurity (Fourth Ross Conference on Obstetric Research)*. Columbus, OH: Ross Laboratories.

Wuitchik, M., Bakal, D., and Lipshitz, J. (1989). The clinical significance of pain and cognitive activity in latent labor. *Obstetrics and Gynecology*, 73(1), 35-42.

Fetal Assessment

Objectives

After reading and studying this chapter, the student should be able to:

1. Identify factors that affect uteroplacental-fetal circulation.

2. Explain the physiology that regulates fetal heart rate.

3. Describe the techniques of electronic fetal monitoring.

4. Demonstrate correct external fetal monitor application.

5. Identify on a sample monitor strip the baseline fetal heart rate, short- and long-term variability, and any periodic changes present. Explain how uterine activity is monitored.

6. Compare the advantages and disadvantages of external and internal fetal monitoring.

7. Discuss the rationale for fetal scalp blood sampling, fetal scalp stimulation, and fetal acoustic stimulation tests.

8. Explain the importance of proper documentation of monitoring findings, using appropriate terminology.

Introduction

Early and informed nursing judgments about fetal heart rate (FHR) data can be crucial to performing timely and appropriate nursing interventions. This chapter begins by discussing the intricate physiologic balance between mother and fetus necessary to maintain fetal health and the various conditions that can jeopardize this balance. It continues by describing the principles of and techniques for using electronic fetal monitoring (EFM) to evaluate the FHR, and it discusses the basic guidelines

for interpreting FHR patterns. Also discussed are other methods for assessing fetal status, such as fetal scalp blood sampling, fetal acoustic stimulation, and fetal scalp stimulation tests.

The chapter concludes with a section on nursing responsibilities associated with fetal monitoring. Included are discussions of documentation using appropriate terminology, client education and support, and the nurse's legal responsibility for the health of the mother and fetus.

Physiologic basis of fetal monitoring

Fetal monitoring provides data about fetal status during the intrapartal period. Hypoxic or nonhypoxic stress on the fetus produces characteristic FHR patterns detectable through electronic monitoring techniques. To detect such patterns accurately, the nurse must understand basic physiologic principles of uteroplacental-fetal circulation and FHR regulation.

Uteroplacental-fetal circulation

During labor, fetal well-being depends on effective oxygen exchange from the maternal circulation through the placenta to the fetus. (For more information, see Chapter 16, Conception and Fetal Development.) Any condition

GLOSSARY

Acceleration: increase in the fetal heart rate (FHR) from the baseline that lasts less than 15 minutes.

Amnionitis: inflammation of the inner layer of the fetal membranes, or amnion.

Baseline fetal bradycardia: baseline FHR below 120 beats/minute.

Baseline fetal heart rate (BHR): resting pulse of the fetus assessed between contractions and without fetal movement. Normal baseline FHR is 120 to 160 beats/minute.

Baseline fetal tachycardia: baseline FHR exceeding 160 beats/minute.

Early deceleration: innocuous waveform deceleration of the FHR that mirrors uterine contractions and typically occurs when the cervix is dilated 4 to 7 cm.

Electronic fetal monitoring (EFM): direct (scalp electrode, intrauterine catheter) and indirect (ultrasound, tocodynamometer) devices that assess the relationship between FHR and uterine contractions.

Fetal scalp blood sampling: test that uses a fetal scalp blood sample to evaluate the fetus's acid-base status during labor. Used as an adjunct to EFM.

Fetal scalp stimulation: test that provides a reassuring sign of fetal well-being during labor by accelerating the FHR with pressure from the examiner's fingers or with application of an Allis clamp to the fetus's head.

Intrauterine pressure catheter: pliable, water-filled tube inserted into the uterus to assess uterine tone and the frequency, duration, and intensity of uterine contractions.

Late deceleration: nonreassuring waveform of the FHR indicating placental insufficiency. Onset occurs after a uterine contraction begins but does not return to baseline until the contraction is over.

Long-term variability: rhythmic fluctuations of 5 to 20 beats/minute above and below the baseline FHR, normally occuring three to five times per minute.

Prolonged deceleration: decrease in the FHR from the baseline lasting several minutes or longer in response to a sudden stimulation of the vagal system, such as uterine tachysystole, anesthetics, or maternal hypotension.

Scalp electrode: small spiral electrode attached to the fetal scalp to provide direct monitoring of the fetal electrocardiogram.

Short-term variability: beat-to-beat changes in the FHR. Normal short-term variability is 2 to 3 beats per amplitude.

Strain gauge: water-filled, pressure-sensitive device connected to an intrauterine catheter that measures intensity, duration, and frequency of contractions.

Tachysystole: contractions occurring closer than every 2 minutes.

Tocodynamometer: externally applied pressure-sensitive device that records the frequency and duration of uterine contractions.

Ultrasound: method of external EFM that sends low-energy, high-frequency sound waves through the abdominal wall in the direction of the fetal heart. After striking the fetal heart wall, these sound waves are deflected through the abdominal wall to the ultrasonic transducer, which relays them to the fetal monitor. They are translated into audible fetal heart tones and FHR waveforms.

Variability: beat-to-beat changes in the FHR that reflect the degree of tonic balance between the sympathetic and parasympathetic nervous systems.

Variable deceleration: nonuniform deceleration pattern indicating cord compression of variable significance; the most common deceleration pattern in labor, usually well tolerated by the fetus.

or factor that disrupts this circulatory route can compromise fetal well-being.

Factors affecting uteroplacental-fetal circulation

Any condition that decreases maternal cardiac output reduces placental blood flow. During labor, uteroplacental-fetal circulation can be affected by maternal position, uterine contractions, placental surface area and diffusion distance, anesthetics, maternal hypertension or hypotension, and cord compression. The nurse's primary goal is to maintain adequate maternal circulation and perfusion to the placenta so that the fetus can receive the needed oxygen and nutrients.

Maternal position

When a client in labor assumes a supine position, two possible conditions can decrease uterine blood flow. In supine hypotensive syndrome, the gravid uterus compresses the vena cava and hinders blood return to the client's heart. As a result, maternal blood pressure and cardiac output decrease, reducing blood flow to the uterus and decreasing placental perfusion. If the aorta becomes compressed, maternal blood pressure may remain normal but blood flow to the uterus is reduced—a phenomenon known as the Posiero effect. To prevent these problems, the nurse must never allow a client to rest in the supine position, even when her blood pressure remains normal. (For additional information and illustration, see Chapter 26, Comfort Promotion during Labor and Childbirth.)

The client's position during labor also affects the frequency and strength of uterine contractions, which can influence uterine blood flow (see below). For example, with the client in a lateral recumbent (side-lying) position, contractions typically are less frequent but stronger; in semi-Fowler's position, they are more frequent but less intense.

Uterine contractions

As the uterus contracts, the spiral arterioles delivering blood to the placenta collapse, decreasing or even cutting off blood flow, depending on the strength of the contraction. This decrease results in lower oxygen availability, which can cause stress on the fetus. A healthy fetus with an adequate oxygen reserve usually can tolerate this stress, but a fetus that is compromised because of a low oxygen reserve may cross the fine line from normal stress to distress. Even a healthy fetus has a limited tolerance to prolonged, repeated episodes of hypoxia caused by uterine hypertonus or tetanic contractions, which may result from oxytocin hyperstimulation or abruptio placentae (premature detachment of the placenta from the uterine wall).

Placental surface area and diffusion distance

Any condition that reduces the surface area of the placenta—such as abruptio placentae or placenta previa—also reduces perfusion. Oxygen diffusion through the placental membrane is impaired by conditions that cause a thickened or edematous membrane, such as diabetes mellitus or Rh disease.

Anesthetics

Use of a regional anesthetic—spinal, epidural, or caudal—during labor can impair normal vasoconstriction of peripheral blood vessels. As these vessels dilate and hold more blood, hypotension develops and less blood returns to the heart, decreasing maternal cardiac output and blood flow to the uterus. In response, the fetus may develop a prolonged deceleration of the heart rate.

Maternal hypertension and hypotension

Maternal hypertension decreases blood flow to the uterus directly, through excessive vasoconstriction. It also reduces the total surface area of the placenta by causing placental infarcts and inhibits placental development by producing a prolonged reduction in blood flow.

Maternal hypotension can result from supine positioning, anesthetic administration, and other factors. Regardless of the cause, however, hypotension can decrease the blood return to the heart, reducing maternal cardiac output and blood flow to the uterus.

Cord compression

A common occurrence during contractions, cord compression temporarily decreases oxygen flow to the fetus. When the contraction subsides, oxygen exchange resumes. This event is analogous to the fetus holding its breath and usually is well tolerated.

Fetal heart rate regulation

The FHR is regulated by the sympathetic and parasympathetic divisions of the autonomic nervous system and chemoreceptors and baroreceptors. The normal range of the FHR is 120 to 160 beats/minute.

Through the vagal reflex, the parasympathetic nervous system controls the FHR and is responsible for its beat-to-beat (moment-to-moment) changes. When the vagal reflex is stimulated, the FHR decreases. Conversely, stimulation of the sympathetic nervous system increases the FHR.

The autonomic nervous system receives information on blood pressure and oxygen status from chemoreceptors (sensory nerve cells) and baroreceptors (pressure-sensitive nerve endings in the walls of the large systemic arteries), which help the autonomic nervous system stabilize blood pressure.

Chemoreceptors detect even minute changes in tissue oxygen levels and trigger the sympathetic nervous system to increase the FHR so that more blood will circulate to the affected area, increasing tissue oxygenation. As a result, fetal blood pressure increases.

Baroreceptors are extremely sensitive to any elevation in blood pressure. An increase in blood pressure provokes baroreceptors to signal the parasympathetic nervous system to rapidly decrease the FHR. As the FHR decreases, so does fetal cardiac output and blood pressure.

Fetal and uterine monitoring

Careful monitoring of fetal and uterine function during labor helps the nurse identify problems before they cause serious complications. Available monitoring methods include manual techniques (fetal heart auscultation and uterine palpation) and internally and externally applied devices for EFM.

Fetal monitoring

The nurse can monitor the FHR through auscultation, using a fetoscope or an ultrasound stethoscope (Doppler blood flow detector), or through EFM. Each method carries distinct advantages and disadvantages.

Fetoscope and ultrasound stethoscope

Auscultating the FHR during labor traditionally has been considered sufficient monitoring for the low-risk client and fetus (NAACOG, 1988). The fetoscope is a special stethoscope that enhances the nurse's ability to hear the fetal heartbeat. One type is attached to a metal band that fits on the nurse's head and conducts sound. The other type is a stethoscope attached to a 3"-diameter weighted bell that is placed on the client's abdomen.

In contrast, the ultrasound stethoscope uses ultra-high-frequency sound waves to detect fetal heartbeats. Typically, this device consists of a headset, a battery charger, a transducer, and an audio unit. The ultrasound stethoscope can be used as early as the tenth week of gestation. (For illustrations of the ultrasound stethoscope and one type of fetoscope, see Chapter 27, The First Stage of Labor.)

According to NAACOG (the organization for obstetric, gynecologic, and neonatal nurses) guidelines, the nurse should perform auscultation for the low-risk client every 60 minutes during the latent phase and every 30 minutes during the active phase of the first stage of labor, and every 15 minutes during the second stage; for the high-risk client, every 30 minutes during the latent phase and every 15 minutes during the active phase of the first stage, and every 5 minutes during the second stage (NAACOG, 1990). Unfortunately, such frequent auscultation is impractical because it requires one-on-one nursing care. Nurses and other personnel who try to follow these guidelines may become frustrated and anxious (Fields and Boehm, 1989).

Another disadvantage of auscultation is that it cannot be used to assess the most important sign of fetal well-being: beat-to-beat variability of the FHR (Parer, 1984). In fact, one-third of obstetric nurses and physicians were unable to recognize significant periodic patterns of fetal distress through auscultation alone (Miller, Pearse, and Paul, 1984). Miller, Pearse, and Paul concluded that although low-risk clients still should be auscultated before and after contractions to attempt to identify abnormal patterns, merely counting audible fetal heartbeats is insufficient to evaluate fetal status thoroughly.

Electronic fetal monitoring

Every method for EFM has advantages and disadvantages that the nurse should understand. When the nurse uses this technology accurately and appropriately, EFM is the most reliable means currently available for assessing fetal status in utero.

Electronic fetal monitoring can be used externally (outside the uterus) or internally (in direct contact with the fetus) to establish a continuous record of the FHR and its relationship to uterine contractions. A heart rate pattern that is normal or otherwise within EFM guidelines is a reliable indicator of fetal well-being. At times, abnormal patterns may occur without indicating fetal distress; however, fetal hypoxia reliably produces changes in the FHR pattern.

External EFM. This technique allows safe, ongoing assessment of the FHR. One widely used method of external EFM is the ultrasound transducer. In this method, a transducer is guided over the client's abdomen to determine the area closest to the fetal heart. (For an illustration of the procedure, see *Psychomotor skills: Applying an external electronic fetal monitor,* page 612.) After placement, the transducer emits low-energy, high-frequency ultrasound waves and directs them through the abdominal wall toward the fetal heart. These ultrasound waves strike the heart wall and are deflected back through the abdominal wall, where the transducer receives them. The transducer then relays the waves to the fetal monitor, which translates them two ways: into a signal that sounds like a heartbeat and into waveform lines on the monitor strip.

Besides being noninvasive, ultrasound poses no apparent risk for the fetus or mother. This method allows the nurse to monitor short-term (but not beat-to-beat) variability, long-term variability, and periodic accelerations and decelerations of the FHR. (See the section on "Fetal heart rate patterns" for more information on these patterns.)

Unfortunately, the monitor can make errors in counting when the FHR falls below 60 beats/minute. It may count both motions of the cardiac cycle (the *lub* and the *dub*), which will falsely double the heart rate, a condition known as doubling. Conversely, with an accelerated FHR of 200 beats/minute or above, the monitor will count only half the beats, a situation known as halving. These problems demonstrate the hazards of relying solely on technology. A nurse who has any question about the accuracy of external EFM should auscultate the FHR to verify the rate.

Another disadvantage of ultrasound involves the belts the client must wear, which can be uncomfortable and usually must be adjusted when the client changes position. Moreover, moving about is limited to the length of the cables hooked to the monitor.

The phonotransducer and abdominal electrodes are other, less used, types of external EFM devices. The

Applying an external electronic fetal monitor

External electronic fetal monitoring (EFM) evaluates fetal heart rate with ultrasound and detects uterine contractions with a tocotransducer. Before applying the monitor, explain the procedure to the client and her family. Have the client void and then assume a semi-Fowler's or side-lying—not supine—position. Turn on the fetal monitor and its speaker. Place both belts under the client's back at about waist level.

Gently tap the diaphragm of the ultrasound transducer to ensure that the unit is operating; if it is, apply a thin coat of gel to the face of the diaphragm. Perform the first and second Leopold's maneuvers to locate the fetus. (For more information on Leopold's maneuvers, see Chapter 27, The First Stage of Labor.)

1 Position the ultrasound transducer in place over the fetal heart and tighten the belt. Verify the location by the tracing on the fetal heart monitor strip.

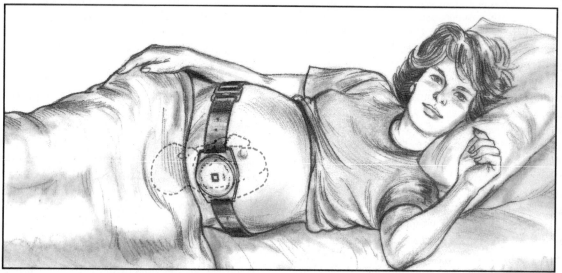

2 Place the tocotransducer over the uterine fundus where it contracts, either midline or slightly to one side. Place your hand on the fundus and palpate for a contraction to verify proper placement. Secure the tocotransducer with its belt, then adjust the pen set-knob so that the baseline reads between 5 and 15 mm Hg on the monitor strip.

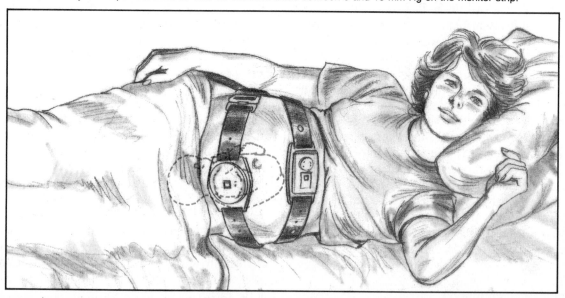

phonotransducer detects the FHR through a microphone placed on the client's abdomen, which amplifies the fetal heartbeat. The abdominal electrodes monitor and record maternal and fetal heartbeats. Both of these methods are less accurate than ultrasound, which has become the most commonly used external monitor.

Internal EFM. Nursing students may wonder why internal EFM is used since external EFM is noninvasive and easier to use. With external EFM, extraneous noises from pulsating maternal vessels and from maternal and fetal movement may interfere with an accurate, clear tracing. The transducer must be repositioned frequently to maintain a clear signal. In contrast, the waveforms produced by internal EFM are not affected by maternal or fetal movement and can produce an accurate tracing of the fetal heartbeat and uterine contractions.

Internal EFM is performed by attaching a small, corkscrew-type spiral electrode to the fetal scalp or buttocks, whichever is the presenting part. The electrode penetrates the presenting part about 1.5 mm and must be attached securely to ensure a good signal. In many health care facilities, nurses with special preparation are allowed to attach these electrodes. (For an illustration of the procedure, see *Psychomotor skills: Applying an internal electronic fetal monitor.*) A plate is attached to the client's leg to hold the wires from the electrode in place. Most clients consider the leg plate less distracting than the belts used with the ultrasound unit.

The spiral electrode picks up the fetal heartbeat and transmits it to the monitor. The monitor transforms the impulse into a fetal electrocardiogram waveform on an oscilloscope screen and a waveform on the printout. These data are more accurate than those provided by external EFM and allow the nurse to track and calculate beat-to-beat variability in the FHR.

Internal EFM with spiral electrodes can be used only when the client's membranes are ruptured, when the cervix is dilated at least 2 cm, and when the presenting part is at least at the −1 station.

Controversies in EFM. In the 1970s, EFM began to be challenged on issues of safety, effectiveness, and impact on the cesarean delivery rate. Since the 1970s, some of these issues have been resolved. What remains to be resolved, however, is the effect of EFM on reducing perinatal mortality and morbidity. As debate continues, EFM has become a standard surveillance tool, prenatally and intrapartally, for the fetus at high risk.

Originally, the safety of internal monitoring generated great concern. Opponents cited the risk of infection from the internal intrauterine catheter and fetal scalp electrodes. Early cases in which the uterus was perforated seemed to confirm opponents' concerns.

PSYCHOMOTOR SKILLS

Applying an internal electronic fetal monitor

Internal electronic fetal monitoring provides the most accurate information for assessing fetal status in utero. The fetal heart rate is monitored via an electrode. The uterine contractions are monitored via an internal catheter connected to a pressure gauge.

The spiral electrode is inserted during a vaginal examination. The electrode is attached to the presenting fetal part, usually the scalp or buttocks.

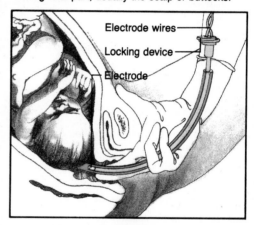

Electrode wires
Locking device
Electrode

The internal catheter is inserted up to the black mark during a vaginal examination and connected to a monitor that interprets uterine contraction pressures.

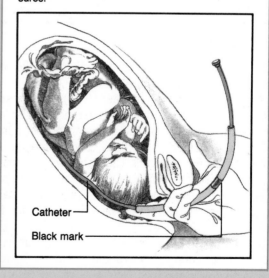

Catheter
Black mark

Indications for electronic fetal monitoring

For many clients, electronic fetal monitoring (EFM) offers advantages over other monitoring methods. High-risk maternal, fetal, pregnancy, and uterine factors that typically call for EFM are listed below.

Maternal factors
- Diabetes
- Pregnancy-induced hypertension
- Hypertension
- Cardiac disease
- Renal disease
- Previous stillbirth

Fetal factors
- Abnormal heart rate on auscultation
- Meconium staining
- Intrauterine growth retardation
- Rh disease

Pregnancy factors
- Third-trimester bleeding
- Premature rupture of the membranes
- Preterm labor
- Postterm labor
- Amnionitis
- Hydramnios or oligohydramnios

Uterine factors
- Induction or augmentation of labor
- Regional anesthesia
- Multiple gestation (more than one fetus)
- Failure of labor to progress

The most common infection related to fetal monitoring is caused by the scalp electrode, but infections have been minor and localized.

Also, Gibbs, Jones, and Wilder (1978) reported that the most important variables in maternal infection are long labor, prolonged ruptured membranes, and numerous vaginal examinations. By itself, fetal monitoring has no effect on the infection rate. The problem of perforating the uterus during the intrauterine catheter procedure can be avoided if personnel introduce the inflexible catheter guide no more than the recommended 1 cm into the uterus.

The rising rate of cesarean deliveries continues to concern health care consumers and providers. Contributing to this rise are such factors as repeat cesarean delivery, dystocia or failure to progress, and breech presentations. However, fetal distress accounts for only a small percentage of the increase in this rate.

On an even broader scale, advocates of natural childbirth commonly have opposed EFM, believing that the less intrusion upon the birth process, the better. This issue is further complicated by physicians' growing fears of malpractice suits. Physicians may feel that if they use EFM technology they will be criticized for dehumanizing the birth process, but if they do not use EFM and fetal complications develop, they risk malpractice suits for not using available technology.

Originally, many families were suspicious of EFM. However, Dulock and Herron (1976) and Beck (1980) conclude that insensitive personnel create more suspicion and hostility than do the EFM procedures. When personnel clearly explain EFM and the rationale for using it, most clients and their families accept it.

Currently, the EFM controversy centers on whether it benefits low- and high-risk pregnant clients. The literature is divided on this issue. Freeman and Garite (1981) report only one intrapartal fetal death among 12,000 deliveries involving EFM. Leveno, et al. (1986) concludes that monitoring all women does not reduce neonatal morbidity in low-risk clients. Wood, et al. (1981) also concluded that low-risk clients do not benefit from EFM. Currently, standard practice advocates continuous monitoring of high-risk clients only. (For a list of high-risk factors, see *Indications for electronic fetal monitoring*.)

Uterine activity monitoring

Like any muscle, the uterus can contract and relax. Its normal resting tone (or baseline tone) is 5 to 15 mm Hg. In the first stage of labor, when the uterus contracts, the tone rises to 50 to 75 mm Hg. During the second stage of labor, when the client does not push, it may rise to 75 to 100 mm Hg with contractions.

Increased uterine activity can result from factors other than normal contractions during labor, including incautious use of oxytocin and abruptio placentae.

Contractions that occur at 3-minute intervals dilate the cervix most effectively and allow sufficient time for the fetus and uterine muscle to reoxygenate. Contractions that occur less than 2 minutes apart or last longer than 90 seconds generally reflect increased uterine activity.

Increased uterine activity can become hyperstimulation, which reduces perfusion to the placenta and can lead to fetal distress. In response to hyperstimulation, the fetus typically displays a prolonged deceleration or late decelerations of the heart rate. Therefore, the nurse must monitor uterine activity as closely as the FHR. Uterine activity can be monitored externally by using palpation or a tocodynamometer or internally with an intrauterine pressure catheter. Telemetry also can be used to monitor the client in labor.

Manual palpation

The manual method of monitoring uterine contractions, palpation requires no special equipment. It does, however, require skill and sensitivity to touch. To palpate uterine contractions, the nurse places the palmar surfaces of the fingers on the top of the uterine fundus where it contracts. (For an illustration, see Chapter 27, The First Stage of Labor.)

During mild contractions, the fundus indents easily and feels like a chin. In moderate contractions, the fundus indents less easily and feels more rigid, like the tip of the nose. With strong contractions, the fundus is firm, resists indenting, and feels like a forehead. The nurse must remember to palpate a set of at least three contractions to obtain sufficient data to evaluate a uterine contraction pattern.

External tocodynamometer

The tocodynamometer, a pressure-sensitive disk, is attached to an elastic belt strapped on the client's abdomen so that the disk lies directly over the fundus. The pressure exerted by uterine contractions is then amplified and relayed to the FHR monitor, which records the frequency and duration of the contractions. (The tocodynamometer does not record the intensity of contractions.)

If the tocodynamometer is not placed appropriately on the fundus, contractions may not be recorded at all. Also, the tighter the belt is strapped, the stronger the contractions appear on the graph, and vice versa.

Internal intrauterine pressure catheter

When oxytocin is used to stimulate labor, or when labor fails to progress normally, most experts recommend use of an internal intrauterine pressure catheter. This device accurately and continuously records uterine tone and the frequency, duration, and intensity of uterine contractions. It can be used only after the cervix has dilated from 2 to 3 cm and the membranes have ruptured.

In this sterile procedure, the nurse assists the physician or nurse-midwife by filling and irrigating the end of a pliable plastic catheter with sterile water. Then the physician or nurse-midwife inserts the catheter through the vagina and into the cervix, alongside the fetus. The catheter is advanced approximately 18″ until its black mark is visible at the introitus. After insertion is completed, the catheter is irrigated again to clear any bubbles or vernix that may interfere with transmission, and taped to the client's leg; the syringe and catheter are attached to their proper outlets on the strain gauge.

Each uterine contraction compresses the water in the catheter. This pressure is relayed through the plastic tubing to an external pressure-sensitive device, which in turn relays the pressure to an attached monitor that records the pressure as mm Hg on the monitor strip.

The contraction is shown on the graph as an inverted "U".

The intrauterine pressure catheter can use various pressure-sensitive devices. One device, the strain gauge, has a plastic dome filled with sterile water that exerts pressure on a membrane within the unit. A more recently developed disposable unit does not require water or a strain gauge. This unit eliminates the time-consuming set-up, irrigation, and calibration required by other types. However, the disposable unit is more expensive and may have to be replaced if the unit is disconnected when the client arises to use the bathroom.

The nurse can speed intrauterine catheter insertion by preparing the equipment in advance—for example, by assembling, irrigating, and calibrating the strain gauge before the catheter is inserted. This gives the nurse time for any necessary troubleshooting.

Telemetry

By using remote monitoring, or telemetry, the nurse can monitor the client in labor as she moves about. External and internal methods are available. For the client with external EFM equipment, a battery-powered, two-way radio transmitter on a shoulder strap allows remote monitoring of the FHR and uterine contractions. The client with internal EFM equipment requires insertion of a transmitter into the vaginal vault after placement of the pressure catheter in the uterus and application of a scalp electrode to the fetal presenting part. Both telemetry methods provide close assessment of the client and allow her to move freely within a specified area and not be confined to bed earlier than she might desire.

Fetal heart rate patterns

Labor and delivery put stress on even the healthiest fetus. Accurate interpretation of a monitor strip of fetal heart patterns can help the nurse determine when a fetus has crossed the line from normal stress to distress. (For more information, see *Reading a fetal monitor strip*, page 616.)

A fetus coping well with the stress of labor typically will exhibit a reassuring FHR pattern; a fetus in distress invariably will demonstrate an abnormal pattern. Fetal distress may reveal itself in various combinations of symptoms: an increasing baseline FHR may indicate that the fetus is attempting to compensate for decreased oxygen reserves; late decelerations indicate placental insufficiency and the need for prompt intervention.

Reading a fetal monitor strip

The monitor strip is divided into two sections. The top section shows the fetal heart rate (FHR), measured in beats/minute (bpm). The nurse reads the strip horizontally and vertically. Reading horizontally, each small square represents 10 seconds. Between each vertical dark line are six squares, representing 1 minute. Reading vertically, each square represents an amplitude of 10 bpm.

The bottom section shows uterine activity (UA), measured in mm Hg. Again, the nurse reads the strip horizontally and vertically. Reading horizontally, each small square represents 10 seconds, with the space between each vertical black line representing 1 minute. Reading vertically, each square represents 5 mm Hg of pressure.

The baseline FHR, the "resting" heart rate, is assessed between uterine contractions and when no fetal movement is occurring. The baseline FHR—normally 120 to 160 beats/minute—serves as a reference for subsequent heart rate readings taken during contractions.

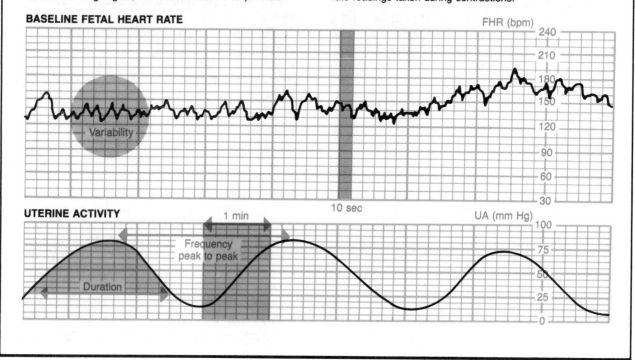

Understanding these and other fetal heart patterns will enable the nurse to know which patterns will not harm the fetus, which patterns necessitate the nurse's intervention, and which patterns require the immediate attention of other health care personnel.

Baseline fetal heart rate

The starting point for all fetal assessment is the baseline FHR. Accurate baseline FHR determination serves as a reference for all subsequent FHR readings taken during labor.

The proper time for establishing the baseline FHR is between uterine contractions and when no fetal movement is occurring. Initially, the nurse establishes the baseline FHR by examining approximately 5 to 10 minutes of the FHR on the monitor strip; the baseline FHR is the average rate between contractions during that 5- to 10-minute period. Once a baseline FHR is established, it does not change unless a new rate is present for 15

minutes. In a full-term fetus, baseline FHR normally ranges between 120 and 160 beats/minute. Deviations from the normal baseline FHR include tachycardia, bradycardia, and increased or decreased variability. (For more information, see *Variations on baseline fetal heart rate,* page 618.)

Baseline tachycardia

A baseline FHR exceeding 160 beats/minute indicates baseline tachycardia. Several factors can produce tachycardia in the fetus. The most common cause is maternal fever, which raises the fetal metabolic rate and, consequently, the baseline FHR. Baseline tachycardia also may be the first sign of intrauterine infection with prolonged rupture of membranes. Another possible cause is maternal anxiety, which releases epinephrine that crosses the placenta and increases the baseline FHR. Drugs that can cause fetal baseline tachycardia when used by the mother include parasympathetic blocking agents, such as atropine and scopolamine, and beta sympathomimetics, such as ritodrine and terbutaline. Baseline tachycardia also may be a response to hypoxia.

Baseline bradycardia

A baseline FHR less than 120 beats/minute is termed baseline bradycardia. A baseline FHR below 120 beats/minute without late decelerations, but with normal beat-to-beat variability, can be reassuring. Baseline bradycardia accompanied by late decelerations and little or no variability is an ominous sign of advanced fetal distress from hypoxia and acidosis.

The rare case of congenital heart block produces a baseline bradycardia of 60 to 80 beats/minute. A fetus with heart block must be delivered in a facility where cardiac surgery is available.

Variability

Variability refers to the beat-to-beat changes in FHR that result from the interaction of the sympathetic nervous system, which speeds up the FHR, and the parasympathetic nervous system, which slows the FHR. It is considered the most important indicator in clinical assessment of fetal well-being.

Variability has two components—long-term and short-term. Long-term variability refers to the larger periodic and rhythmic deviations above and below the baseline FHR. Normal long-term variability ranges from 5 to 20 beats/minute in rhythmic fluctuations, three to five times per minute.

Short-term variability describes the differences in successive heartbeats, as measured by the R-R wave interval of the QRS cardiac cycle. It represents actual beat-to-beat fluctuations in the FHR and the balance between the sympathetic and parasympathetic nervous systems. Short-term variability is classified as present or absent. Normal short-term variability—2 to 3 beats per amplitude—is considered the most reliable single indicator of fetal well-being.

Variability is described as normal, increased, decreased, or absent.

Factors increasing variability. In the healthy fetus, movement accelerates the heart rate and increases long-term variability. This concept serves as the basis for assessing fetal well-being with the nonstress test. This test can be performed weekly, usually after week 32 of pregnancy.

The nonstress test indicates fetal well-being if the fetus can accelerate its heart rate two or more times in 15 minutes in response to a stimulus from contractions or fetal movement; if each acceleration increases 15 beats/minute above the baseline; and if each acceleration lasts 15 seconds or more.

Variability also increases during the second stage of labor, which begins when the cervix is fully dilated

and ends with birth. This increase may be related to a mild hypoxia caused by the increased intensity, duration, and frequency of uterine contractions. As the fetus descends the birth canal, a prolonged deceleration or bradycardia typically results.

Commonly, short- and long-term variability increase when the fetus assumes the occiput posterior position.

When hypoxemia occurs, the fetus responds initially by increasing short- and long-term variability. For example, when uterine contractions occur closer than every 2 minutes or last longer than 90 seconds (a condition known as uterine tachysystole), contractions occur too quickly, preventing complete fetal oxygenation. The fetal stress liberates epinephrine, and variability increases. In this situation, the nurse should reduce the frequency of contractions by decreasing the oxytocin as prescribed and by having the client turn to her left side, which decreases the frequency of contractions.

Factors decreasing variability. Although decreased variability can endanger the fetus, the nurse never should presume fetal distress based solely on a decrease in variability.

Drugs that depress the fetal central nervous system, such as narcotics, or block the action of the fetal parasympathetic nervous system, such as atropine, can decrease variability. When these drugs are administered to the mother, the nurse should expect a decrease in variability and be reassured if no other signs of fetal distress, such as late decelerations, are present.

Fetal dysrhythmias, such as paroxysmal atrial tachycardia and complete heart block, will decrease variability. The sympathetic nervous system becomes dominant and increases the FHR. The nurse should be aware that the higher the FHR, the lower the variability.

Another benign cause of decreased variability is quiet fetal sleep. The fetus normally has sleep-awake cycles lasting 20 to 30 minutes. After a period of normal variability, short- and long-term variability suddenly decrease. This sudden onset, and the absence of such other signs of fetal distress as late decelerations, should reassure the nurse that this is a sleep state, not a sudden catastrophe. When the fetus awakens, the variability reappears just as suddenly.

Two causes of decreased variability that typically do not occur suddenly and are much more dangerous are hypoxia and acidosis. Initially, the fetus may react to hypoxemia with increased heart rate variability. As a continued decrease in oxygen progresses to hypoxia, the heart rate accelerates as the fetus attempts to increase oxygenation. The result is baseline tachycardia and decreased or absent variability. Over time, the lack of oxygen harms the fetal central nervous system. If this cycle of deterioration is allowed to continue, acidosis

Variations on baseline fetal heart rate

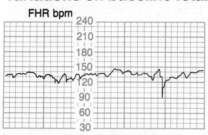

BASELINE FHR 130 BEATS/MINUTE

By properly interpreting baseline fetal heart rate (FHR), the nurse can determine much about fetal well-being. This chart presents possible causes, clinical significance, and nursing interventions associated with baseline tachycardia (FHR above 160 beats/minute persisting for more than 15 minutes) and baseline bradycardia (FHR below 120 beats/minute persisting for more than 15 minutes). The strip at left shows representative baseline FHR; variations on baseline are shown in the chart below.

VARIATIONS ON BASELINE	POSSIBLE CAUSES	CLINICAL SIGNIFICANCE	NURSING INTERVENTIONS
Baseline tachycardia **BASELINE FHR 170 BEATS/MINUTE**	• Early fetal hypoxia • Maternal fever • Parasympathetic agents, such as atropine and scopolamine • Beta-sympathomimetic agents, such as ritodrine and terbutaline • Amnionitis (inflammation of the inner layer of the fetal membrane—the amnion) • Maternal hyperthyroidism • Fetal anemia • Fetal heart failure • Fetal cardiac arrhythmias	Persistent tachycardia without periodic changes usually does not adversely affect fetal well-being—especially when associated with maternal fever. However, tachycardia is an ominous sign when associated with late decelerations, severe variable decelerations, or absence of variability.	Intervene to alleviate the cause of fetal distress and provide supplemental oxygen (7 to 8 liters/minute), as prescribed. Also administer I.V. fluids, as prescribed.
Baseline bradycardia **BASELINE FHR 80 BEATS/MINUTE**	• Late fetal hypoxia • Beta-adrenergic blocking agents, such as propranolol, and anesthetics • Maternal hypotension • Prolonged umbilical cord compression • Fetal congenital heart block	Bradycardia with good variability and without periodic changes is not a sign of fetal distress if the fetal heart rate remains above 80 beats/minute. However, bradycardia caused by hypoxia is an ominous sign when associated with loss of variability and late decelerations.	Intervene to alleviate the cause of fetal distress. Administer supplemental oxygen (7 to 8 liters/minute), start an I.V. line, and administer fluids, as prescribed.

develops and direct myocardial depression of the FHR occurs. At this stage, the fetus will be near death and may display baseline bradycardia.

Periodic changes

Transient accelerations or decelerations from the baseline FHR are called periodic changes and are caused by uterine contractions and fetal movements. They represent the normal rhythmic fluctuations from the fetal resting pulse.

Accelerations

Transient accelerations in the FHR normally are caused by fetal movements and uterine contractions. This type of acceleration typically indicates fetal well-being and adequate oxygen reserve. Accelerations also may be caused by partial umbilical cord compression.

Decelerations

Periodic decelerations from the normal baseline FHR are classified as early, late, or variable, depending on when they occur and their waveform shape. (For more information, see *Common decelerations,* pages 620 and 621.)

Early decelerations. Decelerations that begin early in the contraction are associated with normal FHR variability and are well tolerated by the fetus. They are unaffected by maternal oxygen administration or position changes and require no nursing intervention.

Early decelerations exhibit a uniform waveform shape on the monitor strip, typically mirroring that of the uterine contractions. They arise from pressure on the fontanels produced by uterine contractions when the cervix is dilated 4 to 7 cm. This pressure produces localized hypoxemia that stimulates the chemoreceptors. As the baroreceptors are stimulated, the vagal system decreases the FHR in response. The onset, the lowest point of descent, and the recovery from early decelerations occur exactly in sequence with the contraction.

Late decelerations. These decelerations begin after the beginning of a contraction. The lowest point of a late deceleration occurs after the contraction ends; descent and return are gradual and smooth. The FHR rarely falls more than 30 to 40 beats/minute below the baseline FHR. Late decelerations typically produce U-shaped waveforms.

Usually repetitive, late decelerations occur with each contraction, although in some cases they will occur only with stronger contractions.

Late decelerations are nonreassuring because they indicate uteroplacental insufficiency, which comes from decreased intervillous blood flow. This decreased blood flow leads to inadequate oxygen exchange.

The nurse may counter the underlying cause of uteroplacental insufficiency and may reverse its course by removing it. Maternal hypotension usually can be remedied by changing the client's position to her left side and administering I.V. fluids as prescribed. If oxytocin is overstimulating the uterus, it should be discontinued. Then contractions should occur less frequently, giving the fetus more time to reoxygenate, and the late decelerations may disappear.

However, intrinsic causes of uteroplacental insufficiency usually cannot be reversed. Such conditions as diabetes, pregnancy-induced hypertension, and pregnancy of 42 weeks or more may foster a placenta that is structurally incapable of meeting fetal oxygen needs, particularly during labor.

The nurse who recognizes a late deceleration pattern and intervenes appropriately may help prevent fetal hypoxia and asphyxia. If a second late deceleration occurs, the nurse should notify the physician and intervene to decrease uterine activity by discontinuing oxytocin, maximize uterine perfusion by turning the client on her left side, administer oxygen by mask at a rate of 7 liters/minute, and increase I.V. fluids as prescribed.

If decelerations persist for more than 30 minutes and birth is not imminent, the nurse should alert the physician again and notify other appropriate personnel. A cesarean delivery may be necessary. The need for cesarean delivery depends on the client's parity and degree of cervical dilation. For example, a primiparous client at 2 cm dilation with uncorrectable late decelerations is not a candidate for a vaginal delivery, but a multiparous client at 9 cm dilation possibly could deliver vaginally without jeopardizing the fetus.

Variable decelerations. When fetal movements or contractions compress the umbilical cord, variable decelerations occur. Dramatic and unpredictable, they vary in shape, duration, depth, and timing. To the client and support person, a variable deceleration may seem to indicate that the fetus's heart has stopped. The nurse should reassure them that these decelerations are the most common patterns during labor and usually are no cause for alarm. The nurse should explain that the decrease in FHR is analogous to the fetus holding its breath during a contraction and then resuming breathing.

Variable decelerations seem dramatic, and at times they can resemble early and late deceleration patterns. Cord compression stimulates the chemoreceptors and baroreceptors, causing the FHR to drop rapidly. A deceleration to 60 beats/minute or below is common.

The deceleration in the FHR produces shapes like the letters V, U, or W on the monitor strip. To tolerate these episodes well, the fetus must have sufficient time between contractions to reoxygenate.

In many cases, variable decelerations are preceded and followed by slight accelerations called shoulders. The FHR accelerates slightly, then decelerates suddenly and sharply; the deceleration ends just as suddenly as it begins. Finally, a small acceleration (the other shoulder) occurs before the baseline FHR is reestablished. These shoulders occur because the contraction occludes only the umbilical vein at first. When the umbilical arteries also are occluded, the deceleration occurs. Shoulders are a reassuring sign.

Variable decelerations can be mild, moderate, or severe. The nurse should know the differences but also should realize that certain fetuses can tolerate severe variable decelerations, while other fetuses have difficulties even with mild ones. Therefore, the nurse must

Common decelerations

Decelerations—periodic decreases in fetal heart rate (FHR)—are caused by uterine contractions and fetal movements. This chart illustrates early, late, and variable decelerations, and then lists their possible causes, clinical significance, and appropriate nursing interventions.

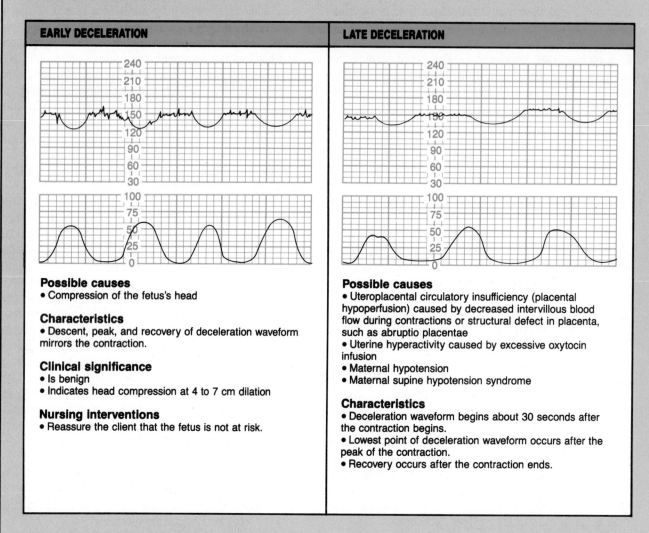

EARLY DECELERATION	LATE DECELERATION

EARLY DECELERATION

Possible causes
• Compression of the fetus's head

Characteristics
• Descent, peak, and recovery of deceleration waveform mirrors the contraction.

Clinical significance
• Is benign
• Indicates head compression at 4 to 7 cm dilation

Nursing interventions
• Reassure the client that the fetus is not at risk.

LATE DECELERATION

Possible causes
• Uteroplacental circulatory insufficiency (placental hypoperfusion) caused by decreased intervillous blood flow during contractions or structural defect in placenta, such as abruptio placentae
• Uterine hyperactivity caused by excessive oxytocin infusion
• Maternal hypotension
• Maternal supine hypotension syndrome

Characteristics
• Deceleration waveform begins about 30 seconds after the contraction begins.
• Lowest point of deceleration waveform occurs after the peak of the contraction.
• Recovery occurs after the contraction ends.

assess the monitor strip according to *reassuring* and *nonreassuring* criteria. A reassuring variable pattern has an abrupt onset and end, the baseline FHR does not increase, and short-term variability does not decrease.

A nonreassuring pattern includes signs of hypoxemia. At first, variability increases, but the baseline FHR remains within normal limits. Eventually, the FHR accelerates to a baseline tachycardia as the fetus tries to compensate for the growing oxygen deficit. Hypoxia becomes more evident as variability decreases. The shape of the variables may become more rounded, and the onset and end smoother, indicating that the central nervous system is adversely affected.

To help correct variable decelerations, the nurse should try to alleviate cord compression by changing the client's position, using the knee-chest, Trendelenburg, or other positions, as needed. (For illustrations, see *Alternate positions for labor* in Chapter 27, The First Stage of Labor.) In most cases, maternal repositioning alleviates cord compression, allowing resumption of oxygen flow and fetal reoxygenation.

If maternal positioning is unsuccessful, the nurse should observe for reassuring and nonreassuring signs. If reassuring signs disappear, the nurse should admin-

Clinical significance
• Indicates uteroplacental insufficiency
• May lead to fetal hypoxia and acidosis, if underlying cause is not corrected

Nursing interventions
• Turn the client on her left side to increase placental perfusion and decrease contraction frequency.
• Increase the I.V. fluid rate to increase intravascular volume and placental perfusion, as prescribed.
• Administer oxygen by mask at 7 liters/minute to increase fetal oxygenation, as prescribed.
• Notify physician or nurse-midwife.
• Assess for signs of the underlying cause, such as hypotension and uterine tachysystole.
• Take other appropriate measures, such as discontinuing oxytocin, as prescribed.
• Explain the rationales for nursing interventions to the client and her support person.

VARIABLE DECELERATION

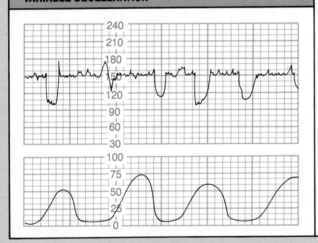

Possible causes
• Umbilical cord compression causing decreased fetal oxygen perfusion

Characteristics
• Deceleration waveform shows abrupt onset and recovery
• Waveform shape varies and may resemble the letter U, V, or W.
• FHR commonly decreases to 60 beats/minute.

Clinical significance
• Is most common deceleration pattern in labor because of contractions and fetal movement
• May indicate cord compression
• Is well tolerated if the fetus has sufficient time to recover between contractions and if the deceleration does not last more than 50 seconds

Nursing interventions
• Help the client change positions. No other intervention is necessary, unless fetal distress is present.
• Assure the client that the fetus tolerates cord compression well. Explain that cord compression affects the fetus the same way that breath-holding affects the client.
• Assess the deceleration pattern for reassuring signs: baseline FHR not increasing, short-term variability not decreasing, abrupt beginning and ending of decelerations, and deceleration duration of less than 50 seconds.
• If assessment does not reveal reassuring signs, notify the physician or nurse-midwife; then start I.V. fluids and administer oxygen by mask at 7 liters/minute, as prescribed.
• Explain the rationales for nursing interventions to the client and her support person.

ister oxygen. If variable decelerations persist, other interventions are necessary. (For more information, see *Nursing research applied: Using amnioinfusion to relieve repetitive variable decelerations*, page 622.)

Prolonged decelerations. Although the nurse must notify the physician as soon as a prolonged deceleration occurs, it does not automatically indicate cord prolapse or uncorrectable fetal distress.

Also known as a reflex bradycardia, prolonged decelerations occur in response to sudden stimulation of the vagal system by a vaginal examination, electrode application, or similar occurrence. They may persist for several minutes or longer. During deceleration, the FHR exhibits normal or increased variabililty. The vagal reflex itself may be caused by sudden hypoxemia with or without accompanying carbon dioxide retention and acidosis.

Other common factors also may trigger the vagal reflex that causes prolonged decelerations. When contractions occur closer than every 2 minutes or the uterus develops hypertonus, the sustained pressure on the fetus triggers the vagal reflex and decelerates the FHR. Variability also may increase. While the stimulus is operating, the FHR remains decelerated, commonly at 60 to 90 beats/minute.

Using amnioinfusion to relieve repetitive variable decelerations

According to recent studies, amnioinfusion has proven consistently effective in relieving persistent and severe variable decelerations after all other interventions have failed. A subsequent study conducted at Sinai Samaritan Health Center in Milwaukee, Wisconsin has supported this finding.

In the two cases cited in the Sinai Samaritan study, both clients presented with preterm premature rupture of the membranes, one at approximately 28 weeks' gestation and the other at 33½ weeks'. One client was febrile, and her amniotic fluid was positive for gram-negative diplococci (later confirmed as *Neisseria gonorrhoeae*). Uterine activity was absent in one client; the other was admitted with regular contractions 5 minutes apart.

In both clients, fetal monitoring showed persistent variable decelerations. These decelerations were reduced significantly by administration of 3,500 to 5,500 ml of normal saline solution through amnioinfusion over a 3-hour period. Both neonates were delivered without complications. Apgar scores were 6 and 3 at 1 minute after birth and 7 and 7 at 5 minutes after birth. The neonate whose mother was febrile during labor showed mild respiratory distress syndrome.

Application to practice

Based on these study results, amnioinfusion appears to decrease variable decelerations during labor. With proper preparation, and as health care facility protocols allow, the nurse could use amnioinfusion to improve the metabolic state of a preterm fetus whose mother experiences premature rupture of the membranes, possibly obviating the need for cesarean delivery.

Galvan, B., Van Mullem, C., and Broekhuizen, F. (1989). Using amnioinfusion for the relief of repetitive variable decelerations during labor. *JOGNN*, 18(3), 222-229.

In addition, such routine procedures as a vaginal examination and fetal scalp electrode application may trigger a prolonged deceleration. The vaginal examination can cause a temporary uterine tachysystole from prostaglandin release caused by manual manipulation of the cervix. Pressure on the fetal head when the scalp electrode is attached can stimulate the vagal reflex.

Prolonged decelerations also can be caused by such drugs as bupivacaine and lidocaine when used for regional (epidural and caudal) and paracervical blocks. These drugs temporarily increase uterine tone and contraction frequency, which can decrease the FHR. Also, maternal supine hypotension syndrome may cause prolonged decelerations.

Maternal pushing in the second stage of labor puts pressure on the fetus's body. This pressure can trigger a vagal reaction, particularly in the last few minutes before birth. This is one way labor personnel know de-

livery is imminent.

When prolonged decelerations occur, the nurse first must assess for cord prolapse or imminent delivery. If the client is receiving oxytocin, the nurse should discontinue the drug as prescribed and perform or assist with a vaginal examination. If the examination reveals a pulsating cord, the nurse should intervene using traditional techniques. (For more information, see *Emergency alert: Cord prolapse* in Chapter 33, Intrapartal Complications.) Katz, et al. (1988) also recommend intervening by rapidly filling the bladder with 500 to 700 ml of normal saline solution to elevate the presenting part and using tocolytics to halt contractions.

If the vaginal examination rules out cord prolapse and imminent delivery, the nurse should assess the client and monitor strip. Uterine hypertonus from oxytocin, anesthetics, or pushing during the second stage of labor can cause prolonged decelerations.

If the deceleration is the result of uterine hypertonus, drugs, or maternal pushing, the nurse should stay with the client and ask another nurse to call the physician, then stop the oxytocin, turn the client on her left side, tell her to stop pushing, administer oxygen by mask, and increase the I.V. fluid rate as prescribed.

In most cases, the deceleration corrects itself in 10 minutes, and the fetus resuscitates itself in 30 to 60 minutes after deceleration ends. During recovery, the FHR shows baseline tachycardia and a few late decelerations. Because tachycardia is a compensatory mechanism that aids fetal reoxygenation, it is a reassuring sign after a prolonged deceleration. The late decelerations verify that the fetus has just experienced hypoxia; they disappear as the fetus recovers.

Other fetal assessment techniques

Although a normal FHR pattern during labor is a reliable indicator of fetal well-being, an abnormal pattern does not always signal distress. Several tests exist to distinguish the fetus that is in danger from the fetus that exhibits an abnormal pattern requiring no intervention. These tests are performed by the physician or nurse-midwife.

Fetal scalp blood sampling test

At times, fetal hypoxia is suggested by a confusing FHR pattern, such as a sustained flat heart rate without late decelerations. In this case, fetal scalp blood sampling—a process for evaluating the fetus's acid-base status—can be used with fetal monitoring to assess fetal status. When vaginal delivery is anticipated within 30 to 60 minutes but the FHR shows uncorrectable late decelerations with normal variability, fetal scalp sampling can indicate that a cesarean delivery may not be necessary.

Fetal scalp stimulation test

Clark, Gimovsky, and Miller (1984) have suggested that more widespread use of the fetal scalp stimulation test could reduce by half the need for fetal scalp blood sampling. A positive (or reactive) response to stimulating the fetal scalp, either with gentle digital pressure or by applying an Allis clamp, is considered a reliable indicator of fetal well-being. A positive response is marked by an acceleration of the FHR by 15 beats/minute for at least 15 seconds.

Fetal acoustic stimulation test

The fetal acoustic stimulation (FAS) test, also called the vibratory acoustic stimulation test, may be a promising alternative to fetal scalp blood sampling. A positive test for FAS eliminates the need for the more invasive and difficult-to-perform scalp sampling procedure.

In FAS, an electrolarynx vibratory device used at 80 decibels is applied to the client's abdomen for 3 seconds. The sound and vibrations cause an accelerated FHR. A positive result, indicated by an FHR acceleration of at least 15 beats/minute above the baseline FHR for at least 15 seconds occurring two or more times within 10 minutes, indicates fetal well-being. Smith, Nguyen, Phelan, and Paul (1986) found that no fetus with a positive test result had a pH less than 7.25, which is considered within the normal range.

Nursing responsibility

According to nursing practice standards, the nurse using EFM when caring for a client in labor is held legally responsible for any procedures performed. This means that the nurse is responsible for recognizing abnormal fetal heart patterns and uterine activity, intervening appropriately, and notifying the physician or nurse-midwife whenever necessary. To meet this responsibility,

the nurse must have received the special preparation needed to perform EFM procedures and interpret results.

The nurse can be held liable for preparing a client for a procedure to which she did not consent. Therefore, once the physician has explained the procedure and informed consent has been obtained, the nurse must make sure that the client fully understands the procedure that will be performed.

If a nonreassuring pattern occurs, standards of care dictate that the nurse notify the physician or nurse-midwife and then intervene appropriately to prevent further deterioration of fetal status. If the physician does not respond in a timely fashion, the nurse must follow the policy established by the health care facility. In most cases, this means informing the nurse-manager, who can intervene as necessary.

Client teaching and support

Childbirth education classes now typically introduce EFM to pregnant clients and discuss its advantages and disadvantages. The nurse should ask the client what she knows about fetal monitoring. The greatest resistance to EFM typically comes from clients who do not understand its purpose. As simply as possible, the nurse should explain how evaluating FHR and uterine contractions can identify possible sources of danger to the fetus, emphasizing that a normal FHR is a highly reliable indicator of fetal well-being.

Also, the nurse should describe how EFM can assist the client during labor and delivery by helping her time the frequency and duration of contractions. While watching the monitor, the client can see contractions begin and know when to begin her paced breathing; she can see when the peak arrives and know that the contraction will dissipate soon; and she can see the descent and know when to take her cleansing breath and relax.

The nurse should explain that EFM allows constant tracking of the FHR; even the nurse who is not in the room can view the tracing on the central display at the nursing station and evaluate the data.

Client teaching should include all the possible situations that may cause her undue anxiety. For example, before attaching the belt of a Doppler ultrasound, the nurse should discuss the kinds of information that this device provides. The client should hear the fetal heartbeat and understand that the normal heart rate varies. If the belt moves, the fetal heart tracing may change and the client may think the heart rate is too fast or slow. Therefore, the nurse should demonstrate how moving the belt can cause a false FHR reading. Turning off the microphone on the monitor will eliminate distracting noises.

Documentation checklist for fetal monitoring

When assessing the fetal monitor strip and documenting findings, the nurse should ask these questions:
• What is the frequency of contractions?
• How long do the contractions last?
• What is their intensity?
• What is the fetal baseline heart rate (BHR)?
• Is the fetal BHR within the normal range?
• If not, is baseline tachycardia or bradycardia present?
• Is long- or short-term fetal BHR variability present?
• Are accelerations present?
• Are decelerations present? If so, are they early, late, variable, or prolonged?
• Based on the monitor readings, have appropriate nursing interventions been performed and documented?
• What was the outcome of the interventions?

An unprepared client may become anxious while viewing variable deceleration patterns on the monitor. To help relieve this anxiety, the nurse should explain variable decelerations, discuss the possible causes of cord compression, and reassure the client that the typical fetus can tolerate it. To demonstrate to the client that the fetus is not endangered by a brief oxygen deficit, the nurse can ask the client or support person to take a deep breath and hold it for 30 seconds, then repeat, and then ask how he or she feels. When the client or support person answers "fine," the nurse can point out that the fetus feels the same.

Applying a fetal scalp electrode and an intrauterine pressure catheter also may cause anxiety about fetal injury. To allay these fears, the nurse should demonstrate the insertion of the scalp electrode so that the client can see that only the tip of the wire slips under the fetal scalp, and explain that the procedure is no more painful than sticking a pin into a thick or calloused area of the finger. The nurse should explain that if the heart rate transmission stops suddenly after the electrode is in place, the electrode has probably fallen off and that this is no cause for alarm.

Before the intrauterine catheter is inserted, the nurse should use an unsterile sample to demonstrate how soft and pliable it is and show the client an illustration of where the catheter is placed in the uterus. The nurse should explain the function of the catheter and the need for data on the strength of contractions, particularly if the client is receiving oxytocin.

Despite the advantages of EFM, the nurse should remember that the client is the focus of the care. She needs to feel that the nurse is monitoring and concerned about her, not a machine. Despite the seeming intrusiveness of technology, the nurse's sensitivity can make even a complicated labor a humane and enriching experience for the client.

Documentation

The monitor strip is considered a vital part of the medical record. Therefore, the nurse must document all assessments, procedures, and interventions on the monitor strip as well as on the chart. If time is short, the nurse should make the monitor strip the primary place to document because it provides a chronological record of events.

Every health care facility should have a manual of terms and abbreviations for EFM. To avoid legal difficulties, the nurse should use only these terms on the chart and the monitor strip in documenting fetal assessments and interventions. For example, the nurse cannot merely describe a late, variable, or early deceleration on the chart. Rather, the nurse should call the deceleration or any periodic change by its specific name in charting and in all communication with the physician. (For a list of points to cover when documenting EFM tracings, see *Documentation checklist for fetal monitoring*.)

Chapter summary

Chapter 25 discussed the physiologic basis of fetal monitoring, described fetal and uterine activity monitoring, explained fetal heart rate patterns and assessment techniques, and discussed nursing responsibilities associated with fetal monitoring, client teaching, and documentation. Here are the chapter highlights.
• Uncompromised uteroplacental-fetal circulation is essential to fetal well-being. It is affected by maternal position, uterine contractions, placental surface area and diffusion distance, anesthetics, maternal hypertension and hypotension, and cord compression.
• Fetal heart rate is monitored with a fetoscope, ultrasound stethoscope, or external or internal electronic devices.
• Uterine activity is monitored with manual palpation, the external tocodynamometer, the internal intrauterine pressure catheter, or telemetry.
• Important FHR patterns include baseline tachycardia and bradycardia, long- and short-term variability, accelerations, and decelerations (early, late, variable, and prolonged).
• Nursing assessment plays a critical role in identifying abnormal FHR patterns that may jeopardize fetal well-being and intervening as necessary.

• Other fetal assessment techniques include three tests: fetal scalp blood sampling, fetal scalp stimulation, and fetal acoustic stimulation.

• The nurse is responsible for teaching the client about activities and equipment that may be used during fetal assessment.

• The nurse must accurately and completely document all nursing activities during the client's care, using nursing diagnoses and terms appropriate to the health care facility.

Study questions

1. Sarah Blackstone, age 29, is admitted to the labor and delivery area in active labor with ruptured membranes. She is at 43 weeks' gestation and has had three previous pregnancies, two of which resulted in births. Her vital signs are normal. What are the indications for EFM?

2. Which type of monitoring would be most appropriate for Mrs. Blackstone? Why?

3. Answer the following questions based on Mrs. Blackstone's monitoring strip below:

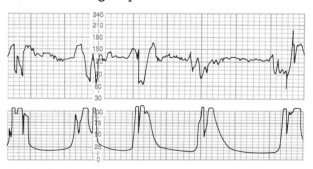

a. What is the baseline fetal heart rate?
b. What is the short- and long-term variability?
c. Which periodic pattern does this strip represent?
d. Is the pattern reassuring or nonreassuring?
e. In what stage of labor is Mrs. Blackstone?

4. Based on Mrs. Blackstone's monitoring strip, which nursing interventions would be appropriate, if any?

5. What are the NAACOG guidelines for auscultation of the FHR that the nurse should be familiar with and use to guide nursing practice?

Bibliography

ACOG. (1989). *Assessment of fetal and newborn acid-base* (Technical Bulletin No. 127.) Washington, DC: Author.

Cunningham, F.G., MacDonald, P., and Gant, N. (1989). *William's obstetrics* (18th ed.). East Norwalk, CT: Appleton & Lange.

Marshall, C. (1985). The art of induction/augmentation of labor. *JOGNN,* 14(1), 22-28.

Fetal monitoring

Blank, J. (1985). Electronic fetal monitoring: Nursing management defined. *JOGNN,* 14(6), 463-467.

Boehm, F., and Fields, L. (1984). Second-generation EFM is waiting in the wings. *Contemporary Ob/Gyn,* 23(3), 179-188.

Clark, S. (1989). Do we still need fetal scalp blood sampling? *Contemporary Ob/Gyn,* 33(3), 75-86.

Clark, S., Gimovsky, M., and Miller, F. (1984). Scalp stimulation test: A clinical alternative to fetal scalp blood sampling. *American Journal of Obstetrics and Gynecology,* 148(3), 274-277.

Fields, L.M., and Boehm, F.H. (1989). Changing issues in FHR monitoring. *Contemporary Ob/Gyn,* 33 (special issue), 145-148.

Freeman, R., and Garite, T. (1981). *Fetal heart rate monitoring.* Baltimore: Williams & Wilkins.

Gibbs, R., Jones, P., and Wilder, C. (1978). Internal fetal monitoring and maternal infection following cesarean section: A prospective study. *Obstetrics and Gynecology,* 52(2), 193-197.

Grylack, L. (1983). To maintain perinatal glucose/insulin homeostasis. *Contemporary Ob/Gyn,* 21(6), 113-124.

Hall, M., and Alexander, C. (1982). Fetal monitoring in a community hospital: Analysis of health maintenance organization fee for service and clinic populations. *American Journal of Obstetrics and Gynecology,* 143(3), 277-285.

Katz, Z., Shoham, Z., Lancet, M., Blickstein, I., Mogilner, B.M., and Zalel, Y. (1988). Management of labor with umbilical cord prolapse: A 5-year study. *Obstetrics and Gynecology,* 72(2), 278-281.

Krebs, H.B., Petres, R.E., and Dunn, L.J. (1983). Intrapartum fetal heart rate monitoring: VII. Atypical variable decelerations. *American Journal of Obstetrics and Gynecology,* 145(3), 297-305.

Lagrew, D., and Garite, T. (1984). Technology 1985: Reviewing the latest in fetal monitoring equipment. *Contemporary Ob/Gyn,* 24(special issue), 91-106.

Laeveno, K., Cunningham, F.G., Nelson, S., Roark, M., Williams, M.L., Guzick, D., Dowling, S., Rosenfeld, C., and Buckley, A. (1986). A prospective comparison of selective and universal electronic fetal monitoring in 34,995 pregnancies. *New England Journal of Medicine,* 315(10), 615-619.

MacDonald, D., et al. (1985). The Dublin randomized controlled trial of intrapartum fetal heart rate monitoring. *American Journal of Obstetrics and Gynecology,* 152(5), 524-539.

Miller, F., Pearse, K., and Paul, R. (1984). Fetal heart rate pattern recognition by the method of auscultation. *Obstetrics and Gynecology,* 64(3), 332-336.

Montgomery, J. (1986). Technology 1987: Advantages of the IU catheter and fetal spiral electrode. *Contemporary Ob/Gyn,* 28 (special issue), 75-84.

Parer, J.T. (1984). Fetal heart rate. In R.K. Creasy and R. Resnik (Eds.), *Maternal/fetal medicine: Principles and practice.* Philadelphia: Saunders.

Queenan, J., Clark, S., Freeman, R., Johnson, T., and Paul, R. (1988). Symposium: Today's high C/S rate: Can we reduce it? *Contemporary Ob/Gyn,* 32(1), 154-166.

Rice, P., and Benedetti, T. (1986). Fetal heart rate acceleration with fetal scalp blood sampling. *Obstetrics and Gynecology,* 68(4), 469-472.

Sarno, A., and Phelan, J. (1988). Intrauterine resuscitation of the fetus. *Contemporary Ob/Gyn,* 32(1), 143-152.

Smith, C., Nguyen, H.N., Phelan, J., and Paul, R. (1986). Intrapartum assessment of fetal well-being: A comparison of fetal acoustic stimulation with acid-base determinations. *American Journal of Obstetrics and Gynecology,* 155(4), 726-728.

Wagner, P., Cabaniss, M., and Johnson, T. (1985). Technology 1986: What's really new in EFM equipment? *Contemporary Ob/Gyn,* 26(special issue), 91-106.

Wood, C., Renou, P., Oats, J., Farrell, E., Beischer, N., and Anderson, I. (1981). A controlled trial of fetal heart rate monitoring in a low-risk obstetric population. *American Journal of Obstetrics and Gynecology,* 141(5), 527-534.

Yeh, S., Diaz, F., and Paul, R. (1982). Ten-year experience of intrapartum fetal monitoring in Los Angeles County–University of Southern California Medical Center. *American Journal of Obstetrics and Gynecology,* 143(5), 496-500.

Zalar, R.W., and Quilligan, E.J. (1979). The influence of scalp sampling on the cesarean section rate for fetal distress. *American Journal of Obstetrics and Gynecology,* 135(2), 239-246.

Nursing responsibilities

Beck, C. (1980). Patient acceptance of fetal monitoring as a helpful tool. *JOGNN,* 9(6), 350-353.

Dulock, H., and Herron, M. (1976). Women's response to fetal monitoring. *JOGNN,* 5(Suppl. 5), 68-70.

Molfese, V., Sunshine, P., and Bennett, A. (1982). Reactions of women to intrapartum fetal monitoring. *Obstetrics and Gynecology,* 59(6), 705-709.

NAACOG. (1988). Statement: Nursing responsibilities in implementing intrapartum fetal heart rate monitoring. Washington, DC: Author.

NAACOG. (1990). OGN nursing practice resource fetal heart rate auscultation. Washington, DC: Author.

Nursing research

Chez, B., Skurnick, J., Chez, R., Verklan, M., Biggs, S., and Hage, M. (1990). Interpretations of nonstress tests by obstetric nurses. *JOGNN,* 19(3), 227-232.

Galvan, B., Van Mullem, C., and Broekhuizen, F. (1989). Using amnioinfusion for the relief of repetitive variable decelerations during labor. *JOGNN,* 18(3), 222-229.

Moenning, R., and Hill, W. (1987). A randomized study comparing two methods of performing the breast stimulation test. *JOGNN,* 16(4), 253-257.

Comfort Promotion during Labor and Childbirth

Objectives

After reading and studying this chapter, the student should be able to:

1. Describe the locations and characteristics of pain typically felt during each stage of labor.

2. Identify factors that affect a client's response to pain during labor.

3. Describe techniques that promote comfort during labor.

4. Discuss nonpharmacologic methods to relieve labor pain.

5. List analgesic and anesthetic agents used to reduce labor pain and discuss their characteristics, administration routes, and adverse effects.

6. Apply the nursing process when caring for a client experiencing labor pain.

Introduction

Few women experience painless labor. In fact, many describe it as intolerable, crushing, grueling, and searing. In a study of 78 primiparous clients, 28% reported moderate pain during labor and childbirth; 37%, severe pain; and 35%, intolerable pain (Nettelbladt, 1976). A larger, international study of primiparous and multiparous clients reported that 15% experienced little or no pain; 35% moderate pain; 30%, severe pain; and 20%, very severe pain (Bonica, 1989).

Pain experienced during normal labor follows a predictable cycle of peaks and valleys. Despite its predictable course, however, each client perceives labor pain as a unique, personal experience based on her physical condition, pain tolerance, and psychological background. The nurse must collaborate with other health care providers to assess the client's perception of pain and the degree of comfort achieved through therapy. This chapter begins by describing the type and location of pain typically experienced during each stage of labor. It then presents assessment considerations for the client experiencing labor pain, psychological and physical comfort measures, nonpharmacologic techniques for pain reduction, and pharmacologic options for pain relief.

Pain during labor

Even though each client responds to pain uniquely, nursing interventions can help reduce pain perception and alter pain response for most clients. To intervene properly, the nurse should understand the type of pain typically experienced during labor, physical and psychological factors that influence pain perception, and how observation of behavior patterns can clarify a client's response to pain.

During the first stage of labor, pain results primarily from cervical effacement and dilation. At 0 to 3 cm of cervical dilation, the client may describe the pain as an ache or discomfort; at 4 to 7 cm, as moderately sharp; at 7 to 10 cm, as severe, sharp, and cramping.

During the second stage of labor, pain results from friction between the fetus and birth canal and from

GLOSSARY

Acupressure: pressure on specific body points to promote energy flow and relieve pain.

Acupuncture: insertion of needles at specific body points to promote energy flow and relieve pain.

Agonist: substance that stimulates physiologic activity at cell receptors that are normally stimulated by naturally occurring substances.

Algesia: hypersensitivity to pain; hyperesthesia.

Analgesia: reduction of pain without loss of consciousness.

Anesthesia: loss of sensation (total or partial) with or without loss of consciousness.

Antagonist: substance that blocks the action of another, such as a drug, by binding to a cell receptor without causing a physiologic response.

Blood-brain barrier: membrane that prevents harmful substances in the blood, such as anesthetic agents, from penetrating brain tissue.

Effleurage: rhythmic, light abdominal stroking used in some forms of massage and in Lamaze childbirth preparation classes. During labor, effleurage can help distract the client and decrease her pain.

Endogenous opiate theory: hypothesis that says natural pain inhibitors found in the central nervous system bind at pain receptor sites and block transmission of pain impulses.

Epidural block: most common regional anesthesia technique, in which an anesthetic agent is injected into the the the epidural space between the dura mater and ligamentum flavum.

Gate control theory: hypothesis that stimulation of larger-diameter, faster-traveling nerve fibers can block pain impulses carried on smaller-diameter, slower-traveling fibers, thus closing a gate that stops or modifies pain transmission.

Inhalation analgesia: anesthetic agent inhaled in small concentrations to produce analgesia without loss of consciousness.

Paracervical block: regional anesthesia technique that blocks nerve conduction on both sides of the cervix, relieving uterine pain during the first stage of active labor.

Pudendal block: regional anesthesia technique used during the second stage of labor to numb the perineum and vagina, primarily for episiotomy repair.

Regional anesthesia: direct nerve block following injection of a local anesthetic agent.

Transcutaneous electric nerve stimulation (TENS): use of electric current to counterstimulate nerve fibers and thus block pain transmission.

pressure on the perineum, bladder, bowel, and uterine ligaments.

During the third stage of labor, pain results from ischemia caused by contraction of uterine blood vessels. Impulses are transmitted as in the first stage—through the sympathetic nervous system to thoracic and lumbar vertebrae (T10 to L1). Cervical dilation may perpetuate pain until the placenta has been expelled. (For illustrations of each stage, see *Pain locations and intensity during labor.*)

Factors that influence labor pain

Many factors affect a client's perception of and ability to cope with pain. These factors may be physiologic, social, or psychological; they include parity, fetal size and position, certain medical procedures, anxiety, fatigue, education level, cultural influence, and coping mechanisms. Knowledge of these influences can help the nurse anticipate, assess, and meet client needs.

Parity
The primiparous client typically experiences longer, more painful labor than the multiparous client, for two reasons. First, the primiparous client's cervix requires greater stretching force because it has never been

stretched. This may require contractions of greater intensity during the first stage of labor. Second, the primiparous client may experience increased anxiety and doubt about her ability to tolerate labor pain, feelings that in themselves may focus attention on the pain. Later in labor, the multiparous client typically experiences more intense contractions than the primiparous client (Bonica, 1989); however, experience and previous cervical changes increase the client's ability to cope.

Fetal size and position
A large fetus may disrupt uterine contractions or arrest active labor. Persistent posterior fetal positions also may disrupt contraction efficiency, prolong labor, or cause severe backache by exerting increased pressure on the sacrum.

Medical procedures
Certain procedures, such as augmentation or induction of labor, may affect a client's response to labor pain. Oxytocin—a drug used commonly to augment or induce labor—reportedly creates stronger, more uncomfortable contractions that peak more abruptly than spontaneous contractions. Other actions that increase discomfort include performing a vaginal examination on a supine client, using a tight abdominal belt to secure a fetal

Pain locations and intensity during labor

The nurse can use the illustrations below to anticipate and monitor the client's pain during labor. In each picture, darker color indicates more intense pain. During most of stage 1, pain centers around the pelvic girdle. During late stage 1 and early stage 2, pain spreads to the upper legs and perineum. During late stage 2 and childbirth, intense pain develops at the perineum.

STAGE 1

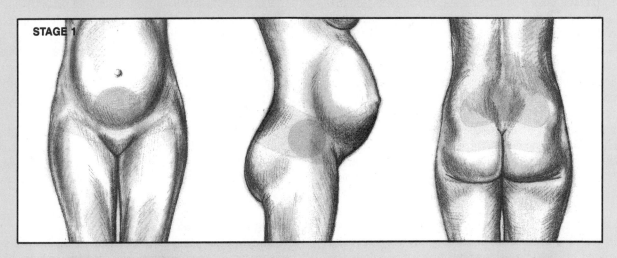

LATE STAGE 1 and EARLY STAGE 2

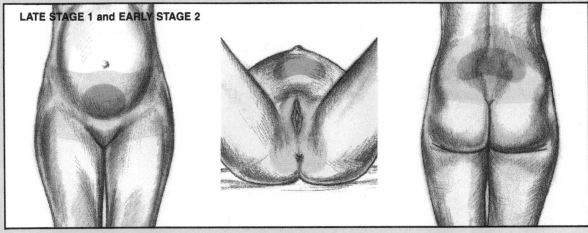

LATE STAGE 2 and DELIVERY

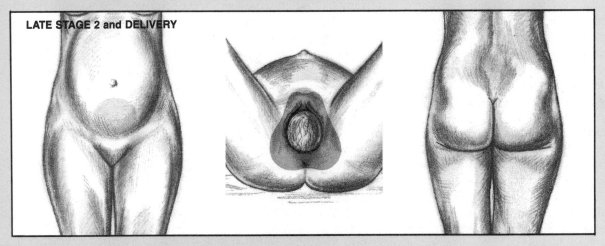

monitor, forbidding a client to change positions or walk, and administering an enema, which may produce intestinal and uterine contractions (Jimenez, 1983).

Anxiety

By impeding normal cervical dilation, excessive anxiety may prolong labor and increase pain perception. An anxious client will experience increased cardiac output and blood pressure, and may face increased risk of the following:

• decreased gastrointestinal function, which can reduce gastric emptying and increase the risk of aspiration

• decreased urinary function, which may result in oliguria

• increased levels of epinephrine and norepinephrine (hormones that typically prepare the body for the "fight or flight" response), which may prolong labor, cause hyperventilation, and result in fetal hypoxia. During sustained pain, norepinephrine can decrease blood flow to the uterus by 35% to 70% (Bonica, 1989). Epinephrine increases vasoconstriction and decreases uterine activity.

• increased plasma levels of cortisol (a steroid hormone secreted by the adrenal cortex), which has been associated with longer labor and decreased uterine activity (Lederman, Lederman, Work, and McCann, 1978).

Some anxious clients—particularly those with little childbirth education—may be especially susceptible to escalating anxiety characterized by the fear-tension-pain cycle (Dick-Read, 1970; Jimenez, 1983). Fear and anxiety increase muscle tension, resulting in vasospasm-induced ischemia, which causes pain. This in turn increases anxiety. Education and preparation for labor may reduce fear and anxiety, thus breaking the fear-tension-pain cycle.

Fatigue

Especially if aggravated by sleep deprivation, fatigue may intensify a client's perception of pain during labor and reduce her coping ability. The client may become more tense and anxious if exhaustion prevents her from using learned pain-reduction methods. An exhausted client in a prolonged latent phase may require sedation to relieve anxiety and induce sleep. Anemia, which may accompany pregnancy, worsens feelings of fatigue.

Education

Clients with childbirth education (physical and psychological) experience less fear, tension, and stress during labor; typically, they require less pain medication. After childbirth, these clients tend to have significantly more positive attitudes toward their neonates (Klusman, 1975; Tanzer and Block, 1987). Further, partners educated in childbirth techniques feel a greater sense of control during labor than those not educated. (See Chapter 21, Family Preparation for Childbirth and Parenting, for more information about education methods aimed at reducing labor pain.)

Culture

A client's cultural background might be expected to influence her behavior during labor, but studies show that culture actually has little effect on how women perceive and react to labor pain; education is the primary factor. Bonica (1989) found that women in Europe, Latin America, Asia, Australia, the Near East, and North America with similar levels of childbirth education exhibited similar verbal, facial, and physical expressions during labor.

The nurse should avoid stereotyping or judging clients by personal standards on such issues as self-control and acceptable modes of expression. Try to view each client's actions according to her own cultural and personal standards.

Coping mechanisms

Normally, people learn to cope with pain through experience, drawing on previously learned coping behaviors when pain recurs. This is one reason why multiparous clients may cope with labor pain more successfully than primparous clients.

Conversely, some painful experiences produce anxiety and fear, possibly affecting the client's self-image and confidence. The nurse should support the client through the pain and remain nonjudgmental.

Behavioral responses to labor pain

Early in labor, during the latent phase, the client typically can respond to teaching and interventions because contractions have not become intensely painful. The transition to active labor, which may be subtle or obvious, typically marks the point when pain alters the client's behavioral responses. She may lose the ability to focus attention, have difficulty following instructions, and forget proper breathing techniques. She also may withdraw from social interaction, yet fear being abandoned or left alone even for brief periods.

By monitoring for reactions common to women in labor, the nurse can gauge the comfort promotion needs of each client. Such reactions include:

• facial grimacing

• muscle tension and grunting (with bearing-down efforts)

• increased blood pressure, pulse rate, and respirations

• desire for personal contact and touch in early active labor

• withdrawal, irritability, and resistance to touch during the transition to active labor.

Based on the client's physical and emotional responses, the nurse may employ various techniques to promote comfort, along with nonpharmacologic and pharmacologic methods of pain relief. The remaining sections of this chapter explain pain assessment during labor, applicable nursing diagnoses, and selection and implementation of comfort promotion and pain-reduction measures.

Nursing care

To provide care for the client in labor, the nurse must be familiar with various nonpharmacologic and pharmacologic pain-relief methods. As always, the nursing process provides a systematic framework for individualized care. (For a care plan on comfort promotion, see *Applying the nursing process: Client with pain related to active labor*, pages 644 and 645.)

Assessment

Assessment of a client experiencing labor pain includes three parts. First is the health history, which investigates any medical factor that could affect the safety or efficacy of pain-reducing pharmacologic agents, plus ongoing questions about the client's pain perception. Second is physical assessment, which includes the client, the fetus, and labor progress. Third is follow-up assessment, performed after implementing pain-relief measures to determine their effectiveness.

Health history
Review the client's medical history, asking specifically about medication allergies and any obstetric problems that could affect the choice of pain-relief methods. Determine how much the client knows about childbirth and pain-relief measures, ask about previous experiences with pain and pain-relieving agents, and assess the client's current pain level and psychological reaction to it.

Check carefully for chronic and acute illnesses that could affect labor progress or place the client at risk, including hypertension (chronic or pregnancy-induced), diabetes mellitus, bleeding disorders, complications of pregnancy, chronic respiratory disease, and severe dehydration. A client with one of these conditions may require such special measures as I.V. fluid administration, cardiac and hemodynamic monitoring, or continual nursing assessment when a pain-relief agent is used

during labor. (For more information on selected disorders, see Chapter 31, High-Risk Intrapartal Clients.)

If the client has pregnancy-induced hypertension (PIH), uteroplacental perfusion may be inadequate and gas exchange may be poor. In mild cases of PIH, most analgesic and anesthetic options remain available as long as fetal assessment reveals no signs of compromise. However, regional anesthesia increases the risk of hypotension, which may cause hypoxia in the client and fetus.

If the client has diabetes mellitus with no evidence of fetal distress, small doses of narcotic analgesics or an epidural block (discussed in detail later in the chapter) may be used for pain relief. The client will require continuous fetal monitoring, glucose surveillance, and vital sign assessment because of an increased risk of PIH.

The client with placenta previa or abruptio placentae may require caesarean delivery. The anesthesia used depends on the presence or absence of active bleeding and fetal distress. Assess for a history of any chronic respiratory disease, which could cause respiratory depression in the anesthetized client. Also note renal or liver disease, which may affect the metabolism of some agents, possibly resulting in toxicity.

Consider the client's obstetric history when assessing the need for pain-relief measures. Pertinent assessment topics include the length of previous labors, the client's perception of previous labor pain, pain-relief measures used in previous labors, and the client's perception of their effectiveness.

Some obstetric problems may recur in successive pregnancies, resulting in longer, more painful labor or possibly necessitating surgical intervention. These include persistent posterior fetal position and cephalopelvic disproportion.

Ask if the client and her partner have attended childbirth education classes. If so, they will have some knowledge of the labor process, coping techniques, and comfort measures. Specifically, assess the client's knowledge of relaxation techniques, positioning, and pharmacologic options for pain relief. Assess the client's reaction to her partner, if he is present. Is he helpful and supportive? Is his anxiety level disturbing to the client?

Physical assessment
When evaluating possible implementation of comfort promotion or pain-relief measures, consider maternal status, fetal status, and labor progress.

Maternal status. At frequent intervals during labor, ask the client to rate her level of pain using a scale from 1 (lowest) to 10 (highest). In addition, observe her spontaneous verbal and nonverbal expressions to assess dis-

FETAL STATUS

Fetal physiologic factors that affect drug choice

Certain fetal body systems, such as the renal system, mature less rapidly than others. Rates of development as well as fetal physiology must be evaluated before the physician or nurse-midwife selects pain-relief agents for the client.

- A fetus with an immature blood-brain barrier has increased risk for high drug concentrations in the central nervous system.
- An immature fetus will have less plasma protein available to bind with analgesic and anesthetic agents. As a result, the plasma concentration of free (active) drug is increased.
- A fetus with an immature liver has insufficient enzymes to metabolize such agents.
- A fetus with an immature renal system cannot excrete analgesic and anesthetic agents.

comfort. Keep in mind that excessive anxiety may impede cervical dilation; a small dose of an analgesic agent may relax an anxious client sufficiently to allow cervical dilation and shorten labor.

Fetal status. Carefully consider fetal age and development before administering prescribed pain-relief agents. An immature fetus has a diminished ability to metabolize analgesic or anesthetic agents used to reduce labor pain; the physician or nurse-midwife must carefully consider fetal status before drug administration. (For specific guidelines, see *Fetal status: Fetal physiologic factors that affect drug choice.*)

Heart rate offers the primary indicator of fetal well-being. Obtain and document baseline fetal heart rate and pattern before pharmacologic measures are instituted. (For more information, see Chapter 25, Fetal Assessment.)

Labor progress. Before implementing prescribed pain-relief measures, consider labor progress. Certain factors, such as side-lying positioning or epidural anesthesia, may slow labor. Also consider contraction intensity, frequency, and duration to help determine the need for pain relief. (For more information, see Chapter 27, The First Stage of Labor.)

Assess cervical dilation to ensure that pharmacologic agents are given at the safest times during labor. Systemic narcotics may be given for analgesia during the first stage of labor, but may prolong labor if administered too early in the latent phase. Antianxiety agents

also may be used in the latent phase to decrease anxiety and fear. Timing is essential to achieve appropriate pain relief without adversely affecting the fetus.

Follow-up assessment

To determine the effectiveness and safety of comfort promotion and pain-relief measures, continue to assess the client and fetus throughout labor. Observe maternal and fetal vital signs frequently (especially respirations), assess the client's cardiovascular response, and watch for such adverse drug reactions as vomiting, itching, and drowsiness.

Pain relief. Assess pain relief continually during nonpharmacologic measures and at 30-minute intervals after analgesic administration. Pain should abate almost immediately after administration of an anesthetic. Assess the duration and degree of pain relief to help anticipate additional pain-relief measures.

Effects on client and fetus. Assess the client's level of consciousness, respiratory rate, blood pressure, and pulse rate. Narcotic analgesics can cause drowsiness that may interfere with effective bearing-down efforts in the second stage of labor. Narcotic analgesics also may produce respiratory depression and hypotension.

To prevent maternal injury, assess for adverse drug reactions (such as nausea and vomiting) and allergic reactions (such as pruritus, urticaria, facial edema, and stridor). Watch for aspiration if a client made drowsy by narcotic analgesics begins to vomit.

After administering pharmacologic agents, assess fetal heart rate according to health care facility protocol. After birth, the neonate's muscle tone, color, and respirations will reflect the effects of pharmacologic agents used on the client. (For more information, see Chapter 36, Care of the Normal Neonate.)

Nursing diagnosis

After assessing the client and fetus, review the findings and formulate nursing diagnoses related to comfort promotion and pain relief. (For a partial list of applicable diagnoses, see *Nursing diagnoses: Comfort promotion.*)

Planning and implementation

The nurse provides or assists with comfort promotion and pain-reduction measures when caring for a client in labor. Methods used to maintain or improve comfort include general comfort measures and relaxation techniques. The client with no childbirth education and little knowledge of labor may need extra attention and help to maintain comfort. Pain reduction may involve nonpharmacologic techniques, pharmacologic agents, or both.

Comfort measures

Intervene to decrease anxiety, promote hygiene, and help the client find comfortable positions that reduce labor pain and facilitate childbirth. Some clients find these actions adequate to maintain comfort throughout labor.

Decrease anxiety. As contractions grow more frequent and intense, anxiety increases. The client may fear withdrawal of support, abandonment, the unknown, or loss of control. Increased epinephrine and norepinephrine levels raise blood pressure and pulse, diminish myometrial activity, exhaust glucose reserves, and decrease adenosine triphosphate synthesis necessary for uterine contractions.

Anxiety also leads to tension, which may cause additional pain. For a client with a nursing diagnosis of *anxiety related to labor pain,* nursing interventions seek to reduce anxiety, thus decreasing blood pressure and heart rate, allowing greater energy production for effective uterine contractions, and reducing muscle tension and the heightened pain perception caused by tension.

The nurse's presence, confidence, attention, and concern help control the client's anxiety. As labor progresses, keep the client informed, teach and reinforce coping strategies, and assure the client that labor is progressing normally. If assessment reveals that labor is not progressing normally, notify the physician immediately. Reassure, encourage, and praise the client throughout labor. If she becomes discouraged or frustrated, reassure her and help her to choose an alternate method of comfort promotion.

Helping the client's partner also may help reduce the client's anxiety. Support the partner's efforts to comfort the client. Offer instructions and assistance as appropriate. (For more information, see Chapter 30, Family Support during the Intrapartal Period.)

Promote hygiene. Nursing interventions to maintain hygiene can increase the client's comfort level by boosting self-esteem, providing distraction, removing an additional source of discomfort (such as wet sheets), and blocking pain perception. For a client with a nursing diagnosis of *self-esteem disturbance related to inability to cope with labor pain or negative perception of behavior,* the nurse may implement the following hygiene measures.

Showers and bathing. Many labor and delivery areas have showers. A warm water massage (hydrotherapy) directed at the client's back promotes relaxation and counterstimulates pain transmission. Provide a stool in the

---

NURSING DIAGNOSES

Comfort promotion

The following list of potential nursing diagnoses are examples of the problems and etiologies that the nurse may encounter when caring for a client in labor. Specific nursing interventions for many of these diagnoses are provided in the "Planning and implementation" section of this chapter.

- Anxiety related to labor pain
- Decreased cardiac output related to epidural anesthesia
- Ineffective airway clearance related to general anesthesia
- Knowledge deficit related to analgesia and anesthesia options
- Pain related to the frequency and intensity of uterine contractions
- Self-esteem disturbance related to inability to cope with labor pain or negative perception of behavior
- Urine retention related to spinal anesthesia

---

shower and a supportive bar for the client to grasp or press against during contractions. Assist the client or ask her partner to assist her in the shower, as needed.

Perineal care. Clean the vulva after the client has a vaginal examination, urinates, or defecates. Provide a sanitary pad and belt to help the client feel secure while walking.

Oral hygiene. Provide frequent mouth care, as necessary. For a dry mouth, offer the client ice chips, mouthwash, or a toothbrush or apply a cool, moistened cloth to her lips. For dry lips, suggest petroleum jelly or lip balm.

Linens and clothing. Change soiled or damp linens and gowns frequently. Offer extra pillows for comfort and socks and additional clothing to prevent chilling. If the client grows warm during active labor, help her remove extra clothing.

Position the client for comfort. For a client with a nursing diagnosis of *pain related to the frequency and intensity of uterine contractions,* suggest that she change positions to enhance comfort. (For more information, see *Alternate positions for labor* in Chapter 27, The First Stage of Labor.) During the latent and early active stages, encourage the client to move about. A client in an upright position will have stronger, more regular, and more frequent contractions because gravity helps align the fetus with the pelvic angle as the uterus tilts forward with each contraction. Maintaining this position may shorten labor and reduce pain and medication requirements (Roberts, 1982).

As labor progresses and an upright position becomes uncomfortable, the client might alternate walking with sitting, side-lying, or kneeling to provide rest and vary the intensity and frequency of contractions. If she must remain in bed during labor because of obstetric or fetal conditions, such as premature rupture of membranes with unengaged presenting part or fetal distress, advise her to assume a side-lying position as often as possible to minimize fetal stress and enhance circulation.

Posterior fetal positions typically prolong labor and cause severe sacral pain (known as back labor). To encourage rotation of the presenting part to an anterior position, thus making the client more comfortable, take the following steps.
• Using Leopold's maneuvers, determine the position of the fetus's back. (For more information, see Chapter 27, The First Stage of Labor.) Direct the client to lie on the same side as the fetus's back with her upper leg propped on pillows.
• Advise the client to assume an all-fours position and to rock her pelvis to encourage fetal rotation and decrease pain. Kneeling or squatting also may be combined with pelvic rocking, but these positions can be uncomfortable and tiring for a client not accustomed to them.
• Suggest that the client straddle a chair or lean on her partner during contractions. During the second stage of labor, encourage her to use a squatting or side-lying position for pushing. Many birthing beds have squatting bars that allow the client to assume more comfortable, efficient positions for childbirth. After a contraction, the client can lean back on a supportive wedge or pillow until her next contraction begins. Squatting increases the pelvic angle by approximately 30% and enhances pushing efforts as the vagina widens and shortens. A side-lying position may slow descent in the second stage of labor, but it provides more effective relief for back pain than squatting.

Relaxation techniques

The goal of relaxation techniques is to reduce anxiety and muscle tension, thus quieting or calming the mind and muscles. Relaxation decreases oxygen consumption, heart rate, respiratory rate, arterial blood lactate concentration, and sympathetic nervous system activity (McCaffery and Beebe, 1989).

Typically, relaxation techniques distract the client from pain, increase her sense of control over the pain, and aid sleep and rest. However, not all techniques succeed with all clients; she may have to try several before finding relief. Even when a relaxation method succeeds, relief from fatigue may last only 5 to 20 minutes. Although these methods may reduce distress, they may not relieve pain. Assess whether and when the client needs analgesia or an anesthetic for pain reduction. If and when this becomes necessary, relaxation techniques may increase effectiveness.

Techniques used to promote relaxation include distraction, progressive muscle relaxation, yawning, controlled breathing, imagery, touch, and music therapy. (For more information on many of these techniques, see Chapter 21, Family Prepration for Childbirth and Parenting.) Ensure that the environment is conducive to relaxation. Remove the telephone, dim glaring lights, and maintain the room temperature at 68° to 70° F. Minimize unnecessary interruptions.

Distraction. Allowing the client to focus on pain or the fear of it can heighten pain perception. Conversely, distraction can decrease pain perception. Distraction from pain requires that the client focus on stimuli other than the pain sensation. For example, a client in labor may shield herself from contraction pain by focusing on music, rocking, singing to herself, visualizing a scene, or changing positions (McCaffery and Beebe, 1989). Early in labor, forms of distraction could include playing cards, reading, playing a board game, or watching television.

Imagery. Using the imagination to develop sensory images may decrease pain intensity, provide distraction from pain, and increase pain tolerance. Suggest ways that the client can develop relaxing images. Encourage her to imagine being in a peaceful place or being massaged by a gentle flow of water. Use words or phrases that convey pain-relieving images (McCaffery and Beebe, 1989).

Progressive muscle relaxation. This method of alternately tensing and relaxing groups of muscles from head to toe can relax the entire body. Relief of muscle tension reduces pain.

Controlled breathing. Deliberate, controlled breathing decreases anxiety, heart rate, blood pressure, and muscle tension; it also increases oxygenation for the client and the fetus. Concentration on breathing may distract the client from her pain. Help her use breathing techniques that work best for her as labor progresses.

Yawning. By stretching the facial muscles, yawning stimulates cardiac activity, increases oxygen in the blood, and expands the lungs. Instruct the client to assume a comfortable position, close her eyes, tense all her muscles, clench her fists, breathe in deeply, and hold it for a few moments. She should yawn as she releases the tension.

Touch. For the typical client, touch conveys a sense of caring and helps aid relaxation. Wiping the client's brow, assisting with effleurage, or massaging her back can reduce tension and increase relaxation. Applying firm pressure may relieve pain. Kneading and stroking muscles improves circulation.

Some clients dislike being touched or massaged, particularly when contractions become more intense or as they enter the transition phase. Be sure to identify which types of touch will help. Light touch, for example, can cause pain in a client under stress because it activates the free nerve endings associated with hair follicles or C fibers (the same pathway as pain transmission). Moderate touch and massage, however, activate the large-diameter A-delta fibers, which close a hypothetical gate to the small pain-carrying C fibers and block the pain message before it reaches the brain. (For more information, see *Theories of pain transmission.*) Examples of this type of touch and massage include hand and foot massage, back rubs, and kneading shoulder and back muscles (Nichols and Humenick, 1988).

Some clients benefit from a specialized technique known as therapeutic touch, which is based on the theory that a universal life energy occupies and sustains every living organism. Obstructions or disruptions in this energy field compromise health and well-being. To practice therapeutic touch, position both hands just above the client's body and become attuned to the energy field with slow, sweeping motions over her body (without touching it). These gentle hand movements free obstructed energy and balance the energy field. Finally, consciously direct energy toward the client (Krieger, 1979.)

Music therapy. Typically, music offers an adjunct to other pain-reducing techniques. It prompts positive associations, aids rhythmic breathing, and distracts the client from environmental noises that might increase anxiety (Hanzer, Lanson, and O'Connell, 1983).

Interventions for the unprepared client

A client with no childbirth education presents a special challenge to the nurse, who must provide information and guide the client through comfort promotion and pain reduction.

If the client has no support person, remain with her and assume the support role. Because the client's anxiety and stress level will be high, teach simple relaxation techniques, including controlled breathing. Do this as early as possible in labor to focus attention and help ensure adequate coping mechanisms for later contractions. Inform the client of what will happen during labor, why, and how long labor may last.

If the client has a support person, focus on the partner's supporting role. Demonstrate touch, massage,

---

Theories of pain transmission

Exactly how pain is transmitted and perceived remains a mystery. However, research involving neurophysiology, psychology, and sociology has contributed to the development of two pain theories that may help explain this complex phenomenon.

Gate control theory
Developed by Melzack and Wall (1965), this theory undergirds many of the pain management techniques used in childbirth preparation, including controlled breathing, distraction, massage, transcutaneous electrical nerve stimulation, and application of heat or cold.

According to this theory, pain transmission can be modified or blocked by counterstimulation. During labor, pain impulses travel from the uterus along small neural fibers (C fibers) in an ascending pathway to the substantia gelatinosa in the spinal column. Nearby transmission cells then project the pain message to the brain. Tactile stimulation—such as massage and application of heat or cold—produces opposing messages that travel along larger, faster neural fibers (A-delta fibers). These opposing messages close a hypothetical "gate" in the substantia gelatinosa, thus blocking the pain message.

The brain will not register pain messages that are blocked by counterstimulation, or the pain perception will be modified. Activities involving the cerebral cortex—such as controlled breathing, distraction, and imagery—also may activate the gating mechanism by sending descending (efferent) impulses through the spinal cord to close the gate at the substantia gelatinosa.

Endogenous opiate theory
In the late 1970s, researchers identified opiate receptor sites in the brain and spinal cord and determined that the central nervous system releases morphinelike substances called endorphins and enkephalins when pain is perceived. These endogenous opiates bind to opiate receptor sites and alter the perception of pain in a manner that is not fully understood. Studies show that women in labor experience elevated endorphin levels (Kimball, 1979).

The endogenous opiate theory sheds light on the pain-reducing effects of acupressure and acupuncture, which also may trigger release of endogenous opiates.

---

and simple breathing patterns. Describe normal labor stages, expected behaviors, and typical interventions, including comfort measures and pain-relieving agents.

If an unprepared client feels out of control, shifting her focus from pain to relaxation techniques may be difficult. To get the client's attention, try such simple techniques as establishing direct eye contact, calling her by name, asking questions, and whispering in her ear. Coach the client through relaxation techniques (particularly controlled breathing) during a contraction; then have her practice the techniques immediately so that she knows how to use them before the next contraction.

Nonpharmacologic pain control

Comfort measures typically fall short of pain relief, which becomes imperative for most clients as labor progresses. Methods to accomplish this goal without using pharmacologic agents include hypnosis, transcutaneous electric nerve stimulation (TENS), and acupressure or acupuncture.

Hypnosis. In this state of altered consciousness, motor control and perception can be influenced by suggestion. The client attains a state of alertness and heightened concentration through imagery, controlled breathing, and other relaxation techniques. Through intense concentration, the client can diminish pain perception. Not all clients respond to hypnosis. In fact, about 40% cannot be hypnotized at all, and about 30% can achieve only a lightly hypnotized state. Only about 30% can achieve a deep state of hypnosis (Melzack, 1984). A client who is interested in using self-hypnosis during labor should consult a professional hypnotist early in the second trimester (Lieberman, 1987). To assist a client with self-hypnosis, encourage the use of relaxation techniques and provide a tranquil environment free from distraction. The client may need up to an hour to achieve a hypnotic state.

TENS. In TENS, electric currents block pain messages by stimulating large-diameter neural fibers. Impulses travel more quickly along the large fibers than along the small-diameter fibers that transmit pain; thus, electrical counterstimulation blocks or modifies pain perception. TENS stimulation also may release endogenous endorphins, which activate opiate receptors in the brain and spinal cord that decreases the client's response to painful stimuli.

Several European clinical trials have focused on women in labor, showing that TENS provided moderate to good pain relief for about 75% of those studied. Most said that it "modulates" the pain or makes it more tolerable (Perez and Hanold, 1988).

Initiate TENS early in the active phase of labor when the client can hold still while the electrodes are applied. Describe the characteristic tingling sensation of TENS, and explain that the unit can be adjusted to enhance pain relief or reduce the tingling. Wash and dry the client's back and apply a water-soluble gel in the region corresponding to T10 through L1 (for the first stage of labor) or S2 through S4 (for the second stage of labor). Place the two electrodes in the appropriate region, one on either side of the spinal cord.

The electrodes usually can stay in place throughout labor. However, if the client complains of pain or irritation, remove them, inspect the skin for redness, and reapply them in a different area. Monitor the client for muscle twitching, which indicates excessive stimulation, and adjust the TENS impulse accordingly. Document the degree of pain relief, any adverse reactions, impulse settings, and times applied and removed.

Never apply TENS electrodes to the client's abdomen because the electrical charge will be too close to the fetus's heart. The electrical impulses produce artifact on fetal tracings obtained with external leads. Even when applied correctly, TENS may disrupt fetal heart rate transmission patterns, particularly when a second unit is applied to the S2 through S4 region. An internal scalp electrode produces the best results when monitoring a fetus during TENS.

Applied and used properly, TENS appears to have no harmful effects on the client or fetus and can reduce the need for analgesia and anesthesia. However, if the client experiences no pain relief or dislikes the tingling sensation, remove the unit and try other pain-reduction measures.

Acupressure and acupuncture. Based on the Chinese theory that energy travels through the body along 12 major pathways or meridians, acupressure and acupuncture seek to reduce pain and enhance well-being by manipulating key points along those meridians (Lieberman, 1987). In acupuncture, the practitioner stimulates selected trigger points with thin needles. In acupressure, the practitioner uses finger pressure instead of needles. Some proponents of the gate control theory believe that acupressure relieves pain by closing the gate of pain transmission at the spinal cord level.

After special preparation, the nurse or support person may perform acupressure on a client during labor to reduce pain in certain areas. For example, pressure on a point in the web between the thumb and index finger may relieve pain in the large intestine area. Pressure approximately 3 inches above the medial malleolus on the medial aspect of the lower leg may relieve pain in the splenic area; pressure on the lateral aspect of the ankle, midway between the lateral malleolus and achilles tendon or just outside the nail bed on the lateral aspect of the fifth toe, may relieve pain in the bladder area.

The practitioner applies pressure to key points with the fingertips or thumbs, using a small circular movement for the first 5 to 10 seconds. Pressure on each point may last up to 1 minute and can be repeated several times during labor. The client should feel a tingling sensation or mild tenderness. The pressure may be slightly uncomfortable but should be tolerable; pain relief should follow. If pain increases, the practitioner should discontinue the technique.

Pharmacologic pain control

Analgesic and anesthetic agents are the two types of pharmacologic pain relief used during labor. (For a summary, see *Drugs used to relieve labor pain*, pages 638 and 639.)

Analgesia refers to pain reduction without loss of consciousness. Although the client may continue to perceive pain, an analgesic agent can make it more tolerable by affecting the peripheral nervous system (by relaxing muscles and increasing blood flow), and the central nervous system (CNS).

Anesthesia refers to partial or complete loss of sensation, sometimes with loss of consciousness. Affecting the entire body or only a region of the body, an anesthetic agent blocks conduction of impulses along pain pathways to the brain.

Regional anesthetic agents are injected into areas surrounding nerves. Types used for labor pain include pudendal block, epidural block, spinal block, saddle block, or paracervical block.

General anesthetic agents render the client unconscious and thus unable to feel pain. These agents may be inhaled or administered I.V. or I.M. Typically, they are used only for emergency cesarean delivery or other surgical interventions because they greatly increase the risk of aspiration, the leading cause of anesthesia-related maternal death.

Ideally, the client should receive information and make choices about pharmacologic options before labor begins. Childbirth education classes typically include such information. The client's obstetrician and anesthesiologist are responsible for describing obstetric analgesia and anesthesia and obtaining written consent to administer these therapies. Provide additional information as needed, including the route of administration, degree and timing of pain relief, impact on labor and the fetus, potential adverse drug reactions, and the effectiveness of the technique selected. In addition, explain how analgesia and anesthesia may interfere with the client's active participation in labor. Describe the immediate and prolonged effects of pharmacologic agents on the neonate. Take steps to ensure that the client's caregivers will support her decision for or against pharmacologic intervention. If a client who planned a "natural" childbirth requires pharmacologic pain relief during labor, help her work through any feelings of guilt or failure and provide reassurance about her decision.

Analgesia. The client may receive an analgesic agent when active labor is established and the cervix begins to dilate. Administration usually takes place via an intravenous or intramuscular injection. (For more information, see *A comparison of analgesia administration routes for a client in labor*, page 640.)

Analgesic agents may cause drowsiness, euphoria, orthostatic hypotension, and dizziness. Use side rails on the bed to ensure client safety if a member of the health care team or a support person cannot be in constant attendance. Caution the client and support person that the client should not get out of bed without a nurse's help.

Categories of systemic analgesic agents used during labor include sedatives, narcotic agonists, mixed narcotic agonist-antagonists, antianxiety agents, and inhalation analgesics.

Sedatives. For the client in the prodromal or latent phase of labor, sedatives allow a few hours of sleep or relaxation before entering active labor. For the client in false labor, sedatives promote rest and stop contractions.

The use of diazepam during labor is not harmful to the client or her fetus unless the dose exceeds 30 mg (Briggs, Freeman, and Yaffee, 1986).

Narcotic agonists. Natural and synthetic opiates, these drugs bind at specific opiate receptor sites in the CNS and alter the client's perception of pain. They depress the CNS, causing drowsiness, euphoria, and reduced respiratory activity. They also stimulate the medullary chemoreceptor trigger zone, producing nausea and vomiting.

Meperidine (Demerol), a synthetic narcotic agonist commonly used during labor, increases pain tolerance and promotes rest between contractions. Administration of meperidine 1 to 3 hours or less before delivery may cause respiratory depression in the neonate. Some researchers also report abnormal reflexes and diminished sucking, alertness, and ability to become and remain quiet for up to 5 days after delivery (Hodgkinson and Hussain, 1982; Cunningham, MacDonald, and Gant, 1989).

Because pain pathways involve transmission via the spinal cord, narcotic agonist administration via epidural catheter is being studied to manage labor pain. Because the drugs act locally on opiate receptors in the spinal cord, this method allows lower doses with greater pain relief and fewer adverse drug reactions than other administration routes. The client still perceives contractions and retains control over the bearing-down efforts.

Adverse reactions to narcotic agonists include nausea, vomiting, pruritus, urine retention, and delayed respiratory depression. After delivery, antiemetics reduce nausea and vomiting, and antipruritics reduce itching. Ambulation improves bladder function.

Regardless of the route of administration, narcotic agonists can cause respiratory depression in the client and neonate. A narcotic antagonist, such as naloxone

(Text continues on page 640.)

Drugs used to relieve labor pain

The following drugs provide analgesia or anesthesia for labor.

CLASS AND DRUG	INDICATION	POSSIBLE ADVERSE EFFECTS	NURSING CONSIDERATIONS
Narcotic agonists			
meperidine, morphine	Alter pain perception	*Maternal:* decreased respirations, orthostatic hypotension, nausea and vomiting, itching, drowsiness *Fetal:* moderate central nervous system (CNS) depression, decreased beat-to-beat variability *Neonatal:* moderate CNS depression, mild behavioral depression	• Review maternal history for drug allergy, substance abuse, chronic respiratory disease, and renal and liver disease. • Frequently assess maternal vital signs, respirations, and level of consciousness • Assess labor stage and progress. • Use continuous electronic fetal heart rate (FHR) monitoring (internal lead), if possible. • Do not administer drug within 2 hours of expected delivery. If birth occurs at time of maximum effect, expect neonatal respiratory depression. Inject naloxone (0.01 mg/kg) into umbilical cord vein or neonate's thigh as prescribed.
Narcotic antagonists			
naloxone	Reverse respiratory depression caused by narcotic toxicity in client or neonate	*Maternal:* may reverse analgesia if given 5 to 10 minutes before delivery, increasing pain perception *Fetal:* none *Neonatal:* may induce withdrawal symptoms in a narcotic-depressed neonate	• Keep resuscitation equipment nearby during administration. • Do not administer to client with known drug dependency. • Develop a plan for alternate pain relief. • Narcotic antagonists will not reverse respiratory depression caused by sedatives, hypnotics, anesthetics, or nonnarcotic CNS depressants.
Narcotic agonist-antagonists			
butorphanol tartrate, nalbuphine	Alter pain perception	*Maternal:* may induce withdrawal symptoms in a narcotic-dependent client; may cause decreased respirations, orthostatic hypotension, nausea and vomiting, itching, drowsiness *Fetal:* moderate CNS depression, decreased beat-to-beat variability *Neonatal:* moderate CNS depression, mild behavioral depression	• Review the client's history for drug allergy, substance abuse, chronic respiratory disease, and renal and liver disease. • Frequently assess maternal vital signs, respirations, and level of consciousness. • Assess labor stage and progress. • Use continuous electronic FHR monitoring (internal lead), if possible.
Tranquilizers			
benzodiazepines (diazepam), phenothiazines (promethazine)	Promote rest and sleep; may reduce anxiety and reduce narcotic requirements	*Maternal:* possible paradoxically increased pain and excitability, especially when given during active labor *Fetal:* decreased beat-to-beat variability; moderate CNS depression, especially with larger doses *Neonatal:* possible hypotonia, decreased feeding, lethargy, and hypothermia	• Review the client's history for drug allergies before administration. • Tranquilizers usually are given only during the first stage of labor; they may have antiemetic effects. • Diazepam readily crosses the placenta. Large doses can affect the neonate for up to 1 week after delivery.

Drugs used to relieve labor pain continued

CLASS AND DRUG	INDICATION	POSSIBLE ADVERSE EFFECTS	NURSING CONSIDERATIONS
barbiturates (secobarbital)	Decrease anxiety during the prodromal or early latent phase of labor	*Maternal:* possible paradoxically increased pain and excitability *Fetal:* none *Neonatal:* possible CNS depression that can persist for several days	• Barbiturates are administered less commonly than other tranquilizers because of their prolonged depressant effects on the neonate. • Barbiturates should be administered only if delivery is not expected for 12 to 24 hours.

Regional anesthetic agents

bupivacaine, lidocaine, chloroprocaine, mepivacaine	Preferred regional method for analgesia and anesthesia during first and second stage of labor; provide anesthesia for vaginal or cesarean delivery; relieve uterine pain (pudendal block relieves perineal pain)	*Maternal:* hypotension (epidural and spinal); delayed analgesia (10 to 20 minutes); one-sided block or ineffective pain relief (spinal); prolonged labor if epidural block given too early; urine retention (epidural and spinal); increased toxicity from vascularity of region (pudendal); hematoma (pudendal); diminished bearing-down efforts (epidural) *Fetal:* transient decreased beat-to-beat variability with lidocaine and mepivacaine; late decelerations; fetal distress secondary to maternal hypotension; about 30% incidence of bradycardia (paracervical) *Neonatal:* CNS depression in presence of severe hypotension; neonatal bradycardia, hypotonia, and decreased responsiveness with accidental fetal intracranial injection (pudendal block)	• Determine baseline maternal vital signs and FHR; assess throughout labor as needed. • Explain procedure and expected feelings as anesthesia is initiated. • *Pudendal:* Assess for diminished bearing-down reflex and fetal symptoms associated with accidental scalp injection. • *Epidural:* Ensure adequate client hydration by administering 500 to 1,000 ml I.V. fluid before injection. Take vital signs every 5 minutes for 30 minutes after injection and report hypotension. Monitor vital signs every 15 minutes throughout continuous epidural infusion. Catheterize if client retains urine. Labor may be augmented with oxytocin if uterine contractions diminish. Assist with positioning and maintain safety (put up side rails). • *Spinal:* Ensure adequate client hydration by administering 500 to 1,000 ml I.V. fluid before injection. Take vital signs every 5 minutes until delivery. Report hypotension, and treat as prescribed. Observe for signs of total spinal block (apnea, unconsciousness, absent blood pressure, absent pulse, pupil dilation). Encourage the client to lie flat for 8 to 10 hours after administration.

General anesthetic agents

halothane, enflurane, thiopental sodium	Anesthesia for cesarean delivery; surgical intervention for obstetric complications, version, extraction, or uterine manipulation	*Maternal:* increased risk of regurgitation and aspiration; increased risk of uterine atony; decreased risk of hypovolemia compared to regional anesthesia *Fetal:* increased risk of fetal CNS depression *Neonatal:* short-term behavioral changes	• Assess for risk of aspiration. Maintain NPO status. • Administer antacid or H_2 blocking agent, as prescribed. • Continuously monitor FHR, especially during induction of anesthesia and in response to anesthesia. • Maintain respiratory support, I.V. fluids, and uterine fundal massage, as necessary, during recovery from anesthesia. • Drowsiness may persist after recovery. Assist with positioning and maintain safety (put up side rails).

A comparison of analgesia administration routes for a client in labor

Listed below are common administration routes for analgesic agents during labor. Subcutaneous and oral routes, rarely used during labor, are not included.

ROUTE, ADVANTAGES, AND DISADVANTAGES	NURSING CONSIDERATIONS
Intravenous *Advantages:* rapid, predictable action; smaller doses than I.M. route *Disadvantages:* requires venous access	• Stop I.V. solutions while injecting analgesia. • Use the port nearest the client. • Inject slowly at the onset of a contraction; blood flow to the uterus and fetus decreases during contractions, minimizing drug transfer to the fetus. • Restart the I.V. slowly to prevent formation of a bolus of analgesia. • If other drugs were mixed with the I.V. solution, flush the line to prevent incompatibility.
Intramuscular *Advantages:* shorter administration time than for I.V.; requires no venous access *Disadvantages:* painful administration	• Inject into a large muscle to promote absorption. • Adjust needle length to accommodate especially thin or obese clients. • Pain relief usually occurs 45 minutes after injection.

(Narcan), may be administered to prevent this. For I.V. administration, use the client's I.V. line or the neonate's umbilical vein; for I.M. administration, use the client's gluteal muscle or the neonate's thigh. Administer these agents cautiously in a drug-dependent client because they may induce withdrawal symptoms.

Mixed narcotic agonist-antagonists. These agents produce an analgesic effect unless narcotics already exist in the client's circulation. In this case, they have an antagonist effect and cause withdrawal. Early withdrawal symptoms include yawning, lacrimation, sweating, mydriasis, piloerection, flushing, tachycardia, tremors, and irritability. If withdrawal occurs, notify the physician immediately to prevent fetal adverse reactions. In equianalgesic doses, butorphanol (Stadol) and pentazocine (Talwin) have shown analgesic effects similar to meperidine (Demerol). Both drugs rapidly cross the placenta and can cause CNS depression in the neonate.

Antianxiety agents. These agents increase narcotic effects while they decrease anxiety and relieve nausea. They do not relieve pain directly. Antianxiety agents used commonly during labor include promethazine (Phenergan), hydroxyzine (Vistaril), and promazine (Sparine). Administer antianxiety agents I.M. or I.V.

Regional anesthesia. By blocking pain transmission without altering consciousness, regional anesthesia allows the client to participate in labor and childbirth while decreasing pain perception and the amount of drug that crosses to the fetus. Many physicians advocate regional anesthesia. Its disadvantages include potential CNS toxicity, hypotension, diminished bearing-down efforts, pruritus, urine retention, nausea, and vomiting.

The physician or anesthesiologist administers the anesthetic with a single, direct injection, several direct injections, intermittent injections, or continuous infusion through an indwelling epidural catheter. Drugs used most commonly include ester-type agents (chloroprocaine hydrochloride, procaine hydrochloride, and tetracaine hydrochloride) and amide-type agents (bupivacaine hydrochloride, etidocaine hydrochloride, lidocaine hydrochloride, and mepivacaine hydrochloride). The choice of agent will differ with the type of anesthetic block used.

Regional anesthesia techniques include local infiltration (including pudendal and paracervical blocks), epidural block, and spinal block. Epidural and spinal blocks carry the risk of hypotension caused by sympathetic blockage. (For illustrations of administration techniques, see *Types of regional anesthesia,* pages 642 and 643.)

Local infiltration. The physician or nurse-midwife may use local infiltration before delivery to perform an episiotomy or after delivery to repair perineal lacerations. This simple method of anesthesia, commonly chosen by prepared clients or clients seeking a more "natural" birth, produces few complications for the client or neonate. The anesthesiologist injects the agent directly into perineal tissue. The client may report a brief burning sensation after injection.

Pudendal block. Another form of local infiltration, this block is used during the second stage of labor to numb the perineum and vagina for delivery, episiotomy repair, or forceps delivery. The pudendal block is especially effective for difficult episiotomies or repairing lacerations after delivery. It does not block pain perceived from uterine contractions, but does decrease bearing-down efforts.

The physician or nurse-midwife injects the drug into the pudendal nerve on each side of the sacrum. Complications include accidental injection into a blood vessel, hematoma, and perforation. If the needle enters the fetus's scalp or cranium, neonatal brachycardia, apnea, and diminished responsiveness may be present after birth.

Paracervical block. Also a type of local infiltration, this technique blocks nerves on either side of the cervix during the active phase of labor, at 4 to 5 cm of dilation. The paracervical block relieves pain stemming from uterine contractions and cervical dilation. Duration of action is approximately 1 hour.

Use of the paracervical block is rare today. Twenty to thirty percent of fetuses develop bradycardia and subsequently may develop fetal acidosis. Also, a risk exists for inadvertent intracranial injection into the fetus.

Epidural block. The most commonly used method of pain relief during labor, the epidural block provides continuous anesthesia during the first and second stages of labor. This type of anesthesia commonly is used during cesarean deliveries. The anesthesiologist injects a local anesthetic agent into the epidural space, located between the dura mater and the ligamentum flavum, at the lumbar region of the spinal column (third to fifth lumbar inner space). Although the client's pelvis and legs feel heavy, she retains some ability to move and bear down.

Continuous epidural infusion is a variation on the epidural block. The client receives continuous infusion of dilute anesthetic agents through an indwelling epidural catheter, a method that maintains continuous drug levels, reduces the amount of drug needed, and decreases the risk of hypotensive crisis (Morrison and Smedstad, 1985). The same precautions should be exercised with the indwelling epidural catheter as with the standard method.

Contraindications for epidural anesthesia include coagulopathy problems, allergic reactions, placental insufficiency, and infection at the puncture site. If a virus, such as herpes, is present on the skin at the site of epidural injection, further dissemination of the virus may occur (Ravindran, 1982). An epidural block should be used with caution if the client has high or low blood pressure. (For more information, see *Emergency alert: Hypotensive crisis.*)

Disadvantages of epidural anesthesia include the need to have skilled anesthesia personnel or a physician on hand to monitor the client and fetus. Further, it may prolong labor, cause difficulty in voiding, increase oxygen use, and increase the risk of forceps delivery because of the client's diminished bearing-down efforts.

Administering epidural anesthesia requires much skill to achieve complete and effective anesthesia; areas of unanesthetized tissue, ineffective anesthesia, or inadvertent spinal anesthesia may result from improper

---

EMERGENCY ALERT

Hypotensive crisis

Hypotensive crisis may occur after spinal or epidural anesthesia because of the spread of the anesthetic agent through the spinal canal. A sympathetic blockade produces marked hypotension from loss of peripheral resistance, decreased venous return, and decreased cardiac output. Decreased placental perfusion occurs with maternal hypotension, resulting in fetal bradycardia.

SIGNS AND SYMPTOMS

- Fetal bradycardia
- Decreased beat-to-beat variability
- Maternal hypotension (20% or greater drop from baseline blood pressure or less than 100 mm Hg systolic)

TREATMENT AND NURSING CONSIDERATIONS

- Turn client to left lateral position to increase uterine perfusion.
- Infuse I.V. fluid rapidly, as prescribed.
- Administer oxygen by mask, as prescribed.
- Elevate the client's legs.
- Notify the anesthesiologist.
- Administer vasopressor (such as ephedrine) I.V. or I.M., as prescribed.
- Stay with the client and monitor blood pressure and fetal heart rate frequently.

---

infusion. Maternal hypotension may occur from sympathetic blockade, producing vasodilation, loss of peripheral resistance, and CNS toxicity. The client may feel chilled from peripheral temperature changes and may experience postpartal urine retention, necessitating catheterization.

Spinal block. This technique resembles the epidural block except that the needle penetrates the meninges and enters the subarachnoid space. The anesthesiologist mixes a single injection of anesthesia with a sample of the client's cerebrospinal fluid and injects it into the third, fourth, or fifth lumbar inner space. The client loses feeling and motor ability in the lower portion of her body. Numbness extends from the umbilicus to the toes for vaginal delivery and from the xiphoid process to the toes for cesarean delivery. A low spinal block, or saddle block, may be used during the second stage of labor if placental extraction or instrumental delivery becomes necessary.

As with an epidural, a spinal block may lead to vasodilation that can cause hypotension and fetal hypoxia. The anesthetic agent could spread, causing a total spinal block, apnea, reduced blood pressure and pulse, and unresponsiveness. Contraindications for spinal block

Types of regional anesthesia

The following chart explains the administration techniques for five types of regional anesthesia.

Local infiltration

Used to numb perineal tissue for episiotomy or laceration repair, this technique involves injection of anesthetic through a 22G needle into the fascia of the perineum. The client may feel a burning sensation. This technique poses no threat to the client, fetus, or neonate.

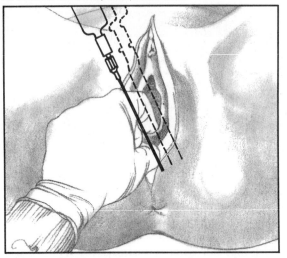

Pudendal block

Used to block perineal and vaginal pain but not uterine contractions during the second stage of labor, this technique involves injection of 3 to 5 ml of anesthetic into the pudendal nerve on each side of the sacrum. The needle crosses the sacrosciatic notch and passes the tip of the ischial spine. Accidental injection into the fetus's scalp or cranium may cause neonatal bradycardia and decreased responsiveness.

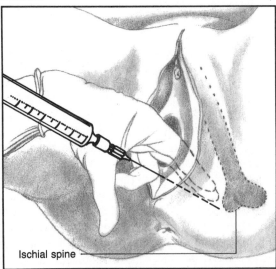

Paracervical block

Used to anesthetize the uterus and cervix during the first stage of labor, this technique involves insertion of an Iowa trumpet into the lateral fornix of the vagina and injection of 5 to 10 ml of anesthetic. The block provides anesthesia through the second stage of labor. Because it is associated with a high incidence of fetal adverse reactions, this technique is used rarely.

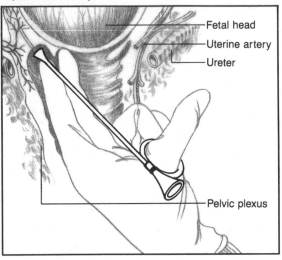

Epidural block

Used to anesthetize the lower half of the body, this technique involves insertion of an 18G stylet into lumbar interspace 3, 4, or 5. Then the tip of the needle is advanced into the epidural space to administer the anesthetic. An epidural block may prolong labor and cause hypotension.

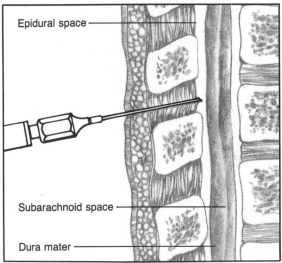

Spinal block

Performed in a similar manner to the epidural block, this technique is used to anesthetize the lower half of the body. However, the needle is advanced somewhat farther, into the subarachnoid space. Thus, the anesthetic is injected directly into spinal fluid. The client loses perception of contractions and ability to bear down. A spinal block to the level of T10 is used for vaginal delivery, to T8 for cesarean delivery.

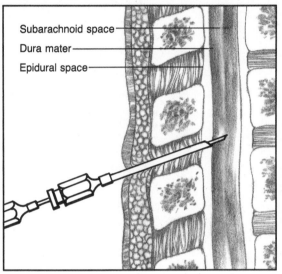

Subarachnoid space
Dura mater
Epidural space

are similar to those for epidural block. Adverse reactions include post-spinal headache, shivering, and urine retention.

Because epidural and spinal anesthesia cause hypotension (produced by vasodilation), I.V. fluids (preferably lactated Ringer's solution) are necessary. Expect to infuse 500 to 1,000 ml of fluid before administration of epidural or spinal anesthesia and to maintain an I.V. infusion for fluid and possible emergency drug administration should hypotension occur. Monitor vital signs every 5 minutes for the first 30 minutes after initiation of epidural anesthesia and every 15 minutes throughout epidural infusion. Monitor vital signs every 5 minutes after administration of spinal anesthesia until delivery, and monitor as prescribed for up to 24 hours after delivery.

Signs and symptoms of anesthesia overdose include circumoral numbness, dizziness, and slurred speech. Maternal and fetal hypoxia may result, causing tachycardia. Be alert for these signs and symptoms, and notify the physician or anesthesiologist if they occur. Treatment of toxicity includes administering oxygen and I.V. fluids.

Administration of epidural or spinal anesthesia requires that the client be placed in a sitting or side-lying position with shoulders parallel and legs slightly flexed to reduce hypotension. Epidural anesthesia does not affect motor pathways but, because the legs are numb, they seem heavy and are difficult to move. A spinal block produces motor paralysis. Ensure the client's safety by using side rails and assisting with position changes.

The client may report feeling cold because of peripheral temperature changes. Provide extra drapes or blankets, as needed.

Postpartal urine retention is common with epidural or spinal anesthesia. Advise the client to empty her bladder before anesthesia administration. Expect to catheterize her if she does not void within 6 hours after delivery.

General anesthesia. Because it requires intubation and increases the risk of aspiration, general anesthesia (where the client loses consciousness) usually is used only when the client undergoes emergency cesarean delivery, intrauterine manipulation, or other surgical intervention. General anesthesia may be attained through inhalation or I.V. drug administration. Inhalation involves high concentrations of the same agents used for inhalant analgesia (nitrous oxide, halothane, and enflurane). The intravenous agent thiopental sodium (Pentothal) produces deep anesthesia and may cause depression in the neonate.

Before anesthesia induction, a nurse anesthetist or anesthesiologist will apply pressure to the client's cricoid

APPLYING THE NURSING PROCESS

Client with pain related to active labor

During labor, the nurse can help minimize client discomfort. The table below shows how the nurse might use the nursing process when caring for the client described in the case history at right. The first column presents history and physical assessment data followed by a paragraph of mental notes. These notes help the nurse make important mental connections among assessment findings, aiding in development of the nursing diagnosis and planning.

The second column lists an appropriate nursing diagnosis; information in the remaining columns is based on this diagnosis. Although not part of the nursing process, a rationale appears for each intervention in the fourth column to explain how it contributes to the care plan.

ASSESSMENT	NURSING DIAGNOSIS	PLANNING
Subjective (history) data • Client states that she and her partner have taken prepared childbirth classes. • Client states that she does not want pain medication. • Client complains of increasing exhaustion. **Objective (physical) data** • Client is crying, writhing, and clenching hands with each contraction. • Vital signs: T 97° F, pulse 110 beats/minute, respirations 34/minute, blood pressure 116/76 mm Hg • Pelvic exam: cervix 4 cm, 100% effaced, engaged occiput, LOA • FHR: 136 beats/minute • Leopold's: longitudinal lie, cephalic presentation **Mental notes** *The client has prepared for natural childbirth. However, at 4 cm, she complains of a great deal of pain and the transition phase, the toughest part, is yet to come. At this time, she needs help implementing relaxation techniques. Also, she may need to consider analgesia; acceptance of analgesia without feelings of guilt will require preparation and support, especially from her partner.*	Pain related to active labor	**Goals** The client will: • remember to use various coping techniques for managing active labor • use imagery, effleurage, breathing, and music therapy to reduce pain • change positions to increase comfort • demonstrate increased ability to cope with contractions.

process during intubation. This occludes the esophagus and reduces the risk of aspiration should the client vomit.

To avoid compressing the vena cava once the tube is in place, move the client from the supine position before anesthesia administration begins. Many obstetric operating room tables provide left lateral tilt capability to displace the gravid uterus off the vena cava. If the table cannot be tilted, insert a wedge beneath the client's right hip. After client positioning, administer oxygen and fluids as prescribed just before anesthesia administration.

Administer a clear antacid—such as sodium citrate—a few hours before surgery to reduce the client's risk of aspiration of acidic stomach contents while anesthetized. If the client requires emergency surgery, the antacid may be administered 30 minutes or less before the procedure. Turning the client from side to side enhances antacid effectiveness and promotes mixing of the antacid with gastric contents. In addition, many anesthesiologists now routinely decrease gastric acidity by administering an H_2 antagonist, such as cimetidine (Tagamet), before surgery.

Because of delayed gastric emptying during pregnancy, the client who requires emergency surgery may be at increased risk for regurgitating, which can cause chemical pneumonitis and death. To reduce gastric volume, some obstetricians forbid clients from drinking anything while in labor.

Because inhalation agents may cause cardiac arrhythmias, monitor maternal electrocardiogram continuously throughout anesthesia administration and during recovery. Uterine atony, also produced by inhalants, may lead to uterine hemorrhage. Fetal and neonatal hypoxia also may occur with deep induction anesthesia, which reaches the fetus in about 2 minutes. If the client received an I.V. anesthetic agent, monitor the neonate closely for depression.

CASE STUDY

Ellen O'Leary, a primagravid client age 30, is admitted to the labor and delivery area. She has been experiencing contractions for 14 hours. Neither she nor her partner has had any sleep.

IMPLEMENTATION		EVALUATION
Intervention Suggest imagery, effleurage, breathing techniques, and music.	**Rationale** Relaxation techniques provide distraction from uterine contractions and increase the client's ability to cope.	Upon evaluation, the client: • demonstrated increased ability to cope with contractions
Provide information on nonpharmacologic options.	Knowledge that various "natural" techniques exist to reduce pain can allay anxiety, increase a sense of control, and promote relaxation.	• changed positions and demonstrated increased comfort • verbalized which techniques increase comfort
Suggest repositioning or walking to increase comfort.	These decrease pain and increase comfort. Walking produces effective, efficient uterine contractions.	• demonstrated behavioral changes, including decreased crying, writhing, and anxiety
Provide information about pharmacologic pain relief options.	Adequate preparation allows the client time to affirm her commitment to natural childbirth or to opt for pharmacologic intervention without excessive guilt.	• exhibited decreased body tension • cooperated with partner • expressed willingness to consider pharmacologic pain relief.

Evaluation

During this step of the nursing process, the nurse evaluates the effectiveness of the care plan by using ongoing subjective and objective criteria. Evaluation findings should be stated in terms of actions performed or outcomes achieved for each goal. The following examples illustrate appropriate evaluation statements for the client experiencing labor pain.

• The client demonstrated knowledge of such comfort promotion techniques as controlled breathing and progressive muscle relaxation.
• The client expressed understanding of pain-relief measures available to her.
• The client reported relief from pain after administration of regional anesthesia.
• Fetal heart rate remained stable after anesthesia administration.
• The client maintained hydration throughout labor.

• The client and neonate displayed normal responsiveness after delivery.

Documentation

The nurse must document all findings and actions taken using the nursing process. Documentation applicable to the client experiencing labor pain includes:
• comfort measures taken and their effectiveness
• analgesic agents administered and their effectiveness
• anesthetic agents administered and their effectiveness
• vital signs
• changes in uterine contractions after drug administration
• changes in fetal heart rate after drug administration.

Chapter summary

Chapter 26 described comfort promotion techniques and pain-reduction methods for the client in labor. Here are the chapter highlights.

• Although labor pain proceeds through a predictable series of peaks and valleys, each client perceives her pain uniquely, based on her physical condition, pain tolerance, and psychological profile.

• Factors that influence the intensity of labor pain include parity, fetal size and position, certain medical procedures, anxiety, fatigue, childbirth education level, culture, and coping mechanisms.

• Comfort measures, support, and reassurance can reduce the client's emotional tension and discomfort. The nurse helps maintain client comfort by decreasing her anxiety, promoting hygiene, positioning the client comfortably, and helping with relaxation techniques.

• Relaxation techniques of benefit during labor include distraction, imagery, progressive muscle relaxation, controlled breathing, yawning, various forms of touch, and music therapy.

• Nonpharmacologic techniques used to minimize and control pain perception in labor include hypnosis, TENS, acupressure, and acupuncture.

• Pharmacologic pain-relief measures should promote maternal analgesia without risk to the client or fetus.

• Analgesics may be initiated when active labor begins, via an intravenous, intramuscular, or subcutaneous route. Drug categories used for analgesia include sedatives, narcotic agonists, mixed narcotic agonist-antagonists, and antianxiety agents.

• Regional analgesia and anesthesia techniques require injection of an anesthetic agent into nerve tissue. Techniques include local infiltration, pudendal block, paracervical block, epidural block, and spinal block.

• General anesthesia, used for cesarean delivery or other surgical intervention, may be administered by inhalation or injection.

Study questions

1. Mrs. Eustaf, age 31, arrives at the labor and delivery area in active labor, 75% effaced and 3 cm dilated. The mother of an active 3-year-old, the client was unable to attend childbirth classes. She says that her labor pains are growing intense, but she prefers to avoid drug-induced pain relief. Decribe nonpharmacologic pain-relief techniques that could help this client.

2. What advantages and risks are associated with systemic medication used for analgesia during labor?

3. What advantages and risks are associated with regional blocks for analgesia or anesthesia during labor?

4. Mrs. Crow, age 40, may receive spinal anesthesia or general anesthesia. How will the nurse's responsibilities and interventions differ with each option?

5. Mrs. Jackson, a primiparous client who has attended childbirth classes, is admitted to the labor and delivery area in early, active labor (4 cm dilated). Crying and visibly anxious, she reports that she cannot cope with the pain of uterine contractions. What can the nurse do to help Mrs. Jackson in this phase of labor?

Bibliography

Bonica, J.U. (1989). Labour pain. In P. Wall and R. Melzack (Eds.), *Textbook of pain* (2nd ed.). New York: Churchhill Livingstone.

Cunningham, R., MacDonald, P., and Gant, N. (1989). *Williams obstetrics* (18th ed.). East Norwalk, CT: Appleton & Lange.

Delke, I., Minkoff, H., and Grunebaum, A. (1985). Effect of Lamaze childbirth preparation on maternal plasma beta-endorphin immunoreactivity in active labor. *American Journal of Perinatology*, 2(4), 317-319.

Dick-Read, G. (1970). *Childbirth without fear.* New York: Harper & Row.

Fenwick, L. (1984). Birthing: Techniques for managing the physiologic and psychosocial aspects of childbirth. *Perinatology/Neonatolgy*, 6, 51.

Jacox, A.K. (1977). *Pain: A source book for nurses and other health professions.* Boston: Little Brown.

Kimball, C. (1979). Do endorphin residues of beta-lipotrophin in hormone reinforce reproductive functions? *American Journal of Obstetrics and Gynecology*, 134(Z), 127-132.

Lederman, R., Lederman, E., Work B.A., and McCann, D.S. (1978). The relationship of maternal anxiety, plasma catecholemines, and plasma cortisol to progress in labor. *American Journal of Obstetrics and Gynecology*, 132(5), 495-500.

Lieberman, A.B. (1987). *Easing labor pain: The complete guide to achieving a more comfortable and rewarding birth.* New York: Doubleday.

Melzack, R., Taenzer, P., Feldman, P., and Kinch, R.A. (1981). Labour is still painful after prepared childbirth training. *Canadian Medical Association Journal,* 125(4), 357-363.

Melzack, R., and Wall, P. (1965). Pain mechanisms: A new theory. *Science,* 150(699), 971-979.

Nettelbladt, P., Fagerstrom, C.F., and Uddenberg, N. (1976). The significance of reported childbirth pain. *Journal of Psychosomatic Research,* 20(3), 215-221.

Nichols, F., and Humenick, S.S. (1988). *Childbirth education: Practice, research, and theory.* Philadelphia: Saunders.

Wolff, B.B., and Langley, S. (1975). Cultural factors and the response to pain: A review. In M. Weisenberg (Ed.), *Pain: Clinical and experimental perspectives.* St. Louis: Mosby.

Nonpharmacologic pain control

DiFranco, J. (1988). Music for childbirth. *Childbirth Educator,* (8), 36-41.

Hanzer, S.B., Lanson, S.C., and O'Connell, A.S. (1983). The effect of music on relaxation of expectant mothers during labor. *Journal of Music Therapy,* 20(2), 50-58.

Klusman, L.E. (1975). Reduction of pain in childbirth by alleviation of anxiety during pregnancy. *Journal of Consulting and Clinical Psychology,* 43(2), 162-165.

Krieger, D. (1979). *The therapeutic touch: How to use your hands to help or to heal.* Englewood Cliffs, NJ: Prentice-Hall.

Melzack, R. (1984). Acupuncture and related forms of folk medicine. In P. Wall and R. Melzack (Eds.), *Textbook of pain.* New York: Churchhill Livingstone.

Tanzer, D., and Block, J.L. (1987). *Why natural childbirth?* New York: Schocken Books.

Velovsky, I., Platonov, K., Ploticher, U., and Shugom, E. (1960). *Painless childbirth through psychoprophylaxis.* Moscow: Foreign Languages Publishing House.

Veran, D., et al. (1982). The clinical significance of a subusoidal FHR pattern associated with alphaprodine administration. *Journal of Reproductive Medicine,* 27, 411.

Wideman, M.V., and Singer, J.E. (1984). The role of psychological mechanisms in preparation for childbirth. *American Psychologist,* 39(12), 1357-1371.

Pharmacologic pain control

Albright, G.A., Joyce, R.H., and Stevenson, D.K. (1986). *Anesthesia in obstetrics* (2nd ed.). Boston: Butterworth.

Bonica, J. (1980). *Obstetric analgesia and anesthesia.* Amsterdam: World Federation of Societies of Anesthesiologists.

Briggs, G., Freeman, R., and Yaffe, S. (1986). *Drugs in pregnancy and lactation* (2nd ed.). Baltimore: Williams & Wilkins.

Gibbs, C.P. (1985). Anesthetic management of the high risk mother. In V.V. Sciaria, R. Depp, and D.A. Eschenbach (Eds.), *Gynecology and obstetrics.* New York: Harper & Row.

Hodgkinson, M.A., and Hussain, F.J. (1982). The duration of effect of maternity administered meperidine on neonatal neurobehavior. *Anesthesiology,* 56, 51-52.

ICEA. (1988, February). ICEA position paper: Epidural anesthesia for labor. *International Journal of Childbirth Education,* 3(1).

Kuhnert, B.R., Linn, P.L., and Kuhnert, P.M. (1985). Obstetric medication and neonatal behavior: Current controversies. *Clinics in Perinatology,* 12(2), 423.

Kuhnert, B.R., Linn, P.L., and Kuhnert, P.M. (1984). Effect of maternal epidural anesthesia on neonatal behavior. *Anesthesia and Analgesia,* 63(3), 301-308.

Morrison, D.H., and Smedstad, K.G. (1985). Continuous epidurals for obstetric analgesia. *Canadian Anesthesiology Society Journal,* 32(2), 101.

Ravindran, R.S. (1982). Epidural analgesia in the presence of herpes simplex virus (type 2) infection. *Anesthesia and Analgesia,* 61(8), 714-715.

Nursing research

Hilbers, S., and Gennaro, S. (1986). Non-pharmaceutical pain relief. *NAACOG Update Series,* Vol. 5. Princeton, NJ: Continuing Professional Education Center.

Jimenez, S. (1983). Application of the body's natural pain relief mechanisms to reduce discomfort in labor and delivery. In *NAACOG Update Series,* Vol. 1. Princeton, NJ: Continuing Professional Education Center.

McCaffery, M., and Beebe, A. (1989). *Pain: Clinical manual for nursing practice.* St. Louis: Mosby.

Perez, P., and Hanold, K. (1988). The use of transcutaneous nerve stimulation in the first stage of labor. In M. Rathi (Ed.), *Current Perinatology.* New York: Springer-Verlag.

Roberts, J. (1982). Which position for the first stage? *Childbirth Educator,* (1), 35.

The First Stage of Labor

Objectives

After reading and studying this chapter, the student should be able to:

1. Differentiate between true labor and false labor.

2. Obtain pertinent health history information during the client's admission to the labor and delivery area.

3. Describe physical assessment techniques used during admission to the labor and delivery area.

4. Interpret laboratory data for the client and fetus.

5. Describe how to assess the client and fetus during the first stage of labor.

6. Implement comfort and support measures for the client and her family.

7. Identify common variations in the first stage of labor and their specific nursing interventions.

8. Describe the impact of cultural background and family support on the childbearing process.

9. Apply the nursing process when caring for a client in the first stage of labor.

Introduction

The first stage of labor begins with the onset of regular, rhythmic uterine contractions that cause progressive cervical changes. It ends with complete cervical dilation of approximately 10 cm. Labor, however, is much more than a physiologic process that allows the fetus to enter the world. It is also the dramatic culmination of the gestational period—a significant life event that represents a pivotal point in the lives of the mother, father, neonate, and other family members. It is a psychological and developmental task that demands rigorous adaptation.

During the first stage of labor, nursing care must meet the client's physical, psychosocial, and cultural needs. To provide this kind of care, nursing responsibilities typically include:

• interpreting history, physical, and laboratory findings and evaluating their possible effects on labor

• assessing the progress of labor and adapting nursing care to meet individual needs

• maintaining client safety through ongoing assessments

• promoting client comfort in a supportive environment that encourages active participation

• recognizing variations in labor and intervening promptly

• teaching the client and her family about the childbirth process and discussing the benefits, risks, and alternatives related to any procedures

• enhancing the client's and support person's self-esteem and childbirth experience by encouraging active participation and development of realistic goals

• integrating the psychosocial and cultural needs of the client and her support person and adapting care to meet individual differences.

This chapter describes how to manage all of these responsibilities. It begins with preadmission care, describing how to gather the health history and physical assessment data needed to evaluate maternal and fetal status and how to distinguish between true and false labor. It also describes how to perform a more detailed, postadmission assessment that includes psychosocial and laboratory study data and how to formulate appropriate nursing diagnoses based on this assessment data.

GLOSSARY

Active phase of labor: second phase of the first stage of labor, when the cervix dilates from 4 to 10 cm. It includes three phases: acceleration, maximum slope, and deceleration (transition). Transition is part of the active phase (7 to 10 cm of cervical dilation).

Amniotomy: artificial rupture of amniotic membranes, performed by a physician or nurse-midwife to enhance or induce labor.

Back labor: labor that occurs when a fetus in the occiput posterior position presses on the sacral nerves during contractions.

Bloody show: blood-tinged vaginal discharge that occurs at the onset of labor when the cervical mucus plug is dislodged and small cervical capillaries break.

Braxton Hicks contractions: irregular uterine contractions that begin in the second trimester and increase in frequency, duration, and intensity as pregnancy progresses. Near term, strong Braxton Hicks contractions may be difficult to distinguish from true labor contractions. Also called false labor contractions.

Breech presentation: intrauterine fetal position in which the buttocks or feet present first.

Caput succedaneum: generalized edema of the fetal scalp, usually caused by cervical pressure on the fetal occiput during labor.

Cephalopelvic disproportion (CPD): condition in which the fetal head is too large or the maternal pelvis too small to permit vaginal birth.

Chorioamnionitis: inflammation of fetal membranes.

Dilation: physiologic increase, widening, or expansion in diameter.

Dilatation: dilation; sometimes used to describe dilation of the cervical os during labor.

Early phase of labor: first phase of the first stage of labor, characterized by the onset of regular contractions and cervical dilation of up to 3 cm. Also called the latent phase of labor.

Effacement: thinning and shortening of the cervix during labor.

Effleurage: light fingertip massage in a circular pattern. During labor, abdominal effleurage can help distract the client and decrease her pain.

Engagement: descent of the fetal presenting part into the maternal pelvis.

False labor: Braxton Hicks contractions.

Ferning: microscopic fern-shaped pattern found in a smear of dried amniotic fluid, indicating rupture of the amniotic membranes.

Fetal scalp sampling: method of detecting fetal hypoxia during labor by measuring the acidity of fetal serum in utero.

First stage of labor: initial stage of labor that begins with the onset of regular, rhythmic uterine contractions and ends with complete cervical dilation of 10 cm.

Hydramnios: excess amniotic fluid associated with congenital neonatal disorders and such maternal disorders as diabetes mellitus. Also called polyhydramnios.

Hyperesthesia: increased sensitivity, usually of the skin, which may occur late in labor.

Leopold's maneuvers: four abdominal palpation maneuvers used to determine the fetal lie, position, and presentation.

Lie: relationship of the fetal long axis to the maternal long axis. May be longitudinal, oblique, or transverse.

Malpresentation: abnormal fetal presentation, such as transverse lie or breech presentation.

Meconium: thick, sticky, green-to-black material that collects in the fetal intestines and forms the first neonatal stool. When present in amniotic fluid, meconium may indicate fetal distress.

Molding: shaping of the fetal head by overlapping of the sutures, which helps the head conform to the birth canal.

Occiput posterior position: variation of the normal fetal position, in which the head enters the pelvic inlet with the occiput facing posteriorly in the oblique diameter, causing back labor.

Position: relationship of the leading fetal presenting part to a point on the maternal pelvis.

Pregnancy-induced hypertension (PIH): abnormal obstetric condition characterized by elevated blood pressure, edema, proteinuria, and exaggerated reflexes.

Presentation: fetal part that enters the maternal pelvis first and can be touched through the cervix. May be cephalic, breech, or shoulder presentation.

Rupture of membranes: rupture of the amniotic sac, followed within 24 hours by labor in 80% of clients.

Station: relationship of the fetal presenting part to the ischial spine of the maternal pelvis.

True labor: characterized by regular contractions that increase in intensity and duration as the intervals between them decrease, along with progressive effacement and cervical dilation.

Then it discusses how to plan and implement initial care and ongoing care, including activities to monitor the client and provide comfort and support. The chapter describes variations in the first stage of labor and concludes with a brief discussion of documentation.

Nursing care before admission

Most women who seek admission and care in the labor and delivery area are in true labor; others are in false labor or very early first-stage labor. Some come for care because they do not know when they should be admitted for labor and delivery. Others know, but are overly anxious or fearful. Still others, exhausted after days of "false starts," want something done to ease their discomfort. A few rely on the health care facility as their sole source of prenatal care.

Before any client can be admitted for care in the labor and delivery area, she must be in true labor or show signs of a medical complication, such as hypertension, that could affect her or the fetus during labor and delivery. To make this determination, the nurse performs an initial assessment that focuses on the imminence of the birth and on fetal stability. This assessment, which includes a brief history and physical examination, should provide sufficient data to distinguish true labor from other conditions that mimic it, such as false labor, urinary tract infection, "terminal pregnancy blues" (generalized physical discomfort and emotional distress near the end of pregnancy), and abruptio placentae (premature detachment of the placenta). However, if delivery appears imminent, omit the preadmission assessment and admit the client immediately.

Initial assessment

Set the tone for the initial assessment by making appropriate introductions and asking the client what name she prefers to be called. Briefly describe nursing activities during this assessment and maintain the client's privacy and confidentiality to gain her trust and ease anxiety.

During the introductory period, observe the client closely to identify clues to her labor status. Postures, facial expressions, or gestures that connote tension, anxiety, or pain may accurately reflect a client's labor prog-

---

CULTURAL CONSIDERATIONS

Response to pain

Although each client has personal beliefs and values, her cultural background may influence her behavior. When caring for a client from a different culture, the nurse should keep the following considerations in mind.

Martinelli (1987) found that the response to pain varies among clients and among cultures. One study of 75 Lamaze-trained clients found that, among ethnic groups, response to labor pain differed significantly—even when anxiety was minimal. Clients from some groups, such as Italians and Hispanics, tended to use body language and expressions freely; those from other groups, such as Vietnamese, Irish, and Native Americans, tended to respond passively and did not openly display discomfort.

To help a client from a different cultural background cope with her pain effectively, be aware of your personal and cultural views and take a nonjudgmental approach. During the health history, identify the client's cultural background and determine how it may affect her response to pain.

---

ress. Perspiration, varying breathing patterns, lack of concentration, and frequent position changes can indicate discomfort or stress during and between contractions. Involuntary grunting or breath holding may signal the onset of the second stage of labor. To help form an accurate initial impression, relate the client's behavior to her cultural background. For example, a client from a culture that frowns on public displays of emotion may lie quietly rather than express her pain verbally or through gestures. (For more information, see *Cultural considerations: Response to pain*.)

If the client is in active labor (second phase of the first stage of labor, when the cervix dilates from 4 to 10 cm), shorten the initial assessment and prioritize the questions. If the client's labor status permits, plan to hold an uninterrupted, systematic health history interview to facilitate the initial assessment and enhance the client's confidence. During the interview, focus on collecting data about her current labor status. Refer to prenatal records, if available, and use the previously documented information. Engage the client's support person in conversation to reduce anxiety, especially if the client is in active labor.

Perform a brief physical examination to determine labor progress and fetal well-being. Be sure to help the client find a comfortable position for the assessment, especially if she is in active labor. Calmly conduct the history and physical assessment between contractions.

Health history

During the initial health history, gather biographical data and investigate the client's health status, health promotion and protection behaviors, and roles and relationships as they relate to her pregnancy, labor, and forthcoming delivery.

To help prioritize this information, obtain health history information in this order:
• biographical data
• expected delivery date
• previous pregnancies and outcomes
• previous labors and deliveries
• contractions
• rupture of amniotic membranes
• bloody show (a pink-tinged or blood-tinged mucus discharge) or vaginal bleeding (a bloody discharge without mucus)
• pregnancy-related health problems
• other health problems
• fetal movements
• prenatal care
• primary caregiver
• support person
• family members or friends.

Also obtain and document any other information required by the health care facility. (For an example, see *Sample labor admission form*, pages 652 and 653.)

Biographical data. Obtain the client's name, address, and other biographical information required by the health care facility.

Particularly note the client's age, because it can affect labor progress and outcome. A client under age 16 may be susceptible to pregnancy-induced hypertension (PIH), precipitous labor, and cephalopelvic disproportion (CPD, a condition in which the fetal head is too large or the mother's pelvis too small to permit vaginal birth). A client over age 35 may be predisposed to uterine dysfunction, premature labor, and placenta previa. (For more information about these concerns, see Chapter 31, High-Risk Intrapartal Clients.)

Health status. After obtaining biographical data, investigate the client's health status, paying particular attention to her current labor status and pertinent obstetric information.

Expected delivery date. Ask the client her expected delivery date or "due date." This information will help in assessing for a preterm or postterm neonate, determining gestational age (fetal age based on the first day of the mother's last menstrual period), and evaluating fetal size. It also will be helpful in planning the client's care. For example, a client who is in labor with a preterm neonate will need rapid assessment, and the neonate may require intensive care.

Previous pregnancies and outcomes. Find out the client's gravidity (number of pregnancies) and parity (number of births). Also determine if any of the pregnancies ended in spontaneous or induced abortions and if all of her children are living. If any of her children are dead, ask about the cause.

Gravidity and parity affect the duration of—and potential for complications in—successive labors. Generally, each labor shortens because the cervix and pelvic soft tissues offer less resistance and the uterus becomes more efficient, which promotes more rapid fetal expulsion. After more than five births, however, the uterus may lose its muscle tone, reducing its efficiency. More than five births may be associated with such complications as abruptio placentae, placenta previa (placental implantation in the uterus so that it covers part or all of the cervix), reduced uterine muscle tone and strength, hemorrhage, perinatal mortality (death sometime between the twenty-eighth week of gestation to the twenty-eighth day after birth), or maternal mortality.

Information about induced or spontaneous abortions helps in planning the client's care. It also reconciles the number of children with the number of pregnancies.

Previous labors and deliveries. Ask the client the date of her last delivery and the length of her last labor—information that can help predict the progress of the current labor and delivery. If the client's last delivery was within the past 10 years and without complications, labor should progress rapidly and smoothly. If the last birth occurred more than 10 years ago, labor may be longer, like that of a primigravid client. (For more information, see Chapter 24, Physiology of Labor and Childbirth.)

As a follow up, inquire about the birth weight of the newborns in previous pregnancies. Also determine if any were born prematurely or required cesarean delivery. Then ask if the client or any of her previous newborns developed complications.

A history of delivering neonates who are large for gestational age (LGA) may indicate gestational diabetes.

(Text continues on page 654.)

Sample labor admission form

During the initial assessment of a client who requests admission for labor, the nurse documents health history data, physical assessment findings, and laboratory test results, if available. Although health care facilities vary in their exact requirements for documentation, most expect the nurse to record the information shown in this form.

OBSTETRIC ADMITTING RECORD

Name _____

Address _____

_____ Telephone _____

BASIC ADMISSION DATA

G	T	P	A	L	LMP		E.D.D.		Age

Date _____ Time _____ : _____ a.m. p.m.

☐ Direct admit ☐ Transport ☐ Other

_____

☐ Ambulatory ☐ Wheelchair ☐ Stretcher

Next of kin _____

Telephone _____

Reason for admission
☐ Onset of labor
☐ Induction of labor
☐ Spontaneous abortion
☐ Cesarean section
  ☐ Primary ☐ Repeat

Observation or evaluation
☐ Fetal status
☐ Medical complication
☐ Obstetric complication
☐ Other _____

Detail reason: _____

_____

_____

ADMISSION PHYSICAL EXAMINATION (Check and detail all positive findings)

Ht	Wt	BP	Temp	Pulse	Resp

System	WNL	Abn	
HEENT	☐	☐	_____
Breasts	☐	☐	_____
Heart and lungs	☐	☐	_____
Abdomen	☐	☐	_____
Extremities	☐	☐	_____
Reflexes	☐	☐	_____

Blood sent _____ : _____ a.m. p.m.

Hgb _____ Hct _____

Urine Alb _____ Glu _____

Other tests _____

_____

_____

_____

_____

Fetal evaluation

Estimated gestation _____ weeks

Fundal height _____

Estimated fetal weight _____

FHR _____

Station _____

Effacement _____

Dilation _____

Position

Presentation
☐ Vertex
☐ Face or brow
☐ Breech (type) _____
☐ Transverse lie
☐ Compound

Nurse _____ Attending _____

CLIENT CARE DATA

Contractions on admission   ☐ None
Frequency _____ Duration _____ Quality _____
Began on _____ at ___ : ___ a.m. p.m.

Membranes on admission   ☐ Intact
☐ Ruptured: Date _____ at ___ : ___ a.m. p.m.
Fluid: ☐ Clear   ☐ Meconium   ☐ Foul-smelling

Vaginal bleeding   ☐ None
☐ Normal show   ☐ Bleeding (describe): _____
_____

Patient has:
☐ Recent URI   ☐ Dentures or caps
☐ Exposure to infection   ☐ Contact lenses
☐ Been vomiting   ☐ Glasses
☐ _____   ☐ _____

Plans for anesthesia   ☐ None planned
☐ Specify type _____
Last oral intake: Date _____ at ___ : ___ a.m. p.m.

Allergies or sensitivities   ☐ None
☐ Specify _____

Current medications ☐ None

Name and type of medication	Last taken	Check if brought in
_____	_____	☐
_____	_____	☐
_____	_____	☐

Procedures ☐ Prep   ☐ Enema (results) _____
☐ Other _____

Miscellaneous: (check which applies)
☐ Smoker   ☐ Non-smoker
☐ Will have support person in labor and delivery
☐ Plans circumcision
☐ Breast-feeding   ☐ Bottle-feeding
☐ Private   ☐ Semi-private   ☐ Rooming in

Physician's name _____
Notified by _____
Date _____ at ___ : ___ a.m. p.m.

SIGNIFICANT PRENATAL DATA

Prenatal education

Yes   No
☐   ☐   Attended classes or received instruction
☐   ☐*   Received prenatal care beginning at
              week _____
☐   ☐*   Records available on admission
*If no, give source of prenatal data: _____
Neonate's physician _____

Lab findings   ☐ None
Blood type and Rh _____
Rubella titre _____
Serology _____
_____
_____

Fetal assessment tests   ☐ None

Date	Test	Result
_____	_____	_____
_____	_____	_____
_____	_____	_____
_____	_____	_____

Latest risk assessment   ☐ No risk noted
☐ At risk   ☐ High risk
1. _____
2. _____
3. _____
4. _____
5. _____

A history of delivering neonates who are small for gestational age (SGA) may indicate premature delivery or intrauterine growth retardation. These problems may recur. A history of cesarean births or complications should alert you to prepare for surgery or close monitoring during a vaginal birth.

Contractions. Ask the client to describe the frequency and duration of her present contractions. Also find out when they began and determine the frequency and duration of those first contractions. Most women focus on their contractions and are eager to describe them. Eliciting this information first shows interest in the client's priorities. More important, it can help predict the client's labor progress and help distinguish true labor contractions from false labor (Braxton Hicks) contractions. (For more information, see *Characteristics of true and false labor.*)

Follow up with questions about the location of pain during the contractions. Ask the client if the location changes when she walks or if she feels rectal pressure during contractions. The location and nature of the pain help differentiate true labor from false labor, urinary tract infections (UTIs), and abruptio placentae. In true labor, the pain typically starts in the back and moves to the front of the fundus as a band of pressure that peaks and subsides. False labor feels like pressure in the abdomen with no regular pattern. UTIs produce a steady suprapubic or flank pain. Abruptio placentae causes constant, acute pain in a rigid, boardlike abdomen. Walking may increase true labor pain, but typically decreases false labor pain. Rectal pressure may indicate a stool-filled bowel or fetal descent and impending delivery.

Rupture of amniotic membranes. Next, determine the condition of the amniotic membranes and, if possible, the amniotic fluid. If the client is unfamiliar with medical terms, word your questions in simpler terms, such as, "Has your bag of waters broken?" Find out when the membranes ruptured and if they broke with a gush or in a trickle. If the client's membranes have ruptured, ask her to describe the amniotic fluid color. Also inquire if the fluid had an odor and if it has been leaking continuously since the membranes ruptured.

In about 10% of pregnant women, the amniotic membranes rupture before labor. In most cases, regular contractions begin within 12 hours of rupture. However, because intact membranes prevent vaginal organisms from entering the uterus, the risk of maternal and perinatal infection increases with the time elapsed between membrane rupture and the onset of contractions.

A client may confuse urinary incontinence, increased vaginal secretions, or the mucus plug (a small mass of mucus that fills the cervical os and is dislodged as labor begins) with rupture of membranes. A gush of water that runs down the legs even after voiding suggests ruptured membranes. Clear or pink-tinged fluid is normal. Green-tinged or yellowish green–tinged fluid signifies passage of meconium (thick, sticky, green-to-black stool of the fetus), a sign of fetal stress that requires immediate assessment. Port wine–colored fluid may indicate bleeding, as in abruptio placentae. Malodorous fluid suggests infection.

Bloody show or vaginal bleeding. Determine if the client has had any bloody show or vaginal bleeding. Increasing bloody show may signal the onset of the second stage of labor. Vaginal bleeding may signal placenta previa or abruptio placentae and subsequent fetal distress.

Pregnancy-related health problems. Return the focus of the interview to the current pregnancy. Ask if the client had any problems, such as bleeding, anemia, infections, or increased blood pressure. Also inquire if she underwent any special tests.

Characteristics of true and false labor

When a client requests admission for labor, the nurse must perform an initial assessment to determine whether she is in true labor. The following chart compares the characteristics of true and false labor.

CHARACTERISTIC	TRUE LABOR	FALSE LABOR
Contractions	Regular and rhythmic	Irregular
Pain	Discomfort that moves from the back to the front of the abdomen	Mild discomfort or pressure in the abdomen and groin; may be relieved by walking
Fetal movement	Unchanged	May intensify
Fetal descent	Progressing	Unchanged
Show	Pinkish mucus, possibly with the mucus plug from the cervix	None
Cervix	Progressing effacement and dilation	Unchanged after 1 to 2 hours

Knowledge of antepartal disorders prepares the health care team to manage possible problems. A history of recurrent UTIs can help differentiate true labor pain from that caused by infection. A history of a sexually transmitted disease (STD), such as gonorrhea, chlamydia, or genital herpes, can help guide the physical assessment and selection of laboratory studies. Special prenatal tests, such as ultrasonography or amniocentesis, can provide information about fetal status or the expected delivery date.

Other health problems. Next, ask if the client has any medical problems, such as diabetes, heart disease, high blood pressure, or kidney disease. A client with a health problem requires close monitoring, especially during labor. Knowledge of the problem will aid in planning intrapartal care.

Fetal movements. Have the client describe current fetal movements and find out if their frequency has changed from the usual rate over the past several days. A fetus usually moves at least 10 times a day. Decreased or absent fetal movements may indicate fetal hypoxia and stress, which require close fetal monitoring.

Health promotion and protection behaviors. Continue the initial assessment by inquiring about the client's antepartal health promotion and protection behaviors.

Prenatal care. First, ask if the client has received regular prenatal care. Between 15% and 30% of women receive no prenatal care; in some geographic areas, the percentage is even higher. Yet lack of prenatal care—or of recent prenatal care—increases the risk of complications and may affect the client's care. For example, a client who has not received care during the second and third trimesters probably will need more explanations and support.

Primary caregiver. If the client has had prenatal care, ask who provided it and where. The client's prenatal records can guide the complete health history and physical assessment. Usually around the client's thirty-sixth week of pregnancy, her physician or nurse-midwife will send copies of her records to the unit where she plans to deliver. (Her records may be less accessible if she delivers in a different health care facility.)

Roles and relationships. Evaluate the roles and relationships that may affect—or be affected by—the client's labor and delivery.

Support person. Ask a question such as, "Will someone be with you during labor?" to help identify the client's support person for inclusion in the plan of care. The support person can remain with the client during the physical assessment unless the person prefers otherwise.

Family members and friends. Ask the client which family members and friends have accompanied her to the unit. This information can help facilitate family support and participation in the client's care. Advising family members and friends of the client's progress and care can help alleviate anxiety and gain their cooperation.

Physical assessment
The initial physical assessment includes evaluation of:
• vital signs
• fetal heart tones
• uterine contractions
• fetal lie (relationship of the fetal long axis to the maternal long axis)
• fetal presentation (fetal part that enters the maternal pelvis first and can be touched through the cervix)
• fetal position (relationship of the leading fetal presenting part to a point on the maternal pelvis)
• engagement (descent of the fetal presenting part into the maternal pelvis)
• estimated fetal weight
• edema and deep tendon reflexes
• amniotic membranes
• cervical changes, fetal descent, and other factors determined by vaginal examination.

Vital signs. For a client in labor, vital signs provide necessary information about maternal and fetal health. They also provide baseline data for future comparisons.

First, check the client's blood pressure, which should range from 90 to 140 mm Hg systolic and from 60 to 90 mm Hg diastolic. A rise of 30 mm Hg systolic and 15 mm Hg diastolic above the client's usual blood pressure may signal anxiety, fear, or PIH, a complication that requires immediate medical attention. Decreased blood pressure may result from shock, maternal exhaustion, or supine hypotension.

Next, take the client's temperature, which normally ranges from 98° to 99.6° F (36.2° to 37.6° C). A temperature elevation may signal dehydration, a serious obstetric infection such as chorioamnionitis (fetal membrane inflammation), or another type of infection, such as a UTI.

Assess the client's pulse rate, which typically ranges from 60 to 90 beats/minute. An elevated pulse rate may be caused by anxiety, pain, infection, dehydration, or drug use.

Auscultating fetal heart tones

The nurse auscultates fetal heart tones to assess the fetal heart rate, which provides information about fetal viability and stress. To auscultate fetal heart tones, follow these guidelines.

1 Place the earpieces of an ultrasound stethoscope in your ears and press its bell gently on the client's abdomen. Start listening at the midline about midway between the umbilicus and the symphysis pubis. As an alternate auscultation method, listen with a fetoscope on your head with the bell extending from the center of your forehead. Then press the bell about ½″ into the client's abdomen. Remove your hands. With either method, move the bell slightly from side to side, if needed, to the point where the heart tones are loudest.

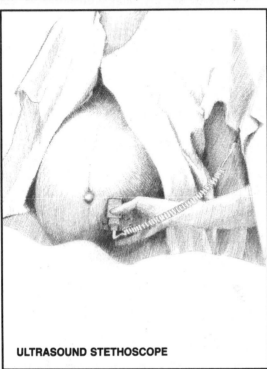

ULTRASOUND STETHOSCOPE

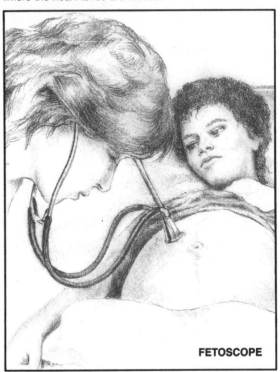

FETOSCOPE

2 Listen throughout several contractions and for at least 60 seconds afterwards to establish the well-being of the fetus. The normal fetal heart rate is 120 to 160 beats/minute. Check the fetal heart rate every 30 to 60 minutes during early labor, every 15 minutes during active labor, and every 5 minutes during the second stage of labor. Remember that heart rate accelerations and decelerations occur periodically during contractions and fetal movements.

3 If fetal heart tones are difficult to hear, perform Leopold's maneuvers to determine the fetal position and find the site where the heart tones are likely to be heard best. Refer to this illustration, which divides the abdomen into quadrants, and start listening at the point indicated by the position. If the fetal heart tones still are not clear, move in the direction indicated by the arrows. The fetus is likely to be in one of the following positions: left sacral anterior (LSA), left occiput anterior (LOA), left occiput posterior (LOP), right sacral anterior (RSA), right occiput anterior (ROA), or right occiput posterior (ROP). For example, with the fetus in a cephalic presentation, fetal heart tones are loudest midway between the client's umbilicus and the anterior superior spine of the ilium; in a breech presentation, tones are loudest at or above the level of the umbilicus.

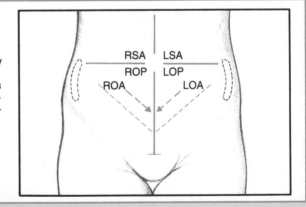

Finally, evaluate the client's respirations, which normally range from 16 to 24 breaths/minute. Increased respirations may indicate hyperventilation, anxiety, pain, or infection. Decreased temperature, pulse, and respirations do not commonly occur during labor.

Fetal heart tones. Assess the fetal heart tones to evaluate fetal well-being. If the health care facility requires, use a fetal heart monitor for this part of the assessment. (For more information, see Chapter 25, Fetal Assessment.) Otherwise, assess the heart tones via auscultation. (For an illustrated procedure, see *Psychomotor skills: Auscultating fetal heart tones*.) A variation from the normal fetal heart rate of 120 to 160 beats/minute may indicate fetal distress.

Uterine contractions. Evaluate the client's contractions to help distinguish true labor from Braxton Hicks contractions. To gather this information, use an external fetal monitor or palpate the client's abdomen, noting the frequency, duration, and intensity of the uterine contractions. Also observe the client during and between contractions to estimate her level of discomfort. (For an illustrated procedure, see *Psychomotor skills: Palpating uterine contractions*.) Ask the client's support person to record the contraction pattern, if possible.

Fetal lie, presentation, and position. Perform Leopold's maneuvers to determine the fetal lie, presentation, and position. (For more information, see Chapter 24, Physiology of Labor and Childbirth. For an illustrated procedure, see *Psychomotor skills: Performing Leopold's maneuvers*, page 658.)

Leopold's maneuvers help detect potential problems, such as breech presentation (where the buttocks or feet present first) or transverse lie (where the fetal long axis is perpendicular to the maternal long axis), that require physician or nurse-midwife evaluation. Also, they help anticipate the course of labor. For example, a client with a fetus in a posterior position probably will have a long, uncomfortable labor with lower back pain. (For more information, see *Variations in the first stage of labor*, page 659.)

Engagement. Palpate the abdomen to verify engagement. After engagement, labor may progress more quickly. In a primiparous client, an unengaged fetus (one that is floating above the pelvis) may indicate CPD. In any client, an unengaged fetus increases the risk of umbilical cord prolapse and warrants close supervision during labor.

PSYCHOMOTOR SKILLS

Palpating uterine contractions

Assessment of uterine contractions by palpation requires no special equipment. It does, however, demand nursing skill and sensitivity to touch. To palpate uterine contractions effectively, the nurse follows these steps.

1 Place the palmar surface of the fingers on the client's uterine fundus and palpate lightly. Note the uterine tightening and abdominal lifting that occurs with contractions. Keep in mind that each contraction has three phases: the increment (building up) phase, the acme (peak) phase, and the decrement (letting down) phase.

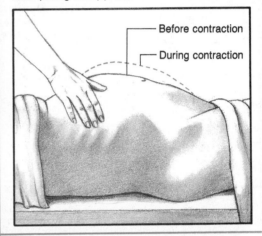

Before contraction
During contraction

2 Palpate during several contractions, determining their frequency, duration, and intensity. To assess frequency, time the period between the beginning of one contraction and the beginning of the next. To evaluate duration, time the period from the onset of uterine tightening to its relaxation. While the uterus is tightened, determine the intensity of the contraction by pressing the fingertips into the fundus. During mild contractions, the fundus indents easily and feels like a chin. In moderate contractions, the fundus indents less easily and feels more rigid, like the tip of a nose. With strong contractions, the fundus is firm, resists indenting, and feels like a forehead.

Estimated fetal weight. Assess the fetal weight by measuring the fundal height. (For more information, see Chapter 19, Care during the Normal Antepartal Period.) Then correlate the estimated weight with the gestational age to identify a fetus that is LGA or SGA.

An LGA estimate may indicate a large fetus or more than one fetus. Alternately, it may indicate hydramnios (excess amniotic fluid), which suggests gestational diabetes and warrants close monitoring during labor. An SGA estimate can result from prematurity or miscal-

Performing Leopold's maneuvers

Leopold's maneuvers allow the nurse's systematic evaluation of the client's abdomen to determine fetal position. Although this palpation technique takes practice to gain proficiency, it is generally reliable except in clients who are obese or who have hydramnios (excess amniotic fluid).

Before performing Leopold's maneuvers, have the client void and lie supine with her abdomen uncovered. To reduce abdominal muscle tension, place a pillow under her shoulders and ask her to draw her knees up slightly. Warm your hands before touching the client's abdomen to avoid startling her or causing discomfort. After she has been prepared, follow these steps.

1 Use the first maneuver to determine which part of the fetus lies in the upper uterus. Facing the client, lightly palpate her upper abdomen with both hands. The head feels round and firm. The buttocks feel softer and have bony prominences.

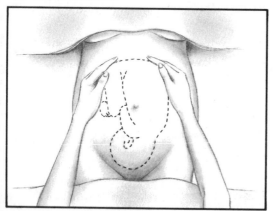

2 Perform the second maneuver to locate the back. Using gentle pressure, palpate the left side of the client's abdomen with the palm of your right hand, while steadying the opposite side with your left hand. Repeat the maneuver with your right hand steadying and your left hand palpating. On one side of the client's abdomen, the back of the fetus should feel firm and smooth; on the opposite side, the extremities should feel like small irregularities or protrusions.

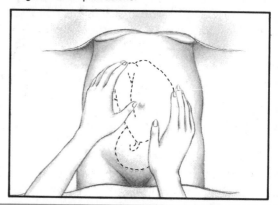

3 Carry out the third maneuver to identify the presenting part (the part of the fetus above the pelvic inlet). Using the thumb and fingers of your dominant hand, grasp the client's abdomen just above her symphysis pubis. The fetal part found here should be the opposite of the one found in the upper abdomen. If the head is palpated and can be moved gently back and forth, it is not yet engaged.

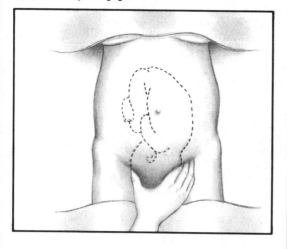

4 Perform the fourth maneuver to determine the descent of the presenting part. Stand facing the client's feet. Then gently move your hands down the sides of the client's abdomen toward her symphysis pubis, noting which side has greater resistance. This resistance is caused by a normal bony prominence of the fetus's head, either the brow (a narrow prominence) or the occiput (a broad prominence). If the head is flexed, the brow will be palpated on the side opposite where the back was identified. If the head is extended, the occiput will be palpated on the same side as the back.

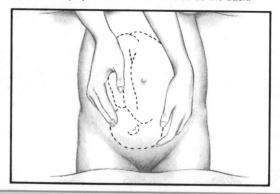

Variations in the first stage of labor

In the first stage of labor, variations may be in the childbirth process, such as premature rupture of membranes (PROM), or may involve the fetus, such as occiput posterior positioning. The nurse must be able to identify such common variations and intervene appropriately.

Premature rupture of membranes

PROM refers to rupture of the amniotic sac before the onset of labor. It occurs in approximately 10% of clients with term pregnancies. Of these, about 80% will begin labor spontaneously within 24 hours. PROM may occur in clients with normal pregnancies, but also commonly occurs in those with multiple gestation, hydramnios, or fetal malpresentation.

When a client reports fluid leakage on admission, obtain a thorough history to rule out such conditions as urinary incontinence, vaginal discharge, or loss of the cervical mucus plug. (For details, see the "Initial assessment" section of this chapter.) To help confirm or rule out PROM, determine the time of occurrence, the time of last sexual intercourse, and the quantity, color, and odor of the fluid.

Then inspect the perineum for obvious fluid leakage. If no fluid is apparent, assist with or conduct a vaginal examination. In addition to the usual vaginal examination equipment, gather a sterile vaginal speculum, sterile cotton swabs, microscope slides, and nitrazine paper.

If specially prepared to perform this procedure, inspect the cervical os through a speculum, using strict sterile technique. Because PROM increases the risk of chorioamnionitis, be especially careful to prevent any contamination. Amniotic fluid pooling in the vaginal vault or oozing from the cervical os signals PROM.

Using a sterile cotton-tipped applicator, take fluid from the cervical os and spread it on a slide to dry. Microscopic evaluation of this fluid can confirm the presence of amniotic fluid—and PROM—through sodium chloride crystallization, or ferning.

Do not insert nitrazine paper into the vagina, because the paper is not sterile. Instead, touch the paper to the speculum blade after removing the speculum from the vagina. The paper will turn bright blue if the fluid is alkaline with a pH of 7.0 to 7.5. Such a positive test result can confirm PROM, although it is less reliable than the microscopic evaluation.

When PROM is confirmed, treatment begins. Some experts believe that the fetus must be delivered within 12 to 24 hours after PROM to prevent chorioamnionitis. This aggressive approach may require induction of labor with oxy-tocin or cesarean birth. Other experts take a more conservative approach, allowing labor to progress naturally. When caring for a client with PROM, use the following interventions:
• Monitor fetal heart tones every 30 minutes. Tachycardia may indicate infection; bradycardia indicates hypoxia, which suggests umbilical cord compression if the membranes have ruptured. (For more information, see Chapter 33, Intrapartal Complications.)
• Evaluate the client's pulse and temperature at least every 2 hours to detect signs of infection (pulse rate over 90 beats/minute or temperature over 99.6° F [37.6° C]).
• Postpone vaginal examinations until after the client begins active labor to avoid introducing infectious organisms.
• Provide frequent perineal care.
• Ensure adequate hydration with oral or I.V. fluids, as prescribed.
• Encourage the client to rest until labor begins.
• Stimulate labor by walking, if the client's condition permits.

Occiput posterior positioning

This fetal malposition occurs when the fetal occiput enters the pelvic inlet posteriorly in the oblique diameter instead of in the transverse diameter. It forces the vertex to press against the sacrum. This prolongs the active phase of labor and makes it more painful, especially in the lower back, producing what is called back labor. The position can cause hypotonic uterine dysfunction (decreased strength of uterine contractions and reduced uterine muscle tone) and, if incomplete rotation occurs, a deep transverse arrest of the fetal head or cephalopelvic disproportion, which may require surgical intervention or forceps delivery. (For information about persistent occiput posterior positioning, see Chapter 31, High-Risk Intrapartal Clients.)

Occiput posterior positioning affects 15% to 30% of all clients. However, given sufficient time and adequate uterine contractions, most fetuses in this position rotate anteriorly. To care for a client with an occiput posterior fetus, take the following steps:
• Help the client change positions frequently to promote fetal rotation.
• Encourage adequate hydration and frequent urination to keep the bladder empty, which provides more room for the fetus to rotate.
• Use sacral massage and counterpressure to relieve lower back pain.
• Administer analgesics to relieve pain, as prescribed.

---

culation of the estimated delivery date. It also can result from a growth-retarded fetus, which requires close monitoring during labor.

Edema and deep tendon reflexes. Inspect and palpate the client's extremities for edema. Slight localized edema of the feet and ankles is normal late in pregnancy. However, edema of the face (especially in the periorbital area and bridge of the nose), hands, or pretibial area may signal generalized edema and PIH, especially if accompanied by brisk deep tendon reflexes or clonus. If these signs are present, notify the physician immediately.

Amniotic membranes. Whether or not the client reported a sudden gush of fluid during the health history, check the amniotic membranes. To do this, inspect the vaginal opening for obvious fluid leakage. If fluid is present, test it with nitrazine paper. A positive test result (in which the paper turns bright blue) may confirm rupture of the amniotic membranes or may indicate nitrazine paper contamination with sterile lubricant, semen, or bloody show.

If the membrane status is in doubt, expect the physician or nurse-midwife to confirm or rule out ruptured membranes by inspecting the cervical os through a speculum and examining the fluid through a microscope. (For more information about cervical inspection, see Chapter 7, Women's Health Promotion.) In a client with ruptured membranes, inspection of the cervical os will reveal oozing, and the microscopic examination will show ferning (a microscopic fernlike pattern produced by sodium chloride crystallization in dried amniotic fluid).

Vaginal examination. The vaginal examination determines the client's labor progress by assessing cervical changes, confirming amniotic membrane status, and evaluating fetal position and descent. If specially educated in this skill, the nurse may conduct the vaginal examination. Otherwise, the nurse assists a physician or nurse-midwife.

To prepare for a vaginal examination, gather the appropriate equipment based on the health care facility's procedures and the maternal and fetal status. For example, if the fetus shows signs of distress, obtain electronic fetal monitoring equipment with an internal catheter or electrode for insertion during the examination. Then help the client into a comfortable lithotomy position and drape her to maintain dignity.

During the examination, talk to the client. Help her relax her vaginal muscles by suggesting conscious relaxation techniques. After the examination, clean the client's perineum and change the disposable pad under her buttocks, as needed. Cover the client with her bed sheet, if she desires. Explain the examiner's findings, as appropriate, and answer any questions.

Immediately document vaginal examination findings. Include the date, time, findings, the examiner's name, and any procedures that were performed, such as an amniotomy (artificial rupture of membranes) or placement of fetal scalp electrode or intrauterine pressure catheter.

With additional preparation, the nurse may conduct a vaginal examination to assess cervical position, dilation, effacement (cervical shortening and thinning), and station (level of the fetal head in relation to the maternal pelvis). (For an illustrated procedure, see *Psychomotor skills: Performing a vaginal examination*, pages 668 and 669.)

Before labor begins, the cervix typically lies in the posterior part of the vagina. During labor, it rotates forward to midposition. A tight muscular band in the vagina may be mistaken for cervical dilation when the cervix actually is closed and posterior. To locate cervical position accurately, palpate the entire vagina with the fingertips.

Dilation, effacement, and station vary as labor progresses. The initial assessment findings will provide a baseline for later evaluations of labor progress and will help in planning the client's care.

If dilation is present without fetal descent, use caution during later vaginal examinations to prevent membrane rupture and umbilical cord prolapse.

Preparation for admission or discharge

Review all of the health history and physical assessment findings to develop a complete clinical picture of the client. Then consider the health care facility's policy for admission. If the client is in true labor or meets the standards for admission, continue to prepare her for delivery. If she is in false labor and she and the fetus are in stable condition, call the physician or nurse-midwife for discharge orders and instructions for the client's return.

For a client who must be discharged, suggest comfort measures and explain medical orders. Keep the client's safety in mind when providing instructions. Suggest that a warm tub bath or shower assisted by a family member can ease discomfort. Propose drinking warm milk or herbal tea and reclining semi-upright with pillows under her knees to promote rest. Encourage hydration with clear liquids and nourishment with light meals rich in carbohydrates. Suggest a massage by the client's support person to promote comfort.

Instruct the client to return to the health care facility if her membranes rupture, if she develops bleeding, if her contractions become more intense, or if she shows signs of infection, such as fever. Also advise her to return if normal fetal movements change dramatically.

Document the client's discharge. Be sure to record the initial assessment findings and recommendations that the client received for follow-up with the health care provider.

After the client is discharged, do not be surprised if she decides to linger in the snack bar or other nearby area, especially if she is a multiparous client in very early labor (which is sometimes difficult to distinguish from false labor) or if she fears a precipitous birth in an uncontrolled environment. The client may base her decision on such factors as her distance from the health care facility, access to transportation, ability to cope with her current status, or her family's concerns and ability to assist her at home.

Nursing care after admission

Clients and their support people enter the labor and delivery unit in widely varying emotional states and degrees of preparedness. Some enter in excited anticipation, armed with extensive preparation through childbirth education classes. Others arrive at the unit with resignation or dread of a painful, unrewarding experience that will bring an unplanned, unwelcome newcomer into their overburdened family. Still others enter in a state of panic-when their well-planned, out-of-hospital birth becomes an obstetric emergency. Others who expected a steady, predictable labor are admitted in frenzy and surprise, faced with a precipitous birth.

Regardless of the family's emotional state or preparation on admission, the nurse should make every effort to create a calm, welcoming environment. This will help decrease their apprehension and stress and promote a more positive childbirth experience.

Orientation

After the client has been officially admitted, acquaint her and her support person with their physical environment. Introduce yourself as the nurse who will care for them, and ask the client and her support person the names they prefer to be called. Remind the client to give any money, jewelry, or other valuables to her family for safekeeping.

To promote relaxation and comfort during labor, many clients bring special items from home, such as pillows, nightgown, fan, radio or tape player, camera, and pictures or personal objects to use as focal points. Help the client and her support person arrange these items to create a personal space that does not block access to the client or equipment. Convey respect for their rights by being nonjudgmental about their preferences, as long as they do not interfere with safety codes or institutional policies.

Orient the client and her support person to the call light, bed adjustment control, equipment to be used, and to the location of the bathroom, lounge, and telephone. A thorough orientation will help reduce their anxiety and convey openness to their needs, encouraging them to participate fully.

An informed consent is obtained before any procedure is performed on a client in labor. The physician or nurse-midwife should inform the client of each procedure's benefits, risks, and alternatives and obtain the consent. Then the nurse should allow time to answer the client's questions and discuss her concerns. If medications or the stress of labor compromises the client's ability to make rational decisions, include her support person or a family member in discussions about care and procedures. Document the client's—or her family's—consent in her records.

Ongoing assessment

After the client is admitted to the labor and delivery area, complete her health history, perform a detailed physical assessment, and collect laboratory data. The assessment data will serve as the basis for developing a care plan for the client and her family.

Health history

This interview supplements the initial health history, which emphasized the client's current labor status, with questions that review all body systems and assess her psychosocial status. If the client's prenatal record includes this information, do not collect it again. If her record is unavailable or if she does not have frequent contractions or severe pain, assess the following areas in this order:
• family history
• medical and surgical history
• activities of daily living
• psychosocial status.

Vary the length of the ongoing health history based on the client's condition. For example, if the client's labor is progressing rapidly, shorten the interview. If the timing of contractions permits, investigate each area.

Family history. Begin by asking the client if anyone in her family has a disorder that may affect her labor and delivery, such as diabetes or hypertension. A client with a family history of these disorders may develop complications during the stress of labor.

Medical and surgical history. Next, determine if the client is allergic to any medications, anesthetics, foods, or other substances. An allergy history is useful in preventing contact with allergens that can add to the client's stress during labor.

Inquire whether the client has ever had a blood transfusion. If so, find out when and determine if it caused any reactions. Particularly note any history of transfusion reactions, which increases the likelihood of a recurrence if the client receives blood during labor.

Ask what kind of surgery the client has had. If she received an anesthetic during surgery, find out which type and how well she tolerated it. Be alert for a history of reproductive organ surgery, which may leave adhesions that can affect labor. The client's experience with spinal anesthesia can help predict how well she will tolerate it during delivery, if needed.

Activities of daily living. Ask the client whether she uses alcohol, cigarettes, or prescription, over-the-counter, or street drugs. If she does, find out how much she consumes daily and when she consumed it last. Use of alcohol or drugs may endanger maternal and fetal health. It also may interfere with labor and the effects of prescribed analgesics or anesthetics, which may require dosage adjustments based on the timing of the last ingestion. Cigarettes reduce fetal weight and produce maternal respiratory congestion, causing difficulty if the client receives a general anesthetic.

Ask when the client had her last food and drink. If general anesthesia is necessary, this information can signal the possibility of vomiting and airway obstruction.

Determine how well the client has been sleeping and resting. The quality and quantity of the client's sleep and rest may determine how much energy she has for labor. A client who has not been sleeping well may benefit from interventions that help her relax, breathe properly, and conserve her energy.

Inquire about the client's weight before becoming pregnant and ask how much weight she has gained during her pregnancy. Note any unusually large weight gain, which could indicate diabetes or hydramnios.

Psychosocial status. For a client in labor, a psychosocial assessment is an important part of her total evaluation. Key factors that influence a client's response to labor include her personality, previously established reaction patterns, and other childbirth experiences. Other influential factors include her relationship with her support person, relationship with her mother, general attitude toward conception, and feelings about the timing of this pregnancy. A client also may be affected by her perception and acceptance of herself as a woman, partner, and mother as well as by various social, cultural, and economic adjustments required during childbearing.

The psychosocial assessment provides information that can be used to enhance the client's coping skills and intervene in self-defeating or stressful behaviors. This will help build her self-confidence, which can promote her sense of control over the process, decrease her stress, and ultimately promote a positive childbirth experience, maternal and fetal well-being, and maternal-infant bonding.

During this part of the health history, observe the client carefully to obtain a full picture of her current psychosocial status. Note how she presents herself for care by considering her general appearance, facial expression, posture, and body language. Also study her verbal and nonverbal cues to help determine how she is coping. For example, a client who appears sad and lethargic may be depressed about having a child.

To assess the client's psychosocial status, pose questions that investigate the following areas.

Cultural or ethnic background. Have the client describe her background. Culture and ethnicity can affect expectations and perceptions of childbirth. For example, some cultures do not allow a male support person during childbirth; others expect his attendance. A culturally sensitive, nonjudgmental nurse can find out what the client expects and try to meet her needs.

Child care considerations. Ask about the client's plans for breast-feeding or bottle-feeding the neonate. If she has not made a decision about feeding, discuss the options with her. If she has made a decision, support it. The client's decision will help determine when to bring the neonate to her for the first feeding. If she wants to breast-feed, plan to put the neonate to the breast shortly after birth. If she wants to bottle-feed, explain that the neonate's first feeding may occur in the nursery. She can administer subsequent feedings.

Discuss child care arrangements. If the client has other children at home, ask how old they are. Also determine if she feels the need for help with child care or household management when she goes home. This information can help predict the client's ability to manage child care and other activities when she returns home. Friends, family members, and older children may help decrease her work load; younger children may increase it. A client discharged shortly after delivery may need referral to a social service or home care nurse agency if she has inadequate help.

Knowledge and concerns about labor and delivery. If the client has attended childbirth education classes, find out which type. This information provides an estimate of her knowledge of labor and delivery and allows proper nursing support for her chosen childbirth method.

To assess the client's understanding of—and worries about—her impending labor and delivery, pose such questions as, "What do you know about labor and delivery?" and "Do you have any concerns or fears about childbirth?"

Knowledge and concerns can affect the client's childbirth experience. Lack of knowledge can lead to nonproductive efforts and stress. To prevent these, provide more information, as needed. A client's ability to cope with childbirth may be hampered by fear of death or trauma to herself or the fetus, fear of a difficult delivery that causes pain and loss of control or self-esteem, or fear of bearing a deformed or stillborn neonate. She also may feel stressed by concerns about her adequacy as a mother, changes in family relationships, or financial problems. Encourage such a client to share her concerns.

Goals for labor and delivery. To obtain this information, ask such questions as, "What are your goals for labor and birth?" or "How would you like your support person to participate?" The client's answers can help determine whether her goals are realistic and flexible and aid in planning for the support person's participation.

Conclude the assessment by finding out what kind of support the client prefers during labor and delivery. Clients vary greatly in the support they want and in their ability to convey their needs to the nurse or support person. Note the client's preferences, and help her support person and family understand them.

Physical assessment

Based on the client's answers during the health history, focus the physical assessment on findings that could affect labor, delivery, and maternal or fetal well-being. The following health history findings require detailed physical assessment:
• Skin rash or lesions, especially on the genitals. These signs may indicate an STD, such as herpes, that could be transmitted to the fetus.
• Jaundice. This sign may signal liver disease, which could reduce the client's ability to clear anesthetics and medications from her body.
• Visual difficulties. These symptoms may result from elevated blood pressure, which occurs in PIH.
• Headaches, dizziness, or syncope. These symptoms also may be linked to PIH.
• Signs and symptoms of upper respiratory tract infections, such as congestion or rhinorrhea (nasal discharge). Such effects may cause problems if the client receives general anesthesia or undergoes intubation. They also may indicate cocaine use.
• Edema. A client with generalized or excessive edema may have PIH or a kidney disorder that may cause labor complications.
• Indigestion, nausea, vomiting, or diarrhea. These gastrointestinal problems can lead to dehydration, which depletes the energy needed for labor.

• Signs and symptoms of dehydration, such as thirst or dry mucous membranes. A dehydrated client will need fluids to maintain her blood volume and prevent further problems.
• Vaginal itching. This symptom may signal a vaginal infection that could be transmitted to the fetus.
• Vulvar varicosities or hemorrhoids. A client with these swollen, tortuous veins should be monitored for pain or thrombosis during labor.
• Dysuria (burning or pain on urination). This symptom suggests a UTI, which could increase the client's discomfort during labor and delivery.
• Problems with back, pelvis, or abduction of legs that involve stiffness, difficulty in moving, or pain. Any of these problems may make the client uncomfortable when in the lithotomy position. Back problems may worsen during labor.
• Varicosities in legs. A client with this condition may develop thrombosis and reduced blood flow to the legs during contractions.
• Calf pain. This symptom may indicate that thrombosis has occurred.

Laboratory studies
Review all of the client's laboratory data. Consider the results of routine antepartal studies, special antepartal tests (if the client has a chronic disease, such as diabetes, or an obstetric concern, such as a genetic disorder), and the routine studies performed on admission to the labor and delivery area. (For additional information, see *Common laboratory studies,* page 664.)

Nursing diagnosis

The nurse reviews all health history, physical assessment, and laboratory test findings. Based on these, the nurse formulates nursing diagnoses for the client, fetus, support person, or other family members, as needed. (For a partial list of possible nursing diagnoses, see *Nursing diagnoses: First stage of labor,* page 665.)

Initial planning and implementation

After assessing the client and fetus, the nurse plans and implements routine admission procedures, such as intravenous (I.V.) fluid infusion and skin preparation. The nurse should prioritize these procedures based on the labor progress, the ease of implementation, and the client's comfort, safety, preference, and need to move about.

Common laboratory studies

To obtain complete assessment data for a client in labor, the nurse must consider the results of routine and special prenatal laboratory studies as well as studies ordered on admission to the labor and delivery unit. The chart below lists commonly ordered studies and describes their significance to the pregnant client.

ROUTINE PRENATAL TESTS

ABO blood typing and Rh typing
Identify blood type and Rh factor—vital information if the client needs a blood transfusion. Also point out potential Rh incompatibility with the fetus if the client is Rh-negative.

Antibody screening test (indirect Coombs' test)
Detects anti-$Rh_o(D)$ antibodies in the client's blood and evaluates the need for $Rh_o(D)$ immune globulin administration.

VDRL test or rapid plasma reagin (RPR) test
Screens for syphilis, which can be transmitted through the placenta to the fetus after the eighteenth week of pregnancy.

Rubella antibodies test
Determines whether the client has antibodies to the disease. If not, she must avoid exposure to rubella during the first trimester to prevent transmittal to the fetus, which could cause anomalies.

Complete blood count
Hemoglobin and hematocrit: Screen for anemia, which may reduce the ability of the blood to carry oxygen to the fetus.
White blood cell (WBC) count with differential: Identifies infections and blood dyscrasias, which could lead to complications when labor stresses the client's body systems.
Platelet count: Assesses clotting mechanisms and alerts to potential bleeding problems during delivery.
Red cell indices: Identify specific type of anemia if hemoglobin and hematocrit are low, and guide specific treatments.

Urinalysis
Albumin: Screens for pregnancy-induced hypertension, renal disease, or kidney disease, which can worsen during pregnancy.
Microscopic analysis: Screens urine for red blood cells, WBCs, casts, epithelial cells, and microorganisms, which may indicate renal disease or infection.

Papanicolaou (Pap) test
Identifies cervical cancer. Also screens for herpes simplex Type 2, which can be transmitted to the fetus during passage through the birth canal.

Gonorrhea culture
Detects gonorrhea, which typically is asymptomatic in women. During childbirth, gonorrhea in the cervix can cause a neonatal eye infection and a serious puerperal infection for the client.

SPECIAL PRENATAL TESTS

Alpha-fetoprotein test
May identify fetal anomalies, such as anencephaly (absence of brain and spinal cord), spina bifida, and other neural tube defects. Very high levels may identify omphalocele (herniation of fetal viscera through the abdominal wall), other anomalies, or fetal death.

Two-hour postprandial plasma glucose test
Evaluates for gestational diabetes.

Hemoglobin electrophoresis
Identifies hemoglobinopathies, such as sickle cell anemia and thalassemia, which may be passed genetically to the fetus.

Hepatitis B surface antigen test
Screens for hepatitis B, which can infect the fetus, producing low birth weight and acute liver changes.

HIV III antibody test
Detects the acquired immunodeficiency syndrome (AIDS) virus, which can be transmitted to the fetus, requiring infection precautions during labor and delivery.

ROUTINE ADMISSION TESTS

Hemoglobin and hematocrit
Track levels of these blood components, because many clients develop anemia, especially late in pregnancy.

VDRL test or rapid plasma reagin (RPR) test
Detects recent infection with syphilis.

Gonorrhea culture
See above.

ABO blood typing and Rh typing
See above. Most health care facilities require these tests on admission of a client who has not had a prenatal workup or whose results are not available.

Urinalysis
Assesses for changes in urine composition, which may occur as pregnancy stresses the kidneys.

NURSING DIAGNOSES

First stage of labor

The following potential nursing diagnoses are examples of the problems and etiologies that a nurse may encounter when caring for a client in the first stage of labor. Specific nursing interventions for many of these diagnoses are provided in the "Planning and implementation" sections of this chapter.

- Altered tissue perfusion: decreased placental, related to maternal position
- Anxiety related to fear of death during childbirth
- Anxiety related to hospital environment
- Impaired gas exchange related to hyperventilation with increasing contractions
- Impaired physical mobility related to electronic fetal monitoring equipment
- Ineffective family coping: compromised, related to client's hospitalization
- Ineffective family coping: compromised, related to client's pain
- Ineffective individual coping related to absence of extended family
- Ineffective individual coping related to lack of family support
- Knowledge deficit related to admission procedures in the labor and delivery area
- Knowledge deficit related to appropriate relaxation techniques
- Knowledge deficit related to obstetric procedures
- Knowledge deficit related to the labor process
- Pain related to uterine contractions
- Potential fluid volume deficit related to restricted oral intake and increased fluid output
- Self-care deficit related to limited mobility during labor

I.V. fluid infusion

Because anesthetics delay gastric emptying and relax the swallowing reflex, which may cause subsequent aspiration, the physician is likely to limit the client's intake to minimum oral fluids and ice chips. However, a client in labor may perspire heavily, breathe rapidly, and urinate frequently, creating the potential for a fluid volume deficit. Therefore, the physician may order continuous I.V. fluid infusion, but its use during labor remains controversial.

Supporters of routine I.V. infusion suggest that it provides safe, adequate hydration and ready access for emergency medications. It also prepares the client for management of labor complications or emergency surgery and for infusion of oxytocin, blood, or blood volume expanders, if needed.

Newton, Newton, and Broach (1988) and other researchers dispute the routine use of I.V.s for clients in labor. Their arguments against nonselective I.V. infusion

include client discomfort, rapid absorption of clear liquids even in labor, placement of the client in the sick role, inhibition of walking, increased risk of phlebitis and sepsis, and potential for accidental fluid overload and induction of neonatal hypoglycemia.

Expect to administer I.V. fluids to a client with a nursing diagnosis of *potential fluid volume deficit related to restricted oral intake and increased fluid output.* Also plan to use this intervention under the following circumstances: maternal exhaustion and dehydration; fetal distress; oxytocin induction or augmentation; grand multiparity (more than five births); history of postpartal hemorrhage; potential for uterine overdistention and atony caused by such factors as multiple gestation, macrosomia, or hydramnios; a life-threatening obstetric or medical condition, such as abruptio placentae, PIH, or diabetes; or potential need for surgery or regional anesthesia.

If an I.V. is ordered, prepare the specified I.V. fluid, such as normal saline or lactated Ringer's solution. Plan to start the I.V. in the client's cephalic vein just above the wrist, if possible. If blood samples have not yet been obtained for laboratory studies, gather the appropriate vials and take samples before starting the I.V. Then infuse the fluid at the prescribed rate.

During the infusion, watch for signs of fluid overload, infiltration, and phlebitis. Also, watch for restlessness or agitation, which can dislodge the catheter.

Skin preparation

A literature review by Mahan and McKay (1983) suggested that complete skin preparation (removal of all pubic hair) contributes to—rather than prevents—infection, primarily because it abrades the skin, creating entry routes for infectious organisms. In most health care facilities, complete skin preparation, or prep, has been omitted or replaced by removal of hair from the lower third of the labia or from around the part of the perineum where an episiotomy or laceration would be repaired. When any type of prep is ordered, perform the procedure according to the health care facility's policy.

Enema administration

For a client in labor, enema administration is no longer a routine procedure. Researchers have found—contrary to previous beliefs—that it does not prevent fecal contamination at birth, that labor is impeded only by severe bowel impaction, that labor stimulation with enemas is ineffective, and that many women have diarrhea during labor so the bowel is relatively empty. They also point out that many clients find enema administration uncomfortable and embarrassing and would prefer to avoid it

(Mahan and McKay, 1983). However, if an enema is ordered, administer it according to the health care facility's policy.

Ongoing planning and implementation

During the first stage of labor, continually monitor the status of the client and the fetus as well as the labor progress. Also provide comfort and support to the client, and plan and implement care for her family.

Do not let any activities interfere with the client's ability to work with her body (efforts to coordinate breathing with contractions) or with her support person's assistance during labor. Instead, encourage the support person's active involvement, use gentle touch and calm verbal assurance to show respect for their efforts, and when appropriate, communicate that all is going well. Repeatedly praise the client's efforts and validate her feelings.

Monitor vital signs

To help provide safe care, evaluate the client's vital signs as often as required by health care facility policy. Taking the phase of labor into account, follow these guidelines:

During the early phase (0 to 3 cm of cervical dilation), assess the client's blood pressure, pulse, and respirations hourly, if no problems are anticipated or discovered. Monitor her temperature every 4 hours throughout labor, unless she has ruptured membranes or a temperature above 99.6° F (37.5° C). In these instances, monitor her temperature every 2 hours while checking her pulse. Be sure to record all findings.

During the active phase of labor (4 to 10 cm of cervical dilation), check blood pressure, pulse, and respirations every hour (if normal). When the client reaches transition, the final part of the active phase of labor (7 to 10 cm of cervical dilation), evaluate more frequently, at least every 30 minutes.

Monitor uterine contractions

The policy of the health care facility—and the physician's or nurse-midwife's orders—will determine exactly how often uterine contractions must be monitored. However, most facilities provide similar guidelines. For example, many state that unless a deviation occurs, the nurse must assess contractions every hour during the early phase and every 30 minutes during the active phase of the first stage of labor.

The facility's policy and physician's or nurse-midwife's orders also will determine whether uterine contractions are monitored by abdominal palpation or electronic fetal monitoring (EFM). Both methods have advantages and disadvantages.

Abdominal palpation requires no special equipment and is noninvasive. When performed by an experienced nurse, it is a reliable way to monitor uterine contractions. (For more information, see *Psychomotor skills: Palpating uterine contractions,* page 657.) However, it is not as accurate as EFM.

EFM provides sensitive, constant, and highly accurate documentation of contractions. It can be external or internal. External EFM is less invasive and usually reliable, but is affected by position and obesity. Internal EFM measures the pressure exerted during contractions more accurately than external EFM, but increases the risk of infection. For EFM to be effective, the equipment must be applied and working properly, the client cooperative, and the nurse skilled at using the equipment and interpreting the data. (For more information, see Chapter 25, Fetal Assessment)

Regardless of the method used, monitor the intensity, frequency, and duration of the contractions. Keep in mind that uterine activity can be affected by maternal exhaustion or dehydration, rupture of membranes, medication, position changes, and increased anxiety. A client with any of these factors needs closer monitoring than usual.

When monitoring contractions, pay careful attention to the relaxation period between them. Resting uterine tonus can become abnormally elevated, making the intensity of the contractions difficult to assess. If palpation reveals that the uterus is not relaxing adequately between contractions, the client may have abruptio placentae or dysfunctional labor. This uterine hypertonicity can decrease placental perfusion, causing severe fetal hypoxia and distress.

Monitor fetal response to labor

Frequently evaluate the fetus to maintain well-being. (For details, see *Fetal status: Fetal evaluations during labor.*) Depending on the health care facility's policies, assess the fetus by auscultating fetal heart tones or using EFM. Each method has advantages and disadvantages.

Auscultation can be performed with an ultrasound stethoscope (Doppler blood flow detector) or fetoscope. This noninvasive technique gives the client more freedom to move. However, it is open to subjective interpretation, making it somewhat less accurate than EFM.

EFM provides a more precise, continuous record of the fetal heart rate and response to contractions than auscultation. Many clients find it more reassuring of fetal well-being and more helpful in anticipating con-

FETAL STATUS

Fetal evaluations during labor

During labor, the nurse must frequently monitor the fetus—as well as the client—to help maintain their health. To assess fetal status accurately, the nurse follows these steps.

• Auscultate the fetal heart rate, rhythm, and response to contractions at least every 30 minutes in the early phase of labor, every 15 minutes during active labor, and every 5 minutes in the second stage of labor. As an alternate technique, evaluate fetal heart rate patterns using an electronic monitor at least every 30 minutes in the early phase of labor, every 15 minutes during active labor, and every 5 minutes in the second stage of labor.
• Note the amniotic fluid color when the membranes rupture.
• Evaluate the results of fetal scalp sampling and pH testing, if prescribed.

tractions and allowing support people to participate in the childbirth experience. Others view it as invasive and unnatural.

External EFM can be restrictive, uncomfortable, and anxiety-producing if a position change or equipment malfunction causes temporary loss of the fetal signal. Internal EFM more accurately records subtleties in fetal response to uterine contractions, improving the health care professionals' ability to respond to a fetus in jeopardy. However, it requires ruptured membranes, which increase the risk of infection, cord accidents, and scalp abscesses. (For more information, see Chapter 25, Fetal Assessment.)

Monitor labor progress

Perform or assist with vaginal examinations, as needed, to monitor cervical dilation, effacement, station, and other indicators of labor progress. (For an illustrated procedure, see *Psychomotor skills: Performing a vaginal examination,* pages 668 and 669.)

The frequency of vaginal examinations generally depends on the client's condition and the nurse's ability to observe the contraction pattern, bloody show, client's behavior, level and location of discomfort, and location of fetal heart tones. If these signs indicate that the labor is progressing normally, vaginal examinations are performed infrequently. If they point to abnormal labor progress, vaginal examinations should be performed regularly.

Vaginal examination frequency also depends on the risk of introducing infection. However, a vaginal examination must be done on admission, before the client receives any medication, when verifying entry into the second stage of labor, when the client develops an increased urge to push, and after spontaneous rupture of membranes. If labor progress is compromised, a vaginal examination can be performed as determined by the health care facility's policy.

Monitor urinary function

Continually evaluate the client's urine output and assess for proteinuria and ketonuria, especially if the client has a nursing diagnosis of *potential fluid volume deficit related to restricted oral intake and increased fluid output.* The client should urinate at least every 2 hours, and her urine should contain no protein or ketones.

During active labor, the client may develop bladder distention with decreased urine output. As the descending fetus compresses the bladder, distention can occur when the bladder contains as little as 100 ml of urine. This increases the client's discomfort, impedes labor progress by preventing fetal descent, and can lead to postpartal UTIs. To detect bladder distention, check for an irregularity in the lower abdomen or a distinct bulge over the symphysis pubis while monitoring uterine contractions and fetal heart tones.

To prevent bladder distention, encourage the client to urinate at least every 2 hours. Help her walk to the bathroom or use the bedpan, and suggest that she listen to running water, pour warm or cool water over her perineum, and perform Kegel exercises. If she still cannot urinate and shows signs of increasing distention, inform the physician or nurse-midwife and obtain an order for straight catheterization.

The presence of protein in urine (proteinuria) may signal the onset of PIH, or it may indicate that the urine was contaminated with vaginal secretions, amniotic fluid, or perspiration. To aid diagnosis of PIH, check for other signs, such as elevated blood pressure, edema, and exaggerated deep tendon reflexes. If you detect these signs, notify the physician or nurse-midwife.

Ketonuria may indicate dehydration or maternal exhaustion. If ketonuria is present, notify the physician or nurse-midwife, and monitor the client and fetus more closely.

Provide comfort and support

During childbirth, the client not only needs physical care but also a supportive human presence, pain relief, acceptance, information, and reassurance. By constantly providing for the client's physical comfort and emotional support, the nurse can meet most or all of these needs.

(Text continues on page 670.)

PSYCHOMOTOR SKILLS

Performing a vaginal examination

During the first stage of labor, a vaginal examination (performed by a specially prepared nurse or physician) provides data about cervical dilation, effacement, station, fetal presentation and position, engagement, and status of the membranes.

When conducting a vaginal examination, the nurse maintains the client's privacy, provides simple guidance, talks with her and her support person, maintains eye contact,

and uses aseptic technique. Taking a gentle, nonassaultive approach, enhance vaginal relaxation by inserting two fingers in the vagina; ask the client to squeeze her vagina around them and then release the tension.

Develop a routine system for collecting the necessary information so that it becomes automatic and efficient during the vaginal examination. To perform the examination, follow these steps.

1 After the client empties her bladder, help her into a comfortable lithotomy position and place a disposable pad under her buttocks. Put on sterile gloves. Then cleanse her perineum with mild soap and water, spreading her labia with your independent hand to avoid contaminating your examining hand.

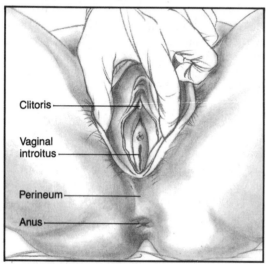

Clitoris

Vaginal introitus

Perineum

Anus

2 Lubricate the index and middle fingers of your examining hand with sterile water or water-soluble jelly. Insert your lubricated fingers slowly into the client's vagina, with the palmar surface down and the rest of the fingers flexed to avoid the rectum.

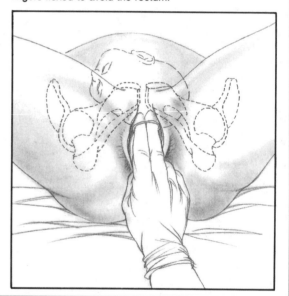

3 Place your other hand on the client's fundus and gently press down. This steadies the fetus and helps press the fetal presenting part against the cervix for examination.

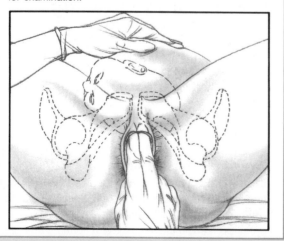

4 Gently rotate the examining fingers while palpating. Identify the fetal presenting part (head, breech, or other part) and position (left, right, anterior, posterior, or transverse).

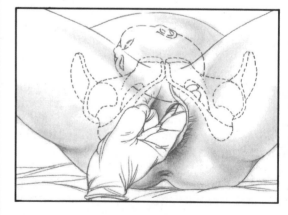

PSYCHOMOTOR SKILLS

Performing a vaginal examination continued

5 Palpate the cervix, noting the centimeters of dilation.

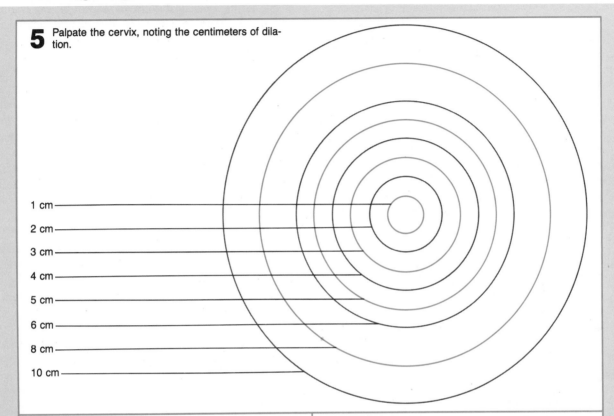

1 cm
2 cm
3 cm
4 cm
5 cm
6 cm
8 cm
10 cm

6 Also note cervical consistency (soft or firm) and degree of effacement.

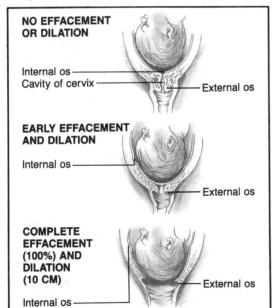

NO EFFACEMENT OR DILATION

Internal os
Cavity of cervix
External os

EARLY EFFACEMENT AND DILATION

Internal os
External os

COMPLETE EFFACEMENT (100%) AND DILATION (10 CM)

External os
Internal os

7 Describe the fetal engagement (descent of the fetal presenting part into the pelvis) and grade the fetal station (the location of the presenting part in relation to the ischial spines of the maternal pelvis). Determine the status of the membranes. Palpation of a bulging slick surface over the presenting part confirms intact membranes.

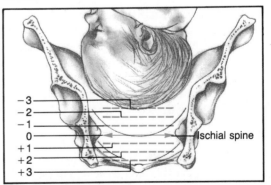

−3
−2
−1
0
+1
+2
+3
Ischial spine

8 Remove your examining hand gently. Allow the client to clean her perineum if she is able to walk to the bathroom. If she is confined to bed, cleanse her perineum and change the disposable underpad.

When caring for a client in the first stage of labor, individualize her care by selecting comfort and support measures that are most effective for her. These measures include creating a supportive atmosphere, promoting good positioning and walking, maintaining hygiene, conserving energy, promoting rest and effective breathing, educating the client and advocating on her behalf, integrating her cultural beliefs and practices, and relieving pain.

All of these measures help reduce the client's anxiety and prevent stress on the fetus. Furthermore, increased maternal anxiety is associated with uterine dysfunction and intrauterine hypoxia that can lead to physiologic disturbances in neonates (Lederman, Lederman, Work, and McCann, 1985; Sosa, Kennell, Klaus, Robertson, and Vrrutia, 1980).

Tailor all comfort and support measures to the client's condition and phase of labor. In early labor, the client may be excited or apprehensive but usually is talkative and sociable. She can be distracted easily with a diversional activity, such as watching television, reading, taking a walk, or even sleeping.

As active labor begins, the client becomes more serious and preoccupied with her contractions. She may become quiet and withdrawn, or panicked and verbal; she may begin to doubt her ability to cope. Companionship and a relaxed, quiet atmosphere can aid her concentration and coping abilities and can promote rest between contractions. Breathing techniques may help her maintain self-control.

During the transition phase, contractions grow rapid and intense. The client becomes self-absorbed, restless, irritable, and hypersensitive and may develop nausea, vomiting, hiccups, belching, or a natural amnesia. Increased perspiration with intermittent chills and hot flashes may sweep quickly over her. She may feel discouraged or panicky. During this phase, do not leave her alone. Provide constant reassurance, firm guidance in using modified breathing techniques, and steadfast physical and emotional support and comfort. Although the transition phase is the most painful, analgesics are used with caution because the amount needed to reduce the pain would depress the fetus and because this phase usually is very brief.

Create a supportive atmosphere. Be sensitive to the family's need to create a supportive environment. Intervene, as needed, to prevent a nursing diagnosis of *ineffective family coping: comprised, related to client's hospitalization, anxiety related to fear of death during childbirth,* or *anxiety related to the hospital environment.* Help the family personalize the environment to enhance the client's comfort, security, and privacy and improve the labor progress by reducing anxiety and pain (Simpkin, 1986).

The ideal labor room is open, airy, private, and free of distracting noises. It conveys respect for the client's privacy and dignity. The room should have adjustable lighting and temperature, a cheerful color scheme, and monitoring equipment.

This ideal environment is common in birthing rooms, labor-delivery-recovery rooms, and alternative birthing centers. It is less common in large public health care facilities or tertiary care centers where most of the clients require sophisticated medical equipment and close supervision. Even under these circumstances, however, the nurse can humanize the environment by maintaining the client's privacy, dimming bright lights (especially during the transition phase), and taking other actions that show concern for the client's comfort.

Promote good positioning and walking. During labor, a client may be confined to bed because of concomitant procedures, such as labor induction, epidural anesthesia, or pain relief through analgesia or sedation; convenience in monitoring maternal and fetal well-being; or the policy of the health care facility. Such a client may have a nursing diagnosis of *impaired physical mobility related to electronic fetal monitoring equipment.* For a client who must remain in bed, help her maintain a lateral—rather than supine—position to enhance labor efficiency, comfort, and safety. (For more information, see *Health promotion through lateral positioning*.)

When allowed freedom of movement, most clients will change positions many times to maximize comfort and enhance labor progress. If the client is not confined to bed, help her find comfortable positions that allow adequate maternal and fetal surveillance. (For more information and illustrations, see *Alternate positions for labor,* page 672.) These interventions will help a client with a nursing diagnosis of *altered tissue perfusion: decreased placental, related to maternal position.*

Also help the client walk around, if possible. Although long walks may tire her, brief walks can decrease pain and improve comfort (Caldeyro-Barcia, 1979). They also can shorten labor by encouraging fetal descent, using gravity to promote application of the presenting part against the cervix, and allowing better alignment of the uterus with the vaginal canal and the presenting part with the cervix (Fenwick and Simkin, 1987).

Contraindications to walking include exhaustion, preterm labor, vaginal bleeding, medication administration, fetal intolerance to labor, an unengaged fetus with cervical dilation or ruptured membranes, fetal malposition, and precipitous labor.

Health promotion through lateral positioning

For many years, health care professionals recommended the supine position for a client in labor. Although this position permits easy monitoring of the client and fetus, it can create problems because it narrows the diameter of the pelvis and the vagina, creates pelvic immobility, increases discomfort, diminishes the intensity of uterine contractions, and does not take advantage of gravity (Fenwick and Simkin, 1987). Most important, this position causes the fetus to compress the client's aorta and inferior vena cava, as shown. This inhibits maternal circulation and leads to maternal hypotension and, ultimately, fetal hypoxia.

Today, the lateral (side-lying) position commonly is used to prevent maternal vessel compression and hypotension. This position promotes maternal and fetal circulation, enhances comfort, increases maternal relaxation, reduces muscle tension, and eliminates pressure points. It also produces stronger—but less frequent—uterine contractions that enhance uterine efficiency and improve cervical dilation (Caldeyro-Barcia, 1979). Pillows can help the client maintain this position, as shown.

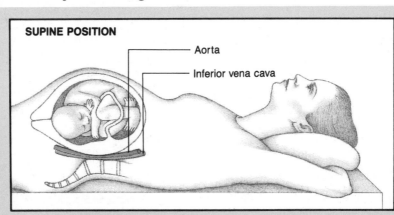

SUPINE POSITION
- Aorta
- Inferior vena cava

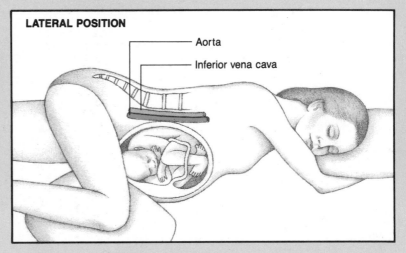

LATERAL POSITION
- Aorta
- Inferior vena cava

Maintain hygiene. During active labor, the client perspires heavily and produces increased vaginal secretions (with intact membranes) or a constant flow of wet, sticky vaginal drainage (with ruptured membranes). These activities can compromise her hygiene, add to her general discomfort, and may result in a nursing diagnosis of *self-care deficit related to limited mobility during labor.*

To maintain hygiene and promote comfort, suggest a warm shower or, if her membranes have not ruptured, a tub bath, to the client who is allowed to walk. As an alternative, perform a sponge or bed bath, providing meticulous perineal care. Change the client's gown and sheets whenever they become saturated. Also change the disposable underpad, especially after a vaginal examination. Frequently wipe the client's face and neck with a cool, clean washcloth, especially during the transition phase. To help her feel fresh, suggest using her own toiletries, if available, and powder her skin or comb her hair.

Provide mouth care during labor. Encouraging the client to brush her teeth or use mouthwash can help freshen her breath, remove any stale taste, and moisten her mouth and throat, which can become dry if oral fluids are restricted. You also can help moisten a dry throat by offering frequent sips of water or allowing her to suck on ice pops, hard candy, or a washcloth saturated with ice water. These techniques are especially effective during the transition phase. To soothe dry, cracked lips, suggest applying lip balm or petrolatum and using lemon and glycerin swabs.

Conserve energy and promote rest. Help the client work with her body by using a conscious relaxation technique, especially if she has a nursing diagnosis of *knowledge deficit related to appropriate relaxation techniques.* (For more information, see Chapter 26, Comfort Promotion during Labor and Childbirth.) This intervention not only will promote the client's self-esteem and sense of control,

Alternate positions for labor

If a client has learned to use certain positions in a childbirth education class, help her and her support person achieve and maintain them. A client in labor rarely is confined to bed and limited to one or two labor positions. In fact, by using alternate positions she can enhance her labor progress, comfort, and safety. If a client has not been taught to use specific positions, suggest several and help her and her support person with them throughout labor. The following illustrations show some common labor positions.

Forward-leaning sitting

For a client with back pain during labor, forward leaning supported by the back of a chair may reduce pain by lifting the weight of the fetus off the spine. Offering some gravity advantage, this position can be used with electronic fetal montoring (EFM) and is a good posture for resting or for a back rub.

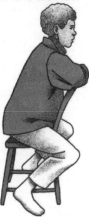

Squatting

By leaning back over her heels with her knees apart, the client can give the fetus as much room in the pelvis as possible. She may need help getting into this position, but once there may find it quite comfortable. Squatting takes advantage of gravity and may relieve backache as well as enhance fetal rotation and descent in a difficult birth. It allows the client to shift her weight for comfort, requires less bearing down, and may increase her urge to push.

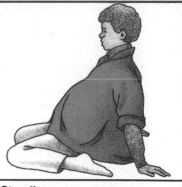

Standing

This position takes advantage of gravity, promotes less painful—but more productive—contractions, and aligns the fetus with the pelvic angle. It also may speed labor and increase the urge to push. If a client prefers to stand, she may lean forward against a wall. Forward leaning offers the same advantages as standing, but may be more restful and may relieve backache.

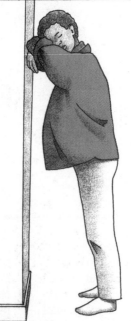

Sitting

A client may find sitting to be the most comfortable position. She may wish to lean against her partner, which allows them to breathe together through the contractions. As an alternative, the client may sit in a chair or in the bed. A good resting position, sitting takes some advantage of gravity and allows EFM.

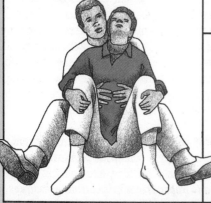

Hands and knees

Getting down on all fours also can relieve low back pain and can take pressure off the umbilical cord and any hemorrhoids. The position may be difficult to get into and out of, but it allows movement and promotes rotation when the fetus is in the occiput posterior position.

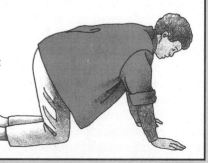

but also will conserve her energy and promote comfort. To promote rest between contractions, maintain a calm, quiet atmosphere and organize nursing tasks to minimize disturbances.

Based on the client's preference, use a gentle or therapeutic touch to promote relaxation. (For more information, see Chapter 26, Comfort Promotion during Labor and Childbirth.) Some clients find these techniques restful and reassuring and respond well even to simple hand-holding. Others find them offensive or intrusive, especially if they develop hyperesthesia (increased sensitivity, usually in the skin).

Use massage to promote relaxation and help the client remain in control. Teach the support person to perform a counterpressure massage on the lower back, sacrum, and buttocks to help ease labor discomfort. During the transition phase, a back or foot massage can be especially effective. Show the client how to use effleurage (a light, fingertip self-massage) on her lower abdomen to decrease pain by providing distraction and increasing circulation. (For more information, see Chapter 19, Care during the Normal Antepartal Period.)

The use of visual imagery, quiet speech, eye contact, and appropriately timed analgesia also can promote rest and conserve energy. So may soft music and a cool breeze created by a hand-held fan, especially during the transition phase. (For more information, see Chapter 26, Comfort Promotion during Labor and Childbirth).

Promote effective breathing. Effective breathing patterns help the client work with her body efficiently and can break the anxiety-pain-hyperventilation cycle that may occur even in a prepared client. They also can help prevent or correct a nursing diagnosis of *impaired gas exchange related to hyperventilation with increasing contractions.*

If the client has learned certain breathing patterns in childbirth education class, reinforce her learning and support her efforts. If she has not attended classes, briefly teach her how to breathe effectively. During early labor, tell her to inhale deeply at the beginning of a contraction and exhale slowly; to take deep, slow, rhythmic breaths through the remainder of the contraction; and to breathe normally between contractions. During active labor, advise her to inhale deeply at the beginning of a contraction and exhale slowly; to take four or five small, shallow breaths during the contraction; and to take four or five deep breaths at the end of the contraction.

Educate and advocate. For each client and her family, provide simple, factual information about such things as labor progress, procedures, and medications. This will decrease the client's fear, tension, and pain and increase

---

CULTURAL CONSIDERATIONS

Using a labor support person

Although each client has personal beliefs and values, her cultural background may influence her behavior. When caring for a client from a different culture, the nurse should keep the following considerations in mind.

Not every culture encourages the use of a labor support person. Even in the United States, a support person has gained wide acceptance only within the past 20 years. The following two examples illustrate how a client's cultural background can affect her ideas about a labor support person—and her nursing care.

In the Orthodox Jewish faith, certain religious laws require modesty to maintain personal dignity. Even a husband, despite his intimate relationship with his wife, is forbidden to observe her directly when she is immodestly exposed. Therefore, if an Orthodox Jewish couple enter the labor and delivery area, the nurse should be sensitive to their beliefs by draping the client appropriately during vaginal examinations and perineal care, and by giving the husband an opportunity to leave the room during care in which his wife's body is exposed (Lutwak, Ney, and White, 1988).

In Dempsey and Gesse's study (1985) of Cuban refugees, most clients expected the father to be present through labor and birth "so he knows what his wife is going through and what will happen." When caring for a Cuban client, the nurse should provide opportunities for the father's involvement whenever possible.

To integrate a client's cultural beliefs into her care, first identify these beliefs by asking open-ended questions, such as, "Would you like any special people or items with you during labor?" or "Would you like anything else now that I've explained our procedures?" By acknowledging the existence of cultural variations, the nurse can incorporate them in the care plan as long as they do not compromise the safety of the client or fetus.

---

her and her support person's confidence in their ability to cope. It also will address nursing diagnoses, such as *knowledge deficit related to the labor process* and *knowledge deficit related to obstetric procedures.*

Advocate on the client's behalf, especially when acute care is needed, as with fetal distress. Continue to encourage the client and her support person to participate in the birth as much as possible. Ultimately, this will enhance their sense of esteem and mastery of the childbirth experience despite the obstacles encountered.

Integrate cultural beliefs and practices. Clients from various cultures may have labor practices and beliefs about childbirth that differ greatly from the nurse's. For example,

---

NURSING RESEARCH APPLIED

A comparison of labor pain in multiparous and primiparous clients

For years, health care professionals believed that multiparous clients felt less pain during labor and delivery than primiparous ones. However, early research results were contradictory. To investigate this phenomenon, Lowe conducted a study on 17 primiparous and 33 multiparous clients in a labor and delivery area. All had normal pregnancies and gave birth vaginally. They varied in their preparation for labor and delivery, use of sedative or analgesic medication, and induction of labor (spontaneous or oxytocin-induced).

The researcher evaluated each client's pain using the McGill pain questionnaire, a survey that rates pain on how a person ranks 20 sets of words that describe the sensory, affective, evaluative, and other aspects of pain. During the first stage of labor, the clients reported pain data in all three phases: early (latent), active, and transitional. They reported on second-stage labor pain immediately after delivery. The researcher found that parity had no overall effect on pain, but discovered that primiparous clients experienced more severe pain than multiparous ones during early labor and less severe pain during the second stage.

Application to practice

The findings of this small, descriptive study suggest that a nurse may need to intervene differently during labor for a primiparous client than for a multiparous one. For any client, the nurse should actively support and enhance confidence in her ability to handle labor, which is based on her perceptions of pain. The nurse must provide strong support to a primiparous client in early labor, when she is especially vulnerable to the effects of increased anxiety and decreased confidence. The nurse needs to help a multiparous client deal with intensifying pain late in the first stage of labor and into the second stage of labor. During this difficult period, the nurse must plan activities carefully to be available to the client.

Lowe, N.K. (1987). Parity and pain during parturition, *JOGNN*, 16(5), 340-346.

---

a client's cultural background may forbid the use of a support person. (For more information, see *Cultural considerations: Using a labor support person*, page 673.)

Be sensitive to the client's beliefs and customs. Find out about her cultural background and individual preferences. Then, based on this information, provide care that shows respect for her health attitudes, beliefs, and behaviors during labor. For a client with a nursing diagnosis of *ineffective individual coping related to absence of extended family*, for example, get family members as involved in the labor process as possible rather than having them wait in another area.

Relieve pain. Labor is physically demanding. Some clients experience extreme pain and other intense physical sensations; others experience merely bothersome cramping. Especially in the active phase of labor, a client may wonder whether she can endure the experience. This can create the classic fear-tension-pain cycle first identified by Grantley Dick-Read in 1945. (For more information, see Chapter 26, Comfort Promotion during Labor and Childbirth.)

For a client with a nursing diagnosis of *pain related to uterine contractions*, try different measures to relieve pain. Use progressive relaxation techniques, biofeedback, acupressure, or visual imagery, along with paced breathing, frequent repositioning, and the emotional and physical assistance of her support person. Or try alleviating her pain through analgesia and anesthesia, depending on safety considerations, labor progress, maternal and fetal well-being, and her preference and coping ability. (For more information, see Chapter 26, Comfort Promotion during Labor and Childbirth, and *Nursing research applied: A comparison of labor pain in multiparous and primiparous clients.*)

Care for the family

Throughout labor, provide care not only for the client and fetus, but also for the family. Each family requires individualized interventions based on needs and childbirth goals. For a family with a nursing diagnosis of *ineffective family coping: compromised, related to the client's pain*, for example, suggest ways for individuals to provide comfort for the client. (For more information, see *Family care: Involvement in labor.*)

Keep in mind that some people choose not to participate in a family member's childbirth experience. The partner may prefer not to be involved; the client may not want her partner to see her during labor. Respect each person's preferences and avoid imposing personal values.

If the client and her partner want to share the experience, acknowledge the partner's importance and offer every opportunity to participate. Involvement in childbirth can increase the partner's self-esteem and lets the partner provide valuable emotional and physical support to the client. In most cases, no one can give better labor support than the client's partner.

The partner's involvement also provides other benefits. Some researchers report that clients use less pain medication when the partner is present during labor. Others have found that labor is shorter when a supportive partner is present. In addition, a man who participates in his child's birth may feel enriched.

If the client's or partner's parents participate in the labor and birth, consider their information needs. In the last 50 years, birthing practices have changed dramat-

---

FAMILY CARE

Involvement in labor

Traditionally, the focus of childbearing has been on the client's role in pregnancy, labor, delivery, and parenting. This focus views childbearing as a physiologic function rather than a developmental role that can be shared. Today, the client may share the labor and birth with her partner or support person as well as other family members, including the neonate's grandparents and siblings. To promote the effective involvement of these people, the nurse can use the following interventions.

For the partner or support person

• Promote confidence in the ability to support the client through this demanding period. If the support person has difficulty accepting what the client is experiencing, offer reassurance that many people find this experience difficult or unpleasant.
• Welcome the support person on admission, using the person's preferred name to encourage relaxation.
• Include the support person in the client's history and physical assessment, if both desire this participation.
• As part of the psychological assessment, evaluate goals for the support person's involvement in childbirth. Keep in mind that involvement may range from being present during labor to active coaching throughout.
• Assess the support person's physical and emotional needs and plan ways to address them during labor.
• Reduce anxiety and feelings of awkwardness by showing concern for the support person's interest and participation in childbirth.
• Make the support person feel important to the client's comfort and support.
• Direct care and support measures if the support person is hesitant or unprepared. Demonstrate or suggest the following comfort activities: hand holding, fanning, wiping the client's face with a cool cloth, offering clear liquids or ice chips, providing a sacral counterpressure massage, and helping her to walk or find a comfortable position with pillows.
• Reinforce the prepared support person's knowledge of conscious relaxation and breathing techniques.
• Facilitate the prepared support person's interaction and foster successful sharing of this intimate, creative experience. Encourage the support person's participation. Do not try to take over or intervene in the support person's style of labor coaching.
• Suggest appropriate times for the support person to take a break to eat, rest, or attend to personal hygiene. This prevents the person from feeling overwhelmed or trapped. Offer to stand in for the support person during breaks. Time these breaks to prevent the disappointment and frustration that may result if birth occurs while the support person is away.
• Help the support person listen to the fetal heart tones, whenever desired.
• Inform the support person of routine changes in fetal heart rate patterns and their significance.
• Assure the support person that frequent monitoring does not indicate an impending problem.
• Keep the support person involved if a crisis arises during labor. Help allay feelings of helplessness and fear by remaining calm and confident, sharing information, and providing reassurance that the health care team is doing everything possible to achieve a healthy outcome.

For the grandparents

• Be sensitive to the impact that unfamiliar and perhaps frightening modern birthing equipment and procedures may have on the grandparents. Explain the equipment and procedures, as needed.
• Regularly inform anxious family members outside the labor and delivery area of the client's progress.
• Advise the family about necessary medical treatments or procedures. Reassure them that the health care team is doing everything possible to provide safe, high-quality care.

For the siblings

• Introduce yourself to the children and the person who will be caring for them and answering their questions.
• Be aware that a child's response to childbirth depends primarily on maturity and interest. Most children included in the experience handle it well.
• Maintain a calm, matter-of-fact attitude to reassure the children that everything is proceeding normally. Most children will assimilate the information casually.

---

ically, requiring the nurse to educate the older generation to aid their understanding and address their concerns.

If the health care facility allows, siblings may participate, which prevents separation anxiety for the children and mother, provides an opportunity to learn about birth, gives a chance to participate in an important family event, and enhances bonding between siblings. Most health care facilities that permit sibling participation require that they be fully prepared in childbirth education classes where they learn about the sights, sounds, and smells of childbirth (Anderson and Del-Giudice, 1983).

Evaluation

To complete the nursing process, evaluate the effectiveness of nursing care by reviewing the goals attained and the family's involvement and satisfaction with the care. State the evaluations in terms of actions performed or

Client with pain related to back labor

The nursing process helps ensure high-quality care for a client in the first stage of labor. The table below shows how the nurse might use the nursing process when caring for the client described in the case history at right. The first column presents history and physical assessment data followed by a paragraph of mental notes. These notes help the nurse make important mental connections among assessment findings, aiding in development of the nursing diagnosis and planning.

The second column lists an appropriate nursing diagnosis; information in the remaining columns is based on this diagnosis. Although not part of the nursing process, a rationale appears for each intervention in the fourth column to explain how it contributes to the care plan.

ASSESSMENT	NURSING DIAGNOSIS	PLANNING
Subjective (history) data • Client says that she is 3 days past her due date. • Client states that this is her first pregnancy. • Client reports that her contractions occur 2 minutes apart and last 45 seconds. • Client reports that her water just broke. • Client describes the pain as "mostly in my back," and says it worsens with contractions. **Objective (physical) data** • Vital signs: temperature 97° F, pulse 112 beats/minute, respirations 32/minute, blood pressure 114/78 mm Hg. • Fetal heart rate: 140 beats/minute. • Uterine contractions: 2-minute frequency, 45-second duration, moderate intensity. • Leopold's maneuvers: vertical lie, occiput posterior presentation, engaged. **Mental notes** *Complaints of back pain that worsens with contractions could indicate fetal occiput posterior positioning, which typically causes an unusually long, uncomfortable labor with lower back pain. If so, the client's husband may be a great help in providing comfort and support.*	Pain related to back labor	**Goals** The client will: • learn to use various coping techniques for managing back labor • use heat or cold to reduce back pain • use various labor positions to foster anterior rotation of the fetus • demonstrate an increased ability to cope with her back labor. The client's partner will: • actively assist her during contractions and back labor.

outcomes achieved for each goal. The following examples illustrate appropriate evaluation statements.
• The client and her family understood admission procedures, equipment, and the expectations of the health care team as evidenced by clear, two-way communication.

• The client used a relaxation method that worked for her during the active phase of labor.
• The support person took effective comfort measures, as evidenced by the client's ability to rest between contractions.

CASE STUDY

Maria Belize, a primiparous client age 23, is admitted to the labor and delivery area with contractions and severe back pain. She walks with difficulty, leaning on her husband. Her respirations are abrupt and rapid, at 32/minute.

IMPLEMENTATION		EVALUATION
Intervention	**Rationale**	Upon evaluation, the client:
Teach the client about the possible causes of back labor and coping strategies that she can use.	Information about back labor gives the client a sense of control over her pain, decreasing her anxiety and pain.	• reported reduced back pain after interventions for back labor were initiated
Assess fetal position.	An occiput posterior fetal position may cause back labor and indicate the need for interventions that favor anterior rotation.	• demonstrated an increased ability to cope with her back labor.
Teach the client to use relaxation techniques and slow, paced breathing (not less than one-half the normal respiratory rate) between contractions.	Relaxation and breathing techniques may help the client relax during labor, reducing her pain.	
Advise the client to increase her respiratory rate (not more than twice the normal rate) and modify her breathing pattern during contractions.	Proper breathing helps maintain relaxation during the later part of labor and prevent hyperventilation.	
Show the client's partner how to apply firm counterpressure with the heel of one hand to the sacral area.	Counterpressure massage can reduce the client's pain and promote her comfort.	
Encourage the client to let her partner know the amount and location of counterpressure that relieves the most pain.	Feedback allows the partner to relieve pain most effectively and prevents feelings of helplessness during a difficult labor.	
Help the client assume a side-lying, upright forward-leaning, or hands-and-knees position.	These positions allow the pressure of the fetus to fall away from the client's back.	
If the fetus is in the occiput posterior position, help the client change positions at least every 30 minutes (from the side-lying to the hands-and-knees to the opposite side-lying position).	Frequent position changes foster anterior rotation of the fetus.	
Apply a warm, moist towel to the client's lower back.	Application of heat may help decrease back discomfort.	
Apply an ice bag or rubber glove filled with ice chips to the client's lower back.	Application of cold may help decrease back discomfort.	

• The support person actively participated in labor by helping the client cope.

Remember that evaluation stimulates continued reassessment—and improvement—of the effectiveness of nursing care throughout the intrapartal period.

Documentation

Based on initial and ongoing assessment findings, the nurse uses the nursing process to formulate nursing diagnoses and then plan, implement, and evaluate the client's care. (See *Applying the nursing process: Client with pain related to back labor.*)

Sample labor progress chart

Throughout the first stage of a client's labor, the nurse must document the labor progress, fetal status, such key events as placement of an internal fetal scalp electrode, and other important data. Although health care facilities may vary in their documentation requirements, most expect the nurse to record information similar to that shown in the sample chart below.

LABOR PROGRESS CHART

Name: MARGARET SMITH
Address: 105 SOUTH STREET
BAR HARBOR, MAINE   Telephone: 555-9801

G	T	P	A	L	EDC	Admit date	Admit time	a.m./p.m.	Age	Blood type and Rh	Page / of /
2	1	0	0	1	1/8/91	1/1/91	4	p.m.	31	O+	

Membranes are ☑ Intact ☐ Bulging ☐ Ruptured / / at : a.m. p.m.
Fluid was ☐ Clear ☐ Meconium ☐ Foul Smelling

	TIME	4 a.m./p.m.				5 a.m./p.m.				6 a.m./p.m.				7 a.m./p.m.				8 a.m./p.m.				a.m./p.m.				a.m./p.m.				a.m./p.m.			
Station Mark X / **Dilation** Mark O		00	15	30	45	00	15	30	45	00	15	30	45	00	15	30	45	00	15	30	45	00	15	30	45	00	15	30	45	00	15	30	45
−4	10																		O														
−3	9																																
−2	8													O																			
−1	7																																
0	6	X				X																											
+1	5					O																											
+2	4	O																															
+3	3													X				X															
	2																																

Effacement % and/or position	80		90			100		100				

Effacement % and/or position: 80 / 90 / 100 / 100

Examined by: H. KANE, MD / HK / HK / HK

Blood pressure: 110/70 / 112/70 / 120/80 / 120/72 / 120/70

FHR: 150 / 160 / 150 / 160 / 150

Contractions
- Frequency: 3-4 / 3 / 2-3 / 2 / 2
- Duration: 45 / 50 / 50 / 50 / 60
- Quality: MOD / MOD / MOD-FIRM / FIRM / FIRM

T: 98
P: 80
R: 18

Medications and key events (use space to sign or initial events)

4:15 p.m. ADMITTED TO LDR # 2 IN ACTIVE LABOR, IV 1000 ml NORMAL SALINE STARTED IN Ⓛ ARM. EXTERNAL FETAL MONITOR APPLIED.
P. Johnson, RN

8:15 p.m. PATIENT PUSHING – PREPARED FOR DELIVERY.
Linda Samuels, RN.

Be sure to document assessment findings and nursing activities as thoroughly and objectively as possible. Thorough documentation not only allows evaluation of the effectiveness of the nursing care plan, but also makes data available to other members of the health care team, which helps ensure consistent care. To document as accurately as possible, make sure the entries describe events exactly, completely, and in chronological order.

Although each health care facility may require documentation of slightly different information, most require the nurse to record the following information on the continuing labor record after initial assessment is completed:
• client's vital signs
• fetal heart rate pattern (variability, baseline, periodic changes, and use of external or internal monitor)
• uterine contraction pattern (intensity, frequency, and duration)
• vaginal examination findings (cervical dilation, effacement, station, position, and status of membranes)
• spontaneous or artifical rupture of membranes and description of amniotic fluid
• application of internal fetal scalp electrode or intrauterine pressure catheter
• client's position changes or behaviors, such as crouching or vomiting
• fluid intake and output
• administration of medications, oxygen, I.V. fluids, and epidural anesthesia
• client's response to treatments received
• presence of family members
• physician or nurse-midwife visits with the client.

(For an example of documentation during the first stage of labor, see *Sample labor progress chart.*)

Chapter summary

Chapter 27 described how to assess and care for the client, fetus, and family during the first stage of labor. Here are the chapter highlights.
• A significant life event, labor is a physiologic, psychological, and sociocultural process.
• Before a client may be admitted to the labor and delivery area, the nurse performs an initial assessment to differentiate true labor from false labor and to obtain baseline information about the labor status. The health history portion of this assessment focuses primarily on obstetric data. The physical assessment portion includes a vaginal examination and evaluation of vital signs, fetal heart tones, uterine contractions, fetal lie, fetal presentation, fetal position, engagement, fetal weight, edema and deep tendon reflexes, and amniotic membrane status.
• The client with true labor contractions is admitted to the labor and delivery area, where the nurse orients her and her support person to the environment and helps them arrange special items from home to create a personalized space.
• After the client is admitted, the nurse performs ongoing assessments. As time permits, the nurse obtains more health history information, collecting data about the client's body systems, past, and psychosocial status. The nurse also performs specific physical assessments based on the health history and reviews laboratory data from routine prenatal, special prenatal, and routine admission tests.
• Initial and ongoing assessment findings serve as the basis for the remaining nursing process steps during labor and delivery.
• Initially, the nurse's planning and implementation may include I.V. fluid administration, as prescribed. Less common procedures include skin preparation and enema administration.
• Ongoing planning and implementation should include monitoring of vital signs, uterine contractions, fetal response to labor, labor progress, and urinary function. It also should include provisions for client comfort and support, such as creating a supportive atmosphere, promoting good positioning and walking, maintaining hygiene, conserving energy, providing for rest, promoting effective breathing, educating the client, advocating on her behalf, integrating cultural beliefs, and relieving pain. In addition, the nurse should plan and implement strategies for family care.
• The nurse should evaluate all care provided to determine how well it achieves goals and meets the client's needs.
• Variations in the first stage of labor include premature rupture of membranes and occiput posterior positioning. The nurse must be prepared to intervene appropriately.
• The nurse thoroughly documents all assessment findings and care in the format required by the health care facility. In most labor and delivery areas, the nurse must record such things as the client's vital signs, fetal heart rate patterns, uterine contraction patterns, and vaginal examination findings as well as application of an internal

fetal scalp electrode or intrauterine pressure catheter, use of medications or oxygen, and presence of family members.

Study questions

1. In the admission section of the labor and delivery area, Faith Martin, a multiparous client age 24, complains of "labor pains coming really fast." What steps should the nurse take to perform an initial assessment of Mrs. Martin and her fetus?

2. In the examination room, Mrs. Martin's membranes rupture spontaneously. How should the nurse intervene to ensure the health of the fetus?

3. How might an occiput posterior fetal position affect a client's labor? How can the nurse promote comfort during this kind of labor?

4. If a client's support person is uncertain about how to comfort her during labor, which techniques might the nurse suggest?

5. Which behavioral clues suggest the transitional phase of the first stage of labor? How can the nurse assist a client through this phase?

Bibliography

Auvenshine, M., and Enriquez, M. (1985). *Maternity nursing: Dimensions of change.* Boston: Jones and Bartlett.

Chagnon, L., and Easterwood, B. (1986). Managing the risks of obstetrical nursing. *MCN,* 11(5), 303-310.

Cunningham, F.G., MacDonald, P.C., and Gant, N.F. (1989). *William's obstetrics* (18th ed.). East Norwalk, CT: Appleton-Century-Croft.

Feldman, E., and Hurst, M. (1987). Outcomes and procedures in low risk birth: A comparison of hospital and birth center settings. *Birth,* 14(1), 18-24.

Fenwick, L., and Simkin, P. (1987). Maternal positioning to prevent or alleviate dystocia in labor. *Clinical Obstetrics and Gynecology,* 30(1), 83-89.

Friedman, E.A. (1978). *Labor: Clinical evaluation and management* (2nd ed.). East Norwalk, CT: Appleton-Century-Croft.

Guidelines for perinatal care (2nd ed.). (1988). Washington, DC: American Academy of Pediatrics and ACOG.

Hoffmaster, J.E. (1983). Labor and intrapartum care. In L.J. Sonstegard, K.M. Kowlaski, and B. Jennings (Eds.), *Women's health, volume II, Childbearing* (pp.109-173). New York: Grune & Stratton.

Horn, M., and Manion, J. (1985). Creative grandparenting: Bonding the generations...participation in the birth experience. *JOGNN,* 14(3), 233-236.

Knuppel, R.A., and Drukker, J. (1986). *High risk pregnancy: Medical management and nursing care.* Philadelphia: Saunders.

Mahan, C.S., and McKay, S. (1983). Prep and enemas: Keep or discard? *Contemporary Obstetrics and Gynecology,* 22(5), 241-248.

Myers, S.T., and Stolte, K. (1987). Nurses' responses to changes in maternity care: Technologic revolution, legal climate and economic changes, part II. *Birth,* 14(2), 87-90.

Pollack, L. (June 1988). Commentary: Reconsidering the risks and benefits of intravenous infusion in labor. *Birth,* 15(2), 80.

Queenan, J.T. (Ed.). (1985). *Management of high risk pregnancy* (2nd ed.). Oradell, NJ: Medical Economics Books.

Sheen, P.W., and Hayashi, R.H. (1987). Graphic management of labor: Alert/action line. *Clinical Obstetrics and Gynecology,* 30(1), 33-41.

Simkin, P. (1986). Stress, pain, and catecholamines in labor: Part 1, a review. *Birth,* 13(4), 227-233.

Standards for obstetric, gynecologic, and neonatal nursing (3rd ed.). (1986). Washington, DC: NAACOG.

Van Lier, D.J., and Roberts, J.E. (1986). Promoting informed consent of women in labor. *JOGNN,* 15(5), 419-422.

Varney, H. (1987). *Nurse-midwifery* (2nd ed.). Boston: Blackwell Scientific Publications.

Whitley, N. (1985). *A manual of clinical obstetrics.* Philadelphia: Lippincott.

Preparation for childbirth

Anderson, S.V., and DelGiudice, G. (1983). *Siblings, birth, and the newborn.* Seattle: Pennypress.

Dick-Read, G. (1987). *Childbirth without fear* (5th ed.). New York: Harper & Row.

Maloni, J.A., McIndoe, J.E., and Rubenstein, G. (1987). Expectant grandparents class. *JOGNN,* 16(1), 26-29.

Nichols, F.H., and Humenick, S.S. (1988). *Childbirth education: Practice, research and theory.* Philadelphia: Saunders.

Phillips, C., and Anzalone, J. (1982). *Fathering, participation in labor and birth* (2nd ed.). St. Louis: Mosby.

Fetal monitoring

Electronic fetal monitoring: Joint ACOG/NAACOG statement. (1988). Washington, DC: NAACOG.

Snydal, S. (1988). Responses of laboring women to fetal heart rate monitoring: A critical review of the literature. *Journal of Nurse-Midwifery,* 33(5), 208-216.

Nursing research

Caldeyro-Barcia, R. (1979). The influence of maternal position on time of spontaneous rupture of the membrane, progress of labor, and fetal head compression. *Birth and the Family Journal,* 6(7), 7-15.

Jones, S.P. (1984). First time fathers: A preliminary study. *MCN,* 9(2), 103.

Lederman, R.P. (1984). *Psychosocial adaptation in pregnancy: Assessment of seven dimensions of maternal development.* East Norwalk, CT: Appleton & Lange.

Lederman, R.P., Lederman, E., Work, B.A., and McCann, D.S. (1985). Anxiety and epinephrine in multiparous women in labor: Relationship to duration of labor and fetal heart rate pattern. *American Journal of Obstetrics and Gynecology,* 153, 870-877.

Lowe, N.K. (1987). Parity and pain during parturition. *JOGNN,* 16(5), 340-346.

Newton, N., Newton, M., and Broach, J. (June 1988). Psychologic, physical, nutritional, and technologic aspects of intravenous infusion during labor. *Birth,* 15(2), 67-72.

Sosa, R., Kennell, J., Klaus, M., Robertson, S., and Vrrutia, J. (1980). The effect of a supportive companion on perinatal problems, length of labor, and mother-infant interaction. *New England Journal of Medicine,* 303(11), 597-600.

Wieser, M.A., and Castiglia, P.T. (1984). Assessing early father-infant attachment. *MCN,* 9(2), 104-106.

Cultural references

Bates, B., and Turner, A.N. (1985). Imagery and symbolism in the birth practices of traditional cultures. *Birth,* 12(1), 29-35.

Dempsey, P.A., and Gesse, T.C. (1985). The childbearing Cuban refugee: A cultural profile. *Urban Health,* 14(5), 32-37.

Dempsey, P.A., and Gesse, T. (1983). The childbearing Haitian refugee: Cultural applications to clinical nursing. *Public Health Reports,* 98(3), 261-267.

Hedstrom, L.W., and Newton, N. (1986). Touch in labor: A comparison of cultures and eras. *Birth,* 13(3), 181-186.

Laderman, C. (1988). Commentary: Cross-cultural perspectives on birth practices. *Birth,* 15(2), 86-87.

Lutwak, R., Ney, A.M., and White, J. (1988). Maternity nursing and Jewish law. *MCN,* 13(1),44-46.

Martinelli, A.M. (1987). Pain and ethnicity: How people of different cultures experience pain. *AORN,* 46(2), 273-281.

Michaelson, K.L. (Ed.) (1988). *Childbirth in America: Anthropological perspectives.* Westport, CT: Bergin & Garvey.

The Second Stage of Labor

Objectives

After reading and studying this chapter, the student should be able to:

1. List characteristics of the onset and progression of the second stage of labor and its typical length for primiparous and multiparous clients.

2. Describe assessment of a client in the second stage of labor.

3. Explain how bearing-down efforts should change as the second stage progresses and how bearing-down efforts may differ among clients.

4. Summarize advantages and disadvantages of various body positions during the second stage of labor.

5. Outline the nurse's responsibilities during delivery and immediately afterward.

6. Apply the nursing process when caring for a client in the second stage of labor.

Introduction

The second stage of labor begins with complete cervical dilation and ends with delivery of the neonate. It requires exhaustive maternal efforts coupled with strong, effective uterine contractions. The client will need substantial emotional support and encouragement. During this highly emotional and stressful period, the nurse must meet the needs of the client, family, and fetus as well as monitor the progress of labor, prepare the environment and equipment needed for delivery, and evaluate the neonate's status after delivery.

This chapter covers characteristics of second stage of labor onset, phases, and duration. Following the

nursing process steps, the chapter then presents assessment topics, nursing diagnoses, and interventions pertinent to the client in the second stage of labor. Finally, the chapter presents guidelines for nursing care of the neonate immediately after delivery. Overall, the chapter gives guidelines for nursing care that is safe and comforting for the client and family during the expulsive phase of labor.

Characteristics of the second stage

The transition from the first to the second stage of labor signals impending birth. The nurse should be aware of the onset of the second stage, of phases typically experienced during this stage, and of expected duration.

Onset

Several characteristics indicate a transition from the first to the second stage of labor, including some or all of the following:

• an increasing urge to push, possibly accompanied by perineal bulging in a multiparous client

• an increase in bloody show, caused by greater cervical dilation

• grunting

• gaping of the anus

GLOSSARY

Anterior "lip": anterior portion of cervix that remains undilated just before complete dilation.

Apgar score: method of evaluating neonatal vigor at 1- and 5-minute intervals after delivery. Ranging from 0 to 10, the score is based on assessment of heart rate, respiration effort, muscle tone, reflex irritability, and skin color.

Birthing chair: specialized chair that allows a woman to give birth in an upright position.

Bonding: feelings of affection or loyalty that bind one person to another in an enduring relationship, as parent to child. Also referred to as attachment.

Crowning: appearance of the fetus's head at the perineum.

Episiotomy: surgical incision made in the perineum to enlarge the vaginal opening for delivery. It is performed to prevent perineal tears, to speed or facilitate delivery, or to prevent excess stretching of perineal muscles and connective tissue.

Fetal presentation: manner in which the fetus enters the pelvic passageway; for example, cephalic, shoulder, or breech.

Fetal station: relationship of the fetal presenting part to the maternal ischial spines.

Multiparous: having given birth to one or more children.

Presenting part: portion of the fetus that first enters the pelvic passageway.

Primiparous: giving birth for the first time.

Second stage of labor: period that begins with complete cervical dilation and ends with delivery of the neonate.

- involuntary defecation
- bulging of the vaginal introitus
- spontaneous rupture of the membranes, if this has not occurred
- abrupt onset of early decelerations (beginning early in the contraction) in fetal heart rate (FHR), possibly caused by compression of the fetus's head during descent into the pelvic canal. (Such FHR changes, although common, should be reported to the physician or nurse-midwife.)

Phases

Some authorities divide the second stage of labor into two distinct phases. The first phase lasts from complete dilation of the cervix until the presenting part reaches the pelvic floor. The second phase lasts from when the presenting part reaches the pelvic floor until birth.

During the first phase, the client may not feel a strong urge to bear down. Typically, these urges are short, manageable, and occur at the peak of each contraction. They may assist in the final retraction of the cervix before fetal descent. During the second phase, the client typically feels an uncontrollable urge to push; during this phase, bearing-down efforts are most effective at expelling the fetus.

Duration

For primiparous clients, the second stage of labor averages 66 minutes, ranging from 48 to 174 minutes. For multiparous clients, the second stage averages 24 minutes, ranging from 6 to 66 minutes (Friedman, 1989). The duration depends on the combined effects of fetal, maternal, psychological, and environmental factors.

Fetal factors that may affect duration include physical condition, size, station, position, molding, rotation, and rate of descent. Maternal factors include parity, labor position, fatigue level, age, degree of expulsive efforts, strength of uterine contractions, size and shape of the bony pelvis, resistance or relaxation of soft tissues, and such obstetric interventions as anesthesia and episiotomy (Cunningham, MacDonald, and Gant, 1989).

Psychological factors that may affect duration include the client's emotional readiness, degree of relaxation, and level of trust in her care providers. The client's preparation for childbirth—from reading, childbirth education classes, information handed down from female relatives, and inner spiritual resources, for example—also affect her reaction to labor, which may influence its duration (Kitzinger, 1984; Peterson, 1984).

Environmental factors, which include bright lights, noise, and hectic activity, may increase the client's anxiety, lengthening labor. A quiet, relaxed environment can shorten labor (McKay and Roberts, 1985; Odent, 1986; van Lier, 1985).

This complex interplay of diverse factors may preclude an accurate prediction of how long the second stage of labor will last, even for a multiparous client. For example, a larger fetus could result in longer labor than the client experienced previously. Conversely, reduced resistance of the cervix and pelvic floor caused by previous delivery could shorten labor despite the larger fetus. Although the client and her family have little control over such physical factors as the size of the fetus or degree of pelvic resistance, they can influence other factors, such as the positions the client assumes during labor.

Some authorities consider abnormal any second stage of labor that lasts longer than 2 hours. However, authorities do not agree on the effect of a prolonged second stage. Some suggest a correlation between a prolonged second stage and infant mortality, postpartal maternal hemorrhage, neonatal seizures, puerperal febril morbidity, and changes in neonatal acid-base status (Hellman and Prystowski, 1952; Minchom, et al., 1987; Wood, Ng, Hounslow, and Benning, 1973). Others have found no difference in neonatal deaths, low 1-minute Apgar scores, and postpartal hemorrhage (Cohen, 1977; Reynolds and Yudkin, 1987).

Although a prolonged second stage of labor (over 2.9 hours in a primiparous client or 1.1 hours in a multiparous client) may indicate a disorder and deserves careful monitoring, it does not necessarily give sufficient reason to terminate labor; if labor is progressing and the fetus displays no signs of distress, some authorities recommend allowing labor to continue until vaginal delivery occurs (Friedman, 1989). The client and fetus should undergo continual monitoring and documentation as labor progresses.

Nursing care

To provide the best possible care, the nurse should apply the nursing process when caring for a client in the second stage of labor.

Assessment

During the second stage of labor, assessment focuses on the client, fetus, and labor progress; it occurs more frequently than during the first stage of labor. As delivery nears, assessment becomes continuous, and the nurse will care for one client exclusively. Beginning early in the second stage and continuing until delivery, the nurse assesses maternal vital signs, cervical dilation, contractions, bearing-down efforts, FHR, fetal descent, amniotic fluid, and the emotional response of the client and support person.

Vital signs

Take vital signs at least every 15 minutes and more often if the client has continuous epidural anesthesia, is hypertensive, or has other complicating conditions. Bearing-down efforts may increase client blood pressure, pulse, and respirations. Take blood pressure as necessary between contractions, but use discretion if pressure

has been stable and birth is imminent. A temperature rise of one degree may occur even in the absence of infection, but a temperature over 100° F should be reported to the physician or nurse-midwife. Dehydration may play a role in temperature elevation.

Cervical dilation

When characteristics of the second stage appear (such as increased bloody show and facial perspiration, decreased restlessness, shaking of the extremities, and involuntary bearing-down efforts), expect a vaginal examination to be performed to confirm dilation and assess the presenting part, fetal station, status of the fetal membranes, and color of the amniotic fluid.

Some clients have a strong urge to bear down before the cervix dilates completely. This can cause edema and tissue damage, and it may impede fetal descent. If examination reveals incomplete dilation and the client has a strong urge, continue to assess dilation every 15 minutes and help the client avoid bearing down. Help her onto her forearms and knees, a position that may decrease the urge to bear down by relieving pressure on the rectum. Instruct her to pant or blow through each contraction until examination reveals that the cervix has receded completely. To maintain her comfort as long as possible in this position, raise the head of the bed and place several pillows under her arms. Some facilities use a large bean bag to support clients in this position.

In some clients, incomplete dilation may be felt as an anterior "lip" on the cervix. This condition stems from uneven pressure of the presenting part on the cervix; all of the cervix recedes except for a small anterior portion. The physician or nurse-midwife may reduce an anterior lip of the cervix manually, using two fingers to ease the cervix over the fetus's head by pressing against it during a contraction. The client can aid reduction by bearing down during the pressing. Keeping the fingers in place during the next contraction will help the physician or nurse-midwife determine whether the lip has been effectively reduced.

Fetal bradycardia to 90 beats/minute may occur for 1 to 2 minutes after manual reduction of the lip. This may result from vagal stimulation and typically resolves on its own. If not, notify the physician or nurse-midwife and initiate standard nursing care for fetal bradycardia. (For more information, see Chapter 25, Fetal Assessment.)

Contractions

Assess the strength, frequency, and duration of uterine contractions every 15 minutes during the second stage. Contractions that have occurred every 2 or 3 minutes may extend to every 5 minutes during this stage, allowing the client to rest between contractions. Some clients have more frequent contractions and report unceasing pain. This pain may relate to increasing pressure from the presenting part and difficulty relaxing between contractions. When the second stage lasts longer than 2 hours, uterine contractions may decrease in strength and frequency. The physician or nurse-midwife should evaluate the need for oxytocin (to stimulate labor) and assess for cephalopelvic disproportion or other abnormalities. (For further discussion, see Chapter 33, Intrapartal Complications.)

If the client has had epidural anesthesia, the support person or nurse may need to cue her when a contraction begins so that she can position herself to bear down.

Bearing-down efforts

Assess the effectiveness of the client's bearing-down efforts and her energy resources as the second stage progresses. Remind her to bear down at the peak of each contraction and to continue bearing down to the end of the contraction to facilitate fetal descent. After assessing the progress of the first few contractions in the second stage, notify the physician or nurse-midwife of the client's status. If descent is delayed, or if the client complains of increased pain, fatigue, or frustration, the physician or nurse-midwife will identify the problem and intervene appropriately.

Although epidural anesthesia can be useful in the first stage of labor, it may create problems for a client in the second stage; the amount of sensory and motor block necessary to relieve pain may reduce, delay, or abolish bearing-down efforts. Moreover, epidural anesthesia may lengthen the second stage and increase the need for forceps or vacuum assistance (Chestnut, Vandewalker, Owen, Bates, and Choi, 1987). If the client's bearing-down efforts produce little descent, even with direct coaching, then the anesthetic agent may have to wear off slightly or be administered in reduced amounts before the client can bear down effectively. Reassure the client that, although the pain will increase somewhat, her improved pushing efforts will help deliver the neonate more quickly.

Fetal heart rate

Assess the FHR more frequently during the second stage of labor than during the first, based on the client's risk status, underlying medical conditions, medications and anesthesic agent used, and any alterations in FHR patterns that arose during the first stage. For a low-risk client, auscultate FHR every 5 minutes or with an electronic fetal monitor, depending on the client's wishes, the physician's or nurse-midwife's preference, and facility policy. Although a standard fetoscope may be used for manual auscultation of FHR, a Doppler ultrasound device typically is less obtrusive (Sleep, Roberts, and Chalmers,

1989). If the client finds repeated FHR auscultation disruptive, consider switching to electronic monitoring. A high-risk client may require electronic monitoring, possibly with an internal scalp electrode to detect fetal distress or beat-to-beat variability. (For more information, see Chapter 25, Fetal Assessment.)

Changes in the FHR become more difficult to interpret during the second stage because they occur more frequently and with more variation than during the first stage (Roberts, 1989). In fact, 50% to 90% of healthy neonates display some abnormality in heart rate during the expulsive phase of labor (Graziano, Freeman, and Bendel, 1980; Krebs, Petres, and Dunn, 1981). Variations in the FHR may result from umbilical cord compression, fetal descent, and maternal bearing-down efforts.

Although few studies focus on the outcomes of second stage FHR changes, Hon and Quilligan (1967) found a correlation between a normal FHR pattern and a normal Apgar score. (Apgar scoring is described in detail later in this chapter.) Specific results of FHR alterations may not be obvious. Usually, however, accelerations pose little danger; decelerations and changes in variability should be monitored closely. (For more information, see *Fetal status: Assessing and managing fetal heart rate changes,* page 686.)

Descent

The fetus normally begins descent during active labor; if descent has not begun by 7 cm of cervical dilation, an abnormality may exist. Failure to descend occurred in approximately 4% of clients in a large sample (Friedman, 1989). Causes included:
• a large fetus (over 4,000 g)
• cephalopelvic disproportion
• fetal malposition, primarily persistent occiput transverse or occiput posterior positions.

Begin assessing descent when cervical dilation is between 7 and 8 cm (usually during the first stage of labor) by measuring the relationship between the fetus's head and the client's ischial spines. Suspect an abnormality if no descent occurs after a primiparous client bears down for 1 hour or a multiparous client bears down for ½ hour. Be careful to distinguish between actual descent and increased swelling of the fetus's scalp, which may give the illusion of descent. (For more information, see Chapter 24, Physiology of Labor and Childbirth.)

Amniotic fluid

Note any change in the color of the amniotic fluid during the second stage of labor because it may indicate fetal distress. When tainted with meconium, amniotic fluid becomes green and may range in consistency from thin

FETAL STATUS

Assessing and managing fetal heart rate changes

Variability in the fetal heart rate (FHR) during the second stage of labor is an indicator of fetal well-being. Yet variations can be difficult to interpret. The nurse can use the following basic guidelines to help interpret and manage FHR changes.

1 Baseline FHR should remain within 20 beats/minute of the rate identified early in labor. A slight decline in this baseline is common, probably resulting from vagal stimulation from increased pressure on the fetus's head during descent into the pelvis.

2 The FHR fluctuates more during the second stage of labor than during the first stage. Accelerations typically have no adverse effect on the neonate. In fact, the absence of accelerations should be investigated.

3 Decreased FHR variability, especially if accompanied by bradycardia, decelerations, or lack of accelerations, may be cause for concern. Decreased FHR variability has been associated with decreased umbilical cord blood pH, which reflects fetal distress.

4 Second-stage FHR decelerations and bradycardia have been reported in 50% to 90% of all FHR tracings and usually produce no lasting adverse effects. In contrast, pronounced or prolonged decelerations require prompt delivery.

5 Terminal bradycardia (FHR below baseline immediately before delivery) is common and probably stems from compression of the fetus's head, vagal stimulation, umbilical cord compression, and impaired uteroplacental perfusion (Ohel, 1978; Herbert and Boehm, 1981). It typically lasts only a few minutes and produces no adverse effects.

6 Scalp stimulation may help in evaluating fetal condition when bradycardia occurs; FHR acceleration in response to stimuli offers a reliable sign of fetal well-being. If the fetus develops bradycardia, the physician or nurse-midwife may press the fetus's scalp with a finger while performing a vaginal examination. If the FHR rises, the fetus is not seriously acidotic. If delivery is not imminent, try raising the FHR by repositioning the client, offering oxygen by mask, and encouraging her to breath through contractions rather than to push (Roberts, 1989).

(1+ or 2+) to thick (3+ or 4+). Thick amniotic fluid may contain particulate meconium. An increase in bloody show, which commonly occurs early in the second stage, may cause pink-tinged amniotic fluid. Port wine–colored fluid may indicate abruptio placentae. Notify the physician or nurse-midwife of any change in amniotic fluid color.

Emotional responses

Assessment of the client's emotional status and that of her support person becomes increasingly important as labor continues. Both may experience fatigue and frustration, especially early in the second stage before the client can bear down. When told that she can push, the client may feel relief and anticipation that labor will end soon. The support person and health care team may feel a surge of renewed energy as well.

Clients may respond in various ways to the sensation of bearing down. Some respond well because bearing down allows them to give in to the urge they feel and do something positive with the pain (van Lier, 1985). These clients may express satisfaction in working hard, receiving positive feedback, and seeing results from their efforts. Others respond poorly to bearing down, especially if the fetus is in a posterior position or if the client fears spontaneous perineal lacerations.

Immediately after delivery, the client may experience a range of emotions and reactions, including relief that the pain has diminished, a sense of achievement, exhaustion, and pleasure or disappointment in the appearance or sex of the neonate.

Nursing diagnosis

Based on continuous assessment and monitoring throughout the second stage of labor, the nurse formulates nursing diagnoses specific to the client, fetus, support person, or other family members, as necessary. (For a partial list of possible nursing diagnoses, see *Nursing diagnoses: Second stage of labor.*)

Planning and implementation

During the second stage of labor, the nurse must plan and act almost simultaneously. After detecting the onset of the second stage and assessing maternal and fetal well-being and labor progress, notify the physician or nurse-midwife of the client's status and of any maternal or fetal complications (such as meconium-stained amniotic fluid, fetal distress, or recent narcotic administration).

As the second stage progresses, the nurse should provide the client with emotional support, coordinate her bearing-down efforts, assist with positioning, monitor hydration, faciliate delivery, and care for the neonate immediately after birth.

Provide emotional support

Especially for the primiparous client, the second stage of labor may result in a nursing diagnosis of *anxiety related to duration of labor* or *ineffective individual coping related to exhaustion.* Help resolve these problems by providing emotional support and reassurance. In addition to emotional needs specific to each client, provide general emotional support to the client by assuring her if labor is progressing normally, that she will not be left alone, and that the physician or nurse-midwife will be summoned at the proper time. Depending on the support person's participation, the nurse's role can range from reassuring to active coaching during the second stage. If the support person participates actively and responds appropriately to the client's efforts, the nurse will need to supply only positive feedback and encouragement.

Provide specific comments as labor progresses; mention when the bulge of the head appears, for example, or comment on the neonate's curly hair. Some clients derive emotional support from seeing their emerging neonate reflected in a well-placed mirror.

Reassure the client that each expulsive effort helps to move her baby down and out. Suggest that the client imagine herself opening and her baby moving down the birth canal and out. Reassure the client by saying what she might be thinking but be too exhausted to express, such as, "You may feel like you are having a bowel movement," or "It may feel like the baby will never come out, but you are making good progress."

Choose words carefully because clients in labor are highly vulnerable and sensitive to suggestions that they are not succeeding. Even mildly critical remarks intended to make the client try harder may be hurtful. Oakley (1980) showed an association between dissatisfaction with the second stage of labor and subsequent postpartal depression (other associated factors included use of an epidural block and instrument deliveries).

The client who becomes exhausted and discouraged during this stage of labor will want to know how much longer the effort must continue. Never try to estimate when birth will occur. Instead, suggest concentrating on and working with the contractions, perhaps by changing position or exhaling forcefully (blowing) instead of pushing through the next one. Encourage the client to rest or doze between contractions. Affirm that labor is hard work that can seem to take forever, but that she is making progress and will get through it. Encourage her to draw energy from her supporters.

Especially during this stage, the client's support person may need emotional support, a brief break, or

---

NURSING DIAGNOSES

Second stage of labor

The following diagnoses address representative problems and etiologies that the nurse may encounter when caring for a client during the second stage of labor. Specific nursing interventions for many of these diagnoses are provided in the "Planning and implementation" section of this chapter.

- Altered patterns of urinary elimination related to epidural anesthesia
- Anxiety related to duration of labor
- Anxiety related to not meeting labor expectations
- Fatigue related to duration of labor, energy expenditure, and possible lack of sleep
- Fluid volume deficit related to restricted fluid intake and fluid loss during labor efforts
- Hopelessness related to prolonged bearing-down efforts that produce little progress
- Impaired tissue integrity related to perineal and vaginal lacerations, or episiotomy
- Ineffective breathing pattern related to painful uterine contractions and bearing-down efforts
- Ineffective individual coping related to exhaustion
- Knowledge deficit related to typical duration of labor
- Pain related to rapid delivery or fetal malposition
- Pain related to uterine contractions, stretching of vaginal and perineal tissues, and childbirth

---

gentle direction. If the client's bearing down does not accomplish quick results, the supporter may need reassurance that the FHR remains normal and that 1 to 2 hours of bearing down is not uncommon. If necessary, suggest such concrete tasks as holding the client's leg, supporting her body in selected positions, massaging her back, offering ice chips, or preparing a cool cloth for her forehead.

Coordinate bearing-down efforts

During painful periods, the client may have a nursing diagnosis of *ineffective breathing pattern related to painful uterine contractions and bearing-down efforts.* Help resolve this problem by coordinating the client's bearing-down efforts.

Early in the second stage of labor, inform the client that she is nearing the time when bearing down will assist with birth. Encourage her to relax and breathe through each contraction until she reaches a point when she cannot help pushing. These early bearing-down efforts will be brief and, as the urge eases, she should resume normal breathing through the rest of the contraction.

As the second stage progresses, bearing-down urges become more intense and aid in expelling the neonate. Encourage the client to bear down with each contraction (Roberts, Goldstein, Gruener, Maggio, and Mendez-Bauer, 1987; Turner, Webb, and Gordon, 1986). Although the nurse need not discourage bearing down early in the second stage, it produces the most pronounced result later in the stage (Roberts, Goldstein, Gruener, Maggio, and Mendez-Bauer, 1987). Never chastise a client who cannot resist the urge to bear down. (For more information, see *Alternative ways of bearing down.*)

If bearing-down efforts produce inadequate results, give positive suggestions for change between contractions, help the client into an alternative position, and encourage her to push through the pain rather than pull back from it. If she pulls back out of fear that she will hurt herself, try placing warm washcloths on the perineum to decrease any burning sensation.

Assist with positioning

In Western society, health care providers typically encourage women to adopt the lithotomy position for delivery. This position maximizes the physician's or nurse-midwife's control over delivery, provides the health care team with the clearest view of the perineum, and allows unhindered access for instrument deliveries or perineal repair. However, despite its almost universal favor in Western health care facilities, the lithotomy position is used infrequently in nonwestern societies. Cross-cultural analyses reveal that almost all societies not influenced by Western medical practices assume some type of upright position for childbirth (Engelmann, 1882; Naroll, Naroll, and Howard, 1961). For the client, squatting, sitting, and other upright positions have distinct advantages, especially for bearing down.

Position changes may be especially helpful for a client with a nursing diagnosis of *pain related to rapid delivery or fetal malposition.* The side-lying position helps slow a rapid delivery and may reduce perineal tension. The forearms-and-knees position can reduce back pain related to labor. When the fetus is in an occiput-posterior position or descends slowly, the client may benefit from a squatting position. If she squats on the toilet, use a flashlight to maintain a steady view of the perineum. Be sure to consider the advantages and disadvantages of a position before suggesting a change to the client. (For more information, see *Advantages and disadvantages of labor positions.*)

If the client assumes a lithotomy position for delivery, maximize her participation and bearing-down efforts by placing two pillows, a bean bag, or a backrest behind her shoulders or at the small of her back. Alternatively, the client can lean against her support person to help maintain a more upright position.

Alternative ways of bearing down

Traditionally, nurses have taught and reinforced the following method of bearing down: the client takes a cleansing breath, exhales, bears down to a count of 10 four times inhaling quickly between counts, and then takes a final cleansing breath. Typically, she assumes a C-shaped position curled around the fetus, holding her knees, with head bent.

Two alternative styles for bearing down include the open-glottis method and the urge-based method. In the former, the client releases air through the glottis while bearing down. Theoretically, this reduces stress on the fetus. In the latter, the client bears down as she feels the urge and in the manner that feels right to her.

Possible effects

Some clinicians believe that these alternative ways of bearing down could prolong the second stage of labor and, in the urge-based method, could lead to hemodynamic changes associated with Valsalva's maneuver (Bassell, Humayun, and Marx, 1980; Roberts, 1980; Yeates and Roberts, 1984; McKay and Roberts, 1985). Sustained bearing-down efforts also may lead to abnormalities in the fetal heart rate (Knauth and Haloburdo, 1986) and depressed Apgar scores (Martinez-Lopez, de la Fuenta, Iniguez, Freese, and Mendez-Bauer, 1984).

However, the few studies that have been done have not shown the adverse effects that clinicians feared (Yeates and Roberts, 1984). In one such study, 31 healthy primiparous clients who had received no formal childbirth education pushed spontaneously without guidance from caregivers. Researchers found that clients made three to five relatively brief (4- to 6-second) bearing-down efforts with each contraction. The number of bearing-down efforts per contraction increased as the second stage progressed. Most efforts were accompanied by the release of air; some included very brief periods of breath holding that lasted less than 6 seconds. The second stage averaged 45 minutes in this study; in no client did it exceed 95 minutes. Fetal heart rate returned to baseline promptly (Roberts, Goldstein, Gruener, Maggio, and Mendez-Bauer, 1987).

Because childbirth educators teach all three bearing-down methods, the nurse should be familiar with each one and work to achieve the most comfortable and effective method for each client.

For some clients, a birthing chair may help maximize comfort while meeting fetal needs and allowing the health care team to monitor maternal and fetal status. (For more information, see *Nursing research applied: Using a birthing chair,* page 691.) Used for bearing down and for delivery, the birthing chair is particularly suitable for primiparous clients because of the longer pushing phase. A tired client who has tried several positions in bed may benefit from the birthing chair's hand grips and back support. The client may assume a side-lying position in the birthing chair, as well as various degrees of upright and recumbent positions. Drawbacks to the birthing chair include a risk of increased blood loss and perineal edema (Sleep, Roberts, and Chalmers, 1989);

Advantages and disadvantages of labor positions

Although the lithotomy position is used most often for delivery, other positions may aid clients during the second stage of labor. These include standing, sitting, forearms and knees, dorsal recumbent, lateral recumbent, and squatting. The following chart describes advantages and disadvantages of each position for the client, fetus or neonate, and health care team.

CLIENT AND FETUS OR NEONATE	HEALTH CARE TEAM
Lithotomy position (on back with knees bent or up on chest)	
Advantages • Leg stirrups may give client a sense of security. **Disadvantages** • Decreased blood flow to the uterus and oxygen to the fetus from the uterus compressing large blood vessels • Less client interaction with fetus and health care team • Increased risk of blood clot formation from stirrups • Decreased ability to push • Sense of vulnerability • Possible aspiration of vomit • Changes in maternal blood flow can cause fetal distress or neonatal depression • Difficult for client to see or hold neonate after birth	**Advantages** • More control of birth situation; useful if client is "out of control" • Easy obstetric intervention • More comfortable, less back strain • Asepsis • Easy to hear fetal heartbeat **Disadvantages** • No easy interaction with client; more difficult to elicit her cooperation
Standing	
Advantages • Reported improved uterine contractibility for first stage • Avoidance of negative hemodynamic changes • Client can watch birth • May increase help of gravity **Disadvantages** • Very tiring; client needs two supporters • Possible increased maternal blood loss, uterine prolapse, and edema of cervix and vulva • Neonate may fall to ground unless "caught"	**Advantages** • Easier interaction with client **Disadvantages** • Difficult to control baby's head and watch perineum • Difficult to assist with delivery
Sitting	
Advantages • Shorter, more comfortable second stage • More efficient for bearing-down efforts • Increases pelvic diameter • Easy to interact with neonate and health care team • Probably causes fewer negative hemodynamic changes **Disadvantages** • Client needs back support • May cause edema of vulva or cervix if prolonged	**Advantages** • Easy access to perineum to control delivery • Easy to intervene (episiotomy, forceps, or pudendal anesthesia) • Easy to hear fetal heart rate **Disadvantages** • Some physicians or nurse-midwives may not want the client's active participation in the birth.
Forearms and knees	
Advantages • No weight on inferior vena cava; may cause less fetal distress • Aids delivery of neonate's shoulder • Relieves pressure on trapped or prolapsed umbilical cord **Disadvantages** • Very tiring • Difficult for client to interact with neonate and health care team • May cause cramps in arms and legs	**Advantages** • Good visualization of perineum and control of delivery • May provide optimal control for breech delivery • May be useful in rotating occiput posterior positions or in delivery of shoulders when they are "tight" **Disadvantages** • Must reorient landmarks and adapt delivery techniques • Usually must turn client to recumbent position for delivery of placenta, repair of lacerations, and rest • Difficult to monitor fetus without fetal scalp electrode

(continued)

Advantages and disadvantages of labor positions continued

CLIENT AND FETUS OR NEONATE	HEALTH CARE TEAM

Dorsal recumbent

Advantages
• May prevent perineal lacerations by causing less tension on perineum
• Less pressure on legs
• Thrombosis less likely to develop because stirrups are not used

Disadvantages
• Same blood flow changes as lithotomy
• Difficult for client to participate in birth
• Decreased ability to push
• Hemodynamic changes may cause fetal distress
• Difficult for client to hold neonate after delivery

Advantages
• Easy access to perineum
• Able to administer pudendal anesthesia or perform episiotomy easily
• Easy to hear fetal heart rate

Disadvantages
• Cannot easily interact with client
• Forceps delivery more difficult because of decreased counterpressure on fetus

Lateral recumbent (on either side with thighs flexed)

Advantages
• Corrects or avoids adverse hemodynamic effects of lithotomy position
• Less tension on perineum
• May help to rotate occiput posterior presentations
• May be helpful in relieving shoulder dystocia
• Comfortable for many clients and conducive to resting between contractions because contractions are less frequent
• Promotes maximum uterine blood flow and fetal oxygenation

Disadvantages
• Less efficient for bearing-down efforts; may be desirable to avoid a precipitious delivery for a multiparous client
• Requires someone to hold leg up for delivery

Advantages
• Conducive for controlled delivery

Disadvantages
• Some practitioners consider position awkward.
• Unable to see and interact with client as easily
• Difficult to repair episiotomy or use forceps
• More difficult to hear fetal heart tones

Squatting

Advantages
• Allows good expulsive effort and shorter second stage
• Pressure of the thighs against the abdomen may aid in expulsion by increasing intra-abdominal pressure and promoting longitudinal alignment of the fetus with the birth canal.
• Increases pelvic bone diameter; anteroposterior diameter of outlet increased by 0.5 to 2 cm; transverse diameter also increased
• Avoids adverse hemodynamic effects of lithotomy position
• Facilitates interaction with neonate and health care team
• Promotes fetal descent and rotation

Disadvantages
• Client's legs can become fatigued, especially if she is not supported.
• Possible increased risk of uterine prolapse because of strenuous bearing-down effort
• May promote increased perineal and cervical edema if prolonged
• Rapid descent and expulsion of fetus may cause vaginal and perineal lacerations.
• Increased blood loss possible
• Rapid expulsion may result in sudden reduction in intracervical pressure and cause cerebral bleeding in the brain of a premature fetus whose skull bones are not yet firm.

Advantages
• Allows some visibility of perineum
• Maximizes bearing-down efforts

Disadvantages
• Cannot intervene easily in this position to help control expulsion of the neonate or aid the delivery with an episiostomy or pudendal nerve block

also, the forearms-and-knees and squatting positions are not feasible. The chair should not be used by a client who has received an epidural block because she will lack the physical control needed to transfer to the chair.

Monitor hydration

A client who shows decreased bearing-down efforts after a period of effective efforts may have a nursing diagnosis of *fluid volume deficit related to restricted fluid intake and fluid loss during labor efforts.* Continue to offer her juice, water, or tea. If bearing down lasts more than 2 hours, start an I.V. line to deliver fluids, as prescribed.

Prepare for delivery

As delivery approaches, nursing responsibilities include making a judgment about when to transfer the client to the delivery room (or when to summon the physician or nurse-midwife), preparing the delivery area, preparing the client, and assisting with delivery.

Transfer to the delivery room. Judging when to transfer a client to the delivery room and when to summon the physician or nurse-midwife is a learned skill. The goal is to allow sufficient time for the client to reach the delivery room before giving birth, but not to allow so much time that the client and staff have an extended wait. Obviously, early arrival is better than delivery of the neonate en route to the delivery room. Typically, a primiparous client should be transferred to the delivery room when about 4 cm of the fetus's head remains visible between contractions. A multiparous client should be transferred before crowning, usually when cervical dilation is between 8 and 10 cm; always consider the client's labor history, current progress, and rate of descent.

Many health care facilities feature combined labor and delivery rooms, where the client labors, delivers, and recovers in the same room with the same staff.

Prepare the delivery area. Make all necessary physical preparations for the impending birth. This includes gathering and setting up needed equipment (including a radiant heat unit, in some cases) and reviewing the client's and physician's or nurse-midwife's wishes for the delivery.

If the client plans to give birth in the labor bed, place extra pads under her buttocks to absorb the blood and amniotic fluid that emerge after delivery. If she will require transfer to a delivery room, ensure that the route contains no obstacles. If delivery occurs en route, be sure the side rails of the bed are raised and that the client remains draped. Try to plan ahead for emergencies; for example, check needed supplies at the start of each day to ensure that all are present and within reach.

NURSING RESEARCH APPLIED

Using a birthing chair

Cross-cultural studies indicate that many women—particularly those from nonwestern societies—prefer to give birth in an upright position. Although use of a birthing chair for delivery is not common in the United States, its use is increasing.

Cottrell and Shannahan (1986) investigated the use of a birthing chair with 55 primiparous clients in normal labor; 22 delivered on a traditional delivery table in the lithotomy position, and 33 used a birthing chair. The researchers found no significant difference between the two groups in the duration of the second stage of labor, duration of bearing-down efforts, amount of blood loss, number of episiotomies, or number of spontaneous lacerations. They did find an increased incidence of perineal swelling in the group that used the birthing chair.

Application to practice

The nurse should realize and respect that most clients do not prefer the lithotomy position. When available, a birthing chair offers clients an alternative. However, the increased risk of perineal swelling requires some precautions. Clients should not be transferred to the birthing chair until fetal descent and involuntary bearing down have begun. This prevents prolonged periods in the birthing chair, which can increase perineal swelling from the pressure of the buttocks against the rim of the chair. Clients should not pull up on the chair's handgrips while bearing down, which also increases pressure. Finally, they should avoid practices that increase venous stasis during the second stage of labor, such as closed-glottis pushing for more than 5 or 6 seconds.

Cottrell, B., and Shannahan, M. (1986). Effect of the birth chair on duration of second stage labor and maternal outcome. *Nursing Research*, 35(6), 364-367.

Know how to operate all delivery room equipment, including stirrups, infant resuscitation equipment, and the bed.

Set up the instrument pack and delivery pack specified by the facility, gloves for the members of the health care team, and any special supplies or equipment requested by the physician or nurse-midwife. Equipment should include the following: a sterile drape to go under the client's buttocks, clamps and scissors for the umbilical cord, a bulb syringe, a dry sterile towel and warm blanket for the neonate, and (usually) a needle holder and syringes. Many health care facilities use a drape pack that contains an abdominal drape, two leggings, and a drape for under the buttocks.

Additional supplies for the neonate may include a radiant heat unit, suctioning equipment with catheters (sizes 5, 8, and 10), oxygen bag and mask (sizes for premature and full-term neonates), laryngoscope with endotracheal tubes (sizes 2.5, 3.0, and 3.5), extra bulb syringes and neonatal suction (DeLee) catheters, feeding tubes, syringes and needles, and neonatal resuscitation drugs, such as naloxone hydrochloride (neonatal injection, 0.02 mg/ml), sodium bicarbonate, epinephrine, 50% dextrose in water, and reagent strips. (For more information, see Chapter 34, Neonatal Adaptation.)

Prepare the client. Do not break the delivery room bed (bend down the lower end so that the client can assume the lithotomy position) until a nurse, physician, or nurse-midwife is in position in case the fetus descends rapidly. Once the client is positioned in the delivery room bed, prepare the perineum by swabbing with an antiseptic solution and, if necessary, by trimming long pubic hairs. (For more information, see *Psychomotor skills: Preparing the perineum*.) A client in the lithotomy position should place her feet in the stirrups or leg holders. Align her knees at equal heights, and check that her legs are abducted at similar angles. Open the drape pack for the physician or nurse-midwife, and assist with draping, as needed. Follow universal blood and body fluid safety precautions throughout delivery.

Prepare the support person for delivery by giving instructions on hand-washing and assisting with gown or scrub suit, boots, cap, and mask according to facility policy.

Assist with delivery. While the physician or nurse-midwife scrubs and dons gown and gloves, adjust lighting as necessary to observe the perineum, which will verify if delivery is imminent. If the client finds bright light distracting, dim the overhead lights but maintain perineal illumination.

As the fetus's head crosses the perineum, perineal tissue may lacerate spontaneously. Perineal damage extensive enough to require sutures occurs in two-thirds of primiparous clients (Sleep, Roberts, and Chalmers, 1989). This spontaneous trauma can cause discomfort to a degree that dominates the experience of early motherhood; sometimes it results in significant disability during the following months and years (Kitzinger, 1984).

To circumvent this potential problem, the physician or nurse-midwife may perform an episiotomy, either midline or mediolaterally. (For more information, see Chapter 26, Comfort Promotion during Labor and Childbirth.) Possible benefits of episiotomy include:

PSYCHOMOTOR SKILLS

Preparing the perineum

After the client assumes the position she will maintain for delivery, the nurse uses an antiseptic solution to clean her perineum of discharge that accumulated during labor. Explain the procedure to the client; assure her that it involves no pain but that the solution may feel cool. Always scrub outward from the vaginal orifice to avoid contaminating it. Always use a fresh sponge when beginning to clean a different area. To clean the perineum, follow these steps.

1 Follow hand-washing protocol. Open a sterile prep tray and either add antiseptic solution to the sterile container or add sterile water to the antiseptic sponges. Expect to use at least six sponges. Don sterile gloves.

2 Use a sponge to scrub gently back and forth from the client's clitoris to her lower abdomen. Apply just enough pressure to remove any discharge.

3 Clean from the outer labia majora up one inner thigh and halfway to the knee. Repeat with another sponge on the opposite leg.

4 Starting at the clitoris, cleanse downward over one labia majora, making one sweep past the anus. Repeat with another sponge on the opposite side.

5 Clean from the top of the vulva downward over the perineum and anus in a single motion.

6 Rinse with sterile water, if desired, by pouring from the vulva downward.

7 Replace the wet pad beneath the client's buttocks with a dry, sterile pad.

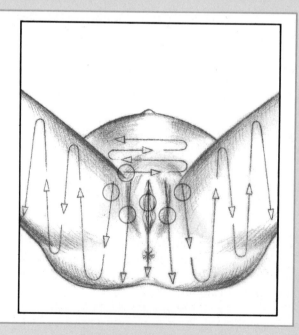

• prevention of damage to the anal sphincter and rectal mucosa (third- and fourth-degree lacerations)
• easier repair and better healing than a spontaneous laceration
• prevention of trauma to the fetus's head
• prevention of serious damage to pelvic floor muscles (Banta and Thacker, 1982).

Authorities disagree on whether the risk of trauma is serious enough to warrant widespread episiotomy use, as currently occurs in Western society (Thacker and Banta, 1983; Sleep, Roberts, and Chalmers, 1989).

The nurse does not assist with the performance or the repair of an episiotomy but should communicate the client's wishes to the physician or nurse-midwife. Further, the nurse should provide care and support during and after an episiotomy.

In theory, prenatal perineal massage by the partner may offer an alternative to episiotomy for reducing perineal damage (Avery and Burket, 1986). In addition, the nurse, physician, or nurse-midwife can "iron out" the perineal tissue firmly with lubricated fingers as the fetus's head moves onto the perineum. Thus far, however, few controlled studies have been conducted to support the claims for perineal massage. Further, some clients may find touch disruptive, particularly because of edema and the increased vascularity of the perineal tissue (Noble, 1983).

Care for the neonate

Immediately after delivery, the physician or nurse-midwife suctions the neonate and ensures an adequate airway and normal breathing. If the amniotic fluid contained meconium, the physician or nurse-midwife would suction immediately after the head appears and before delivering the rest of the body, then assess for aspiration of meconium. After the neonate's delivery, nursing care shifts from the client (now cared for by the physician or nurse-midwife) to the neonate. (For continuing discussion, see Chapter 29, The Third and Fourth Stages of Labor.) Assist with clamping the umbilical cord, perform an initial assessment, dry and wrap the neonate, continue to suction the upper airway as needed, and initiate bonding between the neonate and parents within the first few minutes after delivery.

Clamping the umbilical cord. The physician or nurse-midwife holds the neonate at or below the level of the client's uterus to facilitate transfer of blood until the umbilical cord is clamped. Before clamping, assist with collection of cord blood for analysis according to facility protocol. Typically, the physician or nurse-midwife draws blood from the umbilical vessels into a purple-top (heparinized) tube and stores it in the health care facility refrigerator in case further studies are needed. Blood type and a direct Coombs' test can be obtained from this sample if the client is Rh negative.

To cut the umbilical cord, the physician or nurse-midwife may apply two Kelly clamps (or one Kelly and one plastic clamp) and cut between them. If the physician or nurse-midwife and facility policy permit, ask the client and support person if they would like to cut the cord. (For more information, see *Clamping the umbilical cord,* page 694.)

Assessment. Note the time of birth and the condition of the neonate's airway, amount of mucus, and respiratory efforts. Mucus may be greater following fast descent or cesarean delivery because fetal thorax compression does not force fluid from the respiratory tract. Continue with assessment of the umbilical cord and the neonate's physical condition.

Umbilical cord. Inspect the umbilical cord for obvious abnormalities and verify that it contains two arteries and one vein. The presence of only one artery and one vein has been associated with congenital kidney and cardiac problems. Notify the pediatric personnel of any abnormalities.

Physical examination. Just after the neonate's delivery, perform a quick physical examination to detect obvious congenital anomalies, birthmarks, or bruises associated with delivery. Assign an Apgar score at 1 minute and 5 minutes after delivery, preferably while the neonate lies on the client's abdomen supported by the client, partner, or nurse. (For instructions, see *Assigning an Apgar score,* page 695.) Explain the Apgar score's meaning to the client and her partner. Make note if the neonate passes meconium or urine in the delivery room.

Initiate parent-infant bonding. As soon as the neonate's breathing has been established and the umbilical cord clamped, lay the neonate on the client's abdomen and cover both with a warm blanket. Urge the client and her partner to dry the neonate if necessary while maintaining skin-to-skin contact.

If the neonate's condition warrants placement in a radiant heat unit, position the unit and deliver care within the client's view. Place the dried neonate, unwrapped, on top of a dry blanket. (Radiant heat only warms outer surfaces.) A modified Trendelenburg position will help drain mucus from the airways, if needed.

Assess the client's and partner's response to the neonate. Many new parents feel insecure and will value the nurse's support and instruction. Assist parents if they ask how to hold their infant. Praise them for holding their infant securely and for any other appropriate behavior, such as talking to the infant or observing the

Clamping the umbilical cord

After the physician or nurse-midwife uses sterile scissors to cut the umbilical cord between two Kelly clamps or one Kelly clamp (on the maternal side) and one plastic clamp (on the neonatal side), the nurse must apply a sterile plastic clamp ½" to 1" from the neonate's abdomen. The first clamp then may be removed.

Two types of plastic clamps commonly are used: the Hollister clamp and the Hesseltine clamp. The Hollister clamp has toothed jaws and compresses the cord securely. It requires a special cutting device for removal. The Hesseltine clamp is somewhat less secure; some facilities require the use of two clamps. In either case, the nurse must ensure that the clamp is securely in place because inadvertent unclamping may cause hemorrhage. Typically, nursery personnel remove clamps about 24 hours after birth.

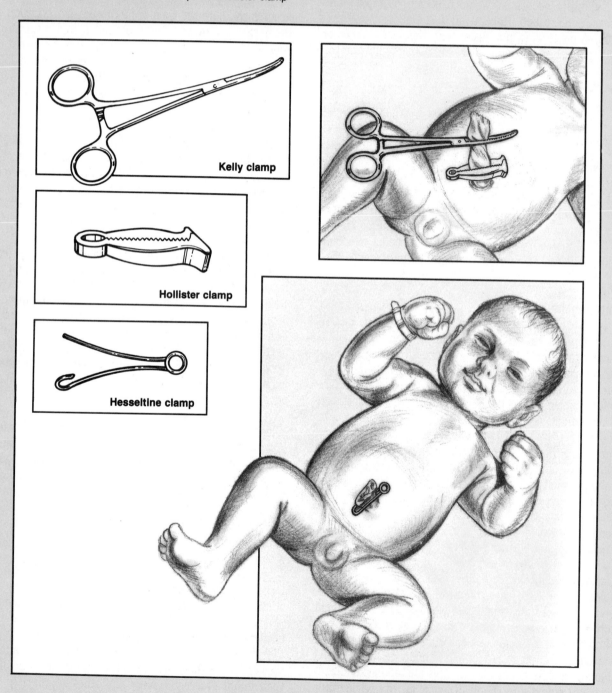

Kelly clamp

Hollister clamp

Hesseltine clamp

Assigning an Apgar score

A method of indicating neonatal vigor, the Apgar score combines the results of five individual assessments: heart rate, respiration, muscle tone, reflex irritability, and color. Typically assigned by the nurse at 1 minute and 5 minutes after the neonate is delivered, the score may reveal the need for resuscitation, confirm trauma during delivery, and indicate congenital anomaly, among other findings. If heart rate is less than 100 beats/minute or respirations are absent, request help and initiate resuscitation immediately.

Assessment steps

Use the guidelines below to assign a score from 0 to 2 in each assessment category. Be sure to follow the appropriate assessment procedures.

Heart rate. Using a stethoscope, count heartbeats for 30 seconds and multiply by 2. Alternatively, feel for a pulse at the base of the umbilical cord or over the heart. If heart rate exceeds 100 beats/minute, give a score of 2. A heart rate under 100 beats/minute warrants a 1, and no detectable heartbeat should receive a 0.

Respirations. After counting and observing, assign a score of 2 for vigorous crying or regular respirations. Irregular, shallow, or gasping respirations score a 1, and absent respiratory effort gets a 0.

Muscle tone. Normally, the neonate's elbows are flexed and thighs and knees drawn up. If the limbs return to this position quickly after being extended, assign a score of 2. If muscles have some tone but do not respond briskly, give a 1. Assign a 0 for flaccid muscles.

Reflex irritability. Insert a bulb syringe into one of the neonate's nostrils or lightly flick the sole of one foot. If the response is a vigorous cry, assign a score of 2. Some motion and weak crying warrants a 1; no response rates a 0.

Color. Observe the skin or mucous membranes for pallor or cyanosis. If the neonate appears completely pink, assign a score of 2 (few neonates receive this score). Acrocyanosis, which refers to bluish hands and feet and applies to most neonates, receives a score of 1. A completely pale or blue neonate receives a score of 0. (In a dark-skinned neonate, check the palms of the hands and soles of the feet to determine pallor or cyanosis.)

Add the scores assigned in each assessment category to arrive at a total Apgar score. The highest score possible is 10; the lowest is 0. Interventions, if necessary, are based on the score.

Interventions

A neonate with a score of 8 to 10 is normal and needs only routine interventions. Aspirate the mouth and nose with a bulb syringe. Dry and wrap the neonate in warm blankets. Perform a brief physical examination.

A score of 5 to 7 indicates mild respiratory, metabolic, or neurologic depression. Stimulate breathing by gently but firmly slapping the soles of the feet or rubbing the spine or sternum. Administer 100% oxygen via bag and face mask. If the neonate shows no improvement and the mother received a narcotic analgesic, expect to administer 0.01 mg/kg of naloxone I.M.

A score of 3 or 4 requires interventions as described above; also, the neonate may require a feeding tube to decompress the stomach. Expect to maintain oxygen administration until the neonate's heart rate exceeds 100 beats/minute and skin is completely pink.

A score of 0 to 2 indicates severe depression and requires immediate intubation and bag ventilation at 40 to 60 breaths/minute with pressures high enough to move the upper chest. Closed chest cardiac massage is performed for bradycardia under 60 beats/minute or cardiac arrest. Resuscitation drugs also are needed.

---

infant's responses. Give feedback about the infant's condition, such as, "The toes and hands are bluish right now but this is typical; they should change to pink within a few hours," or "It is normal for your infant's head to be molded after delivery. It will become more rounded over the next few days."

For photographs of the steps of childbirth, see *Photographic essay on the second stage of labor,* pages 696 and 697.

Evaluation

To complete the nursing process, the nurse evaluates the effectiveness of nursing care by reviewing the goals attained and the outcome of the second stage of labor for the client, support person, and neonate. The nurse also reviews assessment findings, nursing diagnoses, the nursing care plan, and implementation. The following are examples of appropriate evaluation statements.

• After adopting a forearms-and-knees position, the client reported a decrease in the urge to push.
• The support person participated actively in the client's attempts to breathe through contractions.
• The client bore down productively during the final phase of the second stage of labor.
• The client imagined the fetus moving through the birth canal and out.
• The client and her partner expressed appropriate bonding behavior with the neonate immediately after delivery.

(Text continues on page 698.)

Photographic essay on the second stage of labor

The second stage of labor begins with complete cervical dilation and ends with birth. Intense contractions occur every 2 to 3 minutes and last 60 to 90 seconds. For primiparous clients, this stage averages 1 hour; for multiparous clients, 15 minutes. To provide appropriate care for the client, the nruse must be familiar with the steps involved, as shown in the following photographs.

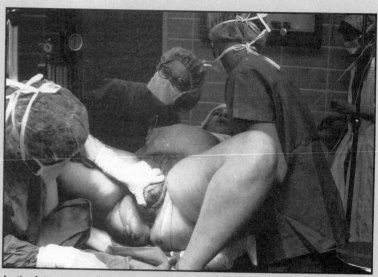

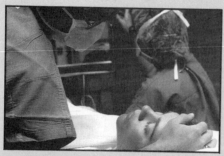

The primary support person and the nurse provide emotional support, coaching, and reassurance to the client entering the second stage of labor. The nurse continuously monitors the client's progress.

As the fetus approaches the perineal floor, the perineum bulges and flattens. As the labia spread, the head appears at the vaginal opening (crowning). At this time, the client should assume an active role and push with each contraction.

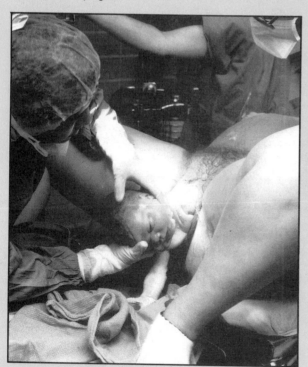

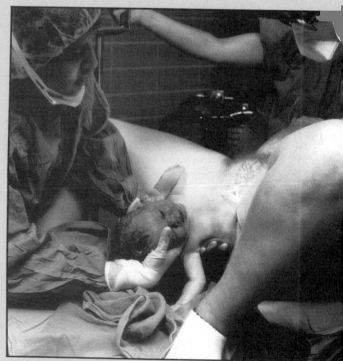

The birth attendant grasps the side of the head and usually applies gentle traction downward to deliver the anterior shoulder, then upward to deliver the posterior shoulder. (In this photograph, the posterior shoulder has emerged first.)

Once the shoulders have emerged, the rest of the body, which is narrower, can slide out with little or no traction needed; but the head and shoulders need support.

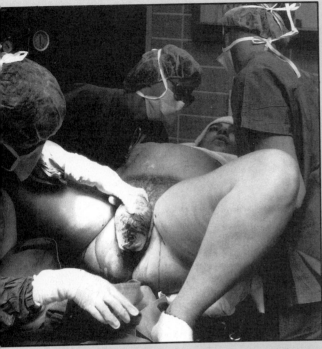

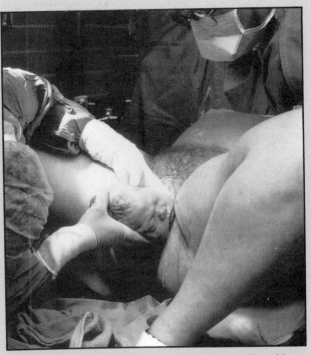

As the fetus's head emerges, it passes over the anterior margin of the perineum; the head then drops down, and the chin lies over the perineum.

To prevent maternal lacerations and damage to the fetus's intracranial area, the birth attendant must control the speed at which the head passes the perineum. When necessary, applying pressure over the perineum can maintain flexion of the head.

External rotation of the head brings the shoulders in line with the anteroposterior diameter of the client's pelvis.

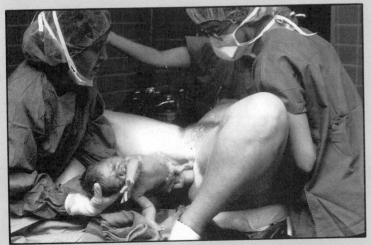

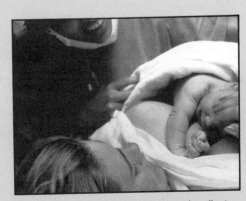

While the birth attendant holds the neonate at or below the level of the client's uterus, the nurse assists with collection of cord blood, if required, and with clamping of the cord before it is cut. The time of the neonate's complete extraction—the time of birth—is recorded.

The nurse initiates bonding between the client and neonate with skin-to-skin contact.

Client with fatigue related to duration of labor

The nursing process helps ensure high-quality care for a client in the second stage of labor. The table below shows how the nurse might use the nursing process when caring for the client in the case history at right. The first column presents history and physical assessment data followed by a paragraph of mental notes. These notes help the nurse make important mental connections among assessment findings, aiding in development of the nursing diagnosis and planning.

The second column lists an appropriate nursing diagnosis; information in the remaining columns is based on this diagnosis. Although not part of the nursing process, a rationale appears for each intervention in the fourth column to explain how it contributes to the care plan.

ASSESSMENT	NURSING DIAGNOSIS	PLANNING
Subjective (history) data • Client states that she has the urge to bear down. • Client reports that she is extremely tired. • Client expresses doubts about her ability to continue. • Client wants to know when labor will end. **Objective (physical) data** • Vital signs: temperature, 99° F; pulse, 110 beats/minute; respirations, 24/minute; blood pressure, 120/80 mm Hg. • Fetal heart rate: 136 beats/minute with regular beat-to-beat variability; mild decelerations at peak of contractions. • Uterine contractions: every 3 to 4 minutes, lasting 70 seconds. • Vaginal examination: cervix completely dilated, 0 station, LOA • Urine: 100 ml, amber color; dipstick shows high ketones, no protein, no glucose. **Mental notes** *Assessment finding indicate that Mrs. Bateman's cervix is completely dilated; however, the fetus is at 0 station and needs to be "pushed" down by the client. Therefore, she needs enouragement and support to help her through the bearing-down stage, which may last for 1 to 2 hours in a primiparous client.*	Fatigue related to duration of labor	**Goals** The client will: • assume a restful position between contractions • assume a position that maximizes bearing-down efforts during contractions • imagine her infant progressing through the birth canal • demonstrate the ability to work toward a goal. The client's support person will: • provide encouragement by giving feedback about progress.

• The client and her partner each held the neonate properly shortly after delivery.
(For a case study that shows how to apply the nursing process to a client in the second stage of labor, see *Applying the nursing process: Client with fatigue related to duration of labor.*)

Documentation

The nurse documents initial and ongoing assessment findings, pertinent characteristics of the client and support person, and all nursing activities and interventions as completely as possible. (For an example of a typical documentation form, see *Documenting the second stage of labor,* pages 700 and 701.)

Although documentation records vary among health care facilities, most require the nurse to document at least the following whenever appropriate:
• vital signs (blood pressure, pulse, temperature)
• vaginal examination findings (cervical dilation, station, position, crowning)
• uterine contractions (duration, frequency, intensity)
• bearing-down efforts
• amniotic fluid (color and amount)
• fluid intake and output
• emotional responses (such as crying, screaming, expressions of fatigue or frustration)

CASE STUDY

Mrs. Bateman, a primiparous client age 35, spent 24 hours in a prolonged latent phase of labor and received morphine sulfate to help her rest. She had an active phase of normal length (4 hours). The client has vomited twice in the past hour and has received no anesthesia; her cervix is completely dilated.

IMPLEMENTATION		EVALUATION
Intervention	**Rationale**	Upon evaluation, the client:
Assure the client that labor is progressing. Remind her of how far she has come and give positive feedback about how well she has done.	When tired, the client may forget how much of the task has been completed. Frequent, specific reminders help to bolster her spirits.	• demonstrated the ability to bear down with each contraction • rested between contrac-
Encourage the client to imagine her infant moving through and out of the birth canal.	Concentrating on a positive image helps distract the client from her frustrations with the duration of labor and level of fatigue.	tions • responded to encour- agement • exhibited labor progress • maintained adequate hy-
Monitor the client's fluid status by consulting with the physician or nurse-midwife; suggest starting an I.V., if appropriate, or increasing the infusion.	Dehydration decreases energy available for bearing-down efforts.	dration.
During her contractions, help the client into a position conducive to bearing-down efforts. If she has no preference, try a semi-sitting position with firm back support.	Position changes can increase the client's comfort level, encourage active participation, and maximize her efforts.	
Between her contractions, help the client into a position that promotes rest and supports her arms and legs.	Rest periods, even short ones, can help the client gather energy for bearing-down periods.	
Minimize noise.	A quiet environment encourages rest between contractions and enhances concentration during contractions.	
Position a mirror so that the client can observe crowning if she wishes. Encourage her to touch the infant's head if she wishes.	Seeing and touching the infant's head offers tangible proof that labor is approaching completion.	

• presence of support person or others
• transfer to delivery room or birthing chair
• perineal preparation
• time of birth (full extraction of neonate)
• names of all people in the room at the time of birth
• fetal heart rate (variability, baseline, periodic changes, use of external or internal fetal monitor)
• episiotomy or lacerations and description of repairs
• positioning and behaviors
• Apgar scores
• resuscitation, if necessary
• passage of meconium or urine
• any neonatal abnormalities or umbilical cord variations
• initial parent-infant bonding.

Chapter summary

Chapter 28 described the second stage of labor. This stage requires great effort from the client and strong support from the nurse. In addition, the nurse must monitor labor progress, assess for abnormalities and impending delivery, and assist with delivery and immediate care for the neonate. Here are the chapter highlights.

(Text continues on page 702.)

Documenting the second stage of labor

Most health care facilities use standard, preprinted forms like the one shown below to document labor and delivery. The form includes space for important details concerning the client and neonate.

Name _____

Address _____

Telephone _____ Labor and delivery support person _____

LABOR SUMMARY

G	T	P	A	L	Blood Type and Rh factor

Position

Presentation
- ☐ Shoulder
- ☐ Cephalic
- ☐ Breech _____
- ☐ Compound

Lie
- ☐ Longitudinal
- ☐ Transverse
- ☐ Oblique

Chronology

EDD _____

	Date	Time
Admit to hospital		
Membranes ruptured		
Onset of labor		
Complete cervical dilation		

Intrapartal events   ☐ None
- ☐ No prenatal care
- ☐ Preterm labor
- ☐ Postterm
- ☐ PROM
- ☐ Meconium
- ☐ Foul-smelling fluid
- ☐ Hydramnios
- ☐ Abruptio placentae
- ☐ Placenta previa
- ☐ Bleeding
- ☐ Hypertension
- ☐ Seizure activity

- ☐ Precipitous labor
- ☐ Prolonged labor
- ☐ Prolonged latent phase
- ☐ Prolonged active phase
- ☐ Prolonged 2nd stage
- ☐ Cephalopelvic disproportion
- ☐ Cord prolapse
- ☐ Extended fetal bradycardia
- ☐ Extended fetal tachycardia
- ☐ Multiple late decelerations
- ☐ Variability _____
- ☐ Anesthesia complications

Monitoring   ☐ None

	FHR	Uterine contractions
External	☐	☐
Internal	☐	☐

Medications during labor   ☐ None

_____

_____

_____

_____

Induction   ☐ None
☐ AROM   ☐ Oxytocin   ☐ PGE$_2$ gel

DELIVERY DATA

Delivery date _____

Method of delivery

Cephalic   ☐ Spontaneous   ☐ Vacuum extraction
        ☐ VBAC   ☐ Low forceps   ☐ Mid forceps

Breech   ☐ Spontaneous   ☐ External rotation
       ☐ Internal rotation

Cesarean ☐ Transverse through skin
        ☐ Transverse through body of uterus
        ☐ Vertical through skin
        ☐ Vertical through lower uterus
        ☐ Transverse through lower uterus

Placenta delivery
☐ Spontaneous   ☐ Manual   ☐ Abnormal adherence
☐ Retained placenta

Cord

Implantation _____

Length _____

Umbilical vessels _____

Cord blood: ☐ to laboratory   ☐ refrigerated
          ☐ discarded
For: ☐ Type   ☐ Coombs'   ☐ VDRL and Rh factor

Episiotomy
☐ None   ☐ Median   ☐ Mediolateral

Laceration
☐ None   ☐ Cervical   ☐ Vaginal
☐ Other _____

DELIVERY DATA continued

Other surgical procedures   ☐ None
☐ Tubal ligation   ☐ Curettage
☐ Other _____

Delivery anesthesia   ☐ None
☐ Local   ☐ Epidural   ☐ Spinal   ☐ General
☐ Other _____

Medications during delivery   ☐ None
_____
_____
_____
_____

NEONATAL DATA

Apgar scores

	1 min	5 min
Heart rate		
Respirations		
Muscle tone		
Reflex irritation		
Skin color		
Totals		

Resuscitation   ☐ None
☐ Oxygen
☐ Bag and mask
☐ Intubation
☐ External cardiac massage
☐ Other
☐ _____ minutes to sustained respiration

Medications   ☐ None
☐ Volume expander
☐ Sodium bicarbonate
☐ Drug antagonists
☐ Erythromycin ½%
☐ AgNo$_3$ 1% or _____
☐ Aqueous vitamin K I.M.
☐ Other _____

Initial neonatal examination
☐ No observed abnormalities
☐ Gross congenital anomalies _____
_____

☐ Meconium staining
☐ Petechiae
☐ Trauma
☐ Other

Basic data
ID bracelet no. _____

Hospital record no. _____

☐ Male   ☐ Female

Birth order: _____ of ☐ ☐ ☐ ☐

Weight _____

Length _____

Transferred: Date   Time

☐ To neonatal nursery
☐ With mother
☐ To NICU

Remarks: _____
_____
_____
_____
_____
_____
_____

Nurse _____

**Physician or
nurse-midwife** _____

Date completed _____

• The second stage of labor, which lasts from complete cervical dilation to delivery, typically takes about 1 hour for primiparous clients and about ½ hour for multiparous clients. Although variations are common, a second stage that takes more than 2 hours may indicate abnormality.

• Indications of the transition from first stage to second stage may include an increasing urge to push, increased bloody show, grunting, a gaping anus, involuntary defecation, bulging of the vaginal introitus, spontaneous rupture of membranes, and early decelerations in the FHR.

• Assessment during the second stage should include vital signs; degree of cervical dilation; the strength, frequency, and duration of contractions; effectiveness of bearing-down efforts; FHR; rate of descent; and color of the amniotic fluid.

• Planning and implementation involves providing emotional support for the client and family, coordinating the client's bearing-down efforts, assisting the client into positions that increase comfort and assist bearing-down efforts, monitoring hydration, preparing for delivery, and caring for the neonate immediately after delivery.

• Nursing care required immediately after delivery includes drying and inspecting the neonate for obvious abnormalities, clamping the umbilical cord, assigning an Apgar score at 1 and 5 minutes, and encouraging parent-infant bonding.

Study questions

1. Mrs. Gatling, a primiparous client age 24, has progressed through the first stage of labor. Her cervix now is dilated fully, and she is bearing down with each contraction. The fetus's head is beginning to distend the perineum. The nurse notes that fetal heart rate (FHR) drops to 60 beats/minute during each contraction and then returns to baseline. How should the nurse respond to this drop in FHR? What factors should be considered in the response? How should the nurse respond if the FHR does not return to baseline?

2. At a shift change, the nurse begins caring for Jennifer Slater, a multiparous client who has been in labor for several hours. Her cervix is dilated fully. She bears down three or four times during each contraction for 5 to 6 seconds each. Should the nurse try to change her method of bearing down? If so, how?

3. Jane Segal, a primiparous client age 38 in the second stage of labor, has received epidural anesthesia. Although she claims to be pushing with each contraction, her efforts have produced little fetal descent after 45 minutes. How should the nurse respond?

4. At 1 minute after delivery, a neonate has a heart rate of 102 beats/minute, shallow respirations, flaccid limbs, moderate reaction to insertion of a bulb syringe in one nostril, and blue hands and feet. What Apgar score should this neonate receive? What response should the nurse make, and why?

Bibliography

Atwood, R.J. (1976). Parturitional posture and related birth behavior. *Acta Obstetrica et Gynecolociea Scandinavica*, 55 (Supplement 57), 1-25.

Banta, D., and Thacker, S.B. (1982). The risks and benefits of episiotomy: A review. *Birth*, 9(Spring), 25-30.

Borell, U., and Fernstrom, I. (1967). The mechanism of labor. *Radiologic Clinics of North America*, 5(1), 73-85.

Butani, P., and Hodnett, E. (1980). Mothers' perceptions of the labor experience. *Maternal-Child Nursing Journal*, 9(Summer), 73-82.

Church, L.K. (1989). Water birth: One birthing center's observations. *Journal of Nurse-Midwifery*, 34(4), 165-170.

Cohen, W.R. (1977). Influence of the duration of second stage labor on perinatal outcomes and puerperal morbidity. *Obstetrics and Gynecology*, 49(3), 266-267.

Cohen, W.R. (1984). Steering patients through the second stage of labor. *Contemporary OB/GYN*, 24(1), 122-141.

Cunningham, F.G., MacDonald, P.C., and Gant, N.F. (1989). *Williams obstetrics* (18th ed.). East Norwalk, CT: Appleton & Lange.

Engelmann, G.J. (1882). *Labor among primitive peoples showing the development of the obstetric science of today* (reprint). New York: AMS Press.

Fitzhugh, M.L., and Newton, M. (1956). Muscle action during childbirth. *Physical Therapy Review*, 36, 805-809.

Friedman, E. (1989). Normal and dysfunctional labor. In W.R. Cohen, D. Acker, and E. Friedman (Eds.), *Management of labor* (pp. 1-18). Rockville, MD: Aspen.

Hellman, L.H., and Prystowski, H. (1952). The duration of the second stage of labor. *American Journal of Obstetrics and Gynecology*, 61, 1223-1233.

Kitzinger, S. (1984). *The experience of childbirth* (5th ed.). New York: Penguin.

Korones, S.B. (1986). *High-risk newborn infants* (4th ed.). St. Louis: Mosby.

Krapohl, A.J., Myers, G.C., and Caldeyro-Barcia, R. (1970). Uterine contractions in spontaneous labor. *American Journal of Obstetrics and Gynecology*, 106(3), 378-387.

McKay, S.R. (1981). Second stage labor—has tradition replaced safety? *AJN*, 81(5), 1016-1019.

McKay, S.R., and Roberts, J.E. (1985). Second stage labor: What is normal? *JOGNN*, 14(2), 101-106.

Mengert, W.E., and Murphy, D.P. (1933). Intra-abdominal pressure created by voluntary muscular effort. *Surgery, Gynecology, and Obstetrics*, 57, 745-751.

Minchom, P., Niswander, K., Chalmers, I., Dauncey, M., Newcombe, R., Elbourne, D., Mutch, L., Andrews, J., and Williams, G. (1987). Antecedants and outcome of very early neonatal seizures in infants born at or after term. *British Journal of Obstetrics and Gynaecology*, 94(5), 431-439.

Nelson, C.C., and Hewitt, M.A. (1983). An Indochinese refugee population in a nurse-midwife service. *Journal of Nurse-Midwifery*, 28(5), 9-14.

Noble, E. (1983). *Childbirth with insight*. Boston: Houghton-Mifflin.

Noble, E. (1981). Controversies in maternal effort during labor and delivery. *Journal of Nurse-Midwifery*, 26(2), 13-22.

Oakley, A. (1980). *Women confined: Towards a sociology of childbirth*. New York: Schocken Books.

Odent, M. (1981). The evaluation of obstetrics at Pithiviers France. *Birth and the Family Journal*, 8(1), 7-15.

Odent, M. (1986). *Birth reborn*. New York: Pantheon.

Peterson, G.B. (1984). *A personal growth approach to childbirth* (2nd ed.). Berkeley, CA: Mindbody Press.

Reynolds, J.L., and Yudkin, P.L. (1987). Changes in the management of labour. *Canadian Medical Association Journal*, 136(10), 1041-1045.

Roberts, J.E., Goldstein, S.A., Gruener, J.S., Maggio, M., and Mendez-Bauer, C.A. (1987). Descriptive analysis of involuntary bearing-down efforts during the expulsive phase of labor. *JOGNN*, 16(1), 48-55.

Roberts, J., and Mendez-Bauer, C. (1980). A perspective of maternal position during labor. *Journal of Perinatal Medicine*, 8(6), 255-264.

Shaw, N.S. (1975). Forced labor: Maternity care in the United States. New York: Pergamon Press.

Sleep, J., Roberts, J., and Chalmers, I. (1989). Care during the second stage of labour. In M.W. Enkin, M.J.N.C. Keirse, and I. Chalmers (Eds.), *A guide to effective care in pregnancy and childbirth*. Oxford, England: Oxford University Press.

Thacker, S.B., and Banta, H.D. (1983). Benefits and risks of episiotomy: An interpretative review of the English language literature, 1860-1980. *Obstetrical and Gynecological Survey*, 38(6), 322-338.

Turner, M.J., Webb. J.B., and Gordon, H. (1986). Active management of labour in primigravidae. *Journal of Obstetrics and Gynaecology*, 7, 79-83.

Ueland, K., and Hansen, J. (1969). Maternal cardiovascular dynamics, Part II: Posture and uterine contractions. *American Journal of Obstetrics and Gynecology*, 103(1), 1-7.

Ueland, K., Novy, M.J., Peterson, E.N., and Metcalf, J. (1969). Maternal cardiovascular dynamics, Part IV: The influence of gestational age on the maternal cardiovascular response to posture and exercise. *American Journal of Obstetrics and Gynecology*, 104(6), 856-864.

Whitley, N. (1985). *A manual of clinical obstetrics*. Philadelphia: Lippincott.

Whitley, N. (1975). Uterine contractile physiology: Application in nursing care and patient teaching. *JOGNN*, 4(5), 54-58.

Winner, W., and Romney, S.L. (1966). Cardiovascular responses to labor and delivery. *American Journal of Obstetrics and Gynecology*, 95(8), 1104-1114.

Wood, C., Ng, K. H., Hounslow, D., and Benning, H. (1973). Time—an important variable in normal delivery. *Journal of Obstetrics and Gynaecology of the British Commonwealth*, 80(4), 295-300.

Maternal position

Bassell, G., Humayun, S.G., and Marx, G.F. (1980). Maternal bearing down efforts—Another fetal risk? *Obstetrics and Gynecology*, 56(1), 39-41.

Caldeyro-Barcia, R.Y. (1978). The influence of maternal position during the second stage of labor. In P. Simlein and C. Reinke (Eds.), *Kaleidoscope of childbearing: Preparation, birth, and nurturing* (pp. 31-42). Seattle Pennypress.

Drahne, A., Prang, G., and Werner, C. (1983). The various positions for delivery. *Journal of Perinatal Medicine*, 10(Supplement 2), 72-73.

Haukeland, I. (1981). An alternative delivery position: New delivery chair developed and tested at Kongsberg Hospital. *American Journal of Obstetrics and Gynecology*, 141(2), 115-117.

Householder, M.S. (1974). A historical perspective on the obstetric chair. *Surgery, Gynecology, and Obstetrics*, 139(3), 423-440.

Humphrey, M.D., Chang, A., Wood, E.C., Morgan, S., and Hounslow, D. (1974). A decrease in fetal pH during second stage of labour, when conducted in the dorsal position. *Journal of Obstetrics and Gynaecology of the British Commonwealth*, 81(8), 600-602.

Irwin, H.W. (1978). Practical considerations for routine applications of left lateral Sims' position for vaginal delivery. *American Journal of Obstetrics and Gynecology*, 131(2), 129-132.

Knauth, D.G., and Haloburdo, E.P. (1986). Effect of pushing techniques in birthing chair on length of second stage labor. *Nursing Research*, 35(1), 49-51.

Kurz, C.S., Schneider, R., and Huch, R. (1982). The influence of the maternal position on the fetal transcutaneous oxygen pressure (tcPO$_2$). *Journal of Perinatal Medicine*, 10(Supplement 2), 74-75.

Leak, W.N. (1955). Position for delivery. *British Medical Journal*, 2, 735-736.

Lehrman, E.J. (1985). Birth in the left lateral position: An alternative to the traditional delivery position. *Journal of Nurse-Midwifery*, 30(4), 193-197.

Liu, Y.C. (1989). The effects of the upright position during childbirth. *Image: Journal of Nursing Scholarship*, 21(1), 14-18.

Martinez-Lopez, V., de la Fuenta, P., Iniguez, A., Freese, U.E., and Mendez-Bauer, C. (1984). Comparison of two methods of bearing down during second stage. Paper presented at the 31st Meeting of the Society for Gynecological Investigation, March 21-24.

McKay, S.R. (1980). Maternal position during labor and birth: A reassessment. *JOGNN*, 9(5), 288-291.

McManus, T.J. (1978). Upright posture and the efficiency of labour. *The Lancet*, 1(8055), 72-74.

Mendez-Bauer, C., Arroyo, J., Garcia-Ramos, C., Menendez, A., Lavilla, M., Izquierdo, F., Villa Elizaga, I., and Zamarriego, J. (1975). Effects of standing position on spontaneous uterine contractility and other aspects of labor. *Journal of Perinatal Medicine*, 3(2), 89-100.

Naroll, F., Naroll, R., and Howard, F.H. (1961). Positions of women in childbirth. *American Journal of Obstetrics and Gynecology*, 82, 943-954.

Newton, M., and Newton, N. (1960). The propped position for second stage of labor. *Obstetrics and Gynecology*, 15, 28-34.

Roberts, J. (1979). Maternal positions for childbirth: A historical review of nursing care practices. *JOGNN*, 8(1), 24-32.

Roberts, J. (1980). Alternative positions for childbirth, Part II: Second stage of labor. *Journal of Nurse-Midwifery*, 25(5), 13-19.

Schneider-Affeld, F., and Martin, K. (1982). Delivery from a sitting position. *Journal of Perinatal Medicine*, 10(Supplement 2), 70-71.

Turner, M.J., Romney, M.L., Webb, J.B., and Gordon, H. (1986). The birthing chair: An obstetric hazard? *Journal of Obstetrics and Gynecology*, 6, 232-235.

Comfort measures

Block, C.R, and Block, R. (1975). The effect of support of the husband and obstetrician on pain perception and control in childbirth. *Birth and the Family Journal,* 2(Spring), 43-50.

Bloom, K.C. (1984). Assisting the unprepared woman during labor. *JOGNN,* 13(5), 303-306.

Chestnut, D.H., Vandewalker, G.E., Owen, C.L., Bates, J.N., and Choi, W.W. (1987). The influence of continuous epidural bupivacaine analgesia on the second stage of labor and method of delivery in nulliparous women. *Anesthesiology,* 66(6), 774-780.

Klusman, L.E. (1975). Reduction of pain in childbirth by the alleviation of anxiety in pregnancy. *Journal of Consulting Clinical Psychology,* 43(2), 162-165.

Scott, J.R., and Rose, N.B. (1976). Effect of psychoprophylaxis (Lamaze preparation) on labor and delivery in primiparas. *New England Journal of Medicine,* 294(22), 1205-1207.

Stevens, R.J. (1976). Psychological strategies for management of pain in prepared childbirth, Part I: A review of the research. *Birth and the Family Journal,* 3(Winter), 157-164.

Tryon, P. (1966). Use of comfort measures as support during labor. *Nursing Research,* 15(2), 109-118.

Fetal effects

Apgar, V. (1966). The newborn (Apgar) scoring system: Reflections and advice. *Pediatric Clinics of North America,* 13(3), 645-650.

Caldeyro-Barcia, R. (1979). The influence of maternal bearing-down efforts during second stage on fetal well-being. *Birth and the Family Journal,* 6(Spring), 17-21.

Caldeyro-Barcia, R. (1979). The influence of maternal position on time of spontaneous rupture of the membranes, progress of labor, and fetal head compression. *Birth and the Family Journal,* 6(Spring), 7-15.

Caldeyro-Barcia, R., Giussi, G., Storch, E., Poseiro, J., LaFaurie, N., Keffenhuber, K., and Ballejo, G. (1981). The bearing-down efforts and their effects on fetal heart rate, oxygenation and acid base balance. *Journal of Perinatal Medicine,* 9(Supplement 1), 63-67.

Graziano, E., Freeman, W., and Bendel, R. (1980). FHR variability and other heart rate observations during second stage labor. *Obstetrics and Gynecology,* 56(1), 42-47.

Herbert, C. and Boehm, F. (1981). Prolonged end-stage fetal heart rate deceleration: A reanalysis. *Obstetrics and Gynecology,* 57(5), 589-593.

Hon, E.H., and Quilligan, E.J. (1967). The classification of fetal heart rate, Part II: A revised working classification. *Connecticut Medicine,* 31(11), 779-784.

Krebs, H., Petres, R. and Dunn, L. (1981). Intrapartum fetal heart rate monitoring, Part V: Fetal heart rate patterns in the second stage of labor. *American Journal of Obstetrics and Gynecology,* 140(4), 435-439.

Ohel, G. (1978). Fetal heart rate in the second stage of labour and fetal outcome. *South African Medical Journal,* 54, 1130-1131.

Roberts, J. (1989). Managing fetal bradycardia during the second stage of labor. *MCN,* 8(6), 41-47.

Nursing research

Andrews, C. (1980). Changing fetal position. *Journal of Nurse-Midwifery,* 25(1),7-12.

Avery, M.D., and Burket, B.A. (1986). Effect of perineal massage on the incidence of episiotomy and perineal laceration in a nurse-midwifery service. *Journal of Nurse-Midwifery,* 31(3), 128-134.

Carr, K.C. (1980). Obstetric practices which protect against neonatal morbidity: Focus on maternal position in labor and birth. *Birth and the Family Journal,* 7(Winter), 249-254.

Cottrell, B., and Shannahan, M. (1986). Effect of the birth chair on duration of second stage labor and maternal outcome. *Nursing Research,* 35(6), 364-367.

Stewart, P., Hillan, E., and Calder, A. (1983). A randomized trial to evaluate the use of a birth chair for delivery. *Lancet,* 1(8337), 1296-1298.

van Lier, D.J. (1985). Effect of maternal position on second stage of labor. Unpublished doctoral dissertation. University of Illinois at Chicago, Health Science Center, Chicago, IL.

Wery, J.L., and Roberts, J.E. (1987). Effects of maternal position on initial interaction with the newborn and subsequent maternal behavior. *Journal of Nurse-Midwifery,* 3(5), 240-243.

Yeates, D., and Roberts, J. (1984). A comparison of two bearing-down techniques during the second stage of labor. *Journal of Nurse-Midwifery,* 29(1), 3-11.

The Third and Fourth Stages of Labor

Objectives

After reading and studying this chapter, the student should be able to:

1. Identify the third and fourth stages of labor.

2. Describe placental separation and delivery.

3. Describe physical assessment during the third stage of labor.

4. Discuss nursing interventions for a client with uterine atony.

5. Explain neonatal assessment and care during the third and fourth stages of labor.

6. Discuss normal assessment findings during the fourth stage of labor.

7. Identify abnormal fourth-stage findings and possible nursing interventions.

8. Select comfort measures to assist the client and her family.

9. Promote bonding between the parents and the neonate.

10. Apply the nursing process when caring for a client during the third and fourth stages of labor.

Introduction

The third stage of labor begins with delivery of the neonate and ends with delivery of the placenta. It may last from a few minutes to 30 minutes. For most clients, this stage occurs without incident and produces a blood loss of less than 500 ml. However, postpartal hemorrhage may occur, signaling an obstetric emergency.

In this stage, the nurse assesses the client for homeostasis, placental status and delivery, and perineal repair. The nurse also evaluates the neonate's adaptation to the extrauterine environment and assesses the family's response to the client and neonate. The nurse must respond quickly to changing circumstances, resetting priorities as needed.

The fourth stage of labor begins after delivery of the placenta and lasts about 1 hour. It marks the beginning of the "fourth trimester" (the first 3 postpartal months), during which the client recovers from the stresses of labor and physiologically returns to a nonpregnant state. During this stage, the client, her partner, and the neonate experience heightened awareness and sensitivity as they further their bonding (Rubin, 1984).

During the third and fourth stages of labor, the client's cultural beliefs can influence her self-care and health promotion measures, interactions with health care professionals, and care of and bonding with the neonate. To provide adequate care, the nurse should become acquainted with the client's cultural beliefs and exercise care to avoid stereotyping her.

In most facilities, the client, her partner or support person, and the neonate remain together during the fourth stage of labor. In others, the neonate may be moved to the nursery while the client remains in the labor and recovery area. Therefore, the type of nursing care needed will depend on facility policy.

Nursing goals for the third and fourth stages of labor relate to the physiologic adaptation and changing needs of the client and her neonate. They typically include:

• maintaining homeostasis of the client and neonate.

• providing necessary equipment, supplies, and medications.

GLOSSARY

Atony: lack of normal tone; uterine atony results in a boggy (soft, poorly contracted) organ and may lead to postpartal hemorrhage.

Episiotomy: surgical incision made in the perineum to enlarge the vaginal opening for delivery; performed to prevent perineal tears, to speed or facilitate delivery, or to prevent excess stretching of perineal muscles and connective tissue.

Fourth stage of labor: period after delivery of the placenta, lasting about 1 hour.

Fundus: rounded portion of the uterus above the level of the fallopian tube attachments.

Hypotonic: having reduced muscle tension; describes a relaxed and poorly contracted muscle.

Involution: retrogressive changes in vital processes or in organs after fulfilling their functions; the return of the reproductive organs to a nonpregnant state.

Lochia: postpartal uterine discharge composed of blood, tissue, leukocytes, and mucus.

Oxytocin: hormone produced by the posterior pituitary gland that causes uterine contractions; also a synthetic hormone (Pitocin) that simulates the actions of the natural hormone.

Postpartal hemorrhage: abnormally large amount (more than 500 ml) of bleeding after delivery, which may be caused by uterine atony, rupture, lacerations, inversion, or hematoma.

Pregnancy-induced hypertension (PIH): group of potentially life-threatening hypertensive disorders that usually develop in the second or third trimester; includes preeclampsia and eclampsia.

Third stage of labor: period that begins with delivery of the neonate and ends with delivery of the placenta.

• promoting bonding and family interaction.
• Initiating breast-feeding, if the client desires.

To meet these goals, nursing activities usually include:
• observing for signs of placental separation
• assisting with placental delivery
• examining the placenta for intactness and number of umbilical cord vessels
• assisting with perineal repair
• observing the neonate's adaptation to extrauterine life, including assessment of respiratory and cardiovascular status
• evaluating the neonate's temperature and keeping the neonate warm
• preparing the neonate for interaction with the parents
• monitoring maternal blood pressure, pulse, and respirations and neonatal heart rate and respirations
• evaluating the amount and character of uterine bleeding
• monitoring uterine location and contractility
• evaluating the suture line if perineal repair was performed
• recognizing abnormal findings and intervening appropriately
• enhancing client and family self-esteem by promoting bonding
• evaluating neonate-parent interaction
• promoting comfort and safety for the client and her neonate
• helping the client meet fluid and nutrient needs
• teaching the family about postpartal recovery and neonatal feeding and care

• addressing the cultural needs of the client and her family, and adapting nursing care to meet those needs
• documenting the client's status and care as well as that of her neonate.

This chapter describes the third and fourth stages of labor and discusses how the nurse provides appropriate care based on careful assessment. It begins immediately after the birth of the neonate, discussing information obtained at the birth. Then it discusses common variations of the placenta and explores related nursing interventions. The chapter describes continuing assessments, clearly distinguishing between normal findings and variations and signs of potential problems. It concludes with a discussion of continuing nursing responsibilities, including promotion of bonding and preparation for discharge.

Nursing care during the third stage of labor

During this stage, the nurse may care for the mother and neonate simultaneously. To provide the best possible care, the nurse should apply the nursing process.

Assessment

Because the third stage of labor is brief, rapidly assess maternal vital signs and the status of the placenta, perineum, fundus, and neonate.

Maternal vital signs

Assess vital signs frequently, reporting changes or abnormal findings to the physician or nurse-midwife immediately. An increasing pulse rate followed by increased respirations and decreased blood pressure may be the first signs of postpartal hemorrhage and hypovolemic shock, which can occur rapidly. These complications are relatively common and typically result from uterine atony and excessive blood loss during placental separation and delivery or from perineal lacerations.

Changes in the client's level of consciousness and vital signs (rising systolic pressure, decreased pulse, and irregular respirations) may indicate increased intracranial pressure caused by rupture of a cerebral aneurysm, which may be precipitated by the increased cardiac output and stress of bearing down during the second stage of labor. However, this complication is rare.

Restlessness, tachypnea, and tachycardia may signal amniotic fluid embolism, another rare complication that may occur when amniotic fluid enters the maternal circulation during placental separation.

Placenta

After delivery of the neonate, watch for these normal signs of placental separation:
• A sudden gush or trickle of blood from the vagina
• Increased umbilical cord length at the vaginal introitus
• Change in the shape of the uterus from discoid (disk-shaped) to globular (globe-shaped)
• Change in the position of the uterus to a location at or above the client's umbilicus.

These signs indicate normal progress of the third stage of labor. They occur when the size of the uterine cavity decreases while the size of the inelastic placental tissue remains constant. As the placental tissue buckles and begins separating from the uterus, bleeding from open decidual arterioles forms a clot between the placental tissue and the uterine wall. This retroplacental clot further shears the placenta from the uterine wall and maintains hemostasis by controlling arteriolar blood flow.

When these signs occur, expect placental delivery shortly. After the placenta separates completely, it descends to the lower uterine segment. Myometrial contractions, which may have subsided temporarily, return at 4- to 5-minute intervals and propel the placenta into the vagina. At this point, the client may push to help expel the placenta. The mechanism for pushing is similar to, but less intense than, that used during the second stage of labor.

Note the mechanism of placental expulsion. The Duncan mechanism (sometimes called the "dirty Duncan") occurs when the dark, rough, maternal side of the placenta appears first. The Schultze mechanism (or "shiny Schultze") occurs when the glistening fetal side appears first. The mechanism of expulsion usually does not affect the client's outcome.

As the placenta is delivered, examine its intactness, number of lobes, texture, and color. Examination of the placenta determines whether fragments remain in the uterus and provides additional information about the neonate's status. Calcifications, discolorations, malformations, cysts, or other abnormalities may indicate poor placental function, explain fetal distress in labor and low birth weight, and indicate the need to evaluate the neonate more thoroughly.

Assess the umbilical cord and its insertion into the placenta. Some cord variations pose potential hazards to the neonate, whereas others are benign. (For more information, see *Placental and umbilical cord variations*, pages 708 and 709.)

Perineum

If the physician or nurse-midwife did not perform an episiotomy, assist with inspection of the perineum for lacerations or edema. Also assist with inspection of the vagina and cervix for lacerations or retained placental fragments.

If the client underwent an episiotomy or sustained lacerations, assist with surgical repair of the tissue by providing adequate light, suture material, a local anesthesia kit (if necessary), and client support. The perineum is stitched in layers to maintain its visual integrity. Assess for an intact suture line, and note the degree of swelling, oozing, or discoloration caused by bruising or hematoma formation.

Fundus

Palpate the fundus to determine its location and consistency. After the placenta is delivered, the fundus normally is midline, 1 to 2 cm below the umbilicus, and firmly contracted. A boggy (soft and poorly contracted) fundus is a sign of uterine atony (lack of muscle tone).

The following factors commonly are associated with uterine atony and the potential for postpartal hemorrhage:
• history of postpartal hemorrhage with previous delivery
• delivery of a large-for-gestational-age neonate
• hydramnios
• multiple fetuses

(Text continues on page 710.)

Placental and umbilical cord variations

After delivery of the placenta, the nurse assesses it carefully, documenting any variations from the norm, such as a placenta that is not intact. The nurse also notes umbilical cord variations, such as unusual insertion into the placenta or an abnormal number of umbilical cord vessels. The illustrations below show some common variations and their significance.

Normal placenta

Normally, the placenta is delivered intact and no fragments remain in the uterus. It has many lobes with smooth, rounded edges and consistent color throughout, indicating adequate tissue perfusion. The placenta at term is flat, cakelike, round or oval, 15 to 20 cm in diameter, and 2 to 3 cm in breadth at its thickest parts. The maternal side is lobulated and the fetal side is shiny. It has no calcifications, discolorations, malformations, cysts, or other abnormalities.

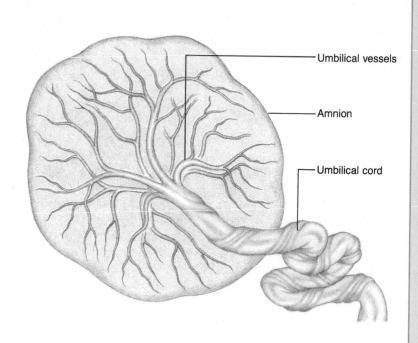

Umbilical vessels

Normal umbilical vessels
The normal umbilical cord contains three vessels: two arteries and one vein.

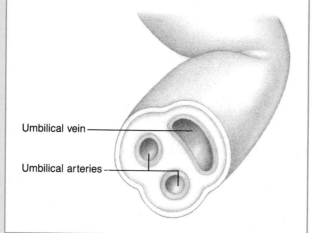

Abnormal number of vessels
Fewer than three umbilical vessels correlates with various congenital anomalies, such as cardiac and renal anomalies.

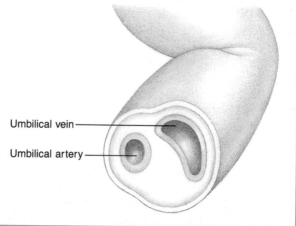

Placental variations

Battledore placenta
In this placental variation, the umbilical cord inserts in the margin (edge) of the placenta. This normal variation occurs in about 10% of gestations.

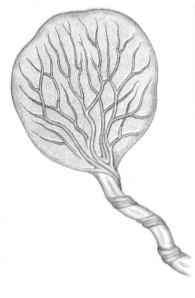

Velamentous insertion
Occurring in about 1% of gestations, a velamentous insertion occurs when the cord vessels branch from the membranes to the placenta. A velamentous insertion poses a danger because, if the membranes rupture, the cord vessels will rupture, leading to fetal hemorrhage. Blood vessels also may rupture, leading to hemorrhage between the amnion and chorion. Compression of the vessels during labor could explain fetal heart rate changes, indicating anoxia.

If velamentous insertion is detected when inspecting the delivered placenta, the danger to the fetus has passed.

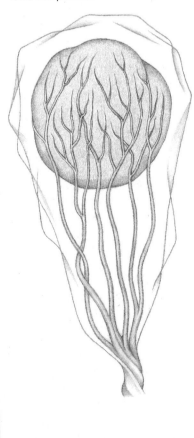

Succenturiate lobe
A succenturiate lobe is an aberrant lobe or entire cotyledon (subdivision of the uterine surface of the placenta) that is separate from the placenta but connected to its main body by blood vessels. Occurring in less than 0.2% of gestations, a succenturiate lobe may tear away from the main portion of the placenta during separation and expulsion. If left in the uterus, a succenturiate lobe can cause postpartal hemorrhage or infection. It also may cause vasa previa (presentation of the cord's blood vessels in front of the fetus's head during labor and delivery). Vasa previa, which also may occur with velamentous insertion, endangers the fetus because the fetus's head can compress the unprotected vessels, reducing fetal oxygen supply. Also, the unprotected vessels may be ruptured easily, leading to life-threatening hemorrhage.

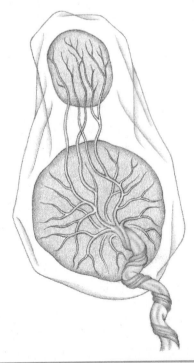

- extended stimulation of labor with oxytocin (Pitocin)
- bladder distention
- traumatic delivery
- grand multiparous client (more than 5 childbirths)
- anesthesia or excessive analgesia.

 If uterine atony is not identified and corrected, post-partal hemorrhage can occur. (For more information, see *Psychomotor skills: Uterine palpation and massage.*)

Neonate

Depending on facility policy, the physician, nurse-mid-wife, or nurse assesses the neonate immediately after delivery by assigning an Apgar score. (For more information, see Chapter 28, The Second Stage of Labor.)

 Continue to assess the neonate throughout the third stage of labor, focusing on evaluation of respiratory and cardiovascular status.

Nursing diagnosis

Based on assessment findings, formulate nursing diagnoses for the client. (For a list of possible nursing diagnoses, see *Nursing diagnoses: Third and fourth stages of labor,* page 717.) Then use the assessment findings and diagnoses to define care priorities during the postpartal period.

Planning and implementation

Routine care includes hygienic care, repositioning and transferring the client to the recovery area (or assisting recovery in the labor-delivery-recovery area), providing neonatal care, and promoting bonding.

Provide hygienic care

At this stage, the client may have a nursing diagnosis of *potential for infection related to perineal laceration* or *potential for infection related to episiotomy.* Immediately after the physician or nurse-midwife has finished inspecting or repairing the perineum, help prevent infection by cleaning the client's vulva with sterile water. Using a wet towel or gauze, wipe from the urethral area to the rectal area. Discard used gauze after each pass. Dislodge and remove dried blood or fecal material, leaving the perineal area free of bacterial contamination.

 Using a downward movement, apply a clean perineal pad. Remove all delivery drapes and immediately place them in a linen hamper.

 To prevent a nursing diagnosis of *potential altered body temperature related to evaporation of perspiration and muscle fatigue,* help the client change from her soiled delivery gown into a clean gown, and cover her with a clean, warm bath blanket. Change her gown even if it is not obviously soiled, because dampness from perspiration can cause chilling.

Reposition and transfer the client

To prevent hip joint dislocation and a nursing diagnosis of *potential for injury related to maternal positioning* or *altered tissue perfusion related to sudden change in pelvic or abdominal blood volume,* pay close attention to body dynamics and homeostasis when repositioning the client. When helping her lower her legs from stirrups or from the flexed position, advise her to bring her legs together and lower them simultaneously.

 A client who has had a local anesthestic and must transfer from the delivery table to a recovery bed will need assistance in moving. Ask another member of the health care team to help stabilize the bed and keep the client's perineal pad in place as you help her move.

 If spinal or epidural anesthesia was used during delivery and the client cannot control her legs, use a draw sheet or roller for the transfer and have other team members assist to ensure client safety.

 After the client has been repositioned, transfer her to the recovery area or allow her to remain in the labor and delivery area, depending on facility policy.

Care for the neonate

While the neonate remains with the mother or parents, provide appropriate care. (For specific nursing care, see *Neonatal status: Third and fourth stages of labor,* page 712.)

Promote bonding

During the third stage of labor, the family may have a nursing diagnosis of *family coping: potential for growth, related to neonate's birth.* For this reason, the neonate's introduction to the parents is paramount. The physician or nurse-midwife places the neonate in the mother's arms even before the cord has stopped pulsating or been cut. A neonate that must remain supine can lie on the mother's abdomen. While assessments and procedures are performed, keep the mother and neonate together.

 Encourage both parents to touch and talk to the neonate immediately. If the parents are afraid to touch the neonate, reassure them. Upon hearing the parents' voices, the neonate should gaze in their direction and may open the eyes fully if they are shaded from the light.

 While the client is being repositioned or transferred to another bed, encourage the father or support person to hold the neonate. If the client plans to breast-feed, allow the father to place the neonate in her arms.

 When the neonate is transferred to a crib, warmer, or the nursery, encourage the father or support person to remain with the neonate and report weight and ac-

Uterine palpation and massage

Through uterine palpation, the nurse can assess the location and firmness of the fundus. Uterine massage can help stimulate uterine contractions, which promote involution and prevent hemorrhage. Also, blood clots may be expelled during uterine massage. To perform uterine palpation and massage, expose the lower abdomen and follow these steps.

1 Place one hand at the level of the symphysis pubis, cupping it against the abdomen to support the fundus and prevent downward displacement. Keep in mind that the elasticity of the ligaments supporting the uterus and the stretching experienced at term place the postpartal uterus at risk for inversion if it is not fixed in place during palpation and massage.

2 Place the other hand at the top of the fundus, cupping it against the abdomen.

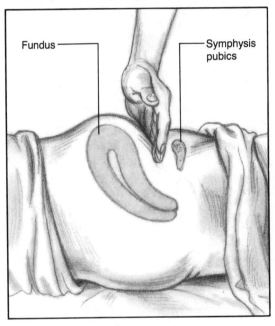

Fundus — Symphysis pubics

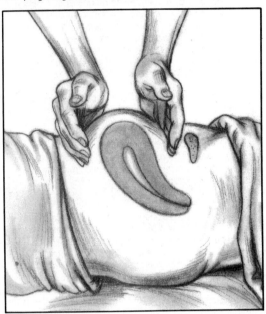

4 To massage the fundus, use the side of the hand above the fundus. Without digging into the abdomen, gently compress and release, always supporting the lower uterine segment with the other hand. Observe for lochia flow during massage.

3 Gently compress the uterus between both hands. Note the level of the fundus above or below the umbilicus in fingerbreadths or centimeters. (One fingerbreadth measures about 1 cm). Also note the firmness of the fundus.

5 Massage long enough to produce firmness. Because the fundus is tender, use only enough pressure to produce desired results without causing discomfort.

---

tivity to the mother. This helps parents and neonate maintain contact and continue bonding.

Evaluation

Before the fourth stage of labor begins, evaluate nursing care provided during the third stage. In many facilities, the delivery nurse continues to care for the mother; in others, another nurse assumes care for the mother after transfer to the recovery area. In either case, evaluate maternal status by reviewing and comparing assessment data and considering the effectiveness of nursing interventions.

The following examples illustrate appropriate evaluation statements:
• The client's placenta was delivered intact.
• The client's fundus was firm.
• The client lost less than 500 ml of blood.
• The neonate adapted appropriately to the extrauterine environment, as shown by stable temperature, heart rate of 120 to 180 beats/minute, and respirations between 40 and 60 with no nasal flaring or grunting.

Third and fourth stages of labor

When caring for the mother during the third and fourth stages of labor, the nurse also must assess and provide care for the neonate.

Assessment

To assess the neonate's respiratory status, count respirations and note skin color. Respirations should range from 40 to 60 breaths/minute. Except for the hands and feet, which may have a blue tinge, the neonate's skin color should be similar to that of the parents.

To assess cardiovascular status, palpate the heart rate or auscultate it through a stethoscope at the point of maximum impulse. The rate should range from 120 to 180 beats/minute, increasing with crying and activity. Palpate the femoral pulse for presence and quality. Lack of a femoral pulse may indicate coarctation of the aorta, a congenital cardiovascular condition.

Assess respiratory and cardiovascular status at 1 and 5 minutes, then at 5-minute intervals unless the situation warrants more frequent assessment. Evaluate the neonate each time the mother is assessed routinely.

Nursing care

An important aspect of care during this time is maintenance of the neonate's temperature. Temperature regulation depends on metabolism of brown fat, which accumulates during the last 3 months of gestation. If hypothermia occurs, the metabolic rate increases to produce heat; this can cause respiratory distress, a condition that can progress to metabolic acidosis and require aggressive intervention. To prevent this, keep the neonate warm.

Dry the neonate thoroughly immediately after delivery. Skin-to-skin contact with the mother provides the warmest environment for the neonate because heat from her body conducts to the neonate. If the mother holds the neonate, cover both with a warm blanket. If she does not, keep the neonate wrapped in warm blankets under a radiant warmer.

The neonate's largest surface area and area of greatest potential heat loss is the head. After drying the scalp, cover it with a stockinet cap or, if facility practice dictates, a plastic bunting head covering.

Other routine neonatal care includes applying identification bands and footprinting, as facility practice dictates. Place a numbered identification bracelet on the neonate's wrist and opposite ankle and on the mother's wrist. Take two sets of neonate footprints, one for the chart and one for the parents. Encourage the support person to participate in footprinting and explain the need for this identification to the mother.

In most facilities, the neonate is weighed and measured in the nursery and receives vitamin K and eye prophylaxis (ophthalmic antiinfective treatment) there as well. Encourage the support person to accompany the neonate and to return to the client and inform her of the neonate's vital statistics. However, if these procedures occur in the delivery area, be prepared to perform them. (For details, see Chapter 36, Care of the Normal Neonate.)

• The client held and gazed at the neonate immediately after delivery.
• The father touched and talked to the neonate.

Documentation

The nurse usually documents assessments and activities of the third stage on the delivery record. The nurse also may be required to complete special forms, such as neonate footprint papers.

Although each health care facility may require documentation of slightly different information, most expect the nurse to record the following on the delivery record:
• episiotomy or laceration repair
• drugs or fluids administered
• time, method, and completeness of delivery of the placenta
• maternal and neonatal vital signs
• interaction between parents and neonate

• maternal status at the time of transfer to the recovery area
• neonatal status at the time of transfer to the recovery area or nursery.

Nursing care during the fourth stage of labor

The nurse uses the nursing process to care for a client during the fourth stage of labor. To interpret assessment data properly and make decisions about care, the nurse must understand the physiology of the recovery period, including shifts in internal pressures and changes in the cardiovascular, respiratory, urinary, reproductive, gastrointestinal, and musculoskeletal systems. (For more information, see Chapter 24, Physiology of Labor and Childbirth.)

Assessment

Maternal status can change rapidly during the fourth stage of labor, and such life-threatening complications as postpartal hemorrhage can occur. Therefore, frequent assessments are necessary. Begin the assessment by reviewing subjective and objective data obtained during the previous stages of labor. (This review has special importance for the nurse providing care in a recovery room separate from the labor and delivery area.) Continue the assessment by collecting current data.

If the neonate stays with the mother during this period, continue to maintain the neonate's warmth and monitor cardiovascular and respiratory status.

Health history

First, review all data obtained on admission and throughout labor and delivery. The following elements of the client's history help interpret fourth stage assessment findings.

Vital signs. Postpartal deviations from the client's baseline can indicate hemorrhage, pregnancy-induced hypertension (PIH), dehydration, or infection.

Obstetric history. The client's gravidity and parity help predict her uterine contractility and response to oxytocic medication. For example, a multiparous client may have inadequate muscle contractility because childbirth commonly causes a loss in uterine muscle tone.

The client's obstetric history can provide other clues about her probable postpartal recovery. For example, a client who experienced postpartal hemorrhage after a previous childbirth has greater risk for hemorrhage after this one (Varney, 1987).

Labor duration and progress. Prolonged labor can lead to uterine atony, particularly if accompanied by many hours of oxytocic stimulation. It also may cause dehydration and exhaustion, which may result in circulatory and musculoskeletal problems. Precipitous labor and delivery can cause uterine atony, predispose the client to hemorrhage, and produce lacerations or cervical tears that may increase blood loss.

Physical assessment

Begin client assessment after the neonate is stabilized and during or immediately after perineal repair. Assess the client's vital signs and level of consciousness.

After any perineal repair is complete and the client has been helped into a more comfortable position, assess postpartal parameters and evaluate her discomfort, recovery from analgesia and anesthesia, and fatigue, hunger, and thirst. Also observe the family's response to the neonate's birth.

Postpartal parameters. During this assessment, evaluate vital signs, fundus, lochia (blood, tissue, and cells shed from the uterus immediately after delivery and continuing for several weeks), perineum, leg pain, and tremors. (For more information, see *Parameters of postpartal assessment*, pages 714 and 715.)

Assess these parameters at least every 15 minutes during the fourth stage. In situations that deviate from the norm, such as a sudden drop in blood pressure or a large increase in bright red lochia, alert the physician or nurse-midwife.

Discomfort. With each assessment during the fourth stage, determine the client's discomfort. Determine the character, intensity, and source of discomfort, such as uterine contractions, laceration repair, or perineal hematoma. Sources of discomfort during the fourth stage of labor directly relate to the length and intensity of labor, the conduct of the delivery, the presence of perineal trauma, and uterine muscle contractility (which affects hemorrhage control). A report of discomfort coupled with physical assessment findings may indicate a problem, such as hematoma formation.

Uterine contractions. Once the placenta has been delivered, the myometrial fibers contract to control blood flow from open vessels at the placental site. Sometimes called afterpains, these contractions are experienced differently by each client. For example, the multiparous client tends to need stronger and longer contractions to firm the uterus than the primiparous client, and those stronger contractions produce more intense afterpains. Postpartal contraction pain also may intensify if oxytocic drugs (Pitocin, Methergine) have been administered to control uterine bleeding.

Episiotomy, laceration repair, or perineal hematoma. A client who has undergone an episiotomy or laceration repair may experience a dull aching or burning sensation from edema and disruption of muscle and nerve tissue. Although some pain is inevitable, severe, throbbing, or increasing pain may signal a serious problem.

An episiotomy, performed during the second stage of labor, can cause great discomfort during the fourth stage. During the second stage, perineal sensitivity is

(Text continues on page 716.)

Parameters of postpartal assessment

For each postpartal assessment parameter, the chart below describes assessment techniques, normal and abnormal findings, and related nursing interventions. During the fourth stage of labor, the nurse must assess these parameters at least every 15 minutes.

PARAMETER AND ASSESSMENT TECHNIQUE	FINDINGS	NURSING INTERVENTIONS
Vital signs Palpation of the pulse for a full minute, observation of respiratory rate and rhythm, and blood pressure auscultation; temperature usually taken 1 hour after birth	*Normal findings* • Pulse within 4 to 17 beats/minute of predelivery rate • Respiratory rate within 2 to 4 breaths of predelivery rate • Systolic and diastolic blood pressure within 10 mm Hg of predelivery pressure	*For a client with normal findings* • Repeat assessments every 15 minutes until the client is stable; then repeat according to facility policy or as prescribed. • Assess for orthostatic changes in blood pressure and increase in pulse if the client reports lightheadedness when rising or walking.
	Abnormal findings • Rapid pulse rate, characteristic of hemorrhage • Pulse rate more than 17 beats/minute slower than predelivery rate, which may indicate heart block or other postpartal cardiac anomaly • Depressed respiratory rate, which can result from medications or anesthesia • Tachypnea, which indicates oxygen need and may result from hemorrhage or shock • Hypotension (less than 10 mm Hg between systolic and diastolic measurements), which may suggest extensive blood loss and impending shock • Hypertension (15 mm Hg increase in diastolic, 30 mm Hg systolic), which may occur with pregnancy-induced hypertension (PIH) • Elevated temperature, which may be caused by dehydration, fatigue, or infection	*For a client with abnormal findings* • Notify the physician or nurse-midwife. • Repeat vital sign assessments at least every 5 minutes along with other assessments • Maintain fluid balance, as needed. • Be prepared to administer oxygen and medications as prescribed. • If hypertension is present, check the client's reflexes. A client with PIH who develops symptoms will show brisk reflexes with ankle clonus.
Fundus Palpation	*Normal findings* • Fundal height between the umbilicus and 1 to 2 cm below the umbilicus • Fundus midline, firm, and about the size of an average cantaloupe	*For a client with normal findings* • Repeat fundal palpation every 15 minutes with other assessments. • Teach the client the significance of a well-contracted uterus. Teach her to palpate her fundus and practice fundal massage.
	Abnormal findings • Boggy (soft, poorly contracted) uterus, deviated from midline and above the umbilicus, which suggests atony, clot retention, or a full bladder	*For a client with abnormal findings* • Massage the fundus until it becomes firm and clots are expressed. • Reassess the fundus at least every 5 minutes. • Encourage the client to void. • Encourage the client who has chosen to breast-feed to begin because nipple stimulation causes the pituitary gland to release oxytocin. • Administer oxytocic medications, if prescribed.

Parameters of postpartal assessment continued

PARAMETER AND ASSESSMENT TECHNIQUE	FINDINGS	NURSING INTERVENTIONS
Lochia Inspection of lochia flow and observation for clots at the perineum while assessing the fundus. Check under the buttocks to ensure that blood is not pooling under the client.	*Normal findings* • Serous fluid with no clots • Scant (1″ stain on perineal pad), light (1″ to 4″ stain), or moderate (4″ to 6″ stain) flow within 15 minutes	*For a client with normal findings* • Repeat the assessment in 15 minutes.
	Abnormal findings • Heavy flow (saturation of one or more perineal pads) in 15 minutes or less, which indicates excessive bleeding and possible uterine atony • A steady trickle of bleeding in a client with a well-contracted uterus, which may indicate cervical, vaginal, or perineal laceration	*For a client with abnormal assessment findings* • Evaluate for uterine atony. • Massage the fundus. • Notify the physician or nurse-midwife, who may need to evaluate the client's condition further.
Perineum Inspection. Remove the perineal pad, position the legs so that the perineum can be observed, and use an adequate light source, such as a flashlight. Alternatively, position the client in the left or right lateral position with the upper leg flexed. Raise the upper buttock slightly to observe the perineum. Ask the client to contract and relax the perineal muscles to assess muscle function. Place a clean pad on the perineum and help the client into a comfortable position.	*Normal findings* • Intact perineum, possibly with slight edema (depending on the duration of the second stage of labor), and painless contraction of perineal muscles (if no episiotomy was performed) • Incision with approximated edges (straight edges meeting without separations), minimal swelling, no discoloration or bleeding from the incision, no discomfort on contraction of perineal muscles, and possible burning sensation in the incision area when voiding (if episiotomy was performed)	*For a client with normal findings* • Maintain cleanliness and comfort if the perineum is intact. • Assess the perineum every 15 minutes in a client with an episiotomy. Place an ice pack on the perineum to increase comfort and decrease edema. Initiate perineal care after assessing the area.
	Abnormal findings • Swelling and discoloration, which may indicate hematoma development • Bleeding, which may indicate unligated blood vessels • Dehiscence (separation of the suture line)	*For a client with abnormal findings* • Report edema, discoloration, or dehiscence immediately to the physician or nurse-midwife. • If signs of hematoma exist, monitor for signs of impending shock, such as restlessness and changes in respirations, pulse, and blood pressure.
Leg pain and tremors Dorsiflexion of the foot. Support the client's thigh with one hand and her foot with the other. Then bend her leg slightly at the knee, and firmly and abruptly dorsiflex the foot.	*Normal findings* • No discomfort in the calf or popliteal space • No ankle clonus	*For a client with normal findings* • Encourage client activity • Repeat this assessment with other assessments every 15 minutes.
	Abnormal findings • Pain in the calf or popliteal space, which may result from a thrombus • Ankle clonus, which may result from PIH	*For a client with abnormal findings* • Report findings to the physician or nurse-midwife. • Obtain elastic stockings and advise the client to wear them as prescribed. • Instruct the client not to massage her legs. • Monitor for signs of embolism, such as shortness of breath, rapid drop in blood pressure, elevated heart rate, ashen coloring, and sweating.

dulled by continuous pressure from the fetal head and by a local anesthetic, which may be injected before the episiotomy. When fetal head pressure is released and normal circulation resumes in the area, the perineum can become extremely tender.

If the client also incurred minor sublabial tears that required no surgical repair, she may experience a burning sensation during voiding, when acidic urine passes over open wounds. Fear of this burning may cause her to postpone voiding, leading to urine retention, bladder distention, and uterine displacement and atony.

Dull aching or burning constitute normal episiotomy pain. Pain that throbs, increases, or does not respond to comfort measures may indicate an abnormality, such as perineal, vulvar, or vaginal hematoma.

A hematoma can form when blood seeps into the tissue because open blood vessels are not closed adequately during episiotomy repair. Characteristically, it swells gradually and reddens or becomes purple. Symptoms may include increasing and throbbing perineal pain, tachycardia, restlessness, and, in severe cases, hypotension.

Cervical and vaginal hematomas pose potential problems during the fourth stage. They produce various discomforts, from a vague inability to achieve comfort to a throbbing sensation in the vagina that cannot be relieved by comfort measures. A hematoma may not be readily apparent on perineal inspection.

Other discomforts. During the fourth stage, the client may experience other discomforts related to second-stage occurrences, such as the exertion and method of pushing, use of regional anesthesia, or positioning during delivery.

The client may experience a dull ache in the sacral area caused by pressure from the fetus's head. If she pushed for an extended time, she may experience discomfort in her abdomen, arms (from holding her legs or a side rail), or upper shoulders and ribs (from curling up and bearing down). If she pushed from her upper chest while contracting her face and neck muscles, she may experience aching behind her eyes and a red or blotchy facial discoloration.

A client who maintained an extended lithotomy position or braced herself with her legs may experience constant leg pain or aches. This pain must be differentiated from that caused by a thrombus or hypertension through assessment for Homan's sign (sharp calf pain with dorsiflexion of the foot), which is not found with muscular aches.

Recovery from anesthesia and analgesia. If the client received an anesthestic or other medications during labor and delivery, evaluate her recovery with each assessment during the fourth stage. As the effects of the drugs begin to dissipate, evaluate the client's condition and response to pain. As numbness from regional or local anesthesia diminishes, she may experience sudden and intense pain in the perineum and at the episiotomy site. Assess the character, intensity, and location of pain, and monitor response to measures such as repositioning and applying ice. These assessments will help distinguish between normal discomfort and pain that signals a problem.

If the client had continuous regional anesthesia, assess the return of motor function to her legs. During each postpartal assessment, note the color and temperature of her legs and toes and her ability to move them.

When the physician or nurse-midwife removes the epidural catheter after discontinuing regional anesthesia, observe and document catheter removal.

If regional anesthesia was employed, observe the lumbar-area puncture site for drainage or bleeding.

If spinal anesthesia was administered, instruct the client to remain supine until motor function returns.

Fatigue, hunger, and thirst. Depending on the duration of labor and the second stage, the client may experience extreme fatigue or exhaustion immediately after delivery. Shaking or tremors may indicate muscle exhaustion or PIH. To differentiate normal postpartal tremors from those caused by PIH, evaluate the client's blood pressure, assess for ankle clonus by dorsiflexing the foot, and assess deep tendon reflexes.

After the neonate is born, the client may feel extremely hungry and thirsty, especially if she was restricted to ice chips or clear fluids during labor and if her labor was long. Keep in mind that labor and delivery consume a great amount of energy and, when preceded by a period of restricted food and fluid intake, may leave a client with a caloric and fluid deficit. Assess nutritional status by testing the first urine with a reagent strip to identify ketones, a sign of fat metabolism caused by insufficient available carbohydrates.

If the client's labor was uncomplicated, honor her requests for food and fluids after delivery. Begin by administering sips of water or clear soda to assess for normal swallowing and for nausea.

Response to birth. Assess the parents' response to the neonate's birth at least once during the fourth stage of labor. Sensitive postpartal assessment of family interaction can provide valuable information that predicts future family interactions.

Bear in mind that responses to birth vary greatly, ranging from joy to relief and from pleasure to withdrawal. Childbirth is a profound physical and emotional experience. Parents may need to reconcile the pain of labor and delivery with the happiness that a child can bring.

The parents' first response to the neonate may be colored by their expectations for a perfect child, experience of pregnancy, culture, the consistency of the actual birth with expectations about it, and the child's normalcy.

Their response to the labor and birth may vary according to their culture, family expectations (including sex and appearance of the neonate), past birth experiences, and overall perspective (Avant, 1988; Choi, 1986; Mercer, 1981; Wadd, 1983; Lee, 1982).

Observe the new family as they experience one another. If they rely on another member, such as a grandmother or aunt, as the primary caregiver, include that member in the bonding experience.

Mother's response. Rubin (1963) describes the progress a mother makes in touching her child. She begins by touching the neonate with her fingertips and proceeds to use her entire hand. The en face position (in which the neonate's face turns toward the mother and they look directly at each other) indicates positive bonding.

The mother may want to count the neonate's fingers and toes to assure herself of her child's normalcy. She may express concern about the neonate's color, breathing, crying, or lack of crying. These concerns reflect the mother's attempt to establish her child's reality and health.

Father's response. Greenberg and Morris (1976) describe the relationship of a father's early contact with his child to his subsequent involvement with the child. The term "engrossment" defines positive bonding between father and child, characterized by tactile, visual, and verbal activities by the father that are directed to the neonate. Touching the neonate's skin, looking closely at the neonate, and expressing feelings of elation all indicate the father's engrossment.

Nursing diagnosis

Carefully review assessment findings and use them to develop appropriate nursing diagnoses. (For a list of possible nursing diagnoses, see *Nursing diagnoses: Third and fourth stages of labor*.)

Planning and implementation

Although the fourth stage of labor is brief and focuses on assessment, planning is necessary and may occur during assessment. During this stage, interventions may include maintaining appropriate maternal positioning and activity, preventing hemorrhage, maintaining hygiene and comfort, maintaining fluid balance, meeting nutritional needs, and promoting bonding.

NURSING DIAGNOSES

Third and fourth stages of labor

The following nursing diagnoses address representative problems and etiologies that a nurse may encounter when caring for a client during the third and fourth stages of labor. Specific nursing interventions for many of these diagnoses are provided in the "Planning and implementation" sections of this chapter.

THIRD STAGE OF LABOR

- Altered tissue perfusion related to sudden change in pelvic or abdominal blood volume
- Decreased cardiac output related to postpartal hemorrhage
- Family coping: potential for growth, related to neonate's birth
- Ineffective breathing pattern related to excess secretions in the neonate
- Ineffective individual coping related to the birth experience
- Impaired gas exchange related to excess secretions in the neonate
- Pain related to perineal trauma
- Potential altered body temperature related to evaporation of perspiration and muscle fatigue
- Potential for injury related to maternal repositioning
- Potential for injury related to neonatal birth trauma

FOURTH STAGE OF LABOR

- Altered nutrition: less than body requirements, related to food restriction and energy expenditure during labor and delivery
- Altered parenting related to unmet expectations about childbirth
- Altered parenting related to unmet expectations about the neonate's capabilities
- Decreased cardiac output related to postpartal hemorrhage
- Fluid volume deficit related to fluid loss from perspiration during labor and delivery
- Fluid volume deficit related to fluid restriction during labor and delivery
- Pain related to difficult labor and delivery
- Pain related to episiotomy
- Pain related to maternal positioning
- Pain related to severe uterine contractions
- Potential for infection related to perineal trauma
- Potential for infection related to perineal laceration
- Potential for infection related to episiotomy

Maintain appropriate maternal positioning and activity

To prevent a nursing diagnosis of *pain related to maternal positioning*, position the client for maximum comfort during her recovery. Adjust her position based on such considerations as the need to prevent postspinal anesthesia headache.

For fundal and perineal assessments, help the client into the supine position. Between assessments, suggest that she assume a semi-Fowler's, high Fowler's, or lateral position, which may be more comfortable and give her a better position from which to view or breast-feed the neonate.

The events of labor and delivery determine the client's activity during the fourth stage. If she experienced an uncomplicated labor and delivery, received little or no analgesia, delivered the neonate with her perineum intact, or delivered with a local anesthetic agent for an episiotomy, she may be able to walk and may appreciate the opportunity.

Before helping the client out of bed for the first time, check her blood pressure. Some clients experience orthostatic hypotension after delivery and may require assistance. For this reason, help her rise slowly to prevent dizziness and weakness, and accompany her on her first walk to prevent a fall.

Expect a client who experienced a long or difficult labor and delivery, received a regional anesthetic, or was heavily medicated during or after delivery to remain in bed and be less active.

Advise a client who experienced postpartal hemorrhage to remain in bed until she stabilizes completely, which may take hours. Take special care to assist her when she first rises from bed.

Prevent hemorrhage

To help prevent a nursing diagnosis of *decreased cardiac output related to postpartal hemorrhage,* monitor the client closely and take measures to prevent uterine atony and hemorrhage. Massage her uterus gently during each assessment, and teach her to do so at regular intervals. If the fundus is boggy, continue massaging until it becomes firm and all clots are expressed.

To prevent uterine atony, administer oxytocin, as prescribed. (For more information, see *Selected major drugs: Fourth stage of labor.*) Encourage breast-feeding, which helps contract the uterus by stimulating the release of endogenous oxytocin.

Encourage voiding to prevent bladder distention, which displaces the uterus and can cause atony. Depending on the client's condition, use the following interventions to prevent bladder distention—and postpartal hemorrhage.
• Provide a bedpan.
• Help the client walk to a bathroom.
• Apply warm water over the perineum to encourage muscle relaxation.
• Use the sound of running water as a psychic stimulant.

• Catheterize the client, if prescribed.
• Encourage fluid intake.

Maintain hygiene and comfort

The client may have a nursing diagnosis of *pain related to severe uterine contractions, pain related to episiotomy, pain related to difficult labor and delivery,* or *potential for infection related to perineal trauma.* For such a client, take measures that increase comfort and promote hygiene, which not only help prevent infection but also enhance comfort. Use the following general interventions to maintain client comfort and hygiene.
• Remove collected secretions, such as lochia and perspiration.
• Teach the client self-care activities that ensure continued cleanliness.
• Provide clean, warm clothing and blankets.
• Change perineal pads and underpads after each assessment or more frequently, if appropriate.
• Clean the perineum at least once during the fourth stage with warm, clear water.
• Teach the client perineal care techniques, including wiping from front to back after urinating or defecating and rinsing the perineal area regularly with warm, clear water.

Uterine contractions. To help relieve discomfort caused by uterine contractions, use the following interventions.
• Administer analgesic agents, as prescribed.
• Reduce the rate of continuous oxytocin infusion, as prescribed.
• Teach abdominal effleurage (light, fingertip massage over the abdomen) to ease the pain of contractions.
• Place a pillow over the client's lower abdomen and help her assume a prone position, if her condition allows. The uterus should contract strongly several times and the pain should subside for a while. When the pain subsides, help the client assume a comfortable position.
• Offer a modified bed bath to remove perspiration and relax sore muscles.
• Offer a back and neck massage to relieve tension and stiffness caused by labor, pushing, or positioning.

Episiotomy, laceration repair, or hematoma. Use the following interventions to help relieve perineal pain.
• Apply an ice pack to the area.
• Apply witch hazel compresses to the area.
• Encourage the client to contract and relax the perineal muscles (Kegal exercises).
• Administer analgesic agents, as prescribed.

Tremors. The following interventions may help relieve discomfort caused by tremors, such as those from chills (unrelated to PIH).

SELECTED MAJOR DRUGS

Fourth stage of labor

This chart summarizes the drugs commonly used during the fourth stage of labor.

DRUG	MAJOR INDICATIONS	USUAL ADULT DOSAGES	NURSING IMPLICATIONS
oxytocin (Pitocin)	Ineffective uterine contractions after delivery of the placenta; heavy amount of lochia	1 to 4 ml (10 to 40 units) in 1,000 ml D_5W or normal saline solution I.V., infused at a rate to control bleeding, usually 20 to 40 milliunits/minute; many clinicians follow with ergonovine maleate or methylergonovine maleate I.M.	• Administer drug I.M. or by I.V. infusion, never by bolus injection. If possible, use an infusion pump or a drip regulator to ensure accurate delivery. • Monitor the client's heart rate, central nervous system (CNS) status, blood pressure, uterine contractions, and blood loss every 15 minutes. • Watch for signs of hypersensitivity, such as blood pressure elevation. In a client who had a long labor accompanied by infusion of oxytocin and large volumes of parenteral fluid, watch for signs of water intoxication, such as edema; oxytocin has an antidiuretic effect. • Use appropriate comfort measures to control pain caused by uterine contractions.
ergonovine maleate (Ergotrate) and methylergonovine maleate (Methergine)	Prevent or control postpartal hemorrhage	For both drugs, 0.2 mg I.M. every 2 to 4 hours to a maximum of five doses.	• Be aware that these drugs may be given if oxytocin does not control postpartal bleeding. • Assess the client's vital signs (especially blood pressure) before administration. • Do not administer this drug before delivery of the neonate because it can cause tetanic contractions. • Do not administer this drug if the client has received epinephrine because the vasoconstrictive effects of both drugs will be cumulative. • Watch for adverse reactions, which may include severe hypertension and signs of cerebral hemorrhage (such as loss of consciousness), myocardial infarction (such as chest pain), and retinal detachment (such as blurred vision). • Monitor the client's blood pressure, pulse rate, uterine contractions, and vaginal bleeding. Report sudden changes in vital signs, frequent periods of uterine relaxation, and any change in lochia character or amount. • Use appropriate comfort measures to control pain caused by uterine contractions.
acetaminophen (Tylenol)	Relief of mild to moderate pain caused by episiotomy or uterine contractions	325 to 650 mg P.O. every 3 to 4 hours as needed	• Assess the client's need for analgesia. Her discomfort may increase with oxytocin administration and development of vaginal or perineal hematoma. • Monitor the client's response to the drug; hypersensitivity (very rare) may cause general malaise, rash, and sweating. *(continued)*

SELECTED MAJOR DRUGS

Fourth stage of labor continued

DRUG	MAJOR INDICATIONS	USUAL ADULT DOSAGES	NURSING IMPLICATIONS
meperidine hydro-chloride (Demerol)	Relief of moderate to severe pain caused by uterine contractions	25 to 100 mg I.M., depending on the client's weight and degree of pain	• Drug should be used only for short-term management of pain. • Assess the client's need for analgesia. Evaluate the drug's appropriateness in relation to the client's vital signs, history of drug sensitivity, and degree of discomfort. • Obtain the client's baseline blood pressure and pulse and respiratory rates before administering this drug. Assess vital signs regularly to determine the client's response to the drug. • Observe for adverse reactions, such as dry mouth, dizziness, and respiratory depression. • Keep naloxone hydrochloride (Narcan) readily available to reverse respiratory depression.
promethazine hy-drochloride (Phenergan)	Adjunct to narcotic administration to sedate client and control nausea related to narcotic administration	12.5 to 25 mg P.O., I.M., or rectally every 4 to 6 hours	• Use with caution in a client with hypersensitivity to this drug or with CNS depression. • Assess the client's need for analgesia and nausea control. Evaluate the drug's appropriateness in relation to the client's vital signs, history of drug sensitivity, and degree of discomfort. • Monitor the client's vital signs and CNS status regularly. • Observe for adverse effects, such as transient hypotension, drowsiness, tinnitus, nervousness, hysteria, blurred vision, seizures, and abnormal movement. • Advise the client to rise slowly, and assist with ambulation.

• Wrap warm blankets around the client's feet or head.
• Provide warm oral fluids if the client's condition warrants.
• Adjust the room temperature.

Maintain fluid balance and meet nutritional needs

During the fourth stage of labor, nursing diagnoses may include *fluid volume deficit related to fluid restriction during labor and delivery, fluid volume deficit related to fluid loss from perspiration during labor and delivery,* or *altered nutrition: less than body requirements, related to food restriction and energy expenditure during labor and delivery.* If the client has one of these nursing diagnoses, employ the following interventions.
• Monitor temperature, pulse rate, and blood pressure and compare them to baseline measurements to estimate the extent of the deficit.
• Provide oral fluids.
• Regulate I.V. fluids as directed by the physician or nurse-midwife.

• Provide nourishment according to the client's preference, if not contraindicated by complications. Assess the appropriateness of her food choices and recommend easily digestible alternatives, if necessary.

Promote bonding

According to Rubin (1984) and other experts, the postpartal client experiences at least 1 hour of heightened awareness and sensitivity to her surroundings, especially to the neonate, unless she received depressant medications. Bonding commonly begins at this time, unless the client is distracted by pain or her environment.

Once the neonate is stabilized, the client may become increasingly concerned about herself. She may wonder why she still looks pregnant, why uterine contractions continue, and why she feels perineal discomfort. These personal concerns may delay bonding.

Rubin (1984) describes the first 1 or 2 days after childbirth as a time of "taking in," when the client exhibits dependent behavior and requires some "mothering" herself. Her needs relate to comfort, nutrition, and sleep, and she may focus on one or all of these during the first hour after delivery.

Nursing interventions can help prevent a nursing diagnosis of *altered parenting related to unmet expectations about childbirth* or *altered parenting related to unmet expectations about the neonate's capabilities.*

Paukert (1982) suggests the following ways to promote family involvement and parent-infant bonding:
• immediate, continuous mother-infant contact
• anticipatory guidance regarding the neonate's needs and abilities
• establishment of an emotionally warm and sensitive environment.

Bonding typically begins during pregnancy as the client relates to the reality of the fetus. Bonding intensifies for both parents when they first see their infant. Typically, the neonate is quiet and alert during the first hour after delivery, and the mother experiences a surge of energy and heightened sensitivity at this time. Afterwards, the neonate and mother may sleep or rest.

Some child development experts place great importance on initial bonding and its role on the future of the parent-neonate relationship (Klause and Kennell, 1982). However, if the immediate postpartal situation does not permit extended contact, assist the family when bonding becomes practical.

Consider the family structure when assisting with bonding. If the client is an adolescent, for example, encourage her mother or other primary caregiver to become involved during bonding.

Immediately after delivery, try promoting mother-infant bonding by encouraging the breast-feeding client to hold the neonate to her breast. During breast-feeding, the mother and infant face each other, have skin-to-skin contact, and interact as the mother responds to the feel, smell, and movement of her infant.

Help the client breast-feed as long as the neonate desires because breast-feeding positively influences bonding, and unrestricted breast-feeding does not cause or increase nipple discomfort (Carvalho, Robertson, and Klaus, 1984). Also, colostrum (yellow fluid secreted by the mammary glands during pregnancy and after childbirth until milk is produced) transmits immunoglobulins, fat-soluble vitamins, calories, and fluid to the neonate. (For more information, see *Nursing research applied: Adequacy of postpartal milk supply.*)

NURSING RESEARCH APPLIED

Adequacy of postpartal milk supply

Mothers continue to cite insufficient milk supply as a major factor in early termination of breast-feeding. To investigate this common problem, Hill and Humenick researched factors that may contribute to a mother's failure to establish a sufficient milk supply. From their research, they developed a model for nursing care during the third and fourth stages of labor.

According to this model, direct and indirect factors may determine adequacy of milk supply. Nursing care can influence several of these factors. Direct factors that affect milk supply and can be influenced during the third and fourth stages of labor include time of first suckling, duration of breast-feeding sessions, neonatal response to suckling, and maternal attitude toward and knowledge of breast-feeding. Indirect factors that can be influenced during these stages include maternal time restraints, comfort, education, and neonatal status and behavior.

Developing an adequate milk supply is key to successful lactation. Prolactin (the hormone responsible for stimulating milk production) is produced in the anterior pituitary gland. During pregnancy, the placental hormone human placental lactogen (hPL) inhibits breast alveoli from producing milk. Immediately after placental delivery, however, hPL diminishes and prolactin can rise almost immediately.

Prolactin production increases when suckling stimulates nerve endings in the nipple. Therefore, the neonate should suckle as soon as possible after birth, preferably within the first hour. Studies show that early and frequent suckling periods stimulate milk production hours sooner than delayed or rigidly scheduled first suckling.

Application to practice
Based on this research, the nurse should assess the client's knowledge of milk production, understanding of early prolactin stimulation, and comfort with and attitude toward breast-feeding. Then the nurse can develop nursing diagnoses and interventions that increase the likelihood of adequate milk production and successful breast-feeding. The following nursing interventions may help prevent insufficient milk supply and early discontinuation of breast-feeding.
• Assess the client's level of knowledge about the importance of initiating breast-feeding during the first 30 minutes after the neonate's birth. Provide information where necessary.
• Position the client in a lateral recumbent or high Fowler's position, with pillow support on the side cradling the neonate's head. If the client wishes to breast-feed on the delivery table or in the delivery position, help her find a position that is comfortable for her and supports the neonate at her breast.
• Encourage the client to continue each breast-feeding session as long as she is comfortable and the neonate appears interested. The more nipple nerve endings are stimulated, the more the prolactin level rises. Brief exposure to suckling, rather than unrestricted suckling, increases nipple trauma. Therefore, encourage the client to gauge the length of each feeding by the neonate's response; when no longer hungry, the neonate will hold the nipple without suckling or will fall asleep.

Hill, P., and Humenick, S. (1989). Insufficient milk supply. *Image: The Journal of Nursing Scholarship, 21*(3), 145-148.

Client with decreased cardiac output related to postpartal hemorrhage

The nursing process helps ensure high-quality care for a client in the third and fourth stages of labor. The table below shows how the nurse might use the nursing process when caring for the client described in the case history at right. The first column presents history and physical assessment data followed by a paragraph of mental notes. These notes help the nurse make important mental connections among assessment findings, aiding in development of the nursing diagnosis and planning.

The second column lists an appropriate nursing diagnosis; information in the remaining columns is based on this diagnosis. Although not part of the nursing process, a rationale appears for each intervention in the fourth column to explain how it contributes to the care plan.

ASSESSMENT	NURSING DIAGNOSIS	PLANNING
Subjective (history) data • Client says to husband, "She has your eyes and my mother's nose, doesn't she?" • Client states, "I'm so hungry, I feel like I haven't eaten in days!" • Client reports, "My bottom stings." **Objective (physical) data** *During labor and delivery:* • Primiparous client. • 16-hour labor. • Vital signs during labor: T 98° F., P 96, R 20, BP 120/60. • Vaginal delivery of large for gestational age (LGA) neonate. • Median episiotomy performed. • Blood loss during delivery 500 ml. • 10 units Pitocin infusing in 600 ml of I.V. fluid. *Currently:* • Vital signs: T 98.2° F., P 88, R 18, BP 120/66. • I.V. solution (labeled to contain 10 units Pitocin) infusing at a rate of 125 ml/hour. • Fundus slightly boggy, located 1 fingerbreadth above umbilicus. • Perineal suture line approximated (straight edges meeting without separations) and intact. • Lochia moderate. • Client holds neonate close to body, exploring her with her fingertips. **Mental notes** *Jennifer is a healthy primiparous client with a long but uncomplicated labor and delivery. LGA delivery, however, is a risk factor for postpartal hemorrhage, and her uterus is slightly boggy. Assessments should focus on other signs of postpartal hemorrhage, and interventions should help prevent it.*	Potential for decreased cardiac output related to postpartal hemorrhage	**Goals** Within 1 hour after delivery, the client will: • have stable vital signs • demonstrate fundal massage • report signs and symptoms of postpartal hemorrhage. The client's husband will: • actively assist her with fundal massage and support.

Evaluation

At the end of the fourth stage of labor, evaluate the effectiveness of nursing care while making a final assessment of the client's stability. The following examples illustrate some appropriate evaluation statements.
• The client's fundus is firm and located 1 cm below the umbilicus.
• The client's perineum is intact.
• The father and other family members held the neonate.
• The neonate opened both eyes fully and responded to the parents' voices.

• The client used effleurage to reduce postpartal discomfort.
• The client began breast-feeding her neonate.

After the fourth stage of labor, a facility with birth areas or units may transfer the client from the birthing room to a room with an adjacent nursery where the neonate will be placed. A more traditional facility may transfer the neonate to a central nursery and move the client to a postpartal room. Finally, if the family wishes to go home, the client and neonate may be discharged a few hours after birth.

CASE STUDY

Jennifer Dalton, a primiparous client age 25, has just given birth to a 9-lb, 2-oz girl after 16 hours of labor. She received a local anesthetic agent for pain control during a median episiotomy. She also received an I.V. infusion of lactated Ringer's solution throughout labor. After delivery of the placenta, 10 units of oxytocin (Pitocin) were added to the remaining 600 ml of solution. Jennifer's husband, Jim, coached her throughout labor and delivery and accompanies her now.

IMPLEMENTATION		EVALUATION
Intervention	**Rationale**	Upon evaluation, the client:
Conduct a complete postpartal assessment every 15 minutes, paying close attention to fundal location and firmness, lochia amount, vital signs, leg pain, and tremors.	During the first hour after delivery, the sudden change in hemodynamics may lead to postpartal hemorrhage, producing restlessness, lightheadedness, heavy lochia, and a boggy uterus. The risk of hemorrhage is greater with a long labor and large neonate because they can reduce uterine muscle contractility.	• had stable vital signs • had moderate lochia • demonstrated fundal massage • repeated the signs and symptoms of postpartal hemorrhage and agreed to report them to a staff member.
Monitor the I.V. infusion.	The I.V. infusion provides fluids and an oxytocic agent to promote uterine contractions. The rate should be maintained or increased in relation to uterine firmness, as prescribed. If the uterus does not respond to the drug, additional medication may be needed.	
Provide oral fluids, as desired.	After delivery, a client may experience thirst because of fluid loss during labor through diaphoresis and fluid restrictions.	
Teach the client and her husband how to massage the fundus. Also explain how breast-feeding helps firm the uterus.	The client must be able to locate the fundus and identify its normal firmness. Massage may be the first and best way to stimulate contractions. An understanding of the relationship between nipple stimulation, oxytocin release, and uterine contractions provides a mechanism for maintaining physiologic stability in the breast-feeding client.	
Teach the client to recognize the signs and symptoms of postpartal hemorrhage.	The client's awareness of signs and symptoms allow her to report potential problems to the nurse immediately.	

Before the transfer occurs, assess the client's ability to leave the delivery area via stretcher or wheelchair and the neonate's stability for transfer in the client's arms or by nursery personnel. Also check the client's and neonate's name bracelets before they are moved. A client who is drowsy from medication should not carry her neonate and may need to be transferred via stretcher with the side rails up.

Documentation

As part of the nursing plan of care, document all nursing care provided as well as the client's response to the care. In addition to a verbal report, a written record will help the postpartal nurse meet the client's individual needs. (For a case study that shows how to apply the nursing process when caring for a client in the fourth stage of labor, see *Applying the nursing process: Client with decreased cardiac output related to postpartal hemorrhage*.)

Although each health care facility may require documentation of slightly different information, most require the nurse to record the following information:
• client's vital signs
• location and consistency of the uterus
• amount and quality of lochia
• condition of perineum
• presence or absence of ankle clonus and calf pain upon dorsiflexion of the client's foot
• parents' response to the neonate's birth
• client discomfort
• reports of fatigue, hunger, or thirst
• urinary status (whether patient has voided)
• drugs, fluids, and food given to the client.

Chapter summary

Chapter 29 described the third and fourth stages of labor. Although relatively brief, these stages are critical periods of physical and psychological adjustment. Nursing care during this time is based on an understanding of the physiologic responses to birth and a complete assessment of the beginning of involution. Nursing interventions are directed toward recognizing deviations that place the client at risk, maintaining comfort and hygiene, and promoting bonding. Here are the chapter highlights.
• The third stage of labor begins with delivery of the neonate and ends with delivery of the placenta. The fourth stage of labor begins after delivery of the placenta and lasts for about 1 hour.
• During the third stage of labor, the nurse assesses maternal vital signs, which may indicate postpartal hemorrhage or other complications; the placenta for intactness, number of blood vessels, and presence of variations; the perineum, which may have been altered by an episiotomy or lacerations; and the fundus, which may indicate uterine atony or postpartal hemorrhage.
• The nurse also assesses the neonate during the third stage of labor, focusing on respiratory, cardiovascular, and temperature status.
• Nursing interventions during the third stage of labor focus on maternal hygiene, repositioning, and possible transfer to the recovery area; neonatal warmth and identification; and bonding for the new family.
• Involution (return to the prepregnant state) begins in the fourth stage of labor. Physiologic changes occur in

the respiratory, cardiovascular, renal, gastrointestinal, and musculoskeletal systems and within the uterus and perineum.
• Assessment during the fourth stage of labor begins with a review of data obtained during previous stages. The nurse performs a physical assessment every 15 minutes, evaluating vital signs, fundus, lochia, perineum, leg pain, and tremors. The nurse also assesses the client's discomfort; recovery from analgesia and anesthesia; fatigue, hunger, and thirst; and response to the neonate.
• Nursing interventions during the fourth stage focus on preventing uterine atony and postpartal hemorrhage through fundal massage, oxytocin administration, initiation of breast-feeding, and prevention of bladder distention.
• If postpartal hemorrhage occurs, nursing interventions include immediately notifying the physician or nurse-midwife, performing continuous fundal massage, increasing oxytocin administration, elevating the client's legs, and administering oxygen.
• The nurse can promote bonding by encouraging the parents to hold the neonate and helping the client breast-feed.
• Other interventions during the fourth stage include maintaining appropriate positioning, activity, hygiene, comfort, fluid balance, and nutrition.
• The nurse must evaluate and document all assessments and care before the client and neonate are prepared for discharge or transferred to another area for continuing care.

Study questions

1. Mrs. Ellen Pendergrast, a primiparous client age 32, has delivered an 8-pound, 2-ounce neonate without complications. What are the immediate priorities in assessing and caring for the neonate?

2. Which findings indicate that Mrs. Pendergrast's placenta has separated? How should the nurse assess the placenta?

3. Mrs. Rosa Palermo, a healthy, multiparous client age 26, had an uncomplicated delivery. How frequently should the nurse assess her during the fourth stage of labor? Which parameters should the nurse assess?

4. Mrs. Palermo has saturated a perineal pad completely in 15 minutes. What could this indicate? How should the nurse intervene?

5. Which nursing interventions can help Mr. and Mrs. Palermo bond with their infant?

Bibliography

Avery, M., Fournier, L.C., and Jones, P.L. (1982). An early postpartum hospital discharge program: Implementation and evaluation. *JOGNN*, 11(4), 233-235.

Cunningham, F.G., MacDonald, P., and Gant, N.F. (1989). *Williams obstetrics* (18th ed.). East Norwalk, CT: Appleton & Lange.

Hangsleben, K. (1983). Transition to fatherhood: An exploratory study. *JOGNN*, 12(4), 264-270.

Leff, E. (1986). Ethics and patient teaching. *MCN*, 11(6), 375-378.

NAACOG. (1986). *Standards for obstetric, gynecologic, and neonatal nursing* (3rd ed.). Washington, DC: Author

Newton, N., Newton, M., and Broach, J. (1988). Psychologic, physical, nutritional, and technologic aspects of intravenous infusion during labor. *Birth*, 15(2), 67-72.

Varney, H. (1987). *Nurse-midwifery* (2nd ed.). St. Louis: Mosby.

Watson, J., Rowe, P., Hansen, J., and Shipes, E. (1987). A time-saving guide to better patient teaching. *Nursing87*, 17(11), 129-136.

Bonding

Anderson, G. (1977). The mother and her newborn: Mutual caregivers. *JOGNN*, 6(5), 50-57.

Avant, K. (1981) Anxiety as a potential factor affecting maternal attachment. *JOGNN*, 10(6), 416-419.

Brodish, M. (1982). Relationship of early bonding to initial infant feeding patterns in bottle-fed newborns. *JOGNN*, 11(4), 248-252.

Gay, J. (1981). A conceptual framework of bonding. *JOGNN*, 10(6), 440-444.

Dean, P., Morgan, P., and Towle, J. (1982). Making baby's acquaintance: A unique attachment strategy. *MCN*, 7(1), 37-41.

Greenberg, M., and Morris, N. (1976). Engrossment: The newborn's impact upon the father. *Nursing Digest*, 4(1), 19-22.

Klaus, M., and Kennell, K. (1982). *Parent-infant bonding* (2nd ed.). St. Louis: Mosby.

Paukert, S. (1982). Maternal-infant attachment in a traditional hospital setting. *JOGNN*, 11(1), 23-26.

Reiser, S. (1981). A tool to facilitate mother-infant attachment. *JOGNN*, 10(4), 294-297.

Virden, S. (1988). The relationship between infant feeding method and maternal role adjustment. *Journal of Nurse Midwifery*, 33(1), 31-35.

Physiologic research

Broach, J., and Newton, N. (1988). Food and beverages in labor. Part II: The effects of cessation of oral intake during labor. *Birth*, 15(2), 88-92.

Gabbe, S. (1988). Current practices of intravenous fluid administration may cause more harm than good. *Birth*, 15(2), 73-74.

Homans, D. (1985). Current concepts: Peripartum cardiomyopathy. *The New England Journal of Medicine*, 312(22), 1432-1437.

Maternal adaptation

Avant, K. (1988). Stressors on the childbearing family. *JOGNN*, 17(3), 179-185.

Bampton, B., Jones, J., and Mancini, J. (1981). Initial mothering patterns of low income black primiparas. *JOGNN*, 10(3), 174-178.

Brown, M., and Hurlock, J. (1977). Mothering the mother. *AJN*, 77(3), 438-441.

Carlson, S. (1976). The irreality of postpartum: Observations on the subjective experience. *JOGNN*, 5(5), 28-30.

Gruis, M. (1977). Beyond maternity: Postpartum concerns of mothers. *MCN*, 2(3), 182-188.

Martell, L., and Mitchell, S. (1983). Rubin's "puerperal change" reconsidered. *JOGNN*, 13(3), 145-149.

Mercer, R. (1981). The nurse and maternal tasks of early postpartum. *MCN*, 6(5), 341-345.

Rubin, R. (1984). *Maternal identity and the maternal experience*. New York: Springer Publishing.

Rubin, R. (1963). Maternal touch. *Nursing Outlook*, 11(11), 828-831.

Rubin, R. (1961). Puerperal change. *Nursing Outlook*, 9(12), 753-755.

Nursing process

Aukamp, V. (1984). *Nursing care plans for the childbearing family*. East Norwalk, CT: Appleton & Lange.

Buckley, K., and Kulb, N. (1983). *Handbook of maternal-newborn nursing*. New York: Wiley Medical.

Harr, B., and Hastings, J. (1981). Parturition care planning. *JOGNN*, 10(1), 54-57.

Honan, S., Krsnak, G., Petersen, D., and Torkelson, R. (1988). The nurse as patient educator: Perceived responsibilities and factors enhancing role development. *Journal of Continuing Education in Nursing*, 19(1), 33-37.

Sherwen, L. (1987). MICC: The maternal-infant core competency project: Report of phase I. *Journal of Professional Nursing*, 3(4), 230-241.

Stevens, K. (1988). Nursing diagnoses in wellness childbearing settings. *JOGNN*, 17(5), 329-336.

Taylor, R. (1987). Making the most of your time for patient teaching. *RN*, 50(12), 20-21.

Tepas, K. (1988). Thermoregulation in newborns. March of Dimes Series 1: The first six hours after birth, Module 1. March of Dimes Birth Defect Foundation.

Tribotti, S., Lyons, N., Blackburn, S., Stein, M., and Withers, J. (1988). Nursing diagnoses for the postpartum woman. *JOGNN*, 17(6), 410-416.

Urbano, M., and Jahns I. (1988). A conceptual framework for nurses' participation in continuing education. *Journal of Continuing Education in Nursing*, 19(4), 182-186.

Watters, N. (1985). Combined mother-infant nursing care. *JOGNN*, 14(6), 478-483.

Cultural references

Broach, J., and Newton, N. (1988). Food and beverages in labor. Part I: Cross-cultural and historical practices. *Birth,* 15(2), 81-85.

Choi, E. (1986). Unique aspects of Korean-American mothers. *JOGNN,* 15(5), 394-400.

Newton, N. (1970). Childbirth and culture. *Psychology Today,* 4(6), 74-75.

Thomas, R., and Tumminia, P. (1982). Maternity care for Vietnamese in America. *Birth,* 9(3), 187-190.

Wadd, L. (1983). Vietnamese postpartum practices: Implications for nursing in the hospital setting. *JOGNN,* 12(4), 252-258.

Nursing research

Carvalho, M., Robertson, S., and Klaus, M. (1984). Does the duration and frequency of early breast-feeding affect nipple pain? *Birth,* 11(2), 81.

Hill, P., and Humenick, S. (1989). Insufficient milk supply. *Image: The Journal of Nursing Scholarship,* 21(3), 145-148.

Lee, G. (1982). Relationship of self-concept during late pregnancy to neonatal perception and parenting profile. *JOGNN,* 11(3), 186-190.

Sheehan, F. (1981). Assessing postpartum adjustment: A pilot study. *JOGNN,* 10(1), 19-23.

Taubenheim, A. (1981). Paternal-infant bonding in the first-time father. *JOGNN,* 10(4), 261-264.

Family Support during the Intrapartal Period

Objectives

After reading and studying this chapter, the student should be able to:

1. Discuss the concept of support and its types.
2. Describe the physical and psychological benefits to the client of support from her family and friends.
3. Describe cultural considerations that the nurse caring for a family during the intrapartal period should acknowledge.
4. Discuss the nurse's role in relating to various support persons.
5. Evaluate the helpfulness of each support person during the intrapartal period.
6. Apply the nursing process when caring for a client as well as family members and friends present during labor and delivery.

Introduction

Although childbirth is a stressful experience for the client, her partner, and other family members, steadfast support by the nurse can help ease emotional stress and physical discomfort during this time. The nurse plays a key role by helping the client's primary support person function effectively. The nurse also provides direct support, as needed, to the client and to involved family members.

This chapter describes various types of support and explores how they can benefit the client during labor. It then outlines sources of support that may be important to the client, including her partner, parents, children, other family members, and friends. Following nursing process steps, the chapter also emphasizes assessment of the client's needs and of the primary support person's preparation and ability and suggests ways to ensure adequate support for all family members involved during the intrapartal period.

Support during labor

Support from trusted family members or friends can help an individual gain, regain, and use personal strength during difficult or challenging periods that demand extra energy and resources (Brown, 1986). Labor and childbirth are such a time. In all but one of 150 cultures studied by anthropologists, a family member or friend provides support for a woman in labor (Raphael, 1976).

Several people may be available to assist a client during labor. Her partner, family members, friends, and health care professionals all care about her physical and emotional needs. In addition, nurses, nurse-midwives, and physicians strive to help the family have a positive experience and one that meets each member's wishes and needs. Whatever their cultural, social, economic, or religious background or configuration, most family members who assist the woman in labor will need the nurse's support.

GLOSSARY

Appraisal support: type of support that includes affirmation and feedback.

Birth culture: beliefs, values, and norms held by a cultural or ethnic group about conception, conditions for procreation and childbearing, the mechanism of pregnancy and labor, and the rules of antepartal and postpartal behavior.

Culture: integrated system of learned (not biologically inherited) beliefs, values, and behaviors characteristic of a society's members.

Emotional support: type of support that includes affection, trust, concern, and listening.

Informational support: type of support that includes advice, suggestions, directives, and other information.

Instrumental support: type of support that includes money, time, and other such resources.

Perceived support: belief that help is available if needed.

Received support: activities performed to assist a person.

Support: feelings of affection, trust, and affirmation as well as the sharing of advice, information, and time between people.

Support person: partner, friend, or family member who provides continuous support during labor and delivery.

Client benefits

Clients who have a continuous support person during labor can benefit physically and psychologically. Consider the following research findings:

• Women with a constant companion during labor had shorter labors and significantly fewer obstetric complications than those with no support person (Sosa, Kennell, Klaus, Robertson, and Urrutia, 1980).

• A constant support person tends to reduce feelings of pain and anxiety, use of labor-inducing drugs, and anesthesia (Hunter, Philips, and Rachman, 1979).

• Women supported during the first stage of labor have more positive feelings about the birth experience and exhibit better coping behaviors than those without support (Peddicord, Curran, and Monshower, 1984).

• A support person provides comfort, reassurance, and assistance with such pain control techniques as breathing exercises, imagery, and distraction (Copstick, Taylor, Hayes, and Morris, 1986).

Individual needs

Although labor and childbirth almost always are associated with pain and anxiety, clients vary in the degree of pain they experience, their tolerance for the pain, and the cultural beliefs that affect their response to the pain. A client who experiences more pain during labor usually will need more support than one who experience less pain. Typically, a primiparous client will experience greater pain and anxiety than a multiparous one (Gaston-Johansson, Fridh, and Turner-Norvell, 1988).

In addition to differences in pain severity and tolerance, clients differ in their verbal and nonverbal response to pain and in their ability to cope with it. The nurse who assesses a client's pain tolerance and coping skills can use the information to formulate specific strategies for direct client support and for use by the primary support person and others.

Types of support

To maximize effectiveness, support should be tailored to a client's specific needs and personality. One client may prefer quiet hand-holding, for example; another may prefer active coaching. Thus, support may take various forms, such as those listed below (House, 1981). The nurse should perform ongoing assessment to ensure that support corresponds to the client's needs and expectations as labor progresses.

Perceived support

The client's belief that support is available should she need it may be more important than the actual availability of support (Sarason and Sarason, 1985). She will perceive support if she feels that people care about her feelings and will help her if asked.

Received support

Referring to specific steps taken by one person to support another, received support may include such actions as touching the client in a caring way, communicating information that she needs, and positioning her to maintain comfort. (For more information, see *Nursing research applied: Support during labor.*) Received support may be included in one of four categories (House, 1981):

• Emotional support. Includes affection, trust, concern, and listening.

• Appraisal support. Includes affirmation and feedback.

• Informational support. Includes advice, suggestions, directives, and other information.

• Instrumental support. Includes money, time, and other such resources.

Sources of support

Mutual confidence, trust, and communication must be present for one person to feel that another is supportive. Although many people may be capable of supporting the client during labor, the typical client prefers to have one trusted person concentrate on her needs, communicate them to others, and provide constant support during labor and delivery.

In North America, the client's partner typically provides support during labor. However, members of some families or cultural groups may prefer a female support person or a family member other than the partner. In some Mexican-American families, for example, a female relative or friend is more likely to act as support person. (For more information, see *Cultural considerations: Selection of a support person,* page 730.) However, the nurse should avoid generalizations and stereotypical thinking about ethnic and cultural preferences. Regardless of who the client selects as support person, important considerations include the person's ability to provide support and the client's and family's satisfaction with that support.

The partner's role

The partner's support can be invaluable to a client in labor. In one study, women claimed that their partners provided more practical support and contributed more to feelings of well-being than the professional staff did (Bennett, Hewson, Booker, and Holliday, 1985). The women in this study stated that their partners helped them by timing contractions, coaching breathing, providing a calming influence, reducing loneliness, and providing helpful distractions. Also, the partner may assist the client by communicating her needs to health care professionals.

The partner can show concern for the client's needs by being understanding, tolerant, supportive, cooperative, available, communicative, and reliable (Lederman, 1984). These feelings should be accompanied by physical actions, verbal communication, and nonverbal communication. Examples of physical actions include giving the client ice chips, rubbing her back, and bringing her items she may want. Verbal support could include coaching breathing or other pain-coping techniques and praising her for her progress. Nonverbal support could include holding her hand and stroking her face.

NURSING RESEARCH APPLIED

Support during labor

A study of 78 women identified the helpfulness of various nursing behaviors during labor. Overall, women rated all nursing behaviors as helpful. However, the six most helpful behaviors (in descending order) included coaching, praising the woman's efforts, providing friendly and personal care, accepting her behavior, treating her with respect, and making her feel cared about as an individual. The four least helpful nursing behaviors included supporting the woman when working with her support person, spending time in the room without performing specific tasks, providing for the needs of the support person, and familiarizing the woman with her surroundings.

Application to practice

These findings provide guidelines for the nurse in planning and implementing care. A client in labor needs nursing support that addresses her psychological needs for self-esteem and that respects her as an individual. Tasks aimed at helping the support person and orienting the client to her surroundings, although necessary at times, are less helpful.

Kintz, D. (1987). Nursing support in labor. *JOGNN,* 16(2), 126-130.

One of the most important aspects of the partner's support efforts is the client's perception of them. In some cases, this perception may exaggerate the amount of support actually provided (Nicholson, Gist, Klein, and Standley, 1983). Thus, the nurse can most accurately assess the partner's achievements by examining the client's responses to the partner's behavior.

Touch is also an important aspect of support. A recent study concluded that touch conveyed sensitivity to the client's need for comfort, pain relief, and alleviation of fear and anxiety (Weaver, 1990).

The partner's feelings may greatly affect that person's support of the client. The partner may find labor and delivery progressively more stressful, a feeling that peaks during delivery (Berry, 1988). Expectations on the partner must be realistic and based on the person's ability to cope with personal stress. The nurse should emphasize that health care professionals will be available to help or to assume the primary job if the partner feels overwhelmed.

A first-time support person may feel more anxiety about the role and may need special assistance from the nurse, especially if the person did not attend childbirth education classes. The nurse may have to coach an inexperienced partner in behaviors that will be helpful to the client during labor. An adolescent partner in particular may need appraisal support (support that includes affirmation and feedback) from the nurse,

Selection of a support person

The nurse should be sensitive to cultural preferences of each client. Especially when the client and nurse have different cultural backgrounds, the nurse needs to be aware of the client's values, beliefs, and practices that may influence her view of appropriate nursing care. When providing support during the intrapartal period, the nurse should be aware of the following cultural variations:

Many Mexican-Americans choose a female relative or friend as a support person rather than a male partner. In the Mexican-American culture, the extended family is an important part of childbirth. The whole family of female relatives who have experience in childbirth may play a prominent role in the education and support of the pregnant woman (Hahn and Muecke, 1987).

Choi (1986) describes Korean-American beliefs and attitudes toward pregnancy, birth, and postpartal practices. She found that many Korean mothers in the United States continued Korean cultural practices. A woman of middle age who has had many sons and much experience in delivering children customarily attends the pregnant woman during labor and delivery. Men and childless women are not permitted in the labor and delivery area.

The birth culture of the Hmong (refugees from Laos) includes many beliefs important for the nurse to recognize. For example, many Hmong women believe that hospitals are unsafe birthing environments (Nyce and Hollingshead, 1984). According to La Du (1982), Hmong women resented hospital treatment, disliked being forced into a supine position, and had their modesty affronted by being shown their deliveries in mirrors.

including reassurance that actions are helpful and supportive to the client.

At times, the partner may become so involved in videotaping or photographing labor and delivery as to neglect the client's needs or even agitate her. The nurse should assess the effect of these activities and moderate them as necessary.

Client's or partner's parents

The client's parents (and her partner's parents) usually assume a role different from that of the partner. Typically, they provide more general support and participate for their own pleasure in the birth experience rather than as primary support persons. For older parents, today's childbirth experience may be markedly different from theirs; they may feel apprehension over current practices. For example, in earlier times, greater numbers of pregnant women were sedated during delivery, and

far fewer fathers witnessed or participated in the birth of their child.

Although some childbirth education classes are designed specifically for the client's or partner's parents, many such parents have no preparation for a support role. They may be uncertain about how to help or how to recognize the kinds of support that their children—now adults themselves—will need during labor. The nurse should assess their needs for instruction about events during labor and delivery.

If the client has no support person, a parent (usually the client's mother) may assume this role. The perceived and received support provided by the client's mother will depend on the quality of their relationship before labor and delivery, on the mother's preparation, and on her ability to cope with her daughter's pain.

Family and friends

In some cultures, female relatives and friends provide support for the client during labor. The partner may take a more passive role or, because of cultural norms, may be forbidden to see the client during labor and delivery.

For some families, childbirth represents a culturally recognized event with extended family members in attendance. Although most families gather in a waiting area, some may wish to participate actively. If family participation is not prohibited by facility policy, the nurse should monitor the family's involvement, keep individuals informed of labor progress, and protect the client from unwanted distractions. Avoid making judgments about family preferences or stereotyping a family based on cultural background. Assess and care for each family in appropriate ways.

Some clients, especially primiparous ones, may plan for family members to participate in childbirth but become uncomfortable when the time arrives. In contrast, other clients may plan only for the partner's participation but find added comfort in participation by additional family members. The nurse should monitor these developments, with the goal of meeting the client's needs.

Client's or partner's children

Occasionally, a client and her partner may wish to have their children witness the birth of a sibling. The couple may feel that group participation will promote family unity. The client may desire the support of older children. At times, a child may ask to view the birth of a new brother or sister.

Although many facilities allow children to attend labor and delivery, most require adherence to specific guidelines. Typically, each attending child must have a support person other than the client's support person.

The child's support person explains what is happening, reassures the child, and removes the child from the area if an emergency develops or if the child becomes frightened. If childbirth takes place at home, one support person may be sufficient for several children because they will be in a familiar environment and can come and go more freely.

Little research has investigated how children are affected by participation in childbirth. Young children may be frightened and may not understand what is happening. One nursing study focused on short-term effects on preschool children who attended the birth of a sibling. Results of this study revealed no significant difference in hostile, affectionate, or regressive behaviors 2 months after the birth (Lumley, 1983). The study also found that many parents who had planned to include a child did not and, of those who did, many failed to provide the requisite support person.

Nursing care

To ensure the client receives proper support during the intrapartal period, the nurse provides care for the client and her family. The nursing process serves as a framework for providing flexible, individualized care. (For a case study, see *Applying the nursing process: Client and support person with knowledge deficit related to inadequate preparation for childbirth*, pages 734 and 735.)

Assessment

During labor and delivery, the nurse should administer sensitive and appropriate care based on the particular needs of the client and her family. This requires a twofold effort: applying clinical knowledge to assess labor progress and using personal skills to assess the client's and family's needs during this physically and emotionally stressful time. Ideally, assessment of the client's and family's support needs should start before labor begins and continue throughout. The nurse should assess the plans and preferences of the client and family as well as the specific needs of each individual involved.

Client preferences
Strive to develop a clear sense of the client's preferences and desires for labor and delivery. One client may have definite ideas about which procedures she does and does not want. Another may make few choices concerning labor and delivery procedures, opting instead to accept the advice of her physician or nurse-midwife and nurse as situations develop. Even if the client has no strong preference about some issues, such as anesthesia or birth position, ask her to specify support options and probable family involvement. Determine who will function as the client's main support person during labor and delivery. Ask if she plans to have other family members or friends present.

Even with careful preparation, conflicts between family preferences and facility policy may arise. To avoid distracting and possibly upsetting the client with a conflict during active labor, thoroughly assess needs and preferences as early as possible.

Primary support person's needs
After determining who will function as the client's primary support person, assess this person's needs and concerns. Assessment should focus on the support person's knowledge about how to assist the client during labor and on personal concerns about labor.

Determine if the support person has had any childbirth preparation, including attending childbirth education classes, reading books on childbirth, viewing videos, or accompanying the client on prenatal health care visits. Even if the client is primiparous, ask if the support person has attended other births. If the client has a strong preference for certain comfort promotion or pain management techniques, assess the support person's knowledge of them.

The length and depth of this assessment depends primarily on the client's stage of labor. Early in labor, ample time should be available for assessment. Later in labor and especially if delivery is imminent, assessment must be shortened or abandoned.

As time allows, assess the support person's goals, expectations, and feelings about labor and delivery. The support person may have a strong desire to photograph the process, which could affect attentiveness to the client's needs. The support person may be nervous about seeing blood or coping with the client's pain. Although discussion of every concern will be impossible, investigate the most critical ones. Discussing feelings and fears may help by itself to allay some of the support person's anxieties.

Although the support person's primary job is to assist the client during labor and delivery, the person also will have individual needs. These needs are complicated further when the client's support person is the expectant father. As labor progresses, the expectant father's attention may shift from the client toward him-

self and the neonate (Leonard, 1977). Lemmer (1987) summarized the needs of an expectant father as follows:
- to be knowledgeable about labor and delivery
- to recognize when to go to the health care facility
- to be kept informed of the client's and fetus's status
- to have a sense of control during labor
- to be able to help relieve the client's pain
- to be able to nurture and support the client
- to have behavioral guidelines during childbirth
- to have a physician or nurse-midwife available
- to be reassured about coaching skills
- to be cared for and nurtured
- to experience personalized care.

Needs and expectations of expectant fathers have many implications for the nurse. Although they can provide powerful and effective support during labor, they experience great personal stress. They are excited and anxious about the neonate's well-being and about providing adequate support; they may need interventions from the nurse.

Cultural beliefs

Assess the client's and family's birth culture for any beliefs and practices that could influence labor and delivery. Birth culture refers to a set of beliefs, values, and norms surrounding the birth process and shared to various degrees by members of a cultural or ethnic group (Hahn and Muecke, 1987). It informs members of the group about the nature of conception, the proper conditions for procreation and childbearing, the mechanism of pregnancy and labor, and the rules and rationales of antepartal and postpartal behavior. The birth culture may influence the client's diet, her response to labor, preferred positions for childbirth, activity restrictions, and family members' roles during childbirth.

Nursing diagnosis

After assessing client preferences, individual support needs, and family members' abilities to support each other, the nurse formulates nursing diagnoses based on these findings. The diagnoses may apply to the client, any or all family members, and other support persons, as necessary. (For a partial list of possible nursing diagnoses, see *Nursing diagnoses: Pregnant client and support person.*)

Planning and implementation

Based on assessment findings and nursing diagnoses, the nurse plans and implements nursing care specific to the client in labor and to her family. Providing care during labor and delivery requires expert clinical knowledge, sensitivity to the family's needs, and excellent

---

NURSING DIAGNOSES

Pregnant client and support person

The nurse may find these examples of nursing diagnoses appropriate for the support person, family, and friends of a client in labor. Specific nursing interventions for many of these diagnoses are provided in the "Planning and implementation" section of this chapter.

- Altered family processes related to change in family roles
- Altered family processes related to lack of adequate support systems
- Altered role performance related to unmet expectations for childbirth
- Anxiety related to insecurity about being helpful to the client in labor
- Anxiety related to lack of ability to reduce the client's pain
- Anxiety related to lack of information about labor progress
- Fear related to real or imagined threat to personal well-being
- Knowledge deficit related to inadequate preparation for childbirth
- Self-esteem disturbance related to uncertainty about the effectiveness of support

---

verbal and nonverbal skills. To ensure adequate and appropriate support for the client in labor, the nurse should assist the primary support person and balance client and family needs.

Assist the primary support person

A support person who helps a client through labor needs assistance from the nurse. A support person with a nursing diagnosis of *knowledge deficit related to inadequate preparation for childbirth* will need even more assistance.

Specific nursing interventions include orienting the support person to the environment, briefly explaining equipment and its use, and informing the support person of the location of restrooms, telephones, and food. Explain that help will be available should the support person need to leave the labor area. With the client's permission, ask the support person to perform such tasks as giving ice chips, performing backrubs, or applying cool cloths. In addition to keeping the support person informed of the client's progress, give brief explanations of potentially disturbing developments during labor, such as bloody show, vomiting, or leg tremors. Avoid using ambiguous or highly technical terms, which may be confusing or frightening.

Remain attentive to the support person's feelings and concerns, keeping in mind the emotional difficulty of watching a loved one in pain. Encourage the support person to focus on the positive aspects of labor rather than on the client's discomfort. Reinforce the importance of support. Emphasize that the support person should avoid asking the client questions during contractions when the client should focus her attention and energy on remaining relaxed. The support person may offer reassuring comments during a contraction but should avoid distracting the client. Demonstrate the gentle and competent care that the client should receive from the support person and health care professionals alike.

Balance client and family needs

In addition to the client and her partner, labor also can affect other family members and support persons, possibly resulting in a nursing diagnosis of **anxiety related to lack of information about labor progress.** Although caring for the client and fetus is the nurse's primary goal and overseeing the primary support person is a secondary goal, the nurse also should try to understand and accept the feelings of family members waiting for the neonate's birth.

In most cases, only the partner attends the delivery, while other family and friends wait nearby. Most family members are content to receive regular reports from the nurse or the partner about how labor is progressing. The nurse should remember, however, that waiting is difficult and, during long labors or periods with little word from the nurse or partner, family members and friends may imagine the worst. When appropriate and with the client's permission, allow family members or friends to make brief visits to the labor area for reassurance and to provide support for the client.

In a stressful situation or an emergency, the nurse may need to ask family members and friends to leave the client's room. Do this carefully and with sensitivity to their feelings. Remember that all visitors, including the support person, may not understand what is happening and may be frightened.

At other times, the nurse may sense that certain family members or friends may be distracting or annoying the client. The client may be uncomfortable having visitors witness her conduct or response to labor. Some relatives may become so engrossed in the birth that they fail to notice their effect on the client. Quietly determine if the client feels distracted or uncomfortable, and tactfully ask if she would prefer to have her visitors leave the labor area. Reassure the client that the nurse is her advocate. The client must live with her family after the birth, putting the nurse—who probably will not see them

again—in a better position to take responsibility for these decisions.

If possible, employ the client's family and friends as resources for continued care and support after the client takes her neonate home (Barnard, 1978). The family's influence will far outlast the nurse's contact with the client.

Evaluation

To complete the nursing process, the nurse evaluates the effectiveness of nursing care by reviewing the support provided for the client, the effectiveness of the primary support person, and the appropriateness of involvement by family members and friends. The following examples illustrate appropriate evaluation statements.
• The support person actively influenced the client's breathing pattern during contractions.
• The support person massaged the client's back and applied a cool cloth to her forehead.
• The support person maintained composure despite discomfort with the client's level of pain.
• Family members expressed gratitude for regular reports on the client's progress.

Documentation

The nurse must document assessment findings, support provided, and nursing activities as thoroughly and objectively as possible. Thorough documentation not only allows evaluation of the effectiveness of the nursing care plan, but also makes data available to other members of the health care team, which helps ensure consistent care. To document as accurately as possible, make sure the entries describe events exactly, completely, and in chronological order.

Although each health care facility may require documentation of slightly different information, the following represent examples of appropriate support-related documentation items:
• client preferences for participation by the primary support person and family members
• statements made by the client and partner about their feelings during labor
• instructions given to the support person
• actions taken by the support person, such as applying a cool cloth to the client's forehead
• client reactions to the support person's assistance
• reports made to the client's waiting family members.

APPLYING THE NURSING PROCESS

Client and support person with knowledge deficit related to inadequate preparation for childbirth

The nursing process helps ensure that the intrapartal client and her support person receive the information they need for childbirth. The table below shows how the nurse might use the nursing process when caring for the client described in the case history at right. The first column presents history and physical assessment data followed by a paragraph of mental notes. These notes help the nurse make important mental connections among assessment findings, aiding in development of the nursing diagnosis and planning.

The second column lists an appropriate nursing diagnosis; information in the remaining columns is based on this diagnosis. Although not part of the nursing process, a rationale appears for each intervention in the fourth column to explain how it contributes to the care plan.

ASSESSMENT	NURSING DIAGNOSIS	PLANNING
Subjective (history) data • Client says neither she nor her mother has attended childbirth education classes. • Client states that she fears labor will be long and painful. • Client says that she wants her mother to stay with her during labor. • Client's mother says she knows nothing about changes in childbirth practices since she had Jane. **Objective (physical) data** • Term pregnancy. • Cervical dilation: 2 cm. • Cervical effacement: 80%. • Fetal station: vertex at −2. • Uterine contractions: every 4 minutes, 30 to 45 seconds' duration, mild intensity. **Mental notes** *Jane has no strategies for handling contractions other than by moaning and becoming tense. Her mother wants to be supportive but lacks information. She has tried to prepare Jane for labor as best she can by relating her own painful experience.*	Knowledge deficit related to inadequate preparation for childbirth	**Goals** The client will: • learn about the course of labor • learn to use various breathing and relaxation techniques to control the effects of contractions • learn positions and activities to help her cope with contractions. The client's mother will: • learn methods to support her daughter in labor • demonstrate active participation in supporting her daughter through labor and delivery.

Chapter summary

Chapter 30 presented aspects of personal support helpful to the client, her partner, and involved family members and friends during labor and delivery. Here are the chapter highlights.

• Support given by a loved one has physical and emotional benefits for the client during labor and delivery.

• Each client and family require various types and amounts of support.

• The client's perception that support is available to her (perceived support) may be more helpful to her emotional well-being than acts of support (received support).

CASE STUDY

Jane, a primigravid client age 16 accompanied by her mother, is admitted to the labor and delivery area in early labor. While getting undressed, gowned, and into bed, Jane has several contractions that she reacts to by grabbing the side of the bed and moaning loudly. Her mother responds by saying to Jane, "This is nothing. They are going to get a lot worse. Having a baby is the worst pain in the world." Jane's mother tells the nurse that she had Jane when she was 15 years old and that she labored alone and unmedicated for 16 hours before Jane was born. She says she is just trying to prepare Jane for the worst.

IMPLEMENTATION		EVALUATION
Intervention	**Rationale**	Upon delivery:
Orient the client and mother to the environment and facility policies.	Information about the environment, policies, labor, and the nurse's role will give the client and her mother a sense of control and help decrease fear and anxiety.	• the client and her mother reported pride in their ability to deal with labor and birth
Keep the client and her mother informed of nursing support during labor.	Sustained human contact is the most critical need of the client in labor and her support person.	• the client, her mother, and her neonate appeared healthy and happy.
Stay with the client and her mother for long periods and, when leaving, inform them how to call the nurse and when the nurse will return.	Information about calling the nurse and when the nurse will return contributes to a sense of control.	
Teach the client to use breathing and relaxation techniques appropriate to her current phase of labor.	Breathing and relaxation techniques should help the client relax, reduce pain, and further labor progress.	
Have the client try different positions and remain as active as possible.	Position changes and activities as tolerated divert the client's focus from labor pain and further labor progress.	
Tell the client to let her mother and the nurse know the effectiveness of breathing and relaxation techniques and the benefits of different positions and alternative activities.	Feedback increases the client's sense of control and prevents her support person from feeling helpless during the episodes of pain.	
Suggest supportive activities for the mother, such as giving praise, administering ice chips, using a cool cloth on the client's face, and timing contractions.	Specific tasks of support enhance the support person's well-being and feelings about being helpful to the client.	
Praise the client and mother often.	Praise enhances the sense of control and feelings of well-being for both.	

• Types of support include emotional, appraisal, informational, and instrumental.

• Common sources of support include the client's partner, their parents, other family members, and friends.

• Support from the partner may be more helpful to the client than support from the nurse.

• The client's primary support person also may need support, particularly as delivery approaches.

• Cultural background may significantly influence how a family participates in labor and delivery.

• While providing direct care for the client and fetus, the nurse also must monitor the needs of support persons and intervene to assist them as necessary.

• Regular updates from the nurse will help to allay the fears of family and friends in the waiting area.

Study questions

1. Jane, a primigravid client age 35 at 41 weeks' gestation, and her husband Bill are admitted to the labor and delivery area. The nurse's admission assessment reveals that Jane and Bill plan for her parents to be present during labor and delivery. Jane's father expresses skepticism about her plans for natural childbirth and breast-feeding. Jane's mother confides that she is anxious about helping Jane with breathing techniques because she was "asleep" during the birth of her own children. What nursing goals and interventions would be helpful for this family?

2. Suki and Kim Thai, a Cambodian couple, are admitted to the labor and delivery area. Suki is age 36 and has 3 children. Although Kim speaks some English, Suki does not. What support strategies could be used with Suki and Kim? What role will culture play in their care?

3. Irving and Silvia Fine are first-time parents. They have read several books about childbirth and have attended childbirth education classes. The couple have no questions and feel confident that they are absolutely prepared. Which strategies might the nurse use with this couple?

Bibliography

Anderberg, G.J. (1988). Initial acquaintance and attachment behavior of siblings with the newborn. *JOGNN*, 17(1), 49-54.

Barnard, K. (1978). The family and you, Part 1. *MCN*, 3(2), 82-83.

Bennett, A., Hewson, D., Booker, E., and Holliday, S. (1985). Antenatal preparation and labor support in relation to birth outcomes. *Birth*, 12(1), 9-16.

Copstick, S.M., Taylor, K.E., Hayes, R., and Morris, N. (1986). Partner support and the use of coping techniques in labor. *Journal of Psychosomatic Research*, 30(4), 497-503.

Fishbein, E.G. (1984). Expectant father's stress—due to the mother's expectations? *JOGNN*, 13(5), 325-328.

Honig, J.C. (1986). Preparing preschool-aged children to be siblings. *MCN*, 11(1), 37-43.

Horn, M., and Manion, J. (1985). Creative grandparenting: Bonding the generations. *JOGNN*, 14(3), 233-236.

House, J. (1981). *Work, stress, and social support*. Reading, MA: Addison-Wesley.

Hunter, M., Philips, C., and Rachman, S. (1979). Memory for pain. *Pain*, 6(1), 35-46.

Leonard, L. (1977). The father's side: A different perspective on childbirth. *The Canadian Nurse*, 73(2), 16-20.

Maloni J.A., McIndoe, J.E., and Rubenstein, G. (1987). Expectant grandparents class. *JOGNN*, 16(1), 26-29.

Peddicord, K., Curran, P. and Monshower, C. (1984). An independent labor-support nursing service. *JOGNN*, 13(5), 312-316.

Raphael, D. (1976). *The tender gift: Breastfeeding*. New York: Schocken Books.

Reading, A.E., and Cox, D.N. (1985). Psychosocial predictors of labor pain. *Pain*, 22(3), 309-315.

Sarason, I.G., and Sarason, B.R. (1985). Social support—insights, from assessment and experimentation. In I.G. Sarason and B.R. Sarason (Eds.), *Social support: Theory, research, and applications* (pp.39-50). Hingham, MA: Kluwer Academia.

Sosa, R., Kennell, J., Klaus, M., Robertson, S., and Urrutia, J. (1980). The effect of a supportive companion on perinatal problems, length of labor, and mother-infant interaction. *The New England Journal of Medicine*, 303(11), 597-600.

Cultural references

Choi, E.C. (1986). Unique aspects of Korean-American mothers. *JOGNN*, 15(5), 394-400.

Hahn, R.A. and Muecke, M.A. (1987). The anthropology of birth in five U.S. ethnic populations: Implications for obstetrical practice. *Current Problems in Obstetrics, Gynecology, and Fertility*, 10(4), 133-171.

La Du, E.B. (1982). A study of the birthing practices of a group of recently immigrated Hmong women. Master's thesis in nursing, School of Nursing, Oregon Health Science University, Portland.

Nyce, J.M., and Hollingshead, W.H. (1984). Southeast Asian refugees of Rhode Island: Reproductive beliefs and practices among the Hmong. *Rhode Island Medical Journal*, 67(8), 361-366.

Nursing research

Berry, L.M. (1988). Realistic expectations of the labor coach. *JOGNN*, 17(5), 354-355.

Brown, M.A. (1986). Social support during pregnancy: A unidimensional or multidimensional construct? *Nursing Research*, 35(1), 4-9.

Collins, B.A. (1986). The role of the nurse in labor and delivery as perceived by nurses and patients. *JOGNN*, 15(5), 412-418.

Gaston-Johansson, F., Fridh, G., and Turner-Norvell, K. (1988). Progression of labor pain in primiparas and multiparas. *Nursing Research*, 37(2), 86-90.

Kintz, D. (1987). Nursing support in labor. *JOGNN*, 16(2), 126-130.

Lederman, R.P. (1984). *Psychosocial adaption in pregnancy*. East Norwalk, CT: Appleton & Lange.

Lemmer, S.C. (1987). Becoming a father: A review of nursing research on expectant fatherhood. *MCN*, 16(3), 261-275.

Lumley, J. (1983). Preschool siblings at birth: Short-term effects. *Birth*, 10(1), 11-16.

Nicholson, J., Gist, N.F., Klein, R.P., and Standley, K. (1983). Outcomes of father involvement in pregnancy and birth. *Birth*, 10(1), 5-9.

Weaver, D.F. (1990). Nurses' views on the meaning of touch in obstetrical nursing practice. *JOGNN*, 19(2), 157-161.

High-Risk Intrapartal Clients

Objectives

After reading and studying this chapter, the student should be able to:

1. Identify conditions that place the client, fetus, or neonate at high risk during labor and delivery.

2. Discuss potential complications that may occur in a high-risk intrapartal client and her fetus or neonate.

3. Adapt nursing care to address the special needs and concerns of selected high-risk intrapartal clients.

4. Describe how to modify the nursing assessment of a high-risk intrapartal client, based on her condition.

5. Describe specific nursing interventions for a high-risk intrapartal client and her fetus or neonate, based on her condition.

6. Recognize emergencies that may arise when caring for a high-risk intrapartal client and describe appropriate nursing interventions.

7. Provide sensitive care for the high-risk intrapartal client's family.

8. Evaluate nursing care for a high-risk intrapartal client.

9. Document significant alterations and nursing interventions accurately when caring for a high-risk intrapartal client.

Introduction

From 10% to 30% of all pregnant clients are high risk; they account for 75% to 80% of perinatal mortality and morbidity (Arias, 1984). Conditions that place a client at high risk include age-related concerns, cardiac disease, diabetes mellitus, infection, substance abuse, pregnancy-induced hypertension (PIH), and Rh isoimmuni-

zation. (For basic information about these conditions, see Chapter 22, High-Risk Antepartal Clients, and Chapter 23, Antepartal Complications.)

High-risk clients fall into two major groups: those with chronic disorders that predispose them to obstetric problems, such as cardiac disease, diabetes mellitus, and substance abuse; and those with pregnancy-related conditions that require special care, such as PIH and Rh isoimmunization.

Added risks

Although childbirth can be a time of change and stress, the emotional and physical demands of labor usually can be managed by the healthy childbearing family. The high-risk intrapartal client may be less well equipped to handle the emotional and physical demands of labor because of her struggle with the uncertainties of the pregnancy outcome. She probably was monitored closely during pregnancy and begins labor keenly aware of the risks for herself, her fetus, or her neonate. Indeed, she may be anxious or frightened about the effects of labor and delivery on her medical or obstetric condition.

Because high risk implies illness or disease, the client may perceive herself as inadequate, may suffer a loss of self-esteem, and may doubt her ability to give birth naturally. She may be unprepared for a positive childbirth experience, believing that cesarean delivery is inevitable or that she or her neonate will die during delivery.

Because the high-risk intrapartal client may believe she is not healthy or normal, her anxieties about pain and the lack of control over labor and delivery may be exaggerated. This anxiety can compound her intrapartal

GLOSSARY

Age-related concerns: health concerns for an adolescent client (under age 19) or a mature client (over age 34) related to maternal, fetal, or neonatal risks during labor and delivery.

Cardiac decompensation: inability of the reserve power of the heart to compensate for impaired valvular functioning.

Cardiac disease: any heart disorder, especially one that places the client at high risk during the intrapartal period.

Cephalopelvic disproportion (CPD): condition in which the fetus's head is too large or the client's pelvis too small to permit normal vaginal delivery.

Chorioamnionitis: inflammation of the fetal membranes, typically caused by infection and producing maternal and fetal tachycardia, fever, uterine and abdominal tenderness, and purulent vaginal secretions.

Diabetes mellitus: endocrine syndrome in which heterogeneous chronic disorders are characterized by altered carbohydrate metabolism caused by inadequate insulin secretion by the beta cells of the islets of Langerhans in the pancreas or by ineffective use of insulin at the cellular level.

Diabetic ketoacidosis (DKA): emergency condition characterized by acidosis and accumulation of ketones in the blood, which results from faulty carbohydrate metabolism. It occurs primarily as a complication of diabetes.

Dystocia: difficult delivery caused by abnormalities in the fetus, client's pelvis, or uterine expulsive powers.

Eclampsia: gravest, convulsive form of pregnancy-induced hypertension characterized by generalized tonic-clonic seizures, coma, hypertension, proteinuria, and edema; occurs between the twentieth week of pregnancy and the end of the first week postpartum.

Erythroblastosis fetalis: serious hemolytic disease of the fetus and neonate that produces anemia; jaundice; liver, spleen, and heart enlargement; and severe generalized edema. Also called hydrops fetalis or hemolytic disease of the newborn.

Hydramnios: excessive amniotic fluid commonly associated with congenital neonatal disorders and such maternal disorders as diabetes mellitus; also called polyhydramnios.

Leiomyoma: benign neoplasm of the uterine smooth muscle that is common in mature clients, can affect fetal growth, and can predispose the client to preterm labor, labor dysfunctions, birth canal obstruction, and postpartal hemorrhage.

Macrosomia: excessively large fetus, weighing over 4,000 g.

Preeclampsia: nonconvulsive form of pregnancy-induced hypertension characterized by increased blood pressure, proteinuria, and edema.

Pregnancy-induced hypertension (PIH): group of potentially life-threatening hypertensive disorders that usually develop in the second or third trimester; includes preeclampsia and eclampsia.

Rh isoimmunization: sensitization of maternal blood antibodies to fetal blood antigens, which can create a serious blood incompatibility during pregnancy and lead to erythroblastosis fetalis.

---

problems because increased maternal anxiety is associated with labor dysfunction, delivery complications, fetal distress, and altered maternal-infant bonding (Gabbe and Main, 1988).

The client and her partner may be frustrated or angry because their childbirth goals are limited. For example, they may not be able to give birth without medical interventions, experience delivery in a birthing room, or be discharged early. The client may worry that her partner will react negatively to her high-risk condition or will perceive her as a failure. Her anxieties may be enhanced by concerns about the neonate's normality and her reactions to it.

In contrast to high-risk clients who invested extra time, expense, and care to produce a healthy pregnancy are those who are at high risk because they received late—or no—prenatal care. In the United States in 1985, 5% of all neonates were born to women who did not receive prenatal care. Such women and their neonates are at high risk because of their socioeconomic status,

poor health, or both. Lack of prenatal care increases the risk of perinatal morbidity and mortality (Brown, 1988).

A high-risk pregnancy has a much higher chance of perinatal complications (problems for the mother and her fetus or neonate). Many high-risk conditions create an unfavorable intrauterine environment that does not support normal fetal growth or oxygenation. The high-risk fetus is especially sensitive to hypoxia, stress, and trauma. Signs of fetal distress, such as fetal heart rate abnormalities and meconium-stained amniotic fluid, may develop more quickly during labor.

For a high-risk neonate, perinatal concerns involve the significant increase in the morbidity and mortality associated with prematurity, postmaturity, or low birth weight (Knupple and Drukker, 1986). These conditions predispose the neonate to birth trauma, perinatal asphyxia, meconium aspiration, hypoglycemia, heat loss, polycythemia, and death (Korones, 1986).

Although the goal of care is a safe, satisfying delivery that produces a normal, healthy neonate, this goal may not be achieved. If a high-risk neonate is born seriously ill, disabled, or without hope for survival, the parents' worst fears are confirmed. If perinatal death or disability occurs, the family will need assistance with coping and grieving. (For more information, see Chapter 39, Care of the Families of High-Risk Neonates.)

Nursing responsibilities

For the high-risk client and her family, the nurse must provide basic intrapartal care. (For more information, see Chapters 27, 28, and 29 on the four stages of labor.) In addition, the experienced nurse must understand the complexities of high-risk labor and delivery, be prepared to participate as an integral member of the perinatal team, and provide specialized care at a critical-care level of specialized practice. These responsibilities should not be undertaken by the beginning nurse. For this kind of care, advanced nursing responsibilities typically include:
• assessing the high-risk intrapartal client and her fetus on admission
• identifying abnormal assessment findings that demand immediate attention and initiating appropriate interventions promptly
• anticipating intrapartal problems by addressing them in the care plan
• promoting a normal labor and delivery and the client's self-confidence in achieving them, whenever possible
• promoting comfort and decreasing anxiety
• assessing labor progress and screening for additional problems
• providing continual information to the client and her family about her care and current status
• explaining the benefits of electronic fetal monitoring and other equipment to decrease the client's anxiety and to gain her acceptance and cooperation
• acknowledging the client's concerns and those of her family to help them cope with this high-risk delivery
• promoting participation and a sense of control by involving the high-risk client and her family in care decisions and goal-setting
• preparing the high-risk family emotionally and physically for cesarean delivery, if needed.

To manage the nursing care of the high-risk intrapartal client, the nurse must perform specialized maternal and fetal monitoring (which demands advanced knowledge and skills), be familiar with the technology used to improve perinatal outcomes, and be ready to provide nursing care as an important part of a specialized perinatal team. To prepare the nurse to handle these responsibilities, this chapter discusses the specialized nursing care for selected high-risk intrapartal clients. For each high-risk condition, the chapter reviews maternal and neonatal risks during delivery. Then it describes how to apply the nursing process when caring

for a high-risk intrapartal client, highlighting specific assessment techniques and interventions for various high-risk conditions. It concludes with a discussion of the documentation necessary to record the specialized nursing care provided.

High-risk conditions

During the intrapartal period, high-risk conditions may include age-related concerns, cardiac disease, diabetes mellitus, infection, substance abuse, PIH, and Rh isoimmunization. They may endanger the client or her fetus or neonate. (For a summary, see *Intrapartal conditions and risks,* pages 740 and 741.)

Age-related concerns

Various age-related factors can place an adolescent client (under age 19) or a mature client (over age 34) at risk during labor and delivery.

Adolescent client

If an adolescent has maintained a healthy, uncomplicated pregnancy, is over age 15, is in good general health, and has had early and consistent prenatal care, adequate nutrition, and family support, she may progress through labor and delivery normally. Her risk for intrapartal problems may be no greater than that for the general population (Hollingsworth, Kotchen, and Felice, 1985).

Even if she has maintained a healthy pregnancy, however, she is likely to be at risk for psychosocial problems during labor and delivery. These are especially common because of unfamiliar surroundings, a sense of isolation, heightened fears and fantasies about labor and delivery, and the forthcoming responsibilities of motherhood.

She also may be at risk for physical problems. A client under age 15 or a multigravid adolescent client over age 15 is at considerably higher risk for poor maternal, fetal, or neonatal outcomes related to birth (Moore, 1989). About 14.5% of neonates born to adolescents under age 15 weigh 2,500 g or less as compared to about 6.9% of neonates born to women in their twenties (Slap and Schwartz, 1989). Low-birth-weight (LBW) neonates of adolescent mothers have higher morbidity and mortality rates. In adolescents, generally smaller stature, lower preconception weight, and insufficient antepartal weight gain contribute to LBW neonates.

Intrapartal conditions and risks

During the intrapartal period, the nurse should be alert to certain conditions that may pose risks for the client and her fetus or neonate, as shown in the chart below.

CONDITION	MATERNAL RISKS	FETAL OR NEONATAL RISKS
Age (adolescent client)	• Abruptio placentae • Uterine dysfunction, which may cause prolonged labor or precipitous birth • Labor arrest • Cesarean delivery related to cephalopelvic disproportion (CPD) or insufficient cervical dilation • Psychosocial problems • Panic related to lack of control	• Low birth weight (LBW) or intrauterine growth retardation (IUGR) • Perinatal asyphxia • Meconium aspiration • Hypoglycemia • Fetal distress caused by reduced perfusion of the fetal-placental unit and insufficient oxygenation • Prematurity • Neonatal infection, especially with a sexually transmitted disease • Neonatal respiratory or central nervous system (CNS) depression
Age (mature client)	• Increased anxiety for neonate • Premature rupture of membranes (PROM) • Preterm labor • Multiple gestation (more than one fetus) • Placenta previa in a multiparous client • Labor dysfunction and postpartal hemorrhage, especially in a client with uterine leiomyoma • Prolonged or arrested labor, which can require oxytocin (Pitocin) administration or cesarean delivery • CPD • Malpositioning	• Chromosomal abnormalities, open neural tube defects, or cardiac defects • LBW or IUGR • Small for gestational age (SGA) or large for gestational age (LGA) • Breech presentation • Perinatal asyphxia • Meconium aspiration • Fetal distress • Stillbirth • Neonatal respiratory or CNS depression
Cardiac disease	• Cardiac decompensation • Congestive heart failure • Pulmonary edema • Maternal death • Preterm labor, if certain cardiac drugs were used	• Fetal hypoxia or asphyxia • IUGR • Increased risk of congenital heart defects
Diabetes	• Preterm labor • Hyperglycemia • Diabetic ketoacidosis • Excessive postpartal bleeding from uterine atony or birth trauma • Hypoglycemia • Hydramnios	• Hydramnios • Congenital malformations • Fetal distress • Fetal death, especially in a client with diabetic ketoacidosis • Macrosomia, which can lead to birth trauma • Neonatal hyperinsulinism leading to hypoglycemia • Respiratory distress syndrome (RDS) • Polycythemia • Hyperbilirubinemia • Hypocalcemia
Infection	• PROM • Premature labor • Fever	• Premature neonate • Neonatal infection or sepsis • RDS • Fetal death

Intrapartal conditions and risks continued

CONDITION	MATERNAL RISKS	FETAL OR NEONATAL RISKS
Substance abuse	• Preterm labor • Precipitous birth • Abruptio placentae • Maternal infection • Psychosocial problems, such as isolation • Interactions between abused substance and drugs administered during delivery	• LBW or SGA neonate caused by IUGR • Premature neonate • Neonatal infection • Congenital malformations • Neonatal withdrawal symptoms
Pregnancy-induced hypertension	• Insufficient perfusion of vital organs, including fetal-placental unit • Seizures, hypertonic uterine activity, and abruptio placentae, if the client develops eclampsia • Preterm labor	• Premature neonate • Toxicity in neonate, if magnesium sulfate was administered to client • IUGR
Rh isoimmunization	• Placental hypertrophy with uteroplacental insufficiency • Chorioamnionitis • Abruptio placentae • Hydramnios, which may cause inefficient contractions • Preterm labor and delivery	• Fetal hypoxia and distress • Anemia • Jaundice • Liver, spleen, and heart enlargement • Anasarca (severe, generalized edema) • Myocardial failure

Of the approximately 5% of pregnant women in the United States who have received little or no prenatal care, about 14% are under age 18 (Brown, 1988). Insufficient prenatal care and other factors may produce an LBW neonate who displays respiratory or central nervous system depression at birth, has a low Apgar score, and is at increased risk for developing sudden infant death syndrome, or SIDS (Institute of Medicine, 1985).

Mature client

Typically, mature primigravid clients are in better health, are better educated and better nourished, and have a higher standard of living than adolescent clients (Jennings, 1987). Although they are at increased risk for some medical and obstetric complications, they typically proceed well through pregnancy and delivery (Acker, 1987), possibly because they tend to seek early prenatal care, are highly motivated and compliant, and receive close monitoring throughout pregnancy and delivery (Queenan, Freeman, Niebyl, Resnik, and Simpson, 1987).

Typically, the mature intrapartal client has been screened prenatally for fetal chromosomal abnormalities, multiple gestation (more than one fetus), gestational diabetes, PIH, appropriate fetal growth, placenta previa, and a tendency for premature labor. A healthy mature client has the same intrapartal nursing needs as a younger client. Her greatest nursing needs will be psychosocial.

For mature clients, aging or obesity are responsible for many intrapartal risks, including diabetes mellitus, gestational diabetes, PIH, chronic hypertension, thrombophlebitis, chronic renal disease, collagen disease, and uterine leiomyoma (benign neoplasm of the uterine small muscle), which can affect labor and delivery (Oats, Abell, Andersen, and Beischer, 1983; Calandra, Abell, and Beischer, 1981). Mature clients also are at higher risk for premature rupture of the membranes (PROM) and preterm labor (Naeye, 1983).

The neonate of a mature client is at increased risk for chromosomal abnormalities (including Down's syndrome), open neural tube defects, and cardiac defects. This is especially significant to nursing care if the client declined prenatal genetic screening or ultrasonography, because she may not be prepared for the birth of a neonate with a disorder.

If the mature client has hypertension or PIH, her neonate is at risk for LBW or intrauterine growth retardation (IUGR) caused by uteroplacental insufficiency. Intrapartal risks for an LBW neonate include increased fetal distress, meconium aspiration, and neonatal depression.

If the client is obese, her neonate may be born with macrosomia from her nutritionally unbalanced diet or from gestational diabetes. Intrapartal concerns for a macrosomic fetus include stillbirth or birth trauma from shoulder dystocia.

One study of infant mortality and maternal age demonstrated that, compared to mothers ages 25 to 29, the risk of neonatal mortality was nearly equal in mothers ages 30 to 34; 18% higher in mothers ages 35 to 39; and 69% higher in mothers ages 40 to 49 (Friede, Baldwin, Rhodes, Buehler, and Strauss, 1988; Berkowitz, Skovron, Lapinski, and Berkowitz, 1990).

Cardiac disease

Maternal cardiac disease complicates nearly 1% of all pregnancies and is a major cause of maternal death in the United States (Greenspoon, 1988). The intrapartal period poses the greatest risk for the client with cardiac disease because the hemodynamic changes of pregnancy peak at this time.

Labor can produce sudden, profound changes in the cardiovascular system. During each contraction, pain and increased venous blood return from the uterus raise cardiac output 20%. Mean arterial pressure rises and is followed by a reflex bradycardia. Uterine contractions can compress the aorta and iliac arteries, forcing more blood to the upper torso and head (Samuels and Landon, 1986).

Intrapartal management of the client with a cardiac disease requires the expertise of an obstetrician, cardiologist, anesthesiologist, and obstetric nurse with critical care skills. The client needs intensive obstetric and cardiac monitoring. Interventions are based on the client's degree of cardiac decompensation (inability of the heart to compensate for impaired functioning). Even a client with minimal activity limitation during pregnancy can experience sudden worsening of the disease during labor. The nurse should be familiar with the normal changes of pregnancy and with the maternal and fetal consequences of cardiac disease. (For more information, see Chapter 22, High-Risk Antepartal Clients.)

Diabetes mellitus

During pregnancy, a client with diabetes mellitus requires close monitoring and management to prevent intrapartal problems. Prevention of hyperglycemia before conception and during pregnancy improves perinatal outcomes but does not remove all risks (Mills, et al., 1988). Uncontrolled diabetes is associated with increased maternal, fetal, and neonatal morbidity and mortality. (For more information about the maternal, fetal, and neonatal effects of diabetes, see Chapter 22, High-Risk Antepartal Clients.)

Uncontrolled diabetes can cause hydramnios (excessive amniotic fluid). It also is associated with hypertensive disorders, such as chronic hypertension and PIH, which affect 15% to 30% of all pregnant clients with diabetes (Cousins, 1987). Women with diabetes also are at risk for preterm labor and, if associated with vascular changes, placental abnormalities.

Neonates of diabetic mothers whose diabetes has not been well controlled have a higher morbidity and mortality rate than those born to nondiabetic mothers. They also are at risk for neonatal hypoglycemia at birth and for macrosomia, which can lead to birth trauma. A neonate of a pregestational diabetic client is at increased risk for congenital malformations, especially if the client's glucose levels were uncontrolled during fetal organ development (Mills, et al., 1988).

Infection

Infections are a major cause of maternal, fetal, and neonatal death. During the intrapartal period, they are more common in clients with premature labor, PROM (especially before 36 weeks' gestation), fever, or fetal death.

The primary perinatal infections are bacterial or viral and are caused by such organisms as group B beta-hemolytic streptococcus, herpes simplex virus (HSV), or hepatitis B virus. (For more information, see Chapter 12, Infectious Disorders, and Chapter 22, High-Risk Antepartal Clients.) They may be transmitted to the fetus through an infected uterus or birth canal and can lead to morbidity or mortality because the fetus's immature immune system cannot fight off these life-threatening organisms. Fungal (candidiasis) or protozoal (trichomoniasis) infections are not potentially fatal (Benoit, 1988).

Many factors can predispose a client to intrapartal infection, including obesity, severe anemia, poor hygiene, uncontrolled diabetes, chronic renal or respiratory disease, and a depressed immune response (Balgobin, 1987). Clients at increased risk for sexually transmitted diseases (STDs), which are the most common intrapartal infections (Cates and Holmes, 1987), constitute a large and varied population, including but not limited to:
• unmarried women
• women under age 24
• women with multiple sex partners, especially with a history of treatment for STDs
• women treated for recurrent vaginitis or a previous STD (Wilson, 1988; Spence, 1989).

During labor, predisposing factors to infection (especially chlamydia) may include preterm labor, prolonged labor, prolonged PROM (rupture that occurs more than

24 hours before labor), use of such invasive equipment as internal fetal scalp electrodes or intrauterine pressure catheters, and multiple vaginal examinations.

Substance abuse

During pregnancy, substance abuse can lead to serious perinatal risks. Substance abusers tend to have un-planned pregnancies or may be uncertain when the preg-nancy began. They may have suboptimal nutrition, smoke heavily, abuse multiple drugs, and seek prenatal care late, if at all (Frank, et al., 1988).

These actions put the substance abuser and her fetus at risk during the intrapartal period. For example, co-caine use during pregnancy causes maternal and fetal vasoconstriction, tachycardia, and elevated blood pres-sure. These effects reduce blood flow to the fetus and can induce uterine contractions (Chasnoff, 1987). Co-caine use also increases the risk of preterm labor, de-livery of an LBW or small-for-gestational-age (SGA) neonate (MacGregor, et al., 1987), and abruptio placen-tae (Burkett, Banstra, Cohn, Steele, and Palow, 1990).

Substance abuse also can cause problems that may affect the antepartal period and lead to intrapartal prob-lems. For example, severe nutritional deficiencies and STDs, which are common among women who abuse drugs, compromise fetal health (Lynch and McKeon, 1990). Substance abuse can produce social isolation, which can affect the client's ability to cope with labor. Use of nonsterile needles can cause maternal infection or embolization, which can affect maternal and fetal health.

Some states have strict laws regarding substance abuse and child protection. For example, if the client used or tested positive for drugs during the antepartal or intrapartal periods, Florida law mandates home en-vironment evaluation and referral of the client for drug treatment before the neonate can be discharged (Florida Statute, 1987).

Pregnancy-induced hypertension

A hypertensive syndrome that occurs during pregnancy, PIH has two forms: preeclampsia (causing hypertension, proteinuria, and edema and possibly causing oliguria, headache, blurred vision, and increased deep tendon re-flexes) and eclampsia (causing convulsions along with the signs of preeclampsia). Affecting about 5% of all pregnancies (Knupple and Drukker, 1986), preeclampsia may progress to eclampsia suddenly or gradually. The client with PIH may be very ill. Failure to recognize and appropriately manage PIH accounts for about 1% of ma-ternal deaths in the United States (Roberts, 1989).

PIH is characterized by insufficient perfusion of many vital organs, including the fetal-placental unit (all fetal and maternal systems that work together to ex-change nutrients, excrete toxins, and perform other func-tions); it is completely reversible with pregnancy termination, but symptoms may remain for 24 to 48 hours after delivery. The client may report sudden weight gain, varying degrees of edema, numbness in her hands or feet, headache, or vision problems—all warning signs of increasing preeclampsia.

The major goal of preeclampsia management is pre-vention of eclampsia. To achieve this goal, the nurse must understand the pathophysiology, progression, and prognosis of the disorder, and must recognize and im-mediately report to the physician the classic signs of preeclampsia. (For more information on PIH, see Chapter 23, Antepartal Complications.)

Rh isoimmunization

Rh isoimmunization refers to sensitization and immune response of maternal blood antibodies to fetal blood an-tigens, which can create a serious blood incompatibility between the two during pregnancy. This can lead to erythroblastosis fetalis (hydrops fetalis or hemolytic dis-ease of the newborn).

Erythroblastosis fetalis is a serious hemolytic dis-ease of the fetus and neonate that produces anemia; jaundice; liver, spleen, and heart enlargement; and an-asarca (severe generalized edema) and may lead to myo-cardial failure. It also may cause placental hypertrophy, which can contribute to fetal hypoxia and death (Knupple and Drukker, 1986) and accounts for a significant per-centage of fetal morbidity and mortality (Queenan, 1985).

Rh isoimmunization results when a client has Rh-negative blood and her fetus has Rh-positive blood. How-ever, this is becoming more rare because most Rh-negative women now receive $Rh_o(D)$ immune globulin (RhoGAM) during antepartal and postpartal care, which provides passive immunization against the Rh antigen.

Today, hemolytic disease of the newborn occurs more commonly when the client develops a sensitivity to other foreign blood antigens. This sensitization is known as nonimmune hydrops fetalis. Maternal factors that con-tribute to development of nonimmune hydrops include multiple gestation; perinatal infections, especially syph-ilis or cytomegalovirus infection; previous transfusion of blood that contained foreign antigens; diabetes mel-litus; thalassemia; or PIH (Sachs, 1987). (For more in-formation about isoimmunization, see Chapter 23, Antepartal Complications.)

Unlike other high-risk intrapartal clients, the client with Rh isoimmunization does not feel ill. However, if she knows the consequences of isoimmunization, she may experience extreme guilt and anxiety because of her body's actions against her fetus. She may have endured frequent invasive tests and close fetal monitoring to prevent fetal death. She may view the intrapartal period as the culmination of a trying time.

Nursing care

Every pregnant client should have been evaluated for medical and obstetric complications before the intrapartal period because early findings can assist health care professionals in correcting deficiencies and avoiding intrapartal complications. Sometimes, however, a high-risk client is first encountered during the intrapartal period or a problem develops late in the pregnancy that goes undetected until admission to the labor and delivery area. In either situation, however, the nurse can use the nursing process to deliver high-quality care.

Assessment

As with any client who seeks admission for labor and delivery, the nurse obtains the high-risk intrapartal client's health history, conducts an abbreviated physical assessment, and assists in collecting specimens for appropriate laboratory tests. (For basic assessment information and procedures, see Chapters 27, 28, and 29 on the four stages of labor.) With a high-risk intrapartal client, however, the nurse must make additional assessments and be prepared to notify the physician of significant findings, as described below.

Health history

When taking a history, keep in mind that a client may perceive a common, normal variation as a problem. (For more information, see *Nursing research applied: Intrapartal complications and childbirth satisfaction.*) Depending on the intrapartal client's condition, adjust the approach to the health history, augmenting the basic interview with appropriate questions. These questions depend on the client's age, disorder, and labor status.

Adolescent client. When assessing an adolescent client, be aware that this may be her first experience in a health care facility. If she is in active labor, she may panic because she is unprepared and feels out of control. She may perceive history questions as unimportant and may be unwilling or unable to answer them because of fear or ignorance. To calm her and obtain the necessary

information, include her support person in the interview and attempt to gain her trust and cooperation. If birth seems imminent, concentrate on the most important history questions and gather data quickly.

After determining her age, parity, and labor status, ask her about length of pregnancy, prenatal care received, and the presence of any complications. This information can direct the physical assessment. Be aware, however, that the adolescent may not know her last menstrual period (LMP), making gestational age assessment and subsequent prediction of IUGR or prematurity inaccurate.

When investigating her obstetric history, particularly note complications that may recur, such as PIH, abruptio placentae, and postpartal hemorrhage. Typically, a young multiparous client has closely spaced pregnancies, rapid labors, and small neonates, all of which predispose her to precipitous (extremely rapid) delivery.

Determine the client's preconception weight and antepartal weight gain. Smaller maternal body size and poor gestational weight gain have been associated with LBW infants, who may not tolerate the stresses of labor well because of poor placental perfusion (Mercer, 1987; Winick, 1989).

Discuss her use of tobacco, alcohol, or drugs—substances that are used by many adolescents. (For more information, see "Substance abuse" later in this section.) These substances can alter fetal and neonatal health.

When evaluating the adolescent client's psychosocial status, be sure to assess her coping methods and support systems. Her ability to cope depends on her developmental stage, preparation for childbirth, family support, and flexibility of the health care team (Corbett and Meyer, 1987). She may need constant support during the intrapartal period.

Mature client. Early in the interview, obtain the mature client's LMP and estimated delivery date, and calculate gestational age because of her increased risk for preterm labor. Also ask about any vaginal fluid leakage, which signifies rupture of amniotic membranes, because the mature client has an increased risk for PROM.

Inquire about any medical or obstetric problems because this information can help guide the plan of care. For example, a client with a chronic medical problem, such as diabetes mellitus or cardiac disease, will need additional specialized intrapartal care.

Determine if the client has a history of infertility. If so, ask how it was treated. Treatment with drugs that stimulate ovulation can predispose her to multiple gestation and accompanying risks, such as premature labor, malpresentation, and dystocia.

Intrapartal complications and childbirth satisfaction

Traditionally, intrapartal complications have been associated with negative perceptions of childbirth, which have been linked to negative perceptions of the neonate and to impaired maternal role attainment. To investigate this phenomenon, researchers examined perceptions of complications in educated primiparous clients and the relationship of these perceptions to their childbirth satisfaction.

Through documentation reviews and personal interviews, researchers found that perceived complications ranged from blood pressure elevations and cesarean delivery to headaches, pruritus, and drops in fetal heart rate. Although many clients perceived complications, most expressed satisfaction with labor and childbirth. Their satisfaction usually was related to how well the experience met their expectations of a smooth, rapid, low-intervention childbirth.

Application to practice

According to this study, many clients perceive common intrapartal events and interventions as unexpected complications. To promote a positive perception of childbirth, the nurse should review aspects of childbirth with clients and discuss the probability of achieving their expectations. During the intrapartal period, the nurse also should continue to discuss perceptions of events as they occur to help clients integrate their expectations with their experiences.

Kearney, M., and Cronenwett, L. (1989). Perceived perinatal complications and childbirth satisfaction. *Applied Nursing Research*, 2(3), 140-142.

Also inquire if she has had any previous spontaneous abortions, has been trying to conceive for a long time, or conceived via artificial insemination. If so, she may be more anxious about this pregnancy outcome and may need close maternal and fetal monitoring during labor, if only to reassure her of normal progress.

Ask if she has had prenatal and genetic screening. For a client who has not been screened, be prepared for the possibility of a neonate with serious chromosomal abnormalities, and plan to alert the neonatal team to the client's history when delivery is imminent. Keep in mind, however, that genetic screening cannot detect all abnormalities; a client who was screened may give birth to a neonate who needs intensive care.

Perform a psychosocial assessment to identify any needs that must be addressed in the plan of care. Determine if the client is anxious about this birth or about other children at home. Find out if she has been managing a high-stress career. Anxiety and stress can affect fetal growth and can increase the risk of complications during labor and delivery (Resnik, 1988).

Assess the client's understanding of her condition and care. A mature primigravid client is likely to have planned her pregnancy and may be knowledgeable about her prenatal health. She may use various community resources, be well-read, and be highly motivated to have a controlled and successful labor and delivery (Winslow, 1987a).

Also evaluate the client's coping skills. They may be well developed, and she may be better able to express her concerns or fears about labor and delivery than a younger client. However, she may have a strong need to be in control (Winslow, 1987b). Such a client may respond well to a nurse who encourages her participation in the plan of care, is sensitive to her needs for adaptation to labor, and supports her role transition.

Cardiac disease. A client with cardiac disease requires careful assessment of cardiovascular status. Inquire if she has recently had difficulty breathing, experienced chest pains or dizzy spells, or has felt increased fatigue. Severe dyspnea, chest pain on exertion, increasing fatigue, or syncope suggest significant cardiac disease or decompensation and should be reported promptly to the physician.

Obtain a complete medication history. Any delay in medication administration during labor and delivery may affect the client's cardiovascular status and general well-being.

Drugs used to treat cardiac disease potentially can harm the fetus and affect the perinatal outcome. Some cardiac medications may have teratogenic effects; others may precipitate preterm labor. Oral anticoagulants are potential teratogens when taken during the first trimester. After the first trimester, they increase the risk of intrauterine bleeding (Hall, Pauli, and Wilson, 1980).

Propranolol, a beta blocker used to treat hypertension and tachyarrhythmias, can cause a constantly high uterine tone (uterine muscle contraction without relaxation) and result in preterm labor (Ueland, 1989). The drug may produce neonatal respiratory depression, sustained bradycardia, and hypoglycemia when taken late in pregnancy or immediately before delivery (Rubin, et al., 1984).

Thiazide diuretics can harm the fetus, especially when used in the third trimester or for extended periods. They may cause severe neonatal electrolyte imbalance, jaundice, thrombocytopenia, and liver damage (Anderson, 1970). However, drugs such as quinidine and the cardiac glycosides are not known to have teratogenic effects or cause problems with use during the third trimester of pregnancy.

Diabetes mellitus. When assessing a diabetic client, determine when she last ate and took insulin. An omitted or reduced insulin dose can cause a surge in blood glucose levels. Insulin deficiency can lead to diabetic ketoacidosis (DKA, an acute complication of diabetes characterized by hyperglycemia, metabolic acidosis, electrolyte imbalance, coma, and possibly maternal and fetal death).

Infection. Because any woman may contract an infectious disease and because it may have grave consequences, assess all intrapartal clients for infection, noting symptoms of, and risk factors for, infection. Early recognition of intrapartal infection allows prompt treatment and helps prevent its spread.

During the admission interview, review the client's history of antepartal illness, possible exposure to STDs, and any treatments received. This information may point to a serious infection, such as an STD, which may be asymptomatic when the disease is most virulent (Krieger, 1984).

Ask the client about recent exposure to colds or viruses or whether she has a persistent cough or fever. Inquire about past or current urinary tract infections, which typically recur during pregnancy. These questions also may uncover evidence of infection.

Also inquire about general signs and symptoms of infection, such as fever, chills, fatigue, and anorexia as well as specific signs and symptoms of upper respiratory, genitourinary, and other infections.

During the client's obstetric history, rule out prolonged PROM, which can lead to chorioamnionitis. Note the onset of labor to rule out prolonged labor, which can predispose the client to infection.

Substance abuse. The admission interview is the ideal time to assess the client for substance use, abuse, or withdrawal. With careful questioning, probe sufficiently to discover if substance abuse is a problem and, if it is, determine the client's current status. This is especially important because the substance abuser may enter the health care facility without revealing her problem (Miller, 1989).

Explore past and present substance use in a nonjudgmental manner. Remember that the substance abuser is likely to be anxious or depressed and to display abrupt behavior changes. She may lack self-confidence and have low self-esteem. If she is afraid, she may be hostile and aggressive.

Begin the history by determining the client's first use of cigarettes, alcohol, and drugs, and then lead to a current substance abuse history. To evoke honest responses, ask nonthreatening questions, such as, "Do you currently drink alcohol or use drugs?"

Review the client's medical history for clues to prior substance abuse, such as serum hepatitis, venous thrombosis, thrombophlebitis, cellulitis, abscess, hypertension, STDs, and human immunodeficiency virus (HIV)

infection (Chasnoff, 1987). Such complications are associated with substance abuse and use of drug equipment.

Pay close attention to the client's complete obstetric history. Substance abuse may have complicated previous pregnancies and may cause problems in this one. Illicit drug use during pregnancy can affect the client and her fetus or neonate.

The client who abuses substances may experience menstrual irregularities or amenorrhea (Confino and Gleicher, 1985). As a result, she may be unaware of her pregnancy until she begins to look pregnant or feel fetal movement. Because of this, determination of gestational age may be difficult, especially if she has not had prenatal care. Maternal nutritional deficiencies and drug exposure in utero can cause IUGR, further complicating gestational age determination (Frank, et al., 1988).

During the history, evaluate the client's feelings about her pregnancy. The substance abuser may have ambivalent feelings about pregnancy. Carefully document her responses and bonding behaviors, such as talking about the fetus and touching her abdomen. This information can help health care professionals make decisions about the neonate's safety.

Pregnancy-induced hypertension. Assess the client for signs and symptoms of PIH, especially those of increasing severity. Expect her to complain of symptoms in various body systems because PIH reduces perfusion to nearly all tissues.

Inquire about the client's pattern of weight gain during pregnancy. A gain of 5 pounds in one week is a warning sign of preeclampsia. Ask about edema of the hands, feet, or face—a common, early sign of preeclampsia. If edema is severe, the client will require further evaluation for other signs of preeclampsia.

Also ask about other signs and symptoms that may suggest PIH. Complaints of tightness and intermittent numbness in her hands and feet indicate ulnar nerve compression from edema. Complaints of epigastric pain or stomach upset may signal hepatic distention, a warning sign of impending preeclampsia. Headache and mental confusion indicate poor cerebral perfusion and may precede seizures. Visual disturbances, such as scotomata, indicate retinal arterial spasm and edema (Roberts, 1989).

Rh isoimmunization. When collecting history data from an isoimmunized client, ask about the antepartal progression of the disorder. She may be extremely knowledgeable about the frequent surveillance of her fetus.

Inquire about her obstetric history, which may provide information about Rh problems. For example, her fetus may be at increased risk for developing erythroblastosis fetalis if she did not receive $Rh_0(D)$ immune globulin during her previous pregnancy.

Also, determine the client's expectations for and concerns about her pregnancy. This information may help guide the nursing care plan.

Physical assessment

During the physical assessment, modify the standard examination to meet the high-risk intrapartal client's needs, and note significant findings that are related to her high-risk condition.

Adolescent client. An adolescent may feel embarrassed or shy about being examined by a "stranger." Her lack of control over her labor may make her feel vulnerable, restricted, and confused. To gain a sense of control over something, she may rebel against the physical assessment and other facility procedures. Provide reassurance, remain calm but firm, and explain each step of the assessment before performing it.

Measure the client's vital signs as accurately as possible. Keep in mind that her anxiety may distort her initial vital signs. Nevertheless, her baseline blood pressure measurement will help detect PIH, and temperature and pulse rate will help detect infection or severe anemia.

Note fundal height, estimate fetal weight, and determine fetal presentation. These assessments can identify LBW, prematurity, malposition, and malpresentation. Alert the physician to any suspicious findings for further evaluation.

Assist with a pelvic examination to determine labor progress, pelvic adequacy, the imminence of delivery, and the possibility of cephalopelvic disproportion (CPD). Gaining her trust is important for this examination. If the client resists this evaluation, expect it to be delayed until she is more settled. Remember that she may perceive a forced pelvic examination as an assault and that she has the right to refuse any procedure.

Mature client. For a mature client, establish a baseline blood pressure and assess for signs and symptoms of PIH. Evaluate fundal height for evidence of SGA or LGA, hydramnios (if she has gestational diabetes or her fetus has an anomaly), or multiple gestation, which are more common in mature multiparous clients.

Ascertain fetal position to detect breech presentation, which occurs more frequently in mature clients (Kirz, Dorchester, and Freeman, 1985).

Cardiac disease. When assessing the client with cardiac disease, be especially alert for dependent edema, crack-les in the lower lung fields, jugular vein distention, cyanosis, clubbing, diastolic murmurs, cardiac arrhythmias, and loud, hard systolic murmurs. Depending on their severity, these findings may indicate cardiac decompensation and must be reported immediately to the physician.

Diabetes mellitus. When assessing the diabetic client, be especially alert for signs of hyperglycemia, such as unusual thirst; increased urine output; and continuous, deep, rapid breathing. Also watch for signs of hypoglycemia, such as faintness, trembling, impaired vision, and changes in level of consciousness.

Infection. When assisting with the physical assessment, be alert for signs of dehydration, maternal or fetal tachycardia, fever, chest congestion, uterine or other abdominal tenderness, costovertebral angle tenderness, perineal lesions, and purulent, malodorous vaginal secretions. These signs suggest infection.

Even if the client displays no obvious signs of infection, be vigilant about following infection control guidelines (Centers for Disease Control, 1987). Assume that any client may be infected with the HIV or hepatitis B virus, and observe universal precautions with every client. (For more information, see Chapter 12, Infectious Disorders.)

Substance abuse. Observe the client's physical appearance for signs of substance abuse. Note drowsiness, lethargy, or a malnourished, gaunt, or untidy appearance. Also note extremely dilated or constricted pupils; track marks, abscesses, or edema in the arms or legs; and inflamed or indurated nasal mucosa.

Pregnancy-induced hypertension. The client's prenatal blood pressure should be compared to her current readings. In preeclampsia, blood pressure increases by at least 30 mm Hg systolic or 15 mm Hg diastolic. If the prenatal blood pressure is unknown, a blood pressure of 140/90 mm Hg after 20 weeks' gestation suggests PIH. Severe preeclampsia exists when blood pressure is 160 mm Hg or more systolic or 110 mm Hg or more diastolic and significant edema and proteinuria are present. However, eclampsia can occur with much lower blood pressure.

Rh isoimmunization. During the physical assessment, observe for signs of chorioamnionitis, such as maternal or fetal tachycardia, fever, uterine or other abdominal tenderness, and purulent vaginal secretions with rupture of the membranes. An isoimmunized client may develop chorioamnionitis if her amniotic fluid becomes contaminated during intrauterine blood transfusions or amniocentesis, which commonly is performed in pregnant clients with Rh problems.

Also note signs of abruptio placentae, such as a painful, taut abdomen, or hydramnios, such as excessive abdominal distention and dyspnea. These obstetric conditions are associated with isoimmunization.

Laboratory tests

Unless otherwise noted, expect to collect all standard admission laboratory tests. (For details, see Chapter 27, The First Stage of Labor.) Consider the client's high-risk condition when reviewing the results.

Adolescent client. During the pelvic examination, specimens to detect STDs and chorioamnionitis, which can cause neonatal complications, may be collected. Expect to collect specimens for all routine laboratory tests if test results are not available on the client's prenatal chart. Expect to obtain blood and urine specimens to test for anemia, STDs, hepatitis, rubella, Rh type and antibody screening, and urinary tract infections, especially if the client has not received prenatal care. Because needles and blood can be frightening to an adolescent client, provide reassurance and support when collecting specimens.

Diabetes mellitus. For a diabetic client, carefully check blood glucose levels, as prescribed. The insulin-dependent diabetic client is at risk for DKA when blood glucose levels approach 300 mg/dl (Hollingsworth and Moore, 1989).

If an elective induction or repeat cesarean delivery is planned, the physician may perform an amniocentesis to determine the lecithin/sphingomyelin (L/S) ratio and phosphatidylglycerol (PG) level. These test results provide information about fetal lung maturity, which helps determine whether a vaginal delivery is possible or cesarean delivery is necessary as well as the timing of delivery.

Infection. Anticipate the laboratory tests ordered for the client with an infection, which may include a complete blood count with differential; erythrocyte sedimentation rate; blood culture; urinalysis; urine culture and sensitivity test; cervical, vaginal, and lesion cultures; chest X-rays; and culture and microscopic evaluation of amniotic fluid. These tests help pinpoint the type and degree of infection.

Substance abuse. Because of the client's life-style, she may have multiple infections and diseases. Expect to perform all routine intrapartal tests as well as tests for hepatitis, tuberculosis, STDs, and HIV infection, as prescribed. If the client admits to substance abuse or shows

its clinical indications, expect a urine toxicology screen to be performed for confirmation, as prescribed.

Pregnancy-induced hypertension. For all intrapartal clients, test a random urine specimen with a protein-sensitive reagent strip to screen for proteinuria, one of the three classic signs of PIH. Be aware that urine contamination with blood or amniotic fluid will cause a false-positive result because these fluids contain protein.

If results indicate proteinuria, expect to collect a 24-hour urine specimen for quantitative analysis, as prescribed. Severe preeclampsia exists when urine protein measures 3+ or 4+ on a reagent strip or 5 g or more (or 300 mg/liter) on a quantitative analysis.

Rh isoimmunization. Lung maturity studies, such as L/S ratio and PG level, may guide plans for an isoimmunized client to have a premature delivery.

Nursing diagnosis

The nurse reviews all health history, physical assessment, and laboratory test findings and then formulates nursing diagnoses appropriate for the high-risk intrapartal client. (For a partial list of possible nursing diagnoses, see *Nursing diagnoses: High-risk intrapartal clients.*)

Planning and implementation

Some nursing interventions for the high-risk intrapartal client are the same as those for any other intrapartal client. For example, the nurse must assess the client and fetus, assist in labor management, promote comfort, assist with delivery, provide emotional support, promote bonding, perform client teaching, and care for the client's family. However, when caring for a high-risk client, the nurse must be prepared to respond to intrapartal emergencies and may need to approach the usual labor and delivery tasks differently and modify normal intrapartal care.

Nursing care in high-risk obstetrics requires advanced nursing knowledge and skills. The nurse must be prepared to participate as an integral member of the perinatal team and work closely with the physician to achieve optimal outcomes. For example, nursing care for the intrapartal client with cardiac disease may require a one-to-one nurse-client ratio. Care for the intrapartal diabetic client focuses on maintenance of euglycemia (normal blood glucose levels) and prevention and identification of fetal distress. For an infected client, intrapartal care calls for prompt, aggressive medical treatment of the infection and planning for immediate care of the neonate to help prevent illness. For a client with PIH, care demands skills and expertise that seek

---

NURSING DIAGNOSES

High-risk intrapartal clients

The following nursing diagnoses address representative problems and etiologies that a nurse may encounter when providing care for a high-risk intrapartal client. Specific nursing interventions for many of these diagnoses are provided in the "Planning and implementation" section of this chapter.

AGE-RELATED CONCERNS	SUBSTANCE ABUSE
• Body image disturbance related to labor and delivery • Decisional conflict related to offering the neonate for adoption • Fear related to labor and delivery • Fear related to lack of control during labor and delivery • Knowledge deficit related to labor and delivery • Self-esteem disturbance related to unexpected cesarean delivery	• Altered nutrition: less than body requirements, related to substance abuse • Fear related to imagined management of labor pain without analgesia • Fear related to removal and loss of neonate by statute • Ineffective individual coping related to lack of family support • Ineffective individual coping related to prospect of prosecution • Knowledge deficit related to infant care • Social isolation related to substance abuse

CARDIAC DISEASE	PREGNANCY-INDUCED HYPERTENSION
• Altered tissue perfusion: cardiopulmonary, related to stress of labor on an abnormal heart • Pain related to labor and delivery	• Altered tissue perfusion: cardiopulmonary, related to elevated blood pressure • Altered tissue perfusion: renal, related to elevated blood pressure • Anxiety related to perinatal outcome • Decreased cardiac output related to vasospasm of PIH • Ineffective family coping: compromised, related to perinatal outcome • Knowledge deficit related to PIH treatments • Potential for injury related to seizures

DIABETES	
• Altered nutrition: less than body requirements, related to increased glucose needs • Anxiety related to high-risk labor and delivery • Fear related to possible congenital malformations from uncontrolled diabetes • Powerlessness related to high-risk condition that threatens maternal and fetal health	

INFECTION	Rh ISOIMMUNIZATION
• Anxiety related to unexpected fetal outcome • Denial related to socially unacceptable infection • Fatigue related to maternal dehydration and exhaustion • Ineffective individual coping related to disruption of bonding • Social isolation related to isolation precautions	• Altered parenting related to the neonate's transfer to the neonatal intensive care unit • Ineffective family coping: compromised, related to lack of opportunity for bonding

---

to detect preeclampsia, prevent eclampsia, and deliver a healthy neonate.

Assess the client and fetus
Although every intrapartal client and fetus should be assessed continuously, the high-risk intrapartal client and fetus may require more frequent or additional types of surveillance, depending on the condition.

Adolescent client. Closely observe the adolescent client for development of PIH, which can be sudden. Pay careful attention to her blood pressure, urine protein levels, degree of edema, and deep tendon reflexes. (For more

information, see "Pregnancy-induced hypertension" later in this section.)

Assess fetal status with intermittent external monitoring so that the adolescent client can get out of bed and be unrestricted, if all parameters are normal. If the client feels threatened by electronic fetal monitoring (EFM), explain that it helps determine her fetus's tolerance of labor. If the fetus shows signs of distress or IUGR, anticipate continuous EFM by internal fetal scalp electrode.

Mature client. Assess vital signs and symptoms to detect impending PIH. Identify evidence of fetal stress by initiating EFM and obtaining a baseline monitor strip. Early detection of fetal distress allows prompt intrapartal treatment.

Cardiac disease. Frequently check the maternal pulse, respirations, and blood pressure, and maintain strict fluid intake and output records, as prescribed. Expect continuous EFM as well as continuous maternal electrocardiogram monitoring; hemodynamic monitoring with an arterial line, central venous pressure, or indwelling pulmonary artery catheter may be ordered as well. Keep resuscitation equipment near the client at all times.

Close observation is particularly important for a client with cardiac disease because she is likely to have a nursing diagnosis of *altered tissue perfusion: cardiopulmonary, related to stress of labor on an abnormal heart* or *altered tissue perfusion: renal, related to intrapartal blood loss.*

Plan to assess the client continuously for at least 24 hours after delivery. Cardiac output increases immediately after delivery, when blood that had been diverted to the uterus reenters the central circulation. A client with cardiac disease who cannot tolerate these postpartal changes may develop decompensation and congestive heart failure. Prompt medical intervention may be required for such a client. Therefore, the nurse must be able to recognize any change and report it immediately to the physician.

Diabetes mellitus. For an intrapartal client with diabetes, expect to observe and report on her fetus, renal and cardiovascular functions, glucose levels, and insulin and glucose infusions.

Assessing the fetus. To detect fetal distress, assess the fetus continuously through EFM and evaluate maternal blood glucose levels hourly. Glucose levels should range from 60 to 100 mg/dl (3.3 to 5.6 mmol/liter). Even short periods of maternal hyperglycemia during labor can lead to neonatal hypoglycemia (Ryan, O'Sullivan, Skylar, and Mintz, 1982).

Assessing renal and cardiovascular functions. If the client has diabetes-related renal disease, anticipate strict recording of her fluid intake and output during labor and delivery. When administering I.V. fluids, expect to use an infusion pump to regulate the exact dosage. Because chronic hypertension usually accompanies renal disease, closely monitor her blood pressure also.

Frequently assess for edema, proteinuria, and hyperactive deep tendon reflexes. Keep in mind that chronic hypertension and PIH are common among diabetics. Carefully evaluate and document these findings. Report abnormal findings promptly to the physician.

A client with a history of cardiovascular complications caused by diabetes requires close cardiac monitoring. Such a client is at high risk for complications and may need follow-up by the critical care team.

Assessing glucose levels and infusions. Expect to check the diabetic client's blood glucose levels carefully during and immediately after the intrapartal period. The physician will attempt to maintain her glucose levels within the target range using a continuous I.V. insulin and glucose regimen. Regimens vary from minimal glucose and no insulin to 5 g of glucose/hour and 1 to 2 units of insulin/hour, adjusted according to hourly glucose levels (Knuppel and Drukker, 1986). Regardless of the insulin regimen used, glucose is necessary to compensate for the energy expenditure of labor (Banerjee, Khew, Saha, and Ratnam, 1971; Jovanovic and Peterson, 1982). Insulin infusion may be needed until delivery of the placenta; glucose, until the client consumes food.

The client who is to have a planned cesarean delivery or induced labor the following morning should be instructed to take nothing by mouth after midnight and to skip her morning dose of insulin.

Check the client's blood glucose levels immediately after delivery and at least every 4 hours thereafter. After the client begins eating, the physician may reinstitute insulin administration when hyperglycemia recurs. The client's antepartal insulin dose serves as a guide to her postpartal dose. Be aware, however, that a lower dose may be prescribed after delivery because of the rapid decline in placental hormones and cortisol, which reduces opposition to insulin.

Infection. Expect to adminster I.V. fluids immediately to improve hydration, reduce fever, and prevent maternal exhaustion (Balgobin, 1987). Use external EFM to avoid further contamination of the fetus. After collecting blood or vaginal cultures to identify the infecting organism, administer I.V. antibiotics, as prescribed. For example, unless contraindicated by the client's allergies, expect to give a broad-spectrum antibiotic combination. Carefully assess maternal and fetal responses to infection treatments during the intrapartal period.

Substance abuse. For a substance abuser, closely assess vital signs for maternal or fetal tachycardia, depressed maternal respirations, and elevated blood pressure.

Pregnancy-induced hypertension. Before delivery, the client must be stabilized and the fetal-placental unit closely monitored. Cardiovascular monitoring with an indwelling pulmonary artery or central venous pressure catheter for the client with severe PIH may be prescribed, especially if she is oliguric. This allows closer monitoring of blood pressure and intravascular volume, which is particularly important with a nursing diagnosis of *altered tissue perfusion: renal, related to elevated blood pressure.*

Determine the client's level of consciousness. As a result of drugs used to treat PIH, she may show depressed vital signs and may sleep between contractions. As long as her respiratory rate is normal, do not be alarmed, but continue to monitor her closely.

The client will require continuous EFM to detect signs of placental insufficiency and evaluate fetal well-being. Keep in mind that the seizures of eclampsia cause maternal hypoxia and can produce fetal bradycardia. After seizures stop, fetal heart rate (FHR) should return to baseline.

Rh isoimmunization. Because abruptio placentae is more common in isoimmunized clients, observe carefully for signs of vaginal bleeding or uterine tetany, such as continuous uterine contractions without relaxation.

During labor, continuous internal EFM with a fetal scalp electrode to monitor FHR and with an intrauterine pressure catheter to monitor uterine contractions may be employed, depending on gestational age and delivery options. Closely observe the FHR for signs of fetal distress or hypoxia. Fetal distress in Rh isoimmunized premature fetuses, especially in the absence of labor, indicates the need for cesarean delivery. Hypoxia may result from placentomegaly, which causes insufficient fetal perfusion. Severe fetal hemolysis may lead to congestive heart failure in the fetus. If an abnormal FHR emerges, expect to assist the physician with fetal scalp sampling to estimate fetal tolerance of labor and to determine if cesarean delivery is required.

Assist in labor management

Expect labor management to be tailored to the high-risk client's needs.

Adolescent client. For an adolescent client, carefully assess labor progress and screen for such problems as uterine dysfunction or labor arrest. The adolescent's immature uterus may have an uncoordinated contraction pattern, and her labor may not progress without augmentation. Because her pelvis may not be fully developed, she may have CPD and a difficult labor.

Mature client. Labor dysfunctions are relatively common in mature clients. Researchers have demonstrated a relationship between advancing maternal age and increasing frequency of labor dysfunctions (Halfar, 1985), labor protraction, and labor arrest (Queenan, Freeman, Niebyl, Resnik, and Simpson, 1987). These dysfunctions may result from decreased efficiency of the aging myometrium or from increased incidence of CPD, uterine leiomyoma, and fetal malposition, such as occiput posterior and occiput transverse (Acker, 1987).

Because of the increased tendency of the mature client to labor dysfunctions, carefully monitor her contraction pattern, which can affect the efficiency of contractions. Also assess fetal position, which can help determine the duration of labor.

If contractions cease and cervical dilation or fetal descent are arrested, anticipate assisting with I.V. fluids, oxytocin (Pitocin) augmentation, and continuous EFM, unless signs of fetal distress or CPD exist. (For more information, see Chapter 33, Intrapartal Complications.)

Cardiac disease. For the client with cardiac disease, keep in mind that maternal position, contractions, and anesthesia can affect cardiovascular status during labor and delivery.

Promote proper positioning for the client with cardiac disease, especially if she has a nursing diagnosis of *altered tissue perfusion: cardiopulmonary, related to stress of labor on an abnormal heart.* She must avoid the supine position because it can increase venous return, stroke volume, and cardiac output and can decrease the heart rate. During labor, encourage use of the lateral recumbent position, which improves cardiac emptying and promotes oxygenation. During delivery, do not elevate the client's legs fully in the lithotomy position because this increases venous return and may overload the heart (Greenspoon, 1988).

Expect to administer antibiotics during labor and delivery to a client with a valvular disorder because of the danger of bacterial endocarditis (Greenspoon, 1988).

Diabetes mellitus. In a client with hydramnios, anticipate a large gush of fluid when the diabetic client's membranes rupture, which can cause umbilical cord prolapse. Be prepared to intervene appropriately. (For more information, see Chapter 33, Intrapartal Complications.)

Substance abuse. Carefully monitor the client's labor progress. Because the substance abuser is at increased risk for precipitous birth, evaluate her labor progress quickly and be prepared for a rapid delivery.

After labor begins, the substance abuser may delay coming to the facility because of fear or may use drugs to ease her labor pains and not realize that delivery is imminent. For these reasons, she is at risk for giving birth outside the facility or en route.

Keep in mind that labor management for a substance abuser is the same as for any other client. Medical management may include early artificial rupture of the membranes. Illicit drug use shortly before delivery increases the risk of fetal distress. Therefore, amniotic fluid must be evaluated for color, such as meconium staining and blood, and quantity. Anticipate continuous EFM to assess fetal well-being.

Pregnancy-induced hypertension. Because a client with eclampsia is likely to be lethargic or semicomatose, she may have a reduced response to uterine contractions. Therefore, expect to monitor her uterine contractions closely, palpating the abdomen frequently.

She may display hypertonic uterine activity and develop vasospasm, which increases the risk of abruptio placentae. A sustained rigid abdomen with severe pain (which the semicomatose client may not notice or report) indicates possible abruptio placentae and must be reported to the physician immediately.

Rh isoimmunization. If the client has hydramnios, her uterine contractions may be inefficient, producing uncoordinated labor patterns with coupling (doubling of inefficient contractions) or hypotonic contractions. For such a client, the physician may rupture the membranes by needling them slowly and carefully. This helps prevent a sudden gush of amniotic fluid, which can cause cord prolapse or vertex malpositioning of the fetus on descent.

Promote comfort
Expect to use nonpharmacologic or pharmacologic comfort measures, as needed, for any intrapartal client. (For more information, see Chapter 26, Comfort Promotion during Labor and Childbirth.) Be aware of the following special considerations for certain high-risk intrapartal clients.

Cardiac disease. For a client with a nursing diagnosis of *pain related to labor and delivery,* keep in mind that labor pains can cause maternal tachycardia and elevate blood pressure, increasing the stress on the heart. Effective analgesia should minimize this effect.

Expect the client to receive regional anesthesia, such as epidural anesthesia, to relieve pain during labor and delivery. Regional anesthesia is particularly useful in a client with cardiac disease because it decreases cardiac output and heart rate and acts as a peripheral vasodilator that reduces venous return to the heart. However, it can cause hypotension, requiring close blood pressure monitoring (Sullivan and Ramanathan, 1985).

Substance abuse. Analgesia for the substance abuser's labor pain will not contribute to her drug problem. However, observe her for interactions between analgesics and illicit drugs. Because the substance abuser commonly is not accompanied by friends or family, provide nonpharmacologic comfort measures and coach her through labor to reduce her feelings of isolation.

Rh isoimmunization. Know that analgesia and anesthesia may be restricted during labor because of fetal immaturity and instability. Be prepared to use nonpharmacologic pain relief measures and to offer labor coaching to the client.

Assist with emergencies
Prepare for and, if necessary, assist with emergencies that may affect the high-risk intrapartal client or her fetus.

Diabetes mellitus. In a client with insulin-dependent diabetes mellitus, poorly controlled blood glucose levels and insulin deficiency can lead to DKA, which can cause intrauterine fetal death (Knuppel and Drukker, 1986). DKA produces maternal acidosis, which causes fetal acidosis and fetal distress. Until prompt treatment restores maternal homeostasis, the client and her fetus will remain in jeopardy. (For more information, see *Emergency alert: Diabetic ketoacidosis.*)

Pregnancy-induced hypertension. A client with PIH always is at risk for eclampsia; prepare to carry out the physician's orders for management. About 5% of clients with preeclampsia develop eclampsia, which is characterized by seizures (Sibai, Lipshitz, and Anderson, 1981). Most seizures occur during the intrapartal period and the first 48 hours of the postpartal period, suggesting that these are the periods in which preeclampsia is most likely to develop into eclampsia (Roberts, 1989). The number of seizures a client experiences can vary from 1 to 20.

Clients most at risk for seizures are those who have not received adequate prenatal care and those with unrecognized PIH of increasing severity. However, no specific signs and symptoms can be used to predict the development of seizures (Sibai, Lipshitz, and Anderson, 1981). Therefore, treatment of all clients with preeclampsia is based on concerns for the few who may develop eclampsia.

For any client with PIH, nursing care includes taking seizure precautions, assisting with prevention or treatment of seizures, and assessing maternal and fetal response to treatment and related disorders.

Taking seizure precautions. To avoid general injury to the client, pad the side rails of her bed. This precaution is particularly important for a client with a nursing diagnosis of *potential for injury related to seizures.* (Never use a padded tongue depressor to keep the client from biting her tongue during a seizure—it is ineffective and may cause further injuries.)

If necessary, establish an airway and administer oxygen. To prevent aspiration of secretions, position the client on her side. If she is oliguric, position her on her left side to increase urine excretion and uterine perfusion.

To reduce the nervous system irritability that usually precipitates seizures, dim the lights and reduce unnecessary noise. Organize care to avoid frequent disturbances. Keep the number of people at her bedside to a minimum, but allow a family member to remain with her. This may help reduce her anxiety and help keep the family informed and involved in her care.

Assisting with prevention or treatment of seizures. Magnesium sulfate ($MgSO_4$) is the treatment of choice for seizures because it is effective and relatively safe, although it can be toxic for the client and fetus. It depresses neuromuscular transmission, which diminishes hyperactive reflexes and prevents seizures. It also reduces cerebral edema and intracranial pressure, which cause mild vasodilation.

Expect to administer $MgSO_4$ I.V. or I.M. For I.V. use, initially give 4 g in a 20% solution slowly over 20 minutes. (To treat seizures, expect to administer 4 g of $MgSO_4$ I.V. over 20 minutes [Knupple and Drukker, 1986].) Follow this I.V. bolus infusion with continuous I.V. infusion of 1 to 2 g/hour, as prescribed.

Although rarely prescribed, $MgSO_4$ may be given I.M. using a deep, Z-track injection in the upper outer quadrant of the buttocks with a 3″, 20G needle. Administer the I.M. loading dose of 5 g injected into each buttock, followed by 5 g every 4 hours in alternating gluteal muscles. If more than 6 hours elapse between doses, expect to give the loading dose again.

Assessing maternal and fetal response to treatment. The therapeutic blood level of $MgSO_4$ is 2.5 to 7.5 mEq/liter; signs of toxicity may appear when the level exceeds 7 mEq/liter (Hayashi, 1986). Monitor the client closely to detect signs of $MgSO_4$ toxicity, such as hypotension, respiratory paralysis, and reduced reflexes. Assess the patellar reflex or, if the client has received epidural anesthesia, the biceps reflex. (Epidural anesthesia may depress the patellar reflex.) Alert the physician if the reflex is absent. Loss of the patellar or other deep tendon reflex may indicate that $MgSO_4$ is approaching toxic levels. However, because this can occur with concentrations lower than the therapeutic level, $MgSO_4$ therapy is not based solely on this observation. At best, the patellar reflex is a gross measure of plasma concentration. Monitor and document deep tendon reflexes every hour for the client receiving $MgSO_4$.

Monitor and document the client's respiratory rate every 15 minutes, and inform the physician if the respiratory rate is depressed. Also note a urine output of less than 25 ml/hour. $MgSO_4$ is excreted by the kidneys, and any renal impairment may lead to magnesium retention and toxicity. Monitor the client's fluid intake and

---

EMERGENCY ALERT

Diabetic ketoacidosis

For a client with diabetes, the stress of labor can trigger ketoacidosis. This form of acidosis is accompanied by ketone accumulation in the blood and can lead to coma and death if not treated promptly. It also can compromise the fetus.

The following chart will help the nurse identify the signs and symptoms of diabetic ketoacidosis and prepare to intervene or assist appropriately. Keep in mind that correction of maternal diabetic ketoacidosis (DKA) should reverse fetal compromise.

SIGNS AND SYMPTOMS

- Hyperglycemia and ketonuria
- Signs of dehydration, such as poor skin turgor, flushed dry skin, oliguria, and confusion
- Hypotension
- Deep, rapid respirations
- Decreased level of consciousness, possibly leading to coma
- Fruity or acetone-like breath odor
- Nausea and vomiting

NURSING CONSIDERATIONS

- Confirm DKA by obtaining arterial blood gas (ABG) levels, as prescribed; using a reagent strip to evaluate the client's urine for ketones; using a reflectometer to monitor blood for a glucose test; and sending for baseline laboratory studies, such as electrolyte and serum blood glucose levels.
- Summon health care team members, including the obstetrician, diabetologist, and internist.
- Record hourly fluid intake and output on a flowsheet.
- Document blood glucose and urine acetone levels, laboratory test results for ABG levels and electrolyte studies, maternal vital signs, and fetal heart rate (FHR)
- Start an I.V. line with an isotonic solution, such as normal saline solution, as prescribed.
- Monitor the client's cardiac status with a bedside ECG monitor, if possible. On an ECG strip, hyperkalemia may produce small P waves, a prolonged PR interval, widened QRS complex, and tall peaked T waves. It can precipitate cardiac arrhythmias and typically occurs in DKA when potassium is pulled from cells into the blood. Attempt to maintain serum potassium in the 4 to 5 mEq/liter range. Expect to draw blood to check serum potassium levels every hour.
- Administer short-acting regular insulin, as prescribed. Before administering insulin, however, ensure that fluid replacement has been initiated.
- Monitory blood glucose levels every hour.
- Administer I.V. glucose only after the client's blood glucose level is at 150 to 200 mg.
- Assess the FHR and variability continuously.

output every hour. Carefully measure and document urine output each hour and before administering a dose of $MgSO_4$. Expect to insert an indwelling urinary catheter for accurate monitoring.

Because $MgSO_4$ is not an antihypertensive drug, expect to continue to monitor the client's blood pressure closely, and record these measurements every 15 minutes. If the blood pressure remains significantly elevated, expect to give a drug such as hydralazine (Apresoline) to control hypertension.

Several drugs may be used in combination to lower blood pressure, induce or augment uterine contractions, and relieve pain. Monitor the client's response to this multiple drug therapy to assess its effectiveness and detect any adverse reactions.

Keep calcium gluconate at the client's bedside in case of $MgSO_4$ overdose. As prescribed, administer 1 g of calcium gluconate in 10 ml of a 10% solution I.V. over 3 minutes.

Expect to continue administering $MgSO_4$ throughout labor and delivery and for at least 24 hours afterward. Document the infusion dosage so that the recovery nurse can continue therapy properly.

Fetal levels of $MgSO_4$ correlate with maternal blood levels. Anticipate continuous fetal monitoring during the intrapartal period. Be aware that $MgSO_4$ therapy may cause a transient loss in beat-to-beat variability with internal fetal monitoring.

Assessing for related complications. A small percentage of clients with eclampsia develop pulmonary edema with a nursing diagnosis of *altered tissue perfusion: cardiopulmonary, related to elevated blood pressure.* To detect this complication, auscultate the client's lungs at least every half hour and monitor her fluid intake and output at least every hour.

According to Roberts (1989), about 20% of clients with PIH are at increased risk for disseminated intravascular coagulation (DIC). Therefore, expect to obtain specimens for clotting studies, and carefully observe all orifices and puncture sites for increased serosanguinous drainage. Report any abnormal findings immediately. If the client shows signs of DIC and spontaneous hemorrhage, prepare for expeditious vaginal or cesarean delivery.

Assist with delivery

A high-risk intrapartal client may have a vaginal or cesarean delivery, depending on her condition and that of her fetus.

Adolescent client. Provide anticipatory guidance for an adolescent client to reduce her anxiety and address a nursing diagnosis of *fear related to labor and delivery.*

To gain her cooperation and reduce her fears, tell her what the delivery room looks like, how she will be positioned, and what she will be asked to do. Answer her questions as simply as possible.

Mature client. For a healthy mature client with no detectable intrapartal risks, expect a vaginal delivery. If labor dysfunction occurs or CPD is identified, prepare for a cesarean delivery, as prescribed.

Kirz, Dorchester, and Freeman (1985) found that mature clients are more likely to need cesarean delivery, although the reasons for them remain unclear. They also found an increased tendency to use epidural anesthesia, which could account for some labor dysfunction.

Kirz, Dorchester, and Freeman (1985) also documented an increased incidence of vacuum extractor and forceps deliveries among mature clients. This could result from decreased efficiency of the aging myometrium, decreased maternal stamina, and increased use of epidural anesthesia.

Anticipate the complications that may arise in the labor and delivery area. If the client has had oxytocin augmentation after a difficult labor, postpartal hemorrhage related to uterine atony may occur. Alert the neonatal team to attend an imminent delivery if assessments suggest neonatal abnormality.

Cardiac disease. During the second stage of labor, bearing down can reduce venous blood flow to the heart by increasing intrathoracic pressure. When the client stops bearing down, cardiac output and blood pressure increase rapidly. Therefore, instruct the client to avoid bearing down in the second stage or expect the physician to use epidural anesthesia, which eliminates the bearing down reflex. After the cervix is dilated fully, labor should progress naturally through the second stage. Uterine contractions usually produce fetal descent; the physician allows it to proceed unless labor continuation would jeopardize the client or her fetus. Keep in mind that some physicians prefer to shorten the second stage by using low forceps or vacuum extraction (Greenspoon, 1988).

If the client with cardiac disease delivers vaginally, expect her blood volume to be redirected to central circulation and cardiac output to increase dramatically. Monitor her closely and observe for abrupt changes in cardiac status.

For a client who undergoes a planned cesarean delivery, expect a blood loss of about 1,000 ml, causing a temporary decrease in cardiac output and blood pressure (Greenspoon, 1988). This client has a nursing diagnosis of *decreased cardiac output related to intrapartal blood loss.*

Prepare for acute neonatal problems because the neonate of a client with cardiac disease has an increased risk of morbidity and mortality. A client with congenital heart disease has an increased risk of giving birth to a neonate with congenital heart disease. Antepartal maternal cyanosis is associated with preterm labor, resulting in LBW or a premature neonate. Maternal cyanosis and tachycardia also may cause hypoxia and fetal death. Keep the neonatal team advised and alert them when birth is imminent so that they can be present in the delivery room (Ueland, 1989).

Diabetes mellitus. If the diabetic client has controlled blood glucose levels during pregnancy and shows no signs of placental insufficiency, anticipate a vaginal delivery after the onset of spontaneous labor. Vaginal delivery at term is preferred with a normal L/S ratio and PG level, indicating fetal lung maturity, and if the fetus shows no evidence of macrosomia or compromise.

Anticipate a difficult delivery if the fetus has macrosomia because it can cause shoulder dystocia and lead to maternal and neonatal birth trauma. If the client experienced a difficult delivery, she may have vaginal and perineal lacerations and excessive postpartal bleeding.

If fetal distress or maternal problems occur, assist with a cesarean delivery if needed. The delivery should be planned carefully to minimize maternal and neonatal morbidity and mortality; the neonatal team should be present at the delivery. (For more information, see *Indications for planned delivery for the diabetic client*, page 757.)

A heel stick of the neonate to obtain a blood sample for glucose testing may be performed in the delivery area. During the intrapartal period, maternal hyperglycemia may lead to neonatal hyperinsulinism and hypoglycemia, causing a rapid drop in the blood glucose level in the first 30 to 60 minutes after birth. Neonatal hypoglycemia may be asymptomatic or produce such signs as twitching, jitteriness, hypotonia, apnea, and seizures. If hypoglycemia is detected, keep the neonate warm until treatment (such as dextrose and water feeding or I.V. glucose therapy) can begin, probably in the neonatal intensive care unit.

Infection. Once an intrapartal bacterial infection is identified, labor induction or augmentation with oxytocin may be prescribed to shorten the diagnosis-to-delivery time to less than 12 hours (Balgobin, 1987). The number of vaginal examinations should be limited and amniotomy should be avoided. Provide meticulous perineal care. Anticipate spontaneous vaginal delivery, depending on the severity of the infection and the maternal and fetal tolerance to labor.

Expect to avoid cesarean delivery in the infected client because it increases the risk of maternal morbidity and postpartal endometritis five- to ten-fold (Balgobin, 1987). However, if the client has active lesions from herpes simplex virus (HSV) infection or has had an HSV genital infection up to 2 weeks before delivery, anticipate a cesarean delivery (if her amniotic membranes have not ruptured). If PROM occurs 4 to 6 hours before the client is admitted, anticipate a cesarean delivery to prevent the fetus from coming into contact with lesions in an infected birth canal.

When anticipating delivery for an infected client, summon the neonatal team so that they are ready for the potentially ill neonate. The neonate may be premature and at increased risk for sepsis; lung maturity problems, such as respiratory distress syndrome, also are likely. If the client received adequate antibiotics for sepsis during labor, the neonate is less likely to have respiratory depression at birth; if not, the neonate may require resuscitation.

Coordinate family care and communicate all pertinent information to the nursery and postpartal teams. After delivery, collect specimens for culture from the mother, neonate, and possibly the placenta, and send them to the laboratory, as prescribed. These cultures may reveal previously undetected infection in the mother and infection transmission to the neonate.

Substance abuse. Work closely with the neonatal team to ensure continuity of care. The neonate of a substance abuser is at increased risk for congenital malformations, prematurity, and IUGR. About two-thirds of neonates born to heroin or methadone users are born with withdrawal symptoms; cocaine-dependent neonates commonly experience painful withdrawal symptoms that may last up to 3 weeks (Landry and Smith, 1987). Anticipate the need for a neonatologist or pediatrician at delivery because the neonate may require resuscitation and intubation.

Pregnancy-induced hypertension. Although PIH resolves shortly after delivery, delivery usually is not desirable until the fetus reaches sufficient maturity. However, delivery will be mandatory in a client whose blood pressure cannot be controlled, whose weight gain (from edema) continues despite bed rest, and whose proteinuria increases. In such a client, delivery is justified even when the estimated gestational age falls below 30 weeks (Knupple and Drukker, 1986).

In an unstable client, cesarean delivery is undesirable because it could contribute to maternal stress and complications. Ideally, the fetal-placental unit is monitored closely, the client is stabilized and monitored closely, and she delivers vaginally.

After the client is stabilized, prepare for vaginal or cesarean delivery, depending on her condition and physician management. Ideally, she would deliver vaginally to avoid the complications of surgery. If the cervix is likely to respond to oxytocin—that is, if it is soft, open, and not posterior in position—and the client and fetus are stable, induced vaginal delivery is preferred. If assessments reveal fetal distress or an estimated fetal weight of less than 1,500 g, cesarean delivery is preferred.

As a result of the stress of PIH, the client may have a shorter labor and a precipitous delivery. Prepare to intervene quickly for such a client.

Alert the neonatal team to be present for delivery, especially if the neonate is premature, which is common in clients with severe preeclampsia. Work with the neonatal team and prepare for care of the neonate.

If the client received $MgSO_4$ during labor, prepare for potential neonatal effects. $MgSO_4$ toxicity may occur in the neonate, producing respiratory depression, hypotonia, and hypotension (Knupple and Drukker, 1986).

Rh isoimmunization. Usually, the isoimmunized client and her physician plan her admission for labor and delivery, preferably in a tertiary care facility that is equipped for intensive care of high-risk neonates. Most experts recommend delivery by 38 weeks' gestation (Queenan, 1985). The results of fetal lung maturity studies, such as L/S ratio and PG level, typically guide plans for delivery. To enhance lung maturity and extrauterine adaptation, the extremely premature fetus may receive glucocorticosteroids and intrauterine blood transfusions before delivery.

Anticipate the labor management and delivery route based on the usual obstetric concerns for a compromised, premature neonate. Expect a vaginal delivery for a fetus in vertex presentation at greater than 35 weeks' gestation. If the cervix is favorable, a trial oxytocin induction may be attempted. Prepare for the probability of a cesarean delivery if the fetus is in a malpresentation (breech) position or is at less than 34 weeks' gestation, if the cervix is unfavorable for induced labor, or if assessment reveals signs of fetal distress. This isoimmunized premature neonate does not tolerate labor well because of severe anemia and decreased oxygenation.

Help coordinate the obstetric and neonatal teams during delivery. If the neonate is affected severely, anticipate resuscitative efforts in the first minutes after delivery.

Provide emotional support

When providing emotional support for a high-risk intrapartal client, plan to deal with specific concerns that may be related to the underlying condition.

Adolescent client. During labor, an adolescent client can become demanding if she fears abandonment and isolation. She may want and need constant support. She may bite, pinch, or cling to the nurse, especially during pelvic examinations. These actions are common in a client with a nursing diagnosis of *fear related to labor and delivery.*

To help the client regain her composure, set limits and maintain a calm, confident approach. Also provide clear directions and descriptions. Elicit the help of her partner or a family member to provide support. Keep in mind, however, that an adolescent client may act out expected roles to gain her family's attention and become more hyperactive and helpless when they are present.

To enhance her coping ability, remain nonjudgmental and provide constant, positive encouragement about her progress and behavior. Direct her primary support person to provide comfort measures and labor coaching to help her through childbirth so that she may recall this event as an accomplishment.

To promote a positive childbirth experience for the adolescent client, emphasize the normality of her experience and promote bonding, which ultimately may enhance the mother-infant relationship.

Throughout labor and delivery, provide supportive coaching and encouragement. Make every effort to decrease the drama and enhance the intimacy and joy of the experience. A client who fears trauma and mutilation from giving birth may have a nursing diagnosis of *knowledge deficit related to labor and delivery.* Such a client may benefit from encouragement to "push the baby out so you can hold the baby in your arms." If the client expresses concern that her body will never be the same and has a nursing diagnosis of *body image disturbance related to labor and delivery,* provide reassurance by explaining what she can expect as she goes through the postpartal period.

Mature client. Involve the mature client and her partner in decisions about her care. This will enhance their sense of autonomy, promote self-esteem, and allow them a greater sense of control. It also may prevent a nursing diagnosis of *fear related to lack of control during labor and delivery.*

If the client and her partner anticipated vaginal delivery but must have cesarean delivery, help them prepare for—and begin to accept—this sudden change in birth plans. Be aware that they may experience loss, grief, anxiety, guilt, feelings of noncontrol, and fear. The client may feel cheated of her anticipated vaginal delivery (Leach and Sproule, 1984). Her partner may experience sadness, apprehension, confusion, and helplessness (Fawcett and Burritt, 1985).

Cardiac disease. For a client with cardiac disease, provide emotional support to relieve anxiety. Explain labor and delivery and tell her what to expect during each stage. Remain at her bedside not only to monitor her health but also to allay anxiety. Address any psychosocial concerns she may have.

Diabetes mellitus. In a diabetic client, normal anxiety about labor and delivery may be compounded by intrapartal concerns about maternal and neonatal well-being. She may develop a nursing diagnosis of *anxiety related to high-risk labor and delivery* or *powerlessness related to a high-risk condition that threatens maternal and fetal health.* The client's anxieties can affect her metabolism and blood glucose levels. To help such a client, provide information and reassurance about her labor status. Answer her questions and offer emotional support.

A diabetic client is likely to be aware of the neonatal risks. During the intrapartal period, all of her fears and concerns may surface as delivery becomes imminent. Because ultrasonography and other tests cannot detect all fetal abnormalities, be prepared for delivery of a neonate with congenital malformations even if the client had normal prenatal test results. Provide support during this period.

Infection. An intrapartal client with an infection will need emotional support because of anxiety for herself and her neonate. If her infection requires isolation precautions, she also may feel isolated or dehumanized because the health care team must wear gowns, gloves, and masks. She may have a nursing diagnosis of *anxiety related to unexpected fetal outcome* or *social isolation related to isolation precautions.* For such a client, provide emotional support and reassurance.

If she has an active HSV infection, she and her partner may be concerned about cesarean delivery and the chance of having a neonate with a potentially fatal infection. While preparing the client for cesarean delivery, provide reassurance and teach her and her partner about the virus and the rationale for surgery.

Also be aware that the client and her partner may harbor guilt, resentment, or embarrassment because of the stigma of this STD. Reassure the client that only the staff responsible for her care will be aware of her diagnosis. The client may invent another, less emotionally charged, reason for cesarean delivery, such as persistent breech or slow labor progress, so that others are not aware of the HSV infection. Such a client may have a nursing diagnosis of *denial related to socially unacceptable infection.* If so, maintain her confidentiality and respect her preferences.

For any client with an infection, explain the disorder and its ramifications, which may include separating her

Indications for planned delivery for the diabetic client

For a diabetic client, the following assessment findings may uncover the need for a planned delivery. Depending on the severity of these findings and the client's condition, planned delivery may include an induced vaginal delivery or a cesarean delivery.

- Fetal distress
- Signs of intrauterine growth retardation, such as inadequate fundal height and abnormal findings on ultrasonography
- Estimated gestation duration greater than 42 weeks
- Pregnancy-induced hypertension
- Signs of markedly failing renal function, such as decreasing urine output
- Macrosomia with a fetus greater than 4,000 g

from her neonate at birth. If so, encourage her to express her frustration and sadness at this prospect (Knupple and Drukker, 1986). This may help prevent a nursing diagnosis of *ineffective individual coping related to disruption of bonding.*

Substance abuse. The substance abuser who is aware of child protection laws may fear prosecution or worry that her neonate will be taken from her. She may have a nursing diagnosis of *ineffective individual coping related to prospect of prosecution* or *fear related to removal and loss of neonate by statute.* If so, try to understand her fears and the difficulty of her decision to seek intrapartal care at the health care facility. Express acceptance of and patience with the client.

The substance abuser who gives birth without the support of her family or friends may have a nursing diagnosis of *social isolation related to substance abuse* or *ineffective individual coping related to lack of family support.* If so, stay with her as much as possible, coach her through labor, and provide reassurance and support.

Rh isoimmunization. Be sensitive to the anxieties and concerns of the isoimmunized client as she faces the birth of a potentially sick, preterm neonate. Technologically advanced antepartal testing may have heightened the client's fears about her neonate's safety. She may be concerned about her neonate's precarious future and may experience a loss of control over the birth if it occurs rapidly and unexpectedly.

The isoimmunized client and her partner may be coping with the transfer of her care from her choice of health care provider and facility to a tertiary care center, which can seem overwhelming and impersonal. If the client is multiparous, she may dwell on previous experiences with Rh isoimmunization. To assist her and her partner, provide attentive care, clear information, and honest reassurance that everything possible is being done to facilitate the safe birth of a healthy neonate.

Promote bonding

For all intrapartal clients, promote maternal-infant bonding, beginning immediately after birth. For certain high-risk intrapartal clients, be aware of the following nursing considerations.

Adolescent client. The adolescent's experience of labor and delivery affects her bonding with her neonate. To promote bonding, express acceptance of, provide support to, and convey respect for the adolescent client.

Adolescents seldom relinquish their neonates for adoption (Brucker and Muellner, 1985). However, if the client chooses to do so, be sure to give her time with her neonate immediately after birth. This brief transition period helps the client begin grieving and allows her to say goodbye to her neonate. It may help her resolve a nursing diagnosis of *decisional conflict related to offering the neonate for adoption.* It also may help her understand her accomplishment as a woman, her ability to manage labor, and her success. This fosters maternal bonding with the neonate and may affect her enjoyment of relationships with future children (Mercer, 1987).

Mature client. Provide opportunities for bonding, which is especially important for the mature client and her family. Because they may have worried and wondered about this neonate, they need reassurance that their child is healthy or anticipatory guidance if the child is not. When promoting bonding, remember to act as the client's advocate and promote family-centered care.

Substance abuse. State laws and social service representatives may determine if the substance abuser can take her neonate home. While her home environment is being evaluated, promote bonding and offer information about the neonate's needs. To help foster early bonding, follow these guidelines:
• Accept the client's condition in a nonjudgmental manner.
• Offer information about the neonate's condition.
• Explain facility policies briefly and directly.
• Encourage contact, such as holding the neonate after birth and planning for nursery visits.

Rh isoimmunization. The isoimmunized client and her partner may not have an opportunity to bond with the neonate immediately after birth. If the client is Rh-negative and has been sensitized, they may have a nursing diagnosis of *altered parenting related to the neonate's transfer to intensive care* or *ineffective family coping: compromised, related to lack of opportunity for bonding.* If so, communicate the need for the client's postpartal follow-up and the potential need for Rh-immunoglobulin, if indicated. Encourage the client's partner to follow the neonate to the intensive care unit to promote bonding, if desired.

Perform client teaching

As needed, provide the high-risk client with appropriate information related to her condition and concerns.

Substance abuse. To establish a safe, healthy environment for the neonate, teach the client about neonatal care, beginning in the delivery area. This is particularly important for a substance abuser with a nursing diagnosis of *knowledge deficit related to infant care.*

Early in the postpartal period, begin to teach her about health promotion. For example, if she has a nursing diagnosis of *altered nutrition: less than body requirements, related to substance abuse,* teach her how to eat a well-balanced diet and obtain low-cost foods that meet her nutritional needs. Arrange appropriate referrrals (for example, to the social worker) to assist her in admission to a drug rehabilitation facility.

Pregnancy-induced hypertension. Briefly explain PIH to help the client understand the need for certain limitations, such as bed rest and possible fluid restrictions and strict adherence to the prescribed treatment. Clear explanations also help allay fears and anxieties, which may produce stress that could increase vasoconstriction. This is particularly important for a client with a nursing diagnosis of *anxiety related to perinatal outcome* or *knowledge deficit related to PIH treatments.*

Care for the family

The family of the high-risk intrapartal client is likely to be very concerned about her and the fetus or neonate. To help them cope with this stressful event, provide sensitive nursing care that is adapted to their needs. (For more information, see *Family care: High-risk intrapartal clients.*)

Cardiac disease. Because the potential for death during childbirth is increased for the client with cardiac disease, her family may feel especially distressed. Therefore, make sure that her family receives constant information and updates about her status, particularly if she is in an intensive care unit and they cannot remain at her bedside.

Pregnancy-induced hypertension. Keep the client and her family informed about all treatments, especially if they have a nursing diagnosis of *ineffective family coping: compromised, related to perinatal outcome.* Because PIH requires administration of various drugs and close monitoring with many machines, it can be frightening for the client and her family.

Evaluation

During the final step of the nursing process, the nurse evaluates the effectiveness of nursing care. The nurse should state all evaluations in terms of actions performed or outcomes achieved for each goal. The following examples illustrate appropriate evaluation statements.

Adolescent client
• The client had an uneventful labor and delivery free of complications.
• The client expressed satisfaction with her decision to keep her neonate or to give up her neonate for adoption.
• The client reported positive feelings and a sense of accomplishment related to her childbirth experience.

Mature client
• The client had an uneventful labor and delivery without complications.
• The client and her partner and family regularly received information about labor progress and fetal status.
• The client began bonding with her neonate immediately after delivery.

Cardiac disease
• The client assumed labor positions that supported cardiac function.
• The client and her partner and family regularly received information about maternal and fetal status.
• The client delivered successfully without further maternal or neonatal complications.

Diabetes mellitus
• The client's blood glucose levels remained within acceptable limits.
• The client displayed no signs of hypoglycemia or hyperglycemia.
• The client delivered a stable neonate.
• The client experienced spontaneous labor at term.
• The client and her family regularly received information about maternal, fetal, and neonatal status.

Infection
• The client verbalized an understanding of the need for infection control techniques.

FAMILY CARE

High-risk intrapartal clients

The family of a high-risk intrapartal client is likely to experience extreme anxiety for her and her fetus during the intrapartal period. Family members may feel left out, isolated from the client, and intimidated by the setting, equipment, and staff. If they focus on the gravity of the client's condition, they may lose sight of the impending celebration of birth.

To help reduce anxiety for the client's family (which may help reduce her anxiety as well), the nurse should be sensitive to their concerns and include a family member in her care if the client chooses. When providing family-centered care, the nurse might use the following interventions.

• Encourage the family member's presence at the client's bedside for reassurance.
• Encourage the family member to use touch or massage to reduce the client's discomfort and anxiety.
• Teach the family member to help the client with relaxation and breathing techniques.
• Instruct the family member to promote comfort by applying a cool cloth to the client's brow or by providing mouth care.
• Allow the family member to fan the client, as needed.
• Keep other family members informed of the client's progress and provide reassurance to them.
• Explain unfamiliar equipment and procedures and the reasons for their use.
• Discuss choices about positioning, analgesia, and anesthesia with the client and family member.
• Clarify and interpret the prescribed treatment for the family, as needed.
• Discuss impending vaginal or cesarean delivery with the client and family member.
• Encourage the family member to take frequent breaks from the bedside to prevent fatigue.
• Incorporate the family's cultural preferences into the care plan whenever possible.
• Attempt to establish realistic childbirth goals with the client and her family. Support their decisions about care.

• The client's family expressed support and concern for the client.
• The client safely delivered a stable neonate.

Substance abuse
• The client received analgesia to relieve labor pain.
• The client expressed an understanding of her labor progress.
• The client demonstrated signs of bonding with her neonate by holding him and gazing at him after birth.

APPLYING THE NURSING PROCESS

Client with altered tissue perfusion: cardiopulmonary, related to vasospasm and elevated blood pressure

The nursing process helps ensure high-quality care for the high-risk intrapartal client. The table below shows how the nurse might use the nursing process when caring for the client described in the case history at right. The first column presents history and physical assessment data followed by a paragraph of mental notes. These notes help the nurse make important mental connections among assessment findings, aiding in development of the nursing diagnosis and planning.

The second column lists an appropriate nursing diagnosis; information in the remaining columns is based on this diagnosis. Although not part of the nursing process, a rationale appears for each intervention in the fourth column to explain how it contributes to the care plan.

ASSESSMENT	NURSING DIAGNOSIS	PLANNING
Subjective (history) data • Client states, "My contractions have been coming every 3 to 4 minutes for the past 2 hours." • Client complains of a severe headache accompanied by vision changes. • Client's prenatal records indicate no unusual medical or family history. • Client states that she has had a normal pregnancy. **Objective (physical) data** • Current vital signs: temperature 98.6° F, pulse 88 beats/minute, respirations 20/minute, blood pressure 140/86 mm Hg. • Prenatal vital signs (from prenatal records): temperature 98.6° F, pulse 88 beats/minute, respirations 20/minute, blood pressure 110/60 mm Hg. • 2+ pitting edema of pretibial area; edematous face and hands. • Brisk deep tendon reflexes (3+; 2 beat clonus evident). • Fundal height of 33 cm. • Estimated fetal weight of 6 to 6½ lbs. • Fetal heart tones within normal limits. • Pelvic examination: 5 to 6 cm cervical dilation, 80% effacement, 0 station. • 2+ proteinuria on a clean-catch urine specimen. **Mental notes** *The client's current blood pressure is much higher than her prenatal baseline measurement of 110/60 mm Hg. Together with headache, edema, 3+ reflexes, and proteinuria, assessment findings suggest pregnancy-induced hypertension (PIH), which may decrease tissue perfusion and endanger the client and her fetus.*	Altered tissue perfusion: cardiopulmonary, related to vasospasm and elevated blood pressure	**Goals:** Upon evaluation, the client will: • have a stable blood pressure • not develop seizures • exhibit normal deep tendon reflexes • display normal fluid balance. Upon evaluation, the fetus will: • have a stable heart rate and normal variability.

Pregnancy-induced hypertension

• The client's blood pressure was stabilized.
• The client's fluid intake and output were balanced.
• The client delivered a stable neonate.
• The client did not develop seizures.
• The client and her neonate remained free of further complications.

Rh isoimmunization

• The client expressed an accurate understanding of her condition and that of her fetus.
• The client delivered a stable neonate.

Documentation

Based on initial and ongoing assessment findings, the nurse uses the nursing process to formulate nursing diagnoses and then plans, implements, and evaluates the client's care. (For a case study that shows how to apply the nursing process when caring for a high-risk intrapartal client, see *Applying the nursing process: Client with altered tissue perfusion: cardiopulmonary, related to vasospasm and elevated blood pressure.*)

Be sure to document assessment findings and nursing activities thoroughly and objectively. Record

CASE STUDY

Mary Bradley, a married, primigravid client age 32, comes to the hospital for admission to the labor and delivery area. She is at 37 weeks' gestation and reports increasing contractions.

IMPLEMENTATION		EVALUATION
Intervention	**Rationale**	Upon evaluation, the client:
Monitor the client's vital signs every 15 minutes.	Frequent assessments can detect increasing blood pressure early.	• had a stable blood pressure of 130/80 mm Hg
Position the client in the left lateral position.	This position enhances placental perfusion and fetal oxygenation.	• remained free of seizures • exhibited normal deep tendon reflexes without clonus
Take seizure precautions.	Precautionary measures help protect the client from injury if seizures occur.	• had adequate fluid intake and output.
Monitor fetal status with continuous electronic fetal monitoring (EFM).	Continuous EFM allows rapid identification of fetal distress, which may be caused by insufficient placental perfusion associated with the vasospasm of PIH.	Upon evaluation, the fetus: • had a stable heart rate of 160 beats/minute and normal variability.
Maintain magnesium sulfate I.V. infusion, as prescribed.	This drug decreases vasospasm and hyperactive reflexes associated with PIH.	
Assess deep tendon reflexes and check for clonus regularly.	These assessments evaluate the effectiveness of treatment.	
Monitor the client's fluid intake and output hourly.	This allows assessment of kidney functioning, which can be compromised by PIH.	
Promote client comfort by assessing her need for pain relief during labor and providing analgesia.	Pain relief helps reduce blood pressure and may help prevent seizures.	
Keep the client and her family informed about maternal and fetal health status.	Such information may decrease their anxiety and reassure them of maternal and fetal health.	

physician management decisions and how nursing care was accomplished. Record all information required by the health care facility. In addition to documentation of basic information, expect to record specific information for a high-risk intrapartal client.

Age-related concerns
• maternal vital signs
• continuous labor progress
• coping responses during labor

• interactions among the client and support person during labor
• fetal heart rate

Cardiac disease
• maternal vital signs
• fluid intake and output
• pulmonary assessment findings
• fetal heart rate

Diabetes mellitus
• maternal vital signs
• fluid intake and output
• blood glucose levels
• insulin and glucose administration

Infection
• maternal vital signs, especially temperature
• fluid intake and output
• character of vaginal secretions, especially color and odor
• fetal heart rate
• client's physiologic response to necessary treatments
• family's response to, and support of, the client

Substance abuse
• fetal heart rate
• maternal vital signs
• maternal contractions and labor progress
• maternal response to analgesia
• interactions between analgesia and illicit drugs
• signs of mother-infant bonding

Pregnancy-induced hypertension
• maternal vital signs, especially blood pressure measurements
• central venous pressure readings
• respiratory assessment findings
• urine reagent strip results
• deep tendon reflexes
• fetal heart rate
• fluid intake and output
• signs of bleeding
• drugs administered and their effects
• $MgSO_4$ levels, if administered

Rh isoimmunization
• fetal heart rate
• signs of maternal bleeding
• maternal vital signs, especially temperature measurements
• maternal labor pattern

Chapter summary

Chapter 31 discussed various high-risk intrapartal conditions and their effects on nursing care of the intrapartal client. Here are the chapter highlights.

• High-risk intrapartal conditions include age-related concerns for adolescent and mature clients, cardiac disease, diabetes, infection, substance abuse, PIH, and Rh isoimmunization. These conditions can increase maternal, fetal, or neonatal mobidity and mortality during labor and delivery.
• The high-risk intrapartal client faces the stress of childbirth compounded with concerns related to the high-risk condition. Because of this, she and her family are likely to be more anxious about her safety and that of her fetus or neonate.
• Many high-risk intrapartal clients have undergone intense prenatal care and vigilant maternal and fetal surveillance.
• Typically, nursing care of a high-risk intrapartal client requires sophisticated nursing skills. It also requires a sound knowledge of the client's high-risk condition, including its etiology, pathophysiology, anticipated medical management, and effects on the client, fetus, and neonate.
• When caring for a high-risk intrapartal client, the nurse obtains a health history, assists with a physical assessment, and collects laboratory test results as for any client who seeks admission for labor and delivery. In addition, the nurse must make specific assessments and be prepared to notify the physician of significant findings. For example, when obtaining a mature client's health history, the nurse may ask if she received infertility treatments, which can cause multiple gestation and attending risks, such as premature labor, malpresentation, and dystocia. During the physical assessment of a client with cardiac disease, the nurse should be alert for dependent edema and other signs of cardiac decompensation. When testing a diabetic client, the nurse should check blood glucose levels carefully, as prescribed.
• Some nursing interventions for the high-risk intrapartal client resemble those for any other intrapartal client. For example, the nurse must monitor the client and fetus, assess labor progress, promote comfort, prepare for delivery, provide emotional support, promote bonding, perform client teaching, and care for the client's family. In addition, the nurse must be prepared to respond quickly to intrapartal emergencies, such as DKA and eclampsia, and may need to approach the usual tasks differently and modify normal intrapartal care.
• Alterations to usual nursing tasks may result from participation as a member of a high-risk perinatal team. The nurse works closely with the physician when re-

stricting analgesia for an isoimmunized client, preventing or arresting seizures in a client with PIH, isolating an infected client from her neonate, and providing support to a substance abuser who may be afraid that a social service agency will take away her neonate.

• The nurse may need to coordinate the perinatal team and must anticipate the care that will be required for the high-risk intrapartal client and her neonate.

• Documentation is critical to nursing care of the high-risk intrapartal client. In addition to recording basic information required by the health care facility, the nurse should document specific interventions related to the client and her neonate.

Study questions

1. Dorothy Langford, age 38, comes to the labor and delivery area prepared to give birth to her first child. For this high-risk client, which intrapartal risks should the nurse assess for and how?

2. At 7:00 a.m., Patricia Kilgalen, a 31-year-old client who is pregnant with her fourth child, arrives for admission to the labor and delivery area. She reports spontaneous rupture of membranes at 2:00 a.m. She has a history of gestational diabetes and has been monitoring her blood glucose four times a day and injecting herself with 20 units of NPH insulin at bedtime. What are the anticipated nursing actions for this client?

3. Mary Jones, age 23, is admitted to the labor and delivery area in the first stage of labor. She has a history of HSV infection and reports an outbreak of lesions 2 weeks ago. After assessing Ms. Jones, what intrapartal care should the nurse anticipate?

4. During the admission interview, Barbara Fein, age 24, reports that she used cocaine regularly during her pregnancy. How can the nurse promote bonding between Ms. Fein and her neonate? Why is this important?

5. Elena Garcia, age 36, is admitted to the labor and delivery area with a blood pressure of 140/90 mm Hg. The nurse suspects PIH. What else should the nurse assess to confirm this suspicion?

Bibliography

Arias, F. (Ed.). (1984). *High-risk pregnancy and delivery.* St. Louis: Mosby.

Avery, P., and Olson, I. (1987). Expanding the scope of childbirth education to meet the needs of hospitalized, high-risk clients. *JOGNN,* 16(6), 418-421.

Bowes, C., and Bowes, W. (1987). Insults to the fetus. In L. Sonstegard, K. Kowalski, and B. Jennings (Eds.), *Women's health: Volume three, Crisis and illness in childbearing* (pp. 91-102). Philadelphia: Saunders.

Brown, S. (1988). Preventing low birthweight. In H. Wallace, G. Ryan, and A. Oglesby (Eds.), *Maternal and child health practices* (3rd ed.; pp.307-324). Oakland, CA: Third Party Pub.

Clark, A., and Affonso, D. (1979). *Childbearing: A nursing perspective* (2nd ed.). Philadelphia: F.A. Davis.

Cohen, H., Green, J., and Cromblehome, W. (1988). Society of Perinatal Obstetrician Abstract Presentation, Las Vegas, Nevada.

Cohen, W. (1989). Preterm labor. In W. Cohen, D. Acker, and E. Freidman (Eds.), *Management of labor* (2nd ed.; pp. 333-367). Rockville, MD: Aspen.

Cunningham, F., MacDonald, P., and Gant, N. (1989). *Williams obstetrics* (18th ed.). East Norwalk, CT: Appleton & Lange.

Gabbe, S., and Main, D. (1988). Reproductive problems associated with lifestyle, work, and hazards in the workplace. In D. Hollingsworth and R. Resnik (Eds.), *Medical counseling before pregnancy* (pp. 97-122). New York: Churchill-Livingstone.

Galloway, K. (1976). The uncertainty and stress of high-risk pregnancy. *MCN,* 1(5), 294-299.

Gleicher, N. (Ed.). (1985). *Principles of medical therapy in pregnancy.* New York: Plenum Medical Book Co.

Ingardia, C. (1986). Additional medical complications in pregnancy. In R. Knuppel and J. Drukker, *High-risk pregnancy: A team approach* (pp.472-479). Philadelphia: Saunders.

Kemp, V., and Page, C. (1986). The psychosocial impact of a high-risk pregnancy on the family. *JOGNN,* 15(3), 232-236.

Knupple, R., and Drukker, J. (1986). *High-risk pregnancy: A team approach.* Philadelphia: Saunders.

Korones, S. (1986). *High-risk newborn infants* (4th ed.). St. Louis: Mosby.

McRae, M., and Mervyn, F. (1989). Contemporary issues in childbirth. In W. Cohen, D. Acker, and E. Friedman, *Management of labor* (2nd ed.; pp. 535-548.). Rockville, MD: Aspen.

Rochat, R., Koonin, L., Atrash, H., and Jewett, J. (1988) Maternal mortality in the United States: Report from the maternal mortality collaborative. *Obsteterics and Gynecology,* 72(1), 90-97.

Schroeder-Zwelling, E. (1988). The unexpected childbirth experience. In F. Nichols and S. Humenick, *Childbirth education: Practice, research and theory* (pp. 303-318.). Philadelphia: Saunders.

Age-related concerns
Acker, D. (1987). Elderly gravida. In E. Friedman, D. Acker, and B. Sachs (Eds.), *Obstetrical decision making* (2nd ed.; pp. 20-21). Philadelphia: B.C. Decker.

Berkowitz, G., Skovron, M., Lapinski, R., and Berkowitz, R. (1990). Delayed childbearing and the outcome of pregnancy. *New England Journal of Medicine*, 322(10), 659-664.

Brucker, M., and Muellner, M. (1985). Nurse-midwifery care of adolescents. *Journal of Nurse-Midwifery*, 30(5), 277-279.

Calandra, C., Abell, D., and Beischer, N. (1981). Maternal obesity in pregnancy. *Obstetrics and Gynecology*, 57(1), 8-12.

Cohen, W., Newman, L., and Friedman, E. (1980). Risk of labor abnormalities with advancing maternal age. *Obstetrics and Gynecology*, 55(4), 414-416.

Corbett, M., and Meyer, J. (1987). *The adolescent and pregnancy.* Boston: Blackwell Scientific Pubs.

Elster, A. (1984). The effect of maternal age, parity and prenatal care on perinatal outcome in adolescent mothers. *American Journal of Obstetrics and Gynecology*, 149(2), 845-847.

Fawcett, J., and Burritt, J. (1985). An exploratory study of antenatal preparation for cesaeran birth. *JOGNN*, 14(3), 244-230.

Friede, A., Baldwin, W., Rhodes, P., Buehler, J., and Strauss, L. (1988). Older maternal age and infant mortality in the United States. *Obstetrics and Gynecolgy*, 72(2), 152-157.

Halfar, M. (1985). Frequency of labor dysfunction in nulliparas over the age of thirty. *Journal of Nurse-Midwifery*, 30(6), 333-339.

Hollingsworth, D., Kotchen, J., and Felice, M. (1985). Impact of gynecologic age on outcome of adolescent pregnancy. In J. Queenan (Ed.), *Management of high-risk pregnancy.* Oradell, NJ: Medical Economics Books.

Institute of Medicine. (1985). *Preventing low birthweight.* Washington, DC: National Academy Press.

Jennings, B. (1987). Mature childbearing. In L. Sonstegard, K. Kowalski, and B. Jennings (Eds.), *Women's health: Volume three, Crisis and illness in childbearing* (pp. 59-64). Philadelphia: Saunders.

Kirz, D., Dorchester, W., and Freeman, R. (1985). Advanced maternal age: The mature gravida. *American Journal of Obstetrics and Gynecology*, 152(1), 7-12.

Leach, L., and Sproule, V. (1984). Meeting the challenge of cesarean births. *JOGNN*, 13(3), 191-195.

McAnarney, E. (Ed.). (1983) *Premature adolescent pregnancy and parenthood.* Orlando, FL: Grune & Stratton.

Magni, G., Rizzardo, R., and Andreoli, C. (1986). Psychosocial stress and obstetric complications: The need for a comprehensive model. *ACTA Obstetrics et Gynecologica Scandinavica*, 65(3), 273-276.

Mansfield, P. (1986). Reevaluating the medical risks of late childbearing. *Women's Health*, 11(2), 37-60.

Mercer, R. (1987). Adolescent pregnancy. In L. Sonstegard, K. Kowalski, and B. Jennings (Eds.), *Women's health: Volume three, Crisis and illness in childbearing* (pp. 47-58.). Philadelphia: Saunders.

Moore, M. (1989). Recurrent teen pregnancy: Making it less desirable. *MCN*, 14(2), 104-108.

Naeye, R. (1983). Maternal age, obstetric complications and the outcome of pregnancy. *Obstetrics and Gynecology*, 61(2), 210-215.

Oats, J., Abell, D., Andersen, H., and Beischer, N. (1983). Obesity in pregnancy. *Comprehensive Therapy*, 9(4), 51-55.

Queenan, J., Freeman, R., Niebyl, J., Resnik, R., and Simpson, J. (1987). Symposium: Managing pregnancy in patients over 35. *Contemporary Ob/Gyn*, 29(5), 180-198.

Resnik, R. (1988). Pregnancy in women aged 35 years or older. In D. Hollingsworth and R. Resnik (Eds.), *Medical counseling before pregnancy* (pp. 14-18). New York: Churchill Livingstone.

Robinson, B. (1988). Teenage pregnancy from the father's perspective. *American Journal of Orthopsychiatry*, 58(1), 45-51.

Singh, S., Torres, A., and Forrest, J. (1985). The need for prenatal care in the United States from the 1980 National Natality Study. *Family Planning Perspectives*, 17(3), 118-124.

Slap, G., and Schwartz, J. (1989) Risk factors for low birth weight to adolescent mothers. *Journal of Adolescent Health Care*, 10(4), 267-274.

Winick, M. (1989). *Nutrition, pregnancy and early intervention.* Baltimore: Williams & Wilkins.

Winslow, W. (1987a). Gravida over thirty-five years of age. In E. Knor (Ed.), *Decision making in obstetrical nursing* (p. 28.). Philadelphia: B.C. Decker.

Winslow, W. (1987b). First pregnancy after 35: What is the experience? *MCN*, 12(2), 92-96.

Cardiac disease

Anderson, J. (1970). The effect of diuretics in late pregnancy on the newborn infant. *ACTA Paediatra Scandinavia*, 59(6), 659-663.

Greenspoon, J. (1988.) Heart disease in pregnancy. In D. Mishell and P. Brenner (Eds.), *Management of common problems in OB/GYN* (pp. 33-40). Oradell, NJ: Medical Economics.

Hall, J., Pauli, R., and Wilson, K. (1980). Maternal and fetal sequelae of anticoagulation during pregnancy. *American Journal of Medicine*, 68(1), 122-140.

Rubin, P., Butters, L., Clark, E., Summer, D., Phil, D., Belfield, A., Pledger, D., Low, R., and Reid, J. (1984). Obstetrical aspects of the use in pregnancy-associated hypertension of the beta-adrenoceptor against atenolol. *American Journal of Obstetrics and Gynecology*, 150(4), 389.

Samuels, P., and Landon, M. (1986). Medical complications. In S. Gabbe, J. Niebyl, and J. Simpson (Eds.), *Obstetrics: Normal and problem pregnancies* (pp. 856-978.). New York: Churchill Livingstone.

Sullivan, J., and Ramanathan, K. (1985). Management of medical problems in pregnancy: Severe cardiac disease. *New England Journal of Medicine*, 313(5), 304-309.

Ueland, K. (1989). Cardiac disease. In R. Creasy and R. Resnik (Eds.), *Maternal-fetal medicine: Principles and practice* (2nd ed.; pp. 746-762.). Philadelphia: Saunders.

Ueland, K., McAnulty, J., Ueland, F., and Metcalf, J. (1981). Special considerations in the use of cardiovascular drugs. *Clinics in Obstetrics and Gynecology*, 24(3), 809-823.

Diabetes mellitus

Banerjee, B., Khew, K., Saha, N., and Ratnam, S. (1971). Energy cost and blood sugar level during different stages of labor and duration of labor in Asiatic women. *Journal of Obstetrics and Gynecology British Commonwealth*, 78, 927-929.

Barrett, A., Stubbs, S., and Mander, A. (1980). Management of preterm labor in diabetic pregnancy. *Diabetolgia*, 18, 365.

Cousins, L. (1987). Pregnancy complications among diabetic women: Review 1965 - 1985. *Obstetrical and Gynecological Survey*, 42(3), 140-149.

Fleischman, A., and Finberg, L. (1983). The infant of the diabetic mother and diabetes in infancy. In M. Ellenberg and H. Rifkin (Eds.), *Diabetes mellitus: Theory and practice* (3rd ed.; pp. 715-725). New York: Medical Examination Publishing Co.

Freinkel, N., Lewis, N., and Akazawa, S. (1984). The honey bee syndrome: Implications of teratogenicity of mannrose in rat-embryo culture. *New England Journal of Medicine*, 310(4), 223.

Freinkel, N. (1980). Gestational diabetes 1979. *Diabetes Care*, 3, 399.

Fuhrmann, K., Reiher, H., Semmler, K., Fischer, F., and Fischer, M. (1983). Prevention of congenital malformations in infants of insulin-dependent diabetic mothers. *Diabetes care*, 6(3), 219-223.

Hare, J., and White, P. (1977). Pregnancy in diabetes complicated by vascular disease. *Diabetes*, 26(10), 953-955.

Hollander, D., Nagey, D., and Pupkin, M. (1987). Magnesium sulfate and ritodrine hydrochloride: A randomized comparison. *American Journal of Obstetrics and Gynecology*, 156(3), 631-637

Hollingsworth, D., and Moore, T. (1989). Diabetes and pregnancy, In R. Creasy and R. Resnik (Eds.), *Maternal-fetal medicine: Principles and practice* (2nd ed.; pp. 925-988). Philadelphia: Saunders.

Jovanovic, L., and Peterson, C. (1982). Optimal insulin delivery for the pregnant diabetic patient. *Diabetes Care*, 5(suppl. 1), 24-37.

Kitzmiller, J. (1982). Diabetic ketoacidosis and pregnancy. *Contemporary Obstetrics and Gynecology*, 10, 142.

Marble, A., Krall, L., Bradley, R., Christlieb, A., and Soeldner, J. (1985). *Joslin's diabetes mellitus* (12th ed.). Philadelphia: Lea & Febiger.

Merkatz, I., Peter, J., and Barden, T. (1980). Ritodrine hydrochloride: A beta mimetic agent for the use in preterm labor. *Obstetrics and Gynecology*, 56, 7.

Mills, J., et al. (1988). Lack of relation of malformation rates in infants of diabetic mothers to glycemic control during organogenesis. *New England Journal of Medicine*, 318(11), 671-676.

Ryan, E., O'Sullivan, M., Skyler, J., and Mintz, D. (1982). Glucose control during labor and delivery. In J. Skyler (Ed.), *Insulin update 1982* (pp. 290-294.). Princeton, NJ: Excerpta Medica.

Infection

Balgobin, B. (1987). Fever in labor. In E. Friedman, D. Acker, and B. Sachs (Eds.), *Obstetrical decision making* (2nd ed.; pp. 232-233). Philadelphia: B.C. Decker.

Benoit, J. (1988). Sexually transmitted diseases in pregnancy. *Nursing Clinics of North America*, 23(4), 937-945.

Cates, W., and Holmes, K. (1987). Sexually transmitted diseases. In J. Last (Ed.), *Public health and preventive medicine* (12th ed.). East Norwalk, CT: Appleton & Lange.

Centers for Disease Control. (1987). Recommendations for prevention of HIV transmission in health care settings. *MMWR*, 36(31), 25-185.

Committee on Infectious Diseases. (1985). Prevention of hepatitis B virus infections. *Pediatrics*, 75(2), 362-364.

Davies, P., and Gothefors, L. (1984). *Bacterial infection in the fetus and newborn infant*. Philadelphia: Saunders.

Eschenbach, D. (1988). Infections and sexually transmitted diseases. In D. Hollingsworth and R. Resnik (Eds.), *Medical counseling before pregnancy* (pp. 249-269). New York: Churchill Livingstone.

Faro, S., and Pastorek, J. (1986). Perinatal infections. In R. Kunupple and J. Drukker (Eds.), *High-risk pregnancy: A team approach* (pp. 74-111). Philadelphia: Saunders.

Gilstrap, L., and Cox, S. (1989). Acute chorioamnionitis. *Obstetrics and Gynecology Clinics of North America*. 16(2), 373-379.

Haggerty, L. (1985). TORCH: A literature review and implications for practice. *JOGNN*, 14(2), 124-129.

Hauer, L., and Dattel, B. (1988). Management of the pregnant women infected with the human imunodeficiency virus. *Journal of Perinatology*, 8(3), 258-262.

Krieger, J. (1984). Biology of sexually transmitted diseases. *Urology Clinics of North America*, 11(1), 15-25.

Centers for Disease Control. (1987). Public health service guidelines for counseling and antibody testing to prevent H.I.V. infection and AIDS. *MMWR*, 36(31), 509-522.

Quinn, P., Butany, J., and Taylor, J. (1987). Chorioamnionitis: Its association with pregnancy outcome and microbial infection. *American Journal of Obstetrics and Gynecology*, 156(2), 379-387.

Spence, M. (1989). Epidemiology of sexually transmitted diseases. *Obstetrics and Gynecology Clinics of North America*, 16(3), 453-470.

Wiley K., and Grohar, J. (1988). Human immunodeficiency virus and precautions for obstetric, gynecologic and neonatal nurses. *JOGNN*, 17(3), 165-168.

Wilson, D. (1988). An overview of sexually transmissible diseases in the perinatal period. *Journal of Nurse-Midwifery*, 33(3), 115-128.

Substance abuse

Acker, D., Sachs, B., Tracey, K., and Wise, W. (1983). Abruptio placentae associated with cocaine use. *American Journal of Obstetrics and Gynecology*, 146(2), 220-221.

Burkett, G., Banstra, E., Cohn, J., Steele, B., and Palow, D., (1990). Cocaine-related maternal death. *American Journal of Obstetrics and Gynecology*, 163(1), 40-41.

Florida Child Abuse Statute 415.503, March 1987.

Frank, D., et. al. (1988). Cocaine use during pregnancy: Prevalence and correlates. *Pediatrics*, 82(6), 888-895.

Landry, M., and Smith, D.E., (1987). Crack: Anatomy of an addiction, part 2. *California Nursing Review*, 9(3), 28.

Lee, C., and Chaing, C. (1985). Maternal fetal transfer of abused substances: Pharmacokinetics and pharmadynamics data. *National Institute of Drug Abuse Research Monograph*, vol. 60, 110-147.

Lynch, M., and McKeon, V. (1990). Cocaine use during pregnancy: Research findings and clinical implications. *JOGNN*, 19(4), 285-292.

MacGregor, S., Keith, L., Chasnoff, I., Rosner, M., Chisum, G., Shaw, P., and Minogue, J. (1987). Cocaine use during pregnancy: Adverse perinatal outcome. *American Journal of Obstetrics and Gynecology*, 157(3), 686-690.

Miller, G. (1989). Addicted infants and their mothers. *National Center for Clinical Infant Programs*, 9(5), 20.

Pregnancy-induced hypertension

Hayashi, R. (1986). Emergency care in pregnancy. In J. Queenan (Ed.), *Management of high-risk pregnancy* (pp. 447-469). Oradell, NJ: Medical Economic Books.

Knupple, R., and Drukker, J. (1986). Hypertension in pregnancy. In R. Knupple and J. Drukker (Eds.), *High-risk pregnancy* (pp. 362-398). Philadelphia: Saunders.

Roberts, J. (1989). Pregnancy related hypertension. In R. Creasy and R. Resnik (Eds.), *Maternal-fetal medicine: Principles and practice* (2nd ed.; pp. 777-823). Philadelphia: Saunders.

Sibai, B., Lipshitz, J., and Anderson, G. (1981). Reassessment of intravenous $MgSO_4$ therapy in preeclampsia-eclampsia. *Obstetrics and Gynecology*, 57(2), 199-202.

Rh isoimmunization

Acker, D. (1987). Rh isoimmunization. In E. Friedman, D. Acker, and B. Sachs (Eds.), *Obstetrical decision making* (2nd ed.; pp. 138-139). Philadelphia: B.C. Decker.

Arias, F., and Johnson, D. (1984). Erythroblastosis fetalis. In F. Arias (Ed.), *High-risk pregnancy and delivery* (pp. 75-90). St. Louis: Mosby.

Lloyd, T. (1987). Rh factor incompatibility: A primer for prevention. *Journal of Nurse-Midwifery,* 32(5), 297-307.

Queenan, J. (1982). Rh immunization. In J. Queenan and J. Hobbins (Eds.), *Protocols for high-risk pregnancies* (pp.133-147). Oradell, NJ: Medical Economics Books.

Queenan, J. (1985). Rh and other blood group immunizations. In J. Queenan (Ed.), *Managment of high-risk pregnancy* (pp. 505-520). Oradell, NJ: Medical Economic Books.

Sachs, B. (1987). Nonimmune hydrops fetalis. In E. Friedman, D. Acker, and B. Sachs (Eds.), *Obstetrical decision making* (2nd ed.; pp. 140-141.). Philadelphia: B.C. Decker.

Nursing research

Kearney, M., and Cronenwett, L. (1989). Perceived perinatal complications and childbirth satisfaction. *Applied Nursing Research,* 2(3), 140-142.

Lederman, R. (1984). Anxiety and conflict in pregnancy: Relationship to maternal health status. *Annual Review of Nursing Research,* 2, 27-61.

Lederman, R. (1986). Maternal anxiety in pregnancy: Relationship to fetal and newborn status. *Annual Review of Nursing Research,* 4, 3-19.

Lederman, R., Lederman, E., Work, B., and McCann, D. (1979). Relationship of psychological factors in pregnancy to progress in labor. *Nursing Research,* 28(2), 94-97.

Scott, D., Oberst, M., and Dropkin, M. (1980). A stress coping model. *Advances in Nursing Research,* 3(1), 9-23.

CHAPTER 32

Special Obstetric Procedures

Objectives

After reading and studying this chapter, the student should be able to:

1. List indications and contraindications for selected obstetric procedures.

2. Describe external and internal version.

3. Summarize methods to induce labor.

4. Explain the types of forceps delivery and the hazards of each.

5. Describe vacuum extraction and situations in which it might be used.

6. Discuss the advantages and disadvantages of episiotomy for the client and the fetus.

7. List the most common reasons for cesarean deliveries in the United States.

8. Prepare a client and family for emergency cesarean delivery.

9. Discuss the potential benefits and complications in vaginal delivery after a previous cesarean delivery.

10. Apply the nursing process when caring for a client and family undergoing a special obstetric procedure.

Introduction

For most healthy clients, labor and delivery proceed normally. Occasionally, however, a client requires special assistance to ensure normal delivery. This assistance could be aimed at changing the fetus's orientation in the uterus, initiating or enhancing uterine contractions, aiding the client in moving the fetus through the birth canal, or delivering the neonate surgically.

To provide the best care possible, the nurse should understand the special obstetric procedures a client may undergo, be able to explain these procedures to the client and her family, and be able to assist as needed. This chapter begins by discussing the following nonsurgical and surgical special obstetric procedures and their indications, contraindications, and risks:

• external and internal version, for rotating a fetus in utero

• labor induction via oxytocin, amniotomy, or prostaglandin gel (PGE$_2$)

• forceps delivery

• vacuum extraction

• vaginal birth after cesarean (VBAC) delivery

• episiotomy

• cesarean delivery.

After describing the procedures, the chapter outlines the nurse's role in caring for the client undergoing a special obstetric procedure and her family.

Nonsurgical procedures

Nonsurgical obstetric procedures, such as external and internal version, labor induction, forceps delivery, vacuum extraction, and VBAC delivery, require the nurse to work closely with the nurse-midwife or physician to ensure a positive outcome for the client and fetus.

GLOSSARY

Amniocentesis: surgical perforation of the uterus and amniotic sac to obtain amniotic fluid for analysis.

Amniohook: instrument used to perform amniotomy.

Amnionitis: inflammation of the amnion, most commonly a complication of premature rupture of the membranes.

Amniotic fluid: fluid within the amniotic sac that allows the fetus to move and cushions the fetus's head and umbilical cord during delivery.

Amniotic sac: inner lining of the uterus that houses the growing fetus and amniotic fluid.

Amniotomy: artificial rupture of the amniotic membranes to enhance or induce labor. Performed by a physician or nurse-midwife.

AROM: artificial rupture of the membranes (amniotic sac).

Augmentation of labor: enhancement of ineffective uterine contractions during labor.

Caput succedaneum: generalized edema of the fetal scalp, usually caused by cervical pressure on the fetal occiput during labor.

Cephalopelvic disproportion (CPD): condition in which the fetus's head is too large or the client's pelvis too small to permit normal vaginal delivery.

Cesarean delivery: surgical incision through the abdominal wall and uterus to deliver the fetus.

Dystocia: difficult delivery caused by abnormalities in the fetus, client's pelvis, or uterine expulsive powers.

Elective induction: initiation of labor for convenience in a term pregnancy.

Episiotomy: surgical incision of the perineum to enlarge the vaginal opening for delivery.

Forceps: two curved blades used to extract the fetus from the birth canal.

Grand multiparity: having had five or more children.

Hypertonia: condition in which the uterus resists stretching.

Indicated or nonelective induction: initiation of labor for medical or obstetric reasons that threaten the health of the fetus or client.

Induction of labor: attempt to speed labor by starting or augmenting uterine contractions.

Laminaria tents: dried hygroscopic seaweed cones used to stretch and soften the cervix.

Oligohydramnios: abnormally small amount of amniotic fluid.

Oxytocin: hormone produced by the posterior pituitary gland that stimulates strong, rhythmic uterine contractions; also, a synthetic hormone (Pitocin) that simulates the actions of the natural hormone.

Precipitous delivery: unusually rapid delivery.

Presenting part: portion of the fetus that first enters the pelvic inlet.

Prostaglandin: naturally occurring hydroxyfatty acid that stimulates uterine contractions.

Ripe cervix: soft, effaced, dilated cervix.

Rupture of membranes: rupture of the amniotic sac, followed within 24 hours by induced or natural labor in 80% of women.

Tetanic uterine contraction: sustained uterine contraction lasting 70 seconds or longer, occurring more than once every 3 minutes and increasing intrauterine pressure to 75 mm Hg or more.

Vacuum extraction: procedure using a cup-shaped suction device applied to the fetus's scalp to provide traction for delivery.

VBAC: vaginal birth after cesarean delivery.

Ventouse: suction cup used in vacuum extraction.

Version: procedure for turning the fetus in utero to a position favorable for delivery.

Version

Two types of version may be performed: external, which is used to rotate the fetus from a breech or shoulder presentation to a cephalic presentation; and internal, which is used to deliver an unengaged second twin by grasping the feet. (For more details and illustrations, see *External and internal version*.)

When external version is performed, the client receives a drug to relax the uterus (such as ritodrine hydrochloride or terbutaline sulfate) and the physician repositions the fetus by manipulating the client's abdomen. Rotating the fetus to a cephalic presentation increases the likelihood of successful vaginal delivery and reduces the probability of cesearean delivery. Performed properly and gently, external version carries little risk for the client or fetus. However, to minimize potential complications, the procedure should be performed:

• late in the third trimester, no earlier than week 36 or 37

• before engagement of the presenting part

• only if amniotic fluid volume is sufficient

• only if the membranes are intact (Cunningham, MacDonald, and Gant, 1989).

External version is more easily accomplished in multiparous clients because their abdominal walls are more relaxed than those of nulliparous clients (Cunningham, MacDonald, and Gant, 1989).

Internal version may be performed to deliver a second twin when the occiput or breech is not over the pelvic inlet and external pressure fails to position a presenting part, or when uterine bleeding occurs. Expect the client to receive an anesthetic agent. The physician reaches one gloved hand through the vagina and cervix and into the uterus, grasps the fetus's legs, and performs a breech delivery. The physician will attempt internal

External and internal version

Version, the manual rotation of the fetus in utero, may be performed externally (the most common method) or internally (only with difficult, second-twin deliveries).

External version

The physician uses slow, steady pressure against the client's abdomen to push the fetus's head toward the pelvic inlet while pushing the buttocks upward. Excessive force may harm the client or fetus. The procedure should be accompanied by continuous external fetal monitoring. Expect the physician to use sonography before and during external version to verify the positions of the fetus and placenta. Also expect that the client will receive no anesthesic agent, because it may mask possible trauma.

BREECH PRESENTATION

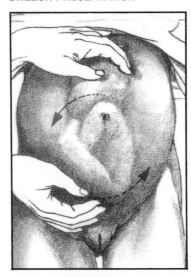

CORRECTED PRESENTATION

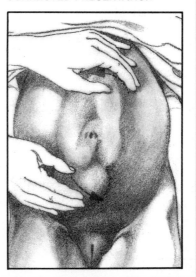

Internal (podalic) version

The physician inserts one sterile, gloved hand through the completely dilated cervix and draws one or both of the fetus's feet toward the birth canal. The physician's other hand applies gentle pressure to the client's abdomen to shift the fetus's head upward. Breech delivery occurs immediately thereafter.

UNENGAGED FETUS

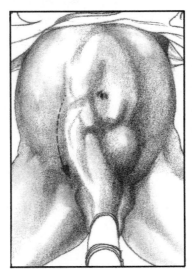

ASSISTED BREECH DELIVERY

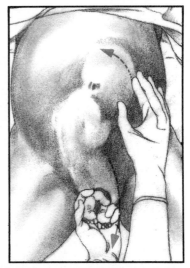

version as a last resort because it places the client and fetus at serious risk for trauma. Failure of either internal or external version may require an emergency cesarean delivery.

A client who knows that her fetus is in a breech position before labor begins may be able to perform version on her own. In one study, women assumed a knee-chest position for 15 minutes, three times a day, for 7 days. In 41% of the women studied, the fetus shifted from a breech to cephalic presentation (Chenia and Crowther, 1987).

Induction of labor

Uterine contractions may be induced through hormone injection or through amniotomy. Induction may be necessitated by an emergency when medical or obstetric problems threaten the health of the client or fetus. The physician also can use labor induction methods to strengthen natural contractions. Occasionally, labor may be induced by choice if the client has a term pregnancy and is free of complications.

The two most common induction methods are intravenous synthetic oxytocin (Pitocin or Syntocinon) infusion and amniotomy. An experimental procedure involves administration of prostaglandin (PGE₂) gel. (For more information, see *Labor induction with PGE₂ gel.*)

Intravenous oxytocin

During natural labor, the posterior lobe of the pituitary gland releases the hormone oxytocin. This hormone stimulates strong, rhythmic contractions of the uterine muscle. Estrogen production increases during pregnancy, which in turn increases the sensitivity of the uterus to minute amounts of oxytocin. Because oxytocin stimulates such a powerful response, the physician can induce labor by infusing minute amounts of it.

Fetal age and cervical readiness are the two major considerations in labor induction. Because menstrual periods can be irregular and the client's memory inaccurate, the physician must carefully measure and document fetal size and maturity (Hacker and Moore, 1986). Clinical criteria of maturity include:
• 39 weeks since the last menstrual period
• documentation of when fetal heart rate (FHR) is first heard using a fetoscope
• an enlarged uterus before the sixteenth calculated week of pregnancy, verified by palpation.

Laboratory criteria of maturity include:
• amniocentesis that determines fetal lung maturity (lecithin/spingomyelin ratio greater than 2)
• fetal biparietal diameter measured by ultrasound
• positive pregnancy test at least 37 weeks previously (Johnson, 1981).

Labor induction with PGE₂ gel

Although still experimental, administration of prostaglandin (PGE₂) as a gel into the cervix, vagina, or extra-amniotic space may induce cervical changes and uterine contractions.

To administer PGE₂ gel extra-amniotically, the physician inserts a catheter through the cervical canal and instills 0.3 to 0.4 mg of the drug. The client remains recumbent for at least 1 hour after administration, and the obstetric team continuously monitors the fetal heart rate and uterine activity. The client's vital signs should be checked every hour for the first 4 hours. Most clients will experience mild uterine contractions.

PGE₂ gel causes few side effects; vomiting, fever, or diarrhea occur in only about 0.2% of cases. The drug almost never hyperstimulates uterine contractions, and fetal effects are minimal (Rayburn, 1989; Cunningham, MacDonald, and Gant, 1989).

In addition, the physician will assess the cervix to determine if it is likely to respond to the induction procedure. A cervix that is soft, effaced, and anterior is felt to be "ripe" and will continue to dilate and efface in response to uterine contractions.

Oxytocin infusion may cause excessive or tetanic uterine contractions that last longer than 70 seconds each, occur more often than once every 3 minutes, and increase intrauterine pressure to more than 75 mm Hg. These excessive contractions may rupture the uterus or rush labor and delivery, resulting in cervical and perineal lacerations. They also may reduce oxygen to the fetus, reducing or disrupting heartbeat.

Excessive contractions or reduced FHR warrants an immediate halt to oxytocin infusion. The oxytocin level will drop by half within about 3 minutes, and the tetanic contractions usually will return to a normal level (Cunningham, MacDonald, and Gant, 1989; Hacker and Moore, 1986).

Oxytocin has a potent antidiuretic action. An infusion of 20 mU/min or more markedly decreases the free water clearance of the kidneys, in turn reducing urine production. Avoid giving the client large amounts of fluid, particularly dextrose 5% in water, during oxytocin infusion to avoid possible water intoxication (Cunningham, MacDonald, and Gant, 1989).

Amniotomy

In this widely practiced but controversial procedure, a physician or nurse-midwife artificially ruptures the amniotic membranes to augment or induce labor. Some call the procedure artificial rupture of the membranes, or AROM. (For an illustration, see *Amniotomy.*)

The physician or nurse-midwife performs the procedure under sterile conditions with the client in the lithotomy position. During and immediately after the procedure, the obstetric team monitors the fetus to ensure that the umbilical cord does not prolapse.

Amniotomy improves the efficiency of uterine contractions because the release of amniotic fluid decreases uterine volume (Oxorn, 1986; Marshall, 1985). Additionally, amniotomy may shorten labor when the client's cervix is soft, dilated, anteriorly positioned, and effaced to some degree. In one study, 40% of women with these characteristics delivered within 4 hours after amniotomy; 85% delivered within 12 hours (Marshall, 1985).

Amniotomy allows earlier detection of meconium-stained amniotic fluid, which can result in fetal pneumonia. It also allows internal probe monitoring of the fetus and uterus.

Because of the advantages of amniotomy, some physicians routinely perform it to increase the efficiency of contractions in a client already in labor.

Despite its benefits and longtime use, amniotomy remains controversial. One reason is that the membranes typically remain intact during natural labor until the second stage of labor (Marshall, 1985). Also, the unbroken amniotic sac cushions the fetus's head and the umbilical cord during delivery. Rupture removes this cushion. The sac also helps dilate the cervix. When the uterus contracts, it pushes the sac into the cervix, increasing fluid pressure and causing dilation. When the membranes rupture, the presenting part of the fetus continues this pressure, which further aids dilation.

One study (Rosen and Peisner, 1987) showed that artificial rupture shortened labor compared to rupture that was naturally delayed until the second stage of labor. Other experts doubt whether amniotomy significantly shortens labor. Whatever the case, Cunningham, MacDonald, and Gant (1989) suggest that no one has shown that a shorter labor is beneficial to the fetus or to the pregnant client.

Other experts contend that the benefits of amniotomy do not outweigh its risks. Marshall (1985) reported that leaving the membranes intact:
• decreases the incidence of FHR decelerations
• reduces fetal acidosis (pH imbalance in the tissue)
• reduces caput succedaneum (edema in and under the fetus's scalp).

If labor does not follow amniotomy immediately, infection may result. One study showed that 23% of fetuses had bacteremia when the client had amniotomy but no immediate labor (Marshall, 1985). Based on this finding, some experts recommend abandoning AROM (Marshall, 1985). Some physicians advocate AROM but without internal monitoring unless the fetus is at risk; they believe the resulting shorter labor enables the client to tolerate pain better (Henderson, 1987). Some experts believe birth should take place no later than 12 hours

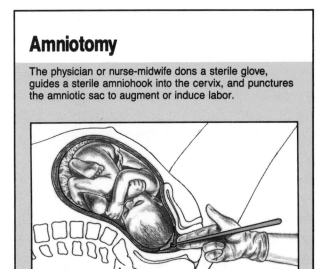

Amniotomy

The physician or nurse-midwife dons a sterile glove, guides a sterile amniohook into the cervix, and punctures the amniotic sac to augment or induce labor.

after AROM to enhance comfort and avoid infection (Marshall, 1985).

If amniotomy fails to induce labor, the physician may initiate oxytocin infusion. If this fails, cesarean delivery may be required.

Forceps delivery

In this procedure, the physician uses two curved, articulated blades to extract the fetus from the birth canal or to rotate the fetus. (For more information, see *Types of forceps*, page 772, and *Forceps delivery*, page 773.)

Fetal station determines the type of forceps used. Low or outlet forceps may be appropriate when the head has reached the perineum (+2 station) and is visibly separating the labia. Forceps can help the client push the fetus out, shortening the second stage of labor. Use of low forceps is relatively safe; complications usually are limited to bruising of the fetus's head and minor perineal, vaginal, or cervical trauma.

If the head is engaged but not visible at the perineum and the vertex of the skull is at the ischial tuberosities, the physician may use mid forceps. However, use of mid forceps is rare because it endangers the client and fetus. Use of high forceps—when the head is unengaged and the vertex of the skull is located above the ischial spines—is extremely rare because of considerable risk to the client and fetus (Oxorn, 1986). Mid or high forceps can fracture the fetus's skull (Korones, 1986). Duker (1985) found that 46% of women who had mid forceps delivery had third-degree perineal lacerations. More than a fifth lost more than 500 ml of blood. Furthermore, use of forceps does not always guarantee delivery. Today,

Types of forceps

The six types of forceps illustrated below (anterior and lateral views) may be used during delivery. Typically, Elliot, Simpson, or Tucker-McLean forceps are used for low or outlet forceps deliveries. The separated shank of the Simpson forceps allows for episiotomy. The solid blades of the Tucker-McLean forceps help prevent head trauma in preterm infants. For rotation and delivery, the physician might choose Kielland, Barton, and Tucker-McLean. Kielland forceps are designed to rotate the fetus from a persistent occiput posterior presentation to a position that accommodates delivery. Barton forceps may be used for mid forceps rotation and delivery of a fetus in the occiput transverse position. The curved shank of the Piper forceps permits traction and flexion of the fetus's head during a breech delivery.

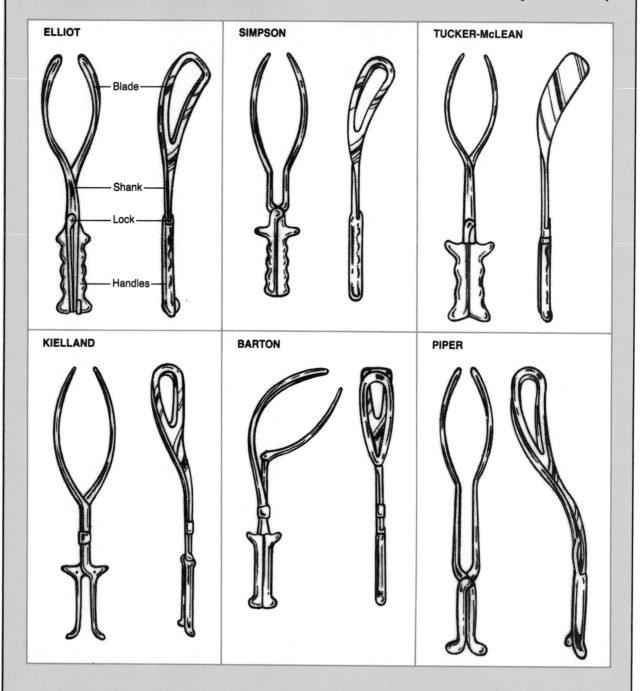

ELLIOT — Blade, Shank, Lock, Handles
SIMPSON
TUCKER-McLEAN
KIELLAND
BARTON
PIPER

Forceps delivery

The physician positions and then locks the blades over the parietal bones in the fetus's skull and pulls the fetus downward and outward through the birth canal during uterine contractions. Once the fetus's head clears the perineum, the rest of the body emerges easily.

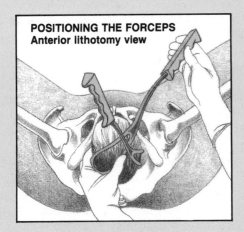

POSITIONING THE FORCEPS
Anterior lithotomy view

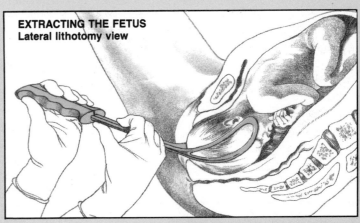

EXTRACTING THE FETUS
Lateral lithotomy view

most physicians perform a cesarean delivery rather than using mid or high forceps (Laub, 1985).

Vacuum extraction

Physicians began experimenting with vacuum extraction as early as 1706, but no acceptable instrument was developed until 1954. That year, a physician developed a mushroom-shaped cup that could hold the fetus's head through negative pressure. Today, this procedure is popular in Europe but less common in the United States (Galvan and Broekhuizen, 1987).

To accomplish vacuum extraction, the physician uses a suction-cup device known as a ventouse. Ventouses are available in several diameters, including 30, 40, 50, and 60 mm. The physician uses the largest cup size possible to minimize trauma to the fetus's scalp, especially to a suture line or fontanel.

The ventouse is attached by tubing to a suction pump. After positioning the ventouse on the fetus's scalp, air is pumped out of the space between the cup and the scalp, creating a vacuum. By pulling a chain or cord attached to the ventouse, the physician draws the fetus through the birth canal. (For an illustration, see *Vacuum extraction*, page 774.)

Those who favor vacuum extraction believe that it decreases delivery time. They also point out that the procedure does not require additional space inside the vaginal canal, as forceps do.

Vaginal birth after cesarean delivery

In VBAC, a client who has had a cesarean delivery attempts to deliver vaginally. This approach offers several advantages over repeated cesarean deliveries:
• family experience of a normal childbirth
• reduced risk of infection and death (Laufer, et al., 1987)
• less discomfort than cesarean delivery
• less recovery time than cesarean delivery
• less cost than cesarean delivery.

Physicians disagree about the extent of the disadvantages in attempting vaginal delivery after an earlier cesarian delivery. One complicating issue is that the reasons for the first cesarean delivery may still be valid. Another is the risk of uterine rupture. Early studies showed that vaginal delivery after an earlier cesarean delivery performed with a low vertical uterine incision commonly led to rupture, massive maternal shock, and extrusion of the fetus into the abdomen. Over the past two decades, however, physicians have used the low transverse incision almost exclusively. Only 0.25% to 0.5% of these scars rupture and, of those that do, about 90% involve only separation of the myometrial covering of the uterus. These ruptures cause no symptoms and little or no bleeding. No deaths have been reported from such a rupture in more than 20 years (Laufer, et al., 1987).

The American College of Obstetricians and Gynecologists (1988) established specific criteria and guidelines for the client attempting VBAC. Although some physicians and facilities continue to avoid the procedure,

Vacuum extraction

The physician applies a ventouse (suction cup device) to the fetus's scalp, removes air to create suction, and pulls to help deliver the fetus.

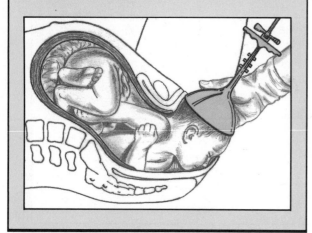

it has become more common. Studies suggest that up to 60% of clients who have had cesarean delivery may wish to attempt vaginal delivery, and of those who do, about 70% complete vaginal delivery successfully (Lipson, 1984).

Criteria for VBAC include:
• previous uterine incision made in the low transverse position
• client desire to try vaginal delivery
• early notification of client's wishes to the physician
• available blood for transfusion
• an obstetric team prepared to perform cesarean delivery if necessary
• physician available during the entire labor
• no client medical problems that contraindicate VBAC.

Controversial areas concerning VBAC include:
• whether a client who has had more than one cesarean delivery should be permitted to attempt VBAC (Some physicians fear that the uterus may be more likely to rupture after multiple incisions.)
• whether a client with a history of cephalopelvic disproportion should try VBAC (Physicians disagree over whether disproportion always recurs.)
• the actual incidence of uterine rupture
• whether oxytocin is safe to administer during VBAC.

(For a summary of indications, contraindications, and risks and complications, see *Summary of selected obstetric procedures,* pages 777 and 778.)

Surgical procedures

During surgical obstetric procedures, including episiotomy and cesarean delivery, the nurse assists the physician or nurse-midwife, as necessary.

Episiotomy

In episiotomy, a procedure used in the United States since the 1920s, the physician cuts the perineum to widen the birth canal, thus minimizing lacerations during delivery.

Episiotomy may be accomplished by two methods. The most common in the United States is a median episiotomy. Using round-tipped scissors, the physician cuts straight downward from the vaginal orifice. In the alternative method—mediolateral episiotomy—the cut angles away from the anus. (For an illustration, see *Types of episiotomy.*)

In 1980, 65% of all deliveries involved an episiotomy (Banta and Thacker, 1982). Nearly 90% of nulliparous clients and about 50% of multiparous clients had episiotomies. Many physicians performed the procedure to help shorten the second stage of labor and minimize injury to the vagina and to the fetus's head. Opponents to widespread episiotomy use have contended that research may not support these alleged benefits (Banta and Thacker, 1982). Bromberg (1986) claimed that the procedure is justified only if an extended laceration seems inevitable.

Before episiotomy takes place, the fetus's head (or buttocks in a breech presentation) should be low enough to keep the perineum stretched. Ideally, it should be bulging and thinned. Waiting until this stage to perform the procedure lessens bleeding because thinner tissue contains fewer blood vessels. However, the physician should make the incision before the muscles supporting the rectum and bladder are severely stretched.

Even with an episiotomy, delivery may extend the incision to the anal sphincter (a third-degree laceration) or to the anal canal (a fourth-degree laceration). These extensions can cause pain, excessive blood loss, suture separation, fistula formation, or even permanent sphincter dysfunction (Borgotta, Piening, and Cohen, 1989). Blood loss usually is greater and repair more difficult and painful with the mediolateral episiotomy because the incision is through thicker tissue.

Avery and Von Arsdale (1987) suggest that clients who massage the perineum during the 6 weeks before delivery may decrease the risk of laceration and the need for episiotomy.

Cesarean delivery

Surgical incision of the abdominal and uterine walls allows cesarean delivery. In the mid-1960s, fewer than 5% of all neonates in the United States were delivered by the cesarean method. By 1987, nearly 25% were delivered by cesarean (Placek, Taffel, and Liss, 1987). Many factors have contributed to the rise in cesarean deliveries.

• Cesarean delivery poses less risk for the client and fetus than high or mid forceps delivery (Cunningham, MacDonald, and Gant, 1989).

• Electronic fetal monitoring allows early detection of fetal distress.

• Physicians express mounting reluctance to deliver breech fetuses vaginally. Most now are delivered by cesarean to minimize fetal injuries (Cunningham, MacDonald, and Gant, 1989).

• Advances in technology, surgical technique, and anesthesia and analgesia have made the procedure safer and more comfortable (Cunningham, MacDonald, and Gant, 1989).

• Pharmacologic and parenteral fluid therapy have significantly reduced such surgical hazards as hemorrhage and infection (Cunningham, MacDonald, and Gant, 1989).

• People no longer think of this procedure as an abnormal event, but rather as an alternative delivery method.

• Changes in health care facility policies allow the client and her partner or other labor support person to participate in cesarean delivery, just as they would in vaginal delivery (Shearer, Shiono, and Rhoads, 1988).

The reasons for cesarean delivery encompass five general categories (Cunningham, MacDonald, and Gant, 1989).

• Dystocia (difficult or abnormal delivery) accounts for about 29% of all cesarean deliveries. The most common cause of dystocia is cephalopelvic disproportion, which results from a large fetus, malpresentation, a contracted pelvis, or—in rare cases—a tumor that blocks the birth canal.

• Previous cesarean delivery is the cause in 35% of all cesarean deliveries.

• Breech presentation prompts 10% of cesarean deliveries. This indication is becoming more common, particularly in nulliparous clients. Although vaginal delivery is still the method of choice, many practitioners consider cesarean delivery safer for breech fetuses.

• Fetal distress is the indication in 8% of all cases.

• Other indications account for the remaining 18% of cesarean deliveries. These include herpes simplex type 2 or condylomata acuminata lesions in the birth canal.

Types of episiotomy

Of the two types of episiotomy used in the United States, the median method is most common because it simplifies repair and minimizes blood loss. The mediolateral episiotomy may prevent extension of the incision into the anal sphincter and rectum.

Episiotomy is performed on the bulging perineum with round-tipped scissors.

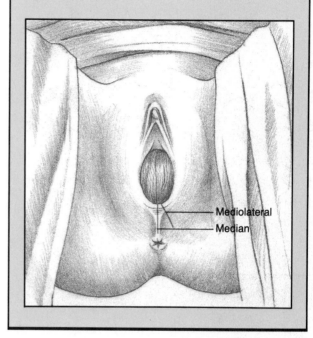

Both are potentially dangerous if transmitted to the fetus during delivery. Condylomatous lesions also may obstruct the birth canal.

All methods of obstetric anesthesia pose some risks for the client and fetus that must be weighed against benefits when choosing an anesthetic agent. Choice of an agent should reflect the circumstances and the client's desires. If the client wishes to witness the delivery, the choice typically is spinal or epidural anesthesia. In an emergency requiring immediate cesarean delivery, a rapid-induction general anesthesia may be the type of choice.

Once the client is anesthetized, the physician selects one of several methods to section the skin of the lower abdomen and the uterine wall. (For more information, see *Types of incisions for cesarean delivery*, page 776.) If time is adequate and the client and fetus are normal, the physician makes a transverse incision at or just below the pubic hairline. The benefits of a transverse incision include:

• only moderate manipulation of the bladder and dissection of supporting structures

• limited blood loss

Types of incisions for cesarean delivery

Skin incisions for cesarean delivery are either vertical or transverse. Uterine incisions are either vertical through the body of the uterus, vertical through the lower uterine segment, or transverse through the lower uterine segment.

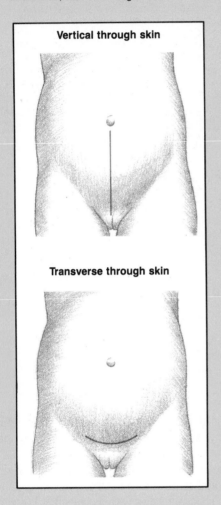

Vertical through skin

Transverse through skin

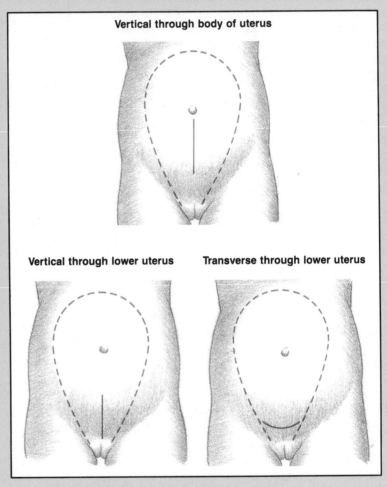

Vertical through body of uterus

Vertical through lower uterus

Transverse through lower uterus

- ease of repair
- limited adherence of bowel or omentum to the incision line
- limited likelihood of rupture during subsequent pregnancies
- barely visible scar.

The potential risks of a transverse incision include:
- extra time
- limited area for extension if more maneuvering space is needed to extract the fetus
- possible extension laterally into major uterine vessels.

The physician may make a low vertical incision in cases of:
- an obese client

- a macrosomic fetus
- multiple gestation (more than one fetus)
- maternal distress (changes in vital signs or uterine bleeding)
- fetal distress (changes in vital signs, especially FHR)
- placenta previa
- abnormal presentation.

Much less common today is the classical incision, in which the physician cuts vertically through the body of the uterus. This type of incision increases the possibility of rupture during subsequent pregnancies.

(For a summary of indications, contraindications, and risks and complications, see *Summary of selected obstetric procedures*.)

Summary of selected obstetric procedures

The following chart outlines some indications, contraindications, and risks and complications for the procedures discussed in this chapter.

PROCEDURE	INDICATIONS	CONTRAINDICATIONS	RISKS AND COMPLICATIONS
Version (external)	• Fetus in noncephalic (shoulder or breech) presentation	• Ruptured amniotic membrane • Cephalopelvic disproportion (CPD) • Oligohydramnios • History of premature labor • Abnormal fetus • Placenta previa • More than one fetus • Maternal obesity	• Fetus's possible return to noncephalic presentation • Client discomfort • Decreased fetal heart rate (FHR) • Premature labor, hemorrhage, premature rupture of membranes • Abruptio placentae • Compression of fetus's spinal cord
Version (internal)	• Emergency need for rapid delivery in breech position only used with second twin	• Lack of anesthesia • No health care team member skilled in internal podalic version (cesarean delivery preferred) • Retracted cervix or contracted, thickened uterus	• Uterine trauma • Lacerations of perineum, vagina, or cervix • Postpartal hemorrhage • Fetal injury
Induction of labor (oxytocin)	• Maternal diabetes • Pregnancy-induced hypertension • Premature rupture of the membranes • Postterm pregnancy • Fetal hemolytic disease • Dead fetus • History of precipitous delivery • Ineffective uterine contractions (only after efforts to reduce tension and promote comfort have failed) • Uterine hypotonia or hypoactivity	• Preterm fetus (unless benefits outweigh risks) • Unripe cervix • Grand multiparity (five or more previous births) • No medical or obstetric need • CPD • Overly distended uterus, as from hydramnios or multiparity • Incoordinate or abnormal contractions • Hypersensitivity to drug • Severe fetal distress • Decreased FHR during contractions • Fetal malposition or malpresentation • Congenital fetal anomalies • When vaginal delivery is contraindicated, such as placenta previa, invasive cervical carcinoma, herpes simplex type 2 in the birth canal, and cord prolapse	• Excessive (tetanic) uterine contractions • Water intoxication with excessive amounts of fluid • Hypersensitivity to drug, resulting in hypertonia • Failure to initiate labor • With laminaria tents, mild pelvic cramping • Small risk of infection with prolonged laminaria insertion
Induction of labor (amniotomy)	• Postterm pregnancy • Insufficient uterine contractions • Medical or obstetric complications	• Preterm fetus, uncertain estimated delivery date • Unripe cervix • CPD • Presenting part unengaged • Placenta previa • Herpes simplex type 2 in birth canal • Fetal malposition or malpresentation • Multiple gestation (more than one fetus) • Hydramnios • Grand multiparity	• Umbilical cord prolapse • Amnionitis • Compression and molding of fetus's head • Failure to initiate labor • Infection
Forceps delivery	• Maternal cardiac or pulmonary disorder • Infection • Maternal exhaustion	• Incomplete cervical dilation • Unengaged presenting part • Fetal malposition or malpresentation	*Low forceps* • Bruises to fetus's head • Trauma to perineum, vagina, or cervix (continued)

Summary of selected obstetric procedures continued

PROCEDURE	INDICATIONS	CONTRAINDICATIONS	RISKS AND COMPLICATIONS
Forceps delivery (continued)	• Motor innervation from epidural or spinal anesthesia • Premature placental separation • Fetal distress • Prolapsed umbilical cord • Failure of descent or rotation	• Intact membranes • CPD • Full bowel or bladder	*Mid forceps* • *Fetal:* fractured skull, epilepsy, cerebral palsy, mental retardation, cephalohematoma, brain damage, intracranial bleeding, respiratory depression and asphyxia, facial paralysis or other neurologic problems, brachial palsy, bruising, cord compression, death • *Maternal:* fractured coccyx; ruptured uterus; lacerations of perineum, vagina, or cervix; hemorrhage; uterine atony; rectal trauma; genital tract infection; bladder injury, atony, or infection
Vacuum extraction	• Similar to forceps delivery	• Preterm fetus • Fetal malposition or malpresentation • Face presentation • CPD • Hydrocephalus or other congenital anomaly • Dead fetus • Incomplete cervical dilation (possible contraindication) • Unengaged head (possible contraindication)	• Lacerations and abrasions of scalp • Cephalohematoma • Intracranial hematoma • Distortion of fetus's head • Caput succedaneum
Vaginal birth after cesarean	• Client desire • Absence of contraindications	• Vertical uterine scar • Multiple gestation • CPD or other medical problem incompatible with vaginal delivery • Estimated fetal weight above 4,000 g	• Uterine rupture with vertical scar • Reasons for previous cesarean may still exist • Infection if membranes have been ruptured 12 hours or more without delivery and without prophylactic antibiotics
Episiotomy	• Insufficient perineal stretching • Rapid, progressive labor • Narrow suprapublic arch and outlet • Preterm fetus weighing under 200 g • Fetus weighing over 4,000 g • Malpresentation	• Presenting part not descended far enough to stretch the perineum	• Pain • Dyspareunia • Infection • Increased blood loss • Altered vaginal shape or size • Extension to anal sphincter or anal canal
Cesarean delivery	• Breech presentation • Fetal distress • Dystocia, possibly caused by CPD, malpresentation, or (rarely) a tumor blocking the birth canal • Previous cesarean delivery • Herpes simplex type 2 in birth canal • Condylomata acuminata in birth canal • Placenta previa, abruptio placentae • Prolapsed umbilical cord • Unsuccessful induction of labor	• Dead fetus • Fetus too premature to survive	• Preterm birth • Anesthesia risk • Aspiration pneumonia • Injury to urinary tract organs or bowel • Bowel obstruction • Dehiscence of surgical wound, leading to evisceration • Infection • Hemorrhage • Thromboemboli

Assessment

Before the client undergoes any obstetric procedure, the nurse should perform an initial assessment that includes the following steps.
• Review the nursing history, or subjective information, focusing on the complications of pregnancy and labor.
• Review the physical assessment performed during admission to the facility. Focus on the client's vital signs; frequency, duration, and intensity of contractions; cervical changes; amniotic fluid; the FHR; and fetal presentation and station.
• Collect additional data to help plan the client's care. Because special obstetric procedures can produce anxiety, especially if unexpected, assess psychosocial aspects of the client and family.
• Continue monitoring during and after any procedure to ensure the safety of the client and fetus and the timely progression of labor.

Health history

Review the entire nursing history for information that may affect the procedure. Pay special attention to the history of the client's previous pregnancies, labors, and deliveries. Also examine the course of the current pregnancy and labor. Note such complications as:
• pregnancy-induced hypertension
• abruptio placentae
• placenta previa
• systemic health problems, such as diabetes, cardiac disease, and anemia.

Notify the obstetric staff of such conditions as premature rupture of membranes or such sexually transmitted diseases as herpes simplex type 2, condylomata acuminata, gonorrhea, syphilis, chlamydia, or acquired immunodeficiency syndrome.

Psychosocial history

Determine the type of labor and delivery preparation the client and family have received. Are they aware of obstetric and special procedures? Do they know why these procedures may be necessary? How do they feel about these interventions? Try to determine how supportive the client's labor partner is to determine if the client may need additional support. Remember that:
• some clients view the need for cesarean delivery as a failure

• some feel that special obstetric procedures conflict with their cultural beliefs
• some may be concerned about logistics, such as finances or caring for other children during their hospitalization.

Offer the client an opportunity to talk about her feelings. The plan of care should reflect any concerns or fears she expresses.

Physical assessment

Collect baseline physical data in the following areas.
• Maternal vital signs, including blood pressure, pulse, respirations, and temperature. Changes in blood pressure and pulse may indicate pregnancy-induced hypertension or signal hemorrhage, a complication that may accompany many obstetric procedures. Changes in blood pressure, pulse, and respirations may indicate pain. Fever may indicate amnionitis, a complication of amniotomy.
• The FHR, including any variability. Take a long, continuous measurement. Some procedures, such as oxytocin infusion, require a 15-minute fetal monitor strip before implementation.
• Contraction frequency, duration, and intensity. This measure will help determine whether amniotomy or oxytocin infusion have successfully increased contraction efficiency.
• Cervical changes, particularly if the client will have induced labor. Assist with a vaginal examination to assess cervical ripeness. Determine effacement, dilation, and consistency of the cervix. If the membranes are ruptured, use extreme caution and meticulously sterile technique when assisting with a vaginal examination.
• Fetal presentation and station. This assessment is important to determine the need for external version. It also helps in measuring labor progress, which may be important in determining the need for forceps or vacuum-extraction. This assessment is vital in the decision to perform amniotomy because the presenting part must be engaged before performing this procedure.
• Condition of the amniotic membranes and fluid. Intact membranes are a prerequisite of amniotomy; ruptured membranes are a contraindication for external version. The color and consistency of leaking amniotic fluid can indicate meconium staining.

Ongoing assessment

To safeguard the client's health and monitor labor progress, continue the assessment during and after labor. The frequency of these checks depends on the procedure used and on the results of the previous assessment. If vital signs approach dangerous levels, assessment should occur frequently.

After delivery, the nurse may be responsible for checking for trauma to the client or neonate as well as other conditions. These assessments vary according to the procedures performed.

Version

During external version, monitor the FHR continuously, and check vital signs every 5 minutes. Also assess the client's comfort level; extreme discomfort may indicate trauma. After the procedure, place the client on bed rest and under observation for several hours. Assess the FHR, vital signs, and uterine contractility every 30 minutes. If the client has had internal podalic version, check for excessive bleeding from perineal, vaginal, or cervical lacerations.

Induced labor

When a client is receiving oxytocin, monitor her vital signs and the FHR and reactivity closely and continuously. Also, before each incremental increase in infusion rate, or once every 15 to 20 minutes, check the frequency, duration, and intensity of contractions.

When contractions occur once every 2 to 3 minutes and last for 50 to 60 seconds, assess cervical changes. The frequency of this assessment depends on the client's history; a multiparous client may proceed more quickly through labor and delivery than a nulliparous client.

Finally, assess urine output to determine any fluid retention problems because these may affect blood pressure.

Amniotomy

Immediately after amniotomy, assess the FHR and characteristics of the amniotic fluid. Then check the FHR at least once every 30 minutes, depending on the stage of labor. Any significant change in the FHR may indicate umbilical cord prolapse; an external fetal monitor can show large variable decelerations during cord compressions. If such changes arise, a vaginal examination should be performed and the nurse-midwife or physician notified immediately.

Check the client's temperature with an oral thermometer every 2 hours to rule out possible infection. A temperature of 100° F (37.8° C) or more warrants hourly temperature assessment.

Forceps delivery

Check the FHR after the physician has applied the forceps but has not yet applied traction to the fetus. A drop in the FHR could indicate compression of the umbilical cord against the fetus's head (Cunningham, MacDonald, and Gant, 1989). Also assess the client's vital signs and comfort level during the procedure.

Immediately after forceps delivery, assess the neonate for cerebral trauma. Observe the client closely for possible tissue trauma, including excessive bleeding, pain, hematoma, and lacerations of the cervix or vaginal walls. Notify nursery personnel and postpartal caregivers that the neonate was delivered by forceps.

Vacuum extraction

Assess the FHR every 5 minutes during vacuum extraction. After delivery, assess the neonate's head for marks, such as an artificial caput succedaneum. Document the marks, and inform the client that they usually disappear within several hours.

VBAC

Assessment of a client attempting VBAC depends on the stage and progress of labor. Pay particular attention to the client's vital signs.

Episiotomy

During the first hour after delivery, observe the incision site for redness, tenderness, swelling, and hematoma. Report any abnormal signs to the physician and document blood pressure, pulse, and any pain the client may have.

Cesarean delivery

Monitor the FHR continuously during preparations for cesarean delivery. During the procedure itself, the nurse anesthetist or anesthesiologist will monitor the client and fetus. Afterward, the physician and nursery staff will assess the neonate and recovery room personnel will monitor the client.

Nursing diagnosis

After reviewing all assessment data, the nurse formulates nursing diagnoses applicable to the client, the fetus, or selected family members. These nursing diagnoses help to direct nursing care for clients undergoing obstetric procedures. (For a partial list of possible nursing diagnoses, see *Nursing diagnoses: Obstetric procedures.*)

NURSING DIAGNOSES

Obstetric procedures

The following potential nursing diagnoses are examples of the problems and etiologies that the nurse may encounter when caring for a client undergoing a special obstetric procedure. Specific nursing interventions for some of these diagnoses are provided in the "Planning and implementation" section of this chapter.

- Altered role performance related to unmet expectations for childbirth
- Anxiety related to fear of death during childbirth
- Anxiety related to uncertain outcome for self and neonate
- Anxiety related to unexpected need for cesarean delivery
- Fatigue related to prolonged labor
- Fear related to real or potential threat to fetus or self
- Fluid volume excess related to oxytocin infusion
- Impaired gas exchange related to required obstetric or special procedure
- Ineffective family coping: compromised, related to unexpected need for obstetric procedure
- Ineffective individual coping related to lack of family support
- Knowledge deficit about obstetric procedure
- Pain related to required obstetric or special procedure
- Pain related to tetanic uterine contractions
- Potential for infection related to AROM
- Potential fluid volume deficit related to restricted oral intake
- Powerlessness related to complications that threaten pregnancy

Planning and implementation

Following the initial assessment of the client and fetus and development of nursing diagnoses, the nurse should plan for and implement obstetric procedures as appropriate. Planning includes preparing the client and initiating nursing activities that take place before, during, and after the procedure. These activities may include starting I.V. infusions, administering oxytocin, preparing for cesarean delivery, and providing psychological support and teaching to the client and family.

Initiate I.V. infusion

The client undergoing a special obstetric procedure may have a nursing diagnosis of *potential fluid volume deficit related to restricted oral intake.* To maintain hydration or administer medicaton, be prepared to start and maintain an I.V. line. Begin all infusions with an 18G or larger needle. If hemorrhage occurs, the client may need blood or blood products.

- A client undergoing external version may need an I.V. tocolytic agent to relax the uterus.
- A client receiving oxytocin requires a specialized I.V. procedure. First, begin an I.V. infusion, then piggyback the medication line onto the main line.
- For cesarean delivery, I.V. infusion maintains hydration, administers anesthesia, and provides an open line in case other medications are needed. Because these clients will remain NPO following delivery, hydration is necessary to prevent fluid volume deficit.

The physician will choose the type of fluid, such as normal saline or Ringer's lactate solution. Maintain a slow "keep vein open" rate if hydration is not compromised. Monitor fluid intake and output, especially during oxytocin infusion, to prevent a nursing diagnosis of *fluid volume excess related to oxytocin infusion.*

Administer oxytocin

A client with ineffective uterine contractions may have a nursing diagnosis of *fatigue related to prolonged labor,* possibly necessitating oxytocin infusion to enhance contractions.

Synthetic oxytocin is available in 1-ml ampules, each of which contains 10 units of the drug, as well as in 0.5 ml ampules and 10-ml multidose vials. As prescribed, add 5 to 10 units of oxytocin to 1,000 ml of an I.V. solution, such as normal saline or lactated Ringer's solution. After adding 10 units of oxytocin to 1,000 ml of I.V. solution, each ml of the resulting solution will provide 10 milliunits (mU) of oxytocin (10 mU/ml).

The recommended starting dose of 0.5 mU/minute should be increased no more than once every 15 minutes, in 1-mU increments. The increases should cease when contractions occur at least every 3 minutes, last 40 to 60 seconds each, and are of adequate intensity. The number of drops/minute will vary according to the type of infusion set used.

Piggyback the oxytocin solution on the primary set as close as possible to the venipuncture site. This allows virtually immediate discontinuation of oxytocin infusion if an emergency occurs while continuing to maintain an open vein. Use an I.V. infusion pump to ensure precise delivery of the solution. Rapid or excessive infusion may result in a nursing diagnosis of *pain related to tetanic uterine contractions.*

Clients typically respond to oxytocin in three phases (Steer and Beard, 1982). During the first phase, called the incremental induction phase, uterine contractions increase as the oxytocin dose increases. When contractions remain constant even when the dose increases, the client has reached the second phase, called the stable induction phase. If the dose continues to increase during this phase, contractions will occur more frequently but weaken. During the third phase, as the oxytocin dose increases further, the uterus relaxes less, possibly reaching a state of hyperstimulation with prolonged contractions. Steer and Beard (1982) suggest that most clients would achieve adequate labor patterns with 4 to 8 mU/minute.

Clients vary in their response to oxytocin. In some, even small amounts may produce hypertonia. In others, the drug fails to induce true labor. Induction should be discontinued if the client fails to achieve regular contractions and cervical dilation within 8 hours. Most clients will become exhausted within that time. The physician may choose to repeat induction the following day, or possibly perform a cesarean delivery (Cunningham, MacDonald, and Gant, 1989; American College of Obstetricians and Gynecologists, 1987).

Protect against infection

A client scheduled for amniotomy has a nursing diagnosis of *potential for infection related to AROM.* To protect against infection, clean the perineum with an antibacterial solution. Provide sterile gloves, a sterile amniohook, and lubricating jelly for the physician or nurse midwife.

Place a clean, absorbent bed liner beneath the client's buttocks before the procedure. Afterward, keep the perineal area clean and dry. Change linens frequently.

Prepare for cesarean delivery

A client who discovers that she must undergo cesarean delivery may have a nursing diagnosis of *fear related to real or potential threat to fetus or self.* To prepare the client and her family for surgery, begin by explaining all steps in the procedure and ensuring that the client has given her written consent. (For related information, see *Nursing research applied: How education affects attitude toward cesarean delivery.*)

Next, take the client to the labor and delivery area or surgical unit, according to facility policy, for physical preparation. This typically includes:
• Abdominal preparation or shaving. Although the actual area of incision may vary, facility policy may instruct the nurse to shave the entire abdomen, beginning below the nipple line and including the pubic area.
• Catheterization. Establish an indwelling urinary catheter with a gravity flow drainage system to prevent bladder distension during surgery.
• Laboratory tests. Obtain the tests ordered by the physician, possibly including complete blood count, electrolytes, and type and cross match for blood replacement.
• I.V. infusion. Begin an infusion with the prescribed solution using a 16G to 18G needle.
• Antacid administration. As prescribed, administer an antacid 15 minutes before anesthesia administration to reduce the complications associated with possible aspiration of gastric contents.
• Positioning. Assist the client into an appropriate position on the delivery or surgical table. Manipulate the table position to prevent the gravid uterus from compressing the inferior vena cava and to help maintain adequate placental perfusion.
• Preparation. Clean the operation site using the recommended antiseptic solution, prepare the support person if one is to attend the delivery, notify the nursery staff and pediatrician, gown and glove the physicians and scrub nurses, check suction and other delivery room equipment for proper functioning, and perform an initial sponge count.
• Assistance. During the procedure itself, assist the surgical team as needed and maintain records as required. Document the starting time of the procedure, the time of delivery, and the completion time. Immediately after delivery, assist in caring for the neonate as needed. (See Chapter 28, The Second Stage of Labor, for more information.)

Provide psychological support

The client may be surprised and dismayed by the need for a special obstetric procedure, especially if it is performed in response to an emergency. The client and family may have little time for mental preparation, which can lead to a nursing diagnosis of *anxiety related to uncertain outcome for self and neonate.* (For a complete nursing care plan, see *Applying the nursing process: Anxiety related to unexpected need for cesarean delivery,* pages 784 and 785.)

To address this nursing diagnosis, provide the client with basic information about the procedure, reassure her that it is safe for the fetus, and offer choices whenever possible to involve her in decisions. Also, listen and respond to her concerns or questions.

A client who has a cesarean delivery may require additional support, especially if it provokes many emotions in her and her support person. Failure to achieve the anticipated vaginal delivery may provoke feelings

How education affects attitude toward cesarean delivery

A recent study indicates that women who had cesarean deliveries and their partners found prenatal education regarding it both helpful and comforting, even when this method was unplanned. Eighty-one couples who enrolled in a Lamaze class read a pamphlet about cesarean delivery and participated in a follow-up discussion about the pamphlet contents. Eighteen of the couples subsequently had cesarean deliveries, and fifteen of those later indicated that they benefited from the preparation.

The researchers then conducted a related study under the same premise, but they solicited responses from all class participants regardless of delivery method. Analysis of the responses revealed that both men and women had a more positive reaction to childbirth, regardless of method, after receiving education. Additionally, the educational program prepared the expectant partners for unanticipated cesarean delivery. The sample included 44 women (mean age: 28.5 years) and 42 men (mean age: 31.5 years). Thirteen of the women, including twelve primiparous women and one multiparous woman, subsequently had cesarean deliveries. Reasons for these deliveries included cephalopelvic disproportion (4), breech presentation (3), fetal distress (3), dystocia (2), and maternal illness and fetopelvic disorder (1).

Application to practice
Although many women and their partners ask for and receive detailed information about unplanned cesarean delivery, many resist this information as a way of coping. This study suggests that the information be included in traditional childbirth education classes, with special attention given to those who appear anxious about cesarean delivery, rather than limiting information only to those who request it. The researchers urge childbirth educators to continue to study the reactions of participants in their classes and explore teaching strategies that will prepare couples for the possibility of a cesarean delivery.

Fawcett, J., and Henklein, J. (1987). Antenatal education for cesarean birth: Extension of a field test. JOGNN, 16(1), 61-65.

associated with grieving, such as anger, denial, and guilt. Acknowledge these feelings. Trite statements, such as, "You're lucky you don't have to go through labor," or "This is better for the baby" may add to the parents' conflicting feelings. The fact that the procedure is best for the fetus will not obviate the client's grief (Schroder-Zwelling, 1988).

One way to help alleviate the client's fears is to allow her some control over her care (Schroder-Zwelling, 1988). For instance, suggest that she and her support person discuss with the anesthesiologist the options for anesthesia. Regional anesthesia allows the client to have many of the same experiences she would have had with a vaginal delivery. It also allows maximum contact between the client and neonate immediately after delivery

(Shearer, Shiono, and Rhoads, 1988). Allowing the client's support person into the delivery room also may improve her feelings about the experience. This way, both can bond with the neonate as soon after delivery as the neonate is awake, active, and able to establish eye contact (Leach and Sproule, 1984).

If the client and her partner have attended childbirth education classes, they are more likely to be prepared for and have a positive attitude toward alternative delivery.

Evaluation

To complete the nursing process, the nurse evaluates the effectiveness of the care plan by reviewing the goals attained and the family's involvement and satisfaction with the care provided. Evaluation should be stated in terms of actions performed or outcomes achieved for each goal. The following examples illustrate appropriate outcome statements.

• Five hours after initiation of oxytocin infusion, the client gave birth vaginally.

• The client exhibited no signs of infection after amniotomy.

• Edema of the neonate's scalp resolved within 48 hours after vacuum extraction.

• The client expressed decreased anxiety when discussing the usual outcomes of cesarean delivery.

• The support person provided psychological support for the client during cesarean delivery.

• The client demonstrated an understanding of the obstetric intervention by cooperating and participating in preparatory activities.

• The client and support person expressed acceptance and understanding of the need for the procedure.

• The FHR showed no serious abnormalities.

Documentation

The nurse documents assessment findings and nursing activities as thoroughly and objectively as possible. Thorough documentation not only allows evaluation of the effectiveness of the care plan but also makes data available to other members of the health care team, which

Anxiety related to unexpected need for cesarean delivery

The nursing process helps ensure high-quality care for the client undergoing a special obstetric procedure and for her family. The table below shows how the nurse might use the nursing process when caring for the client described in the case history at right. The first column presents history and physical assessment data followed by a paragraph of mental notes. These notes help the nurse make important connec-

tions among assessment findings, aiding in development of the nursing diagnosis and planning.

The second column lists an appropriate nursing diagnosis; information in the remaining columns is based on this diagnosis. Although not part of the nursing process, a rationale appears for each intervention in the fourth column to explain how it contributes to the care plan.

ASSESSMENT	NURSING DIAGNOSIS	PLANNING
Subjective (history) data • Client states that she is afraid of surgery. • Client's husband demands angrily, "Why didn't someone tell us that something was wrong? What is going to happen to our baby and to my wife?" **Objective (physical) data** • Childbirth history: gravida II, para I • Allergies and sensitivities: penicillin • Onset of labor: 2 p.m. • Uterine contractions every 2 minutes, lasting 60 seconds and with adequate intensity. • Cephalic presentation. • Cervix dilated 3 cm. • Baseline FHR 140 bpm with decreased variability; late deceleration patterns noted. • Nursing interventions to relieve FHR deceleration ineffective. • Fetal scalp pH: 7.16. • Vital signs at 4:20 p.m.: blood pressure 130/80, pulse 86, temperature 99° F by mouth, respirations 20, FHR 134. • Gestational age of fetus: 40 weeks. • Laboratory data: HCT 38.6, Hb 12.3. • Type and cross match sent. • Prothrombin time: 12.6. **Mental notes** *Because the couple did not anticipate cesarean delivery, they will have little time to plan for it psychologically. The client and her partner may feel threatened by actual or perceived danger to her or to the fetus. The client's husband can offer comfort and support to the client once he copes with the surprise and fear.*	Anxiety related to unexpected need for cesarean delivery	**Goals** The client will: • verbalize an understanding of factual information about preoperative procedures • verbalize fears and concerns for the fetus • express an understanding of reasons for the change in planned delivery. The client's husband will: • provide support for the client by expressing an understanding of the need for cesarean delivery • demonstrate coping behavior by participating appropriately in the client's care.

helps ensure consistent care. To document as accurately as possible, ensure that the entries describe events exactly, completely, and in chronological order.

Each health care facility may require documentation of slightly different information; however, examples of appropriate documentation topics include:
• maternal vital signs
• cervical changes
• FHR
• Time of amniotic sac rupture; amount and color of amniotic fluid
• frequency, duration, and intensity of uterine contractions

• I.V. administration of medications or fluids
• intake and output
• oxytocin dosage
• time of initiation and duration of oxytocin infusion
• description and location of marks left on the neonate's head from forceps delivery
• perineal care delivered after episiotomy
• the client's expressed wish to attempt VBAC
• specific steps taken to prepare the client for cesarean delivery.

CASE STUDY

Maria Gallo, a primiparous client age 28 at 40 weeks' gestation, is admitted for induced labor after spontaneous rupture of the membranes. Upon her admission, presentation was cephalic, and the fetal heart rate (FHR) was normal as read by an external monitor. Induction of labor was initiated with I.V. oxytocin, after which the fetus exhibited distress. The physician has decided to perform an emergency cesarean delivery, leaving the couple confused and frightened.

IMPLEMENTATION		EVALUATION
Intervention Stay with the client and her husband as much as possible.	**Rationale** Anxiety will increase if the client and her husband feel that the nurse is ignoring their fears. Reinforcement supports coping mechanisms, promotes self-confidence, and reduces anxiety.	Upon evaluation, the client and her husband: • verbalized their fears about emergency surgery • verbalized their understanding of the need for emergency surgery • exhibited increased coping skills.
Provide positive emotional support and reinforcement. Encourage the client and her husband to discuss their feelings. Support their attempts to cope with the situation.	Communication can reduce their anxiety.	The client: • stated that she was less fearful with her husband at her bedside in a quiet and calm atmosphere • stated that she expected a successful delivery.
Speak slowly in a calm voice. Reduce stimuli in the client's environment.	The client may be distracted by the noise and confusion related to preparation for emergency surgery. This may cause unnecessary anxiety.	
Answer the client's questions about cesarean delivery.	The couple must understand the current status before they can begin their psychological adjustment.	
Review preoperative procedures, necessary laboratory tests, abdominal preparation, urinary catheter insertion, transfer to the delivery room, and types of anesthesia. Discuss in as much depth as possible what the client will experience postoperatively.	Knowledge will assist the client in preoperative preparation and will reduce her anxiety about postoperative outcomes.	

Chapter summary

Chapter 32 described obstetric procedures required by clients who need special interventions during labor and delivery. Here are the chapter highlights.

• Version is used to rotate the fetus in utero. It may be performed externally when the fetus is in breech or shoulder presentation or internally to provide rapid delivery of a second twin.

• Infusion of synthetic oxytocin is the method employed most commonly to induce labor. During oxytocin administration, the nurse should monitor I.V. fluids and urine output carefully because of the antidiuretic action of the drug.

• Amniotomy, or artificial rupture of the membranes, is widely used in the United States to augment or induce labor. Possible prolapse of the umbilical cord and ascension of pathogens through the vaginal canal are two potential complications that require ongoing nursing assessment.

• Low, or outlet, forceps delivery may be used to assist in delivering a fetus low in the birth canal. Mid and high forceps deliveries are used rarely in the United

States because of the high risk of trauma to the client and fetus.

• In vacuum extraction, the physician applies a suction cup device to the fetus's scalp and traction is applied to the cup to draw the fetus through the birth canal. Unlike forceps, vacuum extraction does not increase the amount of space needed inside the birth canal.

• Commonly performed in the United States, episiotomy is intended to minimize perineal lacerations and fetal head trauma. However, some researchers suggest its widespread use is unnecessary.

• During the past decade, cesarean deliveries in the United States have increased from less than 5% of all deliveries to almost 25%, in part because it now is safer for the client and fetus than such instrument procedures as mid and high forceps deliveries. Cesarean delivery is viewed by physicians as an alternative delivery method.

• Because of advances in cesarean techniques, many clients now have the option of attempting a vaginal delivery after a previous cesarean delivery.

• Most clients and their partners expect a normal labor and delivery. When obstetric interventions are necessary, the couple will need information and guidance to make a sound decision and maintain normal coping strategies. The nurse plays an important role in providing this information and in supporting the client and her partner.

Study questions

1. Mrs. Rita Turner has had three children and now is 35 weeks pregnant with a single fetus. A sonogram has revealed a breech presentation, and her physician has decided to perform external version to rotate the fetus to a cephalic presentation. Which measures should the nurse take before and after the procedure?

2. Ms. Judith Jessie—a primigravid client—was admitted to the labor and delivery area for induced labor. The physician performed an amniotomy. Which actions should the nurse take immediately after amniotomy?

3. Mrs. Maria Carmello has been scheduled for a non-elective oxytocin induction at 37 weeks' gestation. She previously experienced a fetal death at 38 weeks' gestation related to uncontrolled diabetes. What should the nurse look for in assessing Mrs. Carmello's cervix to determine the chances for successful induction?

4. Jane Newman states that she has had one child by cesarean delivery. Now pregnant with her second child, she would like to attempt vaginal delivery. What information does the nurse need to know about VBAC?

Bibliography

American College of Obstetricians and Gynecologists. (November 1987). Induction and augmentation of labor. *Technical Bulletin*, No. 110.

Arms, S. (1975). *Immaculate Deception.* New York: Houghton Mifflin.

Ashford, J. (1986). A history of accouchment force. *Birth*, 13(4), 1550-1985.

Bishop, E. (1964). Pelvic scoring for elective induction. *Obstetrics and Gynecology*, 24(5), 266.

Banta, D., and Thacker, S. (1982). The risks and benefits of episiotomy: A review. *Birth*, 9(1), 25-30.

Borgetta, L., Piening, S., and Cohen, W. (1989). Association of episiotomy and delivery position with deep perineal laceration during spontaneous delivery in nulliparous women. *American Journal of Obstetrical Gynecology*, 160(2), 294-297.

Cunningham, F.G., MacDonald, P.C., and Gant, N.F. (1989). *Williams obstetrics* (18th ed.). East Norwalk CT: Appleton & Lange.

Hacker, N., and Moore, J. (1986). *Essentials of obstetrics and gynecology.* Philadelphia: Saunders.

Henrikson, M., and Wild, L. (1988). A nursing process approach to epidural anagesia. *JOGNN*, 17(5), 316-320.

Hofmeyr, G. (1987). Commentary: Cephalic version and ethnicity. *Birth*, 14(2), 81.

Inturrisi, M., Feleppa, C. and Rosen, M. (1988). Epidural morphine for relief of postpartum, postsurgical pain. *JOGNN*, 17(4), 238-243.

Korones, S.B. (1986). *High-risk newborn infants* (4th ed.). St. Louis: Mosby.

Lumley, J., and Dovey, B. (1987). Do hospitals with family-centered maternity care policies have lower intervention rates? *Birth*, 14(3), 132-134.

Oxorn, H. (1986). *Oxorn-Foote human labor and birth* (5th ed.). East Norwalk, CT: Appleton & Lange.

Placek, P., Taffel, S., and Liss, T. (1987). The cesarean future. *American Demographics*, 9(9), 46-47.

Rosen, M., and Peisner, D. (1987). Effect of amniotic membrane rupture on length of labor. *Obstetrics and Gynecology*, 70, 604.

Induction of labor

Boyan, P., and MacDonald, D. (1988). Commentary: Oxytocin: The need to distinguish between induction and augmentation and between multiparous and primiparous. *Birth*, 15(4), 203.

Curtis, P., and Sofransky, N. (1988). Rethinking oxytocin protocols in the augmentation of labor. *Birth*, 15(4), 199-202.

Food and Drug Administration. New restrictions on oxytocin use. *FDA Bulletin*, 8(5).

Henderson, C. (1987). Artificial rupture of the membranes. *Nursing Times*, 83(38), 63-64.

Jhirad, A. and Vago, T. (1973). Induction of labor by breast stimulation. *Obstetrics and Gynecology*, 41-374.

Johnson, G. (1981). Oxytocics for the Induction of Labor. *March of Dimes*, Series 3, Module 2.

Marshall, C. (1985). The art of induction/augmentation of labor. *Journal of Obstetrics, Gynecological and Neonatal Nursing*, 14(1), 22.

Rayburn, W. (March, 1989). Prostaglandin E$_2$ gel for cervical ripening and induction of labor: A critical analysis. *American Journal of Obstetrics and Gynecology*, 160(3), 529-534.

Salmon, Y., Tan, S., Gen, S., and Kee, W. (1986). Cervical ripening by breast stimulation. *Obstetrics and Gynecology*, 67(1), 21.

Steer, P.J., and Beard, R.S. (1982). Bettering control of oxytocin infusions. *Contemporary OB/GYN*, 19, 117.

Forceps

Duker, L.J., et al. (1985). The midforceps: Maternal and neonatal outcomes. *American Journal of Obstetrics and Gynecology*, 152, 156.

Laub, D.W. (1985). Forceps delivery. *Clinical Obstetrical Gynecology*, June 29, 286.

Vacuum extraction

Galvan, B., and Broekhuizen, F. (1987). Obstetric vacuum extraction. *JOGNN*, 15(4), 242-248.

Episiotomy

Bromberg, M. (1986). Presumptive maternal benefits of routine episiotomy. *Journal of Nurse-Midwifery*, 31(3), 121-127.

Cesarean delivery

Consensus Task Force on Cesarean Childbirth. Cesarean Childbirth. (October, 1981). U.S. Department of Health and Human Services. NIH Publication No. 822067. Bethesda, MD: National Institutes of Health.

Dansforth, D.N. (1985). Cesarean section. *JAMA*, 253(6), 811-818.

Ewy, D., and Youmans, J. (1988). The early parenting experience. In F. Nichols and S. Humenick (Eds.), *Childbirth and education: Practice, research, and theory*. Philadelphia: Saunders.

Leach, L. and Sproule V. (1984). Meeting the challenge of cesarean births. *JOGNN*, 13(3), 191-199.

Schroder-Zwelling, E. (1988). The unexpected childbirth experience. In F. Nichols and S. Humenick (Eds.), *Childbirth and education: Practice, research, and theory*. Philadelphia: Saunders.

Shearer, E., Shiono, P., and Rhoads, G. (1988). Recent trends in family-centered maternity care for cesarean-birth families. *Birth*, 15(1), 3-7.

VBAC

American College of Obstetricians and Gynecologists. (October 1988). Committee on Maternal and Fetal Medicine. *Guidelines for vaginal delivery after cesarean birth*.

Flamm, B.L. (1985). Vaginal birth after cesarean section: Controversies old and new. *Clinical Obstetrical Gynecology*, December 28, 735.

Hemminki, E. (1987). Pregnancy and birth after cesarean section: A survey based on the Swedish birth register. *Birth*, 14(1), 12-17.

Laufer, A., Hodenius, V., Friedman, L., Duncan, N., Guy, C.M., MacPherson, S., and Barrows, N. (1987). Vaginal birth after cesarean section. *Journal of Nurse-Midwifery*, 32(1), 41-47.

Lipson, J. (1984). Repeat cesarean births: Social and psychological issues. *JOGNN*, 13(3), 191-199.

Miller, C. and Sonnemann-Sutter, C. (1985). Vaginal birth after cesarean. *JOGNN*, 14(5), 383-389.

Nursing research

Avery, M., and Von Arsdale, L. (1987). Perineal massage effect on the incidence of episiotomy and laceration in a nulliparous population. *Journal of Nurse-Midwifery*, 32(3), 181-184.

Chenia, F., and Crowther, M. (1987). Does advice to assume the knee-chest position reduce the incidence of breech presentation at delivery? A randomized clinical trial. *Birth*, 14(2), 75-80.

Fawcett, J., and Henklein, J. (1987). Antenatal education for cesarean birth: Extension of a field test. *JOGNN*, 16(1), 61-65.

Rambler, D., and Roberts, J. (1986). A comparison of cold and warm sitz baths for relief of postpartum perineal pain. *JOGNN*, 15(6), 471-474.

CHAPTER 33

Intrapartal Complications

Objectives

After reading and studying this chapter, the student should be able to:

1. Identify factors that place a client and her fetus at risk for intrapartal complications.

2. Assess for signs and symptoms that indicate the potential for or presence of an intrapartal complication.

3. Describe the emotional and psychological needs of a client and her family during an intrapartal complication.

4. Prioritize the needs of a client and fetus during a potentially life-threatening intrapartal complication.

5. Apply the nursing process when caring for a client with an intrapartal complication.

Introduction

Complications that arise during labor raise client fears and may threaten the health and well-being of the client and fetus. The nurse plays a vital role in detecting intrapartal complications, assisting in their resolution, and providing the client with appropriate clinical and emotional care.

This chapter discusses the intrapartal complications the nurse must know about—complications involving the uterus, pelvis, birth canal, placenta, membranes and amniotic fluid, and umbilical cord; systemic disorders of the pregnant client; and complications that center on the fetus. Then, using the nursing process, the chapter investigates appropriate nursing care for each of these complications.

Reproductive system disorders

Many intrapartal complications are caused by reproductive system disorders, which may arise from uterine, pelvic, placental, membrane and amniotic fluid, or umbilical cord factors. To assist the physician, the nurse must understand the physiologic changes associated with these disorders as well as the medical treatment required.

Uterine factors

Many uterine factors can affect the progress of labor. Uterine contractions, the primary power of labor, play a critical role in determining whether labor is normal or dysfunctional. (See *Dysfunctional labor,* page 790, for more information.) Other intrapartal complications related to the uterus include preterm labor, postterm labor, precipitate labor, uterine rupture, uterine inversion, and congenital or structural uterine anomalies.

Dysfunction

Uterine dysfunction may be classified as hypotonic or hypertonic. In hypotonic dysfunction, the more common of the two, contractions grow less frequent and less powerful as labor continues. Eventually, they become too weak to produce adequate cervical dilation. Hypo-

GLOSSARY

Abruptio placentae: premature separation of part or all of the placenta from the uterine wall after the twentieth week of pregnancy and before delivery. Hemorrhage and shock are common complications.

Battledore placenta: benign condition in which the umbilical cord implants at the edge of the placenta.

Coagulopathy: abnormal clotting disorder characterized by hypothrombinemia, hypofibrinogenemia, and subnormal platelet count; caused by a major insult, such as abruptio placentae.

Disseminated intravascular coagulation (DIC): abnormal clotting disorder characterized by hypoprothrombinemia, hypofibrinogenemia, and a subnormal platelet count; caused by a major insult to the body, such as abruptio placentae.

Fourchette: area of the female perineum between the posterior junction of the labia minora and labia majora.

Hypofibrinogenemia: abnormally low fibrinogen (a coagulation agent) in the blood.

Placenta accreta: condition in which part or all of the placenta adheres firmly to the uterine wall.

Placenta increta: condition in which placental villi invade the uterine myometrium.

Placenta percreta: condition in which placental villi penetrate the myometrium to the peritoneal covering of the uterus.

Placenta previa: abnormally low implantation of the placenta so that it encroaches onto the internal cervical os.

Precipitate labor: labor that proceeds very rapidly, usually lasting less than 3 hours.

Puerperium: 6-week period after childbirth.

Transverse lie: presentation in which the long axis of the fetus is perpendicular to that of the mother.

Uterine inversion: abnormal condition in which the uterus is turned inside out, with the internal surface protruding into or beyond the vagina; usually caused by excessive traction on the umbilical cord.

Velamentous: membranous.

---

tonic dysfunction typically occurs during the active phase of labor.

Hypertonic dysfunction, which typically occurs during the latent phase of labor, is characterized by intense, painful contractions unaccompanied by normal cervical dilation.

Preterm labor

When preterm labor cannot be stopped (using techniques described in Chapter 23, Antepartal Complications), delivery should take place in a facility prepared to care for a preterm, potentially high-risk neonate, if possible. If transfer of the pregnant client to such a facility is not possible before delivery, then the neonate may need to be transferred to a neonatal intensive care unit. Ideally, however, client and neonate should reside in the same facility.

Postterm labor

When pregnancy lasts 42 weeks or longer, labor is considered postterm and may cause difficulty if the fetus is large for gestational age—a condition that could result in cephalopelvic disproportion.

Precipitate labor

Characterized by rapid progression, precipitate labor typically lasts less than 3 hours. It may result from decreased resistance of soft tissue in the birth canal or by abnormally strong uterine contractions (Cunningham, MacDonald, and Gant, 1989). Although recent studies suggest that precipitate labor poses no greater risk to the client and fetus than does normal labor (Oxorn, 1986), many experts believe that precipitate labor increases the risk of maternal lacerations and fetal intracranial hemorrhage and asphyxia. Additional risks include unattended delivery, fetal hypoxia from intense uterine contractions, and decreased uterine tone after delivery. (See *Psychomotor skills: Performing an emergency delivery*, page 791, for more information.)

Uterine rupture

A serious medical emergency, rupture of the uterus may occur before or during labor. A complete rupture tears all layers of the uterus, establishing direct communication between the uterine and abdominal cavities. In an incomplete rupture, the myometrium tears, but the peritoneal covering of the uterus remains intact (Oxorn, 1986).

Uterine rupture occurs more frequently after previous cesarean delivery and during prolonged labor, difficult forceps delivery, and oxytocin administration. Although signs and symptoms of uterine rupture vary widely with location and severity, they typically include abdominal pain, vaginal bleeding, hypovolemic shock, and fetal distress. If rupture occurs during labor, contractions may cease.

Uterine inversion

In this rare, potentially life-threatening emergency, the uterus turns inside out so that its internal surface pro-

Dysfunctional labor

When a fetus fails to move out of the uterus and through the birth canal, or when this progression takes an abnormally long time, the client is in dysfunctional labor. (Other terms used to describe dysfunctional labor include dystocia, prolonged labor, and failure to progress.) Experts estimate that dysfunctional labor has a 1% to 7% incidence (Oxorn, 1986). Depending on the circumstances involved, it may threaten the health or life of the client and fetus.

Dysfunctional labor can have any of several causes. Altered uterine muscle contractility can prevent progressive cervical dilation and effacement, thus blocking fetal descent. Altered muscle contractility may result from abnormalities of the uterus or bony pelvis or fetal position and presentation. Administration of narcotic or anesthesic agents in the latent phase, primiparity, and maternal exhaustion are other causes of uterine dysfunction (Oxorn, 1986). In many cases, the cause cannot be identified with certainty.

According to Friedman (1989), the latent phase can be considered prolonged if it exceeds 14 hours for a multiparous client or 20 hours for a nulliparous client.

The most important factors in assessing labor progress are cervical dilation and fetal descent. Without cervical dilation, descent cannot occur. Most nulliparous clients show cervical dilation of at least 1.2 cm per hour during active labor; most multiparous clients dilate by at least 1.5 cm per hour during active labor. Dilation of less than these rates constitutes a prolonged active phase. The active phase is divided into three phases. The acceleration phase occurs when the rate of cervical dilation begins to increase; the phase of maximum slope, when cervical dilation is almost complete; and the deceleration phase, when the rate of cervical dilation slows.

Progression of labor can be depicted by plotting cervical dilation in centimeters against elapsed time. In normal labor, the resulting graph will form an S-shaped curve, as shown below (Friedman, 1989). In dysfunctional labor, the dilation curve will become flattened or strung out.

Effects of prolonged labor on the fetus may include hypoxia, asphyxia, and physical injuries sustained during descent. In many cases, dysfunctional labor is an indication for cesarean delivery.

COMPARISON OF NORMAL AND DYSFUNCTIONAL LABOR PROGRESSION

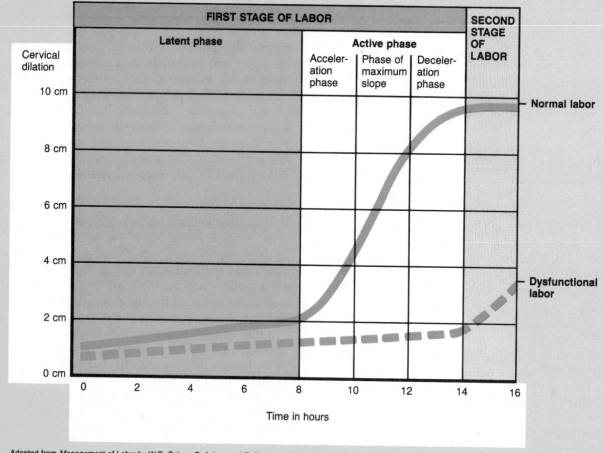

Adapted from *Management of Labor* by W.R. Cohen, D. Acker, and E. Friedman (Eds.), pp. 1-18, with permission of Aspen Publishers, Inc., © 1989.

trudes into or beyond the vagina. Uterine inversion may occur before or after delivery of the placenta. Although the cause may not be apparent, excessive traction on the umbilical cord and attempts to deliver the placenta manually while the uterus is relaxed may be contributing factors. The client may experience significant blood loss and shock. The clearest sign of uterine inversion is the craterlike depression that forms in the abdomen.

Congenital or structural abnormalities

Although uncommon, abnormalities of the uterus, cervix, and vagina may block normal labor and delivery. (For illustrations of these abnormalities, see Chapter 10, Fertility and Infertility.) These abnormalities may range from complete lack of development (agenesis) to development of two separate structures (double cervix or vagina). During embryonic development, the fallopian tubes, uterus, and upper vagina begin to develop at 5 to 6 weeks' gestation. Improper development may produce duplications of all or part of the reproductive structures (Jackson, 1990). The most common abnormality is a septate uterus.

Pelvic factors

Critical to normal fetal descent is the relationship between the size of the pelvis and the size and presentation of the fetus. Complications develop when the pelvis is too small (contracted) to allow normal fetal descent. Additional complications involving fetal descent include lacerations of the vaginal canal and surrounding soft tissues.

Structural contractures

The pelvis may be contracted at the inlet, midpelvis, or outlet, or it may be generally small. This may not be a problem with a small fetus. With a fetus of normal or above normal size, however, contracture may prevent passage.

The client has a contracted pelvic inlet when the anteroposterior diameter measures less than 10 cm or when the diagonal conjugate measures less than 11.5 cm. The client has a contracted midpelvis when the interspinous diameter measures less than 10 cm and a contracted outlet when the interischial tuberous diam-

---

PSYCHOMOTOR SKILLS

Performing an emergency delivery

In cases of precipitate labor, the nurse may be the only health care professional in attendance for the delivery. If this occurs, the nurse should help the client and anyone with her to remain calm and summon additional professional assistance immediately. Never leave the client alone.

1 If delivery takes place at home or in a public location, the first step is to summon assistance or, better yet, to have someone nearby do the summoning. Assistance should include transportation of the client to a health care facility. If delivery occurs in a health care facility before the nurse-midwife or physician arrives, gather a sterile pack or tray containing such sterile equipment as towels, a bulb syringe, a cord clamp, and blankets for the neonate. If time and facilities permit, perform thorough handwashing and don sterile gloves.

2 As the fetus's head reaches and begins to pass the perineum, instruct the client to pant or blow through contractions; forceful bearing down could cause extensive lacerations. To assist her, place one hand gently on the perineum, covering the fetus's head, to prevent a sudden expulsion. Do not attempt to prevent descent forcibly. As the head emerges, immediately break the sac if it is intact. Support the head after it emerges and instruct the client to continue blowing or panting. Check to see if the umbilical cord has wrapped around the fetus's neck and, if so, gently slip it over the head.

If the shoulders do not emerge spontaneously, place gentle traction on the head to help the anterior shoulder slip under the symphysis pubis. Be prepared for the rest of the body to slide out quickly.

3 Wipe the neonate's face dry and use a bulb syringe, if available, to remove fluid and mucus from the mouth and nose. Position the neonate on the client's abdomen, and use blankets to keep the neonate warm at all times.

4 Clamp or tie off the umbilical cord and cut it with sterile equipment. (Unsterilized equipment could lead to a potentially life-threatening infection.) Never pull the cord. The placenta should separate and deliver spontaneously. After placental separation occurs, the shape of the uterus changes from a disk to a globe, the amount of umbilical cord extending from the vagina will lengthen, and a small gush of blood may appear. Urge the client to bear down to help complete delivery of the placenta.

5 Check to see that the client's fundus is firm and, if not, massage it as necessary. A client who breast-feeds her neonate will stimulate oxytocin release that helps keep the fundus firm.

6 Document the events of the delivery, including the time of labor onset and delivery, a description of the birth process, a list of people present, and the sex and condition of the neonate.

eter measures 8 cm or less. A contracted outlet rarely occurs without a contracted midpelvis.

With a normal fetopelvic relationship, uterine contractions gradually rotate the fetus's head to an anterior position that provides the most favorable adaptation between the head and the pelvis. (See Chapter 24, Physiology of Labor and Childbirth, for information on normal pelvic measurements and normal rotational movements.) A contracted pelvis may prevent this internal rotation, possibly placing the fetus's head in the transverse position. As with other causes of arrested fetal descent, this abnormal rotation will impair cervical dilation and may lead to a decrease in the frequency and intensity of uterine contractions.

Lacerations

During delivery, the soft tissues of the birth canal commonly sustain trauma and lacerations of the cervix, vagina, or perineum.

If the client is bleeding heavily after expelling the placenta and her fundus is firm, suspect a cervical laceration. Small cervical lacerations occur commonly during delivery and may not need repair. Severe lacerations, possibly affecting the upper vagina, will require surgical attention. Expect the cervix to be examined after a difficult vaginal delivery.

Lacerations of the lower portion of the birth canal may be classified by severity:
• First-degree lacerations involve the fourchette, perineal skin, and vaginal mucous membranes.
• Second-degree lacerations extend to the fascia and muscles of the perineal body.
• Third-degree lacerations extend to the anal sphincter.
• Fourth-degree lacerations extend to the anal canal.

Placental factors

Placental abnormalities may become apparent during pregnancy, or they may remain undetected until labor or just after delivery (the puerperium). During any stage, they present a major risk to the client and fetus. The most common placental complications include placenta previa, abruptio placentae, and failure of placental separation.

Placenta previa

When the placenta forms near or over the cervical os instead of taking a position higher in the body of the uterus, the client risks mild to potentially life-threatening hemorrhage, depending on the location of the placenta. Four classifications describe this abnormality:
• Complete (or total) placenta previa, where the placenta covers the cervical os completely

• Partial placenta previa, where the placenta covers the os partially
• Marginal placenta previa, where an edge of the placenta meets the rim of the cervical os but does not occlude it
• Low-lying placenta, where the placenta implants in the lower uterine segment and a placental edge lies close to the cervical os.

Placenta previa occurs in 0.4% to 0.6% of pregnancies (Cunningham, MacDonald, and Gant, 1989). Incidence increases with multiparity, previous cesarean delivery, advanced maternal age, twin fetuses, and abnormal fetal lie (Ouimette, 1986).

The main symptom of placenta previa is painless vaginal bleeding after the twentieth week of pregnancy. In some clients, bleeding may not occur until labor begins. When bleeding begins before the onset of labor, it tends to be episodic, beginning without warning, stopping spontaneously, and beginning again later. The client may experience slow, steady bleeding that could affect blood count. Typically, the uterus is soft and nontender.

Diagnosis of placenta previa is based on the client's history, ultrasound examination, and physical assessment. Any pregnant client who reports an episode of painless, vaginal bleeding of sudden onset requires hospitalization and ultrasonography to display the location of the placenta. Laboratory studies should include a complete blood count, coagulation studies, and a type and crossmatch if bleeding is severe. To avoid potentially severe hemorrhage, the client should not have a manual pelvic examination until results of the ultrasound examination are available, especially if the fetus is premature. If the fetus is mature, manual examination should occur only if preparations have been made for immediate delivery. Severe hemorrhage warrants immediate emergency delivery.

Abruptio placentae

In approximately 1 in 75 to 90 pregnancies, some or all of the placenta separates from the uterine wall after the twentieth week of gestation and before delivery (Abdella, Sibae, Hays, and Anderson, 1984). Called abruptio placentae, this condition may threaten the life of the client and fetus. (See *Comparing placenta previa and abruptio placentae* for more information.)

Although the primary cause of abruptio placentae is unknown, the following conditions may contribute to it: maternal hypertension, a short umbilical cord that places traction on the placenta, trauma, a uterine anomaly or tumor, sudden decompression of the uterus, pressure on the vena cava from the enlarged uterus, and dietary deficiency (Cunningham, MacDonald, and Gant, 1989).

Comparing placenta previa and abruptio placentae

By distinguishing between similar placental abnormalities, the nurse can anticipate care measures that the health care team must take.

	PLACENTA PREVIA	ABRUPTIO PLACENTAE
Description	Development of the placenta in the lower uterine segment. Classified according to the degree that it obstructs the cervical os.	Premature separation of some or all of the normally implanted placenta from the uterine wall. Classified according to the type of hemorrhage and degree of separation.
Signs and symptoms	Abdomen appears normal; painless bleeding; uterus soft, except during contractions; fetus palpable; fetal heart tones almost always present; fetal movement not affected.	Abdomen distended, tense, and painful (boardlike); possible concealed hemorrhage; fetus nonpalpable; possible signs of fetal distress; if fetus has died, fetal heart tones absent, no fetal movement.
Management	Bed rest; vaginal or cesarean delivery; vaginal examinations are contraindicated; Trendelenberg position to prevent shock.	Immediate cesarean or vaginal delivery to preserve the life of a live fetus or prevent further bleeding with a dead fetus.
Complications	Hemorrhage; shock; infection; maternal or fetal death.	Hemorrhagic shock; hypofibrinogenemia; disseminated intravascular coagulation; hemorrhage into the myometrium; renal failure (acute tubular necrosis); maternal or fetal death.

Whether an abruption involves a small area of the placenta or total separation, vaginal bleeding after the twentieth week of pregnancy and constant abdominal pain are its classic signs. According to Hurd, Midovnik, Hertzberg, and Levin (1983), additional signs include uterine tenderness or back pain, fetal distress, frequent contractions, hypertonic uterus, preterm labor, and fetal demise. Reliance on bleeding alone for diagnosis may be misleading because the presence and severity of vaginal bleeding may vary with the extent and location of placental separation. For example, vaginal bleeding will occur when a placental edge separates and blood flows between the placenta and uterine wall, escaping through the cervix. Vaginal bleeding will not occur when the center of the placenta separates but the edges remain attached. In this case, hemorrhage severe enough to cause fetal death could be concealed between the placenta and the uterine wall.

Diagnosis of abruptio placentae should be based on the client's history, physical assessment, and ultrasound examination. Most often, a client will report an episode of vaginal bleeding, typically accompanied by continuous abdominal pain. In some cases, she may report uterine contractions. Fetal monitoring may show distress; ultrasound examination may reveal a retroplacental hematoma. Even if ultrasound reveals no bleeding, a tentative diagnosis of abruptio placentae should be made if the client does not have placenta previa (which also would be revealed by ultrasound).

Failure of placental separation

The placenta normally separates from the uterine wall within 10 minutes after fetal delivery. Occasionally, however, placental separation may be delayed—a condition known as retained placenta. Separation may not occur at all—a condition known as abnormal adherence that takes one of three forms: placenta accreta, placenta increta, or placenta percreta.

Retained placenta. When spontaneous placental separation does not occur within 30 minutes after fetal delivery, the nurse-midwife or physician may attempt to remove the retained placenta manually.

Abnormal adherence. In some clients, absence of the decidua basalis allows the placenta to adhere too firmly to the uterine wall. Known as placenta accreta, this condition may occur over the entire placenta or only in a portion of it (Cunningham, MacDonald, and Gant, 1989). In placenta increta, the placental villi invade the myometrium. In placenta percreta, the villi penetrate to the peritoneal covering of the uterus, sometimes causing uterine rupture.

Although the etiology of these conditions is unknown, predisposing factors may include placenta previa, previous cesarean delivery, previous curettage, and multiparity. Incidence of these abnormalities is unknown as well, but placenta accreta is the most commonly reported of the three conditions.

Membrane and amniotic fluid factors

Several complications may arise during labor that are linked to the membranes and amniotic fluid. They include hydramnios, oligohydramnios, premature rupture of the membranes (PROM), and amniotic fluid embolism.

Hydramnios

Normally, amniotic fluid volume equals approximately 1,000 ml at term. In hydramnios, volume reaches or exceeds 2,000 ml and is associated with fetal anomalies, the most common being congenital anomalies of the central nervous and gastrointestinal systems.

Hydramnios occurs in about 0.9% of all pregnant clients; the risk increases in clients with diabetes. In 90% of mild cases, the cause of hydramnios cannot be determined (Hill, Breckle, Thomas, and Fries, 1987). Ultrasonography and physical assessment are used to diagnose this condition.

Oligohydramnios

The counterpart of hydramnios, oligohydramnios refers to an abnormally small amount of amniotic fluid. Its cause is unknown, but a normal reduction in amniotic fluid after week 36 may create or aggravate the condition in postterm pregnancies. Reduced amniotic fluid is associated with maternal hypertension, fetal congenital anomalies, intrauterine growth retardation, and risk to the fetus's life. Experts are unsure about the degree to which fluid may be reduced before such adverse responses occur.

Premature rupture of the membranes

The amniotic sac ruptures before the onset of labor in approximately 10% of clients with term pregnancies, primarily in those with more than one fetus, hydramnios, or fetal malpresentation. About 80% of clients who experience PROM begin labor spontaneously within 24 hours. (For complete information on this disorder, see Chapter 27, The First Stage of Labor.)

Amniotic fluid embolism

A rare obstetric disorder, amniotic fluid embolism has a maternal mortality rate approaching 80% (Clark, 1987). The fetal mortality rate also is high. In this syndrome, amniotic fluid enters the maternal circulation and causes respiratory distress and shock (Oxorn, 1986). Classic symptoms include sudden onset of dyspnea and hypotension, possibly followed by cardiopulmonary ar-

rest. Other significant signs include chest pain; cyanosis; frothy, pink-tinged sputum; tachycardia; and hemorrhage. Coagulopathy affects approximately 40% of clients with this syndrome and may be the cause of death in those who survive the initial hemodynamic insult.

Although it occurs primarily during labor, amniotic fluid embolism has occurred during first and second trimester abortions and even during the postpartal period (Clark, 1987). Most clients who die from this disorder do so within 30 minutes after its onset. Diagnosis is confirmed by cytologic detection of fetal squamous cells and lanugo in a blood sample aspirated through the central line used for hemodynamic monitoring.

Umbilical cord factors

Anomalies involving the umbilical cord typically are not detected until delivery. Some may threaten the fetus's life. Complications that may arise during labor include cord prolapse, abnormal cord length, and abnormal cord implantation.

Cord prolapse

Displacement of the umbilical cord to a position at or below the fetus's presenting part most commonly occurs when amniotic membranes rupture before fetal descent. The sudden gush of fluid carries the long, loose cord ahead of the fetus toward and possibly through the client's cervix and into the vagina. Serious damage may occur when the fetus compresses the cord, interrupting blood flow from the placenta. Factors that increase the risk of cord prolapse include hydramnios, more than one fetus, ruptured membranes, a transverse or breech lie, a small fetus, a long umbilical cord, a low-lying placenta, premature delivery, and an unengaged fetal presenting part.

Umbilical cord prolapse incurs a high infant mortality rate if not detected and treated immediately. Diagnosis of cord prolapse is based on observation of the cord outside the vulva, feeling the cord during a vaginal examination, or observing fetal distress in a high-risk client. (For more information, see *Emergency alert: Umbilical cord prolapse.*)

Abnormal cord length

On average, an umbilical cord measures 55 cm (22"). An excessively long cord raises the risk of knots and prolapse. A short cord may contribute to abruptio placentae, as discussed earlier in the chapter.

EMERGENCY ALERT

Umbilical cord prolapse

If not corrected within 5 minutes, umbilical cord prolapse may cause fetal hypoxia, central nervous system damage, and possible death. Fortunately, rapid assessment and intervention by the health care team can help the client and fetus survive this traumatic event. Discussed below are the signs and symptoms of cord prolapse and appropriate interventions until emergency cesarean or forceps delivery can take place.

SIGNS AND SYMPTOMS

- Client reports feeling the cord "slither" down after membrane rupture
- Visible or palpable umbilical cord in the birth canal
- Violent fetal activity
- Fetal bradycardia with variable deceleration during contractions

NURSING CONSIDERATIONS

- Immediately summon another member of the health care team who can notify the physician and prepare the team for a prompt delivery or emergency surgery.
- Place the client in a Trendelenburg or knee-chest position with her hips elevated, as shown. Either position will shift the fetus's weight off the cord. (Two gloved fingers also can assist in pushing the fetus's presenting part off the cord while the operating room is being prepared.
- Do not attempt to press or push the cord back into the uterus. This may traumatize the cord, stop blood flow to the fetus, or start an intrauterine infection.
- Expect to assist in giving the client supplemental oxygen by face mask at 10 to 12 liters/minute, initiating or increasing I.V. fluids with 5% dextrose in lactated Ringer's solution (to enhance fluid volume and circulation), and sending blood for type and cross-match (if this was not done on admission).
- Expect to assist in monitoring fetal heart tones with an internal fetal scalp electrode on the presenting part.
- Do not attempt to reinsert the cord if it protrudes from the vagina. Instead, lift it with gloved hands and gently wrap it in loose, sterile towels saturated with sterile saline solution.
- Keep the client informed throughout this emergency. Calmly convey the seriousness of the situation and emphasize the importance of cooperation. Reassure the client and her family that the medical and nursing staff will do everything possible to ensure a safe and successful delivery.
- Accompany the client to the operating room, continuing to keep pressure off the cord and monitoring for signs of maternal and fetal distress.

TRENDELENBURG POSITION

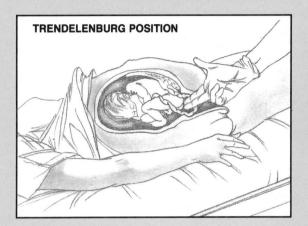

KNEE-CHEST POSITION

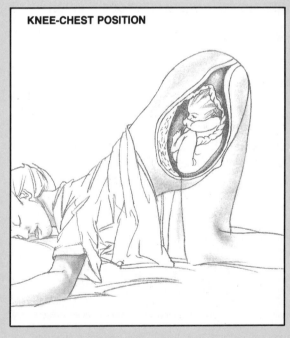

Abnormal cord implantation

Normally, the umbilical cord inserts in the center of the placenta. In a velamentous (membranous) insertion, the cord vessels separate into branches before reaching the placenta and the cord inserts into the membranes rather than the placental disk (Oxorn, 1986). Occasionally with a velamentous insertion, fetal vessels in the membranes cross the internal os and take up a position ahead of the fetal presenting part. This potentially serious condition, known as vasa previa, may be discovered during a pelvic examination when the examiner feels vessels through the cervical os (Cunningham, MacDonald, and Gant, 1989).

Systemic disorders

Complications involving hemorrhage, shock, and disseminated intravascular coagulation (DIC) can occur at any time during labor and delivery.

Hemorrhage and shock

Many factors predispose the client to hemorrage and subsequent shock, including placenta previa, abruptio placentae, uterine rupture, and lacerations during delivery. (See Chapter 44, Postpartal Complications, for a more detailed description.)

Disseminated intravascular coagulation

A pathological form of diffuse rather than localized clotting, DIC leads to massive internal and external hemorrhage as clotting factors (such as fibrinogen) are consumed. Intrauterine fetal death, abruptio placentae, septic shock, or amniotic fluid embolism can initiate normal clotting mechanisms. If these clotting factors are depleted, DIC may occur.

Diagnosis of DIC usually is made by laboratory studies that show a decreased fibrinogen and platelet count, increased prothrombin and partial thromboplastin times, and increased fibrinogen degradation products.

Fetal complications

Many fetal factors can affect the progress of labor, including malpresentation, malposition, macrosomia, shoulder dystocia, and intrauterine fetal death. (For related information, see *Emergency alert: Signs of fetal distress.*)

Malpresentation

When the fetal presenting part is not the head, the condition is known as a malpresentation. Examples of malpresentations include breech, shoulder, and face. (See

---

EMERGENCY ALERT

Signs of fetal distress

Signs of fetal distress indicate that the health—and possibly the life—of the fetus is in jeopardy. For example, meconium-stained or yellow amniotic fluid signals fetal hypoxia, which can lead to anoxia, central nervous system damage, or death. The nurse can use the following chart to identify signs of fetal distress and appropriate interventions.

SIGNS

- Abnormal fetal heart rate pattern, including a heart rate below 120 or above 160 beats/minute, decreased or increased variability, or periodic changes, such as late decelerations or deep, wide, variable decelerations
- Increased or decreased fetal activity
- Meconium-stained or yellow amniotic fluid after membrane rupture

NURSING CONSIDERATIONS

- Help the client into the lateral or knee-chest position to relieve fetal pressure on the vena cava, aorta, or umbilical cord and improve maternal and fetal circulation.
- Supply oxygen to improve oxygenation of the client and the fetus. Administer by face mask at 8 to 10 liters/minute.
- Notify the physician and the surgical team.
- Expect to assist with initiating or increasing I.V. fluids, such as lactated Ringer's solution, to manage hypotension or hypovolemia.
- Expect to discontinue oxytocin immediately (if it is being administered) to improve uteroplacental perfusion.
- Be calm and purposeful when caring for the client. This will help prevent undue fear and anxiety, which could adversely affect uteroplacental perfusion.
- Explain what is happening, and reassure the client to help her gain control and cooperate fully. Keep her family informed and encourage their support.

Chapter 24, Physiology of Labor and Childbirth, for a detailed discussion.)

The most common malpresentation is breech, which occurs in 3% to 4% of births and more frequently in twins (Cunningham, MacDonald, and Gant, 1989; Oxorn, 1986). Currently in the United States, approximately 80% of breech fetuses that reach term are delivered by cesarean (Flanagan, Mulchahey, Korenbrot, Green, and Laros, 1987). However, opinions vary widely on whether cesarean delivery is necessary for such a large percentage of breech fetuses. Many studies have been performed but with no consensus on the proper management of this obstetric problem (Perkins, 1987). Some physicians attempt external version to convert the breech to a vertex presentation. (See Chapter 32, Special Obstetric Procedures, for a description.)

Breech presentation is associated with increased incidence of preterm labor, congenital anomalies, and birth trauma. The major risk to vaginal delivery of a breech fetus is lack of adequate cervical dilation because the buttocks are smaller than the head.

When the head is hyperextended into a face presentation, the chin becomes the presenting part. Although vaginal delivery is possible, the neonate's face will develop marked edema. Internal fetal monitoring is contraindicated because of potential damage to the face, such as skin tearing, infection, scarring, and eye injuries. When the head is midway between extension and flexion, the brow becomes the presenting part. This is a rare presentation and, because it presents the largest cephalic diameter, usually requires cesarean delivery. A transverse lie occurs when the long axis of the mother is perpendicular to that of the fetus and includes shoulder and arm presentations. Either one requires cesarean delivery (Perkins, 1987).

Malposition

Malposition occurs when the fetus's presenting part enters the birth canal in an abnormal position that makes delivery difficult. An example is the persistent occiput posterior position where the occiput of the fetus's head is in one of the posterior quadrants of the maternal pelvis. (See Chapter 26, Comfort Promotion during Labor and Childbirth, for more information.) If the occiput fails to rotate spontaneously to the anterior position, the physician may use forceps to complete the rotation and facilitate delivery. However, forceps deliveries may put the client and fetus at unacceptable risk. (See Chapter 32, Special Obstetric Procedures, for more information.)

Macrosomia

The classic definition of macrosomia is a fetus that weighs more than 4,500 g. This occurs in approximately 1% of births (Oxorn, 1986).

A large fetus does not necessarily preclude vaginal delivery; in fact, many are delivered vaginally or with low forceps. The fetopelvic relationship must be assessed for each client. Predisposing factors for macrosomia include maternal diabetes, multiparity, maternal age over 34, previous macrosomia, maternal height over 67" (170 cm), and maternal weight over 154 lb (70 kg) (Oxorn, 1986).

Shoulder dystocia

In shoulder dystocia, the fetus's head emerges but the anterior shoulder catches on the pubic arch—a rare and usually unexpected condition. Typically in shoulder dystocia, the head emerges and is immediately pulled back tightly against the vulva (Lee, 1987). Predisposing factors include macrosomia, a prolonged second stage of labor, multiparity, prolonged pregnancy, and previous delivery of a neonate weighing more than 4,000 g (Lee, 1987). Because this condition has the potential to cause fetal trauma or death, interventions must be immediate.

Intrauterine fetal death

If fetal activity fails to begin or if it ceases after 20 weeks' gestation, the client should be monitored for fetal heart tones. Absence of fetal heart tones warrants a real-time ultrasound examination to detect heart wall motion. Absence of such motion offers reliable evidence of fetal death.

In more than half the cases of fetal death, the cause cannot be determined. Where the cause is known, however, it may be associated with severe maternal disease, diabetes mellitus, hypertension, abruptio placentae, erythroblastosis fetalis, and umbilical cord accidents.

The death of a fetus is a tragic loss for the couple, possibly compounded by the need to go through labor. Labor usually occurs spontaneously within 2 weeks of the fetus's death. However, an increased risk of a coagulation defect and the severe psychological stress of carrying a dead fetus may prompt the physician to induce labor within a few days of the death. Throughout this time, coagulation studies must be carefully monitored.

(For a case study that shows how to apply the nursing process when caring for a client with intrapartal complications, see *Applying the nursing process: Parental grieving related to the death of the fetus*, pages 802 and 803.)

Nursing care

To provide care to clients with intrapartal complications, the nurse needs to apply knowledge of the disorders within the discipline of the nursing process—a systematic method for gathering data, planning, and intervening. While providing care, the nurse functions in various roles, including teacher, clinician, and advocate.

Assessment

During any labor, but especially one with potential complications, the nurse must monitor carefully both the client and fetus. Assessment may uncover difficulties before they worsen.

Uterine factors

Nursing assessment of the client with hypotonic or hypertonic dysfunctional labor patterns requires continuous, careful monitoring of labor progress and fetal status. To distinguish hypotonic uterine dysfunction from problems caused by cephalopelvic disproportion, the nurse-midwife or physician may perform an amniotomy and initiate internal fetal and uterine monitoring.

When assessing contractions, keep in mind that hypertonic uterine dysfunction typically is seen during the latent phase of labor and is characterized by painful contractions of increased intensity. Though painful, the contractions are not able to produce normal cervical dilation.

Critical assessment criteria for possible preterm or postterm labor include accurate determination of gestational age and estimation of the fetus's size. Gestational age can be determined from the client's history (date of last menstrual period and day of quickening), physical assessment, and ultrasonography. The ultrasound examination also will reveal the fetus's size.

Because a preterm fetus's respiratory system may not be well-developed, the fetus may be sensitive to changes in oxygen supply. Evidence suggests that fetal distress and meconium release occur twice as frequently and meconium aspiration syndrome occurs eight times as frequently in postterm pregnancies as in normal pregnancies (Usher, Boyd, McLean, and Kramer, 1988). Therefore, preterm and postterm pregnancies require careful assessment of fetal well-being, including fetal monitoring according to facility policy.

A client with a history of precipitous labors may not progress through the stages of labor in a normal manner. Because changes may occur rapidly, monitor this client closely.

Assessment of uterine rupture requires careful monitoring of bleeding, fetal status, and the client's vital signs—as well as a review of laboratory test results.

When assessing a client with uterine inversion, carefully monitor blood loss and vital signs to detect shock—an emergency situation. Be prepared to assist other members of the health care team in the attempt to reverse the uterus.

Congenital and structural anomalies are assessed by the nurse-midwife or physician.

Pelvic factors

For a client with structural contractures, assess labor progress, particularly cervical dilation and the frequency and intensity of uterine contractions. Because prolonged labor can endanger the fetus, monitor fetal status closely.

Assess for abnormal bleeding in the client with perineal lacerations.

Placental factors

Assessment of a client with placenta previa includes careful monitoring of bleeding, fetal status, vital signs, and laboratory test results. Assess vaginal bleeding by monitoring the client's perineal and bed pads. Continuous bleeding calls for I.V. fluid replacement; blood transfusions may be needed if hemorrhage occurs. Fetal monitoring may be continuous at first, but after the client's condition stabilizes it may consist of nonstress tests and assessment of fetal heart rate. Vital signs, level of consciousness, skin color and temperature, and pain as well as events preceding the bleeding also are necessary assessment data. Monitor the results of all laboratory tests, which will be performed more frequently if bleeding becomes more severe.

Assessment of a client with abruptio placentae is similar to that for placenta previa. However, because fetal distress is much more likely to occur, fetal assessment must be continuous for a suspected abruption. Also, abruptio placentae can lead to DIC; therefore, monitor the client for signs of this condition. (See "Systemic disorders" below.)

History data of the client may show previous intrauterine fetal death, placenta previa, abruptio placentae, or preeclampsia or eclampsia.

Retained placenta is assessed by measuring the time between fetal and placental delivery; an interval of 30 minutes or more indicates retained placenta. The nurse-midwife or physician assesses for placenta accreta, increta, or percreta.

Membrane and amniotic fluid factors

The client with hydramnios may experience dyspnea during labor and may be comfortable only with the head of the bed elevated. The enlarged uterus also may place additional pressure on the vena cava. Assess the client frequently for supine hypotensive syndrome. The fetus of a client with ogliohydramnios may experience fetal distress from umbilical cord compression and requires close monitoring during labor.

Assessment of a client with PROM includes a thorough history on admission to rule out other possible conditions, such as a urinary tract infection. Determine the time of fluid leakage, the time of last sexual intercourse, and the quantity, color, and odor of the fluid.

The client's perineum also must be inspected for obvious fluid leakage.

Assess vital signs closely in a client with amniotic fluid embolism, particularly respiration and heart rate. Also monitor blood test results, particularly coagulation studies.

Umbilical cord factors

In a client with possible cord prolapse, auscultate fetal heart tones to assess well-being. If the fetus shows any signs of distress, expect to assist with a vaginal examination.

In a client with vasa previa, the nurse-midwife or physician may feel the cord vessels through the cervical os. Abnormal cord length, however, cannot be assessed before delivery.

Systemic disorders

To assess a client who may have DIC, observe for signs of excessive or abnormal vaginal bleeding, hematuria, bleeding from the gums or nose, prolonged bleeding from injection or other trauma sites, petechiae, and ecchymoses. Determine if the client has a history of intrauterine fetal death, abruptio placentae, or preeclampsia or eclampsia. Carefully monitor laboratory test results, particularly coagulation studies.

To assess for hemorrhage and shock, check maternal vital signs frequently for increased heart rate, decreased blood pressure, or widening pulse pressure. Assess vaginal discharge and any increase in vaginal bleeding that would indicate hemorrhage.

Fetal complications

If a client of 20 weeks' gestation or more reports that fetal activity has ceased, monitor fetal heart tones. If none are heard, a real-time ultrasonography is performed to check for heart wall motion. Lack of such motion is reliable evidence of intrauterine fetal death.

Although shoulder dystocia does not occur until delivery, the nurse may assist the nurse-midwife or physician as described earlier. Once malposition, malpresentation, and macrosomia have been diagnosed, continue with careful monitoring of the labor for any further complications.

Nursing diagnosis

After reviewing the assessment data, the nurse formulates appropriate nursing diagnoses for the client, fetus, and family members, as needed. (For a partial list of applicable nursing diagnoses, see *Nursing diagnoses: Intrapartal complications.*)

NURSING DIAGNOSES

Intrapartal complications

The following nursing diagnoses address problems and etiologies the nurse may encounter when caring for the client with intrapartal complications. Specific nursing interventions for many of these diagnoses are provided in the "Planning and implementation" section of this chapter.

- Altered family processes related to the mother's prolonged hospitalization and bed rest
- Anticipatory grieving related to the death of the fetus
- Anxiety related to abnormally prolonged labor
- Anxiety related to uncertain maternal outcome
- Anxiety related to uncertain perinatal outcome
- Dysfunctional grieving related to the death of the fetus
- Fatigue related to prolonged labor
- Ineffective family coping: compromised, related to grieving
- Ineffective individual coping related to exhaustion and anxiety
- Ineffective individual coping related to grieving
- Pain related to abnormally prolonged labor
- Potential for alteration in maternal hemodynamic status caused by hemorrhage
- Potential for fetal compromise related to alteration in the fetal placental unit
- Potential for fetal compromise related to premature delivery and inadequate placental perfusion
- Potential for fetal injury secondary to fetal hypoxia and traumatic delivery
- Powerlessness related to having to carry a dead fetus
- Situational low self-esteem related to the inability to have a normal pregnancy

---

Planning and implementation

Caring for a client and fetus who are experiencing intrapartal complications requires clinical and interpersonal skills.

Uterine factors

The fetus of a client with a hypotonic or hypertonic uterine dysfunction may have a nursing diagnosis of *potential for fetal injury secondary to fetal hypoxia and traumatic delivery.* Continuous, careful monitoring of labor progress and fetal status is essential because fetal hypoxia may occur. Be aware of any signs of fetal distress and be prepared to intervene appropriately.

Caring for the client in preterm labor requires a team approach. An appropriate nursing diagnosis may be *potential for compromised fetus related to premature delivery and inadequate placental perfusion.* The nurse-midwife, physician, and nurse attending the delivery provide care for the client; those with specialized skills in caring for high-risk neonates should provide resuscitation and stabilizing measures for the preterm neonate. If the neonate requires transfer to another facility, keep the client and her family informed of the neonate's condition while providing postpartal and postoperative care.

A client with a history of a precipitous labor will need careful and constant monitoring of fetal and maternal status. Prolonged periods of uterine contractions with decreased periods of uterine relaxation may lead to periods of fetal hypoxia.

The client with a dysfunctional labor pattern may have a nursing diagnosis of *pain related to abnormally prolonged labor.* The client and her support person will need updates on labor progress and the results of all assessments. They may grow physically or emotionally exhausted, discouraged, and anxious. To prevent excessive fatigue, suggest rest periods for the support person during times when someone else can attend the client; tell the support person that the client will not be left alone. Provide information and support, as needed, especially if cesarean delivery becomes necessary.

A client with hypotonic uterine dysfunction may have a nursing diagnosis of *anxiety related to abnormally prolonged labor.* Such a client may receive oxytocin to augment her contractions. Although labor augmentation differs from labor induction with oxytocin, take similar precautions and care for the client as if labor were being induced. (See Chapter 32, Special Obstetric Procedures, for information on labor induction.)

A client with hypertonic uterine dysfunction may have a nursing diagnosis of *ineffective individual coping related to exhaustion and anxiety.* She may be given narcotic analgesia to produce sleep for several hours. Upon awakening, she may have a normal, progressive labor pattern. This intervention is used only if the membranes are intact and no evidence of fetal distress is detected because this treatment delays delivery (Cunningham, MacDonald, and Gant, 1989).

A client with postterm labor may undergo labor induction and, if induction fails, cesarean delivery. A client with preterm labor may have a vaginal or cesarean delivery. Because delivery must be gentle and slow to avoid rapid compression and decompression of the fetus's head as it emerges, an episiotomy may be performed to ensure stable pressure.

A client with preterm labor may have a nursing diagnosis of *anxiety related to uncertain perinatal outcome.* Because a preterm fetus does not tolerate labor and delivery as well as a term fetus, cesarean delivery may be performed, especially if the fetus is in the breech position. This position increases the risk of umbilical cord prolapse and entrapment of the fetus's head by the cervix after the body has emerged (Oxorn, 1986).

If a client experiences uterine rupture, surgical intervention must take place immediately to save the fetus's life and, at times, the client's life. After cesarean delivery, the surgeon will repair the ruptured uterus if it can sustain a future pregnancy or remove it if it cannot. If uterine inversion occurs, immediate interventions must be taken to save the client's life, including blood transfusions and surgical reinversion of the uterus. This emergency situation requires the nurse's assistance.

Some vaginal and cervical anomalies may be repaired surgically; some may not interfere with labor and delivery. Uterine anomalies may contribute to spontaneous abortion, preterm birth, and malpresentation. (For more information, see Chapter 6, Reproductive Anatomy and Physiology.) If these situations occur, be ready to care for the client in the same way as during preterm labor and malpresentation.

Pelvic factors

When caring for a client in labor who has a pelvic condition that may prolong labor, be supportive and alert for impending complications. The client with a contracted pelvis will need constant monitoring of maternal and fetal status because her labor may be arrested. Such a client may have a nursing diagnosis of *fatigue related to prolonged labor.* Keep the client informed of labor progress.

Lacerations of the birth canal may be prevented or minimized by episiotomy. (See Chapter 32, Special Obstetric Procedures, for more information.) A client with lacerations receives the same treatment as one who has had an episiotomy. If the lacerations are third- or fourth-degree, the client should receive nothing by rectum, including suppositories and enemas.

The client with a contracted pelvis may have a nursing diagnosis of *anxiety related to uncertain perinatal outcome.* The client and her support person will need constant updating of the status of her labor. Providing support and reassurance will help them to cope with the possibility of a cesarean delivery. They also will need support and reassurance that they have not failed if a vaginal delivery is impossible.

The client with a contracted pelvis may have a nursing diagnosis of *ineffective individual coping related to exhaustion and anxiety.* When a client has a contracted pelvis, the fetus's presenting part may not engage in the inlet, making cesarean delivery necessary. Even if the presenting part can engage, the fetus may not descend adequately and the cervix may not dilate normally. Rupture of the membranes without adequate engagement creates an open space between the fetus and pelvis, increasing the risk of uterine cord prolapse.

Because labor is prolonged, the client risks exhaustion and intrauterine infection; she also may have a nursing diagnosis of *potential for fetal injury secondary to fetal hypoxia and traumatic delivery.* If the fetus passes through the contracted area, cranial molding can be excessive. Vaginal delivery may require forceps or vacuum extraction.

Placental factors

Placental problems can cause unexpected complications or profuse bleeding that may alarm the client. If placenta previa is diagnosed and the fetus is immature, the client may be hospitalized and on prolonged bed rest. If further bleeding episodes occur, the client may receive an intravenous line with a large-bore intra-catheter for fluid replacement and possible blood product transfusion. She may be transferred to a high-risk perinatal center for further care. The client with placenta previa may have a nursing diagnosis of *anxiety related to uncertain perinatal outcome.* Continuously provide the client and family with updated information to allay anxiety. Assess the coping mechanisms of the client and her family and determine the strength of their support systems; assist family members in verbalizing fears and concerns. Share information to clarify misconceptions and to make them feel involved.

Treatment and interventions for the client with abruptio placentae will depend on the degree of the abruption. Nursing interventions are similar to those for a client with placenta previa; however, fetal status must be monitored continually because fetal distress is more likely with abruptio placentae. In addition, monitor coagulation studies closely because of the risk of DIC.

Be aware of the anxiety that is experienced by the client with placenta previa and her family. The client and family may have a nursing diagnosis of *anxiety related to uncertain maternal outcome.* These feelings will occur not only during an episode of bleeding but until delivery because of the possibility of additional episodes of bleeding. Guidance and teaching will assist the family in dealing with these fears and will provide an understanding of the complication and the necessary interventions.

If the client with abruptio placentae requires emergency procedures, keep the family informed as they occur, and be sensitive to the family's needs during the crisis.

Prepare the client and her family if a cesarean delivery is necessary. They may see it as a disappointment or failure, but that feeling may be balanced by the delivery of a healthy neonate.

Complete and partial previas always warrant cesarean delivery; with marginal previa or a low-lying placenta, a vaginal delivery may be possible. Monitor the client closely during labor because marginal previa may develop into a partial obstruction as the cervix dilates;

prepare the client and her family for either method of delivery.

The client may develop a nursing diagnosis of *potential for alteration in maternal hemodynamic status caused by hemorrhage.* Expect immediate cesarean delivery regardless of the fetus's gestational age. However, if hemorrhage is not severe, bed rest may allow the pregnancy to continue until the fetus is viable or mature. Delivery then may be cesarean or vaginal, depending on the type of previa involved. If hemorrhage occurs, expect to monitor vital signs and fetal status and to administer fluids and blood, as prescribed.

Treatment and interventions for the client with abruptio placentae depend on the degrees of abruption, hemorrhage, and resulting fetal distress. If abruption, hemorrhage, and fetal distress are severe, an appropriate nursing diagnosis would be *potential for compromised fetus related to premature delivery and inadequate placental perfusion.* Emergency delivery is performed regardless of the fetus's gestational age. Support the client and inform her about the measures that will be taken.

When blood loss is not severe and no evidence of fetal distress is found, interventions may be less urgent. If the client is in labor with a full-term fetus, a vaginal delivery may be possible.

If a client's placenta fails to separate spontaneously within 30 minutes after fetal delivery, the physician may attempt to remove it manually (after administering adequate anesthesia or analgesia) by inserting one hand into the uterus and gently peeling the placenta away from the uterine wall. The client may require a dilatation and curretage (D&C) procedure afterward to ensure that all fragments have been removed. She also may receive an oxytocic drug to promote uterine contractions and reduce bleeding.

The treatment of a client with placenta accreta depends on the amount of placenta adhering to the uterine wall and subsequent hemorrhage. A small accreta may be managed by D&C; an oxytocic drug may be used to control bleeding. Total accreta, increta, or percreta require hysterectomy. Nursing care also depends on the amount of adhering placenta, the severity of blood loss, and whether hysterectomy was performed.

Membrane and amniotic fluid factors

The management of hydramnios depends on the severity of the client's symptoms, which may include dyspnea and increased edema of the legs and vulva from increased uterine pressure on the venous system. The client may experience discomfort severe enough to require hospitalization. Amniocentesis may be able to alleviate the discomfort; however, because fluid production continues, relief is temporary.

APPLYING THE NURSING PROCESS

Parental grieving related to the death of the fetus

The nursing process helps ensure high-quality care for a client with intrapartal complications. The table below shows how the nurse might use the nursing process when caring for the client described in the case history at right. The first column presents history and physical assessment data followed by a paragraph of mental notes. These notes help the nurse make important connections among assessment findings, aiding in development of the nursing diagnosis and planning.

The second column lists an appropriate nursing diagnosis; information in the remaining columns is based on this diagnosis. Although not part of the nursing process, a rationale appears for each intervention in the fourth column to explain how it contributes to the care plan.

ASSESSMENT	NURSING DIAGNOSIS	PLANNING
Subjective (history) data • Client has not felt the fetus move for the past 24 hours. • Client has been experiencing mild contractions and has a bloody show. • Client appears nervous but has remained quiet. **Objective (physical) data** • No fetal heart tones. • Ultrasound examination confirms intrauterine fetal death. • Vaginal examination determines that the client is 3 cm dilated, 80% effaced, and at a 0 station. • Client is admitted to the labor unit. **Mental notes** *The emotional responses and coping mechanisms of the client and her husband should be assessed. Physical assessment should include the information that is essential to the care of any client in the first stage of labor, with the exception of fetal assessment. Laboratory values for clotting mechanisms, such as PT, PTT, and fibrinogen levels, must be determined because of the risk of DIC. The couple's support systems, including spiritual or cultural factors that may influence their manner of coping or expressing grief, should be assessed. After the neonate's delivery, the couple may want various types of contact—seeing and holding their child, baptism, or mementos.*	Parental grieving related to the death of the fetus	**Goals** The client and her family will: • progress through labor without increased risk or complications to the mother • ask appropriate questions and receive accurate information • begin their grieving process with the support of the nursing and medical staff • spend as much time as desired with their child • use coping mechanisms that conform with their spiritual beliefs and cultural values.

When ogliohydramnios has been diagnosed before delivery through ultrasonography, prepare the client for possible abnormal fetal appearance, including dry, leathery skin and urinary tract or musculoskeletal anomalies.

A client with PROM may have labor induced if more than 24 hours have passed since membrane rupture; the nurse-midwife or physician bases the decision on fetal and maternal status. If labor is augmented with an oxytocic agent, monitor the I.V. rate and uterine response.

The treatment of a client with amniotic fluid embolism includes maintaining oxygenation and cardiac output as well as managing any coagulation problems, recognizing the symptoms of respiratory distress and shock, and knowing emergency procedures for respiratory and cardiac arrest.

Umbilical cord factors
In a client with potential cord prolapse, a vaginal examination is performed if any signs of fetal distress exist

CASE STUDY

Fay Leary is a 30-year-old gravida 3, para 2 at 38 weeks' gestation. This pregnancy has been uncomplicated. She and her husband Bill are both professionals and they have two children, ages 4 and 6. Fay's previous pregnancies were uncomplicated, and she had spontaneous vaginal deliveries with both children. She has had thorough prenatal care.

IMPLEMENTATION		EVALUATION
Intervention	**Rationale**	Upon evaluation, the client and her husband:
Assure the client and her husband that feelings of shock, anger, and disbelief are normal.	Such strong emotions may be frightening to them. They need to know that this is part of the normal grieving process.	• expressed feelings of anger, disbelief, and sorrow
Tell the couple what you know about the condition.	The client may question whether she could have taken actions to prevent the death.	• held their child and requested footprints and an identification bracelet as keepsakes.
Allow the couple to see and hold their child.	Such contact aids the grieving process, enabling the couple to cope with their loss.	
Provide privacy for the family and prepare them for the physical appearance of their child by describing how the child looks and feels (cold and limp).	The family needs to have adequate time to bond with their child and prevent feelings of shock and additional grief.	
Tell the parents that their child will be on the unit for an extended period. Offer them any available mementos, such as pictures, a lock of hair, footprints, and an identification bracelet. If the parents desire, arrange for baptism.	Some families may decline to see their child at first and then change their decision.	
Continue to provide nursing care to the client after delivery.	Proper care is vital for the client's recovery. Vital signs, the condition of the fundus, and bleeding must be assessed sensitively at appropriate times.	
Avoid such clichés as, "You have other children" or "You can have another baby" or "Everything will be OK." However, do not hesitate to say that you are sorry for their loss.	Clichés prevent honest interpersonal communication between nurse and family.	
Listen to the couple, answer questions honestly, and repeat answers as necessary.	Because of their grieving, they may not recall all they hear and may ask the same question numerous times.	

or when the membranes rupture, especially in a client with twins, a malpresented fetus, or an immature fetus. A nursing diagnosis for a client with a prolapsed cord might be *potential for fetal compromise related to alteration in the fetal placental unit.*

In a client with vasa previa, the examiner may feel the cord vessels through the cervical os. Because rupture of these vessels could cause the fetus to exsanguinate before emergency cesarean delivery could be performed, the client should be kept on bed rest, and the cervical os should not be probed or manipulated. Expect a cesarean delivery.

Abnormal cord length can lead to other complications, such as cord prolapse or abruptio placentae; know the proper nursing care for these complications.

Systemic disorders

The client with potential for hemorrhage and shock and possibly DIC is at risk, as is her fetus. She may have a nursing diagnosis of *potential for alteration in maternal hemodynamic status caused by hemorrhage.* The client with any bleeding condition that could possibly progress to hemorrhage, shock, and DIC should be monitored for coagulation studies.

Treatment of a client with DIC must include treatment of the causative factor as well as aggressive support of blood volume and pressure. The client may require replacement of blood components, such as platelets or fresh frozen plasma (Weiner, 1987). Diagnosis of DIC typically is made by laboratory studies that indicate decreased fibrinogen and platelet count; increased bleeding, prothrombin, and partial thromboplastin times; and increased levels of fibrinogen and fibrin degradation products. Vigilant monitoring of laboratory studies is essential. Prepare the client for the possibility of blood transfusions and component replacement.

A client who understands the seriousness of her condition may have a nursing diagnosis of *anxiety related to uncertain perinatal outcome.* Provide emotional support during emergency procedures.

Fetal complications

A client experiencing any fetal complication requires sensitive, supportive nursing care. The client experiencing a labor complicated with fetal malposition, malpresentation, and macrosomia may have a nursing diagnosis of *pain related to abnormally prolonged labor* or *potential for fetal injury secondary to fetal hypoxia and traumatic delivery.* For more information, see Chapter 26, Comfort Promotion during Labor and Childbirth.

Providing nursing care for the client who has experienced a stillbirth is difficult. Be prepared for widely varying responses from the client and family members. If the client does not display grief, explore her personal feelings of anger and sadness.

A client may have begun labor when she is told her fetus is dead, or she may have known for some time before labor begins. An applicable nursing diagnosis may be *situational low self-esteem related to the inability to have a normal pregnancy.* Be extremely sensitive to the needs of the parents and take cues from them to meet their emotional needs. For example, some parents may need to talk about their loss; others may not. Providing any support or opportunities for grieving that the parents may need is essential. A nursing diagnosis of *anticipatory grieving related to death of the fetus* may apply.

The client with a labor complication of fetal malpresentation may have a cesarean delivery, although some breech presentations can be delivered vaginally. An appropriate nursing diagnosis for such a client may be *anxiety related to uncertain perinatal outcome.* For a client with a fetal malposition, nursing interventions

may assist with these problems. (See Chapter 32, Special Obstetric Procedures, for specific interventions.)

For a client with shoulder dystocia, the nurse-midwife or physician may attempt one of several maneuvers to deliver the shoulders, which may require assistance from the nurse. Downward traction may be applied to the head while an assistant applies moderate suprapubic pressure (Cunningham, MacDonald, and Gant, 1989). If this fails to move the shoulder, the client in a lithotomy position may remove her legs from the stirrups and flex them sharply (with assistance) against her abdomen (McRobert's maneuver) to straighten the sacrum relative to the lumbar spine and possibly free the shoulder (Lee, 1987).

Provide the same nursing care to a client in labor with a known stillbirth as to a client undergoing labor induction. In addition, continuously monitor the client's coagulation studies. Because of the death of the fetus, she may be at risk for DIC.

The death of a fetus is a tragic loss for the parents that can be compounded because the client must still go through labor. A nursing diagnosis of *powerlessness related to having to carry a dead fetus* may apply. Labor usually occurs spontaneously within 2 weeks of the fetus's death. However, the client faces some risks during this period, especially one of developing a coagulation defect. This risk, combined with the psychological stress of carrying a dead fetus, may necessitate inducing labor within a few days of the intrauterine fetal death. Throughout this time, carefully monitor the results of coagulation studies.

Give the parents an opportunity to see and hold their dead child if they wish. Wrap the child in a blanket and prepare the parents for its appearance. Give them as much time as they wish to spend with their child. Offer to provide a lock of hair, footprints, and bracelets; even if the parents decline, gather these things in case they change their minds. A polaroid picture of the child also may be appropriate. Many parents appreciate these simple gestures, which may provide them with the only mementos of their child that they will have.

The parents may want to have their child baptized. All nurses, regardless of their religion, can perform this rite.

Avoid any reassuring platitudes that prevent the parents from expressing their feelings. For example, saying, "You'll be able to have more children" prevents the parents from grieving for this loss. Such phrases protect the health care providers from the parents' expression of grief, but they are not beneficial to the parents. (For more information on helping the parents grieve, see Chapter 39, Care of the Families of High-Risk Neonates.)

Evaluation

During this step of the nursing process, the nurse evaluates the effectiveness of the plan of care. To do this, the nurse evaluates subjective and objective criteria throughout the client's care. Evaluation findings should be stated in terms of actions performed or outcomes achieved for each goal. The following examples illustrate appropriate evaluation statements for the client experiencing intrapartal complications as well as her family:
• The client and her fetus completed labor and delivery safely with little or no additional complications.
• The client and her support person and family received regular updates about her condition and the status of the fetus, as the situation allowed.
• The client's coagulation studies remained within normal limits despite bleeding problems, and DIC was avoided.
• The client remained as comfortable as possible during dysfunctional labor.
• The client and her support person received support and encouragement from the nursing staff during complications.

Documentation

All steps of the nursing process should be documented as thoroughly and objectively as possible. Thorough documentation not only allows the nurse to evaluate the effectiveness of the care plan, but it also makes this information available to other members of the health care team, ensuring consistent care.

When caring for a client with intrapartal complications, include the following points in the documentation:
• maternal vital signs
• maternal contraction rate and intensity
• maternal fluid intake and output
• medications given, time of administration, and effectiveness
• vaginal examinations and results
• vaginal discharge, type, and amount
• laboratory studies and their values
• fetal heart tones, variability, and any abnormal patterns.

Chapter summary

Chapter 33 described complications that may occur during labor and delivery. Here are the chapter highlights.
• Most intrapartal complications are unexpected and may occur without warning. Skilled, knowledgeable nursing care is essential in calming a client's and family's fears and anxieties as they realize that labor is not progressing normally.
• Reproductive system disorders, systemic disorders, and fetal complications may not be detected until labor begins, or they may be identified during the final weeks of pregnancy. These complications may range from having little significance to labor and delivery to threatening the life of the client or fetus. The nurse assists with controlling fears and anxieties concerning the client and fetus while providing complex nursing care.
• In case of fetal death, the nurse assists and comforts the family and allows them to grieve.

Study questions

1. Sally Jones, a 17-year-old visiting from another city, is brought to the emergency department at 34 weeks' gestation and experiencing vaginal bleeding. She reports no abdominal pain; her bleeding started suddenly. What client history should the nurse obtain? What is an applicable diagnosis, and what interventions should the nurse perform?

2. A nurse working the night shift is temporarily alone. Marney Murphy, a 37-year-old multiparous client who says she has been in labor for less than 3 hours, calls for help. The nurse finds the fetus crowning. What should the nurse's initial interventions be? How should they be prioritized?

3. Lisa Sanchez, age 21, has just been admitted to the labor and delivery area with premature rupture of the membranes. An initial monitor strip displays severe fetal distress, and the client reports that she could feel the umbilical cord slide out when the membranes broke. What are the immediate nursing interventions for this client, and what is the rationale for them?

Bibliography

Abdella, T.N., Sibae, B.M., Hays, J.M., and Anderson, G.D. (1984). Perinatal outcome in abruptio placentae. *Obstetrics and Gynecology*, 63(4), 365-369.

Clark, S.L. (1987). Amniotic fluid embolism. In S.L. Clark, J.P. Phelen, and D.B. Cotton (Eds.), *Critical care obstetrics*. Oradell, NJ: Medical Economics.

Cunningham, F.G., MacDonald, P.C., and Gant, N. (1989). *Williams obstetrics* (18th ed.). East Norwalk, CT: Appleton & Lange.

Flanagan, T., Mulchahey, K., Korenbrot, C., Green J., and Laros, R. (1987). Management of term breech presentation. *American Journal of Obstetrics and Gynecology*, 156(6), 1492-1502.

Friedman, E. (1987). Midforceps delivery: No? *Clinical Obstetrics and Gynecology*, 30(1), 93-105.

Friedman, E. (1989). Normal and dysfunctional labor. In W.R. Cohen, D. Acker, and E. Friedman (Eds.), *Management of labor* (pp. 1-18). Rockville, MD: Aspen.

Hill, L.M., Breckle, R., Thomas, M.L., and Fries, J.K. (1987). Polyhydramnios: Ultrasonically detected prevalence and neonatal outcome. *Obstetrics and Gynecology*, 69(1), 21-25.

Hurd, W.W., Midovnik, M., Hertzberg, V., and Levin, J.P. (1983). Selective management of abruptio placentae: A prospective study. *Obstetrics and Gynecology*, 61(4), 467-473.

Jackson, V. (1990). The uterus. In R. Lichtman and S. Papera (Eds.), *Gynecology: Well-woman care* (pp. 261-272). East Norwalk, CT: Appleton & Lange.

Lee, C.Y. (1987). Shoulder dystocia. *Clinical Obstetrics and Gynecology*, 30(1), 77-82.

Ouimette, J. (1986). *Perinatal nursing: Care of the high-risk infant*. Boston: Jones and Bartlett.

Oxorn, H. (1986). *Human labor and birth*. East Norwalk, CT: Appleton & Lange.

Perkins, R.P. (1987). Fetal dystocia. *Clinical Obstetrics and Gynecology*, 30(1), 56-58.

Usher, R.H., Boyd, M.E., McLean, F.H., and Kramer, M.S. (1988). Assessment of fetal risk in postdate pregnancies. *American Journal of Obstetrics and Gynecology*, 158(2), 259-264.

Weiner, C.P. (1987). Disseminated intravascular coagulopathy. In S.L. Clark, J.P. Phelen, and D.B. Cotton (Eds.), *Critical care obstetrics*. Oradell, NJ: Medical Economics.

The Neonate

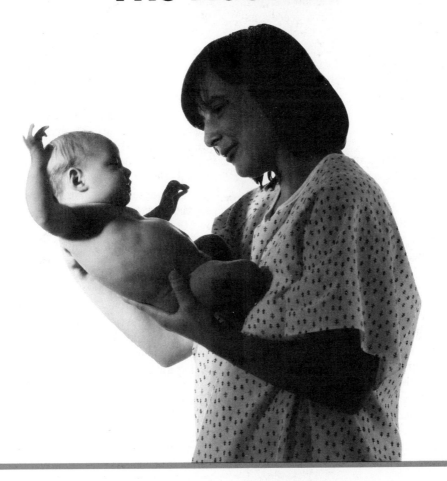

Nursing can enhance the health of our society for years to come by promoting the health of our neonates. Besides possessing the basic skills that ensure neonatal health, the nurse who cares for neonates must be able to help parents learn and adopt health promotion behaviors that improve their children's health and must be able to meet the family's need for information and support in times of stress, such as after the birth of a high-risk neonate.

This unit prepares the nurse to care for normal and high-risk neonates and their families, presenting neonatal care from a family-centered perspective. Transforming abstract theories into family-focused care, it shows how the nurse applies a conceptual framework to clinical practice by adapting effective nursing strategies for individual neonates and their families. In addition to describing how the nurse functions as a member of an interdependent health care team, the unit prepares the nurse to deliver neonatal care within the home, where the nurse can gain valuable insight into the functioning, interrelationships, and resources of the family. The unit also identifies trends in neonatal health care and delineates the problems that pose an increasing threat to future generations—for instance, the growing number of children born with acquired immunodeficiency syndrome (AIDS) or suffering the effects of maternal substance abuse.

The first two chapters in this unit provide a conceptual base for the nurse working with neonates and their families, establishing a theoretical model that can be applied in the various settings described in the remainder of the unit. The five remaining chapters follow a similar format, providing basic information about a specific aspect of neonatal health, then presenting this information in a nursing process framework. To demonstrate how to integrate assessment findings and document nursing care, these five chapters include charts that apply the nursing process to case studies.

Chapter 34
Neonatal Adaptation

Chapter 34 surveys the biological and behavioral changes the neonate experiences during the critical 24 hours following birth, emphasizing the importance of successful adaptation to the extrauterine environment. It begins by discussing the biological characteristics of adaptation, detailing the physiologic adjustments occurring in all body systems. It highlights such important changes as the conversion from fetal to neonatal circulation and onset of independent breathing. It details thermoregulation in the neonate and illustrates neonatal circulation and lung fluid removal within moments of birth.

Next, Chapter 34 discusses the behavioral aspects of neonatal adaptation. It investigates the neonate's interaction with the environment through sensory and behavioral capacities, elaborating on visual and hearing abilities, tactile perception, taste, and smell. The chapter concludes with a description of the periods of neonatal reactivity—a series of distinctive behavioral and physiologic characteristics—and a discussion of neonatal sleep and awake states.

Chapter 35
Neonatal Assessment

Chapter 35 describes the assessment techniques that yield important baseline information about the neonate's physiologic status and adaptation to the extrauterine environment. First, it presents general assessment guidelines, delineating the proper timing and sequence of the various types of assessment. It points out key health history factors to consider and explains how periods of neonatal reactivity may affect physical findings.

Next, Chapter 35 explains how to conduct a brief physical assessment to gather data about the neonate's general appearance, obtain vital signs, and take anthropometric measurements. Then it explores gestational-age assessment. After explaining how a neonate's gestational age helps predict perinatal problems, the chapter identifies the physical and neurologic features that help reveal gestational age. It shows how to correlate gestational age with birth weight, body length, and head circumference.

The chapter then presents the essentials of a complete physical assessment. It highlights assessment of neonatal reflexes and presents a comprehensive chart detailing normal and abnormal head-to-toe assessment findings and listing possible causes of abnormal findings. Chapter 35 concludes by discussing behavioral assessment as a means of exploring the neonate's behavioral state and responses.

Chapter 36
Care of the Normal Neonate

Chapter 36 outlines the nurse's role in ensuring successful neonatal adaptation, helping the family adjust to the neonate, and promoting optimal parent-infant interaction. Using a nursing process framework, it presents pertinent assessment information and nursing diagnoses for the normal neonate.

Chapter 36 then discusses nursing interventions that maintain a stable physiologic status and foster parent-infant bonding. It focuses on measures that ensure neonatal oxygenation, hydration, nutrition, hygiene, safety, and thermoregulation, highlighting interventions that combat cold stress. The chapter presents step-by-step procedures illustrating how to provide routine neonatal care, including bathing, nasal and oral suctioning, administering medications, obtaining a urine specimen, and caring for circumcision and umbilical cord sites.

Chapter 37
Infant Nutrition

Chapter 37 assists the nurse in promoting optimal infant nutrition. After delineating nutrient and fluid requirements for neonates and infants, it discusses the circumstances that impose special nutritional needs and limitations on neonates and infants, and then it reviews nutritional assessment.

Next, Chapter 37 compares and contrasts breast-feeding and formula-feeding, and then it explores the factors that influence parents' choice of infant feeding method. It begins by describing the health benefits of breast-feeding, then reviews the physiology of lactation and the composition of breast milk and examines infant sucking dynamics during breast-feeding. It illustrates the lactating breast and offers step-by-step procedures showing how to assess a neonate's sucking reflex and how to train a neonate to suck properly. Then the chapter provides basic information about formula feeding, describing commercial formulas and equipment, providing formula intake requirements, and detailing nutritional options for the non-breast-feeding infant.

Chapter 37 then presents nursing care for breast-feeding and formula-feeding clients and their infants. It explains how to assess a breast-feeding client's knowledge of feeding techniques and describes how to assess the client's breasts for consistency and nipple condition. For the client using infant formula, the chapter prepares the nurse to assess client knowledge of formula-feeding techniques and infant formula intake requirements. It follows with a discussion of nursing interventions, focusing on general infant-feeding guidelines and client teaching. This section includes detailed client-teaching aids on such topics as breast-feeding positions, initiating breast-feeding, and expressing milk. It touches on drug use during lactation and breast-feeding in special situations, and it offers a breast-feeding schedule for the working mother. Addressing the client using infant formula, the chapter describes interventions that help ensure proper formula preparation and effective burping technique, and it explains how the nurse can promote physical contact between the client and her infant during formula-feeding.

Chapter 38
High-Risk Neonates

Chapter 38 prepares the nurse to care for the high-risk neonate. First, it surveys some important concepts in neonatal intensive care, describing the regionalization of perinatal care and comparing the three levels of perinatal care provided in perinatal care centers. It examines associated ethical and legal issues, including withholding of life-support for the critically ill neonate. Then the chapter focuses on the perinatal problems that lead to high-risk status, ranging from respiratory problems, metabolic disorders, and infection to congenital anomalies and effects of maternal substance abuse. It describes the pathophysiology and etiology of these problems, then highlights the causes and consequences of birth-weight and gestational-age variations, and it discusses child abuse and failure to thrive in the high-risk neonate.

Next, Chapter 38 presents nursing care for the high-risk neonate. It identifies factors that help predict delivery of a high-risk neonate and explains how to assess for each perinatal problem described earlier. After listing pertinent nursing diagnoses for the high-risk neonate, the chapter addresses nursing interventions. Highlighting emergency measures, the chapter features illustrated procedures of neonatal resuscitation and suctioning of an endotracheal tube. It also presents a chart showing indications and nursing considerations for resuscitation drugs. Then Chapter 38 elaborates on general nursing interventions for high-risk neonates, including measures that support oxygenation, thermoregulation, and nutrition. It explains how to prevent or control infection, provide preoperative or postoperative care, and carry out special procedures. The chapter concludes with a discussion of specific medical and nursing management of selected perinatal problems.

Chapter 39
Care of the Families of High-Risk Neonates

Chapter 39 guides the nurse in providing practical and psychosocial support for the family with a high-risk neonate. To establish a theoretical framework for understanding a family's reactions to the birth of a high-risk neonate, the chapter begins by discussing theories of grief and common coping mechanisms.

The chapter then applies these concepts to nursing care. It explains how to assess the parents' socioeconomic and cultural backgrounds, experience with health care facilities, and grieving behavior and coping mechanisms. It describes how to evaluate the family's support systems and examines cultural influences on the expression of grief. After offering pertinent nursing diagnoses, Chapter 39 identifies nursing interventions that help the family deal with their crisis and attain the skills to care for the neonate after discharge. The chapter examines the family's teaching needs and explains how the nurse can bolster the family's internal and external support systems and enhance their bonding with the neonate. Chapter 39 features an examination of nursing measures to support the siblings and grandparents of a high-risk neonate, and it outlines interventions to help families cope with neonatal or fetal death.

Chapter 40
Discharge Planning and Neonatal Care at Home

Chapter 40 addresses discharge planning and home health care services—the tools that extend neonatal care to the home. After delineating the factors that have increased the demand for home health care over the past decade, the chapter discusses the nurse's role in discharge planning and reviews discharge planning systems and resources. It instructs the nurse in assessing the discharge planning needs of the neonate and family, including ways to determine whether the family's circumstances make home health care feasible, and presents a sample discharge planning questionnaire. Next, Chapter 40 explains how to implement the discharge care plan by preparing the parents for the neonate's discharge and helping them select and arrange payment for home health care services.

Chapter 40 then explores home health care in depth, describing available services, equipment, and supplies and reviewing case management of home care. It identifies the types of home health care a neonate may need—routine and basic care for normal, healthy neonates; specialized care for others.

Next, the chapter presents nursing care for the neonate receiving health care at home. It describes the essentials of assessment during the first home visit and on subsequent visits. It focuses on how to evaluate parental knowledge, caregiving skills, and support needs; how to assess whether health care can be delivered safely and adequately in the home; and how to gauge parent-infant interaction. For planning and implementation, Chapter 40 discusses the importance of nursing flexibility and innovation, then addresses such interventions as ensuring parental caregiving knowledge and skills, promoting parent-infant interaction, and helping siblings adjust. Other highlights of Chapter 40 include discussions of nutritional assessment and home nutrition therapy and a chart showing how to assess the neonate requiring special equipment. The chapter includes parent teaching aids on dealing with an infant who has acquired immunodeficiency syndrome and on use of such equipment as a home apnea monitor and nasal cannula for oxygen administration.

CHAPTER 34

Neonatal Adaptation

Objectives

After reading and studying this chapter, the student should be able to:

1. Compare and contrast fetal and neonatal circulation.
2. Identify the unique anatomic structures of fetal circulation.
3. Discuss the status of the integumentary, neurologic, and reproductive systems at birth.
4. Identify the neonate's four defenses against heat loss.
5. Describe the biological adaptations necessary in the hematopoietic, renal, gastrointestinal (GI), hepatic, and endocrine systems to ensure successful transition to extrauterine life.
6. Discuss the capacity of the neonate's immune system to prevent infection.
7. Identify the sensory capacities of the normal neonate.
8. Describe the periods of neonatal reactivity and the physiologic characteristics associated with each.

Introduction

Immediately after delivery, the neonate must assume the life-support functions performed by the placenta in utero. Birth begins a critical 24-hour phase, called the *transitional period*, that encompasses the neonate's adaptation from intrauterine to extrauterine life.

To survive outside the womb, the neonate must successfully navigate the transitional period. Statistics reflect the difficulty of this task: Mortality is higher during this period than at any other time; two-thirds of all neonatal deaths occur in the first 4 weeks after birth (Avery, 1987; March of Dimes, 1985).

The transitional period imposes changes in all body systems and exposes the neonate to a wide range of external stimuli. Conditions that prevent successful adaptation to extrauterine life pose a serious threat. By becoming familiar with the normal events of transition, the nurse may recognize signs of poor adaptation and intervene promptly when they occur.

This chapter begins with a review of the biological characteristics of adaptation during the transitional period, including major changes in every body system. The first section also discusses the importance of neonatal thermoregulation. Next, the chapter describes the behavioral characteristics of adaptation, reviewing the neonate's response to environmental stimulation as well as neonatal sensory capacities. The chapter concludes with a discussion of the periods of neonatal reactivity (a series of behavioral and physiologic characteristics) and neonatal sleep and awake states.

Biological characteristics of adaptation

Crucial physiologic adjustments take place in all body systems after birth. The cardiovascular and pulmonary systems undergo immediate drastic changes as soon as the umbilical cord is clamped and respiration begins. Although cardiovascular and pulmonary changes occur simultaneously, they are discussed separately to facilitate understanding.

GLOSSARY

Acrocyanosis: bluish discoloration of the hands and feet caused by vasomotor instability, capillary stasis, and high hemoglobin levels.

Asphyxia: state of hypoxemia, acidosis, and hypercapnia; strongest stimulus for the first breath.

Bilirubin: yellow bile pigment; a product of red blood cell hemolysis.

Conduction: transfer of heat to a substance in contact with the body; a mechanism of heat loss.

Convection: transfer of heat away from a surface by movement of air currents; a mechanism of heat loss.

Cyanosis: bluish skin discoloration caused by an excess of deoxygenated hemoglobin in the blood.

Ductus arteriosus: tubular connection that shunts blood away from the pulmonary circulation during fetal development.

Ductus venosus: circulatory pathway that allows blood to bypass the liver during fetal development.

Erythropoietin: hormone produced in the kidney that regulates red blood cell production.

Evaporation: conversion of fluid to vapor; a mechanism of heat loss.

Foramen ovale: opening in the interatrial septum that directs blood from the right to left atrium during fetal development.

Functional residual capacity (FRC): volume of air remaining in the lungs after a normal expiration.

Glomerular filtration rate (GFR): volume of glomerular filtrate (a protein-free plasmalike substance) formed over a specific period.

Glucuronyl transferase: liver enzyme necessary for bilirubin conjugation.

Hemoglobin F: hemoglobin produced by fetal erythrocytes; has a higher affinity for oxygen than does adult hemoglobin (hemoglobin A), helping to ensure adequate fetal tissue oxygenation.

Jaundice: yellow skin discoloration caused by bilirubin accumulation in the blood and tissues.

Lipolysis: decomposition of fat.

Neutral thermal environment: narrow range of environmental temperatures at which the least amount of energy is required to maintain a stable core temperature.

Nonshivering thermogenesis: heat production by lipolysis of brown fat; primary method through which the neonate produces heat.

Radiation: transfer of heat from one surface to another without contact between the surfaces; a mechanism of heat loss.

Reflex: involuntary function or movement of any organ or body part in response to a particular stimulus.

Surfactant: phospholipid produced by Type II alveolar cells in the alveolar lining of the lungs; decreases alveolar inflation pressures, improves lung compliance, and provides alveolar stability, thereby decreasing labor of breathing.

Thermoregulation: regulation of body temperature by balancing heat loss and heat production.

TORCH: acronym for a group of viral and nonviral agents that can cause perinatal infections (**T**oxoplasmosis, **O**thers, **R**ubella, **C**ytomegalovirus, and **H**erpes).

Transitional period: period in which the neonate experiences biological and behavioral adaptations to extrauterine life; normally lasts for about 24 hours.

Cardiovascular system

To ensure the neonate's survival, fetal circulation must convert to neonatal circulation during the transitional period. Fetal circulation involves four unique anatomic features that shunt most blood away from the liver and lungs. The *placenta* serves as an exchange organ through which the fetus absorbs oxygen, nutrients, and other substances and excretes wastes (such as carbon dioxide). The *ductus venosus* links the inferior vena cava with the umbilical vein, permitting most placental blood to bypass the liver. The *foramen ovale* and *ductus arteriosus* direct most blood away from the pulmonary circuit. Although a small portion of pulmonary arterial blood enters the pulmonary circuit to perfuse the lungs, the ductus arteriosus shunts most to the aorta to supply oxygen and nutrients to the trunk and lower extremities. (For more information on these structures, see Chapter 16, Conception and Fetal Development.)

Conversion from fetal to neonatal circulation

Beginning at birth, fetal shunts undergo changes that establish neonatal circulation. (For an illustration of blood flow in the neonate, see *Tracing neonatal circulation*.) As the umbilical cord is clamped and the neonate draws the first breath, systemic vascular resistance increases and blood flow through the ductus arteriosus declines. Most of the right ventricular output flows through the lungs, boosting pulmonary venous return to the left atrium. In response to increased blood volume in the lungs and heart, left atrial pressure rises. Combined with increased systemic resistance, this pressure rise results in functional closure of the foramen ovale. (*Functional closure* refers to cessation of blood flow, resulting from pressure changes, that renders a structure nonfunctional.) Within several months, the foramen ovale undergoes *anatomic closure* (structural obliteration from constriction or tissue growth).

Tracing neonatal circulation

With birth comes functional closure of the fetal shunts (ductus venosus, foramen ovale, and ductus arteriosus) that direct blood flow away from the lungs and liver and separate the systemic and pulmonary circulations. As the shunts close, blood flows from the pulmonary arteries to the lungs and through the portal system to the liver. In the large illustration, the darker areas represent regions of high arterial oxygen saturation; the lighter areas, regions of low saturation. The boxed illustrations show the shunts as they previously existed.

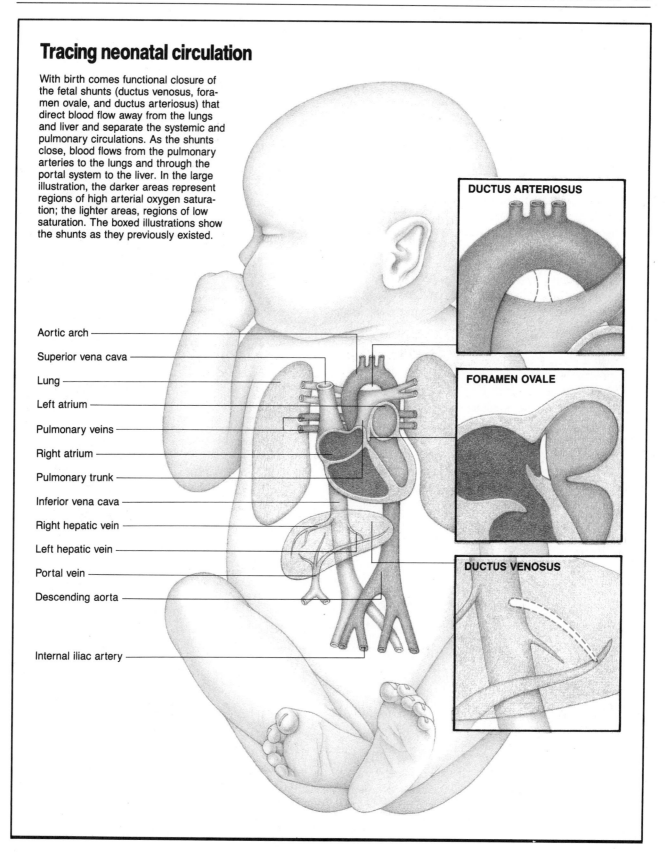

Onset of respiratory effort and the effects of increased partial pressure of arterial oxygen (PaO_2) constrict the ductus arteriosus, which functionally closes 15 to 24 hours after birth. By age 3 to 4 weeks, this shunt undergoes anatomic closure.

Clamping of the umbilical cord halts blood flow through the ductus venosus, functionally closing this structure. The ductus venosus closes anatomically by the first or second week. After birth, the umbilical vein and arteries no longer transport blood and are obliterated.

Because anatomic closure lags behind functional closure, fetal shunts may open intermittently before closing completely. Intermittent shunt opening most commonly stems from conditions causing increased vena caval and right atrial pressure (such as crying); clinically insignificant functional murmurs may result. Also, because shunts allow unoxygenated blood to pass from the right to left side of the heart, bypassing the pulmonary circuit, they may cause transient cyanosis. Both cyanosis and murmurs in the neonate should be carefully monitored and evaluated so that any underlying abnormalities can be detected. (See Chapter 35, Neonatal Assessment, for more information about assessing the neonate's cardiovascular system.)

Blood volume

The blood volume of the full-term neonate ranges from 80 to 90 ml/kg of body weight, depending on the amount of blood transferred from the placenta after delivery. Delayed umbilical cord clamping increases blood volume by up to 100 ml (1 dl), possibly increasing heart rate, respiratory rate, and systolic blood pressure. Changes caused by increased blood volume may persist for about 48 hours, possibly leading to crackles and cyanosis.

Respiratory system

Throughout gestation, biochemical and anatomic respiratory features develop progressively, preparing the fetus for the abrupt respiratory changes brought on by birth. Between weeks 25 and 30 of gestation, Type II pneumocytes (alveolar cells) begin limited secretion of surfactant. A phospholipid, surfactant decreases the surface tension of pulmonary fluids and prevents alveolar collapse at the end of expiration. Reduction of surface tension facilitates gas exchange, decreases inflation pressures needed to open the airways, improves lung compliance, and decreases labor of breathing. (For more information on respiratory system development, see Chapter 16, Conception and Fetal Development.)

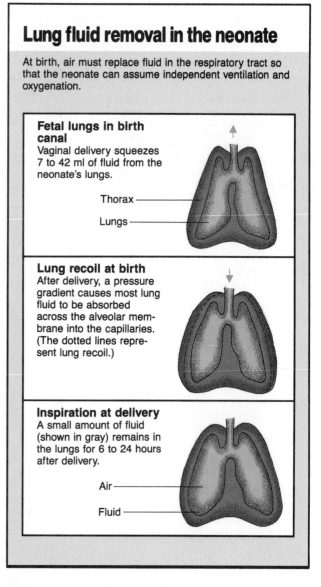

Lung fluid removal in the neonate

At birth, air must replace fluid in the respiratory tract so that the neonate can assume independent ventilation and oxygenation.

Fetal lungs in birth canal
Vaginal delivery squeezes 7 to 42 ml of fluid from the neonate's lungs.

Thorax

Lungs

Lung recoil at birth
After delivery, a pressure gradient causes most lung fluid to be absorbed across the alveolar membrane into the capillaries. (The dotted lines represent lung recoil.)

Inspiration at delivery
A small amount of fluid (shown in gray) remains in the lungs for 6 to 24 hours after delivery.

Air

Fluid

Onset of neonatal respiration

The fetal lungs contain fluid secreted by the lungs, amniotic cavity, and trachea. The fluid volume, which correlates with the neonate's functional residual capacity (FRC), typically reaches 30 to 25 ml/kg of body weight (West, 1985). For the neonate to assume the tasks of ventilation and oxygenation, air must rapidly replace lung fluid. In the healthy neonate, replacement occurs with the first few breaths.

Lung fluid removal. As the neonate's chest squeezes through the birth canal, compression forces out roughly one-third of the lung fluid through the nose and mouth. The pulmonary circulation and lymphatic system absorb the remaining two-thirds after respiration begins.

After the neonate's chest clears the birth canal, elastic recoil pulls 7 to 42 ml of air into the lungs to replace the fluid that was forced out. (For an illustration of the mechanics of lung fluid removal, see *Lung fluid removal in the neonate.*) Consequently, the neonate may cough before the first inspiration. Glossopharyngeal or frog breathing, which involves involuntary muscle contraction, pulls another 5 to 10 ml of air into the lungs. Each breath increases the neonate's FRC.

The time needed to clear the lungs varies from 6 to 24 hours after vaginal delivery of a healthy, full-term neonate (West, 1985). Inadequate lung fluid removal may cause transient tachypnea of the neonate.

Breathing stimuli. Normally, the neonate breathes within 20 seconds of delivery, stimulated by the medullary respiratory center. (For an overview of the factors leading to respiration, see *Stimuli for neonatal respiration.*) Asphyxia—the combination of hypoxemia, hypercapnia, and acidosis—provides the strongest stimulus for the first breath. Before the first breath, the neonate has an arterial oxygen saturation (SaO_2) of only 10% to 20%, reflecting hypoxemia; a partial pressure of arterial carbon dioxide ($PaCO_2$) of approximately 58 mm Hg, reflecting hypercapnia; and an arterial pH of approximately 7.28, reflecting acidosis.

Because the final stage of delivery interrupts gas exchange, even the healthy neonate has some degree of asphyxia at birth. Asphyxia stimulates chemoreceptors in the carotid bodies and aorta. As this stimulation increases, efferent impulses travel to the diaphragm, contracting it. The negative intrathoracic pressure that

Stimuli for neonatal respiration

In response to various stimuli, the neonate draws the first breath within about 20 seconds of delivery. Asphyxia is the most important stimulus for neonatal respiration. However, as the flowchart below shows, other biochemical stimuli also come into play, as do various mechanical, thermal, and sensory factors.

INITIAL STIMULUS		RECEPTOR STIMULATION	RESPONSE
Sensory	Bright lights, touch, pain	Visual, auditory, and proprioceptive chemoreceptors	• Stimulation of medullary respiratory center • Efferent nerve impulses (via spinal cord) • Diaphragmatic contraction
Biochemical	Asphyxia	Aortic and carotid chemoreceptors	
Thermal	Heat loss	Thermal receptors	
Mechanical	Thoracic squeeze, elastic recoil	Stretch receptors	• Glossopharyngeal breathing

RESPIRATION

results draws air into the lungs, increasing intrathoracic volume.

Other stimuli that help trigger breathing include cord occlusion, thermal changes (from rapid heat loss caused by increased energy expenditure), tactile stimulation, and other environmental changes (such as bright lights and noise).

The onset of respiration and lung expansion indirectly decreases pulmonary vascular resistance because of the direct effect of oxygen and carbon dioxide on vessels. As oxygen saturation increases and the PaCO$_2$ value declines, the decrease in pulmonary vascular resistance leads to increased pulmonary blood flow. This further improves oxygen saturation.

Neonatal respiratory function

The respiratory rate varies over the first day, stabilizing by about 24 hours after birth. Maintained by the effects of biochemical and environmental stimulation, the neonate's respiratory function requires:
• a patent airway
• a functioning respiratory center
• intact nerves from the brain to chest muscles
• adequate calories to supply energy for labor of breathing.

Hematopoietic system

Like other body systems, the hematopoietic system is not fully developed at birth. The hematologic features that ensured adequate tissue oxygenation in utero must be replaced by more mature elements after birth.

Red blood cells

Erythropoiesis—production of erythrocytes, or red blood cells (RBCs)—is stimulated by the renal hormone erythropoietin. In the fetus, low oxygen saturation causes erythropoietin release to rise; to ensure adequate tissue oxygenation, RBC production increases. At birth, the increased oxygen saturation that follows the onset of respiration inhibits erythropoietin release, reducing RBC production.

Fetal RBCs have a life span of about 90 days, compared to 120 days for normal RBCs. As fetal RBCs deteriorate, the neonate's RBC count decreases, sometimes resulting in physiologic anemia before stabilization. By age 2 to 3 months, however, the RBC count rises to within acceptable neonatal limits. (For normal neonatal laboratory values, see Chapter 35, Neonatal Assessment.)

Hemoglobin

Blood's oxygen-carrying component, hemoglobin is produced by developing RBCs. After birth, the hemoglobin value decreases simultaneously with the RBC count. Fetal RBCs produce hemoglobin F (fetal hemoglobin), which has a higher affinity for oxygen than hemoglobin A (produced by adult RBCs). This compensatory mechanism helps ensure adequate oxygenation in utero. As RBCs are replaced, hemoglobin A replaces hemoglobin F.

White blood cells

White blood cells (WBCs, leukocytes) serve as the neonate's major defense against infection. WBCs exist in five types: neutrophils, eosinophils, basophils, lymphocytes, and monocytes. Neutrophils account for 40% to 80% of total WBCs at birth; lymphocytes account for roughly 30%. However, by age 1 month, lymphocytes outnumber neutrophils.

Neutrophils and monocytes are phagocytes—cells that engulf and ingest foreign substances. They form part of the mononuclear phagocytic system, which defends the body against infection and disposes of cell breakdown products. Despite the presence of these phagocytic properties, however, the neonate's immature inflammatory tissue response may not localize an infection. (For more information on the neonate's immune response, see pages 820 to 822.)

Thrombocytes

Thrombocytes (platelets) are crucial to blood coagulation. The neonate usually has an adequate platelet count and function. (Brown, 1988; Cloherty and Stark, 1985).

Hepatic system

The neonate's hepatic system—responsible for bilirubin clearance, blood coagulation, carbohydrate metabolism, and iron storage—is immature. Nonetheless, under normal circumstances, it functions adequately.

Bilirubin clearance

A yellow bile pigment, bilirubin is a by-product of heme after RBC breakdown. As RBCs age, they become fragile and eventually are cleared from the circulation by the mononuclear phagocytic system. The iron and protein portions are removed and recycled for further use. After leaving the mononuclear phagocytic system, bilirubin binds to plasma albumin. In this water-insoluble state, it is called indirect (unconjugated) bilirubin.

Indirect bilirubin must be conjugated—converted to direct bilirubin—for excretion. Conjugation occurs in the liver as bilirubin combines with glucuronic acid with the assistance of the enzyme glucuronyl transferase; a water-soluble bilirubin form results. Urobilinogen and stercobilinogen, the bilirubin compounds resulting from breakdown, can be excreted in the urine and stool. (For an illustration of bilirubin clearance, see *Neonatal bilirubin formation and clearance*, page 818.)

Jaundice (icterus). If unconjugated bilirubin accumulates faster than the liver can clear it, the neonate may develop the yellow pallor known as jaundice. Slow or ineffective bilirubin clearance results in some degree of jaundice in approximately half of full-term neonates and 90% of preterm neonates. Fortunately, most full-term neonates avoid toxic bilirubin accumulation because they have adequate serum albumin binding sites and sufficient liver production of glucuronyl transferase. Factors that may increase the risk of unconjugated hyperbilirubinemia (an elevated serum unconjugated bilirubin level) include asphyxia, cold stress (ineffective heat maintenance), hypoglycemia, and maternal salicylate ingestion (Avery, 1987; Maisels, 1987).

Ineffective excretion of conjugated bilirubin may cause conjugated hyperbilirubinemia (an elevated serum conjugated bilirubin level). Always abnormal in the neonate, this condition warrants evaluation.

Jaundice types. Four types of jaundice occur in the neonate—physiologic jaundice, pathologic jaundice, breast milk jaundice (BMJ), and breast-feeding–associated jaundice (BFAJ).

Physiologic jaundice arises 48 to 72 hours after birth. The serum bilirubin level peaks at 4 to 12 mg/dl by the third to fifth day after birth. On average, the bilirubin level increases by less than 5 mg/dl/day. Physiologic jaundice normally disappears by the end of the seventh day (Wilkerson, 1988). Five conditions that may cause physiologic jaundice are decreased hepatic circulation, increased bilirubin load, reduced hepatic bilirubin uptake from the plasma, decreased bilirubin conjugation, and decreased bilirubin excretion.

In contrast, pathologic jaundice occurs within the first 24 hours after birth; the serum bilirubin level rises above 13 mg/dl. Pathologic jaundice may stem from such conditions as blood group or blood type incompatibilities; hepatic, biliary, or metabolic abnormalities; or infection. (See Chapter 38, High-Risk Neonates, for further information on pathologic jaundice.)

BMJ was first identified in the 1960s. Although various causes have been suggested, current theory focuses on increased breast milk levels of the enzyme beta-glucuronidase. Researchers believe this enzyme causes increased intestinal bilirubin absorption in the neonate, thus blocking bilirubin's excretion. BMJ appears as physiologic jaundice subsides (after the seventh day). The serum bilirubin level peaks at 15 to 25 mg/dl between days 10 and 15. BMJ may persist for several weeks or,

rarely, several months. A serum bilirubin level that decreases 24 to 48 hours after discontinuation of breast-feeding confirms the diagnosis.

Controversy exists over whether BMJ warrants treatment. Some physicians and breast-feeding advocates consider treatment unnecessary. Conservative treatment involves temporarily stopping breast-feeding until the bilirubin level declines; this usually takes 24 to 48 hours. The mother should maintain lactation by expressing milk by hand or pump.

BFAJ correlates with the neonate's breast-feeding patterns. The underlying cause of BFAJ is poor caloric intake that leads to decreased hepatic transport and removal of bilirubin from the body. Typically, the neonate who develops BFAJ has not been able to stimulate an early and adequate supply of breast milk. BFAJ usually appears 48 to 72 hours after birth. The serum bilirubin level peaks at 15 to 19 mg/dl by 72 hours. The average serum bilirubin level increases by less than 5 mg/dl/day. Treatment of BMAJ involves measures that ensure an adequate breast milk supply. Wilkerson (1988) recommends breast-feeding the neonate every 2 hours to stimulate the mother's milk production and the neonate's intestinal motility. The mother who quickly identifies signs of hunger in her infant should initiate feeding instead of waiting for the infant to cry vigorously. If the bilirubin level approaches 18 to 20 mg/dl, phototherapy (discussed in Chapter 38, High-Risk Neonates) may be necessary.

Bilirubin encephalopathy (kernicterus). Unconjugated serum bilirubin levels of approximately 20 mg/dl or higher may lead to bilirubin encephalopathy, a life-threatening condition characterized by bilirubin deposition in the basal ganglia of the brain. To assess the risk for bilirubin encephalopathy, the neonate's condition and gestational and chronologic ages must be considered in conjunction with the bilirubin level. The condition may be treated with phototherapy or exchange transfusions (discussed in Chapter 38, High-Risk Neonates).

Blood coagulation

For the first few days after birth, the GI tract lacks the bacterial action to synthesize adequate vitamin K. Vitamin K catalyzes synthesis of prothrombin by the liver, thereby activating four coagulation factors (II, VII, IX, and X). Consequently, the neonate is at special risk for hemorrhage (hemorrhagic disease of the neonate). All neonates now receive a prophylactic injection of vitamin K soon after delivery to help prevent hemorrhage (Glader, 1978; Putnam, 1984).

Neonatal bilirubin formation and clearance

The diagram below shows bilirubin formation and clearance in the neonate. The process begins as mononuclear phagocytes clear aging red blood cells (RBCs) from the circulation. Water-insoluble unconjugated bilirubin must be converted to water-soluble conjugated bilirubin for excretion. This occurs as bilirubin combines with glucuronic acid in the liver.

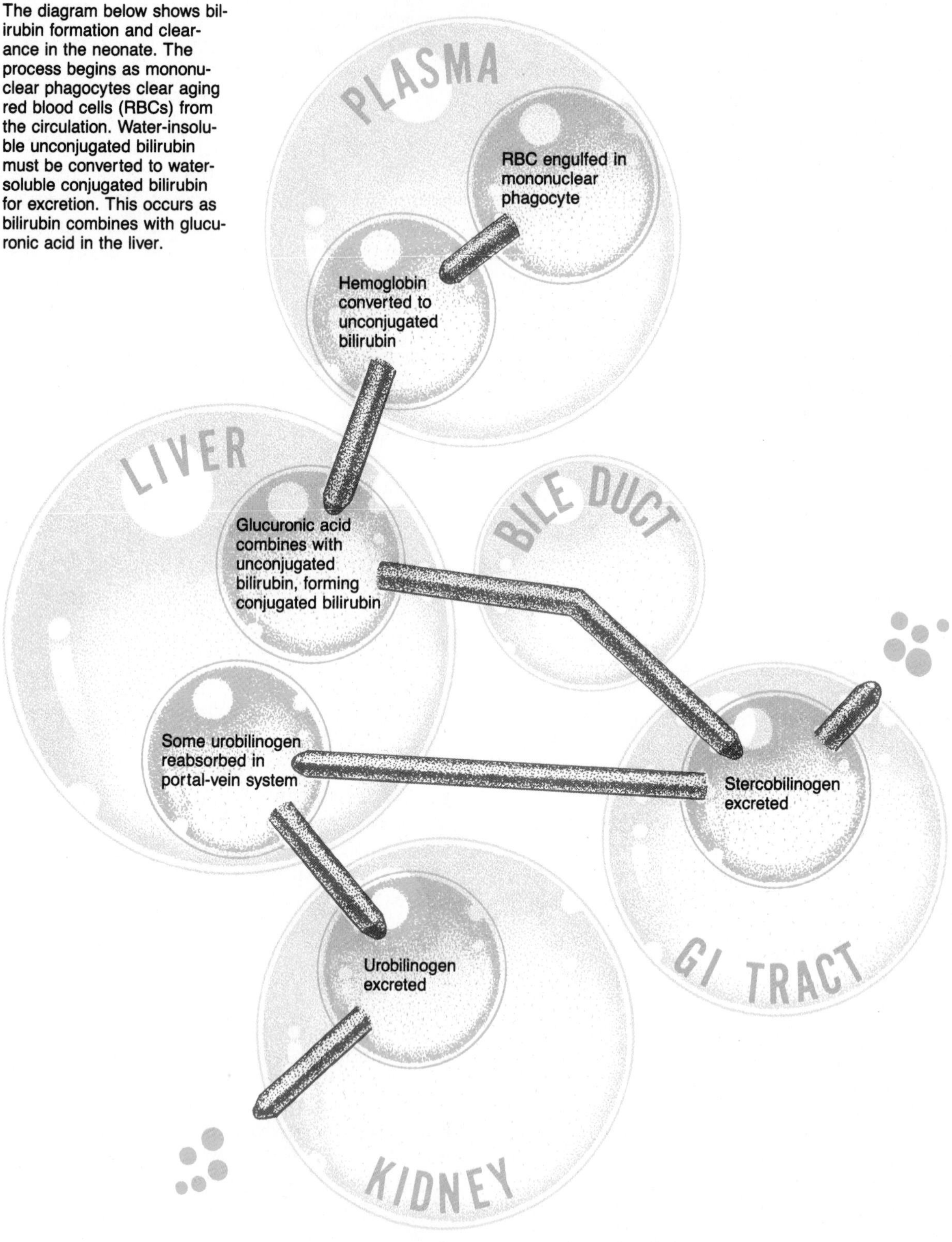

PLASMA

RBC engulfed in mononuclear phagocyte

Hemoglobin converted to unconjugated bilirubin

LIVER

BILE DUCT

Glucuronic acid combines with unconjugated bilirubin, forming conjugated bilirubin

Some urobilinogen reabsorbed in portal-vein system

Stercobilinogen excreted

GI TRACT

Urobilinogen excreted

KIDNEY

Carbohydrate metabolism

The major energy source during the first 4 to 6 hours after birth, glucose is stored in the liver as glycogen. The increased metabolic demands of labor, delivery, and the first few hours after birth cause rapid glycogen depletion (approximately 90% of liver glycogen is used within the first 3 hours). Skeletal muscle glycogen stores also decline rapidly (Streeter, 1986). If the neonate does not receive exogenous glucose, glycogenolysis (breakdown of glycogen into a usable glucose form) occurs. Until the neonate takes in sufficient glucose, glycogenolysis causes release of sufficient glucose into the bloodstream to maintain a serum glucose level of approximately 60 mg/dl. However, such stresses as hypothermia, hypoxia, and delayed feeding may rapidly exhaust glycogen stores, leading to hypoglycemia (Korones, 1986). (For more information on hypoglycemia, see Chapter 38, High-Risk Neonates.)

Iron storage

By term, the liver contains enough iron to produce RBCs until about age 5 months (provided the mother ingested adequate iron during pregnancy). Removed from destroyed RBCs, iron is stored in the liver, then recycled into new RBCs. The neonate must ingest sufficient dietary iron to maintain adequate RBC production.

Renal system

A relatively immature renal system makes the neonate susceptible to dehydration, acidosis, and electrolyte imbalance if vomiting and diarrhea occur (Avery, 1987; Gomella, 1988). The neonate's short, narrow renal tubules inhibit urine concentration and acidification and increase the fraction of excreted amino acids, phosphates, and bicarbonate. Also, the neonate's kidneys are relatively inefficient at secreting hydrogen ions in the tubule to promote acid-base balance.

Glomerular filtration rate

In utero, glomerular perfusion pressure is relatively low and arteriolar resistance high. These conditions contribute to a low fetal glomerular filtration rate (GFR), defined as the volume of glomerular filtrate formed over a specific period. A low GFR limits the kidneys' capacity to excrete excess solutes and regulate body water composition.

In the last trimester of pregnancy, the fetal kidneys undergo tremendous growth and maturation. At 34 weeks of gestation, the GFR—and consequently renal function—improve markedly (Avery, 1987). Thus, neonatal GFR varies with gestational age; the full-term neonate has a higher GFR than the preterm neonate.

The GFR reaches 30% of adult values within the first 2 days of extrauterine life, but it does not attain full adult values until about age 2.

Fluid balance

During the neonate's transition after birth, changes occur in extracellular, intracellular, and total body water volume. At birth, water makes up approximately 70% of the body composition, compared to approximately 58% by adulthood. Extracellular fluid accounts for about 40% of the neonate's total body water. As cell mass increases, this percentage drops; by adulthood, extracellular fluid accounts for 20% of total body water.

The neonate usually voids within 24 hours of birth. The first urine may be dark red and cloudy from urate and mucus (the slight reddish stain has no clinical significance). The neonate's urine usually is odorless; specific gravity ranges from 1.005 to 1.015.

As the neonate's fluid intake increases, urine output increases and urine becomes clear or light straw in color. The breast-fed neonate may require 10 to 12 diaper changes daily. The bottle-fed neonate typically requires about 6 diaper changes daily.

Loss of fluid through urine, feces, insensible (imperceptible) losses, intake restrictions related to small gastric capacity, and increased metabolic rate contributes to a reduction of 5% to 15% of the birth weight over the first 5 days of extrauterine life. However, in the period before the mother's milk supply is established, increased extracellular fluid volume protects the breast-fed neonate from dehydration. The neonate should regain the birth weight within 10 days (Avery, 1987; Ingelfinger, 1985). Typically, the infant doubles the birth weight by age 5 to 6 months and triples it by the first birthday.

GI system

At birth, the neonate must assume the digestive functions previously performed by the placenta—including metabolism of sufficient amounts of water, proteins, carbohydrates, fats, vitamins, and minerals for adequate growth and development.

Gastric capacity

Despite a relatively immature GI system, the healthy neonate can ingest, absorb, and digest nutrients. Gastric capacity is between 40 and 60 ml on the first day after birth; it increases with subsequent feedings. Because of this limited capacity, nutrient needs must be met through frequent small-volume feedings. Gastric emptying time—typically 2 to 4 hours—varies with the volume of the feeding and the neonate's age. Peristalsis is rapid.

Many neonates regurgitate a small amount of ingested matter (1 to 2 ml) after feedings because of an immature cardiac sphincter (a muscular ring constricting the esophagus). Persistent, forceful, or large-volume regurgitation is abnormal and warrants investigation.

GI enzymes

Compared to the adult's intestine, the neonate's is longer relative to body size and has more secretory glands and a larger absorptive surface. The neonate's ability to digest nutrients depends on enzyme action and gastric acidity. The stomach lining consists of chief cells (which secrete pepsinogen and promote protein digestion) and parietal cells (which secrete hydrochloric acid to maintain gastric acidity). Salivary glands secrete only minimal amounts of saliva until age 2 to 3 months, when drooling becomes apparent. Milk digestion begins in the stomach and continues in the small intestine. Secretions from the pancreas, liver, and duodenum aid digestion.

Enzyme deficiencies limit the neonate's absorption of complex carbohydrates and fats. Deficiency of amylase, an enzyme produced in the salivary glands and pancreas, persists until age 3 to 6 months, restricting the conversion of starch to maltose. Deficiency of lipase, which the pancreas secretes in minimal amounts, impedes fat digestion (Avery, 1987). Lipase production increases in the first few weeks after birth.

Vitamin K synthesis

Synthesis of vitamin K through bacterial action is another important GI function. Although initially sterile, the GI tract establishes normal colonic bacteria within the first week after birth, allowing adequate vitamin K synthesis.

Initiation of feedings

In most cases, feedings should begin as soon as the neonate is physiologically stable and exhibits adequate coordination of the sucking and swallowing reflexes. An extended delay before feedings may deplete the neonate's limited glycogen reserves—already taxed by the increased energy demands of the transitional period. This may result in hypoglycemia (reflected by a serum glucose level below 40 mg/dl), which poses a threat to the glucose-dependent brain.

Feedings should be offered by breast or bottle. In some health care facilities, the neonate receives sterile water as the first feeding to verify the sucking and swallowing reflexes without risking aspiration of formula into the airway. One or two swallows of water is sufficient to test the reflexes. (For more information about evaluating the sucking and swallowing reflexes, see Chapter 37, Infant Nutrition.)

Neonatal stools

Initially, the neonate's intestines contain meconium, a thick, dark-green, odorless fecal substance consisting of amniotic fluid, bile, epithelial cells, and hair (from in utero shedding of lanugo—the fine, soft hair covering the fetus's face, shoulders, and back). Typically, the neonate passes the first meconium stool within 24 hours of birth.

After enteric feedings begin, fecal color, odor, and consistency change. Transitional stools usually appear on the second or third day after feedings begin. These greenish brown stools have a higher water content than meconium.

The type of feeding determines the characteristics of subsequent stools. The formula-fed neonate passes pasty, pale-yellow stools with a strong odor. Stools from the breast-fed neonate are golden-yellow, sweet smelling, and more liquid.

The gastric distention that results from food ingestion causes relaxation and contraction of colonic muscles, commonly leading to a bowel movement during or after a feeding. Typically, the breast-fed neonate has more frequent bowel movements than the formula-fed neonate because breast milk digests more rapidly than formula.

Immune system

The immune system is deficient at birth. With delivery comes exposure to substances (for example, bacteria) not normally present in utero. Such exposure activates components of the immune response. The first year is the period of greatest vulnerability to such serious infections as *Hemophilus influenzae*. Bacterial infections (including those caused by group B streptococci and staphylococci) occur in about 2% of neonates; viral infections—such as varicella and cytomegalovirus (CMV)—in about 8% (Berkowitz, 1984).

Immune response

The various elements of the immune system recognize, remember, respond to, and eliminate foreign substances called antigens. Primarily proteins, antigens may invade the body's protective barriers (such as the skin and mucous membranes) or arise from malignant cell transformation.

When local barriers and inflammation fail to fight off antigenic invasion, the immune system initiates a humoral or cell-mediated response. The response is carried out by the mononuclear phagocytic system, which includes cells in the thymus, lymphoid tissue, liver, spleen, and bone marrow. Cells involved in the immune response include lymphocytes (specifically, T cells and B cells), granulocytes, monocytes, RBCs, and platelets.

Humoral immunity. This response is mediated by humoral antibodies. Also called immunoglobulins, these proteins are synthesized in response to a specific antigen. B cells, coated with immunoglobulins, recognize invaders and produce antibodies, which are molecules that react specifically with a matching site on a corresponding antigen. This antigen-antibody reaction activates the complement system, a series of chemical reactions that removes the antigen from the body. Humoral immunity is most important against bacterial and viral reinfections.

Immunoglobulins have one or more molecules, each of which consists of four polypeptide chains. Properties of these chains determine the immunoglobulin's classification.

Immunoglobulin G (IgG). The most abundant immunoglobulin, IgG (gamma globulin) is synthesized in response to bacteria, viruses, and fungal organisms. Maternal IgG, transferred to the fetus via the placenta, confers passive acquired immunity (a short-lived immunity in which no antibodies are produced). Fetal IgG appears by the twelfth week of gestation, with levels increasing significantly during the last trimester.

IgG is active against gram-positive cocci (pneumococci and streptococci), meningococci, *H. influenzae*, some viruses, and diphtheria and tetanus toxins (if the mother has been exposed to these agents). The neonate also has protection against most childhood diseases—including diphtheria, measles, and smallpox—provided the mother has antibodies to these diseases. Because IgG does not act against gram-negative rods (such as *Escherichia coli* and *Enterobacter*), the neonate is more susceptible to infection by these agents.

Passive immunity may interfere with infant immunization by preventing a challenge to the infant's immune system, which ordinarily would cause the immune system to make antibodies to the disease for which the immunization was given. Thus, when the IgG level drops, the infant may contract the disease. For example, an infant may contract pertussis despite receiving the first DPT (diphtheria, pertussis, tetanus) injection.

By about age 3 months, maternally acquired IgG is depleted. By then, however, the body usually produces enough IgG to replace the lost antibodies.

Immunoglobulin M (IgM). The first immunoglobulin produced by antigenic challenge, IgM is the major antibody in blood type incompatibilities and gram-negative bacterial infections. Maternal IgM does not cross the placenta.

By the twentieth week of gestation, however, the fetus produces IgM in response to antigenic exposure. IgM provides active immunity (a long-lasting or permanent immunity resulting from antigenic stimulation through inoculation or natural immunity). High IgM levels in the neonate may signal perinatal infection.

Immunoglobulin A (IgA). The major antibody in the mucosal linings of the intestines and bronchi, IgA appears in all body secretions. It does not cross the placenta and normally is absent in the neonate. Combining with a mucosal protein, IgA is secreted onto mucosal surfaces as a secretory antibody (secretory IgA). Present in breast milk, this substance confers some passive immunity on the breast-fed infant. Secretory IgA also limits bacterial growth in the GI tract.

Cell-mediated immunity. This immune response is most apparent in localized inflammations triggered by fungi, viruses, tissue transplants, and tumors. Various types of T cells carry out cell-mediated immunity. Recognizing a foreign antigen, T cells mobilize tissue macrophages in the presence of migration inhibitory factor. This substance triggers chemical reactions that convert local macrophages into phagocytes and prevent macrophages from leaving the invasion site until they have destroyed the antigen. The breast-fed infant may acquire passive immunity to such diseases as polio, mumps, influenza, and chicken pox through the cell-mediated response.

Congenital infections

Usually, congenital infections—those acquired in utero—result from exposure to such viruses as CMV, rubella, hepatitis B, herpes simplex, herpes zoster, varicella, and Epstein-Barr. However, they also may stem from such nonviral agents as toxoplasmosis, syphilis, tuberculosis, trypanosomiasis, and malaria. Collectively, these viral and nonviral agents are called TORCH—an acronym for toxoplasmosis, others, rubella, CMV, and herpes.

Fetal infection by a TORCH agent follows a systemic maternal infection with placental involvement and fetal spread. TORCH infections can cause a wide range of sequelae, from spontaneous abortion and fetal death to overt or asymptomatic infection at birth. In the early prenatal period, infection by certain TORCH agents (such as rubella and toxoplasmosis) causes disruption of embryogenesis, resulting in severe congenital anomalies (Avery, 1987; Berkowitz, 1984). (For further information on TORCH infections, see Chapter 38, High-Risk Neonates.)

Congenital bacterial infections may arise from bacterial organisms that travel to the fetus through the placenta. Organisms causing such infections include *Lis-*

teria monocytogenes, E. coli, Klebsiella, and *Streptococcus pneumoniae*. The fetus also may become infected by organisms that reach the amniotic cavity via the mother's cervix. Other routes of infection include the fetal skin and mucous membranes, intervillous placental spaces, umbilical cord to the fetal circulation, and respiratory airways (via aspiration). Infectious agents that may take these routes include group B streptococci, *E. coli, L. monocytogenes*, and herpes simplex. An infected neonate may be acutely ill at birth with septicemia, pneumonia, or both (Berkowitz, 1984).

Neurologic system

Although not fully developed, the neonate's neurologic system can perform the complex functions required to regulate neonatal adaptation—stimulate initial respirations, maintain acid-base balance, and regulate body temperature. The neonate's neurologic function is controlled primarily by the brain stem and spinal cord. The autonomic nervous system and brain stem coordinate respiratory and cardiac functions. All cranial nerves are present at birth; however, the nerves are not yet fully sheathed with myelin, a substance essential for smooth nerve impulse transmission.

The neonate has a functioning cerebral cortex, although the degree to which it is used remains unknown. At birth, the brain measures about one-fourth the size of the adult brain. The brain grows and matures in a cephalocaudal (head-to-toe) direction.

The brain needs a constant supply of glucose for energy and a relatively high oxygen level to maintain adequate cellular metabolism (Volpe and Hill, 1987). For this reason, the neonate's oxygenation status and serum glucose levels must be assessed and monitored carefully to detect impaired gas exchange or signs of hypoglycemia.

Nerve tract development

Sensory, cerebellar, and extrapyramidal nerve pathways are the first to develop. This accounts for the neonate's strong sense of hearing, taste, and smell. The cerebellum governs gross voluntary movement and helps maintain equilibrium. The extrapyramidal tract controls reflexive gross motor movement and postural adjustment by regulating reciprocal flexion and extension of muscle groups, thus maintaining smooth, coordinated movement.

Neonatal reflexes

The neonate's reflexes—categorized as feeding, protective, postural, and social—include such primitive reflexes as sucking and rooting (which causes the neonate to turn toward and search for the nipple). Crucial to survival, these reflexes serve as the basis for neonatal

neurologic examination. Persistence of the neonatal reflexes beyond the age at which they normally disappear may indicate a neurologic abnormality. (For information on how to elicit and assess neonatal reflexes, see Chapter 35, Neonatal Assessment.)

Endocrine and metabolic systems

At birth, the endocrine system is anatomically mature but functionally immature. Complex interactions between the neurologic and endocrine systems help coordinate adaptation to extrauterine life. Such interactions take place along three major feedback pathways:
• the parasympathetic–adrenal medulla pathway
• the hypothalamic–anterior pituitary pathway
• the hypothalamic–posterior pituitary pathway (Volpe and Hill, 1987).

Hormonal role in transition

Many extrauterine adaptations are regulated by hormones secreted by the endocrine glands, including growth hormone, thyroid-stimulating hormone, adrenocorticotropic hormone, cortisol, and catecholamines. However, the posterior pituitary gland secretes only a limited amount of antidiuretic hormone (ADH), a substance that limits urine production. Insufficient ADH contributes to the neonate's increased risk of dehydration.

Metabolic changes at birth

Interruption of placental circulation at birth halts the supply of oxygen, nutrients, electrolytes, and other vital substances to the neonate. Withdrawal of maternally supplied glucose and calcium necessitates significant and immediate metabolic changes to ensure successful neonatal adaptation. During the first few hours after birth, serum glucose and calcium levels change rapidly.

Glucose. At birth, the neonate's serum glucose level usually measures 60% to 70% of the maternal serum glucose level. Over the next 2 hours, this level falls, stabilizing between 35 and 40 mg/dl. By 6 hours after birth, however, it usually rises to about 60 mg/dl, unless the neonate experiences cold stress, delayed feeding, metabolic abnormalities, or sepsis.

Calcium. The serum calcium level decreases at birth but usually stabilizes between 24 and 48 hours after birth. A level below 7 mg/dl reflects hypocalcemia. Most commonly, hypocalcemia arises within the first 2 days or at 6 to 10 days after birth. Hypocalcemia may result from hypoxemia, interrupted maternal calcium transfer (early-onset hypocalcemia), or infant formula with an improper calcium-to-phosphorus ratio (later-onset hypocalcemia). In most cases, the full-term neonate given sufficient amounts of the proper formula or breast milk achieves the normal calcium-to-phosphorus ratio of 2:1 (Philip, 1987).

Thermoregulation

Body temperature maintenance—essential for successful extrauterine adaptation—is regulated by complex interactions between environmental temperature and body heat loss and production. The understanding and appropriate management of thermoregulation were among the earliest advances in neonatology.

The neonate has limited thermoregulatory capacity, achieved by body heating and cooling mechanisms. When the neonate can no longer maintain body temperature, cooling or overheating results; exhaustion of thermoregulatory mechanisms brings death. (For a depiction of the progressive effects of hypothermia, see *Dangers of hypothermia in the neonate*.)

As the neonate makes the transition to extrauterine life, the core temperature decreases by an amount that varies with the environmental temperature and the neonate's condition. Initially, the full-term neonate's core temperature falls by approximately 0.54° F (0.3° C)/ minute. Thus, under normal delivery conditions, it may drop 5.4° F (3° C) before the neonate leaves the delivery room.

Maintaining normal body temperature in the neonate can contribute significantly to successful adaptation. Neonatal morbidity and mortality can be favorably influenced by the nurse who takes steps to prevent cold stress. (For interventions that help prevent neonatal heat loss, see Chapter 35, Neonatal Assessment. For a study of the effectiveness of various treatments in preventing heat loss, see *Nursing research applied: A comparison of treatments to prevent neonatal heat loss*, page 824.)

Neutral thermal environment (NTE). Encompassing a narrow range of environmental temperatures, NTE requires the least amount of energy to maintain a stable core temperature. For an unclothed full-term neonate on the first day after birth, NTE ranges from 89.6° to 93.2° F (32° to 34° C). Within this temperature range, oxygen consumption and carbon dioxide production are lowest and core temperature is normal. To maintain body temperature within the NTE, the neonate makes vasomotor adjustments—vasoconstriction to conserve heat and vasodilation to release heat. Environmental temperatures below or above the NTE increase oxygen consumption and boost the metabolic rate—the amount of energy expended over a given unit of time (Gomella, 1988).

Dangers of hypothermia in the neonate

Hypothermia prevention ranks among the most important goals of neonatal nursing care. As shown by the illustration, untreated hypothermia can have grave consequences—culminating in death.

Factors contributing to hypothermia. The following characteristics place the neonate at a physiologic disadvantage for thermoregulation, increasing the risk of hypothermia:

• a large body surface relative to mass
• limited subcutaneous fat deposition to provide insulation
• vasomotor instability
• limited metabolic capacity.

NURSING RESEARCH APPLIED

A comparison of treatments to prevent neonatal heat loss

The neonate not only begins to lose heat at birth but has trouble conserving heat because of the large body surface relative to body mass. Prolonged hypothermia (abnormally low body temperature) in the neonate has been linked with increased mortality, hypoglycemia, higher oxygen consumption, increased anaerobic metabolism, acidosis, bilirubin encephalopathy (kernicterus), and a greater infection risk. Heat loss from the head is particularly dangerous because the neonate's head accounts for almost 21% of the total body surface.

Investigating various methods of minimizing heat loss from the head, researchers compared the effectiveness of three head treatment modalities: no head covering, a stockinette head covering, and a fabric-insulated bonnet. The 90 neonates in the sample were assigned randomly to one of the three treatment groups.

All neonates were cared for under an overhead radiant warmer. Rectal temperatures were recorded 5, 15, and 30 minutes after birth.

Results showed that the fabric-insulated bonnet was most effective in preventing heat loss. The stockinette proved less effective than no head covering at all. Researchers hypothesized that the stockinette not only did not stop heat loss but actually prevented heat gain.

Application to practice

The use of stockinettes in the delivery room is common practice in many health care facilities. However, this study suggests that stockinettes should not be used under a radiant warmer. Although additional research is necessary, these findings should alert the nurse to the potential adverse effects of applying a stockinette to a neonate placed under a radiant warmer.

Greer, P.S. (1988). Head coverings for neonates under radiant heat warmers. *Journal of Obstetric, Gynecologic, and Neonatal Nursing, 17*(4), 265-271.

Mechanisms of heat loss. Heat loss, which begins at delivery, can occur through four mechanisms—evaporation, conduction, radiation, and convection.

• Evaporation. Evaporative heat loss occurs when fluids (insensible water, visible perspiration, and pulmonary fluids) turn to vapor in dry air. The drier the environment, the greater the evaporative heat loss. The pronounced evaporative heat loss occurring with delivery can be minimized by immediately drying the neonate and discarding the wet towels.

• Conduction. This form of heat loss takes place when the skin directly contacts a cooler object—for example, a cold bed or scale. Therefore, any metal surface on which the neonate will be placed should be padded.

• Radiation. A cooler solid surface not in direct contact with the neonate can cause heat loss through radiation. Common sources of radiant heat loss include incubator walls and windows. Occurring even with warm air temperatures, radiant heat loss may be minimized through the use of a thermoplastic heat shield (such as Plexiglas).

• Convection. Heat loss from the body surface to cooler surrounding air occurs through convection. It increases in drafty environments. Thus, a delivery room cooled for the comfort of personnel may cause significant convective heat loss in the neonate.

Defenses against hypothermia. In a cold environment or in other stressful circumstances, the neonate defends against heat loss through vasomotor control, thermal insulation, muscle activity, and nonshivering thermogenesis.

Vasomotor control. Peripheral nervous stimulation activates vasomotor control and metabolic processes to regulate thermal control. The neonate conserves heat through peripheral vasoconstriction and dissipates heat through peripheral vasodilation.

Thermal insulation. Provided by subcutaneous (white) fat, thermal insulation guards against rapid heat loss. The amount of subcutaneous fat determines the degree of thermal insulation. (Subcutaneous fat commonly accounts for 11% to 17% of the full-term neonate's weight.)

Muscle activity. Muscle activity increases heat production. Initially, the neonate reacts to a cold environment with increased movements (often perceived as irritability). For instance, the neonate may assume a tightly flexed posture that reduces heat loss by limiting body surface area.

Whether the neonate can produce heat by shivering remains unknown. Experts now believe the neonate may have some shivering ability. Nonetheless, even if shivering does occur in response to severe cold stress, it does not serve as a major heat source (Avery, 1987; Korones, 1986).

Nonshivering thermogenesis. Defined as the production of heat through lipolysis of brown fat, nonshivering thermogenesis is the neonate's most efficient heat production mechanism because it increases the metabolic rate minimally. A type of adipose tissue, brown fat accounts for up to 1.5% of a full-term neonate's total weight. Named for its brown color—a result of its rich vascular supply, dense cellular content, and numerous nerve endings—brown fat is deposited around the neck, head, heart, great vessels, kidneys, and adrenal glands; between the scapula; behind the sternum; and in the axillae.

The brain, liver, and skeletal muscles take part in nonshivering thermogenesis. In response to heat loss, sympathetic nerves stimulate the release of norepinephrine, the major mediator of nonshivering thermogenesis. Norepinephrine stimulates oxidation of brown fat, causing increased heat production. Heat produced by brown fat oxidation is distributed throughout the body by the blood, which absorbs heat as it flows through fatty tissue.

Integumentary system

The healthy neonate is moist and warm to the touch. Lanugo—fine, downy hair—may appear over the face, shoulders, and back.

As with adults, the neonate's skin serves as the first line of defense against infection. The outermost skin layer, the stratum corneum, is fused with the vernix caseosa. A greasy white substance produced by sebaceous glands, the vernix caseosa coats the fetal skin and protects it from the amniotic fluid. (Because of its protective properties, the vernix caseosa should not be scrubbed off.) With maturation, the stratum corneum becomes an effective protective barrier (Guyton, 1985).

The full-term neonate's skin may appear erythematous (beefy red) for several hours after birth but soon takes on a normal color. In many neonates, vasomotor instability, capillary stasis, and high hemoglobin levels lead to acrocyanosis, characterized by bluish discoloration of the hands and feet. Skin color and circulation usually improve with warming of the hands and feet. (Acrocyanosis should not be confused with central cyanosis, which reflects impaired gas exchange. In central cyanosis, the neonate's skin and mucous membranes turn blue.)

Musculoskeletal system

Ossification (bone development) is incomplete at birth but proceeds rapidly afterward. The neonate's skeleton consists mainly of bone.

Six thin, unjoined bones form the neonate's skull; these bones accommodate subsequent brain and head development. Separating the skull bones are sutures—fibrous joints in which the apposed bones are joined by a thin layer of fibrous connective tissue. Fontanels, soft-tissue areas covered with tough membranes, separate the sutures. Typically, vaginal delivery causes overriding sutures, a spontaneously resolving condition in which the sutures appear to be pushed together.

The muscles are anatomically complete at term birth. With age, muscle mass, strength, and size increase. Increasing muscle strength is crucial to the development of postural control and mobility (Lawrence, 1984).

Reproductive system

The reproductive system is anatomically and functionally immature at birth. However, the female's ovaries contain all potential ova, which decrease in number from birth to maturity by roughly 90%. In approximately 90% of males, the testes have descended into the scrotum by birth, although no sperm appear until puberty.

High maternal estrogen levels may cause transient side effects in the neonate. For example, breast hypertrophy with or without witch's milk (a thin, watery secretion similar to colostrum) may appear in both the male and female neonate. The female may have pseudomenstruation, a mucoid or blood-tinged vaginal discharge caused by the sudden drop in hormone levels after birth (Gomella, 1988). Clinically insignificant, breast hypertrophy and pseudomenstruation resolve spontaneously as the influence of maternal hormones subsides.

Normally, the male neonate has adhesions of the prepuce (penile foreskin) that prevent separation of the prepuce and glans. During fetal development, prepuce tissue is continuous with the epidermal glans covering.

Behavioral characteristics of adaptation

Research on neonatal development in the past 10 to 20 years has shown that the neonate has remarkable sensory, cognitive, and social abilities.

Neonate-environment interactions

The full-term neonate not only perceives the environment but attempts to control it through behavior. Able to see, hear, and differentiate among tastes and smells, the neonate responds to touch and movement, defends against stimulation, and gives signals that, when interpreted by a responsive caretaker, can satisfy the neonate's needs. For example, a neonate uncomfortable in a wet diaper cries; the mother responds by changing the diaper.

The neonate's competencies reflect central nervous system structure, function, and maturity. Als (1982) studied the neonate's ability to interact with the environment through complex regulation of body systems, including autonomic, motor, state-organizational, attentional-interactional, and regulatory functions. As these regulatory systems develop, the neonate's skills repertoire expands. At the same time, interaction with the environment helps the neonate reach a higher level of functioning.

Neonatal sensory capacities

Using the sensory capacities—vision, hearing, touch, taste, and smell—the neonate perceives, interacts with, modifies, and learns from the environment. Combined with the neonate's attractive physical features, these sensory capacities play a major role in the attachment between the neonate and the parents.

Vision

Although the neonate can see, visual acuity is limited to a distance of approximately 9″ to 12″. The neonate has a preference for geometric shapes, such as squares, rectangles, or circles roughly 3″ in diameter. Black and white images hold the neonate's gaze longer than color images (Ludington-Hoe, 1983).

The neonate can conjugate the eyes (move them in unison) at or just after birth. However, immature neuromuscular control limits visual accommodation (the ability to adjust for distance) for the first 4 weeks after birth. Incomplete muscle control of ocular movements sometimes causes transient strabismus (deviation of the eye, or "crossed" eyes). Also, the epicanthal fold covering the inner canthus of the eye may narrow the visible width of the sclera beside the iris, giving a neonate the appearance of having crossed eyes (pseudostrabismus).

The neonate apparently finds the human face intriguing and typically fixes the eyes and gazes intently at a face in proximity, as during feeding or cuddling. Such behavior strongly reinforces parent-neonate attachment.

Visual acuity improves quickly; by age 6 months, adult-level visual acuity is achieved. In the neonate exposed to various pleasing objects in a range of colors, shapes, and contrasts, visual acuity may improve even more rapidly. Placing crib gyms, mobiles, and pictures within view may help stimulate visual development. Because the neonate prefers more color, greater contrast, and more interesting patterns than the light pastels of the traditional nursery, a change in nursery decor and infant clothing may be warranted.

Sensitive to light, the neonate grimaces or frowns and turns the head away from a bright light directed toward the eyes and opens the eyes more readily in a dimly lit room. Thus, by dimming the lights, parents may improve eye contact with the neonate, facilitating attachment.

The neonate responds to movement in the environment, fixing on and following bright or shiny objects soon after birth. For instance, the neonate fixes on and follows a parent's eyes; while gazing at a parent's face, the neonate may appear to imitate that parent's facial expressions, thereby rewarding the parent's response. The ability to fix on and gaze at objects improves rapidly.

Hearing

The neonate can hear at birth. In fact, hearing begins even earlier: The fetus can hear extrauterine sounds (for instance, voices or music) as well as noises originating in maternal body systems, including variable low-pitched sounds in the maternal cardiovascular and GI systems (Kramer and Pierpont, 1976).

Hearing is well established after aeration of the eustachian tube and drainage of blood, vernix caseosa, amniotic fluid, and mucus from the outer ear. Shortly after birth, the neonate turns toward sounds and startles in response to loud noises, such as a ringing telephone, dropped chart, or slammed door. Able to differentiate sounds on the basis of frequency, intensity, and pattern, the neonate responds more readily to sounds below 4,000 Hz. (Human speech usually is between 500 and 900 Hz.)

The neonate responds variously to different vocal pitches. Most women have higher-pitched voices than men and instinctively raise their pitch when talking to an infant. A high-pitched voice attracts the attention of the neonate, who turns toward the sound with increased alertness. In contrast, the lower-pitched male voice seems to have a soothing effect. Mothers commonly make use of this effect by talking in a much lower pitch when trying to calm or console the neonate (Eisenberg, 1965; Redshaw, Rivers, and Rosenblatt, 1985).

Touch

The neonate has well-developed tactile perception, which serves as a stimulus for the first breath. The most sensitive body areas include the face (especially around the mouth), hands, and soles.

Until recently, experts believed that incomplete nerve myelination prevented the neonate from experiencing pain, except perhaps to a limited degree. Current knowledge, however, refutes this assumption. Anand and Hickey (1987) concluded that the pain pathways and cortical and subcortical centers crucial to pain perception are well developed and that the neurochemical systems associated with pain transmission are intact and functional as term approaches. Physiologic changes associated with pain in the neonate include increased blood pressure and pulse during and after a painful procedure. During such a procedure, the neonate's $PaCO_2$ level fluctuates widely and palmar sweating increases. In neonates undergoing painful procedures, researchers also have documented marked hormonal changes—including increased plasma renin levels soon after venipuncture and elevated plasma cortisol levels during and after circumcision without anesthesia. Also, painful stimuli have elicited simple motor responses (flexion and adduction of extremities); distinct facial expressions (pain, sadness, surprise); and characteristic crying. Some preliminary studies suggest that neonates have pain memory as well as pain perception.

Pleasant cutaneous stimulation, on the other hand, induces muscle relaxation—another key factor in parent-neonate attachment. As the mother becomes acquainted with the neonate by lightly touching the face, extremities, and trunk, the neonate's muscle tone and movement decrease and crying stops or declines, reinforcing the mother's attachment (Redshaw, Rivers, and Rosenblatt, 1985).

Handling of the neonate provides sensory stimulation from motion as well as from touch. Such stimulation elicits alertness and orienting responses. These responses, in turn, influence neonatal development and parent-neonate interaction. However, the neonate may tire if handled too much.

Taste
The neonate differentiates among tastes by the first or second day after birth. In response to a tasteless solution (such as sterile water), the neonate's facial expression remains unchanged. A sweet solution, on the other hand, elicits satisfied sucking; a sour solution induces a grimace and cessation of sucking; and a bitter solution provokes an angry facial expression, cessation of sucking, and, frequently, turning away of the head. Breast-feeding mothers also find that neonates prefer bottled breast milk to commercial formula during periods when they cannot nurse (Als, 1982).

Smell
Although little research has been conducted on neonatal olfaction, the neonate is known to react to strong or noxious odors by averting the head from the odor. Sensitivity to olfactory stimuli increases over the first 4 days after birth.

In studies in which neonates smelled breast pads saturated with their mother's milk as well as pads saturated with other human milk, neonates responded to their mother's milk by crying and exhibiting rooting behaviors. A neonate also may be able to recognize the mother's perfume or cologne (Als, 1982).

Characteristic patterns of sleep and activity

During the transitional period, the neonate experiences a series of changes encompassing state of consciousness, behavioral response to stimuli, and physiologic parameters. Various neonate sleep and awake states also have been identified.

Periods of neonatal reactivity

The neonate's initial hours are characterized by a predictable, identifiable series of behavioral and physiologic characteristics (Arnold, 1965). Desmond (1966) described this series collectively as the periods of neonatal reactivity.

All neonates experience the same sequence of periods. However, when each period begins and how long it lasts varies from one neonate to another. Maternal medication, anesthesia, labor duration, and any stress affecting the neonate may influence the duration of a given period.

First period of reactivity
Beginning just after birth, this period lasts roughly 30 minutes. In this phase of intense activity and awareness of external stimuli, the neonate is alert and attentive to the environment and may exhibit vigorous activity, crying, and rapid respiratory and heart rates. The neonate has a strong desire to suckle during this period, so breast-feeding may be initiated. Gradually, the neonate becomes less alert and active and falls asleep.

Neonatal adaptations during this initial period are regulated mainly by the sympathetic nervous system. Irregular respirations, tachypnea, and nasal flaring unrelated to respiratory distress may occur. Other visible features of this period include spontaneous startles, the Moro reflex (in which the neonate extends and moves the limbs away from the body when the head is dropped backward suddenly), grimacing, sucking motions, sudden cries that stop abruptly, fine tremors of the jaw or extremities, blinking, and jerking eye movements.

The first reactivity period provides a good opportunity for early parent-neonate interaction. Studying the attachment of mothers and neonates, Klaus and Kennell (1976) concluded that this is the optimal time for promoting mother-neonate bonding. They referred to this phase as a sensitive period, necessary to some degree for successful mother-neonate attachment. Although the importance of this period to bonding has since been questioned, the work of Klaus and Kennell led to changes in routine obstetric and neonatal nursery care to prevent unnecessary separation of parents and neonate.

The nurse can enhance attachment by allowing the mother and neonate to remain together during this period (provided the neonate is healthy). After drying the neonate and performing initial care, the nurse should allow the parents to see and hold their child. Instillation of prophylactic eye medication should be delayed until after this period so that the neonate's heightened visual awareness can enhance parent-neonate bonding.

Temperature must be monitored and maintained carefully during this period to prevent cold stress. For example, the nurse should carefully dry the neonate or use warmed blankets or overhead warming lights to supply heat and prevent heat loss. Although temperature maintenance should never be forfeited to allow parent-neonate contact, the nurse should keep in mind that skin-to-skin contact between parent and neonate usually maintains the neonate's temperature adequately.

Sleep stage

The neonate typically falls asleep about 2 to 3 hours after birth and remains asleep from a few minutes to 2 to 4 hours. Some authorities classify sleep as a distinct, self-contained period of reactivity. Others consider it a transitional phase bridging the first and second periods.

While asleep, the neonate's respiratory rate increases while the heart rate ranges from 120 to 140 beats/minute. Skin color improves, although some acrocyanosis persists. Because the neonate has little response to external stimuli during the sleep period, attempts at breast-feeding will elicit no response. However, the mother may wish to hold and cuddle her child.

Second period of reactivity

Beginning when the neonate awakens, this period is characterized by an exaggerated response to internal and external stimuli. The heart rate is labile, and episodes of bradycardia and tachycardia occur. The neonate's skin usually appears pink-tinged or ruddy (although skin color naturally varies with racial background). Thick oral secretions frequently cause gagging and emesis. The respiratory rate, ranging from about 30 to 60 breaths/minute, is irregular and may include brief apneic pauses and periodic tachypnea. The neonate usually expels meconium from the GI tract during this period.

The second period may last from 4 to 6 hours. As it ends, the neonate becomes more stable and the respiratory and cardiac rates normalize. A dynamic equilibrium emerges, with the neonate alternating between alert activity and sleep and establishing a pattern of sleeping, crying, activity, and feeding. Although the environment influences the neonate's diurnal and circadian rhythms, temperament also strongly affects behavior.

Nursing measures appropriate for this period include monitoring vital signs, maintaining temperature, and ensuring a patent airway. The nurse also should encourage the parents to get acquainted with their infant at this time. The neonate may exhibit vigorous sucking motions and may appear hungry. (For a discussion of assessment during the two periods of reactivity, see Chapter 35, Neonatal Assessment.)

Sleep and awake states of the neonate

Brazelton (1979) classified the neonate's state of consciousness into six states—two sleep states and four awake states. The sleep and awake states encompass the behavioral states used in the Brazelton Neonatal Behavioral Assessment Scale (BNBAS). Developed by Brazelton to measure a neonate's capabilities, the BNBAS assesses neonatal behavioral responses and elicited responses as well as behavioral states. (For details on the BNBAS, see Chapter 35, Neonatal Assessment.)

The neonate's ability to regulate the state of consciousness reflects central nervous system integrity. The state of consciousness may be affected by medication, hunger, diurnal cycles, stress (such as from noise, pain, and bright lights), and any other physical discomfort. Normally, the neonate in a sleep state responds to stimuli with increased activity, whereas a neonate in the crying state responds with decreased activity.

According to Brazelton, when confronted with external interferences (such as a heel prick or another painful stimulus), the neonate attempts to control the state of consciousness in one of four ways:
• by trying to withdraw physically
• by trying to push away the stimulus with the hands or feet
• by trying to withdraw emotionally (for example, turning away from the stimulus or falling asleep)
• by crying or fussing in an effort to interrupt the stimulus.

State of consciousness serves as a key focus of nursing assessment and as the basis for care of both neonate and parents. The nurse must be sufficiently familiar with neonatal sleep and awake states to recognize the neonate's state and any changes in it. By using this information, the nurse may more skillfully assess the neonate, plan neonatal care, and help promote parent-neonate interaction. (See Chapter 35, Neonatal Assessment, for details on assessing specific sleep and awake states.)

Deep sleep

In this sleep state, the neonate's eyes are closed and no rapid eye movements (REMs) appear. Except for occasional startle reflexes, no spontaneous activity occurs. Respirations are even and regular. The neonate in deep sleep usually cannot be aroused by external stimuli and will not breast-feed. Attempts by the mother to feed the neonate will cause frustration.

Light sleep

During this period, the neonate's eyes are closed and REMs occur. Variable breathing patterns, random movements, and sucking motions typify light sleep. External stimuli may arouse the neonate in this state.

Drowsy state

In this transitional state, the neonate attempts to become fully alert. The eyes may be open or closed and the eyelids may flutter frequently. Muscle movements are smooth, with intermittent spontaneous activity and startles. Tactile or auditory stimuli may evoke a response, but the response may be sluggish until the neonate approaches the next state.

Alert state

In this state, the eyes are open, bright, and shining and the neonate focuses on the source of stimulation. Aware of and responsive to the environment, the neonate makes purposeful movements and shows good eye-hand coordination. The neonate attempts to attain and maintain this state.

The alert state is considered the optimal state of arousal, ideal for parent-neonate contact or breast-feeding initiation. Although only minimally active, the neonate remains alert and responsive to visual and auditory stimulation for prolonged periods. Additional stimulation may cause a change of state (although the response to external stimulation is delayed).

Active state

The neonate's movements increase in this state, and external stimuli cause eye and body movements. The level of this activity increases as the next state approaches.

Crying state

In this state, the neonate responds to both internal and external stimuli. Usually beginning with slight whimpering and minimal activity, the neonate in the crying state typically progresses to increased motor activity, with thrusting movements of the extremities and spontaneous startles. The chance for successful feeding or interaction may improve if the parents or nurse can calm the neonate through such motions as rocking.

Chapter summary

Chapter 34 introduced neonatal adaptation—the transitional period that follows delivery. By becoming familiar with the neonate's normal adaptations during this period, the nurse can more easily identify signs of abnormal adaptation. Here are the key concepts discussed in the chapter.

• The first 24 hours after birth are called the transitional period. During this time, the neonate experiences many biological and behavioral adaptations to extrauterine life.

• At birth, the four unique anatomic features of fetal circulation (the placenta, ductus venosus, foramen ovale, and ductus arteriosus) undergo changes that establish neonatal circulation. The placenta, which serves as the maternal-fetal exchange organ for oxygen, nutrients, and wastes, is removed at birth. The ductus venosus, which shunts most blood from the placenta around the liver to the inferior vena cava, functionally closes as clamping of the umbilical cord eliminates its blood flow. Hemodynamic events triggered by the neonate's initial respirations lead to functional closure of the foramen ovale, an interatrial septum that allows blood to pass from the right to left atrium. The effects of the neonate's initial respirations also cause functional closure of the ductus arteriosus, which during fetal development shunts blood from the pulmonary artery to the descending aorta, away from the lungs.

• The full-term neonate's blood volume typically is 80 to 90 ml/kg of body weight.

• Asphyxia is the strongest stimulus for the first breath. Other breathing stimuli include hypoxia, acidosis, cord occlusion, thermal changes, and tactile stimulation.

• Fetal erythrocytes contain fetal hemoglobin (hemoglobin F), which has a higher affinity for oxygen than adult hemoglobin (hemoglobin A).

• Leukocytes serve as the neonate's main internal defense against infection.

• For several days after birth, vitamin K levels are low because of insufficient bacterial action in the GI tract to synthesize vitamin K. Consequently, the neonate lacks several vitamin K–dependent coagulation factors.

• Before feedings begin, glucose serves as the neonate's major energy source.

• Because of a relatively immature renal system, the neonate is at risk for acidosis, dehydration, and electrolyte imbalance.

• Like the adult, the neonate has two specific immune responses—humoral and cell-mediated.

• The three major classes of immunoglobulins are IgG, IgM, and IgA.

• Neonatal defenses against heat loss include vasomotor control, thermal insulation, muscle activity, and non-shivering thermogenesis.

• Acrocyanosis, a condition characterized by bluish discoloration of the hands and feet, results from vasomotor instability, capillary stasis, and a high hemoglobin level.

• The typical neonate's visual acuity is limited to a distance of 9″ to 12″. The neonate has a preference for black and white geometric shapes.

• Neonatal hearing is well established once the eustachian tube is aerated and the outer ear cleared of vernix, blood, mucus, and amniotic fluid.

• The neonate reacts to pain with physiologic, hormonal, and motor responses.

• The stages of neonatal reactivity represent a predictable series of behaviors and physiologic characteristics.

• The neonate's state of consciousness consists of six states—two sleep states and four awake states. Knowledge of the characteristics of each state improves nursing assessment and care of the neonate and family.

Study questions

1. What are the unique features of fetal circulation?

2. Which conditions trigger closure of the ductus arteriosus?

3. What are the functions of pulmonary surfactant?

4. Which stimuli initiate respirations?

5. Through what process is bilirubin produced and excreted from the body?

6. What is the treatment for breast-milk jaundice?

7. Why is the neonate at risk for hemorrhage?

8. Which factors predispose the neonate to heat loss?

9. What role should the nurse play in caring for the neonate during the transitional period?

10. Which factors account for the neonate's increased infection risk?

11. How do calcium and glucose metabolism change during the transitional period?

12. What are the implications of the periods of reactivity for nursing care of the neonate?

Bibliography

Abrams, G. (1982). Introduction to general pathology: Mechanisms of disease. In S. A. Price and L. M. Wilson (Eds.), *Pathophysiology: Clinical concepts of disease processes* (pp. 5-89). New York: McGraw-Hill.

Avery, G. B. (1987). *Neonatology: Pathophysiology and management of the newborn* (3rd ed.). Philadelphia: Lippincott.

Brown, B. A. (1988). *Hematology: Principles and procedures.* Philadelphia: Lea & Febiger.

Chamberlain, G. (1987). *Lecture notes on obstetrics.* Boston: Blackwell Scientific Publications.

Cloherty, J. P., and Stark, A. R. (1985). *Manual of neonatal care (The Boston manual)* (2nd ed.). Boston: Little, Brown.

Gomella, T. L. (1988). *Neonatology: Procedures, "on-call" problems, diseases, drugs.* Norwalk, CT: Appleton & Lange.

Guyton, A. (1985). *Textbook of Medical Physiology* (7th ed.). Philadelphia: Saunders.

Klaus, M. H., and Fanaroff, A. A. (1986). *Care of the high-risk neonate* (3rd ed.). Philadelphia: Saunders.

Klaus, M. H., and Kennell, J. H. (1976). *Maternal infant bonding.* St. Louis: C.V. Mosby.

Koff, P. B., Eitzman, D. V., and Neu, J. (1988). *Neonatal and pediatric respiratory care.* St. Louis: C.V. Mosby.

Korones, S. B. (1986). *High-risk newborn infants: The basis for intensive nursing care* (3rd ed.). St. Louis: C.V. Mosby.

March of Dimes. (1985). *Report on child health.* White Plains, NY.

Moore, K. (1988). *The developing human* (4th ed.). Philadelphia: Saunders.

Philip, A. G. (1987). *Neonatology: A practical guide.* Philadelphia: Saunders.

Redshaw, M. E., Rivers, R. P. A., and Rosenblatt, D. B. (1985). *Born too early: Special care for your preterm baby.* New York: Oxford University Press.

Streeter, N.S. (1986). *High-risk neonatal care.* Rockville, MD: Aspen.

West, J. B. (1985). *Respiratory physiology—the essentials* (3rd ed.). Baltimore: Williams & Wilkins.

Neonatal physical and behavioral assessment

Als, H., Tronick, E., Adamson, L., and Brazelton, T. B. (1976). The behavior of the full-term but underweight newborn. *Infant Developmental Medicine and Child Neurology, 18,* 590-602.

Berkowitz, I. D. (1984). Infections in the newborn. In M. Ziai, T. Clarke, and T. Merritt (Eds.), *Assessment of the newborn: A guide for the practitioner* (pp. 59-80). Boston: Little, Brown.

Brazelton, T. B. (1973). Neonatal behavior assessment scale. *Clinics in Developmental Medicine,* No. 50. Philadelphia: Lippincott.

Brazelton, T. B. (1979). Behavioral competence of the newborn infant. *Seminars in Perinatology,* 3(1), 35-44.

Eisenberg, R. (1965). Auditory behaviors in the human neonate: Methodological problems. *Journal of Research,* 5, 159-177.

Fantz, R. (1965). Visual perception from birth as shown by pattern selectivity. *Annals of the New York Academy of Science,* 118(21), 793-814.

Foye, H. R. (1984). Capabilities of the human newborn. In M. Ziai, T. Clarke, and T. Merritt (Eds.), *Assessment of the newborn: A guide for the practitioner* (pp. 46-53). Boston: Little, Brown.

Ingelfinger, J. R. (1985). Renal conditions in the newborn period. In J. P. Cloherty and A. R. Stark (Eds.), *Manual of neonatal care* (2nd ed.; pp. 377-394). Boston: Little, Brown.

Lawrence, R. (1984). Physical examination. In M. Ziai, T. Clarke and T. Merritt (Eds.), *Assessment of the newborn: A guide for the practitioner* (pp. 86-111). Boston: Little, Brown.

Ludington-Hoe, S. M. (1983). What can newborns really see? *AJN,* (9), 1286-1289.

Putnam, T. C. (1984). Gastrointestinal bleeding. In M. Ziai, T. Clarke, and T. Merritt (Eds.), *Assessment of the newborn: A guide for the practitioner* (pp. 207-209). Boston: Little, Brown.

Volpe, J. J., and Hill, A. (1987). Neurologic disorders. In G. B. Avery (Ed.), *Neonatology, pathophysiology, and management of the newborn* (pp. 1073-1132). Philadelphia: Lippincott.

Nursing management during transition

Als, H. (1982). Toward a synactive theory of development. Promise for the assessment and support of infant individuality. *Infant Mental Health Journal,* 3(4), 229-243.

Anand, K. and Hickey, P. R. (1987). Pain and its effects in the human neonate and fetus. *New England Journal of Medicine,* 317(21), 1321-1329.

Arnold, H. W., Putman, N. J., Barnard, B. L., Desmond, M. M., and Rudolph, A. J. (1965). Transition to extrauterine life. *AJN,* 65(10), 77-80.

Banta, S. A. (1985). Transition to extrauterine life. *Neonatal Network,* (3)6, 35-39.

Davidson, S. C. (1985). Extrauterine life adaptation. In M. A. Auvenshine and M. G. Enriquez (Eds.), *Maternity nursing: Dimensions of change* (pp. 482-492). Monterey, CA: Wadsworth Health Sciences Division.

Desmond, M. M., and Associates. (1966). The transitional care nursery. *Pediatric Clinics of North America,* 13(3), 651-668.

Glader, B. (1978). Neonatal bleeding: II—Healthy infants. *Perinatal Care,* 2(2), 19-25.

Maisels, I. (1987). Neonatal jaundice. In G. B. Avery (Ed.), *Neonatology: Pathophysiology and management of the newborn* (3rd ed.; pp. 86-111). Philadelphia: Lippincott.

Morin, F. C. (1984). Delivery room resuscitation. In M. Ziai, T. Clarke, and T. Merritt (Eds.), *Assessment of the newborn: A guide for the practitioner* (pp. 12-19). Boston: Little, Brown.

Wilkerson, N. (1988). A comprehensive look at hyperbilirubinemia. *Maternal-Child Nursing,* 13(5), 360-364.

Nursing research

Greer, P.S. (1988). Head coverings for neonates under radiant heat warmers. *JOGNN,* 17 (4), 265-271.

Kramer, L. I., and Pierpont, M. E. (1976). Rocking waterbeds and auditory stimuli to enhance growth of preterm infants. *Journal of Pediatrics,* 88(2), 297-299.

CHAPTER 35

Neonatal Assessment

Objectives

After reading and studying this chapter, the student should be able to:

1. Describe general guidelines to follow when assessing the neonate.

2. Discuss the benefits of allowing parents to observe the neonatal assessment.

3. Identify the proper sequence to use for the comprehensive assessment.

4. Gather appropriate health history information from the prenatal and intrapartal periods.

5. Identify maternal history findings that suggest a gestational-age or birth-weight variation.

6. Discuss the essential elements of neonatal gestational-age, physical, and behavioral assessments.

7. Describe the techniques used to conduct neonatal gestational-age, physical, and behavioral assessments.

8. Describe how the neonate interacts with the environment.

9. Recognize the characteristics of each period of neonatal reactivity and understand how these characteristics may affect assessment findings.

Introduction

The neonate undergoes many physiologic changes during the neonatal period—the first 28 days after birth. To make a successful transition to the extrauterine environment, the neonate must adapt to these changes as smoothly as possible. The nurse plays a critical role in the neonate's transition by conducting a thorough, systematic assessment that provides baseline information

about the neonate's physiologic status and the adequacy of neonatal adaptation.

Besides knowing how to conduct such an assessment, the nurse also must understand the significance of assessment findings. For example, by identifying gestational age, the nurse can determine whether the neonate has a gestational-age variation necessitating special care. Early detection of a potential or actual problem reduces the risk of complications; in some cases, it may mean the difference between life and death.

This chapter begins with an overview of neonatal assessment, including the timing of the various types of assessments—gestational-age assessment, physical assessment, and behavioral assessment. Next, it describes the essential components of these assessments and discusses the techniques used for each. The chapter includes a detailed chart that presents normal and abnormal physical assessment findings.

General assessment guidelines

The nurse must adapt the assessment to the neonate's tolerance, delaying any maneuvers that could compromise the neonate and combining overlapping portions of the various assessments to help conserve the neonate's energy. For instance, gestational-age assessment includes certain characteristics also evaluated during the

GLOSSARY

Appropriate for gestational age: term used to describe a neonate whose birth weight falls between the tenth and ninetieth percentile for gestational age on the Colorado intrauterine growth chart.

Ballard gestational-age assessment tool: tool that examines seven physical (external) and six neuromuscular characteristics to determine a neonate's gestational age.

Brazelton neonatal behavioral assessment scale (BNBAS): tool that determines a neonate's interactive and behavioral capacities.

Cephalocaudal: pertaining to the long axis of the body in a head-to-tail direction.

Dubowitz gestational-age assessment tool: tool that examines 11 physical (external) and 10 neuromuscular characteristics to determine a neonate's gestational age.

En face position: position in which the neonate is held approximately 8" (20 cm) in front of the parent or other observer; allows direct eye contact.

Fetal position: relationship of the landmark on the fetal presenting part to the front, back, and sides of the maternal pelvis.

Fontanel: nonossified area of connective tissue between the skull bones where the sutures intersect; allows molding of the skull for passage through the pelvis during delivery.

Gestational age: estimated age in weeks following conception.

Gestational-age assessment: evaluation of a neonate's physical and neurologic characteristics to determine approximate weeks of fetal development.

Habituation: gradual adaptation to a stimulus through repeated exposure.

Head lag: head position relative to the trunk when the neonate is in a sitting position.

Lanugo: fine hair covering the face, shoulders, and back of the fetus or neonate before 28 weeks' gestation.

Large for gestational age (LGA): term used to describe a neonate whose birth weight exceeds the ninetieth percentile for gestational age on the Colorado intrauterine growth chart.

Mature neonate: neonate of 38 to 42 weeks' gestation; also called term neonate.

Meconium: thick, sticky, green-to-black material that collects in the fetal intestines and forms the first neonatal stool.

Moro reflex: normal neonatal reflex elicited by dropping the neonate's head backward in a sudden motion, resulting in extension and abduction of all extremities, formation of a "C" with the fingers, and adduction, then flexion, of all extremities (as in an embrace).

Motor maturity: maturity of muscle tone and posture, including muscle coordination, muscle movements, and reflexes.

Neonatal adaptation: physiologic and behavioral changes during the first 24 hours after delivery through which the neonate makes the transition from the intrauterine to the extrauterine environment.

Orientation: neonate's ability to respond to visual and auditory stimuli.

Patent ductus arteriosus: abnormal opening between the pulmonary artery and the aorta; results from failure of the fetal ductus arteriosus to close after birth (seen mainly in the preterm neonate).

Periods of neonatal reactivity: predictable, identifiable series of behavioral and physiologic characteristics occurring during the first hours after birth; characterized by distinctive changes in vital signs, state of alertness, and responsiveness to external stimuli.

Poikilotherm: neonate who takes on the temperature of the environment.

Postterm neonate: one born after completion of the forty-second gestational week; also called postmature neonate.

Preterm neonate: one born before completion of the thirty-seventh gestational week; also called premature neonate.

Rooting reflex: normal neonatal reflex elicited by stroking the cheek or corner of the mouth with a finger or nipple, resulting in turning of the head toward the stimulus.

Scarf sign: term describing the distance that the neonate's elbow can be extended across the chest toward the opposite side; an index of gestational age.

Self-quieting behaviors: behaviors the neonate uses to become quiet when crying, including hand-to-mouth movements, fist sucking, and attending to external stimuli (evaluated during the behavioral assessment).

Small for gestational age (SGA): term used to describe the neonate who experienced intrauterine growth retardation and whose birth weight falls below the tenth percentile for gestational age on the Colorado intrauterine growth chart.

Smith's minor anomalies: neonatal physiologic variations (such as abnormal dermal ridges) that may indicate major anomalies (for example, Down's syndrome).

Social behaviors: neonatal responses to others' actions (especially those of caregivers), including smiling, gazing, cuddling, and following voices with the eyes.

Square window sign: term describing the degree to which the neonate's wrist can be flexed against the forearm; an index of gestational age.

(continued)

GLOSSARY continued

Sucking reflex: normal neonatal reflex elicited by inserting a finger or nipple in the neonate's mouth, resulting in forceful, rhythmic sucking.

Synactive theory of development: Als's theory proposing that the neonate continuously interacts with the environment and that the neonate's physiologic status depends on the environmental stimuli received and processed.

Thermoregulation: maintenance of body temperature by complex interaction between environmental temperature and body heat loss and production.

Ventral suspension: term describing the degree to which the neonate extends the back, flexes the arms and legs, and holds the head upright when an examiner positions the neonate prone and places a hand under the chest; an index of gestational age.

Vernix caseosa: grayish white, cheeselike substance, composed of sebaceous gland secretions and desquamated epithelial cells, that covers the near-term fetus and neonate.

---

physical and behavioral assessments; the nurse should examine these characteristics only once. Also, the nurse should allow a neonate who falls asleep during the assessment to sleep undisturbed to recuperate from the stress of birth, then resume the assessment when the neonate awakens.

Assessment sequence

Neonatal assessment proceeds from an immediate determination of the Apgar score to a complete physical assessment.

The immediate assessment—determination of the Apgar score—takes place in the delivery area. The Apgar score is based on five parameters: skin color, heart rate, respiratory rate, muscle tone, and reflex irritability. The cumulative score indicates the neonate's general physical status. (For details on the Apgar score, see Chapter 28, The Second Stage of Labor.)

Once stabilized in the delivery area, the neonate is transferred to the nursery for observation. Some facilities have rooming-in privileges for the mother and neonate after a brief observation. Regardless of the setting, however, the ensuing assessment steps remain the same.

Within the next few hours, the nurse should conduct a complete physical assessment to determine how well the neonate is adapting to the extrauterine environment and to check for obvious problems and major anomalies. This assessment includes evaluation of general appearance, vital sign measurement, and anthropometric measurements.

The nurse then estimates the neonate's gestational age and, if necessary, conducts a formal gestational-age assessment, using a special assessment tool, to determine gestational age precisely. Based on education and experience, the nurse may assist with a behavioral assessment.

Health history

The nurse should obtain a complete history of the prenatal and intrapartal periods from the maternal and delivery room records, then review it for any problems that the client might have experienced during pregnancy.

Determination of preterm or postterm status usually is established by the time of delivery. However, the nurse may want to review the history for factors that increase the risk of a gestational-age variation so that the health care team can anticipate potential perinatal problems more accurately. For instance, the risk of preterm delivery increases with:

• various intrapartal factors, such as multiple gestation (more than one fetus), fetal infection, preeclampsia, premature rupture of the membranes, abruptio placentae, hydramnios (excessive amniotic fluid), placenta previa, and poor prenatal care
• chronic maternal disease, such as cardiovascular disease, renal disease, or diabetes mellitus
• maternal history of abdominal surgery, trauma, uterine anomalies, cervical incompetency, infection, or previous preterm delivery
• maternal age under 18.

With a postterm neonate, the intrapartal history may include weight loss, decreased abdominal circumference, and reduced uterine size—signs of an altered fetal growth pattern (fetal dysmaturity).

The prenatal and intrapartal history also may suggest a birth-weight variation. Such variations include small for gestational age (SGA), defined as a birth weight that falls below the tenth percentile for gestational age on the Colorado intrauterine growth chart, and large for gestational age (LGA), defined as a birth weight that exceeds the ninetieth percentile for gestational age on the growth chart.

Like a gestational-age variation, a birth-weight variation increases the risk of perinatal problems. Women identified as high risk by history or clinical assessment deliver about two-thirds of SGA neonates (Cassady and Strange, 1987). Risk factors for delivery of an SGA neonate include low socioeconomic status, an age under 18 or over 35, multiparity, short stature, low prepregnancy weight, and previous delivery of an SGA neonate.

Typically, the diagnosis of LGA is established during the antepartal period, when fundal height appears disproportionate to gestational weeks. Also, because diabetes mellitus is a leading cause of accelerated intrauterine growth, an elevated maternal serum glucose level may result in an LGA fetus.

Periods of neonatal reactivity

During the first hours after birth, the neonate experiences gradual, predictable changes in physiologic characteristics and behavioral responses, reflecting the periods of neonatal reactivity. The two reactivity periods are separated by a sleep stage (considered a discrete period of reactivity by some authorities).

With each period of reactivity, vital signs, state of alertness, and responsiveness to external stimuli change. The nurse must be able to recognize the characteristics of each period and use them when interpreting assessment findings. (For key features associated with each reactivity period, see *Assessment findings during the periods of neonatal reactivity.*) Although a specific assessment for the period of reactivity is not necessary, the nurse should stay alert for deviations from normal findings because such deviations may signify a disorder. (For more information on the periods of reactivity, see Chapter 34, Neonatal Adaptation.)

Initial physical assessment

During the initial physical assessment of the neonate, the nurse evaluates the neonate's general appearance, assesses vital signs, and takes anthropometric measurements. To prevent the neonate from becoming tired or stressed, the nurse should conduct this assessment as swiftly and systematically as possible.

General appearance

By assessing general appearance, the nurse quickly gauges the neonate's maturity level (a reflection of gestational age) and may detect obvious problems. Features to assess in the general survey include posture, head size, lanugo, vernix caseosa, cry, and state of alertness.

Assessment findings during the periods of neonatal reactivity

The nurse should consider the period of reactivity when assessing the neonate—especially when using the Brazelton neonatal behavioral assessment scale to evaluate behavior. This chart shows the normal assessment findings associated with each reactivity period.

PARAMETER	FIRST PERIOD	SECOND PERIOD
Skin color	Fluctuates from pale pink to cyanotic (blue)	Fluctuates from pale pink to cyanotic, with periods of mottling
Alertness level	Awake and alert, progressing to sleep	Hyperactive, with exaggerated responses
Cry	Rigorous, diminishing as sleep begins	Periodic
Respiratory rate	Up to 80 breaths/minute	40 to 60 breaths/minute, with periods of more rapid respirations
Respiratory effort	Irregular and labored, with nasal flaring, expiratory grunts, and retractions	Usually unlabored
Heart rate	Up to 180 beats/minute	120 to 160 beats/minute, with periods of more rapid beating
Heart rhythm	Irregular, progressing to regular	Irregular as the neonate falls asleep, progressing to regular
Bowel sounds	Absent	Present
Stool	May not be passed	Meconium stool passed
Voiding	Rare	Usually begins
Mucus production	Minimal, diminishing gradually	Present, may be excessive
Sucking reflex	Strong, diminishing as sleep begins	Strong

(For details on normal and abnormal findings when evaluating general appearance, see "Complete physical assessment" later in this chapter.)

Vital signs and blood pressure

After assessing general appearance, the nurse measures vital signs—temperature, respiratory rate, and pulse—and blood pressure (not strictly a vital sign but usually included). For details on how to take neonatal vital signs, see *Psychomotor skills: Taking vital signs.*

Temperature
First, measure the neonate's core (internal) temperature (formerly referred to as rectal temperature). Although axillary temperature also accurately reflects core temperature, many health care professionals question the reliability of axillary temperature in the first 24 hours after birth because of poor peripheral perfusion during this time. However, Bliss-Holtz (1989) found that axillary temperatures are a safe, accurate substitute for rectal temperatures. Comparing rectal, axillary, and inguinal temperatures, the researcher found the greatest discrepancy (0.8° F) between rectal and inguinal temperatures. Rectal and axillary temperatures differed by only 0.2° F.

Axillary temperature should measure 96° to 98° F (35.5° to 36.5° C); it should be approximately 0.2° F—and no more than 1° F—lower than rectal temperature. Skin temperature should measure 0° to 0.9° F (0° to 0.5° C) below axillary temperature. An axillary temperature above 99° F (37° C) reflects hyperthermia or fever; below 96° F (35.5° C), poor peripheral perfusion or prematurity.

External heat or cooling sources may affect the neonate's temperature. Many neonates are poikilotherms, taking on the temperature of the environment. For example, a neonate who is exposed to direct sunlight may experience a rapid increase in core and skin temperatures, becoming restless and irritable. Consequently, room temperature must be kept constant to prevent overheating or excessive cooling of the neonate.

Respiratory rate
The respiratory rate varies with the state of alertness and period of reactivity; thus, it may fluctuate widely in the first hours after birth. After the first period of reactivity (marked by more rapid breathing), the respiratory rate typically measures 40 to 60 breaths/minute. If it exceeds 60 breaths/minute or if the neonate has apneic episodes lasting longer than 15 seconds accompanied by duskiness or cyanosis, the nurse should suspect prematurity, respiratory distress, sepsis, or transient tachypnea. Frequent apneic episodes may occur in the preterm neonate; transient tachypnea is common in the neonate of near-term gestation who was delivered by cesarean. (Unlike vaginal delivery, cesarean delivery does not cause ejection of fetal lung fluid via thoracic squeeze; transient tachypnea results as the fluid is resorbed in the first day or so after birth.)

Pulse
In the first few hours after birth, the heart rate fluctuates from 120 to 180 beats/minute; it may be altered by activity, crying, or a change in the period of reactivity. Typically, the point of maximum impulse occurs at the fourth intercostal space, slightly to the right of the midclavicular line; the apical impulse is shifted slightly to the left.

Blood pressure
Neonatal blood pressure rises during periods of heightened activity; usually, it is relatively high for the first 2 weeks. The most accurate way to measure blood pressure is with a Doppler probe, an electronic instrument that eliminates the need for a stethoscope.

Average systolic blood pressure varies with gestational age. In the term neonate, systolic blood pressure ranges from 63 to 70 mm Hg. In the preterm neonate of 28 to 32 weeks' gestation, it averages about 52 mm Hg; in the preterm neonate of 33 to 36 weeks' gestation, 56 mm Hg. Diastolic pressure in the term neonate ranges from 40 to 50 mm Hg. (For the preterm neonate, the diastolic reading is not a useful parameter because pulse sounds are audible all the way to the zero point on the gauge.)

The nurse should measure blood pressure in both arms and both legs to detect any discrepancy between the two sides or between the upper and lower body. A discrepancy of 10 mm Hg or more between the arms and legs may signal a cardiac defect, such as coarctation of the aorta.

Anthropometric measurements

To take anthropometric measurements (weight, head-to-heel length, head and chest circumference, and crown-to-rump length), the nurse weighs and measures the neonate (as described in *Psychomotor skills: Obtaining anthropometric measurements,* pages 838 and 839.) Birth weight averages 2,500 to 4,000 g (5 lb, 8 oz to 8 lb, 13 oz).

In the term neonate, head-to-heel length averages 45 to 53 cm (18" to 21"); head circumference, 32 to 35 cm (12½" to 13¾"). Chest circumference usually measures about 2 cm less than head circumference, averaging 30 to 33 cm (12" to 13"). Crown-to-rump length approximates head circumference.

PSYCHOMOTOR SKILLS

Taking vital signs

The nurse should measure the neonate's vital signs every 15 minutes for the first hour after birth. If they remain stable during this time, measure them at least every hour for the next 6 hours, then at least once every 8 hours until discharge.

1 Measuring temperature. Place the thermometer in the axilla and hold it along the outer aspect of the neonate's chest, between the axillary line and the arm. Keep the thermometer in place for at least 3 minutes (axillary temperature takes this long to register).

   If the measured axillary temperature is outside the normal range—97.5° to 99° F (36.4° to 37.2° C)—check it again 15 to 30 minutes later. If the temperature still is abnormal, report this finding. A subnormal temperature may indicate infection; an elevated temperature, dehydration. (To ensure consistency of subsequent measurements, document the route used to take the temperature.)

2 Measuring respiratory rate. Count respirations for at least 1 minute. Depending on the period of the neonate's reactivity, the respiratory rate should range from 40 to 80 breaths/minute. An abnormally fast rate (tachypnea) may signal a perinatal problem. A lapse of 15 seconds or more after a complete respiratory cycle (one expiration and inspiration) indicates apnea.

   Assess the neonate's breathing pattern for regularity. An irregular pattern may indicate respiratory dysfunction. Also check for signs of labored breathing, such as uneven chest expansion, nasal flaring, visible chest retractions, expiratory grunts, and inspiratory stridor (a high-pitched sound audible without a stethoscope). In some cases, labored breathing indicates blockage of nasal passages (the neonate is an obligate nose breather).

   To evaluate breath sounds, auscultate the anterior and posterior lung fields, placing the stethoscope over each lung lobe for at least 5 seconds (for a total time of 1 minute). Normally, breath sounds are clear and equal bilaterally. However, immediately after birth, a few crackles (rales) may be audible because of retained fetal lung fluid. Document any abnormal breath sounds.

   Observe the movement of the chest as it rises and falls; it should be symmetrical. Also, determine the ratio between the anterior and posterior diameters of the chest. A ratio exceeding 1 suggests lung hyperinflation or respiratory distress.

3 Assessing pulse. Place the stethoscope over the apical impulse on the fourth to fifth intercostal space at the left midclavicular line over the cardiac apex. Listen for 1 minute to count the pulse and detect any abnormalities in the quality or rhythm of the heartbeat.

   If heart rhythm is irregular, assess whether the irregularity is regular (follows an identifiable pattern) or irregular (lacks an identifiable pattern). This helps identify the type of abnormality present; for example, atrial fibrillation is an irregular rhythm with an irregular pattern.

   Also auscultate for variations from the normal sounds ("lub-dub") of systole and diastole. Determine if the first and second heart sounds are separate and distinct or split into two sounds. Also assess for extra heart sounds and for sounds that seem to stretch into the next sound. Such abnormal sounds may signify a heart murmur, such as from a patent ductus arteriosus (in which blood rushes through the abnormal opening).

4 Taking blood pressure. When using a Doppler probe (an electronic blood pressure monitor), place the cuff directly over the brachial or popliteal artery to ensure an accurate reading; the machine automatically inflates the cuff. For the most accurate reading, keep the cuffed arm or leg extended during cuff inflation. Also observe the color of the extremity; duskiness signifies reduced blood flow.

   When measuring blood pressure by the cuff-and-stethoscope method, make sure to choose the correct cuff size. Cuff width should be half the circumference of the neonate's arm. A cuff that is too large or too small may cause a misleading reading.

   Place the cuff one to two fingerbreadths above the antecubital or popliteal area. With the stethoscope held directly over the chosen artery, hold the cuffed extremity firmly to keep it extended, then inflate the cuff.

   To determine if blood pressure is within the neonate's normal range, compare the readings to baseline values; report any significant deviation.

Gestational-age assessment

Gestational-age assessment determines the neonate's physical and neuromuscular maturity, helping health care providers anticipate perinatal problems associated with preterm or postterm status. Correlation of gestational age with birth weight may suggest perinatal problems related to SGA or LGA status. (For information on specific perinatal problems associated with gestational-age and birth-weight variations, see Chapter 38, High-Risk Neonates.)

   The average full-term gestation lasts about 38 weeks from fertilization, or 40 weeks from the first day of the last menstrual period. Traditionally, gestational age has been calculated from the latter. However, irregular menstrual cycles and fetal growth variations can lead to erroneous calculation.

Obtaining anthropometric measurements

Anthropometric measurements include weight, head-to-heel length, head and chest circumference, and crown-to-rump length. If abnormal, these measurements may indicate a significant problem or anomaly. The nurse should follow the illustrated procedure for taking anthropometric measurements.

1 Measuring weight. Take this measurement before—not after—a feeding, preferably with the neonate undressed. If the neonate must be weighed with clothing or equipment (such as an I.V. armboard), make sure to note this information.

Before the weighing, place one or two pieces of disposable scale paper over the scale to prevent cold stress. When taking the measurement, keep one hand directly above the neonate. However, avoid touching the neonate, which could affect the accuracy of the measurement.

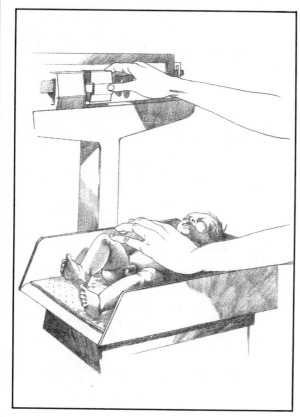

2 Measuring head-to-heel length. Position the neonate supine with legs extended and measure from head to heel. To make this measurement easier, use a length board.

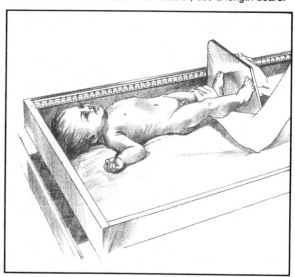

4 Measuring chest circumference. Place a tape measure around the neonate's chest at the nipples. Take the measurement after the neonate inspires, before expiration begins.

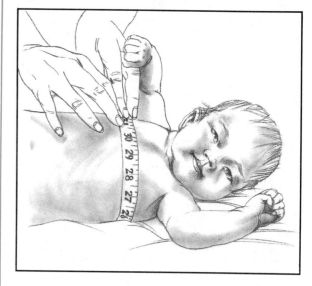

3 **Measuring head circumference.** Place a tape measure securely around the fullest part of the ca-put, from the middle of the forehead to the midline of the back of the skull. Record the result. Keep in mind that if delivery caused molding or swelling of the head, the measured head circumference may be misleading.

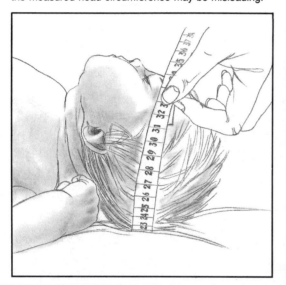

5 **Measuring crown-to-rump length.** With the neo-nate lying on one side, measure from the crown of the head to the buttocks. This measurement should ap-proximate head circumference.

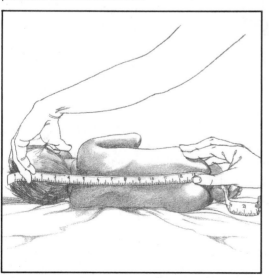

Gestational-age and birth-weight classifications

Previously, health care providers used birth weight alone to classify neonates. However, in the past few decades, as experts recognized the importance of gestational age, new classifications were developed and mortality and morbidity rates identified for each classification. (For more information, see *Classifying the neonate by gestational age and birth weight,* page 840.)

Gestational-age assessment tools

Gestational age should be assessed for any neonate who weighs less than 2,500 g (5½ lb) or who has a suspected alteration in the intrauterine growth pattern. To score gestational age officially using a gestational-age as-sessment tool (a process that typically takes about 10 minutes), the nurse must undergo special preparation. However, even without such preparation, a nurse who is familiar with the progression of fetal characteristics can estimate a neonate's gestational age.

Gestational-age assessment tools rely on external physical features and neurologic maturity—not birth weight—as indices of growth and maturation. Devel-oping in an orderly manner during gestation, external physical features usually are not affected by labor and delivery and thus can be assessed immediately. Evalu-ation of neurologic maturity, however, may have to be postponed for 24 hours or so—especially if the neonate suffered fetal central nervous system depression, which may skew assessment findings.

The most common gestational-age assessment tools are the Dubowitz tool (1970) and the Ballard tool (re-vised in 1988). The Dubowitz tool includes 11 external and 10 neurologic signs. The examiner evaluates and scores each external sign, then totals the scores. After following the same procedure for neurologic signs, the examiner adds the two totals and plots the sum on a graph to identify the neonate's gestational age. (With early client discharge now routine, the Dubowitz tool has become somewhat impractical because the neurologic part of the examination must be delayed.)

The Ballard tool, an abbreviated version of the Du-bowitz tool, consists of 7 physical maturity and 6 neu-romuscular maturity criteria. This tool is refined periodically in response to research. The 1988 revision incorporates criteria for gestational-age assessment of neonates of 20 to 44 weeks' gestation. (For more infor-mation, see *Ballard gestational-age assessment tool,* pages 842 and 843.)

Classifying the neonate by gestational age and birth weight

Organ system maturity depends largely on gestational age. Thus, the greater a neonate's gestational age, the more fully developed the organ systems. At the First World Health Assembly in 1948, the World Health Organization (WHO) defined an "immature" neonate as one weighing 5½ lb (2,500 g) or less; or, if the weight was not specified, one whose gestation lasted less than 37 weeks. In 1950, the WHO Expert Group on Prematurity defined the premature (preterm) neonate as one weighing 2,500 g or less.

However, health care providers recognized that some neonates weighing less than 2,500 g were term or postterm but small for gestational age. Consequently, in 1961, the WHO Expert Committee on Maternal and Child Health redefined the premature neonate as one born before 37 weeks from the first day of the mother's last menstrual period. The committee defined low birth weight (LBW) as 2,500 g or less and subdivided neonates in this category into term and preterm LBW neonates.

In the 1980s, an additional classification—very low birth weight (VLBW)—was added to describe the neonate weighing 500 g to 1,499 g. Most VLBW neonates have a gestational age of 23 to 30 weeks. VLBW neonates have had a tremendous impact on medical research and have sparked important advances in neonatal care—even though they account for only a tiny percentage of neonates. (According to Usher [1987], only 0.87% of live births occur before 31 weeks; VLBW neonates make up just 0.85% of these births.)

Currently, neonates are classified according to the Colorado intrauterine growth chart (shown below). Developed by Battaglia and Lubchenco (1967), this chart correlates gestational age with birth weight. After weighing the neonate and determining gestational age, the examiner plots these two parameters on the graph. The neonate whose weight falls between the tenth and ninetieth percentiles for gestational age on this chart is classified as appropriate for gestational age. One whose birth weight falls outside this range is considered to be small or large for gestational age, with an increased risk for certain perinatal problems. Thanks largely to improved knowledge and technology, however, such a neonate has an improved chance for survival.

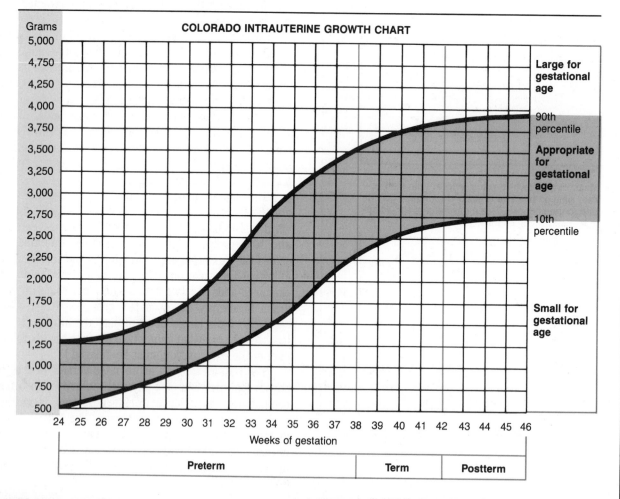

Battaglia, F.C., and Lubchenco, L.O. (1967). A practical classification of newborn infants by weight and gestational age. *Journal of Pediatrics*, 71, 161. Graph used with permission from C.V. Mosby Company.

Assessment of physical features

Certain physical features vary with gestational age and thus reflect neonatal maturity. (These features are called external signs on the Dubowitz tool and physical maturity criteria on the Ballard tool.)

Skin texture, color, and opacity. The preterm neonate has thin, translucent, ruddy skin with easily seen veins and venules (especially over the abdomen). As term approaches, the skin thickens and becomes pinker; also, the number of large vessels visible over the abdomen decreases. The postterm neonate typically has thick, parchmentlike skin with peeling and cracking; few if any blood vessels appear over the abdomen.

Lanugo. Soft, downy hair, lanugo appears at approximately 20 weeks' gestation. From 21 to 33 weeks, it covers the entire body. It begins to vanish from the face at 34 weeks and by 38 weeks may appear only on the shoulders. Lanugo rarely appears after 42 weeks' gestation.

Plantar (sole) creases. Plantar creases should be assessed immediately after birth because the drying effect of environmental exposure causes additional creases to form. The preterm neonate of 34 to 35 weeks' gestation has one or two anterior creases; at 36 to 38 weeks' gestation, creases cover the anterior two-thirds of the sole. In the term neonate, creases appear over both the sole and heel. In the postterm neonate, deeper creases line the entire sole. (For an illustration of this feature and several other physical features, see *How selected physical features progress*, pages 844 and 845.)

Breast size. The examiner assesses breast tissue through observation and palpation. To measure breast tissue, palpate the nipple gently between the second and third fingers. Do not use the thumb and index finger because surrounding skin may be measured inadvertently this way.

Breast tissue and areola size increase with gestation. The areola appears slightly elevated at 34 weeks' gestation. By week 36, a breast bud of 1 to 2 mm is visible; the bud may grow to 12 mm by week 42. Increased breast tissue may indicate subcutaneous fat accumulation from accelerated intrauterine growth (such as occurs in the LGA neonate). In contrast, the SGA or postterm neonate may have decreased breast tissue from inadequate fetal growth or lost fetal weight.

Ear form and firmness. In the preterm neonate of less than 28 weeks' gestation, decreased cartilage distribution prevents the ear from recoiling after it is folded forward against the side of the head and released. The ear appears flat and shapeless until 28 weeks' gestation when incurving of the pinna (the external part of the ear) begins. At 36 weeks' gestation, the upper two-thirds of the pinna are incurved and the pinna recoils instantly. In the term neonate, the pinna has well-defined incurving. The ear of the postterm neonate is firm and set apart slightly from the head.

Genitalia. In the male neonate, the genitalia should be assessed for testicular descent, scrotal size, and number of rugae (skin folds). In the preterm neonate of less than 28 weeks' gestation, the testes remain within the abdominal cavity and the scrotum appears high and close to the body. At 28 to 36 weeks' gestation, the testes can be palpated in the inguinal canal and a few rugae appear. At 36 to 40 weeks' gestation, the testes are palpable in the upper scrotum and rugae appear on the anterior portion. After 40 weeks' gestation, the testes can be palpated in the scrotum and rugae cover the scrotal sac. The postterm neonate has deep rugae and a pendulous scrotum.

The female preterm neonate of 30 to 36 weeks' gestation has a prominent clitoris extending from the labia minora and majora; the labia majora are small and widely separated. (This appearance occasionally complicates sex determination and may upset parents.) At 36 to 40 weeks' gestation, the labia majora are larger, almost covering the clitoris. Labia majora that cover the labia minora and clitoris suggest more than 40 weeks' gestation.

Assessment of neurologic maturity

Assessment of neurologic features (called neurologic signs on the Dubowitz tool and neuromuscular maturity criteria on the Ballard tool) determines the degree of neuromuscular tone—an index of neurologic maturity. Unlike other neurologic characteristics, which develop in a cephalocaudal (head-to-tail) direction, neuromuscular tone begins in the lower extremities and progresses upward.

The Dubowitz neurologic examination initially includes evaluation of posture and of arm and leg recoil. The remaining neurologic criteria are assessed 24 hours after birth to eliminate the effects of maternal analgesia, increased handling from additional assessments, and the normal physiologic fluctuations (such as vital sign changes) of the first few hours.

Correlating gestational age with birth weight

After determining the neonate's gestational age with an assessment tool, the examiner plots the age on the Colorado intrauterine growth chart to correlate it with birth weight. This reveals whether the neonate is SGA, LGA,

Ballard gestational-age assessment tool

To use this tool, the examiner evaluates and scores the neuromuscular and physical maturity criteria, totals the scores, then plots the sum in the maturity rating box to determine gestational age. Unlike portions of the Dubowitz neurologic examination, the Ballard neuromuscular examination can be done even if the neonate is not alert.

	−1	0	1	2	3	4	5
Neuromuscular maturity							
Posture	–						–
Square window (wrist)	>90°	90°	60°	45°	30°	0°	–
Arm recoil	–	180°	140° to 180°	110° to 140°	90° to 110°	<90°	–
Popliteal angle	180°	160°	140°	120°	100°	90°	<90°
Scarf sign							–
Heel to ear							–

Adapted from Maturational Assessment of Gestational Age, © 1988. Used with permission of Jeanne L. Ballard, M.D.

or appropriate for gestational age—information that helps caregivers anticipate perinatal problems.

Correlating gestational age with length and head circumference

The examiner also plots gestational age against length and head circumference on an appropriate growth chart to determine whether these measurements fall within the normal range—the tenth to ninetieth percentile for the corresponding gestational age.

Complete physical assessment

When conducting the complete physical assessment, the nurse may use a systematic, head-to-toe approach tailored to the neonate's size and age, or may assess heart and lung sounds first because these assessments require a quiet neonate. Ensure thermoregulation by placing the neonate under a radiant heat warmer and examining

	−1	**0**	**1**	**2**	**3**	**4**	**5**
Physical maturity							
Skin	Sticky, friable, transparent	Gelatinous, red, translucent	Smooth, pink; visible vessels	Superficial peeling or rash; few visible vessels	Cracking; pale areas; rare visible vessels	Parchment-like; deep cracking; no visible vessels	Leathery, cracked, wrinkled
Lanugo	None	Sparse	Abundant	Thinning	Bald areas	Mostly bald	—
Plantar surface	Heel-toe 40 to 50 mm: −1; <40 mm: −2	>50 mm; no crease	Faint red marks	Anterior transverse crease only	Creases over anterior two-thirds	Creases over entire sole	—
Breast	Imperceptible	Barely perceptible	Flat areola, no bud	Stippled areola; 1- to 2-mm bud	Raised areola; 3- to 4-mm bud	Full areola; 5- to 10-mm bud	—
Eye and ear	Lids fused, loosely: −1; tightly: −2	Lids open; pinna flat, stays folded	Slightly curved pinna; soft, slow recoil	Well-curved pinna; soft but ready recoil	Formed and firm; instant recoil	Thick cartilage; ear stiff	—
Genitalia, male	Scrotum flat, smooth	Scrotum empty; faint rugae	Testes in upper canal; rare rugae	Testes descending; few rugae	Testes down; good rugae	Testes pendulous; deep rugae	—
Genitalia, female	Clitoris prominent; labia flat	Prominent clitoris; small labia minora	Prominent clitoris; enlarging minora	Majora and minora equally prominent	Majora large; minora small	Majora cover clitoris and minora	—
Maturity rating							

Score	−10	−5	0	5	10	15	20	25	30	35	40	45	50
Weeks	20	22	24	26	28	30	32	34	36	38	40	42	44

only one area at a time. For assessments requiring advanced skills, seek appropriate assistance.

Check vital signs before the examination begins; if they are unstable or if the neonate has a temperature below 96° F (35.5° C), do not proceed with the examination. Instead, swaddle the neonate, rewrapping securely. Because the period of reactivity affects assessment findings, record the neonate's behavioral state and age (in hours or days after birth) at the time of the examination.

Assessment of the skin

Examine the neonate's skin for temperature, color, turgor (resiliency), and variations. The skin should feel warm to the touch, with a temperature ranging from 96° to 98° F (35.5° to 36.5° C), or 0.9° F (0.5° C) below core (rectal) temperature.

A reddish hue is normal immediately after birth, reflecting adjustment in central oxygen levels during the transition to the extrauterine environment. However, skin color also reflects the neonate's ethnic heritage. Typically, it deepens with crying and increased motor activity.

How selected physical features progress

Physical features develop in distinctive patterns during gestation. The nurse who is familiar with these patterns can estimate the neonate's gestational age by evaluating some of them, including those described below.

Plantar (sole) creases
As gestation lengthens, plantar creases become deeper and more numerous.

Plantar creases reflecting 34 to 35 weeks' gestation

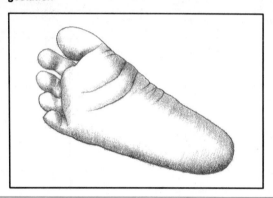

Plantar creases reflecting 36 to 38 weeks' gestation

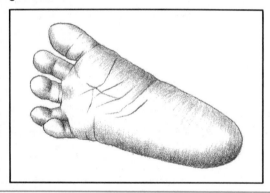

Plantar creases reflecting term birth

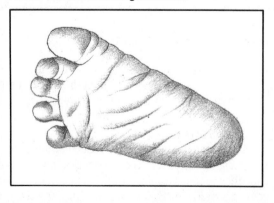

Ear formation and cartilage
The upper two-thirds of the pinna (the portion lying outside the head) show increasing incurving.

Ear formation reflecting 36 weeks' gestation

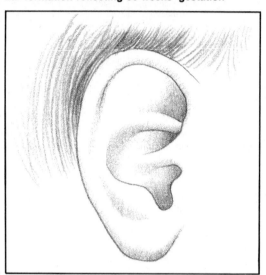

Ear formation reflecting term birth

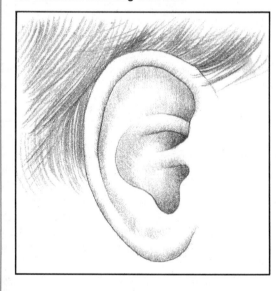

Female genitalia

At about 30 to 36 weeks' gestation, the labia majora are separated widely and the clitoris is prominent (first illustration below). At approximately 36 to 40 weeks, the labia majora nearly cover the labia minora (second illustration). At 40 or more weeks, the labia majora cover the clitoris and labia minora completely (third illustration).

Female genitalia reflecting 30 to 36 weeks' gestation

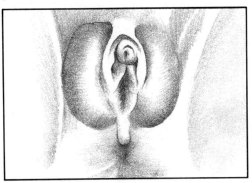

Female genitalia reflecting 36 to 40 weeks' gestation

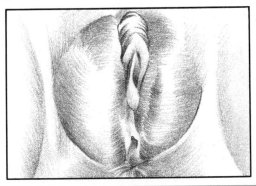

Female genitalia reflecting 40 or more weeks' gestation

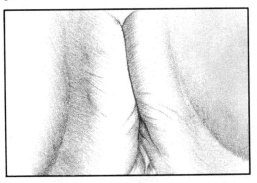

Distinguish ecchymoses (small bluish-purple, hemorrhagic spots) from cyanotic (bluish) discoloration by applying pressure to the affected area. With ecchymoses, the color will remain unchanged; with cyanosis, the area will blanch.

To assess skin turgor, pinch between the thumb and forefinger a small amount of skin along the upper abdominal surface. Then release the skin and observe how quickly it recoils to its original position. If the skin remains tented (elevated), returning to its original position slowly, suspect dehydration.

Palpate the skin to check for edema, which indicates a fluid shift into the extracellular spaces. Document and report any generalized edema, which may indicate a cardiac or renal problem.

Skin variations are common in neonates. Most are minor and do not require treatment.

Assessment of the head and neck

The cranial bones commonly slide over each other during labor and delivery, causing head molding. In the first few hours after birth, the conical, elongated, asymmetrical shape of the molded head may complicate measurement of head circumference. If this happens, the measurement is repeated after head shape normalizes (usually by the end of the first week).

The frontal, sagittal, coronal, and lambdoidal sutures fall between the junction of the skull plates to form the cartilaginous edges of the fontanels—spaces covered by tough membranes between the cranial bones. During the assessment, palpate the suture lines to determine how much the bony edges overlap. Assessment of the anterior and posterior fontanels may reveal a third fontanel along the sagittal suture; in most cases, this represents a normal variation. Two minor fontanels—the mastoid and sphenoidal—rarely have clinical significance.

Hair distribution, texture, and color are other important aspects of the head examination. Unusual hair distribution may represent a minor abnormality.

The neck should appear symmetrical and without webbing and should be flexible enough to allow the head to move freely and equally to each side. Palpate the front of the neck at the midline for the thyroid; also palpate for lymph nodes (which normally cannot be palpated).

To help assess cardiovascular status, palpate the carotid pulses. They should be equal and strong bilaterally. Be sure to use caution when palpating; massage of the carotid artery may stimulate pressure receptors, causing reflex bradycardia (a heart rate below 100 beats/minute).

Smith's minor anomalies

When conducting the physical assessment, the nurse should check for minor anomalies identified by Smith (1988). Resulting from intrauterine factors that impair fetal growth and development, these anomalies always warrant a more thorough investigation. About 90% of neonates with three minor anomalies have one major anomaly; 15% of neonates with one major anomaly have one minor anomaly.

With a thorough understanding of fetal development, the nurse who detects one anomaly can anticipate additional anomalies. For example, if the neonate has a minor anomaly known to occur in the fourth week of gestation, the nurse should conduct a careful assessment of the other structures that develop during that period.

Important areas in which to assess for Smith's minor anomalies include the following.

Hands and feet

Normally, the palms and hands show various dermal ridge patterns, such as radial loops and whorls, and the palm is traversed by two separate lines. Abnormal dermal ridge patterns include ulnar loops on all digits, typifying Down's syndrome (trisomy 21). A single crease traversing the palm (simian crease) also suggests Down's syndrome. Other minor hand and foot anomalies include unequal finger and toe lengths, syndactyly (fusion of two or more digits), polydactyly (extra digits), camptodactyly (bowed digits, usually affecting the fifth finger or toe), clinodactyly (curved digits, also usually affecting the fifth finger or toe), and hypoplastic (shortened or absent) nails.

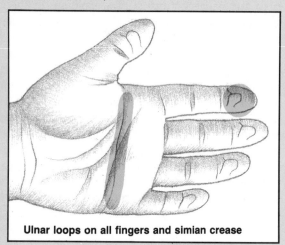

Ulnar loops on all fingers and simian crease

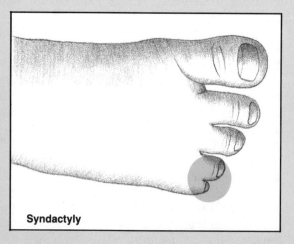

Syndactyly

Eye region

Assess the distance between the eyes, which normally is 2.5 cm. Note hypertelorism (a distance greater than 2.5 cm) or hypotelorism (a distance less than 2.5 cm). Also check for abnormal eye rotation (unexplained eye slanting), inner epicanthal folds (skin folds from the eye to the nasal bridge), and Brushfield's spots in the iris (golden flecks associated with Down's syndrome).

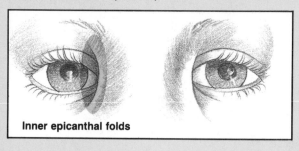

Inner epicanthal folds

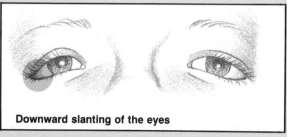

Downward slanting of the eyes

Oral region

High or prominent palatal ridges may signal neurologic impairment, such as cri du chat syndrome or a seizure disorder.

Hair distribution and directional pattern

Abnormal hair swirling (a whorl found higher on the head than normal or a pattern that does not flow in a posterior direction) is associated with microcephaly (an abnormally small head) and other conditions characterized by prematurely arrested brain growth. Abnormal hair growth on the face and eyebrows may be associated with abnormal growth of the facial bones and ears. For example, if an ear is absent, hair will not appear in this area.

Underlying abnormalities in facial and neck bone structure may make hair growth appear more unusual than it is. If the forehead is abnormally short, for instance, the hairline may resemble a widow's peak. If the neck is abnormally short, the occipital hairline may extend to the middle of the posterior neck. Hirsutism (excessive body hair) suggests an endocrine disorder.

(For more information, see *Smith's minor abnormalities,* and *Assessing the fontanels,* page 848.)

Assessment of the face

Examine the neonate's face for symmetry of features and for the characteristics described below.

Mouth, chin, and cheeks

The mouth should appear at the midline; its size should be appropriate for the face. The lips should be sensitive to the touch; gentle stroking should trigger the sucking reflex. The chin normally is slightly receding. The term neonate has fat pads in both cheeks.

Oral cavity

Touch the tongue lightly to check for the normal reaction—a forward tongue thrust. After inspecting the tongue, delay the rest of the oral cavity inspection until near the end of the head-to-toe assessment because this inspection disturbs the neonate. Also, never inspect the oral cavity just after a feeding because this could stimulate the gag reflex, causing vomiting and subsequent aspiration.

When resuming the inspection, position the neonate supine. With a tongue depressor and penlight, inspect for intactness of the hard and soft palates and for Epstein's pearls—small white patches that represent minor variations. Also check the uvula (the skin protruding midline between the tonsils); it should rise when the neonate cries. Finally, assess the amount of salivation; normally, the neonate has moist oral mucous membranes but does not drool constantly.

Eyes

Shortly after birth, the eyelids commonly appear edematous from birth trauma or irritation caused by silver nitrate or erythromycin instillation. In the Caucasian neonate, the sclerae should be clear and white; in other neonates, they may appear slightly yellow. The conjunctivae should be clear and iris color distributed evenly.

If the neonate's eyes are closed during the head-to-toe assessment, delay the eye inspection until the ophthalmic examination (which should be conducted last because it upsets the neonate). When examining the pupils, use a penlight or flashlight and dim the room lights. If this examination must be conducted in an incubator or nursery, shield the neonate's eyes.

The retina should be transparent and intact and the pupils round and centered in the iris. When exposed to light in a darkened room, the pupils should constrict equally bilaterally. If all pupil findings are normal, document them as PERRLA (pupils equal, round, reactive

---

Ears

Preauricular skin tags (extra skin), open sinus tracts appearing as small pinpoint holes on the external ear or preauricular area, rotated or low-set ears, or a smooth or semiround helix may indicate an internal organ abnormality.

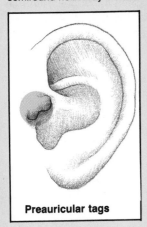

Preauricular tags

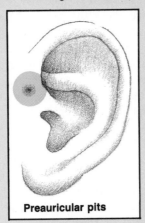

Preauricular pits

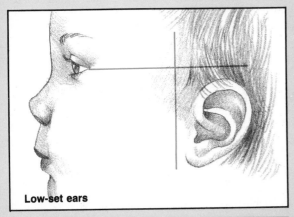

Low-set ears

Genitalia

In the female, labial hypoplasia (failure of the labia to grow) typifies trisomy 18, a congenital condition characterized by severe mental retardation and multiple deformities. In the male, the scrotum may appear to be enveloped in extra skin ("shawl scrotum"), also suggesting trisomy 18.

Other anomalies identified by Smith include:

• skin dimpling, which may result from reduced subcutaneous tissue or the absence of underlying structures (for example, dimples in the sacral area associated with spina bifida)
• open sinus tracts in the sacral area
• pilonidal sinus, an abnormal channel containing a tuft of hair, most commonly found over or near the tip of the coccyx.

Assessing the fontanels

Fontanels are soft-tissue spaces located between the neonate's cranial bones and covered by tough membranes (see the first illustration below). The nurse can palpate them easily by placing two fingers along the suture line (as shown in the second illustration). The anterior fontanel, the larger of the two major fontanels, is situated where the coronal, frontal, and sagittal sutures meet; it closes gradually during the first 18 months. The posterior fontanel, a triangular space situated where the sagittal and lambdoidal sutures meet, typically closes by age 2 to 3 months. However, it may be closed at birth from molding of the head.

FONTANELS AND SUTURE LINES

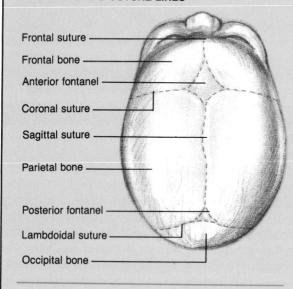

Frontal suture
Frontal bone
Anterior fontanel
Coronal suture
Sagittal suture
Parietal bone
Posterior fontanel
Lambdoidal suture
Occipital bone

PALPATING THE ANTERIOR FONTANEL

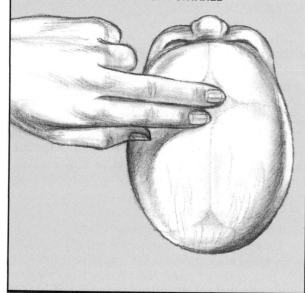

to light, accommodation). To assess for the red reflex, place the penlight or ophthalmoscope directly in front of the pupil and turn on the light; the pupils should appear red bilaterally.

Ears

Inspect the ears for symmetrical shape and size. Skin tags, pinpoint holes, and sinus tracts along the helix or preauricular surface may represent minor abnormalities. Also check the neonate's hearing; a loud noise should elicit the startle reflex or crying.

To perform the otoscopic examination, pull the neonate's ear down and toward the back to straighten the ear canal. (To avoid damaging the neonate's ears, the otoscopic examination should be performed only by an experienced examiner.)

Nose

Because the neonate cannot coordinate tongue movements well, the tongue often falls backward, occluding the oral airway. Consequently, the neonate is an obligate nose breather who depends on patent nares (nostrils). To assess the nares for patency, occlude them one at a time while holding the mouth closed; the neonate should be able to breathe through the open naris. To check for the sneeze reflex, occlude both nares for 1 to 2 seconds; this should trigger sneezing.

Assessment of the thorax

The thoracic cavity should be cylindrical and symmetrical. In the SGA or preterm neonate, expect decreased chest circumference. Normally, chest wall excursion is bilaterally equal.

The ribs should be flexible and symmetrical, with no palpable masses. The xiphoid process may be palpable at the bottom of the sternum; in a thin neonate, it may be visible.

When palpating the clavicles, move the fingers slowly over the anterior clavicular surface. If a mass or lump is detected, try to move the neonate's arm gently while palpating with the other hand. A grating sensation and uneven movement of two juxtaposed bone fragments indicate a fracture (as from delivery trauma).

Assess the amount of breast tissue, as described in the "Gestational-age assessment" section earlier in this chapter. Inspect the nipples for spacing and number. Keep in mind that supernumerary (more than two) nipples may appear as darkened spots just below or beside the natural nipples. A white secretion called witch's milk may appear on breast palpation; typically, this secretion diminishes in the first or second week after birth.

Assessment of the abdomen

The abdomen should have a symmetrical, slightly rounded contour. Peristaltic waves normally are not visible; however, the abdomen should move visibly during breathing. The umbilical cord remnant should appear bluish-white, contain two arteries and one vein (visible immediately after birth), and be free of urine leakage (leakage suggests a fistula from the bladder to the cord).

To palpate the abdomen, begin with gentle pressure and gradually press deeper as the neonate relaxes. (To promote relaxation and comfort during palpation, flex the neonate's legs in the fetal position.) If the neonate has an asymmetrical abdomen, which suggests an internal mass, use great caution during the assessment. Palpation of a Wilms's tumor (a cancerous tumor of the kidney) may cause the tumor to seed to other areas. In the preterm neonate, palpation may reveal a wide separation along the rectus abdominis muscles. This condition, called diastasis recti abdominis, results from abdominal muscle immaturity.

The liver normally lies at the right costal margin. Its sharp edge (which should be palpated no more than 1 cm below the right costal margin) can be felt during inspiration, which lifts the organ forward. The spleen, on the opposite side of the abdomen, is approximately 1 cm below the left costal margin. In the preterm neonate, the spleen is slightly enlarged and thus more easily palpated.

The posterior position of the kidneys makes them less accessible to palpation. If they cannot be palpated with one hand, use bimanual palpation. In this technique, place one hand behind the neonate's back while palpating the abdomen with the fingertips of the other hand. The kidney should be felt between the hands.

Palpate the bladder just above the pubis. Unless it is distended, it should not be visible.

Percuss the abdomen just after the neonate voids to prevent misleading findings. Percussion should reveal tympany below the left costal margin, reflecting a gastric bubble. Most other abdominal areas also should be tympanic. However, dullness should be percussed over the liver, spleen, and bladder. Percussion delineates the borders of these organs to detect enlargement, indicated by increased areas of dullness. Decreased areas of dullness suggest fluid or air where solid tissue is expected.

Finally, auscultate the abdomen for bowel sounds, which normally begin a few hours after birth.

Assessment of the back

To assess the back, position the neonate prone and inspect for spinal alignment, enlargement, and masses. The back should be straight. Examine the sacrum for dimpling or a tuft of hair and observe for bulges. Palpate the vertebral column for enlargement and signs of pain.

Assessment of the anus and genitalia

The perineum should be smooth, without dimpling or extra orifices. The anus should be midline and patent. To test anal patency, put on a disposable glove and gently insert the tip of the little (fourth) finger into the neonate's anus. Assess the anal sphincter by lightly stroking the anus with a cotton-tipped applicator and observing anal constriction—a reaction called the anal wink.

Genital appearance depends on gestational age (as described in the "Gestational-age assessment" section earlier in this chapter). In the term female neonate, the labia majora extend beyond the labia minora to cover the clitoris. A hymenal tag may protrude from the vagina.

To assess the urinary meatus in an uncircumcised male neonate, gently retract the foreskin. If gentle motion does not budge the foreskin, do not force it. Be sure to return the skin to its normal position after inspection; if the foreskin remains retracted, swelling will occur. (Conversely, swelling during the first few days after birth may prevent retraction.) In a circumcised neonate, also check for edema and bleeding.

The meatus may be displaced anywhere along the penile shaft. When displacement is accompanied by a severe chordee—downward bowing of the penis that makes it appear hooded—the neonate's sex may be hard to determine.

Palpate the testes in the scrotal sac by gently squeezing the sac between the forefinger and thumb. If the testes do not appear in the sac, place the forefinger and thumb of the other hand over the inguinal canal to detect them within the canal.

Assessment of the extremities

Inspect the extremities for length, symmetry, and size—relative to each other and to the body as a whole. Normally, the term neonate has a full range of motion, which can be tested either actively or passively. The preterm neonate has limited flexion, especially of the arms. Inspect the hands and feet for number of digits, palmar and plantar creases, and such abnormalities as syndactyly (webbing).

Next, palpate the extremities, noting if the neonate grimaces or cries in response to the examination (possibly indicating fracture). Finally, perform Ortolani's maneuver to check for congenital hip dislocation. (For more information, see *Psychomotor skills: Performing Ortolani's maneuver*, page 850.)

Performing Ortolani's maneuver

To assess the neonate for hip dislocation, the nurse should perform Ortolani's maneuver, as described below.

1 With the neonate supine, grasp the knees by positioning your hands along the outer aspect of the thigh toward the head of the femur, as shown below.

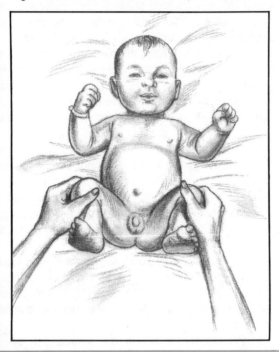

2 Flex the neonate's hips and knees, then abduct them by applying gentle downward pressure, as shown below. If the hip slips out of the acetabulum or makes a clicking or popping sound as it moves through the full range of motion, suspect hip dislocation.

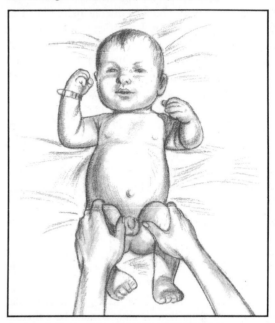

Assessment of neurologic status

When assessing neurologic status, keep in mind that some neurologic characteristics also are evaluated during the gestational-age assessment, which precedes the complete physical assessment. To conserve the neonate's energy, do not reevaluate these characteristics during the complete physical assessment.

First, observe the neonate's posture, which typically reflects fetal positioning, gestational age, or delivery method. The healthy, term neonate has a flexed posture and shows muscle resistance when the examiner extends the extremities. However, with breech delivery or *in utero* positioning, the legs may remain extended for a few days after birth. With some neonates born in a breech position, the legs are flexed back as far as the ears.

Also check for tremors of the extremities. Tremors may stem from hypoglycemia, cold stress, or neurologic immaturity. They may be hard to distinguish from a seizure, which sometimes manifests as a fixed gaze, yawning, or motions resembling sucking, swallowing, or chewing. To distinguish tremors from a seizure, attempt to halt the movement by grasping the involved extremity; tremors will stop, whereas a seizure will continue.

Next, assess reflexes—both localized and mass (full body) reflexes. Localized reflexes include the sucking, rooting, gag, blink, pupillary, grasp, and Babinski reflexes. Mass reflexes include the startle, Moro, fencing, Galant, and stepping reflexes. (For methods used to test reflexes, see *Assessing neonatal reflexes*, page 851.)

Finally, assess the neonate's cry. The cry should be strong and loud, even in a preterm neonate (unless respiratory problems are present). A high-pitched or cat-like cry suggests increased intracranial pressure; a grunting or a low-pitched cry, respiratory distress syndrome; a weak, soft cry, brain damage. Duration of the cry varies with temperament.

Assessing neonatal reflexes

To evaluate neurologic status during the complete physical assessment, the nurse should test neonatal reflexes. The chart below describes testing methods and normal responses. A weak, absent, or asymmetrical response is considered abnormal. Some reflexes (such as the pupillary, blink, and gag reflexes) persist throughout life; others (including the doll's eye, sucking, grasp, Babinski, Moro, fencing, and Galant reflexes) normally disappear a few weeks or months after birth.

REFLEX	TESTING METHOD	NORMAL RESPONSE
Babinski (plantar)	Stroke one side of the neonate's foot upward from the heel and across the ball of the foot.	Neonate hyperextends the toes, dorsiflexes the great toe, and fans the toes outward.
Blink (corneal)	Momentarily shine a bright light directly into the neonate's eyes.	Neonate blinks.
Crawl	Place the neonate prone on a flat surface.	Neonate attempts to crawl forward using the arms and legs.
Crossed extension	Position the neonate supine; extend one leg and stimulate the sole with a light pin prick or finger flick.	Neonate swiftly flexes and extends the opposite leg as though trying to push the stimulus away from the other foot.
Doll's eye	With the neonate supine, slowly turn the neonate's head to the left or right.	Neonate's eyes remain stationary.
Fencing (tonic neck)	With a swift motion, turn the neonate's head to either side.	Neonate extends the extremities on the side to which the head is turned and flexes the extremities on the opposite side.
Galant	Using a fingernail, gently stroke one side of the neonate's spinal column from the head to the buttocks.	Neonate's trunk curves toward the stimulated side.
Grasp	Palmar reflex: Place a finger in the neonate's palm.	Neonate grasps the finger.
	Plantar reflex: Place a finger against the base of the neonate's toe.	Neonate's toes curl downward and grasp the finger.
Moro	Suddenly but gently drop the neonate's head backward (relative to the trunk).	Neonate extends and abducts all extremities bilaterally and symmetrically; forms a "C" shape with the thumb and forefinger; and adducts, then flexes, the extremities.
Pupillary (light)	Darken the room and shine a penlight directly into the neonate's eye for several seconds.	Pupils constrict equally bilaterally.
Rooting	Touch a finger to the neonate's cheek or the corner of mouth. (The mother's nipple also should trigger this reflex.)	Neonate turns the head toward the stimulus, opens the mouth, and searches for the stimulus.
Startle	Make a loud noise near the neonate.	Neonate cries and abducts and flexes all extremities.
Stepping (automatic walking)	Hold the neonate in an upright position and touch one foot lightly to a flat surface (such as the bed).	Neonate makes walking motions with both feet.
Sucking	Place a finger in the neonate's mouth. (The mother's nipple also should trigger this reflex.)	Neonate sucks on the finger (or nipple) forcefully and rhythmically; sucking is coordinated with swallowing.

(For details on normal and abnormal assessment findings and their significance, see *Head-to-toe physical assessment findings*.)

Behavioral assessment

The behavioral assessment allows the nurse to evaluate the neonate's behavioral capacities and interaction with the environment. Experts previously believed that the neonate's behavior was restricted to reflexive reactions to stimuli. However, they now know that the neonate interacts with others as an active participant.

Various tools are available for behavioral assessment. For best results, the assessment should be conducted in a quiet, softly lit setting. Findings must be interpreted in light of the period of reactivity and the neonate's gestational age.

If possible, the nurse should arrange for the parents to observe the assessment so that they can learn firsthand about their child's behavioral and interactive capacities. The nurse also can use this opportunity to assess the parents' behavior and determine the quality of parent-neonate interaction. For example, parental sensitivity and positive follow-up to cues (perceived signals) from the neonate indicate a reciprocal relationship that promotes bonding.

Brazelton neonatal behavioral assessment scale

Developed by pediatrician T. Berry Brazelton in 1973, the Brazelton neonatal behavioral assessment scale (BNBAS) is the most commonly used behavioral evaluation tool. To score the BNBAS reliably, the examiner must take an intensive 2-day course. The nurse without such preparation may want to use the BNBAS as a guideline for assessing neonatal behavior in a more general way, without scoring the neonate.

Areas evaluated by the BNBAS include the neonate's behavioral state (level of wakefulness) and behavioral responses, including elicited responses.

Behavioral state
Begin the BNBAS assessment by observing the neonate's behavioral state (degree of alertness). The neonate experiences six behavioral states.
• Deep sleep is a quiet period during which the neonate makes few or no spontaneous movements; any movements that occur are brief and jerky. No rapid eye movements (REMs) are detected. Respirations are even and regular. The neonate can be aroused from this state only for a few moments.
• In light sleep, the neonate can be aroused and brought to wakefulness easily; REMs can be detected. The arms or legs may move occasionally, and movements are smoother than during deep sleep. The breathing pattern varies as the neonate drifts from light sleep to drowsiness.
• The drowsy state is characterized by an attempt to become fully alert. Movements become more frequent and regular and the eyes open periodically. Although the neonate responds to auditory and tactile stimuli, the response may be sluggish until the next state approaches.
• In the alert state, the neonate seems to be transfixed by external stimuli and has limited motor activity.
• The active state is characterized by regular eye and body movements in response to external stimuli.
• In the crying state, the neonate responds to both internal and external stimuli, cries vigorously and without interruption, and makes thrusting movements.

The neonate should move successively through these states, although the time spent in each may vary widely from one neonate to the next. The sleep-awake pattern also varies, depending on gestational age and other factors. The typical neonate sleeps 10 to 20 hours daily, with deep sleep accounting for only about 4 hours of total sleep. A neonate affected by maternal drug use may have an extremely labile sleep-awake pattern (Blackburn, 1987).

Behavioral responses
Neonatal behavioral responses fall into six categories: habituation, orientation, motor maturity, variations, self-quieting ability, and social behaviors.

Habituation. A protective mechanism, habituation refers to the process of becoming accustomed (habituating) to environmental stimuli, such as noise and light. For example, if one neonate in the nursery starts to cry, a neonate in light sleep will startle initially. If a second neonate then cries, the neonate who was in light sleep may move about. As the other neonates continue crying, the neonate in light sleep gradually becomes less stimulated, reflecting habituation. Normally, habituation occurs after three consecutive presentations of a stimulus (in this example, the continued crying of both neonates is the third presentation).

A neonate's ability to become habituated to a stimulus varies with the behavioral state. Habituation should

(Text continues on page 867.)

Head-to-toe physical assessment findings

Comprehensive physical assessment of the neonate proceeds from head to toe. The chart below shows normal findings, common variations, abnormal findings, and possible causes for each body area. The information in the third and fourth columns is specifically related.

PARAMETER	NORMAL FINDINGS AND COMMON VARIATIONS	ABNORMAL FINDINGS AND POSSIBLE CAUSES	
General appearance and behavior			
Body shape and posture	Well-rounded torso with sufficient subcutaneous tissue and no obvious anomalies	Thin extremities, muscle wasting, loose skin, little or no subcutaneous tissue, obvious anomalies	Malnourishment, fetal stress, congenital defect (such as cleft lip or palate, omphalocele, gastroschisis, meningomyelocele)
	Flexed extremities, bowed legs	Fetal position (fists clenched, arms adducted and flexed, hips abducted, knees flexed)	Prematurity
		Frog position (flexed hips and thighs, extended arms)	Prematurity
		Opisthotonos (acute arching of back, with head bent back on neck, heels bent back on legs, and rigid arm and hand flexion)	Brain damage, birth asphyxia, neurologic abnormality
Muscle tone	Pronounced	Reduced or flaccid	Birth asphyxia, prematurity
	Spontaneous symmetrical movement (possibly slightly tremulous), bilaterally equal flexion and extension	No movement or asymmetrical, irregular, tremulous movement	Birth asphyxia, neurologic dysfunction, prematurity, drug-induced birth injury
Alertness level	Usually easy to console when upset	Decreased alertness, hard to arouse and console	Prematurity, stress, sepsis, neurologic disorder
Cry	Strong	Weak, high-pitched, or absent	Brain damage, neonatal drug addiction, increased intracranial pressure (ICP)
		Raspy	Upper airway problem
		Expiratory grunt during crying	Respiratory distress
Neuromuscular maturity			
Scarf sign	Elbow reaches midline when extended across chest	Elbow extends beyond midline	Prematurity
		Elbow does not reach midline	Postmaturity
Arm recoil	Brisk	Sluggish	Prematurity
Ankle dorsiflexion	0-degree angle	Angle greater than 0 degrees	Prematurity
Popliteal angle	90 degrees or less	Greater than 90 degrees	Prematurity
Heel-to-ear maneuver	Heel reaches only to shoulders	Heel approaches or reaches ear	Prematurity

(continued)

Head-to-toe physical assessment findings continued

PARAMETER	NORMAL FINDINGS AND COMMON VARIATIONS	ABNORMAL FINDINGS AND POSSIBLE CAUSES	
Skin			
Texture	Moist and warm	Gelatinous with visible veins	Prematurity
		Dry, peeling, cracking	Postmaturity
		Edematous, shiny, taut	Kidney dysfunction, cardiac or renal failure
Color	Varies with ethnic background; may deepen with crying and activity • Asian neonate: pink or rosy red to yellow tinge • Black or Native American neonate: pale pink with yellow or red tinge • Caucasian neonate: pale pink to ruddy • Hispanic neonate: pink with yellow tinge Cyanotic discoloration of hands and feet during first 24 hours after birth caused by transition to relatively cool extrauterine environment Reddish tinge just after birth caused by adjustment of central oxygen levels to extrauterine environment	Cyanotic discoloration of hands and feet lasting longer than first 24 hours	Poor peripheral circulation, possibly with cardiac compromise
		Dusky or cyanotic discoloration over entire body	Poor circulation, respiratory compromise
		Plethora (florid complexion), accompanied by elevated hematocrit or hemogloblin level	Polycythemia or blood hyperviscosity
		Pallor	Cardiopulmonary compromise or failure
		Mottling	Prematurity or cardiopulmonary disorder (if associated with cold stress, color changes, bradycardia, or apnea)
	Yellow discoloration (jaundice) arising in first 48 to 72 hours after birth and normally disappearing by the seventh day (physiologic jaundice)	Jaundice on first day after birth (pathologic jaundice)	Isoimmune hemolytic disease (such as Rh or ABO incompatibility), polycythemia, enzyme deficiency, excessive bruising or bleeding, Hirschsprung's disease, pyloric stenosis (or other intestinal obstruction that increases blood supply or shunts blood to liver), maternal diabetes, small-for-gestational-age (SGA) status
Vernix caseosa	Present over entire body	Absent	Severe prematurity
		Minimal or absent	Postmaturity
Lanugo (soft, downy hair)	Sparse or present only on shoulders	Abundant over entire body	Prematurity
		Absent	Postmaturity
Turgor	Adequate (indicated by brisk return of skin to original position after examiner pinches it between fingers)	Poor (indicated by tenting or sluggish return to original position)	Dehydration

Head-to-toe physical assessment findings continued

PARAMETER	NORMAL FINDINGS AND COMMON VARIATIONS	ABNORMAL FINDINGS AND POSSIBLE CAUSES	
Skin variations	Ecchymosis of presenting part Harlequin (clown) sign (pink or reddish skin on one side of body, with color division at midline; caused by vasomotor instability) Mongolian spots (blue-black macules over buttocks, possibly extending to sacral region; most common in dark-skinned neonates) Milia (minute white epidermal cysts caused by sebaceous gland obstruction; commonly seen on face) Miliaria (rash consisting of minute vesicles and papules, resulting from sweat duct blockage; occurs mainly on forehead and in skin folds; also called prickly heat) Erythema toxicum neonatorum (pink, papular rash covering thorax, back, abdomen, and groin; commonly appears within 24 to 48 hours after birth) Nevus flammeus (permanent birthmark; flat, capillary hemangioma ranging from pale red to deep red-purple; also called port wine stain) Telangiectatic nevi (flat, deep pink, localized areas of capillary dilation; typically appear on upper eyelids, across nasal bridge and occipital bone, or along neck; also called stork bite)	Café-au-lait spots (small, light tan macules)	Possible early sign of neurofibromatosis, especially if appearing in group of seven or more
		Meconium staining	Fetal distress
		Petechiae	Hematopoietic disorder
		Cutaneous papilloma (small brownish or flesh-colored outgrowth of skin; also called skin tag)	Possible congenital anomaly
Respiratory system			
Respiratory effort and rhythm	Easy, unlabored effort; abdominal breathing; possible irregular rhythm and apneic episodes lasting less than 15 seconds	Dyspnea; substernal, supracostal, intercostal, or supraclavicular retractions; nasal flaring; stridor; grunting	Respiratory distress
Chest excursion	Symmetrical	Asymmetrical	Diaphragmatic hernia, pneumothorax, phrenic nerve damage
Anteroposterior (AP) diameter	1:1 ratio (almost round)	Ratio > 1:1 (barrel chest)	Poorly developed rib cage and chest musculature, possible prematurity

(continued)

Head-to-toe physical assessment findings continued

PARAMETER	NORMAL FINDINGS AND COMMON VARIATIONS	ABNORMAL FINDINGS AND POSSIBLE CAUSES	
Breath sounds	Clear; equal bilaterally, anteriorly, and posteriorly; crackles during first few hours after birth (unless accompanied by color changes or cyanosis)	Unequal	Pneumothorax or diaphragmatic hernia
		Crackles after first day, rhonchi, expiratory grunts, wheezing	Pulmonary congestion or edema, respiratory distress, pneumonia
Chest percussion	No increase in tympany over lung fields	Increased tympany over lung fields	Lung hyperinflation
Cardiovascular system			
Heart rate and rhythm	120 to 160 beats/minute (higher during active or crying periods); regular	Less than 100 beats/minute (bradycardia) or more than 160 beats/minute (tachycardia)	Prematurity, respiratory compromise, increased cardiac workload, sepsis, congenital heart defect
		Persistent arrhythmias	Congenital heart anomaly
Heart sounds	No audible murmur (however, slight murmur heard over base or left sternal border until foramen ovale closes)	Heart sounds on right side of chest	Possible dextrocardia
		Persistent murmur (usually heard at left sternal border or above apical impulse)	Persistent fetal circulation, congenital heart anomaly
Apical impulse	Located at fourth or fifth intercostal space at midclavicular line; point of maximum impulse located at fourth intercostal space just right of midclavicular line (may shift to the right in first few hours after birth)	Displaced	Cardiac defect or cardiomegaly
Thrill	Absent (except for first few hours after birth)	Present beyond first few hours after birth	Increased cardiac activity
Head and neck			
Head size	Slightly large in proportion to body (average head circumference of term neonate is 32 to 35 cm)	Abnormally small	Microcephaly, caused by congenital syndrome or decreased brain development (such as from intrauterine growth retardation)
		Extremely small	Anencephaly (absent cerebral tissue or absent or minimal skull)
		Abnormally large	Macrocephaly, possibly caused by hydrocephalus (abnormal accumulation of cerebrospinal fluid within cranial vault) resulting from congenital anomaly (such as meningomyelocele, tumor, trauma, or infection)

Head-to-toe physical assessment findings continued

PARAMETER	NORMAL FINDINGS AND COMMON VARIATIONS	ABNORMAL FINDINGS AND POSSIBLE CAUSES	
Fontanels	Anterior fontanel open until age 12 to 18 months; diamond shaped; measures 2 x 3 x 5 cm; located at juncture of coronal, frontal, and sagittal sutures	Premature closure of anterior fontanel	Poor brain development
		Bulging fontanel (usually anterior fontanel)	Increased ICP
	Posterior fontanel open until age 2 to 3 months (may be closed at birth); triangular shaped; measures 1 x 1 x 1 cm; located at juncture of sagittal and lambdoidal sutures	Sunken fontanel	Dehydration
Head and scalp variations	Molding (cranial distortion lasting 5 to 7 days, caused by pressure on cranium during vaginal delivery)	Herniation of brain tissue through skull defect	Encephalocele (congenital or traumatic defect)
		Bradycephalus, premature closure of coronal suture line, increased AP diameter and lateral growth	Anomalies, such as congenital or traumatic defects
		Premature closure of skull sutures (craniosynostosis)	Genetic disorder
		Overriding sutures, caused by excessive pressure on cranium during vaginal delivery	Prematurity
		Localized pitting edema of scalp possibly extending over sutures	Caput succedaneum, caused by pressure on fetal occiput (as during extended labor)
		Forceps marks; edematous or reddened area	Forceps delivery
		Localized scalp swelling	Cephalhematoma (collection of blood between skull and periosteum that does not cross suture lines; commonly caused by forceps trauma; may last up to 8 weeks)
	No masses or soft areas over skull	Masses or soft areas (such as craniotabes) over parietal bones (may be insignificant if no other abnormality exists)	Possible anomaly of internal organs
	No bruits in temporal area over anterior or posterior fontanel	Bruits in vascular areas of head	Cerebral arteriovenous malformation
Head lag	No greater than 10 degrees	Greater than 10 degrees	Hypotonia or prematurity
Hair distribution and texture	Distributed over top of head; single identifiable strands of hair	Fine or fuzzy hair	Prematurity

(continued)

Head-to-toe physical assessment findings continued

PARAMETER	NORMAL FINDINGS AND COMMON VARIATIONS	ABNORMAL FINDINGS AND POSSIBLE CAUSES	
Eyes and eyelids	Symmetrical; aligned with ears, face, nose midline	Wide-eyed, apprehensive look	Postmaturity, SGA status, intrauterine growth retardation
	Eyes spaced approximately 2.5 cm apart	Abnormally wide distance (greater than 2.5 cm) between eyes (hypertelorism)	Fetal hydantoin syndrome (from maternal hydantoin use during pregnancy)
		Abnormally small distance (less than 2.5 cm) between eyes (hypotelorism)	Trisomy 13
	Clear sclera	Yellow sclera	Jaundice (however, slight yellow tinge may reflect only ethnic influence)
		Blue sclera	Osteogenesis imperfecta (fatal genetic syndrome characterized by fragile bones and shortened limbs)
		Scleral hemorrhage	Birth trauma
	Clear conjunctiva	Pink conjunctiva	Conjunctivitis (possibly resulting from silver nitrate or erythromycin instillation)
		Conjunctival hemorrhages	Birth trauma
	Even, bilateral iris color	Gold flecks in iris (Brushfield's spots)	Down's syndrome (trisomy 21), if accompanied by other anomalies
		Coloboma (cleft usually affecting iris, ciliary body, or choroid; extends inferiorly)	Possible congenital malformation of internal organs
	Bilaterally equal pupil reaction to light	Absent or bilaterally unequal pupil reaction to light	Brain damage or increased ICP
	Clear cornea	Hazy, milky cornea	Prematurity; congenital cataract (possibly from congenital rubella)
	Transparent, intact retina	Pigmented retinal areas; tortuous or poorly demarcated retinal vessels	Retinal damage or hemorrhage
	Patent, palpable lacrimal duct	Blocked or absent lacrimal duct	Congenital obstruction
	Positive blink reflex (eyes blink in response to bright light)	Absent blink reflex	Facial nerve paralysis or optic nerve damage
	Positive red reflex (luminous bilateral red appearance of retina)	Absent red reflex	Congenital cataract
	Positive doll's eye reflex (eyes remain stationary when head is moved to left or right)	Absent doll's eye reflex	Trochlear, oculomotor, or abducens nerve damage

Head-to-toe physical assessment findings continued

PARAMETER	NORMAL FINDINGS AND COMMON VARIATIONS	ABNORMAL FINDINGS AND POSSIBLE CAUSES	
Eyes and eyelids (continued)	No eye slant or slant reflecting ethnic background	Pronounced upward eye slant	Down's syndrome
		Downward eye slant	Treacher Collins' syndrome (congenital syndrome characterized by small mandible, beaked nose, and lower lid and external ear malformations)
		"Sunset" eyes (upper lid retraction causing sclera to show above iris)	Hydrocephalus
		Edematous eyelids	Birth trauma or irritation from silver nitrate or erythromycin instillation
		Ptosis (drooping) of eyelids	Oculomotor nerve damage
		Epicanthal folds	Down's syndrome; cri du chat (cat's cry) syndrome
Nose	Located at midline	Located off midline	Congenital malformation or syndrome (such as Apert's syndrome, characterized by premature closure of sutures)
	Appropriate size for face	Beaked	Treacher Collins's syndrome
		Enlarged or bulbous	Trisomy 13
	Patent nares	Nonpatent nares	Nasal obstruction; choanal atresia
		Missing nares	Congenital syndrome or malformation (such as cleft lip)
	Grimace or cry in response to strong odors passed under nose	No response to strong odors passed under nose	Olfactory nerve damage
		Flattened nasal bridge	Congenital syndrome, such as arthrogryposis (characterized by persistent contractures)
	Positive sneeze reflex (indicated by sneezing when both nares are occluded for 1 to 2 seconds)	No response	Possible nonpatent nares
Ears	Symmetrical in size, shape, and placement; top of ear parallel to an imaginary line drawn through the outer and inner canthi of the eye	Low-set, slanted	Congenital syndrome (such as Down's syndrome)
		Pinpoint holes or sinus tracts along preauricular surface	Possible congenital renal anomaly
	Well-curved pinna; rigid cartilage; instant recoil after folding	Flattened or folded pinna; slow recoil	Prematurity

(continued)

Head-to-toe physical assessment findings continued

PARAMETER	NORMAL FINDINGS AND COMMON VARIATIONS	ABNORMAL FINDINGS AND POSSIBLE CAUSES	
Ears (continued)	Positive startle reflex (indicated by startling or crying in response to loud noise)	Absent or minimal startle reflex	Deafness or auditory nerve impairment
	Umbo (cone) of light visible on otoscopic examination; pearl gray, movable tympanic membrane with no bulges (membrane may be covered with vernix caseosa)	Umbo dull or absent; dull, immobile, or red tympanic membrane	Infection
		Blue tympanic membrane	Hemorrhage
		Bulging tympanic membrane	Otitis media (middle ear infection)
Mouth	Symmetrical; appropriate size for face; located at midline	Droops or slants unilaterally when neonate cries or moves mouth	Palsy or damage to seventh cranial or facial nerve, possibly resulting from birth trauma (such as from forceps delivery)
		Birdlike, with shortened vermilion border (exposed red portion of lips) and shortened philtrum (groove from upper lip to nose)	Fetal alcohol syndrome
		Extremely wide (macrostomia)	Metabolic disorder (such as hypothyroidism)
		Unusually small (microstomia)	Down's syndrome
	Lips pink, moist, and formed completely	One or more clefts in upper lip, possibly extending to nasal floor	Cleft lip (congenital anomaly in which maxillary and median nasal processes fail to fuse)
Mucous membranes	Moist and pink	Dry, dusky, or cyanotic	Dehydration, poor oxygenation
	Moderate salivation	Excessive salivation	Tracheoesophageal fistula, esophageal atresia
Palate	Intact with no arching or fissures	Markedly arched	Turner's syndrome
	Epstein's pearls (small, hard, white patches that resolve gradually)	Midline fissure	Cleft palate (congenital anomaly in which two sides of palate fail to fuse; may occur in conjunction with cleft lip)
Tongue	Appropriate size for face	Abnormally large (macroglossia)	Hypothyroidism
		Abnormally small (microglossia)	Congenital syndrome (such as Möbius's syndrome)
	Located at midline	Located off midline	Cranial nerve damage
	Juts forward when touched	Fails to jut forward when touched	Short frenulum
Uvula	Located at midline; rises with crying	Fails to rise with crying	Neurologic dysfunction
Chin	Slightly receding; appropriate size for face	Extremely receding; underdeveloped (micrognathia)	Congenital syndrome (such as Pierre Robin's syndrome)

Head-to-toe physical assessment findings continued

PARAMETER	NORMAL FINDINGS AND COMMON VARIATIONS	ABNORMAL FINDINGS AND POSSIBLE CAUSES	
Oral reflexes	Sucking, swallowing, rooting, and gag reflexes present; sucking and swallowing reflexes well co-ordinated	Absent gag reflex	Neurologic dysfunction
		Absent sucking or rooting reflex	Prematurity or neurologic dysfunction
Neck	Symmetrical	Asymmetrical	Unusual fetal position
	Short, no webbing (excessive skin)	Short and webbed	Down's syndrome
	Full range of motion (head can turn to each side equally)	Partial range of motion or tilting of head to one side (torticollis)	Birth injury; muscle spasm resulting in contraction of sterno-cleidomastoid muscles
	Weak, asymmetrical tonic neck reflex	Strong, asymmetrical tonic neck reflex	Prematurity
		Symmetrical tonic neck reflex	Neurologic dysfunction
	Thyroid located at midline; appropriate in size	Enlarged thyroid	Goiter
		Palpable lymph nodes	Congenital infection
		Palpable neck masses	Cystic hygroma
	Regular, bilaterally equal, strong carotid pulses	Weak or irregular carotid pulses	Cardiac defect or circulatory problem
		Enlarged sternocleidomastoid muscle	Torticollis; birth or fetal injury resulting in sternocleidomastoid hematoma
Thorax			
Clavicles	Even; symmetrical; nontender; without masses or lumps	Uneven; asymmetrical; masses or lumps present	Clavicular fracture; shoulder dystocia (as from birth injury); brachial plexus damage or palsy
Chest circumference	30 to 33 cm (12″ to 13″)	Less than 30 cm	Prematurity or SGA status
		Barrel chest (circumference greater than 33 cm	Respiratory compromise; large-for-gestational-age (LGA) status
Chest excursion	Bilaterally equal	Bilaterally unequal	Phrenic nerve damage
Ribs	Symmetrical, flexible, without masses or crepitus	Asymmetrical	Birth injury or congenital syndrome
		Masses or crepitus present	Fracture or subcutaneous air pocket caused by air leakage resulting from pulmonary dysfunction
Breasts	1 cm of palpable breast tissue	Less than 1 cm (possibly only 5 mm) of palpable breast tissue	Prematurity
	Raised areolas	Flat areolas	Prematurity

(continued)

Head-to-toe physical assessment findings continued

PARAMETER	NORMAL FINDINGS AND COMMON VARIATIONS	ABNORMAL FINDINGS AND POSSIBLE CAUSES	
Breasts (continued)	Horizontally aligned, well-spaced nipples; no extra nipples	Misaligned or supernumerary (more than two) nipples	Possible internal organ anomaly
	Breast hypertrophy, possibly with white nipple discharge (witch's milk) from maternal hormonal influence; appears within the first 2 to 3 days after birth, and usually diminishes during the 1st or 2nd week	Purulent nipple discharge	Mastitis
Xiphoid process	Intact	Absent or depressed	Fracture (may result from resuscitation)
Abdomen			
Shape	Symmetrical; rounded	Asymmetrical	Abdominal mass
		Scaphoid	Diaphragmatic hernia
		Distended	Intestinal obstruction, renal disorder, ascites, edema resulting from congenital renal or cardiac defect, prematurity, fetal hydrops
		Distended left upper quadrant	Pyloric stenosis, duodenal or jejunal obstruction
Abdominal muscles	Strong	Weak	Prune-belly syndrome, possible renal problems (such as hypoplastic kidneys)
		Visible abdominal wall defect over bladder	Bladder exstrophy
	No visible peristaltic waves	Visible peristaltic waves moving in left-to-right direction	Intestinal obstruction (rarely manifests immediately after birth)
Umbilical cord remnant	Bluish white, three vessels (two arteries and one vein) present	Two vessels (one artery and one vein) present	Possible internal congenital anomalies (especially renal anomalies)
		Thick	LGA status
		Small	SGA status or malnourishment
		Red, with discharge	Infection
		Meconium stained	Fetal distress
		Mass (hernia) present, with protrusion of abdominal viscera	Omphalocele
		Hernia	Gastroschisis (congenital fissure of the abdominal wall, not located at umbilical cord insertion site, accompanied by intestinal protrusion)

Head-to-toe physical assessment findings continued

PARAMETER	NORMAL FINDINGS AND COMMON VARIATIONS	ABNORMAL FINDINGS AND POSSIBLE CAUSES	
Abdominal palpation	Abdomen soft, without tenderness or masses	Abdomen tense, rigid, and tender	Intestinal deformity or obstruction
		Masses present	Renal or urinary tract deformity
	Minor separation of rectus abdominis muscles	Wide separation of rectus abdominis muscles (diastasis recti abdominis)	Prematurity
Abdominal auscultation	2 to 4 bowel sounds per minute	Absent bowel sounds	Intestinal obstruction
		More than 4 to 5 bowel sounds per minute (except immediately after feeding)	Intestinal obstruction or hypermotility
	No audible bruit	Bruit over abdominal aorta	Arteriovenous malformation
		Bruit over kidneys	Renal artery stenosis
Abdominal percussion	Tympany over all areas except liver, spleen, and bladder (where dullness is heard)	Increased tympany	Increased fluid or air
		Increased areas of dullness (if liver or spleen is enlarged, dullness extends below costal margins; if bladder is enlarged, dullness extends toward umbilicus)	Mass or enlarged organ at increased area of dullness
Kidneys	Located in lumbar area; right kidney lower than left; 4 to 5 cm long	Enlarged	Polycystic kidney disease
		Both kidneys absent	Potter's syndrome
Liver	Firm	Hard	Liver damage or cardiopulmonary disorder
	Sharp edge of liver palpable just above right costal margin during inspiration	Sharp edge of liver palpable more than 1 cm below right costal margin during inspiration	Enlarged liver (from respiratory distress or congestive heart failure)
Spleen	Palpable 1 cm below left costal margin	Absent or not palpable	Congenital heart defect
		Enlarged	Erythroblastosis fetalis (ABO incompatibility)
Bladder	No visible distention (except just before voiding)	Distended (may be visible above pubic bone)	Urinary tract obstruction or full bladder
Groin	Smooth, no palpable masses	Masses present	Inguinal hernia
	Tympany over gastric bubble, just below left costal margin toward midline	No tympany over gastric bubble	Esophageal atresia or gastric defect
Back			
Spinal column	Straight	Curved	Vertebral misalignment (if caused by fetal position, condition usually resolves gradually)

(continued)

Head-to-toe physical assessment findings continued

PARAMETER	NORMAL FINDINGS AND COMMON VARIATIONS	ABNORMAL FINDINGS AND POSSIBLE CAUSES	
Spinal column (continued)	No visible deviations or defects	Visible defect, such as mass, dimple, or bulge (possibly with tuft of hair)	Spina bifida
		Hernial sac (may be open or covered with portion of spinal cord, meninges, and cerebro-spinal fluid)	Meningomyelocele
		Sinus tracts or pinpoint holes	Pilonidal cysts
	No vertebral enlargement or tenderness	Vertebral bulge, mass, cyst, enlargement, or tenderness	Vertebral fracture, spina bifida, occult meningomyelocele, pilonidal cyst
Buttocks	Symmetrical midline crease	Asymmetrical midline crease	Congenital hip dysplasia
Anus and genitalia			
Anus	Patent, located at midline	Nonpatent or dimpled	Imperforate anus
		Shifted anteriorly or posteriorly	Anal defect
	Anal wink present (indicated by anal sphincter constriction in response to light stroking of anal area)	Anal wink absent	Neurologic deficit
Perineum	Smooth	Dimpled or with extra opening	Urinary or genital malformation; urinary fistula
Female genitalia	Distinguishable as female Enlarged clitoris (from maternal hormonal influence)	Ambiguous genitalia; some structures resembling male genitalia (such as a greatly enlarged clitoris)	Trisomy 18; adrenocortical insufficiency
	Labia majora extend beyond labia minora	Labia majora smaller than labia minora	Prematurity
	Well-formed labia minora	Labia minora larger than labia majora	Prematurity
	Urethral meatus located anterior to vaginal orifice	Displaced urethral meatus	Urinary malformation
	Patent vagina, possibly with discharge or slight bleeding (pseudomenstruation)	Vagina opening completely covered by thickened hymen, possibly with slight bleeding (pseudomenstruation)	Vaginal malformation
Male genitalia	Penis straight; appropriate size for body (2.8 to 4.3 cm long)	Penis curved	Chordee (fibrous constriction of penis)
		Penis enlarged	Renal disorder
	Urinary meatus located at midline, at tip of glans	Urinary meatus displaced to ventral surface	Hypospadias
		Urinary meatus displaced to dorsal surface	Epispadias

Head-to-toe physical assessment findings continued

PARAMETER	NORMAL FINDINGS AND COMMON VARIATIONS	ABNORMAL FINDINGS AND POSSIBLE CAUSES	
Male genitalia (continued)	Urine stream flowing straight from penis	Crooked urine stream or urine leakage from patent urachus (abnormal fetal opening between bladder and umbilicus)	Urinary fistula; phimosis
	Full testes; numerous rugae	Smooth or few rugae	Prematurity
	Darkly pigmented testes	Bluish testes or scrotum	Testicular torsion
		Enlarged or edematous scrotum	Hydrocele or breech delivery
		Dimpled testes	Testicular torsion
	Testes descended on at least one side	Testes not palpable or found high in inguinal canal	Prematurity
Voiding onset	Within first 24 hours	Later than 24 hours	Renal or urinary obstruction or malformation
Arms			
General appearance	Of appropriate length relative to body; bilaterally equal; straight	Shortened or asymmetrical	Maternal diabetes or drug use, congenital syndrome
	Humerus, radius, and ulna symmetrical; no masses present	Humerus, radius, or ulna asymmetrical or absent	Possible syndrome, such as thrombocytopenia-absent radius syndrome
		Mass present on humerus, radius, or ulna	Fracture (as from birth injury)
Range of motion	Full	Limited	Birth injury or trauma
		Limited flexion	Prematurity
		Limited shoulder motion or flexion	Dystocia, brachial plexus damage or palsy
		Limited clavicular motion	Clavicular injury, osteogenesis imperfecta (genetic disorder resulting in fragile bones)
		Limited elbow, wrist, or hand motion	Possible birth injury
Hands and wrists	Hand straight	Hand turned outward	Possible congenital absence of radius
	No simian crease in palm	Simian crease in palm	Down's syndrome
	10 equally spaced fingers; no webbing	More than 10 fingers (polydactyly)	Possible congenital syndrome (such as trisomy 13)
		Webbed fingers, digital tags (syndactyly), unequal finger spacing	Congenital syndrome (such as Apert's syndrome)
	Nails extending beyond nail beds to tips of fingers	Spoon-shaped nails that do not reach beyond nail beds	Congenital syndrome (such as fetal alcohol syndrome)
		Absent nails	Possible congenital absence of radius

(continued)

Head-to-toe physical assessment findings continued

PARAMETER	NORMAL FINDINGS AND COMMON VARIATIONS	ABNORMAL FINDINGS AND POSSIBLE CAUSES	
Hands and wrists (continued)		Meconium-stained nails	Fetal distress
	Nail beds regain pink color equally bilaterally and briskly (within 3 seconds) during capillary refill test	Nail beds remain dusky or regain pink color unequally bilaterally or slowly (longer than 3 seconds)	Poor peripheral perfusion or oxygenation
	Carpal and metacarpal bones of bilaterally equal length; no masses	Carpal and metacarpal bones absent or bilaterally unequal; masses present	Fracture or absence of bone, possibly associated with congenital syndrome
	Strong palmar grasp	Weak palmar grasp	Prematurity
Pulses	Brachial and radial pulses strong and bilaterally equal; equal to femoral pulses	Brachial or radial pulse weak, absent, or bilaterally unequal	Poor peripheral perfusion, possible cardiac defect
Legs			
General appearance	Of apportionate length relative to body; bilaterally equal; straight	Disproportionate length relative to body, short or bilaterally unequal, crooked, internally rotated or bowed	Congenital hip dysplasia
	Fibula, tibia, trochanter, and femur bilaterally symmetrical	Fibula, tibia, trochanter, or femur absent or bilaterally asymmetrical	Fracture or absence of bone (may be associated with congenital syndrome)
		Limited hip motion; audible click heard with Ortolani's or Barlow's maneuver	Congenital hip dysplasia
Femoral pulses	Strong and bilaterally regular	Weak or bilaterally absent	Coarctation of the aorta
		Bounding	Patent ductus arteriosus
Feet	Straight	Turned out (valgus deformity)	Absent fibula, fetal positioning (apparent clubfoot), true clubfoot
		Turned in (varus deformity)	Absent tibia, fetal positioning (apparent clubfoot), true clubfoot
		Pedal edema	Pressure caused by fetal positioning, poor peripheral perfusion, or congenital syndrome (such as Turner's syndrome)
	Plantar creases covering sole	Few plantar creases; may cover only anterior third of sole	Prematurity
	Tarsal and metatarsal bones present and bilaterally equal	Tarsal and metatarsal bones absent or bilaterally unequal	Fracture or absence of bone (may be associated with congenital syndrome)
	10 equally spaced toes; no webbing	More than 10 toes; unequal toe spacing, webbing present	Possible congenital syndrome (such as trisomy 13)
Reflexes	Symmetrical plantar and patellar reflexes (knee jerk)	Absent, weak, or asymmetrical plantar reflex	Neurologic deficit, prematurity
		Absent, weak, or asymmetrical patellar reflex	Neurologic deficit, prematurity

be tested only during deep sleep, light sleep, or the drowsy state. If habituation does not occur after three presentations of a stimulus, the neonate may be hyper-responsive to external stimuli. A slowed or diminished response from the outset of the first presentation (except during deep sleep) suggests lethargy or hyporesponsiveness. These variations commonly reflect neurologic immaturity or impaired neurologic function.

Orientation. This term refers to the neonate's responsiveness to visual and auditory stimuli. For best results, orientation should be tested while the neonate is in the alert or active state.

Normally, the neonate orients to (follows) a visual or auditory stimulus by moving both the head and eyes. No response or lack of head movement is abnormal. Also observe for nystagmus (rapid, darting eye movements) and for gaze aversion after direct eye contact—both normal responses.

A neonate is more responsive to a human face—either real or represented in a picture—than an inanimate object. (This especially is apparent when the neonate is held in the en face—face-to-face—position). If the parents are observing the behavioral assessment, show them how closely their child attends to visual stimuli by holding a brightly colored object, such as a ball, in front of the neonate. As the ball moves from side to side, the neonate's eyes will follow it and the head will turn from side to side.

In response to an auditory stimulus, such as a human voice or noise from a rattle, the neonate typically stops an activity to attend to the sound. If the sound comes from outside the visual field, the neonate will turn toward it. (If the neonate fails to respond, repeat the sound at a different pitch—many neonates alert better to higher pitches.) A sudden or loud stimulus usually causes crying.

Motor maturity. Best assessed with the neonate in the alert state, motor maturity refers to posture, muscle tone, muscle coordination and movements, and reflexes. Evaluate smoothness and equality of arm and leg movements. In the term neonate, asymmetrical or absent movement of an extremity calls for further investigation, as do muscle flaccidity or hypotonia, extreme tremors, and excessive jerking movements.

Keep in mind that the first 24 hours after birth represent a period of progressive changes; thus, motor responses may vary greatly. Neurologic stability typically is established by the third day. However, with early discharge, few neurologic assessments can be delayed until this time. If any abnormalities are detected, the examination must be repeated later.

Variations. This term refers to the frequency of changes in activity level, state, and skin color. Document these changes throughout the behavioral assessment.

Self-quieting ability. To test this, observe how soon and how effectively the neonate self-quiets when crying. Attempts to self-quiet include such behaviors as moving the hands toward the mouth, sucking on the fist, changing position, and attending to auditory or visual stimuli.

If the neonate does not attempt to self-quiet, the nurse or a parent should attempt to console the neonate by singing, talking, rocking, walking, cuddling, or facing the neonate directly. The degree to which this attempt succeeds reflects the neonate's consolability. If the attempt fails to elicit self-quieting, the neonate may be hyperactive or hypersensitive to the environment. Consolability is documented in terms of whether and to what degree the neonate self-quiets after introduction of a visual or an auditory stimulus.

Social behaviors. Neonatal social behaviors include smiling, cuddling, and exhibiting distinct cues. Such cues—signals that indicate the neonate's needs—include crying to be fed and stopping sucking when hunger has been sated. These behaviors should be tested with the neonate in the alert or active state.

Social behaviors are especially important to the parents, who commonly gauge their ability to provide care by their child's response to their actions. During this part of the behavioral assessment, the nurse can demonstrate to the parents that the neonate is an active partner in the relationship, giving as well as responding to cues from the parents. (For a study of the effectiveness of demonstrating the behavioral assessment to parents, see *Nursing research applied: Use of the Brazelton behavioral assessment scale to improve parent-neonate interaction*, page 868.)

Als's synactive theory of development

Extending Brazelton's work, Heidelise Als developed a theoretical model for assessing neonatal behavior based on developmental potential. Als's theory holds that the neonate both shapes and is shaped by the environment, of which the parents form a part. According to Als, whose work spans the last decade, the neonate's physiologic status depends on the environmental stimuli received and processed. Further, neonatal behavior consists of functional subsystems (autonomic-visceral, motoric [motor], and state-attentional), each with distinctive behavioral stress responses.

Use of the Brazelton behavioral assessment scale to improve parent-neonate interaction

According to some experts, early assessment of neonatal behavior improves parent-neonate interaction by enhancing the parents' awareness and understanding of their child's interactive capacities and behavioral characteristics. These experts believe that demonstration of the behavioral assessment to the parents further enhances interaction. The Brazelton neonatal behavioral assessment scale (BNBAS) commonly is used for this purpose. To determine if demonstration of the BNBAS to parents has positive effects on parent-neonate interaction, a researcher reviewed relevant studies conducted since 1977.

Most of the research focused on mothers. One study showed that mothers who had observed the BNBAS knew which behaviors to expect from their neonate. Another found that mothers who had observed the BNBAS first tried to determine the cause when their neonate began to cry; a control group, in comparison, immediately gave their neonate a bottle. Other studies revealed that mothers who learned about their neonate's capacities through the BNBAS more easily identified their child's unique characteristics, responded to their cues more appropriately, and had a more mutual interaction during feeding.

However, one researcher found no significant difference in interaction between mothers who had observed the BNBAS and those who had not. Another researcher found that mothers who had observed the BNBAS did not interact with their neonate differently—although they showed more awareness of neonatal capacities—compared to a control group.

Studies of fathers revealed more mixed results. Forty-two fathers who had been taught to administer the BNBAS demonstrated no significant difference in interaction with their neonate, compared to a control group. However, they did show more knowledge of neonatal behavior, greater satisfaction with their neonate, and more involvement in caretaking. In another study, fathers who had observed the BNBAS scored higher in attitudes toward parenting but did not show a significant increase in caregiving activities. A third study found that first-time fathers who had observed the BNBAS had an improved quality of interaction with their infant at 8 weeks postpartum.

Application to practice
This review of studies indicates that the nurse can help improve parental understanding of neonatal behavior and capacities and thus enhance parent-neonate interaction by demonstrating the BNBAS to the parents. The researcher further recommends that the nurse provide appropriate interventions if any problems are detected during the assessment. For instance, if the BNBAS shows that the neonate rapidly becomes upset by auditory stimuli, the nurse may suggest that the parents minimize noise in the neonate's room. However, Beal cites the need for further research to document the efficacy of the BNBAS as a tool to enhance parent-neonate interaction.

Beal, J.A. (1986). The Brazelton neonatal behavioral assessment scale: A tool to enhance parental attachment. *Journal of Pediatric Nursing,* 1(3), 170-177.

Chapter summary

Chapter 35 described the essential elements of neonatal assessment, including gestational-age, physical, and behavioral assessments. Here are the chapter highlights.

• The nurse must adapt the assessment to the neonate's tolerance, delaying any examination that could compromise the neonate. Also, to conserve the neonate's energy, the nurse should integrate overlapping portions of the various assessments whenever possible.

• In the first few hours after birth, the neonate experiences two distinct periods of reactivity, separated by a sleep stage. Because vital signs, alertness level, and responsiveness to external stimuli change as the neonate enters a new period, the nurse should interpret assessment findings in light of the specific period of reactivity.

• The nurse should perform a brief physical assessment within a few hours after delivery. This assessment includes evaluation of general appearance, vital sign measurements, and anthropometric measurements.

• Within the next few days, or before the neonate is discharged, a comprehensive assessment must be conducted. This assessment includes gestational-age assessment, a complete physical assessment, and behavioral assessment.

• Gestational-age assessment determines the neonate's age in weeks from the time of conception. Gestational-age assessment tools, such as the Ballard and Dubowitz tools, include evaluation of physical and neurologic characteristics.

• The complete physical assessment should proceed systematically from head to toe. To guard against cold stress during this assessment, the nurse should maintain thermoregulation by placing the neonate in a radiant warmer and uncovering only one part of the body at a time. The physical assessment also includes evaluation of neurologic characteristics, such as posture, muscle tone, reflexes, and cry.

• Behavioral assessment reveals the neonate's behavioral capacities and the quality of the neonate's interaction with the environment. The specially prepared nurse may use the Brazelton neonatal behavioral assessment scale to assess neonatal behavior.

Study questions

1. How can the nurse help to ensure thermoregulation when assessing the neonate?

2. How do the periods of reactivity affect assessment findings?

3. Which prenatal and intrapartal history findings suggest a gestational-age or birth-weight variation?

4. Which circumstances warrant precise determination of a neonate's gestational age?

5. What are the two major categories of criteria evaluated with the Dubowitz and Ballard gestational-age assessment tools?

6. Why should the nurse pay special attention to minor abnormalities when conducting the complete physical assessment?

7. What are the advantages of allowing parents to observe the behavioral assessment?

Bibliography

American Academy of Pediatrics and American College of Obstetricians and Gynecologists. (1988). *Guidelines for Perinatal Care* (2nd ed.). Washington DC: Staff.

Carlo, W.A., and Chatburn, R.L. (1988). *Neonatal respiratory care* (2nd ed.). Chicago: Year Book Medical Publishers.

Carter, M.B. (1989). Problems and nursing management strategies related to respiratory distress syndrome in the very preterm baby. *Intensive Care Nursing,* 5(2), 55-64.

Catlett, A.T., and Holditch, D.D. (1990). Environmental stimulation of the acutely ill premature infant: Physiological effects and nursing implications. *Neonatal Network,* 8(6), 19-26.

Cronenwett, L.R. (1985). Parental network structure and perceived support after birth of first child. *Nursing Research,* 34(6), 347-352.

Fonner, C.J., Rushton, C.H., and Fletcher, A.B. (1989). Preparation for neonatal emergencies: A neonatal emergency medication sheet. *Pediatric Nursing,* 15(5), 527-530.

Gordin, P.C. (1990). Assessing and managing agitation in a critically ill infant. *MCN,* 15(1), 26-32.

Hall-Johnson, S.H. (1986). *Nursing assessment and strategies for the family at risk: High-risk parenting* (2nd ed.). Philadelphia: Lippincott.

Hill, A.S., Cochran, C.K., and Dickerson, C. (1989). Nursing care of the infant with erythroblastosis fetalis. *Journal of Pediatric Nursing,* 4(6), 395-402.

Jones, M.A. (1989). Identifying signs that nurses interpret as indicating pain in newborns. *Pediatric Nursing,* 15(1), 76-79.

Kenner, C.A. (1990). Transition to parenthood. In L.P. Gunderson and C.A. Kenner (Eds.), *Care of the 24-25 week gestational age infant* (pp. 159-174). Petaluma, CA: Neonatal Network.

Kimberlin, L.V., Kucera, V.S., Lawrence, P.B., Newkirk, A., and Stenske, J.E. (1989). The role of the neonatal intensive care nurse in the delivery room. *Clinics in Perinatology,* 16(4), 1021-1028.

Montgomery, L.A.V. (1989). An anticipatory support program for high-risk parents: Follow-up results. *Neonatal Network,* 8(3), 31-33.

Newman, C.A. (1990). A survivor against the odds...Care of a very premature baby and his family. *Nursing Times,* 86(13), 48-49.

Penticuff, J.H. (1989). Infant suffering and nurse advocacy in neonatal intensive care. *Nursing Clinics of North America,* 24(4), 987-997.

Pigeon, H.M., McGrath, P.J., Lawrence, J., and MacMurray, S.B. (1989). Nurses' perceptions of pain in the neonatal intensive care unit. *Journal of Pain and Symptom Management,* 4(4), 179-183.

Shapiro, C. (1989). Pain in the neonate: Assessment and intervention. *Neonatal Network,* 8(1), 7-21.

Stang, H., Gunnar, M.R., Snellman, L., Condon, L.M., and Kestenbaum, R. (1988). Local anesthesia for neonatal circumcision. *JAMA,* 259(10), 1507-1511.

Steele, K.H. (1987). Caring for parents of critically ill neonates during hospitalization: Strategies for health care professionals. *Maternal-Child Nursing Journal,* 16(1), 13-27.

Stevens, K.A. (1988). Nursing diagnoses in wellness childbearing settings. *JOGNN,* 17(5), 329-336.

Streeter, N.S. (1986). *High-risk neonatal care.* Rockville, MD: Aspen.

Wilson, J.R.A. (1989). How neonatal nurses report infants' pain. *AJN,* 89(11), 1529-1530.

Wiswell, T.E., Enzenauer, R.W., Holton, M.E., Cornish, J.D., and Hankins, C.T. (1987). Declining frequency of circumcision: Implications for changes in the absolute incidence and male to female sex ratio of urinary tract infections in early infancy. *Pediatrics,* 79(3), 338-342.

Behavioral assessment

Als, H. (1982). Toward a synactive theory of development: Promise for the assessment and support of infant individuality. *Infant Mental Health Journal,* 3(4), 229-243.

Bayley, N. (1965). *Bayley scales of infant development (Infant behavior record).* New York: Psychological Corporation.

Brazelton, T. (1984). *Neonatal behavioral assessment scale* (2nd ed.). Philadelphia: Lippincott.

Davis, D.H., and Thoman, E.B. (1987). Behavioral states of premature infants: Implications for neural and behavioral development. *Developmental Psychobiology,* 20(1), 25-38.

Doll, E.A. (1965). *Vineland adaptive behavior scales.* Circle Pines, MN: American Guidance Service, Inc.

Frankenburg, W.K. (1981). The newly abbreviated and revised Denver developmental screening test. *Journal of Pediatrics,* 99(6), 995-999.

Gestational-age assessment

Ballard, J.L., Novak, K.K., and Driver, M. (1979). A simplified score for assessment of fetal maturation of newly born infants. *Journal of Pediatrics,* 95(5, Pt.1), 769-774.

Ballard, J. (1988). *Maturational assessment of gestational age.* Cincinnati: University of Cincinnati.

Battaglia, F.C., and Lubchenco, L.O. (1967). A practical classification of newborn infants by weight and gestational age. *Journal of Pediatrics,* 71, 159-163.

Cassady, G., and Strange, M. (1987). The small-for-gestational-age (SGA) infant. In G.B. Avery (Ed.), *Neonatology: Pathophysiology and management of the newborn* (3rd ed.; pp. 299-378). Philadelphia: Lippincott.

Dubowitz, L., and Dubowitz, V. (1977). *Gestational age of the newborn.* Reading, MA: Addison-Wesley.

Dubowitz, L.M.S., Dubowitz, V., and Goldberg, C. (1970). Clinical assessment of gestational age in the newborn infant. *Journal of Pediatrics,* 77(1), 1-10.

Usher, R. (1987). Extreme prematurity. In G.B. Avery (Ed.), *Neonatology: Pathophysiology and management of the newborn* (3rd ed.; pp. 264-298). Philadelphia: Lippincott.

Physical assessment

Blackburn, S. (1987). Sleep and awake states of the newborn. In K. Barnard (Ed.), *NCAST learning resource manual* (pp. 25-28). Seattle: University of Washington.

Bliss-Holtz, J. (1989). Comparison of rectal, axillary, and inguinal temperatures in full-term newborn infants. *Nursing Research,* 38(2), 85-87.

Kenner, C., Harjo, J., and Brueggemeyer, A. (1988). *Neonatal surgery: A nursing perspective.* Orlando, FL: Grune & Stratton.

Smith, D.W. (1988). Minor anomalies. In K.L. Jones (Ed.), *Smith's recognizable patterns of human malformation: Genetic, embryologic and clinical aspects* (4th ed.; pp. 662-681). Philadelphia: Saunders.

Nursing research

Beal, J.A. (1986). The Brazelton neonatal behavioral assessment scale: A tool to enhance parental attachment. *Journal of Pediatric Nursing,* 1(3), 170-177.

Brooten, D., Kumar, S., Brown, L.P., Butt, P., Finkler, S.A., Bakewell-Sachs, S., Gibbons, A., and Delivoria-Papadopoulos, M. (1986). A randomized clinical trial of early hospital discharge and home follow-up of very-low-birth-weight infants. *New England Journal of Medicine,* 315(15), 934-939.

Kayiatos, R., Adams, J., and Gilman, B. (1984). The arrival of a rival: Maternal perceptions of toddlers' regressive behaviors after the birth of a sibling. *Journal of Nurse-Midwifery,* 29(3), 205-213.

Kenner, C.A. (1988). *Parent transition from the newborn intensive care unit to home.* Unpublished doctoral dissertation, Indiana University, Indianapolis.

Morgan, J. (1987). What can nurses learn from structured observations of mother-infant interactions? *Issues in Comprehensive Pediatric Nursing,* 10(1), 67-73.

Care of the Normal Neonate

Objectives

After reading and studying this chapter, the student should be able to:

1. Identify the essential components of nursing care of the normal neonate.
2. Identify factors affecting neonatal thermoregulation.
3. Apply the nursing process to nursing care of the normal neonate.
4. Assess the parents' readiness to assume caregiving responsibilities and determine their teaching needs regarding neonatal care.
5. Develop a teaching plan for new parents to promote confidence in their caregiving abilities.
6. Describe nursing strategies that promote a positive parent-infant interaction.

Introduction

The neonate undergoes various physiologic changes during the neonatal period—the first 28 days after birth. To make a successful transition from dependent fetus, the neonate must adapt to these changes effectively, especially during the first 24 hours (known as the transitional period).

The nurse plays a crucial role during the neonatal period by promoting a stable physiologic status. For instance, the nurse maintains oxygenation, hydration, nutrition, elimination, hygiene, and thermoregulation; prevents and detects complications; and ensures environmental safety.

Neonatal nursing care also calls for a family-centered approach that helps ease the neonate's transition to the home and promotes a positive parent-infant in-

teraction. The nurse must assess parent-teaching needs regarding neonatal care and identify risk factors for poor parent-infant bonding. Parent teaching can be enhanced if the nurse serves as a caregiver role model and provides positive reinforcement during the parents' supervised attempts at caring for their child.

While providing care, the nurse must remain aware of cultural differences that may affect the parents' neonatal care decisions—for example, cultural attitudes toward circumcision. Considering these differences when planning, promoting, and implementing holistic neonatal and family care is essential.

This chapter describes how the nurse manages these responsibilities. It begins by describing the data that the nurse collects during ongoing neonatal assessment. Then the chapter discusses how to plan and implement nursing care, highlighting measures that ensure neonatal thermoregulation, safety, and hygiene as well as routine care measures (for instance, umbilical cord care). After describing how the nurse evaluates this care, the chapter concludes with a brief discussion of documentation.

Assessment

During the first few days after the neonate's birth, the nurse should conduct a comprehensive assessment (as described in Chapter 35, Neonatal Assessment).

GLOSSARY

Bonding: process through which an emotional attachment forms, which binds one person to another in an enduring relationship, as between parents and infant. Sometimes called attachment.

Circumcision: surgical removal of the prepuce (foreskin) covering the glans penis.

Incubator: fully enclosed, single-walled or double-walled bed containing a heating source and a humidification chamber.

Neutral thermal environment: range of environmental temperatures that maintains a stable core temperature with minimal caloric and oxygen consumption.

Pathologic jaundice: condition marked by yellow skin discoloration and an increase in the serum bilirubin level (above 13 mg/dl); arising within 24 hours after birth, it results from blood type or blood group incompatibility, infection, or biliary, hepatic, or metabolic abnormalities.

Physiologic jaundice: common condition of the full-term neonate marked by yellow skin discoloration and an increase in the serum bilirubin level (4 to 12 mg/dl); arising 48 to 72 hours after birth and peaking by the third to fifth day, it results from neonatal hepatic immaturity.

Radiant warmer: open bed with an overhead radiant heat source.

Respiratory distress syndrome: acute, potentially fatal neonatal lung disorder (most common in preterm neonates), resulting from surfactant deficiency; characterized by a respiratory rate greater than 60 breaths/minute, lung inelasticity, nasal flaring, expiratory grunts, chest retractions, and peripheral edema.

Smegma: sebaceous secretion that accumulates under the foreskin of the penis and at the base of the labia minora.

Transient tachypnea: neonatal disorder characterized by rapid, shallow breathing (possibly accompanied by cyanosis) that lasts a few hours or days; caused by the retention of fetal lung fluid that follows cesarean delivery.

Vernix caseosa: grayish white, cheeselike substance composed of sebaceous gland secretions and desquamated epithelial cells that covers the near-term fetus and neonate.

Throughout the neonate's hospitalization, however, the nurse should conduct ongoing assessment to ensure optimal neonatal adaptation and to detect changes in the neonate's status.

The nurse evaluates the neonate continually for obvious or subtle changes from baseline clinical findings (including heart and respiratory rate and rhythm, skin color, cry, response to stimuli, alertness level, and irritability level) or laboratory values. The nurse also assesses for indications of neonatal distress. These include:
• abdominal distention
• apprehensive facial expression
• bile-stained emesis
• cyanosis (other than acrocyanosis or periorbital cyanosis)
• excessive mucus production or meconium in the nasal passages
• frequent apneic episodes
• hypotonia during active and alert periods
• jaundice
• labored respirations accompanied by skin or mucous membrane color changes
• lethargy during periods of expected activity
• meconium-stained skin
• persistent, pronounced increase or decrease in heart and respiratory rates from baseline vital signs
• temperature instability.

Such distress could lead to serious complications. (For information on the comprehensive neonatal assessment and a thorough discussion of other characteristics to assess, see Chapter 35, Neonatal Assessment.)

Nursing diagnosis

After gathering assessment data, the nurse reviews it carefully to identify pertinent nursing diagnoses for the neonate. (For a partial list of applicable diagnoses, see *Nursing diagnoses: Normal neonate.*)

Planning and implementation

After assessing the neonate and formulating nursing diagnoses, the nurse develops and implements a plan of care. For the normal neonate, the plan centers on promoting optimal neonatal adaptation and parent-neonate interaction and includes such routine therapeutic interventions as umbilical cord care and vitamin K administration. Nursing goals include:

- ensuring oxygenation
- maintaining thermoregulation
- maintaining optimal hydration and nutrition
- promoting adequate urinary and bowel elimination
- providing hygienic care
- preventing and detecting complications
- ensuring environmental safety
- providing care for the family
- performing routine therapeutic interventions.

The American Academy of Pediatrics (1988) recommends that the neonate be kept in a transitional care or observation area in the nursery during the transition period to allow close observation. Then the neonate may be moved to the mother's room to avoid separating mother and neonate. This area should have oxygen and suction outlets, resuscitation equipment, and multiple electrical outlets with safety grounds.

Ensuring oxygenation

At birth, the neonate must begin breathing through the nose and drawing air into the lungs. Closure of the fetal shunts (ductus arteriosus, ductus venosus, and foramen ovale) after birth changes the circulatory direction and facilitates peripheral circulation and alveolar gas exchange. (See Chapter 34, Neonatal Adaptation, for more information on fetal shunt closure and neonatal respiration.) To ensure successful respiratory adaptation, maintaining adequate oxygenation is crucial.

A few hours after birth, the gastrointestinal (GI) tract begins secreting gastric juices; this leads to increased saliva and mucus production. Mucus production peaks in the first 2 to 3 days after birth. For the neonate with a nursing diagnosis of *ineffective airway clearance related to the presence of mucus,* suctioning with a bulb syringe or sterile catheter may be necessary to prevent aspiration of mucus. A bulb syringe may be kept at the neonate's bedside; clean it with warm, soapy water after each use to reduce the risk of bacterial growth. (For details on how to suction with a bulb syringe, see *Psychomotor skills: Performing routine neonatal care,* pages 880 to 884.)

A suction catheter should be used only if absolutely necessary because suctioning carries a risk of apnea, reflex bradycardia, cardiopulmonary arrest, and laryngospasm. For this procedure, the neonate is placed in a side-lying or prone position. Lubricate the end of the catheter with sterile water, then insert the catheter into the oral cavity without applying pressure. When the catheter reaches the pharynx, apply pressure for 5 seconds, then withdraw. After suctioning the pharynx, suction each naris (nostril). Before each new suctioning attempt, the catheter tip must be lubricated and the catheter rinsed with sterile water.

While suctioning, observe for skin and mucous membrane color changes. If the neonate is attached to a cardiopulmonary monitor, check for changes in the heart and respiratory rates. If the neonate becomes cyanotic (indicated by a bluish color), withdraw the catheter and stop suctioning. The amount and appearance of any secretions and the neonate's tolerance for the procedure should be documented.

An irregular respiratory pattern, including periodic breathing and slight chest retractions, is common in the first few hours after birth while the neonate adapts to the new environment. However, stay alert for changes in the respiratory pattern that persist for several hours or become increasingly severe; these may indicate respiratory distress. If skin or mucous membrane color changes from pink to dusky or cyanotic, check for grunting, nasal flaring, crackles, rhonchi, and other abnormal signs. The neonate with these signs may have a nursing diagnosis of *ineffective breathing pattern related to transition to the extrauterine environment.* Immediately report any significant deviations from normal cardiopulmonary parameters, and assess vital signs continually to help prevent complications.

Maintaining thermoregulation

The term neonate has protective mechanisms to promote heat conservation—layers of adipose tissue and areas of brown fat, most prominent over the scapula and flank. Brown fat supplies fatty acids for heat production (thermogenesis), a process that begins when the neonate starts to lose heat. To maintain a stable core temperature, the body breaks down fats, burns calories, consumes oxygen, and increases the metabolic rate.

The preterm neonate, in contrast, has insufficient adipose tissue and brown fat insulation and may suffer cold stress from heat loss. The posture of the preterm neonate also contributes to heat loss. Unlike the term neonate—who assumes a fetal position to reduce the exposed surface area and thus minimize convective heat loss—the preterm neonate lies flaccid with arms and legs extended, exposing a greater surface area.

Cold stress may occur in any neonate who is exposed to a cold environment without adequate protection or whose caloric expenditure exceeds caloric consumption. When oxygen and nutritional reserves are depleted, the neonate loses protein and muscle tissue as well as weight. Anabolic metabolism ensues, leading to metabolic acidosis.

To stabilize the neonate's body temperature and thus minimize oxygen, caloric, and fat expenditure, maintain a neutral thermal environment. This narrow temperature range maintains a stable core temperature with minimal caloric and oxygen consumption, allowing calories and oxygen to be used for growth and adaptation rather than thermoregulation. (For further information on the mechanisms of heat loss and gain, see Chapter 34, Neonatal Adaptation. For specific nursing measures that help prevent heat loss, see *Preventing heat loss in the neonate.*)

Throughout the neonate's nursery stay, enforce measures to conserve body heat—especially for the neonate with a nursing diagnosis of *potential altered body temperature related to radiant, conductive, convective, or evaporative heat loss.* For example, always keep the neonate dry; a warm, wet neonate loses heat to the surrounding environment through evaporation and convection. Keep the neonate's head covered at all times. The head accounts for 25% of the neonate's total body surface; substantial heat can be lost to surrounding cool surfaces and air through radiation, conduction, and convection unless the head is covered with a blanket, hat, or stockinette. (For more information on neonatal head coverings, see Chapter 34, Neonatal Adaptation.)

Even if the neonate is placed under a radiant warmer and dried to reduce heat loss, wide temperature fluctuations are common in the first few hours after birth. If the neonate has been in an open warmer for 2 to 3 hours and the core (rectal) temperature measures 96.8° (36° C), wrap the neonate in a blanket and place in an open, clear basinette. Monitor skin temperature, which should measure 32° to 32.9° F (0° to 0.5° C) below the core temperature (Carlo and Chatburn, 1988).

Using an incubator or radiant warmer

If the core temperature drops below an acceptable level, keep the neonate in a thermally controlled environment. Depending on health care facility policy, this may necessitate use of an incubator or a radiant warmer. (An incubator is a fully enclosed, single-walled or double-walled bed containing a heating source and a humidification chamber. A radiant warmer is an open bed with an overhead radiant heat source.) Because the neonate requires close observation during the transitional period, keep the incubator or radiant warmer in clear view at all times.

With an incubator, temperature can be controlled externally or servo-controlled by taping a flat probe to the neonate's skin and setting the thermostat to maintain a skin temperature of 96° to 97.7° F (35.5° to 36.5° C). Do not tape the probe to areas of brown fat, such as the scapula and flank; these areas generate more heat, causing a falsely elevated skin temperature reading. With

Preventing heat loss in the neonate

Preventing heat loss is an important part of neonatal nursing care. Heat loss can occur through four mechanisms—conduction, convection, evaporation, and radiation. The chart below describes some nursing measures that help prevent heat loss by each mechanism.

Conductive heat loss

- Preheat the radiant warmer bed and linen.
- Warm the stethoscope before use.
- Wrap the neonate in a warm blanket or allow the mother to hold the neonate to provide the warming effect of skin contact.
- Pad the scale with paper or a preweighed, warmed sheet to weigh the neonate.
- Check the temperature of any surface before placing the neonate on it.

Convective heat loss

- Place the neonate's bed out of direct line with an open window, a fan, or an air-conditioning vent.
- Cover the neonate with a blanket when moving the neonate to another area.
- Raise the sides of the radiant warmer bed to prevent exposing the neonate to air currents.
- Avoid using fans in the delivery room or nursery.

Evaporative heat loss

- Dry the neonate immediately after delivery.
- When the neonate is not in a warming bed, keep the neonate dry and swaddled in warmed blankets.
- Remove wet blankets.
- Delay the bath until the neonate's temperature is stable.
- When bathing the neonate, expose only one body part at a time; wash each part thoroughly, then dry it immediately.
- When assessing the neonate, uncover only the specific area to be assessed.
- Place a cap on the neonate's head in the delivery room.

Radiant heat loss

- Use a radiant heat warmer for initial post-delivery stabilization.
- Place the neonate in a double-walled incubator.
- Keep the neonate away from areas with cold surfaces (such as a cold formula bottle or a window in winter).

a radiant warmer, control the temperature by positioning the skin probe, then setting the thermostat of the bed to maintain a stable skin temperature.

Observing and intervening for cold stress

Signs of cold stress include an accelerated respiratory rate, labored respirations, and an increased metabolic rate accompanied by hypoglycemia (indicating greater use of glucose stores). In the neonate with a nursing diagnosis of *hypothermia related to cold stress*, check for signs of hypoglycemia, such as a serum glucose level below 30 mg/dl before the third day after birth or below 40 mg/dl on or after the third day. (For other laboratory values for the normal neonate, see *Normal neonatal laboratory values,* page 879).

Other signs of hypoglycemia include tremors, seizures, irritability and lethargy (from breakdown of fats and proteins to maintain body heat), and apnea or bradycardia (from changes in arterial oxygen saturation and a shift to anaerobic metabolism). Neurologic immaturity may prevent homeostasis in the hypoglycemic neonate, leading to unstable vital signs.

If the neonate suffers cold stress, rewarm gradually to avoid hyperthermia and its complications; closely observe the neonate and check vital signs every 15 to 30 minutes. Hyperthermia may cause skin reddening, irritability, and an initial increase—then gradual drop—in the heart and respiratory rates, leading to apnea and bradycardia. To prevent complications, report any status changes immediately.

Maintaining optimal hydration and nutrition

Hydration and nutrition are vital to immune system development and maintenance. The American Academy of Pediatrics (1988) recommends that the initial feeding never be delayed more than 6 hours after birth. If the mother plans to breast-feed, the neonate can be put to the breast in the delivery room.

Assessing the adequacy of fluid intake

To maintain adequate output and hydration and help avert a nursing diagnosis of *potential fluid volume deficit related to poor oral intake,* assess fluid intake frequently and compare it to urine output. The term neonate requires a fluid intake of 140 to 160 ml/kg/day to maintain hydration (Streeter, 1986). This requirement increases with illness, preterm birth, and excessive evaporative or radiant fluid loss. Urine output should measure 1 to 2 ml/kg/hour. In the first 24 hours after birth, the neonate may void only once or twice, although output from these first voidings exceeds output from later voidings.

The bottle-fed neonate who requires a diaper change every 2 to 3 hours is receiving adequate fluids. (Diapers should be moderately saturated.) The breast-fed neonate usually voids less frequently but at least six times a day. With any neonate, scanty or infrequent voiding (less than five times a day) suggests impaired fluid intake or a urinary problem. Document this finding and notify the physician.

Assessing for insensible fluid loss

The neonate experiences insensible fluid loss, such as radiant and evaporative fluid loss resulting from the transition to the relatively cool extrauterine environment. For the neonate with a nursing diagnosis of *potential fluid volume deficit related to insensible fluid loss*, assess for and guard against such loss, including that caused by environmental sources. For example, phototherapy (used to treat jaundice) increases GI motility, causing diarrhea and fluid loss in stool. Also, phototherapy increases radiant fluid loss by warming the neonate. (For specific interventions to maintain thermoregulation, see the previous section on "Maintaining thermoregulation.")

Giving the first feeding

For the first feeding, the bottle-fed neonate usually is given sterile water because it is less irritating than formula or glucose water if it is aspirated. (Some facilities suggest an initial sterile water feeding for the breast-fed neonate as well to determine if the neonate is prone to aspiration or other complications.) If the neonate takes the sterile-water feeding without problems, glucose water or formula then may be given. In some facilities, the neonate is given a few milliliters of sterile water followed by 15 to 30 ml of glucose water to prevent hypoglycemia.

During the first feeding, assess the neonate's sucking ability and observe how well the neonate coordinates the sucking, swallowing, and gag reflexes. Immediately after the feeding, check for salivation, mucus production, aspiration, and regurgitation. The neonate produces more saliva and mucus in the first few hours after birth than at later times. Consequently, regurgitation—especially of a combination of mucus and feeding matter—is common. To promote digestion, place the neonate in a right side-lying position, which allows food to move more easily through the stomach and into the GI tract for absorption. This intervention helps prevent a nursing diagnosis of *altered nutrition (less than body requirements) related to decreased oral intake and increased caloric expenditure*.

Continue to check for signs of excessive salivation or mucus production, which may indicate a blind esophageal pouch (esophageal atresia) or a fistula between the esophagus and trachea (tracheoesophageal fistula). A neonate who aspirates or regurgitates copious amounts of mucus or the entire feeding also may have esophageal atresia or a tracheoesophageal fistula.

Regurgitation after a feeding also may indicate an immature cardiac sphincter that allows reflux of feeding matter through the weak muscle. This condition may cause esophageal irritation from acidic gastric juices, possibly leading to aspiration. Projectile vomiting or bile-colored emesis indicates GI blockage. If the vomiting is accompanied by abdominal distention, suspect an intestinal obstruction—a condition that requires immediate intervention.

A neonate with excessive mucus production may require nasopharyngeal suctioning. Be sure to use caution when performing this procedure because it may trigger the gag reflex, causing aspiration.

To prevent aspiration and facilitate digestion, place the neonate in semi-Fowler's position after feeding. The neonate who becomes cyanotic or extremely fatigued during a feeding may have a cardiac or respiratory problem. A respiratory rate above 60 to 80 breaths/minute increases the risk of aspiration.

If aspiration or regurgitation occurs, stop the feeding immediately and allow the neonate to rest before attempting further feeding. Document the incident thoroughly, and report it for further assessment.

Supporting the parents' choice of feeding method

Optimal enteral nutrition may be achieved by breast-feeding, bottle-feeding, or both. Support the parents' choice of feeding method. Their choice may be based on such factors as economic and financial considerations, the mother's occupational status, and sociocultural influences as well as neonatal health implications. (For more information on feeding methods, see Chapter 37, Infant Nutrition.)

Promoting adequate urinary and bowel elimination

Urinary and bowel elimination must be adequate to maintain hydration and nutrition. Elimination patterns are established in the first few days after birth.

Urinary elimination patterns

Although the kidneys begin functioning in utero (fetal urine is the major component of amniotic fluid), the neonate's kidneys do not concentrate urine as effectively as an adult's. The neonate also has an immature glomerular filtration system (restricting elimination of water and solutes) and limited tubular reabsorption (impairing the ability of bicarbonate ions and buffers to maintain the glomerular filtration system at a homeostatic pH).

Monitoring for voiding onset

Despite the limitations described above, voiding should begin by 48 hours after birth. (Some neonates even void on the delivery table.) Over 90% of term neonates void within 24 hours of birth; all but 1% within 48 hours (Kim and Mandell, 1988). Failure to void within 48 hours may indicate a renal disorder, inadequate fluid intake, increased water loss, or fluid retention (edema). The neonate with any of these problems may have a nursing diagnosis of *altered patterns of urinary elimination related to renal immaturity*.

Assessing urine characteristics

Initially, urine should be cloudy and amber (from urinary protein, blood, and mucus); specific gravity should measure 1.005 to 1.015. In the female neonate, blood in the urine represents pseudomenstruation; in the circumcised male neonate, blood originates from the surgical site.

After the first 24 hours or so, urine should appear clear and amber. A specific gravity below 1.005 may indicate excessive fluid loss unless the neonate has been edematous and is eliminating excess fluids. A specific gravity above 1.025 may indicate fluid retention unless the neonate has been dehydrated (in which case it represents an attempt to restore fluid balance).

A deviation from the usual urinary pattern—too few or too many saturated diapers, a high specific gravity, or dilute urine—may warrant a nursing diagnosis of *altered patterns of urinary elimination related to inability to maintain fluid balance.* If the neonate is losing excessive fluids, check skin turgor and assess the fontanels and eye area. With dehydration, skin turgor is decreased and the anterior fontanel and eye orbits appear sunken. Edema, indicated by shiny, taut skin, may suggest fluid retention caused by a cardiac or renal disorder. All of these signs warrant further evaluation to help prevent complications.

Bowel elimination patterns

The first stool (usually passed in the delivery room or within 48 hours after birth) consists of meconium, a thick, dark green, sticky, odorless material made up of amniotic fluid and shed GI mucosal cells. Failure to pass meconium within 48 hours may indicate anal or bowel malformation or Hirschprung's disease (aganglionic megacolon), a congenital disorder characterized by incomplete bowel innervation.

Once feeding patterns have been established, stools change in color and consistency, the GI tract starts to secrete digestive enzymes, and intestinal bacteria (especially *Escherichia coli*) start to colonize. Transitional stools—thinner, lighter green, and seedier than meconium—then appear. After 2 or 3 days, stools change again, taking on distinctive characteristics that vary with the feeding method. (For details on characteristics of the neonate's stools, see Chapter 34, Neonatal Adaptation.)

Feeding method affects stool consistency and output. The stool of a breast-fed neonate is looser and paler yellow than that of a formula-fed neonate. Also, the breast-fed neonate typically passes 2 to 10 stools daily; the formula-fed neonate usually passes one stool daily or every other day.

Assess for deviations in stool pattern or consistency. A neonate with such a deviation may have a nursing diagnosis of *diarrhea related to GI immaturity* or *constipation related to GI immaturity*. If the neonate has diarrhea, a condition that increases fluid loss, assess for signs of dehydration (described above). If the neonate fails to pass stool or passes a hard, ribbon-like stool, suspect an intestinal obstruction. Also assess for abdominal distention, and palpate the abdomen for fecal masses. Observe the neonate during and just after feeding; an abdominal obstruction may cause vomiting and irritability at these times. Report any problem with stools, feedings, and related changes in the neonate's status so that prompt diagnosis and treatment can begin.

Providing hygienic care

Maintaining hygiene is an important aspect of neonatal care. The skin's epidermal layer protects against traumatic injury, helps minimize heat loss, and serves as a barrier against bacterial infection by maintaining the pH of the skin at 4.9.

Bathing the neonate

Because scented, medicated, and harsh soaps can alter the pH of the skin, use only mild soap (or the soap specified by the health care facility) when bathing the neonate. To prevent cross-contamination and bacterial growth, a soap dispenser should be assigned for each neonate. Avoid scrubbing the skin because this may cause abrasions through which microorganisms can enter.

To guard against heat loss during bathing, bathe the neonate only after temperature and vital signs have stabilized—especially if the core temperature is below normal. In the first hour or so after birth, use a soft sterile cotton pad soaked with warm water to remove dried blood, meconium, and debris arising from delivery; then dry the skin thoroughly. Removing these contaminants reduces the risk of infection by the hepatitis B, herpes simplex, and human immunodeficiency viruses (American Academy of Pediatrics, 1988). Also, gently wash off the vernix caseosa, the grayish white substance that covers the skin of the term neonate.

Proceed from head to toe, washing the cleanest areas first to reduce the risk of infection from any contaminated areas and help avoid a nursing diagnosis of *potential for infection related to transition to the extrauterine en-*

vironment. Do not immerse the neonate in a tub; this could cause chilling or infection of the umbilical cord or an unhealed circumcision. During bathing, inspect the neonate's body for such variations as skin tags, unusual hair distribution, palmar creases, and other minor abnormalities. These variations may indicate more serious abnormalities. (For more information, see Chapter 35, Neonatal Assessment.)

Assess the neonate's response to each portion of the bath. For example, a change in appearance or skin color may indicate stress, fatigue, or chilling. (If any of these changes occurs, stop the bath immediately and dry the neonate.) Observe for drainage (exudate), discoloration, swelling, and redness around the eyes, which may signal infection or chemical irritation.

Washing the neonate's hair and scalp may decrease the risk of seborrheic dermatitis (cradle cap)—a potential cause of skin breakdown and infection. However, cradle cap also may occur in a neonate whose hair is washed frequently. The exact cause of this condition remains unknown.

Wash the neonate's face only after feedings, if milk or formula remains on the skin. If necessary, wash the chin and mouth more often. (For an illustrated procedure of techniques used to clean the scalp and face, see *Psychomotor skills: Performing routine neonatal care*, pages 880 to 884.)

After drying the neonate's head and face, wash the rest of the body one part at a time, covering each part immediately after drying it to avoid evaporative heat loss. In the female neonate, clean the perineal region from front to back, proceeding from the cleanest area to the most soiled. In the male neonate, gently clean the penis to remove smegma. Use plain warm water or soapy water followed by a plain warm water rinse. Gently pat the penis dry to avoid causing abrasions. Some health care facilities recommend applying a thin layer of petrolatum gauze or a bactericidal ointment over the circumcision site.

In the uncircumcised male, gently retract the foreskin until encountering resistance, then expose the glans penis. If the foreskin cannot be retracted, do not force it; simply wash the penis as is. Make sure to return a retracted foreskin to its natural position—the neonate's skin is so tight that the foreskin rarely retracts on its own; the glans may become inflamed and swollen if the foreskin is left retracted. Next, lift the scrotal sac—a potential infection source because of accumulated stool—and wash the underlying surface.

Wash the anal region from front to back to avoid cross-contamination from stool and dry the area thoroughly. Also clean the buttocks and genitalia at each diaper change to prevent infection and skin irritation.

Excessive bathing—more frequently than every other day—may dry the skin, increasing the infection risk. Although relatively aggressive washing may be needed to remove the vernix caseosa and dried blood found in natural creases (such as the neck, axillae, and groin), always use care to keep the skin intact.

Ensuring safety during bathing

All neonates have a nursing diagnosis of *potential for injury related to slippage while bathing.* Make sure to maintain a secure grip while bathing the neonate. Support the head, back, and shoulders by placing one hand under the neonate's arm. Using the forearm, support the neonate's back and head; wash with the other hand. Then dry each body part thoroughly. Immediately place the neonate in a bath blanket, making sure the neonate is thoroughly dry. Then redress and swaddle in a dry blanket.

Preventing and detecting complications

To prevent and detect neonatal complications, assess continually, staying alert for subtle changes in the neonate's condition. Document and report any changes immediately. Also monitor laboratory values and report any deviations (see *Normal neonatal laboratory values*). (For a more detailed discussion of complications occurring in neonates, see Chapter 38, High-Risk Neonates.)

Respiratory dysfunction

The most common neonatal complication, respiratory dysfunction may be mild (such as transient tachypnea) or severe (such as respiratory distress syndrome). In a neonate with a nursing diagnosis of *ineffective breathing pattern related to respiratory dysfunction,* stay alert for respiratory distress by assessing for changes in the respiratory rate and effort and checking for accompanying skin color changes, such as duskiness or cyanosis. If cyanosis is present, supplemental oxygen may be necessary. Be sure to allow the neonate to rest between nursing procedures to minimize oxygen consumption. (For additional information about respiratory distress syndrome, which is common among preterm neonates, see Chapter 38, High-Risk Neonates).

Hypocalcemia

The neonate who experienced birth asphyxia, is premature, or was born of an insulin-dependent diabetic mother is at risk for hypocalcemia (a serum calcium level below 7 mg/dl). Hypocalcemia also may occur if enteral feedings must be delayed (such as in the neurologically impaired neonate). Signs of hypocalcemia include twitching of extremities, cyanosis, apneic episodes, seizures, and listlessness. To detect hypocalcemia early and help prevent complications, monitor the serum calcium level. Expect to give enteral or parental calcium supplements to a hypocalcemic neonate.

Physiologic jaundice

Physiologic jaundice (yellow skin discoloration accompanied by an increased serum bilirubin level) is a common neonatal complication resulting from hepatic immaturity. It develops in the full-term neonate 48 to 72 hours after birth. Suspect physiologic jaundice if the neonate's skin appears abnormally yellow. To verify the disorder, apply pressure to the tip of the neonate's nose. With jaundice, a yellow tinge appears instead of the normal blanching as circulation is impeded. (This test is accurate in dark-skinned as well as light-skinned neonates.)

If the neonate has jaundice, pathologic jaundice must be ruled out. Unlike physiologic jaundice, pathologic jaundice develops within 24 hours. (For details on assessing jaundice, see Chapter 35, Neonatal Assessment. For a description of the various forms of physiologic jaundice, see Chapter 34, Neonatal Adaptation. For details on pathologic jaundice, see Chapter 38, High-Risk Neonates.)

Infection

Infection, another common complication, stems from immunologic immaturity. Thorough hand washing significantly reduces the risk of neonatal infection and may help avoid a nursing diagnosis of *potential for infection related to immunologic immaturity.* Before and after performing any nursing procedure, wash the hands. Also emphasize to parents the importance of frequent hand washing and proper hand-washing technique.

Because the neonate does not have localized immune reactions, infection causes only subtle, nonspecific signs. Such signs may include a high, low, or unstable body temperature; a weak or high-pitched cry; pallor; cyanosis; feeding problems or fatigue after feedings; diminished peripheral perfusion causing reduced skin temperature; sudden onset of apneic or bradycardic episodes; and jaundice.

If the neonate has signs that suggest infection, immediately document and report them. Obtain vital signs every 1 to 2 hours, observe closely for behavioral changes, and expect the physician to order a complete diagnostic workup for sepsis. Depending on health care facility policy and updated recommendations from the Centers for Disease Control, isolation procedures may be necessary.

Neonatal ophthalmia, an eye infection caused by *Neisseria gonorrhoea* or *Chlamydia trachomatis,* can be prevented if 1% silver nitrate solution, 1% tetracycline ointment, or 0.5% erythromycin ointment is applied to

Normal neonatal laboratory values

The physician may order various laboratory tests to check for such neonatal complications as infection, hematologic problems, and metabolic disorders (such as hypoglycemia). The chart below shows normal laboratory values for commonly ordered tests. However, because values differ among laboratories, the nurse must check the values for the laboratory used.

TEST	NORMAL VALUES
Hematocrit	51% to 56%
Hemoglobin	16.5 g/dl (cord blood)
Platelets	150,000 to 400,000/mm³
Serum electrolytes Bicarbonate	18 to 23 mEq/liter
Calcium	7 to 10 mg/dl
Carbon dioxide	15 to 25 mEq/liter
Chloride	90 to 114 mEq/liter
Potassium	4 to 6 mEq/liter
Sodium	135 to 148 mEq/liter
Serum glucose	40 to 80 mg/dl
Total protein	4 to 7 g/dl
White blood cell total	18,000/mm³
White blood cell differential Band neutrophils	1,600/mm³ (9%)
Segmented neutrophils	9,400/mm³ (52%)
Eosinophils	400/mm³ (2.2%)
Basophils	100/mm³ (0.6%)
Lymphocytes	5,500/mm³ (31%)
Monocytes	1,050/mm³ (5.8%)

the eyes shortly after delivery. (Tetracycline and erythromycin are less irritating than silver nitrate.) Previously, the medication was administered in the delivery room. However, in many facilities, the procedure now is delayed until the neonate arrives in the nursery. This allows clear vision during the first period of reactivity, facilitating parent-infant bonding. (For details on administering eye medication, see *Psychomotor skills: Performing routine neonatal care,* pages 880 to 884.)

(Text continues on page 884.)

Performing routine neonatal care

During routine neonatal care, the nurse may perform such procedures as cleaning the neonate's scalp and face, suctioning with a bulb syringe, administering I.M injections, instilling eye medications, performing heel sticks, and obtaining urine specimens. The instructions below provide guidelines for these procedures.

Cleaning the scalp and face

The nurse who bathes a neonate should expose only one area at a time, washing and drying thoroughly before exposing the next area. Follow these steps to ensure safety when cleaning the scalp and face.

1 Hold the neonate in the football position, which supports the back and head and frees one hand for bathing.

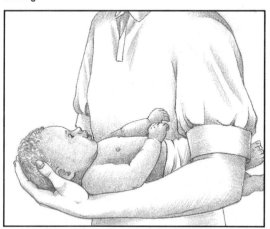

2 If shampooing is necessary, extend the neonate's head slightly while keeping the neonate supine, and tilt the head backward over a small basin. This position allows water to run from the front to the back of the head, preventing soapy water from getting into the neonate's eyes. Gently lather the scalp in a circular motion by hand or with a small cloth or soft brush containing mild, nonmedicated shampoo.

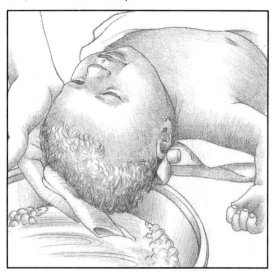

3 To rinse, fill a small cup with tepid water and pour the water over the scalp. Dry the hair quickly and thoroughly with a soft towel to minimize heat loss.

4 To wash the eyes, wrap a small washcloth around one hand so that no ends dangle. (This reduces the risk of dragging a wet cloth across the neonate, which could cause chilling from the dripping water or cross-contamination from contact with a soiled surface.) Moisten the washcloth with water, then gently stroke from the inner aspect of the lacrimal duct to the outer portion of the eyelid.

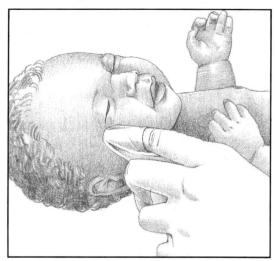

5 Wash the ears by wrapping a cloth around one finger and gently cleaning the external part of the ear (including the posterior portion). Never use a cotton-tipped applicator to clean the ears because this may damage the delicate internal ear structures and lead to infection.

6 To clean the nose, insert the twisted end of a washcloth into the naris (nostril). Remove any crusted matter or nasal secretions at the surface of the nostril. To help detect excessive nasal drainage (which may indicate infection), document any nasal drainage and secretions.

7 Next, wash each side of the face with mild soap.

Suctioning with a bulb syringe

If the neonate has excess mucus in the respiratory tract, the nurse may need to aspirate the mouth and nasal passages using a bulb syringe. To perform this procedure, which demands skill and sensitivity to touch, follow these steps.

1 Depress the bulb to remove air. Then insert the tip of the syringe into the neonate's mouth until it reaches the pharyngeal area.

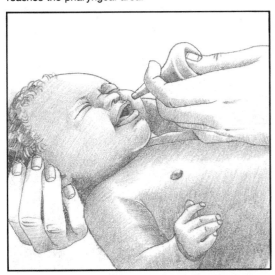

2 Suction one side of the mouth by releasing the bulb end of the syringe. This action pulls the mucus into the tip of the syringe.

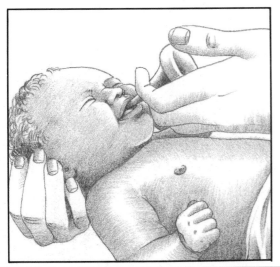

3 Suction the other side of the mouth the same way. Be sure to avoid touching the midline of the throat because this could activate the gag reflex.

4 Finally, suction the nasal passages, one nostril at a time, using the same approach.

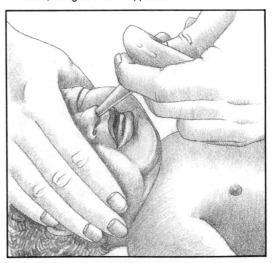

Administering eye preparations

Eye prophylaxis is an essential part of neonatal nursing care. Most states require the administration of 1% silver nitrate ophthalmic solution, 1% tetracycline ointment, or 0.5% erythromycin ointment to prevent ophthalmia neonatorum, a severe eye infection.

To administer the medication, wash the hands thoroughly. Position the neonate securely so that the head remains still. While holding the eyelid open, instill the medication into the conjunctival sac. Repeat with the other eye.

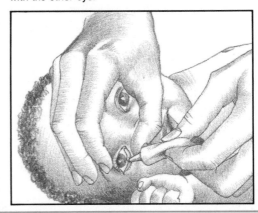

(continued)

Performing routine neonatal care continued

Giving an I.M. injection

When caring for the normal neonate, the nurse may have to administer prophylactic vitamin K or other medications by I.M. injection. In most cases, a 25-gauge (25G), ⅝" needle should be used to allow medication to reach the muscle without causing excessive pain or trauma. A 22G needle is warranted only for thick medications, such as some penicillins.

Before administering any medication, confirm the route, dose, time, and medication, and cross-check the neo-

1 Put on clean gloves to guard against contamination from potentially infected blood. Then examine and palpate the neonate's leg above the knee and below the groin fold to determine how much muscle tissue is present. To find a safe injection site away from the bone and nerves, palpate along the femur. Place two fingers below the groin fold and two fingers above the knee. The thigh surface between these areas contains much muscle tissue and no major blood vessels or nerves, making it a good choice for injection.

The injection may be given along the top of the thigh or in the vastus lateralis, along the side of the thigh above the femur (the shaded area in the illustration). Do not give the injection in the buttocks; because the muscle mass here is not well developed, the needle or medication can enter a major vessel or nerve more easily.

2 To keep the neonate still and reduce tissue trauma, gently restrain the leg. If possible, ask an assistant to help with this; as one person holds the leg, the other can give the injection.

If a pinchable amount of muscle or a large, solid muscle mass is palpated (as in a term neonate), stretch the skin and hold it taut. This reduces the risk of medication entering the subcutaneous tissue. If the muscle is small and soft to a gentle pinch with little palpable mass, gently pinch about 1 cm of skin during needle insertion to allow the injection to reach the muscle mass.

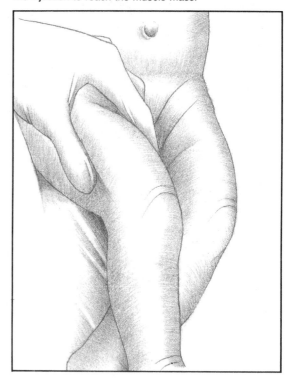

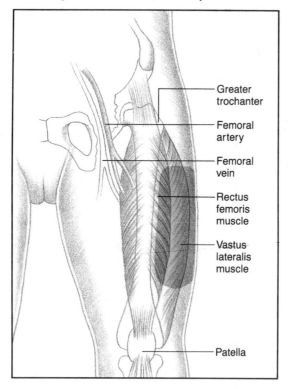

- Greater trochanter
- Femoral artery
- Femoral vein
- Rectus femoris muscle
- Vastus lateralis muscle
- Patella

nate's identification with the medication order and identification bracelet. Also check the neonate's history for reactions to previous medications; although rare, medication or allergic reactions do occur in neonates. Check the

medication record for the previously used injection site. To minimize bruising and increase medication absorption, rotate the injection site from one leg to the other.

To administer the injection, follow these steps.

3 Without releasing the leg, aim the needle at a 90-degree angle toward the thigh. Then, using a quick, darting wrist motion, insert the needle almost down to the hub.

Next, release the skin that has been pinched or stretched. Gently aspirate the plunger to check for a flash of blood. Blood indicates that the needle has pricked a blood vessel; if the medication enters the vessel, an adverse reaction may result. If blood appears, withdraw the needle immediately. Then discard the needle and start the procedure over, using new medication and a new syringe and needle.

If no blood appears, inject the medication steadily by applying gentle pressure on the plunger. When the barrel is empty, withdraw the needle quickly by pulling it straight out (this makes the injection less painful). Do not recap the needle—this may lead to an accidental needle stick. Instead, keep it out of the neonate's reach until it can be discarded.

4 Massage the site with alcohol and soothe the neonate. Besides having a quieting effect, massage increases circulation and enhances medication absorption. In most cases, the site does not need to be covered by an adhesive bandage because any bleeding that occurs is minimal and stops rapidly. Also, removing the bandage might tear the skin, causing more pain than a small injection site.

Performing a heel stick
In some facilities, the nurse who cares for normal neonates is required to perform a heel stick to obtain blood for measurement of glucose level and hematocrit. The blood also is used to test for phenylketonuria, galactosemia, and hypothyroidism.

1 Before beginning, wash the hands and put on gloves. Next, clean the neonate's heel with alcohol and dry with a sterile 2″ x 2″ gauze pad.

2 Choose a capillary site for venipuncture (as shown in the shaded area) to avoid the plantar artery.

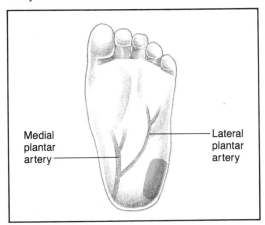

Medial plantar artery   Lateral plantar artery

3 Using the appropriate blade, quickly puncture the heel deeply enough to trigger a free flow of blood. Discard the first drop by wiping it away with another sterile gauze pad.

4 Collect blood into the appropriate capillary tubes. Clean the heel of any blood and cover with a bandage.

(continued)

Performing routine neonatal care continued

Obtaining a urine specimen from a urine collection bag

The nurse may collect a urine specimen from a neonate for routine urinalysis, cultures, specific gravity measurement, or other studies. Follow these steps when using a urine collection bag to obtain the specimen.

1 Remove the diaper and place the neonate in the supine position. With a male neonate, clean the urinary meatus, if soiled, with water and a towelette. Then clean the meatus with povidone-iodine swabs, using one swab for each stroke.

With a female neonate, clean the labia from front to back to avoid contamination from the anal area. Next, clean the urinary meatus with water and a towelette, then with povidone-iodine swabs, again using a front-to-back motion.

2 In an uncircumcised male, retract the foreskin until resistance is met, then clean the glans with povidone-iodine swabs. Release the foreskin, returning it to its natural position. In the circumcised male, clean the glans penis in the same manner.

3 To place the urine collection bag over the urinary meatus, remove the tabs from either side of the bag and uncover the adhesive sides. With a female neonate, apply the bag one side at a time to the labia majora and extend the tab to the femoral (groin) fold.

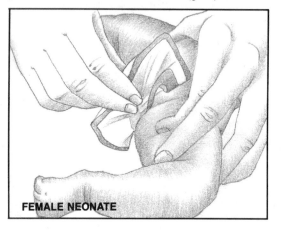

FEMALE NEONATE

With a male neonate, place the bag over the urinary meatus in the same manner, enclosing the penis and scrotum in the bag if possible.

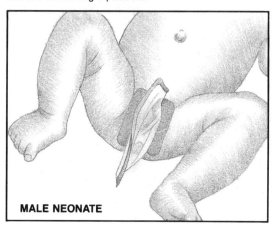

MALE NEONATE

With any neonate, make sure the bag does not cover the anus, because this may contaminate the specimen. After the bag has been positioned, press the tabs in place to ensure a secure fit. If the adhesive does not hold, apply a small amount of benzoin tincture to the skin under the tab to help keep the bag in place. However, use benzoin tincture only if absolutely necessary; the strong adhesion it provides may deter removal of the bag and can cause irritation.

4 Place a clean diaper over the bag and secure it. The diaper holds the bag in place and collects any stool or overflow from the bag.

5 When 1 to 2 ml of urine has been obtained, gently remove the bag and observe for skin irritation. Aspirate the specimen with a syringe, then place the specimen in a sterile plastic tube or culture bottle and send it to the laboratory immediately.

6 Document that a specimen was obtained and sent to the laboratory.

Ensuring environmental safety

Environmental safety is an important concern of neonatal nursing, particularly for the neonate with a nursing diagnosis of *potential for injury related to environmental influences during transition to the extrauterine environment.*

To ensure environmental safety, verify that room lighting is strong enough to allow accurate observation of skin color and respiratory effort, a clock is kept within easy view, and noise is held to the lowest level possible. Also, room temperature should be kept consistent and humidity maintained at 35% to 60% (American Academy of Pediatrics, 1988). Besides promoting thermoregulation, this intervention helps prevent drying of the mucous membranes, which can permit infectious agents to enter the respiratory tract. If necessary, drafts should be sealed off and window shades drawn to minimize neonatal heat loss.

Consider safety when providing all care measures. For instance, after a feeding, position the neonate on the abdomen or the right side to facilitate digestion. Keep the head of the bed elevated approximately 30 degrees to reduce the risk of aspiration. Do not allow pillows, toys, or stuffed animals in the neonate's bed; these items could cause suffocation if they fall onto the neonate's head.

A neonate will move about easily on any flat surface, increasing the risk of falling. Never look away or leave the neonate unattended during weighing or bathing. Before leaving the neonate's bedside, make sure the crib side rails are up and in the locked position.

When the neonate is ready for discharge, confirm that an infant car seat (not a carrier seat, which cannot be locked into place) is available for the trip home. Most states require such seats for children under age 4.

Providing care for the family

Nursing care must involve the entire family—not just the neonate. By facilitating bonding and offering parent teaching, the nurse can help prepare the family for the neonate's discharge.

Promoting parent-infant bonding

Bonding—the reciprocal relationship between parents and infant—may begin even before delivery. For instance, many parents imagine how their child will look and act or may think of the child as male or female. This helps the parents adjust after the neonate's arrival.

How easily a couple makes the transition to parenthood depends on many variables, including their ages, length of time they have been together, previous experience with children, available social support, teaching needs, coping patterns, perception of the neonate, and knowledge of neonatal behavior. Various relationships—between the parents, among the parents and any existing children, and among siblings—also play a role in the assumption of the parenting role.

The parents' perceptions of their parenting abilities also affect bonding. Many new parents have doubts about their ability to care for a dependent person, leading to a nursing diagnosis of *potential altered parenting related to transition to the role of parent.* Through parent teaching, help the parents understand their child's needs and abilities and recognize their child's unique characteristics. For example, call attention to the neonate's positive responses to the parents' initial caregiving attempts. Such responses include recognizing each parent's voice; smiling when a parent smiles; self-quieting when crying or quieting in response to a parent's consoling efforts; and taking feedings well from parents. Seeing these responses usually reassures parents about their parenting skills and reinforces their efforts to care for their child. In turn, as their parenting skills increase, their concerns diminish.

Bonding between parents and infant increases after delivery and continues to grow in the coming days through skin contact. The parents usually examine their child for physical features that link their child with the rest of the family. Immediately after delivery, for instance, the mother typically moves her fingers gently over the neonate's body to mark its boundaries. Putting the neonate to the breast and successfully breast-feeding reinforce the mother's confidence in her ability to nourish her child.

If the parents were unable to see or touch their child in the delivery room, they may fear that bonding will not occur. Reassure them that it will and that the neonate will be ready to interact with them when the sleep phase (which follows the first period of reactivity) ends and the second period of reactivity begins. Also, emphasize the neonate's unique qualities each time the parents interact with their child.

Ask the parents to describe the child they imagined during the pregnancy—for example, a son or daughter, a light-haired or dark-haired child. If their child does not conform to this image, they may need to mourn the loss of the imagined child before they can bond with the real one.

Providing parent teaching

Ongoing parent teaching is an essential part of discharge planning. Such teaching includes bathing, providing cord and diaper rash care, changing diapers, observing stool and voiding patterns, ensuring environmental safety, and integrating the neonate into the family. (For details, see *Parent teaching: Caring for your infant,* pages 886 and 887. For information on discharge planning, see Chapter 40, Discharge Planning and Neonatal Care at Home.)

The nurse also should serve as a caregiver role model for the parents and reinforce their caregiving behaviors. Steele (1987) found that active parental involvement in neonatal care before discharge led to a strong parent-infant bond. If the neonate is rooming-in with the mother or if visiting hours are unrestricted, the parents can observe the nurse caring for the neonate, then practice care in a supervised setting as the nurse offers positive reinforcement and constructive criticism. This promotes the parents' self-confidence.

Encourage the parents to ask questions about the neonate or the required care. Also urge them to interact

PARENT TEACHING

Caring for your infant

Basic infant care techniques include bathing, diaper changing, umbilical cord care, and environmental safety measures. These help ensure your infant's well-being, and they give you an opportunity to learn about your infant's personality and temperament and to bond through close contact. The guidelines and techniques described below will help you provide the best possible care.

Bathing your infant

• Use only nonmedicated, unscented soap. A harsh soap may alter the skin's pH and impair the skin's ability to provide a barrier against infection. Also, be sure to use a mild shampoo, such as a baby shampoo or an unscented product, to reduce the risk of chemical irritation of your infant's eyes from the soap.
• Before bathing your infant, test bath water temperature; it should be warm to the touch.
• Use a firm grasp to hold your infant. Never let go because the infant might slide down in the tub or fall out.
• Do not immerse your infant in a tub until the umbilical cord and circumcision site (if present) have healed be-

cause these are potential infection sites. Wash the umbilical cord and circumcision site with water and pat dry gently. Avoid excessive rubbing.
• The use of powder after a bath is unnecessary and possibly unsafe. Powder particles that disperse into the air may enter the infant's lungs. If these particles are inhaled, they could cause irritation and infection.
• Baby oil after a bath is not recommended. The extra lubrication it provides is unnecessary and may block skin pores. Also, it makes the infant slippery and harder to hold during bathing.

Providing umbilical cord care

• The umbilical cord dries gradually during the first week, then falls off. To clean the cord, gently rub its surface with alcohol swabs or cotton balls saturated with rubbing alcohol. Lift the cord away from the abdomen, then coat the stump or base with alcohol. (This is the area most likely to become infected.)
• Call the physician if you see pus or drainage at the

base of the cord or if the cord remains moist. Pus or drainage may indicate infection. The physician may recommend a 1% silver nitrate solution to dry a moist cord.
• To keep the cord as dry and bacteria-free as possible, fold the diaper down below the cord and avoid giving your infant tub baths.

Changing diapers

• Clean and dry the perineal area, observing for diaper rash (for a girl, always clean the perineal area from front to back; for a boy, always be sure to clean and dry under and around the scrotum). Then place a cloth or disposable diaper on the infant. For a snug fit, wrap the diaper from back to front, then check for gaps at the waist and abdominal areas and around the thighs. (If the diaper is not secure, stool or urine will leak, soiling the infant and bed and possibly causing chilling.) However, make sure the diaper is loose enough to allow the legs to move freely.
• For a boy wearing cloth diapers, fold the diaper so that a double thickness covers the penis. If the infant has been circumcised, allow enough room in front so that

the cloth does not irritate the circumcision site.
• When diapering a girl, keep in mind that urine will fall to the front of the diaper when the infant lies on her stomach and to the back when she is on her back.
• If your infant develops a diaper rash after wearing disposable diapers, consider switching to cloth diapers, which allow air to reach the skin surface and promote healing. However, do not place a disposable diaper over a cloth diaper because this will seal in moisture and may promote bacterial growth.
• If your infant is wearing cloth diapers, use a mild detergent when laundering and rinse these items thoroughly to ensure soap removal.

Caring for your infant's circumcision site

• The circumcision site may appear yellow in light-skinned neonates and lighter than the surrounding skin in dark-skinned neonates. This signifies healing and is not a cause for concern. Observe the circumcision site regularly for pus or bloody discharge, which may indicate delayed healing or infection. If these signs appear, call the physician.

• The rim of the device used for circumcision may remain in place after discharge. Do not be alarmed if you find the rim in your infant's bed; typically, it falls off 3 or 4 days after circumcision. If the rim does not come loose 1 week after the circumcision, call the physician. A retained rim may lead to infection.

(continued)

Caring for your infant continued

Monitoring stool patterns

• Report any changes in your infant's stool pattern or appearance—especially if they are accompanied by fever or behavioral changes, such as irritability or fussiness.
• If your infant cries excessively with a bowel movement or produces small, hard fecal pellets, constipation may be the cause. This problem usually can be corrected by giving additional water between feedings or by introducing fruit juice (if the physician approves).
• In some cases, constipation results from iron supplements or from iron-containing infant formula. If this happens, the physician may recommend that you switch to another formula.

• Diarrhea may result from a particular infant formula, introduction of new foods, teething, or—in the breast-fed infant—changes in the mother's diet. If your infant normally passes stool only once a day but begins to pass loose, watery stools more than 5 times in a 24-hour period, notify the physician. Diarrhea may lead to excess fluid loss.
• In a breast-fed infant, loose, watery stools or a water ring appearing in the diaper around more solid fecal matter may indicate infection. If this sign appears, call the physician. Loose, seedy, dark-green stools with a foul odor suggest an intestinal infection.

Monitoring voiding patterns

• The infant's urine should appear amber and clear. Although usually odorless, it occasionally may take on an ammonia-like odor, which is normal.

• Five diaper changes a day indicate adequate urine output. (The diapers should be at least moderately saturated.)

Ensuring environmental safety

• Maintain adequate temperature and humidity in the infant's room. Keep room temperature at 80° F for the first week, then 75° F. Keep the humidity level at 35% to 70% to maintain moist mucous (nasal) membranes (which serve as an important infection barrier).
• If your infant has nasal secretions that must be removed, remove them with a bulb syringe. Depress the bulb to remove air, then insert the syringe in the infant's

nostrils and release the bulb to withdraw the secretions. This technique adequately removes most nasal secretions without injuring the inside of the nostrils.
• Never prop a formula bottle against the infant because this may lead to inhalation of formula or otitis media (middle ear infection). Bottle propping also eliminates an opportunity for the closeness and touch between you and your infant that is necessary for bonding.

Providing visual and auditory stimulation

• Keep in mind that your infant can see bright objects and will follow a brightly colored ball or a human face. To provide visual stimulation, hang a mobile over the infant's bed. A mobile that turns is better than a stationary mobile because it offers greater variation.
• To provide auditory stimulation or quiet the infant,

place a radio (on low volume) or a music box in the infant's room.
• Because infants can become used to noise, you do not have to reduce the noise level in your home when the infant sleeps. Some infants even sleep better with quiet music in the room.

with the neonate to enhance bonding. For parents with a nursing diagnosis of *anxiety related to lack of confidence in parenting ability,* explain how to detect early signs of potential problems, such as cold stress, infection, and dehydration to help prevent life-threatening complications. The parents may be eager for their child to establish regular sleep-awake and eating patterns. However, inform them that the neonate typically sleeps 10 to 20 hours a day at first. Also emphasize that sleep patterns vary and that a deviation from the typical pattern does not necessarily indicate an abnormality.

Point out that the mother will have an increased need for support after discharge and would benefit by having relatives or friends available to help her. This is especially important for the single mother who may have to serve as the sole caregiver.

Performing routine therapeutic interventions

Routine nursing care of the normal neonate includes umbilical cord care, vitamin K administration, circumcision care, and collection of urine specimens.

Providing umbilical cord care

Immediately after birth, the umbilical cord is moist, making it an excellent breeding ground for bacteria. To avoid a nursing diagnosis of *potential for infection related to umbilical cord healing,* aim to promote drying of the cord and prevent infection. Depending on health care facility policy, one of several methods may be used to clean the cord. The American Academy of Pediatrics (1988) does not recommend a particular method.

The first method entails cleaning the cord by wiping the surface gently with an alcohol swab or a cotton ball saturated with isopropyl alcohol. Pay particular attention to the base of the cord because this area is most likely to become infected. To make sure the base is coated with alcohol, lift the cord away from the abdomen when wiping.

The second method entails use of an antibiotic ointment (such as bacitracin) instead of alcohol to clean the cord. The antibiotic may prevent bacterial growth. However, not all physicians believe such treatment is necessary.

With either method, note any drainage, such as blood, urine, or pus, appearing at the cord. Document and report such drainage so that cultures can be taken and antibiotic therapy initiated, if necessary. Urine leakage may indicate a patent urachus (a fetal structure between the bladder and umbilicus); this condition requires surgical intervention.

Typically, the umbilical cord dries and falls off within the first 2 weeks after birth. Until this happens, fold down the disposable diaper below the cord, turning the plastic layer away from the skin. To keep the area as dry and bacteria-free as possible, avoid giving the neonate tub baths.

Administering vitamin K

The neonate has a vitamin K deficiency, which results partly from lack of intestinal bacterial flora necessary to synthesize vitamin K. Because only small amounts of bacterial flora cross the placenta, this deficiency continues until enteral feedings are established and milk or formula is digested. Without sufficient vitamin K, the liver cannot synthesize coagulation factors II, VII, IX, and X (Streeter, 1986). This deficiency predisposes the neonate to hemorrhage and may lead to a nursing diagnosis of *potential for trauma related to inability to process vitamin K.* Thus, the American Academy of Pediatrics (1988) recommends a prophylactic I.M. injection of 0.5 to 1 mg of vitamin K_1 (phytonadione) during the first hour after birth. (For an illustrated procedure of I.M. injection in the neonate, see *Psychomotor skills: Performing routine neonatal care,* pages 880 to 884.)

Caring for a circumcision site

Circumcision refers to the surgical removal of the prepuce (foreskin) that covers the glans penis. To perform circumcision, the physician may use a device that has two parts—a small, bell-shaped plastic structure with a cylinder-shaped handle that the physician holds during the procedure and a rim that slides over the glans. After securing the rim over the glans and suturing it in place, the physician trims away the foreskin. Because the rim remains in place until the penis heals (about 3 to 4 days), the neonate may be discharged with the rim in place.

Circumcision has become controversial. The traditional rationale for the procedure was that it promotes hygiene and helps prevent penile and cervical cancers, urinary tract infections, and sexually transmitted diseases. However, some medical authorities believe that no known medical reason exists for performing circumcision during the neonatal period. The American Academy of Pediatrics currently is conducting a study on the effects of circumcision.

The main advantage of circumcision is hygienic. The circumcised penis is easier to keep clean and free of smegma, a sebaceous secretion that accumulates under the foreskin. Because the neonate's tight skin makes foreskin retraction difficult, bacterial growth is less common with a circumcised penis. Wiswell, Enzenauer, Holton, Cornish, and Hankins (1987) found an increase in urinary tract infections in male neonates as the circumcision rate declined.

The major disadvantage of circumcision is the pain and discomfort it causes. After circumcision, the neonate cries and has a disturbed sleep-awake pattern. To reduce pain, the neonate may receive a topical anesthetic (Stang, Gunnar, Snellman, Condon, and Kestenbaum, 1988).

Various factors may influence the parents' decision whether to circumcise their child, including religious beliefs, the perception that circumcision is a sign of manhood, and the fear that an uncircumcised male will be stigmatized.

Maintain adequate body temperature by keeping the neonate under a radiant warmer or in a warm room during the circumcision. A circumcision board may be necessary to restrict movement during the procedure. This board has Velcro straps that hold the legs and arms snug, restraining movement without impeding circulation. If this board is used, check capillary refill time (which should be less than 3 seconds), nail bed color (which should be pink), and temperature of extremities (they should feel warm). Loosen the straps for 5 minutes and observe for signs of pressure or irritation. While doing this, gently stroke and talk to the neonate.

If a circumcision board is not used, restrain the neonate's legs by wrapping soft gauze snugly around them and taping them together. Place a rubber band under the tape and leave it exposed. Then attach a safety pin to the rubber band and pin the rubber band to the bed. Use the rubber band under the tab of tape securing the end of the restraint so that the neonate can move the legs about 3″ in all directions.

For the first 1 to 2 hours after circumcision, keep the neonate in a side-lying position and leave the diaper off to reduce irritation and observe the incision for bleeding. If bleeding occurs, grasp the penis gently but firmly with a sterile gauze pad, apply pressure until the bleeding stops, and notify the physician.

Apply petrolatum gauze over the penis to prevent bleeding and encrustation and to serve as a protective layer against abrasion from the diaper. To reduce the risk of contamination from fecal matter or urine—and thereby avoid a nursing diagnosis of *potential for infection related to the circumcision site*—change the petrolatum gauze at each diaper change. The gauze is necessary only for 2 to 3 days after the procedure. The neonate should not be under a radiant warmer once the petrolatum gauze is in place because burning may occur.

Collecting urine specimens

When caring for the normal neonate, urine specimens sometimes must be collected for urine cultures, for routine urinalysis, or to determine urine specific gravity, pH (by dipstick testing), protein, ketones, glucose, bilirubin, or blood.

To obtain urine for a specific gravity measurement or dipstick test, withdraw the specimen from a collection bag (via the covered port at the bottom of the bag) or from a disposable diaper. Both urine collection methods yield accurate results. (For more information, see *Nursing research applied: Comparing values from bagged and aspirated diaper urine specimens*.) For an illustrated procedure of urine specimen collection from a collection bag, see *Psychomotor skills: Performing routine neonatal care*, pages 880 to 884.)

Evaluation

During this step of the nursing process, the nurse evaluates the effectiveness of the care plan by ongoing evaluation of subjective and objective criteria. Evaluation findings should be stated in terms of actions performed or outcomes achieved for each goal. The following ex-

---

NURSING RESEARCH APPLIED

Comparing values from bagged and aspirated diaper urine specimens

Many nurses use a syringe to aspirate urine from a disposable diaper. Unlike the commonly recommended method—placing a plastic collection bag over the perineum and waiting for the neonate to void—this method saves time; usually it yields sufficient urine for testing.

Aspirated diaper specimens have other benefits as well. For instance, a diaper and syringe cost less than a urine collection bag. Also, the method requires fewer resources (no extra equipment is needed to obtain the specimen) and preserves skin integrity (no bag must be applied to the surface of the skin).

Despite these benefits, however, the reliability of aspirated diaper specimens remained uncertain until recently. To determine whether laboratory values from aspirated diaper specimens were as accurate as those from bagged specimens, researchers collected urine specimens from 15 healthy neonates and 10 ill neonates from a Level II neonatal special care unit. The neonates were assigned nonrandomly to either the aspirated diaper specimen group or the collection bag specimen group. Specimens were tested for specific gravity, blood, protein, ketones, and glucose.

Findings revealed no significant differences in laboratory values between the two specimen groups. Also, no significant differences were found in specimens from ill neonates versus those obtained from healthy neonates.

Application to practice

This study supports the use of aspirated diaper urine specimens as a reliable alternative to bagged urine specimens. However, because of the small sample studied, replicated research with an increased sample size may provide further data. Also, study findings are applicable only to one brand of disposable diapers (Pampers); materials in cloth diapers and other disposable diapers may affect laboratory values.

Reams, P. K., and Deane, D. M. (1988). Bagged versus diaper urine specimens and laboratory values. *Neonatal Network*, 6(6), 17-20.

---

amples illustrate appropriate evaluation statements for the normal neonate.

• The neonate did not appear cyanotic or dusky.

• The neonate maintained a stable body temperature of 96° to 97.7° F (35.5° to 36.5° C).

• The neonate voided clear amber urine six times in 24 hours.

• The neonate passed a meconium stool 24 hours after birth.

• The parents exhibited appropriate bonding behavior with their infant.

APPLYING THE NURSING PROCESS

Normal neonate with potential altered body temperature related to heat loss

When caring for the neonate in the nursery, the nurse must guard against neonatal heat loss. The table below shows how the nurse might use the nursing process when caring for the neonate described in the case history at right. The first column presents history and physical assessment data followed by a paragraph of mental notes. These notes help the nurse make important mental connections among assessment findings, aiding in development of the nursing diagnosis and planning.

The second column lists an appropriate nursing diagnosis; information in the remaining columns is based on this diagnosis. Although not part of the nursing process, a rationale appears for each intervention in the fourth column to explain how it contributes to the care plan.

ASSESSMENT	NURSING DIAGNOSIS	PLANNING
Subjective (history) data • Neonate is 2 hours old; Apgar score was 9. • Neonate's mother is a primigravid client, age 22. • Labor and delivery were uneventful. **Objective (physical) data** • Normally developed, average for gestational age. • Color: pink. • Cry: lusty. • Respirations: 40/minute, regular. • Heart rate: 100/minute, regular. • Temperature: 96.8° F. **Mental notes** *Neonate is in the crucial transitional period when he must adapt to the extrauterine environment. As body systems attempt to stabilize, body heat may be lost. Nursing care must support thermoregulation and prevent unnecessary heat loss.*	Potential altered body temperature related to heat loss	**Goals** During the neonate's stay in the health care facility, the neonate will: • avoid heat loss • maintain a steady body temperature • tolerate cleaning of birth fluids from the skin without loss of body heat.

Documentation

All steps of the nursing process should be documented as thoroughly and objectively as possible. Thorough documentation not only allows the nurse to evaluate the effectiveness of the care plan, but it also makes the data available to other members of the health care team, helping to ensure consistency of care. (For a case study that shows how to apply the nursing process when caring for a normal neonate, see *Applying the nursing process: Normal neonate with potential altered body temperature related to heat loss.*)

Documentation for the normal neonate should include:
• vital signs, including temperature, heart rate and rhythm, and respiratory rate and rhythm
• strength and symmetry of peripheral pulses
• capillary refill time
• general appearance

• size and shape of fontanels
• umbilical cord description
• circumcision site description (as appropriate)
• stool and urine passage, including times, amounts, and characteristics
• any abnormal physical or behavioral findings
• parent teaching provided.

Chapter summary

Chapter 36 described nursing care of the normal neonate. Here are the key concepts.
• The nurse conducts ongoing assessment of the neonate to ensure optimal neonatal adaptation and to detect changes in the neonate's status.
• Nursing goals for the normal neonate include ensuring oxygenation, thermoregulation, hydration, and nutrition; promoting adequate urinary and bowel elimination pat-

CASE STUDY

Baby boy Brown was born 2 hours ago to a 22-year-old primigravid mother. The labor and delivery were uneventful; the neonate's Apgar score was 9.

IMPLEMENTATION		EVALUATION
Intervention Keep the neonate dry.	**Rationale** A wet neonate can lose body heat via evaporation and convection.	Upon evaluation, the neonate will: • maintain a temperature of 96° to 97.7° F • lack signs of hypothermia, such as shivering • exhibit normal behavior.
Keep the neonate's head covered.	Heat can be lost from the head via radiation, conduction, and convection.	
Wash the neonate with a small washcloth that is soaked in warm water and wrapped around one hand, uncovering only small areas of the body at a time. Do not immerse the neonate in a tub of water.	Exposing large surface areas allows heat loss via evaporation; tub baths may lead to substantial heat loss.	

terns; providing hygienic care; preventing and detecting complications; ensuring environmental safety; and providing care for the family.

• To promote bonding, the nurse helps the parents identify their child's unique personality and recognize the neonate's responses to the parents. For example, the nurse may point out when the neonate smiles in response to a parent's smile or quiets in response to a parent's attempt at consoling.

• The nurse can ensure sound discharge planning and the neonate's smooth transition to home by assessing the parents' readiness to provide proper cord care, bathing, diaper changes, and environmental safety. Other parent-teaching points include observing for diaper rash and monitoring stool and urine patterns. To help the parents develop confidence in their caregiving abilities, the nurse should have them practice these skills in a supervised setting before the neonate's discharge.

• The nurse must consider cultural and social factors that might influence the parents' attitude toward circumcision and other aspects of neonatal care.

Study questions

1. What is a neutral thermal environment?

2. Which measures should the nurse take to prevent heat loss in the neonate during bathing?

3. Which vital sign changes should the nurse observe for when suctioning the neonate?

4. What are the signs of cold stress?

5. How should the nurse assess the neonate's hydration status?

6. When does voiding onset normally occur?

7. Which measures should the nurse take to ensure environmental safety?

8. Which nursing strategies help promote a positive parent-infant interaction?

Bibliography

American Academy of Pediatrics. (1988). Guidelines for perinatal care (2nd ed.). Washington, DC: American Academy of Pediatrics and American College of Obstetricians and Gynecologists.

Carlo, W.A., and Chatburn, R.L. (1988). *Neonatal respiratory care* (2nd ed.). Chicago: Year Book Medical Pubs.

Kim, M., and Mandell, J. (1988). Renal function in the fetus and neonate. In L.R. King (Ed.), *Urologic surgery in neonates and young infants* (pp. 59-76). Philadelphia: Saunders.

Stang, H., Gunnar, M.R., Snellman, L., Condon, L.M., and Kestenbaum, R. (1988). Local anesthesia for neonatal circumcision. *JAMA,* 259(10), 1507-1511.

Streeter, N.S. (1986). *High-risk neonatal care.* Rockville, MD: Aspen.

Cultural references
Harris, C.C. (1986, Fall). Cultural values and the decision to circumcise. *Image: Journal of Nursing Scholarship,* 18(3), 98-104.

Hardy, D.B. (1987, November/December). Cultural practices contributing to the transmission of human immunodeficiency virus in Africa. *Reviews of Infectious Diseases,* 9(6), 1109-1119.

Nursing research
Bliss-Holtz, J. (1989). Comparison of rectal, axillary, and inguinal temperature in full-term newborn infants. *Nursing Research,* 38(2), 85-87.

Reams, P.K., and Deane, D.M. (1988, June). Bagged versus diaper urine specimens and laboratory values. *Neonatal Network,* 6(6), 17-20.

Steele, K.H. (1987). Caring for parents of critically ill neonates during hospitalization: Strategies for health care professionals. *MCN,* 16(1), 13-27.

Wiswell, T.E., Enzenauer, R.W., Holton, M.E., Cornish, J.D., and Hankins, C.T. (1987). Declining frequency of circumcision: Implications for changes in the absolute incidence and male to female sex ratio of urinary tract infections in early infancy. *Pediatrics,* 79(3), 338-342.

Infant Nutrition

Objectives

After reading and studying this chapter, the student should be able to:

1. Determine the learning needs of the childbearing family regarding infant nutrition.

2. Teach the client how breast milk and infant formula differ in composition and nutritional value.

3. Recognize the impact of nursing interventions on successful feeding outcome.

4. Teach the client positioning techniques that help prevent infant feeding problems.

5. Distinguish research-based interventions for infant nutrition from interventions based on tradition or unfounded assumptions.

6. Describe the nurse's role in identifying and reducing barriers to successful breast-feeding.

Introduction

The rapid physical and developmental growth of the first year necessitates optimal nutrition. Besides playing a crucial part in infant health, nutrition also provides an opportunity for positive feeding experiences and important interactions between infant and caregiver. Parents may view positive feeding experiences and a satisfied infant as a measure of their parenting ability; for the infant, repeated pleasurable feeding experiences help develop trust in the caregiver.

Teaching about infant nutrition is a major role of the nurse who works with young families. By understanding the nutritional needs of the first year, the nurse can provide the client with accurate and practical rationales for feeding recommendations.

This chapter considers the nurse's role in promoting optimal infant nutrition. It begins by describing the infant's nutritional needs. Then it focuses on breast-feeding, highlighting such topics as the physiology of lactation and breast milk composition. Next, the chapter discusses infant formula, including preparation and sucking dynamics. The last section demonstrates how to follow the nursing process steps—assessment, nursing diagnosis, planning, implementation, and evaluation—to individualize nursing care.

Infant nutritional needs

The neonate's immature organ systems and the unparalleled growth of the first year impose special requirements for nutrients and fluids. These factors also limit the types and amounts of foods a neonate can ingest and digest. Recommendations for the introduction of solid foods are based on these limitations.

Nutrient and fluid requirements

As with all diets, the neonate's must contain sufficient amounts of carbohydrates, proteins, fats, vitamins, minerals, and fluids.

GLOSSARY

Colostrum: thin, yellow, serous fluid secreted during pregnancy and the first postpartal days before lactation begins; consists of water, protein, fat, carbohydrates, white blood cells, and immunoglobulins.

Everted nipple: nipple that is turned outward and becomes more graspable with stimulation.

Flat nipple: nipple that is hard to distinguish from the areola; changes shape only slightly with stimulation.

Foremilk: thin, watery breast milk secreted at the beginning of a feeding.

Hindmilk: high-fat breast milk secreted at the end of a feeding.

Inverted nipple: nipple that turns inward; occurs in three types: pseudo-inverted (becomes erect with stimulation), semi-inverted (retracts with stimulation), and truly inverted (inverted both at rest and when stimulated).

Let-down reflex: milk ejection from the breast, triggered by nipple stimulation or an emotional response to the neonate.

Myoepithelial cells: smooth-muscle cells surrounding breast alveoli and ducts; with the let-down reflex, these cells contract and eject milk into breast ductules and sinuses.

Nipple confusion: condition in which the infant does not know how to suck properly from a nipple; caused by frequent nipple changes (such as from use of supplemental bottles during breast-feeding).

Oxytocin: hormone responsible for contraction of smooth muscles surrounding breast alveoli, causing release of breast milk; secreted by the posterior pituitary gland in response to infant sucking on the breast.

Prolactin: hormone causing breast milk production; secreted by the anterior pituitary gland in response to tactile stimulation of the breast.

Rooting reflex: normal neonatal reflex elicited by stroking the cheek or corner of the mouth with a finger or nipple, resulting in turning of the head toward the stimulus.

Energy

Three basic nutrients—carbohydrates, proteins, and fats—supply the body's caloric needs. Carbohydrates should serve as the body's main source of calories. Proteins promote cellular growth and maintenance, aid metabolism, and contribute to many protective substances. Fats provide a concentrated energy storage form, transport essential nutrients (such as fatty acids needed for neurologic growth and development), and insulate vital organs. Carbohydrates, which contain 4 calories per gram, should provide 35% to 55% of the neonate's total calories; fats, which contain 9 calories per gram, 30% to 55%; and proteins, which contain 4 calories per gram, the remaining calories.

Vitamins and minerals

Vitamins regulate metabolic processes and promote growth and maintenance of body tissues. Fat-soluble vitamins (A, D, E, and K) in excess of needs can be stored in the body to some extent and normally are not excreted; therefore, reserves may accumulate. Water-soluble vitamins (C, B_1, B_2, B_6, B_{12}, niacin, folic acid, pantothenic acid, and biotin) are stored only in small amounts. Consequently, if these vitamins are not ingested regularly, deficiencies may develop relatively quickly. (For recommended intake of selected vitamins, see *Daily nutrient requirements for the infant*.)

All major minerals and most trace minerals are essential for a wide range of body functions, including regulation of enzyme metabolism, acid-base balance, and nerve and muscle integrity. Calcium and iron are particularly important for growth—calcium for the rapid bone mineralization of the first year and iron for hemoglobin synthesis.

Fluid

The neonate's difficulty concentrating urine plus a high extracellular water content result in a much greater need for fluid (150 ml/kg/day) compared to the adult (20 to 30 ml/kg/day). By age 1, the daily fluid requirement is roughly 700 ml.

Special considerations

The neonate has limited gastric capacity. Also, fat absorption does not reach adult levels until ages 6 to 9 months. For the first 3 months, limited synthesis of the starch-splitting salivary enzyme ptyalin and absence of pancreatic amylase restrict digestion of complex starches found in solid foods.

Because of the neonate's low glomerular filtration rate (GFR) and difficulty concentrating urine, high renal solute loads may cause fluid imbalance. (Renal solute load is a collective term for solutes that must be excreted by the kidneys.) The major solutes are sodium, potassium, and urea (an end product of protein metabolism). Some commercial infant formulas have a higher renal

Daily nutrient requirements for the infant

The chart below can be used to ensure that the infant's nutritional intake meets growth and developmental needs. (Note: These requirements apply to the normal, healthy infant at age 6 months.)

NUTRIENT	DAILY REQUIREMENT
Protein	14 g
Vitamins	
Vitamin A	375 mcg retinol equivalent
Vitamin B$_6$	0.6 mg
Vitamin B$_{12}$	0.5 mcg
Vitamin C	35 mg
Vitamin D	10 mcg
Vitamin E	4 mg alpha-tocopherol equivalent
Vitamin K	10 mcg
Folate	35 mcg
Niacin	6 mg niacin equivalent
Riboflavin	0.5 mg
Thiamine	0.4 mg
Minerals	
Calcium	600 mg
Iodine	50 mcg
Iron	10 mg
Magnesium	60 mg
Phosphorus	500 mg
Selenium	15 mcg
Zinc	5 mg

Recommended Dietary Allowances, 10th ed., © 1989, by the National Academy of Sciences, National Academy Press, Washington, D.C.

milk contain enough linoleic acid to facilitate myelinization; for this reason, milk that contains less than 2% milk fat is not recommended before age 1.

Sleeping through the night—a significant developmental milestone—usually occurs earlier in the formula-fed infant than in the breast-fed infant. Parents may feel compelled to introduce solid foods early, believing this will lengthen the infant's sleep and help this milestone occur sooner (Wright, 1987). However, before age 3 months, the infant is ill-equipped to ingest solids. The extrusion reflex, in which the tongue pushes out food placed on it, does not diminish until approximately age 4 months. Also, an infant younger than age 3 months lacks the tongue motion needed to pass solids from the front to the back of the mouth. These limitations indicate unreadiness for solid foods.

Nutritional assessment

Weight, length, and head circumference are the major nutritional assessment indices in the infant. In North America, growth charts with standardized measurements for these indices are used to compare an infant to others of the same age. Repeat measurements at various ages show whether the infant is growing at the expected rate. However, current charts are based on formula-fed infants and may be unreliable for exclusively breast-fed infants, who grow rapidly during the first 3 months and more slowly from ages 3 to 6 months (Wood, Isaacs, Jensen, and Hilton, 1988).

The neonate typically loses an average of 10% of the birth weight in the first few days. This may alarm parents, who commonly view weight as a reflection of their infant's health status. However, the formula-fed neonate usually returns to birth weight by day 10 and the breast-fed neonate by 3 weeks (Lauwers and Woessner, 1983; Tulley and Overfield, 1987). Birth weight typically doubles by ages 5 to 6 months and triples by age 1 year. Body length increases by about 50% by age 1; head circumference expands along with the rapidly growing brain.

Infant feeding methods

Choice of an infant feeding method involves more than a simple comparison of the biophysical properties of breast milk and formula. (See *Nutritional and immunologic properties of breast milk and infant formulas,* pages 896

(Text continues on page 899.)

solute load than breast milk. Coupled with the neonate's low GFR, the solutes can cause too much fluid to be excreted, increasing the neonate's fluid needs even more.

Although the basic components of the neurologic system are present at birth, myelinization (development of the myelin sheath that protects nerve fibers) is incomplete. Only breast milk, infant formula, and whole

Nutritional and immunologic properties of breast milk and infant formulas

Health experts recommend breast-feeding over formula-feeding. The chart below compares the nutritional and immunologic properties of breast milk and infant formulas and provides an overview of the health implications of these feeding methods.

COMPONENT AND FUNCTION	BREAST MILK CONTENT	COMMON FORMULA CONTENT	HEALTH IMPLICATIONS AND SPECIAL CONSIDERATIONS
Protein Promotes cellular growth and maintenance	Casein-whey protein ratio of 40:60[A]	Casein-whey protein ratio of 82:18[B] (Some milk-based formulas provide casein-whey ratio closer to that of breast milk.)	Whey proteins are acidified in the stomach; resulting curds are soft and readily digested with minimal energy expenditure. Casein forms tougher, less digestible curd that requires more energy expenditure.
Methionine-cysteine (amino acids) Promote somatic (body tissue) growth	Methionine-cysteine ratio close to 1:1	Methionine-cysteine ratio seven times higher than that of breast milk[C]	More abundant methionine in formulas is poorly tolerated by some infants.[D]
Taurine (an amino acid) Allows early brain and retinal development	Present	Present since 1984[E]	Taurine is an essential amino acid for the neonate; therefore, it must be included in the diet.
Fat Serves as most concentrated calorie source	Breast milk fat content varies throughout the day. Concentration is lowest during the first morning feeding, highest at midmorning, then gradually declines.[F] Fat concentration also increases toward the end of feeding (hindmilk). Breast milk also contains lipase, an enzyme that breaks down triglycerides to fatty acids and glycerol and supplies initial energy before milk reaches the intestine.	Vegetable oils are major fat constituent.	Fat is absorbed to virtually the same degree in breast milk and infant formulas.[G] However, lipase in breast milk provides initial energy supply.
Cholesterol May be needed for synthesis of nerve tissue and bile acids.[H]	Present	Absent	Cholesterol ingestion during infancy may promote synthesis of enzymes linked to cholesterol metabolism, resulting in lower serum cholesterol levels later in life.[I]
Carbohydrate Serves as main calorie source	Lactose is primary carbohydrate in breast milk; small quantities of galactose and fructose also are present.	Lactose is primary carbohydrate in many formulas.	Lactose enhances calcium absorption and metabolizes readily to galactose and fructose, which supply energy for the infant's rapidly growing brain. Lactose promotes lactobacilli growth and increases intestinal acidity. The combination of lactobacilli and an acidic environment helps prevent diarrhea.[J]

[A]Canadian Pediatric Society, 1978; Neville, 1983; Ogra and Greene, 1982. [B]Canadian Pediatric Society, 1978; Casey and Hambridge, 1983. [C]Lawrence, 1985. [D]Ogra and Greene, 1982. [E]Minchin, 1985. [F]Casey and Hambridge, 1983. [H]Lewis, 1986. [I]Canadian Pediatric Society, 1978. [J]Hayward, 1983.

Nutritional and immunologic properties of breast milk and infant formulas continued

COMPONENT AND FUNCTION	BREAST MILK CONTENT	COMMON FORMULA CONTENT	HEALTH IMPLICATIONS AND SPECIAL CONSIDERATIONS
Iron Promotes cellular oxygen transport and storage and carbon dioxide removal; increases resistance to infection	Present in small amounts; high levels of lactose and vitamin C in breast milk facilitate iron absorption.[C]	Present in higher amounts than in breast milk but more poorly absorbed because of lower lactose and vitamin C levels in formulas[C]	Iron in breast milk meets the requirements of an exclusively breast-fed term infant until birth weight triples.[I]
Zinc Promotes cellular growth and repair	Present; zinc-binding ligand (molecule that forms coordinate covalent bonds with metallic ions) in breast milk enhances zinc absorption.[D]	Present in roughly same amount as in breast milk	Zinc is essential for growth and skin integrity and must be included in the neonate's diet.[H]
Calcium, phosphorus, potassium, and **sodium** Calcium promotes bone formation and blood clotting. Phosphorus is involved in bone and tooth formation and other biochemical processes. Potassium and sodium promote fluid and electrolyte balance. Calcium, phosphorus, potassium, and sodium also are renal solutes.	Present	Present in higher amounts than in breast milk	The lower renal solute load of breast milk poses less danger to the infant's immature renal system.[G]
Vitamins Important in various metabolic processes. For example, vitamin D promotes calcium and phosphorus metabolism, vitamin K is crucial to synthesis of coagulation factors, and vitamin E protects retinal and pulmonary cell membranes.	All vitamins, both fat-soluble and water-soluble, present at levels reflecting mother's nutritional status and vitamin intake. Although vitamin D is considered fat-soluble, it has been found in water-soluble as well as fatty portion of breast milk.[K] Vitamin K is present in small amounts. High quantities of vitamin E are present in both colostrum and mature breast milk.	All vitamins present in breast milk in equal or higher amounts.	Vitamin D supplements may be recommended for breast-fed infants to prevent deficiency (rickets), although some authorities question need for this.[L] Vitamin K prophylaxis is recommended at birth for both breast-fed and formula-fed infants to prevent hemorrhagic disease of the newborn.[M]
Fluoride Protects against dental caries	Present in small amounts, which do not increase significantly if mother takes supplements.	Present in controlled amounts	Fluoride supplements at birth are controversial. However, supplements are recommended by age 6 months.[N] Need for supplements may depend on fluoride content of local water. Current fluoride recommendation: 0.25 mg/day if local water supply contains less than 0.3 parts per million.
Thyroid hormone Promotes carbohydrate, protein, and fat metabolism and helps regulate metabolic rate	Present in significant amounts	Present in negligible amounts	Value of breast milk thyroid hormone in protecting against congenital hypothyroidism is unknown.[O]

(continued)

[C]Lawrence, 1985. [D]Ogra and Greene, 1982. [G]American Academy of Pediatrics, 1978. [H]Lewis, 1986. [I]Canadian Pediatric Society, 1978. [K]Lauwers and Woessner, 1983. [L]Fomon, 1987. [M]Shapiro, Jacobson, Armon, Manco-Johnson, Hulac, Lane, and Hathaway, 1986. [N]American Academy of Pediatrics, 1986. [O]Hartman and Kent, 1988.

Nutritional and immunologic properties of breast milk and infant formulas continued

COMPONENT AND FUNCTION	BREAST MILK CONTENT	COMMON FORMULA CONTENT	HEALTH IMPLICATIONS AND SPECIAL CONSIDERATIONS
Immunoglobulins (particularly IgA and IgG) Offer protection against antigens (such as viruses and bacteria) and decrease risk of food allergy. Secretory IgA bathes body surfaces and prevents pathogens from entering the body.[P] IgG increases phagocytosis.[Q]	All immunoglobulins are present in both colostrum and breast milk. Secretory IgA accounts for most IgA during first year of breast-feeding.[R] Breast milk has higher IgA levels than formulas; it also contains antibodies to food proteins and thus may decrease risk of food allergy.[S]	Present in negligible amounts	IgA does not readily cross the placenta and therefore is deficient at birth. IgA levels increase slowly in the infant's first few months.
Lysozymes Protect against micrococci and *Escherichia coli*	Present in amounts up to 3,000 times higher than in cow's milk[C]	Present in minimal amounts	Breast milk lysozymes provide protection up to 6 months after birth as the infant loses transplacentally acquired passive immunity.[R]
Lactoferrin (bacteriostatic and iron-binding protein) Exerts antimicrobial effect by preventing bacteria from obtaining iron necessary for survival	Abundant	Absent	In combination with IgA, lactoferrin in breast milk destroys pathogenic strains of *E. coli* and *Candida albicans*.[T]
Bifidum factor (a nitrogen-containing carbohydrate) Creates unfavorable environment for enteropathic bacteria	Present	Absent	Bifidum factor fosters favorable GI bacterial flora—predominantly *Lactobacillus bifidum*—thus helping to protect against several pathogenic organisms.[G]
Antistaphylococcal factor Resists staphylococci, especially *Staphylococcus aureus*	Present	Absent	Antistaphylococcal factor may promote infant health.
Leukocytes Destroy pathogens by phagocytosis	Present	Absent	Leukocytes may promote infant health.
Interferon Protects against viral infections	Present	Present in negligible amounts	Interferon may promote infant health.
Respiratory syncytial virus (RSV) antibodies Protect against RSV	Present	Present in negligible amounts	RSV antibodies may promote infant health.
Prostaglandins Affect cellular function in all organ systems	Present	Present in negligible amounts	Prostaglandins may promote infant health.
Lactoperoxidase Kills streptococci	Present	Absent	Lactoperoxidase may promote infant health.

[C]Lawrence, 1985. [G]American Academy of Pediatrics, 1978. [P]Marieb, 1989. [Q]Seeley, Stephens, and Tate, 1989. [R]Goldman, Garza, Nichols, and Goldblum, 1982. [S]Hanson, Adlerberth, Carlsson, Castrignano, Hahn-Zoric, Dahlgren, Jalil, Nilsson, and Robertson, 1988. [T]Rumball, 1988.

to 898.) Cultural, psychosocial, and other factors also come into play. Although various health groups have endorsed breast-feeding, many women still choose to use infant formula or to breast-feed only briefly. Consequently, the nurse must be familiar with the basic techniques of both breast-feeding and formula-feeding to work effectively with families of neonates. Also, the nurse must recognize any personal biases toward a particular feeding method and make sure they do not influence the interaction with the family.

Because many clients make infant feeding decisions during pregnancy, the nurse should be prepared to offer guidance at that time to ensure an informed decision. Working with the client after delivery, the nurse helps her gain skills and confidence in the method she has chosen.

Breast-feeding

Breast-feeding is an evolving, interdependent, and reciprocal relationship between mother and infant. Although the reflexes involved are natural, many of the techniques of breast-feeding must be learned by both mother and infant. The nurse who strives to work successfully with the breast-feeding client must have a comprehensive understanding of the physiology of lactation and a genuine commitment to facilitating practices that promote breast-feeding.

Breast-feeding has preventive health potential in both developing and industrialized countries. It has been endorsed officially by the World Health Organization (WHO), the International Pediatrics Association, the American Academy of Pediatrics, and the Canadian Pediatric Society.

Nearly all researchers agree that breast-feeding has health benefits, although they do not concur on the extent of such benefits (Cunningham, 1988; Jason, Nieburg, and Marks, 1984; Kovar, Serdula, Marks, and Fraser, 1984; Kramer, 1988; Leventhal, Shapiro, Aten, Berg, and Egerter, 1986). Several studies show that breast milk has distinct advantages over formulas; in contrast, no studies have reached the opposite conclusion (Baer, 1981). To compare the general benefits and drawbacks of breast-feeding and formula-feeding, see *Comparing infant feeding methods.*)

In North America, an increasing percentage of women are breast-feeding their neonates. Approximately 60% of American women breast-fed in 1985, compared to 25% in 1971 (Fomon, 1987). The trend is similar in Canada, where 79% of women breast-fed in 1984, compared to roughly 25% in the 1970s (Myres, 1988; Tanaka, Yeung, and Anderson, 1987). Internationally, a marketing code for breast milk substitutes established

Comparing infant feeding methods

Despite the health benefits of breast-feeding, some clients may choose formula-feeding. The chart below compares breast-feeding and formula-feeding.

BREAST-FEEDING	FORMULA-FEEDING
• Nutritionally superior to formulas • Promotes immunologic defenses through transfer of maternal antibodies • Less expensive than formula-feeding • Readily available • Promotes development of facial muscles, jaws, and teeth • Aids in maternal uterine involution • May enhance mother-infant bonding • Reduces risk of food allergy	• Allows more accurate measurement of infant intake • Avoids potential need to restrict mother's diet or medications • Lengthens time between feedings • Allows more accurate measurement of infant intake • Lengthens time between feedings • Requires preparation, refrigeration, and storage • Necessitates access to clean water and adequate preparation facilities • May be selected by mothers returning to work

by WHO in 1979 helped promote breast-feeding in developing countries (see *Marketing code for breast milk substitutes,* page 900.)

The U.S. Surgeon General has established as a goal for 1990 that 75% of American women breast-feed at the time of discharge after delivery and that 35% continue to breast-feed by the infant's sixth month (U.S. Department of Health and Human Services, 1984). Canada developed a national program to promote breast-feeding in 1978 (Myres, Watson, and Harrison, 1981).

Physiology of lactation
Lactation operates on a supply-meets-demand basis: The more milk the infant removes, the more milk the breast produces. Hormones control milk production and ejection to make milk available to the infant, as described below.

Milk production. Milk is produced in the breast alveoli—tiny sacs made up of epithelial cells. The female breast has a rich blood supply from which the alveoli extract nutrients to produce milk. The alveoli are situated in lobules—clusters leading to ductules that merge into lactiferous ducts. These larger ducts widen further into ampullae, or lactiferous sinuses, located behind the

Marketing code for breast milk substitutes

In the late 1960s and early 1970s, sales of infant formulas increased and breast-feeding rates dropped among the poor populations of developing countries. Health care professionals concerned about the implications of increased formula-feeding on infant health attributed the changing feeding pattern to aggressive advertising and promotional campaigns by infant formula manufacturers.

In 1979, the World Health Organization (WHO) and UNICEF held an international meeting of government representatives, scientific and health experts, food industry representatives, and such organizations as consumers unions to discuss the issue. The meeting led to an international code for the marketing of breast milk substitutes. At a WHO Assembly in 1981, the code was endorsed by 118 countries of diverse geographic, political, and economic descriptions. (The United States voted against it; Japan, South Korea, and Argentina abstained.)

The code—an attempt to achieve universally acceptable limits of corporate promotion of breast milk substitutes—has been an important document in legitimizing active promotion of breast-feeding. The code's critics, however, contend that no reliable evidence links promotion of infant formula with decreased breast-feeding rates. They also argue that the code represents censorship of scientific and health information and limits the free flow of information.

Here is a summary of the code's provisions.

- Infant formulas should not be advertised to the public.
- No free product samples should be given to mothers.
- Infant formulas should not be promoted in health care facilities.
- Manufacturers should not send company nurses to advise mothers.
- No gifts or personal samples should be given to health care workers.
- Product labels should not include words or pictures (including pictures of infants) that idealize formula-feeding.
- Information given to health care workers about infant feeding should be scientific and factual.
- Information on formula-feeding (including product labels) should include an explanation of the benefits of breast-feeding and the costs and hazards of formula-feeding.
- Unsuitable products, such as sweetened condensed milk, should not be promoted for infants.
- All infant formula products should be of high quality and appropriate for the climate and storage conditions of the country in which they are to be used.

nipple and areola. (For an illustration of the breast structures involved in milk production, see *Physiology of lactation.*)

Lactogenesis—initiation of milk production—begins during the third trimester of pregnancy under the influence of human placental lactogen, a hormone secreted by the placenta. The lactating breast functions in synchrony with maternal hormones; along with effective infant attachment on the breast, these hormones mediate milk flow through the alveoli and ductules.

After delivery of the placenta and the resultant decrease in circulating estrogen and progesterone, the anterior pituitary gland releases prolactin, one of many hormones that stimulate mammary gland growth and development. In response, alveolar secretory cells begin extracting nutrients from the blood and converting them to milk. Initial prolactin production also hinges on tactile stimulation of the nipple-areola junction by infant sucking or milk expression (Neville, 1983).

Prolactin is secreted intermittently throughout the day, with secretion rising markedly during sleep (Neville, 1983) and night feedings (Glasier, McNeilly, and Howie, 1984). Thus, frequent feeding over the entire 24-hour period enhances prolactin secretion and significantly increases milk production (Klaus, 1987). Prolactin secretion also creates a calm, relaxed feeling in the mother, which may enhance mother-infant bonding.

Milk ejection. The hormone oxytocin makes breast milk available to the infant through the let-down reflex. In this reflex, nipple stimulation or an emotional response to the infant causes the hypothalamus to trigger release of oxytocin by the posterior pituitary gland. Myoepithelial cells surrounding the alveoli then contract and eject milk into the ductules and sinuses, making milk available through nipple openings. A conditioned reflex, let-down occurs after 2 to 3 minutes of sucking during the first days of breast-feeding; several let-downs occur over the course of a feeding.

Some women have no symptoms of let-down. Others experience it as a tingling sensation, a momentary pain in the nipple, or a warm rush from the chest wall toward the nipple. In the early postpartal period, other let-down symptoms may include uterine cramps (afterpains), caused by the action of oxytocin on the involuting uterus, and a slight increase in lochia (the vaginal discharge emitted after delivery). Also, the breasts may leak. However, let-down may occur even in the absence of milk leakage: In some women, the sphincters controlling milk expulsion from the lactiferous sinuses to the nipple function so effectively that only active sucking on the breast leads to milk release.

Restricting sucking time—a practice based on the erroneous notion that prolonged sucking causes nipple soreness—can disrupt optimal function of the let-down reflex by preventing the infant from completely emptying the milk ducts. This, in turn, leads to milk buildup and

Physiology of lactation

Milk production takes place in the breast alveoli, tiny glands consisting of epithelial cells. A smooth-muscle layer of myoepithelial cells forms a dense meshwork of overlapping bands ensheathing the alveoli and lactiferous ducts—channels that convey milk to and through the nipples.

From the nutrient-rich blood in surrounding capillaries, alveoli draw the ingredients to make milk. Ten to one-hundred alveoli cluster to form lobules (as shown).

Although distributed throughout the breast, most lobules concentrate in the lower half and toward the axillae against the chest wall.

During pregnancy, the alveoli swell and their cells multiply rapidly. The start of lactation triggers fatty degeneration of cells in the lobule's center; these cells then are eliminated as colostrum corpuscles. Outer alveoli produce milk, which ejects into the cavity remaining in the middle of the lobule.

During pregnancy and lactation, myoepithelial cells multiply and expand. When exposed to oxytocin, a hormone released during breast-feeding, these cells contract, producing a squeezing effect on the lobule that forces milk down the ducts. When breast-feeding ends, myoepithelial cells decline in size and number.

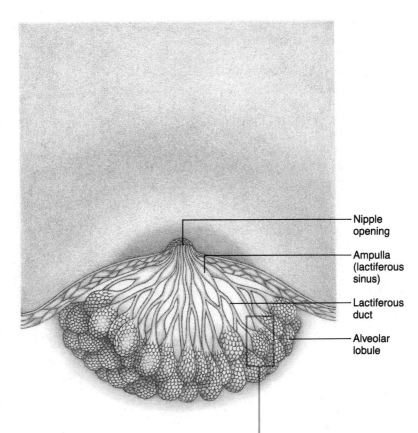

- Nipple opening
- Ampulla (lactiferous sinus)
- Lactiferous duct
- Alveolar lobule

ALVEOLUS

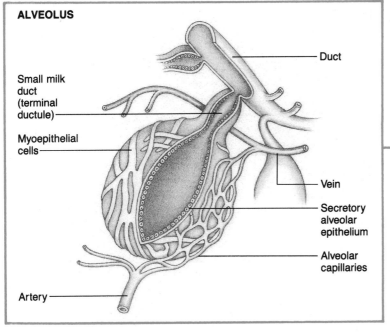

- Duct
- Small milk duct (terminal ductule)
- Myoepithelial cells
- Vein
- Secretory alveolar epithelium
- Alveolar capillaries
- Artery

ALVEOLAR LOBULE

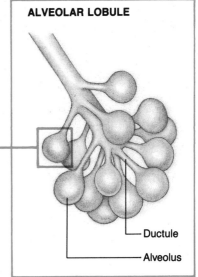

- Ductule
- Alveolus

signals the body to stop producing milk. The breasts become engorged and harden; the nipples may become flat, hindering proper infant attachment. The body responds to engorgement by halting milk production. In the early days of breast-feeding, restricted sucking time may establish a negative feedback system that can lead to insufficient milk production. Also, it may force the infant to feed more often to satisfy hunger.

Breast milk composition and digestion

The composition of breast milk undergoes various changes. Initial feedings provide colostrum, a thin, serous fluid. Unlike mature breast milk, which has a bluish cast, colostrum is yellow (Casey and Hambridge, 1983). However, its color may vary considerably from one woman to the next.

Colostrum contains high concentrations of protein, fat-soluble vitamins, minerals, and immunoglobulins, which function as antibodies. (For more on the immunologic properties of breast milk, see Chapter 34, Neonatal Adaptation.) Colostrum's laxative effect promotes early passage of meconium. Also, the low colostrum volumes produced do not tax the neonate's limited gastric capacity or cause fluid overload.

The breasts may contain colostrum for up to 96 hours after delivery. The maturation rate from colostrum to breast milk varies (Humenick, 1987). With increased breast-feeding frequency and duration in the first 48 hours, colostrum matures to milk more rapidly (Humenick, 1987). This discovery helped disprove the theory that breast-feeding frequency should be limited until mature milk comes in. (However, in some cultures, infants never receive colostrum, as described in *Cultural considerations: Cultural aspects of infant feeding.*)

Breast milk composition also changes over the course of a feeding. The foremilk—thin, watery milk secreted when a feeding begins—is low in calories but contains abundant water-soluble vitamins. It accounts for about 60% of the total volume of a feeding. Next, whole milk is released. The hindmilk, available 10 to 15 minutes after the initial let-down, has the highest concentration of calories for satisfying hunger between feedings.

The rate of milk transfer to the infant varies among mother-infant couples (Woolridge, 1989). Consequently, limiting feeding times or insisting that the woman use both breasts at each feeding may prevent the infant from obtaining the maximum benefit of variable breast milk content.

CULTURAL CONSIDERATIONS

Cultural aspects of infant feeding

When caring for a client whose background is different from yours, keep the following cultural considerations in mind.

Infant feeding practices vary with geography and culture. In Finland, where no infant formula is manufactured, breast-feeding is the norm (Carr, 1989). Some developing countries (for example, Colombia, Brazil, Thailand, and New Guinea) have reversed the recent decline in breast-feeding through vigorous breast-feeding promotion.

Filipinos, Mexican Americans, Vietnamese, and some Nigerians do not give colostrum to neonates; mothers in these groups begin breast-feeding only after milk ejection begins. Some Korean women delay breast-feeding until 3 days after delivery; others begin breast-feeding immediately and breastfeed whenever the infant cries (Choi, 1986).

In Kenya, mothers feed premature neonates only by breast and begin breast-feeding them much earlier than in North America. Kenyans never use gavage tubes and feed neonates from small cups until they are ready to suck (Armstrong, 1987).

The whey proteins that predominate in breast milk lead to formation of soft, easily digested curds. The infant typically digests breast milk within 2 to 3 hours after a feeding and thus may become hungry more often than the formula-fed infant, who typically feeds every 4 hours. In the first few weeks after birth, the breast-fed neonate may feed eight to twelve times every 24 hours.

Infant sucking

The dynamics of sucking on a breast and sucking on an artificial nipple differ dramatically. No frictional movement occurs during breast-feeding (Woolridge, 1986); therefore, it should be painless, provided the infant is properly attached (Minchin, 1985; Royal College of Midwives, 1988). Misinformation about the dynamics of sucking has led to such practices as limiting feeding times. Incorrect infant sucking technique—not prolonged feeding—causes nipple soreness. Some infants must be taught to suck correctly (see *Psychomotor skills: Neonatal sucking reflex,* pages 904 and 905.)

Using images generated by real-time ultrasound studies, investigators have observed the dynamics of breast sucking. Smith, Erenberg, and Nowak (1988) found that the human nipple is a highly elastic structure that elongates to nearly twice its resting length during active feeding. Little change occurs in the nipple's lateral dimension, confirming the theory that the cheeks serve as a passive seal. The researchers also observed that nipple compression between the infant's tongue and palate reduces the tongue's height by half and causes milk ejection.

This sucking pattern was confirmed by Weber, Woolridge, and Baum (1986), who found that the breast-fed infant uses a rolling or peristaltic tongue action in contrast to the squeezing or pistonlike tongue action of the bottle-fed infant. The researchers also noted that the tongue's resting position between bursts of sucking differs in breast-fed and bottle-fed infants.

Intake requirements

A breast-fed infant typically needs to be fed every 2 to 3 hours. During the first 3 to 4 weeks, before the feeding pattern is established fully, parents may wonder if the neonate is receiving adequate nourishment. Signs of adequate intake include 10 to 12 wet diapers in 24 hours, steady weight gain, and contentedness after feeding.

Duration

Despite an increase in breast-feeding rates of women at the time of discharge after delivery, 65% of American women who breast-feed stop before 4 months (Fomon, 1987); 23% of Canadian women stop before 3 months (Tanaka, Yeung, and Anderson, 1987). By anticipating the reasons why a client may choose to stop breast-feeding, the nurse can identify strategies that may help reduce barriers to continued breast-feeding.

Lactation insufficiency (lack of milk) is the most common reason for stopping breast-feeding in the early weeks (Bloom, Goldbloom, Robinson, Stevens, and Houston, 1981; Newman, 1986). The incidence of primary lactation insufficiency is unknown. However, lactation insufficiency most commonly stems from mismanagement of lactation (Newman, 1986; Neifert and Seacat, 1987); this, in turn, may result from such institutional practices as routine supplementation with bottled glucose and water, omission of night breast-feeding until mature milk comes in, and arbitrary feeding schedules. These practices may strain the adaptability of the mother–infant couple and interrupt the interactions necessary for successful breast-feeding (Winikoff, Laukaran, Myers, and Stone, 1986). Also, indiscriminate use of bottles to supplement breast-feeding in the neonate's first days may cause nipple confusion, making the neonate refuse the breast the next time it is offered.

When such problems occur, ready availability of an alternative infant food source may cause the mother to switch to formula rather than try to correct the problems.

Like the client's decision to breast-feed initially, her decision to stop involves many factors, including her age, family or social attitudes toward breast-feeding, and her socioeconomic status or educational level. For example, an adolescent mother may stop breast-feeding when she realizes how much time and energy it requires; a new mother who is the first woman in her family to breast-feed may feel pressured to stop if problems arise.

Maternal ambivalence toward breast-feeding also may play a role (Jones, West, and Newcombe, 1986). However, with proper antepartal teaching, a client may learn to adjust her expectations about breast-feeding and thus avoid becoming so discouraged that she stops when problems occur. For instance, she can learn to anticipate ambivalence and doubt about her ability to breast-feed and to expect such physical discomforts as leaking breasts and frequent feedings.

Hewat and Ellis (1986) compared women who breast-fed for prolonged periods with those who discontinued breast-feeding early. They concluded that those who continued:
• fed their neonates more frequently in the early days of breast-feeding
• showed less anxiety about initial neonatal weight loss and interpreted neonatal behavior in a positive light
• demonstrated a greater ability to relax
• showed more flexibility in their daily routines
• more readily incorporated siblings into the feeding experience
• received more support from their partner.

The nurse can help prevent a poor breast-feeding outcome by advocating institutional practices that promote lactation, teaching the client about the physiology of lactation, providing anticipatory guidance about the normal course of breast-feeding, and making sure the client knows how to obtain information and support after discharge. Although the availability of follow-up support varies, some community health nurses make routine home visits after a neonate's birth. Also, the assistance of a lactation nurse has significantly prolonged breast-feeding during the first 4 weeks and among women of lower socioeconomic status (Jones and West, 1985). Professional and lay breast-feeding support may be available from a lactation consultant or a local LaLeche League group. (For more on breast-feeding support, see *Breast-feeding resource groups*, page 906.)

(Text continues on page 906.)

Neonatal sucking reflex

To determine if the neonate is ready to be put to the breast, the nurse tests for the sucking reflex. If the neonate demonstrates poor sucking, use one of the techniques described here to help train the neonate to suck.

Assessing the sucking reflex

To verify this reflex, the nurse must have freshly washed hands and fingernails as short as possible to avoid injuring the neonate.

1 Stimulate the rooting reflex by stroking the neonate's cheek toward the lips. The neonate should turn toward you.

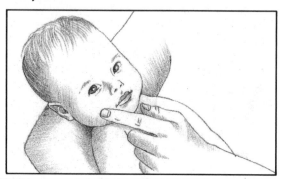

2 Brush your fingertip against the neonate's lips.

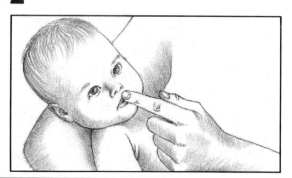

3 Lightly massage the various parts of the gums in this order; outside of the lower gums, top of the lower gums, outside of the upper gums, and top of the upper gums.

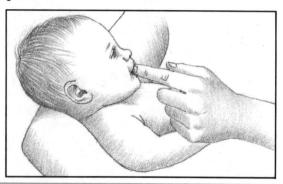

4 Insert your finger, nail side down, in the neonate's mouth and brush your fingertip around the mouth several times. Gently pull down the lower lip; when properly positioned for sucking, you will be able to see the tongue.

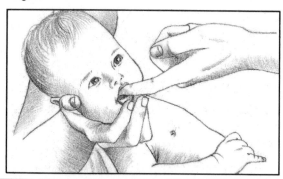

5 Rub the soft palate (at the rear of the mouth) with your index finger to trigger the sucking reflex. Check to see if the tongue extends to the inside of the lower lip (or at least over the lower gum line), indicating proper sucking position. The sides of the tongue should curve around your finger.

Sucking motion should begin at the tip of the tongue and roll backward; you should feel the tongue's rippling against the nail side of your finger. As sucking begins, your finger should be drawn backward until the finger pad touches the soft palate. Sucking should be rhythmic with periodic rests that do not break suction. Choking and other negative responses signal poor sucking. (If you assess poor sucking, you may need to train the neonate to suck properly, as described below.)

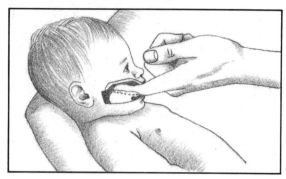

6 The neonate who sucks on your finger 10 to 20 times is ready to breast-feed. To evaluate the sucking pattern during breast-feeding, have the client cup her breast in her hand (as shown here) and insert ¾" to 1" of the areola into the neonate's mouth.

Gently pull down the neonate's lower lip. If the neonate is sucking correctly, you should be able to see the tongue covering the lower gum line and curved around the breast. The areola should be elongated, with the nipple reaching to the back of the mouth.

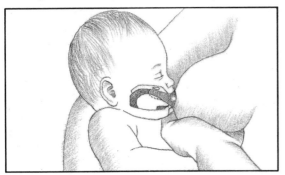

7 Tongue motion should begin at the tip and ripple backward with a wavelike motion that compresses the breast to the palate. The newborn swallows at the end of a tongue ripple (sometimes after each ripple, at other times after several sucks). The vacuum created by the mouth should be strong enough to prevent the neonate from falling off or being pulled off the breast easily.

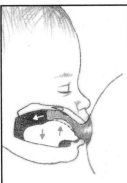

Tongue presses nipple against hard palate, forcing milk from lactiferous ducts and sinuses.

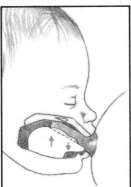

Negative pressure pulls milk toward back of mouth, initiating swallowing.

Training the neonate to suck
Most neonates can be trained to suck properly in two or three feedings.

1 Perform steps 1 through 3 of "Assessing the sucking reflex." Then, insert your finger (nail side down) into the neonate's mouth. Gently rub the hard palate (the rigid portion at the front of the mouth), then the soft palate (at the back of the mouth), to trigger sucking.

As the neonate sucks, gently press forward and down with the nail side of your finger. In an alternating pattern, rub the neonate's hard palate and exert pressure downward and forward. If the neonate responds with the correct sucking motion (as described in step 7 of "Assessing the sucking reflex"), reward with verbal praise and encouragement.

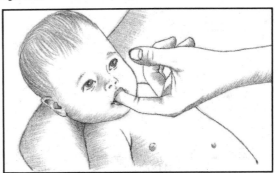

2 For an alternate method, insert the finger, nail side up, and position the finger pad at the point where the tongue starts to slant downward toward the pharynx. Then, gently pull the tongue forward with your finger.

Reward the neonate for proper sucking. Use an eyedropper filled with expressed breast milk or formula. (Use only a hard plastic or glass eyedropper; with the latter, take care not to use excessive pressure, which may cause breakage.) Insert the dropper into the neonate's mouth at a 45-degree angle to the head. If the tongue assumes the correct sucking position, squeeze the dropper to release the milk or formula.

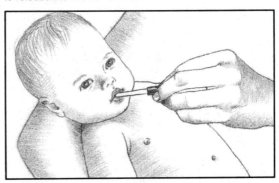

Formula-feeding

Because of the current emphasis on breast-feeding, the client who chooses formula-feeding may feel uncertain about her choice and react defensively if she feels it is being questioned. By recognizing the many factors that go into infant feeding decisions, the nurse can convey respect and offer support to the client who has made an informed decision to formula-feed. Also, by working with the client in the antepartal period, the nurse can help ensure that she receives relevant information in a way that would allow her to revise her choice (Gabriel, Gabriel, and Lawrence, 1986).

   Although choice of specific formula and preparation method are important aspects of formula-feeding, the feeding process goes beyond simply giving the infant a bottle. As with breast-feeding, formula-feeding involves a developing relationship between mother and infant. The nurse who remains aware of this added dimension can provide the family with appropriate anticipatory guidance during the early learning period of infant feeding.

Commercial formulas and equipment
Commercial infant formulas fall into three categories—milk-based, soy-based, and casein hydrolysate-based. (For a comparison of these formula types, see *Nutritional options for the formula-fed infant.*) The American Academy of Pediatrics recommends commercially prepared formulas over other formulas for infants up to age 1 year. Commercial formulas provide all necessary vitamins, so infants receiving them do not require vitamin supplements. However, use of noncommercial formulas necessitates vitamin supplementation.

   Product convenience, personal preference, and economic status influence the client's choice of formula equipment. Commercially available equipment includes glass bottles, boilable plastic bottles, disposable plastic bags (which the preparer places in a hollow plastic holder), and artificial nipples. Because sucking action on the NUK nipple (which is flat and broad) most closely resembles sucking action on the human nipple, some authorities recommend this nipple for breast-fed infants who receive an occasional supplemental bottle.

Infant sucking
Sucking on a regular latex nipple is largely a squeezing action. The bottle-fed infant tends to swallow with every suck at the beginning of a feeding. If milk flow is restricted (for instance, from vacuum buildup that makes the nipple collapse), the suck–swallow ratio may rise to 2:1 or even higher, until sucking stops completely.

Intake requirements
The amount and frequency of formula-feedings vary with infant size, maturity, and activity level. Daily formula intake averages 180 ml/kg.

   Like parents of the breast-fed infant, parents of the formula-fed infant may believe all crying signals hunger. The nurse can help them interpret infant behavior more accurately by reviewing guidelines on feeding frequency. (For formula intake requirements and feeding frequency for infants up to age 1 year, see *Formula guidelines* page 908.)

Digestion
The casein proteins predominating in formula result in tougher, less digestible curds than those in breast milk. Consequently, infant formula takes more time and energy to digest than breast milk. (However, homogenization and heat treatment of commercially prepared formulas have improved curd digestibility somewhat.)

Nutritional options for the formula-fed infant

Although only commercial formulas are recommended for non-breast-feeding infants, a family with a limited budget may use a home formula or another less-than-optimal type of infant nutrition. The table below compares three major types of commercial formulas and three noncommercial variations.

OPTION	RECOMMENDATIONS FOR USE	FORM AND ENERGY CONTENT
Milk-based commercial formula (Enfalac, Similac, SMA, Milumil)	• Infants with no family history of food allergy who receive little or no breast milk	Liquid concentrate, powdered concentrate, ready-to-serve Energy content: 68 kcal/dl
Soy-based commercial formula (Isomil, Nursoy, ProSobee)	• Infants with galactosemia or primary lactase deficiency • Infants recovering from secondary lactose intolerance • Infants with a family history of food allergy but no clinical manifestations • Infants in strict vegetarian families that wish to avoid animal protein formulas	Liquid or powdered concentrate Energy content: 68 kcal/dl
Casein hydrolysate–based commercial formula (Nutramigen, Pregestimil, Alimentum)	• Infants with clinical manifestations of food allergy	Liquid or powdered concentrate Energy content: 68 kcal/dl
Evaporated whole milk formula	• Not recommended; should be used only if family cannot afford commercially prepared formula	Powdered; to lower protein and sodium content, formula must be diluted (one part evaporated milk to two parts water) Energy content: 68 kcal/dl if carbohydrate (such as dextrose or sucrose) is added. Honey and corn syrup are not recommended as additive carbohydrates.
Cow's milk	• Not recommended for infants under age 6 months because of hard-to-digest protein curd, low linoleic acid content, high renal solute load, high mineral content, poorly absorbed butterfat, and risk of GI bleeding (if consumed in large amounts with little solid food) • May be given to infants over age 6 months who consume approximately 180 ml of solid food • Low-fat milk should not be given to infants under age 1 year • Skim milk should be given only to infants over age 1 year who are severely overweight or cannot tolerate higher fat content	Whole, partially skimmed, or powdered Energy content: 69 kcal/dl
Goat's milk	• Not recommended for infants under age 6 months because of hard-to-digest protein curd, low linoleic acid content, high renal solute load, high mineral content, and poorly absorbed butterfat • If used in infant over age 6 months who is consuming approximately 180 ml of solid food, vitamin D and folic acid supplements must be given	Whole, partially skimmed, evaporated, or powdered Energy content: 67 kcal/dl

Adapted with permission of the Minister of Supply and Services Canada, 1989, from Health and Welfare Canada. Publication *Feeding babies: A counselling guide on practical solutions to common infant feeding questions*, 1986.

Formula guidelines

The table below shows recommended formula volume and feeding frequency for infants up to age 1 year who are receiving commercial formula exclusively.

AGE	FORMULA VOLUME PER FEEDING	FEEDINGS PER DAY
1 month	126 ml (4.1 oz)	6
2 months	142 ml (4.6 oz)	5
3 months	161 ml (5.2 oz)	5
4 months	168 ml (5.4 oz)	5
5 months	191 ml (6.2 oz)	4
6 months	179 ml (5.8 oz)	5
7 to 9 months	131 ml (4.2 oz)	5
10 months	136 ml (4.4 oz)	5
11 months	125 ml (4.0 oz)	5
12 months	141 ml (4.5 oz)	4

Adapted from data analysis performed by Ross Laboratories, 1985. Used with permission.

Assessment

The nurse should begin client assessment by collecting general data and then make specific assessments related to the feeding method.

The breast-feeding client and neonate

Ideally, assessment should begin in the early antepartal period as the nurse determines how much the client knows about infant nutrition and breast-feeding techniques. Also, the nurse should evaluate nipple graspability and protractility by determining whether the nipples are slightly everted, flat, or inverted. The slightly everted nipple, the most common type, becomes more graspable when stimulated. A flat nipple is hard to distinguish from the areola and changes shape only slightly when stimulated. Inverted nipples fall into three categories. A pseudoinverted nipple appears inverted but becomes erect with stimulation. A semi-inverted nipple initially appears graspable but retracts with stimulation.

A truly inverted nipple is inverted both at rest and when stimulated.

For the client in the postpartal period, after breast-feeding has begun, the nurse should assess:
• consistency of the breasts (softness, mobility, engorgement, and warmth)
• condition of the nipples (tenderness, abrasions, and discoloration)
• sensations experienced during breast-feeding (such as tingling).

For the breast-feeding neonate, the nurse should assess the sucking reflex before the first feeding because improper sucking will prevent adequate feeding. Clues that the neonate is sucking properly include puffing out of the cheeks and absence of biting. (For details, see *Psychomotor skills: Neonatal sucking reflex*, pages 904 and 905.)

Also assess for signs of lactose intolerance, including abdominal cramps and distention and severe diarrhea. The major carbohydrate in milk, lactose normally is broken down by the enzyme lactase. Lactose intolerance occurs from the absence of lactase in the border of the intestinal villi. Most common among non-Caucasian neonates, lactose intolerance may warrant the use of a soy-based formula, which provides corn syrup solids and sucrose as the primary carbohydrates.

The nurse also should assess for proper client and neonate positioning. The client may assume a sitting or reclining position, bringing the neonate to her. A pillow can be placed under the arms to prevent shoulder elevation, which could cause muscle tension. The client should hold the neonate facing her and level with the breast so that the neonate's neck need not twist or flex.

The nurse should assess the client and neonate during a feeding to determine if the neonate is correctly attached on the breast, as indicated by a wide open mouth with lips curved backward.

Assessment of the client and infant after discharge can promote breast-feeding success. Many life-style adjustments must be made when a neonate joins the family. These adjustments may cause role strain and conflict. Postdischarge nursing assessment may reveal breast-feeding problems caused by such role strain and conflict. (For further information on family adjustment to a neonate's arrival, see Chapter 21, Family Preparation for Childbirth and Parenting.)

The client using infant formula

For the client in the antepartal period, the nurse should assess for:
• knowledge of proper feeding techniques
• understanding of types of formula
• previous experience with infant formula.

Nutritional aid for mothers and infants

In the United States, a government program called the Women, Infants, and Children Nutrition Program (WIC) provides supplemental foods, access to health care, and nutrition education during critical stages of growth and development. Those eligible include pregnant and postpartal women, infants up to age 1 year, and children up to age 5 whom a health care professional has classified as being at nutritional risk. Although federally funded, WIC is administered by states; consequently, eligibility requirements may vary. Further information can be obtained from the Department of Agriculture or from state health departments.

In Canada, access to health care is universal. However, no universal social assistance program exists specifically for mothers and infants. Instead, each Canadian province has its own program. In special cases, government subsidies are available for infant feeding equipment and formulas. Otherwise, a woman receiving social assistance is expected to meet her and her child's nutritional needs with the monthly allowance she receives. Provincial community health nurses employed by the government can provide specific information about health care for Canadian mothers with infants.

Also, the nurse should find out what equipment and facilities the client will use to prepare formula and determine if the client will need financial aid to meet the infant's nutritional needs. (For information on sources of financial aid for mothers of young children, see *Nutritional aid for mothers and infants*.)

For the client in the postpartal period, the nurse should assess bottle and infant positioning during feeding and the client's ability to adjust feeding technique in response to infant cues. The nurse also should inspect the client's breasts for signs of engorgement, such as tenderness, swelling, warmth, hardness, shininess, and redness. (For information on treatment of engorged breasts in the non-breast-feeding client, see Chapter 42, Care during the Normal Postpartal Period.)

Infant factors to assess for include:
• excessive drooling, coughing, gagging, or respiratory distress during feeding (which may indicate tracheal or esophageal fistula, as discussed in Chapter 38, High-Risk Neonates)
• amount of formula the infant takes
• regurgitation after feeding
• mucus in regurgitated matter
• how readily the infant burps
• signs of lactose intolerance (discussed under "The breast-feeding client and neonate.")
• presence of circumoral cyanosis (bluish skin around the mouth) during feeding. This may reflect insufficient oxygen to meet the infant's increased metabolic needs.

Nursing diagnosis

After gathering all assessment data, the nurse must review it carefully to identify pertinent nursing diagnoses for the client or neonate. (For a partial list of applicable diagnoses, see *Nursing diagnoses: Infant nutrition*.)

NURSING DIAGNOSES

Infant nutrition

The following are potential nursing diagnoses for problems and etiologies that a nurse may encounter when caring for a client as she begins to nourish her neonate. Specific nursing interventions for many of these diagnoses are provided in the "Planning and implementation" section of this chapter.

• Altered family processes related to breast-feeding
• Altered family processes related to infant feeding
• Altered nutrition: potential for more than body requirements, related to breast-feeding
• Altered parenting related to infant prematurity and the mother's wish to breast-feed
• Altered role performance related to the new task of breast-feeding
• Altered sexuality patterns related to requirements of the breast-feeding infant
• Anxiety related to change in infant feeding pattern secondary to a growth spurt
• Anxiety related to the ability to breast-feed multiple infants
• Anxiety related to the ability to properly feed the infant
• Body image disturbance related to physiologic changes secondary to breast-feeding
• Ineffective breast-feeding related to improper positioning at the breast
• Knowledge deficit related to breast-feeding
• Knowledge deficit related to formula-feeding
• Pain related to breast engorgement
• Potential fluid volume deficit related to breast-feeding
• Potential for infection related to improper expression and storage of breast milk
• Potential for injury related to improper nipple care
• Sleep pattern disturbance, related to the infant's nutritional needs

Planning and implementation

After assessing the client and formulating nursing diagnoses, the nurse develops and implements a plan of care. For example, if the client has a nursing diagnosis of *knowledge deficit related to breast-feeding*, the nurse should plan what and how to teach her about breast-feeding. Although the plan will depend on the client's abilities, it may include written materials, discussion of proper feeding methods and infant positioning, and client demonstration of breast-feeding.

To anticipate the teaching the client will need, the nurse must consider both short-term and long-term goals. Collaborative planning with the client helps promote goal attainment.

When counseling the client, the nurse should use empathy, warmth, and respect to encourage her to explore her feelings about infant feeding and mothering. Such interaction can build a base for further therapeutic interaction and may enhance the client's responsiveness to specific teaching on infant nutrition.

Care for the breast-feeding client

The nurse's role in working with the breast-feeding client includes teaching of proper feeding techniques and intervention to correct any related problems. The nurse also helps the client deal with physiologic or psychosocial problems related to breast-feeding.

Client teaching
Ideally, teaching about breast-feeding should begin in the antepartal period and continue postpartum until breast-feeding is well established.

Antepartum. In the antepartal period, teaching should focus on practical knowledge that will help the client establish and maintain lactation after delivery. Some general topics that could be incorporated into antepartal teaching include:
• physiologic, emotional, and social factors that influence lactation
• the role of the neonate and the client's partner in breast-feeding outcome
• common breast-feeding problems and possible solutions
• the possibility of continuing to breast-feed after the client returns to work
• the role of support groups or professional services and how to gain access to them.

Antepartal teaching also can help prepare the client to deal with incorrect advice about breast-feeding. Such advice—which may come from friends, relatives, or even health care professionals—typically is based on emotion rather than scientific principles that promote a positive breast-feeding outcome. When initiating breast-feeding, the client is especially vulnerable to such outside interference. To make her less vulnerable, the nurse can establish credibility as a knowledgeable professional during the pregnancy. Then, the nurse may use role-playing techniques, asking the client to predict who might offer advice and having her play the role of each of those persons. Practicing this technique in the antepartal period prepares the client to react rationally to incorrect advice once she begins breast-feeding.

Postpartum. The nurse should encourage the client to take advantage of the neonate's early responsiveness by breast-feeding as soon as possible. For the healthy full-term neonate, no contraindications exist to feeding immediately after delivery. In the first 30 minutes or so after birth, the neonate is highly responsive and eager to suck. Many neonates breast-feed shortly after delivery; all at least make licking or nuzzling motions, helping to stimulate the mother's prolactin production. Also, during this time the client's breasts may be soft and easily manipulated, facilitating proper attachment. Immediate breast-feeding also offers the chance for intimate contact that can enhance mother–neonate bonding and have a positive psychological effect on the parents.

Valid reasons for delaying breast-feeding immediately after delivery include such obvious contraindications as life-threatening illness of the mother or neonate. In less obvious cases, the nurse must exercise good judgment. For example, immediate breast-feeding may be inappropriate if the neonate has anomalies that warrant evaluation, if the mother is heavily sedated or fatigued, or if the neonate has a 5-minute Apgar score of 6 or less.

General breast-feeding guidelines
Although lactation is a natural process, breast-feeding skills must be learned and practiced. The nurse can promote breast-feeding success through timely intervention to correct any problems.

Helping the client initiate breast-feeding. In many cases, the nurse must help the client initiate feeding. However, the client who believes breast-feeding should be entirely natural may feel like a failure for needing help. Especially for a client with a nursing diagnosis of ***knowledge deficit related to breast-feeding,*** the nurse should point out that some infants must learn to breast-feed. Others may need to be wakened for every feeding. (For more information on helping the client initiate breast-feeding, see *Client teaching: Breast-feeding your infant,* pages 912 and 913.)

Providing comfort measures and promoting hygiene. Before a feeding begins, the nurse should meet the client's comfort needs—for example, by having her void or by administering an analgesic, if prescribed. Also, the nurse should encourage her always to wash her hands just before breast-feeding.

Ensuring proper positioning. The nurse should emphasize the importance of correct positioning. The client may breast-feed in three different positions—cradle position, side-lying position, or football hold (described in *Client teaching: Breast-feeding your infant,* pages 912 and 913). Whichever position the client uses, her back and arms should be firmly supported; pillows may be placed under the arm on the breast-feeding side to keep the infant close to the breast.

Help the client into the chosen position and instruct her to hold the infant so that the infant looks down on her breast, then tilt the breast so that the nipple points toward the roof of the infant's mouth. This position typically places the infant's lower lip and jaw well below the nipple.

In the client's eagerness to ensure that breast-feeding goes well, she may lean in toward the infant, believing this facilitates attachment. However, to avoid discomfort, the client should bring the infant toward her instead.

For a client with a nursing diagnosis of ***ineffective breast-feeding related to improper positioning of the infant at the breast,*** the nurse should check for common positioning mistakes, such as placing the infant so low that the neck must hyperextend to grasp the nipple or so high that the neck must flex to grasp it.

Ensuring correct infant attachment. To ensure that the infant is correctly attached on the breast and getting enough nipple tissue to suck properly, instruct the client to cup the breast with her thumb well away from the nipple and fingers. After tickling the infant's lip with the nipple to stimulate rooting, the client should wait for the infant to open the mouth wide (with the tongue pointing downward), then center the nipple in the mouth and pull the infant toward her breast. Sometimes a slight delay before bringing the infant to the breast makes the infant open the mouth wider.

Assess the infant's jaw action to confirm proper attachment. The jaws should move rhythmically (possibly accompanied by slight ear movement). Gumming jaw motions and a clicking sound signal improper attachment. The let-down reflex also confirms proper attachment. If the client lacks the experience to recognize let-down internally from the drawing sensation in the ducts, teach her to place her finger lightly across the top of her breast; with proper attachment, she will feel the drawing sensation externally with her finger.

Establishing a breast-feeding pattern. Advise the client that the infant may need to feed for at least 15 minutes on each breast at each feeding. The client should let the infant complete a feeding on one breast before offering the other (Woolridge, 1989). As milk volume adjusts to the infant's needs, the client may change this pattern several times, offering only one breast at a feeding, then offering both breasts again.

The nurse also should tell the client to expect to breast-feed every 2 to 3 hours during the day and every 4 to 5 hours at night (or sooner, if the infant awakens). On average, the neonate should feed at least once every 3 to 4 hours.

Unless feeding time is extremely long (which may indicate inadequate attachment and let-down), the client should let the infant determine the length of a feeding by continuing to breast-feed until the infant begins to release the nipple. (For information on ending a feeding, see *Client teaching: Breast-feeding your infant,* pages 912 and 913.)

Encouraging night feedings. Because more prolactin is released during night feedings than day feedings, the client should breast-feed at night to take advantage of the nocturnal boost in milk production. This boost proves especially important in the early postpartal period when milk production begins. Early postpartal night feedings also give the mother added experience in handling her breasts and attaching the infant while the breasts are still relatively soft and easily manipulated. Also, increased breast-feeding frequency helps widen and stretch the lactiferous ducts, promoting breast drainage and emptying.

Helping the client cope with growth spurts. Occurring at ages 10 to 14 days, 6 weeks, 3 to 4 months, and 6 months, growth spurts seem much more noticeable in the breast-fed than the formula-fed infant. During a growth spurt,

(Text continues on page 914.)

Breast-feeding your infant

Before you begin breast-feeding, review the guidelines below to gain confidence and help both you and your infant get the most from the experience.

Starting to breast-feed

The first time you breast-feed your infant can be exciting, especially if the infant sucks and feeds properly at once. If your infant does not, however, breast-feeding still can succeed.

During the first days, you and your infant are getting to know each other. Here are some tips that may help.

• No hard and fast rules exist for the first feeding. Do not follow rigid guidelines for feeding times or frequency because these can impede milk production.
• Do not offer the infant a bottle when establishing breast-feeding. Sucking on a nipple differs from sucking on a bottle; nipple confusion may make the infant refuse the breast the next time you offer it.
• Keep the infant in the room with you and breast-feed every 2 to 3 hours or on demand—whichever comes first.
• Feed the infant through the night to help increase milk production.
• Let the infant decide when to stop breast-feeding rather than breaking suction yourself and pulling the infant off the breast. Also, let the infant finish feeding on one breast before offering the other. Keep in mind that reducing breast-feeding time will not prevent sore nipples and may cause milk drainage problems.
• Give yourself and your infant time to develop a mutually satisfying breast-feeding pattern.
• Keep in mind that a breast-fed infant usually needs to be fed more often than a formula-fed infant, so avoid comparing your infant's feeding pattern to that of a formula-fed infant.

Breast-feeding positions

You may use the cradle position, side-lying position, or football hold to breast-feed your infant. By alternating positions, you rotate the infant's position on the nipple to avoid constant friction on the same area.

Cradle position. To use this position—the most common one—sit in a comfortable chair and rest the infant's head in the bend of your arm. You may want to place pillows under your elbow to minimize tension and fatigue. Tuck the infant's lower arm alongside your body so it stays out of the way. The infant's mouth should remain even with your nipple and the stomach should face and touch your stomach.

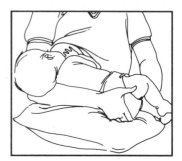

Side-lying position. You may find this position useful for night feedings or if you are recovering from a cesarean section. Lie on your side with your stomach facing the infant's stomach and the infant's head near your breast. Lift your breast; as the infant's mouth opens, pull the infant toward your nipple.

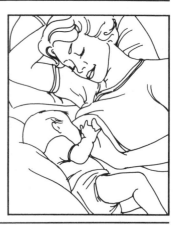

Football hold. This may be the most comfortable position if you have large breasts, if the infant is very small or premature, or if you have had a cesarean section and find other positions uncomfortable. Sit in a chair with a pillow under your arm on the nursing side. Place your hand under the infant's head and bring it close to your breast; place the fingers of your other hand above and below the nipple. As the infant's mouth opens wide, pull the head close to your breast.

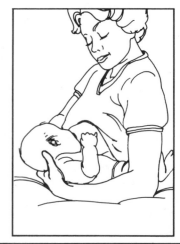

(continued)

CLIENT TEACHING

Breast-feeding your infant continued

Removing the infant from the breast

When removing the infant from the breast to feed from the other breast or to end the feeding, you can use a special technique to minimize pulling or tension on the nipple. Place your little finger in the corner of the infant's mouth, as shown here, and release suction before pulling the infant away.

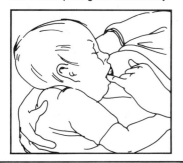

Burping your infant

You may burp your infant in any of the three positions described below. Be sure to place a cloth diaper or pad under the infant's mouth to protect your clothing from any expelled matter.

Upright position. Position the infant upright, with the head resting on your shoulder. Supporting the infant with one hand, pat or rub the infant's back with your other hand.

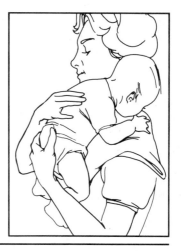

Across your lap. Place the infant face down across your lap. While holding the infant's head with one hand, rub or pat the infant's back with the other.

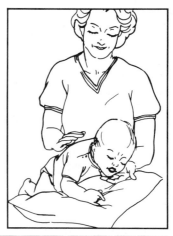

Upright on your lap. With the infant upright on your lap, hold the head from the front with one hand while patting or rubbing the back with the other hand. To help bring up air, gently rock the infant back and forth.

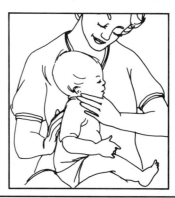

a previously satisfied infant will want to feed much more frequently. The infant's behavior—chewing on fists, crying, and settling only for short periods—may make the client fear that her milk supply is inadequate and that the infant is malnourished. If a growth spurt coincides with the client's return to work, this may raise particular concern about milk supply.

To minimize these fears in the client with a nursing diagnosis of **anxiety related to change in infant feeding pattern secondary to a growth spurt,** point out that the breasts may take up to 48 hours to produce enough milk to meet the increased demands of a growth spurt. The required time may vary somewhat, however, depending on how efficiently the infant feeds and how the client's body responds. (For more information on helping the client deal with fears about her milk supply, see *Client teaching: Coping with fears about your milk supply.*)

Providing nipple and breast care. Usually, the breasts require no care other than daily cleaning with clear water. However, the nipples may become sore, especially during the first days of breast-feeding, necessitating special care.

Nipple soreness. Although proper infant attachment and sucking help prevent nipple soreness, some soreness is common in the first few days or weeks of breast-feeding until the nipples become more elastic. For the client with a nursing diagnosis of **potential for injury related to improper nipple care,** teach about proper infant attachment.

These measures can help relieve sore nipples:
• Apply ice compresses just before feeding (this numbs the nipples and makes them firmer and more graspable).
• Lubricate the nipples with a few drops of expressed milk before the feeding. This helps prevent tenderness as effectively as lanolin-based creams (Hewat and Ellis, 1987; Adcock, Burleigh and Scott-Heads, 1988). Also, such creams have come under question because of possible contamination with pesticides resulting from sheep dipping (FDA, 1988).
• Let the nipples air dry thoroughly after feeding to promote healing and comfort.
• Avoid applying soaps directly to the nipples when washing the breasts.

The value of antepartal nipple preparation in reducing nipple tenderness is controversial. Some breast-feeding experts do not recommend it (Lauwers and Woessner, 1983; Walker and Driscoll, 1989). Others have found the practice helpful (Atkinson, 1978; Storr, 1988). (For a study of nipple preparation as a measure to prevent nipple tenderness, see *Nursing research applied: Prevention of nipple tenderness and breast engorgement.*)

CLIENT TEACHING

Coping with fears about your milk supply

While breast-feeding, you may worry that you are not producing enough milk. At times, you may even fear that your milk supply has stopped. Anxiety about adequacy of milk supply is most common during the first few days of breast-feeding and during your infant's growth spurts, which occur at ages 10 to 14 days, 6 weeks, 3 to 4 months, and 6 months. To prepare for growth spurts, mark them on your calendar so that you can build up your milk supply in advance. Also keep in mind the following points about breast milk.

• Milk supply grows in response to demand: The more milk your infant removes, the more you will produce.
• Expect to breast-feed every 2 to 3 hours while building up your milk supply.
• Use the number of wet diapers to gauge your infant's milk intake. An infant who wets 10 to 12 diapers daily is getting adequate intake.
• Do not skip feedings because that tells your body it does not need to make milk.
• Breast-feed long enough for your infant to receive the rich, more filling hindmilk—about 15 minutes on each breast in the early days.
• Rest as often as possible to increase your milk production. Especially try to rest when your infant is sleeping.
• Accept all offers of help in caring for the infant and doing household chores.
• Offer both breasts at a feeding even if your infant has lately been feeding only at one breast.
• Review your fluid and nutrient intake to ensure that your own needs are met. Remember to drink fluids each time your infant breast-feeds.
• Remember that the need to increase your milk supply during a growth spurt is only temporary.
• Motivate yourself by keeping in mind how much your infant benefits from breast-feeding.

Breast engorgement. Breast engorgement may involve excessive fullness of the breast veins or alveoli. Vascular engorgement occurs in all lactating women as blood flow to the breasts increases to prepare for breast-feeding. However, vascular engorgement commonly is confused with alveolar (milk) engorgement, which refers to alveolar overdistention with milk. Initially, vascular and alveolar engorgement may coincide.

If breast milk is insufficiently removed (as through restricted sucking time, incorrect infant attachment, or improper sucking technique), milk volume will exceed alveolar storage capacity, causing extreme discomfort.

For a client with a nursing diagnosis of *pain related to breast engorgement,* encourage frequent feeding throughout the day and night in the initial days to alleviate engorgement. One study demonstrated that prophylactic breast massage after each feeding in the first 4 days after delivery also helped prevent breast engorgement (Storr, 1988). (See *Nursing research applied: Prevention of nipple tenderness and breast engorgement.*)

Determine the cause of breast engorgement by assessing the client's breast-feeding technique and frequency. Suggest any necessary changes. Because milk engorgement can create serious drainage problems unless treated, teach the client what causes milk engorgement and remind her not to limit feeding time at the first breast offered in the mistaken belief that this will relieve engorgement. If the infant does not feed at the second breast, advise the client to express milk from the second breast, then offer this breast at the next feeding.

To help soften the breasts and facilitate attachment, the client with engorged breasts should express some milk gently before a feeding. Also, the client may massage her breasts after a warm shower or bath (applying mineral oil or a similar lubricant to the hands may make breast massage easier and reduce any discomfort it causes). Cold compresses applied to the breasts between feedings also may reduce discomfort, although no evidence shows that this relieves engorgement (Royal College of Midwives, 1988).

Milk expression. Milk expression by hand or pump may be indicated for a client who needs relief from breast engorgement or who is separated from the infant by infant illness or prematurity or by employment outside the home. Also, milk expression by pump helps improve graspability of flat or retracted nipples.

Hopkinson, Schanler, and Garza (1988) found that women who express their milk can improve milk volume in the early postpartal period by minimizing the interval between delivery and the start of milk expression. They also linked optimal milk production with five or more milk expressions and total pumping time exceeding 100 minutes daily.

Warn the client who has a nursing diagnosis of *potential for infection related to improper expression and storage of breast milk* that expressed milk probably is not sterile. Urge her to minimize bacterial contamination through frequent hand washing, aseptic handling of equipment, and aseptic transfer of her milk to storage containers (McCoy, Kadowski, Wilks, Engstrom, and Meier, 1988).

NURSING RESEARCH APPLIED

Prevention of nipple tenderness and breast engorgement

Nipple preparation as a preventive measure for postpartal nipple tenderness is controversial. Critics of nipple preparation claim that the friction it creates destroys the keratin layer, predisposing the nipple to tenderness. To investigate this theory, Storr (1988) conducted a study of 25 women who served as their own controls by preparing one nipple but not the other. To test the value of breast massage in preventing engorgement, participants also massaged one breast but not the other. Nipple tenderness and breast engorgement were recorded on five-point scales for the first 4 days postpartum. Data analysis revealed that the participants reported less tenderness and engorgement of the prepared, massaged breast.

Application to practice
The findings of this small study challenge the belief that prenatal nipple preparation promotes postpartal nipple tenderness, suggesting instead that such preparation helps prevent nipple tenderness. The study also indicates that breast massage could be recommended as prophylaxis for breast engorgement in the breast-feeding woman.

The nurse can test these findings by replicating the research and validating or disproving the findings. Nipple tenderness and breast engorgement scales can be used to facilitate more accurate descriptions of nipple tenderness.

Storr, G.B. (1988). Prevention of nipple tenderness and breast engorgement in the postpartal period. *Journal of Obstetric, Gynecologic, and Neonatal Nursing,* 17(3), 203-209.

Breast pumps are available as hand-operated, battery-operated, and electric models. (For more information about expressing milk by hand and pump, see *Client teaching: Expressing your milk,* pages 916 and 917.)

Advising the client about supplemental bottles. Some health care facilities continue the outmoded, unscientific practice of giving supplemental bottled fluids to breast-feeding neonates. Besides causing nipple confusion, supplemental bottles given in the early weeks of breast-feeding may interfere with the fragile dynamics of milk supply and demand. The nurse should advise the client to avoid giving supplemental bottles until her milk supply is well established (which typically takes 4 to 6 weeks).

Although some mothers have successfully combined breast-feeding and formula-feeding (Morse and Harrison, 1988), a client who feels she must use formula supplements should be advised to give bottles at a separate time from breast-feeding. This will disrupt the milk supply less than giving a bottle just after breast-feeding.

(Text continues on page 918.)

Expressing your milk

You may express milk when your breasts are engorged, when weaning your infant, or when you want to provide breast milk during periods of separation from your infant. Refer to the guidelines below for milk expression by hand or pump.

Expressing milk by hand
You may want to practice expressing milk by hand at a time when you feel relaxed. The illustrated steps below show the proper expression sequence. Keep in mind that you must squeeze milk from the back of the milk reservoirs forward. To push milk out of nipple openings, start the squeezing motion well behind the areola and move forward. For the final squeeze, keep your fingers behind the areola's outer edge—not on the areola or nipple.

1 Form a "U" with your fingers, as shown here, by placing your thumb above the areola and the other fingers below it.

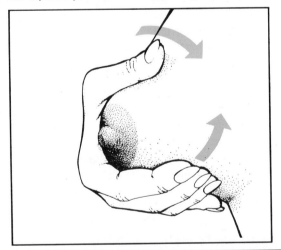

2 While pushing your fingers away from the nipple, squeeze your thumb and fingers together.

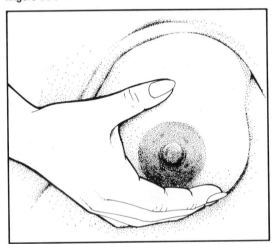

3 Now change direction by squeezing toward the nipple.

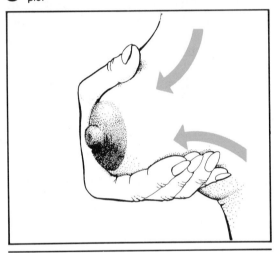

4 Rotate the thumb and fingers a quarter turn around the breast, then return to step 1 and continue until you have rotated 360 degrees around the breast.

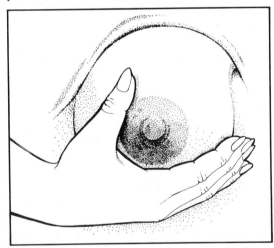

(continued)

Expressing your milk continued

Pumping and storing breast milk

Breast pumps generate a suck-release action via an adapter (flange) that you place over the areola. The adapter presses on milk reservoirs, pushing out milk. Available in pharmacies and maternity shops, breast pumps come in several varieties (see the illustrations). Here are some guidelines to follow when using a breast pump and storing milk.

You can begin pumping breast milk as soon after delivery as you feel well enough. (If your infant was born prematurely, you may begin pumping within 24 hours after delivery.)

First, wash your hands and gather all equipment (make sure the equipment has been thoroughly cleaned). You may want to apply warm, wet washcloths to your breasts or take a warm shower to help release the milk.

Before you begin pumping, stimulate the nipple and areola by rolling the nipple between your thumb and forefinger for a minute or two. This helps trigger the release of milk-producing hormones.

Pump each breast for at least 10 minutes every 3 to 4 hours during the day; at night, pump only if you are awake. Try to pump for a total of at least 100 minutes every 24 hours.

To obtain the most milk, switch breasts several times while pumping. For example, pump for 5 to 8 minutes on each breast, then for 3 to 5 minutes on each breast, and finally for 2 to 3 minutes on each breast.

Transfer milk from the collection bottle to a sterile container (preferably plastic) and refrigerate it immediately. Breast milk can be kept refrigerated for 24 to 48 hours before use.

For longer storage periods (up to 6 months), breast milk must be frozen. Let frozen breast milk thaw in the refrigerator or at room temperature, or set the container in warm water. However, be careful not to overheat it. Once thawed, it must be used within 24 hours. Also, it must not be refrozen.

If you must transport your milk to the hospital, store it in the refrigerator until transport time to prevent bacterial growth. (Some health care facilities may request that you freeze your milk before transporting it. Others freeze it after it arrives.)

Breast pumps

Battery-operated pump. This pump has a battery-operated motor and can be used with one hand. Easy to clean, it is a good choice if you work outside the home or need a breast pump only for short-term use.

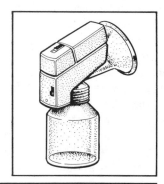

Electric pump. Usually used in hospitals, this pump is efficient and gentle and requires only one hand for operation. It is available as a small, 2-lb model or as a larger model about the size of a small sewing machine (the latter can be rented from a pharmacy or medical supply company).

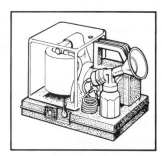

Cylinder pump. This pump has two plastic cylinders, one inside the other, that create gentle suction as you move the cylinder back and forth. Because you must use two hands to operate it, you may find it tiring. Easily cleaned and portable, this pump proves relatively efficient for short-term or intermittent use.

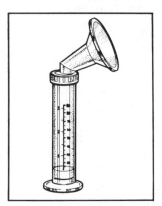

Rubber bulb or bicycle horn pump. To operate this pump, squeeze the rubber bulb, then release it slowly. Although inexpensive, this pump usually is not recommended because of its inefficiency and tendency to cause nipple and areola trauma. Also, sterility cannot be maintained because milk commonly becomes trapped inside the bulb.

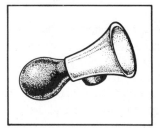

(Parents with a family history of food allergies may wish to avoid any use of formula until the infant's gastrointestinal mucosa has matured and is less susceptible to allergic reactions.)

Ensuring adequate maternal fluid and food intake. Advise the breast-feeding client to maintain a fluid intake sufficient to keep her urine clear and amber. For a client with a nursing diagnosis of *potential fluid volume deficit related to breast-feeding,* provide fluids at each feeding. Also, advise the client to restrict intake of caffeine-containing fluids because caffeine accumulates in the body and transfers to the infant in breast milk, possibly making the infant fussy in the evening.

Although many obstetricians still advise lactating women to consume 500 extra calories daily, the Royal College of Midwives (1988) now recommends that hunger—rather than a rigid caloric requirement—should guide food intake during breast-feeding.

When counseling the client with a nursing diagnosis of *altered nutrition: potential for more than body requirements, related to breast-feeding,* help her establish a well-balanced diet and assure her that she can consume any food in moderation. However, if the infant develops symptoms of food allergy, she may have to restrict some foods. The client with a family history of food allergy may need to modify her diet (ideally, modification should begin during pregnancy).

Advising the client about drug use. Almost any drug the client consumes potentially transfers to the infant through breast milk. However, the client need not necessarily stop breast-feeding during drug therapy. Instead, she should seek her physician's advice. Usually, the breast-feeding woman can safely use therapeutic doses of such drugs as analgesics, antibiotics, stool softeners, and bulk-forming laxatives. On the other hand, potent diuretics, antineoplastic drugs, stimulant laxatives, and radioactive drugs nearly always warrant temporary discontinuation of breast-feeding. Use of oral contraceptives during breast-feeding is controversial. (For recommendations on the use of selected drugs during lactation, see *Drug use during lactation.*)

Promoting family support. The breast-feeding client needs practical and emotional support from those close to her. The client's partner can play an especially key role. Hewat and Ellis (1986) found that mothers of neonates view three types of support from the father as important: physical support (such as helping with housework or other children), verbal reinforcement (such as ensuring the mother that breast-feeding is progressing well), and psychological support or sensitivity to the mother's feelings.

Drug use during lactation

Most drugs ingested by a lactating woman appear in her breast milk. Although many drugs cause no ill effects in the breast-fed infant, some are contraindicated and others should be used with caution. The breast-feeding woman should seek her physician's advice on drug use. However, the nurse may benefit from the general guidelines and partial drug list presented below.

• Because breast milk levels of drugs peak shortly after a drug dose is taken, the client should breast-feed just before or at least 2 hours after taking medication. (Drugs taken every 3 to 6 hours usually reach peak blood and breast milk levels in 1 hour.)

• The premature infant cannot detoxify drugs as well as the full-term neonate and thus is more susceptible to the effects of maternal drugs.

• Medication transferred through breast milk may interact with any drug the infant receives by another route.

• If the client must temporarily stop breast-feeding during drug therapy, she must express her milk by hand or pump to maintain lactation and prevent breast engorgement.

CONTRAINDICATED DRUGS	DRUGS TO USE CAUTIOUSLY
• Bromides • Chloramphenicol • Cyclophosphamide • Diazepam • Diethylstilbestrol • Ergot alkaloids • Gold salts • Indomethacin • Iodides • Methotrexate • Methylergonovine • Radioactive iodine	• Atropine • Barbiturates • Chloral hydrate • Dicumarol • Dihydrotachysterol • Ergonovine • Ethinyl estradiol • Medroxyprogesterone acetate • Methadone • Metronidazole • Nalidixic acid • Nitrofurantoin • Norethisterone • Phenothiazines • Phenylbutazone • Quinine • Senna • Sulfonamides • Thiazide diuretics

Childbirth education groups can serve as a source of support for new parents dealing with role adjustment. For a family with a nursing diagnosis of *altered family processes related to breast-feeding,* urge the partner to provide physical support by helping the client rest when she is establishing her milk supply. Also, encourage the partner to prevent visitors from overwhelming the client in the early breast-feeding days. Further, incorporate the partner in client teaching about such topics as infant positioning and attachment and determining if the infant is getting adequate nourishment.

Grandparents also may be expected to provide support. However, many of today's grandparents formula-fed their infants and thus know little about breast-feeding. Promote grandparent involvement in breast-feeding by developing teaching materials designed specifically for them.

Encouraging cuddling and eye contact. Breast-feeding brings the infant into close contact with the mother, allowing interaction that facilitates attachment. The nurse can encourage such interaction—for example, by suggesting that the client stroke the infant during feeding (especially if the client breast-feeds while lying down, which frees both hands). If the client breast-feeds while sitting, she can make eye contact with the infant.

Breast-feeding in special situations

Few circumstances completely rule out breast-feeding. The nurse with limited exposure to special breast-feeding situations should develop contacts with such groups as the International Lactation Consultant Association (ILCA) or the LaLeche League for information or client referral.

The premature infant. Many premature infants can be breast-fed. Providing breast milk may be the only role the mother of a premature infant is permitted or able to perform; doing so may help her feel she is mothering her infant (Driscoll and Sheehan, 1985). For a client with a nursing diagnosis of *altered parenting related to infant prematurity and the mother's wish to breast-feed,* provide accurate information and ongoing support.

In North America, feeding schedules for premature infants typically are based on infant weight, gestational age, and ability to bottle-feed without signs of distress. However, none of these parameters is a research-based index of readiness to breast-feed (McCoy, Kadowski, Wilks, Engstrom, and Meier, 1988). Some data suggest that the premature infant can coordinate sucking and swallowing earlier for breast-feeding than for bottle-feeding (Meier and Pugh, 1985) and that breast-feeding creates less physiologic stress than bottle-feeding (Meier and Anderson, 1987; Meier, 1988). However, most premature infants breast-feed for shorter durations than full-term neonates (Meberg, Willgraff, and Sande, 1982; Neifert and Seacat, 1988; Pereira, Schwartz, Gould, and Grim, 1984).

Besides coping with the stress of premature delivery, the client who wishes to breast-feed her premature infant but who cannot do so directly must establish and maintain a milk supply by expressing milk.

Multiple infants. Many mothers have successfully breast-fed twins and even triplets and quadruplets (Keith, McInnes, and Keith, 1982). For a client with a nursing diagnosis of *anxiety related to the ability to breast-feed multiple infants,* help instill confidence by relating these findings. However, also promote realistic expectations about the additional time needed to initiate and maintain a milk supply for multiple infants. If the client chooses to breast-feed the infants simultaneously, she may need help in positioning them. Refer her to a Parents of Twins group for support and information if the community has one.

The client with premature multiple infants may have to delay breast-feeding until the infants can tolerate it (Storr, 1989). However, if the infants were born close to term and are permitted to breast-feed, the client should keep them together while breast-feeding to accustom her to breast-feeding multiple infants (Keith, McInnes, and Keith, 1982; Lauwers and Woessner, 1983).

If the client wishes to breast-feed exclusively, this pattern should be initiated in the health care facility. If she plans to supplement breast-feeding with formula, however, advise her that this practice will decrease breast milk production and may create nipple confusion in the infants.

Working outside the home. The client who plans to continue breast-feeding after returning to work will need guidance and support. Although breast-feeding in this circumstance calls for extra commitment and effort, both mother and infant may reap rewards. For instance, knowing that her breast milk is meeting the infant's nutritional and immunologic needs may help ease any misgivings she has about returning to work.

The client may breast-feed at home and pump milk at work, schedule work around feeding times, or wean the infant from work-time feedings. Weaning should be done gradually to avoid adverse effects in both infant and mother. The client who wants to wean may decrease milk production by pumping only minimally, for comfort; as the demand for milk drops, so does milk production. Instruct the client to give the infant a bottle for the feeding that will be eliminated and warn her that her body will probably need several days to adjust to the elimination of each feeding.

Help the working mother devise a breast-feeding schedule that meets her individual needs, especially if she has a nursing diagnosis of *altered role performance related to the new task of breast-feeding.* (For a sample schedule, see *Client teaching: Suggested breast-feeding schedule for the working mother,* page 920.)

The client's work wardrobe should include clothes that can be easily unbuttoned or pulled aside to express milk to feed to the infant later. Breasts may leak in the first few weeks after she returns to work as they readjust to the new schedule. To help prevent or minimize breast leakage, the client can press against the breasts when she feels the tingling that signals let-down. Instruct her to place breast pads in her bra so that milk will not stain clothing and to change the pads frequently to avoid skin irritation from milk. She may prefer to wear patterned fabrics, which disguise milk stains better than solid colors. Taking a sweater and a spare blouse to work will avoid embarrassment caused by milk stains.

Warn the client that anxiety and fatigue caused by her return to work may reduce her milk production for a week or so. Maintaining an adequate fluid intake at work may minimize this problem.

Care for the client using infant formula

For the client who plans to formula-feed her infant, teaching on such topics as formula preparation can begin in the antepartal period. As with breast-feeding, initial formula-feeding experiences can prove crucial for both mother and infant. A positive first feeding experience can enhance maternal confidence and set the right tone for subsequent feedings. The nurse who observes early feedings has a unique opportunity to assess client-infant interaction and, if necessary, provide timely intervention.

Client teaching

The nurse should consider both short-term and long-term goals to anticipate guidance needed by the client who chooses formula-feeding. In the antepartal period, develop varied client teaching methods (perhaps using such items as films and books) to present current recommendations about formula-feeding. Discuss with the client specific feeding situations that might arise and plan a strategy for handling them. For example, ask the client what she would do if a friend or relative told her the infant was not eating enough or if the infant did not sleep through the night as early as a friend's did. Usually, antepartal discussion of growth spurts, of alternatives to early introduction of solid foods, and of support systems is more effective than discussion during the postpartal period, when the client may be fatigued from sleep deprivation and anxiety accompanying new parenthood.

Ensuring proper formula preparation

To teach the client about formula preparation, find out what preparation facilities and equipment will be available as well as which formula the client will use. Where water and refrigeration are readily available, rigorous sterilization practices largely have been replaced with an emphasis on cleanliness of the equipment and preparer. However, a client who lacks easy access to refrigeration and running water may have to modify preparation procedures.

Preparation methods. Four basic methods may be used to prepare infant formula.

Aseptic method. In this method, the preparer sterilizes formula equipment (including the mixing pitcher, measuring spoons, tongs, bottles, nipples, and nipple caps) by boiling it for 10 minutes. After reconstituting the formula according to manufacturer's instructions, the preparer pours the specified amount into each bottle, applies nipples and caps, and stores the bottles in the refrigerator until needed.

Terminal method. The preparer thoroughly washes the equipment and prepares the formula under clean (not sterile) conditions. After pouring reconstituted formula into bottles (with nipples and caps applied loosely), the preparer places the bottles in a pot with a tightly covered lid and boils them for 25 minutes. Once the bottles have cooled slightly, the preparer screws the caps down tightly and refrigerates them. Formula prepared by this method may take up to 2 hours to cool sufficiently to give to the infant.

One-bottle method. Using clean equipment, the preparer reconstitutes enough formula for one feeding, then pours it in a bottle. Prepared formula should be used within 30 minutes; the can containing the remaining unreconstituted formula must be refrigerated.

Clean method. With this method, an entire day's formula is prepared at one time and placed in clean bottles. The preparer reconstitutes the formula, applies clean nipples and caps, and refrigerates the bottles immediately.

General principles. Some common principles are basic to all formula preparation methods. The preparer must use good hand-washing technique—a point to reinforce frequently. Also, before opening the can, the preparer should wash the can opener and the top of the formula can with soap and water.

Prepared formula should be used within 24 hours (or 30 minutes with the one-bottle method). Opened formula cans should be covered with plastic or foil and refrigerated. Equipment used in formula preparation may be cleaned in an automatic dishwasher (providing the temperature reaches 140° F) or in warm, soapy water. However, latex nipples cleaned in a dishwasher may need to be replaced frequently because repeated exposure to heat weakens them. Instruct the client to place latex nipples in a covered basket in the dishwasher to prevent their displacement to the heating element, where they could melt. Also instruct the client to inspect nipples regularly to ensure that no milk particles block the opening, forming a bacterial breeding ground.

Giving the first feeding

No research-based guidelines support delaying formula-feeding. Nonetheless, in many health care facilities, the first feeding is given when the neonate is about 4 hours old. In other facilities, it is given when physiologic and behavioral cues suggest the neonate is ready to feed. Such cues include active bowel sounds, lack of abdominal distention, and sucking and rooting responses to stimulation of the lips. Neonates fed according to these cues are less likely to gag during the first feeding because their sucking and rooting responses are active. In some health care facilities, a nurse—rather than the mother—gives the first bottle (usually sterile water). However, this practice is based on tradition rather than research.

Helping the client with early feedings

Contrary to popular belief, the client using infant formula may require help with early feedings, especially if she has a nursing diagnosis of **knowledge deficit related to formula-feeding.**

Provide comfort measures (such as encouraging voiding and administering an analgesic, if prescribed) and have the client wash her hands before preparing the formula and feeding the infant. Then, help the client to a comfortable position with good back support and instruct her to hold the infant close to her in a semireclining position, with the bottle tilted so that the nipple always is filled with formula. This position minimizes air swallowing and permits air to rise to the top of the infant's stomach.

Some neonates will take an artificial nipple into the mouth readily; others must be coaxed. Instruct the client to stroke the infant's lips gently with the nipple; usually, this causes the mouth to open wide enough for nipple insertion. The first-time mother may be reluctant to place more than the tip of the nipple in the infant's mouth; urge her to insert the nipple further to trigger the sucking reflex.

Instruct the client to check nipple openings by holding the bottle upside down and noting whether formula drips freely from the nipple. (Formula that runs in a continuous stream is flowing too quickly.) The client can assume that nipple openings are the correct size if feedings take roughly 15 to 20 minutes—long enough to meet the infant's nutritional needs without causing fatigue. Warn the client to discard any formula left in the bottle at the end of a feeding because of the risk of bacterial contamination.

Most health care facilities use glass bottles with standard latex nipples; when the infant sucks, air bubbles may appear in these bottles, indicating that the infant is obtaining milk. However, point out that at home, the client may use a feeding system with a collapsible bag in which she cannot see air bubbles move. Instead, she should watch for the bag to collapse gradually—as a sign that the infant is obtaining formula.

Ensuring good burping technique. The infant should be burped after every ounce of formula and again at the end of the feeding. Burping can be done in three positions—upright, across the lap, or upright on the lap (as shown in *Client teaching: Breast-feeding your infant*, pages 912 and 913). Because a neonate's cardiac sphincter does not function fully, the neonate may expel milk along with air; a towel or cloth diaper placed in front of the infant will protect the client's clothing.

Helping the client establish a feeding pattern. Like the breast-fed infant, the formula-fed infant should be fed on a flexible demand schedule, not a rigid regimen. The formula-fed infant may awaken for feedings as often as every 2 hours or as infrequently as every 5 hours; many feed satisfactorily on a 3- or 4-hour schedule. If the client worries that the infant is not getting enough nourish-

Client with a knowledge deficit related to breast-feeding techniques

For the client who plans to breast-feed, the nursing process helps ensure high-quality care and appropriate decision making. The table below shows how the nurse might use the nursing process when caring for the client described in the case history at right. The first column presents history and physical assessment data followed by a paragraph of mental notes. These notes help the nurse make important mental connections among assessment findings, aiding in development of the nursing diagnosis and planning.

The second column lists an appropriate nursing diagnosis; information in the remaining columns is based on this diagnosis. Although not part of the nursing process, a rationale appears for each intervention in the fourth column to explain how it contributes to the care plan.

ASSESSMENT	NURSING DIAGNOSIS	PLANNING
Subjective (history) data • Client states that she has not had much experience with infants. • Client reports that none of her friends or family members has breast-fed. • Client says she has not read any material on breast-feeding. • Client states that she needs "a lot of help with breast-feeding." **Objective (physical) data** • Vital signs: temperature 98° F (36.7° C), pulse 90 beats/minute, respiratory rate 20 breaths/minute and regular, blood pressure 110/78 mm Hg. • Breasts swollen; nipples without cracks or fissures. **Mental notes** *The client is a first-time mother with no knowledge of breast-feeding from family or literature. Openly realizes she needs assistance.*	Knowledge deficit related to breast-feeding techniques	**Goals** Before leaving the health care facility, the client will: • explain breast-feeding techniques • demonstrate proper breast-feeding techniques • explain proper self-care, such as breast care, diet, and medication use • discuss interventions for altered milk production due to illness • discuss milk pumping and storage techniques • discuss the support resources she may use after discharge.

ment, explain that the initial feeding pattern does not necessarily indicate the pattern that will emerge later.

Promoting physical contact. Although formula-feeding allows less intimate contact than breast-feeding, it still provides an opportunity to cuddle the infant. Encourage the client to make eye contact and to vocalize with the infant during feeding.

Encouraging family support. A frequently cited benefit of formula-feeding is that it allows other family members to help with feedings. This help can be particularly valuable if the mother is fatigued. However, encourage family members to do such chores as preparing formula and cleaning formula equipment rather than insisting on giving the infant the bottle—an activity the mother may find relaxing. Siblings may or may not want to assist with feedings; parents should let them decide for themselves, especially in the early feeding days.

For the client with a nursing diagnosis of ***altered family processes related to infant feeding,*** discuss how to spend adequate time with the infant while obtaining help for more tiring chores.

Evaluation

During this step of the nursing process, the nurse evaluates the effectiveness of the plan of care. To do this, the nurse evaluates subjective and objective criteria on an ongoing basis.

Evaluation findings should be stated in terms of actions performed or outcomes achieved for each goal. The following examples illustrate appropriate evaluation statements for the breast-feeding client:
• The client demonstrated appropriate techniques for attaching the infant to the breast.
• The client showed no signs of breast problems, such as sore nipples or excessive engorgement.
• The client expressed an understanding of breast-feeding dynamics.
• The client expressed confidence in her ability to seek help for breast-feeding problems.

CASE STUDY

Sarah Jones, age 23, delivered her first child—a boy weighing 7 lb, 3 oz—5 hours ago. She is about to breast-feed for the first time. As the nurse hands her the neonate, Mrs. Jones says, "How do you breast-feed?"

IMPLEMENTATION		EVALUATION
Intervention Assess the client's level of knowledge about breast-feeding and her prenatal preparation.	**Rationale** Assessment helps provide a baseline from which the teaching plan can be developed.	Upon evaluation, the client: • explained breast-feeding techniques • demonstrated proper breast-feeding techniques • explained proper self-care methods • outlined what steps to take if she becomes ill • demonstrated proper milk pumping techniques • identified support systems available after discharge.
Teach the client about breast-feeding techniques, using short sessions and terms appropriate for her understanding.	The client's individual learning needs will be met.	
Provide the client with pamphlets and names and phone numbers of breast-feeding support groups.	The client can review written materials after her discharge. Support groups can help answer her questions and allay anxiety about breast-feeding.	

The following examples illustrate appropriate evaluation statements for the client who uses infant formula:
• The client expressed an understanding of formula preparation and feeding techniques.
• The client maintained close contact with the neonate during feeding.
• The client expressed confidence in her ability to seek support for feeding problems.

Objective infant criteria include hydration status and weight-gain pattern.

Documentation

All steps of the nursing process should be documented as thoroughly and objectively as possible. Thorough documentation not only allows the nurse to evaluate the effectiveness of the plan of care, but it also makes the data available to other members of the health care team, helping to ensure consistency of care. (For a case study that shows how to apply the nursing process to a client who needs information about breast-feeding, see *Applying the nursing process: Client with a knowledge deficit related to breast-feeding techniques.*)

When assisting a client with breast-feeding, include the following points in the documentation:
• maternal vital signs
• maternal fluid intake and output
• maternal position and comfort level during feeding
• maternal understanding of breast-feeding technique
• maternal understanding of proper infant positioning and ability to achieve proper positioning
• maternal attitude toward breast-feeding
• maternal understanding of dietary needs and breast care
• condition of the nipples and breasts
• infant sucking ability.

When assisting a client with formula-feeding, include the following points in the documentation:

• maternal vital signs
• maternal comfort level when feeding the infant
• maternal understanding of formula preparation
• maternal understanding of normal infant feeding patterns, including amount of formula taken and feeding frequency
• infant sucking ability.

Chapter summary

Chapter 37 described the needs of the childbearing family regarding infant nutrition. Here are the chapter highlights.

• Feeding is an important part of infant care, not only because it provides nutrition but because the reciprocal interactions that take place are important to the infant's psychosocial development and the parent-infant relationship.

• Breast milk and infant formula differ in nutritional value and immunologic properties.

• Unparalleled physical growth takes place during the infant's first year; throughout this period, nutritional requirements change dramatically.

• Feeding methods include breast-feeding and formula-feeding. The nurse should provide the client with appropriate information so that she can make a choice appropriate to her beliefs and life-style.

• Infant feeding can be an emotionally charged issue; many traditional infant feeding practices may not reflect updated knowledge.

• To make breast-feeding mutually satisfying, mother and infant must adjust and integrate their differing—sometimes opposing—needs.

• Nipple abrasion in the breast-feeding client usually can be avoided through correct infant attachment and positioning.

• In the United States and Canada, breast-feeding only recently has become common once again. Thus, the client who breast-feeds may need support and guidance, especially in recognizing the breast-fed infant's frequent feeding requirements.

• The client who chooses formula-feeding may need assistance with early feedings as well as continued support and guidance on infant behavior and feeding recommendations.

Study questions

1. Which details should the nurse include in a nutritional assessment of an infant?

2. How do breast milk and formula differ in nutritional value and immunologic properties?

3. What are some reasons why a client may decide to formula-feed rather than breast-feed?

4. Which physiologic mechanisms are involved in breast milk production?

5. Which institutional practices facilitate milk production in the early postpartal period?

6. Sheila Warren, age 32, is a first-time mother who teaches mathematics at the local high school. All of her friends have breast-fed and have told her how easy and natural it was. Two days after delivery, however, Mrs. Warren has trouble getting her neonate to attach to the breast and suck. Her nipples appear slightly red and she feels frustrated because the neonate will not feed. Which factors should the nurse assess for and what are some appropriate interventions?

7. Deborah Jacobs, age 17, is a single pregnant client no longer involved with the father of her future child. She has not decided how she will feed her infant. Which topics should the nurse discuss with Ms. Jacobs to help her decide which infant feeding method is best suited to her life-style?

8. What challenges does the premature infant pose for the client who wishes to breast-feed?

Bibliography

Finberg, L., Dweck, H., and Krelchmer, N., et al. (1986). Fluoride supplementation. *Pediatrics*, 77(5), 758-761.

Avery, G. B. (1987). *Neonatology: Pathophysiology and management of the newborn* (3rd ed.). Philadelphia: Lippincott.

Carr, C. (1989). A four-week observation of maternity care in Finland. *JOGNN*, 18(2), 100-104.

Health and Welfare, Canada. (1986). Feeding babies: A counselling guide on practical solutions to common infant feeding questions. Minister of Supply and Services, Canada.

Lewis, C. (1986). *Nutrition and nutritional therapy in nursing*. Norwalk, CT: Appleton-Lange.

Marieb, E. (1989). *Human anatomy and physiology*. Redwood City, CA: Benjamin-Cummings.

McWilliams, M. (1986). *Nutrition for the growing years* (4th ed.). New York: Macmillan.

Morse, J., and Harrison, M. (1988). Patterns of mixed feeding. *Midwifery*, 4(1), 19-23.

Myres, A. (1988). Tradition and technology in infant feeding—achieving the best of both worlds. *Canadian Journal of Public Health*, 79(2), 78-80.

Nelms, B., and Mullins, R. (1982). *Growth and development: A primary health care approach*. Englewood Cliffs, NJ: Prentice-Hall.

Pipes, P. (1988). *Nutrition in infancy and childhood* (4th ed.). St. Louis: Mosby.

Seeley, R., Stephens, T., and Tate, P. (1989). *Anatomy and physiology*. Redwood City, CA: Benjamin-Cummings.

Shapiro, A., Jacobson, L., Armon, M., Manco-Johnson, M., Hulac, P., Lane, P., and Hathaway, W. (1986). Vitamin K deficiency in the newborn infant: Prevalence and perinatal risk factors. *Journal of Pediatrics*, 109(4), 675-680.

Tanaka, P., Yeung, D., and Anderson, G. H. (1987). Infant feeding practices: 1984-85 versus 1977-78. *Canadian Medical Association Journal*, 136(9), 940-944.

Winikoff, B., Laukaran, V., Myers, S., and Stone, R. (1986). Dynamics of feeding: Mothers, professionals, and the institutional context in a large urban hospital. *Pediatrics*, 77(3), 357-365.

World Health Organization (1981). International code of marketing of breast-milk substitutes. *WHO Chronicle*, 35, 112-117.

Wright, P. (1987). Hunger, satiety and feeding behavior in early infancy. In R. Boakes, D. Popplewell, and M. Burton (Eds.), *Eating habits, food, physiology and learned behavior* (pp. 75-106). New York: Wiley.

Breast-feeding

Adcock, A., Burleigh, A., and Scott-Heads (1988). Hind milk as an effective topical application in nipple care in the post-partum period. *Breastfeeding Review*, 13, Abstract 68.

American Academy of Pediatrics (1978). Breast-feeding. *Pediatrics*, 62, 591-601.

Baer, E. (1981). Promoting breastfeeding: A national responsibility. *Studies in Family Planning*, 12, 198-206.

Bloom, K., Goldbloom, R. B., Robinson, F. C., Stevens, F. F., and Houston, J. (1982). Factors affecting the continuance of breast feeding. *Acta Paediatrica Scandinavica*, 71(Suppl. 300), 9-14.

Canadian Pediatric Society (1978). Breast-feeding: What is left besides the poetry? *Canadian Journal of Public Health*, 69, 13-20.

Casey, C., and Hambridge, K. (1983). Nutritional aspects of human lactation. In M. Neville and M. Neifert (Eds.), *Lactation physiology, nutrition and breast-feeding* (pp. 199-248). New York: Plenum.

Choi, E. C. (1986). Unique aspects of Korean-American mothers. *JOGNN*, 15(5), 394-400.

Cunningham, A. (1984). Breast-feeding and illness. *Pediatrics*, 74, 416.

Cunningham, A. (1987). Breast-feeding and health. *Journal of Pediatrics*, 110(4), 658-659.

Cunningham, A. (1988). Studies of breastfeeding and infections. How good is the evidence? *Journal of Human Lactation*, 4, 54-56.

Driscoll, J., and Sheehan, C. (1985). Breast-feeding and premature babies: Guidelines for nurses. *Neonatal Network*, 5(1), 18-24.

Food and Drug Administration. (1988, September 13). Lanolin contaminated with pesticides. Talk paper. (T-88-66).

Glasier, A., McNeilly, A., and Howie, P. (1984). The prolactin response to suckling. *Clinical Endocrinology*, 21(2), 109-116.

Goldman, A., Garza, C., Nichols, B., and Goldblum, R. (1982). Immunologic factors in human milk during the first year of lactation. *Journal of Pediatrics*, 100(4), 563-567.

Hanson, L., Adlerberth, L., Carlsson, B., Castrignano, S., Hahn-Zoric, M., Dahlgren, U., Jalil, F., Nilsson, K., and Robertson, D. (1988). Breastfeeding protects against infections and allergy. *Breastfeeding Review*, 13, 19-22.

Hartman, P., and Kent, J. (1988). The subtlety of breast milk. *Breastfeeding Review*, 13, 14-18.

Hayward, A. (1983). The immunology of breast milk. In M. Neville and M. Neifert (Eds.), *Lactation physiology, nutrition and breast-feeding* (pp. 249-270). New York: Plenum.

Hopkinson, J., Schanler, R., and Garza, C. (1988). Milk production by mothers of premature infants. *Pediatrics*, 81(6), 815-820.

Humenick, S. (1987). The clinical significance of breast milk maturation rates. *Birth*, 14, 174-181.

Jones, D., and West, R. (1985). Lactation nurse increases duration of breast-feeding. *Archives of Disease in Childhood*, 60(8), 772-774.

Keith, D., McInnes, S., and Keith, L. (1982). *Breastfeeding twins, triplets and quadruplets: 195 practical hints for success*. Chicago: Center for the Study of Multiple Birth.

Klaus, M. (1987). The frequency of suckling: A neglected but essential ingredient of breast-feeding. *Obstetrics and Gynecology Clinics of North America*, 14(3), 623-633.

Kocturk, T., and Zetterstrom, R. (1988). Breast-feeding and its promotion. *Acta Paediatrica Scandinavica*, 77, 183-190.

Lauwers, J., and Woessner, C. (1989). *Counselling the nursing mother* (2nd ed.). Wayne, NJ: Avery.

Lawrence, R. (1989). *Breastfeeding—a guide for the medical profession* (3rd ed.). St. Louis: Mosby.

Leventhal, J., Shapiro, E., Aten, C., Berg, A., and Egerter, S. (1986). Does breast-feeding protect against infections in infants less than 3 months of age? *Pediatrics*, 78, 896-903.

Meberg, A., Willgraff, S., and Sande, H. (1982). High potential for breastfeeding among mothers giving birth to pre-term infants. *Acta Paediatrica Scandinavica*, 71(4), 661-662.

Meier, P., and Pugh, E. (1985). Breastfeeding behavior of small preterm infants. *MCN*, 10(6), 396-401.

Minchin, M. (1985). *Breastfeeding matters*. Sydney, Australia: George Allen & Unwin.

Myres, A., Watson, J., and Harrison, C. (1981). The national breast-feeding promotion program 1. professional phase—a note on its development, distribution and impact. *Canadian Journal of Public Health*, 72, 307-311.

Neifert, M., and Seacat, J. (1987). Lactation insufficiency: A rational approach. *Birth*, 14(4), 182-190.

Neifert, M., and Seacat, J. (1988). Practical aspects of breast-feeding the premature infant. *Perinatology-Neonatology*, 12(1), 24-31.

Neville, M. (1983). Regulation of mammary development and lactation. In M. Neville and M. Neifert (Eds.), *Lactation physiology, nutrition and breast-feeding* (pp. 103-140). New York: Plenum.

Newman, J. (1986). Breast-feeding: The problem of 'not enough milk'. *Canadian Family Physician*, 32, 571-574.

Nice, F. (1989). Can a breastfeeding mother take medication without harming her infant? *MCN*, 14(1), 27-31.

Ogra, P., and Greene, H. (1982). Human milk and breast feeding: An update on the state of the art. *Pediatric Research*, 16(41), 266-271.

Pereira, G., Schwartz, D., Gould, P., and Grim, N. (1984). Breast-feeding in neonatal intensive care: Beneficial effects of maternal counseling. *Perinatology-Neonatology*, 8(2), 35-42.

Riordan, J., and Countryman, B. (1983). The biologic specificity of breast milk. In J. Riordan, *A practical guide to breastfeeding* (pp. 28-39). St. Louis: Mosby.

Royal College of Midwives (1988). *Successful breastfeeding—a practical guide for midwives.* Oxford: Holywell Press.

Rumball, S. (1988). Structure and function of the human milk protein lactoferrin. *Breastfeeding Review*, 13, 31-32.

Smith, W., Erenberg, A., and Nowak, A. (1988). Imaging evaluation of the human nipple during breast-feeding. *American Journal of Diseases in Children*, 142(1), 76-78.

Storr, G.B. (1989). Breastfeeding premature triplets— one woman's experience. *Journal of Human Lactation*, 5(2), 74-77.

Tulley, M., and Overfield, M. (1987). *Breastfeeding counselling guide.* Raleigh, NC: Lactation Consultants of North Carolina.

U.S. Department of Health and Human Services. (1984). *Report on the surgeon general's workshop on breastfeeding and human lactation* (DDHS Publication No. HRS-D-MC 84-2). Washington, DC: U.S. Government Printing Office.

Walker, M. (1987). How to evaluate breast pumps. *MCN*, 12(4), 270-276.

Walker, M., and Driscoll, J. (1989). Sore nipples: The new mother's nemesis. *MCN*, 14(4), 260-265.

Weber, F., Woolridge, M., and Baum, J. (1986). An ultrasonographic study of the organization of sucking and swallowing by newborn infants. *Developmental Medicine & Child Neurology*, 28(1), 19-24.

Wood, C., Isaacs, P., Jensen, M., and Hilton, H. G. (1988). Exclusively breast-fed infants: Growth and caloric intake. *Pediatric Nursing*, 14(2), 117-124.

Woolridge, M. (1986). The anatomy of infant sucking. *Midwifery*, 2(4), 164-171.

Woolridge, M. (1989, July 8). The physiology of suckling and milk transfer. Paper presented at ILCA Conference, Toronto.

Formula-feeding

Fomon, S. (1987). Reflections on infant feeding in the 1970s and 1980s. *American Journal of Clinical Nutrition*, 46, 171-82.

Jason, J., Nieburg, P., and Marks, J. (1984). Mortality and infectious disease associated with infant-feeding practices in developing countries. *Pediatrics*, 74 (4, Pt. 2), 702-727.

Kovar, M., Serdula, M., Marks, J., and Fraser, D. (1984). Review of epidemiologic evidence for an association between infant feeding and infant health. *Pediatrics*, 74 (4, Pt. 2), 615-638.

Kramer, M. (1988). Infant feeding, infection and public health. *Pediatrics*, 81(1), 164-166.

Minchin, M. (1987). Infant formula: A mass uncontrolled trial in perinatal care. *Birth*, 14(1), 25-33.

Ross Laboratories. (1985). *Formula intake guidelines.* Columbus, OH.

Cultural references

Armstrong, H. (1987). Breastfeeding and low birth weight babies: Advances in Kenya. *Journal of Human Lactation*, 3, 34-37.

Gabriel, A., Gabriel, K. R., and Lawrence, R. (1986). Cultural values and biomedical knowledge: Choices in infant feeding. *Social Science and Medicine*, 23(5), 501-509.

Nursing research

Atkinson, L. (1979). Prenatal nipple conditioning for breast-feeding. *Nursing Research* 28(5), 267-271.

Hewat, R., and Ellis, D. (1984). Breastfeeding as a maternal-child team effort: Women's perceptions. *Health Care for Women International*, 5(5/6), 437-452.

Hewat, R., and Ellis, D. (1986). Similarities and differences between women who breastfeed for short and long duration. *Midwifery*, 2(1), 37-43.

Hewat, R., and Ellis, D. (1987). A comparison of the effectiveness of two methods of nipple care. *Birth*, 14(1), 41-45.

Jones, D., West, R., and Newcombe, R. (1986). Maternal characteristics associated with duration of breast-feeding. *Midwifery*, 2(3), 141-146.

McCoy, R., Kadowski, C., Wilks, S., Engstrom, J., and Meier, P. (1988). Nursing management of breastfeeding for preterm infants. *Journal of Perinatal Neonatal Nursing*, 2(1), 42-55.

Meier, P., and Anderson, G.C. (1987). Responses of small preterm infants to bottle- and breast-feeding. *MCN*, 12(2), 97-105.

Meier, P. (1988). Bottle and breast feeding: Effects on transcutaneous oxygen pressure and temperature in small preterm infants. *Nursing Research*, 37(1), 36-41.

Storr, G.B. (1988). Prevention of nipple tenderness and breast engorgement in the postpartal period. *JOGNN*, 17(3), 203-209.

High-Risk Neonates

Objectives

After reading and studying this chapter, the student should be able to:

1. Define the three levels of neonatal care.

2. Explain the concept of regionalized neonatal care.

3. Identify maternal, antepartal, intrapartal, and fetal factors that increase the risk of perinatal problems.

4. Discuss the physiologic basis for such perinatal problems as hypothermia, fluid imbalance, and hyperbilirubinemia.

5. Identify perinatal problems commonly seen in preterm neonates.

6. Develop nursing diagnoses for neonates with perinatal problems.

7. Discuss the measures used to resuscitate a neonate at delivery.

8. Apply the nursing process when caring for a high-risk neonate.

Introduction

The high-risk neonate is one who has an increased chance of dying during or shortly after delivery or who has a congenital or perinatal problem necessitating prompt intervention. As medicine continues to develop more treatments for perinatal problems, many high-risk neonates who formerly would have died after mere hours or days now survive; many have few or no residual effects of the crisis that marked their first hours after birth.

This chapter begins by describing the levels and regionalization of neonatal care and discussing some ethical and legal concerns surrounding such care. Next,

the chapter describes the etiology and pathophysiology of common perinatal problems. Then it identifies factors that help anticipate a high-risk delivery, highlighting the effects of gestational-age and birth-weight variations on neonatal status. Finally, the chapter shows how to plan and implement nursing care, including both general measures relevant for all high-risk neonates and specific nursing care for selected perinatal problems. The chapter concludes with a brief discussion of documentation.

Neonatal intensive care

Many high-risk neonates require care in a neonatal intensive care unit (NICU). Besides a highly skilled, round-the-clock medical and nursing staff, the NICU offers full life-support, resuscitation, and monitoring equipment and extensive ancillary support staff and services.

Regionalization of care

To ensure the highest quality of care for high-risk neonates, the American Academy of Pediatrics (1988) has established a system of "leveled" regionalized care in which a neonate is referred to the facility with the most appropriate staff and equipment to manage the neonate's specific problems. Ideally, regionalized care allows the most efficient use of resources by eliminating the need

GLOSSARY

ABO blood group incompatibility: isoimmune hemolytic anemia in which a maternal antigen-antibody reaction causes premature destruction of fetal red blood cells (RBCs).

Anencephaly: congenital absence of the cerebral hemispheres in which the cephalic end of the spinal cord fails to close during gestation.

Apnea: absence of spontaneous respirations.

Asphyxia: condition caused by sustained oxygen deprivation and characterized by hypoxemia, hypercapnia, and acidosis.

Bronchopulmonary dysplasia (BPD): lung disease characterized by bronchiolar metaplasia and interstitial fibrosis; associated with oxygen therapy and mechanical ventilation in preterm neonates.

Cleft lip: congenital defect in which one or more clefts appear in the upper lip; caused by failure of the maxillary and median nasal processes to close during embryonic development.

Cleft palate: congenital defect in which a fissure appears in the palatal midline; caused by failure of the sides of the palate to close during embryonic development.

Clubfoot: congenital foot deformity characterized by unilateral or bilateral deviation of the metatarsal bones, causing the foot to appear clublike.

Congenital hypothyroidism: deficiency of thyroid hormone secretion during fetal development or early infancy (also called cretinism).

Congenital hydrocephalus: condition characterized by accumulation of excessive cerebrospinal fluid within the cranial vault.

Dysmaturity: condition of a fetus or neonate being abnormally small for gestational age.

Encephalocele: congenital neural tube defect in which the meninges and portions of brain tissue protrude through the cranium, typically in the occipital area.

Erythroblastosis fetalis: hemolytic anemia of the neonate (Rh or ABO incompatibility) characterized by severe anemia, jaundice, and enlargement of the liver and spleen.

Exchange transfusion: procedure in which the neonate's blood is removed and replaced with fresh whole donor blood to remove unconjugated bilirubin in serum; used to treat hyperbilirubinemia and hemolytic anemia.

Extracorporeal membrane oxygenation (ECMO): technique that maintains gas exchange and perfusion by oxygenating blood outside the body through an arterial shunt; used mainly to treat refractory respiratory failure or meconium aspiration syndrome.

Fetal alcohol syndrome (FAS): syndrome caused by maternal alcohol consumption and characterized by altered intrauterine growth and development, resulting in mental and growth retardation, facial abnormalities, and behavioral deviations.

Galactosemia: hereditary autosomal recessive disorder in which deficiency of the enzyme galactose-1-phosphate uridyltransferase leads to galactose accumulation in the blood.

Gastroschisis: congenital condition characterized by incomplete abdominal wall closure not involving the site of umbilical cord insertion; typically, the small intestine and part of the large intestine protrude.

Gestational age: estimated age in weeks following conception.

Hydramnios: excess amniotic fluid (also called polyhydramnios).

Hyperbilirubinemia: elevated serum level of unconjugated bilirubin.

Hypocalcemia: decreased serum calcium level.

Hypoglycemia: abnormally low serum glucose level.

Imperforate anus: congenital defect characterized by abnormal closure of the anus.

Intrauterine growth retardation: abnormal process in which fetal development and maturation are impeded or delayed by maternal disease, genetic factors, or fetal malnutrition caused by placental insufficiency; seen in the small-for-gestational-age neonate.

Intraventricular hemorrhage (IVH): bleeding into the ventricles.

Inborn error of metabolism: abnormal metabolic condition caused by an inherited defect of a single enzyme or other protein.

Isoimmune hemolytic anemia: disorder in which an antigen-antibody reaction leads to the premature destruction of RBCs.

Large for gestational age (LGA): term used to describe a neonate whose birth weight exceeds the ninetieth percentile for gestational age.

Low birth weight: birth weight of 1,500 to 2,500 g.

Macrosomia: large body size with a high birth weight (4,000 g or more at term).

Maple syrup urine disease: autosomal recessive disorder characterized by an enzyme deficiency in the second step of branched-chain amino acid catabolism.

Meconium: first stool passed by the neonate; thick, dark-green, and sticky.

Meconium aspiration syndrome (MAS): lung inflammation resulting from aspiration of meconium-stained amniotic fluid in utero or as the neonate takes the first few breaths.

Meningomyelocele: congenital neural tube defect in which part of the meninges and spinal cord protrude through the vertebral column.

Microcephaly: congenital anomaly characterized by abnormal smallness of the head relative to the rest of the body and by underdevelopment of the brain, with resulting mental retardation.

Micrognathia: underdevelopment of the jaw, especially the mandible (lower jaw).

GLOSSARY continued

Neonatal mortality: number of deaths per 1,000 live births within the first 28 days after birth.

Necrotizing enterocolitis (NEC): acute inflammatory bowel disorder occurring mainly in preterm neonates.

Neonatal intensive care unit (NICU): nursery that provides the highest level of life-support management, including ventilatory support; heart rate, blood pressure, cardiorespiratory, and blood gas monitoring; I.V. fluid therapy; and experienced round-the-clock medical and nursing care.

Neutral thermal environment (NTE): range of environmental temperatures (89.6° to 93.2° F [32° to 34° C]) that maintains a stable core temperature with minimal caloric and oxygen expenditure.

Oligohydramnios: presence of less than 300 ml of amniotic fluid at term.

Omphalocele: congenital anomaly in which a portion of the intestine protrudes through a defect in the abdominal wall at the umbilicus.

Patent ductus arteriosus (PDA): abnormal opening between the pulmonary artery and the aorta; results from failure of the fetal ductus arteriosus to close after birth.

Pathologic jaundice: condition marked by onset of yellow skin discoloration and a serum bilirubin level above 13 mg/dl within 24 hours after birth; results from blood type or blood group incompatibility, infection, or biliary, hepatic, or metabolic abnormalities.

Phenylketonuria: autosomal recessive disorder characterized by the abnormal presence of metabolites of phenylalanine (such as phenylketone) in the urine.

Placental insufficiency: inadequate or improper functioning of the placenta, leading to a compromised intrauterine environment that jeopardizes the fetus.

Polycystic kidney disease: condition characterized by formation of multiple cysts within the kidney, leading to kidney enlargement and destruction of adjacent tissue.

Polycythemia: abnormal increase in the number of RBCs; in the neonate, it results from maternal-fetal transfusion, delayed umbilical cord clamping, or placental insufficiency.

Posterior urethral valves: congenital anomaly characterized by urinary tract obstruction, hydronephrosis, and an impaired urinary flow.

Postterm neonate: neonate born after completion of week 42 of gestation (also called *postmature* neonate).

Preterm neonate: neonate born before completion of week 37 of gestation (also called *premature* neonate).

Radiant heat warmer bed: open bed with an overhead radiant heat source.

Renal agenesis: congenital absence of one kidney (unilateral renal agenesis) or both kidneys (bilateral renal agenesis).

Respiratory distress syndrome (RDS): acute, potentially fatal neonatal lung disorder resulting from surfactant deficiency; most common in preterm neonates.

Retinopathy of prematurity (ROP): disease of the retinal vasculature associated with oxygen therapy in the preterm neonate (formerly called retrolental fibroplasia).

Rh incompatibility: isoimmune hemolytic anemia in which maternal antibodies cause destruction of fetal RBCs, leading to severe anemia and jaundice in the neonate.

Small for gestational age (SGA): term used to describe a neonate who experienced intrauterine growth retardation and whose birth weight falls below the tenth percentile for gestational age.

Teratoma: congenital tumor consisting of various cell types, none of which normally occur together.

Term neonate: neonate of 38 to 42 weeks' gestation (also called *mature* neonate).

Thermoregulation: maintenance of body temperature by complex interaction between environmental temperature and body heat loss and production.

Very low birth weight: birth weight of 500 to 1,500 g.

for all facilities to acquire the expensive equipment and staff for a NICU.

Every hospital in the United States is assigned to a region and classified according to the level of neonatal care provided. Level 1 care (as in the normal neonatal nursery) is most appropriate for uncomplicated deliveries; level 2 care, for neonates with mild to moderate problems; level 3 (NICU) care, for more serious problems. (For a comparison of staff, equipment, and services in level 1, 2, and 3 facilities, see *Comparing levels of perinatal care,* pages 930 to 932.)

Some neonatal care regions cross state lines; others include only a portion of a single state. Based on their

needs and interdependence, facilities within each region are clustered to form referral networks. Within each region, one facility (or, in some cases, two) is designated as a regional referral center (a level 3 facility). Depending on the specific problems involved, a high-risk neonate who is delivered at a level 1 facility will be transported to a level 2 or level 3 facility.

Obstetric facilities also are classified according to the level of care provided; in some cases, this means that a mother may be cared for in a different facility than her neonate. For example, when no perinatal problems are anticipated, a woman may deliver in a level 1

(Text continues on page 932.)

Comparing levels of perinatal care

To improve the quality of care for high-risk neonates, the American Academy of Pediatrics and the American College of Obstetricians and Gynecologists established guidelines for functions, staff, equipment, facilities, and other resources of levels 1, 2, and 3 perinatal nurseries. The chart below compares these features.

FEATURE	LEVEL 1 CARE	LEVEL 2 CARE	LEVEL 3 CARE
General information			
Function	• Risk assessment • Management of uncomplicated perinatal care • Stabilization of unexpected problems • Initiation of maternal and neonatal transports • Client and community education • Data collection and evaluation	Level 1 functions plus: • Diagnosis and treatment of selected high-risk pregnant clients and neonatal problems • Initiation and acceptance of maternal-fetal and neonatal transports • Education of allied health personnel • Residency education (affiliation)	Levels 1 and 2 functions plus: • Diagnosis and treatment of all perinatal problems • Acceptance and direction of maternal-fetal and neonatal transport • Research and outcome surveillance • Graduate and postgraduate education • System management
Neonates treated	Neonates with uncomplicated, emergency, and remedial problems; asphyxiated neonates requiring immediate resuscitation; large premature neonates without risk factors; neonates with physiologic jaundice.	Neonates meeting level 1 criteria plus those with selected problems, such as: • mild to moderate respiratory distress syndrome (RDS) • suspected sepsis • hypoglycemia • maternal diabetes • post-asphyxiated neonates without life-threatening sequelae	Neonates meeting levels 1 and 2 criteria, plus those with: • prematurity at 24 to 26 weeks' gestation with a birth weight of 500 to 1,250 g • severe RDS • sepsis • severe postasphyxia • symptomatic congenital anomalies of the heart and other organs • special needs (such as total parenteral nutrition or prolonged mechanical ventilation)
Nursery			
Resuscitation equipment and facilities	• 100 foot-candles illumination • Overhead radiant heat • Wall clock • Resuscitation and stabilization equipment • Designated area or room • Full utilities, including suction, oxygen, compressed air, and electrical outlets	Same as level 1	Same as level 1
Admission and observation area	• Located near or adjacent to delivery and cesarean rooms (may be part of maternal recovery area) • Equipment as in resuscitation area	May be located in neonatal or continuing care area	Same as level 2
Neonatal nursery	• Located near postpartal area • Beds and equipment outnumbering obstetric beds by 10% • Resuscitation equipment: one electrical outlet for every two beds; one oxygen, suction, and compressed air apparatus for every five to six beds	Same as level 1	Same as level 1

Comparing levels of perinatal care continued

FEATURE	LEVEL 1 CARE	LEVEL 2 CARE	LEVEL 3 CARE
Continuing care	(For reverse transport from level 2 or 3 facility) • Resuscitation equipment • Four electrical outlets and one oxygen, suction, and compressed air apparatus for every neonate	Located near intermediate nursery	Same as level 2
Intermediate care	Not available	• Located near delivery and intensive care nurseries • Full life support and monitoring, plus resuscitation equipment • Eight electrical outlets, two oxygen outlets, two compressed air outlets, and two suction outlets for every neonate	Same as level 2
Intensive care	Not available	• Available in some facilities • Located near delivery and cesarean rooms	16 to 20 electrical outlets, three to four oxygen outlets, three to four compressed air outlets, and three to four suction outlets for every neonate
Ancillary support			
Operating room	• Technicians on call 24 hours/day; available within 15 to 30 minutes	• Technicians available immediately for emergencies	Same as level 2; may be in delivery room area
Laboratory services • Within 15 minutes	• Hematocrit	• ABGs, blood typing, and Rh determination	• Same as level 2
• Within 1 hour	• Glucose, blood urea nitrogen, creatinine, arterial blood gases (ABGs), routine urinalysis	• Same as level 1, plus electrolytes, coagulation studies, blood available from typing and screening program	• Same as levels 1 and 2, plus special blood and amniotic fluid tests
• Within 1 to 6 hours	• Complete blood count, platelet appearance on smear, blood chemistries, blood typing and cross-matching, Coombs' test, bacterial smear	• Same as level 1, plus coagulation studies, magnesium, urine, electrolytes, and chemistries	• Same as levels 1 and 2
• Within 24 to 48 hours	• Bacterial cultures and antibiotic sensitivity	• Same as level 1, plus liver function test and metabolic screening	• Same as levels 1 and 2
• Within hospital or other available facility	• Viral cultures	• Same as level 1	• Same as level 1, plus available laboratory facilities
Radiography and ultrasound	• Technicians on call 24 hours/day; available within 30 minutes • Technicians experienced in performing abdominal, pelvic, and obstetric ultrasound examinations	• Experienced radiology technicians available immediately in the facility (ultrasound available on call) • Professional interpretation available immediately	Same as level 2 plus: • computed tomography • cardiac catheterization • sophisticated equipment for emergency gastrointestinal, genitourinary, or central nervous sys-

(continued)

Comparing levels of perinatal care continued

FEATURE	LEVEL 1 CARE	LEVEL 2 CARE	LEVEL 3 CARE
Radiography and ultrasound (continued)	• Professional interpretation available on a 24-hour basis • Portable X-ray and ultrasound equipment available to labor, delivery, and nursery areas	• Portable X-ray equipment • Ultrasound equipment available in labor, delivery, and nursery areas	tem studies available 24 hours/day
Blood bank	• Technicians on call 24 hours/day; available within 30 minutes • Performance of routine blood banking procedures	• Experienced technicians available immediately in the facility for blood banking procedures and identification of irregular antibodies • Blood component therapy readily available	Same as level 2 plus: • Resource center for network • Direct-line communication to labor, delivery, and nursery areas

Adapted with permission from the American Academy of Pediatrics (Elk Grove Village, IL) and the American College of Obstetricians and Gynecologists (Washington, DC). *Guidelines for Perinatal care* (2nd ed.). Copyright ©1988.

obstetric facility with a level 1 nursery; if her neonate develops unexpected problems, he or she will require transport to a level 3 neonatal facility. (When a high-risk delivery is anticipated, however, the mother may be transported before delivery to a facility with level 3 neonatal care so that she and her neonate can be together.)

Sometimes, a neonate is returned to the referring facility after treatment in a regional center; this is referred to as reverse transport. Candidates for reverse transport include neonates in whom the problem has resolved completely or neonates who have recovered sufficiently to be managed by the referring facility. Benefits of reverse transport include a decrease in the level 3 neonatal population and, in many cases, closer proximity to the family. (For more information on the regionalization of perinatal care, see Chapter 1, Family Nursing Care: History and Trends.)

Goals of neonatal intensive care

The goals of neonatal intensive care include averting or minimizing complications, subjecting the neonate to as little stress as possible, and furthering parent-infant bonding. To achieve these goals, the NICU staff:
• anticipates, prevents, and detects potential or actual perinatal problems
• intervenes early for identified problems
• carries out care procedures in a way that minimizes disturbance to the neonate
• uses a family-centered approach.

Ethical and legal issues

As treatment advances increase the survival odds for high-risk neonates, debate over various ethical and legal issues grows. Economic factors are intertwined with these issues; as the financial burden of providing medical care for high-risk neonates increases, economic considerations may influence the treatment measures used for a particular neonate.

Resuscitation and life-support decisions

A major ethical and legal dilemma centers on which neonates should be resuscitated—specifically, the gestational age limit below which delivery room resuscitation or other aggressive measures should not be attempted. For example, before 23 weeks' gestation, the respiratory system is too immature to sustain extrauterine survival; thus, some care providers may forgo aggressive measures for a neonate born before this time. Most clinicians use 24 weeks' gestation as the cut-off point because the distance between the fetus's alveoli and arterial capillaries makes gas exchange—and thus extrauterine suvival—difficult before this time. However, in some cases, fetal stress (for instance, from intrauterine growth retardation and certain other conditions) stimulates respiratory development, making extrauterine survival possible and increasing the chance that resuscitation will succeed.

Other specific topics of debate are the number of rounds of resuscitative drugs to administer and the circumstances that warrant ventilatory support and experimental therapies. Some facilities have protocols to address these issues; others rely on physicians to make judgments in individual cases.

A closely related issue concerns the "Do not resuscitate" (DNR) order, which specifies the circumstances under which life support can be withheld legally. In some states, technological support may be discontinued when well-documented evidence strongly suggests that the neonate's condition will not improve. Other states require evidence that supports the poor prognosis, including a flat electroencephalogram for 24 hours in the absence of drugs that depress the central nervous system (CNS).

Quality-of-life considerations
Quality of life becomes a consideration for some high-risk neonates. Many congenital anomalies, for instance, can be corrected by surgery; however, the child may be left with serious disabilities that necessitate costly, lifelong care. For example, neonates with meningomyelocele, a congenital neurologic anomaly, may suffer paralysis despite surgery. In some cases, the physician or parents may believe that the poor quality of life that awaits the child justifies withholding treatment; the expense of lifelong care is a complicating issue.

Decision-making power
Further clouding such dilemmas is the question of who should make care decisions for a neonate. For instance, the choice to allow a severely disabled neonate to die formerly was left mainly to the parents. Now, however, the child's rights sometimes are weighed against the parents'. If caregivers believe that the parents are acting in their own best interests rather than the child's, they may ask the courts to remove the parents as legal guardians. As technology continues to advance, decision making becomes increasingly complex.

Perinatal problems

The most common problems seen in NICUs are prematurity and its sequelae, congenital heart defects, and congenital anomalies requiring emergency surgery (such as omphalocele and tracheoesophageal fistula).

Gestational-age and birth-weight variations

Variations of gestational age (prematurity and postmaturity) and birth weight (small or large size for gestational age) predispose the neonate to various problems. (For information on the causes and consequences of these variations, see *Gestational-age variations*, page 934, and *Birth-weight variations*, pages 935 and 936. For a discussion of ways to help prevent these variations, see *Neonatal mortality*, page 937.)

Respiratory problems

In utero, the placenta supplies oxygen to body tissues; the respiratory arterioles remain partially closed so that blood is diverted through the ductus arteriosus and away from the lungs. At birth, the neonate's lungs must take over the task of providing oxygen for body tissues. For this to happen, lung fluid must be replaced by air and the arterioles must dilate to allow more blood into the lungs. The healthy neonate accomplishes this within seconds. (For an illustration, see Chapter 34, Neonatal Adaptation.)

However, some neonates have trouble initiating respirations or develop respiratory distress after breathing is established. For instance, problems may arise if fluid remains in the lungs or if the blood perfusion of the lungs does not increase; neonates with apnea at birth or a weak respiratory effort (from such conditions as prematurity, asphyxia, or maternal anesthesia) are predisposed to respiratory distress.

Asphyxia and apnea
Asphyxia may occur late in gestation or during delivery. Chemically, this condition is defined as insufficient oxygen in the blood (hypoxemia), excessive carbon dioxide in the blood, and a decreased blood pH. As carbon dioxide accumulates, respiratory acidosis occurs; poor tissue oxygenation leads to buildup of lactic acid, resulting in metabolic acidosis. If hypoxia is prolonged, the foramen ovale and ductus arteriosus—fetal shunts that normally close shortly after delivery—may reopen. This causes a return to fetal circulatory pathways to maintain circulation to the heart and brain.

Asphyxia in a fetus or neonate causes rapid breathing at first. If asphyxia continues, apnea (absence of respirations) ensues, respiratory movements cease, and the heart rate starts to drop. Deep, gasping respirations then begin, the heart rate continues to fall, and blood pressure drops. Respirations weaken progressively until they stop altogether. Because hypoxemia and acidosis cause arteriolar constriction, lung perfusion is poor; consequently, the body cannot be oxygenated.

Without immediate resuscitation, the neonate will die. Complications of prolonged asphyxia include cerebral hypoxia, seizures, intraventricular hemorrhage (IVH), renal failure, necrotizing enterocolitis (NEC), and metabolic imbalances.

(Text continues on page 936.)

Gestational-age variations

Birth before or after full-term gestation markedly increases the risk of perinatal problems. In the past 25 years, advances in research and technology have improved the survival rate dramatically for neonates with gestational-age variations—even extremely preterm neonates.

Preterm neonate

The preterm neonate—the classic high-risk neonate—is one born before completion of the thirty-seventh gestational week. The risks of preterm birth and the associated economic burden are tremendous. Neonatal mortality and morbidity are highest among preterm neonates; each day of prematurity can represent thousands of dollars in medical care and significantly reduces the chance for a positive outcome.

Delivery of a preterm neonate is more likely with any of the following maternal conditions:
• age extreme (under 19 or over 34)
• low socioeconomic status
• poor nutritional status
• poor prenatal care
• exposure to known teratogens (including drugs, alcohol, cigarette smoke, and hazardous chemicals)
• chronic disease (such as cardiovascular disease, renal disease, or diabetes mellitus)
• antepartal trauma, infection, or pregnancy-induced hypertension
• uterine anomalies or cervical incompetency
• a history of previous preterm delivery.

Other predisposing factors include multiple gestation, hydramnios (excessive amniotic fluid), fetal infection, premature rupture of the membranes, abruptio placentae, and placenta previa.

Perinatal problems. General immaturity can lead to dysfunction in any organ or body system. Thus, the preterm neonate risks a wide range of problems, including respiratory distress syndrome, apnea, bronchopulmonary dysplasia, patent ductus arteriosus, ineffective thermoregulation, hypoglycemia, intraventricular hemorrhage, gastrointestinal dysfunction, retinopathy, hyperbilirubinemia, and infection. The preterm neonate also may suffer ineffective development from the effects of intensive medical treatment (such as sensory overload and environmental stress); an immature central nervous system compounds this risk. Also, mother-infant bonding may be jeopardized. (The pathophysiology, assessment, and treatment of the problems listed above are discussed in detail throughout this chapter.)

Postterm neonate

The postterm neonate is one whose gestation exceed 294 days or 42 weeks. Typically, the neonate's weight falls above the ninetieth percentile on the Colorado intrauterine growth chart (discussed in Chapter 35, Neonatal Assessment).

Perinatal problems. Problems associated with postmaturity include fetal dysmaturity syndrome, asphyxia, meconium aspiration, polycythemia, hypothermia, and birth trauma (Fanaroff and Martin, 1987).

Fetal dysmaturity syndrome. Some 20% to 40% of postterm neonates experience placental insufficiency leading to fetal dysmaturity syndrome and a diagnosis of small for gestational age (SGA). After 280 days of gestation, the risk of placental insufficiency, fetal growth retardation, and chronic hypoxia increases. Fetal weight plateaus around the term date until the forty-second week (typically from placental lesion formation and decreased placental weight), then drops rapidly. Placental dysfunction after the forty-second week impairs fetal oxygenation and nutrition and exhausts placental reserves, retarding fetal growth (Resnick, 1989).

Fetal dysmaturity occurs in three forms: chronic, acute, and subacute placental insufficiency. Each form has distinctive manifestations. With *chronic placental insufficiency,* no meconium staining occurs but the neonate appears malnourished, with skin defects and an apprehensive look reflecting hypoxia. *Acute placental insufficiency* leads to a malnourished and apprehensive appearance and green meconium staining of the skin, umbilical cord, and placental membranes. With *subacute placental insufficiency,* the skin and nails are stained bright yellow (from breakdown of green-bile meconium stain), and the umbilical cord, placenta, and placental membranes may be stained greenish brown (Vorherr, 1975).

Asphyxia and meconium aspiration. The postterm neonate has a high risk of birth asphyxia and meconium aspiration. Usher, Boyd, McLean, and Kramer (1988) found that meconium release (defecation) occurs twice as frequently and meconium aspiration syndrome eight times as frequently in postterm neonates than in other neonates. Some researchers suggest that the postterm fetus reacts more dramatically than the term fetus to episodes of asphyxia, experiencing fetal heart abnormalities, gasping, and meconium release.

Oligohydramnios (presence of less than 300 ml of amniotic fluid at term) increases the risk of asphyxia and aspiration by making meconium less diluted and thus unusually thick (Eden, Seifert, Winegar, and Spellacy, 1987). Normally, amniotic fluid volume peaks at 1,000 to 1,200 ml at about 38 weeks' gestation, then decreases rapidly. By week 42, it drops to approximately 300 ml; further decreases occur at 43 and 44 weeks. In the neonate with no congenital anomalies, oligohydramnios confirms postmaturity and has been linked to fetal decelerations (as shown on fetal monitoring strips), bradycardia, or both (Phelan, Plah, Yeh, Broussard, and Paul, 1985).

Other perinatal problems. Intrauterine hypoxia in the postterm fetus may trigger increased red blood cell production, causing polycythemia, which in turn may lead to sluggish perfusion and complications associated with hyperviscosity. Subcutaneous fat deficiency caused by skin wasting predisposes the postterm neonate to hypothermia, despite a mature thermoregulatory system. Thus, a postterm neonate exposed to cold stress may develop respiratory compromise and hypoglycemia (Fanaroff and Martin, 1987).

Delivery complications. The risk of delivery complications increases after 280 days (40 weeks) of gestation. Excessive size may cause a dysfunctional labor and shoulder dystocia, possibly necessitating cesarean delivery. Because of maternal uterine inefficiency and cephalopelvic disproportion, postterm neonates have a higher-than-average rate of surgical deliveries (Boyd, Usher, McLean, and Kramer, 1988).

Birth-weight variations

Like the neonate with a gestational-age variation, one whose weight is inappropriate for the estimated gestational age is at high risk for perinatal problems.

Small-for-gestational-age (SGA) neonate

The SGA neonate is one whose birth weight falls below the tenth percentile for gestational age. SGA status results from intrauterine growth retardation (IUGR), an abnormal process in which fetal development and maturation are delayed or impeded. After prematurity, IUGR is the leading cause of death during the perinatal period (Cassady and Strange, 1987).

Causes of IUGR. IUGR may result from maternal conditions, genetic factors (for example, trisomies), fetal and placental abnormalities, infection, fetal malnutrition caused by placental insufficiency, or exposure to such teratogens as drugs and alcohol.

Maternal conditions. The most common causes of IUGR are maternal conditions that reduce uteroplacental perfusion, such as toxemia, chronic hypertensive vascular disease, and renovascular and cardiac disorders. Maternal hypertension, smoking, renal disease, and diabetes mellitus that progresses to renovascular compromise also can result in IUGR. Ounsted, Moar, and Scott (1985) estimate that the SGA incidence could be reduced by 60% by eliminating such risk factors as smoking and hypertensive disorders.

During early pregnancy, smoking is the most important risk factor for IUGR. Typically, the neonate of a woman who smokes weighs 150 to 200 g less than other neonates. Fetal hypoxia, carbon monoxide poisoning of hemoglobin, and the vascular effects of nicotine have been suggested as smoking-related factors that contribute to IUGR.

The role of maternal nutrition in fetal growth remains unclear. Some researchers minimize its importance while others emphasize it. Those who minimize it point out that despite the high incidence of infertility and spontaneous abortion during famines and wars, only severe maternal starvation during the last trimester has reduced birth weight.

Fetal and placental abnormalities. IUGR can result from infarction, hemangiomas, aberrant cord insertion, single umbilical artery, and umbilical vascular thrombosis. Premature placental separation and other conditions that diminish placental surface area and thus decrease fetal-placental exchange capability also may cause IUGR.

Placental insufficiency. Placental insufficiency is the inadequate or improper functioning of the placenta, leading to a compromised intrauterine environment. Causes of placental insufficiency include systemic diseases (such as diabetes mellitus and infection) and placental abnormalities that impair fetal circulation and compromise fetal nutrition and oxygenation (such as abnormal placental implantation, abnormal cord attachment, and placental membrane abnormalities). Although placental insufficiency is most common in the postterm period, it may occur at any time during gestation. The severity of IUGR arising from placental insufficiency depends on the duration of fetal distress.

Exposure to drugs and alcohol. Maternal use of heroin, cocaine, and methadone significantly reduces the neonate's weight, length, and head circumference at birth (Chasnoff, Bussey, Savich, and Stack, 1986). The neonate of a heroin-addicted mother, for instance, typically is SGA, preterm, and weighs less than 2,500 g. Maternal alcohol consumption may cause fetal alcohol syndrome (FAS). Some neonates show severe manifestations while others appear normal. Besides mental retardation—the most serious and common effect—FAS may reduce the neonate's weight and length at birth (Wright, 1986).

Perinatal problems. Although the SGA neonate may avoid the problems stemming from organ system immaturity seen in the preterm neonate, other perinatal problems may arise.

Asphyxia and meconium aspiration. The SGA neonate who suffered placental insufficiency risks asphyxiation during labor and delivery, as the flow of oxygen and nutrients slows and uterine contractions reduce placental perfusion. Also, the neonate may aspirate meconium that has entered the amniotic sac. Respiratory distress, cyanosis, pulmonary air trapping, pneumothorax, and pulmonary hypertension may result, along with severe asphyxia and cerebral hypoxia (Fanaroff and Martin, 1987).

Organ size variations. Relative to body weight, the SGA neonate has a larger brain and heart than the preterm neonate but smaller adrenal glands and a smaller liver, spleen, thymus, and placenta.

Hematologic and metabolic problems. The SGA neonate may experience hematologic changes from chronic fetal hypoxia, a condition that triggers compensation through increases in red blood cell (RBC) volume (polycythemia) and erythropoietin levels. Polycythemia, in turn, may cause hyperviscosity and sluggish microcirculation perfusion.

Disturbed carbohydrate metabolism and inefficient hepatic gluconeogenesis and glycogenolysis may lead to hypoglycemia. With increased energy requirements but inadequate glycogen and fat reserves, the SGA neonate is predisposed to hypoglycemia (Lubchenco and Koops, 1987). A stressful labor may further deplete already deficient energy reserves.

Long-term problems. An SGA neonate later may suffer developmental, immunologic, and neurologic problems.

Slowed growth and immunologic deficiencies. Growth rate depends on when IUGR occurred and how long it lasted. Commonly, the child who was SGA at birth remains slimmer and shorter than other children of the same gestational age or birth weight. The rate of catch-up growth depends on causative factors and postnatal events. Head growth may equal or exceed weight and height increases.

Impaired fetal skeletal growth may contribute to delayed tooth eruption and enamel hypoplasia. Severely growth-retarded neonates also have an increased incidence of infection, possibly from immunologic deficiency.

Neurologic impairment. IUGR-induced brain damage and its potential effect on neurologic development remains a major medical concern. Most investigators believe IUGR has more serious neurologic consequences in the preterm than the term SGA neonate. Follow-up evaluations in children who experienced IUGR in utero have revealed defects in speech and language comprehension; outcome studies have described hyperactivity, short attention span, poor fine-motor coordination, hyperreflexia, and learning problems. Stunted growth and delayed intellectual or neurologic development were found in children who experienced both short and long periods of IUGR. Other factors that worsen

(continued)

Birth-weight variations continued

the neurologic prognosis include male sex and low socio-economic status, regardless of the severity of compromise (Teberg, Walther, and Pena, 1988).

Large-for-gestational-age (LGA) neonate
The LGA neonate is one whose birth weight exceeds the ninetieth percentile for gestational age. A neonate delivered at term is considered to be LGA if the birth weight exceeds 4,000 g (8 lb, 13 oz). The leading cause of LGA status is maternal diabetes mellitus.

Traditionally, the large neonate was considered a healthy one. However, clinicians now know that the accelerated intrauterine growth of the LGA fetus poses a threat to both mother and neonate during delivery and increases the risk of complications and death in the early neonatal period.

Intrapartal problems. When the membranes rupture, large fetal size and possible high station may result in umbilical cord prolapse. Uterine overdistention from an LGA fetus increases the risk of premature labor. Usually, the physician will initiate labor and delivery before term (once fetal lung maturity has been confirmed) because of the high incidence of unexplained death among term LGA fetuses. If the mother has an adequate pelvis, the physician typically administers oxytocin to induce labor; otherwise, cesarean delivery may be necessary. Shoulder dystocia stemming from cephalopelvic disproportion also may necessitate cesarean delivery, with all the inherent risks.

During vaginal delivery, the neonate's large size may cause birth injury, such as clavicular fracture resulting from shoulder dystocia, skull fracture from increased head size, or other traumatic head injuries (such as cephalhematomas, facial nerve damage, and intracranial bleeding). A difficult delivery also may lead to phrenic nerve damage or brachial plexus palsy.

Perinatal problems. If the mother is diabetic, the neonate may suffer hypocalcemia (possibly from depressed parathyroid function), hypoglycemia (from maternal hyperglycemia that stimulates fetal hyperinsulinism), and polycythemia (from RBC overproduction). Other problems associated with excessive size include congenital anomalies (such as transposition of the great vessels), erythroblastosis fetalis (hemolytic anemia), and Beckwith's syndrome (a hereditary disorder associated with neonatal hypoglycemia and hyperinsulinemia).

If the mother had postconceptional bleeding causing an error in the calculated delivery date, the LGA neonate may be delivered postterm and thus experience respiratory distress from meconium aspiration or intrauterine asphyxiation. The LGA neonate delivered before term to prevent fetal death or intrapartal complications of excessive size may suffer respiratory distress syndrome, hyperbilirubinemia, and other problems linked to prematurity.

Several days after delivery, apneic episodes (cessation of breathing for more than 15 seconds) are common among preterm neonates, many of whom have irregular respiratory patterns from neuronal immaturity. Such episodes may result from acidosis, anemia, hypoglycemia, hyperglycemia, hypothermia, hyperthermia, patent ductus arteriosus (PDA), abdominal distention, regurgitation, sepsis, or IVH. Central apnea (caused by insufficient neural impulses from the respiratory center) and obstructive apnea (resulting from upper airway obstruction) also occur in some preterm and low-birth-weight neonates.

Meconium aspiration syndrome
A lung inflammation, meconium aspiration syndrome (MAS) results from aspiration of meconium-stained amniotic fluid in utero or as the neonate takes the first few breaths after delivery. Meconium staining of amniotic fluid results from fetal asphyxia: In response to asphyxia, intestinal peristalsis increases, the anal sphincter relaxes, and meconium enters the amniotic fluid.

As meconium obstructs the bronchi and bronchioles, it creates a ball-valve effect: Air can enter but not exit the bronchi and bronchioles because meconium acts as a ball, plugging the alveolar sac. Alveoli then become

overdistended; pneumothorax, bacterial pneumonia, or pulmonary hypertension may develop secondarily.

Respiratory distress syndrome
Respiratory distress syndrome (RDS; also called hyaline membrane disease) is characterized by respiratory distress and impaired gas exchange. RDS affects mainly preterm neonates, who have highly pliable and easily overinflated thoracic muscles, weak intercostal muscles, and insufficient surfactant. A lipoprotein synthesized by type II alveolar cells, surfactant is necessary to keep alveoli expanded. Although surfactant production begins at around weeks 22 to 24 of gestation, it is inadequate at this time to prevent alveolar collapse. Surfactant production probably becomes sufficient only after about week 35.

Insufficient surfactant causes alveolar collapse, leading to decreased lung volume and compliance. The resulting atelectasis causes hypoxia and acidosis, which in turn lead to anaerobic metabolism. As lactic acid accumulates in body tissues, myocardial contractility diminishes, impairing cardiac output and arterial blood pressure. Organ perfusion then diminishes; eventually respiratory failure occurs.

Transient tachypnea

This disorder, characterized by transient episodes of tachypnea (accelerated breathing), stems from incomplete removal of fetal lung fluid. Usually accompanied by cyanosis, it affects mainly full-term or nearly full-term neonates born by cesarean delivery (this delivery method eliminates fetal lung compression by the birth canal, which normally helps expel lung fluid).

Bronchopulmonary dysplasia

In this lung disease, the bronchiolar epithelial lining and alveolar walls become necrotic; in some cases, right-sided heart failure develops as a complication. Bronchopulmonary dysplasia (BPD) occurs mainly in preterm neonates as a complication of oxygen therapy or assisted mechanical ventilation—common treatments for RDS. The neonate with BPD typically becomes ventilator-dependent. Low birth weight and overhydration (in a neonate with PDA) may contribute to BPD.

Retinopathy of prematurity

Retinopathy of prematurity (ROP; formerly called retrolental fibroplasia) may lead to blindness. It begins with retinal vasoconstriction, which eventually causes vessels in some portions of the retina to become ischemic. To compensate for ischemia, new capillaries develop to provide oxygen and nutrients to the damaged tissue. However, lacking sufficient structural integrity, the new vessels rupture and hemorrhage. This leads to formation of scar tissue, which grows rigid and shortens, causing traction that results in retinal detachment and eventual blindness. In some cases, however, early retinal changes revert spontaneously, sparing the neonate's vision.

Immature retinal vessels are particularly vulnerable to ROP; the disorder is most common in the preterm neonate of less than 35 weeks' gestation who receives supplemental oxygen. Most experts attribute ROP to high concentrations of administered oxygen leading to an elevated partial pressure of arterial oxygen (PaO_2); even brief PaO_2 elevations have been linked with ROP. However, researchers suspect that coexisting factors must be present. These may include prematurity, blood transfusions, IVH, PDA, apnea, infection, vitamin E deficiency, lactic acidosis, administration of prostaglandin synthetase inhibitors, and prenatal and genetic factors. A study conducted by Subramanian, et al. (1985) shows a link between ROP and continuous exposure to bright lights in the nursery.

The precise PaO_2 level and the duration of the elevation that may cause ROP have not been determined. To minimize the risk, neonatologists now recommend that the PaO_2 level of a neonate receiving oxygen be kept at 60 to 80 mm Hg. (For more information on monitoring

Neonatal mortality

Neonatal mortality refers to the number of deaths per 1,000 live births within the first 28 days after birth. Extremely preterm neonates weighing less than 1,500 g have the highest mortality; as birth weight and gestational age increase, mortality declines. The low-birth-weight neonate—one weighing 1,500 to 2,500 g—is 40 times more likely than the average-weight neonate to die within the first 28 days after delivery (Institute of Medicine, 1985).

Neonatal mortality in the United States has decreased only slightly in this century despite medical advances and improved nutrition and sanitation. In 1986, the United States had the highest neonatal mortality among 20 industrialized nations. In 1988, U.S. neonatal mortality was 9.9%—down from 10.8% in 1987 (National Center for Health Statistics, 1989a). A major cause of the slow pace of the decline in neonatal mortality is the relatively unchanged incidence of low birth weight—6.9% in 1987, compared to 7.5% in 1950 (National Center for Health Statistics, 1989b).

Neonatal mortality is 1.6 times higher among Blacks than Caucasians in the United States, mainly because Blacks have a higher incidence of low birth weight. This mortality gap remains a concern for health authorities, who have responded by devising ways to deal with the problem. In 1985, the Institute of Medicine developed recommendations and strategies for preventing low birth weight, some of which the nurse can help carry out. They include the following:

• Reduce risk factors associated with low birth weight through prepregnancy counseling, expanded reproductive information in health education courses, and improved family planning services.

• Ensure access to early and regular prenatal care for all women by removing social and economic barriers, increasing prenatal services in public health departments, providing transportation and child care services for all clients, and establishing outreach and referral systems to recruit hard-to-reach women.

• Enhance the content of prenatal care by providing for accurate pregnancy dating to detect prematurity and intrauterine growth retardation and expanding the use of ultrasound to identify and prevent low birth weight.

• Implement a public information program to prevent low birth weight by calling national attention to the problem and communicating ways to prevent low birth weight through risk factor avoidance.

the neonate receiving supplemental oxygen, see the "Planning and implementation" section of this chapter.)

All preterm neonates who have received supplemental oxygen should have their eyes examined by the physician before discharge. Abnormal findings are graded I through IV, with I signifying minimal change and IV indicating severe retinal damage and blindness.

Intraventricular hemorrhage

Fragile periventricular capillaries predispose the preterm neonate to IVH, or bleeding into the ventricles of the brain. IVH is associated with increased venous pressure and increased blood osmolarity. RDS also may lead to IVH because it typically causes hypoxia and hypercapnia. (Hypoxia can lead to vessel damage because it interrupts the brain's autonomic regulatory functions, hypercapnia because it causes cerebral vasodilation.)

Necrotizing enterocolitis

An acute inflammatory gastrointestinal (GI) mucosal disease, NEC may develop after hypoxic injury to the bowel at birth or during the early neonatal period. (Most commonly, it arises within the first 2 weeks after birth.) Hypoxia causes shunting of blood away from the GI tract to vital organs; the resulting intestinal ischemia predisposes the bowel to bacterial invasion, leading to necrotic lesions and possible perforation.

NEC has been linked to prematurity, which may predispose the neonate to anoxia and subsequent bowel ischemia. Intrauterine infection, maternal diabetes, multiple gestation, and other conditions that cause fetal stress also may contribute to NEC.

Neonate of a diabetic mother

Long-standing maternal diabetes mellitus or gestational diabetes mellitus (diabetes that arises during pregnancy) may cause various fetal and neonatal complications. Maternal serum insulin and glucose levels typically increase during pregnancy from increased tissue resistance to insulin in response to secretion of human placental lactogen and rising estrogen and progesterone levels. If the glucose level remains elevated, as in poorly controlled diabetes, the fetus responds by producing more insulin to combat hyperglycemia. Continued glucose elevations result in fetal hyperinsulinism, leading to changes in fetal glucose metabolism, growth, and development. Exposure to high glucose levels early in gestational development may have a teratogenic effect, causing various congenital anomalies, including heart defects, sacral agenesis, renal vein thrombosis, and small left colon (Fanaroff and Martin, 1987).

The neonate of a woman with diabetes (sometimes called an infant of a diabetic mother, or IDM) also has an increased risk of asphyxia, prematurity, infection, respiratory distress, severe hypoglycemia, hypocalcemia, hyperbilirubinemia, polycythemia, and neonatal death; unexplained fetal death also is higher than normal in IDMs. Typically, the IDM is large for gestational age (with a birth weight exceeding the ninetieth percentile for gestational age) and thus may suffer birth trauma, such as shoulder dystocia, cephalhematoma, subdural hemorrhage, ocular hemorrhage, or brachial plexus injury (Fanaroff and Martin, 1987).

Previously, large fetal size and the high incidence of fetal death late in gestation led many obstetricians to advise early delivery for pregnant diabetic clients. However, that approach has changed slightly, partly because the fetus affected by maternal diabetes has delayed alveolar maturation and thus cannot synthesize adequate surfactant to establish respirations after delivery. If early delivery is mandatory, however, it typically is scheduled for the thirty-seventh week of gestation.

Metabolic disorders

The most common metabolic disorders in high-risk neonates are hypoglycemia, hypocalcemia, and hyperbilirubinemia and jaundice.

Hypoglycemia

This condition is defined as two serum glucose levels below 35 mg/dl in the first 3 hours, less than 40 mg/dl from 4 to 24 hours, or less than 45 mg/dl from 24 hours to 7 days of age in a term neonate. In a preterm neonate, hypoglycemia is diagnosed when two serum glucose values are below 25 mg/dl during the first 72 hours. Hypoglycemia typically results from prematurity, low birth weight, severe fetal or neonatal stress, or maternal diabetes. Because fetal glycogen is deposited during the last few gestational months, the preterm neonate has deficient glycogen stores; if a stressful event, such as respiratory distress, develops at birth, these stores quickly become depleted. The low-birth-weight neonate has a high metabolic rate and inadequate enzyme supplies to activate glucogenesis—conditions that contribute to hypoglycemia.

Poorly controlled maternal diabetes, on the other hand, triggers increased insulin production by the fetal pancreas (as explained under "Neonate of a diabetic mother"). After birth, the neonate continues to produce high levels of insulin; this facilitates the entry of glucose into muscle and fat cells, rapidly depleting serum glucose. Glucose expenditure during the transition to the extrauterine environment and sudden cessation of maternal glucose when the umbilical cord is clamped further tax the neonate's glucose stores.

Hypocalcemia

Defined as a serum calcium level below 7 mg/100 ml, hypocalcemia typically arises within the first 2 days or at 6 to 10 days after birth. It affects about half of neonates born to women with type I (insulin-dependent) diabetes mellitus. Other risk factors include small-for-gestational-age (SGA) status, prematurity, and birth asphyxia.

During pregnancy, the maternal parathyroid glands attempt to increase the maternal serum calcium level to compensate for loss of the calcium transferred to the fetus. The fetal parathyroid glands respond to this increase by a reduction in function; this in turn may cause hypoparathyroidism and subsequent hypocalcemia. After delivery, the neonatal serum calcium level drops further.

Hyperbilirubinemia and jaundice

Hyperbilirubinemia—an elevated serum level of unconjugated bilirubin—is common among both low-risk and high-risk neonates. It results from overproduction or underexcretion of bilirubin, as from liver immaturity or increased hemolysis. The disorder sometimes leads to jaundice, a yellow discoloration of the skin and sclerae. Types of jaundice include physiologic jaundice, which commonly arises 48 to 72 hours after birth and peaks by the third to fifth day; and pathologic jaundice, which arises secondary to another disorder, appears within the first 24 hours, and is characterized by a serum bilirubin level above 20 mg/dl. Pathologic jaundice, seen mainly in high-risk neonates, results from blood type or blood group incompatibility; infection; or biliary, hepatic, or metabolic abnormalities. (For more information on bilirubin production and excretion and physiologic jaundice, see Chapter 34, Neonatal Adaptation, and Chapter 36, Care of the Normal Neonate.)

The risk of hyperbilirubinemia is greatest in preterm neonates, those who are ill, those with isoimmune hemolytic anemia, and those who experienced a traumatic delivery leading to bruising and polycythemia. Such conditions as hypoxia and hypoglycemia (characterized by bilirubin displacement from binding sites) predispose the preterm neonate to hyperbilirubinemia (Fanaroff and Martin, 1987).

A serum bilirubin level of 15 to 20 mg/dl (or even lower in the preterm neonate) may lead to bilirubin encephalopathy (kernicterus), a condition in which unconjugated bilirubin crosses the blood-brain barrier and accumulates in the brain. This may result in damage to the brain and other organs, such as the kidneys, intestines, and pancreas (Fanaroff and Martin, 1987).

Ineffective thermoregulation

All neonates are in danger of ineffective thermoregulation—particularly hypothermia (an abnormally low body temperature). However, the risk is greatest in the preterm neonate, who has an immature temperature-regulating center, reduced body mass-to-surface ratio, decreased subcutaneous fat, inability to shiver or sweat, and inadequate metabolic reserves.

Hypothermia or hyperthermia (an abnormally high body temperature) can cause dramatic changes in vital signs (including tachycardia or bradycardia, tachypnea, and apnea) and increase energy consumption—especially dangerous in a high-risk neonate. Hypothermia increases oxygen consumption, predisposing the neonate to hypoxia. When hypothermia begins, skin temperature decreases first; without intervention, the core temperature falls and irreversible hypothermia may ensue, leading to death.

The body attempts to compensate for hypothermia by increasing the basal metabolic rate (BMR). If the BMR increases above the normal baseline level, however, energy supplies may become depleted, leading to acidosis. This, in turn, causes changes in subcutaneous tissue; decreased peripheral perfusion may lead to tissue damage and necrosis in the cheeks and buttocks, cessation of GI motility, and internal hemorrhage. Hypoglycemia may occur as glucose is metabolized in an effort to meet cellular energy demands. Less commonly, hypothermia causes coagulation changes (Fanaroff and Martin, 1987).

Other changes that may result from hypothermia include pulmonary vasoconstriction, decreased surfactant production, exacerbation of RDS, and impaired weight gain (Fanaroff and Martin, 1987).

Polycythemia

In this disorder, the number of red blood cells (RBCs) increases, as reflected by a hematocrit elevation. Polycythemia can result from maternal-fetal transfusion, delayed umbilical cord clamping, or placental insufficiency.

As RBCs increase, blood viscosity increases, leading to impaired blood pumping through vessels. Respiratory compromise, cardiac problems, and thrombosis may ensue; hyperbilirubinemia may develop as the excess RBCs are destroyed.

Isoimmune hemolytic anemias

In these disorders (also called erythroblastosis fetalis), RBCs are destroyed prematurely. Two hemolytic anemias occurring in neonates are Rhesus (Rh) incompatibility and ABO blood group incompatibility.

Rh incompatibility

This blood incompatibility, which may cause critical illness in the neonate, occurs when an Rh-negative woman (one who lacks the Rh factor in the blood) carries an Rh-positive fetus. If maternal and fetal blood mix (as from a placental tear, prenatal bleeding, or a previous delivery), the mother may develop antibodies against fetal Rh antigens—a response called Rh sensitization. The antibodies cross the placenta, causing hemolysis of fetal RBCs. The resulting anemia may stimulate release of immature RBCs into the circulation; hemoglobin from hemolyzed RBCs breaks down to bilirubin.

In the fetus, the liver may enlarge to the point where it compresses the umbilical vein, compromising circulation and oxygen delivery. If hypoxia arises, the cardiovascular reserve is depleted rapidly and fluid accumulates, causing ascites. Also, as the liver becomes congested, hepatic protein synthesis may diminish, causing a life-threatening condition called hydrops fetalis, characterized by massive fetal edema (Nicholaides, 1989).

RBC destruction continues after delivery, causing severe anemia and jaundice in the neonate. Fortunately, Rh-negative women now receive Rh_o (D) immune globulin (RhoGAM) within 3 days of a delivery or an abortion. Thus, Rh incompatibility now is rare.

ABO blood group incompatibility

This condition results from an antigen-antibody reaction by maternal RBCs, causing hemolysis of fetal RBCs. ABO incompatibility is most common when the mother has type O blood and the fetus has type A, B, or AB blood. Usually, it causes signs and symptoms similar to but far less severe than those seen in Rh incompatibility. (For more information on Rh and ABO incompatibility, see Chapter 23, Antepartal Complications.)

Effects of maternal substance abuse

Maternal use of alcohol, narcotics, and other chemical substances during pregnancy can have devastating effects on the fetus and neonate.

Fetal alcohol syndrome

This syndrome involves alterations in intrauterine growth and development. A common finding in the NICU, fetal alcohol syndrome (FAS) may lead to growth deficiency, microcephaly, mental retardation, poor coordination, facial abnormalities, behavioral deviations (such as irritability), and cardiac and joint anomalies.

Alcohol crosses the placenta in the same concentration as is present in the maternal circulation. Damage to fetal cells may result from alcohol itself or from acetaldehyde, an alcohol oxidation product. Such damage is not limited to a particular gestational period. Also, researchers cannot pinpoint a safe level of alcohol consumption; even moderate drinking during the first trimester can cause physical characteristics of FAS. Consequently, pregnant women should be advised to avoid all alcohol (Jones, 1986). (Alcoholic beverages now carry labels warning that alcohol ingestion during pregnancy may affect the fetus.)

Drug exposure, addiction, and withdrawal

Maternal drug use during pregnancy is a serious and growing problem. Most drugs cross the placenta, with potentially devastating effects on the fetus. Depending on the stage of fetal development during exposure, maternal narcotic use may cause subtle or profound effects, including congenital anomalies, asphyxia, prematurity, respiratory and cardiac disorders, CNS abnormalities, and death. Intrauterine growth retardation leading to reduced neonatal weight also may occur, possibly from drug-induced slowing of blood flow to the placenta, which reduces nutrient delivery to the fetus. A fetus exposed to such drugs as heroin, cocaine, methadone, or barbiturates also may become addicted and must go through withdrawal after birth.

A pregnant woman who uses drugs also puts her fetus in jeopardy by increasing her risk of poor nutrition, anemia, systemic or local infection, preeclampsia, and exposure to such diseases as human immunodeficiency virus (HIV), the virus that causes acquired immunodeficiency syndrome (AIDS). Intrapartal effects of maternal drug use include fetal distress and preterm delivery. After delivery, the neonate who is going through withdrawal may exhibit behavioral deviations that hinder parent-infant bonding, including irritability, continual crying, and poor feeding.

Ironically, the fetal stress caused by maternal heroin use has one positive consequence: It accelerates respiratory maturation. Consequently, the incidence of respiratory infections and RDS is relatively low among neonates of heroin users (Flandermeyer, 1987).

Maternal use of cocaine—a powerful CNS stimulant causing vasoconstriction, hypertension, and tachycardia—may result in various perinatal problems, depending on the gestational period and duration of exposure. These problems include profound congenital anomalies (such as urogenital anomalies in male neonates), abruptio placentae, altered brain-wave activity, cerebral infarcts (which may develop as late as 40 weeks' gestation), and prune-belly syndrome (characterized by a protruding, thin-walled abdomen; bladder and ureter dilation; small, dysplastic kidneys; undescended testes; and absence of a portion of the rectus abdominis muscle). Death also may occur (Kennard, 1990).

Infection

An infection can be acquired in utero, during labor and delivery, or after birth. The preterm neonate is especially vulnerable to postnatal infection because of reduced transmission of maternal immunoglobulins, including IgM and IgA. Unable to produce antibodies, the preterm neonate also cannot effectively phagocytose foreign proteins or mount a sufficient inflammatory response.

Child abuse and failure to thrive in the high-risk neonate

Potential long-term effects of high-risk status at birth include child abuse and failure to thrive.

Child abuse

While studies have failed to show a clear link between child abuse and preterm birth or chronic illness, both preterm status and congenital anomalies are associated with child abuse. However, the actual cause of abuse usually is secondary; for instance, frustration brought on by the combined pressures of the child's high-risk status and other family circumstances, such as poor financial resources (White, Benedict, Wulff, and Kelley, 1987). Therefore, identifying potential sources of stress and planning interventions to help parents deal with them is a crucial focus of nursing care.

If other factors with a high incidence in child-abuse cases also are present in a high-risk neonate's family, the potential for abuse—and thus the need for further assessment and intervention—may increase. These factors include:
• family or social isolation
• history of family abuse or neglect
• marital problems
• insufficient child-care arrangements
• siblings close in age
• decreased parent-neonate contact in the neonatal intensive care unit (Hunter, Kilstrom, Kraybill, and Loda, 1978).

If indications of a potential problem appear, the nurse should assess further and, as necessary, arrange for follow-up counseling with a nurse specialist in family therapy, a social worker, or other professional to help family members deal with pressures before they lead to child abuse. The nurse who suspects that abuse already has occurred should follow legal requirements and institutional policy for reporting suspected child abuse.

Failure to thrive

In a full-term neonate or infant, failure to thrive is defined as a length and weight below the third percentile. For a preterm neonate or infant whose birth weight was significantly below normal, failure to thrive must be judged in terms of progress; the term should not be applied as long as the infant gains steadily over time, even if length and weight are below the third percentile.

Failure to thrive occurs because the neonate or infant cannot grow and develop normally—for organic reasons, inorganic reasons, or a combination of the two. In *organic* failure to thrive, physiologic problems (some of which may be associated with a high-risk birth) prevent the neonate or infant from digesting or ingesting sufficient nutrients to maintain normal growth. In *inorganic* failure to thrive, diagnosed when no organic cause can be found, the neonate or infant does not develop a bond with the caregiver; even with sufficient intake, the child has poor weight gain and may fail to achieve developmental milestones.

Failure to thrive occurs in high-risk neonates for both organic and inorganic reasons. Not only may a physical defect or repeated illness interfere with growth, but lengthy hospitalization may prevent the formation of a trusting relationship with a permanent caregiver. Likewise, parents who fear that their seriously ill child will die may hold back from forming a normal parent-infant bond.

In the high-risk neonate or infant, lack of steady growth progress, poor eye contact, decreased interaction with the environment, and heightened irritability or lethargy may indicate failure to thrive. If such signs appear, the nurse should report them to the physician while working with the parents to strengthen their bond with the child.

Agents that can infect the fetus or neonate, causing potentially morbid effects, are referred to as TORCH agents. This acronym stands for toxoplasmosis, others, rubella, cytomegalovirus, and herpes. Most TORCH infections are acquired in utero. (For a discussion of maternal TORCH infection, see Chapter 12, Infectious Disorders.)

Cytomegalovirus (CMV) is the most common transplacentally acquired infection; it also can be acquired during delivery. CMV may result in CNS damage, although typically it causes no detectable signs at birth. Rubella, another transplacentally acquired infection, also causes serious sequelae. If acquired during the first trimester, it may result in CNS damage and cardiac defects; after the fourteenth week of gestation, the major sequela is deafness. Other transplacentally acquired infections include measles, chickenpox, smallpox, vaccinia, hepatitis B, HIV, toxoplasmosis, and syphilis. (For details on transplacentally acquired infections, see Chapter 22, High-Risk Antepartal Clients.)

Bacterial pneumonia, which can lead to intrauterine death, may be acquired by the fetus after prolonged rupture of the membranes (more than 24 hours), in which vaginal organisms may migrate upward. Bacterial organisms that can cause intrauterine bacteria pneumonia include nonhemolytic streptococci, *Escherichia coli* and other gram-negative organisms, *Listeria monocytogenes,* and *Candida.*

HIV can be acquired transplacentally at various times in gestation, intrapartally through contact with maternal blood and secretions, and postnatally through breast milk. The neonate with HIV typically has a distinctive facial dysmorphism (malformation) and suffers such problems as interstitial pneumonia, hepatosplenomegaly, recurrent infections, behavioral deviations, and neurologic abnormalities. In many cases, the neonate with HIV is small for gestational age and suffers failure to thrive. (For information on this problem, see *Child abuse and failure to thrive in the high-risk neonate.*)

Infections that can be acquired as the fetus passes through the birth canal include:
• Chlamydia trachomatis, which may lead to conjunctivitis or pneumonia (if secretions pass into the eyes or oropharynx)

• *Neisseria gonorrhoeae*, which may cause ophthalmia neonatorum, an acute purulent conjunctivitis
• herpes simplex virus, which may result in skin vesicles, lethargy, respiratory problems, convulsions, disseminated vascular coagulation, hepatitis, keratoconjunctivitis, and death.

A pregnant client with known herpes simplex virus should be observed closely through frequent cervical cultures to determine whether the virus is active. Active virus at the time of delivery usually warrants cesarean delivery—an approach that has reduced the number of neonatal herpes cases (Hager, 1983).

Congenital anomalies

Many congenital anomalies are life-threatening and warrant immediate intervention and referral to a level 3 nursery. Such disorders include tracheoesophageal malformations, diaphragmatic hernia, choanal atresia, omphalocele, gastroschisis, meningomyelocele, encephalocele, and imperforate anus. Other anomalies do not require immediate treatment but may lead to chronic disability or deformity.

The exact cause of many congenital anomalies remains unknown. Some have been linked to genetic or chromosomal disorders, congenital rubella, exposure to radiation, maternal diabetes, and maternal drug use. Increased maternal age also has been associated with certain anomalies, including the trisomy disorders.

CNS anomalies

More congenital anomalies involve the CNS than any other body system. Some CNS anomalies result in only minimal dysfunction; others have devastating consequences.

Meningomyelocele. In this anomaly (also called spina bifida), part of the meninges and spinal cord substance protrude through the vertebral column; the defect may be covered by a thin membrane. (When only the meninges protrude, the anomaly is called a meningocele.) Meningomyelocele results from defective neural tube formation during embryonic development. Hydrocephalus (discussed below) commonly accompanies the anomaly.

Consequences of meningomyelocele may be severe—for instance, paralysis below the defect. The child's appearance may be noticeably abnormal even after surgical correction.

Encephalocele. In this anomaly, the meninges and portions of brain tissue protrude through the cranium, usually in the occipital area. Typically, it occurs at the midline, through a suture line. Like meningomyelocele, encephalocele results from failure of the neural tube to close during embryonic development, may be accompanied by hydrocephalus, and may lead to paralysis.

Congenital hydrocephalus. In this disorder, excessive cerebrospinal fluid (CSF) accumulates within the cranial vault, leading to suture expansion and ventricular dilation. This anomaly may result from obstruction of the foramen of Monro—a passage allowing communication between the lateral and third ventricles. Hydrocephalus sometimes is associated with meningomyelocele and other neural tube defects, intrauterine infection, meningitis, cerebral hemorrhage, head trauma, or Arnold-Chiari malformation (herniation of the brain stem and lower cerebellum through the foramen magnum into the cervical vertebral canal).

Anencephaly and microcephaly. In anencephaly, the cephalic end of the spinal cord fails to close, causing absence of the cerebral hemispheres. Anencephaly commonly causes stillbirth; if not, the neonate typically lives only a few days.

In microcephaly, the head is abnormally small and the brain underdeveloped, usually resulting in severe mental retardation and motor dysfunction. Microcephaly may result from an inborn error of metabolism (such as uncontrolled maternal phenylketonuria), intrauterine infection, or severe prolonged intrauterine hypoxia. (For a description of some inborn errors of metabolism, see *Inborn errors of metabolism.*)

Teratoma. This tumor, which may be solid or fluid-filled, consists of various cell types, none of which normally occur together. The most common site is the sacrococcygeal area, although the tumor may occur anywhere. Teratoma develops during embryonic development if the primitive streak (a dense area on the central posterior region of the embryonic disk) fails to disappear. This gives rise to a mass that may contain calcium and other tissue fragments, including teeth and hair follicles (visible on X-ray).

Cardiac anomalies

Congenital cardiac anomalies—structural defects of the heart and great vessels—can occur during any stage of embryonic development. Cardiac structures are most susceptible to defects from the third to ninth weeks of gestation. In most cases, the cause remains unknown, although researchers believe that genetic and environmental factors play a role. Defects become noticeable after delivery when fetal circulation normally changes to neonatal circulation.

Congenital cardiac anomalies are classified as acyanotic or cyanotic. Acyanotic defects include atrial septal defect, ventricular septal defect, coarctation of the aorta,

Inborn errors of metabolism

An inborn error of metabolism is a genetic condition in which a defect of a specific enzyme disrupts metabolism and nutrient use. The involved enzyme may not be produced or its action may be blocked by lack of a precursor necessary for a crucial chemical reaction.

The nursing goal for a neonate with an inborn error of metabolism is early detection and prevention of complications. The chart below describes these disorders and presents nursing implications for each.

CONDITION	DESCRIPTION	NURSING IMPLICATIONS
Congenital hypothyroidism	Deficiency of thyroid hormone secretion during fetal development or early infancy. The condition (also known as cretinism) typically stems from defective embryonic development causing absence or underdevelopment of the thyroid gland or severe maternal iodine deficiency; in some cases, it is inherited as an autosomal recessive disorder involving an enzymatic defect in the synthesis of the thyroid hormone thyroxine. Untreated, congenital hypothyroidism can lead to respiratory compromise and persistent physiologic jaundice.	• Signs of congenital hypothyroidism in the neonate include inactivity, jaundice, excessive sleep, hoarse cry, constipation, and feeding problems. • Many states require measurement of thyroid hormone levels at birth to detect congenital hypothyroidism early and thus help minimize mental and physical retardation. The disorder is confirmed by an elevated serum level of thyroid-stimulating hormone (TSH) and a low serum thyroxine (T_4) level. (However, test results may be misleading in the preterm neonate—especially one with respiratory distress syndrome, who typically has abnormal TSH and T_4 levels.) • Treatment involves lifelong administration of L-thyroxine, with periodic dosage adjustments to meet the demands of rapid growth periods. During the neonatal period, thyroxine can be given mixed with several milliliters of formula or crushed and mixed with rice cereal or applesauce when the infant begins eating solid foods.
Galactosemia	Hereditary autosomal recessive disorder in which deficiency of the enzyme galactose-1-phosphate uridyltransferase leads to inability to convert galactose to glucose and subsequent galactose accumulation in the blood. The disorder can be fatal if not detected and treated within the first few days after birth.	• Because the affected neonate cannot tolerate lactose, feeding problems may be the first sign of the disorder. Such problems may include anorexia, diarrhea, vomiting, jaundice, hepatomegaly, growth failure, lack of a red light reflex during eye examination, cataracts, and mental retardation (from elevated fetal galactose levels). Also, birth weight may be somewhat low. With early detection and treatment, these problems may subside. • Diagnosis is confirmed by the galactosemia tolerance test and examination of red blood cells revealing deficient galactose-1-phosphate uridyltransferase activity. • In some cases, galactosemia may be detected in utero by amniocentesis. In such cases, the mother should be placed on a galactose-restricted diet to prevent fetal complications and mental retardation. • Treatment involves lifelong avoidance of galactose-containing foods (milk and milk products).
Maple syrup urine disease	Autosomal recessive disorder characterized by an enzyme deficiency in the second step of branched-chain amino acid (BCAA) catabolism. BCAAs accumulate in the blood and urine, causing severe ketoacidosis soon after birth. Without intervention, the neonate progresses rapidly to death (usually from pneumonia and respiratory failure).	• The neonate typically appears normal at birth but deteriorates within 1 week as respirations become rapid and shallow and the level of consciousness declines. Other signs of the disorder include lethargy, alternating muscle hypotonicity and hypertonicity, brief tonic (rigid) seizures, hypoglycemic manifestations (from altered glucose metabolism), and a maple syrup odor to the urine. • Diagnosis is confirmed by a 2,4-dinitrophenylhydrazine test and serum elevation of the essential amino acids leucine, isoleucine, and valine. • Management involves lifelong dietary restriction of BCAAs and close monitoring of serum leucine, isoleucine, and valine levels. An acute episode warrants peritoneal dialysis.
Phenylketonuria (PKU)	Autosomal recessive disorder characterized by the abnormal presence of metabolites of phenylalanine (such as phenylketone) in the urine. It results from deficiency of phenylalanine hy-	• Most states require PKU screening at birth. The test usually is done within the first 24 to 48 hours after birth. If results are positive, retesting and referral should take place immediately to ensure early treatment. • Obtain blood for the screening test by heel stick. To prevent a false-negative test result, make sure the neonate has received adequate (continued)

Inborn errors of metabolism continued

CONDITION	DESCRIPTION	NURSING IMPLICATIONS
Phenylketonuria (continued)	droxylase, the enzyme responsible for converting the amino acid phenylalanine to tyrosine. Phenylalanine is transaminated to phenylpyruvic acid or decarboxylated to phenylthalanine, which then accumulates in the blood. Prolonged exposure to high serum levels of phenylalanine may cause severe brain damage and mental retardation.	dietary protein and had no contraindications for oral feedings for 24 to 48 hours before the test. • Immediately after diagnosis, the neonate should be given Lafenalac (if the overall condition permits). This formula has a phenylalanine concentration of about 0.5% (in contrast to the 5% found in most infant formulas). • Usually, Lafenalac must be substituted for milk throughout the child's growing periods. Dietary restriction of phenylalanine must continue lifelong. Serum phenylalanine blood levels must be monitored closely throughout childhood. • Provide teaching, nutritional counseling, and emotional support to the neonate's family. Emphasize that the neonate cannot be given substitutions for prescribed food products, especially for Lafenalac. Refer the family to any available support groups for help in coping with the disease. • A woman with PKU who contemplates pregnancy should be warned about the possible effects of an elevated maternal phenylalanine level on the developing fetus (including congenital anomalies and mental retardation).

pulmonic stenosis, and PDA. These anomalies do not interfere with shunting of oxygenated blood from the left to the right side of the heart; the left side continues to eject oxygenated blood, preventing cyanosis. However, pulmonary blood flow to the right ventricle increases, placing the neonate at risk for pulmonary edema and congestive heart failure.

Cyanotic defects include tetralogy of Fallot, transposition of the great vessels, and tricuspid atresia. In such defects, abnormally high pressure in the right side of the heart permits left-to-right shunting of unoxygenated blood. As this blood mixes with oxygenated blood, arterial blood oxygen becomes desaturated. Peripheral perfusion then decreases and cyanosis develops. (For descriptions and illustrations of specific acyanotic and cyanotic defects, see *Congenital cardiac anomalies,* pages 946 and 947.)

Respiratory tract anomalies

The most common respiratory tract anomaly is diaphragmatic hernia. In this defect, the various segments of the diaphragm fail to fuse during embryonic development, causing the abdominal contents to protrude from the abdominal cavity into the thoracic cavity at birth. Diaphragmatic hernia occurs in 1 of every 2,000 births. In the United States, it is twice as common in males as in females (Harjo, Kenner, and Brueggemeyer, 1988).

The defect may be unilateral or bilateral; most commonly, it occurs on the posterolateral aspect of the diaphragm on the left side. In a left-sided defect, the stomach and intestines typically protrude into the thoracic cavity;

protrusion of the liver, spleen, and other abdominal organs is rare.

Most neonates with diaphragmatic hernia have impaired lung development—typically only a lung bud is present (a condition known as hypoplastic lung). This may lead to profound respiratory compromise and death if intervention does not begin immediately after delivery.

GI tract anomalies

These anomalies include tracheoesophageal malformations, abdominal wall defects (omphalocele and gastroschisis), meconium ileus, imperforate anus, and cleft palate and lip.

Tracheoesophageal malformations. Tracheoesophageal malformations, which occur in 1 of every 1,500 live births (Harjo, Kenner, and Brueggemeyer, 1988), result from altered embryonic development of the trachea and esophagus. These anomalies sometimes occur as part of the VACTERL syndrome—vertebral, anal, cardiac, tracheal, esophageal, renal, and limb anomalies. Types of tracheoesophageal anomalies include tracheoesophageal fistula (an abnormal connection between the trachea and esophagus), esophageal atresia (closure of the esophagus at some point), and absence of the esophagus. Usually, tracheoesophageal fistula occurs in tandem with esophageal atresia. In the most common tracheoesophageal malformation, esophageal atresia accompanies distal tracheoesophageal fistula; the upper esophageal section ends in a blind pouch (atresia) that does not connect with the stomach. (For an illustration of this and other types of tracheoesophageal malformations, see *Tracheo-esophageal malformations*, page 948.)

Abdominal wall defects. Omphalocele and gastroschisis occur in approximately 1 of every 7,000 births (Harjo, Kenner, and Brueggemeyer, 1988). In omphalocele, a portion of the intestine protrudes through a defect in the abdominal wall at the umbilicus, in the midline. A thin, transparent membrane composed of amnion and peritoneum typically covers the protruding part. (The membrane sometimes ruptures during delivery and thus may not be visible by the time the neonate is admitted to the NICU.) The defect may be quite large—or small enough to elude detection on brief inspection.

Omphalocele arises during embryonic development when the abdominal contents migrate into the umbilical cord. Normally, at 9 weeks' gestation, the abdominal contents recede from the umbilical cord, regressing into the abdominal cavity; if the contents fail to recede, omphalocele occurs.

Gastroschisis refers to incomplete abdominal wall closure not involving the site of the umbilical cord insertion. Usually, the small intestine and part of the large intestine protrude. No membranous sac covers the protrusion.

Meconium ileus. This intestinal obstruction results from obstruction of the terminal ileum by viscous meconium. Beyond the ileal obstruction, the colon atrophies and narrows in diameter. In at least 95% of cases, it is a sign of cystic fibrosis, a genetic disease resulting from a pancreatic enzyme deficiency.

Imperforate anus. In this malformation, the anus is closed abnormally. Occurring in 1 of every 20,000 live births, the disorder is more common in males than females (Harjo, Kenner, and Brueggemeyer, 1988). It results from persistence of the membrane that separates the lower rectum from the lower aspect of the large intestine. (Normally, this membrane disappears by the ninth week of gestation, leading to formation of a patent tube from the intestine to the rectum.) In many cases, imperforate anus is associated with other defects, such as rectourethral and rectovaginal fistula (both of which permit abnormal evacuation of fecal matter from the rectum).

Imperforate anus occurs as several variants. In anal agenesis, the most common variant, the rectal pouch ends blindly above the surface of the perineum; an anal fistula commonly is present. In anal stenosis, the anal aperture is abnormally small. In anal membrane atresia, the anal membrane covers the aperture, creating an obstruction.

Imperforate anus also may be classified as high or low. In the high form, a fistula links the upper rectal pouch to the bladder, urethra, or vagina. If a fistula is absent, bowel obstruction occurs and the neonate has a large, distended abdomen. In low imperforate anus, intestinal patency may be compromised by a membrane at the anal sphincter level.

Cleft palate and cleft lip. These congenital defects, which occur in 1 of every 1,000 live births (Harjo, Kenner, and Brueggemeyer, 1988), sometimes result from chromosomal abnormalities. Cleft palate occurs when the sides of the palate fail to fuse during embryonic development, leading to a fissure in the palatal midline. The fissure may be complete, extending through both the hard and soft palates into the nasal cavities, or incomplete.

In cleft lip (harelip), one or more clefts appear in the upper lip. This anomaly results from failure of the maxillary and median nasal processes to close during embryonic development. The defect, which is more common in males than females, may be unilateral or bilateral and sometimes occurs in conjunction with other anomalies. It commonly accompanies cleft palate.

Genitourinary tract anomalies

Genitourinary tract anomalies include renal agenesis, polycystic kidney disease, posterior urethral valves, and external genital ambiguity.

Renal agenesis. One of the most common congenital anomalies in males, renal agenesis may be unilateral (absence of one kidney) or bilateral (absence of both kidneys). The bilateral form (also called Potter's association) is incompatible with life and typically causes stillbirth or death during the neonatal period; autopsies of neonates with bilateral renal agenesis show hypoplastic lung and multiple pneumothoraces. With unilateral agenesis, the single kidney enlarges to maintain normal renal function.

Polycystic kidney disease. In this disorder, which occurs as an autosomal recessive disease in the neonate and as an acquired disease in the adult, multiple cysts form within the kidney. As the cysts enlarge, adjacent tissue is destroyed. At birth, the neonate with polycystic kidney disease typically suffers renal failure, respiratory distress, congestive heart failure, and hypertension.

Posterior urethral valves. This anomaly, which occurs only in males, causes urinary tract obstruction, hydronephrosis, impaired urine flow, and (when untreated) profound renal damage. Typically, the obstructing valves are exaggerations of two mucosal folds that normally are continuous with the lower end of the urethera where the ejaculatory ducts open.

Congenital cardiac anomalies

Abnormalities during fetal development may cause structural defects of the heart and great vessels. These defects probably stem from a combination of genetic or chromosomal disorders and environmental factors. Maternal alcoholism, malnutrition, rubella, or diabetes mellitus may contribute to cardiac anomalies. In the illustrations, blood flow is indicated by arrows—red arrows for adequately oxygenated blood, black arrows for poorly oxygenated blood.

Atrial septal defect

In this defect, an abnormal opening in the atrial septum allows blood to shunt from the left to right atrium. In many cases, it results from failure of the foramen ovale to close. Increased blood flow to the right heart and pulmonary arteries causes the right ventricle and atrium to enlarge.

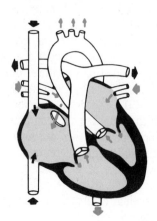

Coarctation of the aorta

This anomaly obstructs preductal or postductal blood flow, causing increased pressure in the left ventricle. To compensate, collateral circulation develops, enhancing blood flow from the proximal arteries and bypassing the obstructed area.

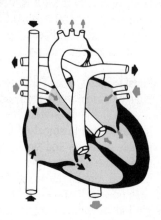

Pulmonic stenosis

This defect may be characterized by poststenotic dilation of the pulmonary trunk and concentric hypertrophy of the right ventricle, which cause a systolic pressure differential between the right ventricular cavity and pulmonary artery.

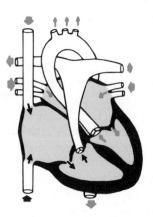

Tetralogy of Fallot

This anomaly consists of four defects—ventricular septal defect, overriding aorta, pulmonic stenosis, and right ventricular hypertrophy. Hemodynamic changes depend on the severity of these defects and may range from a left-to-right shunt to a right-to-left shunt, in which unoxygenated blood from the right ventricle enters the aorta directly.

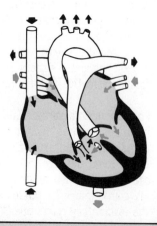

Transposition of the great vessels

In this anomaly, the pulmonary artery arises from the left ventricle and the aorta from the right ventricle, preventing the pulmonary and systemic circulations from mixing. Without associated defects that allow these circulatory systems to mix—such as a patent ductus arteriosus or septal defect—the neonate will die.

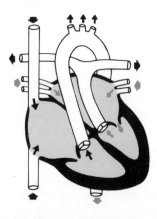

Ventricular septal defect
In this defect, an abnormal opening in the ventricular septum allows oxygenated blood to flow from the left to right ventricle; blood recirculates through the lungs and pulmonary artery. If the defect is large, pulmonary vascular resistance increases, causing elevated pulmonary and right ventricular pressures.

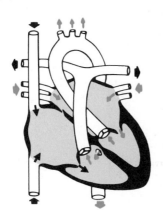

Patent ductus arteriosus
This anomaly occurs when the ductus arteriosus—a tubular connection that shunts blood away from the fetus's pulmonary circulation—fails to close after birth. Blood then shunts from the aorta to the pulmonary artery.

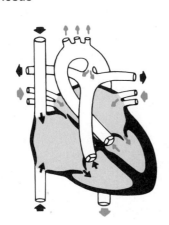

Tricuspid atresia
In this defect, which usually is accompanied by an atrial or ventricular septal defect (both shown), the tricuspid valve is absent or incomplete, preventing the flow of blood from the right atrium to the right ventricle. Right atrial blood then shunts through an atrial septal defect into the left atrium.

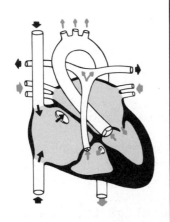

External genital ambiguity. This problem may reflect a developmental defect, genetic abnormality, or hormonal influences. In some cases, it complicates determination of the neonate's sex. In males, genital ambiguity typically stems from a developmental abnormality. In females, a common cause is congenital adrenal hyperplasia, a condition stemming from blockage of cortisol precursors (enzymes that convert cholesterol to cortisol). The resulting corticotropin deficiency leads to increased secretion of cortisol precursors and androgens and subsequent masculinization of the female external genitalia.

Musculoskeletal anomalies
The most common congenital musculoskeletal anomaly is clubfoot (talipes). This deformity involves unilateral or bilateral deviation of the metatarsal bones; talus deformation and a shortened Achilles tendon give the foot a clublike appearance. Clubfoot sometimes is associated with other anomalies, such as meningomyelocele.

The second most common musculoskeletal disorder is congenital hip dysplasia. This disorder occurs more commonly in females.

Assessment

In many—perhaps most—cases, delivery of a high-risk neonate can be predicted from the maternal health history or from antepartal or intrapartal data. For instance, fetal distress (signaled by an abnormal fetal heart rate, meconium-stained amniotic fluid, or a fetal scalp blood pH below 7.25) warns strongly of a high-risk delivery. Thus, anticipation and preparation can help prevent or minimize perinatal problems. When a client is due to deliver, check the calculated date of delivery and review the history for factors that help predict neonatal outcome. (For more information, see *Risk factors for perinatal problems,* page 949.)

If a high-risk neonate is expected, a brief assessment immediately after delivery verifies the endangered status, as when the neonate fails to breathe spontaneously or has central cyanosis or an inadequate heart rate. Poor 1-minute and 5-minute Apgar scores also may confirm or suggest high-risk status. In some cases, however, a perinatal problem is not discovered until a complete examination is conducted several hours or days later. (For a detailed discussion of neonatal assessment, see Chapter 35, Neonatal Assessment.)

Tracheoesophageal malformations

Tracheoesophageal malformations result from incomplete separation of the trachea and esophagus during the first trimester of pregnancy. Among the most serious surgical emergencies in neonates, they require immediate correction. In many cases, they are accompanied by other congenital anomalies. Common variations of tracheoesophageal malformations are illustrated here.

Esophageal atresia with distal tracheoesophageal fistula is the most common variation.

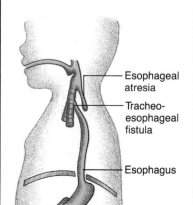

Esophageal atresia

Tracheoesophageal fistula

Esophagus

In **esophageal atresia without tracheoesophageal fistula,** the upper esophageal portion ends in a blind pouch, the upper and lower esophageal portions do not connect, and the trachea and esophagus are not linked by a fistula.

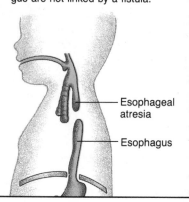

Esophageal atresia

Esophagus

Tracheoesophageal fistula without esophageal atresia (sometimes called an H-type tracheoesophageal fistula) is characterized by an intact esophagus and a connection between the trachea and esophagus.

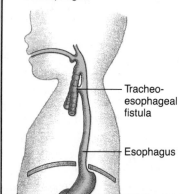

Tracheoesophageal fistula

Esophagus

In some cases, **esophageal atresia** occurs with a **proximal fistula.**

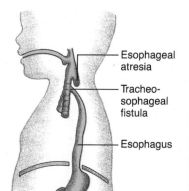

Esophageal atresia

Tracheoesophageal fistula

Esophagus

Esophageal atresia sometimes occurs with a **double** (proximal and distal) **fistula.**

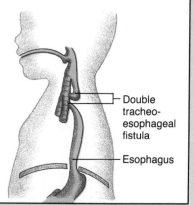

Double tracheoesophageal fistula

Esophagus

Gestational-age and birth-weight variations

In many cases, maternal, antepartal, and intrapartal factors give advance warning of these problems—particularly preterm or postterm status. If the neonate weighs less than 2,500 g or has a suspected alteration in the intrauterine growth pattern, gestational age should be determined from a thorough gestational-age assessment, then correlated to birth weight. (For infor-

mation on gestational-age assessment, see Chapter 35, Neonatal Assessment.)

Maternal, antepartal, and intrapartal history

The preterm neonate is the classic high-risk neonate, making prematurity the leading predictor of high-risk status. Prematurity and postmaturity usually can be anticipated from maternal, antepartal, and intrapartal data; the calculated delivery date; and ultrasound evaluation. For example, maternal weight loss, decreased abdominal circumference, and reduced uterine size during pregnancy may indicate an altered fetal growth pattern reflecting postterm gestation; ultrasound can be used to estimate gestational weeks.

The diagnosis of large for gestational age (LGA) typically comes during the antepartal period, when fundal height appears disproportionate to gestational weeks (and ultrasound determines exact fetal size.). Also, because maternal diabetes mellitus is a leading cause of accelerated intrauterine growth, this condition suggests an LGA fetus.

About two-thirds of SGA neonates are born to women with SGA-associated risk factors (Cassady and Strange, 1987). Consequently, check the maternal history for such factors as low socioeconomic status, age extreme, increased parity, short stature, low prepregnancy weight, and previous delivery of an SGA neonate.

Neonatal findings

After delivery, assess the neonate for physical signs of gestational-age and birth-weight variations as well as perinatal problems associated with these variations. For example, the preterm neonate may appear inactive, with extended positioning at rest, splayed legs, and arms held away from the body. The respiratory pattern typically is irregular, possibly with apneic episodes. Other signs of prematurity include translucent, ruddy skin; visible blood vessels; absent skin folds (from decreased subcutaneous fat); thick vernix caseosa, especially around the neck and thighs; prominent lanugo across the back and face; long, thin fingers with soft, pliable nails; sparse or absent breast tissue; and immature external genitalia.

Physical examination of the postterm neonate typically reveals macrosomic (excessively large) features. Some postterm neonates also have green, brown, or yellow meconium staining of the skin, nails, umbilical cord, or placental membranes. A postterm LGA neonate may show signs of birth trauma and hypoglycemia. With a postterm SGA neonate, expect dry, cracked, wrinkled skin with decreased subcutaneous fat; no visible vernix caseosa or lanugo; skin maceration; long, thin arms and legs; long nails; and full hair growth.

Although birth weight must be correlated with gestational age to verify SGA or LGA status, assess for associated physical signs and perinatal problems if either problem is suspected. The typical SGA neonate has loose, dry skin with diminished skinfold thickness; reduced breast tissue (from soft-tissue wasting); skin wasting in the buttocks and thighs; widened skull sutures with large fontanels; and shortened crown-to-heel, femoral, and foot lengths (from bone growth failure). In a neonate with these findings, also check for congenital anomalies, which are 10 to 20 times more common in SGA neonates than normal neonates.

Risk factors for perinatal problems

The health care team can anticipate a neonate's high-risk status from the maternal, antepartal, or intrapartal history or from certain neonatal conditions present at birth.

MATERNAL RISK FACTORS

- Age over 34 or under 19
- Alcohol or drug use during pregnancy
- Chronic illness (including diabetes mellitus, anemia, hypertension, kidney disease, or heart disease)
- Cigarette smoking
- Death of a previous fetus
- Death or illness of a previous neonate
- Exposure to toxic chemicals, radiation, or other hazardous substances or conditions
- Exposure to infection during pregnancy
- Family history of a genetic disease (such as Down's syndrome)
- Hereditary disease
- Isoimmunization
- Low socioeconomic status
- More than seven previous pregnancies
- Poor prenatal care
- Previous multiple fetuses
- Short interval between pregnancies (less than 18 months)

ANTEPARTAL RISK FACTORS

- Abruptio placentae
- Accelerated fetal growth
- Fetal surgery
- First-trimester bleeding
- Hydramnios
- Intrauterine growth retardation
- Multiple fetuses
- Placenta previa
- Pregnancy-induced hypertension
- Premature rupture of the membranes

INTRAPARTAL RISK FACTORS

- Abnormal fetal presentation
- Cesarean delivery
- Fetal distress (as indicated by late decelerations and decreased beat-to-beat variability)
- Maternal anesthetics or analgesics
- Prolonged labor
- Umbilical cord prolapse
- Use of forceps during delivery

NEONATAL RISK FACTORS

- Abnormal placental weight or appearance
- Cardiorespiratory depression
- Congenital anomaly
- Low Apgar score
- Lack of spontaneous respirations
- Meconium-stained amniotic fluid
- Prematurity
- Postmaturity
- Small or large size for gestational age
- Unusual number of umbilical vessels

With the LGA neonate, assess for signs of birth injury, congenital anomalies, hypoglycemia, and polycythemia. If the LGA neonate is preterm, check for signs of respiratory distress and hyperbilirubinemia. With a postterm LGA neonate, expect respiratory distress from meconium aspiration syndrome or asphyxiation. With the LGA neonate of a diabetic mother, check for signs of hypoglycemia and hypocalcemia.

Respiratory problems

Signs of a respiratory problem may be obvious, immediate, and life-threatening, such as with birth asphyxia or apnea, or may arise hours, days, or even weeks later.

Asphyxia and apnea
The cardinal sign of asphyxia is deep gasping or failure to breathe spontaneously at delivery. Associated signs include a slow heart rate, abnormally low blood pressure, poor muscle tone, and poor reflexes. To help anticipate birth asphyxia, check for such risk factors as maternal diabetes, infection, pregnancy-induced hypertension, or anesthesia; more than one fetus; prolonged labor; prolapsed umbilical cord; abruptio placentae; placenta previa; prolonged rupture of the membranes; meconium-stained amniotic fluid; oligohydramnios; hydramnios; umbilical cord compression; placental insufficiency; abnormal fetal heart rate patterns; isoimmunization; delivery complications; excessive fetal size; abnormal presentation; or neonatal prematurity, postmaturity, or congenital anomalies.

Apneic episodes commonly manifest as rapid respirations punctuated by brief pauses. Hypoxemia, cyanosis, and bradycardia may ensue. With central apnea, expect absence of respiratory efforts and muscle flaccidity. With obstructive apnea, expect respiratory motions accompanied by hypoxemia and bradycardia, (from inability to draw air into the lungs).

Meconium aspiration syndrome
In MAS, signs of respiratory distress may be mild, moderate, or severe. The neonate typically appears barrel chested because of an increased anteroposterior chest diameter (from bronchial obstruction by meconium or tension pneumothorax). Skin and nails may be meconium stained.

Respiratory distress syndrome
Signs of RDS may appear at delivery or within a few hours. They include tachypnea (a respiratory rate over 60 breaths/minute), labored respirations, grunting, nasal flaring, cyanosis, and chest retractions. The neonate may become restless and agitated (probably from the increas-ing $PaCO_2$ level) and show fatigue even after simple care procedures. Complex procedures, such as endotracheal suctioning, may thoroughly exhaust the neonate's limited energy reserves, leading to bradycardia and hypoxia.

The likelihood of RDS may be determined antenatally from analysis of amniotic fluid lipids; a lecithin-sphingomyelin ratio below 2 and a phosphatidylglycerol level below 3% suggest fetal lung immaturity and a high risk for RDS.

RDS affects mainly preterm neonates. Other risk factors include maternal diabetes mellitus, infection, or hemorrhage; maternal steroid or analgesic use; more than one fetus; abruptio placentae; umbilical cord prolapse; meconium-stained amniotic fluid; fetal distress; and breech presentation.

Transient tachypnea
Tachypnea—alone or accompanied by hypoxemia, cyanosis, grunting, and chest retractions—is the hallmark of this disorder. Cesarean delivery and term or near-term gestation are common history findings.

Bronchopulmonary dysplasia
Because BPD typically occurs as a complication of treatment for RDS, signs usually arise after supplemental oxygen administration or mechanical ventilation. The severity of these signs reflects the degree of disease progression and pulmonary dysfunction. Expect nasal flaring, retractions, tachypnea, and grunting. However, the first clue to BPD may be difficulty weaning the neonate from a ventilator. As the disease progresses, carbon dioxide retention and pulmonary secretions increase and crackles can be auscultated. Bronchospasm may result from bronchial smooth muscle hypertrophy. Typically, the neonate's condition worsens and oxygen dependency occurs. (Conversely, decreased oxygen dependency may be the earliest sign of recovery.)

Retinopathy of prematurity

Ophthalmoscopic examination of the neonate with ROP reveals a proliferation of dilated, tortuous retinal vessels; edema; and retinal detachment.

Intraventricular hemorrhage

Typically, IVH causes bulging fontanels, increasing head size, hypotonia, forceful vomiting, downward eye deviation, seizures, lethargy, and extreme irritability. Also assess for generalized signs of hemorrhage, including temperature instability, bradycardia, increasing respiratory distress, apnea, and hypotension.

Necrotizing enterocolitis

Signs of NEC may be generalized—for instance, apnea, hypothermia, lethargy, and irritability—or restricted to the GI tract. GI signs include abdominal distention and tenderness; absent bowel sounds; visible distended, rope-like bowel loops; vomiting; increased gastric residual matter; bloody stools; and feeding problems. Also, stools may contain positive reducing substances—various forms of glucose in abnormal amounts—which indicate impaired intestinal carbohydrate absorption caused by NEC-induced tissue damage.

Determine the neonate's glucose level from a copper reduction tablet test and perform a guaiac test to check for occult blood in the stool. X-ray evidence of pneumatosis (air within the intestinal walls), adynamic ileus (intestinal obstruction caused by reduced intestinal motility), thickened bowel walls, and free air in the peritoneum or portal system confirm the diagnosis.

Neonate of a diabetic mother

Typically, this neonate is macrosomic, with a birth weight in the upper percentile range for gestational age. The face is round with chubby cheeks and the skin is ruddy to bright red. Signs of hypoglycemia and hypocalcemia (discussed below) may be present; however, over half of neonates of diabetic mothers have asymptomatic hypoglycemia. Assess for signs of birth trauma, such as bruising, ecchymosis, and shoulder dystocia (sometimes manifested as a flaccid or unusually positioned arm).

For the neonate whose mother had questionably or poorly controlled diabetes during pregnancy, assess for signs of hypoglycemia and check blood-glucose levels using a glucose oxidase dipstick at delivery and 30 minutes afterward.

Metabolic disorders

Signs of metabolic disorders range from extremely mild to severe.

Hypoglycemia

Signs of hypoglycemia include apnea or bradycardia, seizures, irregular respirations, cyanosis, irritability, listlessness, lethargy, tremors, feeding problems, vomiting, hypotonia, and a high-pitched cry. Also, neurologic immaturity may prevent homeostasis in the hypoglycemic neonate, leading to unstable vital signs. However, some hypoglycemic neonates are asymptomatic.

Besides maternal diabetes, risk factors for hypoglycemia include prematurity, SGA status, severe isoimmune hemolytic anemia, and birth asphyxia.

A glucose oxidase dipstick value below 25 mg/100 ml indicates hypoglycemia and warrants a venous blood sample to confirm the diagnosis. Hypoglycemia is confirmed by a blood-glucose level below 40 mg/dl before the first day after birth or below 45 mg/dl on or after the third day.

Hypocalcemia

The hypocalcemic neonate may have seizures, irritability, hypotonia, poor feeding, a high-pitched cry, and signs associated with hypoglycemia. Suspect hypocalcemia in the neonate of a diabetic mother. Other at-risk neonates include those who are preterm or SGA and those who experienced birth asphyxia.

To assess for hypocalcemia, attempt to elicit Chvostek's sign by tapping the skin over the sixth cranial nerve (in front of the ear); unilateral contraction of the muscles surrounding the eye, nose, and mouth indicates tetany, a sign of hypocalcemia. A serum calcium level below 7 mg/100 ml confirms the diagnosis.

Hyperbilirubinemia and jaundice

The neonate with hyperbilirubinemia has yellow skin and sclerae. For the most accurate assessment, apply pressure over the tip of the neonate's nose; a yellow tinge appearing as circulation returns indicates jaundice.

With pathologic jaundice (the more dangerous jaundice form), the serum bilirubin level rises above 13 mg/dl within the first 24 hours after delivery. Transcutaneous bilirubinometry (reflective photometry) sometimes is used as a screening tool for hyperbilirubinemia. This method detects bilirubin levels through the skin and is considered superior to observation of the skin or sclera color alone. However, its accuracy may be reduced in neonates with dark skin.

With severe hyperbilirubinemia (bilirubin encephalopathy), signs vary with the disease phase. Phase 1 signs include hypotonia, vomiting, lethargy, a high-pitched cry, a poor sucking reflex, a decreased or absent Moro reflex, and diminished flexion. During phase 2, spasticity develops; this may take the form of opisthotonus, a prolonged, severe muscle spasm in which the back arches acutely, the head bends back on the neck, the heels bend back on the leg, and the arms and hands flex rigidly at the joints.

In phase 3, spasticity diminishes, the sclera shows above the iris (a condition called "sunset" eyes), and seizures may occur. During phase 4, gastric, pulmonary, and CNS hemorrhages may develop (these problems also may occur during phase 2). A neonate who survives phase 4 usually has residual effects, such as mental retardation, cerebral palsy, and sensory alterations, such as deafness and poor visual acuity or blindness.

Ineffective thermoregulation

Hypothermia (a body temperature below 99.5° F [37.5° C]) causes an accelerated respiratory rate, labored respirations, an increased metabolic rate, and signs of hypoglycemia (indicating greater use of glucose stores).

Hyperthermia (a core temperature above 99.5° F may cause skin reddening, dehydration, irritability, and an initial rise, then gradual drop, in the heart and respiratory rates.

Polycythemia

The neonate with polycythemia may have such signs as tachypnea, cyanosis, convulsions, jaundice, and pleural and scrotal effusions. However, most polycythemic neonates are asymptomatic (Cassady and Strange, 1987).

Isoimmune hemolytic anemia

When isoimmunization has occurred in utero, antepartal ultrasound evaluation may reveal fetal hepatomegaly and hydramnios; fetal monitoring may detect an abnormal heart rate pattern caused by tissue hypoxia at the level of the medulla oblongata (which controls cardiac function via the autonomic nervous system).

The neonate with Rh incompatibility typically is anemic at birth, as indicated by pale mucous membranes, and has massive generalized edema; with severe disease, expect pathologic jaundice, congestive heart failure, an enlarged liver and spleen, and generalized ascites. The neonate with ABO incompatibility may have anemia at birth and develop hyperbilirubinemia after delivery.

Effects of maternal substance abuse

The neonate with FAS may have cardiac anomalies, decreased joint mobility, behavioral deviations, kidney defects, labial hypoplasia, and distinctive facial features. The latter include short palpebral fissures (eye openings); ptosis (drooping eyelids); strabismus (eye muscle deviation); a thin, smooth upper lip with a long philtrum (vertical groove) above it; a short, upturned nose; and a receding jaw. Behavioral deviations include irritability, excessive crying, and poor feeding.

The neonate affected by maternal drug abuse may have muscle tremors, twitching, or rigidity, with inability to extend the muscles; seizures; temperature instability; GI disturbances, including vomiting and diarrhea; tachycardia; tachypnea; diaphoresis with mottling over the extremities; and excessive sneezing and yawning. If the mother used heroin or methadone during pregnancy, the neonate may be SGA or have a low birth weight with cardiorespiratory depression at delivery.

Assessing for neonatal drug withdrawal

The neonate whose mother used such drugs as narcotics, barbiturates, or cocaine during pregnancy may be addicted at birth and go through withdrawal. Classic signs of neonatal drug withdrawal are listed below.

VITAL SIGN DEVIATIONS

- Profound diaphoresis
- Skin mottling
- Tachycardia or bradycardia (depending on the drug involved)
- Tachypnea
- Temperature instability (fever followed by hypothermia)

NEUROMUSCULAR SIGNS

- Absent or strong sucking reflex (may be poorly coordinated with swallowing reflex)
- Exaggeration of other neonatal reflexes
- Difficulty extending muscles
- Jerky movements
- Muscle rigidity with flexion
- Muscle twitching
- Seizures
- Tremors

BEHAVIORAL SIGNS

- Decreased sleep periods and lengthened awake periods
- Dislike for cuddling and close body contact
- Frequent or prolonged sneezing or yawning
- High-pitched or weak cry
- Inconsolability
- Irritability

GASTROINTESTINAL SIGNS

- Frequent vomiting
- Increased gastrointestinal motility, with diarrhea and rapid (possibly visible) peristalsis

---

Typically, the behavior pattern of the drug-addicted neonate is disorganized, with marked fussiness and irritability (which may be exacerbated by eye contact), prolonged periods of high-pitched crying, and poor consolability. Normal neonatal reflexes, especially the Moro reflex, are highly exaggerated. The sucking reflex is strong and the neonate may suck on the hands and fists frequently. However, sucking may be poorly coordinated with swallowing, impairing feeding. Sleep periods may be abnormally short; unlike the normal neonate, who spends more time asleep than awake, the addicted neonate may have a sleep-awake ratio of 1 to 3.

Signs of drug withdrawal typically begin about 12 to 48 hours after birth. (For a list of these signs, see *Assessing for neonatal drug withdrawal.*) As withdrawal progresses, these signs worsen. Try to verify that the mother used drugs during pregnancy if neonatal drug addiction or withdrawal is suspected. However, keep in mind that some women may deny or misrepresent drug use.

If the neonate's mother used I.V. drugs, an HIV test should be done. Maternally conferred IgG may interfere with the accuracy of an HIV antibody test for the first few months after birth; therefore, an HIV antigen test is preferred. Assess for signs of HIV infection, including facial dysmorphism, hepatosplenomegaly, interstitial pneumonia, subtle neurologic abnormalities, behavioral changes, and recurrent infection.

Infection

The neonate with an infection may be SGA at birth, with a nonspecific rash, pallor, hypotonia, jaundice, lethargy, hyperthermia, or hypothermia. Other common signs accompanying infection include apnea or tachypnea, tachycardia or bradycardia, abdominal distention, hepatomegaly, splenomegaly, seizures, diarrhea, occult blood in the stool, and bleeding disorders. The behavior pattern may be abnormal and the reflexes diminished; poor feeding may cause failure to thrive.

With an intrapartally acquired infection, the neonate may not appear ill at birth but will show gradual deterioration in vital signs over the next 6 to 12 hours. However, with group B streptococcal infection—a commonly acquired intrapartal infection—the neonate may have dyspnea and cyanosis and appear quite ill. However, RDS and congenital cardiac anomalies can cause similar signs and must be ruled out. The following laboratory results suggest perinatal infection:
• an increased number of immature cells, as shown by the white blood cell (WBC) differential
• a WBC count above 20,000/mm³, reflecting leukocytosis (an abnormal increase in the number of WBCs)
• an absolute neutrophil count exceeding 60%
• a thrombocyte count below 100,000/mm³ with an abnormally high reticulocyte count.

A neonate who acquired HIV intrapartally may be preterm or SGA, with an abnormally small head and distinctive facial features. (For an illustration of these features, see *Facial dysmorphism in the neonate with human immunodeficiency virus.*) Disorders seen in neonates with HIV infection include oral candidiasis (thrush) and lymphoid interstitial pneumonitis. Later, such problems as lymphadenopathy, chronic diarrhea, viral and bacterial infections, *Pneumocystis carinii* pneumonia, and parotid gland enlargement may occur.

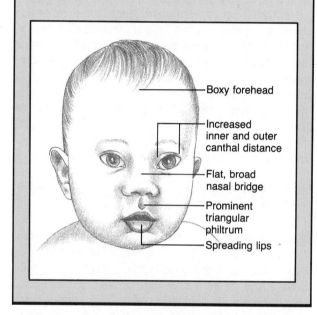

Facial dysmorphism in the neonate with human immunodeficiency virus

The neonate who acquired the human immunodeficiency virus (HIV) transplacentally may have the facial features shown here.

- Boxy forehead
- Increased inner and outer canthal distance
- Flat, broad nasal bridge
- Prominent triangular philtrum
- Spreading lips

Because maternal HIV antibodies are transferred to the fetus, a neonate whose mother has the virus may test positive for HIV antibodies even when not infected. Consequently, an HIV culture or antigen test must be used to confirm infection.

Congenital anomalies

Antepartal factors suggesting congenital abnormalities include increased or decreased amniotic fluid volume. For example, hydramnios (excess amniotic fluid) may accompany tracheoesophageal anomalies; oligohydramnios (insufficient amniotic fluid) may signify a genitourinary tract anomaly. If a congenital anomaly is discovered in one body system, other systems should be investigated thoroughly because congenital anomalies commonly occur in tandem.

CNS anomalies
Most CNS anomalies are apparent even on rapid inspection.

Meningomyelocele. Most commonly, this anomaly appears in the lumbosacral region of the vertebral column. CSF may leak through the defect. Sometimes it is covered only by a thin, membranous sac; otherwise, nerve tissue is exposed. In less obvious cases, the defect manifests as a slight indentation or dimple over the lumbosacral region, detected on palpation; sometimes the indentation is covered by a mole with hair follicles. Such a dimple or mole should be reported for further evaluation. If meningomyelocele is detected, also check for associated anomalies, such as hip dislocation, knee and foot deformities, and hydrocephalus.

If the defect appears above the lumbosacral region, the lower extremities may lack sensation and movement and the bladder and bowel may lack innervation, causing impaired bladder and bowel function. To assess bowel innervation, test for an anal wink by lightly stroking the anus with a cotton-tipped applicator; absence of anal sphincter constriction indicates lack of bowel innervation.

Encephalocele. Suspect this defect when the meninges protrude through the cranium. The defect may be covered with skin or membrane and may be accompanied by hydrocephalus, paralysis, and seizures.

Hydrocephalus. The neonate with this abnormality has an enlarged head with an excessive diameter (the occipitofrontal circumference typically exceeds the ninetieth percentile by 2 cm). Wide or bulging fontanels, a shiny scalp with prominent veins, and possible separation of the suture lines are common. Also check for downward eye slanting caused by increased intracranial pressure, and for "sunset" eyes (appearance of the sclera above the iris), reflecting upper lid retraction. (For an illustration of this condition, see *Assessing congenital hydrocephalus*.)

Associated findings include an abnormal heart rate (usually bradycardia), apneic episodes, vomiting, irritability, excessive crying, and reduced alertness.

Anencephaly and microcephaly. Suspect anencephaly if the neonate lacks a forehead and has a minimal posterior cranium. Suspect microcephaly if head circumference is more than three standard deviations below the average for age, sex, race, and gestational age (Brann and Schwartz, 1987); the forehead is narrow and receding; the occiput (back of the head) is flattened; and the vertex (top of the head) is pointed.

Teratoma. This tumor may be visible on inspection of the sacral area; it may be completely or partly external.

Cardiac anomalies
A heart murmur, which can be assessed on auscultation, is common to most cardiac anomalies. Other general

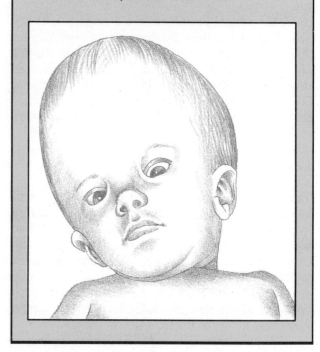

Assessing congenital hydrocephalus

This congenital disorder causes head enlargement with prominent scalp veins; "sunset" eyes (appearance of the sclera above the iris) also are characteristic.

signs of cardiac anomalies include diminished capillary refill time, tachypnea, dyspnea, and tachycardia.

With acyanotic defects, cyanosis usually is absent. Atrial and ventricular septal defects may cause no signs at birth (although a systolic murmur is possible with the atrial defect). PDA causes a continuous or systolic heart murmur, increased heart pulsation (a heartbeat palpable over the precordium), tachycardia, tachypnea, hepatomegaly, bounding pulses, a palpable thrill over the suprasternal notch, bounding peripheral pulses, widened pulse pressure, and signs of respiratory distress or congestive heart failure (CHF), such as increasing respiratory effort, crackles or other moist breath sounds, feeding intolerance, fatigue, and decreasing urine output.

Coarctation of the aorta also may cause CHF as well as systolic hypertension in the arms, systolic hypotension in the legs, weak or absent femoral pulses, and a systolic ejection murmur at the left sternal border.

With cyanotic cardiac defects, expect cyanosis, especially during hypoxic spells. With tetralogy of Fallot, also expect dyspnea and a continuous murmur heard across the back. Transposition of the great vessels may cause tachypnea, poor feeding, dyspnea, and a soft murmur at the midsternal border. With tricuspid atresia, a systolic murmur at the second intercostal space along the left border may be auscultated. Expect signs of CHF with transposition and tricuspid atresia.

Respiratory tract anomalies

Cyanosis and respiratory compromise are the first signs of diaphragmatic hernia; the more severe the defect, the greater the respiratory compromise. The chest typically appears asymmetrical and the abdomen concave (from lack of abdominal contents). Substernal, intercostal, and suprascapular retractions typically occur over the unaffected side. The neonate typically is tachypneic, with a respiratory rate of at least 80 breaths/minute.

Record the neonate's temperature and assess pulse and respirations. Also, auscultate breath sounds over the entire chest wall; expect diminished or absent breath sounds on the affected side. A decrease or other change in breath sounds usually signifies gastric distention, which can lead to further respiratory compromise. Depending on the extent of the defect, heart sounds may be displaced.

GI tract anomalies

Except for meconium ileus, signs of these anomalies are obvious.

Tracheoesophageal malformations. In almost half of affected neonates, the maternal history includes hydramnios. After delivery, suspect a tracheoesopagheal malformation if the neonate has labored breathing, chest retractions, nasal flaring, cyanosis, or frothy secretions. Difficulty inserting a nasogastric tube and choking or aspiration during oral feedings are other suggestive signs.

Abdominal wall defects. Omphalocele and gastroschisis are apparent from the protruding intestine (see *Assessing omphalocele*). Evaluate the defect for signs that the exposed viscera are becoming dry or infected. Also observe for fluid loss through the defect, which may be considerable, and for signs of gastric distention (such as a distended abdomen). If the neonate has omphalocele, examine carefully for associated anomalies, which frequently accompany this defect.

Meconium ileus. This disorder manifests as abdominal distention, bilious vomiting, and distended bowel loops in the right lower quadrant (found on palpation).

Imperforate anus. This anomaly usually is obvious at delivery, although in some cases it is detected only during an attempt to take a rectal temperature. With a complete defect, the anus appears as a dimple in the perineal skin; an incomplete defect may manifest as a narrow opening

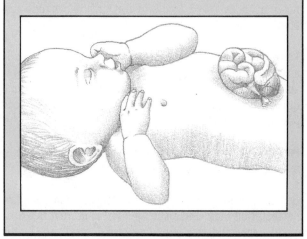

Assessing omphalocele

In this congenital anomaly, a portion of the intestines protrudes through a defect in the abdominal wall around the umbilicus. The herniated matter may be covered by a thin membrane.

where the anus should appear. If this anomaly is accompanied by bowel obstruction, the abdomen will be distended. The neonate typically does not pass meconium; however, sometimes meconium passes through a fistula or misplaced anus.

The level of the defect commonly is diagnosed by abdominal X-rays. A lateral abdominal X-ray with the neonate inverted distinguishes high from low imperforate anus: if air appears below a line drawn from the pubis to the sacrococcygeal junction (with a marker placed over the rectum), the defect is low. Air appearing above the line indicates a high defect.

Cleft palate and cleft lip. Except when the cleft affects the soft palate only, these anomalies are obvious. (For a description, see "Cleft palate and cleft lip" in the "Perinatal problems" section earlier in this chapter.) The neonate may have difficulty sucking, with expulsion of milk or formula through the nose. With cleft lip, the neonate may have signs of localized infection in the oral cavity, causing a fever, crying, and irritability.

Genitourinary tract anomalies

An anomaly involving the kidneys commonly causes acute renal failure, as reflected by oliguria or anuria. In many cases, the neonate has associated signs, such as hypoplastic lungs or GI defects.

Renal agenesis. Maternal oligohydramnios during pregnancy is a predictor of this anomaly; fetal ultrasound examination can confirm it before delivery. With bilateral renal agenesis, stillbirth occurs or the neonate dies within a few days after birth. Check for Potter facies: low-set ears; prominent skin folds beneath the eyes; a small, flattened nose; and a small chin and mandible with excessive skin folds. Oliguria or anuria within the first 48 hours after birth is diagnostic of this disorder. Skeletal anomalies that sometimes accompany renal agenesis include bowed legs and flat or broad hands and feet.

Polycystic kidneys. A protruding abdomen and greatly enlarged kidneys suggest this disorder; the liver also is enlarged. Fluid buildup may cause signs of acute renal failure, such as oliguria or anuria, edema, and blood pressure fluctuations.

Posterior urethral valves. A dribbling urine stream in a male neonate suggests this defect.

Genital ambiguity. In the affected female, androgen hypersecretion may cause such genital abnormalities as a small penis and the beginning of a scrotal sac. In the male, genital abnormalities may include abnormally small or undescended testes, hypospadias, and incomplete scrotal fusion.

The nurse who detects ambiguous genitalia should notify the physician immediately so that genetic evaluation can begin. Sex determination not only permits prompt treatment of the underlying adrenal disorder but may help reduce parental anxiety. Definitive sex determination may take up to 2 weeks. Meanwhile, review the prenatal history, especially noting any maternal exposure to hazardous environmental substances, and check the family history for associated problems.

Musculoskeletal anomalies

Clubfoot may be mild to severe and occurs in several varations. In equinovarus, the most common form, the heel turns inward from the midline of the leg, the foot is plantarflexed, the inner border of the foot is raised, and the anterior part of the foot is displaced so that it lies medial to the vertical axis of the leg. Other forms of clubfoot include calcaneovalgus, metatarsus adductus, and metatarsus varus.

If the neonate has an obvious foot deformity, first rule out "apparent clubfoot" (caused by fetal positioning) by taking the foot through the full range of motion. If the foot does not revert to a natural position with manipulation, suspect true clubfoot.

NURSING DIAGNOSES

High-risk neonate

The following are potential nursing diagnoses for problems and etiologies that a nurse may encounter when caring for a high-risk neonate. Specific nursing interventions for many of these diagnoses are provided in the "Planning and implementation" section of this chapter.

- Altered family processes related to the birth of a high-risk neonate and the adjustments necessitated by the neonate's condition and hospitalization
- Altered growth and development related to functional immaturity, prolonged environmental stress, a congenital anomaly, or lack of stimulation appropriate for gestational age and physical status
- Altered nutrition: less than body requirements, related to increased caloric requirements, respiratory distress, gastrointestinal immaturity, a weak sucking reflex, or metabolic dysfunction
- Fluid volume deficit related to renal immaturity or increased fluid loss
- Hypothermia related to an immature temperature-regulating center, decreased body mass-to-surface ratio, reduced subcutaneous fat, inability to shiver or sweat, and inadequate metabolic reserves
- Impaired gas exchange related to surfactant deficiency and altered alveolar function
- Ineffective airway clearance related to inability to expel excess secretions
- Ineffective breathing pattern related to respiratory and neurologic immaturity
- Potential altered parenting related to the neonate's condition, difficulty coping with a less-than-perfect neonate, and enforced separation of neonate and parents
- Potential aspiration related to meconium in amniotic fluid
- Potential impaired skin integrity related to frequent invasive procedures
- Potential for infection related to immunologic immaturity, altered ventilation, ineffective airway clearance, or frequent invasive procedures
- Potential for injury related to lack of cushioning from inadequate subcutaneous fat

---

Nursing diagnosis

After gathering all assessment data, the nurse must review it carefully to identify pertinent nursing diagnoses for the neonate. (For a partial list of applicable diagnoses, see *Nursing diagnoses: High-risk neonate*.)

Planning and implementation

Once a fetus or neonate is identified as high risk (such as when fetal distress has been detected late in pregnancy), initial intervention should focus on preventing complications and death. Some high-risk neonates require emergency interventions; others, such as those with relatively minor congenital anomalies, are fairly stable at birth but require prompt treatment to prevent complications.

Emergency intervention

In most cases, the need for resuscitation at delivery can be anticipated from maternal, antepartal, or intrapartal factors (as discussed in the "Assessment" section of this chapter). Immediately after delivery, the neonate must be evaluated to determine the need for resuscitation. Depending on the neonate's condition and response to each resuscitative measure, neonatal resuscitation typically involves some combination of the following:
- free-flow oxygen
- positive-pressure ventilation (PPV)
- closed-chest cardiac massage
- gastric decompression
- emergency drugs
- endotracheal intubation.

Preparation for resuscitation
Before every delivery, verify that emergency equipment and supplies are present, in working order, and ready to use; ideally, all items should be double-checked. This helps avert problems during resuscitation, when replacement of a missing supply or malfunctioning part could cause a dangerous treatment delay. (For a list of equipment and supplies, see *Resuscitation equipment and supplies.*)

Resuscitation personnel
Every delivery should be attended by at least one person skilled in all resuscitation techniques and another person who is an experienced resuscitation assistant. When asphyxia is likely, a third person also should be present in the delivery room to manage the mother so that the resuscitators can attend solely to the neonate.

Before performing resuscitation on a neonate, an inexperienced nurse should observe a skilled nurse per-

Resuscitation equipment and supplies

To help ensure the most effective resuscitation, the nurse should be familiar with the delivery room equipment and supplies listed below.

Bag-and-mask equipment
- face masks (sizes 0.1 and 2)
- infant resuscitation bag (anesthesia bag or self-inflating bag) capable of delivering 90% to 100% oxygen
- oxygen delivery unit with adjustable fraction of inspired oxygen, humidification source, flowmeter, tubing, pressure gauge or pressure-release (pop-off) valve (40 to 60 cm H_2O)
- oropharyngeal airway (sizes 000, 00, and 0)

Emergency drugs and solutions
- dextrose 10% in water
- epinephrine 1:10,000
- naloxone 0.02 mg/ml
- normal saline solution
- sodium bicarbonate 4.2% (5 mEq/10 ml)
- volume expander (albumin, normal saline solution, or lactated Ringer's solution)

Intubation equipment
- endotracheal tubes with adapters (sizes 2.5, 3, 3.5, and 4 mm)
- extra bulbs and batteries
- gloves
- laryngoscope with straight blades (sizes 0 and 1)
- Magill forceps
- wire stylet for tubes
- scissors

Suction equipment (80 to 100 mm Hg)
- bulb syringe
- DeLee mucus trap
- mechanical suction machine
- suction catheters (#5, #6, #8, and #10 Fr.)

Other items
- adhesive tape
- blood pressure cuff and gauge
- cardiorespiratory monitor
- clock or timer
- electrocardiograph electrodes
- I.V. solution and tubing
- water-soluble lubricating jelly (such as K-Y jelly)
- nasogastric tube
- radiant warmer resuscitation bed (preheated)
- sterile gloves
- sterile water
- stethoscope
- syringes (tuberculin 3, 5, and 10 ml)
- umbilical artery catheter tray (including #3.5 and #5 Fr.)

forming the procedures, then practice on a mannequin to the point of proficiency. The first few times the nurse resuscitates a neonate, close supervision is mandatory.

Resuscitation procedure

Initial neonatal evaluation and subsequent resuscitative measures are based on respirations, heart rate, and skin color—not on the 1-minute Apgar score (American Heart Association and American Academy of Pediatrics, 1987). Waiting until the end of the first minute to start resuscitation makes the procedure more difficult and increases the chance for brain damage and death. With a severely asphyxiated neonate, a delay is especially dangerous. (However, Apgar scores *should* be used to help determine whether resuscitative measures are effective.)

Like any resuscitation, the goal of neonatal resuscitation is to ensure the ABCs—airway, breathing, and circulation. Resuscitation follows an orderly sequence; after each intervention, the team quickly evaluates the neonate's condition and response to the intervention, then decides which further measures, if any, are necessary.

The next few paragraphs present a brief overview of the resuscitation sequence as it relates to evaluation of the neonate. (For a detailed description of the steps used in resuscitation, see *Psychomotor skills: Resuscitating a neonate.*)

Respirations. If the neonate lacks spontaneous respirations, PPV with a bag and mask must begin immediately. If the neonate is breathing (as indicated by chest movements), the resuscitation team moves on, evaluating heart rate.

Heart rate. If the heart rate is below 100 beats/minute, closed-chest cardiac massage (chest compression) typically begins as PPV continues. (PPV should be initiated whenever the heart rate is below 100, even if the neonate has spontaneous respirations.) If the heart rate is above 100 beats/minute, the team evaluates skin color.

Skin color. If the neonate has central cyanosis, reflecting lack of oxygen in the blood, the team administers free-flow oxygen by holding the end of an oxygen tube close to the neonate's nose or by holding an oxygen mask over the neonate's mouth and nose.

Special considerations

Although most neonates respond to PPV and chest compressions, some require other measures.

Gastric decompression. Bag-and-mask ventilation forces air to enter the stomach, which can prevent full lung expansion, cause aspiration of gastric contents, and lead to abdominal distention (which impedes breathing). Consequently, when bag-and-mask ventilation is required for more than 2 minutes, an orogastric tube must be inserted

Resuscitating a neonate

The neonate with birth asphyxia or another form of cardio-pulmonary compromise needs immediate resuscitation after delivery. The guidelines below, which describe the essential steps in neonatal resuscitation, reflect the recommendations of American Heart Association and American Academy of Pediatrics (1987).

Suctioning the airway

1 Dry the neonate and place on a firm surface under a preheated radiant warmer. Extend the neck slightly to the "sniff" position. To maintain this position, place a rolled towel or blanket under the shoulders to raise them 3/4" to 1" off the surface.

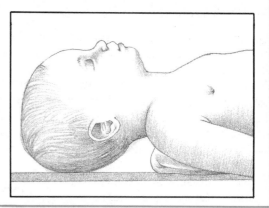

2 Using a soft catheter, mechanical suction, or a bulb syringe, suction the mouth, then the nose, to remove blood, meconium, or other matter. If the neonate has copious oral secretions, turn the head to the side to facilitate suctioning. To avoid stimulating the vagal reflex, which could cause bradycardia or apnea, avoid suctioning too vigorously or for more than 10 seconds.

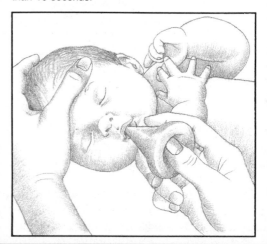

Administering positive-pressure ventilation

1 If drying, suctioning, or other tactile stimulation (such as tapping the soles or rubbing the back) does not induce respirations immediately, begin positive-pressure ventilation with a bag and mask at once. Attach the resuscitation bag to an oxygen source and select a mask of the correct size (size 0 for the preterm neonate, size 1 for the term neonate). Connect the mask to the resuscitation bag.

2 Standing at the neonate's side or head, apply the mask so that it covers the neonate's nose and mouth, with the edge of the neonate's chin resting within the rim of the mask. To obtain an airtight seal, use light downward pressure on the rim to apply the mask.

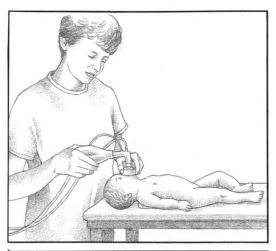

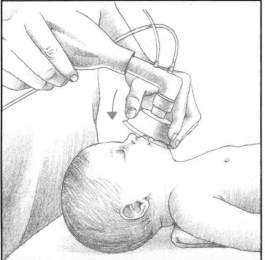

3 Check the seal and the ventilation technique by ventilating two or three times and watching for chest movement. (Make sure to squeeze the bag with the fingertips only, not the entire palm.) The neonate's chest should rise slightly, as in a shallow breath. A deep breath indicates that the lungs are being overinflated from excessive pressure on the bag.

If the neonate's chest does not rise, suspect an inadequate seal, a blocked airway, or insufficient pressure delivered by the bag. Correct these problems by reapplying the mask; repositioning the neonate's head; checking for secretions and suctioning, if necessary; or increasing the pressure to 20 to 40 cm H_2O or until the pop-off valve activates.

4 If the chest rises slightly, give an initial ventilation of 15 to 30 seconds with 100% oxygen at a rate of 40 ventilations/minute. Initial breaths may require a pressure of up to 40 cm H_2O; for subsequent ventilations, use only the minimum pressure necessary to move the chest.

5 Subsequent actions depend on the heart rate. Check the heart rate with a cardiac monitor (if a monitor is not available, listen to the apical beat with a stethoscope or feel the umbilical pulse at the base of the cord). To estimate the 1-minute heart rate, count the heartbeat for 6 seconds and multiply by 10.
• If the heart rate is above 100 beats/minute and the neonate is breathing spontaneously, discontinue bag-and-mask ventilation and provide gentle stimulation (for instance, by rubbing the skin). Monitor the neonate to assess for stabilization.
• If the heart rate is above 100 beats/minute but the neonate is not breathing spontaneously, continue to ventilate at a rate of 40 breaths/minute.
• If the heart rate is 60 to 100 beats/minute and increasing, continue to ventilate. If the heart rate is between 60 and 100 but *not* increasing, continue to ventilate and verify that the chest is moving properly and that 100% oxygen is being delivered.
• If the heart rate is less than 60 beats/minute or between 60 and 80 beats/minute and *not* increasing, another member of the team must start closed-chest cardiac massage (chest compressions) at once while the first resuscitator continues to ventilate.

(continued)

PSYCHOMOTOR SKILLS

Resuscitating a neonate continued

Performing chest compressions

1 To ensure the best outcome, resuscitation team members should position themselves so that each can work effectively without hindering the other.

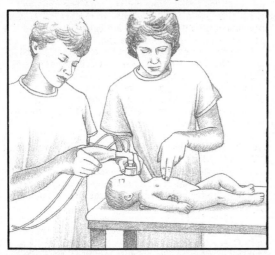

2 The resuscitator who administers chest compressions may use either the thumb method or the two-finger method.

For the **thumb method,** place both thumbs side-by-side over the midsternum, with the hands encircling the chest and the fingers supporting the neonate's back (illustration at left). If the neonate is very small, one thumb can be placed over the other (illustration at right).

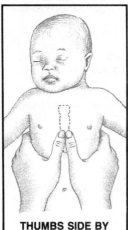

THUMBS SIDE BY SIDE

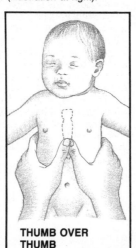

THUMB OVER THUMB

For the **two-finger method,** place the tips of the middle finger and the ring or index finger over the midsternum in the midline while supporting the neonate's back with the other hand.

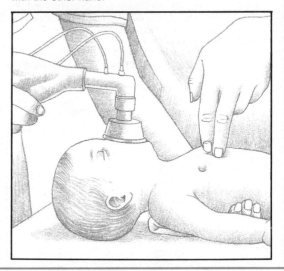

3 With either method, depress the sternum ½" to ¾", then release the pressure to allow the heart to refill; keep the thumbs or fingertips in contact with the sternum at all times, even during the release. Deliver 120 compressions/minute (one compression equals the downward stroke plus the release). When delivering compressions, take care not to squeeze the chest with the whole hand or apply pressure to the xiphoid process.

4 To determine if chest compressions are effective, one resuscitator should check the pulse after 30 seconds of compressions, then periodically (by counting for 6 seconds). Once the neonate's heart rate reaches 80 beats/minute, chest compressions should be discontinued. However, ventilations should continue until the heart rate exceeds 100 beats/minute and the neonate is breathing spontaneously.

If the heart rate is below 80 beats/minute, chest compressions and ventilation must continue; in some cases, emergency drugs are administered at this point. If the neonate still shows no response, resuscitation continues until the physician decides to stop it.

Resuscitation drugs

For the neonate with no detectable heartbeat at delivery, the physician typically orders emergency drugs immediately (along with bag-and-mask ventilation and chest compressions). Drugs also are indicated for a neonate whose heart rate remains below 80 beats/minute despite adequate bag-and-mask ventilation and chest compressions. The chart below summarizes indications and nursing considerations for drugs recommended for neonatal resuscitation by the American Heart Association and American Academy of Pediatrics (1987).

DRUG	INDICATIONS	NURSING CONSIDERATIONS
dopamine	Poor peripheral perfusion, thready pulses, and continuing signs of shock after administration of epinephrine, a volume expander, and sodium bicarbonate	• Administer as a continuous I.V. infusion in a prepared solution. • Use an infusion pump to control the infusion rate.
epinephrine	Heart rate of 0 or heart rate below 80 beats/minute after 30 seconds of ventilation with 100% oxygen and chest compressions	• Prepare 1 ml 1:10,000 dilution in a syringe for I.V. or endotracheal administration. • Administer rapidly.
sodium bicarbonate	Metabolic acidosis	• Prepare two prefilled syringes (10 ml) or draw 20 ml into a syringe for I.V. administration. • Give over at least 2 minutes.
naloxone hydrochloride (neonatal narcan)	Severe respiratory depression in a neonate whose mother received a narcotic no more than 4 hours earlier	• Draw 2 ml 0.02 mg/ml dilution into a syringe for I.V., I.M., subcutaneous, or endotracheal administration. • Inject rapidly.

to suction gastric contents; the tube is left in place throughout resuscitation to vent air.

Emergency drugs. Drugs may be administered if the neonate fails to respond to bag-and-mask ventilation and chest compressions. Such drugs typically are administered via the umbilical vein or, in some cases, through a peripheral vein (such as a scalp or extremity vein) or an endotracheal tube. (For information on drugs recommended for use in neonatal resuscitation, see *Resuscitation drugs.*)

Endotracheal intubation. This intervention, which should be performed only by an experienced intubator, is indicated when diaphragmatic hernia is suspected, when the neonate requires prolonged ventilation, or when prolonged bag-and-mask ventilation proves ineffective.

Endotracheal intubation also is necessary when MAS is suspected. If the amniotic fluid contains thick meconium—a sign of asphyxia experienced in utero—the neonate has a nursing diagnosis of *potential for aspiration related to meconium in the respiratory tract.* As soon as the neonate's head is delivered, the mouth, oropharynx, and hypopharynx must be suctioned with a flexible suction catheter. Immediately after delivery, an experienced intubator visualizes the larynx with a laryngoscope, then intubates the trachea and suctions any meconium from the lower airway—preferably by applying suction to an endotracheal tube. After the tube has been inserted, continuous suction is applied as the tube is withdrawn. This procedure is repeated until no more meconium is suctioned.

Post-resuscitation care

After resuscitation, observe the neonate closely for signs of respiratory distress, including cyanosis, apnea, tachypnea, and inspiratory retractions. Blood pressure and perfusion are other key indicators; if either is inadequate, expect to administer volume expanders to reverse shock.

If an endotracheal tube is in place, observe for tube dislodgement, signs of tube obstruction, and associated complications, such as pneumothorax. To monitor tube placement, check tube length (from the point where it leaves the mouth to the connection point) and assess for equal bilateral breath sounds and symmetrical chest expansion.

If the neonate was severely asphyxiated at delivery, the physician may want to maintain serum glucose at 100 to 150 mg/dl; expect to administer dextrose 10% in water and monitor the serum glucose level. Also monitor the hematocrit and assess renal status by measuring fluid intake and checking for abrupt weight changes, which may signal renal complications of asphyxia. Ensure thermoregulation by keeping the neonate under a radiant warmer and monitoring skin temperature.

If the neonate requires transport to a level 3 nursery, make preparations according to institutional protocol and notify the nursery of the impending admission as soon as possible so that staff and necessary equipment can be mobilized.

General nursing guidelines

Although the neonate's condition will dictate the specifics of nursing care, the same nursing goals apply to all high-risk neonates: Ensure oxygenation, ventilation, thermoregulation, nutrition, and fluid and electrolyte balance, prevent and control infection, and provide developmental care. Neonates who must undergo surgery will require preoperative and postoperative stabilization. In some cases, the nurse also must carry out special procedures. Throughout neonatal care, offer emotional support and teaching to the parents to help them cope with their child's condition.

Supporting oxygenation and ventilation

Most neonates who have been successfully resuscitated—as well as many other high-risk neonates—need supplemental oxygen to prevent or correct hypoxia. Supplemental oxygen can be administered by hood, nasal cannula, or continuous positive-airway pressure (CPAP); it always should be warmed and humidified. To avoid a nursing diagnosis of *impaired gas exchange related to surfactant deficiency and altered alveolar function* or *ineffective breathing pattern related to respiratory and neurologic immaturity*, be alert to neonates who require additional ventilatory support in the form of mechanical ventilation.

The goal of supplemental oxygen therapy is to maintain a PaO_2 of 60 to 80 mm Hg. A higher level may lead to ROP; a lower level, to profound hypoxia and CNS problems (including cerebral hemorrhage and brain damage). Record the fraction of inspired oxygen (FiO_2) as a percentage (however, for the older neonate who is receiving oxygen by nasal cannula, FiO_2 may be recorded in liters/minute). FiO_2 ranges from 21% (the oxygen concentration in room air) to 100%.

Because oxygen is a drug, the nurse must be familiar with its potential adverse effects and ways to avoid them. For instance, to prevent or minimize the risk of ROP, always administer oxygen at the lowest concentration that will correct hypoxia, using an oxygen analyzer to determine the actual concentration of delivered oxygen.

To ensure therapeutic efficacy and avoid oxygen toxicity, monitor the neonate's oxygenation status continuously with a noninvasive technique, such as transcutaneous oxygen pressure ($tcPO_2$) monitoring or pulse oximetry. With a $tcPO_2$ monitor, the probe measures oxygen diffusion and carbon dioxide perfusion across the skin; with pulse oximetry, the probe measures beat-to-beat arterial oxygen saturation. Be sure to place the probe in a well-perfused area. $TcPO_2$ readings should range from 50 to 80 mm Hg; oximetry readings should be no less than 90% (Chatburn and Carlo, 1988).

However, $tcPO_2$ or oximetry values alone are not adequate; they must be correlated with simultaneously obtained arterial blood gas (ABG) samples drawn every 3 to 4 hours. To obtain ABG samples, use a heparinized syringe; place the samples on ice to prevent oxygen and carbon dioxide diffusion.

Oxygen hood and nasal cannula. An oxygen hood, which fits over the neonate's head, can deliver up to 100% oxygen and allows easy access to the rest of the neonate's body for care procedures. A nasal cannula delivers oxygen concentrations above room air (21%); typically, it is used for a neonate with BPD or a congenital cardiac defect (the minimal equipment involved allows frequent cuddling and other stimulation).

CPAP. CPAP usually is implemented if the PaO_2 level of a neonate receiving an FiO_2 of 60% or higher drops below 60 mm Hg. CPAP delivers air at a constant pressure throughout the respiratory cycle, keeping the lungs expanded at all times to reduce shunting and improve oxygenation. CPAP may be delivered via a nasopharyngeal tube or an endotracheal tube inserted through the mouth or nose. Some neonatologists believe a nasal tube is more secure than an oral tube. However, prolonged nasal intubation may cause anterior naris (nostril) damage and deviation or nasal septal erosion. An excessively long oral tube, on the other hand, may become kinked. With either tube, take steps to avoid accidental extubation.

During CPAP therapy, monitor the neonate's vital signs, blood pressure, and respiratory effort; stay especially alert for tachycardia, tachypnea, and arrhythmias.

Mechanical ventilation. Mechanical ventilation usually is used instead of CPAP if any of the following criteria are present:
• PaO_2 level below 50 mm Hg with administration of 100% oxygen (Goldsmith and Karotkin, 1988)
• $PaCO_2$ level above 80 mm Hg
• arterial pH below 7.2.

During mechanical ventilation, assess the neonate's vital signs, breath sounds, chest movement, respiratory effort, and oxygenation status every hour. When assessing breath sounds, keep in mind that in a mechanically ventilated neonate, breath sounds normally are loud and high-pitched. However, extremely high-pitched sounds may signal excessive secretions. A pitch decrease, in contrast, may reflect atelectasis or pulmonary air leakage.

As necessary, suction the endotracheal tube to maintain a patent airway, making sure to apply suction only while removing the catheter. If possible, use a suctioning remethod that does not necessitate interruption of mechanical ventilation. (For step-by-step instructions for one such method, see *Psychomotor skills: Suctioning an endotracheal tube*, page 964.) Report any change in the amount or consistency of secretions.

Be sure to assess endotracheal tube positioning and patency regularly; a tube resting along the tracheal wall may impair ventilation. Also check ventilator function periodically, making sure all alarms are working. Assess the system for leaks.

Maintaining thermoregulation

An essential part of care for all neonates, thermoregulation is particularly crucial to the high-risk neonate, whose oxygen and energy reserves may be depleted rapidly by illness. The preterm neonate especially is at risk for cold stress because of limited subcutaneous fat, an extremely high surface-to-mass ratio, inability to shiver, and minimal brown fat (a type of fat that provides body heat).

Heat loss may result from radiation, conduction, evaporation, or convection (as discussed in Chapter 34, Neonatal Adaptation). A neonate who suffers heat loss and subsequent cold stress may experience peripheral vasoconstriction, hypoglycemia, reduced cerebral perfusion, metabolic acidosis, exacerbation of RDS, decreased surfactant production, impaired kidney function, GI disturbances, hypoglycemia, and, ultimately, death.

A first step in preventing hypothermia is to minimize cooling at delivery; such cooling may delay adequate thermoregulation for hours. During the initial examination and resuscitation, the neonate should be placed under a radiant heat warmer. Wrap the neonate in a plastic bag or thermal foil blanket as soon as possible after resuscitation, and then transfer the neonate to an incubator or radiant warmer bed. The practice of drying the neonate thoroughly after birth has been found to cause cold stress (Perlstein, 1988).

Because heat loss from the neonate's head is considerable, keep the neonate's head covered at all times. Also, warm the hands before touching the neonate to prevent conductive heat loss through handling. (For a detailed discussion of specific nursing measures that promote thermoregulation, see Chapter 36, Care of the Normal Neonate.)

Neutral thermal environment. Throughout care, aim for a neutral thermal environment (NTE), a narrow range of environmental temperature (89.6° to 93.2° F [32° to 34° C] that maintains a stable core (rectal) temperature with minimal caloric and oxygen expenditure. Although NTE may prove hard to achieve, certain measures may help prevent a nursing diagnosis of *hypothermia related to an immature temperature-regulating center, decreased body mass-to-surface ratio, reduced subcutaneous fat, inability to shiver or sweat, and inadequate metabolic reserves.* For instance, use of a warmed, humidified incubator with an air temperature of 96.8° F (36° C) helps maintain proper skin temperature (Perlstein, 1987).

Thermoregulation during transport. Special measures must be taken if the neonate requires transport to another facility. Causes of heat loss during transport include poor heat retention in the transport bed, radiant heat loss within the transport vehicle, and drafts as the transport bed passes through unheated corridors or as the door or hood to the transport bed is opened to place the neonate inside. To help minimize the risk of cold stress from these causes, provide an NTE before transport (for instance, by protecting the neonate from heat loss during examinations or care procedures). Also, wrap the neonate before transport or place a warming mattress in the transport bed to enhance its heating capacity.

Providing adequate nutrition

The accelerated metabolic rate and energy expenditure of the high-risk neonate may lead to a nursing diagnosis of *altered nutrition: less than body requirements, related to increased caloric requirements, respiratory distress, GI immaturity, a weak sucking reflex, or metabolic dysfunction.* Respiratory distress, for instance, increases caloric requirements 50% to 75%; the metabolic response to surgery, by 30% (Kaempf, Bonnabel, and Hoy, 1989).

The preterm neonate may need 104 to 130 calories/kg/day, compared to the normal healthy neonate, who requires 100 to 120 calories/kg/day. However, caloric requirements change over time and should be adjusted depending on the neonate's tolerance.

For the high-risk neonate who can take nourishment by mouth, breast milk is the preferred nutritional form. (For a related study, see *Nursing research applied: Comparing the effects of breast-feeding and bottle-feeding on transcutaneous oxygen pressure in preterm neonates*, page 965.) If the neonate cannot receive breast milk, the physician may order a special high-calorie infant formula to provide 24 or 27 calories/oz (in contrast to the 20 calories/oz in standard formulas). In some cases, a neonate may begin feedings with half-strength formula and

Suctioning an endotracheal tube

When a neonate requires endotracheal intubation, the nurse must suction the tube frequently to maintain a patent airway. A common suctioning procedure is described below. Before, during, and after suctioning, assess the neonate's skin color, heart rate, respirations, and breath sounds.

1 Follow standard hand-washing technique, then assemble the following equipment:
- sterile gloves
- injectate (warmed to 98.6° F [37° C])
- normal saline solution for tracheal instillation and catheter clearance
- suction catheter (5 or 6 Fr. for endotracheal tubes with a 2.5-mm or 3.0-mm internal diameter; #8 Fr. for an endotracheal tube with a 3.5-mm internal diameter)
- suction apparatus, with negative pressure set to 80 mm Hg for a flow of 4.8 liters/minute
- servo-controlled heat exchanger apparatus to warm saline solution to 98.6° F.

2 Connect the suction catheter to the tubing of the negative-pressure source. Then draw 0.5 ml of normal saline solution (warmed to 98.6° F by the servo-controlled heat exchanger) into a syringe.

3 Inject 0.5 ml of the warmed saline solution into the endotracheal tube.

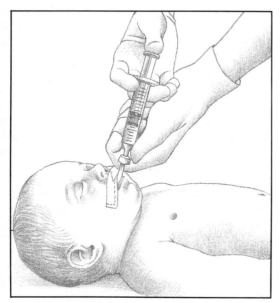

4 Wait 6 seconds for secretions to liquefy.

5 Insert the suction catheter without negative pressure until it just clears the tip of the endotracheal tube. Using a rotating motion and applying continuous negative pressure, withdraw the catheter, taking no more than 10 seconds. The entire procedure should take no longer than 10 seconds. Reestablish ventilation for at least 6 seconds.

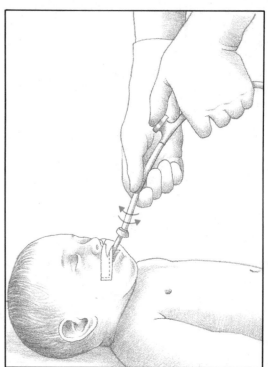

6 Repeat suctioning by inserting the suction catheter without negative pressure until the catheter just clears the tip of the endotracheal tube.

7 Using a rotating motion and applying continuous negative pressure, remove the suction catheter taking no longer than 10 seconds.

8 Immediately reestablish ventilation.

gradually increase to three-quarters-strength, then full-strength.

Enteral nutrition (gavage feedings). To avoid aspiration resulting from a weak sucking reflex, uncoordinated sucking and swallowing, or respiratory distress, many high-risk neonates must be fed enterally, typically through a tube passed through the nose or mouth into the stomach. (However, some neonates must be fed through a surgically placed gastrostomy tube.)

Although a nasogastric tube typically is used to provide enteral feedings, some neonatologists prefer a nasojejunal or orojejunal tube. A nasojejunal tube is passed from the nose through the stomach to the jejunum; an orojejunal tube is passed from the mouth to the jejunum. Because of a possible link between jejunal tubes and NEC, some authorities do not recommend them for neonates weighing less than 2,000 g (Moyer-Mileur, 1986). Nonetheless, jejunal tubes are used with increasing frequency in neonates with gastric reflux and a high risk for aspiration pneumonia. With either tube, placement usually is confirmed by X-ray and aspirate pH values.

If intermittent bolus feedings are prescribed, a tube is passed with each feeding; continuous feedings are administered through an indwelling tube. Typically, the delivery rate for enteral feedings is increased at 12-hour intervals; the increase must be gradual to avoid complications associated with poor feeding tolerance, such as dehydration, diarrhea, vomiting, and abdominal distention. Monitor the neonate closely for these signs.

Check tube placement every 4 hours; remove the tube immediately if the neonate begins to choke or cough or becomes cyanotic—signs that the tube has entered the trachea. To prevent aspiration, keep the mattress elevated 30 degrees for 30 minutes after intermittent bolus feedings and at all times for continuous feedings.

To check gastric residual matter, aspirate gastric contents every 4 hours by attaching a syringe containing 0.5 to 1 ml of air to the tubing. Inject the air while listening through a stethoscope over the epigastric area for a rush of air. Note the color, amount, and consistency of gastric contents; more than 15 ml of matter aspirated before a feeding may signal poor tolerance of feedings.

Parenteral nutrition. This method, in which nutrients are administered by the I.V. route, may be required by the preterm or postsurgical neonate who cannot tolerate oral or enteral feedings. Parenteral nutrition requirements depend on birth weight and diagnosis. For many high-risk neonates, a solution of dextrose 5% or 10% in water (80 to 100 ml/kg/day) is initiated in the delivery room or soon after transfer to the NICU. Electrolytes typically are added to the solution 24 hours after delivery; the

---

NURSING RESEARCH APPLIED

Comparing the effects of breast-feeding and bottle-feeding on transcutaneous oxygen pressure in preterm neonates

To determine how feeding method affects oxygenation, transcutaneous oxygen pressures ($tcPO_2$) of five small preterm neonates were monitored during bottle-feeding and breast-feeding. The neonates, who served as their own controls, were bottle-fed by nurse-researchers or breast-fed by their mothers. Data were collected from the first oral feeding until discharge. Monitoring began 10 minutes before each feeding and continued for 10 minutes afterward. Seventy-one feeding sessions were videotaped and monitored.

Results showed that $tcPO_2$ and temperatures differed during bottle-feeding and breast-feeding. Qualitative $tcPO_2$ differences occurred in all neonates. In the breast-fed neonates, $tcPO_2$ fluctuated cyclically near the baseline during sucking bursts and rest periods. In the bottle-fed neonates, $tcPO_2$ values:
• decreased during intake
• returned to or near baseline (recovery) as sucking ceased
• reached a plateau or neared baseline when the neonate rested or burped
• decreased gradually within 10 minutes after the feeding.

As the neonates matured, those who were bottle-fed had a more pronounced and compact $tcPO_2$ pattern because of more rapid sucking and longer sucking bursts. The $tcPO_2$ pattern of the breast-fed neonates flattened near a normal baseline. (Dissimilar $tcPO_2$ patterns during breast-feeding and bottle-feeding ruled out a quantitative comparison.)

No neonate experienced hypothermia during a feeding; breast-fed neonates became warmer (although their temperatures stayed within a normal range) because of the increased feeding time, close contact with the mother's breasts, and the warmer temperature of breast milk.

Application to practice

This study casts doubt on the common assumption that breast-feeding is more stressful than bottle-feeding for preterm neonates. Because $tcPO_2$ reflects tissue oxygenation, $tcPO_2$ reductions during bottle-feeding suggest that the sucking and swallowing pattern used with this feeding method interrupt ventilation and lead to greater and more sustained hypoxemia than occurs with breast-feeding. The $tcPO_2$ decline was most pronounced in neonates weighing less than 1,500 g, suggesting poor integration of breathing and feeding. In contrast, the $tcPO_2$ pattern during breast-feeding suggests that this feeding method causes fewer ventilatory interruptions.

These findings call into question the current practice of restricting breast-feeding in preterm neonates until successful bottle-feeding is established. Because of the small sample studied, however, results must be replicated before they can be applied to clinical practice.

Meier, P. (1988, January-February). Bottle- and Breast-feeding: Effects on transcutaneous oxygen pressure and temperature in preterm infants. *Nursing Research, 37*(1), 36-41.

most commonly administered electrolytes are sodium and potassium chloride.

Monitor urine and serum glucose levels carefully during parenteral nutrition to prevent glycosuria and hyperglycemia; if these conditions develop, expect to reduce the dextrose concentration. For the preterm neonate, hyperglycemia is confirmed by a glucose oxidase dipstick or heelstick glucose value above 150 mg/100 ml.

If the neonate will not be fed orally for more than 3 days, expect the physician to order total parenteral nutrition (TPN), which provides adequate carbohydrates, amino acids, lipids, glucose, vitamins, and electrolytes for growth and development. When caring for the neonate who is receiving TPN, monitor the serum glucose level with a glucose oxidase dipstick and the urine glucose level with a copper reduction tablet or glucose oxidase dipstick. Obtain hematocrit and serum electrolyte and urea levels to assess how well the neonate is tolerating TPN. (Required laboratory values vary from one facility to another; however, expect to obtain calcium, phosphate, magnesium, alkaline phosphate, protein, and transaminase levels at least weekly.)

Any substance with a dextrose concentration above 12.5% must be administered via a central line (such as an umbilical vessel catheter); peripheral administration of fluids with a higher dextrose concentration can cause tissue swelling, necrosis, and cellular death at the infusion site. When administering parenteral nutrition via a central line, maintain meticulous aseptic technique and clean the infusion site according to institutional protocol to minimize the risk of contamination. Also, make sure the line remains intact to prevent the introduction of organisms that may cause systemic infection. Keep the dressing over the insertion site occlusive; if it appears loose, change it immediately.

In some facilities, blood cultures and cultures from the infusion site are obtained routinely; in others, cultures are required only if infection is suspected. With the extremely preterm neonate, who has limited vascular volume, avoid obtaining blood cultures unless an infection is suspected.

Maintaining fluid and electrolyte balance

Renal immaturity, small fluid reserves, a high metabolic rate, and pronounced insensible fluid losses make even the normal, healthy neonate susceptible to fluid and electrolyte imbalance. Perinatal problems—especially those causing diarrhea, vomiting, or high fever—and surgery can further upset fluid balance in the high-risk neonate, leading to a nursing diagnosis of *fluid volume deficit related to renal immaturity or increased fluid loss.*

Both clinical and environmental conditions influence fluid requirements. For example, congestive heart failure, certain renal disorders, and use of a thermal blanket or mist tent reduce the fluid requirement. On the other hand, the neonate who is receiving phototherapy has a greater need for fluid, as does one with respiratory distress or blood loss. Likewise, use of a radiant warmer increases fluid needs by enhancing insensible fluid losses. After surgery, a neonate is particularly vulnerable to fluid volume deficit—not only is hypovolemia a natural response to surgery, but the neonate loses blood during surgery and loses insensible fluids in the cool, dry operating room. To counter environmental conditions that promote insensible fluid loss, provide an NTE whenever possible.

I.V. fluid requirements for the high-risk neonate range from 60 to 200 ml/kg/day. To maintain fluid balance, give sufficient fluids to maintain a urine output of about 1 ml/kg/hour and a specific gravity of 1.005 to 1.012. However, if gastric compression is used, give additional fluids, as prescribed, to counter gastric fluid losses.

Measure fluid intake and urine output hourly for each shift, and at 24-hour intervals by using a urine collection bag or by weighing diapers. Weigh the neonate daily, using the same scale if possible, and compare fluid intake to output for each shift and at 24-hour intervals. Also monitor laboratory data (hematocrit, blood pH, and serum electrolyte, blood urea nitrogen, creatinine, and uric acid levels) to evaluate acid-base status. Assess urine specific gravity with each voiding or at least every 4 hours.

Stay alert for signs of fluid deficit and fluid excess; the latter is most likely with a cardiac or renal problem. (For signs of fluid deficit and excess, see *Assessing fluid status*.)

Assess the neonate's electrolyte status by monitoring serum electrolyte levels. As a general rule, serum sodium should approximate 133 to 146 mmol/liter; serum calcium, 6.1 to 11.6 mg/dl; serum potassium, 4.6 to 6.7 mmol/liter; and serum chloride, 100 to 117 mmol/liter.

Preventing and controlling infection

Nearly all high-risk neonates have a nursing diagnosis of *potential for infection related to immunologic immaturity, altered ventilation, ineffective airway clearance, or frequent invasive procedures.* Consequently, take the following precautions to help minimize the risk of infection.

• Practice meticulous handwashing. Scrub for 3 minutes before entering the nursery and wash hands frequently throughout caregiving activities. After providing care, perform a 1-minute scrub.

Assessing fluid status

Various factors place the high-risk neonate in danger of fluid imbalance—particularly fluid volume deficit. To assess for fluid volume deficit or excess, check for the signs listed below.

Signs of fluid volume deficit (dehydration)
- Dry mucous membranes
- Elevated hematocrit, hemoglobin level, and blood urea nitrogen value
- Increasing heart and respiratory rates
- Low-grade fever
- Poor skin turgor
- Slightly decreased blood pressure
- Sunken eyeballs or fontanels
- Urine output less than 1 ml/kg/hour
- Urine specific gravity above 1.013
- Weight loss

Signs of fluid volume excess (overhydration)
- Chronic cough
- Crackles
- Dyspnea
- Edema
- Increasing central venous pressure
- Rhonchi
- Tachypnea
- Urine output exceeding 5 ml/kg/hour

• Pay meticulous attention to asepsis during all care procedures. Maintain sterile technique during invasive procedures, such as suctioning and drawing blood from arterial lines. As permitted by facility protocol, use triple-dye alcohol or an antimicrobial agent when caring for the umbilical cord and any puncture sites.

• Make sure all equipment used for neonatal care is sterile or has been cleaned thoroughly. A stethoscope should be assigned to each neonate to prevent cross-contamination, and health care providers should refrain from using their own equipment when providing neonatal care.

• Avoid wearing rings and other jewelry. Many facilities also prohibit nursery staff from using hand lotions, which serve as a breeding ground for pathogenic organisms.

• Wear gloves and follow other universal precautions when changing diapers and performing other activities involving contact with body secretions.

• If an I.V. line is in place, document the appearance of the I.V. site every 30 minutes to 1 hour, depending on the solution being given. If redness or swelling appears, indicating infiltration, the infusion site may have to be changed. However, never stop a glucose or calcium infusion abruptly without immediately restarting it because this may cause serum glucose or calcium levels to fluctuate widely.

• When bathing the neonate, use mild soap and wash only creases and soiled areas. Avoid harsh chemicals, such as alcohol and povidone-iodine, and carefully rinse the neonate's skin after using any irritating substance.

• Maintain an intact skin barrier—especially if the neonate has a nursing diagnosis of *potential impaired skin integrity related to frequent invasive procedures*—by using as little tape as possible to secure I.V. catheters, urine collection containers, feeding tubes, and other equipment (tape removal may peel off the epidermis). Also, first apply an adhesive removal pad when removing ECG leads.

• To help prevent pressure-point breakdown, change the neonate's position, provide range-of-motion exercises, and place the neonate on sheepskin or a waterbed. Assess the skin for redness (especially over bony prominences), which indicates poor circulation to the reddened area. To guard against skin tears and scrapes when turning or moving the neonate, apply a protective transparent covering over elbows, knees, and other vulnerable joints.

• Evaluate all visitors for signs of infection.

• Any staff member with active herpes simplex lesions (those that have not reached the crusting stage) should refrain from working in the nursery. Even after lesions have crusted, the person should wear gloves and wash hands before and after contact.

To detect infection early, assess the neonate regularly for such systemic signs as hypothermia or hyperthermia, lethargy, jaundice, petechiae, respiratory distress, purulent drainage from the eyes or umbilical site, and subtle behavioral changes. Also check for signs of localized infection from the umbilical and I.V. sites.

If the neonate has potential signs of infection, place in an incubator and, if possible, an isolation room to protect other neonates. Expect the physician to prescribe prophylactic antibiotics (typically ampicillin and gentamicin) and a septic workup, which routinely includes cultures of blood, CSF, and urine; a chest X-ray; serum electrolyte analysis; and a complete blood count (CBC) with differential.

Once culture and sensitivity test results determine the infectious organism, the physician may change the antibiotic prescribed; in most cases, a combination of antibiotics is used. If the physician prescribes gentamicin, obtain peak and trough serum blood levels after the third dose to detect or prevent adverse drug effects; obtain a trough level 30 minutes before administering the next dose and a peak level 30 to 45 minutes afterward. Antibiotic therapy typically continues for 10 days, with reevaluation at the end of the course.

During antibiotic therapy, assess the neonate for signs of drug-induced nerve damage, including palsy, decreased arm or leg mobility, and tremors; also check for behavioral changes, which could signal decreased tolerance of antibiotic therapy. Monitor fluid intake and output every 4 to 8 hours, and notify the physician if output falls below normal.

For a group B streptococcal infection, monitor blood pressure, including mean arterial pressure. Decreasing blood pressure may warrant administration of plasmanate to expand blood volume and correct the shock response resulting from this infection. Unless immediate aggressive interventions begin, this infection carries a mortality rate as high as 90% (Christensen, Rothstein, Hill, and Hall, 1985; Nelson, Merenstein, and Pierce, 1986).

Providing developmental care and environmental support

Research from the past 20 years shows that the neonate is aware of surroundings and responds to sensory stimulation. Within the past decade, health care providers increasingly have aimed to establish a developmentally appropriate environment for the high-risk neonate by reducing detrimental stimulation, providing appropriate stimulation during caregiving activities, and teaching parents how to provide appropriate stimulation.

To reduce environmental noise, for example, eliminate loud music and loud talking near the neonate and make sure doors, trash-can bottoms, and incubator portholes are padded. Also, dim the lights and minimize handling of the neonate. When trying to arouse the neonate, use a soft voice and call the neonate by name.

For the neonate with a nursing diagnosis of *altered growth and development related to functional immaturity, prolonged environmental stress, and lack of stimulation appropriate for gestational age and physical status,* nursing interventions include:
• initiating direct-care procedures only when the neonate is alert
• providing rest periods between activities
• encouraging parents to interact with the neonate in ways that promote optimal development
• providing tactile, auditory, visual, and vestibular stimulation (handling) according to the neonate's tolerance. Activities that provide such stimulation include gentle stroking, caressing (especially during feeding), talking, singing, calling the neonate by name, playing a tape of the parents' voices, promoting eye contact with visitors, displaying pictures and designs near the neonate, holding the neonate in a ventral (face-down) position during burping, and stroking the back until the neonate burps. Also, continually assess the neonate's response to stimulation.

Ensuring preoperative and postoperative care

For the neonate who requires surgery, preoperative nursing care includes monitoring vital signs, maintaining a patent airway, assessing respiratory status, en-suring fluid balance, and maintaining adequate nutrition (as with enteral or parenteral feedings). Depending on the neonate's specific problems, other measures may be warranted—for example, providing gastric decompression via a nasogastric tube; preventing trauma, heat loss, and infection at a defect site (such as with encephalocele or gastroschisis); and administering broad-spectrum antibiotics.

After surgery, check vital signs for the first 24 hours—every 15 minutes for the first hour, every 30 minutes for the next 2 hours, every hour for the next 4 hours, then every 2 hours. Maintain patency of the airway and any airway tubes by suctioning frequently and checking for signs of respiratory distress. Support oxygenation and ventilation by giving supplemental oxygen or maintaining mechanical ventilation, as appropriate, and by turning the neonate from side to side every few hours.

Ensure fluid and electrolyte balance by monitoring fluid intake and output and checking serum electrolyte levels. If the neonate must be fed through a gastrostomy tube, give feedings by slow gravity drip. If possible, have the neonate suck on a pacifier to stimulate the sucking and swallowing reflexes.

Maintain skin integrity at the surgical site by cleaning frequently (as specified by facility protocol) and observing for signs of infection, such as skin breakdown, erythema, edema, or bloody or purulent drainage. To prevent disruption of the suture line, use restraints if necessary.

If a nasogastric tube is present for postoperative gastric decompression (to prevent stress on the surgical site), tape the tube to the neonate's face. Irrigate the tube frequently to ensure patency and drainage, and connect it to low-intermittent suction.

If a chest tube is present, check for patency of the system by observing for a consistent flow of bubbles in the underwater seal container. Auscultate breath sounds frequently; diminishing breath sounds may signal a developing pneumothorax.

If a colostomy was performed (as with certain GI defects), check the amount, color, and consistency of stools. When changing dressings, avoid applying undue friction when cleaning around the stoma. Check for skin breakdown and bleeding near the stoma.

For the neonate recovering from surgery for a neurologic anomaly, check neurologic status frequently by assessing pupil size and response, level of consciousness, behavior and activity levels, motor function, and firmness of fontanels. Also evaluate for signs of increased intracranial pressure (such as lethargy, a high-pitched cry, and "sunset" eyes) and measure head circumference daily. Monitor fluid intake and output and observe extremities for mottling and poor capillary refill.

After surgery for a cardiac anomaly, frequently assess vital signs, breath sounds, and results of ABG analysis and blood tests (especialy hematocrit and hemoglobin values). Maintain electronic cardiorespiratory monitoring and assess urine output hourly.

Carrying out special procedures

Many high-risk neonates require phototherapy or exchange transfusion to treat hyperbilirubinemia; a few require extracorporeal membrane oxygenation (ECMO). General nursing measures during phototherapy and exchange transfusions focus on maintaining body temperature, proper timing of care to avoid unnecessary stress, and assessing oral intake, urine output, and stools. With any of the procedures described in this section, observe the neonate closely for respiratory compromise. The neonate with hyperbilirubinemia is at risk for asphyxia and respiratory distress; the neonate who requires ECMO commonly has preexisting respiratory distress.

Phototherapy. In this procedure, used to treat hyperbilirubinemia, the neonate is placed unclothed approximately 18″ under a bank of lights for several hours or days until the serum bilirubin level drops to within acceptable limits. Phototherapy lights decompose bilirubin in the skin through oxidation, facilitating biliary excretion of unconjugated bilirubin. (For an illustration, see *Phototherapy unit*.)

Nursing responsibilities. To prevent retinal damage, an opaque mask must be placed over the neonate's eyes. Make sure that the mask is tight enough to stay in place but not so tight that it impedes circulation or puts pressure on the eyeballs (direct pressure may cause reflex bradycardia). Also, keep the genitals covered with a mask or small diaper to catch urine and stool while leaving the skin surface open to the light. Observe for signs of pressure caused by eye and genital coverings. Turn the neonate every 2 hours to relieve pressure on the knees, hips, and other joints and to allow exposure of all skin surfaces.

Turn off the phototherapy lights for 2 to 5 minutes at least every 8 hours to assess the eyes for irritation or redness and help the neonate establish a normal sleep-awake pattern (phototherapy may lengthen sleep). Monitor the number and consistency of stools; bilirubin breakdown increases gastric motility, resulting in loose stools that can cause skin excoriation and breakdown. Be sure to clean the neonate's buttocks after each stool to help maintain skin integrity.

Check the serum bilirubin level every 4 to 8 hours to determine if phototherapy is effective, and frequently assess skin and sclera color to check the degree of jaundice. Also estimate fluid losses and check for de-

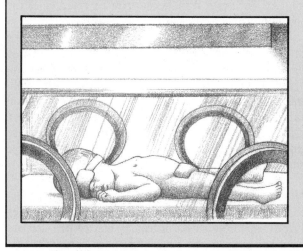

Phototherapy unit

As this illustration shows, the neonate undergoing phototherapy is placed under phototherapy lights unclothed, except for eye and genital coverings. Fluorescent lights, daylight lamps, blue lights, or special high-intensity quartz lamps may be used. The nurse should turn the neonate every 2 hours to expose all body surfaces to the lights.

hydration, which occurs as GI hypermotility pulls fluids into the intestines; if dehydration occurs, notify the physician. To minimize insensible fluid losses, place the neonate in an incubator if possible, and provide I.V. fluids, as prescribed.

Complete exchange transfusion. Hyperbilirubinemia that does not respond to phototherapy may necessitate a complete exchange transfusion. In this procedure, the neonate's blood is removed via an umbilical catheter and replaced with fresh whole donor blood to remove the unconjugated bilirubin in the serum. The procedure carries a risk of transfusion reaction and subsequent death.

To minimize the risk of cardiovascular complications, isovolumetric exchange transfusion may be used. In this method, both the umbilical vein and umbilical artery are catheterized: One catheter is inserted into the umbilical artery and another into the umbilical vein. A three-way stopcock is placed at the end of each catheter and a syringe is connected to the arterial catheter at the junction of the stopcock; the arterial catheter will serve as the site for blood withdrawal. After the neonate's blood is withdrawn, warmed whole blood is administered via the venous catheter.

In the most common isovolumetric technique, 5 to 10 ml of the neonate's blood are removed and the same amount of warmed donor blood administered via the venous catheter over at least 2 minutes. Withdrawing or administering blood at a faster rate may lead to life-threatening arrhythmias. Half-way through the exchange transfusion, calcium gluconate is administered to prevent hypocalcemia and consequent cardiac irritability.

The procedure takes 1 to 2 hours, depending on the volume of blood exchanged and the neonate's condition. (The volume of blood to be exchanged typically is calculated by multiplying kilograms of body weight by 180 ml.) An exchange transfusion may be repeated if the serum bilirubin level continues to rise.

In some facilities, fetal exchange transfusion is used to treat isoimmune hemolytic anemia in utero. In this technique, introduced by Liley (1963), fetal blood is withdrawn and donor blood administered through an umbilical artery catheter. Although fetal exchange transfusion can predispose the fetus to infection and hemorrhage, it has proven successful. Fetal transfusions usually are carried out at regional centers with little risk to the mother and a success rate of 65% to 70% (Pringle, 1989).

Nursing responsibilities. For several hours before an exchange transfusion, withhold oral intake to decrease the risk of aspirating saliva or feeding matter (the neonate must be strapped into a supine position during the procedure, increasing the aspiration risk). Also, obtain a blood sample for laboratory analysis of the total and conjugated serum bilirubin levels.

Donor blood should be checked by two staff members to verify that it is the correct blood. During the transfusion, vital signs are assessed every 5 to 15 minutes; a running total of the amount of blood administered and withdrawn is kept. The best way to accomplish this is for an assistant to call out the amounts—for example, by stating "5 ml of blood out" and "5 ml of blood in." The exact time of blood administration and withdrawal should be documented. The heart and respiratory rates displayed on the monitor should be noted and the cardiac monitor observed for arrhythmias, which may signal poor tolerance of the transfusion.

When the procedure is completed and the catheter is withdrawn, assess the infusion site for bleeding; expect to transfer the neonate to the phototherapy unit. For the next several hours, monitor the neonate closely for signs of complications, such as metabolic acidosis, hypothermia, circulatory overload, electrolyte disturbances, air embolism, arrhythmias, infection, and hypoglycemia.

Check serum bilirubin levels every 4 to 8 hours to determine if the exchange transfusion was effective. (Always draw blood with the phototherapy lights off to prevent misleading laboratory results.) Approximately 4 hours after the transfusion, check serum electrolyte and glucose levels; if these levels are below normal, a corrective I.V. solution may be ordered.

ECMO. In major neonatal centers, ECMO may be used to maintain gas exchange and perfusion during preoperative management of diaphragmatic hernia or for selected neonates with refractory respiratory failure or MAS. In this technique, the neonate's blood is oxygenated outside the body through an arterial shunt to maintain ventilation and oxygenation; this permits cardiopulmonary recovery at low FiO_2 levels and ventilator settings.

In the neonate, ECMO usually involves venoarterial bypass, in which a cannula is inserted into the right atrium via the right internal jugular vein and the aortic arch is cannulated via the right common carotid artery. Blood circulates through tubing via a pumping device, then through a membrane oxygenator. After blood is oxygenated, it flows through a heating device and into the carotid cannula. The neonate continues on mechanical ventilation during ECMO, with ventilator settings reduced to the minimum level required.

Nursing responsibilities. A specially trained nurse perfusionist typically manages the neonate during ECMO, drawing blood samples for ABG analysis hourly from the neonate and at specified intervals from the ECMO circuit. This nurse also monitors laboratory values (including CBC, platelet count, hemoglobin, hematocrit, and serum electrolytes) and adjusts the heparin drip, as needed, to maintain optimal clotting times.

The nurse assigned to the neonate should change the neonate's position and check vital signs frequently. Weigh dressings under the neonate's neck and assess for blood leakage at the cannulation site. Be sure to monitor fluid intake and output and $tcPO_2$ or pulse oximetry readings frequently. Also, check neurologic status hourly; suction the endotracheal tube and collect tracheal aspirate, as prescribed.

Supporting the family and promoting parent-infant bonding

The birth of a critically ill neonate creates a crisis for family members. Provide emotional support to the family throughout the neonate's stay but especially during each parent's first visit to the NICU—a potentially overwhelming experience. Explain the use of monitors and other supportive equipment to lessen the intimidating effect these machines can have. To help the parents adjust to their child's appearance, emphasize the neonate's normal features.

The parents may be especially anxious if their child is being cared for in a regional center located far from their home. For the family with a nursing diagnosis of *potential altered parenting related to the neonate's condition, difficulty coping with a less-than-perfect neonate, and enforced separation,* make sure to keep communications open and pay special attention to the family's needs. Encourage the parents to visit frequently; if this is not possible, ask them to keep in touch with the NICU staff by telephone. Give them the names and telephone numbers of the physician, primary nurse, social worker, and other contact persons, such as parent support group representatives.

To promote parent-infant bonding, encourage the parents to contribute to their child's environment by attaching a small family item, such as a family photograph, to the neonate's bed. Allow the parents to touch and hold their child whenever possible and provide them with simple caregiving tasks, such as diaper changes. Point out how their child responds to their presence, voice, and touch, and show them how to offer appropriate sensory stimulation so that they can take an active role in their child's development—a measure that enhances their self-esteem. (For a detailed discussion of nursing care for the neonate's family, see Chapter 39, Care of the Families of High-Risk Neonates.)

If the neonate's problem has an underlying genetic cause, refer the parents for genetic testing, as appropriate. Throughout nursing care, consider the neonate's discharge planning needs to ease the transition to the home. (For information on discharge planning and home care for the high-risk neonate, see Chapter 40, Discharge Planning and Neonatal Care at Home.)

Management of selected perinatal problems

This section presents an overview of the management of selected problems seen in high-risk neonates. (For a summary of treatments used for all of the perinatal problems discussed in this chapter, see *Medical management of perinatal problems*, pages 972 and 973.)

Respiratory problems

Serious respiratory depression at birth calls for immediate resuscitation (as discussed earlier). After resuscitation, monitor the neonate's cardiopulmonary status and skin temperature. Obtain blood samples for ABG analysis at least every 4 hours (or as needed); obtain samples for serum electrolyte analysis on admission and 24 hours after delivery. Monitor arterial blood pressure at least every 2 hours; stay alert for subtle changes, which may signal an impending change in respiratory status.

For RDS, standard interventions include administration of supplemental oxygen and positive-pressure ventilation. If the severity of RDS has not been determined, the neonate typically is given supplemental oxygen or positive-pressure ventilation (CPAP or positive end-expiratory pressure). Assess the neonate every 30 minutes during this therapy.

To help prevent RDS, exogenous surfactants may be administered to preterm neonates via an endotracheal tube to stimulate surfactant production (Jobe, 1988). However, this experimental treatment is available only in selected regional centers. Antenatally, several approaches are available. For instance, ritodrine may be administered to prevent premature labor and delivery before the fetal lungs have matured; subsequent lecithin-sphingomyelin ratios are determined to assess fetal lung maturity. If the pregnancy is threatened at 28 to 32 weeks, betamethasone or another glucocorticoid may be given 24 hours before delivery to stimulate fetal surfactant production. (For a case study that shows how to apply the nursing process when caring for a neonate with respiratory problems, see *Applying the nursing process: Preterm neonate with impaired gas exchange related to surfactant deficiency and altered alveolar function*, pages 978 and 979.)

Necrotizing enterocolitis

For NEC, parenteral nutrition is necessary to allow the bowel to rest. A temporary colostomy may be performed. A portion of localized necrotic bowel may be excised; widespread bowel necrosis may necessitate massive bowel resection, with resulting short-gut syndrome, a condition characterized by impaired nutrient digestion. Expect to administer antibiotics to control secondary infection.

Neonate of a diabetic mother

Assess for signs of birth trauma (for example, by evaluating mobility, especially in the upper extremities), correct any fluid or electrolyte imbalances, and assess for complications stemming from widely fluctuating serum glucose, calcium, and bilirubin levels. Also monitor the neonate's vital signs, $tcPO_2$ or pulse oximetry values, and ABG values. (For specific interventions associated with hypoglycemia, hypocalcemia, and hyperbilirubinemia, see the "Metabolic disorders" section below.)

Metabolic disorders

For hypoglycemia, if the neonate has no other problems, early feedings may be initiated to counteract the glucose imbalance. In other cases, expect to give glucose I.V., as 3 ml/kg of dextrose 10% in water. (The use of dextrose 25% to 50% in solution is contraindicated because it can cause vascular damage leading to ischemic necrosis.)

For hypocalcemia, expect to administer I.V. or oral supplemental calcium. The typical I.V. dosage is 24 mg/kg/day; the typical oral dosage, 75 mg/kg/day (Kliegman and Wald, 1986). When administering calcium by slow infusion, check the pulse frequently to detect bradycardia. Assess the infusion site every 30 minutes for signs

Medical management of perinatal problems

Management of a perinatal problem may involve any or all of the measures specified in the chart below. (For details on nursing care for a neonate with some of these problems, see the "Planning and implementation" section of this chapter.)

Birth asphyxia

- Immediate resuscitation followed by supplemental oxygen, continuous positive-airway pressure (CPAP), or mechanical ventilation

Meconium aspiration syndrome

- Immediate resuscitation, with endotracheal intubation and suctioning of the lower airway

Episodic apnea

- Treatment of the underlying disorder (such as intracranial hemorrhage or hypoglycemia)
- Aminophylline or theophylline to stimulate respirations
- CPAP

Respiratory distress syndrome

- Supplemental oxygen, CPAP, or mechanical ventilation, with close monitoring of oxygenation status
- Preventive therapies, such as maternal betamethasone administration to stimulate fetal surfactant production or administration of exogenous surfactant to the neonate

Transient tachypnea

- Oxygen administration (or, rarely, CPAP or mechanical ventilation) with close monitoring of oxygenation status

Bronchopulmonary dysplasia

- Close monitoring of oxygenation status during supplemental oxygen therapy
- Gradual weaning from mechanical ventilation
- Nutritional support (typically enteral or parenteral feedings)
- Fluid restriction and diuretics to prevent pulmonary edema

Retinopathy of prematurity

- Close monitoring of oxygenation status during supplemental oxygen therapy
- Frequent ophthalmologic evaluations
- Reduced intensity of nursery lighting
- Cryosurgery

Intraventricular hemorrhage

- Supportive treatment, typically including vitamin K, platelets, and anticonvulsant medication
- Reduced environmental stimulation and handling
- Close monitoring of neurologic status

Necrotizing enterocolitis

- Colostomy
- Parenteral nutrition
- Antibiotics

Neonate of a diabetic mother

- Treatment of associated birth trauma
- Correction of associated metabolic and electrolyte imbalances

Hypoglycemia

- Early oral feedings or I.V. glucose (typically as dextrose 10% in water)
- Close monitoring of serum glucose level

Hypocalcemia

- Supplemental calcium (typically as I.V. or oral calcium gluconate)

Hyperbilirubinemia and jaundice

- Early, frequent feedings
- Phototherapy
- Exchange transfusion

Polycythemia

- Partial exchange transfusion

Ineffective thermoregulation

- Maintenance of neutral thermal environment
- Gradual rewarming (1°/hour)

Rh incompatibility

- Complete exchange transfusion with Rh-negative red blood cells, sometimes followed by phototherapy
- Close monitoring of hematocrit and serum bilirubin level

ABO blood group incompatibility

- Correction of hyperbilirubinemia (as with phototherapy)
- Close monitoring of hematocrit and serum bilirubin level

Fetal alcohol syndrome

- Developmental care
- Reduced environmental stimulation
- Enteral feedings if the neonate has incoordinated sucking and swallowing

Drug exposure, addiction, or withdrawal

- Developmental care
- Reduced environmental stimulation
- Enteral feedings, if the neonate has incoordinated sucking and swallowing
- Swaddling and frequent feedings to decrease irritability and tremors
- Phenobarbitol to control seizures (for a neonate going through drug withdrawal)

Infection

- Antibiotics
- Infection control measures (including universal precautions)

Meningomyelocele

- Surgery
- Proper positioning

Medical management of perinatal problems continued

Encephalocele

- Surgery
- Proper positioning

Congenital hydrocephalus

- Surgical placement of a ventriculoperitoneal or ventriculoatrial shunt
- Proper positioning

Microcephaly

- Supportive treatment
- Anticonvulsant medications

Teratoma

- Surgical tumor excision
- Proper positioning

Cardiac anomalies

- Palliative or corrective surgery
- Diuretics or digoxin to control congestive heart failure
- Supportive therapy (such as I.V. fluids and iron supplements to correct anemia)

Diaphragmatic hernia

- Respiratory support
- Gastric decompression
- Extracorporeal membrane oxygenation
- Surgical restoration of abdominal contents to their proper anatomic position
- Postsurgical endotracheal intubation and chest tube placement
- Antibiotics

Tracheoesophageal malformations

- Surgical separation of the trachea and esophagus (with gastrostomy tube placement to prevent aspiration and provide access for feedings)
- Continuous low-pressure suction of blind pouch
- Oxygen therapy

Omphalocele or gastroschisis

- Oxygen therapy
- Immediate positive-pressure ventilation followed by I.V. fluid administration
- Coverage of defect with sterile dressings (to keep tissues moist and reduce heat loss)
- Gastric decompression
- Surgical reduction of defect or creation of pouch around herniated abdominal contents to reduce tissue swelling (with placement of gastrostomy tube to provide access for feedings)

Meconium ileus

- Enemas and fluid administration
- Ileostomy

Imperforate anus

- Gastric decompression
- Colostomy

Cleft palate and cleft lip

- Later surgical repair
- Use of special nipple for feeding
- Close monitoring for ear infection

Unilateral renal agenesis

- Surgical removal of affected kidney (If other kidney is functional, surgery may not be necessary.)

Polycystic kidney disease

- Surgical removal of the affected kidney
- Gastric decompression
- Dialysis
- Antibiotics for urinary tract infection

Posterior urethral valves

- Surgical correction of the obstruction
- Placement of nephrostomy tube or stent for drainage
- Open fetal surgery for temporary relief of obstruction (if diagnosed antepartally)

Genital ambiguity

- Hydrocortisone (if caused by congenital adrenal hyperplasia)
- Later surgical reconstruction of external genitalia

Clubfoot

- Corrective shoes, casts, or braces
- Later corrective surgery, if necessary

---

of infiltration, which may cause tissue necrosis and sloughing. Monitor the serum calcium level every few hours, or according to institutional policy. Once the serum calcium level stabilizes, draw daily blood samples.

For hyperbilirubinemia, the treatment depends on the serum bilirubin level. If the level is elevated only moderately or begins to fall by the fourth or fifth day after birth, the physician may order only early, frequent feedings, which increase intestinal motility and thus speed bilirubin excretion. However, persistent or severe hyperbilirubinemia commonly warrants phototherapy or complete exchange transfusion to prevent bilirubin encephalopathy.

The serum bilirubin level at which these treatments are ordered depends on the physician, institutional policy, and the neonate's gestational age and condition. Some physicians initiate treatment when the bilirubin level measures 15 to 20 mg/100 ml; others wait until it reaches 20 mg/100 ml. (However, the preterm neonate may receive prophylactic phototherapy.) The nurse caring for a neonate undergoing phototherapy or exchange transfusion should perform the measures described earlier under "Special procedures."

Polycythemia

For an asymptomatic neonate, the physician may order only close observation and monitoring of the serum bilirubin level and fluid status. For a symptomatic neonate, a partial exchange transfusion may be ordered.

Isoimmune hemolytic anemia

Care for the neonate with Rh or ABO incompatibility treatment centers on correcting anemia, managing hyperbilirubinemia, and preventing complications. Typically, these disorders warrant exchange transfusion followed by phototherapy.

To prevent Rh isoimmunization, expect the physician to administer prophylactic anti-D immunoglobulin (RhoGAM) to a woman with Rh-negative blood during the twenty-eighth week of pregnancy (Fanaroff and Martin, 1987) and within 48 to 72 hours of delivery of an Rh-positive neonate. (For more information on prevention of Rh isoimmunization, see Chapter 22, High-Risk Antepartal Clients.)

Effects of maternal substance abuse

For FAS, no treatment exists because the structural damage occurs in utero. Supportive management focuses on developmental care and environmental support. If the neonate has poorly coordinated sucking and swallowing reflexes, expect to give enteral feedings to prevent aspiration; physical therapy also may be implemented to help alleviate this problem.

For the neonate who is addicted to maternal drugs or going through drug withdrawal, nursing goals include:
• ensuring adequate nutritional intake
• improving coordination of the sucking and swallowing reflexes
• reducing irritability by minimizing environmental stimulation
• avoiding abrupt movements near the neonate
• promoting a normal sleep-awake cycle to prolong sleep
• stabilizing body temperature.

To reduce tremors and extraneous movement, swaddle the neonate and touch the tremulous area firmly and calmly. To minimize muscle rigidity or hypertonicity, bathe the neonate in warm water, massage gently, and swaddle in a flexed position. Do not leave the neonate in a supine position that maintains muscle extension or stiffness.

For the neonate going through withdrawal, treatment varies with the health care facility and the substance involved. Seizures may be controlled with phenobarbital (5 to 8 mg/kg/day).

Congenital anomalies

For a potentially life-threatening congenital anomaly, immediate interventions must begin; the neonate may require corrective surgery within hours. Specific management varies with the anomaly and the neonate's condition.

Meningomyelocele. This condition calls for surgery—perhaps within a few hours after birth. The surgeon removes the herniated tissue and covers the defect with surrounding skin.

Before surgery, if the defect is open, cover it immediately with warm saline-solution compresses and plastic wrap. To reduce pressure on the defect and minimize tissue damage, position the neonate to avoid pressure on the defect; be sure to support the defect when moving the neonate.

After surgery, place a rolled towel under the neonate's hips to maintain the legs in a relaxed position. Observe the suture line for signs of CSF leakage and infection, indicated by redness or swelling. Closely monitor neurologic status and assess movement; lack of movement suggests neurologic damage (from the anomaly or surgery). Also monitor for skin mottling, coolness of the legs and arms, decreased capillary refill, and reduced muscle tone.

Prevent contamination of and trauma to the wound and stay alert for signs of infection (particularly meningitis). To prevent fecal contamination of the suture line, tape a cup or a plastic diaper lining to the lower part of the surgical dressing to cover the anus. Because surgery for this disorder may cause hydrocephalus, check head circumference daily.

If the neonate's bladder function is disturbed, monitor fluid intake and output and observe for bladder distention. With lack of innervation (neurogenic bladder), an indwelling catheter may be necessary both before and after surgery. However, in some facilities, the Credé method is used to remove urine from the urethra. In this method, gently roll the fingers from the umbilicus toward the symphysis pubis; pushing on the bladder forces urine into the urethra for elimination. (However, be aware that this method may cause infection from reflux of urine from the lower urinary tract to the bladder.)

Encephalocele. This defect must be closed surgically, necessitating removal of external brain tissue. Surgery may cause such problems as paralysis, mental retardation, or even death.

Preoperatively, position the neonate to avoid pressure on the defect. To prevent infection at the defect, administer antibiotics, as prescribed; cover the defect if CSF leakage occurs. Postoperatively, monitor neurologic status and vital signs frequently; assess motor function in all extremities. If the neonate cannot breathe independently, support respirations by maintaining mechanical ventilation. Inspect the dressing for drainage or CSF leakage; to avoid serious neurologic complications, maintain its sterility. Avoid placing the neonate on the suture site.

Congenital hydrocephalus. This disorder typically warrants surgical placement of a ventriculoperitoneal shunt (or, rarely, a ventriculoatrial shunt). The shunt drains CSF from the dilated ventricle into the peritoneal cavity or atrium for absorption and removal; it must be revised periodically as the child grows.

Preoperatively, keep the neonate comfortable. To prevent apnea caused by backward head movement, position the neonate on one side and keep the head of the bed flat or slightly elevated. Postoperatively, maintain suture line integrity and observe for signs of CSF leakage and infection.

To monitor for increasing intracranial pressure, measure and record head circumference once during each shift. As head circumference decreases, discomfort should subside and oral feedings may begin slowly. Also assess for suture line integrity, check the alertness level, and note how well the neonate tolerates enteral or oral feedings.

Teratoma. In most cases, this tumor is excised within the first 28 days after birth. The surgical procedure depends on the tissue involved and the amount of associated tissue. If the tumor is in the sacrococcygeal area, the coccyx may be removed along with the tumor to avoid tumor recurrence. (The nursing measures described below apply mainly to a neonate with a sacrococcygeal tumor.)

Before surgery, position the neonate to minimize pressure on the affected area. After surgery, assess neurologic function by observing movement and color of the legs. Also assess the appearance and amount of drainage from the incision site. Keep the neonate prone, and place sheepskin under the knees to prevent skin irritation and breakdown. To assess for urine retention, measure urine by weighing diapers; if urine output diminishes, notify the physician. Take measures to help prevent infection and minimize stress on the incision line; if necessary, use loose leg restraints to prevent suture line trauma.

Cardiac anomalies. Treatment may be medical or surgical, depending on the specific defect. For an acyanotic defect, corrective surgery may be delayed in favor of symptomatic treatment. For instance, indomethacin, a synthetic prostaglandin inhibitor, may be administered I.V. to close a PDA. However, if this defect is accompanied by severe CHF, the duct is ligated surgically.

For temporary or palliative surgical treatment of an atrial or ventricular septal defect, a band may be placed around the pulmonary artery to decrease blood flow into the pulmonary circulation and alleviate CHF. Other treatments are aimed at managing CHF and include diuretic therapy and digoxin to support cardiac output. When the child is older, a patch graft may be placed to correct the defect.

Surgical correction of coarctation of the aorta, attempted during the toddler or preschool years, involves resection of obstructed blood flow through placement of a graft over the stenotic area; the two segments then are anastomosed on either side of the stenosis.

With a cyanotic defect, palliative surgery typically is performed during the neonatal period. For example, balloon septostomy may be used to open atrial shunts or an artificial graft may be placed. Palliative medical treatments aim to prevent complications of hypoxemia— for instance, iron supplements may be given to correct anemia and fluids and nutritional therapy to prevent fluid overload or dehydration. (Oxygen administration will not improve the neonate's color because cyanosis does not result from pulmonary compromise.) A temporary shunt may be placed to increase pulmonary blood flow.

Nursing goals for the neonate with a congenital cardiac anomaly include maintaining adequate cardiopulmonary function and preventing complications. The neonate will require intensive, expert care and close monitoring. Assess for cyanosis, heart murmurs, arrythmias, absent or unequal pulses, and respiratory distress, and monitor daily weight and fluid intake and output.

Diaphragmatic hernia. Although recent changes in surgical technique have decreased mortality from this anomaly, the neonate with a diaphragmatic hernia poses a challenge for the health care team. Gastric decompression is necessary to relieve gastric distention caused by pressure over the stomach and decreased intestinal motility. The sooner the defect is corrected, the better the prognosis. Surgery for diaphragmatic hernia involves transthoracic or transabdominal incision to restore the abdominal contents to their proper anatomic position. The surgeon pulls the outer skin layers to cover the abdominal wall defect.

Unfortunately, surgical repair does not guarantee survival. If the neonate has respiratory complications or if the unaffected lung is compromised and the affected lung is hypoplastic, the prognosis is guarded at best.

Preoperatively, the main nursing goal is to stabilize and support respiration. Expect to administer prophylactic antibiotics and I.V. fluids; as prescribed, give dextrose 10% in water for the first 24 hours after birth. As appropriate, obtain samples for CBC, WBC differential, serum electrolyte levels, and ABG analysis.

Postoperatively, stay alert for signs of complications, such as a right-to-left shunt, pneumothorox, and pulmonary arterial hypertension. Maintain airway patency, respiratory support, and fluid and electrolyte balance. Auscultate breath sounds every 1 to 2 hours to detect a developing pneumothorax, indicated by diminished breath sounds. Check the incision site every 1 to 2 hours for signs of leakage or infection. As ordered, institute feedings gradually once the neonate no longer requires ventilatory assistance.

The neonate probably will require endotracheal intubation; perform endotracheal suctioning and maintain ventilatory support, as needed. To help reinflate the lung on the affected side, a chest tube also is placed. Maintain chest tube patency: monitor chest tube drainage every hour and make sure to move the contents away from the chest wall toward the collection system to maintain patency. Be sure to monitor the amount and color of drainage. If chest tube patency appears questionable or drainage suddenly increases or decreases markedly, notify the physician.

Tracheoesophageal malformations. Surgical intervention is necessary to separate the trachea and esophagus and to maintain the patency of each structure. The surgical procedure used depends on the specific malformation. A gastrostomy tube commonly is inserted during surgery to prevent gastric reflux and aspiration pneumonia. Some neonates also require cervical esophagostomy to drain saliva and mucus from an atretic area (this procedure is performed only when no tracheoesophageal fistula is present).

Nursing goals include maintaining a patent airway and ensuring fluid and electrolyte balance before and after surgery. Preoperatively, if a blind pouch has been diagnosed, observe secretions for color and amount. As ordered, insert a nasogastric tube and connect it to the blind pouch to provide continuous low-pressure suction and prevent aspiration. Check tube patency hourly, and assess vital signs every 1 to 2 hours.

Oxygen therapy may be required if the neonate's breathing effort increases or if cyanosis develops. A warmed mist, delivered by an oxygen hood or through a closed incubator, may be used to thin secretions. Monitor vital signs, respiratory effort, skin color, appearance of the I.V. infusion site, and the amount of secretions suctioned.

Postoperative nursing interventions resemble those used for the neonate with diaphragmatic hernia, except that no chest tube is present. Turn the neonate every 2 hours to prevent atelectasis. If the neonate can tolerate it, perform nasopharyngeal suctioning with a marked catheter, as ordered, to a depth just short of the suture line to help prevent suture perforation during suctioning.

If the nasogastric tube remains in place for gastric decompression, maintain its patency by inserting 2 ml of air every 2 hours. If cervical esophagostomy was performed, maintain skin integrity by cleaning the skin, applying petroleum jelly to create a waterproof barrier, and applying a secretion-absorbing dressing every 4 hours. Diminished secretions suggest that the stoma is closing, necessitating surgical dilatation with a soft rubber catheter.

Keep the neonate in an upright position before and after surgery—for instance, by using a cholasia chair, which allows the neonate to remain upright after feeding to prevent reflux of secretions. Maintain patency of the gastrostomy tube by inserting 2 ml of air every 2 to 4 hours (gravity drainage typically is used). Also, note how well the neonate tolerated medical and nursing procedures, and assess the appearance of secretions, the neonate's breathing effort, and skin color.

Once enteral feedings begin, assess the neonate's tolerance for them. Any aspirate found before the next feeding may indicate impaired intestinal activity; make sure to document and report this finding.

Bottle feedings typically can begin once an intact suture line is verified. Expect to begin bottle feedings gradually with a clear electrolyte solution, such as Pedialyte. Give feedings slowly to prevent aspiration and gastric distention. Methylene blue, a dye, commonly is added to feedings to reveal suture line leakage. If a fistula is present, this dye appears in the chest tube; dye appearing only in the gastrostomy tube means that the suture line is intact.

If the esophagus has been pulled taut and stretched to make the ends meet, gastrostomy feedings may be needed and the surgeon may perform dilatation with increasing catheter sizes several weeks after surgery. When these feedings begin, evaluate how well the neonate tolerates them. A dusky skin color or choking during feedings may indicate fistula leakage; increased mucus may indicate stenosis around the surgical site.

Abdominal wall defects. The neonate with gastroschisis or omphalocele requires immediate intervention in the delivery room—ventilatory support followed by peripheral line placement for I.V. fluid administration. As soon as possible, cover the defect with sterile gauze dressings moistened with warm normal saline solution; place plastic wrap on top of the dressings to help keep tissues moist and reduce heat loss. Maintain gastric decompression with a nasogastric tube.

Corrective treatment of a small defect involves complete or primary surgical reduction. In the operating room, the bowel and protruding tissues are inspected for trauma that could cause loss of GI contents and bacterial wound contamination. If the protruding contents are too large to return to the abdominal cavity, a silastic pouch is placed around them. Later, keep this pouch (now referred to as a silo) suspended from the top of the incubator to help reduce tissue swelling and facilitate eventual return of the abdominal contents to the abdominal cavity. Position the neonate supine and moisten the silo with povidone-iodine every 8 hours (or as specified by facility protocol).

If the defect is large, the reduction must be performed in stages to prevent excessive pressure on the diaphragm and resulting complications, such as respiratory compromise and tissue hypoxia. In some cases, reduction may be performed in the NICU; in others, the neonate must return to the operating room.

The nursing goal is to minimize the risk of infection and maintain the herniated tissue and organs in optimal condition. Be sure to maintain sterile technique throughout caregiving procedures. Before surgery, keep the dressings sterile and moist and evaluate for skin breakdown from supine positioning. If appropriate, place an air mattress or sheepskin under the neonate to minimize skin breakdown.

After the neonate's final surgical closure, expect to administer feedings through a gastrostomy tube. Begin feedings gradually and increase the volume based on the neonate's tolerance. Usually, a central line also must be inserted for administration of parenteral nutrition, which will continue for several days or weeks.

Monitor for changes in respiratory status and vital signs (especially during the immediate postoperative period), and assess tolerance of feedings once these begin. Also evaluate the appearance of the defect, checking closely for signs of infection. To assess for circulatory compromise caused by pressure from the defect, check capillary refill in the legs.

Imperforate anus. The neonate with this anomaly requires surgical restoration of the anal canal to achieve urinary and bowel continence. For a low defect, a peripheral anoplasty typically is performed during the neonatal period. For an intermediate defect, a colostomy is performed in most cases, with further surgery performed several months later. A high defect always necessitates a colostomy.

Nursing goals include preventing gastric distention and dehydration. Preoperatively, nursing measures depend on the severity of the defect. Expect to maintain gastric decompression and initiate I.V. therapy.

Postoperatively, position the neonate on the stomach or side. Maintain gastric decompression until 24 hours before feedings are to begin. If anoplasty was performed, assess the site for skin breakdown, redness, and drainage. Clean it regularly and after every stool; avoid taking rectal temperatures or examining the rectum. To minimize stool formation until the incision heals, delay feedings at least 24 hours after surgery.

If the neonate has a colostomy, assess the suture line and skin around the stoma for color, swelling, and drainage; check for separation of the suture line. As needed, change the dressing to prevent infection, and change the colostomy bag to prevent leakage.

Cleft palate and cleft lip. Surgical repair of these anomalies usually is delayed to prevent disruption of facial growth and tooth-bud formation. However, it must occur early enough so that the defect does not interfere with speech development. Repair of cleft lip (cheilorrhaphy, or Z-plasty) commonly takes place when the child is 3 months old; repair of cleft palate (by joining of the palatal segments) typically is performed when the child is 9 to 15 months old.

Ensure adequate nutrition before and after surgery because air leaks around the cleft and nasal regurgitation typically cause feeding problems. Many neonates with cleft lip can be breast-fed (except after surgery); the mother may provide breast milk she has pumped. With cleft palate, a feeding neonate requires a syringe or cleft palate feed or a special elongated nipple (such as a Martin's nipple). When using an elongated nipple, be sure to place it far into the mouth—but not far enough to induce gagging. Burp the neonate frequently while feeding because cleft lip or palate causes swallowing of much air during feeding. To prevent aspiration of feeding matter through the palatal opening and the nares, elevate the head of the bed or place the neonate in an infant seat or on the stomach after feedings.

The neonate's abnormally short eustachian tubes provide easy access for nasal and oral bacteria, increasing the risk of ear infection. To help reduce this risk, clean the nose and oral cavities after feedings, and assess frequently for fever, irritability, and other signs of ear infection. To remove excess formula, rinse the neonate's mouth with water after feedings.

Be sure to teach the parents how to provide the special care their child requires. Cleft palate and lip can cause long-term speech, dental, hearing, and other problems, so the nurse should refer parents to appropriate professionals for follow-up care.

Polycystic kidney disease and posterior urethral valves. A polycystic kidney is removed surgically. Before surgery, monitor the neonate for infection (especially of the urinary tract). Afterward, maintain gastric decompression and monitor urine output, urine specific gravity, and dipstick for blood every 2 hours. Report any decrease in urine output.

With posterior urethral valves, the obstruction is corrected surgically and a nephrostomy tube or stent is

(Text continues on page 980.)

APPLYING THE NURSING PROCESS

Preterm neonate with impaired gas exchange related to surfactant deficiency and altered alveolar function

For the high-risk neonate, the nursing process helps ensure high-quality care and appropriate decision making. The table below shows how a nurse might use the nursing process when caring for the neonate described in the case history at right. The first column presents history and physical assessment data followed by a paragraph of mental notes. These notes help the nurse make important mental connections among assessment findings, aiding in development of the nursing diagnosis and planning.

The second column lists an appropriate nursing diagnosis; information in the remaining columns is based on this diagnosis. Although not part of the nursing process, a rationale appears for each intervention in the fourth column to explain how it contributes to the care plan.

ASSESSMENT	NURSING DIAGNOSIS	PLANNING
Subjective (history) data • Mother is age 17, a gravida 3. • Mother had premature rupture of the membranes (6 hours) and a 4-hour labor. • Fetal heart rate: 150 to 160 beats/minute. • Apgar scores: 3 at 1 minute, 7 at 5 minutes. **Objective (physical) data** • Nasal flaring, audible grunting, moderate substernal retractions, and diminished breath sounds on admission to the NICU. • Apical pulse: 160 beats/minute. • Respiratory rate: 72 breaths/minute. • Axillary temperature: 97.4° F. • Blood pressure: 40/20 mm Hg. • Weight: 950 g. • Gestational age: 27 weeks. • ABG values: pH 7.25, PaO_2 40 mm Hg, $PaCO_2$ 55 mm Hg. **Mental notes** *Gestational age of 27 weeks classifies the neonate as preterm and thus at risk for respiratory distress syndrome (RDS) resulting from pulmonary immaturity. Also, vital signs and other objective data reflect respiratory problems. Oxygen and suctioning equipment should be kept on hand.*	Impaired gas exchange related to surfactant deficiency and altered alveolar function	**Goals** During the neonate's stay in the NICU, she will: • exhibit a respiratory rate of 40 to 60 beats/minute • maintain a patent airway • resolve signs of RDS • demonstrate clear bilateral breath sounds • maintain an arterial pH of 7.35 to 7.45, a PaO_2 of 60 to 80 mm Hg, and a $PaCO_2$ of 25 to 35 mm Hg.

CASE STUDY

Amy Stone was born at 27 weeks' gestation weighing 950 g. She was intubated in the delivery room and given bag-and-mask ventilation for 6 minutes. After resuscitation, she was admitted to a level 3 (NICU) nursery.

IMPLEMENTATION		EVALUATION
Intervention	**Rationale**	Upon evaluation, the neonate:
Review significant maternal, antepartal, and intrapartal data; review the neonate's Apgar scores and resuscitative measures at delivery.	Maternal, antepartal, and intrapartal factors can affect neonatal outcome; Apgar scores reflect the neonate's initial adaptation and verify the need for resuscitation.	• exhibited a respiratory rate of 40 to 60 beats/minute
Assess the neonate for signs of respiratory distress—tachypnea (a respiratory rate above 60 breaths/minute), nasal flaring, retractions, grunting, diminished breath sounds, cyanosis, and apnea. A respiratory rate above 60 breaths/minute	Tachypnea indicates respiratory distress; nasal flaring reflects an attempt to boost oxygen intake; retractions indicate decreased lung compliance; grunting is an attempt to prevent alveolar collapse; diminished breath sounds may signal areas of lung collapse or fluid accumulation; cyanosis and apnea reflect $PaCO_2$ elevation.	• demonstrated no nasal flaring, grunting, or tachypnea and showed only mild chest retractions (if any) • demonstrated clear bilateral breath sounds • maintained a patent airway • demonstrated acceptable PaO_2, and $PaCO_2$.
Suction the neonate's nares and oropharynx carefully, as needed.	Suctioning helps maintain a patent airway by relieving obstruction caused by mucus and other fluids.	
Maintain a neutral thermal environment (NTE) and an axillary temperature of 97.7° to 98.8° F (36.3° to 37.1° C).	Maintaining an NTE and an axillary temperature within this range reduces the risk of cold stress.	
Administer oxygen as needed and prescribed.	Supplemental oxygen helps combat hypoxia.	
Monitor the amount of oxygen administered by recording the fraction of inspired oxygen (FiO_2) every hour.	High FiO_2 with high ventilator pressures can cause or contribute to bronchopulmonary dysplasia and retinopathy of prematurity.	
Use transcutaneous oxygen ($tcPO_2$) monitoring or pulse oximetry to monitor the neonate's PaO_2 and $PaCO_2$.	These techniques allow constant noninvasive monitoring of PaO_2 and $PaCO_2$, thereby reducing the need for frequent blood samples.	
Monitor arterial blood gas (ABG) values as needed and correlate results with $tcPO_2$ or pulse oximetry results.	Correlation establishes the diagnosis of RDS. Assesses oxygenation status.	
Review chest X-rays.	X-rays show areas of atelectasis caused by RDS.	
Determine if the neonate has adequate gagging and sucking reflexes.	If these reflexes are absent, the neonate may aspirate secretions.	
Position the neonate on the abdomen or the side.	An abdominal or side-lying position allows optimal chest expansion to facilitate secretion drainage and helps maintain a patent airway.	
Organize nursing care to promote optimal rest and minimize stimulation of the neonate.	More rest and less stimulation decrease oxygen consumption and the metabolic rate.	

placed to drain the ureter that has been anastomosed around the stenotic area. Sometimes, temporary relief of the obstruction is achieved antenatally with open fetal surgery. This procedure has the highest reported success rate of any fetal surgery attempted (Pringle, 1989).

Nursing goals include maintaining fluid and electrolyte balance and supporting respiration (hypoplastic lungs accompany some renal problems). If surgery is scheduled, preoperative nursing care centers on maintaining fluid and electrolyte balance. Assess intake and output every 4 to 8 hours, and check urine specific gravity every 4 hours. Support respiratory efforts, as needed, by maintaining oxygen therapy or assisted ventilation.

Assess the neonate before and after surgery for signs of acute renal failure, such as oliguria or anuria, edema, blood pressure fluctuations, and cardiopulmonary compromise secondary to fluid accumulation. Take postoperative measures to prevent infection. Also, assess for signs of respiratory compromise, decreased urine output, and drainage from the nephrostomy tube or stent. Evaluate renal status by comparing vital sign measurements with baseline values. Also compare fluid intake and output from the previous 24 hours to detect any difference.

Observe and evaluate output from any nephrostomy tube or stent. To help prevent infection, protect the dressing at the suture line and observe this site closely. Keep all dressings dry; as needed, replace dressings at the suture line and around tubes.

Genital ambiguity. If genital ambiguity stems from congenital adrenal hyperplasia, hydrocortisone is given to arrest the disorder; with severe adrenal hyperplasia, hydrocortisone must be administered immediately to prevent acute adrenocorticol failure—a fatal condition. Later, surgical reconstruction of the external genitalia may be attempted.

Expect to assist in genetic testing and determination of the neonate's underlying problem if this has not been established. Providing support to the family is a nursing priority. Refer them to a psychiatrist or other professional for help in coping with this problem. Also, advise them to select a unisex name for their child. Some professionals encourage parents to delay the announcement of their child's birth until the sex can be determined; others believe that a delay exacerbates parental anxiety.

Clubfoot. Typically, corrective shoes, casts, or braces are used as soon as possible to correct the deformity. If these measures fail, surgery may be performed when the child is several years old. Inform the parents of the need for early and continual medical evaluation to avoid problems when the child begins to walk.

Congenital hip dysplasia. Treatment involves pressing the femoral head against and into the acetabulum. This pressure allows formation of an adequate socket before ossification is complete. To abduct and externally rotate the leg and flex the hip, a triangular pillow is applied over the diaper. At a later date, the neonate typically is placed in a spica cast.

Evaluation

During this step of the nursing process, the nurse evaluates the effectiveness of the care plan by ongoing evaluation of subjective and objective criteria. Evaluation findings should be stated in terms of actions performed or outcomes achieved for each goal. The following examples illustrate appropriate evaluation statements for the high-risk neonate.

• The neonate's vital signs improved.
• The neonate maintained an adequate core temperature.
• The neonate's cardiopulmonary status improved or remained within acceptable limits.
• The neonate maintained fluid and electrolyte balance, as evidenced by adequate urine output, no signs of dehydration or fluid overload, and acceptable serum electrolyte levels.
• The neonate tolerated feedings.
• The I.V. infusion site remained free of signs of infiltration.
• Skin integrity remained intact.
• The neonate's parents showed positive coping mechanisms in response to their child's problem.
• The neonate's parents know how to obtain appropriate counseling and support.

For the neonate with respiratory problems, these additional evaluation statements may be appropriate.
• Signs of increased breathing effort diminished.
• The neonate's ABG and $tcPo_2$ or pulse oximetry values approached normal limits.
• The neonate had no episodes of apnea.

For the neonate with infection, this additional evaluation statement may be appropriate.
• The neonate showed a positive response to antibiotic therapy, as evidenced by improved vital signs and reductions in behavioral deviations, high-pitched crying, and temperature instability.

For the neonate with hyperbilirubinemia or isoimmune hemolytic anemia, these additional evaluation statements may be appropriate.

• The serum bilirubin level decreased to normal or near-normal limits.
• Jaundice diminished, as evidenced by improved skin and sclera color.
• The neonate was free of complications, such as transfusion reaction or infection, after exchange transfusion.

For the neonate who underwent surgery, these additional evaluation statements may be appropriate.
• The neonate's vital signs remained normal.
• No signs of postoperative complications appeared.
• The suture line remained intact.
• The incision site remained clean and free of redness or swelling.

Documentation

All steps of the nursing process should be documented as thoroughly and objectively as possible. Thorough documentation not only allows the nurse to evaluate the effectiveness of the care plan, but it also makes this information available to other members of the health care team, helping to ensure consistency of care.

Documentation for the high-risk neonate should include the following points:
• vital signs and alertness level
• changes in status
• serum bilirubin, calcium, and glucose levels
• fluid intake and output
• stool characteristics
• tolerance for feedings
• location and appearance of any I.V. infusion site
• presence of any gastric distention
• presence of an indwelling nasogastric tube
• amount and appearance of secretions obtained by suctioning
• tolerance for medical and nursing procedures
• parents' level of acceptance of their child's problem.

For the neonate with respiratory problems, documentation also should include the following points:
• breathing effort
• any apneic episodes
• administration route and FiO_2 of supplemental oxygen (if given)
• ABG and $tcPO_2$ or pulse oximetry values
• ventilator pressure, rate, and positive end-expiratory pressure settings (if the neonate is on a mechanical ventilator).

For the neonate with a diagnosed infection, documentation also should include the following points:

• behavioral and physical changes indicative of infection
• the time when antibiotic therapy began and ended
• response to and tolerance of antibiotic therapy
• any cultures or blood samples taken.

For the neonate receiving phototherapy, documentation also should include the following points:
• number of stools
• skin turgor
• skin and sclera color
• amount and color of urine.

For the neonate who underwent exchange transfusion, documentation also should include the following points:
• tolerance for the procedure
• neurologic status.

For the neonate who underwent surgery, documentation also should include the following points:
• preoperative and postoperative vital signs
• the time when feedings were instituted
• tolerance for feedings
• respiratory effort
• appearance and amount of drainage from the incision site
• appearance of the suture line
• presence of bladder distention
• need for Credé's maneuver.

Chapter summary

This chapter described nursing care for the high-risk neonate. Here are the chapter highlights.
• Neonatal care is delivered in level 1, 2, and 3 nurseries; the level reflects the intensity of care provided. Many high-risk neonates require level 3 (intensive) care.
• Regionalization of neonatal care promotes high-quality care and allows the most efficient use of resources.
• The goals of neonatal intensive care include anticipation of perinatal problems, early intervention, and minimal disturbance of the neonate.
• In many cases, the birth of a high-risk neonate can be anticipated from maternal history findings or from antepartal, intrapartal, or fetal factors.
• Prompt recognition of actual or potential perinatal problems in the delivery room helps avert long-term complications.
• A gestational-age or birth-weight variation predisposes the neonate to perinatal problems. The preterm neonate is particularly at risk because general immaturity can cause dysfunction in any organ or system.

• Common problems seen among high-risk neonates include respiratory dysfunction, metabolic disorders, and congenital anomalies.

• Neonatal resuscitation proceeds in an orderly sequence, with each succeeding step based on the neonate's condition and response to the previous measure.

• When caring for a neonate receiving supplemental oxygen or mechanical ventilation, the nurse should monitor the neonate's oxygenation status continuously.

• Maintaining thermoregulation and ensuring fluid balance are particularly important for the high-risk neonate, who is at increased risk for hypothermia and fluid volume deficit.

• The nurse caring for a high-risk neonate must follow strict infection control guidelines.

• Developmental care has taken on increasing importance in the NICU. To provide such care, the nurse should reduce detrimental stimulation and provide appropriate stimulation according to the neonate's tolerance.

• The nurse should evaluate all care to determine the neonate's response to interventions and progress toward goals and must document assessment findings and nursing activities thoroughly.

Study questions

1. Which steps can the nurse take to identify the high-risk neonate?

2. Which maternal history findings suggest a potential perinatal problem?

3. Barbara Jenkins, born 2 hours ago, is exhibiting classic signs of respiratory distress. What are these signs?

4. What is the function of pulmonary surfactant in respiration?

5. How can the nurse help prevent complications of oxygen therapy in neonates?

6. Lina Lissman was born at 42 weeks' gestation weighing only 1,600 g. Describe some problems she may face as a postterm SGA neonate, and identify appropriate nursing assessment and interventions.

7. Born at 36 weeks' gestation, Marcus Glisson is a preterm neonate and thus is predisposed to hypothermia.

What are the physiologic reasons for this predisposition, and which nursing interventions can help prevent hypothermia?

Bibliography

Aloan, C.A. (1986). *Respiratory care of the newborn: A clinical manual.* Philadelphia: Lippincott.

American Academy of Pediatrics. (1988). *Guidelines for Perinatal Care* (2nd ed.). Chicago: Author.

American Heart Association and American Academy of Pediatrics. (1987). *Textbook of Neonatal Resuscitation.* Dallas.

Brann, A., and Schwartz, J.F. (1987). Developmental anomalies and neuromuscular disorders. In A. A. Fanaroff and R. J. Martin (Eds.), *Neonatal-perinatal medicine* (p. 540). St. Louis: Mosby.

Carlo, W.A., and Lough, M. (1988). *Neonatal Respiratory Care* (2nd ed.). Chicago: Year Book Medical Publishers.

Chatburn, R.L., and Carlo, W.A. (1988). Assessment of neonatal gas exchange. In W.A. Carlo and M. Lough (Eds.), *Neonatal Respiratory Care* (2nd ed.). Chicago: Year Book Medical Publishers.

Christensen, R.D., Rothstein, G., Hill, H., and Hall, R. (1985). Fatal early onset group B streptococcal sepsis with normal leukocyte counts. *Pediatric Infectious Disease Journal,* 4(3), 242-245.

Cummings, M.R. (1988). *Human Heredity: Principles and Issues* (pp. 382-383). St. Paul: West Publishing.

Duff, R.S., and Campbell, A.G.M. (1973). Moral and ethical dilemmas in the special-care nursery. *New England Journal of Medicine,* 289, 890-894.

Fanaroff, A.A., and Martin, R.J. (1987). *Behrman's neonatal-perinatal medicine: Diseases of the fetus or infant.* St. Louis: Mosby.

Goldsmith, J.P. and Karotkin, E.H. (1988). *Assisted ventilation of the neonate* (2nd ed.). Philadelphia: Saunders.

Hager, J.J. (1983). Characteristics and management of pregnancy in women with genital herpes simplex virus infection. *American Journal of Obstetrics and Gynecology,* 145, 784.

Harjo, J., Kenner, C., and Brueggermeyer, A. (1988). Alterations in effective breathing patterns. In C. Kenner, J. Harjo, and A. Brueggermeyer (Eds.), *Neonatal Surgery: A nursing perspective.* (pp. 79-120). Orlando, FL.: Grune & Stratton.

Harjo, J., Kenner, C., and Brueggermeyer, A. (1988). Alterations in the gastrointestinal system. In In C. Kenner, J. Harjo, and A. Brueggermeyer (Eds.), *Neonatal Surgery: A nursing perspective.* (pp. 121-189). Orlando, FL.: Grune & Stratton.

Harrison, M.R., Golbus, M.S., and Filly, R.A. (1984). *The unborn patient.* Orlando, FL: Grune & Stratton.

Hastreiter, A.R. (1988). Cardiovascular disease in the neonate. *Clinics in perinatology,* 15(3).

Hodson, W.A., and Truog, W.E. (1988). *Critical care of the newborn* (2nd ed.). Philadelphia: Saunders.

Jobe, A. (1988). *Surfactant replacement therapy.* Workshop presented at the National Perinatal Association Conference, Perinatal Health: Facing the 21st Century, San Diego, CA.

Kaempf, J.W., Bonnabel, C., and Hoy, W.W. (1989). Neonatal nutrition. In G.B. Merenstein and S.L. Gardner (Eds.), *Handbook of Neonatal Care* (p. 185). St. Louis: Mosby.

Kenner, C., Harjo, J., and Brueggemeyer, A. (1988). *Neonatal surgery: A nursing perspective.* Orlando, FL: Grune & Stratton.

Klaus, M.H., and Fanaroff, A.A. (1986). *Care of the high risk neonate.* Philadelphia: Saunders.

Kliegman, R.M., and Wald, M.K. (1986). Problems in metabolic adaptation: Glucose, calcium, and magnesium. In M.H. Klaus and A.A. Fanaroff (Eds.), *Care of the High Risk Neonate* (3rd ed.). Philadelphia: Saunders.

Liley, A.W. (1963). Intrauterine transfusion of foetus in hemolytic disease. *British Medical Journal,* 5365, 1107-1109.

Lough, M.D., Doershuk, C.F., and Stern, R.C. (1985). *Pediatric respiratory therapy* (3rd ed.). Chicago: Year Book Medical Publishers.

Lough, M.D., Williams, T.J., and Rawson, J.E. (1979). *Newborn respiratory care.* Chicago: Year Book Medical Publishers.

Merenstein, G.B., and Gardner, S.L. (1989). *Handbook of neonatal care.* St. Louis: Mosby.

McPherson, S.P. (1990). *Respiratory therapy equipment* (4th ed.). St. Louis: Mosby.

Moyer-Mileur, L.J. (1986). Nutrition. In N.S. Streeter (Ed.), *High-risk neonatal care* (p. 276). Rockville, MD: Aspen.

Nelson, S.N., Merenstein, G.B., and Pierce, J.R. (1986). Early onset group B streptococcal disease. *Journal of Perinatology,* 6, 234.

Nicolaides, K.H. (1989). Studies on fetal physiology and pathophysiology in Rhesus disease. *Seminars in Perinatology,* 13(4), 328-337.

Perlstein, P.H. (1988). The thermal environment. In A.A. Fanaroff and R.J. Martin (Eds.), *Behrman's neonatal-perinatal medicine: Diseases of the fetus or infant.* St. Louis: Mosby.

Philip, A.G.S. (1985). Noninvasive neonatal diagnosis. *Clinics in Perinatology,* 12(1).

Pringle, K.C. (1989). Fetal diagnosis and fetal surgery. *Clinics in Perinatology,* 16(1), 13-22.

Sammons, W.A.H., and Lewis, J.M. (1985). *Premature babies: A different beginning.* St. Louis: Mosby.

Sansone, D.M., and Grundy, E.E. (1986). *Newborn respiratory care: An equipment/lab manual.* Englewood Cliffs, NJ: Brady.

Streeter, N.S. (1986). *High-risk neonatal care.* Rockville, MD: Aspen.

Stern, L. (1987). The respiratory system in the newborn. *Clinics in Perinatology,* 14(3), 433-754.

Subramanian, K.N.S., Glass, P., Avery, G.B., Kolinjavadi, N., Keys, M.P, Sostek, A.M., and Friendly, D.S. (1985). Effect of bright light in the hospital nursery on the incidence of retinopathy of prematurity. *New England Journal of Medicine,* 313(7), 401-404.

Thibeault, D.W., and Gregory, G.A. (1986). *Neonatal pulmonary care* (2nd ed.). East Norwalk, CT: Appleton & Lange.

Weil, W.B., Bartholome, W.B., Bell, W.R., Diamond, E.F., and Fost, N.C. (1983). *American Academy of Pediatrics policy statement: Treatment of critically ill newborns.* Chicago: American Academy of Pediatrics.

Birth-weight and gestational-age variations

Boyd, M.E., Usher, R.H., McLean, F.H., and Kramer, M.S. (1988). Obstetric consequences of postmaturity. *American Journal of Obstetrics and Gynecology,* 158(2), 334-338.

Brar, H.S., and Rutherford, S.E. (1988). Classification of intrauterine growth retardation. *Seminars in Perinatology,* 12, 2-10.

Cassady, G., and Strange, M. (1987). The small-for-gestational-age (SGA) infant. In G.B. Avery (Ed.), *Neonatology: Pathophysiology and management of the newborn* (pp. 299-378). Philadelphia: Lippincott.

Chasnoff, I.J. (1988). Drug use in pregnancy: Parameters of risk. *Pediatric Clinics of North America,* 35(6), 1403-1412.

Creasy, R.K., and Resnick, R. (1989). Intrauterine growth retardation. In R.K. Creasy and R. Resnick (Eds.), *Maternal-fetal medicine: Principles and practice* (2nd ed.; pp. 547-564). Philadelphia: Saunders.

Eden, R.D., Seifert, L.S., Winegar, A., and Spellacy, W.N. (1987). Perinatal characteristics of uncomplicated postdate pregnancies. *Obstetrics and Gynecology,* 69, 296-299.

Lubchenco, L.O., and Koops, B.L. (1987). Assessment of weight and gestational age. In G.B. Avery (Ed.), *Neonatology: Pathophysiology and management of the newborn* (3rd ed.; pp. 235-257). Philadelphia: Lippincott.

Ounsted, M., Moar, V.A., and Scott, A. (1985). Risk factors associated with small-for-date and large-for-dates infants. *British Journal of Obstetrics and Gynecology,* 92, 226-232.

Phelan, J.P., Plah, L.P., Yeh, S.Y., Broussard, P. and Paul, R.H. (1985). The role of ultrasound assessment of amniotic fluid volume in the management of the post-date pregnancy. *American Journal of Obstetrics and Gynecology,* 151, 304-308.

Resnick, R. (1989). Post-term pregnancy. In R.K. Creasy and R. Resnick (Eds.), *Maternal-fetal medicine: Principles and practice* (2nd ed.; pp. 505-509). Philadelphia: Saunders.

Teberg, A.J., Walther, F.J., and Pena, I.C. (1988). Mortality, morbidity, and outcome of the small-for-gestational age infant. *Seminars in Perinatology,* 12, 84-94.

Usher, R.H., Boyd, M.E., McLean, F.H., and Kramer, M. S. (1988). Assessment of fetal risk in postdate pregnancies. *American Journal of Obstetrics and Gynecology,* 158, 259-264.

Vorherr, H. (1975). Placental insufficiency in relation to postterm pregnancy and fetal postmaturity. *American Journal of Obstetrics and Gynecology,* 123(1), 67-103.

Wright, J. (1986). Fetal alcohol syndrome. *Nursing Times,* 34-35.

Endotracheal suctioning

Gunderson, L.P., McPhee, A.J., and Donovan, E.F. (1986). Partially ventilated endotracheal suction in newborns with respiratory distress syndrome. *American Journal of Diseases of Children,* 14(5), 462-466.

Zmora, E., and Merritt, R. (1980). Use of side-hole endotracheal tube adaptor for tracheal aspiration. *American Journal of Diseases of Children,* 134, 250-254.

Failure to thrive and child abuse

Hunter, R.S., Kilstrum, N., Kraybill, E.N., and Loda, F. (1978). Antecedents of child abuse and neglect in premature infants: A prospective study in a newborn intensive care unit. *Pediatrics,* 61(4), 629-635.

White, R., Benedict, M.I., Wulff, L., and Kelley, M. (1987). Physical disabilities as risk factors for child maltreatment: A selected review. *American Journal of Orthopsychiatry,* 57(1), 93-101.

Maternal substance abuse

Anderson, R.C. (1986). The effects of alcohol consumption during pregnancy. *American Association of Occupational Health Nurse Journal,* 34(2), 88-91.

Bates, C.K. (1988). Medical risks of cocaine use. *Western Journal of Medicine,* 148(4), 440-444.

Bowen, O.R., and Sammons, J.H. (1988). The alcohol-abusing patient: A challenge to the profession. *JAMA,* 260(15), 2267-2270.

Braude, M.C., Szeto, H.H., Kuhn, C.M., Bero, L., Ignar, O., Field, E., Lurie, S., Chasnoff, I.J., Mendelson, J.H., Zuckerman, B., Hingson, R., Frank, D., Parker, S., Vinci, R., Kayne, N., Morelock, S., Amaro, H., Kyei-Aboage, K., and Howard, J. (1987). Perinatal effects of drugs of abuse. *Federation Proceedings,* 46(7), 2446-2453.

Chappel, J.N. (1987). Alcohol and drug dependencies: How to spot; What steps to take. *Consultant,* 27(4), 60-64, 66, 71.

Chasnoff, I.J., Burns, W.J., Schnoll, S.H. and Burns, K.A. (1985). Cocaine use in pregnancy. *New England Journal of Medicine,* 313, 666-669.

Chasnoff, I.J., Bussey, M.E., Savich, R., and Stack, C.M. (1986). Perinatal cerebral infarction and maternal cocaine use. *Journal of Pediatrics,* 108(3), 456-459.

Chasnoff, I.J., Burns, K.A., and Burns, W.J. (1987). Cocaine use in pregnancy: Perinatal morbidity and mortality. *Neurotoxicology and Teratology,* 9(4), 291-293.

Cherukuri, S, Minkorff, H., Feldman, J., Parekh, A., and Glass, L. (1988). Cohort study of alkaloidal cocaine "crack" in pregnancy. *Obstetrics and Gynecology,* 72(2), 147-151.

Critchley, H.O.D., Woods, S.M., Barson, A.J., Richardson, T., and Leberman, B.A. (1988). Fetal death in utero and cocaine abuse. Case report. *British Journal of Obstetrics and Gynecology,* 95, 195-196.

Doberzak, R.M., Shanzer, S., Senie, R.T., and Kandall, S.R. (1988). Neonatal neurologic and electroencephalographic effects of intrauterine cocaine exposure. *Pediatrics,* 113, 354-358.

Flandermeyer, A.A. (1987). A comparison of the effects of heroin and cocaine abuse upon the neonate. *Neonatal Network,* 6(3), 42-48.

Gunby, P. (1988). Warning label required for alcohol containers, *Journal of the American Medical Association,* 260(21), 3109.

Jones, K.L. (1986). Fetal alcohol syndrome. *Pediatrics in review,* 8(4), 122-126.

Kennard, M. J. (1990). Cocaine use during pregnancy: Fetal and neonatal effects. *Journal of Perinatal and Neonatal Nursing,* 3(9), 53-63.

Madden, J.D., Payne, R.F., and Miller, S. (1986). Maternal cocaine abuse and effect on the newborn. *Pediatrics,* 77(2), 209-211.

Pinto, F., Torrioli, M.G., Tempesta, E., and Fundaro, C. (1988). Sleep in babies born to chronically heroin addicted mothers. A follow up study. *Drug and Alchohol Dependence,* 21, 43-47.

Schneider, J.W., and Chasnoff, I.J. (1987). Cocaine abuse during pregnancy: Its effects on infant motor development—A clinical perspective. *Topics in Acute Care and Trauma Rehabilitation,* 2(1), 59-69.

Smith, J. (1988). The dangers of prenatal cocaine use. *MCN,* 13, 174-179.

Neonatal mortality

Institute of Medicine. (1985). *Preventing low birth weight.* Washington, DC: National Academy Press.

National Center for Health Statistics. (1989, March 28). *Monthly vital statistics report—Births, marriages, divorces, and deaths for 1988.* U.S. Dept. of Health and Human Services Publication No. (PHS) 89-1120. Hyattsville, MD: U.S. Public Health Service.

National Center for Health Statistics. (1989, June 29). *Monthly vital statistics report—Advance report of final natality statistics, 1987.* U.S. Dept. of Health and Human Services, 38, (3). Hyattsville, MD: U.S. Public Health Service.

Nursing research

Cabal, L., Devaskar, S., Siassi, B., Plajsteck, C., Waffarn, G., Blanco, C., and Hodgman, J. (1979). New endotracheal tube adaptor reducing cardiopulmonary effects of suctioning. *Critical Care Medicine,* 7, 552-555.

Meier, P. (1988, January-February). Bottle- and Breast-feeding: Effects on transcutaneous oxygen pressure and temperature in preterm infants. *Nursing Research,* 37(1), 36-41.

Care of the Families of High-Risk Neonates

Objectives

After reading and studying this chapter, the student should be able to:

1. Identify concerns of the family of a high-risk neonate.

2. Identify the stages of grief as they apply to the family of a high-risk neonate.

3. Describe nursing interventions that help the family cope with a high-risk neonate.

4. Implement strategies to encourage parent interaction with a high-risk neonate.

5. Understand cultural differences in family responses to the crisis created by the birth of a high-risk neonate.

6. Identify interventions that provide support to the family of a neonate who dies.

Introduction

With the birth of a high-risk neonate (one who is preterm or very ill), family members experience a sense of loss. Even the family of a preterm neonate who becomes healthy enough to leave the neonatal intensive care unit (NICU) within a few weeks must work through some grief at the loss of the expected "perfect" child before they can bond strongly to the imperfect one. The family of a neonate with a chronic illness or congenital anomaly must find ways to cope with long-term grief and develop strategies to provide the special care the condition will require (and perhaps to balance these care needs with those of other children). If the neonate is stillborn or dies within a few hours or days after birth, family members must complete their bonding with the neonate, then

detach themselves gradually so they can focus again on the family's life and needs.

In such situations, nursing care must meet the family's psychosocial as well as physical needs. To provide this kind of care in the first weeks after the birth of a high-risk neonate, the nurse must:

• understand the function of grief

• recognize the stages of grief in individual family members

• assess how family members are responding to and coping with the crisis of the high-risk neonate

• identify and implement strategies to help family members cope

• help family members identify support systems that can provide further help

• teach family members about the condition and care of the high-risk neonate

• maintain empathetic contact with family members as they work to integrate care of the high-risk neonate into family life.

This chapter explains how the nurse can help the family deal with their own needs as well as those of the high-risk neonate. It begins by describing typical responses of family members to the birth of a high-risk neonate. It defines the stages of grief, explaining how family members typically progress through them and how the experience and expression of grief may vary according to individual situations and cultural norms. The chapter then shows how to use the nursing process to help the family cope with the birth of a high-risk neonate, form a bond with the neonate, and begin to deal with long-term concerns. This section also includes in-

---

GLOSSARY

Anticipatory grief: sadness in anticipation of loss.
Bonding: process through which an emotional attachment forms, which binds one person to another in an enduring relationship, as between parents and infant.
Coping mechanism: mechanism by which a person handles stress and anxiety.
Grief: intense sadness experienced after the loss of a valued person or object.
Grief process: cycle that follows a loss; the Kübler-Ross model progresses from denial through anger, bargaining, and depression to acceptance (stages may overlap or regress and may be repeated many times before acceptance is complete).

Mourning: actions or expression of grief.
Pathologic mourning: mourning that does not lead to resolution of grief.
Perinatal period: period extending from the twenty-eighth week of gestation to the end of the fourth week after birth.
Preterm neonate: neonate born before completion of the thirty-seventh week of gestation.
Tertiary care center: facility capable of providing care for the most critically ill neonates; has highly technological equipment and specially trained personnel.

---

terventions that help the family deal with perinatal and fetal death.

Family reactions

To the family, the birth of a high-risk neonate may seem like a tragedy. Over the course of the pregnancy, they built expectations of a child whose features would reflect their own, whose abilities they could nurture, and whose interests they would share. With the neonate's birth, the family experiences the loss of the "perfect" child of their dreams. They must deal with that loss and the grief it causes and find ways of adjusting their expectations and plans to match the reality of the child born to them.

To understand the feelings experienced by the family of a high-risk neonate—and thus better anticipate their needs—the nurse must be familiar with the stages of grief and the coping mechanisms family members may use to deal with their sense of loss.

Grief

Because of the enormity of a perinatal loss, parents and other family members must adapt slowly to the situation—or experience overwhelming anxiety and pain. The degree of parental feelings of grief do not correlate with the severity of the neonate's condition (Benefield, Leib, and Reuter, 1976).

Before the family can accept their loss, they must progress through several stages of grief. Various researchers and theorists have developed concepts of grieving. Among the most influential is that of Kübler-Ross (1969), who proposed that a person encountering death or another type of loss progresses through five stages: denial, anger, bargaining, depression, and acceptance. Sahu (1981) and other authorities apply these stages specifically to perinatal loss. Based on studies by Bowlby (1961) and Parkes (1970) as well as on original research, thanatologist Glen Davidson (1984) describes four phases, or dimensions, of grief that survivors of loss may move among: shock and numbness, yearning and searching, disorientation, and reorganization.

Regardless of the grief model used, the nurse should regard the stages of grief as descriptive rather than clearly defined. Rather than progressing through the stages in an orderly manner, the parents and other family members may experience aspects of several stages at once or may regress to a stage previously experienced.

Denial

In this first stage, the parents attempt to deny the reality or seriousness of their child's condition; this allows them to hope that the child may improve. They cannot let go abruptly of the hopes and dreams they developed during the pregnancy. By postponing recognition of their child's condition, they protect themselves until they are ready to face and cope with the situation.

Anger

As awareness of the situation develops, the parents progress to this stage. Anger may take the form of resentment, bitterness, rage, blaming, or envy of others with healthy neonates. Needing to hold something or someone accountable for their child's condition, parents may direct their anger outward. For instance, they may accuse members of the health care team of not caring properly for their child; or they may accuse each other of some past action that caused the situation—for example, the mother's smoking during pregnancy. Some parents, especially those who cannot express their anger, may direct their feelings inward, becoming depressed and guilt-ridden as they blame themselves for their child's condition.

Bargaining

During this stage, a parent may be willing to do anything that might help the neonate or delay the perinatal loss. Bargaining may involve religious beliefs ("I'll go to church every Sunday if God will let my baby get better") or the desire to try new forms of medical therapy.

Depression

In this stage, feelings of hopelessness, powerlessness, or despair predominate. Some depressed parents put their feelings into words; others become noncommunicative and wish to be left alone. Still others, such as the previously well-groomed parent who begins neglecting his or her appearance, signal depression through behavior. As long as it does not continue for an excessive time, this stage represents real progress toward acceptance because it signals recognition of the neonate's situation and its potential impact on the present and future.

Acceptance

This final stage, which takes most people at least several months and can take as long as 2 years to achieve, is marked by resumption of normal daily activity and diminishing preoccupation with the loss (Lindemann, 1944). Parents whose child has died continue to experience sadness when they remember their loss; at certain times, such as the anniversary of the child's birth or death, they again may pass through denial, anger, and depression (all usually less acute) before returning to acceptance. However, they manage to incorporate the memory of their loss into their lives and move on.

For the family of a child who survives with a chronic disability, however, complete acceptance may be difficult or even impossible to achieve. The chronic condition necessitates continual adaptation and coping; the disability and the limitations it places on the child's life remain a constant cause of sorrow (Lemons, 1986). Olshansky (1962) termed this persistent effect *chronic sorrow.*

Coping mechanisms

Parents may use various coping mechanisms to deal with the sadness and worry they feel for a high-risk neonate. Denial and anger, the first and second stages of grief, are coping mechanisms; so are withdrawal (one manifestation of depression, the fourth stage) and guilt (the

form anger takes if it turns inward). A fifth method of coping is intellectualizing.

Denial

Shock and disbelief are the most common first reactions to the birth of a high-risk neonate (Tarbert, 1985). Although denial serves a protective purpose for a brief time, as long as parents cling to denial they cannot participate in care decisions or make realistic plans. Should the neonate die, they may be unable to grieve successfully.

Anger

Anger and hostility may succeed denial as parents attempt to deal with their shock (Brooten, et al., 1988). Needing a way to feel power over their situation, parents may direct their anger against the health care team, blaming them for their child's condition.

Guilt

Many parents of a high-risk neonate try to cope with their powerlessness through guilt, telling themselves that they did something to cause their child's abnormality or failed to do something to prevent it (Cordell and Apolito, 1981). Like denial and anger, guilt is a mechanism parents must move beyond to function effectively.

Withdrawal

Parents who have progressed to the stage of depression in the grief process may withdraw emotionally to protect themselves from the anticipated pain of losing their child. Even though they may visit regularly, they invest little energy into building a parent-child relationship.

Intellectualizing

Some parents attempt to retreat from the painful emotions they feel by searching for meaning in the situation; knowing about such matters as blood values and oxygen levels can give them something to focus on. These parents need the assurance of receiving accurate information and having their questions answered carefully, but they also may need help to refocus on the neonate.

Assessment

For an accurate assessment of the family of a high-risk neonate, the nurse must thoroughly assess family members and evaluate the support systems available to them.

During the assessment, the nurse should keep in mind the various stages of grief; this helps identify the family's need for practical and emotional support. Because parents usually are the family members most closely involved with the neonate, this chapter focuses mainly on them. However, the nurse should not overlook the neonate's siblings, grandparents, and other close family members.

Parents

Already upset by the arrival of a high-risk neonate, parents may feel further stress within the NICU, with its sophisticated equipment, flashing monitors, buzzing alarms, and hurrying staff members. For this reason, the nurse should try to conduct the assessment in a quiet, unhurried, and straightforward manner; this helps to calm parents and reassure them that the health care team is concerned for their well-being.

Assessment of the parents should include the following:
• age, experience as parents, and history of previous childbirths
• understanding of and feelings about the neonate's condition
• concerns about the neonate's care
• family and home care arrangements
• response to the NICU
• grieving behavior and coping mechanisms.

Age, experience, and history

Find out the parents' age and their experience as parents. Young or first-time parents may have little experience dealing with illness. Especially if they are young enough to require parenting themselves, they may feel particularly inadequate about coping with a high-risk neonate.

Ask about any family history of problem pregnancies or deliveries. Parents who have experienced a previous perinatal illness or death may fear or believe that the past problem and this one are related. Even if their anxiety is inappropriate, it may impair their ability to cope with their neonate. On the other hand, parents whose earlier pregnancies and deliveries were problem-free may have trouble accepting that this delivery has produced a high-risk neonate.

To determine whether genetic counseling might be advisable eventually, look for indications of a genetic cause for the neonate's condition. Ask about the presence, in this or previous generations, of such conditions as inherited disorders, metabolic disorders, or chromosomal disorders. Even if parents are not aware of any history of these problems, such a condition in the neonate suggests a genetic link (Fibison and James, 1985).

Understanding and feelings

Ask parents what they understand about their child's condition and how it makes them feel. Although grief and anxiety are natural reactions to the delivery of a neonate who is preterm or born with a severe illness or an obvious physical anomaly, parents may feel perinatal loss for other reasons as well. Because of the value society places on physical beauty, any physical irregularity may cause great anxiety. (Even the birth of a neonate who is healthy but not of the desired sex or whose physical features differ from the expected ones can result in a sense of loss.) Knowing the cause of the parents' grief is essential in planning interventions to help them deal with it; even if their grief seems out of proportion, it is real and must be addressed.

Here and throughout the assessment, stay alert for signs of stress developing between the parents. For example, if only one parent has been given some information, the other may feel excluded. If the mother has not been able to see the neonate since the delivery, she may resent what feels to her like exclusion; also, her idea of the neonate's condition may be incorrect. The father, meanwhile, may feel he is protecting her by not describing the condition in detail.

Concerns about care of the neonate and its effects

To determine where counseling and teaching can decrease anxiety, explore the parents' feelings about their ability to care for their child. They may express doubt about being able to care for their child at home and may worry about financial consequences of giving up work days to spend time with their child and about long-term medical expenses.

Also look and listen for signs of emotional discomfort. A parent who feels anxious and powerless may have trouble absorbing and putting into practice information about caregiving. A parent who hesitates to participate in simple neonatal care may be establishing emotional distance from the neonate.

Family and home care arrangements

Ask parents about arrangements they have made for care of other children at home and other family concerns. Even parents who have made adequate care arrangements may worry that they are short-changing their other children. Assess whether they need help allocating their time or arranging care for the children.

Ask parents how their other children are responding to the birth of a high-risk neonate. Under these circumstances, an older child's relationship with the parents may change (Trahd, 1986). However, parents may not be aware of this in the first days and weeks, when the neonate holds so much of their attention. Most parents probably realize that siblings are likely to feel neglected or jealous because of the disruptions in routine and the time parents spend at the NICU. However, parents may not be aware of other feelings the high-risk neonate may evoke, including fear and guilt that they somehow are responsible for the neonate's illness. Asking what responses parents have noticed may help them relate better with their other children and also will help focus teaching plans for preparing the neonate's siblings to visit the NICU.

Response to the NICU

Ask parents what previous experience they have had with health care facilities. The less experience they have, or the less recent their experience, the more unsettling they may find the NICU and the more help they may need in understanding that many of the procedures and equipment that seem extraordinary actually are routine.

The apparent ease with which the NICU staff functions may increase parents' doubts about their own ability to provide care, especially if no one explains what is happening and why. To plan ways to make parents more comfortable in the NICU, ask how much they understand about the equipment being used to help their child and invite questions about the care being given.

Also assess the effect of the NICU location on the developing parent-infant bond and on the relationship between the parents. For most parents, the ideal situation is an NICU located within the mother's obstetric unit. Here, both parents can visit the neonate in the first few days after delivery with little or no trouble. However, if the neonate must be transferred to a distant tertiary care facility, only the father may be able to visit for the first several days. Ask whether the mother was able to spend time with the neonate before the transfer and what effect the transfer has had on each parent. Particularly if the mother did not see the neonate before the transfer, she may feel isolated and resentful of the father's greater contact (Consolvo, 1984); the father, meanwhile, may feel uncomfortable in the primary parent role in which circumstances have placed him.

If the NICU is relatively far from the home, neither parent may be able to visit frequently. Assess for signs that the parents' lack of physical contact is delaying parent-infant bonding. Without such bonding, their interest and motivation may not be strong enough to meet their child's long-term needs.

Grieving behavior and coping mechanisms

Throughout the neonate's hospitalization, parents typically exhibit signs of grief. Determine each parent's grief stage (as described in the "Family reactions" section). However, keep in mind that grief expression may depend somewhat on cultural background. (For details on this topic, see *Cultural considerations: Variations in grief expression,* page 990.)

Also determine which coping mechanism each parent is using—denial, anger, guilt, intellectualizing, or withdrawal. (Remember, though, that coping mechanisms may vary from day to day or even moment to moment.) Accurately identifying the coping mechanisms that parents use is crucial to planning nursing interventions that respond to their needs.

To assess for denial, look for signs that parents are denying the reality of the neonate's condition. Normally, parents move beyond denial on their own, so assess for signs that this transition is occurring; if it is not, they may require help.

If parents exhibit anger or hostility (such as toward the health care team), assess for any misunderstanding of the neonate's condition. Keep in mind that angry parents usually are reacting to the situation and rarely feel real hostility toward health care personnel.

Clues that a parent is using guilt to cope include such obvious statements as, "It's all my fault" as well as more subtle indications, such as utterances beginning with "If only I..." In guilt statements, listen for misunderstandings of the causes of the neonate's condition.

Parents who focus on the cause of their child's condition more than on the neonate as a person are using intellectualizing as a coping mechanism. These parents may ask many questions about their child's treatment and seem hesitant to focus on the child.

Assess for withdrawal by observing how the parents relate to their child. Withdrawn parents may not touch or hold their child or may look away while doing so.

Support systems

Coping with the birth of a high-risk neonate is not something that one parent—or even both—can handle alone. Parents need help from various sources. The nurse should assess parents for the support systems they use actively and for their awareness of other potential sources of support.

Family and friends

For most parents, the first line of support comes from within the family. In a two-parent family, the partners typically form each other's base of support. If one parent is unavailable—for example, as in the case of a single mother—another family member or a close friend may assume the support role. Assess parents to determine which family members or close friends make up their

---

Variations in grief expression

To evaluate grieving behavior accurately in a family that has experienced or anticipates a neonate's death, the nurse must be aware of any cultural customs that may affect grief expression. However, the nurse should assess carefully before drawing conclusions. Although some cultures are associated with characteristic grieving behaviors, practices change over time. Also, a person born into one culture but socialized in another may be influenced by elements of both.

Black Americans, Mexican Americans, and Arabs tend to display grief openly. Chinese and Japanese cultures frown on public display of emotion; consequently, members of a traditional Chinese or Japanese family may not respond to the nurse's encouragement to communicate their feelings, although they may grieve quietly at home. Members of certain Native American tribes also may not express grief openly. Also, some may refuse to visit a dying neonate out of fear of modern medicine or "evil spirits" (York and Stichler, 1985).

Some Hispanic cultures regard public expression of grief as acceptable for the mother but not the father, in whom such expression is considered a sign of weakness. (Of course, such attitudes may show up in any family, regardless of culture.) In a few cultures, handling of the body is part of the formalized expression of grief.

In certain Asian cultures, where one does not give up hope for survival until death has occurred, anticipatory grief (sadness in anticipation of a neonate's expected death) is considered inappropriate (Manio and Hall, 1987). Also, not all cultures perceive a neonate's death as a tragic event (York and Stichler, 1985). For example, in Korean tradition, more concern is focused on the parents than on the dead neonate; as adults, the parents are considered more important members of the family and society than the neonate, whose life had just begun (Choi, 1986).

Although both individual and culturally shaped expressions of grief deserve respect and support, family members occasionally need guidance to avoid manifestations or attitudes that might harm themselves or others. For example, in some Asian cultures, the mother may be blamed for causing the neonate's condition by something she did or ate (Manio and Hall, 1987); in such a case, the nurse and physician must do their best to help the mother and family understand the true cause and to dissolve any feelings of guilt or blame.

The following religious beliefs can affect the amount of grief family members feel and the practices they follow after a neonate's death:
• belief in an afterlife
• acceptance of death as God's will
• belief that the soul returns to the ancestors or reincarnates in another body
• belief that spirits control illness and death
• belief in the value of religious rituals for the dead.

support base and how nursing care can assist the supporters.

Ask about the relationship between the neonate's parents and grandparents. In many cases, grandparents can provide both emotional and practical support. Be aware, however, that grandparents may require some assistance to function most effectively as support persons for the parents. (For a related study, see *Nursing research applied: Parents' and grandparents' reactions to the birth of a preterm neonate.*)

Other support sources
Beyond the circle of family and friends, additional support may be available to parents through religious practices, cultural customs, and support groups consisting of other parents.

Religious practices. The birth of a high-risk neonate may pull the parents back to their religious roots. They may find comfort in speaking with a member of the clergy, reading scripture, or participating in religious services. Assess parents for their interest in seeing a chaplain or their own priest, minister, or rabbi. Ask whether they would like any religious practices to be observed for their neonate; members of some Christian churches, for example, may wish to have their child baptized. Even parents who might not think of asking for such support may use it if they know it is available.

Cultural customs. If cultural identity is important to the family, they may derive additional support from observing traditional care customs with their child. In assessing cultural customs, however, bear in mind that although cultural norms exist, variations do occur. Also, the beliefs one generation holds to strongly may be less important to a second or third generation. Athough an overall awareness of such beliefs is helpful, assess the parents for their own beliefs as individuals.

Begin the cultural assessment by asking about the main elements of values and beliefs the parents hold and the customs these values dictate regarding childbirth in general and the birth of a high-risk neonate in particular. Then focus on specific care concerns parents may want addressed.

Support groups. Assess parents for their awareness of parent-to-parent support groups—including national organizations, local groups, and groups associated with the health care facility.

NURSING RESEARCH APPLIED

Parents' and grandparents' reactions to the birth of a preterm neonate

Although many neonatal intensive care units (NICUs) use a family-centered approach, the "family" typically is limited to the neonate's parents. The needs and responses of additional family members rarely have been addressed. Thus, although grandparents may be regarded as ideal sources of support for the neonate's parents, they get little help in dealing with their own feelings.

To explore the feelings and perceptions of grandparents and parents to the birth of a preterm neonate—and thus improve intergenerational care in the NICU—the researchers conducted a retrospective exploratory survey of 83 grandparents and 50 parents of preterm neonates who had spent 6 to 12 weeks in an NICU. Subjects answered a questionnaire consisting of open-ended and fixed-response items. The questionnaires given to grandparents and parents were similar in content.

Findings showed that about one-third of both the grandparents and parents felt that the neonate looked worse than expected, and that mothers were the group most unprepared for the appearance of the NICU. One-third of the grandparents expressed negative views of the appearance of the NICU and of the neonate's suffering.

Grandparents and parents had differing perceptions of NICU grandparental visiting policies. Although 61% of parents believed that the health care facility restricted grandparent visits, only 25% of the grandparents felt that their visiting privileges had been restricted. These restrictions evoked anger in 19% of the mothers and 6% of grandmothers. Also, about half of the respondents believed grandparents' activities had been restricted during their visits to the NICU; about 25% of parents and 7% of grandparents disliked these restrictions. During their visits, 57% of grandparents entered the neonate's room, 40% were allowed to touch the neonate, and 20% were allowed to hold the neonate.

All four groups (mothers, fathers, grandmothers, and grandfathers) indicated they had felt intense anxiety about the neonate's condition, but parents reported much more intense fear than did grandparents. Grandmothers experienced such emotions as shock and grief, although less intensely than mothers.

For both parents and grandparents, the spouse was the main source of emotional support. However, one-third of the mothers indicated that they received less emotional support than they needed—a greater percentage than for grandparents and fathers. Most parents sought out and received information about the neonate from nurses, physicians, or experienced parents. Grandparents, on the other hand, relied on the parents for information.

Seventy percent of grandparents identified specific concerns they had about the neonate's parents, including their ability to cope with the situation, physical and emotional strain, and the financial implications of their child's hospitalization. Nearly half of the grandmothers identified concerns about their ability to cope and about the emotional strain they experienced. Parents and grandparents had similar concerns about the neonate; however, compared to parents, grandparents were less concerned about the neonate's survival than about the neonate's intellectual development.

Application to practice
The findings of this study suggest that nurses could intervene more effectively to provide family-centered care by being more sensitive to the unique needs of grandparents after the birth of a preterm neonate. For example, giving grandparents access to accurate information might relieve some of the burden on the parents to provide information about the neonate's status. Also, opportunities for emotional support and education might help decrease grandparents' anxiety and thus help them support the neonate's parents; this, in turn, would reaffirm the grandparents' important role in the family. The authors indicate the need for prospective study and a larger sample size to explore the responses and experiences of extended family members to the birth of a preterm neonate.

Blackburn, S., and Lowen, L. (1986). Impact of an infant's premature birth on the grandparents and parents. *JOGNN*, 15(2), 173-178.

Nursing diagnosis

After gathering assessment data, the nurse must review it carefully to identify pertinent nursing diagnoses for the family. (For a partial list of applicable diagnoses, see *Nursing diagnoses: Family of a high-risk neonate*, page 992.)

Planning and implementation

After assessing the family and formulating nursing diagnoses, the nurse develops and implements a plan of care. The goal of nursing care is to help the family develop the understanding, skills, and confidence to give competent care after the neonate's discharge. Thus, the nurse should plan interventions to help them deal with the crisis of a high-risk neonate and to meet the neonate's needs. Such interventions should focus on the neonate's

---

NURSING DIAGNOSES

Family of a high-risk neonate

The following are potential nursing diagnoses for problems and etiologies that a nurse may encounter in caring for the family of a high-risk neonate. Specific nursing interventions for many of these diagnoses are provided in the "Planning and implementation" section of this chapter.

- Anticipatory grieving related to the prospect of the neonate's death
- Anxiety related to the neonate's condition and unknown outcome
- Defensive coping related to the seriousness of the neonate's condition and long-term implications
- Denial related to immediate and long-term implications of the neonate's condition
- Ineffective family coping: compromised, related to family disorganization secondary to the neonate's condition
- Ineffective individual coping related to family disorganization secondary to the neonate's condition
- Ineffective individual coping related to the stress of a preterm birth
- Knowledge deficit related to the hospital course and care of the high-risk neonate
- Parental role conflict related to limited opportunities to care for the neonate
- Potential altered parenting related to poor parent-infant bonding
- Powerlessness related to the health care environment and limited interaction with the neonate

---

physical and developmental needs and the family's practical and emotional needs.

Whenever possible, involve family members in planning. This not only helps ensure that they can carry out the planned interventions, but it also makes them active participants in their child's care. Such involvement particularly helps the family with a nursing diagnosis of *powerlessness related to the health care environment and limited interaction with the neonate.*

Interventions for the family of a high-risk neonate fall into four main categories:
- providing information
- strengthening support systems
- teaching caregiving skills
- enhancing parent-infant bonding.

Depending on the neonate's status, the nurse also may need to help the family plan for their child's discharge or help them cope with their child's death.

Provide information

Two nursing diagnoses that apply to almost every family of a high-risk neonate are *knowledge deficit related to*

the hospital course and care of a high-risk neonate and *anxiety related to the neonate's condition and unknown outcome.* Nursing care is essential in helping the family with either diagnosis. In many cases, the family relies mainly on the nurse—not just for information but for help in understanding that information. Although the physician initially may identify the neonate's medical condition to the parents and may speak with them regularly, the nurse typically provides daily reports and thus may be the person to whom parents turn with questions.

The more thorough the parents' understanding, the better equipped they will be to cope with the crisis and achieve the eventual goal of adequate caregiving at home. To give them the most complete picture possible, cover the following topics:
- the neonate's medical condition, its cause (if known), and its long-term implications
- potential length of stay and probable course of treatment in the NICU
- ways parents can enhance their contact with their child
- ways parents can participate in their child's care.

Present, reinforce, and reinterpret
Such factors as familiarity with health care facilities, previous experience with health problems, and emotional state affect parents' ability to comprehend information the health care team gives them. Thus, adapt teaching strategies to parents' needs and assess the parents' comprehension frequently.

Recognize emotional blocks to understanding. Especially during denial, the first stage of grief, parents may not absorb all the information they receive about their child's condition. Although parents with a nursing diagnosis of *denial related to the immediate and long-term implications of the neonate's condition* can be frustrating to work with, the problem arises from grief. Acknowledge the parents' feelings, but persist, presenting the information in small chunks and reinforcing it patiently. Eventually, parents will move beyond denial and begin to take in the facts.

Review and clarify. Even after progressing past denial, parents may need help to grasp their child's condition fully. Try to be present whenever the physician talks with them, and review any new information with them afterward to clarify uncertainties and correct misunderstandings. Invite their questions, and encourage them to talk over what they have learned.

Once parents become hungry for information, they may seek it constantly—for example, in conversation with other parents with children in the NICU. Listen for

CULTURAL CONSIDERATIONS

Incorporating cultural customs into the neonate's care routine

When caring for a client from a different culture, the nurse should keep the following considerations in mind.

Although nearly all parents feel intimidated during their first visit to the neonatal intensive care unit (NICU), those who have deep religious beliefs or belong to an ethnic group with strong cultural identity and traditional health practices may feel particularly uncomfortable. To help reduce their anxiety, the nurse should find out if their customs include any health-related practices (for example, folk remedies). Practices that pose no health threat, or that can be modified so they do not, can be incorporated fairly easily into the neonate's care routine.

For instance, to prevent the escape of spirits or the entrance of "bad air" into the body, mothers in some Hispanic cultures wrap their child in an abdominal binder or cover the umbilical stump with a coin (Zepeda, 1982). Neither custom can be permitted as is—the binder could restrict breathing or cause vomiting and a coin covering an incompletely healed stump could cause infection. However, the nurse may suggest covering the stump with a dry, sterile dressing; if necessary, a cauterizing agent, such as silver nitrate, can be applied to heal the stump rapidly before the neonate's discharge.

Various folk remedies involve protection from evil spirits by such means as medallions, crosses, special clothes, prayer cards, and candles. If having such items near their child would comfort the parents, the nurse may tape them to the wall, hang them on the outside of the crib, or place them on a nearby table. As long as the candles remain unlit, even they can be placed near the neonate.

Parents with deep religious beliefs may welcome the opportunity to place devotional objects near their child. The nurse may tape religious medals or scapulars to an armboard, diaper, or crib frame or place pictures or books on a nearby table.

Augment spoken information. To give parents a clearer idea of neonatal care procedures, use any available illustrations or photographs. Also, provide information booklets, written in lay terms, that address the neonate's condition. (Several national support groups, such as the March of Dimes, publish such booklets.) As they read this material at home, they may develop a better understanding of what they have been told.

Reassure parents about their responses. Parents may need help in understanding what is happening to them emotionally. Explain that anxiety, fear, anger, and guilt are common among parents of high-risk neonates. To provide further reassurance and help them deal with their feelings, discuss the stages of grief.

Familiarize parents with the NICU

To most parents, the NICU is an alien and frightening environment. To make them feel more comfortable, describe the neonate's care routine, identifying each piece of equipment used and explaining its purpose. Be aware that anything attached to the neonate—even a temperature probe taped to the abdomen—may look threatening. If a new piece of equipment is introduced after the parents' first visit, explain its purpose and operation. Also encourage parents to enliven their child's surroundings with photographs or toys. If they have other children, suggest that parents ask them to draw pictures to tape near their child's incubator or crib. (For further suggestions on personalizing the NICU, see *Cultural considerations: Incorporating cultural customs into the neonate's care routine.*)

Outline the course of treatment

As far as possible, explain the probable course the neonate's treatment will take and the time that may be involved. In the case of a preterm neonate, for example, explain that feedings may need to be instituted slowly and that physical growth probably will be slow but steady unless unexpected complications arise. Prepare parents for the chance that their child may need oxygen therapy or assisted ventilation at some point.

Be realistic

An insistent question among parents of high-risk neonates is whether their child will survive. A problem that the health care team regards as minor may seem to parents like a sign of impending death. While not playing down the likelihood of death if the neonate's condition is life-threatening, do not minimize the chance for survival, either. Advise parents that although the usual hospital course of a high-risk neonate is unstable at best, the health care team may be surprised by the amount of fight in even the smallest and sickest neonate.

---

such conversations, and intervene if necessary to clarify differences so that parents do not expect their child to have the same course of illness as another with a different diagnosis or maturity level.

Recognize parents' concerns. In seeking information, parents' main concerns may differ from those of the health care team. For example, they may focus on their child's long-term problems before short-term problems have been overcome. During parents' conversations with the physician and in review sessions afterward, make sure they receive the information they need, but also support them by noting and following up on their concerns.

Maintain communication

For the parents with a nursing diagnosis of *potential altered parenting related to poor parent-infant bonding*, foster attachment and reduce anxiety by letting them know by frequent communication that they are welcome partners in their child's care. Even if the parents visit frequently, encourage them to phone daily. Initiate calls to them from time to time simply to give progress reports or to check with them about points brought up in their last visit. Include news of milestones achieved by their child, such as a weight gain, as well as a condition update.

If parents live so far away that daily phone calls are too costly, write them a note every few days to give them a sense of their child's course between one visit and the next. If possible, occasionally include a photograph of their child.

Strengthen support systems

The family of a high-risk neonate needs a tremendous amount of support—to deal with their feelings, to balance their responsibilities and reorganize their routines, to allocate their time and energy, and to find ways to cope with the practical and financial burdens of caring for their child. The nurse should plan interventions that help parents make good use of the support sources they know of and identify other potential sources.

Enhance parents' support systems

Ensure that parents make the best possible use of familiar support systems by encouraging them to communicate with each other and by providing opportunities for them to discuss their feelings.

Promote communication between parents. Even if the parents normally serve as each other's greatest source of emotional support, their ability to meet each other's needs may fall short in a crisis. Also, they may move through grief at vastly different rates. However, one parent may assume that the other is at the same stage; when that assumption proves wrong, anger and resentment on both sides may result. To counter this potential, urge them to keep communication open.

Provide openings to discuss feelings. When parents visit their child, invite them to express their feelings. Such a comment as, "You must feel overwhelmed by all this" may release a flood of feelings. If one parent speaks but not the other, ask the silent parent what his or her reactions are.

Given an opening for honest discussion, parents may find common ground in their concerns and a sense of relief at not being alone. Even if they are not at the same stage of grief, one may be able to affirm the other's feelings as something he or she went through. If parents cannot reach common ground in their perceptions, urge them to find another family member—a grandparent, for example—who is understanding and supportive. Likewise, encourage a single parent to look to another family member or close friend for support.

Especially in the first few days after the neonate's birth, the parents' needs may differ. The mother, physically weakened and perhaps feeling isolated from other family members and from her child while in the maternity unit, may not have her usual control of her feelings. She may depend heavily on the father's visits for emotional support; between these visits, she may feel particularly alone. Even after her discharge, such feelings may persist because of her separation from her hospitalized child.

The father, too, needs support. The comfort he provides to the mother may drain his reserves. Should he believe he must be strong in crisis, he may be reluctant to reach out to other family members. His sense of isolation may increase further if friends and coworkers lack sympathy for any life-style changes he makes in response to family needs (Battles, 1988).

Each parent may feel so overwhelmed by the situation as to be unaware of the emotional drain made on the other. Help them open up to each other and discuss their feelings, which can strengthen understanding between them.

Also encourage parents to find time alone together—perhaps something as simple as a regular stop at a coffee shop on the way home from a visit to the NICU. Such an occasion, away from the pressures of home and hospital, may help them replenish their mental and emotional reserves.

Encourage family support

Among the most important interventions by the nurse caring for the family of a high-risk neonate are those that promote interaction among all family members. The family can be the strongest source of support for individual family members in a crisis. Conversely, physical or emotional isolation of any one member from the rest may put tremendous stress on all members and on the family as a whole.

Help siblings cope. Unless their needs receive attention, siblings of a high-risk neonate may face lifelong problems in dealing with the changes such a birth creates. Communication problems may develop (Scheiber, 1989), and siblings may experience conflicting feelings about the neonate.

Besides helping parents balance the needs of the neonate and siblings for attention, make sure they are aware of the feelings siblings may be experiencing. For

Caring for the siblings of a high-risk neonate

Siblings of a high-risk neonate need special attention to make them feel like important family members. To help siblings cope with a visit to the neonatal intensive care unit (NICU) or the death of the neonate, the nurse may refer to the guidelines below.

When siblings visit the NICU

Many facilities permit siblings to visit the NICU in an effort to help them understand and feel more sympathetic about the neonate's special needs. Contrary to popular belief, sibling visits do not increase the incidence of infection in neonates (Wranesh, 1982); nor do siblings develop emotional problems from visiting (Consolvo, 1987).

Before the visit, siblings should be prepared through a joint teaching effort by the nurse and the parents. For preschoolers (ages 2 through 4), the nurse should concentrate on explaining basic information about the neonate's condition and the NICU in simple, direct terms. For children ages 5 and older, the scope can be widened to include possible ways their roles in the family may change (parents should offer specific ideas about this) and how they may be able to participate in the neonate's care. Parents may want to show older children how to perform simple caregiving tasks during their visit.

For siblings of any age, the nurse may suggest that they contribute an item to the neonate's environment—perhaps a drawing or toy—that can be placed near the neonate's crib. This helps siblings develop an attachment to the neonate and reinforces their own identity within the family.

Any time siblings visit, the nurse should make sure they have an opportunity afterward to express their thoughts and ask follow-up questions. The more matter-of-fact their understanding becomes, the better they will be able to cope and the less of a stranger the neonate will seem to them when the neonate is discharged.

Helping siblings cope with a neonate's death

Although children mourn when a neonate sibling dies, they do so differently from an adult. Even though they may feel sad, for instance, they may continue to play (Trouy and Ward-Larson, 1987). For various reasons—unresolved fears of abandonment, guilt over the neonate's death, and inability to understand their parents' expressions of grief—children typically have a harder time than adults in expressing grief. Consequently, they may need help in understanding what has happened and in dealing with it.

Although the nurse or social worker can provide advice and perhaps written materials to help siblings deal with death, the nurse should urge parents to take charge of explaining the neonate's death to siblings. Doing so can help parents regain confidence in their parenting ability (Gardner and Merenstein, 1989) and can reassure siblings that their parents still care and watch out for them.

In helping siblings understand a neonate's death, the nurse should keep in mind their limitations and needs. Preschoolers do not view death as permanent; no matter how often they are told that their little brother or sister is not coming back, the point may not sink in completely. Also, they may believe that a bad thought they had about the neonate caused the death. In contrast, school-age children may understand the permanence of death but probably will have many questions about death itself.

All children, but especially younger ones, may be shaken to see a parent crying. If this occurs, reassure them that grown-ups can feel sad and that letting the sadness out by crying or talking about it is beneficial.

Children may ask the same questions repeatedly, either because they need confirmation of what they were told or because some new angle for looking at the neonate's death and its consequences has occurred to them. All children have a basic need for clear, honest information about the neonate's death and for straightforward answers to their questions. Thus, the nurse and parents should avoid evasive explanations that the neonate has been "taken away" or "gone to sleep"; these explanations can create misunderstandings and nightmares that the same thing may happen to them.

---

example, siblings may become fearful as they sense their parents' fear. If they are not old enough to understand the neonate's health problem or if no one explains it to them, they may fear "catching" the same ailment. In many cases, siblings fear that the neonate will take their mother away from them.

Siblings also may feel guilt over the neonate's condition. Not wanting to share the parents' attention with another child, for example, a sibling earlier may have wished that the birth would not occur and now may fear that the neonate's condition is a punishment for that wish. Preschool-age children, who believe that their thoughts have the power of actions (Gardner and Merenstein, 1989), are particularly likely to feel guilty.

Jealousy and anger may occur as siblings see how much of the parents' time and energy the neonate has captured. To regain some attention for themselves, they may display signs and symptoms similar to those of the ill neonate. If the siblings are staying with friends or relatives while the mother is hospitalized, they may be angry with the neonate for disrupting their home life.

Using terms the siblings can understand, explain to them the neonate's condition. Also, urge the parents to let siblings visit and care for the neonate and reassure them that their lives will not change drastically. (For more information about nursing interventions for siblings, see *Caring for the siblings of a high-risk neonate*.)

Encourage closeness between parents and other family members. Let parents know that they are not expected to spend every possible moment with the neonate. Discuss with them their own needs and those of children at home, and help them set priorities for meeting these needs along with the neonate's.

For a family with a nursing diagnosis of *ineffective family coping: compromised, related to family disor-*

Supporting the grandparents

When talking with grandparents of a high-risk neonate or preparing them for a visit to the neonatal intensive care unit (NICU), the nurse must keep in mind that they not only share many of the parents' difficulties in coping with the birth of a high-risk neonate but may feel an extra burden because of their role in the family.

Like the parents, grandparents usually form a picture of an anticipated "perfect" child, whose loss they now must grieve. To avoid still more pain, they may feel some urge to stay at an emotional distance and so lessen the sense of loss should the neonate die.

Because they also are parents, grandparents may feel guilty about the neonate's condition, blaming themselves for failing to give advice to the parents that could have resulted in the birth of a healthier neonate. Along with their sorrow for the neonate, they feel the pain of watching their own child's grief and worry. Also, although they may wish to help, grandparents may feel even more overwhelmed than parents by the NICU and have more trouble imagining themselves contributing effectively to the neonate's care.

The nurse should assure the grandparents that they can provide much welcome support. Some facilities present classes designed specifically to help grandparents support the parents (Horn and Manion, 1985). If the parents approve, encourage the grandparents to take part in caring for the neonate, perhaps with coaching by the parents. Also, if the grandparents are present when the physician or nurse speaks with the parents, urge them afterward to help the parents understand the information given.

At home, grandparents can provide even more help by relieving the parents of some of their parenting tasks (Blackburn and Lowen, 1986). This helps assure parents that the other children are in good hands while they visit the neonate or attend to other responsibilities.

ganization secondary to the neonate's condition, help parents explore ways of scheduling regular family time together at home and of making sure that birthdays and other special occasions are not neglected. Suggest, for example, that parents ask grandparents or other relatives to help with housekeeping chores so that when parents are home they can devote attention and energy to family interaction, not just to home care.

Encourage family members to interact with the neonate. Help parents plan ways to include grandparents, siblings, and other family members in visits to the NICU. If the neonate is stable and the facility's physical layout and policies permit, suggest bringing the whole family together in a private area near the NICU. If no such area is available but sibling visits are permitted, family members can take turns visiting the neonate; the time they spend together in the waiting area may provide the chance for them to interact with and support one another. Grandparents and older, responsible siblings also may take part in the

neonate's care. (For more information on enhancing the role of grandparents when a high-risk neonate is born, see *Supporting the grandparents.*)

Make parents aware of support groups

Inform parents of support groups available within the facility, locally, and nationally. Many facilities with NICUs have parent or family support groups, organized by parents or the nursing or social services staff. Parent-to-parent support groups in particular can provide emotional support and practical advice. Parents who take part in these groups can discuss their concerns, learn how parents of neonates with similar problems have coped, and find out about available community resources. If an in-house support group is available, let parents know its meeting time and place.

National support groups include those tied to a specific problem, such as spina bifida, and those with a more general scope, such as the March of Dimes. Provide parents with names, addresses, and phone numbers for local chapters (or, if no local group exists, national headquarters). Many national groups provide practical help. For instance, the United Way and the March of Dimes may provide funding for medical care, equipment, and transportation for follow-up care. Encourage parents to talk with the facility's social worker about applying for such assistance.

Teach caregiving skills

To promote parenting skills and parent-infant bonding, the nurse should involve parents in their child's care. With few exceptions, parents can provide some care for even the sickest neonate (Kelting, 1986). Although some parents welcome the chance to do this, others express doubts. These doubts may reflect insecurity about their own abilities or reluctance to establish a relationship with the neonate. If parents are uncomfortable with the idea of becoming caregivers, recognize their fears and work toward overcoming them. To do this, begin with the simplest procedures and increase the parents' participation only as they indicate readiness.

Increase the family's comfort level

To help the parents feel comfortable around their child, arrange for the neonate and parents to be together as much as possible. Take the mother to the NICU as soon as she has recovered sufficiently from delivery; if the neonate's health status permits, let the mother hold as well as see her child for a few minutes. Encourage her to touch her child if she seems hesitant.

Whenever parents come to the NICU, help them feel physically close to their child—for instance, by arranging chairs to let them comfortably see and touch their child. When their child is in a quiet but alert state, in which interaction is least stressful, encourage the parents to use gentle touch to get acquainted. Try to provide privacy and minimize interruptions at this time.

Involve parents in basic care

As the neonate's condition permits, encourage the parents to perform basic care. For instance, if the neonate is stable, invite the parents to participate in feeding. Show them how to hold their child during and after feeding, and explain how to perform simple mouth care. If the mother is considering breast-feeding, explain that giving breast milk may be beneficial physically and psychologically to both her child and her (Steele, 1987). Even if the neonate cannot suckle, the mother can provide breast milk she has pumped.

If the neonate must be gavage-fed, show the parents how to assist by holding the feeding tube or cylinder or by pouring the milk into the container. Invite them to supply a pacifier for their child to use between feedings.

Bathing the neonate can be a special time for parents. For the first bath with parents present, explain any special precautions they must take and encourage parents to watch their child respond to gentle touch; on future occasions, parents may give the bath with minimal supervision.

Diapering provides another opportunity for parents to strengthen their caregiving skills and perhaps also a chance to make some care decisions. Even if the neonate's fecal output must be monitored carefully, parents can change the diaper, weighing it themselves or saving it for a staff member to weigh. Offer parents their choice of several diaper ointments and creams, and encourage them to apply whatever they choose with a gentle touch.

As parents become more familiar with neonatal care needs, encourage them to rely less on staff supervision during caregiving—for example, suggest that they perform routine bottle- or breast-feeding on their own. The more successfully they function on their own as caregivers, the more confident they will feel when caring for their child at home.

An ideal way to enhance and evaluate parents' caregiving ability is to observe them as they care for their child. Such supervision also may decrease anxiety in parents before discharge and may prove particularly helpful if the neonate has complex care needs. Many facilities provide this experience by means of a care-by-parent unit. In this arrangement, one or both parents live with the neonate for 18 to 36 hours in a private room within or near the NICU.

Involve parents in developmental care

To help parents participate in developmental care, which can reduce some physical and mental limitations re-

sulting from high-risk birth, suggest that they bring in items that stimulate vision and hearing, such as brightly colored toys or mobiles, tape recordings of family members' voices, or toys that make soothingly rhythmic sounds. Devices that mimic the sound of the maternal heartbeat are especially effective in calming a fussy neonate.

Invite participation in decision making

Ask parents how they would like their child's daily care routine to be adjusted to give them maximum participation. For example, they may ask that bath time be set for when they can be present and routine medical procedures scheduled to avoid interfering with visiting time. Accommodate the parents' desires as much as possible; if something will not fit in, explain the problem to them.

Involve parents in decision making on as many levels as possible, both simple and complex. Even when the physician must make the final decision, help them to understand the options and the reason for the physician's choice so that they become partners in the decision.

Enhance parent-infant bonding

Parents whose neonate is critically ill or separated from them for long periods may show poor bonding with the neonate for several years (Plunkett, Meisels, Stiefel, Pasick, and Roloff, 1986). However, to withstand the rigors of caregiving for a high-risk neonate, they must develop a strong bond. The nurse can promote bonding by continuing to encourage frequent visiting, caregiving, phone calls, and other interaction. Also, give the parents the fullest possible picture of their child's characteristic behavior, including patterns of fussiness and wakefulness, so that they know what to expect once their child is discharged. Such advance knowledge minimizes strains on parent-infant bonding. (For a case study that shows how to apply the nursing process when caring for the family of a high-risk neonate, see *Applying the nursing process: Parents with ineffective individual coping related to the stress of a preterm birth*, pages 1002 and 1003.)

Plan for the neonate's discharge

As technological advances have increased survival rates, many high-risk neonates who only a few years ago would have lived hours or days now survive and eventually go home with their parents. However, some require complex, demanding, and expensive care for years—perhaps the rest of their lives. Nursing care for the family of a high-risk neonate should aim to ensure that the family will know how to provide this level of care.

Preparation of the family for the neonate's discharge requires an evaluation of their concerns and any weaknesses in their caregiving ability. The nurse must look not only for the skills they demonstrate but for any persisting fears—understandable as they face the prospect of taking over care of a neonate whose life so far has been supported by advanced equipment. For example, they may fear that they will not recognize signs of a sudden downturn until too late. (For details on planning for a neonate's discharge, see Chapter 40, Discharge Planning and Neonatal Care at Home.)

Evaluate readiness to assume care

To determine whether the family needs further nursing intervention before the neonate's discharge, evaluate the parents for their emotional and practical readiness to assume primary care. Discharge to a poorly prepared family could result in such problems as failure to thrive or abuse of the neonate by a family member.

Although careful teaching can prepare most parents to be effective caregivers, some parents need more than this. Carefully evaluate the parents' ability and motivation to care for their child, and inform the physician if they display any of the following behaviors as the neonate's discharge date nears:
• delay in arranging for medical-support equipment in the home
• infrequent calls or visits to the NICU
• apparent lack of interest in giving simple care to their child in the NICU.

Explain further care needs and options

Make sure parents understand which kinds of continuing care their child will require after discharge. (For information on care needs related to specific conditions, see Chapter 40, Discharge Planning and Neonatal Care at Home.)

For parents whose child is likely to remain technologically dependent for life, the availability of health services is a major concern—not just whether they exist but whether they are affordable and available nearby. Help parents identify facilities in their area that offer continuing support, and encourage them to enlist the social worker's help in applying for funds from institutional, governmental, and support-group sources.

Help the family deal with death

If the neonate has a poor prognosis or if death appears imminent, the nurse can help the family deal with the prospect of death as well as the event itself. Fetal loss and stillbirth also warrant special nursing interventions.

Perinatal death

The kinds of interventions family members need before and after a neonate's death depend somewhat on the relationship they have formed with the neonate and on the stage of grief they are in. To facilitate a healthy resolution of grief, carry out measures that help family members complete their bond with the neonate. Some family members experience a brief denial phase after the death of a high-risk neonate; others skip denial and show signs of anger, guilt, or despair.

Prepare the family for the neonate's death. Even if the parents have spent little time with their child, their emotional bond probably has been developing since pregnancy. To resolve their grief, they must complete their bonding with the neonate as their child and a member of their family, building memories to sustain them in the future.

To promote bonding, encourage the parents to name their child (if they have not done so already). As they look at the child, point out physical features that resemble those of family members; this may help them put their thoughts about their child into words (Krone and Harris, 1988). Find out whether they want the child to be baptized or to receive some other blessing, and make appropriate arrangements. If possible, let them hold their child; otherwise, encourage gentle touching and stroking.

Also plan interventions to help family members deal with their grief. For family members in denial, do not attempt to force them past denial, but provide and reinforce clear, accurate information about the child's condition.

For family members feeling anger, provide the opportunity to vent feelings. However, if one family member blames another for the child's condition, point out that in most cases, preterm birth, neonatal illness, and birth defects result from a combination of factors. Even if the action of one or both parents seems to have been the immediate cause, laying blame serves no purpose.

Use similar reasoning to help family members put aside guilt, a form of self-targeting anger. Although the mother is more likely to express feelings of guilt—remembering a week of unauthorized dieting or a single glass of wine—the father may feel guilt for not being committed enough to the mother's care while she was pregnant.

Anticipatory grieving can occur during the fourth stage of grief—depression and withdrawal. If the neonate is in critical condition and not expected to live, the parents may begin grieving by withdrawing from the neonate (Lindemann, 1944). Even if the parents say nothing, reduced attention to their child may signal that they have begun to withdraw.

Anticipatory grieving and emotional withdrawal may occur briefly or continue throughout the neonate's hospitalization. Although these behaviors can ease pain when an anticipated perinatal death occurs, they also can create problems in bonding if the neonate survives. For the family with a nursing diagnosis of *anticipatory grieving related to the prospect of the neonate's death,* make sure the parents' understanding of their child's condition is not bleaker than the situation warrants, and inform them that even critically ill neonates may recover.

Make arrangements for the death. Keep parents informed of changes in their child's condition. Assure them that the staff will do its best to let them know when death appears near so that they can be with their child.

Before the family arrives, dress the neonate in regular baby clothing (some units keep a supply of baby clothes to use if the parents have not provided any). If family members will be permitted to hold their child, have a receiving blanket ready for wrapping the neonate; later, parents may wish to have the blanket as a keepsake.

When the family arrives, provide as much privacy as possible. Move the neonate to a private area (or at least to the quietest corner of the NICU). Post a sign near the entrance to this area, alerting staff to the family's need for quiet. When no additional medical intervention is planned, let the family spend the last few moments alone with the neonate.

Provide support after the death. Family members need support to cope with the immediate reality of their child's death and to deal with their grief. After the neonate has died, the nurse should give family members all the time they need to say goodbye to and hold the child.

If the family was absent at the time of death, check with the physician about notification procedure. Some physicians prefer to inform the family personally rather than by telephone. Offer to be present to give support when the family is notified. (For information about organizations that help bereaved parents cope with perinatal loss, see *Resources for dealing with perinatal loss.*)

Prepare the body. If the family arrived after the neonate died, prepare the body for them to see. Wash, dress, and wrap the neonate in a way that displays positive features and covers disfigurements. With the physician's permission, remove all tubes and lines (except where removal might affect the outcome of an autopsy); disconnect, tie off, and secure those lines under the clothing while the family visits. Remove drainage stains and tape marks; cover surgical wounds or puncture sites with small dressings.

Place the wrapped body in a cool area until just before the family arrives. Then, before presenting the body to them, wrap it in warmed linens, which will transfer some of the warmth to the neonate's skin.

Resources for dealing with perinatal loss

The grief and loss experienced by the family of a neonate who dies last far longer than the brief time most neonatal nurses are in contact with the family. Consequently, the nurse should be aware of support groups that can help family members deal with their loss in the months and years to come.

Pregnancy and Infant Loss Center (PILC)
1421 E. Wayzata Boulevard, Suite 40
Wayzata, MN 55391
612-473-9372

Founded in 1983 by a group of bereaved parents, this national organization works to promote an environment in which families can participate in healthy grieving, helps families find and use their own support networks, provides information and education to professionals, and serves as parent advocate after the death of a high-risk neonate. PILC makes referrals to local support groups, publishes a quarterly newsletter, distributes literature on perinatal bereavement, and gives workshops and in-service programs.

Resolve Through Sharing
La Crosse Lutheran Hospital
1910 South Avenue
La Crosse, WI 54601
608-791-4747

This comprehensive hospital-based perinatal bereavement program provides guidelines for professionals caring for families who have experienced miscarriage, ectopic pregnancy, stillbirth, or neonatal death. It aims to ensure consistent, sensitive care for grieving family members. Its activities include nationwide educational and certification programs for childbirth educators.

Source of Help in Airing and Resolving Experiences (SHARE)
St. Elizabeth's Hospital
211 South 3rd Street
Belleville, IL 62222
618-234-2415

This organization aims to ensure support for parents from the time they anticipate a problem by helping them to express grief and related emotions. It maintains a national listing of relevant resources and helps parents contact local support groups and other resources, such as fertility specialists and printed materials. SHARE publishes a bimonthly newsletter for caregivers and families and presents workshops throughout the United States and abroad.

Preserve mementos. To provide the family with tangible memories of the neonate, assemble a memory packet, including such items as photographs, a lock of hair, the identification bracelet, a footprint, caps, and blankets. If the family does not wish to take these items home, let them know that the packet will be kept in case they want it later; when they are past the initial shock, these mementos may help them through grief.

Help with funeral arrangements. For some parents, making funeral arrangements for their child is calming; focusing on the task at hand helps them accept their loss and deal with their grief. Recognize, however, that parents who have never before experienced the death of a close relative may need help to identify what needs to be done; particularly distraught parents may be unable to face the task at all. Discuss with them—or have the chaplain or social worker discuss—possible funeral and burial choices (including having the hospital take care of the body, if that option is available).

If the parents' reactions to the death are so intense that they cannot make arrangements, call on a family support source, such as a grandparent, to help out. (However, do not seek help if parents can do their own planning; a well-meaning relative or friend who takes over may deprive parents of tasks that would help them resolve grief.)

Even if the parents can make their own arrangements, talk with other family members about ways to help them out at home. Relatives may think they should remove all signs of preparation for the child's birth—crib, toys, clothing—and keep the mother so busy once she comes home that she has no chance to think about her loss. Explain that such tasks as packing up these items may help parents come to terms with their loss. Suggest that offering an afternoon's child care or other practical help might be more appropriate.

Help with resolving grief. Between experiencing and accepting their child's death, parents go through a lengthy internal struggle. The aim of nursing interventions during this period is twofold: help maintain basic family functioning and help family members work through grief to a healthy resolution.

Identify and intervene in dysfunctional grief. Be familar with signs of dysfunctional grief. After their child's death, parents may experience disorganization and physical ailments. For instance, various studies show that the risk of disease increases during bereavement. Parkes (1970) described psychosomatic pain, especially chest pain, among bereaved adults. Mourners also have a higher risk of serious illness than nonmourners (Lindemann, 1944; Rees and Lutkins, 1967). Lynch (1979) found a twofold risk of myocardial infarction in mourners compared to nonmourners and, depending on the region in which they lived, a threefold risk of gastrointestinal cancer.

Some bereaved parents may be unable to eat, sleep, or make decisions; they may seem caught up in anger at the health care team or depression about their inability to produce a healthy child. In some cases, they may fail to cope with everyday experiences or to meet their own and their children's basic needs.

To assess for these problems, monitor the parents' physical appearance, if possible. Also, talk with them frequently about how they are managing home affairs, and be ready to call in a friend or relative who can help keep the family functioning until the parents can resume their normal roles. Suggest that they undergo a physical examination approximately 4 months after the loss to ensure early detection of any physical problems associated with bereavement. (For more information about dysfunctional grief, see *Pathologic mourning.*)

Counter misunderstandings. Because family members may pass through the stages of grief at different rates, misunderstandings may arise. Most commonly, the mother's grief takes longer to resolve. Her attachment may be greater because of the special bond she developed with the fetus during pregnancy. Thus, she may find grief resolution more difficult. The father, meanwhile, may seem to have distanced himself from the dead neonate. His grief may not be evident, even though his sense of loss may be great.

To help reduce misunderstandings, teach the parents about the grief stages and encourage them to communicate with each other about their feelings—not only about the loss of their child, but about the pressures they feel in its aftermath. The father, for example, may explain that although the loss is painful for him, he feels he must be stoic, fearing that the same people who sympathize with the mother's expression of grief would disapprove of his. If the parents have trouble understanding each other, suggest that they talk together with the social worker, chaplain, or another counselor.

Also talk with other family members. As they reach their own points of grief resolution, they may become impatient with the mother (or both parents) for being "preoccupied" with the child's death. When the mother attempts to discuss her feelings, for example, other family members may urge her to stop dwelling in the past. They even may encourage her to start a "replacement" child before she is ready to consider another pregnancy.

To avert such well-meaning intrusion, discuss with other family members the individuality of grieving. Assure them that 6 weeks of acute mourning are by no means unusual, that full resolution of grief may take 2 years, and that accepting the mother's feelings will help her resolve her grief.

Pathologic mourning

Ultimately, grief results in healing. When the process is completed, family members can resume normal functioning, remembering the dead neonate with sorrow but able to move on. In a few cases, however, mourning (the outward expression of grief) becomes pathologic—most commonly when a parent tries to suppress grief (Gardner and Merenstein, 1989) instead of letting the process work through. The family member may never reach resolution without intervention by a professional skilled in grief counseling.

The nurse who cares for the family of a neonate who has died should stay alert for indications that a family member is fighting recognition of grief. If any of the following signs or symptoms appear, alert other members of the health care team and refer the family member to an expert:
• agitated depression
• changes in relationships with family or friends
• hostility toward specific individuals
• illness that may be psychosomatic (for example, chronic fatigue and headache)
• inability to function productively
• loss of social-interaction patterns
• overactivity with no sense of loss
• schizophrenia-like formality of manner
• symptoms resembling those of the neonate.

Fetal death

Because parents can begin bonding with a child as soon as they are aware of a pregnancy, the death of a fetus can be as traumatic as the death of a neonate. Nursing interventions similar to those provided after a neonate's death can help parents who suffer a fetal loss; however, depending on when in the pregnancy the fetal loss occurs, opportunity to provide such interventions may be limited. Thus, the timing and circumstances of the fetal loss guide nursing interventions.

First-trimester fetal death. With a first-trimester loss (usually a spontaneous abortion), the mother may have been unaware of the pregnancy—and she may not be hospitalized for treatment. If she simply is treated in the physician's office, little opportunity exists for nursing intervention; yet she may need such intervention.

On the other hand, if the mother was aware of the pregnancy, she and her partner may have begun their emotional investment; if so, they will need to grieve. Unfortunately, family and friends may minimize a first-trimester fetal loss, believing that the pregnancy cannot have meant that much yet, and thus fail to give parents support. Nursing interventions in this situation include affirming the parents' right and need to grieve, explaining the stages of grief to them, and encouraging them to communicate with and support each other.

Second-trimester fetal death. Fetal death at this stage typically results in spontaneous abortion. In most cases, the parents were aware of the pregnancy and had invested themselves emotionally in the forthcoming birth. Nursing interventions include helping the parents express their grief, explaining the stages of grief, and encouraging them to communicate with each other and other family members.

Third-trimester fetal death. As pregnancy progresses and parents invest more time and energy in the fetus, bonding with the expected child increases. Thus, third-trimester fetal loss may be quite traumatic. The mother may have to go through labor to expel the fetus, adding to the trauma. Parents in this situation need much support from each other, other family members, and friends. Nursing interventions may include suggesting that they pack up whatever clothes, toys, and other items they had begun accumulating for the expected child to help them complete their bonding. Although this may be a difficult task, it can help parents face their loss and express their feelings (Limbo and Wheeler, 1986).

Stillbirth

Stillbirth—the death shortly before or during delivery of a fetus that had been expected to live—is a wrenching experience as happy anticipation suddenly vanishes. If fetal death occurs before labor begins, the parents also must deal with feelings of helplessness as they wait for delivery to occur. Because grieving will be easier if they complete their bonding, encourage the parents to look at, touch, and hold the stillborn neonate. Also, provide solitude as they say goodbye to their child.

Evaluation

During this step of the nursing process, the nurse evaluates the effectiveness of the care plan by ongoing evaluation of subjective and objective criteria. Evaluation findings should be stated in terms of actions performed or outcomes achieved for each goal. Keep in mind that while the neonate is hospitalized, the nurse may have difficulty evaluating the effect of care for the family, because full results of some interventions may not be apparent until after the neonate is discharged.

The following examples illustrate appropriate evaluation statements for the family of a high-risk neonate.

APPLYING THE NURSING PROCESS

Parents with ineffective individual coping related to the stress of a preterm birth

For the family of a high-risk neonate, the nursing process can reduce stress and increase confidence in the ability to provide neonatal care. The table below shows how the nurse might use the nursing process when caring for the family described in the case history at right. The first column presents history and physical assessment data, followed by a paragraph of mental notes. These notes help the nurse make important mental connections among assessment findings, aiding

in development of the nursing diagnosis and planning.

The second column lists an appropriate nursing diagnosis; information in the remaining columns is based on this diagnosis. Although not part of the nursing process, a rationale appears for each intervention in the fourth column to explain how it contributes to the care plan.

ASSESSMENT	NURSING DIAGNOSIS	PLANNING
Subjective (history) data • Parents report their first pregnancy produced a healthy neonate at term. • Parents state that they have no previous experience with preterm neonates. • Parents report feelings of anxiety. • Parents describe changes in eating and sleeping habits. • Parents state that they have noticed changes in family interactions. **Objective (physical) data** • Neonate is hospitalized 30 miles from the family home. • Parents cry when discussing the neonate's condition. • Parents appear restless. **Mental notes** *Changes in the parents' eating and sleeping habits and in family interactions could be caused by anxiety, which in turn may stem from lack of experience with high-risk neonates, concern about their son's condition and chances for survival, the complexity and expense of his health care, and distress at their separation from him. The neonate's grandparents, who live nearby, might prove helpful in helping teach the parents how to care for the neonate and in taking care of the older child while the parents visit the neonate.*	Ineffective individual coping related to the stress of a preterm birth	**Goals** Before the neonate is discharged, the parents will: • demonstrate verbal and nonverbal behaviors that indicate decreased anxiety • identify strategies to help them cope with stress • use appropriate support systems and resources • provide for the basic needs of the family as a unit as well as individual family members • show confidence when providing neonatal care.

• The parents demonstrated specific caregiving skills required by their neonate during and after hospitalization.
• The parents identified and used available support sources during and after the neonate's hospitalization.
• The parents' verbal and nonverbal behaviors reflected at least a moderate level of comfort in meeting the neonate's physical and emotional needs.
• The parents demonstrated an understanding of and used appropriate coping mechanisms.
• The parents expressed grief in a constructive manner.
• The parents demonstrated an accurate perception of the neonate's condition and have realistic expectations.

Documentation

The nurse should document all steps of the nursing process as thoroughly and objectively as possible. Thorough documentation not only allows the nurse to evaluate the effectiveness of the care plan, but it also makes this information available to other members of the health care team, helping to ensure consistency of care.

Documentation for the parents of a high-risk neonate should include:
• signs of individual expressions of grief
• length and frequency of visits to the neonate
• nature of the interaction with the neonate

CASE STUDY

Jonathan Hawley, age 9 days, was born at 30 weeks' gestation; his preterm status puts him at high risk for various health problems. His parents live 30 miles from the hospital. Jonathan has one older sister, age 2. Both sets of grandparents live near the Hawleys.

IMPLEMENTATION		EVALUATION
Intervention Encourage the parents to communicate their feelings about their child with each other.	**Rationale** Maintaining open communication helps to prevent and correct any misunderstandings or misconceptions between the parents, reducing stress and anxiety.	Upon evaluation, the parents: • demonstrated a reduced anxiety level • reported improved sleeping and eating habits • appeared calm when handling their child • used appropriate support systems • showed appropriate coping mechanisms.
Encourage the parents to use family resources to help cope with stress.	Help from other family members and friends during a crisis adds stability that can help the parents cope with this unsettling situation.	
Provide information to the parents about their child's condition, including medical status, equipment used, and future concerns.	Such information helps reduce the parent's anxiety about their child's condition.	
Provide an atmosphere that encourages open communication between the parents and nurse.	Ongoing, open communication between the nurse and parents fosters trust.	
Encourage the parents to participate actively in their child's care.	Caring for their child increases the parents' confidence and self-esteem and helps prepare them for specific caregiving skills they will need after the child's discharge. It also enhances parent-infant bonding as parents come to know their child better and learn to meet the child's physical and emotional needs.	

• ability to express feelings about the neonate
• ability to identify and provide for the neonate's care needs
• ability to accept help and advice from the health care team
• verbal expression of coping ability
• expression of comfort with caring for the neonate at home
• willingness to make necessary arrangements for home care
• ability to identify appropriate follow-up medical care for the neonate
• contact with the deceased neonate if perinatal death has occurred.

Documentation for the neonate with regard to family interaction should include the following points:

• physiologic response to parents' care, including response to feeding and simple caregiving activities
• eye contact and other signs of interaction with parents
• response to interaction by the parents (for example, "Takes feeding easily from mother; no vomiting after eating; quiet after feeding").

Chapter summary

Chapter 39 described how to care for family members after the birth of a high-risk neonate. Here are the chapter highlights.

• Loss and grief occur in families that experience a real or perceived loss of the neonate. Death of the neonate or birth of a neonate who is preterm, severely ill, or afflicted with a physical or mental anomaly or disability may trigger these responses.

• The stages of grief described by Kübler-Ross include denial, anger, bargaining, depression, and acceptance. Completion of grieving can take a year or more; family members may progress through the stages at different rates and may experience facets of two or more stages at once.

• Initially, the nurse must assess the parents, grandparents, and siblings for ability to cope emotionally and practically with the birth of a high-risk neonate. Factors to assess include family history; understanding of the neonate's condition; familiarity with the health care environment; home and family needs; and support from such sources as other family members, religious practices, and cultural customs.

• Later nursing assessment focuses on the developing relationship between the family and the neonate, the family's acquisition of neonatal care skills, and use of coping mechanisms.

• Nursing intervention includes providing accurate, consistent information to family members; establishing communication with them; strengthening family support systems and interaction between family members and the neonate; teaching caregiving skills; enhancing parent-infant bonding; and planning for the neonate's discharge.

• In the event of a neonate's death, nursing interventions include providing emotional support, arranging a quiet area for the family to say goodbye to the neonate, collecting mementos for the family, and encouraging the family to complete their bonding with the neonate.

Study questions

1. Ann Davis is crying at the bedside of her child, whose congenital anomaly will necessitate repeated hospitalizations and lifelong care. Which interventions can the nurse use to help her express her grief?

2. Neonate Tim Keller has been transferred to the tertiary NICU. If the parents cannot visit him more than once a week, which interventions might the nurse suggest to encourage parent-infant bonding?

3. Teresa Brown has been transferred to a private room for the remainder of her stay after the death of her 2-day-old child. Her sister, who is taking care of the family's two other children, mentions that she is planning to pack away all the baby clothes and furniture before Teresa is discharged. How should the nurse respond?

4. Elena Morales, a recent immigrant from Central America, cries frequently when talking about her preterm child, who is on respiratory support. Her husband Carlos displays no particular emotion in talking about their child. What can the nurse do to investigate if Carlos is suppressing his emotions and risking pathologic mourning?

Bibliography

Als, H. (1986). A synactive model of neonatal behavioral organization: Framework for the assessment of neurobehavioral development in the premature infant and for support of infants and parents in the neonatal intensive care environment. In J. K. Sweeney (Ed.), *The high-risk neonate: Developmental therapy perspectives. Physical and Occupational Therapy in Pediatrics*, 6(3/4), 3-55.

Aukamp, V. (1987). A field study to identify nursing diagnoses for childbearing families. In A.M. McLane (Ed.), *Classification of nursing diagnoses: Proceedings of the 7th NANDA conference*. St. Louis: Mosby.

Cubberley, D.A. (1987). Diagnosis of fetal death. *Clinical Obstetrics and Gynecology*, 30(2), 259-267.

Dignan, P.S.J. (1987). Genetics and pregnancy loss: Value of counseling between pregnancies. In J.R. Woods and J.L. Esposito (Eds.), *Pregnancy loss: Medical therapeutics and practical considerations*. Baltimore: Williams & Wilkins.

Fibison, W.J., and James, S.R. (1985). Developmental implications of heredity. In S.R. Mott, N.F. Fazekas, and S.R. James (Eds.), *Nursing care of children and families: A holistic approach*. Menlo Park, CA: Addison-Wesley.

Hack, M., and Breslau, N. (1986). Very low birth weight infants: Effects of brain growth during infancy on intelligence quotient at 3 years of age. *Pediatrics*, 61(4), 629-635.

Hunter, R.S., Kilsrom, N., Kraybill, E.N., and Loda, F. (1978). Antecedents of child abuse and neglect in premature infants: A prospective study in a newborn intensive care unit. *Pediatrics*, 61(4), 629-635.

Kennell, J.H., and Klaus, M.H. (1980). Parenting in the premature nursery. In E.J. Sell (Ed.), *Follow-up of the high-risk newborn: A practical approach*. Springfield, IL: Charles C. Thomas.

Lawhon, G. (1986). Management of stress in premature infants. In D.J. Angelini, C.K. Whalen Knapp, and R.M. Gibes (Eds.), *Perinatal/neonatal nursing: A clinical handbook*. Boston: Blackwell Scientific Publications.

Leventhal, J.M., Egerter, S.A., and Murphy, J.M. (1984). Reassessment of the relationship of perinatal risk factors and child abuse. *American Journal of Diseases of Childhood,* 138(11), 1034-1039.

Minde, K., Trehub, S., Corter, C., Boukydis, C., Celhoffer, L., and Marton, P. (1978). Mother-child relationships in the premature nursery: An observational study. *Pediatrics,* 61(3), 373-379.

Plunkett, J.W., Meisels, S.J., Stiefel, G.S., Pasick, P.L., and Roloff, D.W. (1986). Patterns of attachment among preterm infants of varying biological risk. *Journal of the American Academy of Child Psychiatry,* 25(6), 794-800.

Rivers, A., Caron, B., and Hack, M. (1987). Experience of families with very low birth-weight children with neurologic sequelae. *Clinical Pediatrics,* 26(5), 223-230.

Sahin, S.T. (1987). The physically disabled child. In S.H. Johnson (Ed.). *Nursing assessment and strategies for the family at risk: High-risk parenting.* Philadelphia: Lippincott.

Schraeder, B.D. (1980). Attachment and parenting despite lengthy intensive care. *MCN,* 5(1), 37-41.

Sell, E.J., Gaines, J.A., Gluckman, C., and Williams, E. (1985). Early identification of learning problems in neonatal intensive-care graduates. *American Journal of Diseases of Childhood,* 139(5), 460-463.

Steele, N. F. and Harrison, B. (1986). Technology-assisted children: Assessing discharge preparation...ventilator assisted children. *Journal of Pediatric Nursing,* 1(3), 150-158.

Stein, M. (1987). The usefulness of nursing diagnoses in neonatal intensive-care units. In A.M. McLane (Ed.), *Classification of nursing diagnoses: Proceedings of the 7th NANDA conference.* St. Louis: Mosby.

Thompson, M.H., and Khot, A.S. (1985). Impact of neonatal intensive care. *Archives of Disease in Childhood,* 60(3), 213-214.

Wranesh, B.L. (1982). The effect of sibling visitation on bacterial colonization rate in neonates. *JOGNN,* 11(4), 211-213.

Cultural references

Bampton, B., Jones, J., and Mancini, J. (1981). Initial mothering patterns of low-income black primiparas. *JOGNN,* 10(3), 174-178.

Leininger, M.M. (1985). Transcultural care diversity and universality: A theory of nursing. *Nursing and Health Care,* 6(4), 208-212.

Manio, E.B., and Hall, R.R. (1987). Asian family traditions and their influence in transcultural health care delivery. *Children's Health Care,* 15(3), 172-177.

Tripp-Reimer, T., Brink, P. J., and Saunders, J. M. (1984). Cultural assessment: Content and process. *Nursing Outlook,* 32(2), 78-82.

York, C.R., and Stichler, J.F. (1985). Cultural grief expressions following infant death. *Dimensions of Critical Care Nursing,* 4(2), 120-127.

Zepeda, M. (1982). Selected maternal-infant care practices of Spanish-speaking women. *JOGGN,* 11(6), 371-374.

Families in crisis

Battles, R.S. (1988). Factors influencing men's transition into parenthood. *Neonatal Network,* 6(5), 63-66.

Blackburn, S., and Lowen, L. (1986). Grandparents in NICUs. *MCN,* 11, 190-192.

Consolvo, C.A. (1984). Nurturing the fathers of high-risk newborns. *Neonatal Network,* 2(6), 27-30.

Consolvo. C.A. (1987). Siblings in the NICU. *Neonatal Network,* 5(5), 7-12.

Eager, M. (1977). Long-distance nurturing of the family bond. Butterworth Hospital, Grand Rapids, MI, Part 3. *MCN,* 2(5), 293-294.

Eager, M., and Exoo, R. (1980). Parents visiting parents for un-equaled support. *MCN,* 5(1), 35-36.

Edwards, K.A., and Allen, M.E. (1988). Nursing management of the human response to the premature birth experience. *Neonatal Network,* 6(5), 82-86.

Erdman, D. (1977). Parent-to-parent support: The best for those with sick newborns. *MCN,* 2(5), 291-292.

Fajardo, B. (1988). Brief intervention with parents in the special care nursery. *Neonatal Network,* 6(6), 23-30.

Goodman, N.T., (1982). Children are family, too! *Nursing Management,* 13(6), 52-54.

Hawkins-Walsh, E. (1980). Diminishing anxiety in parents of sick newborns. *MCN,* 5(1), 30-34.

Horn, M., and Manion, J. (1985). Creative grandparenting: Bonding the generations. *JOGNN,* 14(3), 233-236.

Johnson, S.H. (1986). *Nursing assessment and strategies for the family at risk: High-risk parenting* (2nd ed.). Philadelphia: Lippincott.

Kelting, S. (1986). Supporting parents in the NICU. *Neonatal Network,* 4(6), 14-18.

Lemons, P.M. (1986). Beyond the birth of a defective child. *Neonatal Network,* 5(3), 13-20.

Murray, R., Zentner, J., Brockhaus, J., Brockhaus, R., and Sullivan, E.P. (1989). The family--basic unit for the developing person. In R.B. Murray and J.P. Zentner (Eds.), *Nursing assessment and health promotion strategies through the life span.* East Norwalk, CT: Appleton & Lange.

Scheiber, K.K. (1989). Developmentally delayed children: Effects on the normal sibling. *Pediatric Nursing,* 15(1), 42-44.

Steele, K.H. (1987). Caring for parents of critically ill neonates during hospitalization: Strategies for health-care professionals. *MCN,* 16(1), 13-27.

Tarbert, K.C. (1985). The impact of a high-risk infant upon the family. *Neonatal Network,* 3(4), 20-23.

Trahd, G.E. (1986). Siblings of chronically ill children: Helping them cope. *Pediatric Nursing,* 12(3), 191-193.

Varner, B., Ossenkop, D. and Lyon, J. (1980, November-December). Prematures, too, need rooming-in and care-by-parent programs. *MCN,* 5, 431-432.

Waechter, E. (1970). The birth of an exceptional child. *Nursing Forum,* 9(2), 202-216.

Walwork, E., and Ellison, P. H. (1985). Follow-up of families of neonates in whom life support was withdrawn. *Clinical Pediatrics,* 24(1), 14-20.

Grief

Backer, B.A., Hannon, N., and Russell, N.A. (1982). *Death and dying: Individuals and institutions.* New York: Wiley.

Beckey, R.D., Price, R.A., Okerson, M., and Riley, K.W. (1985). Development of a perinatal grief checklist. *JOGNN,* 14(3), 194-199.

Benefield, D.G., Leib, S.A., and Reuter, J. (1976). Grief response of parents after referral of the critically ill newborn to a regional center. *New England Journal of Medicine,* 294(18), 975-978.

Benefield, D.G., Leib, S.A., and Vollman, J.H. (1978). Grief response of parents to neonatal death and parent participation in deciding care. *Pediatrics,* 62(2), 171-177.

Bowlby, J. (1961). Process of mourning. *International Journal of Psychoanalysis,* 42, 317-340.

Cordell, A.S., and Apolito, R. (1981). Family support in infant death. *JOGNN,* 10(4), 281-285.

Davidson, G.W. (1984). *Understanding mourning: A guide for those who grieve.* Minneapolis: Augsburg Publishing House.

Douma, C., and First, S. (1986). Management of bereaved parents. In D.J. Angelini, C.M. Whelan Knapp, and R.M. Gibes (Eds.),

Perinatal/neonatal nursing: A clinical handbook. Boston: Blackwell Scientific Publications.

Freitag-Koontz, M. J. (1988). Parents' grief reaction to the diagnosis of their infant's severe neurologic impairment and static encephalopathy. *Journal of Perinatal and Neonatal Nursing*, 2(2), 45-57.

Gardner, S.L., and Merenstein, G.B. (1986). Perinatal grief and loss: An overview. *Neonatal Network*, 5(2), 7-15.

Gardner, S.L., and Merenstein, G.B. (1989). *Handbook of neonatal intensive care.* St. Louis: Mosby.

Garland, K.R. (1986, a). Grief: The transitional process. *Neonatal Network*, 5(3), 7-10.

Garland, K.R. (1986, b). Unresolved grief. *Neonatal Network*, 5(3), 29-37.

Grubb-Phillips, C.A. (1988). Intrauterine fetal death: The maternal bereavement experience. *Journal of Perinatal and Neonatal Nursing*, 2(2), 34-44.

Hodge, D.S., and Graham, P.L. (1985). Supporting bereaved parents: A program for the NICU. *Neonatal Network*, 4(3), 11-18.

Kavanaugh, R.E. (1974). *Facing death.* New York: Viking.

Klingbeil, C.G. (1986). Extended nursing care after a perinatal loss: Theoretical implications. *Neonatal Network*, 5(3), 21-28.

Krone, C., and Harris, C.C. (1988). The importance of infant gender and family resemblance within parents' perinatal bereavement process: Establishing personhood. *Journal of Perinatal and Neonatal Nursing*, 2(2), 1-11.

Kübler-Ross, E. (1969). *On Death and Dying.* New York: Macmillan.

Limbo, R.K., and Wheeler, S.R. (1986). *When a baby dies: A handbook for healing and helping.* Holmen, WI: Harsand Press.

Lindemann, E. (1944). Symptomatology and management of acute grief. *American Journal of Psychiatry*, 101: 141-148.

Lynch, J.J. (1979). *The broken heart: The medical consequences of loneliness.* New York: Basic Books.

Miles, M.S. (1985). Helping adults mourn the death of a child. *Issues in Comprehensive Pediatric Nursing*, 8(1-6), 219-241.

Mina, C.F. (1985). A program for helping grieving parents. *MCN*, 10(2), 118-121.

Null, S. (1989). Nursing care to ease parents' grief. *MCN*, 14(2), 84-89.

O'Donohue, N. (1979, September-October). The perinatal bereavement crisis: Facilitating the grief process. *Journal of Nurse-Midwifery*, 24(5), 16-19.

Olshansky, S. (1962, April). Chronic sorrow: A response to having a mentally defective child. *Social Casework*, 43, 190-193.

Opirhory, G.J. (1979, May-June). Counseling the parents of a critically ill newborn. *JOGNN*, 8(3), 179-182.

Parkes, C.M. (1970). "Seeking" and "finding" a lost object: Evidence from recent studies of the reaction to bereavement. *Social Science and Medicine*, 4(2), 187-201.

Rees, W.D., and Lutkins, S.G. (1967). The mortality of bereavement. *British Medical Journal*, 4(570), 13-16.

Sahu, S. (1981). Coping with perinatal death. *Journal of Reproductive Medicine*, 26(3), 129-132.

Schiff, H.S. (1987). *The bereaved parent.* New York: Crown Publications.

Solnit, A., and Stark, M. (1961). Mourning and the birth of a defective child. *Psychoanal. Study Child*, 16:523-537.

Thomas, N., and Cordell, A.S. (1983). The dying infant: Aiding parents in the detachment process. *Pediatric Nursing*, 9(5), 355-357.

Trouy, M.B., and Ward-Larson, C. (1987). Sibling grief. *Neonatal Network*, 5(4), 35-40.

Woods, J.R., and Esposito, J.L. (1987). *Pregnancy loss: Medical therapeutics and practical considerations.* Baltimore: Williams & Wilkins.

Young, R.K. (1977). Chronic sorrow: Parents' response to the birth of a child with a defect. *MCN*, 2(1), 38-42.

Nursing research

Blackburn, S., and Lowen, L. (1986). Impact of an infant's premature birth on the grandparents and parents. *JOGNN*, 15(2), 173-178.

Brooten, D., Gennaro, S., Brown, L.P., Butts, P., Gibbons, A.L., Bakewell Sachs, S., and Kumar, S.P. (1988). Anxiety, depression, and hostility in mothers of preterm infants. *Nursing Research*, 37(4), 213-216.

Choi, E.C. (1986). Unique aspects of Korean-American mothers. *JOGNN*, 15(5), 394-400.

Gennaro, S. (1985). Maternal anxiety, problem-solving ability, and adaptation to the premature infant. *Pediatric Nursing*, 11(5), 343-348.

Discharge Planning and Neonatal Care at Home

Objectives

After reading and studying this chapter, the student should be able to:

1. Understand why the demand for home health care for neonates has increased in the past decade.

2. Define discharge planning, describe its goals, and identify the personnel and resources typically involved in planning for a neonate's discharge.

3. Discuss discharge planning needs of both the neonate and the family.

4. Recognize the financial implications of home health care for the family.

5. Describe methods the nurse may use to prepare parents for the neonate's discharge.

6. Describe the home health care needs of neonates with specific perinatal problems.

7. Discuss community resources that support home health care for neonates.

8. Apply the nursing process when caring for a neonate in the home.

Introduction

For increasing numbers of neonates, health care has been extended to the home. In the past decade, dramatic changes in health care—economic pressures, advances in the treatment of high-risk neonates, and the desire by families for more active participation in health care—have led to a growing demand for home health care and other community-based services.

Philosophical changes within the neonatal health care community also have played a role. For example, early discharge is now standard for normal healthy neonates. For the nurse working within the setting of a health care facility, early discharge means less time to plan for the neonate's discharge—yet a greater need for thorough discharge planning. For the nurse who makes postdischarge visits to the home, early discharge may mean a longer period of follow-up with a greater need for family support and individualized attention.

Also, high-risk neonates who survive their initial problems and become medically stable commonly require further treatment at home. Many have multiple chronic problems that call for specialized, complex home care; some depend on monitors and other technological devices. In 1988, for example, an estimated 10,000 American families experienced the birth of a catastrophically ill child (National Association of Children's Hospitals and Related Industries, Inc., 1989). Thus, home health care for neonates has become increasingly complex as well as common. The long-term success of the sophisticated technology now available for home use may hinge on how effectively the nurse and other health care professionals can extend their specialized knowledge and skills to the home.

To meet the challenges of home health care, the nurse must have expert assessment skills—sophisticated and holistic in scope, yet specific. Discharge planning must be the focus of care from the time of the neonate's admission to the nursery. As the main liaison between the family and health care providers, the nurse must possess a wealth of knowledge about neonatal and pediatric home health care and act as family advocate in determining the appropriateness of this care.

GLOSSARY

Apnea monitor: device that sounds an alarm when breathing or heartbeat stops or when the respiratory or heart rate drops below a preset level.

Child life therapist: professional who uses play activities to help ill children cope with their illness and medical environment.

Discharge planning: formulation of a plan by the health care team, client, family, and appropriate outside agencies to ensure that the client's physical and psychosocial needs are met after discharge.

Home health aide: person trained to provide personal care, such as bathing, dressing, and feeding, for the client at home.

Home health care: services, supplies, and equipment provided to a client in the home to maintain or promote physical, mental, and emotional health.

Respite care: care provided by a secondary caregiver to relieve the primary caregiver; may be required for several hours to several weeks.

Tertiary care facility: perinatal care facility that offers the most advanced technological and specialty care for neonates referred within a specific region.

This chapter discusses both preparation for and delivery of home health care for neonates. The first section describes discharge planning, which takes place within the health care facility. It delineates the nurse's role in discharge planning, discusses resources the nurse uses in discharge planning, and explains how to identify the discharge planning needs of the neonate and family. The second section of the chapter describes how the nurse provides health care in the home for both the normal and special-needs neonate. After describing the concept of case management and selection of home health care services and suppliers, this section demonstrates how to follow the nursing process steps—assessment, nursing diagnosis, planning, implementation, and evaluation—when caring for a neonate at home. The chapter concludes with a brief discussion of documentation.

Discharge planning

Discharge planning involves the formulation of a program by the health care team, client, family, and appropriate outside agencies to meet the client's physical and psychosocial needs after discharge. Discharge planning for a neonate prepares the neonate and family (or other primary caregivers) for care at home or in another health care facility.

The American Nurses' Association (1975) defines discharge planning as "that part of the continuity of care...designed to prepare the client for the next phase of care, whether it be self care, care by family members, or care by an organized health care provider."

All clients have the right to planned continuity of care after discharge. When effective, discharge planning improves both the continuity and cost-effectiveness of care. In response to fiscal restraints and pressure from third-party payers, most health care facilities now emphasize discharge planning.

Nurse's role

The nurse's role in discharge planning is delineated in the standards of neonatal nursing established in 1986 by NAACOG, the organization for obstetric, gynecologic, and neonatal nurses.

• The nurse develops the discharge plan, making referrals as necessary to help the family cope with the neonate's condition.
• The nurse helps integrate the neonate into the family.
• The nurse provides the family with health education to promote neonatal and infant care.
• The nurse initiates and participates in neonatal care conferences with the family and other members of the health care team.

Discharge planning systems

Although nurses are responsible for the health care aspects of discharge planning, some health care facilities have centralized discharge planning conducted by social workers or by a combination of social workers and nurses. With this system, the discharge planning department receives a list of new admissions every morning and identifies those neonates who will need extensive discharge planning.

Other facilities have a decentralized system, in which the nurse who works most closely with the client is responsible for discharge planning; as necessary, this nurse consults with other professionals for help with special aspects of planning, such as obtaining financial assistance.

The high-risk screen, a popular tool used by admitting offices, categorizes clients according to the intensity of their discharge planning needs. Most commonly, it is used in centralized discharge planning systems to "red-flag" and prioritize clients. In primary or secondary perinatal care facilities, the high-risk screen is used at nursery admission to identify:

• preterm neonates
• neonates of adolescent mothers
• neonates of mothers who used drugs or other substances during pregnancy
• neonates with no insurance coverage.

The use of high-risk screens is less helpful in a tertiary (intensive care) facility, where almost every neonate fits the high-risk category.

Discharge planning resources

Discharge planning requires close collaboration among health care team members. In most cases, the nurse can refer the family to any professional for discharge planning assistance (although in some cases a physician's order is required for a referral to a specialist from another discipline). Typically, in-facility resource personnel involved in discharge planning include:

• clinical nurse specialist
• physician
• social worker
• financial counselor
• speech, hearing, occupational, and physical therapists
• utilization review nurse
• dietitian
• respiratory therapist
• child life therapist.

For example, the nurse would collaborate with a social worker when planning the discharge of a preterm neonate of an unwed mother who rarely visits and is undecided about keeping her child. In this case, the nurse documents lack of visits by the mother and any conversations with other family members; the social worker determines whether the child should be discharged to another family member or to foster care if the mother chooses not to keep the child.

Complex discharge

For help with a complex discharge, particularly on weekends or holidays when other resource personnel may be unavailable, the nurse may refer to unit discharge planning manuals. Also, some facilities have parent libraries that offer information at the layperson's level on diseases, medical procedures, child development, and community resources; toy libraries may be available to lend toys adapted for children with special needs. For help in identifying appropriate home care resources within the community, a community nurse may prove invaluable.

Nurses and other professionals who are experts in discharge planning may belong to the American Association for Continuity of Care. This organization holds annual conferences and state-level meetings where members share information. The legislative arm lobbies for continuity-of-care issues at the national level.

Family involvement

To enhance their commitment to and confidence in the discharge plan, the neonate's parents should be allowed to participate actively in discharge planning and set realistic goals mutually with the health care team. The Joint Commission on Accreditation of Healthcare Organizations (JCAHO) stipulates that the medical record document the parents' involvement in discharge planning (1989). To help ensure parental involvement, the nurse may use a questionnaire, such as the one shown in *Discharge planning questionnaire*, page 1010.

Identifying discharge planning needs

To help avoid a delay in discharge once the neonate is medically ready, the nurse or other discharge planner should begin family preparation and arrangements for needed services at the time of delivery or, at the latest, by the time the neonate is admitted to the nursery. The nurse assesses the discharge planning needs of both the neonate and parents, using information from the nursing admission assessment and from ongoing assessment. (For details on gathering relevant data from admission information, see *Admission assessment*, page 1011.)

Neonatal needs

Assess the scope and complexity of the neonate's physical care needs, which may vary from routine care and arrangements for follow-up medical visits for the normal neonate to complex, high-technology care for the special-needs neonate. Identify the neonate's primary caregiver and at least one secondary caregiver who will be responsible for care in the primary caregiver's absence. Also determine which community agencies may need to be involved in home health care, which equipment and supplies will be required at home, and whether the home is adequate and safe for health care. To determine the latter, consider arranging for a predischarge home visit by a community health nurse.

Parental needs

To determine the parents' discharge planning needs, assess their:

• ability and willingness to care for the neonate at home
• ability to bond with the neonate

Discharge planning questionnaire

To help assess the neonate's and family's discharge planning needs, the nurse may ask the parents (or other primary caregiver) to complete a questionnaire, such as the one shown here.

1. What is your name and your relationship to the infant?

_____

2. During which times of day will you be able to visit your infant here at the health care facility?

_____ Mornings   _____ Nights

_____ Afternoons   _____ Not sure

_____ Evenings

3. How will you get here to visit your infant?

_____ Own car   _____ Relative or friend
                             will bring

_____ Public   _____ Other
       transportation

4. Who will be caring for your infant after discharge?

_____ Mother   _____ Friend

_____ Father   _____ Day care

_____ Babysitter   _____ Other

_____ Relative

5. Who will be able to help you with your infant's care at home?

_____ Spouse   _____ Other

_____ Relative   _____ No one available

_____ Friend

6. What kinds of help do you think your family will need to care for your infant at home?

_____

_____

7. Would you like to see a social worker who can help your family work out problems you might be having while your infant is in the health care facility?

_____ Yes   _____ No

8. Do you have any questions about your insurance coverage for your infant's home care?

_____ Yes   _____ No

9. Would you like to see a financial counselor to discuss your insurance coverage or to obtain information on applying for financial assistance?

_____ Yes   _____ No

10. Please indicate if you would like to see any of these professionals.

_____ Chaplain   _____ Dietitian

_____ Child life therapist _____ Other

Adapted with permission from Children's Hospital Medical Center, Cincinnati.

- understanding of growth and development
- knowledge of neonatal and infant care techniques
- physical and psychosocial support systems
- need for additional caregivers
- stress level
- medical insurance and financial resources
- psychosocial adaptation to the changing family structure.

Assessing the feasibility of home care

Although caring for the neonate at home may sound ideal, this is not always best for the neonate or family. The parents and health care team must consider many factors when determining the most appropriate postdischarge care setting, especially if the neonate has special needs.

Neonate's health status. Usually, the neonate must be in stable condition to be cared for at home. If the neonate will need high-technology equipment or extensive professional services, a final decision on the suitability of home care should be delayed until the neonate is medically stable. Continuing instability or the need for frequent laboratory tests usually necessitates institutional care.

Parental willingness and ability. For home care to succeed, the parents must be willing and able to take on primary responsibility for the neonate's health care. Some parents—those who are ill themselves, for instance—are unable physically to care for a child. Others cannot afford to quit a job to stay home with the neonate, particularly if the employer pays for medical insurance. Home care also may be out of the question if the neonate needs complex or frequent care—a situation requiring two or more caregivers so that one can relieve the other.

The nurse should not assume that all parents want to care for a special-needs child at home. Some parents feel intimidated by medical equipment and overwhelmed by the demands of providing complex care. Some are unwilling to add the burden of health care to their other responsibilities or to make the necessary life-style changes to accommodate complex home care. A few parents, unable to cope with an uncertain future, are unsuited psychologically to caring for a special-needs child.

In some cases, parents express the desire to care for the neonate at home but repeatedly fail to attend learning sessions; this may indicate that they have unexpressed concerns about their ability to provide home care. Other parents are willing but lack the ability to learn caregiving skills.

Practical and psychosocial support. The parents of a special-needs child must have sufficient physical and psychosocial support to cope with home health care. Yet these parents may not get the support they need. The U.S. General Accounting Office (1989) identified lack of information about available services or a resource person to contact when parents need help with home care as among the most common reasons why families with special-needs children have trouble obtaining support services.

Ideally, friends and other family members should be available to help care for other children and perform household chores. Respite for the parents also is crucial; a secondary caregiver who is trained in the required skills should be available to relieve the parents periodically from caregiving.

Psychosocial support is particularly important; parents of chronically ill children perceive less social support than parents of well children (Ferrari, 1986). Knowing that someone understands what the parents are going through, cares about them, and is available to offer emotional support can help the parents withstand the emotional rigors of caring for a special-needs child.

Cost considerations. In the United States, cost is a major issue when planning for discharge. Most major insurers provide only minimal coverage, if any, for home care even

Admission assessment

To obtain sufficient information to formulate a discharge plan, the nurse may want to use information obtained from the neonate's parents by an admission assessment tool, such as the one shown here. Each question is accompanied by a rationale that explains how the answer might affect the neonate's discharge planning needs.

Is this your first child?
Rationale: For parents of a first child, teaching of routine neonatal care is essential. However, all parents can benefit from a review of routine neonatal care.

Where does your family live?
Rationale: A family living in a rural area may have trouble obtaining follow-up care at a tertiary perinatal center for a special-needs neonate. Also, certain high-technology home care services may not be available in isolated areas.

Who will be the caregiver at different times of the day?
Rationale: Secondary caregivers and babysitters may need to learn special care techniques.

How do you plan on paying for home health care?
Rationale: For the neonate with a chronic illness or an anticipated long-term need for home health care, public and private insurers may cover only some costs, if any. Thus, the family will need financial counseling about alternative financial sources.

Is your family experiencing much stress right now? How extensive is your family's support system?
Rationale: To provide a safe environment for home care, the family may need help to minimize stress or enhance their support systems before the neonate's discharge. For the family with significant stress or little support, a referral to a social service agency may be necessary.

How much do you know about your child's medical condition?
Rationale: General teaching usually can begin soon after the neonate's admission to the nursery. (However, predicting what the neonate's condition will be at discharge or exactly which equipment and services will be needed at home may be impossible.)

though home care usually costs significantly less than institutional care of comparable duration. Also, few insurers will pay for home care if it costs more than institutional care—a situation that may occur with a special-needs child who requires one-to-one nursing care.

When home care is covered by insurance, the family may have to pay a yearly deductible of $100 to $500 before the insurer will begin to reimburse 80% of the

Alternatives to home care

Alternatives for neonates and infants who require continued medical care but cannot be discharged to the home vary with local and state laws and with financial reimbursement methods. In some regions, foster care for special-needs neonates is available. However, some state Medicaid programs do not reimburse for care provided in foster homes if the foster-home program is poorly regulated.

Although some special-needs neonates might be eligible for nursing home placement, many nursing homes do not accept pediatric clients or lack the high-technology equipment and skilled care some neonates, such as those dependent on a tracheostomy or ventilator, require. Thus, for lack of an alternative, some neonates must remain in the tertiary health care facility.

However, some new alternative care arrangements have been established. The Children's Home of Pittsburgh, for instance, has a transitional infant care program that serves as a bridge between neonatal intensive care units and the home. Infants receive medical and nursing care while parents, who are provided with live-in facilities, are trained to become competent and confident in their child's care.

Also, some regions now have day health care settings, called prescribed pediatric extended care (PPEC) facilities, which expedite the discharge of special-needs children. These facilities provide individualized nursing and supportive care while the parents work as well as respite care when a parent is ill or needs a break from caregiving. The homelike, normalcy-oriented setting allows children to interact with their peers and eliminates the need for parents to hire private-duty nurses at home. Care in PPEC facilities is about two-thirds as expensive as in-home skilled nursing care (Pierce, Freedman, and Reiss, 1987).

charges. Also, some insurers cover only certain types of equipment; for instance, they may pay for durable medical equipment, such as enteral feeding pumps, but not for disposables, such as the feeding bags and tubes used with such pumps. Moreover, most third-party payers limit the amount they will reimburse yearly for home nursing services; the average $5,000 limit would cover just 1 week of around-the-clock nursing care at $30/hour (this amount includes indirect costs as well as the nurse's wage). Many special-needs children nearly exhaust their lifetime maximum insurance benefits before discharge; further medical costs may devastate the family financially. This is a major concern for U.S. citizens, legislators, and health care providers and has sparked the introduction of catastrophic health care legislation.

Hidden costs usually are not reported in comparisons of institutional and home health care expenses; however, such costs can be substantial. Hidden costs include lost income when a family member must take time off from work to care for the child, higher home electricity bills (such as when the neonate requires me-

chanical ventilation), modifications of the home or family vehicle to accommodate special equipment, and transportation to and from physician appointments.

Other factors. The family considering home care must have transportation for follow-up medical visits. Also, the home environment must be suitable for caregiving, with adequate space to store supplies and set up equipment. Preferably, it also should have indoor plumbing, refrigeration, electricity, and a telephone (or easy access to one). Availability of services also must be considered. For instance, private-duty nurses may not be available in rural areas.

Supporting the family's decision. The nurse and other members of the health team must be willing to support the family's informed decision regarding the neonate's placement. This is particularly important if the parents are considering an alternative care setting and have unresolved doubts about their moral, ethical, and legal obligations to their child; reinforcement of these doubts by the nurse could cause overwhelming parental guilt. (For information on options for placement of the special-needs child, see *Alternatives to home care*.)

Likewise, the nurse should avoid imposing personal values on the parents. A parent's unkempt appearance or unhealthful life-style, for instance, may offend the nurse; lack of toilets and running water in the home may not conform to the nurse's view of a safe, healthful home environment. However, make an effort to maintain objectivity when considering whether such deficiencies represent real threats to the child's health and safety. After all, many children thrive even in the harshest environments. Also, the nurse who tries to "make the picture perfect" stands a good chance of encountering repeated disappointments and may have trouble establishing a positive relationship with the family. In any event, making referrals to the appropriate social service agencies and other resources fulfills the nurse's responsibility.

On the other hand, if the parents seem incapable of responsible parenting and their behavior or attitude suggests that the neonate will be neglected or abused after discharge, the nurse should consider notifying a social worker, who may attempt to have the court place the neonate in protective custody.

Ongoing assessment of discharge planning needs
Obviously, the nurse cannot assess all discharge planning needs at the time of nursery admission but must continue to assess these needs throughout the neonate's stay in the health care facility. As new needs arise, they must be incorporated into the discharge plan.

Many health care facilities conduct ongoing assessment of discharge planning needs during weekly discharge planning rounds and regularly scheduled client care conferences in addition to daily nurse-physician rounds. Topics discussed in these forums typically include the parents' understanding of and attitude toward the neonate's condition, the parents' coping ability and capacity to provide adequate care at home, the home environment, the family's need for support services and community resources, and the neonate's readiness for discharge.

Discharge planning rounds. During discharge planning rounds, each client on the unit is discussed briefly by a multidisciplinary team consisting of nurse, physician, social worker, occupational or physical therapist, dietitian, child life therapist, and perhaps a utilization review nurse and financial counselor. The team discusses assessment findings and ways to meet the neonate's and family's discharge planning needs.

Each team member is assigned specific tasks. The physician, for instance, typically will record which pediatrician or other primary care physician the parents have chosen for postdischarge care. The nurse will provide parent teaching (such as how to perform cardiopulmonary resuscitation [CPR], if appropriate), and make referrals to home health care companies. The social worker will determine if friends or other family members will be available to help with household tasks. The financial counselor will determine if the family's medical insurance covers private-duty home nursing care and, if so, to what dollar limit.

This discussion is documented in the client progress notes. In subsequent days or weeks, members of the health care team report on their assignments and work to finalize the discharge plan.

Client care conference. This forum, usually used to discuss a single client in depth, aids in the development and implementation of the discharge plan for the neonate who requires special planning. For some special-needs neonates, several such conferences may be required. The nurse may call the conference to conduct prospective planning or to discuss a new development or health crisis. To minimize the miscommunication and differences of opinion that can arise when several professionals are involved in a client's care, all major health care team members should take part in the conference; to help ensure continuity of care, the neonate's private physician also should attend. Usually, the parents are invited to attend, at least for the summary.

The physician or primary nurse usually chairs the conference, describing the neonate's current situation and requesting clarification and consensus on the plan of care. The nurse should ensure that the parents are supported rather than intimidated at the conference and

that any questions or concerns they bring up are addressed adequately. As with discharge planning rounds, the client care conference is summarized by the primary nurse and recorded in the neonate's medical record.

Implementing the discharge plan

To implement the discharge plan, the nurse prepares the parents by teaching them about the care the neonate will require, helps them select a home health agency and order medical equipment and supplies, arranges for follow-up medical visits, makes appropriate referrals to community health services and other resources, and verifies that a family support system is in place by the time the neonate is discharged.

For the neonate with special needs, the American Academy of Pediatrics (1984) recommends that the discharge plan include a primary care physician, a case coordinator, a defined backup system for medical emergency care, verification of family access to a telephone, and a means of monitoring and adjusting the care plan as necessary. If the neonate requires special equipment, some health care facilities require that the equipment be brought there and used to check its operation and familiarize the parents with it.

Preparing the parents for the neonate's discharge

The nurse must ensure that the parents learn caregiving skills before the neonate's discharge. Besides routine neonatal and infant caregiving techniques, teaching topics may include emergency interventions, signs and symptoms of medical problems, use of special equipment, the purpose and adverse effects of medications, and names of people to contact when the parents have questions.

Use of written, standardized teaching plans ensures that teaching content is congruent over time and among professionals; however, when using such plans, make sure to individualize them so that they are relevant to the family's unique situation. Also, provide adequate learning time, making allowances for such problems as tardiness or missed appointments because of work responsibilities, lack of transportation, or difficulty finding a babysitter.

During parent preparation, keep in mind the various factors that can affect a parent's readiness and ability to learn: anxiety, previous experiences with illness, physical and mental capacities, cultural and ethnic background, language, family relationships, and motivation. As necessary, adjust the teaching plan around these factors. Because many parents are under stress when learning new information or skills and may not absorb information completely, be sure to reinforce verbal teaching with printed materials written at a fourth-grade reading level; preferably, these materials should have pictures or diagrams. Topics covered in such handouts should include illnesses, medications, special procedures, and well-baby care. (Use of written teaching materials also makes documentation of teaching more efficient and consistent.)

Besides verbal and written instruction, another useful teaching strategy is demonstration. Asking for a return demonstration of skills demonstrated by the nurse gives parents the chance to practice these skills and allows the nurse to check for evidence of their caregiving competence and confidence.

Videotapes are increasingly used as a teaching tool because they allow demonstration of skills with maximum consistency of content. Many nurses find that one-on-one teaching time is reduced when parents have seen a videotape. Many videotaped teaching resources are available for parents.

Selecting home health care services

Over the past 10 years, the home health care industry has seen phenomenal growth. However, not every agency or company that describes itself as a home health care service specializes in neonatal or pediatric care. The discharge planning staff should steer the parents toward agencies and companies with neonatal and pediatric expertise.

To avoid problems with reimbursement that could delay the neonate's discharge, the nurse should aim for early identification of the home health care services the neonate will need. (For specific information on home health care services, see the "Home health care" section of this chapter.)

Planning for payment of home health care

If third-party payment is unavailable, refer the family to a financial counselor for information on alternative funding sources, such as private, religious, local, and national associations and foundations, as well as specialized support groups, such as the March of Dimes Foundation.

Arranging for follow-up care

Verify that the parents know the dates and times of scheduled follow-up medical visits; this information should be supplied to them in writing. Also make sure they will have transportation for these visits. If they do not have transportation, refer them to a social worker, who can inform them of transportation services. Also make sure the parents know whom to call with questions and concerns about the neonate's health care. To evaluate the effectiveness of the discharge plan and to provide emotional support, arrange to call the parents a few days after the neonate's discharge.

Preparing discharge instructions

Discharge instructions may take the form of written materials, such as booklets and printed instruction sheets for specific diseases, medication, or equipment; however, be sure to individualize such materials. Give discharge information to the parents early enough to allow them to read it, absorb it, and come up with questions that can be answered before the neonate's discharge, while the health care team is most accessible. Make sure to give parents emergency numbers to keep by the telephone at home. However, tell them that they are welcome to place nonemergency calls to ask any questions that may arise.

Send a copy of the discharge instructions and information about the neonate's status at discharge to the private physician's office and to the health care agency that will follow the child at home. If the parents received teaching handouts, also send a copy of these to the home health care agency to ensure continuity of care.

Documenting the discharge plan

The JCAHO (1989) stipulates that the discharge plan be recorded in the client's medical record; this promotes continuity of care, provides a communication link for other team members, and serves as a reference for legal and other purposes. Make sure the medical record includes:

• assessment of the neonate's needs, problems, capabilities, and limitations
• evidence of parental participation in discharge planning
• evidence of parental learning of information provided
• availability of recommended services for the family
• the neonate's medical status at discharge
• the actual discharge plan, including prescribed medications, follow-up medical appointments, and any referrals to community agencies.

Home health care

Home health care—the services, supplies, and equipment provided to a client at home—helps to maintain or promote a client's physical, mental, or emotional health. Home health care can reduce the cost of neonatal care while providing support to the family.

Studies show that home health care can be safe and cost-effective even for high-risk neonates. Brooten, et al. (1986) randomly assigned low-birth-weight neonates to two groups. One group was discharged according to routine nursery criteria. The second group was discharged an average of 11 days earlier and weighed 200 g (7 oz) less; a perinatal nurse specialist provided evaluation and parent teaching and support for this group before discharge, during home visits 1 week after discharge, and periodically afterward. The researchers found no difference between the groups in number of rehospitalizations or in physical and mental growth and development, but health care costs per neonate in the group discharged earlier were $18,560 lower than for the other group.

Home health care also may improve mother-infant interaction. Norr, Nacion, and Abramson (1989) studied interaction between low-income, inner-city mothers and their neonates in three groups:
• simultaneous early discharge of mother and neonate (24 to 47 hours after delivery)
• early discharge of the mother, with discharge of the neonate after 48 hours
• simultaneous conventional discharge of mother and neonate (48 to 72 hours after delivery).

The selection criteria ensured that only low-risk mothers and neonates were discharged early. A nurse and community aide visited the simultaneous early-discharge group 1 to 2 days after discharge to conduct physical examinations and phenylketonuria and bilirubin testing; provide standard teaching on health, safety, and infant growth and development; and discuss the mothers' concerns. The researchers found stronger mother-infant bonding, fewer maternal concerns, and greater maternal satisfaction with postpartal care in this group, with no increase in maternal or neonatal morbidity in the first 2 weeks after discharge. However, all of the subjects in this study required careful health monitoring, and the mothers needed considerable teaching during the first month at home.

As these studies suggest, including a perinatal nurse specialist in a home health care program helps ensure that the parents receive expert advice and that neonatal problems are prevented or detected early through comprehensive assessment. In regions where perinatal nurse specialists are not available, home nurse generalists must maintain conscientious communication with nurse specialists and physicians to provide continuity of care.

Home health care services, equipment, and supplies

Home health care services may be provided by public agencies or private companies. Equipment, supplies, and other products used for home care typically are obtained from private companies. The tremendous expansion in home health care has led to increased competition among providers of services and products. However, many services are geared to geriatric clients; therefore, careful selection is crucial.

Services
Formerly, home health care was the nearly exclusive province of the public health nurse, who provided not only illness care but health promotion and comprehensive family care. However, the passage of Medicare and Medicaid legislation led to dramatic changes in payment and provision systems and in client eligibility for home care. As physicians' roles in home care enlarged, such care became less comprehensive and more narrowly focused on illness care. Currently, professionals who may provide home health care include nurses, physicians, social workers, dietitians, and speech, hearing, occupational, and physical therapists. Many clients also require home health aides and homemaker services.

Nurses involved in home health care include public or community health nurses, private-duty nurses, and nurses from home care departments of local hospitals or for-profit (proprietary) home health care companies. These nurses and other professionals can be hired through a public, proprietary, or hospital-based agency.

A certified home care nursing agency (which may be run privately or publicly) is one that is subject to certain standards of care and has been certified for Medicare reimbursement. Such an agency can provide nurses for intermittent visits and also may provide speech, hearing, occupational, and physical therapists; homemakers; and home health aides. Many certified agencies also can supply private-duty or hourly nurses for families who have private insurance or can pay directly for nursing care.

Equipment and supplies
Home health care equipment and supplies can be obtained from durable medical equipment companies, surgical pharmacies, and home infusion therapy services. Selection of a vendor should take into account the company's pediatric experience and the range of equipment and supplies provided. Optimally, the vendor should offer preventive maintenance, free loaner equipment during repairs, 24-hour availability for emergency service, and prompt response to service calls.

Durable medical equipment companies provide respiratory equipment, such as oxygen tanks, mechanical ventilators, and apnea monitors; most also can supply hospital beds (but usually not cribs), wheelchairs, phototherapy equipment, enteral feeding pumps, and other supplies for home use. These companies usually employ a nurse or respiratory therapist to manage the home use of their equipment. Home infusion therapy services can provide home chemotherapy, pain control therapy, an-

Criteria for home mechanical ventilation

The decision to care for a mechanically ventilated neonate at home is a difficult one. The parents must undergo extensive predischarge teaching, and the neonate's prolonged need for complex care creates an enormous emotional and financial drain on the family. Also, home assessment of the mechanically ventilated neonate can be challenging. In the health care facility, blood gas analysis, transcutaneous monitoring, and pulse oximetry help the health care team assess the neonate's ventilatory requirements. At home, where these evaluative mechanisms usually are not available, management is based on skin color, absence or presence of signs of respiratory compromise, and, in some cases, apnea monitoring.

On the other hand, the ventilator-dependent neonate who is cared for at home usually has a decreased infection risk, greater socialization, and better stimulation for growth and development (Donar, 1988).

Ahmann (1986) identifies the following criteria for mechanical ventilation at home.

- The neonate must have a stable underlying disease and continued inability to be weaned from mechanical ventilation.
- The neonate must be able to maintain an adequate nutritional intake, as measured by consistent growth and development.
- The parents must have a positive attitude, motivation, and willingness to make a 24-hour commitment to their neonate's care.
- The family must have access to a community source for equipment and supplies, emergency care, and home nursing personnel and must have the financial resources to support the cost of prolonged, complex care.
- The home must support the mechanical and electrical needs of the ventilator and have adequate space for caregiving activities and storage of equipment and supplies.

tibiotic therapy, and enteral feedings. For neonates and infants, home infusion therapy is used mainly to deliver total parenteral nutrition.

Case management

Case management is a system whereby a single person manages a client's care, helping to prevent duplication of services, to decrease costs (by assuring timely services and preventing complications), and to promote continuity of care. In the home care setting, the case manager may be responsible for advising the family on the services they need, arranging for nurses and equipment, arranging for payment of services, solving problems, and visiting the family regularly. For home care,

the community health nurse is especially well-suited to serve as case manager.

Ironically, case management has become so popular that several case managers may be assigned to a family—perhaps one from the insurance company, another from the home health agency, and yet another from developmental services. However, not every family requires case management; many need information only and can act as their own case managers. Case management is most helpful for parents who lack the ability or means to coordinate their child's care and for those whose child has multiple needs necessitating the involvement of several agencies and support services (U.S. General Accounting Office, 1989).

Neonatal home health care needs

The trend toward early discharge has increased the need for home health care for both normal, healthy neonates and special-needs neonates. (For information on when mechanical ventilation may be appropriate, see *Criteria for home mechanical ventilation*. For indications for nutritional therapy and applicable nursing considerations, see *Home nutrition therapy*.)

Routine and basic care

For the normal, healthy neonate, home health care typically involves assessment of the neonate and teaching, counseling, and support for the family. Areas of particular interest to the nurse include the neonate's nutritional status, healing of the umbilicus and circumcision site, feeding patterns, urinary and bowel elimination patterns, and sleep-awake patterns. As necessary, the nurse may draw blood samples for various laboratory tests (such as serum bilirubin analysis).

The nurse also assesses the parents' ability to provide routine care (such as bathing, feeding, diapering, stimulation, and cord and circumcision care) and perform basic health care procedures (such as taking rectal temperature, administering vitamins and medications, and suctioning with a bulb syringe).

Some otherwise healthy neonates require phototherapy at home for the treatment of jaundice or an elevated serum unconjugated bilirubin level. Phototherapy, which involves exposure of the neonate's skin to various lights, previously necessitated continued hospitalization. The significant cost of the treatment in this setting and the enforced separation from parents led practitioners to attempt home phototherapy (Hartsell, 1986; Heiser, 1987). Home phototherapy with supportive teaching for parents is a safe, satisfactory intervention that produces substantial savings for families, health care facilities, and insurance providers (Heiser, 1987).

Home nutrition therapy

The neonate who cannot ingest sufficient nutrients orally or whose gastrointestinal (GI) tract cannot be used for nutritional replenishment may require enteral or parenteral (I.V.) nutrition therapy at home to ensure adequate nutrition.

Enteral nutrition
The preferred method for nutritional support, enteral nutrition is the administration of nutrients through a feeding tube to the GI tract. Besides helping to maintain GI function, enteral therapy has fewer risks and costs less than parenteral nutrition. Enteral therapy may be required to supplement oral feedings or to supply the total caloric intake for the neonate with a vomiting disorder (such as gastroesophageal reflux), an inadequate sucking reflex (for instance, from prolonged mechanical ventilation), or a respiratory or cardiac disorder that reduces the energy available for oral feeding.

Administration routes. High-risk neonates usually receive enteral nutrition through a nasogastric (NG) tube or an orogastric tube—methods known as gavage feeding. In some cases, however, a gastrostomy tube is used. Gavage feeding commonly is used for intermittent or short-term home use but also may be appropriate for long-term home use. The tube may be made of polyurethane, polyvinyl chloride, or silicone (Silastic) material. Although Silastic tubes are more expensive than ones made of harder plastic, they are preferred for home use because they are easier to insert and cause less irritation to the GI mucosa. For home use, they can be reused after washing with soap and water.

Gastrostomy feedings necessitate surgical placement of a tube in the abdomen to deposit feedings directly into the stomach. Gastrostomy feedings are the preferred method for long-term home enteral nutrition.

Administration methods. The method used to administer gavage or gastrostomy feedings depends on the neonate's GI tolerance. Bolus feedings can be given by gravity through a syringe attached to the tube; larger volumes are introduced into the stomach at a rate similar to that of normal sucking on a breast or bottle. Some high-risk neonates given bolus feedings experience feeding intolerance, manifested as diarrhea or vomiting. Bolus feedings are contraindicated in neonates or infants with a history of gastroesophageal reflux (unless the cardiac sphincter has been repaired) because they may precipitate regurgitation or aspiration.

With continuous feedings, a pump and administration set are used to deliver small volumes of formula continuously. Although continuous feedings usually are tolerated better than bolus feedings, they restrict the neonate's mobility because the pump and tubing must remain attached to the neonate. However, scheduling most feedings at night minimizes the need to restrict daytime activities (if appropriate, oral feedings can be given during the day). Because the family must rent the pump and buy the tubing, continuous feedings are relatively expensive.

Enteral nutrition formulas. The high-risk neonate may need a high-calorie enteral nutrition formula (27 to 30 calories/oz) to meet energy and growth demands. Some of these formulas are hyperosmolar, however, and may cause diarrhea and subsequent weight loss.

Parenteral nutrition
Parenteral nutrition refers to the I.V. administration of fluids containing glucose, amino acids, electrolytes, vitamins, and minerals in specific proportions necessary for growth. In most cases, parenteral nutrition is administered as total parenteral nutrition (TPN), a nutritionally complete form usually delivered through a central venous catheter inserted into a large neck or chest vessel. Many neonates and infants receive a combination of TPN and enteral nutrition.

Candidates for parenteral therapy include neonates who cannot receive adequate food through the GI tract. For instance, neonates with congenital GI anomalies, such as omphalocele (protrusion of an intestinal portion through an abdominal wall defect at the umbilicus) or gastroschisis (protrusion of an intestinal portion through a defect elsewhere in the abdominal wall), may have suffered significant small intestine loss during surgery or may have developed multiple obstructions secondary to adhesions. Thus, they may be unable to tolerate any enteral formula.

Nursing considerations
• For enteral feedings, teach the parents to position the neonate prone, with the shoulders at least 30 degrees higher than the feet, and to maintain the neonate in this position for at least 20 minutes after the feeding.
• If the neonate has gastroesophageal reflux, inform the parents that the head must remain higher than the stomach to reduce the risk of aspiration. If appropriate, teach them how to use a special harness to maintain proper positioning, with the head of the crib elevated 30 to 45 degrees.
• To help prevent aspiration of enteral feedings, show the parents how to aspirate stomach contents to check for residual matter before feedings. Also teach them how to use a stethoscope to auscultate air insertion through the tube when checking tube placement before feedings.
• Make sure the parents know how to prepare and administer feedings. For example, teach them to warm the formula to room temperature. Explain how to attach the filled drip set to the tube and regulate the flow using the clamp or pump. Advise them to burp the neonate periodically and at the end of the feeding and to position the neonate on the right side afterward.
• Instruct the parents to call the physician if the feeding tube becomes blocked or dislodged; insertion of a new tube may be necessary.
• Teach the parents how to provide skin care around the tube insertion site or stoma. Advise them to tape the NG tube without applying upward pressure against the nostril. Instruct them to clean the neonate's nose or stoma with soap and water (or the prescribed solution) and to keep the area dry.
• Instruct the parents how to prepare a high-calorie enteral formula, if ordered; proper preparation helps minimize diarrhea. Make sure they know how to assess for diarrhea and other complications of tube feedings, such as vomiting, aspiration of feeding matter (from improper tube position), abdominal cramps (from rapid feeding administration), and skin breakdown around the stoma of the gastrostomy tube.
• Mouth care is especially important for infants who are fed enterally or parenterally. Instruct the parents to swab the neonate's mouth with moistened sponge-tipped swabs or gauze to keep it clean and moist and to apply white petrolatum to the lips to help prevent drying and cracking.
• Instruct the parents to weigh the child regularly to monitor nutritional status.

Candidates for home phototherapy typically include term neonates who tolerate oral feedings well and lack underlying hemolytic disease. Also, the parents must be willing and able to manage this treatment at home and to arrange for serial laboratory bilirubin testing.

Specialized care

Besides routine and basic care, the high-risk or special-needs neonate requires sophisticated, complex care at home. Such care may involve apnea monitoring, suctioning, chest physiotherapy, oxygen therapy, tracheostomy care, mechanical ventilation, enteral or parenteral nutrition, medication administration, and developmental stimulation programs.

The typical neonate who requires specialized home care is preterm or low birth weight and has one or some combination of the following disorders: respiratory distress, bronchopulmonary dysplasia, apnea of prematurity, patent ductus arteriosus, hearing or visual impairment, hydrocephalus, intraventricular hemorrhage, seizures, or necrotizing enterocolitis. Congenital anomalies and the effects of maternal substance abuse also may necessitate specialized home care. (For information on the pathophysiology and management of these and other perinatal disorders, see Chapter 38, High-Risk Neonates.)

Psychosocial support is a key aspect of home care for the family of the special-needs neonate. The transition from the intensive care unit to the home can be stressful for parents; although they are relieved that their child is well enough to be discharged, they also may have doubts and fears about their ability to provide care at home.

Assessment

Before the first home visit, the nurse should review the discharge plan to become acquainted with the neonate's hospital course, discharge medications, and care instructions and to determine the parents' caregiving skills, confidence level, and teaching and support needs.

First home visit

Make every effort to establish a rapport so that the parents will feel free to discuss their concerns openly. Avoid medical jargon and be attentive and nonjudgmental as the parents discuss their concerns. Keep in mind that the home, unlike the health care facility, is the family's territory; an intrusive, domineering approach here could make the family resent the nurse's presence.

Obtain baseline information about the neonate's physical status, growth, and development, and make a preliminary assessment of the parents' caregiving knowledge and skills and the family's support system.

Also assess the home environment and the family's emergency plans, and confirm that any required equipment is functioning properly and that all needed supplies are present. Obtain information for insurance and other financial matters, and have the parents sign any necessary forms. At this visit and all subsequent visits, ask the parents what their main concerns are and then address these concerns.

Also obtain a health history and perform a physical assessment; however, if this will take more time than the family can spare, the history may be obtained gradually over subsequent visits. For the high-risk neonate, gear the physical assessment toward the specific condition, as described below under "Assessment of the special-needs neonate."

If the neonate is taking medications, review the dosages and schedules with the parents. If the schedules are inconvenient, with nighttime doses and many separate dosage times, consider asking the physician to modify them.

Parental caregiving knowledge and skills. Assess the parents' ability to perform routine and basic neonatal health care. Also evaluate their ability to provide any specific interventions, such as phototherapy, that the neonate requires. If the neonate needs specialized care, such as enteral or parenteral feeding, apnea monitoring, or oxygen therapy, assess the parents' understanding of the purpose of this care and the proper operation of equipment and medical supplies; make sure they know how to examine the neonate for problems related to the use of such equipment. (For detailed assessment information, see *Assessment guidelines for the neonate who requires special equipment.*) If premixed solutions are required, such as for nutritional therapy, verify that the family has a refrigerator for solution storage; if not, find out if the home infusion therapy service can supply refrigeration, and if so, whether they will charge for this.

Support system. Although the hospital discharge planning staff makes a preliminary assessment of the support system that may be available to the family after discharge, the home health care nurse has the advantage of assessing the support system in action, determining its extent and reliability. The major support needs of the family caring for a special-needs child at home are physical support for caregiving and household tasks, respite care, and psychosocial support.

Physical support. Assess how much physical support the parents need and how much they are receiving. Many parents of special-needs children must rely on help from friends and relatives because few community support agencies are geared toward the special-needs child.

Assessment guidelines for the neonate who requires special equipment

The chart below shows key assessment guidelines if the neonate requires special medical equipment. Before the first home visit, the nurse should obtain the health history to review the reason for the equipment and the neonate's hospital course. On each home visit, verify that all equipment is functioning properly; conduct a rapid review of functional patterns and body systems, then focus the assessment on the neonate's specific problem.

EQUIPMENT AND INDICATIONS	HEALTH HISTORY AND PHYSICAL ASSESSMENT DATA	PARENTAL KNOWLEDGE AND SKILLS	EQUIPMENT-RELATED DATA
Apnea monitor Apnea of prematurity, respiratory compromise, tracheostomy use, acute drug withdrawal, family history of apnea or sudden infant death	• Vital signs • Respiratory status • Frequency and duration of predischarge apneic episodes, need for resuscitation after an episode, and any associated signs or precipitating factors • Postdischarge history of pallor, cyanosis, or hypotonia • Postdischarge history of apnea or bradycardia alarms, their frequency and duration, and type of stimulation required to arouse the neonate	• Understanding of apnea and purpose of monitor • Knowledge of correct monitor settings • Operation of monitor • Safety precautions; proper response to monitor alarms • Ability to keep an accurate apnea log • Knowledge of infant CPR procedure	• Presence of all needed supplies in the home, including lead wires, patches, and an instruction manual • Use of grounded outlet for monitor • Appropriateness and accuracy of monitor settings • Proper monitor placement (on a hard surface at the bedside with sufficient ventilation behind and above monitor) • Correct placement of electrodes (they must contact sides of chest wall)
Oxygen therapy Respiratory or cardiac disorder	• Vital signs • Respiratory status • Skin color changes, such as peripheral cyanosis and signs of respiratory distress	• Understanding of purpose and use of oxygen therapy • Competence and confidence in using equipment • Knowledge of safety precautions	• Accuracy of concentration and liter flow • Use of recommended equipment • Correct number of hours of daily oxygen therapy • Proper equipment function • Adequate supply level of oxygen source • Use of a humidity source (if prescribed) and proper humidifier function and settings • Proper use of prescribed delivery method (such as cannula or mask)
Tracheostomy Upper airway obstruction, respiratory failure from mechanical or neurologic problems, chronic aspiration, long-term mechanical ventilation	• Vital signs • Respiratory status • Quality, color, viscosity, and odor of tracheal secretions • Condition of skin at tracheostomy site	• Purpose of tracheostomy • Indications for suctioning (such as when the neonate has wheezing breath sounds, when bubbling of secretions can be heard in the airway, and when the neonate shows signs of respiratory distress) • Competence and confidence in performing tracheostomy care (such as routine daily cleaning of the tracheostomy site, daily changing of tracheostomy ties, suctioning, and tube insertion and removal) • Knowledge of modified cardiopulmonary resuscitation procedure	• Proper use of humidification source (such as compressor with a nebulizer or cascade, room humidifier, or tracheostomy humidifying filter) • Correct size of tracheostomy tubes and suction catheter

(continued)

Assessment guidelines for the neonate who requires special equipment continued

EQUIPMENT AND INDICATIONS	HEALTH HISTORY AND PHYSICAL ASSESSMENT DATA	PARENTAL KNOWLEDGE AND SKILLS	EQUIPMENT-RELATED DATA
Mechanical ventilator Respiratory disorder	• Vital signs (compare observed respiratory rate against ventilator rate) • Skin color, respiratory pattern, and rise and fall of chest with each breath	• Understanding of ventilator's purpose, function, and operation • Ability to assess for signs of respiratory distress, fatigue, and periorbital edema • Ability to prevent atelectasis through frequent positioning changes, hyperinflation, chest physiotherapy, and suctioning • Ability to check for proper ventilator function and settings • Knowledge of proper response to ventilator alarms • Ability to use other equipment the neonate requires (such as oxygen therapy or apnea monitor)	• Proper ventilator settings • Correct bellows functioning • Alarm lights on • Connections secure • Tubing unkinked • Humidifier filled • Availability of backup power supply (such as batteries or a generator)
Enteral or parenteral nutrition therapy Inability to ingest adequate calories by mouth	• Nutritional status (such as growth parameters and daily tube or I.V. intake) • Skin condition around tube or I.V. insertion site	• Knowledge and ability to prepare and administer feedings correctly • Ability to assess for proper tube placement before each tube feeding (using a stethoscope to auscultate air insertion through tube) • Ability to identify such problems as tube dislodgement and nasal irritation • Knowledge of proper interventions for tube dislodgement • Ability to identify and troubleshoot equipment problems • Ability to provide mouth care and assess and intervene for complications of tube feedings (such as vomiting, diarrhea, aspiration of feeding matter, and abdominal cramps) or parenteral nutrition (such as air embolism, infection, metabolic problems, and fluid extravasation) • Understanding of special positioning requirements during feedings	• Correct function of feeding pump • Appropriateness of feeding technique; enteral or I.V. formula; placement, size, and type of tube; administration method; feeding frequency and duration; and neonate positioning • Availability of refrigeration for storage of feeding solutions • Adequate home sanitation to allow sterile procedures required for nutritional therapy

Meals On Wheels, for example, provides hot meals for people physically unable to cook for themselves but not for parents struggling with an ill child. Also, many insurance companies reimburse homemaker services for adults who cannot physically maintain their homes but not for parents of ill children, on the grounds that the parents are physically able to perform household tasks.

Also assess whether the parents have a realistic attitude toward their need for physical support. Many parents are reluctant to ask for help, feeling that they should be able to care for their special-needs child round the clock while keeping house, attending to other children, and meeting their personal needs.

Respite care. Determine whether a secondary caregiver is available. The parents of a child who requires high-technology or other complex care need occasional respite, or relief, from caregiving but may have trouble finding it. Some regional perinatal centers provide respite care. Also, respite care is available through various community programs; however, the caregivers provided by these programs rarely are trained to care for special-needs neonates or infants. On the other hand, friends and relatives may be intimidated by the idea of caring for a child who depends on medical equipment; although wishing they could help, they may worry that they will not know what to do if something happens and that the child will die while in their care.

Thus, many parents of special-needs children discover that only a nurse is comfortable with, or capable of, caring for their child. But hiring a nurse to provide a few hours of respite care costs at least five times as much as a regular babysitter. Consequently, parents may forego respite care and never take a break from caregiving. Eventually, this can take a toll on the parents' health as well as the couple's relationship and other family relationships.

Psychosocial support. Determine if the parents are aware of support groups and other resources that can provide psychosocial support, especially if their neonate has special needs. Members of parent support groups have had first-hand experience in caring for special-needs children and can offer advice on which problems to anticipate, how to cope with problems, and where to find special supplies or services. For instance, Sick Kids Need Involved People (SKIP) is a support group for families of technology-dependent children, particularly those requiring tracheostomies and ventilatory support. Founded in 1980, it promotes specialized pediatric home care for medically fragile children. (For a study of the effects of belonging to a parent support group, see *Nursing research applied: How membership in a support group affects parents of chronically ill children.*)

Home environment. Assess whether the home has adequate facilities and space for caregiving. For the special-needs neonate, check for sufficient electrical outlets and adequate shelving or other storage arrangements for supplies (however, make sure supplies are not stored directly over the neonate's bed). Determine whether the family might benefit by installing ramps to allow easier movement of the child and equipment into and out of the house. Also observe for evidence that home health care may be disrupting family functioning; if so, assess whether the parents should consider converting a downstairs room into the child's bedroom to give them privacy from home health personnel.

Emergency plan. Determine if the family has a good emergency plan. A telephone is essential; if the home lacks one, find out if the parents have made other arrange-

---

NURSING RESEARCH APPLIED

How membership in a support group affects parents of chronically ill children

To determine how psychosocial support affects parental needs, 159 families of children with chronic conditions were asked to complete surveys revealing specific needs related to their child's condition. Forty percent were members of a parent support group (denoted as PSG); 60% did not belong to such a group (denoted as NPSG). Among the PSG subjects, the mean age of the child was 5.7 years and the mean family income was $20,000 to $25,000; 92% were part of a two-parent family. Among the NPSG subjects, the mean age of the child was 7.3 years and the mean family income was $15,000 to $20,000; one-third were single parents.

The PSG subjects identified a greater need than NSPG subjects for help with their child's medical expenses (perhaps their higher income made them ineligible for external assistance). They also had a greater need for information on sex education, sexuality, and obtaining emergency babysitting.

NPSG parents, in contrast, needed more basic information, such as on immunizations and routine child care, the chance of having another child with the same problem, and parent support groups. The researchers suggest that until these basic needs are addressed, these parents will have difficulty progressing to higher-level needs.

Application to practice
This study suggests that the nurse can better serve the parents of children with chronic conditions by becoming familiar with support groups and incorporating such information into nursing interventions. The nurse should identify families who are not involved in a support group and provide them with basic information as well as offer to make a direct referral to a support group. Establishing and maintaining a support group also can be an important nursing intervention. More research is needed to determine the most effective time to make a referral and to identify the services that support groups provide most effectively.

Rawlins, P., and Horner, M. (1988). Does membership in a support group alter needs of parents of chronically ill children? *Pediatric Nursing*, 14 (1), 70-72.

---

ments for obtaining help in an emergency. To help ensure prompt emergency intervention, verify that they have notified the police and fire departments in writing about their child's condition, medications, and treatments as well as the names of the child's health care providers and the health care facility to transport the child to in an emergency. Likewise, the parents should notify the telephone and electric companies requesting placement on a priority service list, advance notification of anticipated interruptions, and priority reinstatement of service after unexpected interruptions.

Also make sure parents and all other caregivers know how to administer infant CPR correctly and when to seek immediate medical attention for a problem. Check whether CPR instructions are posted near the neonate's bed and a list of emergency telephone numbers is located near all telephones.

Subsequent home visits

Once the nurse has established a rapport with the family and made baseline assessments, assessment during later visits should focus on detecting changes in the neonate's physical status, observing the parents' caregiving skills for improvement, and assessing parent-infant interaction. For the high-risk or special-needs neonate, also assess specific aspects of the neonate's condition (as described below under "Assessment of the special-needs neonate") and observe how the neonate's care is affecting other family members.

Physical status. Take vital signs and assess for changes in the neonate's condition. For the neonate receiving phototherapy, assess for signs of treatment efficacy, such as improved color of the skin and mucous membranes. Also check for dehydration, an adverse effect of phototherapy, which may manifest as lethargy, poor feeding, and excessive, watery stools.

Parental caregiving skills. As the parents become more familiar and comfortable with neonatal care, expect their caregiving skills to improve. A deficiency in skills warrants additional teaching sessions.

Parent-neonate interaction. The home is a good environment in which to observe parent-neonate interaction, which is crucial to child growth and development. In some cases, the nurse may use a specific assessment tool to assess the mother-neonate relationship. Also note the degree of eye contact between parent and neonate and observe how frequently the mother fondles, kisses, and vocalizes with the neonate. Keep in mind that problems in parent-infant bonding sometimes manifest in neonatal or infant behavioral problems, such as sleep disturbances, feeding disorders, failure to gain weight, and refusal to cuddle or feed. (For more information on assessing parent-infant interaction, see Chapter 43, Psychosocial Adaptation of the Postpartal Family.)

Assessment of the special-needs neonate

For the special-needs neonate, augment routine assessment with an investigation tailored to the specific problem.

Respiratory disorder. Measure the pulse, respiratory rate, and temperature. A change from baseline values when unrelated to crying, position changes, feeding, or activity may signal cardiac or respiratory compromise. Auscul-

tate the lungs, noting the general quality of breath sounds and checking for adventitious sounds.

Assess the skin color and respiratory pattern, and note any signs of respiratory distress, such as pallor, cyanosis, nasal flaring, chest retractions, edema, or diaphoresis. Ask the parents if they have noted irritability, appetite loss, or other signs of respiratory distress, such as color changes. Assess respiratory secretions for amount, consistency, color, and odor; suspect infection if secretions are foul-smelling, yellowish green, or more copious or viscous than normal. Also assess for medication efficacy and adverse effects; be sure to ask the parents whether they have noticed the latter.

Determine whether the parents understand respiratory anatomy and physiology as well as the pathophysiology, signs and symptoms, and course of the underlying respiratory disease and the purpose of each intervention. Also find out if they know how to assess the neonate's respiratory status.

The neonate with respiratory compromise is predisposed to respiratory infections; simple colds can rapidly progress to fulminant viral pneumonia, bronchopneumonia, respiratory syncytial virus, reactive airway disease, or bronchospasm. Assess whether the parents can identify signs of respiratory infection, such as irritability, fever, cyanosis, increased respiratory distress, pallor, tachypnea, increased oxygen requirements, increased secretions, cough, and poor feeding.

A respiratory disorder can compromise the neonate's nutritional status; therefore, be sure to assess nutritional intake and growth. (For information on evaluating nutritional status, see *Assessing the neonate's nutritional status.*)

If the neonate is receiving nebulized medications, assess the parents' administration skills. Also, if appropriate, observe them as they perform chest physiotherapy, assessing whether they position the neonate correctly and use proper percussion techniques. Also observe the parents as they suction the neonate (performed after chest physiotherapy). Suctioning may be done with a bulb syringe or a catheter. In some cases, a suction machine is used at home; assess whether the parents know how to use this equipment properly. (For information on supplemental oxygen therapy, see *Comparing oxygen delivery systems,* page 1024.)

Neurologic problem. In hydrocephalus, excessive cerebrospinal fluid (CSF) accumulates within the cranial vault, leading to suture expansion and ventricular dilation. The neonate discharged with hydrocephalus may have a surgically placed ventricular shunt to drain excess CSF from the ventricles to a distal compartment, such as the peritoneum.

Assessing the neonate's nutritional status

Prematurity and other perinatal problems can retard neonatal growth and development; the poor oral motor skills that result can cause impaired oral feeding, placing the neonate at risk for malnutrition and feeding problems. The neonate with a cardiac or respiratory disorder is at special risk for poor nutritional status; this neonate has an increased caloric requirement (because so much energy is expended in breathing) but a reduced tolerance for the labor required to ingest food. Other causes of poor nutritional status include:
• prolonged intubation (as with mechanical ventilation), which may cause oral hypersensitivity and refusal to feed
• reflux vomiting from gastroesophageal reflux, in which gastric contents flow upward into the esophagus, leading to loss of nutrients and calories
• medications that affect nutritional requirements.

To assess a feeding disorder, the nurse should monitor growth characteristics, review the neonate's nutritional history, and observe a feeding. (For help in assessing some feeding disorders, the nurse may need to consult with a speech or occupational therapist or a dietitian.)

Growth characteristics
Obtain serial measurements of weight, length, and head circumference. Measure weight regularly, using a balance beam scale, and plot the result on a growth chart. For the first 3 months, an infant should gain 30 g (1 oz) daily.

Measure length (the distance from the base of the heel to the top of the head) with the neonate supine on a flat surface. While an assistant (such as a family member) holds the measuring tape even with the top of the neonate's head, stretch the tape alongside the neonate, straightening the hips and knees.

To determine if the neonate's growth is adequate, plot measured length on the growth chart and correlate it to measured weight. Head circumference, an index of brain growth, also should be measured regularly and plotted on a growth chart.

Nutritional history
Obtain a nutritional history, which includes the neonate's overall health status, medical problems, feeding history (including any feeding-related problems), medications, and nutritional supplements. Ask the parents to keep a diet log, recording specific information about feeding times and the types and precise amounts of food or fluid given. When assessing nutritional status, review log entries for the previous 1 to 7 days, noting any vomiting or other feeding-related problems.

Observation of feeding
Observe the neonate's oral motor skills and sucking ability and check for such problems as poor coordination of sucking and swallowing, neck hyperextension during feeding, oral hypersensitivity (manifested by resistance to touching of the mouth), food refusal, feeding lethargy, and respiratory compromise during feeding. For the neonate with frequent vomiting, try to determine the cause. Vomiting may result from overfeeding, reflux disorders, and inadequate burping.

Before the first home visit, review the neonate's health history for shunt location, serial head circumference measurements, neurologic status, and prognosis. On each visit, measure head circumference, noting any abnormally rapid increase. Assess the neonate's mental status (orientation level, alertness, and behavior). Check range of motion of the neck, and assess eye movements for nystagmus, convergence, and ability to follow. Also evaluate the fontanels, which should be flat and soft, and palpate the sutures, which should not be split or overlapped.

Assess for shunt obstruction and infection, which may manifest in fontanel tenseness or bulging, increased head circumference, irritability, vomiting, appetite changes, sleepiness, and sunset eyes (upper lid retraction causing the sclera to show above the iris). Infection may cause fever, erythema, and tenderness along the shunt tract.

Determine if the parents understand the purpose of the shunt and know how to check the fontanel to assess for shunt obstruction and infection. Also make sure they know when to call the physician (such as for rapidly increasing head circumference, irritability, vomiting, or hypoglycemia, hypocalcemia, and decreased alertness).

The preterm and low-birth-weight neonate are predisposed to seizures. A symptom rather than a disease in itself, a seizure may stem from such conditions as intraventricular hemorrhage, head trauma, or drug withdrawal. A neonate with seizures usually is discharged on anticonvulsant therapy, which typically continues until the child is at least 6 months old.

Before the first home visit, review the health history for the type of seizure the neonate has experienced, seizure signs observed, postseizure behavior, and medications. During each visit, assess vital signs, alertness level, and motor and ocular responses to stimulation. Ask the parents whether they have observed signs of a seizure. (Preferably, they should keep a seizure log.) A subtle seizure may manifest as eyelid fluttering, nystagmus, drooling, tongue thrusting, lip smacking, tonic limb positioning, bicycling movements of the legs, or apnea. Also assess whether the parents can differentiate a seizure from jitteriness (unlike seizures, jittery movements commonly subside when the limbs are restrained.)

Determine whether the parents know how to assess the neonate's neurologic status and behavior, care for the neonate during a seizure, observe activity during and after the seizure, and provide emergency interventions (including CPR) for apnea. Also assess whether they know when to seek medical attention (such as when a seizure is prolonged), and evaluate their understanding of anticonvulsant medication—its regimen, potential adverse effects, and the need to avoid abrupt discontin-

Comparing oxygen delivery systems

Oxygen therapy can be provided in the home through various delivery methods and systems. The liter flow or oxygen concentration required usually determines the delivery method used. Delivery methods include nasal cannula or catheter, oxyhood, tent, high-flow mask, and nebulizer. The cannula, which provides a direct flow of oxygen to the nares (nostrils), is the most common oxygen delivery system for home use. It imposes the fewest restrictions on a child attempting to interact with the environment; attaching extension tubing (up to 50′) to the can-

nula allows the child to move freely from room to room. However, the cannula can become dislodged from the nares with extensive manipulation; use of self-fastening (Velcro) straps and adhesive dressings can reduce this risk by securing the cannula in the proper position.

Oxygen delivery systems include the oxygen concentrator, cylinder oxygen, and liquid oxygen. The chart below compares the advantages and disadvantages of these systems.

Oxygen concentrator (separates oxygen from ambient air; provides low-flow oxygen)	**Cylinder oxygen** (oxygen stored in cylinder)	**Liquid oxygen** (oxygen stored in liquid state under pressure)
Advantages • Cost-effective for the neonate who needs continuous low-flow oxygen *Disadvantages* • Cannot be used with a high-flow mask or nebulizer • Requires electricity • Requires an oxygen cylinder as a backup in case of malfunction or power failure • Bulky • Noisy • Emits heat	*Advantages* • Cost-effective for the neonate who requires high-flow oxygen or intermittent oxygen for up to 12 hours/day • Can be used with a high-flow oxygen mask, a nasal cannula, a nasal catheter, or a nebulizer • Portable when a small cylinder is used *Disadvantages* • Requires a humidification source if the flow must exceed ¾ liter • Must be used with caution and kept in a stand or cart; the safety cap must be fastened securely in case the neonate falls	*Advantages* • Cost-effective for the neonate who needs continuous low- to moderate-flow oxygen • Usually can be used with any oxygen delivery method • Smaller and more lightweight than other oxygen systems • Refillable portable units available when the neonate is transported outside the home *Disadvantages* • Humidification source required if the flow will exceed ¾ liter • May cause burns if oxygen comes into contact with skin during transfer from a stationary to portable unit • Must be used in an upright position

uation (which could cause seizures). Make sure they know how often blood samples will be required for blood drug level monitoring and understand that stressful events (such as immunizations, infections, fever, and emotional stress) may trigger a seizure. Determine their knowledge of safety precautions, such as secure positioning, and make sure they understand that the child's neurologic outcome may remain undetermined for some time.

Visual or hearing impairment. Conditions leading to visual impairment include retinopathy of prematurity (ROP) and rarely, congenital cataracts. A retinal disorder seen mainly in preterm and low-birth-weight neonates treated with oxygen therapy for respiratory distress, ROP can be detected as early as 6 weeks after birth. A congenital cataract is an opacification of the lens associated with such disorders as trisomy 13 and 18, galactosemia, and rubella syndrome. Many visually impaired neonates have multiple physiologic problems, including respiratory and neurologic compromise.

A neonate who receives oxygen therapy typically undergoes ophthalmologic examination before discharge. However, ROP usually is not detectable until after the neonatal period. Therefore, before the first home visit, be sure to review the medical records to determine if the neonate received oxygen therapy and is at risk for ROP.

During the first visit, perform a vision screening, examining the lids, pupils, sclera, and conjunctivae. Note any lesions, discharge, and unequal or absent pupillary reaction to light. Also assess for nystagmus, strabismus, and red reflex. Evaluate the neonate's ability to focus on an object placed 8″ to 10″ directly ahead and to follow objects moving horizontally. If the results of this screening suggest a problem, refer the child to an ophthalmologist.

For the neonate with a previously diagnosed visual impairment, assess the parents' understanding of the condition and their awareness of home stimulation programs. Such programs may involve placement of mobiles and colorful toys in the crib, shaking a colorful noisemaker, or slowly moving an object from side to side in front of the neonate.

A hearing impairment is associated with such factors as low birth weight, congenital or perinatal infection, severe birth asphyxia, hyperbilirubinemia, exposure to high levels of environmental noise, chronic maternal illness, and malnutrition. The impairment may be unilateral or bilateral, may vary from mild to profound, and may involve low-frequency sound, high-frequency sound, or both. Depending on the auditory structures involved, a hearing impairment also may be classified as conductive (involving structures of the outer and middle ear), sensorineural (involving malformation of or damage to inner ear structures), or mixed (a combination of conductive and sensorineural).

A hearing impairment may not be detected before discharge. If a hearing problem is suspected, conduct an informal auditory behavioral screening, which determines responses to noisemakers with known intensity and frequency. If the results of this examination suggest a problem, refer the child for a complete audiologic and medical evaluation.

If a hearing impairment already has been diagnosed, find out if the child is wearing a hearing aid and whether the parents are aware of the benefits of a home stimulation program, which can teach them how to provide an optimal auditory environment and use alternative communication methods

Acquired immunodeficiency syndrome (AIDS).
Every neonate born to a woman infected with human immunodeficiency virus (HIV) carries the mother's HIV antibodies. This complicates neonatal diagnosis because a neonate who tests positive for HIV at birth may not actually be infected. To make a definitive diagnosis, the physician must determine if the child is producing HIV antibodies, indicating true HIV infection; this may take up to 15 months (Cruz, 1988).

Keep in mind that signs and symptoms of HIV infection may not appear until age 6 months to 2 years. A distinctive facial dysmorphism can help with early detection, as can persistent oral candida infections and diaper rash from diarrhea. Other suggestive findings include failure to thrive, severe bacterial infections, chronic parotid swelling, and pulmonary lymphoid interstitial pneumonitis. Sometimes central nervous system abnormalities are the only signs of HIV infection. For instance, the neonate may be microencephalic with delayed cognitive and motor functioning. In some cases, the brain is affected directly; at least 50% of affected neonates have encephalopathy (Cruz, 1988).

If AIDS is suspected, perform a complete physical assessment of the neonate. If AIDS already has been diagnosed, assess the parents' ability and willingness to care for their child at home, especially if a parent also has AIDS or abuses drugs. Determine how much the parents know about the disease and the care required for the neonate (such as management of life-threatening opportunistic infections). Also find out if they know which precautions are necessary to prevent disease spread to other family members; a misinformed caregiver may be afraid of catching the disease through casual contact and thus avoid the neonate, placing the neonate at risk for inadequate care and sensory deprivation. (For home care guidelines, see *Parent teaching: When your infant has AIDS,* page 1026.)

Effects of maternal substance abuse. The neonate affected by maternal substance abuse during pregnancy may remain in the health care facility until drug withdrawal is achieved. However, if this problem somehow eludes detection before discharge, the home health nurse who suspects it should check for such suggestive signs as abnormal reflex responses, marked irritability, continual high-pitched crying, poor feeding, muscle tremors, twitching, or rigidity with inability to extend the muscles. (For details on assessing for neonatal drug addiction or withdrawal, see Chapter 38, High-Risk Neonates).

Assess parent-neonate interaction, which may be jeopardized if the neonate is irritable or unconsolable. Also assess the parents' ability and willingness to care for their child; like the parents of the neonate with AIDS, this neonate's parents may be unstable, with poor caregiving and parenting skills.

Assessment of the family of the special-needs neonate
For the family of the special-needs neonate, discharge may herald a new crisis. Already grieving over the loss of the anticipated "perfect" child, they must now confront the challenge of providing complex care on their own. To ensure family-centered nursing care during this stressful transition, assess family members for the following factors, found by Wegener and Aday (1989) to increase the risk of stress in family members of special-needs neonates:
• discontinuous medical care of the neonate
• financial problems
• many extended family members living in the household
• lack of a designated nurse–case manager at the time of the neonate's discharge.

Also evaluate the parents for signs of grief and determine the coping mechanism each parent is using. Expect the parents to show signs of exhaustion and possibly marital strain. Assess siblings for overt or covert signs of jealousy and resentment of the neonate. Also explore family dynamics, strengths, and weaknesses.

When your infant has AIDS

To care for your infant with AIDS, you will need to follow certain safeguards. Because of a weakened immune system, the child is more vulnerable to infection by germs that most children can fight off. Also, although AIDS cannot be transmitted through casual contact, you and other family members should avoid coming into direct contact with the infant's blood and body fluids. The precautions below can help ensure the safety of your infant as well as the rest of the family.

• Instruct all family members to wash their hands before eating and after using the toilet.
• To prevent the infant from developing an intestinal infection, use premixed commercial formulas, or prepare formula with pasteurized milk and milk products. Do not put the infant to bed with a bottle of milk or juice because bacteria grow rapidly in these fluids.
• Do not feed the infant directly from a jar; bacteria from the mouth may spoil the food that remains in the jar. Refrigerate opened jars and use the food within 24 hours.
• Cook or peel fruits and vegetables and cook meats thoroughly before giving them to the infant.
• Use a dishwasher or wash dishes in hot, sudsy water and air dry them.
• If possible, use disposable diapers. When changing diapers, wear disposable gloves; place used diapers in a sealed plastic bag.
• Keep diaper-changing areas separate from food preparation and serving areas. After each diaper change, clean the changing surface with a 1:10 solution of household bleach and water. (Be sure to wear disposable gloves when doing this.)
• Reserve separate towels and washcloths for the infant.
• Launder items soiled with the infant's blood or body fluids separately from the family laundry, and use hot sudsy water. The rest of the infant's laundry can be washed with other household laundry.
• Flush the infant's body wastes down the toilet and keep the infant's trash in a closed plastic container. Place needles and other sharp objects in an impenetrable container and arrange for their disposal.
• If you have a pet in the house, keep the animal's waste products away from the infant; do not allow animals that may bite or scratch to come near your child.

Parental grief and coping mechanisms. The parents of a neonate with a chronic or disabling condition must pass through the stages of grief to deal with the loss of the "perfect" child and accept the real one. These stages typically include denial, anger, bargaining, depression, and acceptance. Like anyone faced with a stressful situation, parents of high-risk neonates also use certain coping mechanisms—denial, anger, withdrawal, guilt, and intellectualizing—to deal with their feelings. If possible, determine which stage of grief each parent is in and which coping mechanism each parent is using. (For details on assessing the stages of grief and coping mechanisms, see Chapter 39, Care of the Families of High-Risk Neonates.)

If the neonate has a chronic condition, assessment of the parents in subsequent months or years may uncover chronic sorrow, a phenomenon first described by Olshansky (1962). The intensity of chronic sorrow varies from person to person and over time; it may disappear temporarily, only to recur. To assess for chronic sorrow, observe for sadness, fear, anxiety, anger, guilt, ambivalence, helplessness, or hopelessness. Keep in mind, however, that some parents conceal their sorrow; a few even try to suppress it to cope with the grim reality they face, seeming unduly optimistic about their child's condition.

Effect on the couple's relationship. Many parents of special-needs children report a strengthening of the marital relationship over time (Thomas, 1987). Also, studies show that parents of a special-needs child do not necessarily experience reduced marital satisfaction or have a shorter marriage duration. Nonetheless, the child's condition undoubtedly causes tremendous stress within the relationship, especially at first. Some couples may choose to stay together even though they do not derive support or enjoyment from the relationship.

Assess for both overt signs of marital stress, such as arguments, and more subtle indications, such as terse conversation and reluctance to acknowledge the partner's presence. If stress is apparent or suspected, consider tactfully suggesting that the couple see a marriage counselor.

Effect on siblings. Siblings of chronically ill children may be ill-informed about the nature of the neonate's illness. Also, they may be unsure of what others expect of them and feel that their own identify is threatened. Anger, guilt, and resentment are common (Seligman, 1987). To help prevent or detect these problems, assess siblings for signs of behavioral changes and maladaptation—jealousy and resentment of the neonate, aggressive behavior, fear, guilt, and anger. (For more information on assessing sibling reactions to the birth of a high-risk neonate, see Chapter 39, Care of the Families of High-Risk Neonates.)

Nursing diagnosis

After gathering assessment data, the nurse must review it carefully to identify pertinent nursing diagnoses for the neonate. (For a partial list of applicable diagnoses, see *Nursing diagnoses: Neonate receiving nursing care at home.*)

Planning and implementation

For the nurse who provides intermittent home visits, nursing goals include managing or correcting any problems detected during assessment and ensuring that the parents (or other primary caregivers) are providing safe, appropriate care. (For information about routine neonatal care, see Chapter 36, Care of the Normal Neonate. For nursing interventions for specific perinatal problems, see Chapter 38, High-Risk Neonates. For parent-teaching information on some specific equipment, see *Parent teaching: Using a home apnea monitor,* page 1028, and *Parent teaching: When your infant is receiving oxygen by nasal cannula,* page 1029.

Nursing care in the home calls for flexibility and innovation. Be patient and understanding about interruptions in teaching sessions and unanticipated household events. If the family has a diagnosis of *altered family processes related to the arrival of a new family member or household disruption caused by the neonate's care,* help them devise individualized solutions to such problems as cramped quarters, inadequate storage space for equipment and supplies, and too few electrical outlets.

A key nursing intervention is to ensure that the neonate has a source of primary pediatric care, that all of the neonate's care is coordinated, and that the family's resources are adequate to provide appropriate, ongoing care. If necessary, help the family obtain a pediatrician; also facilitate communication and coordination among care providers. If the home lacks indoor plumbing, running water, hot water, or electricity, make sure a social service agency has been contacted. Besides city and county social services departments, resources for financial assistance include:
• state children services programs
• federal Special Supplemental Food Program for Women, Infants, and Children, Aid to Dependent Children program, and Aid to Dependent Families and Children program
• Salvation Army
• religious organizations and charities.

Be prepared to help the family through sudden financial crises triggered by the neonate's care requirements. For example, mechanical ventilation may increase monthly electric bills substantially; if necessary, refer the family to a social service agency to arrange for emergency financial assistance to pay these bills, or help them contact the electric company to make special payment arrangements.

NURSING DIAGNOSES

Neonate receiving nursing care at home

When caring for a neonate at home, the nurse may find these examples of nursing diagnoses appropriate. Specific nursing interventions for many of these diagnoses are provided in the "Planning and implementation" section of this chapter.

FOR THE NEONATE

• Altered growth and development related to impaired oral feeding and inadequate calorie intake
• Altered nutrition: less than body requirements, related to immature gastrointestinal function or inefficient feeding patterns
• Impaired physical mobility related to restrictions imposed by feeding tubes or I.V. lines
• Impaired skin integrity: potential, related to the presence of feeding tubes or I.V. lines
• Ineffective airway clearance related to pooling of secretions
• Potential for infection related to respiratory compromise
• Sensory-perceptual alteration: auditory, related to perinatal infection
• Sensory-perceptual alteration: visual, related to retinopathy of prematurity

FOR THE FAMILY

• Altered family processes related to the arrival of a new family member or household disruption caused by the neonate's care
• Anxiety related to the neonate's constant care needs or the demands of delivering complex, specialized care
• Grieving related to loss of the anticipated healthy neonate
• Ineffective family or individual coping related to the stress of caregiving procedures or fear that the neonate will die
• Knowledge deficit related to the neonate's medical condition or neonatal caregiving skills

---

Ensuring parental caregiving knowledge and skills

For parents with a nursing diagnosis of *knowledge deficit related to the neonate's medical condition or neonatal caregiving skills,* reinforce discharge teaching about the underlying disease and the care required. An effective way to do this is to observe the parents as they care for the neonate, then demonstrate any aspect of their care that is incorrect and ask for a return demonstration.

A parent may feel overwhelmed by the responsibility of providing care, even when the neonate's care needs seem fairly simple to the nurse. The parent's reaction may lead to a nursing diagnosis of *ineffective family or individual coping related to the stress of caregiving*

Using a home apnea monitor

Because your infant has had problems breathing, the doctor has determined that a home apnea monitor is necessary. The monitor will alert you to changes in your infant's heart rate or absence of breathing. By following the steps below, you can help ensure your infant's well-being when the monitor is in use.

General guidelines
• Prepare the home environment for monitoring—for instance, by providing a sturdy surface for the monitor and by displaying emergency telephone numbers (such as for the doctor and monitor dealer or vendor) in a prominent place.
• Make sure other family members know how to use the monitor.
• If your monitor has electrodes, make sure the respirator indicator goes on each time your infant breathes. If it does not, move the electrodes slightly until it does.
• If the apnea or bradycardia alarm goes off, check the color on the inside of the infant's mouth. If it is bluish and the infant is not breathing, try to stimulate breathing by calling loudly, then touching the infant. Use gentle touch at first, then stronger stimulation as necessary; do not shake the infant. If the infant does not respond, initiate cardiopulmonary resuscitation (CPR).
• A loose-lead alarm may indicate a dirty electrode, a loose electrode patch, a loose belt, a disconnected or malfunctioning wire, or monitor malfunction. If this alarm sounds, see the equipment manual for instructions.
• Periodically review CPR and other life-saving techniques you have been taught. Make sure that everyone who cares for your infant knows these techniques.
• Notify the local police, ambulance company, telephone company, and electric company that your infant is on an apnea monitor. Also make sure the pediatrician and visiting nurse know about the monitor.
• For two useful booklets—*A Manual for Home Monitoring* and *At Home with a Monitor*—write to the Sudden Infant Death Syndrome Alliance, 10500 Little Patuxent Parkway, Suite 420, Columbia, MD 21044 or call 1-800-221-SIDS.

procedures or fear that the neonate will die. Even when the parents' caregiving skills are deficient, convey a sense of trust and confidence in their eventual ability to care for the child adequately at home.

Keep in mind that the addition of a dependent new family member can be enormously stressful, possibly resulting in a nursing diagnosis of *anxiety related to the*

neonate's constant care needs or the demands of delivering complex, specialized care. Reassure the parents that negative as well as positive feelings are bound to arise during the immediate postdischarge period; if necessary, refer them for counseling or other support resources to ease the neonate's transition to the home. Also, to reduce the burden presented by the neonate's care demands, encourage the parents to seek and accept any offers of help.

Promoting positive parent-neonate interaction

If parent-neonate interaction suggests poor bonding, reinforce teaching about neonatal behavioral states, communication cues, growth and developmental patterns, and sleep-awake patterns. (For details on these topics, see Chapter 43, Psychosocial Adaptation of the Postpartal Family.) If poor interaction seems to stem from parental disappointment or grief over the neonate's medical condition or physical appearance, encourage the parents to express their feelings freely, without fear of being judged as bad people or bad parents.

In some cases, poor parent-child interaction or parental failure to provide proper care may reflect child neglect or abuse. The nurse who suspects this should contact the local child protective services agency.

Helping siblings adjust

The addition of a new family member may cause siblings to feel neglected and unloved, especially if the neonate's care is demanding and time-consuming. If family assessment reveals sibling behavioral changes or maladaptation, urge the parents to help siblings understand the neonate's condition and express their fears and concerns, and to reassure siblings that they are not the cause of the neonate's illness. Also encourage the parents to let siblings participate in the neonate's care at a level appropriate for each sibling's developmental stage; this can help the sibling feel more involved in and important to the family. (However, if a sibling is assuming too much caregiving responsibility, point out to the parents that the sibling may need more time to be a child.) Also urge the parents to spend some time alone with each sibling regularly to convey the feeling that the sibling has a special place in the family.

Evaluation

During this step of the nursing process, the nurse evaluates the effectiveness of the care plan by ongoing evaluation of subjective and objective criteria. Evaluation findings should be stated in terms of actions performed or outcomes achieved for each goal. The following examples illustrate appropriate evaluation statements for the neonate receiving care at home:

When your infant is receiving oxygen by nasal cannula

The doctor has prescribed oxygen therapy by nasal cannula for your infant. To improve the safety and effectiveness of this treatment, refer to the guidelines below.

Setting up the system

1 Make sure you have a nasal cannula, tubing, skin tape, oxygen tank, and humidifier (if prescribed). Also, keep a spare cannula available to use when the original one is being cleaned.

2 Fill the humidifier with sterile distilled water and attach it to the flowmeter.

3 Attach the flowmeter to the oxygen source and connect the cannula to the system.

4 To apply the cannula, slip it over the infant's head so that the nasal prongs curve inward toward the face. Tape the cannula to each cheek to secure it.

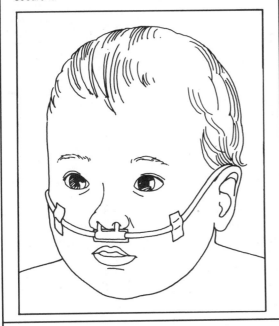

5 Adjust the flowmeter to the prescribed rate.

Maintaining hygiene

• Once a week, or whenever the cannula appears dirty, wash it with soap and water; let it dry for 24 hours. Make sure no water remains in the cannula after cleaning, because this could block the flow of oxygen.
• Every day, remove the humidifier from the oxygen source, empty the remaining water from the tank, and clean it with equal parts water and hydrogen peroxide.

Ensuring safety

• Store the oxygen container upright and secure it to prevent it from falling (which may cause a leakage in the system).
• Keep the tank away from direct sunlight and do not store grease, oil, or other flammable materials nearby. Keep a fire extinguisher nearby.
• Keep the oxygen tank at least 5 feet from heat sources and electrical devices and ban smoking near the oxygen tank.
• Make sure the electrical equipment is properly grounded.
• Turn off both the volume regulator and flow regulator when oxygen is not in use to prevent oxygen leakage.
• Do not use alcohol-based or oil-based substances (such as petroleum jelly or baby oil) on your infant, because these substances are highly flammable.
• Dress the infant in flame-retardant clothing.
• Weaning from supplemental oxygen must be done gradually, as instructed by the doctor. Never discontinue oxygen therapy abruptly; this may cause serious harm to your infant.
• Notify the police and fire departments that oxygen tanks are in the home.

• The neonate's physiologic status remained stable, with no changes in vital signs since the last visit.
• The neonate maintained a satisfactory nutritional status based on a defined weight gain.
• The home environment is safe and adequate for the neonatal care required.

• The family has sufficient resources to care for the neonate at home.
• All appropriate items required for the neonate's care are present in the home.
• Medical equipment is functioning properly.
• The parents provide the required care in a competent and confident manner.

APPLYING THE NURSING PROCESS

Parent with a knowledge deficit related to apneic episodes

During discharge planning, the nursing process helps ensure high-quality care. The table below shows how the nurse might use the nursing process when caring for the parent of the neonate described in the case history at right. The first column presents history and physical assessment data followed by a paragraph of mental notes. These notes help the nurse make important mental connections among assessment findings, aiding in development of the nursing diagnoses and planning.

The second column lists an appropriate nursing diagnosis; the information in the remaining columns is based on this diagnosis. Although not a part of the nursing process, a rationale appears for each intervention in the fourth column to explain how it contributes to the care plan.

ASSESSMENT	NURSING DIAGNOSIS	PLANNING
Subjective (history) data • Mother states she is afraid her child will have apneic episodes at home and may die of sudden infant death syndrome (SIDS). • Mother asks questions about SIDS and home apnea monitoring. **Objective (physical) data** • Neonate is a white male, age 3 weeks, who was born at 35 weeks' gestation weighing 2,500 g. • Neonate is eating well and will be ready for discharge soon. • Vital signs: rectal temperature 99.6° F; pulse 138/minute; respirations 30/minute; blood pressure 110/68 mm Hg. • Neonate has two or three apneic events daily, each lasting 20 to 25 seconds; sometimes his face turns pale to slightly bluish. Neonate resumes breathing after gentle stimulation. These events are not accompanied by bradycardia. **Mental notes** *Because of the mother's lack of experience with neonates and her single marital status, she is markedly anxious about the neonate's apneic episodes. However, she is able to provide gentle stimulation, when required, to revive him.*	Knowledge deficit related to apneic episodes	**Goals** By the time the neonate is discharged, the mother will: • show an understanding of the causes and treatment of apnea of prematurity • show an understanding of SIDS and its relationship to apnea • demonstrate infant observation techniques and infant cardiopulmonary resuscitation (CPR) • express an understanding of the benefits and risks of home apnea monitoring.

• The family shows a positive adjustment to the responsibility of providing complex care for their special-needs neonate.

Documentation

All steps of the nursing process should be documented as thoroughly and objectively as possible. Thorough documentation not only allows the nurse to evaluate the effectiveness of the care plan, but it also makes this information available to other members of the health care team, helping to ensure consistency of care. (For a case study that shows how to apply the nursing process when caring for the family of a neonate receiving nursing care at home, see *Applying the nursing process: Parent with a knowledge deficit related to apneic episodes.*)

Documentation of a home nursing visit should include:
• the neonate's physiologic status, including vital signs

• the neonate's nutritional status based on a defined weight gain
• the parents' ability to provide the required care
• the parents' ability to cope with neonatal care responsibilities and the neonate's condition
• the parents' understanding of the neonatal care required.

Chapter summary

Chapter 40 discussed preparation for and delivery of home health care for neonates. Here are the chapter highlights.
• Over the past decade, economic pressures, the move toward early discharge of neonates, the desire by families

CASE STUDY

Brian Klingefelt was born 3 weeks ago, at 35 weeks' gestation, with apnea of prematurity. His mother Susan, age 24, is an unmarried primiparous client. Brian is becoming more stable and his mother is being prepared for his discharge. However, he continues to experience apneic episodes and will require home apnea monitoring.

IMPLEMENTATION		EVALUATION
Intervention	**Rationale**	Upon evaluation, the mother:
Teach the mother about the disease process, causes, and treatment of apnea of prematurity, and provide appropriate teaching handouts.	An understanding of apnea of prematurity and its treatment can help allay the mother's anxiety.	• was able to explain the causes and treatment of apnea
Contact a clinical nurse specialist to consult with the mother about SIDS and its relationship to apnea.	Teaching the mother that apnea of prematurity is not a strong risk factor for SIDS will help reduce her anxiety.	• showed that she understands the relationship of SIDS to apnea • expressed an understanding of the purpose of
Provide information on home apnea monitors.	Knowledge of how to use an apnea monitor and respond to monitor alarms also will make the mother less fearful.	a home apnea monitor • demonstrated infant CPR and observation techniques.
Schedule a class in infant CPR with the mother and other caregivers; have them give return demonstrations of CPR.	Return demonstration of infant CPR reinforces newly learned procedures.	
Teach the mother and other caregivers how to assess the neonate for signs of apnea, such as changes in skin color, respiratory pattern, and movements.	Knowing how to recognize signs of respiratory compromise and respond appropriately helps reduce anxiety.	

for more active participation in health care, and advances in the treatment of high-risk neonates have increased the need for home health care. Studies show that home care can be safe and cost-effective even for high-risk neonates.

• The discharge plan is a joint effort by the health care team, client, family, and appropriate outside agencies to meet a client's physical and psychosocial needs after discharge.

• Discharge planning should begin when the neonate is delivered or, at the latest, by nursery admission. The nurse continues to assess the neonate's and family's discharge planning needs until the neonate is discharged.

• Within the health care facility, resource personnel used in discharge planning may include a clinical nurse specialist; physician; social worker; financial counselor; occupational, speech, hearing, and physical therapists; utilization review nurse; dietitian; respiratory therapist; and child life therapist.

• To prepare the parents for the neonate's discharge, the nurse teaches them caregiving skills, emergency interventions, signs and symptoms of medical problems, use of special equipment, and names of people to contact when they have questions. Teaching strategies may incorporate verbal and written instruction, demonstration, and videotapes.

• Neonatal home health care needs range from routine well-baby care for the normal, healthy neonate to complex, high-technology care for the special-needs neonate. The latter may involve apnea monitoring, suctioning, chest physiotherapy, oxygen therapy, tracheostomy care, mechanical ventilation, enteral or parenteral nutrition, medication administration, and developmental stimulation programs.

• Establishing a rapport with the family and avoiding a domineering approach are priorities for the home health nurse. Besides evaluating the neonate's physical status, the nurse should assess the parents' caregiving knowledge and skills, parent-neonate interaction, the home environment, the family's support system, the family's emergency plans, and the functioning of any required equipment.

• The family of a special-needs neonate requires physical support (such as for caregiving and household tasks), respite care, and psychosocial support.

• Goals for the home health nurse include managing or correcting any problems detected during assessment; ensuring that the parents (or other primary caregivers) are providing safe, appropriate care; supporting parent-infant interaction; and helping family members adjust to the neonate.

Study questions

1. What is the nurse's role in discharge planning?

2. Which factors should the health care team and family take into account when determining the feasibility of home care?

3. Which methods might the health care team use to conduct ongoing assessment of discharge planning needs?

4. Samuel Yang, age 23 days, is scheduled for discharge. However, he will require a feeding tube and tracheostomy tube at home. Which factors should the nurse consider when helping his parents choose a home health care agency and medical equipment supplier?

5. What are some sources of financial assistance for neonatal home health care that the nurse should discuss with Samuel's parents?

6. Which items should the nurse include when documenting Samuel's discharge plan?

7. What are some benefits of early discharge and home health care for neonates?

8. What role does the case manager play in home health care?

9. Which interventions can the nurse take to help siblings adjust to the birth of a special-needs neonate?

Bibliography

Discharge planning and home health care

Ahmann, E. (1986). *Home care for the high risk infant: A holistic guide to using technology.* Rockville, MD: Aspen.

American Nurses' Association (1975). *Continuity of care and discharge planning programs* (p. 3). New York: Author

Anderson, G.C. (1986). Pacifiers: The positive side. *MCN,* 11(2), 122-124.

Arenson, J. (1988). Discharge teaching in the NICU: The changing needs of NICU graduates and their families. *Neonatal Network,* 6(4), 29-52.

Chavez, R.A., and Schwab, S.V. (1988). Model program: Pediatric extended care. *Children's Health Care,* 16(4), 296-298.

Joint Commission for Accreditation of Healthcare Organizations (1989). *The joint commission 1990 AMH accreditation manual for hospitals* (p. 131). Chicago: Author.

Krajewski, D.M. (1989). Primary team nursing in pediatric home care. *Caring,* 8(5), 46-48.

NAACOG. (1986). *Standards for obstetric, gynecologic, and neonatal nursing* (3rd ed.; p. 32). Washington, DC: Author.

National Association of Children's Hospitals and Related Institutions, Inc. (1989). Fact sheet on catastrophically ill children. In *Pediatric nursing, forum on the future: Looking toward the 21st century.* Proceedings and report from an invitational conference, May 16-17, 1988 (p. 9). Pitman, NJ: Anthony J. Jannetti.

National Institutes of Health. (1986). Infantile apnea and home monitoring. *Consensus conference development statement,* 6(6). Washington, DC: Author.

Norr, K., Nacion, K., and Abramson, R. (1989). Early discharge with home follow-up: Impacts on low-income mothers and infants. *JOGGN,* 18(2), 133-141.

Office of Technology Assessment. (1987). Technology-dependent children: Hospital versus home care (excerpt). *Caring,* 6(10), 58-60.

U.S. General Accounting Office. (1989, June). *Health care—Home care experiences of families with chronically ill children* (GAO-HRD-89-73) (p. 3). Washington, DC: Author

Wegener, D.J., and Aday, L.A. (1989). Home care for ventilator-assisted children: Predicting family stress. *Pediatric Nursing,* 15, 371-376.

Special-needs neonate

American Academy of Pediatrics Ad Hoc Task Forces on Home Care of Chronically Ill Infants and Children. (1984). Guidelines for home care of infants, children, and adolescents with chronic disease. *Pediatrics,* 74, 434-436.

American Academy of Pediatrics Joint Committee on Infant Hearing. (1982). Position Statement. *Pediatrics,* 70(3), 496-497.

Aranda, J.V., et al. (1983). Apnea and control of breathing in newborn infants. In L. Stern (Ed.), *Diagnosis and management of respiratory disorders in the newborn.* Reading, MA: Addison-Wesley.

Bancalari, E., and Gerhardt, T. (1986). Bronchopulmonary dysplasia. *Pediatric Clinics of North America,* 33(1), 1-23.

Brown, L.W. (1984). Home monitoring of the high-risk infant. *Clinics in Perinatology,* 11(1), 85-100.

Cruz, L.D. (1988, November). Children with AIDS: Diagnosis, symptoms, care. *AORN Journal,* 48, 893-910

Donar, M.E. (1988). Community care: Pediatric home mechanical ventilation. *Holistic Nursing Practice, 2*(2), 68-80.

Ellison, P.H. (1984). Management of seizures in the high-risk infant. *Clinics in Perinatology, 11*(1), 175-188.

Ensher, F.L., and Clark, D.A. (1986). *Newborns at risk: Medical care and psychoeducational intervention.* Rockville, MD: Aspen.

Eviatar, L. (1984). Evaluation of hearing in the high-risk infant. *Clinics in Perinatology, 11*(1), 153-173.

Friendly, D.S. (1987). Eye disorders in the neonate. In G.B. Avery (Ed.), *Neonatology: Pathophysiology and management of the newborn* (3rd ed.; pp. 1298-1316). Philadelphia: Lippincott.

Handy, C.M. (1989). Patient centered high-technology home care. *Holistic Nursing Practice, 3*(2), 46-53.

Hartsell, M.B. (1986). Home phototherapy. *Journal of Pediatric Nursing, 1*(4), 282-283.

Heiser, C.A. (1987). Home phototherapy. *Pediatric Nursing, 13*(6), 425-427.

Jackson, D.F. (1986). Nursing care plan: Home management of children with BPD. *Pediatric Nursing, 12*(5), 342-348.

Kenney, M.M. (1987). Hospital to home: Care of the child with a tracheostomy. *Neonatal Network, 6*(1), 21-24.

Olshansky, S. (1962, April). Chronic sorrow: A response to having a mentally defective child. *Social Casework, 43*, 190-193.

Pesquera, K. (1988). Nutrition monitoring in pediatric home care. *Caring, 7*(6), 32-33.

Pierce, P.M., Freedman, S.A., and Reiss, J.G. (1987). Prescribed pediatric extended care (PPEC): A new link in the continuum. *Children's Health Care, 16*(1), 58.

Sauve, R.S., and Singhal, N. (1985). Long-term morbidity of infants with bronchopulmonary dysplasia. *Pediatrics, 76*(5), 725-733.

Schreiner, M.S., Donar, M.E., and Kettrick, R.G. (1987). Pediatric home mechanical ventilation. *Pediatric Clinics of North America, 34*(1), 47-60.

Seligman, M. (1987). Adaptation of children to a chronically ill or mentally handicapped sibling. *Canadian Medical Association Journal, 136*(12), 1249-1252.

Swanson, J.A., and Berseth, C.L. (1987). Continuing care for the preterm infant after dismissal from the neonatal intensive care unit. *Mayo Clinic Proceedings, 62*(7), 613-622.

Thomas, R.B. (1987). Family adaptation to a child with a chronic condition. In M.H. Rose and R.B. Thomas (Eds.), *Children with chronic conditions* (p.39). Orlando: Grune & Stratton.

Torrence, C. (1985). Neonatal seizures. Part II: Recognition, treatment and prognosis. *Neonatal Network, 4*(2), 21-28.

Tyson, J.E., and Metze, H. (1989). Bronchopulmonary dysplasia. In H.F. Eichenwald and J. Ströder (Eds.), *Current therapy in pediatrics—2.* Toronto: B.C. Decker.

Volpe, J.J. (1977). Neonatal seizures. *Clinics in Perinatology, 4*(1), 43-63.

Webb, L.Z., et al. (1982, July-August). Developmental care in the neonatal ICU. *Dimensions of Critical Care Nursing, 1*(4), 221-231.

Family needs

Ferrari, M. (1986). Perceptions of social support by parents of chronically ill versus healthy children. *Children's Health Care, 14*, 26-31.

Jessop, D.J., and Stein, R.E.K. (1989). Meeting the needs of individuals and families. In R.E.K. Stein (Ed.), *Caring for children with chronic illness* (pp. 63-74). New York: Springer.

Klaus, M.H., and Kennell, J.H. (1986). *Maternal-infant bonding.* St. Louis: Mosby.

Lyman, R., Wurtele, S., and Wilson, D. (1984). Psychological effects on parents of home and hospital apnea monitoring. *Journal of Pediatric Psychology, 10*(4), 439-448.

Saylor, C.F., Purohit, D.M., Ford, M., Norris, D., and McIntosh, J. (1989). Children's health care: Brief report—Anxiety in mothers of infants on apnea monitors. *Child Health Care, 18*(2), 117-120.

U.S. General Accounting Office. (1989, June). *Health care—Home care experiences of families with chronically ill children* (GAO-HRD-89-73) (p. 3). Washington, DC: Author

Wills, J.M. (1983). Concerns and needs of mothers providing home care for children with tracheostomies. *MCN, 12*(2), 89-107.

Young, L.Y., Creighton, D.E., and Sauve, R.G. (1988). The needs of families of infants discharged home with continuous oxygen therapy. *JOGNN, 17*(3), 187-193.

Nursing research

Brooten, D., Kumar, S., Brown, L., Butts, P., Finkler, S., Bakewell-Sachs, S., Gibbons, A., and Delivoria-Papadopoulos, M. (1986). A randomized clinical trial of early hospital discharge and home follow-up of very-low-birth-weight infants. *New England Journal of Medicine, 315*(15), 934-939.

Rawlins, P., and Horner, M. (1988). Does membership in a support group alter needs of parents of chronically ill children? *Pediatric Nursing, 14*(1), 70-72.

UNIT SIX

The Postpartal Period

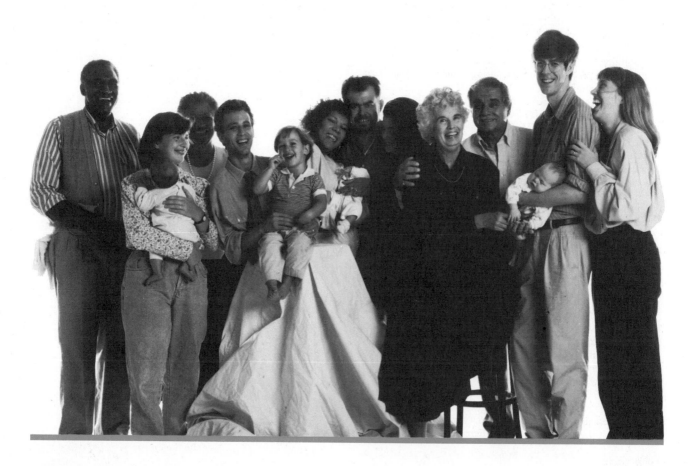

The postpartal period typically brings exhilaration to the client and her family—but it can pose challenges as well. The client confronts physiologic challenges as she recovers from pregnancy and delivery while coping with a demanding neonate. She also faces psychosocial challenges, such as the task of adapting to her role as new mother, readjusting her relationship with her partner, and dealing with an altered body image. Other family members face similar challenges as they strive to adapt to changes in their roles and in the overall family structure.

This unit explains how the nurse meets the physiologic, psychosocial, and teaching needs of the postpartal family by providing specific nursing measures, knowledge, counseling, and support. It describes the anatomic and physiologic changes that restore the body to a nonpregnant state, and it discusses nursing care to promote a full postpartal recovery. Taking a family-centered approach, it explains how the nurse helps individual family members adjust to changes in their roles, tasks, and responsibilities while promoting optimal adaptation to childbirth and the new family structure. The unit also covers such trends as home nursing care for the postpartal client.

Chapter 41
Physiology of the Postpartal Period

Chapter 41 surveys the client's physiologic changes that occur in the first 6 weeks after delivery. Using a body systems approach, it describes the changes that restore the reproductive system to a nonpregnant state, highlighting uterine involution, endometrial regeneration, amount and duration of lochia, and cervical contraction. It summarizes postpartal changes involving the vagina, external reproductive structures, pelvic support structures, and breasts. It illustrates postpartal changes in fundal height and onset of milk production through nipple stimulation and features a chart comparing the duration and appearance of lochia during the three stages of lochial discharge.

Next, the chapter explores postpartal endocrine changes, focusing on the rapid decline in placental hormones, the complex hormonal interplay leading to resumption of the menstrual cycle and ovulation, and the return of the endocrine glands to their normal size. Then it summarizes postpartal reversal of pregnancy-related changes in other body systems. Highlights of this summary include a discussion of the postpartal decrease in blood volume; reversal of pregnancy-induced varicose conditions; coagulatory stimulation during the early postpartal period; and gradual reversal of pregnancy-related anatomic and functional changes of the urinary, gastrointestinal, and musculoskeletal systems.

Chapter 42
Care during the Normal Postpartal Period

Chapter 42 prepares the nurse to help the postpartal client make a full, healthy recovery after delivery and achieve optimal adaptation to the birth of her child. It discusses the elements of a thorough postpartal assessment, stressing the need for ongoing evaluation of vital signs, comfort level, rest and sleep patterns, psychosocial status, and all body systems. It highlights assessment of the uterus and lochia to evaluate uterine involution and detect potential signs of hemorrhage, and it offers illustrated procedures showing how to determine fundal position and evaluate the condition of the perineum.

After providing pertinent nursing diagnoses for the postpartal client, Chapter 42 explains how to plan and implement nursing care. It highlights nursing measures that promote uterine involution and prevent hemorrhage; explains how to reduce discomfort from uterine contractions and perineal pain; discusses nursing activities that promote respiratory stability and bowel elimination; and tells how to prevent postpartal hematologic, gastrointestinal, and neurologic complications. Next, it outlines appropriate client teaching—especially important when early discharge is anticipated. It includes a chart comparing the indications, dosages, and nursing implications for drugs used during the postpartal period. It also offers guidelines for providing perineal care and presents client-teaching aids on postpartal exercises and self-care after discharge. Finally, the chapter presents pertinent evaluation and documentation data for the postpartal client.

Chapter 43
Psychosocial Adaptation of the Postpartal Family

Chapter 43 examines the role of the nurse in helping the postpartal family adjust to the changes resulting from childbirth. It begins by discussing the transition to parenthood, defining the main components of parenting and describing parenting tasks. Then it elaborates on the elements of parent-infant bonding, examining how early contact and neonatal behavioral and sensory capacities affect bonding.

Next, the chapter investigates parent-infant interaction and the factors that influence it. It describes optimal conditions for interaction, focusing on the effects of neonatal attentiveness and temperament. Then it discusses the communication cues and patterns that mold the developing parent-child relationship. After elaborating on the various forms of verbal and nonverbal interaction between parent and neonate, Chapter 43 explores the adaptation of each family member to childbirth. It delineates the phases of maternal adaptation, discusses the factors that affect parental adaptation, and describes sibling adaptation.

Then the chapter presents nursing care to promote family adaptation. It describes some important tools used to evaluate maternal adaptation and assess the mother-infant relationship. After explaining how to evaluate maternal emotional status and assess mother-infant bonding and interaction, the chapter tells how to evaluate paternal and sibling adaptation and gauge parental caregiving skills. It presents relevant nursing diagnoses, then presents nursing interventions that promote parent-infant bonding, ease the transition to parenthood, and promote adaptation of all family members. The chapter features guidelines on helping the disabled client adapt to parenthood. It concludes by explaining how to evaluate and document care related to psychosocial adaptation of the postpartal family.

Chapter 44
Postpartal Complications

Chapter 44 prepares the nurse to anticipate, prevent, and (when necessary) manage common postpartal complications. It delineates the pathophysiology and etiology of common postpartal complications, including puerperal infection, postpartal hemorrhage, birth canal injuries, vascular complications, urinary tract infections, diabetes mellitus, and postpartal mood swings.

Next, the chapter delineates nursing care for the client with a postpartal complication. It explains how to assess for each complication, presents relevant nursing diagnoses, and discusses planning and implementation. It offers tables detailing the risk factors for puerperal infection, postpartal hemorrhage, and postpartal mood swings; provides a scale that the nurse can use to evaluate perineal healing; and features a client-teaching aid on self-care for mastitis. Finally, the chapter identifies appropriate evaluation and documentation for the client with a postpartal complication.

Chapter 45
Maternal Care at Home

Chapter 45 discusses the nurse's role in providing home health care for the postpartal client, describing how such care helps ensure a full recovery and helps family members adapt to their new roles. It describes the advantages of home care, including enhancement of family-centered care, a more relaxed caregiving atmosphere, and the opportunity to develop greater mutual trust and provide more relevant care. It delineates strategies that improve the success of home nursing care, such as cooperating closely with other care providers, planning ahead, building rapport, and incorporating the client's preferences and cultural customs into nursing care.

Next, Chapter 45 applies the nursing process to care of the postpartal client at home, emphasizing how to adapt nursing care to the home setting. It discusses the benefits of assessment in the home, such as the ability to gather first-hand data about the client's and family's beliefs, customs, and preferences. After reviewing some drawbacks to home assessment, the chapter describes the history and physical data the nurse should gather to assess the client's postpartal recovery. Then it tells how to evaluate the client's psychosocial sta-

tus—including adaptation to her new role, interaction with the neonate, and emotional well-being—and how to assess the home for safety, adequacy, and psychosocial environment. After presenting pertinent nursing diagnoses, Chapter 45 provides planning and implementation for the postpartal client at home. It explains how to develop a nursing contract with the client to establish mutual goals and provides a sample contract. Then it focuses on nursing measures that promote postpartal recovery, help the client adapt to the maternal role, promote parenting skills, enhance the couple's relationship, and help siblings adapt. It features detailed nursing interventions for postpartal mood swings. The chapter concludes by describing how to evaluate and document care provided to the postpartal client at home.

Physiology of the Postpartal Period

Objectives

After reading and studying this chapter, the student should be able to:

1. Discuss the process of uterine involution.
2. Compare and contrast uterine involution in the primiparous and multiparous client.
3. Describe the normal progress of lochia.
4. Discuss the postpartal restoration of normal hypothalamic-pituitary-ovarian function.
5. Identify the hemodynamic events that restore blood volume to the nonpregnancy level.
6. Describe the postpartal return of normal physiologic function of all body systems.
7. Identify specific pregnancy- and delivery-related changes that may not resolve completely.

Introduction

Throughout pregnancy, gradual changes occur in all body systems. The most pronounced changes are those affecting the reproductive system and the hormonal processes that regulate its function. During the postpartal period (puerperium), these changes resolve; eventually, each body system returns to a nonpregnant state.

Although officially defined as a 6-week period, the postpartal period spans the time between delivery and the resumption of normal physiologic function. Thus it may vary greatly, especially among lactating clients. The client's physical capabilities and body image must adapt to postpartal changes and the restorative processes accompanying them. The nurse who understands such changes can assess the client more proficiently and make scientifically grounded decisions, facilitating the client's return to optimal health.

This chapter describes the anatomic and physiologic alterations that restore the body to a nonpregnant state. It begins with the reproductive and endocrine systems, highlighting the dramatic postpartal uterine and hormonal changes. The chapter continues with a description of the postpartal status of each body system.

Reproductive system

The reproductive system recovers from pregnancy and childbirth in a unique and efficient manner. However, some structures retain permanent effects.

Uterus

After delivery of the fetus and placenta, the uterus undergoes profound and dramatic changes leading to its return to a nonpregnant state. These changes, which involve both the myometrium (uterine muscle) and endometrium (uterine lining), take place through physiologic mechanisms not common to other organs.

Involution

The myometrium resumes a normal size through involution. A gradual process, involution results from muscle contractions and autolysis—self-disintegration or self-digestion of cells or tissue.

GLOSSARY

Alveolus: secretory unit of the mammary gland in which milk production takes place.

Anovulatory: failure of the ovary to produce, mature, or release an ovum (as in an anovulatory menstrual cycle).

Autolysis: self-disintegration or self-digestion of tissue or cells.

Basal metabolic rate: rate at which cells use oxygen; lowest metabolic rate that preserves physiologic function.

Cervical canal: structure extending from the external cervical os to the interior of the uterus.

Colostrum: thin, yellow, serous fluid secreted by the breasts during pregnancy and the first postpartal days before lactation begins; consists of water, protein, fat, carbohydrates, white blood cells, and immunoglobulins.

Corpus luteum: spherical yellowish tissue that grows within the ruptured ovarian follicle after ovulation and secrets progesterone.

Cystocele: herniation of the urinary bladder into the anterior vaginal wall.

Decidua: epithelial tissue of the endometrium during pregnancy.

Decidua basalis: portion of the decidua directly beneath the implanted ovum, attached to the myometrium.

Diastasis recti abdominis: separation of the rectus abdominis muscles at the midline.

Endometrium: mucous membrane lining of the uterus, a portion of which forms the decidua during pregnancy.

Enterocele: herniation of the intestine into the posterior portion of the vagina.

Fundus: rounded portion of the uterus above the level of the fallopian tube attachments.

Golgi body: complex membranous intracellular structure whose elements consist of flattened sacs (also called Golgi complex or Golgi apparatus).

Hyalinization: conversion into a glasslike substance.

Lactation: synthesis and secretion of milk from the breasts.

Lactogenesis: initiation of breast milk production.

Let-down reflex: milk ejection from the breast triggered by nipple stimulation or an emotional response to the neonate.

Lochia: vaginal discharge after delivery occurring in three distinct stages.

Myometrial contractions: postpartal uterine contractions that reduce uterine size (also called afterpains).

Myometrium: uterine muscle.

Oxytocin: hormone secreted by the posterior pituitary gland that stimulates uterine smooth-muscle contractions and breast milk ejection.

Oxytocin receptors: cellular structures in the breast that are sensitive to the effects of oxytocin.

Postpartal period: approximately 6-week period following delivery during which the anatomic and physiologic changes resulting from pregnancy resolve (also called puerperium).

Prolactin: hormone causing breast milk production; secreted by the anterior pituitary gland in response to tactile stimulation of the breast.

Rectocele: herniation of the rectum into the vagina.

Rugae: transverse folds in the vaginal mucosa.

Uterine involution: gradual return of the uterus to a nonpregnant size and condition after delivery.

Vaginal introitus: entrance to the vagina.

Immediately after delivery of the placenta, strong myometrial contractions (afterpains) shrink the uterus to the size of a grapefruit—a reduction of roughly half from the immediate predelivery size. This rapid shrinkage forces the uterine walls into close proximity, causing the center cavity to flatten.

Myometrial contractions are irregular in both timing and strength. A multiparous client usually experiences stronger, more uncomfortable contractions than a primiparous client—probably because uterine muscles lose elasticity with each pregnancy. Also, a lactating client has stronger contractions than a nonlactating client because oxytocin, a hormone that helps regulate milk ejection, stimulates uterine muscles.

Uterine involution is rapid and steady. Just after delivery, the uterus weighs 1,000 to 1,200 g; 1 week later, it weighs 500 g. By 6 weeks postpartum, the uterus has returned to its normal nonpregnant weight of 50 to 70 g (Cunningham, MacDonald, and Gant, 1989).

Uterine size decreases along with uterine weight. One hour after delivery, the fundus of the uterus (the rounded portion above the level of the fallopian tube attachments) is palpable at or just above the umbilicus. Each day thereafter, the uterus becomes smaller so that the fundus is palpable about one fingerbreadth lower than on the previous day (see *Postpartal changes in fundal height and uterine cell size*). By 2 weeks postpartum, the uterus has returned to the pelvic cavity and no longer can be palpated as an abdominal organ. Although never regaining its nulliparous size and shape, the uterus usually resumes a nonpregnant size and contour by 6 weeks postpartum.

Through autolysis—the second mechanism leading to involution—hypertrophic uterine cells return to a nonpregnant shape and size. The by-products of autolyzed cellular protein are absorbed and excreted by the

Postpartal changes in fundal height and uterine cell size

After delivery, uterine involution—the process that returns the uterus to a normal size—advances so rapidly that the level of the fundus is one fingerbreadth lower than on the previous day. Autolysis (self-destruction) of hypertrophic uterine muscle cells aids involution. The illustration also compares the size of uterine muscle cells in the pregnant, postpartal, and nonpregnant uterus.

FUNDAL HEIGHT

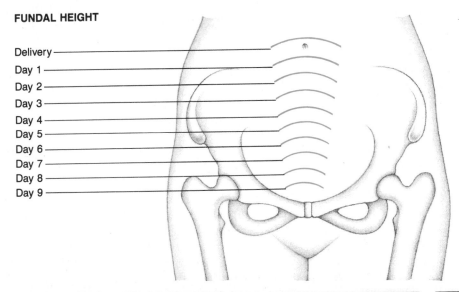

Delivery
Day 1
Day 2
Day 3
Day 4
Day 5
Day 6
Day 7
Day 8
Day 9

UTERINE INVOLUTION

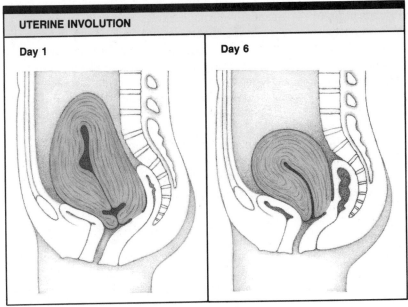

Day 1

Day 6

UTERINE MUSCLE CELLS

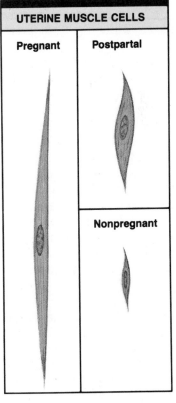

Pregnant

Postpartal

Nonpregnant

renal system. Because autolysis reduces uterine cell size so efficiently, the number of uterine cells after delivery remains unchanged from pregnancy.

Endometrium

During the postpartal period, healing and regeneration restore normal endometrial structure and function. As the placenta and membranes separate from the uterine wall at delivery, the decidua basalis (the decidual portion directly beneath the implanted ovum attached to the myometrium) remains in the uterine cavity.

In the early stages of involution, myometrial contractions compress blood vessels throughout the decidua and at the placental site, leading to hemostasis (arrest of bleeding). Contractions in the arteriolar walls immediately after delivery enhance hemostasis. Veins and arterioles at the placental site also undergo hyalinization. Hyaline thickening narrows the vessel lumen, leading to microscopic vascular changes and a more stable hemostasis.

After the first 2 or 3 postpartal days, the decidua basalis differentiates into two distinct layers. Occlusion of decidual blood vessels leads to necrosis of the superficial layer, which is sloughed off as part of the lochial discharge (see "Lochia"). The deeper decidual layer (basal layer) remains attached to the uterine wall.

By 7 days postpartum, endometrial glands begin to regenerate within the basal layer; by 16 days postpartum, the endometrium is completely restored except at the placental site. Involution of the placental site and restoration of normal tissue here take longer than in the rest of the endometrium.

As the placental site heals, regenerating endometrial tissue slowly and progressively replaces the decidua basalis. Immediately after delivery, the decidua basalis at the placental site measures 8 to 9 mm thick; by 8 days postpartum, it has shrunk by half. At 8 weeks, it measures approximately 2 mm and still has not healed completely. Healing occurs gradually and without scarring. If healing were less efficient and the placental site became scarred, the area available for implantation of a fertilized ovum would be significantly reduced, limiting the number of future pregnancies.

Fallopian tubes

Postpartal changes in the fallopian tubes take place mainly at the cellular level. During the first few weeks after delivery, many clients show acute inflammatory changes in the cells lining the fallopian tubes but lack symptoms of inflammation (such as fever and tenderness). Inflammation, which may stem from cellular debris that has collected within the lumen of the tubes, resolves without treatment and causes no damage.

The fallopian tubes also show the effects of changing hormone levels. With the sudden sharp drop in the estrogen level after delivery, epithelial cells lining the tubes take on a menopausal appearance, displaying atrophy and decreased numbers of ciliated cells. These changes are most pronounced at 2 weeks postpartum. With a gradual return to normal hormonal balance by 6 to 8 weeks postpartum, epithelial cells return to the condition seen in the early follicular phase of the menstrual cycle, with an increase in ciliated cells to help propel the ovum.

Isthmus

Softened and elongated during pregnancy, the isthmus resumes its normal size and consistency over the first few postpartal weeks. As it does so, it returns to its normal location between the uterine body and internal cervical os.

Lochia

The amount and duration of lochia—postpartal vaginal discharge—correlate with endometrial healing and regeneration. Generally, clients who have cesarean deliveries exhibit a lighter lochial flow of shorter duration than those who deliver vaginally—probably because some of the uterine debris found in lochia is removed manually during cesarean delivery.

In all clients, lochial flow occurs in three distinct stages (see *Stages of lochia*). Although rates of lochial discharge vary among clients, normal parameters for the amount and duration of lochia during each stage have been established. Lochia rubra, the first stage, typically lasts for the first 4 postpartal days and contains a mixture of mucus, tissue debris, and blood.

As uterine bleeding subsides, lochia becomes paler and more serous, entering the second stage. Called lochia serosa, this pink or brownish discharge persists for 5 to 7 days postpartum.

Between 7 and 14 days postpartum, sloughing at the former placental site may cause a sudden temporary increase in lochial flow or even bleeding. This self-limiting condition should last no more than 1 to 2 hours.

The final stage of lochial discharge is lochia alba, a creamy white, brown, or colorless discharge consisting mainly of serum and white blood cells (WBCs). Lochia alba usually diminishes after the third postpartal week but may persist for 6 weeks or longer.

Certain lochial variations are considered normal and do not signify a postpartal complication. Also, a client's perception of her lochial flow may differ from that of a trained examiner. In a study by Oppenheimer, Sherriff, Goodman, Shaw, and James (1986), some women reported a persistent lochia serosa at 6 weeks postpartum without complications or adverse effects; also, some stated that they did not experience lochia alba. Other findings of this study suggest that lochial flow increases with delivery of a large neonate, decreases with parity, and is not affected by breast-feeding.

On the other hand, lochia is considered abnormal if it contains large clots (as large as or larger than a dime) or tissue fragments (pieces of tissue, not the tissue debris normal to lochial flow). Also, lochia should not have a foul or offensive odor and should not relapse to a previous stage.

Cervix

In a client who delivered vaginally, cervical muscle tone is poor and the cervix and lower uterine segment are thin and collapsed. Examination of the external os reveals lacerations and bruising—usually more pronounced in the primiparous than the multiparous client.

The external os contracts slowly; on the second and third days after delivery, it remains flaccid and open approximately 2 to 3 cm. By the end of the first week, the os has contracted to 1 cm and cervical tone has improved, making admission of one finger difficult. At this point, cervical edema and hemorrhage have subsided markedly and the cervical canal (the structure extending from the external os to the interior of the uterus) has begun to reform as the cervix thickens.

Although the cervix resumes its normal functional anatomy by 6 to 12 weeks postpartum, it never regains its nulliparous appearance. The external os remains widened and linear, compared to the tiny circular os of the nulliparous client. Occasionally, the os appears fish-mouthed, particularly in cases of significant cervical trauma during delivery.

Blood and lymphatic vessels

During the postpartal period, extrauterine blood vessels decrease to a normal size and large intrauterine vessels are replaced by smaller vessels. The size and number of lymphatic vessels also decrease to normal.

Vagina

After vaginal delivery, the vagina is smooth-walled and somewhat enlarged, with poor muscle tone and significant edema. Gradually, it shrinks and the edema subsides. By the third postpartal week, rugae reappear within the vaginal walls. These rugae may remain permanently flattened to varying degrees, never returning to the nulliparous state (characterized by numerous mucosal infoldings). Consequently, the vaginal canal rarely resumes its nulliparous size.

Stages of lochia

Lochia progresses through three stages, each with distinctive characteristics that reflect progressive endometrial healing.

STAGE	USUAL DURATION	DESCRIPTION
Lochia rubra	1 to 4 days postpartum	Bloody, possibly with some mucus, tissue debris, and small clots. May have a slightly fleshy odor.
Lochia serosa	5 to 7 days postpartum	Pink-brown, serous, odorless
Lochia alba	1 to 3 weeks postpartum	Creamy white, brown, or almost colorless. May have a slightly stale odor.

The vaginal epithelium also undergoes notable postpartal changes. Vascular and well-lubricated during pregnancy because of estrogen increase, the epithelium becomes fragile and atrophic by the third or fourth postpartal week. In the nonlactating client, atrophy resolves by 6 to 10 weeks postpartum as estrogen normalizes. However, because the estrogen level remains low during lactation, the breast-feeding client may continue to experience symptoms of vaginal atrophy, such as decreased vaginal lubrication and diminished sexual response.

External structures

The clitoris and labia may remain permanently enlarged to some extent—a residual effect of the cellular hypertrophy, enhanced vascularity, and increased fat deposits occurring with pregnancy. After vaginal delivery, the vaginal introitus remains edematous and sometimes ecchymotic. Lacerations may appear on the introitus and perineum, even if an episiotomy was not performed.

Without such complications as hematoma or infection, the perineum heals rapidly. Usually, the introitus and perineum resume a nonpregnant state by 6 weeks postpartum. However, in cases of extreme musculofascial relaxation, extensive laceration, or inadequate perineal repair, the introitus may show residual gaping; typically, this change is permanent. Nonetheless, muscular contraction exercises, such as Kegel exercises, may help the introitus (as well as the vagina) approximate a nonpregnant state. (For information on these exercises, see Chapter 21, Family Preparation for Childbirth and Parenting.)

Pelvic muscular support structures

Uterine support structures, such as the broad and round ligaments, stretch significantly during pregnancy as the uterus expands. During vaginal delivery, the support structures of the uterus, vagina, urethra, and bladder undergo trauma. Although laxity of these structures improves gradually, some pelvic relaxation may persist beyond the postpartal period, causing any of the following conditions:
• uterine prolapse (sliding of the uterus into the vaginal canal)
• cystocele (herniation of the bladder into the vagina)
• rectocele (herniation of the rectum into the vagina)
• enterocele (herniation of the intestine into the posterior portion of the vagina).

Because the effects of stretching are cumulative, the likelihood of permanent relaxation of pelvic muscular support increases with each pregnancy and delivery.

Breasts

The breast changes initiated during pregnancy—nipple and areola enlargement, maturation of lobes and ducts, and increased vascularity—progress after delivery, particularly in the lactating client. The size of breast cells and the number of oxytocin receptors (cellular structures sensitive to the effects of oxytocin) also increase.

In the first 2 postpartal days, breast alveoli (tiny sacs made up of epithelial cells) enlarge and display substantial amounts of rough endoplasmic reticulum and Golgi bodies (membranous intracellular structures); the reticulum and Golgi bodies play key roles in milk production. The alveoli—the basic secretory units of the breast—are the site of milk production. Surrounded by a capillary network, alveoli cluster in groups of 10 to 100 to form lobules. Each lobule is drained by a lactiferous duct. The breast contains 15 to 20 lactiferous ducts, which merge at the nipple and areola to allow emptying of the breast. (For more information on the anatomy of the lactating breast, see Chapter 37, Infant Nutrition.)

Lactation—synthesis and secretion of breast milk—results from an interaction among several hormones. Alveolar growth and development is regulated by estrogen, progesterone, human placental lactogen (hPL), prolactin, cortisol, and insulin. Estrogen stimulates the release of prolactin and sensitizes the mammary gland to prolactin action. However, in combination with progesterone, estrogen inhibits prolactin. The profound drop in serum estrogen and progesterone levels after delivery of the placenta removes this inhibition, allowing prolactin to stimulate lactogenesis (initiation of milk secretion) within the alveoli.

How nipple stimulation affects milk production

Nipple stimulation triggers a series of events leading to milk production, as shown in the diagram below.

Dopamine, a neurotransmitter originating in the hypothalamus, also inhibits prolactin (hence its alternate name, prolactin-inhibiting factor). However, nipple stimulation overcomes this inhibition. When the neonate sucks on the nipple, nerve endings in the areola transmit sensory messages to the hypothalamus that cause dopamine production to diminish; this removes prolactin inhibition. (For details on this hormonal interaction, see *How nipple stimulation affects milk production*. For further information on lactation and breast-feeding, see Chapter 37, Infant Nutrition.)

In some cases, such as when the client chooses to bottle-feed her neonate, lactation must be suppressed. (For information on methods of suppression, see Chapter 42, Care during the Normal Postpartal Period.) With suppression, absence of sucking and emptying of the breasts usually leads to breast involution and cessation of lactation within 1 week. No longer stimulated, alveolar cells flatten and stop secreting milk; within 24 hours, cellular organelle structure begins to take on a more normal configuration, with a decrease in rough endoplasmic reticulum and Golgi bodies. Mammary blood flow decreases, leading to further involution. Over the next 3 months, connective and adipose tissue replaces glandular tissue, although the breast retains some increased glandular tissue. As involution nears completion, the breasts typically resume their nonpregnancy size. However, a mild alteration in breast shape may be permanent.

Endocrine system

Like the reproductive system, the endocrine system undergoes profound postpartal changes. Many of these changes interrelate with those of the reproductive system.

Placental hormones

With delivery of the placenta, levels of circulating placental hormones drop rapidly. The serum estrogen level plunges sharply in the first 3 hours after delivery, then more gradually until the seventh postpartal day, when it reaches its lowest level. In the nonlactating client, estrogen begins to rise to a normal level at approximately 2 weeks postpartum. In the lactating client, the rise is delayed, leading to such problems as vaginal mucosal atrophy (the estrogen level increases gradually when breast-feeding frequency decreases).

Serum progesterone falls below normal luteal-phase levels by the third postpartal day. After the first week, progesterone cannot be detected in the circulation until ovulation returns. However, it may not resume a normal pattern for several menstrual cycles. A study by Poindexter, Ritter, and Besch (1983) suggests that progesterone production normalizes slowly over three to four cycles. Consequently, the first few postpartal menstrual cycles may be irregular and shorter than normal.

The two remaining placental hormones—hPL and human chorionic gonadotropin (hCG)—also rapidly diminish. Reyes, Winter, and Faiman (1985) found that circulating hCG—the hormone measured in most standard pregnancy tests—disappears within 8 to 24 hours after delivery in both lactating and nonlactating clients. The decline is so pronounced that by the end of the first postpartal week a urine pregnancy test is negative. Neither hCG nor hPL is produced until a subsequent pregnancy.

Pituitary hormones

Levels of thyrotropin and adrenocorticotrophic hormone, which increase during pregnancy to help maintain the corpus luteum, drop to nonpregnancy levels in the postpartal period. Antidiuretic hormone (ADH, or vasopressin), no longer needed in larger amounts to maintain fluid balance, also diminishes.

In the nonlactating client, serum prolactin typically drops to a nonpregnancy level by 3 weeks postpartum. In the lactating client, it remains elevated into the sixth week and sometimes beyond, depending on breast-feeding frequency. The client must breast-feed at least six times daily to maintain this elevation; otherwise, prolactin falls to a normal level within 6 months.

Levels of circulating follicle-stimulating hormone (FSH) and luteinizing hormone (LH) remain low for the first 2 weeks postpartum. FSH levels are identical in lactating and nonlactating clients. However, low estrogen levels in lactating clients reduce ovarian sensitivity to FSH, making ovulation less likely.

Hypothalamic-pituitary-ovarian function

Resumption of the menstrual cycle is coordinated by hormones secreted by the hypothalamus (gonadotropin-releasing hormone [GnRH]), pituitary gland (FSH and LH), and ovaries (estrogen and progesterone). Although a period of amenorrhea normally follows delivery, experts do not concur on its physiologic basis or the mechanism that reestablishes a normal cycle. Some attribute postpartal amenorrhea to a GnRH deficiency, others to pituitary insensitivity to GnRH, and still others to a hormonal deficiency involving the hypothalamus, pituitary gland, and ovaries.

Among nonlactating clients, the average time before the return of ovulation is about 10 weeks; menstruation typically resumes by 7 to 9 weeks. Thus, for most nonlactating clients, the first postpartal menstrual period may be anovulatory.

Lactation delays the return of a normal menstrual cycle; the length of the delay depends on breast-feeding duration and frequency. Thus, a client who breast-feeds for 6 months will have longer-lasting amenorrhea than one who breast-feeds for 4 weeks. Likewise, six or more daily breast-feeding sessions decrease the chance for a normal menstrual cycle.

Return of ovulation in lactating clients also varies. For both lactating and nonlactating clients, an increased interval before the first postpartal menstrual period increases the likelihood of an ovulatory cycle. Thus, the longer a client breast-feeds, the greater the chance that the first postpartal cycle will be ovulatory. (However, poor nutritional status during lactation may delay resumption of normal hypothalamic-pituitary-ovarian function.)

Reversal of other changes

No longer stimulated by an increased estrogen level, the pituitary, thyroid, and parathyroid glands resume their normal size after delivery. Thyroxine, thyroxine-binding plasma proteins, and parathyroid hormone decrease to a nonpregnancy level. Corticosteroid levels, elevated during pregnancy by reduced renal excretion of cortisol, also fall. Nonpregnancy levels may resume as early as 1 week postpartum; by the sixth week, all clients have normal serum cortisol levels.

The rapid decline in estrogen, progesterone, cortisol, and hPL leaves insulin relatively unopposed (not blocked) in the early postpartal period compared to late pregnancy. Also, for the first few postpartal days, the serum glucose level, which decreases during pregnancy, remains low. Consequently, clients with diabetes mellitus have a greatly reduced need for exogenous insulin; some require none. As hormone levels begin to stabilize, the need for exogenous insulin returns and the insulin requirement approximates the nonpregnancy dosage.

Respiratory system

The postpartal period typically brings complete resolution of pregnancy-related respiratory changes and associated complaints, such as shortness of breath, chest and rib discomfort, and decreased tolerance for physical exertion.

Reversal of anatomic changes

Anatomic changes in the thoracic cavity and rib cage, caused by increasing uterine size, reverse gradually after delivery. Thus, full lung expansion returns and the rib cage regains a normal diameter. As the estrogen level declines, vascularization of the respiratory tract—increased by pregnancy—also resumes a nonpregnancy status.

Reversal of functional changes

As the serum progesterone level declines, oxygen demand decreases, and the uterus no longer impinges on the diaphragm, the following changes occur, restoring normal respiratory function.
• Tidal volume (the amount of air exchanged with each breath), minute volume (the amount of air expelled from the lungs per minute), and vital capacity (the amount of air expelled after maximum inspiration) decrease to nonpregnancy values.
• Functional residual capacity (the amount of air remaining in the lungs after normal, quiet inspiration) rises to nonpregnancy values.

Resumption of normal acid-base balance and oxygen saturation

Shifting hormone levels after delivery cause reversal of the mild hyperventilation of pregnancy. Thus, arterial oxygen partial pressure (PaO_2) decreases, arterial carbon dioxide partial pressure ($PaCO_2$) increases, and the bicarbonate level rises. As the respiratory rate falls to a nonpregnancy level, $PaCO_2$ elimination and red blood cell (RBC) oxygen-carrying capacity normalize, reducing serum pH.

Postpartal hormonal changes also restore a normal respiratory stimulus. Thus, the $PaCO_2$ threshold needed to stimulate respiration increases.

Cardiovascular system

After delivery, the cardiovascular system exhibits few subjectively noticeable changes as it resumes a nonpregnancy status.

Reversal of anatomic and auscultatory changes

Cardiac enlargement and displacement reverse as the uterus resumes its normal size and position. Abnormal heart sounds—a result of the anatomic and hemodynamic changes caused by pregnancy—also resolve in the postpartal period.

Reversal of hemodynamic changes

Altered significantly by pregnancy, blood volume and cardiac output quickly resume a nonpregnancy status after delivery. Blood pressure and pulse undergo less dramatic changes.

Blood volume

Increased approximately 45% during pregnancy, blood volume drops sharply just after delivery. Within 4 weeks, it returns to a nonpregnancy level as the following events occur.
• Blood loss during delivery immediately reduces blood volume. Normal vaginal delivery leads to an average blood loss of 500 ml; cesarean delivery, 1,000 ml or more. The increase in blood volume during pregnancy allows the body to withstand this substantial loss. However, excessive blood loss at delivery may delay functional recovery (as described in *Nursing research applied: Return of normal daily function after delivery*.)
• After delivery, extravascular fluid shifts to the circulation, leading to a plasma volume increase that helps offset blood loss at delivery. This fluid then is excreted by the renal system—first in large amounts, later more gradually, as postpartal diuresis occurs.
• Delivery of the placenta reduces the size of the maternal vascular bed by 10% to 15%. Thus, a smaller blood volume is needed for tissue perfusion.
• The vasodilatory effects of hormonal tissue disappear after delivery, reducing the amount of blood required to maintain adequate tissue perfusion and blood pressure.

Cardiac output

Markedly increased during pregnancy, cardiac output remains high for 48 hours postpartum, then declines gradually to a nonpregnancy level. Studying this decline, Robson, Hunter, Moore, and Dunlop (1987) found that by 24 weeks postpartum, cardiac output has fallen an average of 33%, reaching normal nonpregnancy levels. (The decline is similar in lactating and nonlactating clients.) Most of the decrease occurs as early as 2 weeks postpartum.

Blood pressure and pulse

Immediately after delivery, blood pressure readings should differ only slightly, if at all, from readings taken during the third trimester of pregnancy. A decrease may indicate uterine hemorrhage or excessive blood loss at delivery; an increase may signal a pre-eclamptic tendency, especially if accompanied by headache or visual changes. According to Robson, Hunter, Moore, and Dunlop (1987), blood pressure readings typically remain relatively stable in the first 12 weeks postpartum, then

---

NURSING RESEARCH APPLIED

Return of normal daily function after delivery

A recent study examined women's postpartal readiness to resume household, social, and occupational activities as well as assume responsibility for care of a neonate. The researchers investigated the effect of delivery method on the rate of postpartal recovery and examined the role of other variables in a woman's perceptions of her recovery.

The subjects were 70 women of various occupations who had delivered full-term neonates within the previous 5 years. Thirty had delivered vaginally, 40 by cesarean delivery. Each woman completed a questionnaire from which researchers measured the impact of childbirth on functional ability by comparing predelivery and postpartal activity levels.

The study found that delivery method significantly affected functional recovery. At the end of the traditional 6-week postpartal period, 72% of the women who had delivered vaginally reported normal energy levels, compared to only 34% of those who had undergone cesarean delivery. Among both groups combined, only 51% felt that their usual energy and functional levels had returned by 6 weeks postpartum.

Women in both groups resumed occupational activities at the time specified by their employers, although many did so out of obligation rather than increased energy. Age, parity, and neonatal complications had no effect on recovery and return to normal activities. However, postpartal complications, such as infection and excessive blood loss, significantly decreased the activity level.

Application to practice

The results of this study indicate that although postpartal physiologic changes generally resolve within 6 weeks, recovery of functional ability may take much longer. The nurse who is aware of the time lag between physiologic and functional recovery can provide more realistic anticipatory guidance to pregnant and postpartal clients and can serve as client advocate to minimize demands on new mothers. A nurse working in an occupational health setting may use the information revealed by this study to recommend maternity policies that mutually benefit the postpartal client, her family, and her employer. Further, the nurse should inform a client who has undergone cesarean delivery that she may need an extended time to recover her functional ability.

Tulman, L., and Fawcett, J. (1988). Return of functional ability after childbirth. *Nursing Research*, 37(2), 77-81.

---

increase gradually until the twenty-fourth week when nonpregnancy readings return.

For 7 to 10 days after delivery, transient bradycardia (a heart rate of 50 to 70 beats/minute) may occur. This finding is normal and may result from the decrease in cardiac work load that follows delivery. On the other hand, tachycardia (a heart rate above 100 beats/minute) warrants investigation because it may reflect hypovolemia—especially in a client with a low RBC count or a decreasing hemoglobin level.

Reversal of varicose conditions

Varicose conditions of the legs, anus (hemorrhoids), or vulva may arise during pregnancy from diminished venous return of the legs, pressure exerted by the fetus, and straining during labor and delivery. In many clients, these conditions improve significantly or regress completely after delivery. However, signs and symptoms become more pronounced with each pregnancy. If problems persist after the postpartal period, surgery may be required.

Hematologic system

Levels of blood constituents may vary in the postpartal period. Coagulation, enhanced during pregnancy and delivery, normalizes gradually. However, coagulatory stimulation induced by labor and delivery increases the risk of thromboembolism.

Red blood cell parameters

Immediately after delivery, the hemoglobin level and hematocrit vary from one client to the next, as does the RBC count. Generally, for a client who delivered vaginally without complications, these values remain near predelivery levels despite normal blood loss at delivery. (This phenomenon results from hemoconcentration—packing of blood cells—which follows postpartal diuresis.) In a client who underwent cesarean delivery, increased blood loss may cause RBC parameters to fall slightly just after delivery.

In a healthy client with adequate nutrition, all RBC parameters typically will return to nonpregnancy levels by 6 weeks postpartum. A significant or progressive decrease in these parameters in the first few postpartal days is abnormal and may indicate excessive or continued blood loss.

White blood cell count

The WBC count increases in the first 10 to 12 days postpartum, possibly rising as high as 25,000/mm³ (the increase is mainly in granulocytes). Although this change reflects a normal stress response, it may complicate diagnosis of a postpartal infection, which also increases the WBC count.

Serum electrolytes

Serum potassium and calcium levels, which rise during pregnancy, fall rapidly to nonpregnancy values after delivery because of the fluid shift and subsequent diuresis.

Coagulation factors

Postpartal changes in coagulation factors are gradual. Throughout pregnancy, levels of coagulation factors I (fibrinogen), VII, IX, and X rise progressively; during late pregnancy, fibrinolysis (destruction of blood clots) diminishes. These circumstances place the pregnant client at a progressively increasing risk for thromboembolic disorders.

Delivery stimulates the coagulation system, increasing this risk even further in the early postpartal period. Studying the rate at which coagulation factors normalize after delivery, Dahlman, Hellgren, and Blomback (1985) found that these factors remain significantly elevated for the first 2 to 3 weeks postpartum, then fall gradually, approaching nonpregnancy levels after 6 weeks. The platelet count returns to a nonpregnancy level by 2 weeks postpartum. However, traumatic delivery, infection, or prolonged immobility may delay the return to normal levels.

Urinary system

Pregnancy affects both the anatomic structure of the urinary tract and the function of the urinary system; delivery may contribute to certain anatomic changes. Unlike most other body systems, the urinary system may show the effects of pregnancy and delivery well into—and even beyond—the postpartal period.

Reversal of anatomic changes

At delivery, fetal passage through the pelvis and vagina causes varying degrees of trauma to the urethra and bladder. A normal amount of trauma leads to edema and microscopic bleeding. Delivery complications (such as precipitous delivery or forceps instrumentation) may cause increased trauma, leading to laceration of the urethra and meatus. With cesarean delivery, the potential for surgical trauma of the bladder is a possibility.

Delivery trauma accompanied by anesthesia (especially spinal or epidural anesthesia) may impair bladder tone. If this occurs, the bladder may lose sensitivity, resulting in a diminished voiding urge. This contributes to postpartal urine retention.

Postpartal diuresis may cause bladder overdistention, possibly resulting in muscle damage, atony, and urinary tract infection (from stasis and urine retention). Without such complications, however, the lower urinary tract resumes normal function within 1 or 2 weeks as edema and diuresis resolve, although bladder distention may persist for 3 months.

Typically, dilation of the renal pelvis, calyces, and ureters begins in the first trimester and progresses as pregnancy advances. Slowing urine passage through the ureters, dilation causes distention of the renal pelvis. Within the first 12 to 16 weeks postpartum, dilation resolves gradually, although some mild dilation may persist for years (Jaffe, 1985). Urinary frequency, urgency, and other symptoms caused by pressure on the bladder from increasing uterine size resolve after delivery.

Reversal of functional changes

Pregnancy increases the renal plasma flow and the glomerular filtration rate (GFR). In late pregnancy, the GFR begins a gradual decline that continues into the postpartal period. Usually, the GFR returns to a nonpregnancy level by 6 weeks postpartum. Renal plasma flow also normalizes.

Urinalysis

Mild proteinuria, caused by excretion of protein by-products of uterine involution, is common after delivery but should disappear by 6 weeks postpartum. Glycosuria, another common postpartal finding, usually resolves by the end of the first week.

Gastrointestinal system

With the gastrointestinal (GI) tract no longer obstructed by the expanding uterus and hormone levels declining rapidly, the GI tract quickly resumes normal function after delivery.

Appetite

After vaginal delivery, most clients are extremely hungry from lack of food intake and the exertion of labor and delivery—especially if little or no anesthesia was used.

Appetite tends to subside to a normal level in 1 to 2 days, although a breast-feeding client may maintain an increased appetite and food intake while breast-feeding.

After cesarean delivery, the client whose appetite return is less pronounced may be started on a clear liquid diet and gradually advanced to a regular diet as GI function returns.

Bowel motility and evacuation

During pregnancy, GI motility is inhibited by the high serum progesterone level (which relaxes intestinal smooth muscle, decreasing peristalsis) and by increasing uterine size (which compresses the intestines). With delivery resolving both factors, normal peristalsis and bowel function usually return rapidly. However, bowel motility may remain sluggish in cases of intestinal manipulation during cesarean delivery or use of anesthetic or analgesic agents.

Typically, bowel evacuation normalizes once bowel motility is restored. Nonetheless, the first bowel movement may be delayed until 2 to 3 days postpartum for reasons unrelated to intestinal function. For example, abdominal muscle tone may be so poor that the client cannot attain sufficient pressure to evacuate the bowel. Also, the client may avoid bowel evacuation, fearing it will cause pain or damage the episiotomy. Residual dehydration from labor and the subsequent decrease in the fluid content of the stool also may impair bowel evacuation. In many cases, a stool softener, laxative, suppository, or enema must be used to reestablish normal bowel function.

Reversal of other changes

Gallbladder emptying, slowed during pregnancy, increases after delivery, reducing the risk of gallstones. The bile flow, hepatic work load, and hepatic blood flow decrease to nonpregnancy levels, and liver function studies should no longer be abnormal.

Musculoskeletal system

Although pregnancy-related changes in the musculoskeletal system reverse after delivery, joints and muscles may show some residual effects.

Reversal of postural and joint changes

As pregnancy advances, increasing body weight and the shift in the center of gravity subject the musculoskeletal system to significant stress. Also, estrogen, progesterone, and relaxin (a hormone released by the corpus luteum during pregnancy) relax the joints, decreasing their stability. Abdominal distention exaggerates the lordotic (forward) curvature of the lumbar spine and loosens pelvic joints.

Delivery removes the mechanical strain on the musculoskeletal system and halts secretion of relaxin. Over the first 6 to 8 postpartal weeks, posture returns to normal and structural changes reverse gradually. However, foot enlargement—caused by the effects of relaxin on foot joints as well as weight gain and dependent edema—may persist. Thus, increased foot and shoe size tend to be a permanent reminder of pregnancy.

Reversal of muscular changes

Enlargement of breast and abdominal wall muscles during pregnancy weakens these structures. Although the damage is not permanent, many clients have trouble regaining satisfactory muscle tone in these areas.

During the third trimester, the rectus abdominis muscles may separate, causing diastasis recti abdominis. This condition sometimes can be corrected by postpartal abdominal exercises. However, it may persist indefinitely unless adequate muscle tone is restored. Poor abdominal muscle tone may contribute to back strain and complaints of low backache.

Effects of regional anesthesia

Regional (spinal or epidural) anesthesia used during delivery may cause transient musculoskeletal effects, including decreased sensation and function in the lower extremities. However, these effects usually disappear within 8 to 12 hours.

Integumentary system

Pregnancy-related skin changes resolve completely or partially after delivery as hormone levels decrease and the skin no longer is stretched.

Reversal of hormone-related changes

During the postpartal period, pigmentation changes caused by pregnancy—including chloasma (also called melasma, or mask of pregnancy) and linea nigra (a dark midline streak on the abdomen)—reverse gradually. However, they may never disappear completely.

Pregnancy may stimulate pigmented nevi (colored moles), causing them to enlarge or change color or leading to formation of new nevi. These changes tend to regress after delivery. Nevi that do not resume their prepregnancy appearance warrant further evaluation. Nipple darkening, also caused by pregnancy, reverses partially in the postpartal period. Any increased acne associated with pregnancy also resolves as hormone levels stabilize.

Pregnancy-related hirsutism also regresses (however, coarse hairs that arose during pregnancy tend to remain). Some clients complain of excessive hair loss from the head after delivery. This is a compensation for the below-normal loss during pregnancy; the postpartal loss is merely catching up with the loss that would have taken place without pregnancy. The catch-up process ends roughly 6 to 12 months postpartum.

Some vascular skin conditions observed in pregnant clients mimic those accompanying liver disease, such as spider angiomas and palmar erythema. Stemming from enhanced subcutaneous blood flow (caused by the increased serum estrogen level), these conditions disappear soon after delivery as the estrogen level falls.

Changes in the mucous membranes during pregnancy—epistaxis (nosebleed), nasal edema with congestion, and bleeding of the gums—reverse as the estrogen level decreases. Some pregnant clients develop gingivitis, sometimes with small vascular nodules at the gum line. This condition, called epulis gravidarum, usually regresses within 1 to 2 months postpartum (Gabbe, Niebyl, and Simpson, 1986).

Striae (stretch marks) result from increased corticosteroid levels and mechanical stretching of the skin during pregnancy. These harmless marks commonly appear over the abdomen, back, thighs, and breasts. As body size normalizes, striae shrink and fade from dark red to silvery-white within a year after delivery. Although they become less apparent, they never disappear completely.

Diaphoresis

In the first 2 to 3 days postpartum, many clients experience episodes of profuse diaphoresis (sweating). Associated with the postpartal fluid shift, diaphoresis is a normal mechanism that helps the renal system excrete excess fluid and waste products. It should resolve within the first postpartal week.

Other systems

Metabolic, neurologic, and immunologic changes brought on by pregnancy reverse rapidly after delivery.

Metabolic system

Throughout pregnancy, the basal metabolic rate (BMR)—the lowest rate of metabolism that preserves physiologic function—rises until delivery, when it measures approximately 20% above normal. (The increase primarily reflects fetoplacental demands and the greater cardiac work load.) After delivery, the BMR decreases rapidly, approaching nonpregnancy levels by 5 to 6 days postpartum.

Neurologic system

Neurologic effects of pregnancy, which may range from minor to extremely bothersome, rarely linger after delivery.

Entrapment neuropathies

Among the most common neurologic changes caused by pregnancy, entrapment neuropathies are nerve compression disorders usually caused by fluid retention. As soft tissue becomes edematous, it exerts pressure on nerves within the tissue, causing such symptoms as numbness, tingling, and loss of function. For example, in carpal tunnel syndrome, the median nerve in the wrist is compressed. With the disappearance of edema after delivery, entrapment neuropathies usually resolve. In rare cases, surgery is required to release an entrapment.

Reversal of other changes

Other neurologic complaints during pregnancy include tension headache and syncopal or near-syncopal episodes. These conditions are associated with stress, decreased rest, poor nutritional status, increased blood glucose levels, and hormonal changes accompanying pregnancy. As delivery eliminates these factors, tension headaches and syncopal episodes diminish. With proper postpartal nutrition and rest, they disappear completely.

Immunologic system

Inhibited during pregnancy to prevent the body from rejecting the fetus as foreign matter, the immune system resumes normal function during the postpartal period. However, a client lacking the Rh factor (an antigenic substance usually found in RBCs) who delivers an Rh-positive neonate may become sensitized to the Rh antigen in neonatal RBCs and may produce Rh antibodies directed against the sensitizing antigen; this could cause problems in subsequent pregnancies. To prevent this, an Rh-negative client must receive Rh_o (D) immune globulin (RhoGAM) at 28 weeks of pregnancy and again within 72 hours after delivery. (For a complete discussion of Rh sensitization, see Chapter 23, Antepartal Complications.)

Chapter summary

Chapter 41 described the postpartal physiologic processes that restore the body to a nonpregnant state. Here are the key concepts.

• Pregnancy affects all body systems to varying degrees. Each system returns to a nonpregnant state during the postpartal period. However, some pregnancy-related changes do not reverse completely.

• The rapid drop in serum estrogen and progesterone levels after delivery triggers reversal of many pregnancy-related changes.

• Within 6 weeks after delivery, the uterus returns to an approximately normal size and shape through involution. This process involves uterine muscle contractions and self-destruction of uterine cells.

• The superficial lining of the uterus becomes necrotic and is sloughed off after delivery.

• Lochia (postpartal vaginal discharge) progresses through three stages—lochia rubra, lochia serosa, and lochia alba.

• In a breast-feeding client, breast development continues after delivery. Prolactin stimulates milk production in the breast alveoli; oxytocin causes contraction of the alveoli, which leads to ejection of milk toward the nipple.

• In a nonlactating client or a client who discontinues breast-feeding, the breasts undergo involution, possibly becoming engorged for 1 to 2 days. With absence of sucking and emptying of the breast, milk production ceases within 1 week.

• In the nonlactating client, menstruation usually returns in 7 to 9 weeks, although the first period may be anovulatory. In the lactating client, the return of menstruation is delayed, depending on the duration and frequency of breast-feeding.

• Anatomic and functional changes in the respiratory system resolve with delivery as hormone levels decrease and the thoracic cavity and rib cage are no longer affected by the pregnant uterus.

• The coagulation system, enhanced by pregnancy, is stimulated further in the early postpartal period, increasing the risk of thromboembolism.

• Some changes in the urinary system, such as dilation of the renal pelvis, calyces, and ureters, may persist beyond the postpartal period.

• Gastrointestinal function quickly returns to normal, although bowel evacuation may be delayed for several postpartal days.

• Weakened breast and abdominal wall muscles require exercise to restore muscle tone in these areas.

• Some integumentary changes caused by pregnancy, such as linea nigra and striae, may not reverse completely after delivery.

Study questions

1. What is the expected condition of the uterus, breasts, and lochia in a breast-feeding client 24 hours after delivery?

2. During a prenatal class, a gravida 2, para 1 client, age 28, asks if she will experience the same changes during recovery from this delivery as she did with her first delivery. After gathering information about her first postpartal experience, how should the nurse answer her?

3. A postpartal client experiences painful uterine contractions 36 hours after delivery. How should the nurse explain the reason for these contractions?

4. What role does sucking on the breast play in lactation?

5. A nonlactating gravida 1, para 1 client, age 18, asks when she can expect her menstrual period to resume and whether it will be like her previous periods. How should the nurse respond?

6. Which changes resulting from pregnancy and childbirth may never reverse completely?

Bibliography

Cunningham, F., MacDonald, P., and Gant, N. (Eds). (1989). *Williams obstetrics* (18th ed). East Norwalk, CT: Appleton & Lange.

Dahlman, T., Hellgren, M., and Blomback, M. (1985). Changes in blood coagulation and fibrinolysis in the normal puerperium. *Gynecologic Obstetric Investigation,* 20(1), 37-44.

Gabbe, S., Niebyl, J., and Simpson, J. (1986). *Obstetrics: Normal and problem pregnancies.* New York: Churchill Livingstone.

Jaffe, D. (1985). Postpartum evaluation of renal function. *Clinical Obstetrics and Gynecology,* 28(2), 298-309.

Karp, R., Greene, G., Smiciklas-Wright, H., and Scholl, T. (1988). Postpartum weight change: How much of the weight gained in pregnancy will be lost after delivery? *Obstetrics and Gynecology,* 71(5), 701-707.

Oppenheimer, L., Sherriff, E., Goodman, J., Shaw, D., and James, C. (1986). The duration of lochia. *British Journal of Obstetrics and Gynecology,* 93(7), 754-757.

Poindexter, A., Ritter, M., and Besch, P. (1983). The recovery of normal plasma progesterone levels in the postpartum female. *Fertility and Sterility,* 39(4), 494-498.

Raisanen, I. (1988). Plasma levels and diurnal variation of B-endorphin, B-lipotropin and corticotropin during pregnancy and the early puerperium. *European Journal of Obstetrics and Gynecology and Reproductive Biology,* 27(1), 13-20.

Reyes, F., Winter, J., and Faiman, C. (1985). Postpartum disappearance of chorionic gonadotropin from the maternal and neonatal circulations. *American Journal of Obstetrics and Gynecology,* 153(5), 486-489.

Robson, S., Hunter, S., Moore, M., and Dunlop, W. (1987). Haemodynamic changes during the puerperium: A Doppler and M-mode echocardiographic study. *British Journal of Obstetrics and Gynecology,* 94(11), 1028-1039.

Nursing research

Tulman, L., and Fawcett, J. (1988). Return of functional ability after childbirth. *Nursing Research,* 37(2), 77-81.

Care during the Normal Postpartal Period

Objectives

After reading and studying this chapter, the student should be able to:

1. Identify the physiologic and psychosocial components of postpartal nursing care.

2. Describe safety, comfort, rest, and exercise requirements for the postpartal client.

3. State the indications, actions, and dosages for specific medications used in the postpartal period.

4. Use the nursing process to plan appropriate and individualized care for the postpartal client.

5. Design a teaching plan to meet the needs of the postpartal client and her family.

6. Prepare the client and her partner for independent functioning as parents after discharge.

Introduction

The postpartal period is a time of both exhilaration and stress. Although the client is engrossed in her neonate and eager to share her good news with family and friends, she also faces new physical, emotional, and financial challenges. She may have concerns about the changes that motherhood will bring and may feel anxious about the new relationship she and her partner must develop as they adapt to their roles as parents.

Caring for the postpartal client offers the nurse an opportunity to promote a full and healthy recovery from delivery while helping the client and her partner make an optimal adaptation to the birth of their child. As early discharge after delivery becomes increasingly common, skillful implementation of the nursing process takes on greater importance as a way for the nurse to meet the client's physiologic, psychosocial, and teaching needs.

This chapter discusses the nurse's role in caring for the postpartal client. It begins with assessment of vital signs and body systems, including signs of poor postpartal recovery. Then it discusses how to plan and implement care, highlighting measures that help ensure the client's smooth transition to a nonpregnant status. It includes client teaching aimed at preventing postdischarge problems. After describing how to evaluate postpartal nursing care, the chapter concludes with a brief discussion of documentation.

Assessment

Just after delivery, the physiologic changes brought on by pregnancy and delivery begin to reverse. The nurse must monitor the progress of the client's transition to a nonpregnant status, staying alert for signs of poor transition as well as complications of pregnancy and delivery.

Postpartal assessment begins with a review of the antenatal, labor, and delivery records. The nurse on the postpartal unit should make sure this information has been included in the report from the nurse who transferred the client from the recovery unit. Then, throughout the client's stay, the nurse must measure vital signs, determine the client's comfort level, assess rest and sleep patterns, and evaluate the status of all body systems.

GLOSSARY

Colostrum: thin, yellow, serous fluid secreted during pregnancy and the first postpartal days before lactation begins; consists of water, protein, fat, carbohydrates, white blood cells, and immunoglobulins.

Breast engorgement: excessive fullness of the breasts resulting from temporary lymphatic and venous stasis; occurs during the early part of the lactation cycle.

Diastasis recti abdominis: separation of the rectus abdominis muscles at the midline.

Episiotomy: surgical incision in the perineum to enlarge the vaginal opening for delivery; performed to prevent perineal tears, speed or facilitate delivery, or prevent excess stretching of perineal muscles and connective tissue.

Fundus: rounded portion of the uterus above the level of the fallopian tube attachments.

Homans' sign: pain in the calf on dorsiflexion of the foot, indicating superficial thrombosis or thrombophlebitis.

Kegel exercises: isometric exercises in which the muscles of the pelvic diaphragm and perineum are contracted voluntarily (also called pubococcygeus exercises); help increase contractility of the vaginal introitus and improve urine retention.

Lochia: vaginal discharge after delivery occurring in three distinct stages; composed of blood, tissue, leukocytes, and mucus.

Morbid temperature: oral temperature exceeding 100.4° F (38° C) that persists for 2 successive days after delivery, excluding the first 24 hours.

Myometrial contractions: postpartal uterine contractions that reduce uterine size (also called afterpains).

Myometrium: uterine muscle.

Oxytocin: hormone secreted by the posterior pituitary gland that stimulates uterine smooth-muscle contractions and breast milk ejection.

Perineum: the region between the vulva and anus; bounded in the front by the pubic arch and the arcuate ligaments, in the back by the tip of the coccyx, and laterally by the inferior rami of the pubis and ischium and the sacrotuberus ligaments.

Postpartal period: approximately 6-week period following delivery during which the anatomic and physiologic changes resulting from pregnancy resolve (also called puerperium).

Secundines: placenta and membranes expelled after delivery (afterbirth).

Uterine atony: poor uterine muscle tone.

Uterine subinvolution: failure of the uterus to return to a nonpregnant size and condition after delivery.

Uterine involution: gradual return of the uterus to a nonpregnant size and condition after delivery.

Vital signs

Careful monitoring and evaluation of vital signs yields valuable information about the client's status. Obtain complete vital signs—temperature, pulse, and respiratory rate—and measure blood pressure every 15 minutes for the first hour after delivery, then every hour for the next 4 hours or until vital signs are stable. Thereafter, obtain vital signs every 4 hours until 24 hours after delivery, then every 8 hours until discharge.

Temperature

Measure the client's temperature orally. A slight temperature elevation from mild dehydration, caused by labor and delivery, is common during the first 24 hours after delivery. However, suspect infection if the client has a morbid temperature, defined by the Joint Committee on Maternal Welfare as one that exceeds 100.4° F (38° C) for 2 successive days after delivery, excluding the first 24 hours (Gibbs and Weinstein, 1976).

Pulse

The pulse may remain normal for an hour or so after delivery. During the first postpartal rest or sleep, which usually occurs 2 to 4 hours after delivery, the pulse rate typically decreases, possibly slowing to 50 beats/minute (bradycardia). This condition may persist for several days without ill effects and probably results from supine positioning and such normal physiologic phenomena as the postpartal increase in stroke volume and reduction in vascular bed size.

On the other hand, an abnormally rapid pulse (tachycardia) may be an early sign of excessive blood loss—especially if the pulse is thready and the client has such signs as pallor, an increased respiratory rate, and diaphoresis. (However, transient tachycardia may occur during periods of excitement, incisional discomfort, or severe uterine contractions; usually, it is not a cause for concern.)

Respiratory rate

Although the respiratory rate rarely changes significantly after delivery, it may drop slightly (along with the pulse rate) during the first postpartal sleep or if the client received a narcotic during labor. Like the pulse rate, the respiratory rate increases slightly during periods of excitement or discomfort. If it increases significantly, however, suspect uterine hemorrhage.

Blood pressure

Postpartal blood pressure should not differ significantly from the client's average reading under normal circumstances. A gradual but persistent drop in blood pressure suggests excessive blood loss. A persistent elevation, especially when accompanied by edema, proteinuria, headache, blurred vision, and hyperactive reflexes, suggests pregnancy-induced hypertension (PIH), a potentially life-threatening disorder. Although most common during the antepartal period, PIH sometimes arises after delivery. To ensure prompt intervention, immediately report suspicious signs and symptoms to the physician.

Keep in mind that certain drugs used during labor and delivery or the postpartal period may affect blood pressure. For instance, oxytocin, ergonovine, and methylergonovine may increase blood pressure; bromocriptine, used to suppress lactation, may decrease it.

Comfort level

Comfort is essential to the client's postpartal recovery and adaptation to the role of new mother. However, even if she has uterine cramps, breast tenderness, or perineal discomfort, she may be too excited by the birth of her child to complain of discomfort. Stay alert for covert clues to discomfort, such as a change in vital signs, restlessness, inability to relax or sleep, facial grimaces, and a guarding posture.

Rest and sleep patterns

Fatigue is common during the first week after delivery. The tiring last few weeks of pregnancy, the exhausting work of labor and delivery, and dramatic hormonal changes contribute to postpartal fatigue. Assess the client's rest and sleep patterns continually, keeping in mind that individual requirements for rest and sleep vary.

Reproductive system

Assess the uterus, lochia, and perineum every 15 minutes for the first hour after delivery, then hourly for at least 4 hours. Thereafter, assess every 8 hours until discharge.

Uterus

Immediately after the placenta is delivered, uterine involution should begin. A gradual process that restores the uterus to a nonpregnant state, involution involves contractions of the myometrium (uterine muscle) and self-disintegration of cells or tissue. (For more information on the physiology of uterine involution, see Chapter 41, Physiology of the Postpartal Period.)

Assessment of the uterus helps in evaluating the progress of involution. Uterine muscle tone should be sufficient for muscles to compress vessels, thereby controlling bleeding.

To ensure accurate assessment of the uterus, ask the client to void beforehand. Then locate the fundus—the rounded portion of the uterus above the level of the fallopian tube attachments. Just after delivery, the fundus should be located at or slightly above the midline at the level of the umbilicus. Each day thereafter, it should descend approximately 1 cm (about one fingerbreadth) toward the symphysis pubis (the slightly movable interpubic joint of the pelvis), until about the tenth postpartal day, when it is no longer palpable as an abdominal organ. (For assessment details, see *Psychomotor skills: Postpartal assessment techniques,* page 1055.)

Next, assess the consistency of the uterus. It should feel firm. A soft, pliable (boggy) uterus indicates uterine atony (poor muscle tone). This condition, which may lead to hemorrhage, most commonly results from bladder distention or uterine enlargement (such as in the client with hydramnios or one who gives birth to a very large neonate or more than one neonate). Uterine enlargement causes overstretching of muscle fibers, which then cannot contract effectively to compress vessels. Other risk factors for uterine atony include a prolonged or accelerated labor (both of which exhaust uterine muscles), general anesthesia, or administration of magnesium sulfate (for example, to stop premature labor or to prevent or control seizures in a client with PIH).

If the client has a boggy uterus, determine if it is caused by bladder distention. After delivery, the bladder may fill rapidly from postpartal diuresis, which eliminates the excess tissue fluid that accumulated during pregnancy as well as any I.V. fluids administered during labor. If bladder distention is responsible for the boggy uterus, expect the uterus to be displaced upward and to the right (above the symphysis); also expect an increased lochial flow. Be sure to review the client's labor and delivery history to check the time and amount of the last voiding or catheterization.

If the client had a cesarean delivery, take great care when assessing the uterus. With a slow, gentle motion, press on the abdomen toward the uterus, avoiding sutures or staples. Inspect the incision site every 15 minutes for the first hour, once an hour for the next 4 hours, then at least once every 8 hours. Evaluate the site for color, warmth, edema, discharge, degree of approximation (distance between the edges of the incision), and the condition of sutures, staples, dressing, or supportive abdominal binder.

Lochia

After the client has delivered, lochia should begin to flow from the vagina. Normally, lochia progresses through stages marked by changes in its appearance. During the first stage, lochia rubra, the discharge is bright red; this stage lasts for approximately 4 days. On about the fifth postpartal day, lochia serosa, the second stage, should begin. This pinkish, serous discharge typically extends through the seventh day. During the second and third postpartal weeks, the creamy white, brown, or colorless discharge known as lochia alba should be present.

Assess the type and amount of lochia. Lochia should progress through the stages described above without relapsing to an earlier stage. Evaluate the consistency of the discharge. Lochia should never contain large clots, tissue fragments, or membranes. If such material is passed, save all specimens for further evaluation. Also note the odor; normally, lochia has a fleshy, not foul, odor. A foul odor may signal infection (as may absence of lochia).

Jacobson (1985) suggests the following classifications to describe the amount of lochia:
• scant: blood appears on a tissue only when the vaginal area is wiped or the stain on the perineal pad is less than 1″ long
• light: the stain on the perineal pad measures 1″ to 4″ long
• moderate: the stain on the perineal pad is 4″ to 6″ long
• heavy: the pad becomes saturated within 1 hour.

If the client has a heavy lochial flow, begin a pad count to determine the amount of discharge more precisely. Record the number of pads used and the degree of saturation of each pad. To make lochial assessment more accurate, obtain the client's cooperation by teaching her about the lochial stages, including how to monitor them and how to describe consistency and amount.

Expect a relatively light lochial flow in the post-cesarean client because the uterine contents are evacuated thoroughly during this procedure. In contrast, lochial flow may be slightly heavier during and after breast-feeding sessions from the effects of oxytocin, a hormone released during breast-feeding (the uterine contractions stimulated by oxytocin lead to expulsion of excess lochia). Also, lochial flow increases when the client rises from a lying to a standing position; lochia may escape down the legs as accumulated discharge and small clots are released. Tell the client to expect this so she will not become alarmed when it happens. To prevent her clothing from becoming stained, provide a hospital gown and disposable slippers.

Perineum

For accurate assessment of the perineum, arrange for adequate lighting and position the client properly; elevate the head of the bed no more than 30 degrees.

An episiotomy or perineal laceration should appear to be healing with no exudate; the site should be clean and not excessively tender. Assess the approximation of the incision or wound and check for such abnormalities as redness, warmth, tenderness, edema, ecchymosis, discharge, and hemorrhoids. If the perineum is ecchymotic, exquisitely painful, and grossly discolored, with a collection of blood under the skin surface, suspect a hematoma and report this to the physician.

Breasts

Breast inspection is an important part of nursing assessment during the first few days after delivery. With the client supine and her bra removed, inspect the breasts for symmetry of size and shape. Then palpate in a circular direction as during a standard breast examination. Start by palpating the outer breast tissue, then move the fingers 1 cm toward the center of the breast and repeat. Continue with this pattern until all breast regions have been examined, noting any masses (which may indicate infection or a blocked milk duct). If the breasts are tense, warm, boardlike, and painful, suspect breast engorgement, which results from transient lymphatic and venous stasis. To help determine appropriate interventions, assess the extent of engorgement. Also inspect the nipples for erectility, cracking, and soreness.

If the client has chosen to breast-feed her neonate, determine if she is at the appropriate stage in the lactation cycle, based on the number of days after delivery. For example, on the first and second days after delivery, colostrum should be secreted from the breasts and the client should be able to breast-feed comfortably every 2 to 4 hours. Also, she should be drinking an extra quart of fluids, increasing her food intake by 500 calories over her basic daily caloric needs, and wearing a support bra; the nipples should be free of cracks and reddened areas.

By the second or third postpartal day, the breast-feeding client should begin to feel tingling and throbbing in her breasts and notice some release of mature milk when her breasts are stimulated or when she hears her neonate cry. Mature milk is bluish, whereas colostrum is yellow. Be sure to document this finding.

Urinary system

Assessment of urinary elimination patterns is a key component of postpartal nursing assessment. Despite rapid urine production and bladder filling after delivery, many clients have difficulty voiding. For example, the client with severe perineal and urethral discomfort may

PSYCHOMOTOR SKILLS

Postpartal assessment techniques

Through careful assessment, the nurse can help ensure a normal postpartal recovery and may prevent complications. The guidelines below describe techniques the nurse may use to assess fundal position, evaluate the condition of the perineum, and detect thrombophlebitis.

Assessing fundal position

To assess the position of the fundus—an index of the progress of uterine involution—place the right hand at the symphysis pubis (the base of the uterus) to support the uterus while palpating the fundus with the left hand.

Document fundal height in centimeters from the umbilicus. For instance, if the fundus is located 1 cm below the umbilicus, record this as *U-1*. Also note the consistency of the uterus (for instance, firm or boggy).

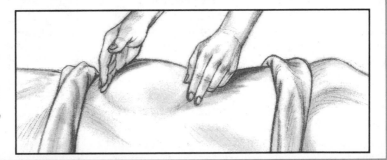

Inspecting the perineum
To evaluate for healing of an episiotomy or perineal lacerations, inspect the perineum regularly, using the following technique.

Verify adequate lighting, put on disposable gloves, and position the client appropriately. For example, if she has a right mediolateral episiotomy, position her on the right side. If she has a midline episiotomy, position her supine with knees flexed.

For optimal visualization in a side-lying client, flex the top leg upward at the knee. Standing behind her, gently lift the upper buttock to expose the perineum and anus.

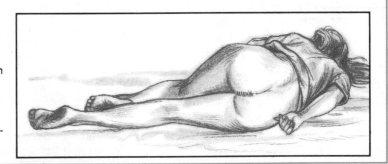

Eliciting Homans' sign

Coagulatory stimulation increases the risk of thromboembolism during the postpartal period. To assess for superficial thromboembolism, attempt to elicit Homans' sign.

Position the client supine. With one hand supporting her knee, lift the leg and dorsiflex the foot (bend it upward) toward the ankle. If this maneuver causes pain, suspect superficial thromboembolism. (Deep-vein thrombosis may not cause a positive Homans' sign.)

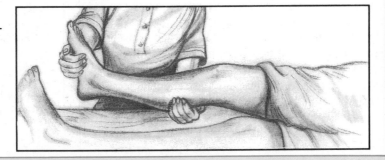

not be able to relax the perineal muscles sufficiently to void; in the postcesarean client or a client who received regional anesthesia, the bladder may lack sensitivity to pressure, impairing the urge to void.

Failure to void within 6 to 8 hours after delivery may cause excessive uterine bleeding because bladder distention prevents uterine contractions and subsequent vessel compression. When voiding finally does occur after a delay, it may be incomplete, with substantial urine remaining in the bladder. This condition, called urinary stasis, may contribute to urinary tract infection.

To evaluate the client's bladder, palpate the suprapubic area. A full bladder is distended above the symphysis and can be palpated readily as a soft, movable mass. A uterus that is boggy, elevated, and deviated to one side supports the suspicion of a full bladder.

Once the client is ambulatory and can perform satisfactory self-care, determine her urine output pattern. Note the time of each voiding and the amount voided, and ask if her bladder feels empty afterward. Also find out if she is experiencing urinary frequency, burning, or urgency.

Cardiovascular system

The hypervolemia of pregnancy protects the postpartal client to some extent from the detrimental effects of blood loss during delivery. However, if the client has lost more than 500 ml of blood, suspect uterine hemorrhage. Commonly, hemorrhage has a sudden onset. To ensure early detection and avert serious consequences, be sure to monitor vital signs and assess her lochia carefully. (For more information on assessing hemorrhage, see *Emergency alert: Postpartal hemorrhage*, and Chapter 44, Postpartal Complications.)

Respiratory status

Assess the client's respiratory rate, rhythm, and depth. Respiratory assessment is especially important if the client had a prolonged labor or a complicated or surgical delivery or if she received an anesthesia that causes decreased sensation and motor activity. Because these circumstances increase the risk of respiratory complications, check for altered breathing patterns and poor gas exchange by auscultating the lungs every 4 hours for adventitious sounds, such as crackles (rales) and rhonchi. Evaluate the breathing pattern regularly until the respiratory rate normalizes and the lungs are free of adventitious sounds.

EMERGENCY ALERT

Postpartal hemorrhage

A leading cause of maternal mortality, postpartal hemorrhage demands prompt recognition and intervention to avert grave consequences. Normal blood loss at delivery is less than 500 ml; the nurse should suspect hemorrhage if the client's estimated blood loss exceeds 500 ml. Keep in mind that hemorrhage is not always obvious; sometimes it manifests as a slow but steady trickle of blood.

Postpartal hemorrhage commonly stems from uterine atony (poor muscle tone), lacerations of the cervix or vagina, or disseminated intravascular coagulation. Several weeks after delivery, the most common cause of hemorrhage is retention of placental fragments (secundines).

The nurse who suspects hemorrhage should notify the physician immediately, then continually monitor the client's vital signs, assess the condition of the uterus, and evaluate the amount and character of lochia. Refer to the chart below to help identify signs of postpartal hemorrhage and prepare for appropriate interventions.

SIGNS

- Boggy (soft, pliable) uterus
- Excessively large uterus located above the umbilicus at the midline (must be differentiated from a uterus displaced to the right, which results from bladder distention)
- Excessive lochia, possibly containing large blood clots with or without tissue fragments
- Lochia that flows in a steady trickle
- Increased pulse and respiratory rate with decreased blood pressure (however, these signs may not arise until later, when shock occurs)

NURSING CONSIDERATIONS

- Gently massage the uterus to stimulate contractions.
- Rapidly infuse oxytocin I.V. or administer carboprost, ergonovine, or methylergonovine by I.M. injection, as prescribed and necessary.
- Assess lochial flow to estimate the type and amount of blood loss and to detect any clots or tissue fragments. If lochia is bright red and flows in a slow trickle and the fundus is firm and located at the midline, suspect cervical or vaginal laceration as the cause of hemorrhage.
- Inspect for accumulated blood posterior to the perineum by turning the client from side to side and checking for blood on bed sheets and the perineal pad.
- Position the client flat on her back to facilitate circulation to vital organs.
- Make sure the blood bank has typed and cross-matched the client for possible blood replacement.
- As necessary, prepare the client for surgery.

Hematologic system

Usually, a complete blood count is performed 24 to 48 hours after delivery. Typically, the white blood cell (WBC) count is elevated, sometimes reaching 25,000/mm³—especially if the client had a prolonged labor. Although the exact cause of this increase is unknown, Cunningham, McDonald, and Gant (1989) suggest it may result from the pronounced energy expenditure and stress of labor and delivery. Consequently, an elevated WBC count is not a reliable marker of postpartal infection. However, when accompanied by other potential infection signs, it may help to confirm an infection.

Compare the postpartal hemoglobin level and hematocrit to the corresponding predelivery levels. If the postpartal hemoglobin level is more than 3 g/dl below the predelivery level, the client is at risk for anemia; if it is 5 g/dl or more below the predelivery level, suspect heavy blood loss.

If the delivery was uncomplicated, measurement of coagulation factors usually is not necessary. Levels of coagulation factors I, VII, IX, and X, which normally increase during pregnancy, should fall to prepregnancy levels within a few weeks after delivery. Nonetheless, hypercoagulability—a result of decreased plasma volume—predisposes the postpartal client to thromboembolic disease. To check for this condition, which most often affects the lower extremities as thrombophlebitis, have the client lie supine with both legs extended. Inspect the legs for symmetry of shape and size, and palpate the thighs and calves to detect areas of warmth, edema, tenderness, redness, or hardness. Then attempt to elicit Homans' sign (pain in the calf when the foot is dorsiflexed).

Gastrointestinal status

Assess the client's progress toward reestablishing normal bowel function, documenting this progress daily. Bowel sounds should resume gradually on the first postpartal day. To determine the presence and quality of bowel sounds, assess the abdomen carefully in all four quadrants. Keep in mind that the postcesarean client may have diminished bowel sounds accompanied by abdominal distention and lack of peristalsis (from immobility, surgical manipulation, and anesthesia).

Assess abdominal shape, consistency, and tone. During the postpartal period, the abdomen typically is slightly distended and soft with poor muscle tone. Hydramnios, a very large neonate, or more than one neonate may cause even more pronounced distention. The client with a distended abdomen may notice an increased abdominal girth and complain of discomfort caused by flatus (gas) accumulation. This condition typically arises on the second postpartal day and is accompanied by absent or diminished bowel sounds. Keep in mind that absent or diminished bowel sounds may indicate paralytic ileus—a decrease or cessation of intestinal peristalsis resulting from anesthesia or manipulation during surgery.

Inspect the rectal area for hemorrhoids, which may cause redness, discomfort, and itching. Hemorrhoids may arise during pregnancy or from the expulsive effort of labor and delivery. Usually, they disappear in the first few postpartal weeks. Document the presence of hemorrhoids and any associated signs and symptoms.

Neurologic system

If the client complains of headache, check for other signs and symptoms associated with PIH—edema, proteinuria, blurred vision, decreased blood pressure, and hyperactive reflexes. Try to determine the onset, intensity, duration, and location of the headache and find out if any specific factors seem to trigger or relieve it. Keep in mind that in a client who received some types of regional anesthesia, such as a spinal block, headache may result from loss of cerebrospinal fluid through the dural puncture site—a condition called postspinal headache.

During the first 4 hours after delivery, the client who received regional anesthesia should regain full sensory and motor function. Occasionally, however, residual neurologic effects may occur. To assess for the return of sensation and movement, ask the client to move her lower extremities and to report the level of feeling present. (As sensation and motor function return, the client may report a heightened awareness of discomfort and may need further evaluation to determine the need for pain relief.)

Musculoskeletal status

Assess breast and abdominal muscle tone, which commonly is diminished from overstretching and the effects of increased hormone levels during pregnancy. In some cases, the abdomen has become so stretched that the rectus abdominis muscles, which lie side-by-side, separate at the midline. This condition, called diastasis recti abdomini, rarely warrants treatment. However, the physician may want to follow up by ordering periodic measurement of the separation.

Many postpartal clients are concerned about poor muscle tone and eager to regain their prepregnancy figure. When conducting the assessment, provide an opening for the client to express such concerns and recommend appropriate exercises (as discussed in the "Planning and implementation" section of this chapter.)

Immune system

Detection of postpartal infection is a primary nursing concern. In most cases, such infection involves the reproductive system. Besides regularly assessing the client's temperature (as discussed above under "Vital signs"), observe closely for subtle signs and symptoms of infection, such as chills, malaise, and pallor. (Keep in mind that an elevated WBC count is not a reliable infection marker during the postpartal period.) Also review the client's chart for risk factors for puerperal infection, such as prolonged labor, prolonged time since rupture of the membranes, vaginal or cervical lacerations, and retention of placental fragments. (For details on assessing for postpartal infection, see Chapter 44, Postpartal Complications.)

The client who received regional anesthesia has an increased risk of infection because of the invasive administration route used. Carefully and regularly inspect the spinal or epidural site for redness, warmth, edema, pain, and tenderness; promptly report any of these signs to the physician.

Also review the client's chart to assess her Rh status and rubella status. If either is questionable, take the actions described in the "Planning and implementation" section of this chapter.

Psychosocial status

The postpartal nurse has a unique opportunity to assess the client's and her partner's response to childbirth and to evaluate their interaction with the neonate. Typically, they focus initially on the neonate's sex, size, and facial similarities to their older children or to other relatives. Many facilities provide a place on the nursing record to describe parent-neonate interaction. If so, be sure to document this regularly. (For a complete discussion of psychosocial assessment, see Chapter 43, Psychosocial Adaptation of the Postpartal Family.)

Nursing diagnosis

After gathering assessment data, the nurse must review it carefully to identify pertinent nursing diagnoses for the client. (For a partial list of applicable diagnoses, see *Nursing diagnoses: Postpartal client*.)

NURSING DIAGNOSES

Postpartal client

The following are potential nursing diagnoses for problems and etiologies that the nurse may encounter when caring for a client during the postpartal period. Specific nursing interventions for many of these diagnoses are provided in the "Planning and implementation" section of this chapter.

- Altered patterns of urinary elimination related to perineal and urethral edema and ecchymosis
- Anxiety related to new role development
- Constipation related to poor intestinal tone, diminished food intake, and immobility
- Fatigue related to pregnancy, labor, and delivery
- Impaired physical mobility related to bedrest, anesthesia, or inability to ambulate
- Impaired skin integrity related to the perineal wound
- Ineffective breathing pattern related to immobility following cesarean delivery
- Knowledge deficit related to self-care or parenting skills
- Pain related to the perineal wound, uterine contractions, or breast engorgement
- Potential for injury related to blood loss, fatigue, limited food intake, or medication effects
- Sleep pattern disturbance related to hospitalization and caring for the neonate around the clock
- Social isolation related to sensory deprivation or separation from home, family, and friends

---

Planning and implementation

After assessing the client and formulating nursing diagnoses, the nurse develops and implements a plan of care. For example, for a client with a nursing diagnosis of *impaired skin integrity related to the perineal wound,* aim to prevent perineal infection through measures that promote perineal hygiene.

When the client arrives on the postpartal unit, identify her by checking her identification band carefully. In many facilities, the postpartal client has an individual identification bracelet and a bracelet with a number that corresponds to the number on her neonate's bracelet; to ensure accuracy, check both bracelets.

Provide a brief orientation to the unit, including such information as where the bathroom, telephone, and personal supplies are located and what time meals are served. Review visiting hours rooming-in policy. If visiting hours are limited, promote client compliance by explaining that such limits are imposed for the client's and neonate's well-being. Also make sure the client understands why visitors must comply with infection-prevention measures, such as washing hands and putting on cover gowns before handling the neonate.

Ensuring safety

Various factors may contribute to weakness and light-headedness for the first few hours after delivery, leading to a nursing diagnosis of *potential for injury related to blood loss, fatigue, limited food intake, or medication effects.* Consequently, advise the client to call for help when getting out of bed for the first time. Also show her how to raise or lower the bed rails. To prevent injury to the neonate, caution her against falling asleep in bed with the neonate.

If the client received regional anesthesia, she may have impaired motor or sensory function in the lower extremities. To guarantee safety, make sure all functions have returned to a satisfactory level before helping her out of bed.

Providing for adequate sleep and rest

For an hour or so after delivery, the client may be too excited to sleep or rest, despite her fatigue. Within a few hours, however, she may fall into a deep, although short, sleep. This sleep is especially crucial for the client who is recovering from a cesarean delivery or a prolonged, difficult labor and delivery. For the client with a nursing diagnosis of *fatigue related to pregnancy, labor, and delivery,* help determine rest and sleep requirements and encourage her to limit visitors and telephone calls. If necessary, ask visitors to leave the client's room when she feels tired to allow her to sleep.

The client may choose to have the neonate room-in with her. If she is undecided about rooming-in, inform her that this arrangement does not necessarily disrupt sleep. Keefe (1988) found that clients whose neonates spent the night in the nursery slept no longer or better than those whose neonates roomed-in.

Promoting uterine involution and preventing hemorrhage

The uterus should have sufficient tone after delivery to contract effectively so that vessels are compressed and involution proceeds normally. If the client has a boggy, or atonic, uterus, monitor her vital signs closely because hemorrhage can have a sudden onset. Interventions for uterine atony may vary with the underlying cause.

Facilitating voiding
If uterine atony stems from bladder distention (as indicated by a boggy uterus that is displaced upward and to the right), make every effort to keep the client's bladder empty. Within the first 4 hours after delivery, encourage her to walk to the bathroom; if she is confined to bed, offer a bedpan. Other nursing interventions that promote spontaneous voiding include turning on the faucet in the client's bathroom, irrigating the perineum, placing the client's hands in water, and providing plenty of fluids.

If the client cannot relax the perineal muscles sufficiently to void (as with severe perineal and urethral discomfort), she may have a nursing diagnosis of *altered patterns of urinary elimination related to perineal and urethral edema and ecchymosis.* Failure to void within 8 hours of delivery necessitates urinary catheterization, as does bladder distention. Fortunately, many clients regain normal urinary elimination patterns after just a single catheterization.

If the client requires catheterization, be sure to use sterile technique to minimize the risk of infection. Also, conduct this procedure with extreme gentleness, offering appropriate explanations. Catheterization during the early postpartal period causes more discomfort than usual because of the edematous, bruised condition of the bladder, urethra, urinary meatus, labia, and perineum.

Massaging the uterus
When uterine atony does not stem from bladder distention, gentle massage of the uterus may be sufficient to stimulate uterine contractions, restoring firm tone. The nurse also may teach the client how to massage her own uterus. However, emphasize that she must do this gently to avoid overstimulation, which could prevent contractions.

Administering oxytocin
If massage fails to induce contractions, expect to administer an I.V. oxytocin preparation or I.M. carboprost. (For more information about these and other drugs administered to postpartal clients, see *Selected major drugs: Drugs used during the postpartal period,* pages 1060 and 1061.) If hemorrhage occurs despite drug therapy, expect the client to undergo surgical exploration and evacuation of the uterus. (For a complete discussion of interventions for postpartal hemorrhage, see Chapter 44, Postpartal Complications.)

Relieving discomfort from uterine contractions

The severity of uterine contractions, or afterpains, typically varies with parity. In the primiparous client, af-

SELECTED MAJOR DRUGS

Drugs used during the postpartal period

This chart summarizes the major drugs currently used during the postpartal period.

DRUG	MAJOR INDICATIONS	USUAL ADULT DOSAGES	NURSING IMPLICATIONS
bromocriptine (Parlodel)	Prevention of postpartal lactation	2.5 mg P.O. twice daily with meals for 14 to 21 days	• Monitor blood pressure. Transient hypotension may occur during the first 3 days of therapy. • Check for seizure activity. • Advise the client to use contraceptive methods other than oral contraceptives during treatment. • Warn the client to use caution when ambulating. • Do not initiate therapy sooner than 4 hours after delivery and not until signs have stablized.
carboprost (Prostin/M15)	Postpartal hemorrhage from uterine atony that does not respond to conventional management	250 mcg deep I.M.; may repeat dose at 15- to 90-minute intervals; maximum total dosage should not exceed 2 mg	• Obtain vital signs; assess the amount and character of lochia and the condition of the fundus. • Administer cautiously to a client with cervical lacerations. • Watch for adverse gastrointestinal (GI) effects. • Do not administer I.V.
codeine	Mild to moderate postpartal pain	15 to 60 mg P.O. every 3 to 4 hours as needed (usually given with 325 to 650 mg of acetaminophen)	• Monitor respiratory and circulatory status and bowel function. • Observe the client for drowsiness; make sure she is alert when caring for her neonate.
diphenhydramine (Benadryl)	Nighttime sedation	25 to 50 mg P.O. at bedtime	• Observe the client for drowsiness; make sure she is alert when caring for her neonate. • Assess the client for nausea and dry mouth.
docusate sodium (Colace)	Stool softener	50 to 300 mg P.O. daily or until bowel movements are normal	• Assess the client for bowel activity, mild abdominal cramping, and diarrhea.
ergonovine maleate (Ergotrate Maleate)	Prevention or treatment of postpartal hemorrhage from uterine atony or subinvolution	0.2 mg I.M. every 2 to 4 hours to a maximum of five doses; or 0.2 mg I.V. (only for severe uterine bleeding). After initial I.M. or I.V. dose, may give 0.2 to 0.4 mg P.O. every 5 to 12 hours for 2 to 7 days.	• Monitor blood pressure, pulse rate, and uterine response. Report sudden changes in vital signs, frequent periods of uterine relaxation, and any change in the character or amount of lochia. • Dilute I.V. preparation to a volume of 5 ml with normal saline solution, and administer over at least 1 minute while blood pressure and uterine contractions are monitored. • Contractions begin 5 to 15 minutes after P.O. administration, 2 to 5 minutes after I.M. injection, or immediately after I.V. injection. They may continue 3 hours or more after P.O. or I.M. administration, 45 minutes after I.V. injection.
ibuprofen (Motrin)	Mild to moderate postpartal pain	400 mg P.O. every 4 to 6 hours	• Assess the client for signs and symptoms of GI irritation, such as nausea, vomiting, diarrhea, and gastric discomfort. • Warn the client not to take more than 1.2 g/day without consulting her physician.

SELECTED MAJOR DRUGS

Drugs used during the postpartal period continued

DRUG	MAJOR INDICATIONS	USUAL ADULT DOSAGES	NURSING IMPLICATIONS
meperidine (Demerol)	Moderate to severe postpartal pain (such as after cesarean delivery)	50 to 150 mg P.O., I.M., or S.C. every 3 to 4 hours; or by continuous I.V. infusion, 15 to 35 mg/hour as needed or around the clock	• Monitor the client's pulse rate. • Check for signs of central nervous system (CNS) depression, such as drowsiness or lethargy. Make sure the client is alert when caring for her neonate. • Assess the client's pain level. • To avoid toxic metabolites, give the smallest effective dosage.
methylergonovine (Methergine)	Prevention and treatment of postpartal hemorrhage from uterine atony or subinvolution	0.2 mg I.M. or I.V. every 2 to 4 hours for a maximum of 5 doses. After the initial I.M. or I.V. dose, may give 0.2 to 0.4 mg P.O. every 6 to 12 hours for 2 to 7 days.	• Monitor and record blood pressure, pulse rate, and uterine response. Report any sudden change in vital signs, frequent periods of uterine relaxation, and any change in the character or amount of lochia. • Decrease the dosage if severe cramping occurs. • Contractions begin 5 to 15 minutes after P.O. administration, 2 to 5 minutes after I.M. injection, and immediately after I.V. injection. They continue 3 hours or more after P.O. or I.M. administration, 45 minutes after I.V. administration.
morphine	Severe pain (such as after cesarean delivery)	4 to 15 mg S.C. or I.M. May be injected by slow I.V. infusion (over 4 to 5 minutes) diluted in 4 to 5 ml of water for injection.	• Monitor for respiratory depression and hypotension. • Check for signs of CNS depression, such as drowsiness or lethargy. Make sure the client is alert when caring for her neonate. • Drug may be injected into the epidural space for prolonged pain relief. Monitor the client for delayed respiratory depression (up to 24 hours after administration). • If the client has pruritus after I.V. or epidural administration, expect to give antihistamines.
oxytocin (Pitocin)	Reduction of postpartal bleeding after expulsion of the placenta	1 to 4 ml (10 to 40 units) in 1,000 ml of dextrose 5% in water or normal saline solution I.V., infused at a rate necessary to control bleeding (usually 20 to 40 milliunits/minute); or 10 units I.M.	• Administer by I.V. infusion, not I.V. bolus injection. • Monitor and record uterine contractions, heart rate, and blood pressure every 15 minutes. • Assess the amount and character of lochia and the condition of the fundus. • Check for increased pulse rate in response to pain from contractions.
simethicone (Mylicon)	Flatulence, functional gastric bloating (such as after cesarean delivery)	40 to 125 mg after each meal and at bedtime	• Make sure the client chews tablets thoroughly before swallowing. • Assess the client for bowel activity and abdominal distention.

terpains may not be noticeable; in the multiparous client, they may cause severe discomfort. Because breast-feeding promotes the release of oxytocin (which stimulates contractions), the breast-feeding client typically has more severe afterpains during and after feeding sessions. For the client with a nursing diagnosis of *pain related to uterine contractions*, expect to administer a mild analgesic (such as acetaminophen with codeine) or a nonsteroidal anti-inflammatory drug (such as ibuprofen).

Reducing perineal discomfort

Perineal lacerations or an episiotomy may cause considerable pain, possibly leading to a nursing diagnosis of *pain related to the perineal wound.* An ice pack applied to the perineum in the first few hours after delivery helps soothe the area by constricting vessels and reducing the vascular response of inflammation. The nurse may use a commercial perineal ice pack or may make a simple pack by filling a latex glove with small ice cubes and knotting it at the top. After preparing the ice pack, cover it with a small towel, dressing, or washcloth, and tape the closure. (The covering prevents trauma to tender perineal tissues while allowing sufficient cold to penetrate.) Then place the pack between the perineum and the perineal pad.

Warmth may be applied to the perineum 12 to 24 hours after delivery. Warmth causes vasodilation, which relieves discomfort and edema and promotes the local inflammatory response by hastening the arrival of leukocytes and antibodies at the site. A warm sitz bath can provide the necessary warmth. Typically, the client takes this treatment three or four times daily, with each bath lasting 15 to 20 minutes, until the discomfort has diminished or the perineum has healed. To ensure that the client can self-administer the bath correctly, provide complete instructions. (For more information on sitz baths, see *Psychomotor skills: Providing perineal care.* For a study comparing the efficacy of warm and cold sitz baths, see *Nursing research applied: A comparison of treatments for postpartal perineal discomfort.*)

A topical spray or ointment also may be applied to relieve perineal discomfort. A topical spray may be an anesthetic, which provides local pain relief, or a steroid, which reduces edema and promotes healing. To apply a topical spray, shake the can thoroughly, then aim the stream at the perineal wound from a distance of 8″ to 10″. To apply a topical ointment, use an applicator or a gloved finger. Beginning at the edge of the vaginal introitus, apply the ointment to the wound in a downward or outward direction. Repeat topical applications at intervals specified by the physician or manufacturer.

Occasionally, the physician or nurse-midwife may order perineal heat lamp treatments, which promote perineal comfort and healing through a drying effect. Place the heat lamp between the client's legs, at least 18″ from the perineum. For client safety, limit treatments to the prescribed length, use a bulb no brighter than 40 watts, and make sure the bedclothes remain clear of the lamp. Also, make sure the lamp is positioned securely and cannot fall onto the client.

PSYCHOMOTOR SKILLS

Providing perineal care

Perineal pain is a major source of postpartal discomfort. If severe, it may prevent voiding, necessitating catheterization. The guidelines below describe care the nurse can administer to help relieve perineal pain.

Preparing a sitz bath

A sitz bath relieves discomfort and promotes healing of the perineum. In the method described below, the equipment includes a portable sitz bath basin and a container (such as a bag or reservoir) with tubing.

1 Fill the sitz bath basin with warm to hot water until it is half to three-quarters full. If facility policy allows, add 1 oz of witch hazel, which has a drying effect. (If the client has perineal edema or is using topical analgesia, keep water temperature moderate because these circumstances decrease perineal sensitivity to temperature.)

2 Lift the toilet seat and place the filled basin on top of the toilet. Close the clamp on the bag, then fill the bag half full. Open the clamp to release any air in the tubing, then close it.

3 Hang the bag above the level of the client's head; in many facilities, the bag can be hung from a hook on the bathroom wall. Then thread the tubing from the bag through the opening in the back of the basin and clip it onto the bottom of the sitz bag (most basins have a small notch where the tubing is clipped).

4 Instruct the client to sit on the basin. Then open the clamp to let water flow from the bag into the basin. Instruct the client to sit on the basin for 15 to 20 minutes, or as specified by the physician.

5 After the treatment has ended, empty the basin and bag and clean and rinse the basin, bag, and tubing.

Using a water and disinfectant spray

To help relieve perineal discomfort, the nurse may use a water and disinfectant spray (such as the Surgigator) or may teach the client how to use one. As the client sits on the toilet, hold the nozzle a few inches from the perineum. Direct the flow against the perineum, taking care not to let the nozzle touch the skin. After the treatment, gently blot-dry the perineum, working from front to back.

Other measures that may be used to reduce perineal discomfort include mild analgesia (such as oxycodone, propoxyphene, or codeine with acetaminophen), witch hazel compresses, and a commercial water and disinfectant spray (such as the Surgigator or Hygenique).

To keep the perineal region clean, show the client how to use a perineal irrigation, or squirt, bottle after each voiding. The client fills the bottle with warm water, then aims it at the perineum to rinse off any urine or lochia remaining on the surface.

Ensuring lactation suppression

For the client who chooses to bottle-feed her neonate, lactation is suppressed through drug therapy or a natural method. With either method, lactation ceases within 1 week.

Drug therapy typically involves bromocriptine. A synthetic ergot alkaloid derivative, bromocriptine inhibits secretion of prolactin, a hormone that stimulates milk production. If the client is receiving this drug, monitor for such adverse reactions as fatigue, dizziness, hypertension, hypotension, and seizures; contact the physician immediately if these problems arise. Advise her to finish all the medication in her prescription if no adverse reactions occur.

In the natural method of lactation suppression, the client must avoid any stimulation of the breasts and nipples and wear a tight, support bra or breast binder. The client who has just delivered may prefer this method over taking a drug; for the client who wishes to discontinue breast-feeding after several weeks or months, this method is the only available option.

Promoting respiratory stability

Monitor the client's respiratory rate and effort. For the postcesarean client, who may have a nursing diagnosis of *ineffective breathing pattern related to immobility following cesarean delivery,* carry out measures that promote effective breathing patterns, thereby reducing the risk of pneumonia or atelectasis. For instance, have her cough and deep-breathe hourly; remind her to turn every 1 to 2 hours to promote oxygenation and prevent skin breakdown. Also, within a few hours after delivery, teach her how to use an incentive spirometer. This device maintains lung expansion and mobilizes secretions. One type, consisting of a mouthpiece and a chamber containing one or two balls, also allows the client to participate actively in her care because she can monitor the progress of her efforts—as her inspirations become stronger, she can make the ball rise progressively higher in the chamber.

NURSING RESEARCH APPLIED

A comparison of treatments for postpartal perineal discomfort

Nurses have used various strategies to help reduce perineal discomfort from episiotomy pain. The warm sitz bath, one of the most commonly used interventions, promotes healing by enhancing vasodilation, which improves circulation.

However, several researchers theorized that a cold sitz bath may reduce discomfort more effectively than a warm sitz bath—by producing local anesthesia, reducing edema, and decreasing intracellular metabolism. To test this theory, they studied 40 women in the first 24 hours after delivery; all of the women had episiotomies.

The subjects were assigned randomly to two groups. One group took a cold sitz bath, with water temperature ranging from 61.9° to 65° F (16.6° to 18.3° C), followed 6 hours later by a warm sitz bath, with a water temperature of 98° to 112° F (36.7° to 44.4° C). The second group took the sitz baths in reverse order. Before and after each bath, the women rated their pain on a scale.

Results showed that immediately after the cold sitz bath, all women experienced significantly better pain relief. However, the two groups showed no statistical difference in long-term pain relief. The researchers also noted that many women were unwilling to participate in the study because they did not want to try a cold sitz bath or had been satisfied previously with a warm sitz bath.

Application to practice
The results of this study suggest that the nurse may recommend a cold sitz bath for more effective short-term relief of perineal pain during the postpartal period. However, the nurse must keep in mind that the client may have a clear preference in this matter and should not be pressured to take a cold sitz bath.

Ramler, D., and Roberts, J. (1986). A comparison of cold and warm sitz baths for relief of postpartum perineal pain. *JOGNN,* 15(6), 471-474.

Preventing hematologic complications

If the client has a subnormal hemoglobin level and hematocrit, she may be in danger of anemia from blood loss. For a severely anemic client, expect the physician to order a blood transfusion. In less serious circumstances, provide a diet rich in iron to help prevent anemia, and teach the client about dietary iron sources.

Because the postpartal client—especially the multiparous client—is at risk for thrombophlebitis, stress the importance of early, moderate exercise (such as walking in the hallway). Unless the client received high doses of analgesias or anesthesias during labor and delivery, she should be able to walk around within a few hours of delivery. Also, instruct her to wear foot coverings that do not constrict the knee, to elevate her legs on a stool from time to time when sitting (to prevent blood stasis in the calves), and to avoid crossing her legs at the knee.

Promoting bowel elimination

Although bowel function usually returns to normal rapidly after delivery, various factors may hinder bowel elimination. To help avoid a nursing diagnosis of *constipation related to poor intestinal tone, diminished food intake, and immobility,* encourage early ambulation, plenty of fluids, and a well-balanced, high-fiber diet. For example, encourage the client to walk to the bathroom within 4 to 6 hours after delivery and to walk around the postpartal unit. Also advise her to act on any urge to defecate, taking adequate time to sit on the toilet at the time when her bowel movements normally occur. If she is reluctant to attempt a bowel movement out of fear that it will tear open her episiotomy suture line, reassure her that she will not damage the repaired wound by bearing down gently. If exercise and diet do not improve bowel elimination, the physician may order a stool softener, such as docusate, or a stimulant laxative, such as a bisacodyl suppository.

After the first few postpartal hours, the client may be hungry and thirsty. Provide cool liquids and a light meal, regardless of the time of day, and encourage the client to drink 1 or 2 quarts (four to eight 8-oz glasses) of fluid daily to replace fluids lost during labor and delivery.

Relieving abdominal distention and flatus accumulation

The postcesarean client may complain of abdominal distention accompanied by flatus accumulation. Interventions for this problem include insertion of a rectal tube to help expel flatus in the distal colon or suppositories to promote bowel activity and subsequent flatus expulsion. Also, the physician may order simethicone, which reduces flatus formation.

Encourage early ambulation and slow resumption of oral intake, beginning with ice chips and progressing to a liquid, then regular, diet. Advise the client to avoid carbonated beverages and gas-forming foods (such as cabbage, asparagus, and brussels sprouts).

Relieving hemorrhoidal discomfort

If the client has hemorrhoids, assure her that the acute discomfort should last only 2 to 3 days. In the meantime, apply soothing witch hazel compresses soaked in ice chips, use an anesthetic or steroid-based cream, or administer anti-hemorrhoidal suppositories. Other measures that help relieve hemorrhoidal discomfort include

mild analgesias, sitz baths, and a side-lying position. Sometimes the hemorrhoid discomfort can be reduced by pushing the inflamed tissues back into the rectum with a finger cot or a gloved, lubricated finger; if appropriate, teach the client how to do this herself.

Avoiding neurologic complications

The client who received spinal anesthesia may develop postspinal headache. If so, position her flat; or, if she is permitted to lie on her side, make sure her head is elevated no more than 30 degrees. Make sure she remains supine for 8 to 10 hours after anesthesia administration. Monitor her response to positioning; if she reports that the headache has worsened, lower the head of the bed. Because fluid replacement helps prevent postspinal headache, monitor fluid intake in a client at risk for this problem.

When headache results from PIH, interventions may include bed rest and administration of magnesium sulfate or sedatives. (For details on nursing interventions for the client with PIH, see Chapter 44, Postpartal Complications.)

Correcting musculoskeletal deficits

Beginning immediately after delivery, suggest mild exercises to improve muscle tone, such as arm, head, and shoulder raises or deep abdominal breathing with contraction of the abdominal muscles. Within a few days of delivery, the client may begin abdominal exercises, alternately contracting and relaxing the abdominal muscles. Advise her to reduce or stop exercising if lochial flow increases or if she becomes uncomfortable or fatigued. (For more information on postpartal exercises, see *Client teaching: Postpartal exercises,* and "Implementing client teaching" below.)

Ensuring adequate immunologic status

If the client has signs and symptoms of postpartal infection, expect to administer antibiotics and to carry out measures to minimize or reverse any precipitating factors, such as anemia. (For complete nursing interventions for the client with postpartal infection, see Chapter 44, Postpartal Complications.)

To prevent isoimmunization (development of antibodies against $Rh_o(D)$ antigens), all Rh-negative pregnant clients now receive Rh immune globulin (RhoGAM) during or near the twenty-eighth week of pregnancy. Cord blood is sampled after delivery to determine the neonate's Rh status. If the neonate is Rh-positive, make sure the client receives an additional RhoGAM injection within 72 hours of delivery, even if she received a pre-

CLIENT TEACHING

Postpartal exercises

Exercises can help strengthen abdominal and pelvic muscle tone, restore normal abdominal contour and lung capacity, strengthen the chest wall to help support breast tissue, and correct postural problems caused by pregnancy. The exercises described below commonly are recommended for the postpartal period. If your doctor approves, you probably can begin them within a few days of delivery. Follow your doctor's guidelines on the number of repetitions for each exercise; also, if you experience serious or continuing discomfort, report this right away.

Abdominal breathing

Lie on your back with your knees bent. Inhale through your nose, allowing your abdomen to expand.

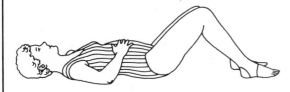

Then exhale slowly through your mouth while contracting your abdomen. Make sure your shoulders and neck do not move during this exercise.

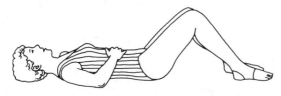

Pelvic tilt

Lie on your back with your knees bent.

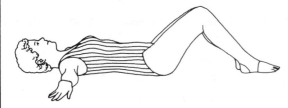

Press the small of your back against the floor while tightening the stomach and buttocks. Hold this position for several seconds.

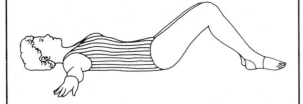

Chin-to-chest raise

Lie on your back with your knees bent. Keeping your shoulders as flat as possible, raise your chin and try to touch it to your chest. Hold this position for a few seconds, then return to the starting position.

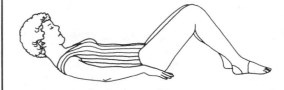

Sit-ups

Lie on your back with your knees bent.

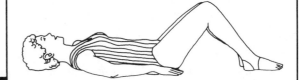

Raise your head and shoulders and reach for your knees with arms outstretched until you achieve a partial sitting position (your waist should remain on the floor).

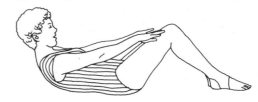

Then slowly lower your head and shoulders back to the starting position.

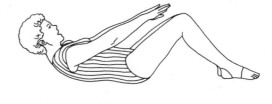

(continued)

Postpartal exercises continued

Hip raise
Lie on your back with your knees bent, arms at your side, and feet flat on the floor. As you push down with your feet, slowly raise your hips up off the floor. Slowly return to the starting position.

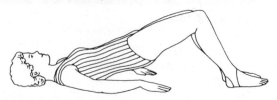

Chest strengthening
Lie on your back and extend your arms straight out to the sides.

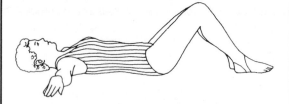

Keeping your elbows straight, bring your hands together above your chest. Return to the starting position.

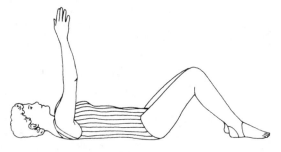

With your elbows bent, clasp your hands together above your chest. Press your hands together for 3 seconds, then relax.

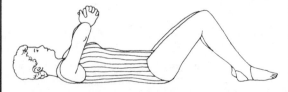

Knee rotations
Lie on your back with your knees bent.

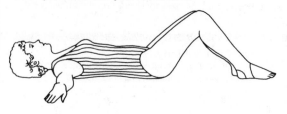

Bring your knees together, then rotate them slowly to the left until they touch the floor (or as far as is comfortable).

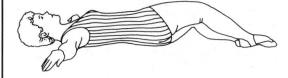

Next, rotate them to the right, again trying to touch the floor. Keep your shoulders flat on the floor and your feet stationary throughout this exercise.

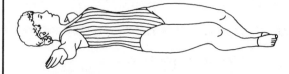

Kegel exercises
These exercises improve vaginal tone and help prevent stress incontinence and hemorrhoids. To perform them, contract the perineal muscles for several seconds, then relax them.

If you are not sure which muscles to contract and relax, do this exercise while urinating. After the urine begins to flow, attempt to stop the urine stream; as you do this, the perineal muscles contract. Then allow the urine to flow freely again; as you do this, the perineal muscles relax.

Although you can perform these exercises at any time (no one can see you doing them), you may want to continue to do them while urinating because this lets you monitor your progress. As muscle tone improves, your contractions will become stronger and you will be able to stop the urine stream more easily.

natal injection. (For more information on preventing isoimmunization, see Chapter 23, Antepartal Complications.)

If the client's antenatal rubella titer test revealed that she lacks immunity (indicated by a titer less than 1:10), she should be immunized before discharge. If she will receive the live vaccine (Meruvax II), warn her to avoid becoming pregnant for 3 months after immunization.

Promoting psychosocial adaptation

Postpartal hospitalization provides the client and her partner with an opportunity to adjust to their new role as parents and to review and receive information and feedback about the childbirth experience. The nurse should encourage the client to express her feelings—both positive and negative—about the experience. This helps prepare her for motherhood and future pregnancies (Konrad, 1987) and may avoid a nursing diagnosis of *anxiety related to new role development.* (If the client does not have a partner, identify a support person with whom she can share her feelings.) If appropriate, suggest that the client's partner participate in a fathers' support group to help him learn child care skills and coping strategies and to provide a forum where he can express his feelings (Taubenheim and Silbernagel, 1988).

Provide the client with positive feedback about her behavior during labor and delivery and her ongoing acquisition of parenting skills. If she has a negative perspective about the childbirth experience based on a misperception, provide a brief explanation to clarify the situation and promote positive feelings.

If the client is an adolescent, she poses a special challenge. To promote psychosocial adaptation, the nurse must understand adolescent behavior—especially the drive for independence, which plays a major role in adolescent judgment and decision making. A nonjudgmental approach—essential to developing a positive relationship with this client—may necessitate self-exploration of the nurse's own feelings and attitudes toward adolescent sexuality, pregnancy, and motherhood. (For further information on promoting psychosocial adaptation of the postpartal client, see Chapter 43, Psychosocial Adaptation of the Postpartal Family.)

Implementing client teaching

The trend toward early discharge (within 24 to 48 hours of delivery) has made postpartal client teaching increasingly important—yet difficult to complete. Client teaching may be carried out by the postpartal nurse or a nurse who provides follow-up care at home after early discharge.

Client preparation for independent function in her new role begins during pregnancy but intensifies after delivery. To facilitate client teaching, determine the client's reading and comprehension levels, and provide appropriate videotapes, films, pamphlets, or booklets to reinforce the teaching. Later, ask her to give return demonstrations to assess her skills.

Teaching should focus on self-care and neonatal care. The former include such topics as postpartal danger signs, rest, nutrition, and exercises. (For details on some of these topics, see *Client teaching: Self-care after discharge,* page 1068. For information on neonatal care topics, see Chapter 36, Care of the Normal Neonate, and Chapter 37, Infant Nutrition.)

Especially for the client with a nursing diagnosis of *knowledge deficit related to self-care or parenting skills,* consider using both individual and group teaching. During individual teaching, summarize important points in writing, perhaps listing them in a pamphlet that the client can take home to review. Also, keep in mind that creative teaching strategies make learning more enjoyable. For instance, Coleman (1987) developed a board game that a group of new mothers can play to help them learn about neonatal care.

For the multiparous client, provide opportunities for teaching and discussion of topics of specific interest. Hiser (1987) found that most concerns of multiparous clients after discharge are affective rather than psychomotor. Appropriate affective topics might include how the client can meet the needs of other children, find time for herself, and regain a positive body image while caring for her neonate.

Postpartal examination
Make sure the client knows that she must visit the physician 4 to 6 weeks after delivery for the postpartal examination. To reinforce this information, provide a written reminder. Also review danger signs the client should watch for after discharge. Advise her to call the physician if any of these signs arise.

Breast care
Regardless of the infant feeding method the client is using, teach her to inspect her breasts daily, using a circular palpation pattern. This also is a good time to stress the importance of the monthly breast self-examination. (For more information on client teaching for the breast-feeding client, see Chapter 37, Infant Nutrition.)

With the bottle-feeding client, who must suppress lactation, inform her that she may notice an occasional release of milk and may experience some breast fullness and discomfort until milk production ceases. Instruct her to drink adequate, but not excessive, amounts of

---

CLIENT TEACHING

Self-care after discharge

As you recover from delivery and welcome a new child into your life, you may experience dramatic physical and emotional changes. The guidelines below will help ensure your well-being during this challenging period.

Postpartal warning signs

If you have any of the following problems after discharge, notify your doctor promptly:
• heavy vaginal bleeding or passage of clots or tissue fragments
• a fever of 100.2° F or higher for 24 hours or longer
• a red, warm, painful area in either breast
• excessive breast tenderness not relieved by a support bra, pain pills, or warm or cool compresses
• pain on urination or voiding of only small amounts of urine
• a warm, red, tender area on either leg, especially the calf.

Hygiene, rest, and nutrition

• When using a sanitary belt and perineal pad, attach the front tab on the pad first and wear the pad with the blue line away from your body. To prevent contamination from fecal organisms, apply and remove the pad from front to back. Change the pad every 4 hours.
• Before emptying your bladder or moving your bowels, remove the perineal pad, using a front-to-back motion. Afterward, use a perineal squirt or spray bottle to cleanse the perineum. Wipe or pat the area gently with toilet tissue, again moving from front to back, then apply a fresh pad.
• After voiding or moving your bowels, wipe from front to back, then wash your hands thoroughly.
• Take a shower daily. Once the perineum has healed, you may take tub baths.
• Avoid sexual intercourse and do not place anything in your vagina (including tampons and douches) until after the postpartal examination (if your doctor advises).
• Rest frequently during the day, especially if you must awaken during the night to care for your infant.
• Consume a nourishing diet—at least 2,200 calories daily (2,500 calories if you are breast-feeding). Include foods from all four food groups. If you have trouble moving your bowels, add high-fiber foods (such as fresh fruits and vegetables, bran, and prunes) to your diet.

---

fluids. For severe breast discomfort, recommend a mild analgesia or application of ice packs. Also instruct her to wear a snug bra day and night for the first few weeks after discharge and to wash her breasts daily with mild soap and water when she showers or bathes. Warn her not to let the shower stream run directly onto her breasts because this could stimulate them, causing lactation.

Rest and sleep requirements

Advise the client to anticipate increased sleep and rest requirements after discharge. Also counsel her to have realistic expectations of herself, her neonate, and her family. Some clients assume that they will be able to resume their usual schedule immediately, preparing all meals or returning to full-time work at home or at the office. Such expectations may prevent satisfactory adjustment to the new role. Consequently, recommend that the client limit her activities to caring for herself and the neonate for the first week after discharge, then increase other activities gradually over the following weeks.

If the client has limited support and must be self-sufficient after discharge, help her set priorities and reasonable goals so that she can get adequate rest. Also urge her to ask a friend or relative to help during the first week or two at home if possible. Such a person could assist with laundry, shopping, and care of older children.

Resumption of sexual activity

If the client does not ask when she can resume sexual intercourse, provide an opening—for instance, by saying, "Many clients are not sure when they can safely resume sexual intercourse and have questions about birth control." Inform her that she should avoid sexual intercourse until the physician has conducted the postpartal examination and evaluated her condition. If her postpartal recovery is satisfactory, the physician probably will inform her that she may resume sexual intercourse at that time. However, advise her that intercourse must be gentle at first because the vaginal and perineal areas may remain tender. Also, she may need to use a lubricant because postpartal hormonal changes may cause vaginal dryness.

Caution the client that she can become pregnant during the postpartal period—whether or not she is breast-feeding. Identify her need for family planning information by determining how she and her partner would feel about another pregnancy occurring so soon after this one. Based on her teaching needs, review family planning methods and refer the client to appropriate follow-up resources. (For information on this topic, see Chapter 9, Family Planning.)

Postpartal exercises

Provide the client with teaching materials on exercises. Also, inform her that after the postpartal examination the physician may approve more vigorous exercise, such as paced walking, swimming, and low-impact aerobics. If appropriate, recommend a community exercise program supervised by an experienced teacher.

For the client with especially poor abdominal tone, institute a teaching plan focusing on improving body tone before discharge or refer her to a postpartal exercise program.

Community resources

Despite the advantages of early discharge—lower health care facility costs, reduced exposure to pathogens, and enhanced parent-infant bonding (Jansson, 1985)—the practice has some drawbacks. Home visits to clients who were discharged early have uncovered breast-feeding problems, transitory depression, fatigue, neonatal icterus, and poor parent-infant bonding. To help prevent or minimize such problems, inform the client about community resources that can help her and her partner make a more satisfactory adjustment to parenthood. In many regions, for example, community health nurses make home visits to provide guidance, support, and counseling as well as assess the health of the client and neonate. The nurse also may offer information and support through follow-up telephone calls.

Preparing the client for discharge

When the client is ready for discharge, make sure she has sufficient supplies, such as perineal pads, a 24-hour supply of infant formula (if necessary), and satisfactory clothing for the neonate. If the family is having financial problems, refer them to a social worker, who may be able to provide some of these items.

At discharge, make sure the client is escorted from the building according to facility protocol; many facilities require that she be taken to a specific exit by wheelchair. To ensure that she and the neonate are in satisfactory condition when leaving, do not let her leave the facility's property unless escorted by appropriate hospital staff.

If the family plans to go home by automobile, make sure an infant car seat or restraint is available; in many states, such a seat is required by law. Inform the parents that studies show that an adult's lap is not a safe place for the neonate to ride (Kidwell-Udin, Jacobson, and Jensen, 1987). In fact, a neonate held on the lap may suffer fatal injury in an accident.

Evaluation

During this step of the nursing process, the nurse evaluates the effectiveness of the care plan by ongoing evalution of subjective and objective criteria. Evaluation findings should be stated in terms of actions performed or outcomes achieved for each goal. The following examples illustrate appropriate evaluation statements for the postpartal client:

• The client maintained vital signs within a normal range.
• The client's uterus remained firm and the fundus descended 1 cm toward the symphysis each day.
• The client voided about 400 ml of urine 2 to 4 hours after delivery.
• The client had a normal lochial flow with no large clots, tissue fragments, or membranes.
• The client demonstrated adequate healing of the episiotomy, with no exudate.
• The client ambulated within 2 hours of vaginal delivery.
• The client had normal bowel sounds on the first postpartal day.
• The client showed positive interaction with the neonate.
• The client knows how to care for her perineum.
• The client demonstrated how to apply and remove perineal pads correctly.
• The client can determine whether her lochial flow is normal.
• The client knows how and when to examine her breasts.
• The client can state danger signs to stay alert for after discharge.

APPLYING THE NURSING PROCESS

Client with altered patterns of urinary elimination related to perineal and urethral edema and ecchymosis

When caring for the postpartal client, the nursing process helps ensure high-quality care and appropriate decision making. The table below shows how the nurse might use the nursing process when caring for the client described in the case history at right. The first column presents history and physical assessment data followed by a paragraph of mental notes. These notes help the nurse make important mental connections among assessment findings, aiding in development of the nursing diagnosis and planning.

The second column lists an appropriate nursing diagnosis; the information in the remaining columns is based on this diagnosis. Although not part of the nursing process, a rationale appears for each intervention in the fourth column to explain how it contributes to the care plan.

ASSESSMENT	NURSING DIAGNOSIS	PLANNING
Subjective (history) data • Client states she feels as if she needs to void. • Client complains of severe perineal pain. • Client states she has not voided since a catheter was inserted about 1 hour before delivery. **Objective (physical) data** • Bladder palpable above symphysis pubis. • Steady trickle of lochia. • Edematous, discolored perineum and urethra. • Boggy uterus. • Fundus displaced above and to the right of the umbilicus. **Mental notes** *The client's boggy, displaced uterus suggests bladder distention, which can prevent uterine contractions and lead to hemorrhage. Although the client feels the urge to void, she cannot relax sufficiently because of severe perineal and urethral discomfort. Nursing care must focus on promoting urinary elimination.*	Altered patterns of urinary elimination related to perineal and urethral edema and ecchymosis	**Goals** Before leaving the hospital, the client will: • empty her bladder independently • express decreased perineal discomfort • demonstrate an understanding of uterine involution.

• The client can state when to return to her physician for the postpartal examination.
• The client knows which activity levels are appropriate in the early weeks after discharge.

Documentation

All steps of the nursing process should be documented as thoroughly and objectively as possible. Thorough documentation not only allows the nurse to evaluate the effectiveness of the care plan, but it also makes this information available to other members of the health care team, helping to ensure consistency of care. (For a case study that shows how to apply the nursing process when caring for a postpartal client, see *Applying the nursing process: Client with altered patterns of urinary elimination related to perineal and urethral edema and ecchymosis.*)

Documentation for the postpartal client should include:
• location and condition of the fundus
• amount, color, and consistency of lochia
• appearance of the perineum, episiotomy, or surgical incision
• physical findings from the examination of the breasts and extremities
• bowel and bladder elimination status
• client's comfort level and any necessary interventions to improve it
• client's activity level and rest and sleep patterns
• nature of the client's interaction with the neonate
• client teaching provided and the client's understanding of this teaching

CASE STUDY

Anna Conrad, a primigravid client age 26, delivered a 7 lb 2 oz male 6 hours ago under epidural anesthesia. Palpation reveals a boggy fundus located 2 cm above and to the right of the umbilicus. Ms. Conrad reports that she changed her perineal pad 30 minutes ago; now it is saturated.

IMPLEMENTATION		EVALUATION
Intervention	**Rationale**	Upon evaluation, the client:
Initiate measures that help the client void spontaneously, such as running water over the perineum, turning on the faucets in the bathroom, and encouraging her to walk.	Spontaneous voiding eliminates the need for catheterization and the associated risk of infection.	• voided 650 ml spontaneously • demonstrated a midline fundus located at the level of the umbilicus • showed a moderate lochial flow • expressed an understanding of involution.
Administer analgesia, as prescribed, and evaluate its effectiveness.	Elimination of perineal discomfort can help the client relax sufficiently to void spontaneously.	
If the client cannot void, insert a urinary catheter, using sterile technique, as prescribed.	Catheterization relieves bladder distention, a condition that places the client at risk for postpartal hemorrhage.	
Explain the process of uterine involution and emphasize the importance of voiding.	A well-informed client more actively participates in her care.	

• client's ability to use sitz baths and other perineal comfort measures
• client's use of a support bra.

Chapter summary

Chapter 42 described nursing care during the normal postpartal period. Here are the chapter highlights.
• In the first 24 hours after delivery, the client normally may have a slight temperature elevation. After this time, however, a persistent elevation may indicate an infection, which the nurse must report and investigate immediately.

• Approximately 2 to 4 hours after delivery, the client's pulse typically decreases as the result of normal physiologic phenomena.
• Decreased blood pressure may reflect excessive blood loss, as from uterine hemorrhage; increased blood pressure may indicate PIH.
• The uterus should follow a predictable course of movement during involution. At all times, the fundus should feel firm and be located at the midline. A soft, or boggy, fundus suggests uterine atony; this in turn could lead to hemorrhage. To stimulate uterine contractions, the nurse may massage the uterus gently.
• The nurse should monitor lochial discharge, noting its consistency and any deviation from the normal progression through the lochial stages—lochia rubra, lochia serosa, and lochia alba.
• The nurse should make every attempt to keep the client's bladder empty. If the client cannot void because of pain, edema, or the effects of anesthesia, catheterization may be necessary.

• Excitement, excessive blood loss, or medications used during labor and delivery may compromise respiratory status during the postpartal period. The postcesarean client is at increased risk for respiratory problems because of immobility and the effects of anesthesia.

• Hypercoagulability resulting from decreased plasma volume places the postpartal client at increased risk for thromboembolism. To minimize this risk, the nurse should encourage early ambulation.

• The nurse can help promote spontaneous bowel movements by providing a high-fiber, well-balanced diet; encouraging increased fluid intake and early exercise; and advising the client to heed the urge to defecate.

• The nurse may suggest mild exercise shortly after delivery to improve muscle tone and improve lung expansion. Later, the physician may recommend a more comprehensive postpartal exercise program.

• The nurse should assess the client's interaction with the neonate and, if appropriate, document this information in the client's chart.

• With the increasing incidence of early discharge, the nurse must assess the client's learning needs quickly and effectively and implement an appropriate teaching plan. Postpartal teaching topics include postdischarge danger signs, resumption of sexual activity, family planning, postpartal exercises, rest and sleep requirements, and community resources.

Study questions

1. At 4 hours postpartum, Mrs. Sigma, a multiparous client age 38, has a boggy uterus that is displaced above and to the right of the umbilicus. Which interventions should the nurse carry out?

2. Which factors may affect the severity of uterine contractions (afterpains)?

3. Six days after delivery, Cindy Chu, a multiparous client age 28, has lochia rubra and pronounced episiotomy pain. Also, she is breast-feeding and complains of nipple pain. What else should the nurse check during the assessment, and which nursing interventions are appropriate for this client?

4. Mrs. Della Rosa, age 23, is a primiparous client. At 3 hours postpartum, she has a slight temperature elevation (99.9° F); however, her blood pressure has remained stable. What is the likely cause of the temperature elevation, and how should the nurse follow the client's condition?

5. Sandy Stead, age 16, will be discharged in 18 hours. What should the nurse include in a teaching plan to prepare her to care for herself upon returning home?

Bibliography

Assessment

Clark, A. (1978). *Culture, childbearing, health professionals.* Philadelphia: F.A. Davis.

Cunningham, F., MacDonald, P., and Gant, N. (1989). *Williams obstetrics* (18th ed.). East Norwalk, CT: Appleton & Lange.

Gibbs, R.S., and Weinstein, A.J. (1976). Puerperal infection in the antibiotics era. *American Journal of Obstetrics and Gynecology,* 124(7), 769-787.

Jacobson, H. (1985). A standard for assessing lochia volume. *MCN,* 10(3), 174-175.

Rutledge, D.L., and Pridham, K.F. (1987). Postpartum mothers' perceptions of competence for infant care. *JOGNN,* 16(3), 185-194.

Intervention

Avant, K.C. (1988). Stressors on the childbearing family. *JOGNN,* 17(3), 179-185.

Coleman, T. (1987). Untrivial pursuit. *MCN,* 12(5), 346-347.

Ferguson, H. (1987). Planning letter-perfect postpartum care. *Nursing87,* 17(5), 50-51.

Fullar, S.A. (1986). Care of postpartum adolescents. *MCN,* 11(6), 398-403.

Gay, J.T., Edgil, A.E., and Douglas, A.B. (1988). Reva Rubin revisited. *JOGNN,* 17(6), 394-399.

Hampson, S. (1989). Nursing interventions for the first three postpartum months. *JOGNN,* 18(2), 116-122.

Jansson, P. (1985). Early postpartum discharge. *AJN,* 85(5), 547-550.

Kidwell-Udin, P., Jacobson, D., and Jensen, R. (1987). It's never too soon to teach car safety. *MCN,* 12(5), 344-345.

Konrad, C.J. (1987). Helping mothers integrate the birth experience. *MCN,* 12(4), 268-269.

Nice, F.J. (1989). Can a breastfeeding mother take medication without harming her infant? *MCN,* 14(1), 27-31.

Phillips, C.R. (1988). Rehumanizing maternal-child nursing. *MCN,* 13(5), 313-318.

Rubin, R. (1975). Maternal tasks in pregnancy. *MCN,* 4, 143-53.

Rubin, R. (1984). *Maternal identity and the maternal experience.* New York: Springer.

Taubenheim, A.M., and Silbernagel, T. (1988). Meeting the needs of expectant fathers. *MCN,* (13)2, 110-113.

Vezeau, T.M., and Hallsten, D.A. (1987). Making the transition to mother-baby care. *MCN,* 12(3), 193-198.

Nursing diagnosis

Tribotti, S., Lyons, N., Blackburn, S., Stein, M., and Withers, J. (1988). Nursing diagnoses for postpartum women. *JOGNN,* 17(6), 410-416.

Nursing research

Hiser, P.L. (1987). Concerns of multiparas during the second postpartum week. *JOGNN,* 16(3), 195-203.

Humenick, S., and Bugen, L.A. (1987). Parenting roles: Expectation versus reality. *MCN,* 12(1), 36-39.

Keefe, M.R. (1988). The impact of infant rooming-in on maternal sleep at night. *JOGNN,* 17(2), 122-126.

Ramler, D., and Roberts, J. (1986). A comparison of cold and warm sitz baths for relief of postpartum perineal pain. *JOGNN,* 15(6), 471-474.

Ruff, C.C. (1987). How well do adolescents mother? *MCN,* 12(4), 249-253.

Storr, G.B. (1988). Prevention of nipple tenderness and breast engorgement in the postpartal period. *JOGNN,* 17(3), 203-209.

Psychosocial Adaptation of the Postpartal Family

Objectives

After reading and studying this chapter, the student should be able to:

1. Identify the components and tasks of parenting.
2. Discuss the importance of parent-infant bonding.
3. Describe how neonatal behavior affects bonding.
4. Explain the currently accepted view on the effects of early parent-neonate contact.
5. Describe the optimal conditions for parent-neonate interaction.
6. Identify appropriate parental responses to neonatal communication cues.
7. Identify synchronous reciprocity in parent-neonate interaction.
8. Discuss the phases of maternal adaptation to parenthood.
9. Describe the adjustment of the father, siblings, and grandparents to the birth of a new family member.
10. Apply the nursing process when caring for the postpartal family.

Introduction

The birth of a child creates major changes in the family. Family members—especially the parents—must adjust to changes in their roles, tasks, and responsibilities. The family as a whole also must adapt to meet the demands of the dependent neonate and the changing needs of individual members.

The nurse can help the postpartal family make a healthy transition to the changing family structure by offering knowledge, assistance, and support. Serving as a resource person, the nurse teaches the family about the components of healthy parent-neonate interaction, explains the neonate's characteristics and needs, helps the family meet those needs, and provides emotional support and guidance.

This chapter begins with a discussion of the transition to parenthood. The chapter then describes how parents typically become acquainted with the neonate and develop a positive attachment and bonding; this section is highlighted by a discussion of the effects of early parent-neonate contact. Next, the chapter discusses typical features of parent-neonate interaction, including such concepts as communication cues and reciprocity. It then describes how individual family members adapt to the arrival of a new family member, including factors that may help or hinder successful adaptation. The chapter concludes by demonstrating how to apply the nursing process to promote psychosocial adaptation of the postpartal family. A brief discussion of documentation is included.

Transition to parenthood

Parenting is a complex process encompassing various tasks, attitudes, and responsibilities through which a mature adult takes on the care of a dependent child.

GLOSSARY

Acquaintance: knowledge about another person that results from interaction; a prerequisite of parent-infant bonding.

Bonding: process through which an emotional attachment forms, which binds one person to another in an enduring relationship, as between parents and infant; sometimes called attachment.

Cognitive-affective skills: aptitude that links mental processes with emotions.

Cognitive-motor skills: aptitude that links mental processes with physical activity.

Communication cue: verbal or nonverbal message intended to elicit a response in the receiver.

Dyad: unit consisting of a pair of individuals in a close relationship.

En face position: position in which the neonate is held approximately 8″ (20 cm) in front of the parent or other observer; allows direct eye contact.

Engrossment: close face-to-face observation between parent and neonate (used to describe father-infant interaction).

Entrainment: phenomenon in which a neonate or an infant moves in rhythm to adult speech.

Reciprocity: process in which a neonate gives cues and the parent or other caregiver interprets, then responds to, these cues.

Synchrony: interaction in which each party acts and reacts in a manner appropriate to the cues given.

The parent-child dyad, or unit, is the most basic and complex relationship within the family, profoundly affecting the child's development. According to Klaus and Kennell (1982), the foundation for all other relationships developed during the child's lifetime is established within the parent-child relationship. Erikson (1959) proposed that the emergence of basic trust between parent and child during infancy is essential to the child's ability to develop successful relationships.

The birth of a child impels a parent to put aside the role of perceived carefree person and move toward a more responsible, caregiving role. How successfully the parent does this determines how well parenting tasks and responsibilities are performed. Each person has a preconceived concept of parenting based on childhood experiences, values, cultural and ethnic background, philosophy, and desires.

Besides taking on the role of parent to the new child, a parent in a couple relationship must successfully negotiate parenting tasks and responsibilities with the partner to adapt to the changing family structure. Also, the couple's relationship must accommodate the parent-child relationship; if the couple have other children, they also must help them adjust to the arrival of a new family member. At the same time, the parents must redefine their relationship to each other to meet the family's changing needs; this can prove challenging because the birth of a child reduces the couple's time alone together.

Components of parenting

According to Steele and Pollack (1987), parenting involves two principal components—cognitive-motor skills and cognitive-affective skills.

Cognitive-motor skills link mental processes with physical activities, as in physical caregiving tasks. These skills typically must be learned. Examples of cognitive-motor skills used by new parents include diapering, bathing, and feeding.

Cognitive-affective skills link mental processes with feelings or emotions, as in nurturing and other skills that reflect an awareness of and concern for the child. Because cognitive-affective skills establish the caregiving environment, they strongly influence both the way in which the parent performs cognitive-motor skills and the child's emotional response to the parent's care.

Parenting tasks

To make a smooth transition to parenthood, a person must accomplish certain tasks. Some tasks are psychological—for instance, reconciling the real child with the "fantasy" child the parent imagined before and during pregnancy. Some parents have trouble accepting the sex or characteristics of the real child if they differ from those of the imagined child; before they can move into their new roles, they must grieve for the loss of the fantasy child. (See Chapter 39, Care of the Families of High-Risk Neonates, for details on grieving.)

Other tasks parents must accomplish include gaining competence in caregiving skills, providing a safe environment for the neonate, becoming sensitive to neonatal communication cues, learning how to respond appropriately to the neonate's needs, establishing the neonate's place within the family, and helping other family members adjust to the neonate's arrival.

Acquaintance, attachment, and bonding

The development of a healthy parent-child relationship in the early postpartal days and weeks increases the chance for optimal child growth and development. Poor attachment and bonding can lead to such disorders as vulnerable child syndrome, child abuse, failure to thrive, and a disturbed parent-child relationship (Klaus and Kennell, 1982).

During the immediate postpartal period, parents and neonate typically become *acquainted*—they interact to gain information about each other. Acquaintance behaviors include eye contact, touching, verbalizing, and exploring (Klaus and Kennell, 1983). Acquaintance is a prerequisite of attachment and bonding.

Although the terms *attachment* and *bonding* now are used interchangeably to describe the process in which parent and child form an enduring relationship, earlier theorists offered varying definitions. For instance, Brazelton (1978) defined bonding as the initial mutual attraction between parent and child and attachment as the long-term process of maintaining the relationship. Klaus and Kennell (1976) described attachment as a unique relationship between two people that is specific and enduring.

Mercer (1983) defined attachment as a "process in which an affectional and emotional commitment or bonding...is formed and is facilitated by positive feedback to each partner through a mutually satisfying experience." According to Stevenson-Hinde and Parkers (1982), attachment begins during pregnancy and intensifies in the early postpartal period; once established, it is constant and consistent.

Preconditions for attachment

The quality of parent-child attachment is influenced by such variables as parental endowments, cultural practices, and the parent's relationship with his or her mother and father (Klaus and Kennell, 1982). Mercer (1983) identified preconditions that must be present for a healthy parent-child attachment to develop naturally:
• emotional health on the part of the parent
• adequate social network that includes family and friends
• competent parental communication and caregiving skills
• parental access to the child
• temperamentally suitable parent-child match.

Effects of neonatal behavior and sensory capacities on attachment

Over the past several decades, various studies have disproved that the neonate is a passive recipient of actions. Research by Brazelton (1974, 1978), Korner (1967), and Blauvelt and McKenna (1961) shows that the neonate interacts with and helps to shape the environment; Piaget (1976) also proposed that the neonate actively participates in his or her development. Thus, the quality of parent-child attachment is shaped partly by neonatal behavior and sensory capacities.

Behavioral categories

Bowlby (1969) theorized that neonatal behavior is organized into five relatively independent categories: sucking, crying, following with the eyes, clinging, and smiling. Elicited by specific stimuli, these behaviors evoke a response from the caregiver. (For more information on neonatal behavior, see Chapter 35, Neonatal Assessment.)

Sensory capacities

The neonate interacts with the environment through the senses. According to Garland (1978), "at no time in life is a person more sensorially aware than at the time of birth." The manner and level at which parent and neonate receive, process, and assimilate sensory stimulation and send back a message based on this stimulation profoundly affect the way they interact and form an attachment.

All senses play a role in attachment. For example, Klaus, et al. (1972) and Lang (1972) found that mothers felt closer to their neonates after eye contact with them; Klaus and Kennell (1976) reported that by the sixth day after birth, neonates can distinguish by odor their own mother's breast pad from the breast pads of other women. (For details on neonatal sensory capacities, see Chapter 34, Neonatal Adaptation.)

Effects of early contact on attachment

Research has yet to determine the value of early mother-neonate contact on long-term attachment. (Research on father-infant attachment has begun only recently.) Studies of other mammals suggest that such contact is necessary to attachment (Bowlby, 1969); human studies conducted or analyzed by Klaus, et al. (1972) suggest that early contact promotes attachment.

Until the mid-1970s, maternity and nursery policies emphasized separation of mother and neonate, delayed initiation of breast-feeding, and placed restrictions on parental visits to neonates in intensive care nurseries. However, based on research findings from the 1960s through the 1980s, many health care facilities have reversed such policies and now encourage early parent-neonate contact.

The groundwork for this change was laid by Desmond, Rudolph, and Phitaksphraiwan (1966). After observing term neonates during the first hours after birth, the researchers reported that the neonate exhibits a distinctive series of behavioral and physiologic characteristics, termed periods of neonatal reactivity. From studies of mother-infant attachment and separation, Klaus, Kennell, Plumb, and Zuehlke (1970) concluded that the first period of reactivity—the first 30 to 60 minutes after delivery—is a sensitive time that may be crucial to mother-infant attachment. (For more information on periods of reactivity, see Chapter 34, Neonatal Adaptation.)

The first studies of Klaus, et al. (1972) involved small samples from a specific population. For example, the subjects of one study were 14 poor, unmarried primiparous women who had 1 hour of contact with their nude neonates within 3 hours of delivery, then spent 5 hours each day with their neonates for the next 3 days. The researchers found that after 1 month, these mothers engaged in more fondling, en face (face-to-face) interaction, and soothing behaviors and were more attentive to their neonates than mothers who had not had early extended contact with their neonates.

However, the findings of other researchers seemed to contradict those of Klaus, et al. In a series of studies, de Chateau and Wiberg (1977a) found that 22 middle-class Swedish primiparous women who had 15 minutes of extra skin-to-skin contact after delivery did not show stronger bonding or increased competency or affection toward their neonates compared to 20 primiparous women who had not had early contact.

In 1982, Lamb raised questions about the methodology Klaus and Kennell used, casting doubt on their conclusions about the long-term value of early contact on parent-child attachment. However, Lamb felt that the researchers' work might support some beneficial short-term effects of early contact.

Lamb's work was welcomed by some health care providers, who were concerned that the emphasis on early contact caused parental guilt and anxiety when such contact was impossible, such as when a neonate needed immediate medical care. Today, most health care facilities encourage early contact based on experts' belief that such contact may promote optimal attachment, even if it is not essential. The American Medical Association (1977) has urged health care professionals to support early parent-neonate interaction.

Parent-neonate interaction

Positive interaction between the parents and neonate promotes healthy bonding. Such interaction depends on the ability of both parties to send, receive, and interpret messages correctly.

Optimal conditions for interaction

The best time for interaction is when both the parent and neonate are rested, focused, and attentive; preferably, the neonate should be in a quiet, alert state. The first period of reactivity may be such a time.

Health also is important. Prematurity or illness may restrict the neonate's ability to interact. Likewise, if the mother is fatigued or suffering postpartal discomfort or complications, her desire, energy, and attention for interacting may be limited. Under these conditions, bonding may take longer to achieve.

Neonatal attentiveness and temperament

By altering the degree of attentiveness to stimuli, the neonate can affect the interaction with the parent. A neonate who is attentive and responsive rewards the parent's interactive efforts; this in turn encourages the parent to continue such interaction. Thus, the more attentive and responsive the neonate, the more frequently the parent will interact.

Temperament also plays a part. A neonate who smiles frequently, eats well, is easy to console, and remains alert for long periods is more pleasant to interact with than one who is irritable and hard to console.

Communication cues, reciprocity, and synchrony

The neonate presents predictable, behaviorally organized communication cues that reflect neonatal needs and normally elicit a response from the parent or other caregiver. Prematurity, illness, temperament, and other factors can affect a neonate's ability to send communication cues.

Parental sensitivity to neonatal cues is essential to the developing parent-child relationship. As part of this relationship, parents also exhibit communication cues that elicit a response from the neonate. Parents typically vary in their ability to interpret neonatal cues and respond appropriately.

Communication cues can be verbal or nonverbal. Verbal cues used by neonates include crying and cooing;

nonverbal cues include reaching movements, facial expressions, staring, and gaze aversion. For example, a neonate who averts the gaze and turns away from a stimulus is indicating either boredom or overstimulation (Field, 1978). By refusing to focus on the person offering stimulation, the neonate signals that he or she does not want additional stimulation at that time.

The process by which the neonate gives cues and the parent interprets and responds to these cues is known as reciprocity. Through reciprocity, the interaction is maintained and the parent-neonate relationship develops. Reciprocity may take several weeks to develop.

Appropriate action and reaction to cues by parents and neonate is called synchrony (Censullo, Lester, and Hoffman, 1985.) A synchronous, reciprocal interaction is mutually rewarding. Ideally, mother and neonate establish synchrony within the first few weeks of delivery. (For an example of reciprocity, see *Reciprocity in parent-neonate interaction*.)

Verbal communication and entrainment

At first, parent-neonate communication takes on unique qualities. In most mother-neonate couples studied by Lang (1972), mothers spoke to their neonates in a high-pitched voice as they held them in the en face position. To soothe a neonate, parents frequently speak softly and slowly; to gain the neonate's attention, they use fast, high-pitched speech. Parents also use such games as "peek-a-boo" to communicate with their neonate verbally.

Healthy neonates move in rhythm with adult speech (Condon and Sander, 1974). This phenomenon, known as entrainment, is essential to parent-infant bonding, rewarding the parent and encouraging further communication. Entrainment continues as the child learns speech.

Nonverbal interaction

To interact nonverbally, parents may imitate the neonate's facial expressions. This helps the neonate develop communication skills by demonstrating that the parent responds to nonverbal interaction and that nonverbal behaviors have a meaning between people.

Rubin (1963) found that initial touching between mother and neonate progresses in a typical pattern. First, the mother touches the neonate with her fingertips only; then she progresses to whole-hand touching, and finally embraces the neonate with her arms. Primiparous and multiparous women demonstrate the same progression, although the latter progress to the embrace more rapidly.

Rodholm and Larsson (1979) found that fathers use the same touching pattern; in a later study, they found that medical students also used this pattern, even though they were not related to the neonates with whom they were interacting. These findings suggest that such touching is a human behavior pattern not restricted to parents.

Family adaptation to childbirth

As family members begin their relationship with the neonate, family relationships, interactions, and life-style must be adjusted. The adjustments each individual makes influence the welfare of the family as a whole.

Maternal adaptation

Many factors affect the mother's adaptation to the birth of a child. Energy level, attitude, degree of confidence in caregiving skills, and psychological status can help or hinder adaptation. For instance, a client who is exhausted from labor and delivery may lack the energy to interact with her neonate, and one who lacks experience with children may feel overwhelmed by the challenges of providing child care.

Adaptation phases

Rubin, one of the first nurses to study parental behavior, identified three phases of behavior that occur as a woman adapts to the parental role (1963): taking in, taking hold, and letting go. These phases establish a framework for understanding maternal adaptation; however, they must now be viewed from a wider perspective. Maternity and neonatal care policies and procedures have changed since Rubin conducted her research, as have family expectations about the childbirth experience. In particular, the length of time spent in each phase now is much shorter than Rubin observed it to be, especially if the mother has early contact with the neonate. Also, because of the current emphasis on early discharge, the nurse probably will not see clients progress to the third stage.

Taking in (dependent) phase. Immediately after delivery, the client usually is exhausted and dependent on others to meet her needs for nourishment, rest, and comfort. Because she focuses on her own needs, she may not initiate contact with the neonate. Also, she may be excited and eager to talk about the childbirth experience, reviewing the events and seeking details from others so that she can integrate them into reality. Rubin proposed that this phase lasts 1 to 2 days after delivery;

Reciprocity in parent-neonate interaction

The diagram shows how the neonate's communication cues trigger a response from the parent and the parent's cues trigger a response from the neonate. Known as reciprocity, this process helps maintain parent-neonate interaction and promotes a healthy parent-child relationship.

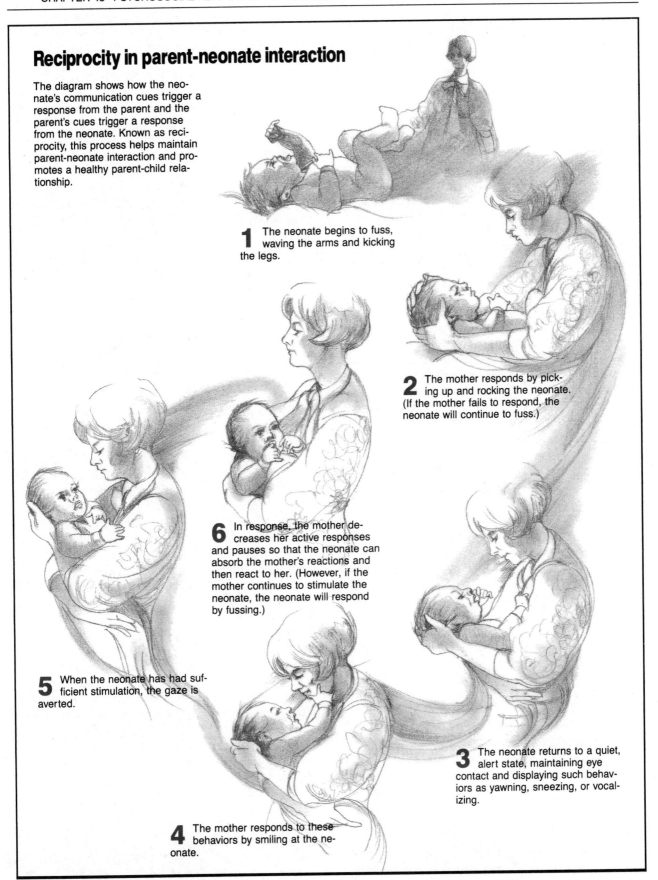

1 The neonate begins to fuss, waving the arms and kicking the legs.

2 The mother responds by picking up and rocking the neonate. (If the mother fails to respond, the neonate will continue to fuss.)

6 In response, the mother decreases her active responses and pauses so that the neonate can absorb the mother's reactions and then react to her. (However, if the mother continues to stimulate the neonate, the neonate will respond by fussing.)

5 When the neonate has had sufficient stimulation, the gaze is averted.

3 The neonate returns to a quiet, alert state, maintaining eye contact and displaying such behaviors as yawning, sneezing, or vocalizing.

4 The mother responds to these behaviors by smiling at the neonate.

today, the nurse should expect it to last just a few hours because of early discharge and other factors.

Taking hold (dependent-independent) phase. In this phase, the client vacillates between seeking nurturing and acceptance for herself and seeking to resume an independent role. In an attempt to regain control of her body, she may express concerns about her breast-feeding ability and bowel and bladder control. As her energy and comfort levels increase, her focus shifts from herself to the neonate. She seeks positive feedback and reassurance about her caregiving skills and performance as a mother and responds to teaching with enthusiasm. However, she may become discouraged easily if she feels incompetent as a caregiver. According to Rubin, this phase lasts from 3 days to 8 weeks postpartum; however, its duration may be much shorter now.

Letting go (interdependent) phase. During this final phase, the client gives up obsolete roles (such as that of a childless woman) and takes on the new role of mother. Also, she begins to accept the neonate as an individual separate from herself. As her mothering and caregiving abilities become more established, she gains confidence; her dependency on others lessens, and interdependency on family members or a support system takes over. This phase typically is marked by stress as the client and other family members reorganize tasks, responsibilities, and schedules.

Paternal adaptation

As the father's role and tasks within the family have evolved to include more active participation in child care and nurturing, researchers have begun to investigate paternal adaptation and father-neonate interaction. Results of recent studies of paternal adaptation refute earlier theories that minimized fathers' feelings for their neonates. For instance, Greenberg and Morris (1974) described engrossment between first-time fathers and neonates during early contact; observing their neonates en face, the fathers appeared to be preoccupied and absorbed. Engrossment may promote father-infant bonding.

As described earlier, fathers use the same progressive touching pattern typical of mothers. Also, they tend to talk rapidly in response to such neonatal behaviors as vocalization, whereas mothers are more likely to touch the neonate. When both parents are with the neonate, the father touches, vocalizes, and holds the neonate more than the mother does but smiles at the neonate less (Park, 1979).

Keller, Hildebrandt, and Richards (1985) found that 6 weeks after delivery, fathers who had extended early contact with their children showed more en-face behavior, participated more actively in care, and reported a more positive adjustment to fatherhood than those who had not had such contact. A study by Jones (1981) revealed that fathers who had voluntarily held their neonate within 1 hour after delivery showed more nonverbal behavior toward the neonate 1 month later. Clarke-Stewart (1978) found that fathers more frequently initiated play than mothers, whereas mothers more frequently dominated caregiving activities.

The opportunity to attend care classes or otherwise receive instructions on bathing, feeding, and diapering helps acquaint fathers with their neonates. Bills (1980) and Giefer and Nelson (1981) found that participation in such classes increased fathers' comfort level in handling and caring for their neonates. Fathers who had attended classes also reported greater father-child affectional bonds (Bills, 1980).

Factors affecting parental adaptation

Various factors may affect the ease with which a parent adapts to the birth of a child.

Maternal age

The mother's age affects her capacity for bonding as well as her readiness to assume the maternal role. For example, the adolescent mother usually lacks an established identity and a secure relationship with the neonate's father. Faced with parenting tasks and responsibilities in addition to the typical adolescent concerns of school and social life, she may feel overwhelmed and may begin to resent the child. Also, she has dependency needs of her own and usually is not mature enough to assume a full maternal role or meet her child's financial needs. Her support system may be inadequate and her friends and family may not be ready to accept her as a parent.

In contrast, the mother over age 30 may have planned her pregnancy carefully. Her adaptation to parenthood usually is relatively smooth because she is more likely to have had varied life experiences, an established career, a sound economic base, and a secure relationship with the neonate's father. Nonetheless, the older mother is at risk for social isolation, especially if few of her friends are having children. Her own parents may be too old or ill to help with child rearing. Also, her career may suffer if she tries to juggle parenthood with work responsibilities; this could lead to role conflict. Further, her energy level may be lower than that of a younger mother and she may have trouble coping with the physical demands of motherhood.

Personal aspirations

A woman who is heavily involved with her career and who unintentionally becomes pregnant may resent or fail to anticipate the demands of parenthood. Thus, she may be unwilling or unable to devote adequate time and energy to the parent-child relationship. At the other extreme, a woman who has waited many years for a wished-for child may ignore her own needs and invest herself totally in her child.

Like new mothers, fathers may find that parenthood interferes with personal aspirations. A father who initially agrees to share child-care tasks, for example, may have second thoughts once he realizes the demands involved. Unless the couple can negotiate parenting tasks and responsibilities successfully, the couple's relationship may be jeopardized, which in turn will create problems in the parent-child relationship.

Other factors

The level of support available to the family can affect parental adaptation. A woman with many established relationships and extensive social support usually has an easier time adjusting to the role of new mother than one who is isolated.

Poor economic status can hinder adaptation. The family with limited finances may be unable to obtain necessities for the child, which makes them more vulnerable to stress and sets the stage for problems in the couple's relationship and the parent-child relationship.

A sensory, mental, or physical disability can add extra challenges to parenthood.

Adaptation of other family members

The adaptation of close family members, such as siblings and grandparents, to the birth of a child has important implications for the family as a whole as well as for individual family members.

Siblings

Siblings must assume new roles when a brother or sister is born. Jealousy is a normal reaction to the attention the neonate receives. In an attempt to regain a parent's attention, the sibling may revert to infantile behavior or display hostility or aggression toward the neonate. Eventually, as the sibling spends time with the neonate, these reactions usually diminish.

Early sibling-neonate interaction seems to occur in a pattern. Nearly all siblings (96.7%) look at the neonate, focusing on the head and face; a slightly lower percentage (86.7%) touch the neonate (Marecki, et al., 1985). However, more studies are needed to improve the understanding of sibling interaction and bonding. (For a study of sibling behavior on first contact with a new brother

or sister, see *Nursing research applied: Initial sibling-neonate interaction*.)

Grandparents

The arrival of the first grandchild heralds a new status and role for the parents of the neonate's mother and father; the new grandparents' self-image must change accordingly. Most people look forward to the arrival of a grandchild. However, a few resent it because it signifies the passage of time and drives home the reality of aging.

A grandchild's arrival can provide the opportunity for the grandparent to become closer to his or her child

---

NURSING RESEARCH APPLIED

Initial sibling-neonate interaction

A recent study examined acquaintance and attachment behaviors of 30 children, aged 17 months to 11 years, during their initial contact with a sibling neonate. Acquaintance behaviors include eye contact, touching, verbalizing, and exploring; attachment behaviors include kissing and gazing. The children were permitted to interact spontaneously with their sibling neonates. The researcher observed the interaction and interviewed the parents before or after the visit.

Results showed that the siblings demonstrated more acquaintance behaviors than attachment behaviors. Initially, siblings were subdued, relaxing only after receiving reassurances from their mother. (In fact, the siblings interacted more with their mother than with the neonate.) Most children gazed, then smiled, at the neonate.

Behavior varied with age. The younger children most commonly touched the neonate's head; older children touched the arms and legs first. Some children in the youngest group (aged 17 months to 4 years) showed negative behaviors, such as rejecting or ignoring the mother, demanding that the neonate be moved away from the mother, or touching the neonate aggressively.

Siblings who had developed a prenatal relationship with the neonate showed a higher frequency of attachment behaviors than those who had experienced a previous loss of a relationship, such as the death of a family member or pet or the parents' divorce. Also, the freedom to interact spontaneously with the neonate seemed to promote acquaintance, whereas certain parental behaviors seemed to delay acquaintance. For example, when parents took photographs, forced the sibling to touch the neonate, or recounted a painful delivery, siblings averted their gaze or moved away from the neonate.

Application to practice

The results of this study underline the importance of mother-sibling reunion after childbirth. The study also suggests that the nurse should provide an environment that fosters spontaneous interaction between siblings and neonates and offer anticipatory guidance to parents concerning the troubled behaviors that might be expected of younger children on early contact with a sibling neonate. However, because of the small sample size, no definitive conclusion can be drawn from this research.

Anderberg, G.J. (1988). Initial acquaintance and attachment behavior of siblings with the newborn. *JOGNN*, 17(1), 49-54.

(the neonate's parent). Also, a grandparent can add extra significance to the arrival of the new family member by sharing family stories with the neonate's siblings; this in turn helps the siblings to adapt.

Nursing care

To help the postpartal family adapt to the birth of a neonate, the nurse uses an understanding of attachment and bonding as well as family theory. (For information on family theory, see Chapter 2, Family Structure and Function.) The nursing process provides a systematic framework for organizing information and applying interventions when caring for the postpartal family.

Assessment

Initial psychosocial assessment focuses on the client. Eventually, however, the nurse should broaden the assessment to include the father and other family members, such as siblings and grandparents.

Assessment tools
Tools used to assess maternal adaptation and the mother-child relationship include the neonatal perception inventory (NPI) and the maternal-infant observation scale. Developed by Broussard in 1964, the NPI screens for problems in maternal adaptation during the neonatal period and may suggest the need for further evaluation. The maternal-infant observation scale, created by Avant in 1975, is used to evaluate the mother-infant relationship. (For details on these tools, see *Psychosocial assessment tools*.)

The Brazelton neonatal behavioral assessment scale (BNBAS) evaluates the neonate's behavioral capacities and interaction with the environment. Allowing the parents to observe while the BNBAS is administered may enhance parent-neonate interaction and bonding. (For details on the BNBAS, see Chapter 35, Neonatal Assessment).

Evaluating maternal emotional status
The client's emotional status can affect her interaction with the neonate and her adaptation to her role. To assess emotional status, evaluate the client's mood, attitude, energy level, feelings about the childbirth experience, level of confidence in caregiving, and sense of satisfaction with her neonate. Immediately after delivery, most clients have a positive mood and attitude from the joy and excitement they feel over the birth of the child. However, fatigue may set in quickly, and the client may seem disinterested in her neonate. To distinguish fatigue from disinterest, assess mother-neonate interaction just after the client awakens from a nap and has more energy for interaction.

A client who feels overwhelmed by becoming a mother may seem withdrawn. With such a client, check for other signs that indicate a potential for maladaptive parenting, such as depression, low self-esteem, lack of support, and a seeming preoccupation with physical discomfort.

Continue to assess the client's emotional status throughout her stay. Be sure to check for signs and symptoms of postpartal "blues," such as crying spells, irritability, insomnia, and poor appetite. When these problems persist for more than 2 weeks and impair the client's ability to cope with daily activities, she may have postpartal depression, a more serious disorder. In rare cases, postpartal psychosis develops; signs and symptoms of this disorder may include severe depression and suicidal impulses. The neonate may be at risk for neglect or abuse from the client's gross distortion of reality, delusions, confusion, agitation, and flight of ideas (Hamilton, 1982).

Although early discharge makes unlikely the nurse's detecting of postpartal depression or psychosis, the nurse who detects postpartal emotional problems should expect the client to be referred to a counselor, psychiatric nurse clinician, or a psychiatrist for early treatment. (For more information on postpartal depression and psychosis, see Chapter 45, Maternal Care at Home.)

Assessing mother-infant interaction
Observe the client and neonate together, and assess their interaction. If possible, observe during a feeding session because this is when the mother and neonate are most likely to interact. To ensure accuracy, assess interaction on at least two occasions; if the client is fatigued or in discomfort during one assessment, her behavior may give a false impression.

Note the amount of eye contact between the client and neonate. Does the client pay more attention to the observer or the neonate? Also note whether she holds the neonate close or at a distance, and assess the quality of her touch. Does she stroke, kiss, and fondle the neonate, or is her touch rough, quick, and unaffectionate? Does she talk to, smile at, or sing to the neonate when changing the diaper? These behaviors show that the client acknowledges the neonate's presence and seeks a response.

Listen to the client talk to her neonate. Does she speak directly in a soothing or playful way? If her tone

Psychosocial assessment tools

The neonatal perception inventory (NPI) and the maternal-infant observation scale are screening aids that the nurse can use to reveal disorders in maternal adaptation or in the mother-infant relationship. Although these tools are not diagnostic instruments, they serve as screening aids that may indicate the need for further investigation.

Neonatal perception inventory

The NPI examines the mother's perception of six neonatal behaviors: crying, feeding, spitting up, sleeping, elimination, and predictability. The tool consists of four forms; the client fills out two forms on each of two separate occasions. On the first or second day postpartum, the client fills out the NPI "average baby" form based on her perception of how the average neonate behaves; then she fills out the NPI

"your baby" form on which she anticipates her own neonate's behavior. At 4 weeks postpartum, she fills out two similar forms; on the "your baby" form, she rates her neonate's actual behavior. Scores show whether the client has a positive or negative perception of her neonate. Results of the forms administered 4 weeks postpartum are more predictive of later childhood development behaviors than those obtained earlier (Broussard, 1978).

NEONATAL PERCEPTION INVENTORY–AVERAGE BABY

How much crying do you think the average baby does?
☐ a great deal   ☐ a good bit   ☐ moderate amount   ☐ very little   ☐ none

How much trouble do you think the average baby has in feeding?
☐ a great deal   ☐ a good bit   ☐ moderate amount   ☐ very little   ☐ none

How much spitting up or vomiting do you think the average baby does?
☐ a great deal   ☐ a good bit   ☐ moderate amount   ☐ very little   ☐ none

How much difficulty do you think the average baby has in sleeping?
☐ a great deal   ☐ a good bit   ☐ moderate amount   ☐ very little   ☐ none

How much difficulty do you think the average baby has with bowel movements?
☐ a great deal   ☐ a good bit   ☐ moderate amount   ☐ very little   ☐ none

How much trouble do you think the average baby has in settling down to a predictable pattern of eating and sleeping?
☐ a great deal   ☐ a good bit   ☐ moderate amount   ☐ very little   ☐ none

NEONATAL PERCEPTION INVENTORY–YOUR BABY

How much crying do you think your baby will do?
☐ a great deal   ☐ a good bit   ☐ moderate amount   ☐ very little   ☐ none

How much trouble do you think your baby will have feeding?
☐ a great deal   ☐ a good bit   ☐ moderate amount   ☐ very little   ☐ none

How much spitting up or vomiting do you think your baby will do?
☐ a great deal   ☐ a good bit   ☐ moderate amount   ☐ very little   ☐ none

How much difficulty do you think your baby will have sleeping?
☐ a great deal   ☐ a good bit   ☐ moderate amount   ☐ very little   ☐ none

How much difficulty do you think your baby will have with bowel movements?
☐ a great deal   ☐ a good bit   ☐ moderate amount   ☐ very little   ☐ none

How much trouble do you think your baby will have settling down to a predictable pattern of eating and sleeping?
☐ a great deal   ☐ a good bit   ☐ moderate amount   ☐ very little   ☐ none

(continued)

Psychosocial assessment tools continued

Maternal-infant observation scale

This screening tool helps assess mother-infant interaction and bonding. To administer it, the examiner sits quietly in the client's room for 15 minutes during a feeding and observes for 20 seconds out of each minute. The examiner then adds the frequency counts for behaviors in the "Affectionate behavior subscale," "Proximity maintaining subscale," and "Caretaking behavior subscale," and obtains the overall attachment score by adding up these subscores.

MATERNAL-INFANT OBSERVATION SCALE																
Date: _____ Time: _____ TV on? _____ Others present? _____																
Time in minutes	1	2	3	4	5	6	7	8	9	10	11	12	13	14	15	Subtotal
Affectionate behavior subscale																
Positions infant en face																
Looks at infant																
Talks (sings, coos to infant)																
A-T-L (assessory touch-love)																
Kisses infant																
Smiles at infant																
Touches with fingertips only																
Touches with fingertips and palms																
Subscale total																
Proximity maintaining subscale																
Holds infant																
Maintains close contact with infant																
Encompasses infant																
Keeps infant on her knees																
Subscale total																

is demanding or rejecting, assess this again on a subsequent occasion; if it continues, try to identify the cause.

Find out if the client worries about the neonate when the two are apart and if she believes the neonate knows her voice and notices her presence. Also pay close attention to the client's comments about the neonate. Does she express pleasure and satisfaction with the way her child is feeding? Note whether and how she talks about the neonate's characteristics. Does she use "claiming" expressions, such as, "He's got his daddy's eyes"? The client who claims her child has reconciled the real child with the "fantasy" child and has placed the child within the family context; this shows that interaction has begun.

Other indications of claiming include referring to the neonate as "my baby" or "our baby" and calling the neonate by name rather than "it."

Also listen for attribution of negative personality traits to the neonate—for example, such statements as, "This baby is so stubborn; she just won't breast-feed." Lack of interaction also may be signaled by such comments as, "He's mad at me today" or, "She doesn't like me." In some cases, the client may state that the neonate prefers to be held by someone other than herself. Expression of continued disappointment with the neonate's gender or physical appearance also warns of a relationship at risk.

Time in minutes	1	2	3	4	5	6	7	8	9	10	11	12	13	14	15	Subtotal
Caretaking behavior subscale																
Nurses infant																
Bottle-feeds infant																
Burps infant																
Undresses, uncovers, or diapers infant																
Subscale total																
Mother's attention																
(+) Complete attention on infant																
(−) Distracted at times																
(−) Easily distracted																
Subscale total																
Mother's initial receiving of infant																
(+) Reaches for infant																
(−) Passively accepts																
(−) Postpones																
Subscale total																
Overall attachment score (add 5 subtotals)																

Adapted with permission from P.K. Avant (1982). Maternal-infant Observation Scale. *Analysis of current assessment strategies in the health care of young children and childbearing families*, pp. 172-173. Copyright 1982, S. Humenick, University of Wyoming, Laramee.

To help evaluate the client's feelings about her neonate, ask the client questions. (For examples of relevant assessment questions, see *Assessing psychosocial adaptation*, page 1086.)

If the assessment uncovers a lack of interaction, suspect parental maladaptation and refer the client and neonate for consultation with a qualified counselor.

Evaluating maternal sensitivity and response to neonatal communication cues

Observing how the client responds to the neonate's communication cues yields further information about the developing mother-infant relationship. Note how long the client takes to respond to the neonate's cues; ignoring the neonate may indicate a problem. Also evaluate the appropriateness of the client's responses. Some mothers cannot differentiate among communication cues that signal hunger, fatigue, the need to be held, the need for eye contact, and the need for a soothing or stimulating voice. If she misinterprets cues or overstimulates or understimulates the neonate, the interaction may be asynchronous. Aim to detect asynchrony early and intervene promptly before such behaviors become entrenched.

Signs that the client is responding inappropriately to communication cues include forcing or refusing eye contact with the neonate or stimulating a tired neonate.

Assessing psychosocial adaptation

Depending on the client's and family's circumstances, the nurse may use questions similar to those shown below to determine how the client feels about her neonate and how she perceives her family's responses to the birth of the neonate. Rationales are given to explain the purpose of asking each question.

How do you feel about being a parent to this infant?
Rationale: This question gives the client a chance to express her concerns about parenting. The answer may reveal problems in bonding or in adaptation to the parental role. The remaining questions may help pinpoint some of her concerns.

How do you feel about your infant's behavior?
Rationale: If the client perceives the neonate as troublesome or abnormal, mother-infant interaction may be in jeopardy and the neonate may be at risk for abuse.

Does your infant look the way you expected?
Rationale: If the client perceives the neonate as unattractive or as having the "wrong" features, interaction may be compromised.

How do you feel about having a boy (or girl)?
Rationale: If the client was anticipating a child of the opposite sex, she will need to grieve over the loss of the fantasy child before she can bond with the real child.

Is the infant's father pleased with the infant?
Rationale: The client who receives support from the neonate's father has a better chance for a healthy adaptation to the parenting role.

Does the infant's father plan on helping you at home?
Rationale: The father who participates in child care or household tasks shows positive adaptation to his new role and tasks; this in turn may promote the client's adaptation.

How do you feel about having someone help you at home?
Rationale: Rejection of help or other indications of possessiveness toward the neonate may signify a problem in adaptation.

How do your other children feel about this infant?
Rationale: This question gives the client a chance to express any concerns she may have about the neonate's siblings. If the siblings are having problems adjusting to a new brother or sister, the client may need help coping.

What have the baby's grandparents said about this infant?
Rationale: Failure of the grandparents to accept the neonate or to offer emotional support to the client may create problems for the client adapting to the parental role.

For example, she may talk to the neonate too much, too little, or at the wrong time. Also, she may overfeed or underfeed the neonate, hold the neonate too much or too little, or tickle or bounce a fatigued neonate. Ignoring the neonate also shows lack of sensitivity to neonatal communication cues and needs.

Assessing maternal adaptation
Assess whether the client is progressing normally through the stages of adaptation—taking in, taking hold, and letting go. Also determine whether she uses a consistent, intelligent approach toward her neonate, such as by asking questions about neonatal care and evaluating the effectiveness of her caregiving attempts.

Ask the client how her family feels about the neonate; the feelings of other family members can affect how the client perceives herself. For instance, the new mother tends to view others' acceptance of the neonate as acceptance of herself as a woman and mother. Such acceptance helps her adapt to the maternal role. On the other hand, if the neonate has an abnormal or unusual appearance that upsets family members, the client may interpret their response as a rejection of her.

Evaluating paternal adaptation
To provide family-centered care, assess the adaptation of all family members, not just the client. The father's emotional status and adaptation to parenthood are particularly important. Because he usually serves as the client's main support person, his responses and behavior can play a key role in the client's adaptation to parenthood.

Many fathers have a great need to talk about the childbirth experience and their feelings but have no chance to do so except with the client. Thus, stay alert for signs that the father wants to unburden himself. If he had planned to participate actively in the birth but could not do so because of labor or delivery complications, assess for signs that he feels angry or disappointed.

Also determine the father's level of knowledge about neonatal behavior and care. Even if he will not be the primary caregiver, inadequate information about the neonate or lack of confidence in providing care can limit his interactions with the neonate.

Evaluate the father's expectations about the client's postpartal recovery and his understanding of the time and energy involved in caring for a neonate. Unrealistic expectations may lead to resentment, poor father-child interaction, and problems in the couple's relationship. For instance, if he is anticipating a rapid resumption of the client's normal energy level and desire for sexual activity, he may become resentful if her postpartal recovery takes longer than expected.

Also check for signs that the father is disappointed with the neonate's sex or is upset over a minor physical aberration. These feelings may jeopardize father-child interaction and cause the client to feel that he does not accept her as a woman or mother.

Assessing sibling adaptation
Observe the siblings as they interact with the neonate, checking for hostility, aggression, and jealousy. Also assess how the client and her partner deal with these problems.

Identifying support systems
Determine how much emotional and practical support is available to the client both within and outside the family. The client with adequate practical and emotional support is more likely to adapt well to the maternal role. Evidence of such support includes visits, phone calls, gifts, and flowers. Also find out who will be available to help with child care or household tasks after discharge. In some cases, new parents fail to anticipate the need for help and then feel overwhelmed when the demands of child care become obvious.

Determining parental caregiving skills
To determine how much teaching the parents will need to gain competence in caring for the neonate, find out about their previous child-care experience and observe them as they provide care. With new parents, inexperience may be obvious. If the parents are experienced, however, do not automatically assume they are adept at giving care. Instead, ask them if they would like a refresher course, and give them the chance to ask questions.

Nursing diagnosis

After gathering assessment data, the nurse must review it carefully to identify pertinent nursing diagnoses for the postpartal family. (For a partial list of applicable diagnoses, see *Nursing diagnoses: Postpartal family*, page 1088.)

Planning and implementation

After assessing the postpartal family and formulating nursing diagnoses, the nurse develops and implements a care plan. Nursing goals that promote psychosocial adaptation of the postpartal family include:
• promoting interaction
• helping parents assess the childbirth experience
• easing the transition to parenthood
• promoting psychosocial adaptation in special-needs clients

• promoting paternal adaptation
• supporting sibling adaptation
• promoting grandparent adaptation
• reducing social isolation
• ensuring postdischarge care.

Promoting interaction
Unless the neonate needs immediate medical intervention, arrange for the parents to interact with the neonate immediately after delivery to take advantage of the neonate's enhanced receptivity at this time. Optimally, eye prophylaxis should be delayed to allow the neonate to make eye contact with the parents. Urge the parents to get acquainted with the neonate by cuddling, touching, and exploring the neonate's body. If appropriate, encourage the client to initiate breast-feeding at this time.

For the remainder of the client's stay, increase the chance for positive interaction by providing postpartal comfort measures (as described in Chapter 42, Care during the Normal Postpartal Period). Make sure the client gets sufficient rest so that she has enough energy to interact with the neonate; if possible, bring the neonate to the client just after she has had a nap.

Teach the parents about neonatal behavioral states and the periods of neonatal reactivity, and encourage interaction when the neonate is in a quiet, alert state. During their times together, provide privacy and freedom from distractions.

Helping the parents interpret their neonate's behavior also enhances interaction. Teach them about neonatal communication cues, behavioral capacities, growth and development patterns, and sleep and awake patterns. Also explain the concepts of reciprocity and synchrony, and show the parents how to respond appropriately to the neonate's cues. Explain that they—not the neonate—are responsible for interpreting cues and responding appropriately.

A client who openly compares her fantasy child with her real child may have a nursing diagnosis of *dysfunctional grieving related to loss of the fantasy child*. Because grieving is a prerequisite of acceptance and bonding, encourage her to express her feelings. This can help her avoid a nursing diagnosis of *potential altered parenting related to disappointment over the neonate's sex or appearance*.

Helping parents assess the childbirth experience
To help the parents come to terms with and integrate the childbirth experience into their lives, give them the opportunity to talk about it. This is especially important if complications arose or if they feel disappointed about some aspect of the experience.

Help the parents understand and accept both positive and negative feelings. If they have doubts about

Postpartal family

For the postpartal family, the nurse may find the following nursing diagnoses appropriate:

- Altered family processes related to the neonate's birth
- Anxiety related to the stress of the changing family structure and the transition to parenthood
- Dysfunctional grieving related to loss of the fantasy child
- Family coping: potential for growth, related to the birth of a new family member
- Ineffective individual coping related to parenting tasks and responsibilities
- Knowledge deficit related to parenting tasks, infant care, and community resources
- Parental role conflict related to the birth of a new family member
- Potential altered parenting related to disappointment over the neonate's sex or appearance
- Social isolation related to the demands of caring for a neonate or an infant

their performance during labor and delivery, offer reassurance. If they have questions, answer these as completely as possible, referring, if necessary, to the labor and delivery records.

Easing the transition to parenthood

Stress is a normal reaction to the birth of a child and the challenging new roles and responsibilities that come with it. Thus, all clients have a potential nursing diagnosis of *anxiety related to the stress of the changing family structure and the transition to parenthood.* To help ease anxiety, teach the client about neonatal characteristics and care, and provide information, encouragement, and support.

Mood swings, brought on partly by hormonal fluctuations, may contribute to anxiety in the postpartal client. Explain that such swings are normal and expected, and encourage the client to cry if she feels the urge. If she seems to want to talk, act as an interested listener.

The client who lacks caregiving experience may have a nursing diagnosis of *ineffective individual coping related to parenting tasks and responsibilities* or *knowledge deficit related to parenting tasks, infant care, and community resources.* When teaching this client about caregiving tasks, use a supportive approach; the seeming ease with which a nurse performs neonatal care may reinforce the client's feelings of inadequacy. Supervise

her as she cares for the neonate, offering praise and encouragement. Express confidence in her ability to cope with new tasks. (For details on parent teaching related to caregiving activities, see Chapter 36, Care of the Normal Neonate.)

Promoting psychosocial adaptation in special-needs clients

Special-needs clients include adolescent and older clients and those with sensory, mental, or physical disabilities.

Expect the adolescent client to have a greater need for teaching about neonatal and infant care. Ask how she plans to care for her child after discharge; if her arrangements seem inadequate, refer her to the appropriate resources.

The first-time mother over age 30 may feel anxious about her caregiving skills and her changing role. Particularly if she gave up a career to have a child, she may have a nursing diagnosis of *parental role conflict related to the birth of a new family member.* Urge this client to express her feelings about becoming a mother; if appropriate, refer her for counseling.

The disabled client will need individualized nursing care to ease the transition to parenthood. (For appropriate nursing interventions, see *Helping the disabled client adapt to parenthood.*)

Promoting paternal adaptation

Make sure to include the father in nursing interventions, such as by inviting him to child-care demonstrations and giving him the opportunity to express his feelings and concerns. If he has questions about the events of childbirth or the mother's or neonate's condition, offer clarification. Also stay alert for signs that he feels inadequate as a labor partner, husband, or father. If such signs arise, reassure him that many new fathers have these doubts.

Offer anticipatory counseling so that the father knows what to expect in the months ahead. Topics that may be appropriate to include are resumption of sexual activity, the expected course of the mother's postpartal recovery, and the need to provide practical and emotional support at home.

Supporting sibling adaptation

Many siblings feel uncertain or jealous when a brother or sister is born. To help siblings adjust and thus avoid a nursing diagnosis of *altered family processes related to the neonate's birth,* urge the parents to let siblings visit the neonate in the health care facility (if facility policy allows). Be aware that studies have failed to support the notion that sibling visits increase the risk of neonatal infection (Solheim and Spellacy, 1988).

Encourage the client to call siblings on the telephone frequently and to spend uninterrupted time with them

Helping the disabled client adapt to parenthood

Most disabled clients can develop a full, rewarding parenting role. Nursing care for these clients and their families necessitates extra creativity, empathy, and emotional support, with emphasis on communication and individualized interventions.

Vision-impaired client
Although a vision-impaired client cannot make eye contact with her neonate, she can use other senses and their senses to develop a bond. Give her the opportunity to touch, hear, and smell the neonate. Be sure to provide a thorough orientation to the surroundings, since the health care facility is an unfamiliar environment.

To help the client feel comfortable and confident when performing physical caregiving tasks, describe the motions involved. For example, when teaching her how to wrap the neonate in a blanket, describe this process step by step. Have her feel the position of the blanket and neonate at each stage, then guide her as she performs the actions, giving her ample time to become familiar with each step through touch.

Hearing-impaired client
When working with a hearing-impaired client, first determine if she can read lips or use sign language. The nurse who does not know sign language should seek help from a knowledgeable resource person. In some cases, a magic slate or tablet and pen can be used to communicate. (Be aware that federal law stipulates that facilities receiving federal funds must provide alternative ways of communicating with hearing-impaired clients.)

Although the client cannot hear her neonate, she may be able to feel sound vibrations. If she can vocalize, encourage her to do so with the neonate. Also consider recommending that she obtain a device that converts sound waves into a flashing light signal; this device can be placed on the nursery door at home to alert the client when the child is crying.

Mentally impaired client
A multidisciplinary team approach incorporating family and community support is required to address the needs of this client and her child. Unless severely impaired, the mentally impaired client can learn caregiving skills. If her social, communication, daily living, and independent living skills have not been assessed, refer her to the appropriate professional for evaluation.

If the client functions well enough to care for her neonate, implement a thorough plan for teaching child care tasks, taking into account her best learning method. Keep the teaching environment free from distractions, and ask the client to give return demonstrations of skills taught. Use an appropriate teaching pace, and if necessary, repeat teaching points.

Be sure to identify support resources and incorporate them into discharge planning. If the client lacks adequate support, help her make contact with a local support group, such as a parenting group. Refer her to a community health nurse or visiting nurse for follow-up assessment of her daily living skills.

Physically disabled client
Many parents with physical disabilities are quite creative in performing caregiving tasks. Base interventions on the client's particular strengths and weaknesses. For example, a client with psychomotor dysfunction may require referral to an occupational therapist, adaptation of the home environment, and an assistant caregiver until a comfortable and safe caregiving routine has been established.

---

when they visit. Also, instruct her to watch for overt and subtle signs of sibling jealousy. Overt signs include hitting or throwing objects at the neonate; subtle signs include attempting to take the neonate out of the crib or covering the neonate with toys.

Promoting grandparent adaptation
Encourage the parents to include the grandparents in their new family life because grandparents can serve as key support persons. However, keep in mind that changes in maternity and infant care practices over the past few decades may create conflicts between parents and grandparents. If such conflicts arise, help resolve them by providing teaching to grandparents and incorporating extended family issues in parenting classes. Also recommend that grandparents attend grandparent classes offered by the health care facility or community. Topics typically included in such classes include modern childbirth practices, parenting techniques, and the grandparent role.

Although many grandparents enjoy participating in caregiving, the nurse should not assume that all grandparents want to participate. Follow their lead in this matter, offering caregiving instruction only if they express a desire for it.

Grandparents also can help siblings adjust to the birth of the neonate. Encourage them to give siblings extra attention and a chance to express their feelings about the birth of a new family member. To help perpetuate a sense of family continuity, suggest that they relate family history to the siblings, including telling siblings about their parents' births.

Reducing social isolation
To cope with the responsibilities of parenthood after discharge, the client will need a social support network to avert a nursing diagnosis of *social isolation related to the demands of caring for a neonate or an infant.* Especially if the client is a single mother and lacks such a network, help her develop one by referring her to com-

---

Postpartal family with dysfunctional grieving related to loss of the fantasy child

For the postpartal family, the nursing process helps ensure high-quality care and appropriate decision making. The table below shows how the nurse might use the nursing process when caring for the client described in the case history at right. The first column presents history and physical assessment data followed by a paragraph of mental notes. These notes help the nurse make important mental connections among assessment findings, aiding in development of the nursing diagnosis and planning.

The second column lists an appropriate nursing diagnosis; information in the remaining columns is based on this diagnosis. Although not part of the nursing process, a rationale appears for each intervention in the fourth column to explain how it contributes to the care plan.

ASSESSMENT	NURSING DIAGNOSIS	PLANNING
Subjective (history) data • Client states, "I'm very disappointed. We didn't get the son we wanted, and I'm too old to have another baby." • Client says the neonate "isn't even cute, like my other girls were." • Client's husband holds the neonate only for brief periods. **Objective (physical) data** • Client is a multiparous client age 39; her husband is age 40. • Labor and delivery were normal. • Lochia rubra is present. • Uterus is enlarged but responsive to massage. **Mental notes** *Mrs. Samuels is disappointed that her fourth child is a girl; her husband's behavior suggests that he shares her disappointment. Close, repeated assessment of her interaction with the neonate, followed by appropriate intervention, will be necessary to ensure that her attitude does not jeopardize mother-infant bonding.*	Dysfunctional grieving related to loss of the fantasy child	**Goals** The client and husband will: • express their feelings of loss • discuss their disappointment over the neonate's sex • accept the neonate as she is • show appropriate bonding behaviors.

munity resource groups. Many communities have single-parent support groups.

Ensuring postdischarge care

Make sure the client knows when and where to go for postpartal medical care. The 6-week postpartal examination not only allows the physician or nurse-midwife to assess her postpartal recovery, but it also gives health care providers the chance to evaluate her psychosocial adaptation. (For more information on postdischarge postpartal care, see Chapter 42, Care during the Normal Postpartal Period, and Chapter 45, Maternal Care at Home.)

Evaluation

During this step of the nursing process, the nurse evaluates the effectiveness of the care plan by ongoing evaluation of subjective and objective criteria. Evaluation findings should be stated in terms of actions performed or outcomes achieved for each goal. The following examples illustrate appropriate evaluation statements for the postpartal family.

• The client had early contact with the neonate and showed positive bonding behaviors, such as fondling, kissing, and cuddling.
• The client expressed her feelings about the childbirth experience.
• The client expressed an understanding of the best times to interact with the neonate.
• The client began to reconcile the fantasy child with the real child and showed signs that she accepts the neonate.
• The client has responded appropriately to neonatal communication cues.
• The client showed increasing proficiency and confidence in caregiving skills.
• The client allowed the neonate's siblings to visit the neonate and called them on the telephone several times during her stay.
• The father expressed realistic expectations for the client's postpartal recovery.
• The neonate's grandparents gave support and encouragement to the parents and siblings.

CASE STUDY

Mrs. and Mr. Samuels, ages 39 and 40, respectively, have just had their fourth child and their fourth daughter. Labor and delivery were uneventful. Mr. Samuels attended, as he did for the previous three deliveries.

IMPLEMENTATION		EVALUATION
Intervention Spend unhurried time with the client and her husband.	**Rationale** An unhurried approach will allow adequate time for the client and her husband to express their feelings.	Upon evaluation, the client and her husband: • expressed disappointment that their fourth child is a girl • expressed guilt about having those feelings • showed an understanding that their disappointment and associated guilt are normal feelings • began to establish appropriate bonding with the neonate, as indicated by their behavior.
Encourage the client and her husband to express their feelings about the neonate; remain nonjudgmental as they do so.	A nonjudgmental attitude gives the client and her husband the opportunity to express their feelings honestly.	
Observe the client and her husband as they interact with the neonate.	Observation can reveal whether the client and her husband are accepting or rejecting the neonate.	
Be aware of the possible need for referral to a psychiatric nurse clinician or counselor.	A rapid discharge may necessitate speedy referrals so that home care follow-up occurs.	

Documentation

All steps of the nursing process should be documented as thoroughly and objectively as possible. Thorough documentation not only allows the nurse to evaluate the effectiveness of the care plan, but it also makes this information available to other members of the health care team, helping to ensure consistency of care. (For a case study that shows how to apply the nursing process when caring for the postpartal family, see *Applying the nursing process: Postpartal family with dysfunctional grieving related to loss of the fantasy child*.)

Documentation of nursing care for the postpartal family should include the following points:
• signs of positive bonding, or lack of such signs
• the quality of parent-neonate interaction
• client's ability to interpret and respond appropriately to neonatal communication cues
• evidence of reciprocity and synchrony in parent-neonate communication
• client's progression through the stages of maternal adaptation
• client's emotional status, including any signs of postpartal depression
• father's emotional status and adaptation to parenthood
• client's caregiving skills
• availability of practical and emotional support after discharge
• adaptation of siblings and grandparents to the neonate's birth.

Chapter summary

Chapter 43 discussed psychosocial adaptation of the postpartal family. Here are the chapter highlights.
• Parenting is a complex process with emotional and physical components. A person's perception of parenting is based on childhood experiences, values, cultural and ethnic background, philosophy, and personal desires.

• The birth of a neonate necessitates changes in family interrelationships and in tasks, responsibilities, and life-styles of individual family members.

• The quality of parent-infant interaction has important implications for the future of the parent-child relationship and the child's psychological development.

• Early parent-neonate contact promotes but probably is not essential to bonding.

• Maternal adaptation to the parental role occurs in three phases: taking in (dependent) phase, taking hold (dependent-independent) phase, and letting go (interdependent).

• Although father-neonate interactions and adaptation to the paternal role have not been studied thoroughly, research suggests that fathers have intense feelings toward their neonates and that early father-neonate contact eases the adjustment to parenthood.

• Sibling jealousy is a normal reaction to the birth of a new family member and usually diminishes over time.

• Grandparents can help the postpartal family adapt to childbirth by giving emotional support and helping with child care. However, nursing interventions may be necessary to resolve conflicts between parents and grandparents over child-care practices.

• Although nursing assessment and interventions focus on the mother because she is the primary client, the nurse should incorporate other family members into the nursing process.

• Nursing goals for the postpartal family include promoting bonding and interaction, helping parents come to terms with childbirth, easing the transition to parenthood, and supporting sibling and grandparent adaptation.

Study questions

1. What are the components and tasks of parenting?

2. How do neonatal capacities and behavioral traits affect the quality of parent-neonate interaction?

3. What are some optimal conditions for parent-neonate interaction?

4. How do synchrony and reciprocity contribute to parent-neonate communication?

5. Mrs. Duncan, age 24, and Mr. Duncan, age 25, have just had their first child. Which factors should the nurse assess to determine how well they are adapting to the birth of their child?

6. When observing Mrs. Duncan with her neonate, the nurse notices signs of poor mother-infant bonding and inappropriate maternal interpretation of neonatal communication cues. What are examples of such signs?

7. Which nursing interventions should the nurse carry out to enhance Mrs. Duncan's interaction with her neonate and promote more effective maternal-infant communication?

8. On a visit to the nursery, Johnny Garcia, age 5, pinches his new baby brother. Which interventions should the nurse use to help his parents deal with his feelings of jealousy over the addition of a new family member?

9. What role can grandparents play in the psychosocial adaptation of the postpartal family?

Bibliography

Blauvelt, H., and McKenna, J. (1961). Mother-neonate interaction capacity of the human newborn for orientation. In B.M. Forss (Ed.), *Determinates of infant behavior*, Vol. 1. New York: Wiley.

Condon, W.S., and Sander, L.W. (1974). Synchrony demonstrated between movements of the neonate and adult speech. *Child Development*, 45(2), 456-462.

de Chateau, P. (1976). Neonatal care routines: Influences on maternal and infant behavior and on breastfeeding. Thesis. Umea, Sweden.

Lang, R. (1972). *Birth book*. Ben Lomond, CA: Genesis Press.

Mead, G.H. (1934). *Mind, Self and Society*. Chicago: University of Chicago Press.

Mechanic, D. (1978). *Medical sociology* (2nd ed.) New York: Free Press.

Piaget, J. (1976). *Psychology of intelligence*. Lanham, MD: Littlefield.

Scott, L. (1988). *Time out for motherhood*. Los Angeles: Jeremy P. Tarcher.

Mother-infant bonding

American Medical Association. (1977, December 4-7). *Statement on parent and newborn interaction*. Presented at the meeting of the House of Delegates, Chicago.

Avant, P.K. (1980). Maternal attachment and anxiety: An exploratory study. *Dissertation Abstracts International*, 40, 165 B. University Microfilms No. 79-15863.

Avant, P.K. (1982). Anxiety as a potential factor affecting maternal attachment. *JOGNN*, 6, 416.

Brazelton, T.B., et al. (1974). The origin of reciprocity: The early mother-infant interaction. In M. Lewis and L.A. Rosenblum, (Eds). *The origins of behavior*, Vol. 1: The effect of the infant on its caregiver. New York: Wiley.

Broussard, E.R., and Hartner, M.S.S. (1970). Maternal perception of the neonate as related to development. *Child Psychiatry and Human Development*, 1(1), 16-25.

Broussard, E.R., and Hartner, M.S.S. (1971). Further considerations regarding maternal perception of the newborn. In J. Hellmuth (Ed.), *Exceptional infant, Vol. 2, Studies in abnormalities*. New York: Brunner/Mazel.

Broussard, E.R. (1978). Psychosocial disorders in children: Early assessment of infants at risk. *Continuing Education for the Family Physician*, 8(2), 44-57.

Cohler, B.J., Grunebaum, H.U., Weiss, J.L., Hartman, C.R., and Gallant, D.S. (1976). Child care attitudes and adaptation to the maternal role among mentally ill and well mothers. *American Journal of Orthopsychiatry*, 46(1), 123-134.

de Chateau, P. (1976). Neonatal care routines: Influences on maternal and infant behavior and on breastfeeding. Thesis. Umea, Sweden.

de Chateau, P. (1976). The influence of early contact on maternal and infant behavior in primiparae. *Birth and the Family Journal*, 3(4), 149-155.

de Chateau, P., and Wiberg, B. (1977a). Long-term effect on mother-infant behavior of extra contact during the first hour post partum, I. First observation at 36 hours. *Acta Paediatrica Scandinavica*, 66(2), 137-143.

de Chateau, P., and Wiberg, B. (1977b). Long-term effect on mother-infant behavior of extra contact during the first hour post-partum, II. Follow-up at three months. *Acta Paediatrica Scandinavica*, 66(2), 145-151.

Frommer, F.A., and O'Shea, G. (1973). Antenatal identification of women liable to have problems in managing their infants. *British Journal of Psychiatry*, 123(573), 149-156.

Klaus, M.H, Jerauld, R., Kreger, N.C., McAlpine, W., Steffa, M., and Kennell, J.H. (1972). Maternal attachment: Importance of the first postpartum days. *New England Journal of Medicine*, 286(9), 460-463.

Klaus, M.H., and Kennell, J.H. (1976). Human maternal and parental behaviors. In M.H. Klaus, J.H. Kennell, (Eds.). *Maternal-infant bonding*. St. Louis: Mosby.

Klaus, M.H., and Kennell, J.H. (1982). *Parent-infant bonding* (2nd ed.). St. Louis: Mosby.

Klaus, M.H., and Kennell, J.H. (1983). *Bonding: The beginnings of parent-infant attachment*. St. Louis: Mosby.

Klaus, M.H., Kennell, J.H., Plumb, N., and Zuehlke, S. (1970). Human maternal behavior at the first contact with her young. *Pediatrics*, 46(2), 187-192.

Korner, A.F. (1967). Individual differences at birth: Implications for early experience and later development. *Journal of the American Academy of Child Psychiatry*, 6, 676-690.

Lamb, M.E. (1982). Early contact and maternal-infant bonding: One decade later. *Pediatrics*, 70(5), 763-768.

Porter, R.H., Cernoch, J.M., and McLaughlin, F.J. (1983). Maternal recognition of neonates through olfactory cues. *Physiology and Behavior*, 1(30), 151-154.

Porter, R.H., Cernoch, J.M., and Perry, S. (1983). The importance of odors in maternal-infant interactions. *MCN*, 12(3), 147-154.

Rubin, R. (1961). Maternal behavior. *Nursing Outlook*, 9, 682.

Rubin, R. (1963). Maternal touch. *Nursing Outlook*, 11(11), 828-831.

Father-infant bonding

Clarke-Stewart, K. (1978). And daddy makes three: The father's impact on mother and young child. *Child Development*, 49(2), 466-478.

Field, T. (1978). Interaction behaviors of primary versus secondary caretaker fathers. *Developmental Psychology*, 14(2), 183-184.

Giefer, M.A., and Nelson, C. (1981, November/December). Principles and practice. A method to help new fathers develop parenting skills. *JOGGN*, 10(6), 455-457.

Greenberg, M., and Morris, N. (1974). Engrossment: The newborn's impact upon the father. *American Journal of Orthopsychiatry*, 44(4), 520-531.

Keller, W.D., Hildebrandt, K.A., and Richards, M.S. (1985). Effects of extended father-infant contact during the newborn period. *Infant Behavior and Development*, 8(3), 337-350.

McDonald, D.L. (1978). Paternal behavior at first contact with the newborn in a birth environment without intrusions. *Birth Family Journal*, 5(Fall), 123-132.

Park, R.D. (1979). Perspectives on father-infant interaction. In J.D. Osofsky (Ed.), *The handbook of infant development*. New York: Wiley.

Rodholm, M., and Larsson, K. (1979). Father-infant interaction at the first contact after delivery. *Early Human Development*, 3(1), 21-27.

Parental adjustment

Bell, R.Q., and Harper, L.V. (Eds.). (1980). *Child effects on adults*. Lincoln, NE: University of Nebraska Press.

Brim, O.G. (1960). Personality development as role learning. In I. Iscoe and H. Stevenson (Eds.), *Personality development in children*. Austin: University of Texas Press.

Brim, O.G. (1966). Socialization through the life cycle. In O.G. Brim and S. Wheeler, S. (Eds.), *Socialization after childhood: Two essays*. New York: MacMillan.

Brim, O.G. (1977). Adult socialization. In D.L. Sills, (Ed.), *International encyclopedia of the social sciences* (pp. 555-562) New York: Free Press.

Desmond, M.M., Rudolph, A., and Phitaksphraiwan, P. (1966). The transitional care nursery: A mechanism for preventive medicine in the newborn. *Pediatric Clinics of North America*, 13(3), 651-668.

Erikson, E.H. (1959). Identity and the life cycle: Selected papers. In *Psychological issues*, Vol. 1, No. 1, New York: International Universities Press.

Fraiberg, S. (1980). *Clinical studies in infant mental health: The first year of life*. New York: Basic Books.

Friedman, M.M. (1981). *Family nursing: Theory and assessment*. East Norwalk, CT: Appleton & Lange.

Garland, K.R. (1978, July-September). Factors in neonatal attachment, Part 1: Keeping abreast. Newborns are people, too! *Journal of Human Nurturing*, 206-213.

Haley, J. (1963). *Strategies of psychotherapy*. Philadelphia: Saunders.

Hamilton, G.H. (1982). Psychosis of pregnancy, *American Journal of Orthopsychiatory*, 49, 330.

Heiss, J. (1976). An introduction to the elements of role theory. In J. Heiss (Ed.), *Family roles and interaction: An anthology* (2nd ed.). Chicago: Rand McNally.

Steele, B., and Pollack, C. (1987). A psychiatric study of parents who abuse infants and small children. In R.E. Helfer and R.S. Kempe (Eds.), *The battered child* (4th ed.). Chicago: University of Chicago Press.

Ventura, J.N. (1986, March/April). Parent coping, a replication. *Nursing Research, 35*(2), 77-80.

Parent-infant bonding

Bills, B.J. (1980, September/October). Enhancement of parental-newborn affectional bonds. *Journal of Nurse-Midwifery, 25*(5), 21-26.

Bowlby, J. (1969). *Attachment.* New York: Basic Books.

Brazelton, T.B. (1973). *Neonatal behavioral assessment scale.* Philadelphia: Lippincott.

Brazelton, T.B. (1974). Does the neonate shape his environment? In D. Bergsman (Ed.), *The infant at risk.* White Plains, NY: National Foundation of the March of Dimes.

Brazelton, T.B. (1978, Winter). The remarkable talents of the newborn. *Birth Family Journal, 5,* 187-191.

Mercer, R.T. (1983). Parent-infant attachment. In L.J. Sonstegard (Ed.), *Women's Health, Vol. 2, Childbearing.* New York: Grune & Stratton.

Stevenson-Hinde, J. and Parkers, C.M., (1982). *The place of attachment in human behavior.* New York: Basic Books.

Grandparent adjustment

Horn, M. and Manion, J. (1984, May/June). Creative Grandparenting: Bonding the Generations. *JOGGN, 14*(3), 233-236.

Maloni, J., McIndoe, J.E., and Rubenstein, G. (1987, January/February). Expectant grandparents class. *JOGGN,* 26-29.

Olson, M.L. (1981, November/December). Fitting grandparents into new families. *MCN, 6*(6), 419-421.

Nursery care

Kennell, J., and Klaus, M. (1971). Care of the mother of the high risk infant. *Clinics in Obstetrics and Gynecology, 14*(3), 926-954.

Rambo, B. (1984). *Adaptation nursing: Assessment and intervention.* Philadelphia: Saunders.

Roy, C. (1984). *Introduction to nursing: An adaptation model* (2nd ed.). Englewood Cliffs, NJ: Prentice-Hall.

Sibling adjustment

Marecki, M., et al. (1985, September/October). Early sibling attachment. *JOGNN, 14*(5), 418-423.

Nursing research

Anderberg, G.J. (1988). Initial acquaintance and attachment behavior of siblings with the newborn. *JOGGN, 17*(1), 49-54.

Censullo, M., Lester, B., and Hoffmann, J. (1985). Rhythmic patterning in mother-newborn interaction. *Nursing Research, 34*(6), 342-346.

Jones, C. (1981). Father to infant attachment: Effects of early contact and characteristics of the infant. *Research in Nursing and Health, 4,* 183-192.

Solheim, K., and Spellacy, C. (1988). Sibling visitation: Effects on newborn infection rates. *JOGGN, 17*(1), 43-48.

Ventura, J.N. (1986, March/April). Parent coping, a replication. *Nursing Research, 35*(2), 77-80.

Postpartal Complications

Objectives

After reading and studying this chapter, the student should be able to:

1. Identify the major causes of puerperal infection.
2. Describe common causes of and treatments for postpartal hemorrhage.
3. Discuss postpartal nursing management of a client with pregnancy-induced hypertension.
4. Name the assessment data that suggest thrombophlebitis.
5. Describe nursing considerations for a diabetic client during the postpartal period.
6. Recognize a client at risk for a postpartal psychiatric disorder.
7. Understand the postpartal care needs of a substance-abusing client.
8. Apply the nursing process when caring for a client with postpartal complications and document appropriately.

Introduction

The postpartal period—the 6-week period following delivery—is a time of significant physiologic and psychological stress. Fatigue caused by labor, blood loss during delivery, and other conditions brought on by childbirth can cause complications—some of them critical—in the postpartal client. Prevention of such complications is a major focus of nursing care. Once a complication occurs, of course, the nurse must work to promote the client's recovery and ensure that the problem does not jeopardize the developing mother-neonate relationship.

This chapter focuses on common postpartal complications and related nursing care. It begins by discussing the physiology and etiology of postpartal complications, then shows how to apply the nursing process when providing care for the client with a complication. The chapter concludes with a brief discussion of documentation.

Puerperal infection

Puerperal infection—an infection of the reproductive tract occurring during the postpartal period—is a leading cause of childbearing-associated death throughout the world (Cunningham, MacDonald, and Gant, 1989). Labor and delivery reduce resistance to infection by bacteria normally found in or on the body. Most puerperal infections result from such bacteria as beta-hemolytic streptococci, staphylococci, and coliform. However, various other organisms may play a role.

Because the duration of labor and the incidence of infection are directly proportional, prolonged labor increases the risk of puerperal infection (Eschenbach and Wager, 1980). Also, rupture of the amniotic sac may

GLOSSARY

Bacteremic shock: type of shock that occurs in septicemia (systemic infection of the bloodstream) when endotoxins are released from certain bacteria; also called septic shock.

Central venous pressure: pressure within the superior vena cava; represents the pressure under which blood returns to the right atrium.

Chorioamnionitis: inflammation of the fetal membranes; a predisposing factor for puerperal infection.

Cystitis: bladder inflammation producing dysuria, urinary frequency and urgency, hematuria, and other urinary symptoms.

Cystocele: herniation of the urinary bladder through the vaginal wall.

Dehiscence: spontaneous opening of a surgical wound (such as an episiotomy).

Depression: abnormal emotional state characterized by exaggerated feelings of sadness, melancholy, dejection, worthlessness, and hopelessness that are inappropriate and out of proportion to reality.

Disseminated intravascular coagulation (DIC): abnormal clotting disorder characterized by hypoprothrombinemia, hypofibrinogenemia, and a subnormal platelet count; caused by a major insult to the body, such as abruptio placentae.

Dyspareunia: painful or difficult intercourse.

Eclampsia: gravest convulsive form of pregnancy-induced hypertension, affecting one of every 200 clients with preeclampsia; characterized by generalized tonic-clonic seizures, coma, hypertension, proteinuria, and edema; occurs between the twentieth week of pregnancy and the end of the first postpartal week.

Fistula: abnormal passage between two internal organs or from an internal organ to the body surface.

Hematoma: collection of extravasated blood trapped in the tissues of the skin or in an organ resulting from trauma or incomplete hemostasis, as after surgery.

Hydramnios: excessive amniotic fluid associated with congenital neonatal disorders and such maternal disorders as diabetes mellitus.

Hypovolemia: abnormally diminished volume of circulating fluid.

Levator ani: one of a pair of muscles of the pelvic diaphragm that stretches across the bottom of the pelvic cavity supporting the pelvic organs; separates into the pubococcygeus and the iliococcygeus.

Major depressive episode: disorder of emotional origin that is sometimes precipitated by childbirth; characterized by depressed mood, markedly diminished interest or pleasure in activities, significant weight loss or gain, insomnia or hypersomnia, psychomotor agitation, fatigue, feelings of worthlessness or excessive or inappropriate guilt, diminished ability to think, or recurrent thoughts of

death; at least five of these symptoms must be present and at least one of the five must be either depressed mood or loss of interest.

Mastitis: inflammation of the breast.

Pessary: device inserted into the vagina to treat uterine prolapse, uterine retroversion, or cervical incompetence.

Postpartal hemorrhage: large amount (more than 500 ml) of bleeding after delivery, which may be caused by uterine atony, rupture, lacerations, inversion, or hematoma.

Postpartal period: approximately 6-week period following delivery during which the anatomic and physiologic changes resulting from pregnancy resolve (also called the puerperium).

Preeclampsia: nonconvulsive form of pregnancy-induced hypertension characterized by the onset of acute hypertension, proteinuria, and edema after the twenty-fourth week of gestation.

Pregnancy-induced hypertension: group of potentially life-threatening hypertensive disorders that may develop in the second or third trimester; includes preeclampsia and eclampsia.

Proteinuria: presence in the urine of abnormally large amounts of protein, usually albumin.

Puerperal infection: infection of the reproductive tract occurring during the postpartal period.

Pyelonephritis: acute inflammation of the ureters and kidneys, commonly caused by *Escherichia coli;* produces the effects of cystitis plus fever, chills, flank pain, and other signs and symptoms.

Retained placenta: condition in which the placenta remains in the uterus 30 minutes after the second stage of labor.

Salpingitis: inflammation or infection of the fallopian tube.

Thrombophlebitis: formation of a thrombus (clot) in response to inflammation of the vein wall.

Toxic shock syndrome: severe illness caused by a bacterial infection; has been associated with improper tampon use and typically causes sudden high fever, vomiting, diarrhea, myalgia, vaginal redness or discharge, skin rash, and sore throat.

Urinary tract infection: infection of one or more structures of the urinary tract; most commonly caused by gram-negative bacteria.

Uterine atony: poor uterine muscle tone.

Uterine inversion: abnormal condition in which the uterus is turned inside out so that the internal surface protrudes into or beyond the vagina; usually caused by excessive traction on the umbilical cord.

Uterine involution: gradual return of the uterus to a nonpregnant size and condition after delivery.

Uterine subinvolution: failure of the uterus to return to a nonpregnant size and condition after delivery.

Uterine prolapse: downward displacement of the uterus in which the cervix may protrude from the vagina.

allow bacterial entry (normally, the intact amniotic sac acts as a barrier, preventing bacteria from ascending into the uterine cavity). Intrauterine manipulation during delivery of the fetus and placenta also can result in infection (Cunningham, MacDonald, and Gant, 1989), as can contamination by health care personnel during vaginal examination in the second stage of labor.

Types of puerperal infection

A puerperal infection develops from a local lesion or its extension. With a local lesion, the infection remains within the original infection site. The vagina, the cervix, a hematoma, an episiotomy, and any other wounds (such as a laceration of the vulva, vagina, or perineum) are potential entry points for pathogenic organisms. An operation incision (such as from a cesarean delivery) also may be the source of infection; the mortality rate from puerperal infection is two to four times higher after cesarean than after vaginal delivery (Petetti, 1985).

Extension of the original lesion occurs when a localized infection spreads to other areas via the blood or lymphatic vessels, leading to such infections as salpingitis, parametritis, peritonitis, or thrombophlebitis. (For an illustration of the routes of some types of puerperal infection, see *Extension of puerperal infection*, pages 1098 and 1099.)

Localized wound infections
A localized infection may arise from a repaired external or internal wound. With infection of an external wound, such as an episiotomy, the apposing wound edges become edematous and separate; the wound then exudes pus and possibly sanguineous matter. An internal wound, such as a vaginal laceration, may become infected directly or by extension from the perineum. In this case, the vaginal mucosa becomes edematous and red; necrosis and sloughing follow. Cervical infection, which typically develops from a cervical laceration, may serve as the origin for a more distant infection.

Endometritis
After placental delivery, the placental attachment site is less than 2 mm thick, contains many small openings, and is infiltrated with blood, making it highly vulnerable to bacterial penetration; the remaining decidua also is susceptible to bacteria. Endometritis, the resulting infection, may involve the entire mucosa and sometimes impedes uterine involution (gradual return of the uterus to a nonpregnant size and condition).

Salpingitis
Commonly caused by gonorrheal organisms, this infection develops from bacterial spread into the lumen of the fallopian tubes. It usually manifests during the second week postpartum.

Parametritis
This infection, also called pelvic cellulitis, involves the retroperitoneal fibroareolar pelvic connective tissue; severe cases may involve connective tissue of all pelvic structures. Transmission may occur via lymphatic vessels from an infected cervical laceration or from a uterine incision or laceration. In some cases, however, parametritis represents ascent of an infection that began in a cervical laceration.

Peritonitis
This infection of the peritoneum arises in the same manner as parametritis. Generalized peritonitis poses a grave threat; bowel loops may become bound together by purulent exudate and abscesses may develop in various pelvic sites.

Thrombophlebitis
This venous inflammation occurs when a puerperal infection spreads through veins—usually the ovarian veins, which drain the upper part of the uterus. In thrombophlebitis, a thrombus, or clot, forms and attaches to the vessel wall. The condition is known as pelvic thrombophlebitis when it involves the uterine and ovarian veins and as femoral thrombophlebitis when it involves the femoral, popliteal, or saphenous veins. (For more information on thrombophlebitis, see the "Vascular complications" section of this chapter.)

Bacteremic (septic) shock
Parametritis, peritonitis, or thrombophlebitis may lead to systemic infection of the bloodstream, resulting in bacteremic shock. In this condition, vascular resistance decreases, causing a severe blood pressure decline and the threat of imminent death. Bacteremic shock most frequently stems from gram-negative organisms.

In toxic shock syndrome (TSS), a form of bacteremic shock, *Staphylococcus aureus* enters the bloodstream through microulcerations, or small abrasions, in the vaginal or cervical mucosa. Because vaginal and cervical lacerations are common during vaginal delivery, the postpartal client is at increased risk for developing TSS. (For details on TSS, see Chapter 13, Gynecologic Disorders.)

Extension of puerperal infection

A puerperal infection may arise from a localized infection that spreads through the blood or lymphatic vessels. Infection routes in three types of puerperal infections are illustrated.

PARAMETRITIS
Infection spreads via lymphatic vessels to the retroperitoneal fibroareolar pelvic connective tissue.

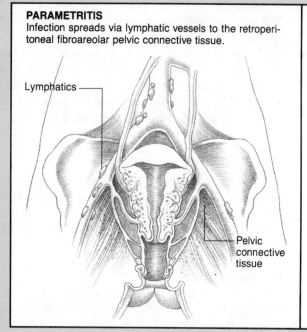

Lymphatics

Pelvic connective tissue

PERITONITIS
Infection spreads via lymphatic vessels to the peritoneum.

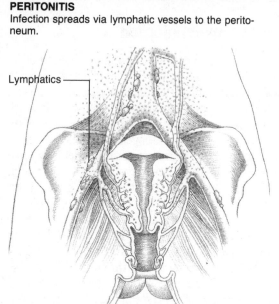

Lymphatics

Postpartal hemorrhage

Postpartal hemorrhage occurs when a client loses more than 500 ml of blood during or after the third stage of labor. Postpartal blood loss is particularly dangerous because it is hard to quantify or, in some cases, collects in the uterus, remaining occult. Blood loss commonly is underestimated at the time of delivery because precise measurement is difficult; actual loss usually is twice that of estimated loss (Cunningham, MacDonald, and Gant, 1989).

Postpartal hemorrhage may occur early or late. Early (or immediate) postpartal hemorrhage arises within 24 hours after delivery; it occurs in approximately 5% of postpartal clients (Cunningham, MacDonald, and Gant, 1989). Late (or delayed) hemorrhage develops 2 days to 6 weeks postpartum and occurs in approximately 0.1% of postpartal clients (Danforth and Scott, 1986).

Causes

Any condition that results in trauma during childbirth can lead to postpartal hemorrhage. The most common causes are uterine atony (poor muscle tone); lacerations of the vagina, cervix, perineum, or labia; and retained placental fragments.

Uterine atony

This condition may stem from uterine enlargement, such as with hydramnios (excessive amniotic fluid), multiple gestation (more than one fetus), or delivery of a very large neonate. As the uterus enlarges, its muscle fibers become overstretched and cannot contract effectively to compress vessels; thus the uterus continues to bleed, setting the stage for hemorrhage.

Other causes of uterine atony include a prolonged or accelerated labor (both of which exhaust uterine muscles), general anesthesia (which relaxes muscles), or administration of magnesium sulfate (for instance, to stop premature labor). Also, the client with a history of postpartal hemorrhage has an increased risk for uterine atony.

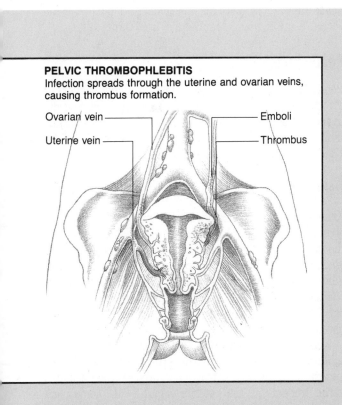

PELVIC THROMBOPHLEBITIS
Infection spreads through the uterine and ovarian veins, causing thrombus formation.

Ovarian vein

Uterine vein

Emboli

Thrombus

Lacerations

Laceration of the vagina, cervix, perineum, or labia provides a potential hemorrhage site. A cervical laceration is particularly likely to hemorrhage because of increased cervical vascularity during pregnancy and immediately after delivery. Perineal and vaginal lacerations also may contribute to postpartal blood loss. However, these wounds are more likely to cause long-term damage by weakening the perineal muscles, which may necessitate later surgery. (For more information on lacerations, see the section on "Birth canal injuries.")

Retained placental fragments

Retained placental fragments, which sometimes adhere to the uterus, can cause hemorrhage by impeding uterine contraction. In some cases, the entire placenta remains in the uterus at least 30 minutes after the second stage of labor (a condition known as retained placenta). Retained placental fragments are the major cause of late postpartal hemorrhage.

Other causes

Postpartal hemorrhage also may result from various other conditions.

Hematoma. This collection of extravasated blood forms when blood escapes into the connective tissue beneath the skin of the external genitalia (vulvar hematoma) or beneath the vaginal mucosa (vaginal hematoma).

Episiotomy dehiscence. An episiotomy may dehisce (split open) in response to such factors as pressure caused by a vaginal hematoma. Also, a client who is obese or who has diabetes mellitus is more susceptible to episiotomy dehiscence because these conditions impair healing.

Uterine inversion. Hemorrhage immediately follows this condition, in which the uterus is turned inside out. (For more information on uterine inversion, see Chapter 33, Intrapartal Complications.)

Uterine subinvolution. Uterine atony, retained placental fragments, or postpartal endometritis may cause this condition, in which the uterus fails to return to a nonpregnant size and condition after delivery.

Sequelae

A few clients who recover from severe postpartal hemorrhage suffer anterior pituitary gland necrosis, or Sheehan's syndrome. (For details on this condition, see *Postdelivery anterior pituitary necrosis*, page 1100.) Other potential sequelae of postpartal hemorrhage include transfusion reactions, hepatitis, and renal failure from prolonged hypotension.

Birth canal injuries

Many clients suffer lacerations of the vagina and cervix during childbirth; also, labor and delivery normally cause changes in the position of pelvic structures.

Vaginal and perineal lacerations

Lacerations of the anterior vagina near the urethra are relatively common intrapartal events (Cunningham, MacDonald, and Gant, 1989). Typically, these injuries

Postdelivery anterior pituitary necrosis

Approximately 15% of clients who survive severe hypovolemic shock associated with postpartal hemorrhage develop postdelivery anterior pituitary necrosis (Cunningham, MacDonald, and Gant, 1989). In this condition (also called Sheehan's syndrome or pituitary insufficiency), the pituitary gland becomes ischemic and necrotic, resulting in:
• failure to lactate
• loss of pubic and axillary hair
• breast and genital atrophy
• oligomenorrhea or amenorrhea
• fatigue.

The severity of signs and symptoms depends on the extent of pituitary damage. If 10% of the pituitary gland remains functional, the client can maintain a relatively normal status (Cunningham, MacDonald, and Gant, 1989). Treatment usually involves thyroid hormone, cortisone, and estrogen replacement, along with a diet high in protein and carbohydrate to counter weight loss and muscle wasting.

are accompanied by perineal lacerations; a deep perineal laceration may involve the anal sphincter and extend through the vaginal walls. Lacerations of the middle and upper thirds of the vagina, less common than anterior lacerations, usually result from forceps delivery; these wounds may lead to copious blood loss.

Cervical lacerations

Cervical lacerations up to 2 cm long are common during childbirth (Cunningham, MacDonald, and Gant, 1989). Normally, they heal uneventfully within 6 to 12 weeks and cause no further problems; however, the external os remains elongated permanently.

Deep cervical lacerations, an occasional result of precipitous labor, may lead to serious hemorrhage because of increased vascularity of the cervix and fragility of surrounding tissues. The tear may involve one or both sides of the cervix, possibly reaching up to or beyond the vaginal junction. Primiparous clients typically suffer more cervical lacerations than multiparous clients (Monheit, Cousins, and Resnik, 1980).

Levator ani injuries

The levator ani is one of a pair of muscles that lies across the pubic arch and pelvic diaphragm, supporting the perineal floor. Injury to this muscle results from over-

distention of the birth canal; this in turn may cause muscle fibers to separate or decrease in tone. When this happens, the pelvis becomes relaxed; urinary incontinence may develop if the pubococcygeal muscle is involved (Cunningham, MacDonald, and Gant, 1989).

Pelvic joint injury

Pelvic immobility and subsequent joint injury may occur if the client's legs are positioned improperly during delivery or if she remains in stirrups for a prolonged period. (For more information on this problem, see Chapter 29, The Third and Fourth Stages of Labor.)

Pelvic relaxation

Exaggeration of the normal relaxation of pelvic support structures during childbirth may cause displacement of the uterus and other pelvic structures. Uterine prolapse (downward displacement) occurs in varying degrees. In mild prolapse, the cervix descends below its normal position in the vaginal canal; in moderate prolapse, the cervix reaches the introitus; in severe prolapse, the entire uterus protrudes from the vagina.

Enterocele (prolapse of the intestine into the posterior vaginal wall), cystocele (prolapse of the bladder into the anterior vaginal wall), and urethrocele (prolapse of the urethra into the anterior vaginal wall) sometimes accompany uterine prolapse. The combination of marked cystocele and uterine prolapse may cause obstruction of the lower ureter, with resulting hydronephrosis and renal dysfunction. (For more information on uterine displacement, see Chapter 13, Gynecologic Disorders.)

Fistula

An abnormal passage, a fistula may follow a traumatic delivery, such as a difficult forceps delivery or a delivery in which pressure is exerted during slow fetal descent. The fistula may be vesicovaginal or rectovaginal. A vesicovaginal fistula is an opening between the vagina and the urinary tract (urethra, bladder, or ureter); urine passes into and discharges from the vagina. A rectovaginal fistula is an opening between the rectum and vagina in which flatus and stool may be discharged through the vagina. This type of fistula usually forms after unsuccessful repair of an episiotomy or laceration; although a portion of the anal sphincter heals after repair, the area above the sphincter may break down.

Vascular complications

Vascular complications of the postpartal period include pregnancy-induced hypertension and venous thrombosis.

Pregnancy-induced hypertension

Pregnancy-induced hypertension (PIH) refers to hypertensive disorders that develop between the twentieth week of pregnancy and the end of the first postpartal week. Preeclampsia refers to hypertension with albuminuria or edema. Eclampsia occurs in a client who has preeclampsia and involves seizures, possibly with coma; untreated, eclampsia usually is fatal.

Although the cause of PIH is unknown, inadequate prenatal care may be a contributing factor. Other possible predisposing factors include primigravidity, multiple gestation, preexisting diabetes mellitus or hypertension, and hydramnios. (For a detailed discussion of PIH, see Chapter 23, Antepartal Complications.)

Venous thrombosis

Venous thrombosis (thrombus formation in a vein) affects less than 1% of postpartal clients (Easterling and Herbert, 1986). Various conditions predispose the postpartal client to this disorder: increased levels of certain blood-clotting factors; greater platelet number and adhesiveness; release of thromboplastin substances from deciduous tissues, placenta, and fetal membranes; and increased fibrinolysis inhibition. Hydramnios, preeclampsia, cesarean delivery, and immobility are additional risk factors. Since early ambulation has become the norm, the frequency of venous thrombosis has decreased dramatically.

When venous thrombosis occurs in response to inflammation of the vein wall, it is known as thrombophlebitis. When no inflammation is present, it is termed phlebothrombosis. In thrombophlebitis, the thrombus is attached firmly to the vein wall; it is less likely to break away and form a life-threatening pulmonary embolus than in phlebothrombosis, in which the thrombus is attached more loosely.

Typically, thrombophlebitis lasts 4 to 6 weeks, with symptoms subsiding gradually. In severe cases, potentially fatal abscesses develop. Thrombophlebitis is most common in a superficial vein (superficial thrombophlebitis) but may develop in a deep leg vein (deep-vein thrombophlebitis). Typically, superficial thrombophlebitis manifests on the third or fourth postpartal day.

Other postpartal complications

Other complications of the postpartal period include mastitis, urinary tract disorders, diabetes mellitus, substance abuse, and postpartal psychosis.

Mastitis

This inflammation of the breast, which occurs in 2% to 3% of breast-feeding clients, involves the tissue around the nipple and sometimes the periglandular connective tissue as well (Cunningham, MacDonald, and Gant, 1989). The most common cause is infection by *S. aureus* bacteria; other causative organisms include beta-hemolytic streptococci, *Haemophilus influenzae, H. parainfluenzae, Escherichia coli,* and *Klebsiella pneumoniae.* The pathogenic organism usually enters through a crack or abrasion in the nipple (however, mastitis can occur even in clients with intact nipples). Frequent breast-feeding helps prevent mastitis.

Urinary tract disorders

Because of normal postpartal diuresis, urine production increases markedly in the first 48 hours after delivery; urine output typically measures 500 to 1,000 ml/voiding (Eschenbach and Wager, 1980). This increase in urine production heightens the risk of urinary tract infection. Other conditions that are common during the postpartal period, such as increased bladder filling and reduced sensitivity to the voiding urge, also may lead to urinary tract problems.

Cystitis
This inflammatory condition of the bladder and ureters may result from retention of stagnant urine in the bladder, catheterization, or bladder trauma during delivery. Usually, the infecting organisms ascend from the urethra to the bladder, then spread to the kidneys.

Pyelonephritis
This diffuse pyogenic inflammation of the pelvis and parenchyma of the kidney occurs when a bladder infection spreads to the ureters and kidneys; it begins in the interstitium and rapidly extends to the tubules, glomeruli, and blood vessels.

Bladder distention

This condition may follow urine retention, which results from increased bladder capacity and decreased sensitivity to the voiding urge (such as from bladder edema or anesthetics used during delivery). Also, the client with a distended bladder may void incompletely, leading to urine stasis—a condition that fosters bacterial growth and subsequent urinary tract infection. Bladder distention, in turn, may prevent uterine contractions and subsequent vessel compression, causing hemorrhage.

Urinary incontinence

Urinary incontinence may result from bladder distention with overflow or from relaxation of the pelvic floor muscles.

Diabetes mellitus

Diabetes mellitus refers to a group of endocrine disorders characterized by impaired carbohydrate metabolism secondary to insufficient insulin secretion or resistance to insulin by target tissue. Because pregnancy alters carbohydrate metabolism and increases the need for insulin, the blood glucose level may be difficult to control during pregnancy. Thus, a pregnant client with previously stable diabetes may suffer complications. (For a detailed discussion of diabetes in pregnant clients, see Chapter 22, High-Risk Antepartal Clients.)

In the early postpartal period, the diabetic client may need little or no exogenous insulin because the rapid postpartal decline in placental hormones and cortisol reduces opposition to insulin. However, as hormone levels begin to stabilize, the need for exogenous insulin increases. Throughout the postpartal period, the insulin dosage must be readjusted to achieve diabetic control in clients with insulin-dependent and noninsulin-dependent diabetes. Clients diagnosed with gestational diabetes usually resume a normal glucose status postpartally.

Substance abuse

In some clients, substance abuse is not detected until the postpartal period, when the neonate shows neurobehavioral abnormalities or other effects of maternal substance abuse. The reason is twofold: Many pregnant substance abusers do not seek prenatal care, and even if signs of substance abuse manifest earlier, the client may deny her problem because of fear of possible legal and social ramifications. (For a discussion of the effects of maternal substance abuse in neonates, see Chapter 38, High-Risk Neonates.)

Postpartal psychiatric disorder

Childbirth can sometimes precipitate a major depressive episode. In many cases, the client with a major depressive episode must be admitted to a psychiatric hospital for treatment.

Nursing care

The nurse uses the nursing process to assess the client for postpartal complications and to intervene appropriately.

Assessment

Thorough assessment with specific attention to the client's history necessary for early detection of a postpartal complication, which can help avert critical sequelae.

Puerperal infection

Review the client's history for risk factors (for details, see *Risk factors for puerperal infection*). Because puerperal infection is associated with temperature elevation, obtain vital signs regularly. Suspect an infection if the client has a morbid temperature, defined by the Joint Committee on Maternal Welfare as one that exceeds 100.4° F (38° C) for 2 successive days after delivery, excluding the first 24 hours (Gibbs and Weinstein, 1976). However, be aware that a low-grade fever is common postpartally; during the first 24 hours after delivery, it most likely represents spontaneous sloughing of necrotic decidua and blood from the uterine cavity, not infection.

Be sure to note any complaints of chills, malaise, or generalized pain or discomfort because these signs and symptoms commonly accompany infection. Assess uterine tone and fundal height, and evaluate lochial discharge, noting the amount, color, consistency, and odor. Also obtain information about the client's sleep and rest patterns and hydration and nutritional status.

Laboratory analysis typically reveals an elevated white blood cell count and an increased erythrocyte sedimentation rate if infection is present. Blood and vaginal cultures may be analyzed to isolate the causative organism; however, isolation typically proves difficult because a blood or vaginal culture may become contaminated by various microorganisms, and a vaginal culture may become contaminated by blood.

Risk factors for puerperal infection

The nurse should stay alert for signs and symptoms of infection in a postpartal client with any of the risk factors presented below.

PRENATAL RISK FACTORS

- Anemia
- History of venous thrombosis
- Lack of prenatal care
- Poor nutrition

INTRAPARTAL RISK FACTORS

- Cesarean delivery
- Chorioamnionitis (fetal membrane inflammation)
- Episiotomy
- Forceps delivery
- Numerous vaginal examinations during labor, especially after rupture of the membranes
- Intrauterine fetal monitoring
- Lacerations of the vaginal wall or perineum
- Prolonged rupture of membranes

POSTPARTAL RISK FACTORS

- Inadequate infection control
- Postpartal hemorrhage
- Retained placental fragments

Localized wound infection. Inspect for localized areas of edema, erythema, and tenderness; purulent drainage; gaping of wound edges; and dysuria. Stay alert for complaints of pain in a specific area. Lochial evaluation can be important; in a localized episiotomy infection, for instance, lochia may have a foul odor and appear yellow.

Endometritis. Check for a fever (which may range from low-grade to 103° F [39.4° C]), malaise, lethargy, anorexia, chills, a rapid pulse, lower abdominal pain or uterine tenderness, and severe afterpains. Lochia may range from normal to foul-smelling, scant or profuse, and bloody to serosanguineous and brown.

Parametritis. Besides the signs and symptoms seen in endometritis, this condition may cause a prolonged, sustained fever and tenderness on one or both sides of the abdomen.

Peritonitis. The clinical picture presented by peritonitis also resembles that of endometritis. Other possible findings include vomiting, diarrhea, anxiety, tachycardia, shallow respirations, and bowel distention. Also check for abdominal guarding, rigidity, and rebound tenderness.

Thrombophlebitis. Assess for tenderness, warmth, and redness in a portion of the vein, low-grade fever, and possibly a slight increase in the pulse. Try to elicit Homan's sign by dorsiflexing the foot; pain in the calf with this maneuver may signify thrombophlebitis. (For more information on assessing for thrombophlebitis, see "Vascular complications" later in this section).

Bacteremic shock. In the client who has a suspected or diagnosed infection, stay alert for fever, confusion, nausea, chills, vomiting, and hyperventilation. In early shock, arterial blood gas (ABG) measurements typically reflect respiratory alkalosis. Later, the client becomes apprehensive, restless, irritable, and thirsty; flushing, tachycardia, tachypnea, hypothermia, and anuria are typical. ABG findings may show a progression to metabolic acidosis with hypoxemia.

Besides ABG analysis, the physician will order various studies to verify the diagnosis and guide intervention—hematologic tests, leukocyte analysis, creatinine and blood urea nitrogen tests, central venous pressure, pulmonary artery and wedge pressures, and hemodynamic values.

Postpartal hemorrhage

This condition can progress to shock, so be sure to assess the client carefully and thoroughly. Because hemorrhage usually can be predicted, review the client's history for such predisposing conditions as a prolonged labor or prenatal anemia. (For other predisposing conditions, see *Anticipating postpartal hemorrhage,* page 1104). Also note the client's weight and frame size; a small-framed client is more likely than one with a larger frame to suffer hemorrhage. If possible, quantify blood loss, keeping in mind that a loss exceeding 500 ml is ominous.

Early postpartal hemorrhage may manifest either as a large gush or as a slow, steady trickle of blood from the vagina. Even a seemingly innocuous trickle may lead to significant blood loss, which becomes increasingly life-threatening.

Late postpartal hemorrhage usually has a sudden onset; shock may ensue rapidly. When this occurs, immediate intervention is crucial to prevent cardiac arrest and death. Because late postpartal hemorrhage typically occurs after discharge (up to 1 month postpartum) and without warning, it can be especially dangerous to the unsuspecting client.

To detect trends that may reveal deteriorating status in a client with significant blood loss, measure vital signs regularly and assess skin turgor and color. A serious hemorrhage may cause the skin to turn pale and clammy. It also may trigger chills, visual disturbances, and a rapid, thready pulse. However, keep in mind that pulse and blood pressure may not change significantly until

---

Anticipating postpartal hemorrhage

To ensure early detection of hemorrhage, the nurse should review the client's chart carefully for the following predisposing factors:

- Cesarean delivery
- Delivery of a large neonate
- Forceps or mid forceps rotation at delivery
- Hematoma
- Hydramnios
- Intrauterine manipulation
- Lacerations of the birth canal
- Magnesium sulfate use during labor
- Manual removal of the placenta
- Multiparity
- More than one fetus
- Premature placental separation
- Previous postpartal hemorrhage
- Prolonged labor
- Retained placental fragments
- Uterine atony
- Uterine inversion
- Uterine subinvolution

---

the client loses more than 10% of her blood volume. At this point, compensatory mechanisms triggered by hemorrhage fail and shock ensues; signs and symptoms then vary according to the stage of shock (as described earlier under "Bacteremic shock.")

Determining the cause of hemorrhage. In a client with excessive vaginal bleeding, try to determine the cause to help guide intervention. For instance, assess uterine tone; a firmly contracted fundus rules out uterine atony and suggests an unrepaired cervical laceration as the cause of bleeding.

If the client has severe perineal pain with sensitive ecchymosis, suspect vulvar hematoma as the cause of hemorrhage. A vaginal hematoma, on the other hand, manifests as severe rectal pain and pressure and inability to void. Be aware that a vaginal hematoma is more difficult to visualize than a vulvar hematoma.

To assess for episiotomy dehiscence, another possible cause of hemorrhage, carefully inspect the area surrounding the episiotomy sutures and assess general perineal healing at least three times daily. Pain, a gaping suture line, and a reddened, edematous episiotomy suggest dehiscence.

Signs and symptoms of uterine subinvolution, which also may lead to hemorrhage, include a large, noncontracted uterus positioned above the umbilicus, prolonged

lochial discharge, backache, and a heavy sensation in the pelvis.

Birth canal injuries

Injury to the birth canal may cause a wide range of signs and symptoms. To prevent further complications, these problems must be detected promptly. Review the client's history, especially the intrapartal records, for risk factors, which include:
- prolonged labor with protracted descent
- delivery of a large neonate
- abnormal fetal presentation
- cesarean, forceps, version, or vacuum extraction delivery
- previous history of cesarean delivery, traumatic delivery, uterine surgery, or postpartal hemorrhage
- uterine retroversion or anomaly.

Other key factors to assess for include the amount and color of vaginal bleeding, level of consciousness, subjective expressions of well-being, vital sign measurements and patterns, and fundal height and tone. Stay alert for signs of impending shock.

Perineal and vaginal lacerations. An extensive perineal laceration usually is apparent; this wound may bleed and interfere with normal voiding. The Redness, Edema, Ecchymosis, Discharge, Approximation (REEDA) scale may be used to assess the condition of the perineum. (For details on this tool, see *Using the REEDA scale*.) A vaginal laceration may bleed and is visible on pelvic examination.

Cervical lacerations. Signs and symptoms of a deep cervical laceration include bright red (arterial) vaginal bleeding with a firmly contracted uterus. The cervix appears lacerated, edematous, bruised, and ulcerated.

Levator ani injury. When the client resumes sexual intercourse, she may report a reduction in pleasure. Urinary incontinence may occur if the pubococcygeal muscle also was involved. If the injury caused weakening of the perineal floor, intercourse may be painful (a condition called dyspareunia).

Pelvic relaxation. Uterine prolapse is visible on vaginal examination. To help determine the degree of prolapse, the examiner may ask the client to bear down during the examination. Also, the client may report a sensation of a lump in the vagina during prolonged standing or straining. If the cervix is irritated or eroded from its descent, vaginal discharge may occur (although this may be masked by lochial discharge). With cystocele and urethrocele, the client may retain urine, which may lead to frequency and urgency on urination and other signs and symptoms of urinary tract infection.

Using the REEDA scale

To evaluate perineal healing after an episiotomy or laceration, the nurse may use the Redness, Edema, Ecchymosis, Discharge, Approximation (REEDA) scale. This scale, which provides a means for objective assessment, evaluates the five components of healing (as its name suggests). Daily documentation allows tracking of the healing. The total score may range from 1 to 15; the higher the total, the worse the condition of the perineum.

POINTS	REDNESS	EDEMA	ECCHYMOSIS	DISCHARGE	APPROXIMATION
0	None	None	None	None	Closed
1	Within 0.25 cm of incision bilaterally	Perineal, less than 1 cm from incision	Within 0.25 cm bilaterally or 0.5 cm unilaterally	Serous	Skin separation 3 mm or less
2	Within 0.5 cm of incision bilaterally	Perineal or vulvar, between 1 and 2 cm from incision	Between 0.25 and 1 cm bilaterally or between 0.5 and 2 cm unilaterally	Serosanguineous	Skin and subcutaneous fat separation
3	Beyond 0.5 cm of incision bilaterally	Perineal or vulvar, greater than 2 cm from incision	Greater than 1 cm bilaterally or 2 cm unilaterally	Bloody, purulent	Skin, subcutaneous fat, and fascial layer separation
SCORE					
				TOTAL	

Davidson, N. (1974). REEDA: Evaluating postpartum healing. *Journal of Nurse-Midwifery,* 19(2), 6-9. Used with permission.

Pelvic relaxation may cause stress incontinence (involuntary discharge of urine on coughing, laughing, sneezing, or straining). Diagnosis of stress incontinence can be made on pelvic examination by manually restoring and maintaining the normal posterior urethrovesical angle to check for deformity (reflected by an increased angle).

Fistula. Vesicovaginal fistula causes involuntary discharge of urine from the vagina. Rectovaginal fistula causes involuntary discharge of flatus and stool from the vagina.

Vascular complications
Evaluate the client for evidence of PIH and venous thrombosis.

PIH. Usually, signs and symptoms of PIH subside rapidly after delivery. However, in the high-risk client, monitor blood pressure closely during the first 24 hours postpartum. Suspect PIH if systolic pressure rises at least 30 mm Hg and diastolic pressure increases at least 15 mm Hg above the baseline value. Be aware that an increase in blood pressure may signify an impending seizure.

With mild preeclampsia, expect generalized edema and proteinuria in addition to hypertension. With severe preeclampsia, blood pressure increases more sharply and the client typically complains of a severe, persistent headache and visual disturbances, such as blurring. She also may have epigastric pain, hyperreflexia (exaggerated reflexes), vomiting, apprehensiveness, photophobia, and sensitivity to noise.

Inspect the client's hands and feet for edema, which may make visualization of the joints impossible. Be sure to assess fluid intake and urine output; the latter may drop below 30 ml/hour even if the client is receiving I.V. fluids. Weigh the client daily to assess postpartal diuresis.

Promptly report urine output below 30 ml/hour, proteinuria, and other suggestive findings to the physician. In the preeclamptic client, blood volume may increase without an accompanying increase in hemoglobin; thus, an accurate hemoglobin measurement is important. The physician usually orders clotting studies to rule out disseminated intravascular coagulation (DIC), a grave bleeding disorder resulting from damage to the vessel wall. Such damage is a characteristic feature of preeclampsia (Cunningham, MacDonald, and Gant, 1989) and may predispose the client to DIC. (For a more detailed discussion of clinical findings in PIH, see Chapter 23, Antepartal Complications.)

Venous thrombosis. Check the client's history for the following risk factors:

- obesity
- age over 40
- parity greater than three
- previous history of venous thrombosis
- anemia
- heart disease
- venous stasis from prolonged inactivity, such as after anesthesia and surgery.

With superficial thrombophlebitis, the affected vessel feels hard and thready or cordlike and is extremely sensitive to pressure. The surrounding area may be erythematous and feel warm; the entire limb may be pale, cold, and swollen. The client may have a low-grade fever.

In a client with suspected DVT or one who is at risk for DVT, perform a general assessment, including temperature measurement. Stay alert for complaints of cramping or aching pain in a specific region, especially if that region appears stiff, swollen, and red. Attempt to elicit Homan's sign; however, be aware that a negative Homan's sign does not rule out DVT. Other manifestations of DVT include malaise, edema of the ankle and leg with taut, shiny skin over the edematous area, fever, and chills. Measure leg, calf, and thigh circumferences to document any edema.

When the popliteal vein is involved, expect pain in the popliteal and lateral tibial areas; with anterior and posterior tibial vein involvement, the entire lower leg and foot are painful. Inguinal pain suggests femoral vein involvement; lower abdominal pain, iliofemoral vein involvement.

Pulmonary embolism, a potential complication of venous thrombosis, may manifest as sudden onset of dyspnea accompanied by diaphoresis, pallor, confusion, and a blood pressure decrease. The client may complain of chest pain accompanied by anxiety, tachycardia, and weakness. If these signs and symptoms occur, notify the physician immediately. Prompt initiation of therapy improves the chance for recovery.

Other postpartal complications

Assess the client for evidence of mastitis, urinary tract disorders, diabetes mellitus, substance abuse, and postpartal psychiatric disorder.

Mastitis. Signs and symptoms of mastitis typically do not arise until 2 to 3 weeks after delivery. A portion of the breast is firm, tender, reddened, and warm; axillary lymph nodes may become enlarged. The client reports chills, malaise, headache, nausea, and aching joints. Typ-

ically, the body temperature measures 102° to 104° F (38.8° to 40° C). A culture of breast milk or the neonate's throat will identify the causative organism; elevated leukocyte and bacterial counts indicate infectious mastitis (Niebyl, 1985).

Urinary tract disorders. With cystitis, expect urinary urgency and frequency, dysuria, discomfort over the bladder area, hematuria, and a low-grade fever. With pyelonephritis, expect urinary urgency, dysuria, nocturia, cloudy urine, chills, and flank pain accompanied by a temperature of 102° F or higher.

Bladder distention causes a boggy (soft) uterus that is displaced upward and to the right. Bladder distention with overflow is characterized by frequent voiding of small amounts (less than 75 ml/voiding).

Diabetes mellitus. If the client's history indicates that she has diabetes, be aware that she is at increased risk for developing other postpartal complications, including infection, hemorrhage, hypoglycemia, and hyperglycemia. Also, because of cardiovascular degeneration, the risk of preeclampsia is four times greater in diabetic clients than in the general population (Gilbert and Harmon, 1986).

Infection in the diabetic client typically involves the urinary tract; the vagina also is vulnerable because of altered pH and glycosuria, conditions conducive to bacterial growth (Gilbert and Harmon, 1986). If the client had a cesarean delivery, monitor her closely for infection at the incision site and the indwelling catheter site. If she delivered vaginally, assess episiotomy healing and evaluate lochia for signs of infection (such as foul odor or a yellow or greenish color).

Also assess for signs of hemorrhage; its risk in the diabetic client stems from her predisposition to hydramnios and fetal macrosomia (large fetal size). These conditions cause uterine overdistention, which in turn may lead to uterine atony and subsequent postpartal hemorrhage.

Hyperglycemia or hypoglycemia may develop as plunging levels of placental hormones alter postpartal glucose metabolism. Psychological stressors, such as strong postpartal emotions, and the physical work of labor contribute to glucose alterations. To detect hyperglycemia, assess for thirst, hunger, weight loss, and polyuria. Left untreated, hyperglycemia may lead to diabetic ketoacidosis. Also check for indications of hypoglycemia—tremulousness, cold sweats, piloerection, hypothermia, and headache. Confusion, hallucinations, bizarre behavior, and, ultimately, seizures and coma may occur in late hypoglycemia.

Substance abuse. Because postpartal hospital stays are shorter than ever, remain alert for and report possible signs of substance abuse. These signs fall into three categories: physical, psychosocial, and obstetric.

Physical signs of substance abuse include chronic nasal congestion, dilated pupils, anorexia nervosa, tachycardia, irregular pulse, and needle marks on the skin. Physical signs in the neonate also may suggest substance abuse. (For information on assessing the effects of maternal substance abuse in neonates, see Chapter 38, High-Risk Neonates.)

Psychosocial signs include memory loss, frequent mood swings, hostile or violent behavior, low self-esteem, and a drastic change in financial or social status.

Suggestive obstetric findings include a previous preterm delivery, history of abruptio placentae, hypertension, precipitous delivery, and previous delivery of a low-birth-weight neonate.

The substance-dependent client may develop cardiovascular and central nervous system complications. Cocaine and certain other vasoconstrictive drugs may cause a transient increase in blood pressure, which may be mistaken for preeclampsia.

Abusing multiple substances is common and may complicate assessment, hindering anticipation of maternal and neonatal needs. To help detect any drugs ingested in the previous few hours or days, the physician may order toxicologic urine and blood screening. When assessing a client suspected of abusing drugs, try to establish a rapport and convey a caring, nonjudgmental attitude. If she admits to abusing substances, attempt to elicit the following information:
• extent and type of substance abused
• any substance abused by the client's partner
• previous participation in a substance-abuse treatment program
• degree of a commitment to stop substance abuse.

Postpartal psychiatric disorder. This disorder usually arises after discharge. However, a review of the client's history may help anticipate a problem.

Signs and symptoms of postpartal major depressive episode, the most serious postpartal psychiatric disorder, include depressed mood, markedly diminished interest or pleasure in activities, significant weight loss or gain, insomnia or hypersomnia, psychomotor agitation, fatigue, feelings of worthlessness or excessive or inappropriate guilt, diminished ability to think, and recurrent thoughts of death. At least five of these symptoms must be present and at least one of them must be either depressed mood or loss of interest (DSM-III-R, 1987). The client may demonstrate a lack of bonding with the neonate, or she may express overt hostility and a desire to harm herself. She may feel unable to love her neonate and may lose her ability to cope with family life and its everyday tasks.

Psychosocial assessment

If the client has a diagnosed postpartal complication, conduct a thorough psychosocial assessment to determine:
• how well she is coping with the complication
• whether the complication is affecting her ability to care for and bond with the neonate
• how the complication is affecting her family.

To help determine psychosocial status, urge the client to express her feelings about the delivery and her plans for the neonate's arrival at home. Assess the adequacy of family support that will be available during the first 2 postpartal weeks.

Evaluation of mother-neonate interaction is an important part of the psychosocial assessment and should be conducted over more than one observation period. Dyadal nursing care, in which a single nurse (per shift) cares for both the client and neonate, maximizes this assessment. (For details on psychosocial assessment, see Chapter 43, Psychosocial Adaptation of the Postpartal Family.)

Nursing diagnosis

After gathering all of the assessment data, the nurse must review it carefully to identify pertinent nursing diagnoses for the client. (For a partial list of applicable diagnoses, see *Nursing diagnoses: Postpartal complications*, page 1108.)

Planning and implementation

After assessing the client and formulating nursing diagnoses, the nurse develops and implements a care plan. Nursing goals include preventing or detecting complications early, carrying out appropriate interventions, and providing emotional support and teaching to the client and her family to help them cope with the situation.

Providing emotional support is especially important if the client has a nursing diagnosis of **anxiety related to perceived health status.** For the client with a nursing diagnosis of **knowledge deficit related to the etiology and treatment of the postpartal complication,** explain the cause of the complication, the expected course, and the planned treatments.

Puerperal infection

For the client with a nursing diagnosis of **potential for infection related to broken skin or traumatized tissue,** prevention is the best intervention. Careful aseptic technique, especially thorough hand washing, is crucial. To

NURSING DIAGNOSES

Postpartal complications

The following are potential nursing diagnoses for problems and etiologies that the nurse may encounter when caring for a client with a postpartal complication. Specific nursing interventions for many of these diagnoses are provided in the "Planning and implementation" section of this chapter.

- Altered health maintenance related to decreased capacity for deliberative and thoughtful judgment
- Altered tissue perfusion: peripheral, related to hypovolemia
- Anxiety related to perceived health status
- Body image disturbance related to birth canal injury
- Fluid volume deficit related to active postpartal hemorrhage
- Ineffective breast-feeding related to an interrupted breast-feeding schedule or inability to initiate breast-feeding
- Ineffective individual coping related to a deficit in problem-solving skills
- Knowledge deficit related to aseptic technique and perineal hygiene
- Knowledge deficit related to dietary and insulin requirements
- Knowledge deficit related to the etiology and treatment of the postpartal complication
- Pain related to birth canal injury
- Potential altered parenting related to interrupted mother-infant bonding
- Potential for infection related to broken skin, traumatized tissue, and altered blood glucose level
- Potential for infection related to a fistula, uterine prolapse, or venous stasis
- Potential for injury related to dislodgement of a blood clot
- Potential for injury related to seizure secondary to eclampsia
- Potential for violence: self-directed or directed at others, related to postpartal psychiatric disorder
- Sexual dysfunction related to altered body structure secondary to a birth canal injury
- Sleep pattern disturbance related to the need for frequent monitoring

prevent cross-contamination among clients, make sure each client has her own sanitary supplies and that non-disposable items are cleaned after each use.

Also teach the client techniques that help prevent infection. (Client teaching is important even if an infection already is diagnosed.) For instance, although the closed vulva protects the birth canal from bacterial invasion after delivery, the client must maintain perineal hygiene to preserve this barrier. To prevent contamination of the vagina with rectal bacteria, instruct her to use a front-to-back motion when applying perineal pads and cleansing the vulvar and perineal area.

For the client with a diagnosed infection, expect to administer antimicrobial and antipyretic therapy. The physician will choose an antibiotic based on the location and severity of the infection, the causative organism, and the client's physiologic status. Usually, the physician takes an aggressive treatment approach, choosing a broad-spectrum antibiotic because blood and vaginal cultures rarely identify specific causative organisms in puerperal infection. Many clients require a combination of oral and I.V. antibiotics.

The physician also may order analgesics to help relieve general malaise, headache, and backache. For a localized wound infection, the physician may incise the infected area or remove sutures to promote drainage.

Independent nursing actions for the client with a puerperal infection focus on alleviating signs and symptoms and helping to meet the client's psychosocial needs. Thus, be prepared to carry out comfort measures, ensure adequate rest, and provide a relaxed, quiet environment to counter malaise. To promote healing, provide sitz baths or a perineal heat lamp, if prescribed. Teach the client how to clean and change the dressing over the infected area and how to remove and apply perineal pads properly, using a front-to-back motion. Also, ensure a fluid intake of 2,000 ml/day.

Allow the client and neonate to spend as much time together as possible. If she has a nursing diagnosis of *knowledge deficit related to the etiology and treatment of the postpartal complication,* teach her and her family about her condition and treatment, and provide emotional support and encouragement. To help them work through anxiety and discouragement, encourage them to express their feelings.

Postpartal hemorrhage

Early identification and prompt, aggressive intervention are necessary to avert grave consequences of hemorrhage. As with puerperal infection, prevention is the optimal defense. (For a case study that shows how to apply the nursing process when caring for a client with a postpartal complication, see *Applying the nursing process: Client with a fluid volume deficit related to active postpartal hemorrhage,* pages 1114 and 1115.)

Prevention strategies. Prevention hinges on averting or treating underlying causes of hemorrhage. To detect retained placental fragments, the nurse-midwife or physician will inspect the delivered placenta for completeness; missing pieces warrant uterine exploration.

After placental separation, the physician may order an oxytocic drug to prevent uterine atony, another potential cause of hemorrhage. When administering an oxytocic drug, monitor vital signs and uterine contractions every 15 minutes. Gentle uterine massage also helps to stimulate uterine contractions (as described in Chapter 42, Care during the Normal Postpartal Period). If oxytocic therapy and uterine massage fail to stimulate contractions, expect surgical exploration and evacuation of the uterus.

To prevent hemorrhage from a deep cervical laceration, immediate suturing is necessary. However, perfect repair is difficult, and suturing sometimes causes further complications (such as cervical inversion and exposure of the endocervical glands).

Blood loss from a hematoma commonly is underestimated, so be prepared for the possibility of hemorrhage in the client with a vulvar or vaginal hematoma. (Small hematomas, however, usually reabsorb naturally.) To prevent serious blood loss from a hematoma, the physician may incise and evacuate, or drain, the hematoma. Because incision and evacuation may cause infection, be sure to practice aseptic technique and teach the client how to perform perineal hygiene, especially if she has a nursing diagnosis of *knowledge deficit related to aseptic technique and perineal hygiene.*

To prevent serious hemorrhage from episiotomy dehiscence, the physician will incise and drain the area. If dehiscence results from an infection, the physician will order antibiotic therapy. Aseptic technique, frequent perineal pad changes, and careful hygiene are critical in the treatment of dehiscence.

If the client has suffered uterine inversion, blood replacement and surgical reinversion are needed to save the client's life. (For more information, see Chapter 33, Intrapartal Complications.)

To avert hemorrhage from uterine subinvolution, the physician may prescribe oxytocic agents to stimulate uterine contraction or increase uterine tone. Curettage may be performed to remove retained placental tissue. Because breast-feeding stimulates uterine contractions, thereby aiding involution, encourage the client to begin or continue breast-feeding (if she has chosen this feeding method).

General interventions. When caring for the client with postpartal hemorrhage, be sure to conduct frequent, careful observations to detect status changes early. Closely monitor the following:
• vital signs
• fundal status, the amount and frequency of uterine massage administered, and any blood clots expressed
• number of perineal pads used, the percentage of pad saturation, and the time required to saturate the pad (weigh pads to assess blood loss)
• amount, color, consistency, and odor of lochia
• fluid intake and urine output (output should measure at least 30 ml/hour).

Check the client's level of consciousness frequently and report any changes to the physician. Be sure to maintain fluid replacement carefully because the client will have a nursing diagnosis of *fluid volume deficit related to active postpartal hemorrhage.* When administering oxytocic therapy, check I.V. lines for patency, and document the effectiveness of therapy. Also document central venous pressure (CVP) recordings and perform CVP maintenance. As prescribed, type and crossmatch blood in anticipation of transfusion or surgery.

Because this client has a nursing diagnosis of *altered tissue perfusion: peripheral, related to hypovolemia,* be prepared to carry out the following measures:
• Increase the existing I.V. infusion rate or start an I.V. drip to boost circulating blood volume, as prescribed.
• Assist with insertion of a CVP line (if one was not inserted earlier).
• Administer an I.V. oxytocic agent (such as oxytocin [Pitocin] or methylergonovine [Methergine]), as prescribed.
• Give supplemental oxygen at 6 liters/minute, as prescribed.
• Insert a urinary catheter, as prescribed.
• Lower the head of the bed, and position the client supine.
• Monitor the client's vital signs, urine output, blood loss, and general condition.
• Massage the fundus gently but firmly.
• Draw blood for a complete blood count; type and crossmatch the client's blood for possible transfusion, as prescribed.
• Monitor vital signs every 5 to 15 minutes.
• Provide simple, appropriate explanations to the client to allay her anxiety.
• Keep a count of perineal pads applied, and document the percentage of saturation and saturation time.

Birth canal injuries
Any birth canal injury may cause fatigue. Thus, group nursing procedures together to promote sleep and rest. Also, help the client participate in her recovery to the extent that she can. To help avoid a nursing diagnosis of *sexual dysfunction related to altered body structure secondary to a birth canal injury,* teach her how to perform Kegel exercises to strengthen pelvic floor muscles. (For information on these exercises, see Chapter 42, Care during the Normal Postpartal Period.)

Depending on their size and location, some perineal and vaginal lacerations heal on their own. For the client with a nursing diagnosis of *pain related to birth canal injury,* provide pain relief measures and teach the client how to manage pain through the use of sitz baths, topical or oral medications, and distraction. (For a related study, see *Nursing research applied: Comparison of heat and cold application to the perineum after an episiotomy or laceration.*) If the client has difficulty voiding, insert an indwelling catheter, as prescribed, until healing begins.

An extensive perineal or vaginal laceration that bleeds profusely requires suturing, as does a deep cervical laceration. Because of their location, labial lacerations are difficult to repair and cause much discomfort during healing.

For a levator ani injury, medical and nursing management vary depending on the severity of the injury as well as the emotional impact on the client and family. In some cases, surgery is necessary; in others, the injury heals spontaneously.

For uterine prolapse, the physician manually repositions the uterus in the pelvis and may insert a pessary to elevate it and support the ligaments. Usually, the physician inserts the pessary initially, then the client removes it before going to bed and reinserts it each morning. Teach her how to insert the pessary correctly; instruct her to wash it with a mild antiseptic solution and to rinse it thoroughly before each insertion.

For a vesicovaginal fistula, the physician will attempt surgical repair. After surgery, the bladder must be drained for 10 days via an indwelling catheter. If surgical repair is not possible, the physician will order continuous bladder drainage because spontaneous closure of the fistula sometimes occurs. For a rectovaginal fistula, management involves surgical repair and antibiotic therapy. Because this client may have a nursing diagnosis of ***body image disturbance related to birth canal injury,*** be sure to provide emotional support. Passage of urine or stool through a fistula can make this injury particularly stressful for the client.

Vascular complications

Skilled nursing intervention for the postpartal client with PIH or venous thrombosis can help avert a negative outcome of these complications.

PIH. Nursing management for preeclampsia and eclampsia focuses on preventing seizures and monitoring signs and symptoms of these disorders. The ultimate goal is to stabilize the client's status by intervening appropriately, providing optimal environmental conditions, and promoting psychosocial adjustment.

Nursing interventions. If the client was diagnosed as preeclamptic during pregnancy, the physician may order I.V. magnesium sulfate postpartally to decrease the seizure threshold, provide sedation, and dilate blood vessels. (See Chapter 23, Antepartal Complications, for a detailed discussion of nursing care for the client receiving mag-

---

NURSING RESEARCH APPLIED

Comparison of heat and cold application to the perineum after an episiotomy or laceration

A warm sitz bath is the traditional method used to relieve postpartal perineal discomfort. After trauma, heat application increases local arteriolar dilation and blood flow, promoting wound healing and providing analgesia. Cold application, on the other hand, constricts vessels, resulting in decreased blood flow and local bleeding; cold also reduces edema. Because of these effects, some investigators have proposed that cold therapy may promote earlier trauma resolution and more effective pain relief.

To test this hypothesis, the researcher randomly assigned 90 postpartal women to one of three treatment groups—warm perineal pack, cold perineal pack, or warm sitz bath. The treatments, which were administered in the first 24 hours postpartum, lasted 20 minutes. All of the subjects had perineal discomfort from an episiotomy, laceration, or both.

The subjects rated their perineal discomfort before treatment, immediately afterward, and 30 minutes, 1 hour, and 2 hours later. An examiner (who did not know which treatment group the subject was in) objectively assessed the condition of the perineum before each treatment and 2 hours afterward, using the Redness, Edema, Ecchymosis, Discharge, Approximation (REEDA) scale.

The study found no significant differences in REEDA scores among the three treatment groups. However, in the eight subjects whose edema worsened during the study period, seven had received either a warm pack or a warm sitz bath. This finding suggests that heat may increase perineal edema. Also, the researcher suggests that the cold packs might have been more effective in reducing edema had a less absorbent covering been used or treatment time extended. The small sample size and lack of sufficient time between treatment and objective assessment also may have limited the detection of significant differences among the three groups.

Application to practice

Because REEDA scores correlated with subjective reports of pain, this study supports the use of the REEDA scale to assess perineal condition. Also, although the findings do not show that cold application is superior to warmth in relieving perineal discomfort, the researcher's use of an objective tool to evaluate perineal condition makes this study suitable as an objective baseline with which future researchers can compare their findings. Future studies perhaps should aim to investigate the effectiveness of cold packs applied for an extended time, beginning immediately after delivery.

Hill, P. D. (1989). Effects of heat and cold on the perineum after episiotomy/laceration. *JOGNN*, 18(2), 124-129.

---

nesium sulfate.) A narcotic also may be prescribed. Immediately report any change in the client's condition.

Usually, the preeclamptic client will not receive oxytocic agents postpartally because of their hypertensive qualities; therefore, make sure to massage the uterus frequently to promote uterine contractions. Also encourage frequent voiding to keep the bladder empty and thus help avoid uterine atony.

The eclamptic client has a nursing diagnosis of *potential for injury related to seizure secondary to eclampsia.* To help ensure client safety in case of a seizure, make sure bed rails are padded, an airway is at the bedside, and emergency equipment (including oxygen and suction apparatus) is readily available. During a seizure, do not attempt to force open the client's mouth. Strong muscle contractions prevent the jaws from opening without injury; also, the client may bite off a portion of any object in her mouth and aspirate it during the seizure. After the seizure is over, move the tongue aside with a tongue depressor and insert an oral airway.

Environmental management. Maintaining an optimal environment is crucial for the client with PIH. Minimize external stimulation by keeping the room dark and removing the telephone and television; the ring of a telephone or a flickering image on the TV screen may cause a seizure. Keep visitors to a minimum and visits short. Once the client shows signs of improvement, external stimuli can be reintroduced gradually.

When providing care, be thorough and efficient so as to disturb the client as little as possible. For instance, group together vital sign checks, hanging of I.V. solutions, dressing changes, pain assessments, and other routine nursing procedures. As soon as the client's condition improves, extend the time between vital sign checks.

Psychosocial management. The client who is not critically ill probably will express concern about her own and the neonate's physical safety, leading to a nursing diagnosis of *anxiety related to perceived health status.* Assure her that her condition is not permanent and probably will reverse. If the neonate is in the neonatal intensive care unit (NICU), encourage her to keep in touch with the NICU staff by telephone. Urge family members to visit the nursery so that they can tell the client about the neonate. If possible, place a photograph of the neonate at the client's bedside.

On the other hand, if the client is too ill or too sedated to inquire about the neonate or even to remember the delivery, suggest that the nurse who attended during labor and delivery talk to her to help her understand the circumstances.

Venous thrombosis. Preventing and detecting pulmonary embolism are the highest priorities when caring for the postpartal client with venous thrombosis who has a nursing diagnosis of *potential for injury related to dislodgement of a blood clot.* Monitor the client for dyspnea, a low-grade fever, tachycardia, chest pain, a productive cough, pleural friction rub, and signs of circulatory collapse. As prescribed, administer an anticoagulant, and monitor for therapeutic efficacy and adverse effects of the drug. Observe closely for signs of bleeding, and teach the client about the drug's purpose, adverse effects, and interactions with any other medications she is receiving. For thrombophlebitis, also expect to administer antibiotics.

Do not massage or rub the affected extremity and caution the client never to do this, especially if she has phlebothrombosis. Because the thrombus is loosely attached to the vessel wall, rubbing can dislodge it, increasing the risk of embolism.

Management of the client with superficial thrombophlebitis typically involves local heat application, elevation of the affected limb, bed rest, analgesics, and use of elastic stockings to help prevent blood from pooling in the legs. If these interventions are ineffective, the physician may prescribe an anticoagulant. For DVT, treatment typically includes I.V. heparin therapy, bed rest, analgesics, elevation of the affected limb, and elastic stockings.

Once symptoms subside, the client can resume ambulation gradually. Instruct her to wear elastic support stockings and to perform prescribed leg exercises. Caution her not to stand or sit for long periods and to avoid crossing her legs because this reduces circulation. Make sure she knows how to identify signs and symptoms of thrombus formation, and advise her to call the physician when they occur. Also teach her how to manage symptoms and relieve pain. For instance, warm, moist soaks increase circulation to the affected area, and analgesics provide pain relief. Throughout her stay in the health care facility, encourage her to visit with the neonate frequently to promote bonding.

Other postpartal complications

Nursing care for these widely varying complications depends on the specific disorder. For example, in cases where the client abuses substances or has postpartal psychosis, a multidisciplinary management approach is particularly important.

Mastitis. Because this infection usually manifests after discharge, teach the client how to prevent and detect mastitis when preparing her for discharge. The first line of defense against mastitis is prevention of cracked nipples. Advise the client not to use soap or alcohol to clean the nipples because these substances have a drying effect. Instead, instruct her to use plain water, allow the nipples to air dry, then apply a breast cream that does not contain lanolin. To avoid undue tension on the tissues, instruct her to remove the neonate from her breast carefully at the end of a feeding session. Because mastitis also may result from milk duct blockage and resulting milk stasis, advise the client to breast-feed frequently and to call the physician if her breasts become severely engorged.

Treatment for mastitis includes a full course of organism-specific antibiotic (usually lasting 10 days), bed rest for at least 48 hours, close monitoring, and client teaching. (See *Client teaching: Self-care for mastitis.*)

An untreated breast infection may result in an abscess, necessitating surgery. Even after surgery, however, the client usually can continue breast-feeding with no ill effects (Niebyl, 1985; Tully and Overfield, 1989). However, teach or remind her how to place the neonate's mouth carefully on the nipple. If postoperative breast-feeding is contraindicated, advise her to pump her breasts for several days until breast-feeding can resume. This may avert a nursing diagnosis of *ineffective breast-feeding related to an interrupted breast-feeding schedule or inability to initiate breast-feeding.*

Urinary tract disorders. Expect to administer antimicrobial therapy, provide comfort measures (such as sitz baths), and apply topical antiseptics. Catheterization may be necessary to prevent stagnant urine from accumulating in the bladder. Ensure a fluid intake of more than 3,000 ml/day, and record fluid intake and output. As prescribed, collect urine specimens for culturing.

Diabetes mellitus. Caring for the postpartal diabetic client can be challenging because her blood glucose level may fluctuate widely, causing rapid changes in her exogenous insulin requirement. Medical management focuses on returning the client gradually to her prepregnancy insulin dosage. (The postpartal insulin dosage typically is half, or even less, of the prepregnancy dosage.) The client may return to her prepregnancy dosage within 48 hours to 1 month postpartum, although this varies with the intrapartal course of the disease (Robertson, 1987).

Nursing care centers on monitoring serial blood glucose measurements and observing for signs of hypoglycemia and hyperglycemia, preventing or controlling complications of diabetes, and teaching the client about her insulin needs. Also, ensure proper nutrition and promote mother-infant bonding (as described in Chapter 43, Psychosocial Adaptation of the Postpartal Family).

Monitoring blood glucose. Monitor the client's blood glucose level every 4 hours or more frequently, as needed. Instruct her to call for help immediately if she notices signs or symptoms of hypoglycemia or hyperglycemia. If hyperglycemia occurs, monitor urine for ketones every 4 hours.

CLIENT TEACHING

Self-care for mastitis

To help ensure a complete recovery from mastitis, follow the guidelines below.

- Breast-feed your infant at least every 2 or 3 hours.
- Begin breast-feeding with the affected breast and continue with this breast until it feels completely soft.
- To allow your breast to empty completely, do not wear a brassiere or other restrictive clothing when breast-feeding.
- Breast-feed in different positions during each feeding session to promote full drainage of all milk ducts.
- Immediately before each feeding, apply a warm, wet washcloth to the affected area. Repeat this as often as desired.
- Gently massage the affected area while you breast-feed.
- Express by hand or pump any milk your infant does not remove from your breast.
- Increase your daily fluid intake by several glasses.
- Rest as much as possible, and ask your family and friends for help with other children and household chores.
- Contact the physician if your infant develops diarrhea (this may mean that your mastitis medication should be changed) or if you do not feel better after 48 hours of antibiotics and breast-feeding.

This teaching aid may be reproduced by office copier for distribution to clients. © 1991, Springhouse Corporation.

Preventing or controlling complications. This client has a nursing diagnosis of *potential for infection related to broken skin, traumatized tissue, and altered blood glucose level.* To help detect infection, monitor the client's temperature at least every 4 hours for the first 24 hours postpartum, and notify the physician if it reaches 100.4° F (38° C) or more. To prevent hemorrhage, assess uterine tone and fundal height; evaluate lochia amount, color, and odor; check perineal pad saturation; and monitor bladder status. Good perineal hygiene and frequent hand-washing are imperative infection control practices.

Client teaching. Make sure the client understands the expected postpartal changes in her dietary and insulin requirements, especially if she has a nursing diagnosis of *knowledge deficit related to dietary and insulin requirements.* Emphasize that she should remain flexible and patient because postpartal diabetes control may be difficult to achieve, causing frustration and anger. Also, stress that she should not consider herself "cured" of diabetes if she is able to go a day or two without insulin and eat a regular diet during the postpartal period.

Because insulin does not enter breast milk, the client can breast-feed if she wishes (Gilbert and Harmon, 1986). However, caution her that the additional 300 to 500 calories/day required to maintain breast-feeding will necessitate insulin adjustments, as may altered postpartal sleeping and eating patterns. Also inform her that the glucose content of breast milk rises along with the maternal blood glucose level.

If the client had gestational diabetes, advise her to have a follow-up oral glucose tolerance test 6 to 8 weeks postpartum. Inform her that she may develop gestational diabetes in future pregnancies, and advise her to seek prenatal care early if she becomes pregnant again.

Substance abuse. The substance-abusing postpartal client requires a multidisciplinary treatment approach. Besides the nurse and physician, a social worker, child protection worker, and community health worker may be involved in her care. Treatment depends on her willingness to admit her problem and comply with a drug treatment program, such as Alcoholics Anonymous or Narcotics Anonymous.

The client may be difficult to care for—irritable, manipulative, angry, defensive, and fearful. If necessary, set limits on acceptable behavior. However, remain non-judgmental and avoid exacerbating any guilt the client may feel about her substance abuse, especially if her neonate is congenitally malformed or suffering other effects of maternal substance abuse.

Substance abuse may complicate accurate pain assessment and relief. To be effective, any analgesic administered must be equianalgesic to that of the substance (or substances) the client is accustomed to taking. Furthermore, creative nonpharmacologic pain relief methods, such as distraction, music therapy, and biofeedback, may prove challenging. However, having the client rate her pain on a scale of one to ten may aid efforts to evaluate the effectiveness of pain medication. Also, when possible, group together nursing procedures to decrease stimulation and increase rest for the client. Be aware, too, that care is more likely to be effective when provided consistently by a familiar staff.

Keep in mind that a substance-dependent client will not recover from her addiction during her short postpartal stay, even if she wants to. Treatment takes time, and its success depends greatly on the client's commitment and the treatment approach. (The client who received methadone before delivery should remain on the drug during the postpartal period. To establish trust and prevent drug withdrawal, make sure she receives the correct methadone dosage at the right time.)

For information about community substance abuse treatment programs, call the national drug treatment referral hotline (1-800-662-HELP), or urge the client to call this number. Provide the client with the telephone number of a crisis intervention or parent support hotline and arrange for follow-up medical care for both the client and neonate. This is especially important if the client has a nursing diagnosis of *ineffective individual coping related to a deficit in problem-solving skills* or *altered health maintenance related to decreased capacity for deliberative and thoughtful judgment.*

Breast-feeding concerns. If the client expresses a desire to breast-feed, explain to her that the substance or substances she has been using may appear in her breast milk. If she seems likely to continue her substance abuse after discharge, explain the dangers to the neonate of breast-feeding under these conditions.

Legal and ethical considerations. The increasing problem of maternal substance abuse has sparked debate on such issues as the rights of substance-abusing clients and their neonates and the responsibilities of all parties involved in their care. Medical ethicists, the legal and legislative communities, and health care professionals are debating such controversial topics as:
• whether a substance-abusing mother should be held legally accountable if her neonate suffers neurobehavioral abnormalities
• whether a neonate should be placed in a home where known substance abuse has occurred before and may occur again
• whether a woman who abuses substances is sufficiently stable emotionally to meet the physical and psychosocial needs of her neonate.

Most states allow a substance-abusing client to be discharged from the health care facility with her neonate unless she has previously abused a child or health care professionals have sufficient reason to believe the neonate is at high risk for neglect or abuse. Early consultation with a social worker can initiate child welfare visits if the neonate is determined to be at high risk for abuse or neglect; a history of substance abuse usually is sufficient documentation to initiate such visits.

Postpartal psychiatric disorder. Supportive therapy, such as psychiatric consultation, should begin as early as possible. Many clients require hospitalization and psychotropic drugs. Electroconvulsant therapy may be used as a last resort (Theesen, Alderson, and Hill, 1989).

Allow the client to express her feelings freely, and respond in a supportive, empathetic manner. To give her a sense of control, encourage her to participate in her

Client with a fluid volume deficit related to active postpartal hemorrhage

During the postpartal period, the nursing process helps ensure high-quality nursing care. The table below shows how the nurse might use the nursing process when caring for the client described in the case history at right. The first column presents history and physical assessment data followed by a paragraph of mental notes. These notes help the nurse make important connections among assessment findings, aiding in development of the nursing diagnosis and planning.

The second column lists an appropriate nursing diagnosis; information in the remaining columns is based on this diagnosis. Although not part of the nursing process, a rationale appears for each intervention in the fourth column to explain how it contributes to the care plan.

ASSESSMENT	NURSING DIAGNOSIS	PLANNING
Subjective (history) data • Client reports that she feels constant pelvic pressure. • Client says she feels as though her vaginal flow is "gushing." • Client reports feeling light-headed and dizzy. • Client states that she bled heavily after her last delivery. **Objective (physical) data** • Temperature: 98.6° F. • Pulse: 118 beats/minute. • Respiration: 16 breaths/minute. • Blood pressure: 90/50 mm Hg. • Two perineal pads saturated within 10 minutes of application. **Mental notes** *A soft, boggy uterus indicates uterine atony. The client's vital signs, subjective feelings, and her copious vaginal bleeding suggest hemorrhage. The neonate's large size and a past history of postpartal hemorrhage predispose the client to hemorrhage.*	Fluid volume deficit related to active postpartal hemorrhage	**Goals** During the client's stay in the postpartal unit, she will: • demonstrate normal uterine tone • show decreased vaginal bleeding • regain normal vital sign measurements.

care and the neonate's care as much as possible. Recognize and reinforce all positive parenting behaviors.

If the client's behavior warrants a nursing diagnosis of *potential for violence: self-directed or directed at others, related to postpartal psychiatric disorder,* notify the physician at once and, if necessary, initiate appropriate emergency procedures, as specified by facility policy. Make sure she remains under observation at all times.

Evaluation

During this step of the nursing process, the nurse evaluates the effectiveness of the care plan by ongoing evaluation of subjective and objective criteria. Evaluation

findings should be stated in terms of actions performed or outcomes achieved for each goal. The following examples illustrate appropriate evaluation statements for the client with a postpartal complication:

• The client's verbal and nonverbal behavior reflected an increased comfort level.

• The client's vital signs improved or remained within normal limits.

• The client demonstrated adequate wound healing.

• The client was able to interact with her neonate.

• The client demonstrated how to perform perineal hygiene.

For the client with a puerperal infection, these additional evaluation statements may be appropriate:

CASE STUDY

Tisha Williams, a 29-year-old gravida 3, para 3 client, is admitted to the postpartal unit. Her neonate weighing 4,200 g was born 1 hour ago. Two perineal pads were applied immediately before her transfer to the unit; now they are completely saturated. Examination reveals a boggy (soft) uterus.

IMPLEMENTATION		EVALUATION
Intervention	**Rationale**	Upon evaluation, the client:
Review the client's labor and delivery course.	A review of the labor and delivery records will reveal factors that place the client at high risk for postpartal hemorrhage.	• demonstrated a firm fundus • showed a decreased lochial flow, as indicated by 75% saturation of the peri-neal pad within a 4-hour period
Administer an oxytocic agent, as prescribed, and evaluate and document its effectiveness.	Oxytocic agents stimulate uterine contractions; as the uterus contracts, blood vessels are compressed and blood loss decreases.	• demonstrated normal vital signs.
Massage the fundus until it feels firm.	Massage stimulates uterine contractions, helping to reverse uterine atony.	
Assess the uterus regularly, noting its consistency.	Regular uterine assessment is necessary to determine the effectiveness of oxytocic therapy and uterine massage.	
Monitor lochia, noting its color and amount.	An accurate record of the amount of lochia helps quantify blood loss; evaluation of lochial color may help determine the source of bleeding.	
Monitor vital signs every 15 minutes until the client is stable.	Vital sign patterns, or trends, are more important than a single reading. During hypovo-lemic shock, as from hemorrhage, the pulse increases while the blood pressure declines.	
Explain all procedures to the client.	If the client understands the rationale for treatments, she is less likely to feel anxious.	

• The client's temperature is normal and drainage is no longer purulent.
• The client expressed an understanding of infection control measures.

For the client with postpartal hemorrhage, these additional evaluation statements may be appropriate:
• The client's uterine tone improved.
• The client's lochial flow decreased to within normal limits.

For the client with a birth canal injury, this additional evaluation statement may be appropriate:
• The client demonstrated knowledge of pelvic floor exercises.

For the client with PIH, these additional evaluation statements may be appropriate:

• The client's blood pressure declined to within normal limits.
• The client remained free of seizures.
• The client maintained normal reflexes (2 +).
• The client's edema decreased.
• The client maintained a urine output greater than 30 ml/hour.

For the client with venous thrombosis, these additional evaluation statements may be appropriate:
• The client's condition remained stable, with no signs of pulmonary embolism.
• The client walked increasing distances without pain.
• The client's leg circumference decreased.

• The client expressed an understanding of the purpose, dosage, and adverse effects of anticoagulant medication and the necessity for continued medical supervision.

For the client with diabetes, these additional evaluation statements may be appropriate:
• The client's blood glucose level remained within normal limits.
• The client showed no signs or symptoms of hypoglycemia or hyperglycemia.
• The client remained free of infection.
• The client expressed an understanding of the effects of nutrition, rest, and breast-feeding on her insulin requirements.

For the substance-abusing client, these additional evaluation statements may be appropriate:
• The client acknowledges that she has been abusing substances.
• The client expressed readiness to enter an appropriate treatment program.

Documentation

All steps of the nursing process should be documented as thoroughly and objectively as possible. Thorough documentation not only allows the nurse to evaluate the effectiveness of the care plan, but it also makes this information available to other members of the health care team, helping to ensure consistency of care.

Documentation for the client with a postpartal complication should include the following:
• the client's vital signs
• color, amount, consistency, and odor of lochia
• percentage of perineal pad saturation and time required for saturation
• the client's comfort level
• laboratory results
• changes in status
• the location and appearance of any I.V. lines
• the client's ability to care for and interact with the neonate
• the client's feelings about her condition
• effect of the client's condition on her family.

For the client with a puerperal infection, also document:
• appearance of the affected area
• the client's understanding of the treatment course.

For the client with postpartal hemorrhage, also document:

• fluid status, including intake and output, every 8 hours for at least 24 hours postpartum
• uterine tone and bladder status
• effectiveness of ocytocic therapy
• CVP measurements.

For the client with a birth canal injury, also document:
• bowel status, including the presence or absence of bowel sounds and bowel movements
• fundal height
• uterine tone.

For the client with PIH, also document:
• fluid intake and urine output
• signs of edema
• status of deep tendon reflexes
• presence of urinary protein
• daily weight
• consciousness level.

For the client with venous thrombosis, also document:
• clotting times and other laboratory values, such as prothrombin time and partial thromboplastin time.

For the client with diabetes mellitus, also document:
• serial blood glucose levels
• insulin administered
• signs or symptoms of hypoglycemia or hyperglycemia
• signs or symptoms of preeclampsia, infection, or hemorrhage
• client teaching about diet, exercise, insulin dosage and schedule, blood glucose monitoring schedule, signs and symptoms to report to the physician, and the need for regular follow-up medical care.

For the substance-abusing client, also document:
• signs and symptoms of drug withdrawal or continued drug use during hospitalization
• response to prescribed analgesics
• extent of the client's interaction with the neonate, her partner, and the health care team
• absence or presence of signs of mother-infant bonding
• expressions of willingness to be treated for substance abuse.

For the client with a postpartal psychiatric disorder, also document:
• the client's verbal and nonverbal behavior toward the neonate
• the client's perception of her parenting ability
• referral to or contact with other health practitioners, such as a psychiatrist
• treatment plans
• conferences with the client's support persons.

Chapter summary

Chapter 44 discussed nursing care of clients with postpartal complications. Here are the chapter highlights.

• Puerperal infection is potentially life-threatening, but prompt recognition and intervention may prevent grave consequences. The infection may remain localized to a specific part of the reproductive tract or may spread to more distant sites. A morbid temperature is the hallmark of puerperal infection.

• Postpartal hemorrhage can occur early or late in the postpartal period. Difficulty in quantifying blood loss sometimes delays recognition of hemorrhage. However, in many cases, hemorrhage can be predicted from such risk factors as uterine atony (and its underlying causes), lacerations, retained placental fragments, and uterine inversion. Identifying the cause of hemorrhage is essential to treatment.

• Changes in pelvic support structures resulting from injury to the birth canal may be permanent. Such trauma is possible during any delivery but may be compounded by a prolonged labor and the use of instruments. For the client with pelvic relaxation, Kegel exercises are a key intervention to strengthen the pelvic floor.

• Stasis, increased levels of certain blood-clotting factors, and other postpartal conditions may cause venous thrombosis and the attendant risk of pulmonary embolism. Common treatments include anticoagulant medication, bed rest, analgesics, use of antiembolism stockings, local heat, and elevation of the affected limb.

• In the postpartal client with diabetes mellitus, fluctuating blood glucose levels can pose a management challenge. Diabetes also increases the risk of other postpartal complications, such as infection, hemorrhage, and PIH. Thus, prevention of these complications is an important part of nursing care.

• The postpartal client who abuses substances is more readily identified now than previously. The nurse should stay alert for cardiovascular and central nervous system complications in this client; if she is addicted, she may experience withdrawal symptoms. A multidisciplinary health care approach can best meet the client's varied needs.

• A postpartal psychiatric disorder rarely manifests before discharge. Treatment typically involves psychiatric evaluation, hospitalization, and medication; in rare cases, electroconvulsant therapy is needed.

• Other complications that may arise during the postpartal period include mastitis, PIH, diabetes mellitus, and such urinary tract disorders as cystitis, pyelonephritis, bladder distention, and urinary incontinence.

Study questions

1. What are the major types of puerperal infection?

2. How much blood must a postpartal client lose to warrant a diagnosis of postpartal hemorrhage?

3. Which important points should be included in a discharge teaching plan for a client with thromboembolic disease?

4. What are the physical, obstetric, and psychosocial signs of substance abuse?

5. Stacy Gruening, a primigravid client, has just been admitted to the postpartal unit. The client had saturated one perineal pad with bright red blood by the time she reached the unit. In addition to frequent monitoring for further bleeding, what other signs and symptoms should the nurse check for during assessments of Ms. Gruening?

6. During the initial assessment of Ms. Gruening, the nurse notes that her uterus becomes firm after fundal massage and is displaced to the right. How should the nurse intervene?

Bibliography

Brunner, L.S., and Suddarth, D.S. (1988). *Textbook of medical-surgical nursing* (6th ed.). Philadelphia: Lippincott.

Cunningham, F., MacDonald, P., and Gant, N. (1989). *Williams obstetrics* (18th ed.). East Norwalk, CT: Appleton & Lange.

Danforth, D.N., and Scott, J.R. (Eds.). (1986). *Obstetrics and gynecology* (5th ed.) Philadelphia: Lippincott.

Gilbert, E.S., and Harmon, J.S. (1986). *High-risk pregnancy and delivery: Nursing perspectives.* St. Louis: Mosby.

Gordon, M. (1989). *Manual of nursing diagnosis 1988-1989.* St. Louis: Mosby.

Monheit, A.G., Cousins, L., and Resnik, R. (1980). The puerperium: Anatomic and physiologic readjustments. *Clinical Obstetrics and Gynecology, 23*(4), 973-984.

Birth canal injuries

Davidson, N. (1974). REEDA: Evaluating postpartum healing. *Journal of Nurse-Midwifery*, 19(2), 6-9.

Postpartal hemorrhage

Bastin, J.P. (1989). Action STAT! Postpartum hemorrhage. *Nursing89*, 19(2), 33.

Rigby, P.G. (1987). Bleeding: Symposium on bleeding disorders in pregnancy. *American Journal of Obstetrics and Gynecology*, 156(6), 1422-1425.

Wahl, S.C. (1989). Septic shock: How to detect it early. *Nursing89*, 19(1), 52-59.

Puerperal infection

Eschenbach, D.A., and Wager, G.P. (1980). Puerperal infections. *Clinical Obstetrics and Gynecology*, 23(4), 1003-1037.

Gibbs, R.S., and Weinstein, A.J. (1976). Puerperal infection in the antibiotics era. *American Journal of Obstetrics and Gynecology*, 124(7), 769-787.

Gilstrap, L.C., and Cunningham, F.G. (1979). The bacterial pathogenesis of infection following cesarean section. *Obstetrics and Gynecology*, 53(5), 545-549.

Petetti, D.B. (1985). Maternal mortality and morbidity with cesarean delivery. *Clinical Obstetrics and Gynecology*, 28(12), 763.

Wager, G.P. (1983). Toxic shock syndrome. *American Journal of Obstetrics and Gynecology*, 146(1), 93-102.

Wolf, P.H., Perlman, J., and Fortney, J. (1987). Toxic shock syndrome. *JAMA*, 258(7), 908.

Vascular complications

Chesley, L. (1978). Eclampsia: The remote prognosis. *Seminar on Perinatology*, 2(1), 99-111.

Other postpartal complications

American Psychiatric Association. (1987). *DSM-III-R: Diagnostic and statistical manual of mental disorders* (3rd ed., rev.). Washingon, DC: Author.

Bodendorfer, T.W., Briggs, G., and Gunning, J. (1979). Obtaining drug exposure histories during pregnancy. *American Journal of Obstetrics and Gynecology*, 135(4), 490-494.

Carmack, B.J., and Corwin, T.A. (1980). Nursing care of the schizophrenic maternity patient during labor. *MCN*, 5(2), 107.

Chasnoff, I., Burns, W., and Schnall, S. (1985). Cocaine use in pregnancy. *New England Journal of Medicine*, 313(11), 666-669.

Cregler, L., and Mark, H. (1986). Special report: Medical complications of cocaine abuse. *New England Journal of Medicine*, 315(23), 1495-1499.

Easterling, W., and Herbert, W. (1986). The puerperium. In D.N. Danforth and J.R. Scott (Eds.), *Obstetrics and gynecology* (5th ed.). Philadelphia: Lippincott.

Hollander, P., and Maeder, E.C. (1985). Diabetes in pregnancy no longer a barrier to successful outcome. *Postgraduate Medicine*, 77(2), 137-146.

Landry, M., and Smith, D.E. (1987). Crack: Anatomy of an addiction, part 2. *California Nursing Review*, 9(3), 28.

Leveno, K.J., and Whalley, P.J. (1980). Dilemmas in the management of pregnancy complicated by diabetes (symposium on diabetes mellitus). *Medical Clinics of North America*, 66(6), 1325-1346.

Little, B.B., Snell, L., Klein, V., and Gilstrap, L. (1989). Cocaine abuse during pregnancy: Maternal and fetal implications. *Obstetrics and Gynecology*, 73(2), 157-160.

MacGregor, S.N., Keith, L., and Chasnoff, T. (1987). Cocaine use during pregnancy: Adverse perinatal outcome. *American Journal of Obstetrics and Gynecology*, 157(3), 686-690.

Madden, J.D., Payne, T.F., and Miller, S. (1986). Maternal cocaine abuse and effect on the newborn. *Pediatrics*, 77(2), 209-211.

Mercer, R.T., and Ferketich, S.L. (1988). Stress and social support as predictors of anxiety and depression during pregnancy. *Advances in Nursing Science*, 10(2), 26-39.

Niebyl, J. (1985). When the nursing mother has mastitis. *Contemporary OB/GYN* 29(2), 31-32.

O'Hara, M.W., Neunaber, D.J., and Zekoski, E.M. (1984). Prospective study of postpartum depression: Prevalence, course, and predictive factors. *Journal of Abnormal Psychology*, 93(2), 158-161.

Oxorn, H. (1986). *Oxorn-Foote human labor and birth* (5th ed.). East Norwalk, CT: Appleton & Lange.

Phillips, K. (1986). Neonatal drug addicts. *Nursing Times*, 82(12), 36-38.

Robertson, C. (1987). When your pregnant patient has diabetes. *RN*, 50(11), 18-22.

Stuart, G.W., and Sundeen, S.V. (1987). *Principles and practice of psychiatric nursing* (3rd ed.). St. Louis: Mosby.

Theesen, K., Alderson, M., and Hill, W. (1989). Caring for the depressed obstetric patient. *Contemporary OB/GYN*, 33(2), 123-129.

Tully, M., and Overfield, M. (1989). Breastfeeding: A handbook for hospitals. Indiana: Mead Johnson Nutritionals.

Watson, J.P., Elliott, S.A., Rugg, A.J., and Brough, D. (1984). Psychiatric disorder in pregnancy and the first postnatal year. *British Journal of Psychiatry*, 453-462.

White, P. (1980). Classification of diabetes, 1978. In K. Niswander (Ed.)., *Manual of obstetrics*. Boston: Little, Brown.

Woods, J.R., Plessinger, M.A., and Clark, K.E. (1987). Effect of cocaine on uterine blood flow and fetal oxygenation. *JAMA*, 257(7), 957-961.

Nursing research

Hill, P.D. (1989). Effects of heat and cold on the perineum after episiotomy/laceration. *JOGNN*, 18(2), 124-129.

Maternal Care at Home

Objectives

After reading and studying this chapter, the student should be able to:

1. Identify the advantages of caring for postpartal clients at home.

2. Discuss the factors involved in planning for a postpartal home nursing visit.

3. Develop a contract or nursing care plan for a postpartal client receiving care at home.

4. Help the postpartal client and her partner improve their parenting skills.

5. Discuss nursing interventions appropriate for a client with postpartal depression.

Introduction

Labor and delivery last a comparatively short time but parenthood lasts a lifetime. Although much help is available to bring a child into the world, many parents are left on their own shortly after a neonate's birth. Increasingly, clients are leaving the health care facility within 24 hours of delivery, with no further contact with health care professionals for 3 to 6 weeks.

However, current trends may help to address this problem. More health care professionals now recognize that a neonate's birth necessitates adaptation by the entire family over an extended period. Also, consumers are demanding more personalized care than health care facilities traditionally have provided. Moreover, escalating health care costs and changing reimbursement policies have made early discharge more common; early discharge may increase the need for comprehensive fol-

low-up care at home. Thus, postpartal follow-up has increasingly become a nursing intervention.

Most early discharge programs have been developed within the last decade. Earlier, the average length of stay after delivery was 10 days; a reduction to 3 or 5 days was seen as radical. Today, a client may be discharged as early as 2 hours postpartum. In most cases, however, early discharge takes place 24 to 48 hours after delivery. Early discharge does not increase the risk of life-threatening complications. Norr and Nacion (1987) found no differences in the types and amount of morbidity between clients discharged early and those discharged later.

Thus, nurses now offer continued support for childbearing families in the home. The challenge for the home care nurse is to ensure continuity of care and maintain a high quality of care while taking advantage of the benefits of the home setting. By allowing a broader perspective for understanding the postpartal family, nursing care in the home enhances family-centered care. Also, because most clients are more relaxed in their own surroundings than in an institutional setting, mutual trust can be established quickly.

At home, the nurse can incorporate the realities of the client's home situation into all aspects of care, making that care holistic and more relevant. For the client, home care means that daily routines and schedules are dictated not by health care facility policy but by the family's normal activities and requirements. Most clients sleep better at home than in the health care facility and benefit from the freedom to choose their own food and visiting hours.

GLOSSARY

Contract: written or verbal agreement between the nurse and the client that spells out the goals of nursing care and specifies what each party will do to accomplish these goals.

Early postpartal discharge: discharge from the health care facility 2 to 72 hours after delivery.

Family-centered care: philosophical approach to health care that proposes that childbirth affects the entire family; incorporates such practices as paternal and sibling participation in childbirth and alternative birth settings.

"Fitting in the missing pieces": psychological process in which the client reviews the events of childbirth to help incorporate the experience into her self-concept and identity as a person and a mother.

Formative evaluation: process in which the nurse and client judge progress toward goals during home care visits.

Home nursing visit: provision of nursing care in a client's home.

Maternity blues: postpartal disorder characterized by transient mood alteration involving crying episodes and sadness (also called "baby blues"); usually lasts 1 to 10 days.

Postpartal depression: postpartal mood swings marked by tearfulness, despondency, feelings of guilt and inadequacy, and inability to cope; may last from a few weeks to a year or more.

Postpartal period: approximately 6-week period following delivery during which the client's anatomic and physiologic changes resulting from pregnancy resolve (also called *puerperium*).

Summative evaluation: process in which the nurse and client judge progress toward goals after home care visits are discontinued.

This chapter shows how the nurse can provide support in the home to help ensure a full postpartal recovery and help parents adapt to their new roles. The chapter begins by describing strategies that make home nursing care more effective. Then it describes how the nurse applies the nursing process when providing care at home, including ways of adapting standard nursing assessment methods and interventions to the home setting. The chapter concludes with a brief discussion of documentation.

Nursing strategies

The key to the success of home health care is close cooperation between health professionals within the health care facility and those providing care at home. The home care nurse should obtain a copy of the discharge plan and review it carefully before the first home visit. (For a discussion of discharge planning and an overview of home health care, see Chapter 40, Discharge Planning and Neonatal Care at Home.)

Although most assessment methods and interventions used in the home are similar to those used in the health care facility, home care calls for thorough planning coupled with a flexible, innovative approach. Also, because the nurse is a guest in the client's home, es-

tablishing rapport and showing a regard for family customs and routines take on paramount importance.

Planning ahead

Unavoidable disruptions and distractions add an element of uncertainty to the home visit. Telephone calls and unplanned visits by relatives and friends may cause interruptions; noise made by children, televisions, and stereos may break the concentration needed in a teaching session. However, careful timing of visits can minimize this problem. For instance, the nurse can schedule visits when the client is least likely to have visitors or when older children are in day care or school.

Setting specific appointment times and verifying them the day before helps ensure that the client will be at home when the nurse arrives. To reduce travel time, arrange to visit several clients living in the same area on the same day; get clear directions to the home and keep a road map in the car.

Establishing rapport

To provide family-centered care, establish a rapport based on mutual trust. Unlike the health care facility, the home is the family's territory; the family's unwritten rules, not health care facility policy, dictate acceptable behavior. Recognize and respect family beliefs, customs, and routines.

Keep in mind that some people are uncomfortable when a stranger comes into the home. To put the client at ease, begin the first visit by making introductions, then clarify the purpose of the visit and describe the services the nurse can provide. Determine whether the client requested the visit herself or was referred by a third party. If she was referred, find out if she understands the reason for the referral; a client who does not know why the nurse is there may refuse to share information freely or even to become involved in the process. If this happens, explore the reasons for refusal. Perhaps she simply does not know how home nursing visits can help her; or maybe the problem that triggered the referral has been resolved.

Be aware, too, that some clients may be ashamed of their homes, perceiving the nurse as socially superior to them (or perhaps believing that the nurse sees herself as superior). On the other hand, some clients may believe they are superior to the nurse or may perceive home care as a service meant for a lower socioeconomic group. To help dispel these feelings, maintain a friendly but professional manner and convey a caring attitude; also offer an accurate, complete description of the purpose and nature of home nursing visits.

The informality of a home visit can lead to role confusion, particularly in the less experienced nurse who confuses friendship with the professional helping relationship. To avoid this problem, keep in mind that the nursing role, unlike friendship, is goal directed; together with the client, the nurse continually evaluates progress toward goal achievement. To gain a clearer perspective on a relationship with a client, consider taking a colleague along on a home visit or reviewing the case with a colleague.

Be sure to consider how the client's cultural background may be affecting her postpartal recovery and her general life-style. Understanding and accepting the client's cultural beliefs and customs enhances the nurse-client relationship; also, the client will understand interventions and teaching more readily if they are congruent with her cultural beliefs. (If the client is from another country and has inadequate English language skills, teaching materials may have to be adapted or a translator used.)

Explore the client's culturally related beliefs about childbirth, postpartal recovery, and child rearing. For example, in some cultures, the mother rests while female friends or the neonate's grandparents assume child care responsibilities. Keep in mind that for some cultures, routine Western postpartal practices—early ambulation, exercise, showering, and warm sitz baths—may seem incomprehensible or even dangerous. In certain non-Western cultures, women may remain in seclusion, follow dietary restrictions, carefully time their exposure to heat and cold, and limit their activity. In a few cultures, women are considered impure during the postpartal pe-

riod and must follow certain rituals to avoid spreading the impurities (Greener, 1989).

Assessment

For the postpartal client at home, a complete assessment includes a history, physical examination, psychosocial assessment, evaluation of mother-neonate interaction, and home assessment. However, not all clients may wish to be examined or to answer questions about their personal relationships; thus, the nurse must be sensitive to the client's right to refuse. (For specific questions on psychosocial assessment, see *Postpartal psychosocial assessment,* page 1122.)

Assessment in the home has important advantages. If the client was discharged early, thorough assessment is particularly important to detect postpartal complications. Also, assessment in the home yields in-depth data about the client's family, life-style, beliefs, values, customs, and interests and information available only indirectly in an institutional setting. In the home, for instance, the nurse has a first-hand view of the responsibilities of a client who has several preschool-age children; to the nurse in the health care facility, these responsibilities are less obvious.

If other family members are home during the assessment, the nurse can observe family interactions. The effects of relatives, friends, neighbors, and even household pets also can be incorporated into the assessment. By observing the family over time through serial home visits, the nurse gains greater insight into the client and her family, the safety and cleanliness of the home, and the degree to which the parents are providing a stimulating environment for child development.

Despite these advantages, assessment at home poses special problems. For instance, outside the institutional setting, which legitimizes and formalizes the caregiver's role, the client might find some assessment procedures embarrassing or an invasion of privacy. Also, the nurse cannot simply close the curtain for privacy when examining the client, as in the health care facility.

To avoid infringing on the client's or family's privacy or personal space, use sensitivity, tact, and creativity. Let the client choose the best time and location for personal discussions and potentially embarrassing assessment procedures, and obtain her verbal permission before beginning the assessment. If other members of the household are within hearing range, maintain confidentiality by conducting the assessment in another part

Postpartal psychosocial assessment

To assess the postpartal client's psychosocial status and adaptation to the maternal role, explore her feelings by asking such questions as those shown here. Remember to keep all questions open-ended. If a client hesitates to answer any question, clarify and reword it; if she still seems resistant, go to the next question.

Daily activities

- How well are you managing your daily activities?
- How do you feel about your appetite and the amount of sleep you are getting?
- How would you rate your effectiveness in managing your responsibilities?

Impact of childbirth events

- What thoughts and feelings do you have when you look back at your childbirth experience?
- How do you think you handled the experience?
- What aspects of the experience stand out in your mind and why?

Mother-infant interaction

- How do you feel about yourself as a mother?
- How do you think your infant feels about you as a mother?
- What thoughts and feelings do you have when you are with your infant?
- What concerns do you have about your infant's health and safety? How do you handle these concerns?

Social activities and support

- In what stage are you in resuming your social activities and responsibilities with other adults?
- How is your relationship with your infant's father?
- Since delivery, which social activities have you engaged in that were pleasurable? Which were not pleasurable?

Self-esteem

- How would you rate yourself right now in terms of goodness?
- How well do you feel you are adjusting?
- What thoughts and feelings have you had about your physical attractiveness since the delivery?
- What is your predominant mood these days?
- How do you view your future?

Adapted with permission from Affonso, D. D. (1987). Assessment of maternal postpartum adaptation. *Public Health Nursing, 4*(1), 12.

of the home or tactfully asking others to move to another room for a few minutes.

History

The nurse who has had no previous contact with the client should review the antepartal and intrapartal records carefully; a telephone call to the person who made the referral also can be helpful. Also review the client's history of previous pregnancies, noting any spontaneous or therapeutic abortions or stillbirths, the delivery method for each, and any complications.

When reviewing the immediate past pregnancy and delivery, note:
- whether it was a planned or unplanned pregnancy
- the extent of the client's prenatal care
- exposures during pregnancy (such as smoking, alcohol, drugs, X-rays, communicable diseases, and occupational hazards)
- hospital admissions or problems during pregnancy, such as bleeding or infection.

Assess the client's breast-feeding experience, if relevant, and ask about family planning and contraceptive use. Also question her about her sleeping and eating patterns and comfort level. If subsequent visits occur, ask her to relate her main concern.

Physical examination

To assess the client's postpartal recovery and help detect or prevent complications, conduct a brief physical examination that focuses on evaluating postpartal recovery. During the examination, teach the client about postpartal physiologic changes and show her how to assess her progress toward recovery.

In the first few days after delivery, obtain vital signs, staying alert for a temperature above 100.4° F (38° C), which may signify infection. Note any increase in the pulse or respiratory rate or any decrease in blood pressure, which may indicate uterine hemorrhage.

Conduct a review of body systems to check for expected reversal of the changes that took place during pregnancy. To assess uterine involution, palpate the fundus; by the tenth day postpartum, it should no longer be palpable as an abdominal organ. Determine whether lochia is progressing through the normal stages; examine the perineum to determine if an episiotomy or laceration is healing properly. Check the breasts for engorgement, lactation stage, and nipple condition. (For a complete discussion of the postpartal physical examination, see Chapter 42, Care during the Normal Postpartal Period.)

Psychosocial status

Ideally, obtain a psychosocial history, keying in on such topics as psychological problems after previous deliveries, the client's social support systems, and any recent or current family stress. Also assess the client's economic status, review her work history, and ask about her child care plans.

Be aware, however, that psychosocial assessment may be difficult for nurse and client alike. The client may have trouble expressing her feelings or may feel that the nurse's questions are intrusive or unnecessary; the nurse may feel uncomfortable about asking such questions. To make this assessment less stressful, acknowledge and understand personal values and beliefs about childbirth and families, and convey a nonjugmental attitude. If the client is willing to provide information to and explore her feelings with the nurse, the nurse's psychosocial assessment can help focus nursing interventions.

To adapt to her new role, the client must relive and understand the events of childbirth so that she can incorporate them into her life and self-concept—a process described by Affonso (1977) as "fitting in the missing pieces." Most postpartal clients express satisfaction and positive feelings; some, though, have ambivalent feelings, which may indicate conflicts that could compromise postpartal adaptation. Assess for other potential signs of poor adaptation, such as disinterest in the neonate, adults, or adult activities; lack of social participation; and social isolation.

The postpartal client may experience mood swings and emotional lability. To check for these problems, ask the client to describe her moods and feelings; be alert to extremes, such as elation and depression. (If appropriate, obtain further information about her moods from family members.) If she complains of fatigue, ask openended questions to determine its degree, what she believes is causing it, her ability to perform normal daily activities, and her feelings about her condition.

When assessing psychosocial status, stay alert for signs of postpartal mood swings; usually arising after discharge, these are more likely to be discovered by the home care nurse than the nurse in the health care facility. The cause of such mood swings is unknown. However, researchers suspect physiologic factors, such as changing hormonal levels and genetic predisposition. (For a study of the effects of the neonate's gestational age on maternal postpartal emotional status, see *Nursing research applied: Anxiety and depression in mothers of term and preterm neonates.*)

Postpartal mood swings may manifest as maternity blues, as a more severe alteration in mood swings, or as a major depressive episode.

NURSING RESEARCH APPLIED

Anxiety and depression in mothers of term and preterm neonates

To determine if a neonate's gestational age affects maternal emotional status, a researcher compared levels of anxiety and depression in 41 mothers of preterm neonates with those of 41 mothers of term neonates; the mothers were matched for age, parity, delivery method, and race. Before discharge, all subjects completed two questionnaires measuring anxiety and depression; after discharge, they completed the same questionnaire weekly for the next 6 weeks.

The results indicated that although all subjects experienced heightened anxiety and depression in the first week postpartum, mothers of preterm neonates were significantly more anxious and depressed than their full-term counterparts. However, no differences were found between the two groups over the next 6 weeks. Parity and delivery method had no bearing on anxiety and depression levels.

Application to practice
This study suggests that supportive nursing interventions are important for all postpartal clients, not just those with preterm neonates. A better understanding of how depression and anxiety change over time may help the nurse provide anticipatory guidance during the first postpartal weeks. Interventions directed toward validating the normalcy of postpartal anxiety and depression can help the postpartal client adapt to her new role.

Gennaro, S. (1988). Postpartal anxiety and depression in mothers of term and preterm infants. *Nursing Research,* 37(2), 82-85.

Maternity blues ("baby blues"), a transient mood alteration, is characterized by sadness, crying episodes, fatigue, and low self-esteem. Usually arising within the first 3 weeks postpartum, it is experienced by 50% to 80% of postpartal clients (Hopkins, Marcus, and Campbell, 1984). Typically, it is self-limiting, lasting from 1 to 10 days (Condon and Watson, 1987).

A more severe alteration in mood swings occurs in approximately 20% of postpartal clients and manifests as tearfulness, despondency, feelings of guilt and inadequacy, and inability to cope with neonatal care. Generalized fatigue and complaints of ill health also are common. Signs and symptoms typically arise within a few weeks of delivery and may last from a few weeks to a year or more (Hopkins, Marcus, and Campbell, 1984).

Major depressive episode, a severe form of depression, occurs in approximately 0.1% of postpartal women and in many cases requires hospitalization (Hopkins, Marcus, and Campbell, 1984). A client with a major depressive episode will have at least five of the following symptoms: depressed mood, markedly diminished interest or pleasure in activities, significant weight loss or weight gain, insomnia or hypersomina, psychomotor ag-

---

Evaluating the client's home

To assess the safety, adequacy, and psychosocial environment of the client's home, the nurse should determine the answers to such questions as those shown below.

- How many rooms do the client and her family occupy? Has the addition of the neonate caused crowding?
- Does the family own or rent the home or apartment? Is the cost of housing burdensome to the family?
- Does the home have adequate heat, lighting, and ventilation to care for the neonate and client safely?
- Are floors and stairs in safe condition?
- Does the neonate have a crib that meets safety standards? Does the client have a comfortable chair and a quiet place in which to breast-feed?
- Are safety hazards present that might impose a danger to the client or neonate, such as missing stair railings or uncovered electrical outlets?
- Does the home have running water and refrigeration? Can the client safely prepare and store formula for the neonate?
- Is the bathroom sanitary? Does it have a toilet, towels, and soap so that the client can carry out perineal care?
- How many bedrooms does the home have? Does the neonate sleep in the same room as the parents, in the parent's bed, or in another room?
- How do family members feel about their home? Do they consider it adequate for the needs of their growing family?

---

itation, fatigue or loss of energy, feelings of worthlessness, diminished ability to think, and recurrent thoughts of death. At least one of the symptoms of this psychiatric disorder is depressed mood or loss of interest or pleasure (DSM-III-R, 1987).

Mother-infant interaction

In the home, the nurse can observe mother-infant interaction over time and within the natural setting, taking into account the effects of other family members and the home surroundings. An optimal time to observe is during a feeding session, when the client and infant are most likely to interact closely. (For more information on assessing mother-infant interaction, see Chapter 43, Psychosocial Adaptation of the Postpartal Family.)

Home environment

Determine if the home is conducive to safe, adequate care of the client and neonate and whether it promotes positive psychosocial adaptation. For example, check for safety hazards and availability of basic necessities, such as water, electricity, and heat, and assess whether the client can obtain privacy in the home. (For details on home assessment, see *Evaluating the client's home.*)

Nursing diagnosis

After gathering all of the assessment data, the nurse must review it carefully to identify pertinent nursing diagnoses for the client. (For a partial list of applicable diagnoses, see *Nursing diagnoses: Postpartal client receiving nursing care at home.*)

NURSING DIAGNOSES

Postpartal client receiving nursing care at home

For the postpartal client who is receiving nursing care at home, the nurse may find the following nursing diagnoses appropriate. Specific nursing interventions for many of these diagnoses are provided in the "Planning and implementation" section of this chapter.

- Altered family processes related to the birth of a neonate
- Altered role performance related to postpartal mood swings
- Altered sexuality patterns related to a painful episiotomy or fear of conception
- Fatigue related to the need to care for the neonate throughout the night
- Impaired home maintenance management related to the demands of caring for the neonate
- Ineffective individual coping related to adaptation to the maternal role
- Knowledge deficit related to neonatal care
- Pain related to the perineal wound
- Potential altered parenting related to postpartal mood swings
- Situational low self-esteem related to loss of the prepregnancy figure
- Sleep pattern disturbance related to frequent demands of the neonate or infant
- Social isolation related to the neonate's constant care demands

Planning and implementation

After assessing the client and formulating nursing diagnoses, the nurse develops and implements a care plan. Nursing goals for the postpartal client receiving care at home include promoting postpartal recovery, helping the client adapt to the maternal role, promoting parenting skills, enhancing the couple's relationship, and helping siblings adapt to the birth of a new family member. Depending on the number of visits the nurse will make, meeting all of these goals may be a challenge.

Although the nurse may set tentative goals before a visit, definite goals should be established mutually with the client at the beginning of each visit. Mutual goal-setting ensures that the client understands goals; this in turn helps her to accomplish them. One way to set goals mutually is to develop a contract with the client that describes each goal and specifies exactly what the nurse and client will do to meet it. The contract may be verbal or it may be written and signed by the nurse and client; in some cases, the nurse may want to include the contract in the written care plan. (See *Sample contract for home care*, page 1126.) The nurse should keep in mind, however, that a contract may not be appropriate for the client who wants a less active role in her care.

Even if the contract is formalized in writing, it is not static. Together with the client, the nurse should reevaluate the contract continually and renegotiate, modify, or terminate it as necessary as well as ensure that goals and time limits for meeting them are realistic.

To deal with newly emerging needs, the nurse also should be prepared to change goals at the last minute to address a sudden crisis. Suppose, for instance, that the nurse plans to teach neonatal care skills to a client with a nursing diagnosis of *knowledge deficit related to neonatal care.* On arrival, however, the nurse finds the client in tears because the neonate kept her up all night. In this case, the nurse should postpone interventions for the long-term goal (correcting the knowledge deficit) and set new, short-term goals to deal with the client's immediate need for rest.

The nurse should plan each visit carefully in relation to the tentative goal set for the visit. If physical examination is planned, arrive with any equipment that will be needed. Forgetting a stethoscope, for instance, could mean that the goal for that visit remains unmet; scheduling another visit could be costly and time-consuming.

As appropriate, refer the client to community resources, such as self-help groups or parenting classes. Some prenatal instruction classes, for instance, include a fourth trimester class to discuss parenting.

Promoting postpartal recovery

If assessment reveals postpartal complications or delayed postpartal recovery, intervene as appropriate, referring the client to a physician if necessary. For example, after inspecting the episiotomy site, the nurse may determine that the client has a nursing diagnosis of *pain related to the perineal wound.* In this case, recommend a sitz bath three or four times daily, with each bath lasting 15 to 20 minutes. If the client does not know how to administer this treatment, provide teaching. Other interventions for perineal discomfort include application of a topical anesthetic spray or ointment, a mild oral analgesic, or witch hazel compresses. (For details on these treatments, see Chapter 42, Care during the Normal Postpartal Period.)

Helping the client adapt to the maternal role

To help avoid a nursing diagnosis of *ineffective individual coping related to adaptation to the maternal role,* use interventions that help the client regain control of her life. Begin by encouraging her to talk about the events of childbirth and her feelings about the experience. This is especially important if she experienced unanticipated labor or delivery events or if the neonate had medical problems; in this case, the client may need to grieve for the lost fantasy of the perfect childbirth or the perfect child before she can adapt to her new role. Be aware that many postpartal clients are afraid to admit that they feel confused and upset; if necessary, give her "permission" to talk about these issues.

To help the client accept and deal with her feelings, maintain a nonjudgmental attitude. If she seems angry, allow her to express this and help her deal with her anger constructively. Urge her to cry if she feels like it; tears can be healing and help relieve stress.

Offer praise and reassurance for her efforts to fulfill her responsibilities. If she feels overwhelmed by the tasks of her new role as parent, help her break down large tasks into smaller, more manageable parts. Keep in mind that a new mother needs some mothering herself, so encourage her to nurture and pamper herself, paying attention to her own needs as well as the neonate's.

Teach the client who is having trouble adapting to her new role because of a nursing diagnosis of *situational low self-esteem related to loss of the prepregnancy figure* about proper diet and exercise. To help avoid a nursing diagnosis of *sleep pattern disturbance related to frequent*

Sample contract for home care

A written contract, such as the one shown below, may be useful for the nurse caring for the postpartal client at home. Formulated jointly by the nurse and client, such a contract ensures mutual goal-setting and promotes close collaboration between nurse and client.

Client name _____

GOAL: The client will exercise once a day and rest periodically throughout the day.

RESPONSIBILITIES	COMPLETION DATE
The client will:	
• discuss and explore the problem (the need for rest and improved muscle tone) with the nurse	
• reassess her desire for performing household tasks	
• take the phone off the hook and nap when the infant naps	
• seek help with caregiving or household tasks from her spouse, relatives, and friends	
• consider hiring a babysitter	
• carry out the recommended postpartal exercise regimen once a day	
• read materials supplied by the nurse.	
The nurse will:	
• offer support and encouragement	
• make a home visit when the spouse is at home to discuss division of household labor	
• provide information about babysitting resources	
• discuss guidelines for selecting a babysitter	
• supply instructions for recommended postpartal exercises	
• give suggestions for obtaining adequate rest.	

EVALUATION: The client reports that she feels more rested and is carrying out the recommended exercise regimen.

Client's signature _____   Nurse's signature _____

Date _____

---

demands of the neonate, advise her to sleep when the neonate sleeps.

If other family members are home during visits and are open to participating in teaching sessions, they may be included. For example, discuss with them the client's need for rest, and urge them to offer her physical and emotional support. This may necessitate an exploration of the division of household labor to determine which partner takes care of the neonate, looks after other children, buys groceries, prepares and cleans up after meals, cleans the house, and does the laundry. If the client now does most of these chores, suggest that other family members help relieve her of some of them.

If the client has a nursing diagnosis of *potential altered parenting related to postpartal mood swings,* refer her for counseling or therapy. Also, because sleep deprivation may contribute to postpartal mood swings, help her plan ways to get adequate rest—for instance, by finding a babysitter. Errante (1985) found that most cases of postpartal mood swings respond to time and therapy. (For other ways to help this client, see *Nursing interventions for postpartal mood swings,* page 1128.)

For the client with a nursing diagnosis of *social isolation related to the neonate's constant care demands,* help her develop contacts within the community and refer her to appropriate community resources, such as counseling services, self-help groups, and babysitting services (sponsored by many churches).

If the client plans to return to work outside the home, give her an opportunity to discuss her feelings about this. Many parents seek approval for their decisions from health care professionals; provide emotional support to help the client feel better about her decision. As necessary, refer her to community resources, such as day care centers, and offer guidelines for selecting a day care provider. Advise her to consider the provider's personality, age, experience with infants, and fee and the availability of references and transportation. If the parents decide to use a babysitter, suggest that they hire one on a trial basis and invite the person to the home to meet them and to care for the child in their presence (Rothenberg, Hitchcock, Harrison, and Graham, 1983).

If the client is apprehensive about leaving her child with a day care provider, point out the benefits of this. For example, the child may gain independence and trust in others; the day care provider may help the client see the child from a different perspective and may suggest alternative ways of dealing with behaviors that are unfamiliar to the inexperienced mother.

(For a case study that shows how to apply the nursing process when caring for the postpartal family, see *Applying the nursing process: Client with altered role performance related to postpartal mood swings* ["maternity blues"], pages 1130 and 1131.)

Promoting parenting skills

In the past, the extended family provided opportunities for learning about parenting; new parents could rely on advice and assistance from their parents and other relatives. Today, families are smaller and members of the extended family may be dispersed across the country. Also, with more women working outside the home and one-parent families increasing, many parents lack parenting skills and may have a nursing diagnosis of *knowledge deficit related to neonatal care.*

To increase their competence and confidence in caring for the neonate, reinforce discharge teaching of neonatal caregiving skills and provide information about infant growth and development. As appropriate, recommend fourth trimester classes, which offer anticipatory guidance and provide a forum for parents to share

their concerns. Also teach the parents about their neonate's capacities and behavioral traits (as described in Chapter 35, Neonatal Assessment).

Most new parents also benefit from discussing their concerns with other parents, as in a parent support group. Besides offering first-hand knowledge and advice from experienced parents, a parent support group helps new parents feel that they are not alone in their concerns and that their child is not the first to behave in unexpected ways (Rothenberg, Hitchcock, Harrison, and Graham, 1983). Help the parents contact parent support groups by providing information and telephone numbers.

Enhancing the couple's relationship

The birth of a neonate leads to wide-ranging changes in family dynamics and interrelationships. The nurse who makes home visits can help the family adapt to these changes. By introducing the topic and letting family members know that such changes and the feelings associated with them are expected, the nurse may be able to begin a dialogue that helps them cope with the changes and express their feelings about them.

Typically, the client and her partner have trouble finding time alone together during the early postpartal period. To help them deal with this problem, arrange to see them together during a visit and have them explore the changes that have taken place in their relationship and responsibilities since the neonate's birth. Do not focus only on problems; encourage them to see the strengths of their relationship as well.

Ask the couple what they each enjoy most about their new role as parents, what they find most difficult about being parents, and how they expected the neonate's birth to affect their roles and relationships. Also ask how their relationship has changed and how they would like it to be. Point out that changes in a relationship affect both partners; the neonate's father may feel driven to work harder out of a sense of increased responsibility, whereas his partner may want him to help with child care. Each may feel that the other has the easier job. Discussing the division of household labor, as described earlier, may help clarify or resolve inequities in household responsibilities.

The birth of a child usually alters the couple's sexual relationship. Fischman, Rankin, Soeken, and Lenz (1986) found that the frequency of and desire for sex declines during the postpartal period. However, be aware that the couple may be embarrassed to ask questions about sex. Consequently, approach the topic gently by asking them to describe the changes that have taken place in their relationship, then asking, "And what about sex?" Urge them to share their feelings about sex with each

Nursing interventions for postpartal mood swings

Chalmers and Chalmers (1986) have delineated four areas of concern for the client with postpartal mood swings, sometimes described as postpartal depression—the overwhelming nature of neonatal care, the meaning of motherhood, self-concept, and the relationship with her partner. The chart below shows nursing interventions to help the client deal with each concern.

CLIENT CONCERN	INTERVENTION
Overwhelming nature of neonatal care The time involved in caring for a neonate may seem overwhelming to the new mother. Her concept of herself as a mother may hinge on her ability to feed the neonate and cope with the neonate's crying; when feeding does not go well or the neonate is fretful, she feels she has failed.	• Mobilize the client's support system. • "Mother" the client. • Explore child care options. • Refer the client to a support group. • Teach the client various approaches to coping with a crying neonate. • Solicit the partner's support. • Advise the client to sleep when the neonate sleeps. • Instruct the client to break down large tasks into small, manageable parts. • Give positive reinforcement for a job well done.
Meaning of motherhood For the client with postpartal mood swings, the romanticized view of motherhood that she may have developed during pregnancy is replaced by feelings of confinement, isolation, and lack of time to herself. She feels overwhelmed by the responsibilities of being a mother 24 hours a day and may feel guilty about neglecting her partner and other children.	• Help the client grieve over the loss of her fantasies about motherhood. • Encourage the client to express her anger. • Help the client make social contacts so that she can share her concerns with other mothers. • Help the client find time to spend with her other children.
Self-concept After delivery, a client's self-concept may undergo dramatic changes. Disappointment related to the childbirth experience—for instance, an unexpected cesarean delivery—may lead to feelings of failure and guilt. Weight gain and poor muscle tone may cause the client to feel overweight and unattractive. In some clients, role conflicts lead to resentment and depression. For instance, the client may resent the neonate for interrupting her career; or if the client is compelled by economic circumstances or peer pressure to return to her job, she may feel guilty about leaving the child with someone else.	• Review the events of childbirth with the client and help her accept, understand, and integrate the experience. • Provide diet counseling. • Teach the client how to perform postpartal exercises, such as leg rolls, abdominal breathing, and arm raises, to help her regain her prepregnancy figure and thereby enhance her self-esteem. • Encourage the client to find time for herself.
Relationship with her partner The birth of a new family member triggers many changes in the couple's relationship. The neonate's constant care demands may restrict the couple's freedom, impose on their privacy, alter their sexual relationship, and result in general lifestyle changes. Also, the client may have role expectations that her partner cannot—or will not—fulfill.	• Reinforce the strengths of the relationship. • Provide counseling about resumption of sexual intercourse and family planning. • Explore the division of household labor and suggest changes, if necessary. • Encourage the partners to communicate openly.

other, emphasizing that many postpartal couples have concerns about sex.

Some clients are reluctant to resume sex out of fear of discomfort, leading to a nursing diagnosis of *altered sexuality patterns related to a painful episiotomy or fear of conception.* If this is the case, point out that intercourse usually can resume once the perineum has healed, bleeding has stopped, and the partners feel ready.

However, caution the client that the first intercourse after childbirth may be somewhat painful because of perineal tenderness or vaginal dryness induced by hormonal changes. Recommend the use of lubricating jelly and positions that do not put pressure on the episiotomy site (if one is present), especially for the first postpartal intercourse.

If the client is afraid to resume sex out of fear of conception, provide teaching about family planning. Keep in mind that because oral contraceptives are contraindicated during breast-feeding, the breast-feeding client who used this contraceptive method before pregnancy may have special teaching needs in the early postpartal weeks.

Fatigue sometimes is a factor in reduced postpartal sexual activity. The couple may be so exhausted by caring for the neonate that they cannot become aroused or fall asleep as soon as they relax. Lack of privacy and interruptions by a crying neonate can contribute to a loss of interest in sex; if the client feels unattractive, low self-esteem and depression may compound the problem.

To enhance the couple's sexual relationship, encourage them to take the time to put romance back in their relationship. Point out that the resumption of sex should be based on planning, not left to luck and spontaneity; a rushed encounter can be unsatisfying for both partners. Suggest, for instance, that they plan to take the neonate to the babysitter's house for an evening, or that the client plan rest periods during the day so that she has the energy for sex in the evening.

Helping siblings adapt

Siblings may react to the birth of a neonate with jealousy, anger, and other negative behaviors, which may lead to a nursing diagnosis of *altered family processes related to the birth of a neonate.* Help the parents deal with this problem by advising them to spend time alone with each sibling and to let siblings participate in neonatal care. (For more information on promoting sibling adaptation, see Chapter 43, Psychosocial Adaptation of the Postpartal Family.)

Evaluation

During this step of the nursing process, the nurse evaluates the effectiveness of the care plan by ongoing evaluation of subjective and objective criteria. Evaluation findings should be stated in terms of actions performed or outcomes achieved for each goal.

For postpartal home visits, the nurse makes two types of evaluations. Formative, or ongoing, evaluation takes place at the end of each visit as the nurse reviews mutually set goals and determines whether the client met the goals. Later, when the nurse and client decide to discontinue home visits, the nurse conducts summative evaluation.

The following examples illustrate appropriate evaluation statements for the client receiving nursing care at home:
• The client's postpartal recovery is progressing normally, without complications.
• The client and her partner show competence and confidence in neonatal caregiving skills.
• The client has begun a postpartal exercise regimen.
• Other family members provide physical support with household tasks and neonatal care so that the client can obtain adequate rest.
• The client shows a positive adaptation to the maternal role.
• The client and her partner discuss their concerns and feelings with each other.
• Other family members demonstrate a healthy adjustment to the birth of the neonate.

Documentation

All steps of the nursing process should be documented as thoroughly and objectively as possible. Thorough documentation not only allows the nurse to evaluate the effectiveness of the care plan, but it also makes this information available to other members of the health care team, helping to ensure consistency of care.

Documentation is particularly important for the client who receives nursing care at home; if care continues over an extended period, other health care professionals are likely to be involved. When nursing visits are terminated, the nurse should prepare a discharge summary.

Documentation of care should include the following points:
• progress of the client's postpartal recovery
• client's adaptation to her new role
• date of any contracts used in the nursing process as well as the goal, proposed nursing interventions, and proposed client and nursing actions specified by the contract
• client's neonatal caregiving skills
• adaptation of other family members to the neonate's birth.

Client with altered role performance related to postpartal mood swings ("maternity blues")

During the postpartal period, the nursing process helps ensure high-quality care. The table below shows how the nurse might use the nursing process when caring for the client described in the case history at right. The first column presents history and physical assessment data followed by a paragraph of mental notes. These notes help the nurse make connections among assessment findings, aiding in development of the nursing diagnosis and planning.

The second column lists an appropriate nursing diagnosis; information in the remaining columns is based on this diagnosis. Although not part of the nursing process, a rationale appears for each intervention in the fourth column to explain how it contributes to the care plan.

ASSESSMENT	NURSING DIAGNOSIS	PLANNING
Subjective (history) data • Client says she is experiencing mood swings and tearful periods. • Client states she feels extremely fatigued. • Client expresses an inability to cope with the care of her neonate and reports that she feels guilty about this. **Objective (physical) data** • Client appears unkempt; came to the door wearing a nightgown at 2 o'clock in the afternoon. • Client appears sad and does not maintain eye contact during conversation. • Client began to cry when revealing her feelings. **Mental notes** *"Maternity blues" is common in the first few weeks after delivery. Associated signs and symptoms typically include low self-esteem and fatigue. Assessment of the availability of family support and interventions to increase support are essential to helping the client cope with her feelings.*	Altered role performance related to postpartal mood swings	**Goals:** Within the next 4 weeks, the client will: • express more positive feelings about herself and her new role as mother • perform neonatal care with increasing ease and confidence • demonstrate more energy in caring for herself, the neonate, and other family members.

Chapter summary

Chapter 45 discussed maternal care at home. Here are the chapter highlights.
• Providing nursing care for postpartal clients at home is both challenging and rewarding. As postpartal health care facility stays become shorter, the nurse can fill the gap in support that the client may experience when assuming the parental role.
• Home visits call for planning and a flexible, innovative approach. The nurse may have to deal with such problems as distractions, client resistance, and nursing role confusion.

CASE STUDY

Cindy Mooradian, a primiparous client age 32, was discharged with a full-term male neonate. Within 1 week after discharge, she began to feel depressed and fatigued. Her husband returned to work immediately after her discharge and her mother and mother-in-law have not been able to visit.

IMPLEMENTATION		EVALUATION
Intervention Instruct the client to rest or sleep when the neonate rests or sleeps.	**Rationale** Increased rest and sleep help minimize fatigue.	Upon evaluation, the client: • expressed a positive attitude about herself and the parenting role • reported that she feels more rested • demonstrated increasing ease and confidence when caring for the neonate.
Encourage and help the client find time for herself.	Taking time for herself helps restore the client's self-esteem.	
Teach the client postpartal exercises (such as leg rolls, arm raises, and abdominal breathing).	Postpartal exercises improve the client's body image, enhancing self-esteem.	
Provide emotional support.	Emotional support helps the client feel better about herself.	
Teach the client various ways to cope with a crying neonate, such as gently rocking the neonate, singing or speaking soothingly, or playing soft music.	Constructive ways of dealing with a crying neonate help lessen anxiety.	
Instruct the client to break down large tasks into small, manageable parts.	Several small tasks seem less overwhelming than one large task and help the client feel that she has the situation under control.	
Encourage the client to express her feelings and make contacts with other new mothers.	Discussing her concerns with other new mothers reduces the client's sense of isolation and provides adult stimulation.	
Provide positive reinforcement for a job well done.	Positive reinforcement promotes self-esteem.	
Solicit the partner's support in helping the client cope with her new role and responsibilities.	The partner's involvement and support can reduce the client's fatigue by making her responsibilities seem less overwhelming.	
Urge the client to grieve for the lost fantasy of motherhood.	Grieving helps the client accept her situation and evaluate it more realistically.	

• Assessment in the home can provide the nurse with important information about the client's needs, including life-style, beliefs, values, and interests. However, the nurse must respect family customs and practices and may have to find creative ways to ensure client privacy.
• The home setting can enhance sharing and interaction between the nurse and client; use of a contract can promote the client's participation in a self-help program..

• Nursing interventions focus on helping the client and her partner adapt to their new roles as parents, teaching them parenting and caregiving skills and helping the family maintain or resume positive interrelationships.
• Encouraging the client to relive the childbirth experience and explore her feelings associated with it is an important nursing functions. Through counseling, teaching, and support, the nurse can help her incorporate these feelings into her new self-concept.

• Postpartal mood swings commonly are encountered by the home care nurse; mild forms usually respond well to nursing interventions.

Study questions

1. How does early discharge increase the need for home nursing visits?

2. What are the main advantages of home nursing care for the postpartal client?

3. Which strategies help ensure the success of home nursing care?

4. On a home visit with Mrs. Cortez and her neonate 2 days after delivery, the nurse finds that the home does not have running water. Why does this pose a problem to the new mother? Besides availability of running water, what other environmental features should the nurse assess?

5. Mrs. Thompson greets the nurse with downcast eyes and a flat affect. What other signs should the nurse look for to determine if the client is having trouble adapting to her new role or may be experiencing postpartal mood swings?

6. How can the use of a contract enhance the nursing process for both the client and nurse?

7. Nine weeks after delivery, Mrs. Samuels, age 24, reports that she is concerned because she and her husband have not resumed sex. How should the nurse intervene to help them?

Bibliography

Balzer, J.W. (1988). The nursing process applied to family health promotion. In M. Stanhope and J. Lancaster (Eds.), *Community health nursing: Process and practice for promoting health* (2nd ed.; pp. 371-386). St. Louis: Mosby.

Fischman, S.H., Rankin, E.A., Soeken, K.L., and Lenz, E.R. (1986). Changes in sexual relationships in postpartum couples. *JOGNN*, 15(1), 58-63.

Flagler, S. (1988). Maternal role competence. *Western Journal of Nursing Research*, 10(3), 274-285.

Gorrie, T.M. (1986). Postpartal nursing diagnosis. *JOGNN*, 15(1), 52-56.

Greener, D.L. (1989). Transcultural nursing care of the childbearing woman and her family. In J.S. Boyle and M.M. Andrews (Eds.), *Transcultural concepts in nursing care*. Glenview, IL: Scott Foresman.

Hampson, S.J. (1989). Nursing interventions for the first three postpartum months. *JOGNN*, 18(2), 116-122.

Harrison, M.J., and Hicks, S.A. (1983). Postpartum concerns of mothers and their sources of help. *Canadian Journal of Public Health*, 74(5), 325-328.

Hiser, P.L. (1987). Concerns of multiparas during the second postpartum week. *JOGNN*, 16(3), 195-203.

Loveland-Cherry, C. (1988). Issues in family health promotion. In M. Stanhope and J. Lancaster (Eds.), *Community health nursing: Process and practice for promoting health* (2nd ed.; pp. 387-398). St. Louis: Mosby.

Rothenberg, B.A., Hitchcock, S., Harrison, M.L., and Graham, M. (1983). *Parentmaking: A practical handbook for teaching parent classes about babies and toddlers*. Menlo Park, CA: Banster.

Stevens, K.A. (1988). Nursing diagnoses in wellness childbearing settings. *JOGNN*, 17(5), 329-336.

Stolte, K.M. (1986). Nursing diagnosis and the childbearing woman. *MCN*, 11(1), 13-15.

Tegtmeier, D., and Elsea, S. (1984). Wellness throughout the maternity cycle. *Nursing Clinics of North America*, 19(2), 219-227.

Early discharge

Norr, K.F., and Nacion, K. (1987). Outcomes of postpartum early discharge, 1960-1986: A comparative review. *Birth*, 14(3), 135-141.

Lemmer, C.M. (1987). Early discharge: Outcomes of primiparas and their infants. *JOGNN*, 16(4), 230-236.

Postpartal assessment

Affonso, D.D. (1987). Assessment of maternal postpartum adaptation. *Public Health Nursing*, 4(1), 9-16.

Cropley, C. (1986). Assessment of mothering behaviors. In S.H. Johnson (Ed.), *Nursing assessment and strategies for the family at risk* (2nd ed.; pp. 15-40). Philadelphia: Lippincott.

Hans, A. (1986). Postpartum assessment: the psychological component. *JOGNN*, 15(1), 49-51.

Postpartal mood swings

Affonso, D.D. (1977). Missing pieces: A study of postpartum feelings. *Birth and the Family Journal*, 4(4), 159-164.

Affonso, D.D., and Domino, G. (1984). Postpartum depression: A review. *Birth*, 11(4), 231-245.

American Psychiatric Association (1987). *DSM-III-R: Diagnostic and statistical manual of mental disorders* (3rd ed., rev.). Washington, DC: Author.

Chalmers, D.E., and Chalmers, B.M. (1986). Postpartum depression: A revised perspective. *Journal of Psychosomatic Obstetrics and Gynaecology*, 5, 93-105.

Condon, J.T., and Watson, T.L. (1987). The maternity blues: Exploration of a psychological hypothesis. *Acta Psychiatrica Scandinavia*, 76(2), 164-171.

Errante, J. (1985). Sleep deprivation or postpartum blues? *Topics in clinical nursing,* 6(4), 9-18.

Hopkins, J., Marcus, M., and Campbell, S.B. (1984). Postpartum depression: A critical review. *Psychological Bulletin,* 95(3), 498-515.

Kraus, M.A., and Redman, E.S. (1986). Postpartum depression: An interactional view. *Journal of Marital and Family Therapy,* 12, 63-74.

Kruckman, L., and Asmann-Finch, C. (1986). *Postpartum depression: A research guide and international bibliography.* New York: Garland.

Petrick, J.M. (1984). Postpartum depression: Identification of high-risk mothers. *JOGNN,* 13(1), 37-40.

Nursing research

Blackburn, S., Lyons, N., Stein, M., Tribotti, S., and Withers, J. (1988). Patients' and nurses' perceptions of patient problems during the immediate postpartum period. *Applied Nursing Research,* 1(3), 141-142.

Censullo, M., Lester, B., and Hoffman, J. (1985). Rhythmic patterning in mother-newborn interaction. *Nursing Research,* 34(6), 342-346.

Gennaro, S. (1988). Postpartal anxiety and depression in mothers of term and preterm infants. *Nursing Research,* 37(2), 82-85.

Perry, S.E. (1983). Parents' perceptions of their newborn following structured interactions. *Nursing Research,* 32(4), 208-212.

APPENDICES, MASTER GLOSSARY, INDEX

APPENDICES

NAACOG Standards for the Nursing Care of Women and Newborns

The eight universal standards together encompass the field of nursing care of women and newborns. The first three are the universal standards of nursing practice; health education and counseling; and policies, procedures, and protocols. The remaining five are generic standards that relate to all aspects of nursing. They include professional responsibility and accountability, utilization of nursing personnel, ethics, research, and quality assurance.

Standard I: Nursing practice

Comprehensive nursing care for women and newborns focuses on helping individuals, families, and communities achieve their optimum health potential. This is best achieved within the framework of the nursing process.

Standard II: Health education and counseling

Health education for the individual, family, and community is an integral part of comprehensive nursing care. Such education encourages participation in, and shared responsibility for, health promotion, maintenance, and restoration.

Standard III: Policies, procedures, and protocols

Written policies, procedures, and protocols clarify the scope of nursing practice within the health care setting and delineate the qualifications of personnel authorized to provide care to women and newborns.

Standard IV: Professional responsibility and accountability

Comprehensive nursing care for women and newborns is provided by nurses who are clinically competent and accountable for professional actions and legal responsibilities inherent in the nursing role.

Standard V: Utilization of nursing personnel

Nursing care for women and newborns is conducted in practice settings that have qualified nursing staff in sufficient numbers to meet patient care needs.

Standard VI: Ethics

Ethical principles guide the process of decision making for nurses caring for women and newborns when personal or professional values conflict with those of the patient, family, colleagues, or practice setting.

Standard VII: Research

Nurses caring for women and newborns utilize research findings, conduct nursing research, and evaluate nursing practice to improve the outcomes of patient care.

Standard VIII: Quality assurance

Quality and appropriateness of patient care are evaluated through a planned assessment program using specific, identified clinical indicators.

Source: NAACOG. (1990). *NAACOG Standards for the Nursing Care of Women and Newborns*, 4th ed. (Advanced release). Washington, DC: NAACOG.

APPENDIX

2

NANDA Taxonomy of Nursing Diagnoses

A taxonomy for classifying nursing diagnoses has evolved over several years. The following list is grouped around nine human response patterns endorsed by the North American Nursing Diagnosis Association, as of summer 1990.

PATTERN 1. Exchanging: A human response pattern involving mutual giving and receiving

1.1.2.1. Altered nutrition: more than body requirements

1.1.2.2. Altered nutrition: less than body requirements

1.1.2.3. Altered nutrition: potential for more than body requirements

1.2.1.1. Potential for infection

1.2.2.1. Potential for altered body temperature

1.2.2.2. Hypothermia

1.2.2.3. Hyperthermia

1.2.2.4. Ineffective thermoregulation

1.2.3.1. Dysreflexia

1.3.1.1. Constipation

1.3.1.1.1. Perceived constipation

1.3.1.1.2. Colonic constipation

1.3.1.2. Diarrhea

1.3.1.3. Bowel incontinence

1.3.2. Altered urinary elimination

1.3.2.1.1. Stress incontinence

1.3.2.1.2. Reflex incontinence

1.3.2.1.3. Urge incontinence

1.3.2.1.4. Functional incontinence

1.3.2.1.5. Total incontinence

1.3.2.2. Urinary retention

1.4.1.1. Altered (specify type) tissue perfusion (renal, cerebral, cardiopulmonary, gastrointestinal, peripheral)

1.4.1.2.1. Fluid volume excess

1.4.1.2.2.1. Fluid volume deficit

1.4.1.2.2.2. Potential fluid volume deficit

1.4.2.1. Decreased cardiac output

1.5.1.1. Impaired gas exchange

1.5.1.2. Ineffective airway clearance

1.5.1.3. Ineffective breathing pattern

1.6.1. Potential for injury

1.6.1.1. Potential for suffocation

1.6.1.2. Potential for poisoning

1.6.1.3. Potential for trauma

1.6.1.4. Potential for aspiration

1.6.1.5. Potential for disuse syndrome

1.6.2. Altered protection

1.6.2.1. Impaired tissue integrity

1.6.2.1.1. Altered oral mucous membrane

1.6.2.1.2.1. Impaired skin integrity

1.6.2.1.2.2. Potential impaired skin integrity

PATTERN 2. Communicating: A human response pattern involving sending messages

2.1.1.1. Impaired verbal communication

PATTERN 3. Relating: A human response pattern involving establishing bonds

3.1.1. Impaired social interaction

3.1.2. Social isolation

3.2.1. Altered role performance

3.2.1.1.1. Altered parenting

3.2.1.1.2. Potential altered parenting

(continued)

NANDA Taxonomy of Nursing Diagnoses continued

3.2.1.2.1. Sexual dysfunction

3.2.2. Altered family processes

3.2.3.1. Parental role conflict

3.3. Altered sexuality patterns

PATTERN 4. Valuing: A human response pattern involving the assigning of relative worth

4.1.1. Spiritual distress (distress of the human spirit)

PATTERN 5. Choosing: A human response pattern involving the selection of alternatives

5.1.1.1. Ineffective individual coping

5.1.1.1.1. Impaired adjustment

5.1.1.1.2. Defensive coping

5.1.1.1.3. Ineffective denial

5.1.2.1.1. Ineffective family coping: disabling

5.1.2.1.2. Ineffective family coping: compromised

5.1.2.2. Family coping: potential for growth

5.2.1.1. Noncompliance (specify)

5.3.1.1. Decisional conflict (specify)

5.4 Health-seeking behaviors (specify)

PATTERN 6. Moving: A human response pattern involving activity

6.1.1.1. Impaired physical mobility

6.1.1.2. Activity intolerance

6.1.1.2.1. Fatigue

6.1.1.3. Potential activity intolerance

6.2.1. Sleep pattern disturbance

6.3.1.1. Diversional activity deficit

6.4.1.1. Impaired home maintenance management

6.4.2. Altered health maintenance

6.5.1. Feeding self-care deficit

6.5.1.1. Impaired swallowing

6.5.1.2. Ineffective breast-feeding

6.5.1.3. Effective breast-feeding

6.5.2. Bathing or hygiene self-care deficit

6.5.3. Dressing or grooming self-care deficit

6.5.4. Toileting self-care deficit

6.6. Altered growth and development

PATTERN 7. Perceiving: A human response pattern involving the reception of information

7.1.1. Body image disturbance

7.1.2. Self-esteem disturbance

7.1.2.1. Chronic low self-esteem

7.1.2.2. Situational low self-esteem

7.1.3. Personal identify disturbance

7.2. Sensory or perceptual alterations (specify—visual, auditory, kinesthetic, gustatory, tactile, olfactory)

7.2.1.1. Unilateral neglect

7.3.1. Hopelessness

7.3.2. Powerlessness

PATTERN 8. Knowing: A human response pattern involving the meaning associated with information

8.1.1. Knowledge deficit (specify)

8.3. Altered thought processes

PATTERN 9. Feeling: A human response pattern involving the subjective awareness of information

9.1.1. Pain

9.1.1.1. Chronic pain

9.2.1.1. Dysfunctional grieving

9.2.1.2. Anticipatory grieving

9.2.2. Potential for violence: self-directed or directed at others

9.2.3. Post-trauma response

9.2.3.1. Rape-trauma syndrome

9.2.3.1.1. Rape-trauma syndrome: compound reaction

9.2.3.1.2. Rape-trauma syndrome: silent reaction

9.3.1. Anxiety

9.3.2. Fear

APPENDIX

3

Neonatal Weight Conversion Table

The nurse can use the table below to convert a neonate's weight from customary units (pounds and ounces) to metric units (grams), or from metric to customary. The left column shows pounds; the top row shows ounces. The remaining numbers indicate grams.

Converting from customary to metric units
For a neonate weighing 4 pounds, 8 ounces, determine the weight in grams by finding *4 pounds* in the left column.

Next, find *8 ounces* in the top row. The intersecting number (2041) is the neonate's weight in grams.

Converting from metric to customary units
For a neonate weighing 4224 grams, find *4224* in the gram section. Read across to the left column (*9 pounds*), then read upward to the top row (*5 ounces*) to determine the neonate's weight in customary units (9 pounds, 5 ounces).

Ounces																
Pounds	0	1	2	3	4	5	6	7	8	9	10	11	12	13	14	15
0	—	28	57	85	113	142	170	198	227	255	283	312	340	369	397	425
1	454	482	510	539	567	595	624	652	680	709	737	765	794	822	850	879
2	907	936	964	992	1021	1049	1077	1106	1134	1162	1191	1219	1247	1276	1304	1332
3	1361	1389	1417	1446	1474	1502	1531	1559	1588	1616	1644	1673	1701	1729	1758	1786
4	1814	1843	1871	1899	1928	1956	1984	2013	2041	2070	2098	2126	2155	2183	2211	2240
5	2268	2296	2325	2353	2381	2410	2438	2466	2495	2523	2551	2580	2608	2637	2665	2693
6	2722	2750	2778	2807	2835	2863	2892	2920	2948	2977	3005	3033	3062	3090	3118	3147
7	3175	3203	3232	3260	3289	3317	3345	3374	3402	3430	3459	3487	3515	3544	3572	3600
8	3629	3657	3685	3714	3742	3770	3799	3827	3856	3884	3912	3941	3969	3997	4026	4054
9	4082	4111	4139	4167	4196	4224	4252	4281	4309	4337	4366	4394	4423	4451	4479	4508
10	4536	4564	4593	4621	4649	4678	4706	4734	4763	4791	4819	4848	4876	4904	4933	4961
11	4990	5018	5046	5075	5103	5131	5160	5188	5216	5245	5273	5301	5330	5358	5386	5415
12	5443	5471	5500	5528	5557	5585	5613	5642	5670	5698	5727	5755	5783	5812	5840	5868
13	5897	5925	5953	5982	6010	6038	6067	6095	6123	6152	6180	6209	6237	6265	6294	6322
14	6350	6379	6407	6435	6464	6492	6520	6549	6577	6605	6634	6662	6690	6719	6747	6776
15	6804	6832	6860	6889	6917	6945	6973	7002	7030	7059	7087	7115	7144	7172	7201	7228

(Grams)

APPENDIX

4

Temperature Conversion Table

The nurse can use this table to determine Fahrenheit (°F) and Celsius (°C) temperature equivalents. Alternatively, temperatures can be converted with the following formulas.

To convert from °F to °C:	To convert from °C to °F:
°F = (°C × 1.8) + 32	°C = (°F − 32) ÷ 1.8

DEGREES FAHRENHEIT	DEGREES CELSIUS	DEGREES FAHRENHEIT	DEGREES CELSIUS
93.2	34.0	101.5	38.6
93.6	34.2	101.8	38.8
93.9	34.4	102.2	39.0
94.3	34.6	102.6	39.2
94.6	34.8	102.9	39.4
95.0	35.0	103.3	39.6
95.4	35.2	103.6	39.8
95.7	35.4	104.0	40.0
96.1	35.6	104.4	40.2
96.4	35.8	104.7	40.4
96.8	36.0	105.2	40.6
97.2	36.2	105.4	40.8
97.5	36.4	105.9	41.0
97.9	36.6	106.1	41.2
98.2	36.8	106.5	41.4
98.6	37.0	106.8	41.6
99.0	37.2	107.2	41.8
99.3	37.4	107.6	42.0
99.7	37.6	108.0	42.2
100.0	37.8	108.3	42.4
100.4	38.0	108.7	42.6
100.8	38.2	109.0	42.8
101.1	38.4	109.4	43.0

APPENDIX

5

1990 Nutritional Guidelines and Weight Table

The U.S. government has revised five of its seven dietary guidelines for Americans. The revisions reflect the use of a health-based definition for desirable weight, a focus on the total diet, and a focus on specific foods in the diet.

Guidelines

Modifications in the dietary guidelines address the intake of calories, fat, cholesterol, sodium, complex carbohydrates, and fiber. Excess intake of the first four and insufficient intake of the last two have been linked with obesity, heart disease, high blood pressure, stroke, diabetes, and some forms of carcinomas. Summaries of the specific recommendations follow.

Eat a variety of foods.

Because no single food can supply all nutrients in the amounts needed, a nutritious diet must contain a variety of foods. More than 40 nutrients are required to maintain health, including vitamins, minerals, amino acids, certain fatty acids, and sources of calories. To ensure variety, select foods daily from the five major food groups:

- vegetables
- fruits
- breads, cereals, rice, and pasta
- milk, yogurt, and cheese
- meats, poultry, fish, dry beans and peas, eggs, and nuts.

   Many pregnant women, women of childbearing age, teenage girls, and young children need an iron supplement. Also, some pregnant or breast-feeding women may need supplements to meet their increased requirements for other nutrients.

Maintain healthy weight.

Excess or inadequate weight increases the risk of developing health problems. Excess weight has been linked with hypertension, heart disease, stroke, diabetes mellitus, certain carcinomas, and other problems. Inadequate weight is associated with osteoporosis in women and an increased risk of early death in both sexes.

   A healthy weight depends on how much of the weight is fat, where the fat is located, and whether the person has weight-related problems or a family history of such problems. Healthy weight cannot be determined exactly; researchers are trying to develop more precise ways to describe it. However, the following guidelines can help the nurse judge whether a client's weight is healthy.

• *A weight within the range in the table for the client's age and height.* The table allows higher weights for people ages 35 and older compared to younger adults because research suggests that slightly increased weight among older people

is not associated with health risks. The weight ranges given here are likely to change based on ongoing research. Also, the table shows weights in ranges because people of the same height with equal amounts of body fat may differ in amount of muscle and bone. The higher weights in each range are suggested for people with more muscle and bone. Weights above the range are unhealthy for most people; weights below the range may be healthy for some small-boned people but have been linked to health problems.

• *Body shape.* For adults, health depends on body shape as well as height. Research suggests that excess abdominal fat poses a greater health risk than excess fat in the hips and thighs.

   To assess body shape, find the waist-to-hip ratio. First, measure around the waist near the navel as the client stands relaxed. Then measure around the hips, over the buttocks where they are largest. Divide the waist measurement by the hip measurement to find the ratio. A ratio above 1 suggests a greater risk for several diseases.

Choose a diet low in unsaturated fat, saturated fat, and cholesterol.

Most health experts recommend that Americans eat less fat—both unsaturated and saturated fat—and cholesterol. Populations with high-fat diets have more obesity and certain types of carcinomas; high amounts of saturated fat and cholesterol increase the risk of cardiac disease. Also, with a low-fat diet, the variety of foods needed for nutrients can be consumed without exceeding caloric needs because fat contains more than twice the calories of an equal amount of carbohydrates or protein. A diet low in saturated fat and cholesterol can help maintain a desirable blood cholesterol level. (A blood cholesterol level above 200 mg/dl increases the risk of heart disease.)

   For adults, dietary fat should account for 30% or less of the total calories needed for healthy weight; saturated fat should provide less than 10% of calories. Because animal products are the source of all dietary cholesterol, eating less fat from animal sources will help lower both saturated fats and cholesterol.

Choose a diet with plenty of vegetables, fruits, and grain products.

Americans and other populations with diets low in dietary fiber and complex carbohydrates (such as starch) and high in fat tend to have more heart disease, obesity, and some carcinomas. To help ensure a varied diet, increase dietary fiber and carbohydrate intake, and decrease dietary fat in-

(continued)

1990 Nutritional Guidelines and Weight Table continued

take, adults should eat at least three servings of vegetables, two servings of fruits, and six servings of grain products daily. Preferably, most dietary fiber should come from foods rather than supplements.

Use sugar in moderation.

Sugar and most foods containing large amounts of sugar are high in calories and low in essential nutrients. Therefore, most healthy people should eat these foods in moderation; people with low caloric needs should eat them sparingly. Sugar also contributes to tooth decay.

Use salt and sodium in moderation.

Most Americans consume more salt and sodium than they need. In populations with diets low in sodium, hypertension is less common than in the United States. Restriction of dietary salt and sodium may help reduce the risk of hypertension and usually helps decrease blood pressure in people with hypertension.

Drink alcoholic beverages in moderation, if at all.

Alcoholic beverages provide calories but little or no nutrients; they are linked with many health problems and accidents and can be addictive. Therefore, they should be consumed in moderation, if at all. The following individuals should not consume any alcoholic beverages:
• pregnant women or women trying to conceive
• people who plan to drive or engage in other activities requiring attention or skill
• people taking medications
• people who cannot limit their alcohol intake.

Weight table

The following table reflects ongoing research, which presently suggests that people can carry somewhat more weight as they age without added health risk. Because people of the same height may differ in muscle and bone makeup, weights are shown across a range for each height.

| HEIGHT* | WEIGHT IN POUNDS† | |
	Ages 19 to 34	Ages 35 and over
5'0"	97-128	108-138
5'1"	101-132	111-143
5'2"	104-137	115-148
5'3"	107-141	119-152
5'4"	111-146	122-157
5'5"	114-150	126-162
5'6"	118-155	130-167
5'7"	121-160	134-172
5'8"	125-164	138-178
5'9"	129-169	142-183
5'10"	132-174	146-188
5'11"	136-179	151-194
6'0"	140-184	155-199
6'1"	144-189	159-205
6'2"	148-195	164-210
6'3"	152-200	168-216
6'4"	156-205	173-222
6'5"	160-211	177-228
6'6"	164-216	182-234

*without shoes
†without clothes

Source: U.S. Department of Agriculture, U.S. Department of Health and Human Services (1990). *Nutrition and Your Health: Dietary Guidelines for Americans* (3rd ed.). Washington, DC.

APPENDIX

6

Selected Resources for the Disabled Pregnant Client

A disability is defined as an impairment that limits major activities, such as hearing, seeing, or walking. Millions of women of childbearing age in the United States alone are disabled. Until recently, a disabled woman was discouraged from having a child; her family and friends worried that the neonate would inherit the disability and that the woman might be unable to care for the child. Health care professionals knew little about the effects of pregnancy, labor, and childbirth on the disabled woman's body.

Despite such discouragement, growing numbers of disabled women have chosen to become parents. To help provide a safe delivery and postpartal period for the disabled client and her neonate and to ensure the psychosocial well-being of the client and her partner, the nurse must be familiar with management techniques to use with the disabled client. These techniques involve client teaching, treatment planning, nursing care, and related subjects. The following resources can provide details.

AUDIOVISUALS

Arthritis Patient Services
1945 Randolph Road
Charlotte, NC 28207
704-331-4878

Eric Miller Company
Professional Video Programs
P.O. Box 443
114 Forrest Avenue
Narberth, PA 19072
215-667-3360

Multi-Focus, Inc.
1525 Franklin Street
San Francisco, CA 94109-4592
1-800-821-0514
415-673-5100

ORGANIZATIONS

American Association of Spinal Cord Injury Nurses
75-20 Astoria Boulevard
Jackson Heights, NY 11370
718-803-3782

American Foundation for the Blind
15 West 16th Street
New York, NY 10011
212-620-2000

American Occupational Therapy Association, Inc.
1383 Picard Drive
Rockville, MD 20850
301-948-9626

Arthritis Foundation
P.O. Box 19000
Atlanta, GA 30326
404-872-7100

Canadian Paraplegic Association
520 Sutherland Drive
Toronto, Ontario
Canada M4G 3V9
416-422-5644

International Childbirth Education Association
P.O. Box 20048
Minneapolis, MN 55420
612-854-8660

La Leche League International
9616 Minneapolis Avenue
Franklin Park, IL 60131
708-455-7730

Muscular Dystrophy Association
810 7th Avenue
New York, NY 10019
1-800-223-6333

National Head Injury Foundation
333 Turnpike Road
Southboro, MA 01772
1-800-444-6443

National Information Center on Deafness
Gallaudet University
800 Florida Avenue, NE
Washington, DC 20002
202-651-5051

National Multiple Sclerosis Society
205 E. 42nd Street, 3rd Floor
New York, NY 10017
212-986-3240

National Rehabilitation Information Center
8455 Colesville Road, Suite 935
Silver Spring, MD 20910-3319
301-588-9284

National Spinal Cord Injury Association
600 W. Cummings Park
Suite 2000
Woburn, MA 01801
1-800-962-9629
617-935-2722

Courtesy of Wilma Asrael, OTR, MHDL, ACCE.

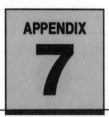

APPENDIX

7

Support Resources for Families with Special-Needs Neonates

The nurse may wish to refer families with special-needs neonates to some of the following organizations for specific advice and coping techniques.

BIRTH DEFECTS

Association of Birth Defect Children, Inc.
Orlando Executive Park
5400 Diplomat Circle
Suite 270
Orlando, FL 32810
407-629-1466

March of Dimes Birth Defects Foundation
1275 Mamaroneck Avenue
White Plains, NY 10605
914-428-7100

CEREBRAL PALSY

United Cerebral Palsy Associations, Inc.
1522 K Street, Suite 1112
Washington, DC 20005
800-USA-5UCP

Canadian Cerebral Palsy Association
880 Wellington Street, Suite 612
City Centre
Ottawa, Ontario
Canada K1R 6K7
613-235-2144

CRANIOFACIAL ABNORMALITIES

American Cleft Palate–Craniofacial Association
1218 Grandview Avenue
Pittsburgh, PA 15211
412-481-1376

Cleft Lip and Palate Program
Hospital for Sick Children
555 University Avenue
Toronto, Ontario
Canada M5G 1X8
416-598-6019

CYSTIC FIBROSIS

Cystic Fibrosis Foundation
6931 Arlington Road, #200
Bethesda, MD 20814
301-951-4422

Canadian Cystic Fibrosis Foundation
2221 Yonge Street, Suite 601
Toronto, Ontario
Canada M4S 2B4
416-485-9149

DOWN'S SYNDROME

National Down Syndrome Society
666 Broadway
New York, NY 10012
212-460-9330

Down Syndrome Association of Metropolitan Toronto
P.O. Box 490
Don Mills, Ontario
Canada M3C 2T2
416-690-2503

HYDROCEPHALUS

National Hydrocephalus Foundation
22427 South River Road
Joliet, IL 60436
815-467-6548
(For a Canadian organization, see the Spina Bifida and Hydrocephalus Association of Ontario, below.)

INTRAVENTRICULAR HEMORRHAGE (IVH)

IVH Parents
P.O. Box 56-1111
Miami, FL 33256-1111
305-232-0381

MENTAL RETARDATION AND DELAYED DEVELOPMENT

Association for Retarded Citizens of the United States
2501 Avenue J
Arlington, TX 76006
817-640-0204

Canadian Association for Community Living
York University Kinsmen Building
4700 Keele Street
Downsview, Ontario
Canada M3J 1P3
416-661-9611

PHYSICAL DISABILITIES

National Easter Seal Society, Inc.
70 East Lake Street
Chicago, IL 60601
312-726-6200

Easter Seals Canada
45 Sheppard Avenue, East
Suite 801
Toronto, Ontario
Canada M2N 5W9
416-250-7490

RARE DISORDERS

National Organization for Rare Disorders
P.O. Box 8923
New Fairfield, CT 06812
800-999-NORD
203-746-6518

Lethbridge Society for Rare Disorders
100-542-7 Street, South
Lethbridge, Alberta
Canada T1J 2H1
403-329-0665

PARENTS OF PREMATURE AND HIGH-RISK INFANTS

Parent Care, Inc.
101½ South Union Street
Alexandria, VA 22314
703-836-4678

PHENYLKETONURIA (PKU)

PKU Parents
c/o Dale Hilliard
8 Myrtle Lane
San Anselmo, CA 94960
415-457-4632

SEVERE HANDICAPS

(TASH) The Association for Persons with Severe Handicaps
7010 Roosevelt Way NE
Seattle, WA 98115
206-523-8446

Support Resources for Families with Special-Needs Neonates continued

SIBLING SUPPORT

A.J. Pappanikou Center on Special Education and Rehabilitation
991 Main Street, Suite 3A
East Hartford, CT 06108
203-282-7050

SICKLE CELL DISEASE

National Association for Sickle Cell Disease
4221 Wilshire Boulevard, Suite 360
Los Angeles, CA 90010
800-421-8453
213-936-7205

Canadian Sickle Cell Society
1076 Bathurst
Toronto, Ontario
Canada M5R 3G8
416-537-3475

SPINA BIFIDA (MENINGOMYELOCELE)

Spina Bifida Association of America
1700 Rockville Pike
Suite 250
Rockville, MD 20852
301-770-SBAA

Spina Bifida and Hydrocephalus Association of Ontario
55 Queen Street East
Suite 300
Toronto, Ontario
Canada M5C 1R6
416-364-1871

TECHNOLOGY-DEPENDENT CHILDREN

SKIP: Sick Kids Need Involved People
990 Second Avenue
New York, NY 10022
212-421-9160

TURNER'S SYNDROME

Turner's Syndrome Society
York University
Administrative Studies Building
Room 006
Downsview , Ontario
Canada M3J 1P3
416-736-5023

VISUAL AND AUDITORY DEFICITS

American Society for Deaf Children
814 Thayer Avenue
Silver Spring, MD 20910
301-585-5400 (international office)

Helen Keller National Center for Deaf-Blind Youths and Adults
111 Middle Neck Road
Sands Point, NY 11050-1299
516-944-8900

APPENDIX

8

Guidelines to Prevent H.I.V. Transmission

Human immunodeficiency virus (HIV), which causes acquired immunodeficiency syndrome (AIDS), is transmitted through sexual contact, exposure to blood and blood components, and perinatally from mother to neonate. The rising incidence of HIV infection increases the nurse's risk of exposure to blood of clients infected with HIV. To prevent exposure to blood and avoid infection, the nurse should follow universal and environmental precautions.

Universal precautions
Because medical history and examination cannot identify all clients infected with HIV, the nurse must take steps to prevent possible transmission. Use the following universal blood and body-fluid precautions when caring for all clients, especially during emergency care situations in which the client's infection status is unknown and the risk of blood exposure is increased.

1. When contact with a client's blood or body fluid is likely, use appropriate barrier precautions to prevent skin and mucous membrane exposure. Don gloves before touching a client's blood or body fluids, mucous membranes, or nonintact skin; before touching items or surfaces soiled with blood or body fluids; and before performing vascular access procedures. Change gloves after contact with each client. Wear a mask and protective eyewear or a face shield during procedures likely to generate droplets of blood or body fluids; wear a gown or apron during procedures likely to generate splashes of these fluids. If a glove is torn or a needlestick or other injury occurs, don a new glove as soon as the client's safety permits; remove the needle or item involved in the accident from the sterile field.

2. Wash hands and other skin surfaces immediately and thoroughly after any contact with blood or body fluids. Always wash hands immediately after removing gloves.

3. Take precautions to prevent injuries from needles and other sharp objects during and after procedures, when cleaning used instruments, and when disposing of used needles. To prevent needlesticks, do not recap used needles or manipulate them by hand in any manner. Place used disposable needles, scalpel blades, and other sharp objects in puncture-resistant containers (which should be located as close as possible to the work area). Place large-bore reusable needles in a puncture-resistant container to be transported for reprocessing.

4. To minimize the need for emergency mouth-to-mouth resuscitation, ensure that mouthpieces, resuscitation bags, or other ventilation devices are available wherever resuscitation procedures are likely.

5. A nurse with exfoliative dermatitis or exudative lesions should refrain from direct client care and from handling client care equipment.

6. A pregnant nurse should strictly follow all precautions to minimize the risk of HIV transmission; because HIV can be transmitted perinatally, the fetus also is at risk for infection.

These precautions apply to blood and any body fluid containing visible blood. Occupational transmission of HIV to health care workers by blood has been documented; infection control therefore focuses on preventing exposure to blood.

Universal precautions also apply to semen and vaginal secretions, which have been implicated in the sexual transmission of HIV. The risk of occupational transmission is not known because exposure to semen is limited and gloves are worn routinely during vaginal examinations.

Universal precautions also apply to tissues, cerebrospinal fluid, synovial fluid, pleural fluid, peritoneal fluid, pericardial fluid, and amniotic fluid. HIV has been isolated in some of these substances, but HIV transmission by them is undocumented.

These precautions do not apply to feces, nasal secretions, sputum, sweat, tears, urine, and vomitus (unless they contain visible blood). Although HIV has been isolated in some, the transmission rate of HIV through them is very low or nonexistent. Human breast milk has been implicated in perinatal transmission of HIV, but universal precautions need not be taken because the neonate is infected after breast-feeding, not from the type of incidental exposure the nurse can expect. (However, wear gloves if exposure to breast milk is frequent.) Universal precautions do not apply to saliva because of the extremely low risk of infection, but follow general infection control practices—such as wearing gloves when examining mucous membranes—to minimize the risk further.

Environmental precautions
No environmental mode of HIV transmission has been documented. HIV survival outside the human body is brief, particularly in the concentrations typically found in a client's blood. Therefore, no changes in the recommended sterilization, disinfection, or housekeeping procedures are required. Take the following precautions during the care of all clients.

1. Follow the currently recommended sterilization and disinfection procedures for all client care equipment; these procedures are adequate to sterilize or disinfect instruments and other items contaminated by blood or other body fluids.

Before reusing them, sterilize instruments or devices that enter a client's sterile tissue or vascular system or that transport blood. Sterilize or disinfect items that touch intact mucous membranes. Use germicides registered with the U.S. Environmental Protection Agency as sterilants for sterilization or high-level disinfection, depending on contact time.

Thoroughly clean medical instruments and devices requiring sterilization or disinfection before exposing them to the germicide. Follow the manufacturer's specifications for compatibility of the device with the germicide.

HIV is inactivated rapidly when exposed to common commercially available germicides, even at low concentrations. In addition, a solution of sodium hypochlorite (household bleach) prepared daily makes an effective and inexpensive germicide, although it may not be compatible with certain medical devices. Concentrations between 1% and 10% are

Guidelines to Prevent H.I.V. Transmission   continued

effective, depending on the amount of organic material on the surface to be cleaned.

2. Because walls, floors, and other environmental surfaces are not associated with HIV infection, extra measures to disinfect or sterilize them are not necessary. However, routine cleaning and removal of soil is recommended. Schedules and methods vary according to area, type of surface to be cleaned, and amount and type of soil present. Horizontal surfaces in client care areas usually are cleaned regularly when soiling or spills occur and when a client is discharged; vertical surfaces should be cleaned only if visibly soiled.

3. Use chemical germicides approved for use as hospital disinfectants to decontaminate spills of blood and other body fluids. In client care areas, remove visible material first and then decontaminate the area; in laboratories, flood the contaminated area with a liquid germicide before cleaning, then decontaminate with fresh germicide. Wear gloves when cleaning and decontaminating.

4. Hygienic storing and processing of linen is sufficient to prevent HIV infection from soiled linen. Handle soiled linen as little as possible and bag it at the location it was used; do not agitate it unnecessarily or sort or rinse it in client care areas. Place linen soiled with blood or body fluids in leak-proof bags. Linen should by washed with detergent in hot water (at least 160° F) or with suitable chemicals in cooler water.

5. Hospital waste has not been shown to be more infective than residential waste. To reduce any possibility of waste causing disease in the outside community, identify potentially infective wastes that should receive special precautions or disposal methods. These include microbiology laboratory waste, pathology waste, and blood or blood components. Such wastes should be incinerated or autoclaved before disposal in a sanitary landfill. Pour large amounts of blood, secretions, or excretions down a drain leading to a sanitary sewer; other infectious wastes can be ground and flushed into the sewer. Although potentially infective, items that have contacted blood, secretions, or exudates usually do not require the disposal methods listed above.

Strict adherence to these precautions will reduce exposure to blood and other substances possibly infected with HIV, thereby reducing the risk of transmission. Remember that these precautions do not eliminate the need for other disease-specific isolation precautions, such as isolation for pulmonary tuberculosis or enteric precautions for infectious diarrhea.

Source: U.S. Department of Health and Human Services. (1989). *Guidelines for prevention of transmission of human immunodeficiency virus and hepatitis B virus to health-care and public safety workers.* Washington, DC: U.S. Government Printing Office.

MASTER GLOSSARY

ABO incompatibility: condition in which the mother's blood type is O and the neonate's blood type is either A, B, or AB.

ABO blood group incompatibility: isoimmune hemolytic anemia in which a maternal antigen-antibody reaction causes premature destruction of fetal red blood cells.

Abortion: spontaneous or induced termination of pregnancy before the fetus reaches the age of viability.

Abruptio placentae: premature separation of part or all of the placenta from the uterine wall after the twentieth week of pregnancy and before delivery; hemorrhage and shock are common complications.

Abuse: physical violence directed against one person by another who lives in that household, typically resulting in serious physical and psychological damage to the person; also called battering or domestic or family violence.

Acceleration: increase in the fetal heart rate from the baseline that lasts less than 15 minutes.

Accommodator: person who learns best from personal experience and hands-on demonstration.

Acquaintance: knowledge about another person that results from interaction; a prerequisite to parent-infant bonding.

Acquired immunodeficiency syndrome (AIDS): life-threatening disease that disables the immune system, rendering the body susceptible to opportunistic infection; present when an individual with human immunodeficiency virus (HIV) infection develops Kaposi's sarcoma, extrapulmonary cryptococcosis, *Pneumocystis carinii* pneumonia, or other designated diseases.

Acrocyanosis: bluish discoloration of the hands and feet caused by vasomotor instability, capillary stasis, and high hemoglobin levels.

Acrosome: membranelike covering on the head portion of a spermatozoon.

Active listening: close evaluation of body language and voice inflection to supplement verbal communication.

Active phase of labor: second phase of the first stage of labor, when the cervix dilates from 4 to 10 cm; includes three phases: acceleration, maximum slope, and deceleration (transition).

Acupressure: pressure on specific body points to promote energy flow and relieve pain.

Acupuncture: insertion of needles at specific body points to promote energy flow and relieve pain.

Adjuvant therapy: treatment in addition to the primary treatment.

Affirmation: technique used to reinforce a client's abilities, efforts, and self-esteem.

Age-related concerns: health concerns for an adolescent client (under age 19) or a mature client (over age 34) related to maternal, fetal, or neonatal risks during labor and delivery.

Agonist: substance that stimulates physiologic activity at cell receptors that are normally stimulated by naturally occurring substances.

Alcoholism: pathologic pattern of alcohol use marked by cognitive, behavioral, and physiologic symptoms that indicate inability to reduce intake, continued use despite adverse consequences, tolerance, and specific withdrawal symptoms; also called alcohol dependence.

Algesia: hypersensitivity to pain; hyperesthesia.

Allantois: diverticulum in the caudal end of the embryo; allantoic blood vessels help form those of the umbilical cord.

Alleles: pair of genes that may be different from each other but occupy corresponding sites (loci) on homologous chromosomes.

Alveolus: secretory unit of the mammary gland in which milk production takes place.

Ambivalence: conflicting feelings.

Amenorrhea: absence of menses.

Amino acids: building blocks of protein; divided into 9 essential amino acids (which the human body cannot make and must be provided in the diet) and 11 nonessential amino acids (which the body can make from the essentials in the diet).

Amnihook: instrument used to perform amniotomy.

Amniocentesis: prenatal needle aspiration procedure for obtaining amniotic fluid for analysis.

Amnionitis: inflammation of the inner layer of the fetal membranes, or amnion; most commonly a complication of early rupture of membranes.

Amniotic fluid: fluid within the amniotic sac that allows the fetus to move and cushions the fetus's head and umbilical cord during delivery.

Amniotic sac: membrane that surrounds the fetus, contains amniotic fluid, and eventually lines the chorion.

Amniotomy: artificial rupture of the amniotic membranes, performed by a physician or nurse-midwife to enhance or induce labor.

Amphetamine: drug that stimulates the sympathetic nervous system.

Analgesia: reduction of pain without loss of consciousness.

Androgen: class of hormone that stimulates the development of male secondary sex characteristics, such as facial hair and increased musculature.

MASTER GLOSSARY continued

Androgyny: combination of male and female characteristics in the same individual.

Anemia: blood disorder characterized by a change in red blood cells or decreased hemoglobin, which may be related to a deficiency of iron, vitamin B_{12}, or folic acid.

Anencephaly: congenital absence of the cerebral hemispheres in which the cephalic end of the spinal cord fails to close during gestation.

Anesthesia: loss of sensation (total or partial) with or without loss of consciousness.

Anorexia nervosa: eating disorder characterized by a morbid fear of weight gain and by self-starvation.

Anovulation: failure of the ovaries to produce, mature, or release ova.

Antagonist: substance that blocks the action of another, such as a drug, by binding to a cell receptor without causing a physiologic response.

Anteflexed uterus: normal position in which the uterine corpus flexes forward at an acute angle.

Antepartal period: period during pregnancy and before labor and delivery.

Anterior "lip": anterior portion of the cervix that remains undilated just before complete dilation.

Anteverted uterus: normal position in which the uterine corpus flexes forward at a less acute angle than an anteflexed uterus.

Anthropometry: science that deals with measurement of the size, weight, and proportions of the human body.

Antibody: protein produced in the body in response to invasion by a foreign agent (antigen); reacts specifically with the antigen.

Anticipatory grief: sadness in anticipation of loss.

Antigen: foreign substance that stimulates the immunologic system to formulate mechanisms with which to fight against it (antibody).

Apgar score: method of evaluating neonatal vigor at 1- and 5-minute intervals after delivery; ranging from 0 to 10, the score is based on assessment of heart rate, respirations, muscle tone, reflex irritability, and skin color.

Apnea: absence of spontaneous respirations.

Apnea monitor: device that sounds an alarm when breathing stops or drops below a preset level.

Appraisal support: type of support that includes affirmation and feedback.

Appropriate for gestational age: term used to describe a neonate whose birth weight falls between the tenth and ninetieth percentile for gestational age on the Colorado intrauterine growth chart.

AROM: artificial rupture of membranes (amniotic sac).

Asphyxia: condition caused by sustained oxygen deprivation and characterized by hypoxemia, hypercapnia, and acidosis.

Assessment: systematic collection of subjective and objective data about a client's health status; a step in the nursing process.

Assimilator: person who learns best by assembling small bits of information gathered from various sources.

Asynclitism: lateral flexion of the fetus's head toward either the symphysis pubis (anterior asynclitism) or sacrum (posterior asynclitism) during labor.

Atony: lack of normal tone; uterine atony produces a boggy (soft, poorly contracted) organ and may lead to postpartal hemorrhage.

Atrophic vaginitis: inflammation in a short, dry, somewhat inelastic vagina, as may occur in a postmenopausal woman.

Attachment: process in which parent and child form an enduring relationship; sometimes differentiated from bonding.

Attitude: relationship of the parts of the fetus to one another.

Augmentation of labor: enhancement of uterine contractions from ineffectual to effectual during labor.

Autolysis: self-disintegration or self-digestion of tissue or cells.

Autosome: general term for any chromosome except a sex chromosome.

Azoospermia: absence of sperm in semen.

Back labor: labor that occurs when a fetus in the occiput posterior position presses on the sacral nerves during contractions.

Bacteremic shock: type of shock that occurs in septicemia (systemic infection of the bloodstream) when endotoxins are released from certain bacteria; also called septic shock.

Ballard gestational-age assessment tool: assessment tool that examines seven physical (external) and six neuromuscular characteristics to determine a neonate's gestational age.

Ballottment: passive movement of the fetus elicited during pelvic examination in the fourth and fifth months of pregnancy.

Barbiturate: nonnarcotic, sedative drug that can cause physical and psychological dependence.

Basal body temperature (BBT) method: natural contraceptive method that predicts a client's fertile period by monitoring her daily BBT (the lowest body temperature of a healthy individual while awake).

Basal metabolic rate: rate at which cells use oxygen; lowest metabolic rate that preserves physiologic function.

Baseline fetal bradycardia: baseline fetal heart rate below 120 beats/minute.

Baseline fetal heart rate: resting pulse of the fetus assessed between contractions and without fetal movement; normal baseline fetal heart rate is 120 to 160 beats/minute.

Baseline fetal tachycardia: baseline fetal heart rate exceeding 160 beats/minute.

MASTER GLOSSARY continued

Battledore placenta: benign condition in which the umbilical cord implants at the edge of the placenta.

Bicornate uterus: Y-shaped or heart-shaped uterus.

Bilirubin: yellow bile pigment; a product of red blood cell hemolysis.

Biofeedback: relaxation technique that uses electronic monitoring of the heart rate, temperature, and muscle contractions to teach the client to gain control over involuntary physical responses to stress.

Biparietal diameter: greatest transverse distance between the two parietal bones.

Biphasic pattern: sharp midcycle rise in basal body temperature followed by a return to the baseline.

Birth culture: beliefs, values, and norms held by a cultural or ethnic group about conception, conditions for procreation and childbearing, the mechanism of pregnancy and labor, and the rules of pre- and postnatal behavior.

Birthing chair: specialized chair that allows a client to give birth in an upright position.

Blastocyst: embryo precursor just after the morula stage.

Blastomere: daughter cell formed by mitosis just after fertilization of an ovum.

Blood-brain barrier: membrane that prevents harmful substances in the blood, such as anesthetic agents, from penetrating brain tissue.

Bloody show: blood-tinged vaginal discharge that occurs at the onset of labor when the cervical mucus plug is dislodged and small cervical capillaries break.

Body image: mental image of one's physical appearance, posture, gestures, personality, attitudes, and self-concept, and one's perception of others' reactions to that image.

Body language: nonverbal signals, such as facial expression, gestures, and body position.

Bonding: process through which an emotional attachment forms, which binds one person to another in an enduring relationship, as between parents and infant; sometimes called attachment.

Braxton Hicks contractions: painless uterine contractions that occur at irregular intervals throughout pregnancy but become more noticeable as term approaches; also called false labor contractions.

Brazelton neonatal behavioral assessment scale (BNBAS): assessment tool that determines a neonate's interactive and behavioral capacities.

Breast engorgement: excessive fullness of the breasts resulting from temporary lymphatic and venous stasis; occurs during the early part of the lactation cycle.

Breast self-examination (BSE): procedure by which a woman assesses her breasts and accessory structures for signs of abnormality.

Breast shield: device worn late in pregnancy to draw out inverted nipples in preparation for breast-feeding.

Breech presentation: fetal position in which the buttocks or feet present first.

Bronchopulmonary dysplasia (BPD): lung disease characterized by bronchiolar metaplasia and interstitial fibrosis; associated with oxygen therapy and mechanical ventilation in preterm neonates.

Bulimia: eating disorder characterized by binge-purge cycles, depression, and self-deprecation.

Calorie: measurement of heat (energy); also called kilocalorie or kcal.

Cancer: malignant neoplasm that invades surrounding tissue and metastasizes to other body regions.

Capacitation: process of spermatozoon activation that includes structural change in the acrosome.

Caput succedaneum: generalized edema of the fetal scalp, usually caused by pressure on the fetal occiput during labor or vacuum extraction.

Carbohydrate: energy source providing 4 calories/g; found in the diet in the form of starches, sugars, and fiber (which provides no calories).

Carcinoma: malignant epithelial neoplasm (cancer) that tends to invade surrounding tissue and metastasize to distant regions of the body.

Carcinoma in situ: malignant neoplasm within surface epithelium that has not invaded deeper tissues.

Cardiac decompensation: inability of the reserve power of the heart to compensate for impaired valvular functioning.

Cardiac disease: any heart disorder, especially one that places the client at high risk during the intrapartal period.

Cardinal movements of labor: series of positional changes that occur as the fetus passes through the pelvis; progression includes descent, flexion, internal rotation, extension, external rotation (restitution and shoulder rotation), and expulsion.

Carrier: person who has one normal and one abnormal gene at corresponding loci, when the abnormal gene is not expressed phenotypically; expression may occur in offspring if male and female carriers each transmit the abnormal gene.

Central venous pressure: pressure within the superior vena cava; represents the pressure under which blood returns to the right atrium.

Cephalocaudal: pertaining to the long axis of the body in a head-to-tail direction.

Cephalopelvic disproportion: condition in which the fetus's head is too large or the birth canal too small to permit normal vaginal delivery.

Cervical canal: structure extending from the external cervical os to the interior of the uterus.

Cervical cap: cup-shaped, flexible rubber device that fits over the cervix, is used with a spermicide, and acts as a barrier to spermatozoa.

MASTER GLOSSARY continued

Cervical conization: removal of a cone-shaped piece of cervical tissue for analysis or treatment; also called cone biopsy.

Cervical dysplasia: abnormal development of cervical tissue.

Cervical mucus test: examination of cervical mucus for color, consistency, stretchiness, and quantity—all of which normally change throughout the menstrual cycle in response to hormonal stimulation; can predict a client's fertile period.

Cervical stenosis: narrowing of the canal between the cervical os and lower uterine corpus.

Cesarean delivery: surgical incision through the abdominal wall and uterus to deliver the fetus.

Chemotherapy: treatment with anticancer drugs.

Childbirth exercises: activities designed specifically to tone and strengthen muscles stressed during pregnancy, labor, and childbirth.

Child life therapist: professional who uses play activities to help ill children cope with their illness and environment.

Chlamydia: sexually transmitted disease (STD) caused by *Chlamydia trachomatis,* which is typically asymptomatic; the most common STD in the United States.

Chloasma: pigment changes that typically appear on cheeks, temples, and forehead during pregnancy; also called melasma.

Chorioamnionitis: inflammation of the fetal membranes, typically caused by infection and producing maternal and fetal tachycardia, fever, uterine and other abdominal tenderness, and purulent vaginal secretions.

Chorionic villus sampling (CVS): prenatal diagnostic procedure for obtaining fetal tissue from the villous area of the chorion.

Chromosome: microscopic, threadlike structure in the cell nucleus that contains genetic information arranged in a linear sequence.

Chronic hypertension: persistently elevated arterial blood pressure that is present and observable before pregnancy, diagnosed by 20 weeks' gestation, or that extends past 42 days postpartum.

Chronic hypertension with superimposed pre-eclampsia: hypertension that is present and observable before pregnancy and that is complicated by the hypertensive syndrome associated with pre-eclampsia.

Circumcision: surgical removal of the prepuce (foreskin) covering the glans penis.

Civil action: lawsuit addressing the rights and duties of private persons; typically, one person sues another for monetary damages.

Cleansing breath: deep, relaxed breath before and after any patterned breathing during labor.

Cleft lip: congenital defect in which one or more clefts appear in the upper lip; caused by failure of the maxillary and median nasal processes to close during embryonic development.

Cleft palate: congenital defect in which a fissure appears in the palatal midline; caused by failure of the sides of the palate to close during embryonic development.

Climacteric: period of physiologic and psychological changes that occur toward the end of a female's reproductive years and includes a premenopausal, menopausal, and postmenopausal phase that may last up to 20 years; a male also may experience a climacteric stage as sexual activity decreases with age.

Clubfoot: congenital foot deformity characterized by unilateral or bilateral deviation of the metatarsal bones, causing the foot to appear clublike.

Clustering: process of grouping related assessment data to identify broad client needs; the nurse may then consult the NANDA taxonomy to choose an appropriate diagnostic category that addresses those needs.

Coagulopathy: abnormal clotting disorder characterized by hypothrombinemia, hypofibrinogenemia, and subnormal platelet count; caused by a major insult, such as abruptio placentae.

Cocaine: central nervous system stimulant derived from coca leaves that produces euphoria and anesthetizes nerve endings.

Cognitive-affective skills: skills that link mental processes with emotions.

Cognitive-motor skills: skills that link mental processes with physical activity.

Coitus interruptus: natural contraceptive method in which the male withdraws his penis from the vagina immediately before ejaculation; also called the withdrawal method.

Colostrum: thin, yellow, serous fluid secreted by the breasts during pregnancy and the first postpartal days before lactation begins; consists of water, protein, fat, carbohydrates, white blood cells, and immunoglobulins.

Colposcopy: examination of cervical and vaginal tissue using a colposcope for magnification.

Communication cue: verbal or nonverbal message intended to elicit a response in the receiver.

Conception: onset of pregnancy, starting with fertilization of an ovum and ending with its implantation in the uterine wall.

Conceptus: products of conception, including fetal membranes, placenta, and pre-embryo, embryo, or fetus.

Conditioned response: reaction acquired through training and repetition, as employed in the psychoprophylactic method of childbirth education.

Condom: sheath made of thin rubber, collagenous tissue, or animal tissue that is worn over the penis during intercourse to prevent sperm from entering the uterus.

MASTER GLOSSARY continued

Conduction: transfer of heat to a substance in contact with the body; a mechanism of heat loss or gain.

Condyloma: wartlike growth on the external genitals, vagina, cervix, or anus that may become an invasive cervical lession; caused by the human papillomavirus; also known as a venereal wart.

Condylomata acuminata: sexually transmitted disease caused by human papillomavirus infection, which produces wartlike anogenital lesions.

Congenital anomaly: abnormality present at birth; particularly, a structural abnormality that may be genetically inherited, acquired during gestation, or caused during delivery.

Congenital heart defect: one of five common defects: atrial septal defect or ventricular septal defect, tetralogy of Fallot, patent ductus arteriosus, valvular abnormality, or coarctation of the aorta.

Congenital hydrocephalus: condition characterized by accumulation of excessive cerebrospinal fluid within the cranial vault.

Congenital hypothyroidism: deficiency of thyroid hormone secretion during fetal development or early infancy; also called cretinism.

Consanguinity: kinship; blood relationship.

Consent: voluntary act in which one person agrees to an action by another person; not all consent given is informed consent.

Contraceptive sponge: doughnut-shaped device made of soft, synthetic material that contains spermicide.

Contract: written or verbal agreement between the nurse and the client that spells out the goals of nursing care and specifies what each party will do to accomplish these goals.

Contraction: involuntary and intermittent tightening or shortening of uterine muscle fibers that leads to cervical dilation, effacement, and fetal descent.

Contract learning: process in which the nurse and client agree on goals and anticipated outcomes before teaching begins.

Convection: transfer of heat away by movement of air currents; a mechanism of heat loss or gain.

Converger: person who learns best from applying abstract concepts to life experience.

Coping: process by which an individual deals with stress, solves problems, and makes decisions.

Coping mechanism: conscious response to stress that allows an individual to confront a problem directly and solve it.

Corona radiata: layer of granulosa cells that adheres to the zona pellucida before fertilization of an ovum.

Corpus luteum: spherical yellowish tissue that grows within a ruptured ovarian follicle after ovulation and secretes progesterone.

Couvade symptoms: pregnancy symptoms in an expectant father.

Crisis: period of instability or disorganization that follows failure of normal coping skills; risk is highest when a stressful event coincides with a crucial stage in family development.

Crossing-over: exchange of corresponding segments between homologous chromosomes while the chromosomes are paired during the first meiotic division.

Crowning: appearance of the fetus's head at the perineum.

Cryosurgery: treatment that destroys tissue by applying extreme cold.

Cryotherapy: therapeutic use of cold; may be used to treat condylomata acuminata by freezing—and destroying—the lesions.

Culdocentesis: use of a needle puncture or incision to remove intraperitoneal fluid (blood and purulent drainage) through the vagina.

Culture: integrated system of learned beliefs, values, and behaviors characteristic of a society's members.

Cyanosis: bluish skin discoloration caused by an excess of deoxygenated hemoglobin in the blood.

Cycle of violence: common pattern of abuse; it has three phases (increasing tension, abusive episode, and kindness and contrition) and may vary in intensity and duration for each couple.

Cystitis: inflammatory condition of the urinary bladder and ureters characterized by dysuria, urinary frequency and urgency, hematuria, and other symptoms; may be caused by bacterial infection, calculus, or neoplasm.

Cystocele: herniation of the urinary bladder through the anterior vaginal wall.

Decidua: epithelial tissue of the endometrium during pregnancy.

Decidua basalis: portion of the decidua directly beneath the implanted ovum, attached to the myometrium.

Defendant: person against whom a lawsuit is brought.

Defense mechanism: unconscious response to stress that distorts reality and allows an individual to avoid, rather than directly cope with, an anxiety-producing situation.

Dehiscence: spontaneous opening of a surgical wound (such as an episiotomy).

Delirium tremens (DTs): acute, sometimes fatal psychotic reaction to alcohol withdrawal that occurs in about 5% of withdrawing alcoholics and usually lasts 2 to 4 days; characterized by fever, tachycardia, hypertension or hypotension, vivid hallucinations, seizures, and combativeness.

Denial: defense mechanism that involves refusal to acknowledge thoughts, feelings, desires, impulses, or facts that are consciously intolerable.

Dependent edema: interstitial accumulation of excess fluid in the lowest portions of the body.

MASTER GLOSSARY continued

Diabetes mellitus: endocrine syndrome in which heterogeneous chronic disorders are characterized by altered carbohydrate metabolism caused by inadequate insulin secretion by the beta cells of the islets of Langerhans in the pancreas or by ineffective use of insulin at the cellular level.

Diabetic ketoacidosis: emergency condition characterized by acidosis and accumulation of ketones in the blood, which results from faulty carbohydrate metabolism; occurs primarily as a complication of diabetes.

Diagnosis-related group (DRG): one of 470 groups of related diagnoses, each of which has an estimated length of hospital stay and cost; in the prospective payment system, DRGs are the basis for reimbursement by many private insurance companies and federal insurance programs.

Diaphragm: dome-shaped, flexible rubber device with a thick rim that contains a spring; it fits over the cervix, is used with a spermicide, and prevents pregnancy by blocking sperm passage into the uterus.

Diastasis recti abdominis: separation of the rectus abdominis muscles at the midline.

Dilatation: dilation; sometimes used to describe dilation of the cervical os during labor or to refer to an external means of dilation, such as drugs or instruments.

Dilatation and curettage (D & C): surgical method of pregnancy interruption that requires cervical dilation and uterine scraping with a metal curette to remove the products of conception; may be used as part of the treatment for endometriosis or as follow-up to an incomplete abortion.

Dilatation and evacuation (D & E): surgical method of pregnancy interruption that requires extreme cervical dilation and evacuation of uterine contents by large-bore suction equipment and crushing instruments.

Dilation: progressive widening of the external cervical os; also called dilatation.

Dimpling: breast skin puckering or depression, possibly caused by an underlying growth; also called retraction.

Diploid: having a full set of homologous chromosomes (46), as normally found in somatic cells.

Discharge planning: formulation of a program by the health care team, client, family, and appropriate outside agencies to ensure that the client's physical and psychosocial needs are met after discharge.

Displacement: defense mechanism that transfers emotions from an anxiety-producing object to a less threatening object.

Disseminated intravascular coagulation (DIC): abnormal clotting disorder characterized by hypoprothrombinemia, hypofibrinogenemia, and a subnormal platelet count; caused by a major insult to the body, such as abruptio placentae.

Diverger: person who learns best by creating new ideas after sharing experiences with others.

DNA: deoxyribonucleic acid; the chemical that carries genetic information.

Dominant: capable of genetic expression when a gene is present on only one of a pair of homologous chromosomes.

Doula: lay person who provides support during labor.

Down's syndrome: disorder in which birth defects are caused by an extra number 21 chromosome; also called trisomy 21.

Dubowitz gestational-age assessment tool: assessment tool that examines 11 physical (external) and 10 neuromuscular characteristics to determine a neonate's gestational age.

Ductus arteriosus: tubular connection that shunts blood away from the pulmonary circulation during fetal development.

Ductus venosus: circulatory pathway that allows blood to bypass the liver during fetal development.

Dyad: pair of individuals in a close relationship.

Dysmaturity: undernourished fetus or neonate that is abnormally small for gestational age.

Dysmenorrhea: painful menstruation; a possible contraindication to intrauterine device (IUD) use.

Dyspareunia: painful or difficult intercourse; may result from vaginal dryness associated with menopause.

Dystocia: difficult delivery caused by fetal factors, such as malpresentation, malposition, macrosomia, and intrauterine fetal death; the client's pelvis; or uterine expulsive powers.

Dysuria: painful or difficult urination.

Early deceleration: innocuous waveform deceleration of the fetal heart rate that mirrors uterine contractions and typically occurs when the cervix is dilated 4 to 7 cm.

Early phase of labor: first phase of the first stage of labor, characterized by the onset of regular contractions and cervical dilation of up to 3 cm; also called the latent phase of labor.

Early postpartal discharge: discharge from the health care facility 2 to 72 hours after delivery.

Eclampsia: gravest, convulsive form of pregnancy-induced hypertension, affecting one of every 200 clients with preeclampsia, characterized by generalized tonic-clonic seizures and coma; occurs between the twentieth week of pregnancy and the end of the first postpartal week.

Ectocervix: outer portion of the cervix lined with squamous epithelium.

Ectoderm: outermost of the three primary germ cell layers of the embryo.

Ectopic pregnancy: implantation of the fertilized ovum outside the uterine cavity.

EDD: expected date of delivery.

MASTER GLOSSARY continued

Educational pelvic examination: assessment technique that allows the client to view her genitals and cervix through a hand mirror as they are identified by the examiner.

Effacement: progressive thinning and shortening of the cervix during labor.

Effleurage: relaxation technique that uses light, rhythmic fingertip massage over the abdomen during labor; can help distract the client and decrease her pain.

Ejaculation: forceful expulsion of semen through the penile urethra.

Elective abortion: termination of pregnancy by choice before the age of viability.

Elective induction: initiation of labor for convenience in a term pregnancy.

Electronic fetal monitoring (EFM): direct (scalp electrode, intrauterine catheter) and indirect (ultrasound, tocodynamometer) devices that assess the relationship between the fetal heart rate and uterine contractions.

Embryo: developing organism after the pre-embryonic stage and before the fetal stage, usually occurring during weeks 4 through 8.

Emotional support: type of support that includes affection, trust, concern, and listening.

Empty nest syndrome: pattern of emotions that characterize a family whose children have recently left home.

En face position: position in which the neonate is held approximately 8″ (20 cm) in front of the parent or other observer; allows direct eye contact.

Encephalocele: congenital neural tube defect in which the meninges and portions of brain tissue protrude through the cranium, typically in the occipital area.

Endocervix: inner portion of the cervix.

Endoderm: innermost of the three primary germ cell layers of the embryo.

Endogenous opiate theory: hypothesis that natural pain inhibitors found in the central nervous system bind at pain receptor sites and block transmission of pain impulses.

Endometrial biopsy: test in which a sample of endometrial tissue is analyzed to determine the condition of the endometrium or help identify the phase of the menstrual cycle.

Endometriosis: abnormal condition in which endometrial tissue grows and functions outside the uterine cavity.

Endometrium: mucous membrane lining of the uterus, a portion of which forms the decidua during pregnancy.

Engagement: descent of the fetal presenting part into the maternal pelvis; the widest diameter of the fetal presenting part is at or below the level of the ischial spines.

Engrossment: close face-to-face observation between parent and neonate; sometimes used to describe father-infant interaction.

Enterocele: herniation of the intestine into the posterior portion of the vagina.

Entrainment: phenomenon in which a neonate or an infant moves in rhythm to adult speech.

Epidural block: most common regional anesthesia technique, in which an anesthetic agent is injected into the epidural space between the dura mater and ligamentum flavum.

Episiotomy: surgical incision in the perineum to enlarge the vaginal opening for delivery; performed to prevent perineal tears, speed or facilitate delivery, or prevent excess stretching of perineal muscles and connective tissue.

Erythroblastosis fetalis: serious hemolytic disease of the fetus and neonate that produces anemia; jaundice; liver, spleen, and heart enlargement; and severe generalized edema; also called hydrops fetalis or hemolytic disease of the newborn.

Erythropoietin: hormone produced in the kidneys that regulates red blood cell production.

Ethics: discipline that attempts to identify, organize, analyze, and justify human acts by applying certain moral principles to a given situation.

Ethnicity: affiliation with a group of people classified according to a common racial, national, linguistic, or cultural origin or background.

Ethnocentrism: belief that one's own cultural standards are superior.

Etiology: causal or contributing factor or factors.

Evaluation: determination of how successfully care plan goals have been met; a step in the nursing process.

Evaporation: conversion of fluid to vapor; a mechanism of heat loss.

Everted nipple: nipple that is turned outward and becomes more graspable with stimulation.

Exchange transfusion: procedure in which the neonate's blood is removed and replaced with fresh whole donor blood to remove unconjugated bilirubin in serum; used to treat hyperbilirubinemia and hemolytic anemia.

Expressivity: extent to which signs of a gene reveal themselves.

Extracorporeal membrane oxygenation (ECMO): technique that maintains gas exchange and perfusion by oxygenating blood outside the body through an arterial shunt; used mainly to treat refractory respiratory failure or meconium aspiration syndrome.

Facilitator: person whose skill, aptitude, or experience eases the performance of a task.

False labor: Braxton Hicks contractions.

MASTER GLOSSARY continued

Family-centered care: philosophical approach to health care that proposes that childbirth affects the entire family; incorporates such practices as paternal and sibling participition in childbirth and alternative birth settings.

Family functions: purposes for which the family exists and tasks necessary to attain those purposes; includes physical survival, sustenance, personal nurturing, education, and the passing on of values and beliefs.

Family pattern: overall organization of family relationships regardless of roles adopted by each member.

Family theory: set of assumptions and hypotheses that provides a reference point for studying and understanding the family.

Fat: energy source providing 9 calories/g; found in the diet in meat, dairy products, vegetable oils, and miscellaneous foods.

Father image: each man's concept of himself as a father, shaped from childhood memories of his own father, other role models, revision of his father image through other children, literature, and his imagination.

Female circumcision: religious or cultural procedure that removes a portion of the clitoris and labia.

Ferning: microscopic, fern-shaped pattern found in a smear of dried amniotic fluid, indicating rupture of the amniotic membranes.

Fertility awareness method: any of four natural contraceptive methods based on identification of fertile and infertile periods during the menstrual cycle and avoidance of intercourse during fertile periods.

Fertilization: penetration of a female gamete by a male gamete.

Fetal alcohol syndrome: syndrome caused by maternal alcohol consumption; characterized by altered intrauterine growth and development that results in mental and growth retardation, facial abnormalities, and behavioral deviations.

Fetal lie: relationship of the long axis of the fetus to the long axis of the mother.

Fetal-placental unit: umbilical cord, placental layers, and chrorionic villus—through which placental transfer occurs.

Fetal position: relationship of the landmark on the fetal presenting part to the front, back, and sides of the maternal pelvis.

Fetal presentation: manner in which the fetus enters the pelvic passageway; for example, cephalic, shoulder, or breech.

Fetal scalp blood sampling: test that uses a fetal scalp blood sample to evaluate the fetus's acid-base status during labor; used as an adjunct to electronic fetal monitoring.

Fetal scalp stimulation: test that provides a reassuring sign of fetal well-being during labor by accelerating the fetal heart rate with pressure from the examiner's fingers or with application of an Allis clamp to the fetus's head.

Fetal station: relationship of the fetal presenting part to the maternal ischial spines.

Fetus: developing organism that forms after the embryonic stage from around week 9 through delivery.

Fibrin: insoluble protein formed from fibrinogen that is essential for blood clotting.

Fibrinogen: protein clotting factor in blood plasma that is converted to fibrin by the action of thrombin.

Fibroid: benign, slow-growing uterine neoplasm.

First stage of labor: stage of labor that begins with the onset of regular, rhythmic uterine contractions and ends with complete cervical dilation of 10 cm.

Fistula: abnormal passage between two internal organs or from an internal organ to the body surface.

"Fitting in the missing pieces": psychological process in which the client reviews the events of childbirth to help incorporate the experience into her self-concept and identity.

Fixation: defense mechanism that stops development because of inability to resolve an issue.

Flashback phenomenon: auditory and visual hallucinations related to a previous frightening or pleasurable experience; may result from use of a psychoactive drug.

Flat nipple: nipple that is hard to distinguish from the areola; changes shape only slightly with stimulation.

Folic acid deficiency anemia: blood disorder in which immature red blood cells fail to divide, become enlarged, and decrease in number.

Follicle-stimulating hormone (FSH): anterior pituitary hormone; in women, it stimulates follicular growth; in men, it promotes spermatogenesis.

Fontanel: nonossified area of connective tissue between the skull bones where the sutures intersect; allows molding of the fetal skull for passage through the pelvis during delivery.

Foramen ovale: opening in the interatrial septum that directs blood from the right to left atrium during fetal development.

Forceps: two curved blades used to extract the fetus from the birth canal.

Foremilk: thin, watery breast milk secreted at the beginning of a feeding.

Formative evaluation: process in which the nurse and client judge progress toward goals during home care visits.

Fourchette: area of the female perineum between the posterior junction of the labia minora and labia majora.

MASTER GLOSSARY continued

Fourth stage of labor: period after delivery of the placenta, lasting about 1 hour.

Functional residual capacity (FRC): volume of air remaining in the lungs after a normal expiration.

Fundus: rounded portion of the uterus above the level of the fallopian tube attachments.

Funic souffle: blowing sound heard as fetal blood courses through the umbilical cord.

Galactorrhea: flow of breast milk unrelated to breast-feeding.

Galactosemia: hereditary autosomal recessive disorder in which deficiency of the enzyme galactose-1-phosphate uridyltransferase leads to galactose accumulation in the blood.

Gamete: male or female reproductive cell (spermatozoon or ovum).

Gamete intrafallopian transfer (GIFT): procedure in which oocytes (incompletely developed ova) are taken from the ovary, mixed with spermatozoa, and then instilled into the distal end of the fallopian tube; with GIFT, fertilization takes place in vivo (in the woman's own body).

Gametogenesis: developmental process by which spermatozoa and ova are formed.

Gastroschisis: congenital condition characterized by incomplete abdominal wall closure not involving the site of umbilical cord insertion; typically, the small intestine and part of the large intestine protrude.

Gate control theory: hypothesis that stimulation of larger-diameter, faster-traveling nerve fibers can block pain impulses carried on smaller-diameter, slower-traveling fibers, thus closing a gate that stops or modifies pain transmission.

Gene: self-reproducing biological unit of heredity; located at a specific locus (site) on a particular chromosome.

Genotype: individual's genetic constitution; may refer to the total genetic constitution or to specific alleles at a locus.

Gestational age: estimated age in weeks following conception.

Gestational-age assessment: evaluation of a neonate's physical and neurologic characteristics to determine approximate weeks of fetal development.

Gestational diabetes: type of diabetes first diagnosed during pregnancy, which may be asymptomatic except for impaired glucose tolerance test values; also called gestational diabetes mellitus.

Gestational edema: generalized interstitial accumulation of excess fluid (face, hands, sacrum, abdomen, ankles, tibia) after 12 hours of bed rest or a weight gain in excess of 2 kg (4 to 4½ lb) per week; the edema may be less significant than the weight gain.

Gestational hypertension: elevated blood pressures present on two occasions at least 6 hours apart characterized by systolic and diastolic pressure equal to or exceeding 140/90 mm Hg or a rise of 30 mm Hg systolic or 15 mm Hg diastolic above the client's baseline values.

Gestational proteinuria: protein in the urine just after labor recorded on two or more occasions at least 6 hours apart in a clean-catch or catheter-obtained specimen; protein must be 300 mg/liter or greater in a 24-hour specimen, or greater than 1 g/liter in a random daytime sample.

Glomerular filtration rate (GFR): volume of glomerular filtrate (a protein-free plasmalike substance) formed over a specific period.

Glucuronyl transferase: liver enzyme necessary for bilirubin conjugation.

Goal: desired outcome of nursing care that guides formation and implementation of nursing interventions.

Golgi body: complex membranous intracellular structure whose elements consist of flattened sacs; also called Golgi complex or Golgi apparatus.

Gonorrhea: sexually transmitted disease, caused by *Neisseria gonorrhoeae,* that may be asymptomatic or may produce vaginal discharge, urinary symptoms, dyspareunia, and menstrual irregularities.

Graafian follicle: mature ovarian vesicle located near the ovarian surface that contains an ovum; in response to hormonal stimulation during the menstrual cycle, the ovum matures and the vesicle ruptures.

Grand multiparity: having had more than five children.

Grief: intense sadness experienced after the loss of a valued person or object.

Grief process: cycle that follows a loss; the Kübler-Ross model progresses from denial through anger, bargaining, and depression to acceptance; stages may overlap or regress and may be repeated many times before acceptance is complete.

Habituation: gradual adaptation to a stimulus through repeated exposure.

Hallucinogen: psychotomimetic drug that alters consciousness and causes hallucinations.

Haploid: having only one-half of a set of homologous chromosomes (23), as normally found in gametes.

Health care facility: organization that provides health care services based on societal and client demands.

Health care provider: health care facility, agency, or professional that delivers services to clients.

Health maintenance organization (HMO): group practice that charges a flat fee for each insured client, regardless of the extent or type of services the group provides; emphasizes provision of government-mandated services that help maintain health and reduce inpatient hospital stays.

MASTER GLOSSARY continued

Hematocrit: volume percentage of red blood cells in whole blood.

Hematoma: collection of extravasated blood trapped in the tissues of the skin or in an organ, resulting from trauma or incomplete hemostasis, as after surgery.

Hemoglobin: protein in red blood cells that transports oxygen.

Hemoglobin F: hemoglobin produced by fetal erythrocytes; has a higher affinity for oxygen than does adult hemoglobin (hemoglobin A), helping to ensure adequate fetal tissue oxygenation.

Herpes genitalis: sexually transmitted disease caused by the herpes simplex virus; characterized by recurrent outbreaks of genital blisters that progress to shallow, painful ulcers.

Heterozygote: individual with two different alleles at a corresponding loci on homologous chromosomes.

Hindmilk: high-fat breast milk secreted at the end of a feeding.

Hirsutism: excessive body hair; in women, its distribution follows a masculine pattern.

Hoffman's exercises: areola-stretching technique designed to facilitate breast-feeding by breaking adhesions and allowing inverted nipples to become more protractile.

Homan's sign: pain in the calf on dorsiflexion of the foot, indicating superficial thrombosis or thrombophlebitis.

Home health aide: person trained to provide personal care, such as bathing, dressing, and feeding, to the client at home.

Home health care: services, supplies, and equipment provided to a client in the home to maintain or promote physical, mental, and emotional health.

Home nursing visit: provision of nursing care in a client's home.

Homologous chromosomes: matching pair of chromosomes.

Homozygote: individual with identical alleles (normal or abnormal) at corresponding loci on homologous chromosomes.

Hormone replacement therapy: use of estrogen by itself or with progestin to relieve menopausal symptoms.

Hot flash: transient sensation of warmth over the upper chest, face, and extremities caused by vasomotor disturbances associated with menopause.

Human immunodeficiency virus (HIV): retrovirus that can lead to acquired immunodeficiency syndrome (AIDS), which compromises the body's immune system and renders it susceptible to opportunistic infections.

Hyalinization: conversion into a glasslike substance.

Hydramnios: excessive amniotic fluid associated with congenital neonatal disorders and such maternal disorders as diabetes mellitus; also called polyhydramnios.

Hymen: fold of membranous tissue that occludes or partially blocks the vaginal orifice.

Hyperbilirubinemia: elevated serum level of unconjugated bilirubin.

Hyperemesis gravidarum: abnormal prenatal condition characterized by excessive nausea or vomiting leading to dehydration and starvation.

Hyperemia: increased amount of blood.

Hyperesthesia: increased sensitivity, usually of the skin, which may occur late in labor.

Hyperglycemia: abnormally high serum glucose level.

Hyperplasia: increase in cell number.

Hyperplastic obesity: condition characterized by an increase in the number of fat cells.

Hypertonia: condition in which the uterus resists stretching.

Hypertrophic obesity: condition characterized by an increase in the size of fat cells.

Hypertrophy: increase in cell size.

Hypocalcemia: decreased serum calcium level.

Hypofibrinogenemia: abnormally low fibrinogen (a coagulation agent) in the blood.

Hypoglycemia: abnormally low serum glucose level.

Hypotonic: having reduced muscle tension; describes a muscle that is relaxed, not well contracted.

Hypovolemia: abnormally diminished volume of circulating fluid.

Hysterectomy: surgical removal of the uterus, which may be performed through an abdominal or vaginal incision.

Hysterosalpingography: X-ray film of the uterus and fallopian tubes to detect uterine abnormalities and assess tubal patency.

Hysteroscopy: visual examination of the uterus through a hysteroscope (illuminated tube) that has been passed through the vagina; during this procedure, the client can be sterilized by passing silicone through the hysteroscope and using it to occlude the fallopian tubes.

Imagery: relaxation technique in which the client focuses on a mental representation of a real or imagined place; also called visualization.

Imperforate anus: congenital defect characterized by abnormal closure of the anus.

Implantation: attachment of the blastocyst to the uterine wall; occurs 6 to 7 days after fertilization of the ovum.

Implementation: nursing actions that carry out interventions described in the nursing care plan to achieve established goals; a step in the nursing process.

In vitro fertilization: procedure during which oocytes are taken from the ovary, mixed with spermatozoa, and fertilized and incubated in a glass petri dish; up to four viable embryos then are placed in the woman's uterus.

MASTER GLOSSARY continued

Inborn error of metabolism: abnormal metabolic condition caused by an inherited defect of a single enzyme or other protein.

Incompetent cervix: condition in which the cervix will not maintain a pregnancy to term.

Incontinence: inability to control urination or defecation.

Incubator: fully enclosed, single-walled or double-walled bed containing a heating source and a humidification chamber.

Indicated or nonelective induction: initiation of labor for medical or obstetric reasons that threaten the health of the fetus or client.

Induction of labor: attempts to speed labor by starting or augmenting uterine contractions.

Infertility: inability to conceive after 1 year of regular intercourse without contraception or inability to carry a pregnancy to birth.

Informational support: type of support that includes advice, suggestions, directives, and other information.

Informed consent: legal rule in which a client is entitled to receive certain information about a proposed course of treatment or surgery; usual required information includes risks, benefits, and alternatives.

Inhalation analgesia: anesthetic agent inhaled in small concentrations to produce analgesia without loss of consciousness.

Instrumental support: type of support that includes money, time, and other such resources.

Intervention: action performed by the nurse to implement the nursing care plan.

Intrapartal period: period during labor and delivery.

Intrauterine device (IUD): plastic contraceptive device that contains copper or progesterone and is inserted in the uterine cavity; may prevent pregnancy by altering endometrial physiology and inhibiting implantation of the fertilized ovum.

Intrauterine growth retardation: abnormal process in which fetal development and maturation are impeded or delayed by maternal disease, genetic factors, or fetal malnutrition caused by placental insufficiency; seen in the small-for-gestational-age neonate.

Intrauterine pressure catheter: pliable, water-filled tube inserted into the uterus to assess uterine tone and the frequency, duration, and intensity of uterine contractions.

Intraventricular hemorrhage: bleeding into the ventricles.

Inverted nipple: nipple that turns inward; occurs in three types: pseudoinverted (becomes erect with stimulation), semi-inverted (retracts with stimulation), and truly inverted (inverted both at rest and when stimulated).

Involution: retrogressive changes in vital processes or in organs after fulfilling their functions; return of the reproductive organs to a nonpregnant state.

Iron deficiency anemia: blood disorder in which a lack of iron leads to production of smaller (microcytic) red blood cells, reducing oxygen transport throughout the body.

Isoimmune hemolytic anemia: disorder in which an antigen-antibody reaction leads to premature destruction of red blood cells.

Isoimmunization: development of antibodies in response to isoantigens (blood group antigens).

Jaundice: yellow skin discoloration caused by bilirubin accumulation in the blood and tissues.

Karyotype: chromosome complement arranged by relative size, centromere position, and staining pattern and depicted by photomicrograph.

Kegel exercises: isometric exercises in which the muscles of the pelvic diaphragm and perineum are contracted voluntarily (also called pubococcygeus exercises); helps increase contractility of the vaginal introitus and improve urine retention.

Ketosis: condition characterized by an abnormally high concentration of ketone bodies in body tissues and fluids; also called ketoacidosis.

Klinefelter's syndrome: disorder caused by an extra X chromosome in the male (XXY).

Labor: process that occurs from the onset of cervical effacement and dilation to delivery of the placenta.

Lactation: synthesis and secretion of milk from the breasts.

Lactogenesis: initiation of breast milk production.

Lactose intolerance: condition in which an individual lacks sufficient lactase (the enzyme necessary to break down lactose, or milk sugar); symptoms include diarrhea, abdominal cramps, and flatulence after ingesting milk or milk products.

Laminaria tents: dried hygroscopic seaweed cones used to dilate the cervix.

Lanugo: fine hair covering the face, shoulders, and back of the fetus or neonate before 28 weeks' gestation.

Laparoscopy: visual examination of the internal abdomen through a laparoscope (illuminated tube) inserted into the abdomen via a 1″ (2.5-cm) incision; during this procedure, a woman's reproductive organs can be assessed for causes of infertility, or sterilization can be performed by ligating the fallopian tubes through the laparoscope.

Laparotomy: 4″ to 5″ (10- to 13-cm) abdominal incision below the umbilicus; during this procedure, female sterilization can be performed by crushing, ligating, banding, or electrocoagulating the fallopian tubes.

MASTER GLOSSARY continued

Large for gestational age (LGA): term used to describe a neonate whose birth weight exceeds the ninetieth percentile for gestational age on the Colorado intrauterine growth chart.

Late deceleration: nonreassuring waveform of the fetal heart rate indicating placental insufficiency; occurs after a uterine contraction begins but does not return to baseline until the contraction is over.

Learned helplessness: belief that one is powerless and unable to act independently.

Learning style: mode of receiving and recalling information preferred by the client; for example, memorization, observation, interaction, or experimentation.

Leiomyoma: benign neoplasm of the uterine smooth muscle that is common in mature clients; can affect fetal growth and predispose the client to preterm labor, labor dysfunctions, birth canal obstruction, and postpartal hemorrhage.

Leopold's maneuvers: four abdominal palpation procedures used to determine the fetal lie, position, and presentation.

Let-down reflex: milk ejection from the breast triggered by nipple stimulation or an emotional response to the neonate.

Levator ani: one of a pair of muscles of the pelvic diaphragm that stretches across the bottom of the pelvic cavity, supporting the pelvic organs; separates into the pubococcygeus and the iliococcygeus.

Liability: obligation to pay monetary damages in a civil action.

Libido: psychic energy or instinctual drive associated with sexual desire, pleasure, or creativity.

Lie: relationship of the fetal long axis to the maternal long axis; may be longitudinal, oblique, or transverse.

Lightening: subjective sensation the client may feel as the fetus descends into the pelvic inlet and changes the shape and position of the uterus near term.

Linea nigra: dark line extending from the umbilicus or above to the mons pubis.

Linkage: association of genes located on the same chromosome, resulting in a tendency for some nonallelic genes to be associated in inheritance.

Lipolysis: decomposition of fat.

LMP: first day of the last menstrual period.

Lochia: vaginal discharge after delivery occurring in three distinct stages; composed of blood, tissue, leukocytes, and mucus.

Locus: the specific site of a particular gene in a chromosome (plural, loci).

Long-term variability: rhythmic fluctuations of 5 to 20 beats/minute above and below the baseline fetal heart rate, normally occurring 3 to 5 times per minute.

Low birth weight: birth weight of 1,500 to 2,500 g.

Lumpectomy: breast cancer surgery that removes only the lump; usually followed by radiation therapy.

Luteal phase: second half of the menstrual cycle from ovulation to menstruation.

Luteinizing hormone (LH): anterior pituitary hormone that stimulates ovulation and corpus luteum development.

Lymphedema: excess fluid collected in tissues of the hand and arm when lymph nodes or vessels are removed or blocked.

Macrosomia: excessively large fetus, typically weighing over 4,000 g.

Major depressive episode: disorder of emotional origin that sometimes is precipitated by childbirth; characterized by depressed mood, markedly diminished interest or pleasure in activities, significant weight loss or gain, insomnia or hypersomnia, psychomotor agitation, fatigue, feelings of worthlessness or excessive or inappropriate guilt, diminished ability to think, or recurrent thoughts of death; at least five of these symptoms must be present and at least one of the five must be either depressed mood or loss of interest.

Malformation: developmental defect.

Malpractice: form of negligence action brought against such professionals as nurses, physicians, lawyers, and accountants that alleges failure to meet applicable standards, thus causing harm.

Malpresentation: abnormal fetal presentation, such as transverse lie or breech presentation.

Mammogram: X-ray used to diagnose and evaluate breast lesions.

Maple syrup urine disease: autosomal recessive disorder characterized by an enzyme deficiency in the second step of branched-chain amino acid catabolism.

Marijuana: commonly abused drug obtained from the flowering tops, stems, and leaves of the hemp plant; also called cannabis sativa, weed, grass, pot, or tea.

Mastectomy: surgical removal of the breast.

Mastitis: inflammation of the breast.

Maternity blues: postpartal disorder characterized by transient mood alteration involving crying episodes and sadness (also called "baby blues"); usually lasts 1 to 10 days.

Maturational crisis: intensification of problems or symptoms linked to the developmental level of an individual or family.

Mature neonate: neonate of 38 to 42 weeks' gestation; also called term neonate.

Meconium: thick, sticky, green-to-black material that collects in the fetal intestines and forms the first neonatal stool; when present in amniotic fluid, may indicate fetal distress.

MASTER GLOSSARY continued

Meconium aspiration syndrome (MAS): lung inflammation resulting from inhaling meconium-stained amniotic fluid in utero or when the neonate takes the first few breaths.

Meditation: relaxation technique that achieves an altered state of consciousness by slow deep-breathing and focusing on a single mental stimulus.

Megaloblastic anemia: blood condition in which immature blood cells become abnormally large, possibly because of nutrient deficiencies.

Meiosis: specialized form of cell division that produces gametes.

Menarche: onset of menses, usually occurring between ages 12 and 13.

Meningomyelocele: congenital neural tube defect in which part of the meninges and spinal cord protrudes through the vertebral column.

Menopause: cessation of menses with the decline of cyclic hormonal production and function, usually between ages 40 and 60; may begin at an earlier age—for example, after surgical removal of the uterus, ovaries, or both.

Menorrhagia: abnormally heavy or long menstrual flow; also called hypermenorrhea.

Menstruation: cyclic discharge of blood and mucosal tissue from the uterus between menarche and menopause, except during pregnancy or lactation.

Meralgia paresthetica: tingling and numbness in the anterolateral portion of the thigh caused by entrapment of the lateral femoral cutaneous nerve in the area of the inguinal ligaments.

Mesoderm: middle layer of the three primary germ layers of the embryo.

Metastasis: transfer of disease from one part of the body to another via the lymphatic system or bloodstream.

Methadone: synthetic narcotic used in detoxification programs to replace heroin.

Metrorrhagia: bleeding or spotting between menstrual periods.

Microcephaly: congenital anomaly characterized by abnormal smallness of the head relative to the rest of the body and by underdevelopment of the brain, with resulting mental retardation.

Micrognathia: underdevelopment of the jaw, especially the mandible (lower jaw).

Mid-life crisis: questions of self-esteem during middle adulthood related to the perceived loss of beauty, youth, and physical power.

Minerals: nonorganic substances necessary for normal body functioning; those needed in large amounts, such as calcium, phosphorus, sodium, and magnesium, are called macrominerals; those needed in small amounts, such as iron, iodine, zinc, and fluoride, are called microminerals, trace minerals, or trace elements.

Minilaparotomy: 3/4″ to 1¼″ (2- to 3-cm) abdominal incision above the pubis; during this procedure, female sterilization can be performed by crushing, ligating, banding, or electrocoagulating the fallopian tubes.

Mitosis: cell division characteristic of all cell types except gametes.

Mitral valve prolapse: cardiac disease in which the mitral valve leaflets protrude into the atrium during ventricular systole.

Mittelschmerz: abdominal pain near the ovaries during ovulation; a symptom that may help predict fertile periods in the sympto-thermal contraceptive method.

Molding: shaping of the fetal head by overlapping of the sutures, which helps the head conform to the birth canal.

Monophasic pattern: relatively flat basal body temperature that does not vary more than 0.05° F each day.

Monosomy: absence of one chromosome of a homologous pair.

Montrice: trained professional support person during labor.

Morbid temperature: oral temperature exceeding 100.4° F (38° C) that persists for 2 successive days after delivery, excluding the first 24 hours.

Morning-after contraceptive: oral medication given 24 to 72 hours after sexual intercourse to prevent conception; typically used in emergencies, such as rape, condom breakage, or expulsion of an intrauterine device.

Moro reflex: normal neonatal reflex elicited by dropping the neonate's head backward in a sudden motion, resulting in extension and abduction of all extremities, formation of a "C" with the fingers, and adduction, then flexion, of all extremities (as in an embrace).

Morula: small mass of cells formed after a zygote undergoes several mitotic divisions.

Mosaicism: two or more cell lines that differ genotypically but develop from a single zygote; an error that occurs during mitosis.

Mother image: each woman's concept of herself as a mother, shaped from childhood memories of her own mother, other role models, revision of her mother image through other children, literature, and her imagination.

Motivation: incentive or reason to act.

Motor maturity: full development of muscle tone and posture, including muscle coordination, muscle movements, and reflexes.

Mourning: actions or expression of grief.

Mucus plug: protective mucus barrier that blocks the cervical canal during pregnancy; caused by estrogen stimulation.

Multiparous: having given birth to one or more children.

MASTER GLOSSARY continued

Music therapy: relaxation technique that uses musical sounds to alter physiologic responses to stress.

Mutation: any permanent inheritable change in DNA.

Myoepithelial cells: smooth-muscle cells surrounding breast alveoli and ducts; with the let-down reflex, these cells contract and eject milk into breast ductules and sinuses.

Myometrial contractions: postpartal uterine contractions that reduce uterine size; also called afterpains.

Myometrium: uterine muscle.

Myotonia: increased muscle tension that causes voluntary and involuntary muscle contractions; a physiologic response to sexual stimulation.

Nagele's rule: method of calculating the expected date of delivery (EDD) using a client's first day of the last menstrual period (LMP).

Necrotizing enterocolitis: acute inflammatory bowel disorder occurring mainly in preterm neonates.

Negligence: failure to act as a reasonable person would given similar training, experience, and circumstances.

Neonatal adaptation: physiologic and behavioral changes during the first 24 hours after delivery through which the neonate makes the transition from the intrauterine to the extrauterine environment.

Neonatal intensive care unit (NICU): nursery that provides the highest level of life-support management, including ventilatory support; heart rate, blood pressure, cardiorespiratory, and blood gas monitoring; I.V. fluid therapy; and experienced round-the-clock medical and nursing care.

Neonatal mortality: number of deaths per 1,000 live births within the first 28 days after birth.

Neonatal social behaviors: neonatal responses to actions by caregivers and others, such as smiling, gazing, cuddling, and following voices with the eyes.

Neoplasm: benign or malignant growth with uncontrolled or progressive cell multiplication; also called tumor.

Neuromuscular dissociation: relaxation technique that uses tension and relaxation of specific muscle groups to develop awareness of muscle tension.

Neutral thermal environment: narrow range of environmental temperatures at which the least amount of energy is required to maintain a stable core temperature.

Nicotine: addictive alkaloid found in tobacco.

Nipple confusion: condition in which the infant does not know how to suck properly from a nipple; caused by frequent nipple changes (such as from use of supplemental bottles during breast-feeding).

Nipple inversion: inturning or depression of the nipple.

Noncompliance: failure to act in accordance with requests, instructions, demands, or requirements.

Nondisjunction: failure of homologous chromosomes or chromatids to separate during mitosis or meiosis, resulting in daughter cells that contain unequal numbers of chromosomes.

Nonpitting edema: condition in which pressure does not leave a depression despite interstitial accumulation of excess fluid.

Nonshivering thermogenesis: heat production by lipolysis of brown fat; primary method through which the neonate produces heat.

Notochord: rod-shaped structure that defines the primitive axis of the body and forms the central developmental point of the axial skeleton.

Nuclear family: traditional family structure that includes father, mother, and their biological children.

Nulliparous: never having given birth to a child.

Nursing care plan: written guide to a client's care encompassing the assessments, nursing diagnoses, planning, goals, and interventions throughout the course of care; the plan is revised and updated as needed.

Nursing diagnosis: descriptive statement identifying actual or potential client health problems that can be resolved or diminished by nursing care; a step in the nursing process.

Nursing process: systematic problem-solving method that forms the framework for nursing practice; consists of five steps: assessment, nursing diagnosis, planning, implementation, and evaluation.

Nutrient density: concentration of nutrients in relation to calories in a diet.

Obesity: body weight of 20% or more above ideal weight.

Objective data: information about a client's health status obtained through physical assessment and diagnostic study results.

Occiput posterior position: variation of the normal fetal position, in which the head enters the pelvic inlet with the occiput facing posteriorly in the oblique diameter, causing back labor.

Oligohydramnios: presence of less than 300 ml of amniotic fluid at term.

Oligospermia: abnormally low number of spermatozoa in semen.

Omentectomy: removal of all or part of the fold of the omentum, a portion of the peritoneum that extends from the stomach to adjacent organs.

Omphalocele: congenital anomaly in which a portion of the intestine protrudes through a defect in the abdominal wall at the umbilicus.

Oogenesis: process by which ova develop.

Oophorectomy: removal of one or both ovaries.

Operant conditioning: repeated rewards that encourage specific behaviors.

Opiate: narcotic drug derived from opium (such as codeine, morphine, and heroin) that may relieve pain or induce sleep.

MASTER GLOSSARY continued

Oral contraceptive: hormonal compound (estrogen, progestin, or both) that is taken by mouth and inhibits ovulation.

Orgasmic platform: engorged lower third of the vagina during the sexual response cycle.

Orientation: neonate's ability to respond to visual and auditory stimuli.

Osteoporosis: decreased bone mass, occurring most commonly in menopausal women.

Out-of-phase endometrium: discrepancy of 2 or more days between the ovulatory date, cycle date, and histologic date of the endometrium.

Ovaries: female gonads; glands located on each side of the pelvis that contain ova and secrete the hormones estrogen and progesterone.

Ovulation: maturation and discharge of an ovum from the ovary in response to hormonal stimulation during the menstrual cycle.

Ovum: female gamete (plural, ova).

Oxytocin: hormone secreted by the posterior pituitary gland that stimulates uterine smooth-muscle contractions and breast milk ejection; also, a synthetic hormone (Pitocin) that simulates the actions of the natural hormone.

Oxytocin receptors: cellular structures in the breast that are sensitive to the effects of oxytocin.

Paced breathing: learned breathing technique that aids relaxation and helps the client maintain control during labor contractions; may be slow, modified, or patterned.

Papanicolaou (Pap) test: cytologic study of stained exfoliated cells to detect and diagnose certain conditions in the female reproductive tract, particularly premalignant and malignant conditions, such as cancer of the vagina, cervix, and endometrium.

Paracervical block: regional anesthesia technique that blocks nerve conduction on both sides of the cervix, relieving uterine pain during the first stage of active labor.

Parity: obstetric classification of a woman by the number of births and stillbirths that occur after 28 weeks of gestation.

Patent ductus arteriosus: abnormal opening between the pulmonary artery and the aorta; results from failure of the fetal ductus arteriosus to close after birth (seen mainly in the preterm neonate).

Pathologic jaundice: condition marked by yellow skin discoloration and an increase in the serum bilirubin level (above 13 mg/dl); arising within 24 hours after birth, it results from blood type or blood group incompatibility, infection, or biliary, hepatic, or metabolic abnormalities.

Pathologic mourning: mourning that does not lead to resolution of grief.

Peau d'orange: orange-peel-like appearance of breast skin caused by edema.

Pediculosis pubis: sexually transmitted disease caused by *Phthirus pubis* (lice) infestation, which produces mild to severe pruritus in areas covered by pubic or other types of hair.

Pedigree: diagram of a family tree depicting occurrence of one or more traits in the various family members.

Pelvic examination: assessment of the external and internal genitalia by inspection and palpation.

Pelvic inflammatory disease (PID): infection of the oviducts, ovaries, and adjacent tissue; may result from intrauterine device use or a sexually transmitted disease.

Pelvis: bony structure made up of the sacrum, coccyx, and innominate bones; passageway through which the fetus travels during labor.

Penetrance: frequency with which a gene manifests itself in phenotypes of individuals with that gene.

Perceived support: belief that help is available if needed.

Perimenopausal: occurring during the climacteric stage.

Perinatal period: period extending from the twenty-eighth week of gestation to the end of the fourth week after birth.

Perineum: region between the vulva and anus; bounded in front by the pubic arch and the arcuate ligaments, in back by the tip of the coccyx, and laterally by the inferior rami of the pubis and ischium and the sacrotuberus ligaments.

Periods of neonatal reactivity: predictable, identifiable series of behavioral and physiologic characteristics occurring during the first hours after birth; characterized by distinctive changes in vital signs, state of alertness, and responsiveness to external stimuli.

Peripartum cardiomyopathy: cardiac disease in which the left ventricle functions abnormally during the last month of pregnancy or first 6 postpartal months.

Pessary: device inserted into the vagina to treat uterine prolapse, uterine retroversion, or cervical incompetence.

Phenotype: observable expression of a genetically determined trait.

Phenylketonuria: autosomal recessive disorder characterized by the abnormal presence of metabolites of phenylalanine (such as phenylketone) in the urine.

Physiologic jaundice: common condition of the full-term neonate marked by yellow skin discoloration and an increase in the serum bilirubin level (4 to 12 mg/dl); arising 48 to 72 hours after birth and peaking by the third to fifth day, it results from neonatal hepatic immaturity.

Pica: consumption of nonfood items.

MASTER GLOSSARY continued

Pitting edema: condition in which pressed tissues leave a small depression or pit; caused by interstitial accumulation of excess fluid.

Placenta accreta: condition in which part or all of the placenta adheres firmly to the uterine wall.

Placenta increta: condition in which placental villi invade the uterine myometrium.

Placenta percreta: condition in which placental villi penetrate the myometrium to the peritoneal covering of the uterus.

Placenta previa: abnormally low implantation of the placenta so that it encroaches onto the internal cervical os.

Placental insufficiency: inadequate or improper functioning of the placenta leading to a compromised intrauterine environment that jeopardizes the fetus.

Plaintiff: person who initiates a lawsuit.

Planning: one step in the nursing process that includes setting and prioritizing goals for each nursing diagnosis, formulating interventions to help the client achieve these goals, and developing the nursing care plan.

Pleiotropy: multiple signs and symptoms caused by one or two genes.

PLISSIT model: description of four levels of sexual counseling: permission, limited information, specific suggestions, and intensive therapy.

Poikilotherm: neonate who takes on the temperature of the environment.

Polar body: small, nonfunctional cell produced along with a functioning ovum during oogenesis.

Polycystic kidney disease: condition characterized by formation of multiple cysts within the kidney, leading to kidney enlargement and destruction of adjacent tissue.

Polycystic ovary disease: endocrine disturbance in which continued ovarian stimulation from luteinizing hormone causes anovulation and polycystic ovaries; also called Stein-Leventhal syndrome.

Polycythemia: abnormal increase in the number of red blood cells; in the neonate, it results from maternal-fetal transfusion, delayed umbilical cord clamping, or placental insufficiency.

Polydipsia: excessive thirst; a characteristic symptom of diabetes mellitus.

Polymenorrhea: increased frequency of menstrual bleeding.

Polyphagia: excessive hunger; a characteristic symptom of diabetes mellitus.

Polypharmacy: practice of taking different drugs simultaneously in varying dosages.

Polyuria: excessive urine excretion; a characteristic sign of diabetes mellitus.

Position: relationship of the leading fetal presenting part to a point on the maternal pelvis.

Postcoital examination: assessment of spermatozoa survival in cervical mucus after sexual intercourse.

Posterior urethral valves: congenital anomaly characterized by urinary tract obstruction, hydronephrosis, and impaired urine flow.

Postpartal hemorrhage: abnormally large amount (more than 500 ml) of bleeding after delivery, which may be caused by uterine atony, rupture, lacerations, inversion, or hematoma.

Postpartal period: approximately 6-week period following delivery during which the anatomic and physiologic changes resulting from pregnancy resolve; also called puerperium.

Postterm neonate: neonate born after completion of week 42 of gestation; also called postmature neonate.

Pre-embryo: developing organism from implantation through week 3, when—according to most authorities—the organism becomes an embryo.

Precipitate labor: labor that proceeds very rapidly, usually lasting less than 3 hours.

Precipitous delivery: unusually rapid delivery.

Preeclampsia: nonconvulsive form of pregnancy-induced hypertension characterized by the onset of acute hypertension, proteinuria, and edema after the twenty-fourth week of gestation; called eclampsia when it includes seizures and coma.

Preferred provider organization (PPO): group practice similar to a health maintenance organization, except that the insured client has the option of receiving care from a provider outside the group for a somewhat higher fee; PPO services are not government-mandated.

Pregnancy-induced hypertension (PIH): group of potentially life-threatening hypertensive disorders that may develop in the second or third trimester; includes preeclampsia and eclampsia.

Premenstrual syndrome (PMS): cyclic cluster of signs and symptoms, such as breast tenderness, fluid retention, and mood swings, that usually occurs after ovulation and before or during menses.

Presentation: fetal part that enters the maternal pelvis first and can be touched through the cervix; may be cephalic, breech, or shoulder.

Presenting part: portion of the fetus that first enters the pelvic passageway.

Preterm neonate: neonate born before completion of the thirty-seventh week of gestation.

Preterm neonate: neonate born before completion of the thirty-seventh week of gestation; also called premature neonate.

Primary infertility: failure to conceive by a couple in which the woman has never been pregnant.

Primiparous: giving birth for the first time.

Primitive streak: small aggregation of cells at the caudal end of the embryo that offers early evidence of the embryonic axis.

MASTER GLOSSARY continued

Professional standards review organization (PSRO): organization that reviews the quality, usage, and type of services offered by a health care facility.

Programmed learning: teaching strategy where the nurse asks nonthreatening follow-up questions after each teaching session; may include computer-aided learning.

Progressive muscle relaxation: systematic muscle contraction and relaxation to reduce tension.

Projection: defense mechanism that involves attributing to someone else traits that are unacceptable in oneself.

Prolactin: hormone causing breast milk production; secreted by the anterior pituitary gland in response to tactile stimulation of the breast.

Prolonged deceleration: decrease in the fetal heart rate from the baseline lasting several minutes or longer in response to a sudden stimulus of the vagal system, such as uterine tachysystole, anesthetics, or maternal hypotension.

Prospective payment system (PPS): reimbursement system for health care services that allows a specific amount of money for a specific diagnosis, no matter how many days the client is hospitalized.

Prostaglandin: naturally occurring hydroxyfatty acid that stimulates uterine contractions.

Protein: energy source, essential in various body functions, that provides 4 calories/g; can be complete (providing all 9 essential amino acids in the proportion needed for growth) or incomplete.

Proteinuria: presence in the urine of abnormally large amounts of protein, usually albumin.

Protractility: state of nipple protrusion rather than inversion.

Psychoprophylactic method: childbirth preparation technique developed by Ferdinand Lamaze that emphasizes concentration, relaxation, and education.

Psychosis: major mental disorder of organic or emotional origin characterized by extreme personality derangement or disorganization; commonly accompanied by severe depression, agitation, regressive behavior, illusions, delusions, and hallucinations so severe that the individual loses touch with reality, cannot function normally, and usually requires hospitalization.

Puberty: developmental stage early in adolescence when reproductive ability begins and secondary sex characteristics develop.

Pudendal block: regional anesthesia technique used during the second stage of labor to numb the perineum and vagina, primarily for episiotomy repair.

Puerperal infection: invasion by microorganisms of the reproductive tract during the postpartal period.

Puerperium: 6-week period after childbirth.

Pyelonephritis: acute inflammation of the ureters and kidneys, commonly caused by *Escherichia coli;* produces the effects of cystitis plus fever, chills, flank pain, and other signs and symptoms.

Quickening: first awareness of fetal movement, typically felt after 16 to 20 weeks.

Radiant warmer: open bed with an overhead radiant heat source.

Radiation: transfer of heat from one surface to another without contact between the surfaces; a mechanism of heat loss or gain.

Rape: sexual intercourse without consent, achieved through the use of threats, force, intimidation, or deception; requires penile penetration of the vagina.

Rape examination kit: commercially prepared kit that includes everything needed for rape examination and evidence collection.

Rape-trauma syndrome: group of symptoms that results from rape and includes an acute phase, outward adjustment phase, and a reorganization phase; also a nursing diagnosis approved by the North American Nursing Diagnosis Association.

Rationalization: defense mechanism that involves creation of reasons to justify painful or unacceptable situations or actions.

Reaction formation: defense mechanism that involves behaving in a way exactly opposite to an unconscious wish.

Received support: activities performed to assist a person.

Recessive: incapable of genetic expression unless the responsible allele is carried on both members of a pair of homologous chromosomes.

Reciprocity: process in which a neonate gives cues and the parent or other caregiver interprets, then responds to, the cues.

Recommended dietary allowances (RDAs): specific quantities of essential nutrients for different ages, sexes, and conditions judged adequate to maintain nutritional status of nearly all healthy people by the Food and Nutrition Board of the National Academy of Sciences.

Rectocele: herniation of the rectum into the vagina.

Reflex: involuntary function or movement of any organ or body part in response to a stimulus.

Refractory period: time after an orgasm when restimulation and orgasm are not possible for a man.

Regional anesthesia: direct nerve block following injection of a local anesthetic agent.

Regionalization of care: system that avoids costly duplication of services and ensures availability of essential services in a geographical area; hospitals and special facilities, such as neonatal intensive care units and trauma units, are classified as primary, secondary, and tertiary health centers, depending on the facilities and personnel available, the population served, the number of beds in the facility, and other criteria.

MASTER GLOSSARY continued

Regression: defense mechanism of retreat to an earlier developmental phase to reduce the demands of maturity.

Renal agenesis: congenital absence of one kidney (unilateral renal agenesis) or both kidneys (bilateral renal agenesis).

Repression: defense mechanism of unconscious exclusion from the conscious mind of painful impulses, desires, or fears.

Respiratory distress syndrome: acute, potentially fatal neonatal lung disorder (most common in preterm neonates), resulting from surfactant deficiency; characterized by a respiratory rate greater than 60 breaths/minute, lung inelasticity, nasal flaring, expiratory grunts, chest retractions, and peripheral edema.

Respite care: care provided by a secondary caregiver to relieve the primary caregiver; may be required for hours or weeks.

Respondeat superior: legal rule under which an employer is held legally responsible for negligence or malpractice committed by an employee functioning within the scope of employment.

Retained placenta: condition in which the placenta remains in the uterus 30 minutes after the second stage of labor.

Retinopathy of prematurity (ROP): disease of the retinal vasculature associated with oxygen therapy in the preterm neonate; formerly called retrolental fibroplasia.

Retroflexed uterus: position in which the uterine corpus flexes toward the rectum and the cervix lies in the normal position.

Retroverted uterus: position in which the uterine corpus flexes toward the rectum at a less acute angle than a retroflexed uterus.

Rh incompatibility: isoimmune hemolytic anemia in which maternal antibodies cause destruction of fetal red blood cells, leading to severe anemia and jaundice in the neonate.

Rh isoimmunization: sensitization of maternal blood antibodies against fetal blood antigens, which can create a serious blood incompatibility during pregnancy and can lead to erythroblastosis fetalis.

Rheumatic heart disease: cardiac disease in which an untreated streptococcal infection leads to bacterial invasion and alteration of the mitral or tricuspid valve.

Rhythm method: natural contraceptive method that predicts a fertile period by analyzing the length of eight previous menstrual cycles; also called calendar method.

Ripe cervix: soft, effaced, dilated cervix.

Risk management: steps taken to minimize either the chance of injury or the harm that occurs.

Role: set of repetitive behaviors adopted consciously or unconsciously that provides consistency in family relationships and accomplishment of tasks.

Rooting reflex: normal neonatal response elicited by stroking the cheek or corner of the mouth with a finger or nipple, resulting in turning of the head toward the stimulus.

Rugae: transverse folds in the vaginal mucosa.

Rupture of the membranes: rupture of the amniotic sac, followed within 24 hours by labor in about 80% of women.

Salpingitis: inflammation or infection of the fallopian tube.

Salpingo-oophorectomy: surgical removal of the fallopian tubes and ovaries.

Scabies: sexually transmitted disease caused by *Sarcoptes scabiei* (itch mite) infestation, which produces papular lesions and extreme pruritus along body creases in such areas as the axillae, breasts, and genitals.

Scalp electrode: small spiral electrode attached to the fetal scalp to provide direct monitoring with a fetal electrocardiogram.

Scanning: technique for relieving stress by identifying and then relaxing tense muscles.

Scarf sign: term describing the distance that the neonate's elbow can be extended across the chest toward the opposite side; an index of gestational age.

Second stage of labor: period that begins with complete cervical dilation and ends with delivery of the neonate.

Secondary infertility: failure to conceive by a couple in which the woman has been pregnant before but now cannot conceive or carry a pregnancy to term.

Secretory phase: first half of the menstrual cycle from menstruation to ovulation.

Secundines: placenta and membranes expelled after delivery; the afterbirth.

Self-care: active and assertive participation in attaining one's health care goals.

Self-differentiation: personal growth characterized by identification of one's abilities, actions, and relationships with others.

Self-esteem: degree to which one values oneself.

Self-quieting behaviors: actions the neonate uses to quiet the self when crying, including hand-to-mouth movements, fist sucking, and attending to external stimuli (evaluated during the behavioral assessment).

Semen: white, viscous secretion of male reproductive organs consisting of spermatozoa and nutrient fluids ejaculated through the penile urethra.

Sexual assault: penetration of any orifice by the penis, other male appendage, or an object without consent, achieved through the use of threats, force, intimidation, or deception.

Sexuality: ongoing process of recognizing, accepting, and expressing oneself as a sexual being.

MASTER GLOSSARY continued

Sexually transmitted disease (STD): disorder acquired through vaginal, anal, or oral intercourse.

Short-term variability: Beat-to-beat changes in the fetal heart rate (FHR); normal short-term variability is 2 to 3 beats/minute from the baseline FHR.

Sibling rivalry: competition between siblings for parental love and approval.

Sickle cell anemia: autosomal recessive blood disorder in which hemoglobin molecules become sickle- or crescent-shaped, which affects their oxygen-carrying capacity and causes vessel obstruction.

Situational crisis: intensification of problems or symptoms linked to a traumatic event.

Small for gestational age (SGA): term used to describe a neonate who experienced intrauterine growth retardation and whose birth weight falls below the tenth percentile for gestational age on the Colorado intrauterine growth chart.

Smegma: sebaceous secretion that accumulates under the foreskin of the penis and at the base of the labia minora.

Smith's minor abnormalities: neonatal physiologic variations, such as abnormal dermal ridges, that may indicate major anomalies (for example, Down's syndrome).

Somatic complaints: physical symptoms caused by psychological concerns.

Spectatoring: phenomenon in which an individual imagines observing himself or herself during sexual activity.

Spermatogenesis: process by which spermatozoa develop.

Spermatozoon: male gamete (plural, spermatozoa).

Spermicide: chemical substance that kills spermatozoa; the active ingredient in contraceptive foams, creams, suppositories, and jellies.

Spinnbarkeit: stretchiness of cervical mucus at ovulation; caused by estrogen.

Spontaneous abortion: abrupt termination of pregnancy from natural causes before the age of viability.

Spousal rape: sexual intercourse that results from threats, physical force, or intimidation by the woman's spouse or partner.

Square window sign: term describing the degree to which the neonate's wrist can be flexed against the forearm; an index of gestational age.

Staging: categorization of neoplasms by their extent and spread from the original site to other body regions.

Standards of care: acts that a reasonable person would have performed or omitted under specific circumstances; conduct against which the defendant's actions are judged in a malpractice case.

Standardized nursing care plan: care plan developed for a group of clients with similar physical, emotional, or learning needs that reflects common standards of care.

Station: relationship of the fetal presenting part to the maternal ischial spine.

Sterilization: process that terminates fertility, rendering an individual unable to reproduce.

Strain gauge: water-filled, pressure-sensitive device connected to an intrauterine catheter that measures intensity, duration, and frequency of uterine contractions.

Striae gravidarum: pink streaks in the skin caused by separated connective tissue; typically appear on the breasts, abdomen, buttocks, or thighs and turn silvery after childbirth; also called stretch marks.

Subjective data: assessment information obtained from the client and others with intimate knowledge of the client, typically through interviews.

Substance abuse: maladaptive pattern of continued substance use despite knowledge of impaired social, occupational, psychological, or physical functioning caused or exacerbated by the substance; abused substances can include nicotine (in tobacco), alcohol, and legal and illegal drugs.

Substance dependence: cluster of cognitive, behavioral, and physiologic symptoms that indicate impaired control of substance use as evidenced by tolerance and withdrawal symptoms.

Sucking reflex: normal neonatal reflex elicited by inserting a finger or nipple in the neonate's mouth, resulting in forceful, rhythmic sucking.

Summative evaluation: process in which the nurse and client judge progress toward goals after home visits are discontinued.

Support: feelings of affection, trust, affirmation, and the sharing of advice, information, and time between people.

Support person: partner, friend, or family member who provides continuous support during labor and delivery.

Surfactant: phospholipid produced by Type II alveolar cells in the alveolar lining of the lungs; decreases alveolar inflation pressures, improves lung compliance, and provides alveolar stability, thereby decreasing effort in breathing.

Sympto-thermal method: natural contraceptive method that predicts fertile periods based on basal body temperature, cervical mucus changes, and such symptoms as mittelschmerz and changes in libido.

Synactive theory of development: Als's theory proposing that the neonate continuously interacts with the environment and that the neonate's physiologic status depends on the environmental stimuli received and processed.

Synchrony: interaction in which each party acts and reacts in a manner appropriate to the cues given.

Synclitism: state in which the fetal biparietal diameter is parallel to the plane of the maternal pelvic inlet.

MASTER GLOSSARY continued

Syphilis: sexually transmitted disease caused by *Treponema pallidum,* which produces painless, papular lesions (chancres) and may progress through various stages to heart damage, seizures, and death.

T₄ lymphocyte: type of lymph cell that is vital to the body's immune response.

Tachysystole: contractions occurring more frequently than every 2 minutes.

Tail of Spence: extension of breast tissue, which projects from the upper outer quadrant of the breast toward the axilla; also called the axillary tail.

Tenesmus: persistent, ineffectual spasms of the rectum or bladder accompanied by the desire to empty the bowel or bladder.

Teratoma: congenital neoplasm consisting of various cell types, none of which normally occur together.

Term neonate: neonate of 38 to 42 weeks' gestation; also called mature neonate.

Tertiary care facility: perinatal care facility that offers the most advanced technological and specialty care for critically ill neonates referred within a specific region.

Testes: male gonads; reproductive glands contained in the scrotum that produce spermatozoa and the androgenic hormone testosterone.

Tetanic uterine contraction: sustained uterine contraction lasting 70 seconds or longer, occurring more than once every 3 minutes, and increasing intrauterine pressure to 75 mm Hg or more.

Therapeutic abortion: termination of a pregnancy for medical reasons (physiologic or psychological) before the age of viability.

Therapeutic communication: interaction that focuses on attaining client goals rather than on the mutual pleasure received from social communication.

Therapeutic empathy: ability to view experiences, emotions, and thoughts from a client's perspective and to use that knowledge to build the client's awareness and help set goals.

Thermoregulation: maintenance of body temperature by complex interaction between environmental temperature and body heat loss and production.

Third stage of labor: period that begins with complete delivery of the neonate and ends with delivery of the placenta.

Thrombophlebitis: formation of a thrombus (clot) in response to inflammation of the vein wall.

Tocodynamometer: externally applied pressure-sensitive device that records the frequency and duration of uterine contractions.

TORCH infections: acronym for a group of infections, including toxoplasmosis, other infections (chlamydia, group B beta hemolytic streptococcus, syphilis, and varicella zoster), rubella, cytomegalovirus, and herpesvirus type 2.

Touch therapy: relaxation technique that uses tactile stimulation to alter perceptions of discomfort during labor.

Toxic shock syndrome (TSS): rare, potentially fatal, multisystem disorder caused by a toxin secreted by *Staphylococcus aureus;* has been associated with improper tampon use and typically causes sudden high fever, vomiting, diarrhea, myalgia, vaginal redness or discharge, skin rash, and sore throat.

Toxicity: quality or quantity of a substance that makes it poisonous.

Transcutaneous electric nerve stimulation (TENS): use of electric current to counterstimulate nerve fibers and thus block pain transmission.

Transient tachypnea: neonatal disorder characterized by rapid, shallow breathing (possibly accompanied by cyanosis) that lasts a few hours or days; caused by the retention of fetal lung fluid that follows cesarean delivery.

Transitional period: time during which the neonate experiences biological and behavioral adaptations to extrauterine life; normally lasts about 24 hours.

Transverse lie: presentation in which the long axis of the fetus is perpendicular to that of the mother.

Trichomoniasis: sexually transmitted disease caused by *Trichomonas vaginalis,* which is characterized by vaginal discharge, urinary symptoms, and vulvar edema, pruritus, and tenderness.

Trisomy: presence of an extra chromosome in a diploid cell.

Trophoblast: layer of ectoderm on the outside of the blastocyst that implants the embryo in the uterine wall and forms the chorion, amnion, and chorionic villi.

True labor: characterized by regular contractions that increase in intensity and duration as the intervals between them decrease, along with progressive effacement and cervical dilation.

Tumescence: swelling, as when the penis or breasts swell during sexual activity.

Ultrasound: method of external electronic fetal monitoring that sends low-energy, high-frequency sound waves through the abdominal wall in the direction of the fetal heart; waves are translated into audible fetal heart tones and fetal heart rate waveforms.

Univeral precautions: infection control measures that treat all blood and body fluids as potentially infectious.

Urethritis: urethral inflammation caused by a lower urinary tract infection, which produces the same effects as cystitis.

Urinary tract infection: invasion by microorganisms of one or more structures of the urinary tract; most commonly caused by gram-negative bacteria.

MASTER GLOSSARY continued

Uterine atony: poor uterine muscle tone.

Uterine inversion: abnormal condition in which the uterus is turned inside out so that the internal surface protrudes into or beyond the vagina; usually caused by excessive traction on the umbilical cord.

Uterine involution: gradual return of the uterus to a nonpregnant size and condition after labor and delivery.

Uterine prolapse: downward displacement of the uterus from its normal position in the pelvis.

Uterine souffle: blowing sound heard with a stethoscope as blood flows through the uterine arteries to the placenta.

Uterine subinvolution: failure of the uterus to return to a nonpregnant size and condition after labor and delivery.

Vacuum curettage: surgical method of pregnancy interruption that requires cervical dilatation and suction equipment to evacuate the uterine contents.

Vacuum extraction: procedure using a cup-shaped suction device applied to the fetus's scalp to provide traction for delivery.

Vaginal introitus: entrance to the vagina.

Vaginitis: vaginal inflammation that may be caused by fungi, protozoa, or bacteria.

Variability: beat-to-beat changes in the fetal heart rate that reflect the degree of tonic balance between the sympathetic and parasympathetic nervous systems.

Variable deceleration: nonuniform deceleration pattern indicating cord compression of variable significance; the most common deceleration pattern in labor, usually well tolerated by the fetus.

Varicosity: enlarged, tortuous area of a vessel; in pregnancy, typically venous varicosities of the legs, rectum, or vulva.

Vasectomy: male sterilization procedure that requires cutting and tying or cauterizing of part of the vas deferens.

Vasocongestion: blood vessel engorgement and increased blood flow to tissues; a physiologic response to sexual stimulation.

VBAC: vaginal birth after cesarean delivery.

Vegetarian: individual who avoids all animal products (vegan), all but eggs and milk (lacto-ovo vegetarian), all but poultry (pollo-vegetarian), or all but fish (pesco-vegetarian).

Velamentous: membranous.

Ventouse: suction cup used in vacuum extraction.

Ventral suspension: term describing the degree to which the neonate extends the back, flexes the arms and legs, and holds the head upright when an examiner positions the neonate prone and places a hand under the chest; an index of gestational age.

Vernix caseosa: grayish white, cheeselike substance composed of sebaceous gland secretions and desquamated epithelial cells that covers the near-term fetus and neonate.

Version: procedure for turning the fetus in utero to a position favorable for delivery.

Very low birth weight: birth weight of 500 to 1,500 g.

Viability: age and weight at which the fetus is capable of surviving outside the uterus (usually 24 weeks and 50l g).

Vitamins: compounds needed in small amounts for normal body functioning; may be fat-soluble (stored in fat) or water-soluble (incapable of being stored by the body).

Vulvitis: vulvar inflammation, which may be caused by fungi, protozoa, bacteria, other organisms, chemical irritation, or allergic reaction.

Womb name: nickname by which expectant parents refer to the fetus during pregnancy.

Zona pellucida: noncellular layer covering the surface of a mature ovarian follicle.

Zygote: diploid cell formed by the union of a haploid ovum and spermatozoon; develops into an embryo.

INDEX

i refers to an illustration; t refers to a table.

Q

XYZ

i refers to an illustration; t refers to a table.